Handbook of
ATTACHMENT

SECOND EDITION

Theory, Research, and Clinical Applications

Edited by
JUDE CASSIDY
PHILLIP R. SHAVER

THE GUILFORD PRESS
New York   London

With respect and gratitude
for the pioneering work
of John Bowlby and Mary Ainsworth

© 2008 The Guilford Press
A Division of Guilford Publications, Inc.
72 Spring Street, New York, NY 10012
www.guilford.com

looseeeqiq

Printed in the United States of America

This book is printed on acid-free paper.

Last digit is print number: 9   8   7   6   5   4   3   2   1

Library of Congress Cataloging-in-Publication Data

Handbook of attachment : theory, research, and clinical applications / Edited by Jude Cassidy, Phillip R.
Shaver.—2nd ed.
        p. cm.
    Includes bibliographical references and index.
    ISBN 978-1-59385-874-2 (hardcover)   ISBN 978-1-60623-028-2 (paperback)
    1. Attachment behavior.   2. Attachment behavior in children.   I. Cassidy, Jude.   II. Shaver, Phillip R.
    BF575.A86H36 2008
    155.9′2—dc22
                                                                        2008006573

About the Editors

Jude Cassidy, PhD, is Professor of Psychology at the University of Maryland and Director of the Maryland Child and Family Development Laboratory. Her research focuses on attachment, social and emotional development in children and adolescents, social information processing, peer relations, and early intervention. Dr. Cassidy serves as coeditor of the journal *Attachment and Human Development*. She is a Fellow of the American Psychological Society, and received a Boyd R. McCandless Young Scientist Award from the American Psychological Association.

Phillip R. Shaver, PhD, is Distinguished Professor of Psychology at the University of California, Davis. He has coauthored and coedited numerous books and has published over 200 scholarly journal articles and book chapters. Dr. Shaver's research focuses on attachment, human motivation and emotion, close relationships, personality development, and the effects of meditation on behavior and brain. He is a member of the editorial boards of *Attachment and Human Development*, *Personal Relationships*, the *Journal of Personality and Social Psychology*, and *Emotion*. Dr. Shaver is a fellow of both the American Psychological Association and the Association for Psychological Science. He received a Distinguished Career Award from the International Association for Relationship Research and is currently President of that organization.

Contributors

Kathleen E. Albus, PhD, Center for Promotion of Child Development through Primary Care, Baltimore, Maryland

Joseph P. Allen, PhD, Department of Psychology, University of Virginia, Charlottesville, Virginia

Karen Appleyard, PhD, Center for Child and Family Policy, Duke University, Durham, North Carolina

Jay Belsky, PhD, Institute for the Study of Children, Families and Social Issues and School of Psychology, Birkbeck University of London, London, United Kingdom

Lisa J. Berlin, PhD, Center for Child and Family Policy, Duke University, Durham, North Carolina

Kelly K. Bost, PhD, Department of Human and Community Development, University of Illinois at Urbana–Champaign, Urbana, Illinois

Inge Bretherton, PhD, Department of Human Development and Family Studies, University of Wisconsin, Madison, Wisconsin

Preston A. Britner, PhD, Department of Human Development and Family Studies, University of Connecticut, Storrs, Connecticut

Elizabeth Carlson, PhD, Institute of Child Development, University of Minnesota, Minneapolis, Minnesota

Jude Cassidy, PhD, Department of Psychology, University of Maryland, College Park, Maryland

James A. Coan, PhD, Department of Psychology, University of Virginia, Charlottesville, Virginia

Judith A. Crowell, MD, Division of Child and Adolescent Psychiatry, Department of Psychiatry and Behavioral Sciences, Stony Brook University Medical Center, Stony Brook, New York

Michelle DeKlyen, PhD, Center for Research on Child Well-Being, Princeton University, Princeton, New Jersey

Mary Dozier, PhD, Department of Psychology, University of Delaware, Newark, Delaware

Byron Egeland, PhD, Institute of Child Development, University of Minnesota, Minneapolis, Minnesota

R. M. Pasco Fearon, PhD, Department of Psychology, University of Reading, Reading, United Kingdom

Brooke C. Feeney, PhD, Department of Psychology, Carnegie Mellon University, Pittsburgh, Pennsylvania

Judith A. Feeney, PhD, School of Psychology, University of Queensland, Queensland, Australia

Peter Fonagy, PhD, Psychoanalysis Unit, Department of Clinical, Educational, and Health Psychology, University College London, and Anna Freud Centre, London, United Kingdom

Nathan A. Fox, PhD, Child Development Lab, Department of Human Development, University of Maryland, College Park, Maryland

R. Chris Fraley, PhD, Department of Psychology, University of Illinois at Urbana–Champaign, Champaign, Illinois

Carol George, PhD, Department of Psychology, Mills College, Oakland, California

George Gergely, PhD, Institute for Psychological Research, Hungarian Academy of Sciences, Budapest, Hungary, and Anna Freud Centre, London, United Kingdom

Pehr Granqvist, PhD, Department of Psychology, Uppsala University, Uppsala, Sweden

Mark T. Greenberg, PhD, Prevention Research Center, Pennsylvania State University, University Park, Pennsylvania

Karin Grossmann, PhD, Department of Psychology, University of Regensburg, Regensburg, Germany

Klaus E. Grossmann, PhD, Department of Psychology, University of Regensburg, Regensburg, Germany

Amie Ashley Hane, PhD, Department of Psychology, Williams College, Williamstown, Massachusetts

Cindy Hazan, PhD, Department of Human Development, Cornell University, Ithaca, New York

Erik Hesse, PhD, Department of Psychology, University of California, Berkeley, California; Center for Child and Family Studies, Leiden University, Leiden, The Netherlands

Myron A. Hofer, MD, Department of Psychiatry and Sackler Institute for Developmental Psychobiology, Columbia University, New York, New York

Carollee Howes, PhD, Psychological Studies in Education Program, Graduate School of Education and Information Studies, University of California, Los Angeles, California

Deborah Jacobvitz, PhD, Department of Human Ecology, College of Natural Sciences, University of Texas at Austin, Austin, Texas

Susan M. Johnson, EdD, Department of Psychology, University of Ottawa, and Ottawa Couple and Family Institute, Ottawa, Ontario, Canada

Kathryn A. Kerns, PhD, Department of Psychology, Kent State University, Kent, Ohio

Heinz Kindler, PhD, Deutsches Jugendinstitut, München, Germany

Lee A. Kirkpatrick, PhD, Department of Psychology, College of William and Mary, Williamsburg, Virginia

Roger Kobak, PhD, Department of Psychology, University of Delaware, Newark, Delaware

Alicia F. Lieberman, PhD, Child Trauma Research Project, University of California, San Francisco, and San Francisco General Hospital, San Francisco, California

Karlen Lyons-Ruth, PhD, Department of Psychiatry, Harvard Medical School, Cambridge, Massachusetts

Stephanie Madsen, PhD, Department of Psychology, McDaniel College, Westminster, Maryland

Carol Magai, PhD, Department of Psychology, Long Island University, Brooklyn, New York

Robert S. Marvin, PhD, Mary D. Ainsworth Child–Parent Attachment Clinic and Department of Psychology, University of Virginia, Charlottesville, Virginia

Mario Mikulincer, PhD, School of Psychology, Interdisciplinary Center, Herzliya, Israel

Jonathan J. Mohr, PhD, Department of Psychology, George Mason University, Fairfax, Virginia

Joan K. Monin, PhD, Department of Psychology, Carnegie Mellon University and University Center for Social and Urban Research, University of Pittsburgh, Pittsburgh, Pennsylvania

Kristine A. Munholland, MSW, PhD, Kaiser Permanente Hospice, Portland, Oregon

H. Jonathan Polan, MD, Department of Psychiatry, Weill Medical College of Cornell University and Division of Developmental Psychobiology, New York State Psychiatric Institute, Columbia University, New York, New York

Michael Rutter, MD, Social, Genetic and Developmental Psychiatry Centre, Institute of Psychiatry, King's College London, London, United Kingdom

Abraham Sagi-Schwartz, PhD, Center for the Study of Child Development, University of Haifa, Haifa, Israel

Phillip R. Shaver, PhD, Department of Psychology, University of California, Davis, California

Jeffry A. Simpson, PhD, Department of Psychology, University of Minnesota, Minneapolis, Minnesota

Arietta Slade, PhD, Department of Clinical Psychology, City University of New York, New York, New York, and Yale Child Study Center, Yale University, New Haven, Connecticut

Judith Solomon, PhD, Children's Hospital, Oakland, California

Susan Spieker, PhD, Department of Family and Child Nursing, Center on Human Development and Disability, University of Washington, Seattle, Washington

L. Alan Sroufe, PhD, Institute of Child Development and Department of Psychiatry, University of Minnesota, Minneapolis, Minnesota

K. Chase Stovall-McClough, PhD, Child Study Center, Institute for Trauma and Stress, New York University School of Medicine, New York, New York

Stephen J. Suomi, PhD, Laboratory of Comparative Ethology, Eunice Kennedy Shriver National Institute of Child Health and Human Development, National Institutes of Health, Bethesda, Maryland

Mary Target, PhD, Psychoanalysis Unit, Department of Clinical, Educational, and Health Psychology, University College London, and Anna Freud Centre, London, United Kingdom

Ross A. Thompson, PhD, Department of Psychology, University of California, Davis, California

Marinus H. van IJzendoorn, PhD, Center for Child and Family Studies, Leiden University, Leiden, The Netherlands

Brian E. Vaughn, PhD, Department of Human Development and Family Studies, Auburn University, Auburn, Alabama

Nancy S. Weinfield, PhD, Westat, Inc., Rockville, Maryland

Charles H. Zeanah, MD, Institute for Infant and Early Childhood Mental Health, Tulane University Health Sciences Center, New Orleans, Louisiana

Debra Zeifman, PhD, Department of Psychology, Vassar College, Poughkeepsie, New York

Peter Zimmermann, PhD, Department of Psychology, University of Dortmund, Dortmund, Germany

Preface

It seems unlikely that either John Bowlby, when he first wondered about the relation between maternal deprivation and juvenile delinquency, or Mary Ainsworth, when she answered an advertisement in a London newspaper to work as a postdoctoral researcher with Bowlby, dreamed for a moment that their theoretical efforts would spawn one of the broadest, most profound, and most creative lines of research in 20th-century (and now 21st-century) psychology. But that is what happened. Anyone who today conducts a literature search on the topic of "attachment" will turn up more than 10,000 entries since 1975, and the entries will be spread across scores of physiological, clinical, developmental, and social psychology journals; will include numerous anthologies; and will deal with every stage of life from infancy to old age.

In the fields of social and emotional development, attachment theory is the most visible and empirically grounded conceptual framework. In the growing clinical literature on the effects of early parent–child relationships, including troubled and abusive relationships, attachment theory is prominent. In the rapidly expanding field of research on close relationships in adolescence and adulthood—including the study of romantic,

marital, or "pair-bond" relationships—attachment theory is one of the most influential approaches. Among researchers who study bereavement, Bowlby's volume on loss is a continuing source of insight and intellectual inspiration.

Moreover, attachment theory is one of the best current examples of the value of serious, coherent theorizing in psychology. It is a model of the process by which scientists move back and forth between clear conceptualizations and penetrating empirical research, with each pole of the dialectic repeatedly influencing the other over an extended period. Attachment theory today is in many respects similar to attachment theory 30 years ago, but it has become much more specific and deeply anchored in a wide variety of research methods, and it is being extended in important new directions as a result of careful and creative research. Because the theory was remarkably insightful and accurate to begin with, and because Ainsworth was such an effective researcher, the initial studies inspired by the theory were largely supportive of the theory's basic ideas, but they were also surprising and provocative in certain respects. The theory encountered considerable criticism at first, as any new scientific theory should. Yet the many honors accorded to Bowlby and Ainsworth toward the ends of their careers symbolize the considerable respect their work now engenders.

One problem created by the enormous literature on attachment, and by the theory's continual evolution in the light of new research, is that few scholars and researchers are familiar with the entire picture that is emerging. In order to make optimal use of the theory as a researcher, clinician, or teacher, one has to know what Bowlby and Ainsworth originally said; what subsequent research has revealed; which measures of attachment have been developed as well as what they actually measure; and what recent theoretical and empirical developments contribute to the overall "story" of attachment relationships and personality development. The purpose of the present volume is to satisfy these important professional needs. The book will prove useful to anyone who studies attachment processes; who uses attachment theory in clinical work; or who teaches courses and seminars that touch on, or focus on, attachment. It will be an excellent single resource for courses devoted to attachment theory and research.

The first edition of the *Handbook of Attachment*, published in 1999, has been extensively read, frequently cited, and influential in affecting research and clinical applications of attachment theory and research. We have been deeply gratified by the field's response to the volume; it has inspired everything from graduate seminars and clinical discussion groups to theoretical debates, major new research programs, and systematic tests of clinical interventions. Because psychology in general has moved energetically in the direction of neuroscience and behavioral genetics, there are many new findings to incorporate into an expanded theory. Because federal granting agencies have become increasingly interested in advancing "translational" research—research that moves basic research findings into the realm of clinical applications—there is a great deal of new information about intervention procedures and outcomes.

We have dealt with the many new developments in two ways. First, we have added entirely new chapters to the volume—on social neuroscience, affect regulation, attachment in the middle childhood years, foster care, divorce, and attachment issues in an aging population. Second, we have successfully asked authors of the previous chapters, or new authors who have taken over the territories covered by the original chapters, to retain what is historically and theoretically valuable from the first edition, but to alter the chapter content and structure vigorously where needed to convey what has changed over the past decade. In most of the chapters, large proportions of the subtopics covered and references cited are new. None of the first edition's chapters remains unchanged, and some have been entirely reworked.

The first section, "Overview of Attachment Theory," provides an updated primer on the theory. The first two chapters correspond roughly to the first and second volumes of Bowlby's trilogy, *Attachment and Loss*. Jude Cassidy, in Chapter 1, explains the central construct of attachment, and Roger Kobak and Stephanie Madsen, in Chapter 2, explain Bowlby's and Ainsworth's ideas about the emotional effects of disruption in attachment relationships. In Chapter 3, Phillip R. Shaver and R. Chris Fraley revisit the issues of loss and grief that Bowlby addressed in the third volume of *Attachment and Loss*. They show that despite many interesting new issues, challenges, and controversies in bereavement research, Bowlby's ideas stand up well and remain influential among both researchers and clinicians. Chapter 4 deals with what is perhaps the best-known part of the theory: Bowlby's and Ainsworth's conceptions of individual differences in the quality of attachment during childhood. Nancy S. Weinfield, L. Alan Sroufe, Byron Egeland, and Elizabeth Carlson summarize what has been discovered, especially in their own influential studies at the University of Minnesota, about the consequences of early attachment patterns. Their chapter illustrates the great value of long-term longitudinal studies. In Chapter 5, Inge Bretherton and Kristine A. Munholland examine the concept of "internal working models," which attachment theorists since Bowlby have used to explain the coherence and continuity of attachment patterns. The chapter contains much new information about the nature and structure of working models, including what is being learned from methods associated with cognitive neuroscience. Although there is obviously no way to replace Bowlby's and Ainsworth's seminal publications with a single section of a single volume, the initial five chapters of this handbook will provide readers—both those new to the field and those experienced in it—with a useful theoretical foundation.

The second section of the volume, "Biological Perspectives," stems from Bowlby's reliance on ethology and primate research in the creation of attachment theory. Bowlby derived many of his ideas from what today might be called psychobiology and evolutionary psychology, and his borrowing from those fields has been repaid with seminal hypotheses that can be tested in studies of primates and other mammals. In Chapter 6, Jeffry A. Simpson and Jay Belsky show how attachment theory fits with other midrange theories in evolutionary biology and psychology—theories that were not available when Bowlby formulated his theory. Just as child–parent relations made more sense when placed by Bowlby into an evolutionary, cross-species comparative framework, attachment theory itself makes more sense when viewed in the context of other neo-Darwinian evolutionary theories. Simpson and Belsky also argue that the major attachment patterns delineated by Ainsworth (secure, avoidant, and ambivalent) may represent different evolved strategies for increasing reproductive success in particular kinds of physical and social environments.

Chapter 7 marks a shift from the broad evolutionary considerations of the previous chapters to a review by H. Jonathan Polan and Myron A. Hofer of specific, systematic experimental studies of attachment-related behavioral and physiological processes in rats. Under these authors' high-powered analytic microscope, many remarkable details of attachment and separation responses become visible, and the notion of an attachment behavioral system becomes more complex. Their chapter is made new partly by an expansion of research on the effects of social experiences on gene expression. This new emphasis in research on psychobiological development shows up in various places in this new edition of the Handbook. In Chapter 8, Stephen J. Suomi shows that many of Bowlby's ideas about attachment and separation processes in humans, which were strongly affected by his reading of primate research, have been tested and elaborated in more detail in recent experimental and field-observational studies of rhesus monkeys and other primates. Two of the largest contributions of this research have been to reveal the interplay of infant temperament (now attributable to specific genes and gene polymorphisms) and parenting skills in determining the long-range behavioral outcomes of parenting, and to document the intergenerational transmission of attachment orientations—a process also probed in recent studies of humans.

In Chapter 9, Brian E. Vaughn, Kelly K. Bost, and Marinus J. van IJzendoorn show that the nature and effects of temperament have been more difficult to specify in humans than in rhesus monkeys. There is still no agreement on a single definition of, or conceptual framework for characterizing, human temperament, and no clear picture of the supposed association between individuals' temperaments and the nature of their attachment relationships. But there is growing specificity in measuring temperament, linking it with genes, and mapping its independent contributions to emotional and social development. The updated chapter shows that neither attachment constructs nor temperament constructs are likely to subsume the other; instead, many phenomena of basic and clinical interest are affected by both kinds of factors. In Chapter 10, Nathan A. Fox and Amie Ashley Hane explain how researchers have used a variety of psychophysiological assessment techniques to supplement and explain behavioral indicators of attachment processes. The authors discuss various surface psychophysiological measures (e.g., electroencephalography, skin conductance, heart rate), but also measures of hormones and neurochemicals used in attachment studies. In Chapter 11, James A. Coan integrates findings from the new field of social neuroscience, which relies heavily on brain imaging technology. Coan looks simultaneously at concepts and perspectives in attachment theory and in social neuroscience, and begins to create a framework that can include both.

The third section of the volume, "Attachment in Infancy and Childhood," begins with Robert S. Marvin and Preston A. Britner's explanation in Chapter 12 of the normative development of the attachment behavioral system across the lifespan. In Chapter 13, Jay Belsky and R. M. Pasco Fearon show that child–parent attachment patterns need to be viewed in social and developmental context; a particular relationship in a child's life, no matter how central, is unlikely to exist and have influences independently of other important relationships and ecological factors. Chapter 14 begins with the premise that caregiving is not restricted to parents, and that parents therefore are not children's only attachment figures. In this chapter, Carollee Howes and Susan Spieker examine attachment in the context of multiple caregivers—first considering children's attachments to other-than-mother caregivers, and then describing child–mother attachment relationship quality when children participate in day care programs, where they may develop attachment relationships with nonparental caregivers.

In Chapter 15, Lisa J. Berlin, Jude Cassidy, and Karen Appleyard explore the influence of early attachment on several kinds of affectional bonds: those with siblings, friends, romantic partners, and children. They also consider the large body of research on the influence of early attachments on children's important relationships that often do not meet Bowlby's criteria for affectional bonds: relationships with peers (as opposed to relationships with friends). Ross A. Thompson, in Chapter 16, discusses the complex issues that must be considered in efforts to understand why infant attachment sometimes does and sometimes does not predict later functioning; he provides a detailed review of the many longitudinal studies of attachment in infancy and childhood. In Chapter 17, Kathryn A. Kerns examines various ways of measuring attachment in the middle childhood years—a time when children typically still rely heavily on parental attachment figures, but also form important relationships with other adults and with peers. In Chapter 18, Judith Solomon and Carol George explain how quality of attachment has been measured in infancy and childhood. The authors show both that a complex construct has been successfully measured, with many scientific payoffs, and that much remains to be done to extend the measurement of attachment beyond infancy and to assure that it is measured in multiple, convergent ways.

The fourth section, "Attachment in Adolescence and Adulthood," contains chapters growing out of Bowlby's early contention that attachment characterizes humans "from the cradle to the grave." Chapter 19, by Joseph P. Allen, considers both the normative developmental changes in attachment and the meaning of individual differences in attachment phenomena during adolescence. The chapter includes identification and discussion of a series of "developmental transformations," each of which reflects critical changes in the attachment system during adolescence. This is an example of an important area of attachment research that has become increasingly well formulated since the first edition of the *Handbook of Attachment* was published. In Chapter 20, Debra Zeifman and Cindy Hazan argue that pair bonds between adult lovers and marital partners are true attachments, and that they can best be understood in terms of attachment theory. Chapter 21, by Judith A. Feeney, is a review of much of the recent research by personality and social psychologists that has grown out of the theoretical perspective explained by Zeifman and Hazan. Jonathan J. Mohr, in Chapter 22, offers a related and comprehensive examination of attachment in same-sex romantic relationships. He explores the evolutionary basis of same-sex attraction and the relevance

of the attachment system for same-sex relationships. He also reviews research that sheds light on attachment processes in these relationships, and shows how examination of attachment in same-sex relationships makes a unique contribution to understanding attachment processes more broadly. In Chapter 23, Mario Mikulincer and Phillip R. Shaver summarize the large and growing body of research on attachment and affect regulation in adulthood. From the beginning, Bowlby emphasized that emotions, emotion regulation, and psychological defenses are core aspects of attachment. Research related to this emphasis in the theory has grown considerably in recent years, adding a new bridge between basic research and clinical applications. In Chapter 24, Carol Magai examines the emerging area of research on attachment issues in middle and later life, when aging parents are often cared for by their middle-aged offspring. This reversal of roles in the context of major stresses related to aging, declining health, and death arouses many needs and emotions related to attachment that are of great interest to basic researchers, clinicians, and social policymakers. These topics will become increasingly important as the average age of people in all industrial societies continues to increase.

The remaining two chapters in this section deal with the complex measurement issues that have arisen as different kinds of researchers, with different theoretical and applied agendas, have measured attachment and attachment orientations in different ways in adolescence and adulthood. In Chapter 25, Erik Hesse provides a detailed conceptual analysis of the Adult Attachment Interview (AAI), explaining its origins and revisions and the fascinating literature it has spawned. Chapter 26, by Judith A. Crowell, R. Chris Fraley, and Phillip R. Shaver, places the AAI in the context of other adult attachment measures, several of which are designed to assess patterns of attachment in close relationships other than those between children and parents.

The fifth section of the volume, "Psychopathology and Clinical Applications of Attachment Theory and Research," contains chapters reflecting the strong roots of attachment theory in clinical psychology and psychiatry, and the contributions that the theory and associated research are making to clinical work. Despite the fact that Bowlby—a psychiatrist and psychoanalyst who treated patients throughout his career—based his original ideas on clinical observations, and despite the fact that Ainsworth was also trained as a clinician, until recently it has been developmental and social psychologists rather than clinical psychologists who have found attachment theory and research of greatest relevance. Bowlby and Ainsworth themselves viewed their work as having important clinical applications, and both were interested in improving clinical treatment. Both were pleased, late in their careers, when clinicians increasingly found their work useful.

The first four chapters in this section focus on psychopathology, and the next four examine attachment theory in relation to specific therapeutic perspectives. In Chapter 27, Michelle DeKlyen and Mark T. Greenberg provide a systematic and detailed examination of the connection between attachment and psychopathology in childhood. The inclusion in this section of Chapter 28, Karlen Lyons-Ruth and Deborah Jacobvitz's examination of attachment disorganization, follows from recent studies of attachment and psychopathology suggesting that individuals with disorganized attachment are at particular risk for psychopathology. The chapter examines the developmental origins, correlates, and outcomes of attachment disorganization, and reviews data and theoretical models linking disorganized attachment with adult violence, trauma, and maltreatment. The new research in this area will be especially fascinating to clinicians and clinical researchers. In Chapter 29, Mary Dozier and Michael Rutter discuss attachment issues associated with foster care and adoption. In foster care and in some cases when older children are adopted, new parents have an opportunity to affect the development of a child whose prior attachment history was likely to have been troubled. In Chapter 30, Mary Dozier, K. Chase Stovall-McClough, and Kathleen E. Albus examine attachment and psychopathology in adulthood.

Next are chapters describing the contributions that attachment theory and research are making to specific forms of therapy. In Chapter 31, Lisa J. Berlin, Charles H. Zeanah, and Alicia F. Lieberman describe contributions to infant–parent psychotherapy and other interventions with infants and young children. In Chapter 32, Arietta Slade describes contributions, especially of research using the AAI, to individual psychotherapy with adults. Chapter 33, by Peter Fonagy, George Gergely, and Mary Target, provides an overview of the complex relations between attachment theory and psychoanalytic theory, suggesting points of both substantial contact and significant divergence. This chapter lays out in detail the authors'

work on the importance of "reflective functioning" or "mind-mindedness" in maintaining adult attachment security and fostering security in children. In Chapter 34, Susan M. Johnson describes contributions of attachment theory and research to family and couple therapy.

The final section of the volume, "Systems, Culture, and Context," provides a sampling of the many topic areas into which attachment theory and research have been extended. In Chapter 35, Carol George and Judith Solomon examine caregiving behavior—the biologically based behavior (closely intertwined with attachment behavior) that Bowlby claimed must be understood in order to ensure a thorough understanding of attachment. Chapter 36, by Karin Grossmann, Klaus E. Grossmann, Heinz Kindler, and Peter Zimmermann, reconsiders the role of the exploratory behavioral system, as well as what Ainsworth called the "attachment–exploration balance." Chapter 37 deals with a frequently asked question about attachment processes: Are they essentially the same or importantly different across cultures? Marinus H. van IJzendoorn and Abraham Sagi-Schwartz review studies conducted around the world and show that although many of the parameter settings of the attachment behavioral system vary in understandable ways as a function of cultural context, the system itself is recognizably the same. Pehr Granqvist and Lee A. Kirkpatrick, in Chapter 38, show that attachment theory and research shed new light on a variety of religious phenomena. Chapter 39, by Brooke C. Feeney and Joan K. Monin, examines ways in which attachment theory and research add to our understanding of divorce, which has important emotional effects on divorcing adults and their children. In Chapter 40, Michael Rutter discusses implications of attachment theory and research for public policy, especially policies concerning child care.

This is a volume of huge scope, with thousands of references, and it has taken many talented people's time and dedication to bring it to fruition. Our first thanks go to the international cast of chapter authors—busy people all—who agreed not only to write for the volume, but also to tailor their chapters to our specific needs. As you will see, the chapters are not like ones in the usual anthologies, in which authors simply spell out their own ideas and research programs without much regard for what other authors in the same book are saying. Here, each author or set of authors looks seriously at the history of the area under discussion and explains how work in that area is progressing, what new conclusions are being drawn, and how the work might be applied. In many places the authors refer to other chapters in the volume, making it easier to see how different topics are connected. Many of the chapters were vetted by colleagues, and all were carefully commented upon and edited by both of us. Several of the chapters went through multiple drafts. The chapter authors, all people with considerable experience and their own high standards, were remarkably cooperative with our editorial plans and interventions. We believe that the book is unusually approachable, readable, and understandable as a result.

We had wonderful assistance from the professionals at The Guilford Press. Seymour Weingarten, Editor-in-Chief, helped conceptualize the first edition and get us involved with it; he then remained incredibly supportive, patient, and enthusiastic throughout the process. Carolyn Graham and Judith Grauman were enormously helpful on a daily basis, responding quickly and helpfully to our many queries. We were fortunate in having the stellar Marie Sprayberry serve once again as our copyeditor. Laura Specht Patchkofsky was our multitalented production editor. Paul Gordon designed a lovely cover. Behind the scenes of any large and long effort such as this one, there are scores of other professionals who quietly do excellent work without ever personally meeting the beneficiaries of their labor. We thank them, sincerely, as a group.

We are also extremely grateful to our families. It's not easy to study and write about attachment every day while telling your own family members that you'll be with them in a while, when the urgent editorial tasks are finished. The contradiction between sensitivity and responsiveness to chapter authors and sensitivity and responsiveness to your loved ones is palpable. Certainly it is enlightening and personally gratifying for people who study attachment to experience its ramifications in everyday life.

Finally, we wish to thank each other. Collaborating on a large project like this one is somewhat like running a family business. It requires open, honest communication about both shared and divergent opinions. Over the years of working on this book, we have been guests in each other's homes; eaten some great conference meals together; discussed every chapter in great detail; and begun to collaborate on research, not just on book editing. It's rare for two professors at universities thousands of miles apart to sustain such a good and deep working relationship, especially when we come from different parts of psychology and conduct different kinds of research. Sharing conceptual and editing problems, thoughts about attachment theory and research, computer screens in different cities, and reactions to the book as it developed has been extremely rewarding. We heartily congratulate and thank each other.

As we did with the first edition, we dedicate this volume to the memories of John Bowlby and Mary Ainsworth. They not only had great ideas, which they were able to transform into excellent research; they provided a model of how people can work together to create a large intellectual edifice that has many beneficial consequences for other professionals and the people whose lives they work to improve.

JUDE CASSIDY
PHILLIP R. SHAVER

Contents

PART V. PSYCHOPATHOLOGY AND CLINICAL APPLICATIONS OF ATTACHMENT THEORY AND RESEARCH

PART VI. SYSTEMS, CULTURE, AND CONTEXT

PART I

OVERVIEW OF ATTACHMENT THEORY

CHAPTER 1

The Nature of the Child's Ties

JUDE CASSIDY

John Bowlby's work on attachment theory can be viewed as starting shortly after his graduation from Cambridge University, with the observations he made when he worked in a home for maladjusted boys. Two boys, both of whom had suffered disruptions in their relationships with their mothers, made important impressions on him. Bowlby's more systematic retrospective examination, published over a decade later as "Forty-Four Juvenile Thieves: Their Characters and Home Life" (Bowlby, 1944), as well as the observations of others (Bender & Yarnell, 1941; Goldfarb, 1943), convinced him that major disruptions in the mother–child relationship are precursors of later psychopathology. Bowlby's observations led not only to his belief that the child's relationship with the mother is important for later functioning, but also to a belief that this relationship is of critical immediate importance to the child. Bowlby, along with his colleague James Robertson, observed that children experienced intense distress when separated from their mothers, even if they were fed and cared for by others. A predictable pattern emerged—one of angry protest followed by despair (Robertson & Bowlby, 1952). Bowlby came to wonder why the mother is so important to the child.

At the time, the two widely accepted theories that offered explanations for the child's tie to the mother were both secondary-drive theories. Psychoanalytic and social learning theorists alike proposed that an infant's relationship with the mother emerges because she feeds the infant (e.g., Freud, 1910/1957; Sears, Maccoby, & Levin, 1957), and that the pleasure experienced upon having hunger drives satisfied comes to be associated with the mother's presence. When Bowlby was first developing attachment theory, he became aware of evidence from animal studies that seriously called this perspective into question. Lorenz (1935) noted that infant geese became attached to parents—even to objects—that did not feed them. Harlow (1958) observed that infant rhesus monkeys, in times of stress, preferred not the wire-mesh "mother" that provided food, but the cloth-covered "mother" that afforded contact comfort. Soon systematic observations of human infants were made, and it became evident that babies too became attached to people who did not feed them (Ainsworth, 1967; Schaffer & Emerson, 1964). Years later, Bowlby recalled that

> this [secondary-drive] theory did not seem to me to fit the facts. For example, were it true, an infant of a year or two should take readily to whomever feeds him, and this clearly is not the case. But, if the secondary drive dependency theory was inadequate, what was the alternative? (1980b, p. 650)

Because he found himself dissatisfied with traditional theories, Bowlby sought a new explanation through discussion with colleagues from such fields as evolutionary biology, ethology, developmental psychology, cognitive science, and control systems theory (Bowlby, 1969/1982). He drew upon all of these fields to formulate the innovative proposition that the mechanisms underlying the infant's tie to the mother originally emerged as a result of evolutionary pressures. For Bowlby, this strikingly strong tie, evident particularly when disrupted, results not from an associational learning process (a secondary drive), but rather from a biologically based desire for proximity that arose through the process of natural selection. Bowlby (1958, 1960a, 1960b) introduced attachment theory in a series of papers, the first of which was "The Nature of the Child's Tie to His Mother." All of the major points of attachment theory were presented there in at least rudimentary form, providing, as Bretherton (1992) noted, "the first basic blueprint of attachment theory" (p. 762). These ideas were later elaborated in Bowlby's trilogy, *Attachment and Loss* (1969/1982, 1973, 1980a).

A member of Bowlby's research team during this period of initial formulation of attachment theory was a developmental psychologist visiting from Canada, Mary Salter Ainsworth. Her serendipitous connection with Bowlby—a friend had shown her a newspaper advertisement for a developmental research position—proved fortunate for the development of attachment theory. Ainsworth conducted two pioneering naturalistic observation studies of mothers and infants in which she applied the ethological principles of attachment theory as a framework. One of these investigations was conducted in the early 1950s in Uganda; the other was carried out in the early 1960s in Baltimore. These inquiries provided the most extensive home observation data to date and laid the foundation for Ainsworth's contributions to attachment theory, as well as for Bowlby's continued formulations. Ainsworth later created an assessment tool, the "Strange Situation," that triggered the productive flowering of the empirical study of individual differences in attachment quality—the research that is largely responsible for the place of attachment theory in contemporary developmental psychology.

The present chapter summarizes Bowlby's initial ethological approach to understanding the child's tie to the mother, along with elaborations based on more recent research and theorizing. First, I discuss the biological bases of attachment,

describing the evolutionary roots of attachment behavior, the attachment behavioral system and its organization, the role of context in the system's operation, the role of emotion, the role of cognition, and individual differences in attachment. Next, I examine the attachment system in relation to other behavioral systems: the exploratory, fear, sociable, and caregiving systems. Third, I consider the nature of the child's attachment bond to his or her attachment figures, and describe how attachments differ from other affectional bonds. Finally, I discuss multiple attachments. Although Bowlby's idea that attachment is a lifespan phenomenon was present in his earliest writings (e.g., Bowlby, 1956), his principal focus was the tie to the mother during childhood, and I maintain that focus in this chapter.

BIOLOGICAL BASES OF ATTACHMENT BEHAVIOR

The most fundamental aspect of attachment theory is its focus on the biological bases of attachment behavior (Bowlby, 1958, 1969/1982). "Attachment behavior" has the predictable outcome of increasing proximity of the child to the attachment figure (usually the mother). Some attachment behaviors (smiling, vocalizing) are signaling behaviors that alert the mother to the child's interest in interaction, and thus serve to bring her to the child. Other behaviors (crying) are aversive, and bring the mother to the child to terminate them. Some (approaching and following) are active behaviors that move the child to the mother.

An Evolutionary Perspective

Bowlby proposed that during the time in which humans were evolving, when they lived in what he called "the environment of evolutionary adaptedness," genetic selection favored attachment behaviors because they increased the likelihood of child–mother proximity, which in turn increased the likelihood of protection and provided survival advantage. In keeping with the evolutionary thinking of the time, Bowlby emphasized survival of the species in his earliest theoretical formulations. By the time he revised *Attachment* (Volume 1 of his trilogy, *Attachment and Loss*; Bowlby, 1969/1982), he noted that advances in evolutionary theory necessitated a framework within which for all behavioral systems, including attachment, "the ultimate outcome to be attained is always the survival of the genes an individual is carrying" (p. 56). (For a more extensive discussion of attachment and this notion of "reproductive fitness," see Simpson & Belsky, Chapter 6, this volume.)

Many predictable outcomes beneficial to the child are thought to result from the child's proximity to the parent (Bowlby, 1969/1982). These include feeding, learning about the environment, and social interaction, all of which are important. In the environment of evolutionary adaptedness, infants who were biologically predisposed to stay close to their mothers were less likely to be killed by predators, and it was for this reason that Bowlby referred to protection from predators as the "biological function" of attachment behavior.[1] Because of this biological function of protection, Bowlby considered infants to be predisposed particularly to seek their parents in times of distress. In a basic Darwinian sense, then, the proclivity to seek proximity is a behavioral adaptation in the same way that a fox's white coat on the tundra is an adaptation. Within this framework, attachment is considered a normal and healthy characteristic of humans throughout the lifespan, rather than a sign of immaturity that needs to be outgrown.

The Attachment Behavioral System

Attachment behaviors are thought to be organized into an "attachment behavioral system." Bowlby (1969/1982) borrowed the behavioral system concept from ethology to describe a species-specific system of behaviors that leads to certain predictable outcomes, at least one of which contributes to reproductive fitness. The concept of the behavioral system involves inherent motivation. There is no need to view attachment as the by-product of any more fundamental processes or "drive." Children are thought to become attached whether their parents are meeting their physiological needs or not. This idea is supported by evidence indicating that in contrast to what secondary-drive theories lead one to expect (e.g., Freud, 1910/1957; Sears et al., 1957), attachment is not a result of associations with feeding (Ainsworth, 1967; Harlow, 1962; Schaffer & Emerson, 1964). Furthermore, findings that infants become attached even to abusive mothers (Bowlby, 1956) suggest that the system is not driven by simple pleasurable associations. Bowlby's notion of the inherent motivation of the attachment system is compatible with Piaget's (1954) formulation of the inherent motivation of the child's interest in exploration.

Central to the concept of the attachment behavioral system is the notion that several different attachment behaviors are organized within the individual in response to a particular history of internal and external cues. Sroufe and Waters (1977) emphasized that the attachment behavioral system is "not a set of behaviors that are constantly and uniformly operative" (p. 1185). Rather, the "functional equivalence" of behaviors is noted, with a variety of behaviors having similar meanings and serving similar functions. As Bowlby (1969/1982) noted, "whether a child moves toward a mother by running, walking, crawling, shuffling or, in the case of a thalidomide child, by rolling, is thus of very little consequence compared to the set-goal of his locomotion, namely proximity to mother" (p. 373). The behaviors chosen in a particular context are the ones the infant finds most useful at that moment. With development, the child gains access to a greater variety of ways of achieving proximity, and learns which ones are most effective in which circumstances. Indeed, as Sroufe and Waters pointed out, this organizational perspective helps to explain stability within the context of both developmental and contextual changes. Thus an infant may maintain a stable internal organization of the attachment behavioral system in relation to the mother over time and across contexts, yet the specific behaviors used in the service of this organization may vary greatly. Thus, whereas a nonmobile infant may be expected to cry and reach out to the mother for contact, a mobile child may achieve the same goal of establishing contact by crawling after her.

This emphasis on the organization of the attachment behavioral system also helps to explain its operation in a "goal-corrected" manner. Unlike certain reflexes that, once activated, maintain a fixed course (e.g., sneezing, rooting), the attachment behavioral system enables the individual to respond flexibly to environmental changes while attempting to attain a goal. Bowlby used the analogy of a heat-seeking missile: Once launched, the missile does not remain on a preset course; rather, it incorporates information about changes in the target's location and adjusts its trajectory accordingly. Similarly, the infant is capable of considering changes in the mother's location and behavior (as well as other environmental changes) when attempting to maintain proximity to her. And the flexible use of a variety of attachment behaviors, depending on the circumstances, affords the infant greater efficiency in goal-corrected responses. For instance, an infant may see the mother starting to leave in an unfamiliar environment and may desire to increase proximity to her. The infant may begin by reaching for her and then following her (changing course as she moves); if this fails, calling or crying may be initiated.

Bowlby's approach to the organization of attachment behavior involves a control systems perspective. Drawing on observations of ethologists who described instinctive behavior in animals as serving to maintain them in a certain relation with the environment for long periods of time, Bowlby proposed that a control systems approach could also be applied to attachment behavior. He described the workings of a thermostat as an example of a control system. When the room gets too cold, the thermostat activates the heater; when the desired temperature is reached, the thermostat turns the heater off. Bowlby described children as wanting to maintain a certain proximity to their mothers. When a separation becomes too great in distance or time, the attachment system becomes activated, and when sufficient proximity has been achieved, it is terminated. Bowlby (following Bretherton, 1980; see Bowlby, 1969/1982) later described the attachment system as working slightly differently from a thermostat—as being continually activated (with variations of relatively more or less activation), rather than being completely turned off at times. According to Bowlby, the child's goal is not an object (e.g., the mother), but rather a state—a maintenance of the desired distance from the mother, depending on the circumstances. Bowlby described this idea of behavioral homeostasis as similar to the process of physiological homeostasis, whereby physiological systems (e.g., blood pressure and body temperature) are maintained within set limits. Like physiological control systems, a behavioral control system is thought to be organized within the central nervous system. According to Bowlby, the distinction between the two is that the latter is "one in which the set-limits concern the organism's relation to features of the environment and in which the limits are maintained by behavioral rather than physiological means" (p. 372).

The Role of Context

The child's desired degree of proximity to the parent is thought to vary under differing circumstances, and Bowlby (1969/1982) was interested in understanding how these different circumstances contribute to relative increases and decreases in activation of the attachment system. Thus he described two classes of factors that contribute to ac-

tivation of the attachment system, both of which are conditions indicating danger or stress. One relates to conditions of the child (such as illness, fatigue, hunger, or pain). The other relates to conditions of the environment (such as the presence of threatening stimuli); particularly important are the location and behavior of the mother (such as her absence, withdrawal, or rejection of the child). Interaction among these causal factors can be quite complex: Sometimes only one needs to be present, and at other times several are necessary. In regard to relative deactivation of the attachment system, Bowlby made it clear that his approach had nothing in common with a model in which a behavior stops when its energy supply is depleted (e.g., Freud, 1940/1964). In Bowlby's view, attachment behavior stops in the presence of a terminating stimulus. For most distressed infants, contact with their mothers is an effective terminating stimulus. Yet the nature of the stimulus that serves to terminate attachment behavior differs according to the degree of activation of the attachment system. If the attachment system is intensely activated, contact with the parent may be necessary to terminate it. If it is moderately activated, the presence or soothing voice of the parent (or even of a familiar substitute caregiver) may suffice. In either case, the infant is viewed as using the mother as a "safe haven" to return to in times of trouble. In sum, proximity seeking is activated when the infant receives information (from both internal and external sources) that a goal (the desired distance from the mother) is exceeded. It remains activated until the goal is achieved, and then it stops.

The Role of Emotion

According to Bowlby (1979), emotions are strongly associated with attachment:

> Many of the most intense emotions arise during the formation, the maintenance, the disruption, and the renewal of attachment relationships. The formation of a bond is described as falling in love, maintaining a bond as loving someone, and losing a partner as grieving over someone. Similarly, threat of loss arouses anxiety and actual loss gives rise to sorrow; whilst each of these situations is likely to arouse anger. The unchallenged maintenance of a bond is experienced as a source of joy. (p. 130)

It is likely that these affective responses originally resulted from evolutionary pressures. An infant predisposed to experience positive emotions in relation to an attachment and sadness with its loss may actively work to maintain attachments, which contribute in turn to the infant's enhanced reproductive fitness.

Bowlby also viewed emotions as important regulatory mechanisms within attachment relationships, noting, for instance, that anger and protest, as long as they do not become excessive and destructive, can serve to alert the attachment figure to the child's interest in maintaining the relationship (Bowlby, 1973; see Kobak & Madsen, Chapter 2, this volume). More recently, attachment theorists have noted the ways in which the regulation of emotions is used in the service of maintaining the relationship with the attachment figure, and they have noted that individual differences in attachment security have much to do with the ways in which emotions are responded to, shared, communicated about, and regulated within the attachment relationship (Cassidy, 1994; Cassidy & Berlin, 1994; Cassidy & Kobak, 1988; Kobak & Duemmler, 1994; Thompson & Meyer, 2007; see also Kobak & Madsen, Chapter 2; Bretherton & Munholland, Chapter 5; and Thompson, Chapter 16, this volume).

The Role of Cognition

Drawing on cognitive information theory, Bowlby (1969/1982) proposed that the organization of the attachment behavioral system involves cognitive components—specifically, mental representations of the attachment figure, the self, and the environment, all of which are largely based on experiences. Bretherton (1991) suggested that repeated attachment-related experiences could become organized as scripts, which would in turn become the building blocks of broader representations (see also Vaughn et al., 2006). (This emphasis on the importance of an individual's actual experiences was another way in which Bowlby's theory differed from that of Freud, who emphasized instead the role of internal fantasies.) Bowlby referred to these representations as "representational models" and as "internal working models." According to Bowlby, these models allow individuals to anticipate the future and make plans, thereby operating most efficiently. (There is in fact evidence that even young children are capable of using representations to make predictions about the future; see Heller & Berndt, 1981.) The child is thought to rely on these models, for instance, when making decisions about which specific attachment behavior(s) to

use in a specific situation with a specific person. Representational models are considered to work best when they are relatively accurate reflections of reality, and conscious processing is required to check and revise models in order to keep them up to date. Extensive discussion of these cognitive models is provided by Bretherton (1990; Bretherton & Munholland, Chapter 5, this volume) and by Main, Kaplan, and Cassidy (1985); see also Baldwin (1992) for a review of similarities between these models and a variety of constructs within the literatures on developmental, social, clinical, and cognitive psychology. Bowlby (1969/1982, 1973, 1979, 1980a) also discussed the role within the attachment system of other cognitive processes, such as object permanence, discrimination learning, generalization, nonconscious processing, selective attention and memory, and interpretative biases.

Individual Differences

In extending the biological emphasis of Bowlby's initial theorizing, Main (1990) proposed that the biologically based human tendency to become attached is paralleled by a biologically based ability to be flexible to the range of likely caregiving environments. This flexibility is thought to contribute to variations associated with quality of attachment. Whereas nearly all children become attached (even to mothers who abuse them; Bowlby, 1956), not all are securely attached. Striking individual differences exist. Secure attachment occurs when a child has a mental representation of the attachment figure as available and responsive when needed. Infants are considered to be insecurely attached when they lack such a representation. Bowlby's early clinical observations led him to predict that just as feeding does not cause attachment in infants, so individual differences in feeding (e.g., breast vs. bottle feeding) do not contribute to individual differences in attachment quality. In one of his earliest writings, Bowlby (1958) predicted that the important factor is "the extent to which the mother has permitted clinging and following, and all the behavior associated with them, or has refused them" (p. 370). This prediction has since gained empirical support (e.g., Ainsworth, Blehar, Waters, & Wall, 1978; see also De Wolff & van IJzendoorn, 1997). (Theoretical issues related to individual differences in attachment security are discussed in detail by Weinfield, Sroufe, Egeland, & Carlson, Chapter 4, this volume.)

ATTACHMENT IN RELATION
TO OTHER BEHAVIORAL SYSTEMS

The attachment behavioral system can be fully understood only in terms of its complex interplay with other biologically based behavioral systems. Bowlby highlighted two of these as being particularly related to the attachment system in young children: the exploratory behavioral system and the fear behavioral system. The activation of these other systems is related to activation of the attachment system. Activation of the fear system generally heightens activation of the attachment system. In contrast, activation of the exploratory system can, under certain circumstances, reduce activation of the attachment system. As any parent knows, providing a novel set of car keys can at least temporarily distract a baby who wants to be picked up, as long as the infant's attachment system is not intensely activated. These two behavioral systems are discussed in this section, as are the sociable and caregiving behavioral systems.

The Exploratory System

The links between the exploratory behavioral system and the attachment behavioral system are thought to be particularly intricate. According to Bowlby, the exploratory system gives survival advantages to the child by providing important information about the workings of the environment: how to use tools, build structures, obtain food, and negotiate physical obstacles. Yet unbridled exploration with no attention to potential hazards can be dangerous. The complementary yet mutually inhibiting nature of the exploratory and attachment systems is thought to have evolved to ensure that while the child is protected by maintaining proximity to attachment figures, he or she nonetheless gradually learns about the environment through exploration. According to Ainsworth (1972), "the dynamic equilibrium between these two behavioral systems is even more significant for development (and for survival) than either in isolation" (p. 118).

The framework that best captures the links between the attachment and exploratory systems is that of an infant's use of an attachment figure as a "secure base from which to explore"—a concept first described by Ainsworth (1963) and central to attachment theory (Ainsworth et al., 1978; Bowlby, 1969/1982, 1988). On the basis of her observa-

tions during the infant's first year of life, Ainsworth referred to an "attachment–exploration balance" (Ainsworth, Bell, & Stayton, 1971). Most infants balance these two behavioral systems, responding flexibly to a specific situation after assessing both the environment's characteristics and the caregiver's availability and likely behavior. For instance, when the infant experiences the environment as dangerous, exploration is unlikely. Furthermore, when the attachment system is activated (perhaps by separation from the attachment figure, illness, fatigue, or unfamiliar people and surroundings), infant exploration and play decline. Conversely, when the attachment system is not activated (e.g., when a healthy, well-rested infant is in a comfortable setting with an attachment figure nearby), exploration is enhanced. Thus attachment, far from interfering with exploration, is viewed as fostering exploration. Bowlby (1973) described as important not only the physical presence of an attachment figure, but also the infant's belief that the attachment figure will be available if needed. A converging body of empirical work, in which maternal physical or psychological presence was experimentally manipulated, has provided compelling evidence of the theoretically predicted associations between maternal availability and infant exploration (Ainsworth & Wittig, 1969; Carr, Dabbs, & Carr, 1975; Rheingold, 1969; Sorce & Emde, 1981).

The Fear System

The fear behavioral system is also thought to be closely linked to the attachment system. For Bowlby, the biological function of the fear system, like that of the attachment system, is protection. It is biologically adaptive for children to be frightened of certain stimuli. Without such fear, survival and reproduction would be reduced. Bowlby (1973) described "natural clues to danger"—stimuli that are not inherently dangerous, but that increase the likelihood of danger. These include darkness, loud noises, aloneness, and sudden looming movements. Because the attachment and fear systems are intertwined, so that frightened infants increase their attachment behavior, infants who find these stimuli frightening are considered more likely to seek protection and thus to survive to pass on their genes. The presence or absence of the attachment figure is thought to play an important role in the activation of an infant's fear system, such that an available and accessible attachment figure makes the infant much less susceptible to fear, and there is evidence that this is so (Morgan & Ricciuti, 1969; Sorce & Emde, 1981). In fact, even photographs of the mother can calm a fearful infant, as can "security blankets" for children who are attached to such objects (Passman & Erck, 1977; Passman & Weisberg, 1975). The fear behavioral system is discussed more extensively by Kobak and Madsen (Chapter 2, this volume).

The Sociable System

A complete understanding of the attachment behavioral system rests on an understanding of its distinction from the sociable (or "affiliative") behavioral system.[2] Although Bowlby did not discuss this behavioral system as extensively as he did some others, he did point out, as have other theorists, that the sociable system is distinct from the attachment behavioral system. Bowlby (1969/1982) wrote,

> "Affiliation" was introduced by Murray (1938): "Under this heading are classed all manifestations of friendliness and goodwill, of the desire to do things in company with others." As such it is a much broader concept than attachment and is not intended to cover behavior that is directed towards one or a few particular figures, which is the hallmark of attachment behavior. (p. 229)

According to Ainsworth (1989), it is "reasonable to believe that there is some basic behavioral system that has evolved in social species that leads individuals to seek to maintain proximity to conspecifics, even to those to whom they are not attached or otherwise bonded, and despite the fact that wariness is likely to be evoked by those who are unfamiliar" (p. 713). Harlow and Harlow (1965) described the "peer affectional system through which infants and children interrelate ... and develop persisting affection for each other" as an "affectional system" distinct from those involving infant and parents (p. 288). Bronson (1972) referred to affiliation as an "adaptive system" present in infancy and separate from attachment. Bretherton and Ainsworth (1974) examined the interplay among several behavioral systems in infants, including the sociable and the attachment systems, and Greenberg and Marvin (1982) examined this interplay in preschool children. Hinde (1974) described nonhuman primates' play with peers, which he identified as different from

mother–child interaction, as "consum[ing] so much time and energy that it must be of crucial adaptive importance" (p. 227).

The sociable system is thus defined as the organization of the biologically based, survival-promoting tendency to be sociable with others. An important predictable outcome of activation of this system is that individuals are likely to spend at least part of their time in the company of others. Given evidence from the primate literature that individuals in the company of others are much less likely to be killed by predators (Eisenberg, 1966), it seems reasonable to assume that humans too would derive the important survival advantage of protection from associating with others. The sociable system is likely to contribute to an individual's survival and reproductive fitness in other important ways: Primates biologically predisposed to be sociable with others increase their ability to gather food, build shelter, and create warmth; they learn about the environment more efficiently; and they gain access to a group of others with whom they may eventually mate (see Huntingford, 1984, for a review). Strong evidence of the importance of the sociable system for the development of young nonhuman primates comes from several studies, most notably those of Harlow and his associates (e.g., Harlow, 1969), in which monkeys reared with their mothers but without peers were seriously hindered in their social development and could not mate or parent effectively (see also Miller, Caul, & Mirsky, 1967).

Observations of both humans and other primates clearly show differences between the attachment and sociable systems in what activates behavior, in what terminates behavior, and in the way behaviors are organized (Bretherton & Ainsworth, 1974; Harlow, 1969; Vandell, 1980). The sociable system is most likely to be activated when the attachment system is not activated. According to Bowlby,

> A child seeks his attachment-figure when he is tired, hungry, ill, or alarmed and also when he is uncertain of that figure's whereabouts; when the attachment-figure is found he wants to remain in proximity to him or her and may want also to be held or cuddled. By contrast, a child seeks a playmate when he is in good spirits and confident of the whereabouts of his attachment-figure; when the playmate is found, moreover, the child wants to engage in playful interaction with him or her. If this analysis is right, the roles of attachment-figure and playmate are distinct. (1969/1982, p. 307)

Lewis, Young, Brooks, and Michalson (1975) interpreted their observations of pairs of 1-year-olds and their mothers similarly: "Mothers are good for protection, peers for watching and playing with" (p. 56).

The Caregiving System

In one of his earliest writings, Bowlby (1956) pointed out that further understanding of attachment could be gained from examination of the mother's tie to her infant. Bowlby later (1984) wrote briefly about "parenting behavior" from a biological perspective as "like attachment behavior, … in some degree preprogrammed" (p. 271). He described the biologically based urge to care for and protect children, yet he simultaneously viewed individual differences in the nature of parenting as emerging largely through learning. Although Bowlby wrote little about this topic, his ethological perspective, his ideas about interrelated behavioral systems, and his interest in attachment-related processes across the lifespan lend themselves readily to an elaboration of the parental side of what he (Bowlby, 1969/1982) called the "attachment–caregiving social bond." Solomon and George (1996; George & Solomon, 1996; see also George & Solomon, Chapter 35, this volume) have filled this void, writing in detail about the "caregiving system." As George and Solomon (Chapter 35, this volume, Note 1) state, it is difficult to delineate precisely which aspects of parenting behavior should be considered part of the caregiving system. I propose that the term "caregiving system" be used to describe a subset of parental behaviors—only those behaviors designed to promote proximity and comfort when the parent perceives that the child is in real or potential danger. The chief behavior within this system is retrieval (Bowlby, 1969/1982); others include calling, reaching, grasping, restraining, following, soothing, and rocking.[3]

Just as the child's interactions with the parent involve more than the attachment system (e.g., a child may approach the father not for comfort but for play), so other parental systems may be activated during interactions with the child (Bowlby, 1969/1982). These various behavioral systems can all be viewed as enhancing the child's survival and reproductive fitness (e.g., teaching, feeding, playing). A parent may be differentially responsive to a child when each of these different parental behavioral systems is activated (e.g., sensitive when teaching or feeding, yet insensitive when the caregiving system is activated). The predominance of

each of these parental behavioral systems varies considerably both across and within cultures. For instance, as Bretherton (1985) pointed out, among Mayan Indians in Mexico, mothers rarely serve as playmates for their infants but are quite available and responsive as caregivers (Brazelton, 1977). Similarly, Ainsworth (1990) noted that "the mothers of Ganda babies who were securely attached to them almost never played with them, even though they were highly sensitive caregivers" (p. 482; see also van IJzendoorn & Sagi-Schwartz, Chapter 37, this volume). Within-culture variation exists as well: Within a particular culture, one mother may be a readily available attachment figure, yet stodgy and inept in the role of playmate; another mother may be comfortable in interaction with her children only in her roles as teacher or coach when attention is focused on a task or skill, and may be uncomfortable with attachment-related interactions. Main, Hesse, and Kaplan (2005) have proposed that such parental discomfort (anxiety) may emerge when infant behavior interferes with parents' ability to preserve "the state of mind that had seemed optimal for maintenance of the relationship to their own parents during childhood" (p. 292). (For additional discussion of the ways in which particular parents experience discomfort when faced with particular infant behavior, see Cassidy et al., 2005.)

As is the case with the child's attachment system, the predictable outcome of activation of the caregiving system is parent–child proximity, and the biological function is protection of the child. In most cases, both parent and child work together to maintain a comfortable degree of proximity. If the child moves away, the parent will retrieve him or her; if the parent moves away, the child will follow or signal for the parent to return. Following Bowlby's (1969/1982) thinking, it seems likely that when the caregiving system is relatively activated, the child's attachment system can be relatively deactivated; attachment behaviors are not needed, because the parent has assumed responsibility for maintaining proximity. If the caregiving system is not relatively activated, then the child's attachment system becomes activated, should the context call for it. This is one reason why the mother's leaving is particularly disturbing to a child and particularly likely to activate attachment behavior. This "dynamic equilibrium" (Bowlby, 1969/1982, p. 236) contributes to understanding the notion of the mother's providing "a secure base from which to explore." The mother's monitoring of infant–mother proximity frees the infant from such monitoring and permits greater attention to exploring. For instance, if, when visiting a new park, a mother actively follows the infant in his or her explorations, the infant is much more likely to cover a wide area than if the mother sits on a bench talking with friends. Empirical support for this proposition comes from a study in which the simple act of a mother's diverting her attention away from the infant to a magazine in a brief laboratory procedure reduced the quality of infant exploration (Sorce & Emde, 1981).

Yet parent and child do not always agree on what distance between them is acceptable. For example, a mother's fear system may be activated and prompt her to retrieve an infant whose activated exploratory system leads him or her to prefer to move away. Parents and their children may also differ in terms of how their priorities guide activation of their behavioral systems. For instance, when an infant's attachment system is activated in the presence of the mother, the infant's sole wish is for her to respond. Although such infant behavior is usually a powerful activating stimulus for the mother's caregiving system, the mother may choose among several competing needs and may or may not provide care (Trivers, 1974). The child's concern is immediate and focused; the mother's concerns may be more diffuse and long-range. The mother may have to leave the infant to work to support the family (in which case activation of her food-getting behavioral system has taken precedence over her caregiving system). Or she may have several children to whose needs she must attend. Main (1990) has proposed that from an evolutionary perspective, maternal insensitivity to a particular child may be useful to the mother if it maximizes the total number of surviving offspring (see also Simpson & Belsky, Chapter 6, this volume).

As is true for many behavioral systems, activation of the caregiving system results from both internal and external cues. Internal cues include presence of hormones, cultural beliefs, parental state (e.g., whether the parent is tired or sick), and activation of other parental behavioral systems (e.g., exploratory, food-getting, fear). External cues include state of the environment (e.g., whether it is familiar, whether there is danger, whether others are present and who these others are), state of the infant (e.g., whether the infant is sick or tired), and behavior of the infant (e.g., whether he or she is exhibiting attachment behavior). Activation of the caregiving system has crucial implications for the infant, who cannot otherwise survive.

Ethologists have suggested that infants therefore have evolved characteristics that serve to activate the caregiving system: their endearing "babyish" features (the large rounded head with the high forehead, the small nose) and their thrashing arm movements. Attachment behaviors, of course, motivate parents to respond; even aversive behaviors, such as crying, typically motivate parents to provide care in order to terminate them. Given that an infant's attachment system is activated by stimuli that indicate an increased risk of danger (e.g., loud noise, looming objects), a parent who increases proximity when a child's attachment behavior is activated increases the likelihood of being able to protect the child, should the danger prove real. Similarly, when the parent perceives or expects danger that the child does not, parental proximity also increases the likelihood of survival. Thus it is likely that the close link between the child's attachment and fear systems is paralleled by a close link between the parent's caregiving and fear systems, such that when a parent's fear system is activated, so too is his or her caregiving system.

Fear is only one of the powerful emotions likely to be linked to the caregiving system. Just as attachment is associated with powerful emotions (Bowlby, 1979), so is the caregiving system. These emotions may in fact be as strong as any an individual experiences in his or her lifetime. The birth of a first child (which establishes the adult as a parent) is often accompanied by feelings of great joy; threats to the child are accompanied by anxiety; the death of a child brings profound grief. This intertwining of the caregiving system with intense emotions may result from selective pressures during evolution: Enhanced reproductive fitness may result when, for instance, a parent's anxiety about threats to a child prompts the parent to seek effective interventions.

The role of parental soothing as a component of the caregiving system merits consideration. Why would a parent who safely holds a crying child out of reach of a large barking dog continue to comfort the child? Why would a parent pick up a distressed child whom the parent perceives to be in no danger? What could be the role of such soothing behaviors? I propose that soothing behaviors serve indirectly to facilitate the parent's monitoring of potential or real dangers to the child. Parental provision of contact usually comforts a distressed child. If the child continues to be distressed for a substantial time following contact, there may be another threat of which the parent is unaware. Through continuing attempts to soothe the child, the parent gains information about threat to the child. The parent may not realize, for instance, that the child has a painful splinter in his or her foot. Furthermore, there are many ways in which inconsolable crying (beyond early infancy) can signal serious health problems. And a parent will not know whether crying is inconsolable unless the parent attempts to console.

Further research is needed to illuminate additional aspects of the caregiving system. First, given that there are times when the child's distress does not stem from activation of his or her attachment system, research could examine whether it is best to consider parental behavior in response to such distress as part of the caregiving system. For instance, it seems plausible that a child may get upset because his or her exploratory system is frustrated, and that the child's distress prompts the mother to pick the child up and comfort him or her. It may be that the mother's behavior then contributes to the child's attachment-related expectations about the mother's likely responses to his or her distress, and thus to the formation of the child's representational model of the mother. Second, research is needed to determine how separate the caregiving system is from other parental systems, and whether it is only the caregiving system that affects the child's attachment system. Third, it is unclear whether it is best to think of a single parental caregiving system in humans or of separate maternal and paternal caregiving systems. Harlow has proposed separate maternal and paternal systems in primates (Harlow, Harlow, & Hansen, 1963; see also Grossmann, Grossmann, Kindler, & Zimmermann, Chapter 36, this volume). If two separate systems exist in humans, there must be considerable overlap, even though genetic, hormonal, and cultural factors may contribute to differences in the specific characteristics of these systems.[4]

THE ATTACHMENT BOND

Whereas "attachment behavior" is behavior that promotes proximity to the attachment figure, and the "attachment behavioral system" is the organization of attachment behaviors within the individual, an "attachment bond" refers to an affectional tie. Ainsworth (1989) described an attachment bond not as dyadic, but rather as characteristic of the individual, "entailing representation in the internal organization of the individual" (p. 711). Thus this bond is not one between two people; it is

instead a bond that one individual has to another individual who is perceived as stronger and wiser (e.g., the bond of an infant to the mother). A person can be attached to a person who is not in turn attached to him or her; as described below, this is usually the case with infants and their parents.[5]

The attachment bond is a specific type of a larger class of bonds that Bowlby and Ainsworth referred to as "affectional bonds." Throughout the lifespan, individuals form a variety of important affectional bonds that are not attachments. To make it completely clear what an attachment bond is, one needs to delineate what it is not. Ainsworth (1989) described the criteria for affectional bonds, and then the additional criterion for attachment bonds. First, an affectional bond is persistent, not transitory. Second, an affectional bond involves a specific person—a figure who is not interchangeable with anyone else. This bond reflects "the attraction that one individual has for another *individual*" (Bowlby, 1979, p. 67, original emphasis). For instance, the sadness associated with the loss of a close friend is not lessened by the fact that one has other close friends. Bowlby emphasized specificity when he stated: "To complain because a child does not welcome being comforted by a kind but strange woman is as foolish as to complain that a young man deeply in love is not enthusiastic about some other good-looking girl" (1956, p. 58). Third, the relationship is emotionally significant. Fourth, the individual wishes to maintain proximity to or contact with the person. The nature and extent of the proximity/contact desired vary as a function of a variety of factors (e.g., age and state of the individual, environmental conditions). Fifth, the individual feels distress at involuntary separation from the person. Even though the individual may choose separation from the figure, the individual experiences distress when proximity is desired but prevented. In addition to these five criteria, an additional criterion exists for an attachment bond: The individual seeks security and comfort in the relationship with the person (Ainsworth, 1989). (The attachment is considered "secure" if one achieves security and "insecure" if one does not; it is the seeking of security that is the defining feature. See also Hinde, 1982; Weiss, 1982.) It is this final criterion that leads attachment researchers to refer to "parental bonds" to children and "child attachments" to parents: When the roles are reversed and a parent attempts to seek security from a young child, it is "almost always not only a sign of pathology in the parent but also a cause of it in the child" (Bowlby, 1969/1982, p. 377). (The situation is viewed differently later in life, when a middle-aged offspring takes care of an increasingly infirm and dependent parent; see Magai, Chapter 24, this volume.)

The existence of an attachment bond cannot be inferred from the presence or absence of attachment behavior. To begin with, it is important to remember that most behaviors can serve more than one behavioral system (Bretherton & Ainsworth, 1974; Sroufe & Waters, 1977). Thus, for instance, every approach does not serve the attachment system; even though approach can be an attachment behavior, it can also be an exploratory or sociable behavior. Yet it is also the case that distressed infants separated from their mothers may seek comfort from strangers (Ainsworth et al., 1978; Bretherton, 1978; Rheingold, 1969), and approach in that context is considered attachment behavior. Nonetheless, an enduring attachment bond of an infant to a stranger cannot be assumed to exist, and it is thus possible for an infant to direct attachment behavior to an individual to whom he or she is not attached. Some babies will stop crying when comforted by a stranger, but observations in the Strange Situation reveal that this comfort is generally not as satisfying as that provided by the mother (Ainsworth et al., 1978).

Similarly, even during a period when the child is directing no attachment behavior to the parent, the child is still attached. When, for instance, a contented child is in comfortable surroundings with the mother present, the attachment system is not likely to be activated to a level that triggers attachment behavior. Thus activation of attachment behavior is largely situational; it may or may not be present at any given time. The attachment bond, however, is considered to exist consistently over time, whether or not attachment behavior is present. Bowlby (1969/1982) pointed out that even the cessation of behavior during a long separation cannot be considered an indication that the attachment bond no longer exists.

The strength of attachment behaviors is sometimes mistakenly regarded as reflecting the "strength" of the attachment bond. There are striking variations in strength of activation of attachment behaviors across contexts and across children. Yet no evidence exists that these variations in themselves map onto variations in child–mother attachment in any meaningful way. According to Ainsworth (1972),

> to equate strength of attachment with strength of attachment behavior under ordinary nonstressful cir-

cumstances would lead to the conclusion that an infant who explores when his mother is present is necessarily less attached than one who constantly seeks proximity to his mother, whereas, in fact, his freedom to explore away from her may well reflect the healthy security provided by a harmonious attachment relationship. (p. 119)

Ainsworth characterized individual differences in relationships with an attachment figure as variations in quality rather than in strength. Similarly, it is a mistake to label as "very attached" a young child who clings fearfully to the mother; such attachment behavior may reflect insecure attachment or secure use of the mother as a safe haven, depending on the context.

Given that the strength of attachment behaviors should not be confused with the strength of an attachment bond, is strength nonetheless a useful dimension on which to consider an attachment bond? One might assume that Bowlby's proposition that children develop "attachment hierarchies" (discussed in the following section) implies that some attachments are stronger than others. Although Bowlby himself did occasionally use this terminology—for example, "How do we understand the origin and nature of this extraordinarily strong tie between child and mother?" (Bowlby, 1988, p. 161)—such usage was relatively rare, particularly when he was comparing one attachment with another (when doing so, he referred instead to "secure" and "insecure" attachments). Ainsworth (1982a) suggested that Hinde's (1979) notion of "penetration," as opposed to notions of either strength or intensity, may provide a more useful framework for characterizing an attachment bond. According to Hinde, penetration is a dimension of relationships that describes the centrality of one person to another's life—the extent to which a person penetrates a variety of aspects of the other person's life. Ainsworth pointed out that the concept of penetration is particularly useful when considering the changing nature of a child's attachment to the parent as the child grows older. She proposed that it may be more appropriate not to talk of the bond as becoming "weaker," but rather as characterizing a relationship that penetrates fewer aspects of the growing child's life as he or she comes to spend more time away from the parents and to develop new relationships.

For Bowlby (1969/1982), there are two important propositions about the nature of the attachment bond within the larger context of a relationship. First, the attachment bond reflects only one feature of the child's relationship with the mother: the component that deals with behavior related to the child's protection and security in time of stress. The mother not only serves as an attachment figure, but may also serve as playmate, teacher, or disciplinarian. These various roles are not incompatible, and it is possible that two or more may be filled by the same person. Thus, for example, a child may direct attachment behavior to the mother when he or she is frightened, and yet at other times may interact with her in ways relatively unrelated to attachment (e.g., play). Consequently, it would be a mistake to label as an attachment behavior a child's approach to the mother in order to engage in peekaboo. As Bretherton (1980) noted, a behavior may serve different behavioral systems at different times, even when it is directed to the same individual. Yet it is important to note that even though a mother may be a frequent playmate for her 5-year-old, it does not negate the fact that this relationship is essentially characterized as an attachment relationship. Bowlby summarized his position on this issue as follows:

> A parent–child relationship is by no means exclusively that of attachment–caregiving. The only justification, therefore, for referring to the bond between a child and his mother in this way is that the shared dyadic programme given top priority is one of attachment–caregiver. (p. 378)

Second, an attachment bond cannot be presumed to exist even though a relationship may contain an attachment component. As noted earlier, the fact that a 1-year-old distressed about separation from the mother will direct his or her attachment behaviors to a friendly stranger does not mean that the relationship with the stranger involves an attachment bond. This is true even in more ongoing relationships, such as relationships with peers. A young child may routinely direct attachment behavior to a close friend and feel comfort in the friend's presence (particularly in a context such as school, when a parent is not present) without that relationship's involving an attachment bond. This is evident from the fact that the loss of such a friend usually does not have the devastating effects on the child that loss of a true attachment figure (e.g., a parent) has. Thus, even though children may at times turn to friends for comfort (Hazan & Zeifman, 1994), these friendships need not be attachment relationships.

MULTIPLE ATTACHMENTS

Bowlby stated three principal propositions about multiple attachments in infancy. First, most young infants are thought to form more than one attachment. According to Bowlby (1969/1982), "almost from the first, many children have more than one figure to whom they direct attachment behavior" (p. 304).[6] Indeed, empirical observations have revealed that the majority of children become attached to more than one familiar person during their first year (Ainsworth, 1967; Schaffer & Emerson, 1964). According to Bowlby, "responsiveness to crying and readiness to interact socially are amongst the most relevant variables" (p. 315) in determining who will serve as an attachment figure. In most cultures, this means that the biological parents, older siblings, grandparents, aunts, and uncles are most likely to serve as attachment figures. Generally, the mother's role as an attachment figure is clear. The father is also particularly likely to become an additional attachment figure early in the infant's life. Observational studies have revealed that fathers are competent caregivers (Belsky, Gilstrap, & Rovine, 1984), and that children use their fathers as attachment figures (Ainsworth, 1967). Ainsworth (1967) noted the special infant–father relationship that sometimes emerged in Uganda:

> It seemed to be especially to the father that these other attachments were formed, even in the cases of babies who saw their fathers relatively infrequently. One can only assume that there was some special quality in the father's interaction with his child—whether of tenderness or intense delight—which evoked in turn a strength of attachment disproportionate to the frequency of his interaction with the baby. (p. 352)

Furthermore, there is evidence that individual differences in quality of infant–father attachment are related to paternal behavior: Infants are more likely to be securely attached to fathers who have been sensitively responsive to them (see van IJzendoorn & De Wolff, 1997, for meta-analytic findings). Evidence has also emerged that siblings (Stewart & Marvin, 1984; Teti & Ablard, 1989) and day care providers (Ahnert, Pinquart, & Lamb, 2006) can serve as attachment figures. In unusual and stressful situations, infants can even become attached to other infants (see Freud & Dann's [1951] observations of child survivors of a concentration camp). Howes and Spieker (Chapter 14, this volume) provide an extensive discussion of multiple attachment figures.

Second, although there is usually more than one attachment figure, the potential number of attachment figures is not limitless. Bretherton (1980, p. 195) has described the infant as having a "small hierarchy of major caregivers," which is in contrast to the larger group of individuals with whom the infant has other sorts of relationships (Weinraub, Brooks, & Lewis, 1977). Marvin, VanDevender, Iwanaga, LeVine, and LeVine (1977) reported that most Hausa infants observed in Nigeria were attached to no more than three or four attachment figures; Grossmann and Grossmann (1991) reported similar observations for a sample of German infants.

Third, although most infants have multiple attachment figures, it is important not to assume that an infant treats all attachment figures as equivalent, or that they are interchangeable; rather, an "attachment hierarchy" is thought to exist. According to Bowlby (1969/1982), "it is a mistake to suppose that a young child diffuses his attachment over many figures in such a way that he gets along with no strong attachment to anyone, and consequently without missing any particular person when that person is away" (p. 308). Bowlby proposed that this strong tendency for infants to prefer a principal attachment figure for comfort and security be termed "monotropy" (see also Ainsworth, 1964, 1982b).[7] Bowlby cited as evidence of this phenomenon the tendency of children in institutions to select, if given the opportunity, one "special" caregiver as their own (see Burlingham & Freud, 1944). Ainsworth (1982b) described responses to major separations from and losses of attachment figures as further support for the idea that a hierarchy exists: "The child would tolerate major separations from subsidiary figures with less distress than comparable separations from the principal attachment figure. Nor could the presence of several attachment figures altogether compensate for the loss of the principal attachment figure" (p. 19).[8] (For similar findings, see Heinicke & Westheimer, 1966.)

Also consistent with this hierarchy notion are data from observational studies of both mothers and fathers, which show that most infants prefer to seek comfort from their mothers when distressed; in the mother's absence, however, an infant is likely to seek and derive comfort and security from other attachment figures as well (Kagan, Kearsley, & Zelazo, 1978; Lamb, 1976a, 1976b, 1978; Rut-

ter, 1981; see also Ainsworth, 1967; Schaffer & Emerson, 1964). For a review of the relatively few experimental studies examining attachment hierarchies, and a discussion of the relevant methodological issues, see Colin (1996). See also Kobak, Rosenthal, and Serwik (2005) for data and a discussion of attachment hierarchies in middle childhood, and Kobak, Rosenthal, Zajac, and Madsen (2007) for a discussion of how attachment hierarchies are transformed during adolescence.

What determines the structure of an infant's attachment hierarchy? Colin (1996) listed a likely set of contributing factors: "(1) how much time the infant spends in each figure's care; (2) the quality of care each provides, (3) each adult's emotional investment in the child, and (4) social cues" (p. 194). To this list, I would add that the repeated presence across time of the figure in the infant's life, even if each encounter is relatively brief, is likely to be important.

Why would monotropy have evolved as a tendency of human infants? Neither Bowlby nor Ainsworth addressed this question. I propose three possibilities here, all of which may operate simultaneously. The fact that there may be multiple ways in which the tendency toward monotropy contributes to infant survival and reproductive fitness increases the likelihood of its emerging through genetic selection. First, the infant's tendency to prefer a principal attachment figure may contribute to the establishment of a relationship in which that one attachment figure assumes principal responsibility for the child. Such a relationship should increase the child's likelihood of survival by helping to ensure that care of the child is not overlooked. This system seems more practical than the alternative, wherein a large number of caregivers have equal responsibility for a large number of offspring; this latter system might leave any individual child "falling between the cracks."

Second, monotropy may be most efficient for the child. When faced with danger, the child does not have to make a series of assessments and judgments about who may be most readily available, most responsive, and best suited to help. Rather, the child has a quick, automatic response to seek his or her principal attachment figure.

Third, monotropy may be the child's contribution to a process I term "reciprocal hierarchical bonding," in which the child matches an attachment hierarchy to the hierarchy of the caregiving in his or her environment. Evolutionary biologists writing on parental investment (e.g., Trivers, 1972) have suggested that adults vary in their investment in offspring largely as a function of the extent to which this investment contributes to the transmission of the adults' genes (i.e., their reproductive fitness). Following this reasoning, it should be most adaptive for the child to use as a principal attachment figure the person who, correspondingly, is most strongly bonded to him or her (i.e., the person who provides the most parental investment and has the most to gain—in terms of reproductive fitness—from the baby's healthy development). In most cases, it is the biological mother who has the greatest biological investment in the child. With the exception of an identical twin, there is no one with whom the child shares more genes than the mother (50%). Although the biological father and siblings also share 50% of their genes with a child, their investments are nonetheless considered to be less, because (1) only the mother can be certain of a true biological connection; (2) the mother devotes her body and bodily resources to the infant for 9 months of pregnancy and often nurses the child for a considerable period thereafter; and (3) the mother has fewer opportunities to produce additional offspring than fathers and siblings do. If this process of reciprocal hierarchical bonding exists, it may help to explain not only monotropy, but also, in part, why the biological mother is generally the principal attachment figure.

The infant's selection of the principal attachment figure occurs over time, and it is important to consider why it takes a period of time for this centrally important attachment to crystalize rather than happening immediately, as it does in some other mammals. Jay Belsky (personal communication, October 2007) has proposed two possible explanations, in addition to the obvious fact that human newborns do not possess the skills needed to form attachments because of their immature status at birth. First, the mother may not survive childbirth; many surely did not do so during our ancestral past. Second, the infant needs to be able to discern which individual is making the intensive investment upon which he or she is so dependent—a judgment that is likely to take some time.

Given the existence of multiple attachments, what is the course of their development across the lifespan? As noted earlier, two or three attachments usually develop during the infant's first year. These are usually with other family members or other people closely involved in the child's care. By middle childhood, when the child is spending more time with people outside the family, oppor-

tunities for new attachments may arise. In adolescence and young adulthood, individuals usually begin to develop attachments to sexual partners. Although attachments to parents typically remain throughout life, the later attachments may become the most central ones in the individual's adult life.

When considering multiple attachments, theorists are faced with several sets of questions. One of these has to do with similarities versus differences in quality across different attachments (i.e., concordance rate). To what extent are a child's attachments to different caregivers similar? Studies examining concordance rate yield inconsistent results. Some studies reveal independence of attachment across caregivers (Belsky & Rovine, 1987; Grossmann, Grossmann, Huber, & Wartner, 1981; Main & Weston, 1981); some studies reveal similarity of attachment across caregivers (Goossens & van IJzendoorn, 1990; Steele, Steele, & Fonagy, 1996); and two meta-analytic studies have revealed significant but weak concordance between attachment to mother and attachment to father (Fox, Kimmerly, & Schafer, 1991; van IJzendoorn & De Wolff, 1997; see Berlin, Cassidy, & Appleyard, Chapter 15, this volume, for additional discussion of concordance of attachment quality across parents).

Another question relates to the integration of multiple attachments. If a child's attachments are similar, he or she may develop a consistent set of internal working models of attachment figures, him- or herself, and relationships. Yet what if the child is faced with attachments that contribute to conflicting models? What if the child's experiences with one parent contribute to a model of the attachment figure as sensitively responsive and of the self as worthy of such care, but negative experiences with the other parent contribute to very different models? If differing models of attachment figures eventually become integrated, how does this happen? In relation to models of the self, Bretherton (1985) asked over two decades ago: "Is an integrated internal working model of the self built from participation in a number of nonconcordant relationships? If so, how and when? Or are self models, developed in different relationships, only partially integrated or sometimes not at all?" (p. 30). Researchers have made little progress in answering these questions.

Still another question about multiple attachments relates to the issue of how these different attachments influence children's functioning. It could be that the attachment to the principal attachment figure, usually the mother, is most influential. On the other hand, it could be that one attachment is most influential in some areas and another is most influential in other areas. Or perhaps having at least one secure attachment, no matter who the attachment figure is, serves as a protective factor to facilitate the child's functioning across areas. Relatively little empirical work has addressed these possibilities, given that most research examining the sequelae of attachment focuses only on infant–mother attachment. The research that is available suggests that when a child is securely attached to one individual and insecurely attached to another, the child behaves more competently when the secure relationship is with the mother than when it is with the other attachment figure (Easterbrooks & Goldberg, 1987; Howes, Rodning, Galluzzo, & Myers, 1988; Main et al., 1985; Main & Weston, 1981; Sagi-Schwartz & Aviezer, 2005). These same studies indicate, however, that the best-functioning individuals have two secure relationships, while the least competent children have none. van IJzendoorn and Sagi-Schwartz (Chapter 37, this volume) review the cross-cultural data and report similar evidence that multiple secure attachments enhance children's functioning; more extensive discussion of models of the influence of multiple attachments can be found in that chapter.

SUMMARY

This chapter has addressed the issues that Bowlby presented in his initial ethological approach to understanding the nature of a child's tie to the mother. Bowlby's observations led him to be dissatisfied with the explanations provided by existing theories and prompted him to consider alternative explanations. Drawing on the thinking of evolutionary biologists, cognitive scientists, control systems theorists, and developmental psychologists, he initiated what proved to be one of the earliest neo-Darwinian theories of evolutionary psychology, tackling the problem of the ways humans evolved to master the primary task of genetic transmission: survival through infancy and childhood to reproductive age (see Simpson & Belsky, Chapter 6, this volume). This chapter has begun with a description of the biological bases of attachment and of how attachment may have evolved. I have then described the connections between the attachment behavioral system and other behavioral systems. Finally, I have provided a description of

attachment and other affectional bonds and discussed the issue of multiple attachments. In general, Bowlby and Ainsworth's original ideas have held up well, while providing a remarkably fruitful foundation for related ideas and studies. Those ideas have yielded the huge research literature reviewed in the present volume, and the torrent of new ideas, studies, and research methods shows no sign of letting up.

Other issues and concepts central to the early formulation of attachment theory are covered elsewhere in this volume: The developmental course of attachment is described by Marvin and Britner (Chapter 12) and by Zeifman and Hazan (Chapter 20); issues related to separation and loss are considered by Kobak and Madsen (Chapter 2) and by Shaver and Fraley (Chapter 3); theory about individual differences in attachment quality is addressed by Weinfield and colleagues (Chapter 4); and attachment-related communication and representations associated with individual differences are discussed by Bretherton and Munholland (Chapter 5).

ACKNOWLEDGMENTS

The writing of this chapter was supported by Grant Nos. RO1-MH50773 from the National Institute of Mental Health and RO1-HD36635 from the National Institute of Child Health and Human Development. Additional support was provided by a sabbatical from the Department of Psychology, University of Maryland at College Park.

NOTES

1. As Bowlby (1988) noted in his final collection of lectures, later revisions to evolutionary theory contain the thinking that demarcation of a "principal" biological function (i.e., Bowlby's initial selection of protection) is unnecessary; the multiple benefits of attachment all contribute to its conveying an evolutionary advantage.
2. See Greenberg and Marvin (1982; see also Ainsworth, 1989) for discussion of the advantages of the term "sociable system" rather than "affiliative system." For data and more extensive discussion related to the interplay of the sociable system with other behavior systems, see discussions by Ainsworth et al. (1978), Bretherton (1978), Bretherton and Ainsworth (1974), Cassidy and Berlin (1999), and Greenberg and Marvin (1982).
3. This perspective differs somewhat from that of Bowlby. Bowlby (1969/1982, p. 240) described "maternal retrieval behavior" as distinct from other parenting

behavior, with the former having the predictable outcome of proximity and the biological function of protection. It is unclear, however, what for Bowlby would constitute a behavioral system. The position taken here is that retrieval is the parental equivalent to child proximity seeking; it is a behavior, not a behavioral system. The relevant behavioral system would be what here is called the "caregiving system," which includes a variety of behaviors, one of which is parental retrieval of the child. This perspective, along with Solomon and George's perspective, also differs from that proposed by Bretherton and her colleagues (Bretherton, Biringen, & Ridgeway, 1991). Their view incorporates the notion of a "parental side of attachment," in which the parent's bond to the child is considered part of the attachment system, in part because of its great emotional power.

4. Within the modern evolutionary perspective, the existence of separate maternal and paternal caregiving systems is readily understood. Both mothers and fathers are concerned with their own reproductive fitness. Yet, because mothers and fathers may differ substantially in the extent to which the survival of any one child enhances this fitness, their parenting behavior may differ. Compared to fathers, mothers have more to gain in terms of reproductive fitness from each child, for several reasons (e.g., mothers' certainty about parental status, shorter reproductive lifespan, longer interchild intervals, and greater energy expenditure per child [during pregnancy and lactation]; see Trivers, 1972).

5. Consensus is lacking about terminology related to the attachment bond. The description provided here is Ainsworth's (1989) and reflects Bowlby's most common usage. Yet in the second edition of the first volume of his trilogy, *Attachment and Loss*, Bowlby (1969/1982) described a bond as "a property of two parties," and labeled the child–parent bond as the "attachment–caregiving" bond (p. 377). In contrast to the implied notion of an "attachment relationship," Ainsworth (1982b) stated:

> That there is a "relationship" between mother and child, in Hinde's (1979) sense, from the time of the infant's birth onward, and that the nature of this relationship stems from the interaction between them, is not to be gainsaid, but neither the mother-to-infant bond nor the emergent infant-to-mother attachment seems to me to comprehend all the important aspects of this relationship. (p. 24)

Bretherton (1985) also pointed out the limits of considering an attachment a "property of two parties": "A representational view of relationships ... underscores that the two partners have, in another sense, two relationships: the relationship as mentally represented by the attached person and by the attachment figure" (p. 34). Ainsworth (personal communication, 1986) suggested that the most appropriate way to consider an "attachment relationship" is as a "shorthand" des-

ignation for "a relationship in which the attachment component is central" (see also Ainsworth, 1990).

6. There has been some confusion over Bowlby's position on this issue. Lamb, Thompson, Gardner, and Charnov (1985), for instance, mistakenly stated, "Bowlby was firmly convinced that infants were initially capable of forming only one attachment bond" (p. 21). In fact, from his earliest writings on (1958, 1969/1982), Bowlby described the role of multiple attachment figures. Bowlby (1969/1982) noted that "it has sometimes been alleged that I have expressed the view ... that mothering 'cannot be safely distributed among several figures'" (Mead, 1962). No such views have been expressed by me" (p. 303).

7. Starting with his earliest writings, Bowlby (e.g., 1958) used the term "principal attachment-figure" or "mother-figure" rather than the term "mother." This usage underscored Bowlby's belief that although this figure is usually the biological mother, it is by no means necessarily so. From the beginning, Bowlby recognized that the figure's status (father, adoptive parent, grandmother, aunt, nanny) is less important than the nature of the figure's interactions with the infant.

8. One of the most moving passages of Bowlby's writing illustrates how one attachment figure can be more centrally important to a child's well-being than others:

> About four weeks after mother had died, [4-year-old] Wendy complained that no one loved her. In an attempt to reassure her, father named a long list of people who did (naming those who cared for her). On this Wendy commented aptly, "But when my mommy wasn't dead I didn't need so many people—I needed just one." (Bowlby, 1980a, p. 280)

REFERENCES

Ahnert, L., Pinquart, M., & Lamb, M. E. (2006). Security of children's relationships with nonparental care providers: A meta-analysis. *Child Development*, 74, 664–679.

Ainsworth, M. D. S. (1963). The development of infant–mother interaction among the Ganda. In B. M. Foss (Ed.), *Determinants of infant behavior* (Vol. 2, pp. 67–112). New York: Wiley.

Ainsworth, M. D. S. (1964). Patterns of attachment behavior shown by the infant in interaction with his mother. *Merrill–Palmer Quarterly, 10,* 51–58.

Ainsworth, M. D. S. (1967). *Infancy in Uganda: Infant care and the growth of attachment*. Baltimore: Johns Hopkins University Press.

Ainsworth, M. D. S. (1972). Attachment and dependency: A comparison. In J. L. Gewirtz (Ed.), *Attachment and dependency* (pp. 97–137). Washington, DC: V. H. Winston.

Ainsworth, M. D. S. (1982a). *Attachment across the lifespan*. Unpublished lecture notes, University of Virginia.

Ainsworth, M. D. S. (1982b). Attachment: Retrospect and prospect. In C. M. Parkes & J. Stevenson-Hinde (Eds.), *The place of attachment in human behavior* (pp. 3–30). New York: Basic Books.

Ainsworth, M. D. S. (1989). Attachments beyond infancy. *American Psychologist, 44,* 709–716.

Ainsworth, M. D. S. (1990). Some considerations regarding theory and assessment relevant to attachments beyond infancy. In M. T. Greenberg, D. Cicchetti, & E. M. Cummings (Eds.), *Attachment in the preschool years: Theory, research, and intervention* (pp. 463–488). Chicago: University of Chicago Press.

Ainsworth, M. D. S., Bell, S. M., & Stayton, D. J. (1971). Individual differences in Strange-Situation behavior of one-year-olds. In H. R. Schaffer (Ed.), *The origins of human social relations* (pp. 17–52). New York: Academic Press.

Ainsworth, M. D. S., Blehar, M., Waters, E., & Wall, S. (1978). *Patterns of attachment: A psychological study of the Strange Situation.* Hillsdale, NJ: Erlbaum.

Ainsworth, M. D. S., & Wittig, B. A. (1969). Attachment and exploratory behaviour of one-year-olds in a strange situation. In B. M. Foss (Ed.), *Determinants of infant behaviour* (Vol. 4, pp. 111–136). London: Methuen.

Baldwin, M. W. (1992). Relational schemas and the processing of social information. *Psychological Bulletin, 112,* 461–484.

Belsky, J., Gilstrap, B., & Rovine, M. (1984). The Pennsylvania Infant and Family Development Project: I. Stability and change in mother–infant and father–infant interaction in a family setting at one, three, and nine months. *Child Development, 55,* 692–705.

Belsky, J., & Rovine, M. (1987). Temperament and attachment security within the Strange Situation: An empirical rapprochement. *Child Development, 58,* 787–795.

Bender, L., & Yarnell, H. (1941). An observation nursery. *American Journal of Psychiatry, 97,* 1158–1174.

Bowlby, J. (1944). Forty-four juvenile thieves: Their characters and home life. *International Journal of Psycho-Analysis, 25,* 19–52, 107–127.

Bowlby, J. (1956). The growth of independence in the young child. *Royal Society of Health Journal, 76,* 587–591.

Bowlby, J. (1958). The nature of the child's tie to his mother. *International Journal of Psycho-Analysis, 39,* 350–373.

Bowlby, J. (1960a). Grief and mourning in infancy. *Psychoanalytic Study of the Child, 15,* 3–39.

Bowlby, J. (1960b). Separation anxiety. *International Journal of Psycho-Analysis, 41,* 1–25.

Bowlby, J. (1969/1982). *Attachment and loss: Vol. 1. Attachment.* New York: Basic Books.

Bowlby, J. (1973). *Attachment and loss: Vol. 2. Separation: Anxiety and anger.* New York: Basic Books.

Bowlby, J. (1979). *The making and breaking of affectional bonds.* London: Tavistock.

Bowlby, J. (1980a). *Attachment and loss: Vol. 3. Loss: Sadness and depression.* New York: Basic Books.

Bowlby, J. (1980b). By ethology out of psycho-analysis: An experiment in interbreeding. *Animal Behavior, 28,* 649–656.

Bowlby, J. (1984). Caring for the young: Influences on development. In R. S. Cohen, B. J. Cohler, & S. H. Weissman (Eds.), *Parenthood: A psychodynamic perspective* (pp. 269–284). New York: Guilford Press.

Bowlby, J. (1988). *A secure base.* New York: Basic Books.

Brazelton, T. B. (1977). Implications of infant development among the Mayan Indians of Mexico. In P. H. Leiderman, S. R. Tulkin, & A. Rosenfeld (Eds.), *Culture and infancy* (pp. 151–187). New York: Academic Press.

Bretherton, I. (1978). Making friends with one-year-olds: An experimental study of infant–stranger interaction. *Merrill–Palmer Quarterly, 24,* 29–52.

Bretherton, I. (1980). Young children in stressful situations: The supporting role of attachment figures and unfamiliar caregivers. In G. V. Coelho & P. I. Ahmed (Eds.), *Uprooting and development* (pp. 179–210). New York: Plenum Press.

Bretherton, I. (1985). Attachment theory: Retrospect and prospect. In I. Bretherton & E. Waters (Eds.), Growing points of attachment theory and research. *Monographs of the Society for Research in Child Development, 50*(1–2, Serial No. 209), 3–38.

Bretherton, I. (1990). Open communication and internal working models: Their role in the development of attachment relationships. In R. A. Thompson (Ed.), *Nebraska Symposium on Motivation: Vol. 36. Socioemotional development* (pp. 59–113). Lincoln: University of Nebraska Press.

Bretherton, I. (1991). Pouring new wine into old bottles: The social self as internal working model. In M. Gunnar & L. A. Sroufe (Eds.), *Minnesota Symposium on Child Psychology: Vol. 23. Self processes in development* (pp. 1–41). Hillsdale, NJ: Erlbaum.

Bretherton, I. (1992). The origins of attachment theory: John Bowlby and Mary Ainsworth. *Developmental Psychology, 28,* 759–775.

Bretherton, I., & Ainsworth, M. D. S. (1974). Responses of one-year-olds to a stranger in a strange situation. In M. Lewis & L. A. Rosenblum (Eds.), *The origins of fear* (pp. 131–164). New York: Wiley.

Bretherton, I., Biringen, Z., & Ridgeway, D. (1991). The parental side of attachment. In K. Pillemer & K. McCartney (Eds.), *Parent–child relations through life* (pp. 1–22). Hillsdale, NJ: Erlbaum.

Bronson, G. (1972). Infants' reactions to unfamiliar persons and novel objects. *Monographs of the Society for Research in Child Development, 37*(3, Serial No. 148).

Burlingham, D., & Freud, A. (1944). *Infants without families.* London: Allen & Unwin.

Carr, S. J., Dabbs, J., & Carr, T. S. (1975). Mother–infant attachment: The importance of the mother's visual field. *Child Development, 46,* 331–338.

Cassidy, J. (1994). Emotion regulation: Influences of attachment relationships. In N. Fox (Ed.), The development of emotion regulation. *Monographs of the Society for Research in Child Development, 59*(2–3, Serial No. 240), 228–249.

Cassidy, J., & Berlin, L. J. (1994). The insecure/ambivalent pattern of attachment: Theory and research. *Child Development, 65,* 971–991.

Cassidy, J., & Berlin, L. J. (1999). Understanding the origins of childhood loneliness: Contributions of attachment theory. In K. J. Rotenberg & S. Hymel (Eds.), *Loneliness in childhood and adolescence* (pp. 34–55). New York: Cambridge University Press.

Cassidy, J., & Kobak, R. (1988). Avoidance and its relation to other defensive processes. In J. Belsky & T. Nezworski (Eds.), *Clinical implications of attachment* (pp. 300–323). Hillsdale, NJ: Erlbaum.

Cassidy, J., Woodhouse, S., Cooper, G., Hoffman, K., Powell, B., & Rodenberg, M. S. (2005). Examination of the precursors of infant attachment security: Implications for early intervention and intervention research. In L. J. Berlin, Y. Ziv, L. M. Amaya-Jackson, & M. T. Greenberg (Eds.), *Enhancing early attachments: Theory, research, intervention, and policy* (pp. 34–60). New York: Guilford Press.

Colin, V. L. (1996). *Human attachment.* New York: McGraw-Hill.

De Wolff, M. S., & van IJzendoorn, M. H. (1997). Sensitivity and attachment: A meta-analysis on parental antecedents of infant attachment. *Child Development, 68,* 571–591.

Easterbrooks, A., & Goldberg, W. (1987). *Consequences of early family attachment patterns for later social–personality development.* Paper presented at the biennial meeting of the Society for Research in Child Development, Baltimore.

Eisenberg, J. F. (1966). The social organization of mammals. *Handbuch Zoologie, 8,* 1–92.

Fox, N. A., Kimmerly, N. L., & Schafer, W. D. (1991). Attachment to mother/attachment to father: A meta-analysis. *Child Development, 62,* 210–225.

Freud, A., & Dann, S. (1951). An experiment in group upbringing. *Psychoanalytic Study of the Child, 6,* 127–168.

Freud, S. (1957). Five lectures on psycho-analysis. In J. Strachey (Ed. & Trans.), *The standard edition of the complete psychological works of Sigmund Freud* (Vol. 11, pp. 3–56). London: Hogarth Press. (Original work published 1910)

Freud, S. (1964). An outline of psycho-analysis. In J. Strachey (Ed. & Trans.), *The standard edition of the complete psychological works of Sigmund Freud* (Vol. 23, pp. 139–207). London: Hogarth Press. (Original work published 1940)

George, C., & Solomon, J. (1996). Representational models of relationships: Links between caregiving and attachment. *Infant Mental Health Journal, 17,* 198–216.

Goldfarb, W. (1943). The effects of early institutional care on adolescent personality. *Journal of Experimental Education, 12,* 106–129.

Goossens, F. A., & van IJzendoorn, M. (1990). Qual-

ity of infants' attachments to professional caregivers: Relations to infant–parent attachment and daycare characteristics. *Child Development, 61,* 832–837.

Greenberg, M., & Marvin, R. S. (1982). Reactions of preschool children to an adult stranger: A behavioral systems approach. *Child Development, 53,* 481–490.

Grossmann, K., & Grossmann, K. E. (1991). Newborn behavior, early parenting quality, and later toddler–parent relationships in a group of German infants. In J. K. Nugent, B. M. Lester, & T. B. Brazelton (Eds.), *The cultural context of infancy* (Vol. 2, pp. 3–38). Norwood, NJ: Ablex.

Grossmann, K. E., Grossmann, K., Huber, F., & Wartner, U. (1981). German children's behavior towards their mothers at 12 months and their fathers at 18 months in Ainsworth's Strange Situation. *International Journal of Behavioral Development, 4,* 157–181.

Harlow, H. F. (1958). The nature of love. *American Psychologist, 13,* 673.

Harlow, H. F. (1962). The development of affectional patterns in infant monkeys. In B. M. Foss (Ed.), *Determinants of infant behavior* (Vol. 1, pp. 75–88). New York: Wiley.

Harlow, H. F. (1969). Age-mate or affectional system. In D. S. Lehrman, R. A. Hinde, & E. Shaw (Eds.), *Advances in the study of behavior* (Vol. 2, pp. 334–383). New York: Academic Press.

Harlow, H. F., & Harlow, M. K. (1965). The affectional systems. In A. M. Schrier, H. F. Harlow, & F. Stollnitz (Eds.), *Behavior of non-human primates* (Vol. 2, pp. 287–334). New York: Academic Press.

Harlow, H. F., Harlow, M. K., & Hansen, E. W. (1963). The maternal affectional system of rhesus monkeys. In H. R. Rheingold (Ed.), *Maternal behavior in mammals* (pp. 254–281). New York: Wiley.

Hazan, C., & Zeifman, D. (1994). Sex and the psychological tether. In K. Bartholomew & D. Perlman (Eds.), *Advances in personal relationships: Vol. 5. Attachment processes in adulthood* (pp. 151–177). London: Jessica Kingsley.

Heinicke, C., & Westheimer, I. (1966). *Brief separations.* New York: International Universities Press.

Heller, K. A., & Berndt, T. J. (1981). Developmental changes in the formation and organization of personality attributions. *Child Development, 52,* 683–691.

Hinde, R. A. (1974). *Biological bases of human social behavior.* New York: McGraw-Hill.

Hinde, R. A. (1979). *Towards understanding relationships.* London: Academic Press.

Hinde, R. A. (1982). Attachment: Some conceptual and biological issues. In C. M. Parkes & J. Stevenson-Hinde (Eds.), *The place of attachment in human behavior* (pp. 60–70). New York: Basic Books.

Howes, C., Rodning, C., Galluzzo, D. C., & Myers, L. (1988). Attachment and child care: Relationships with mother and caregiver. *Early Childhood Research Quarterly, 3,* 703–715.

Huntingford, F. (1984). *The study of animal behavior.* London: Chapman & Hall.

Kagan, J., Kearsley, R., & Zelazo, P. (1978). *Infancy: Its place in human development.* Cambridge, MA: Harvard University Press.

Kobak, R. R., & Duemmler, S. (1994). Attachment and conversation: Toward a discourse analysis of adolescent and adult security. In K. Bartholomew & D. Perlman (Eds.), *Advances in personal relationships: Vol. 5. Attachment processes in adulthood* (pp. 121–149). London: Jessica Kingsley.

Kobak, R., Rosenthal, N., & Serwik, A. (2005). The attachment hierarchy in middle childhood: Conceptual and methodological issues. In K. A. Kerns & R. A. Richardson (Eds.), *Attachment in middle childhood* (pp. 71–88). New York: Guilford Press.

Kobak, R., Rosenthal, N., Zajac, K., & Madsen, S. (2007). Adolescent attachment hierarchies and the search for an adult pair bond. *New Directions in Child and Adolescent Development, 117,* 57–72.

Lamb, M. (1976a). Effects of stress and cohort on mother–infant and father–infant interaction. *Developmental Psychology, 12,* 435–443.

Lamb, M. (1976b). Interactions between two-year-olds and their mothers and fathers. *Psychological Reports, 38,* 447–450.

Lamb, M. (1978). Qualitative aspects of mother– and father–infant attachments. *Infant Behavior and Development, 1,* 265–275.

Lamb, M., Thompson, R. A., Gardner, W. P., & Charnov, E. L. (1985). *Infant–mother attachment.* Hillsdale, NJ: Erlbaum.

Lewis, M., Young, G., Brooks, J., & Michalson, L. (1975). The beginning of friendship. In M. Lewis & R. A. Rosenblum (Eds.), *Friendship and peer relations* (pp. 27–60). New York: Wiley.

Lorenz, K. E. (1935). Der Kumpan in der Umvelt des Vogels. *Journal of Ornithology, 83,* 137–213, 289–413.

Main, M. (1990). Cross-cultural studies of attachment organization: Recent studies, changing methodologies, and the concept of conditional strategies. *Human Development, 33,* 48–61.

Main, M., Hesse, E., & Kaplan, N. (2005). Predictability of attachment behavior and representational processes at 1, 6, and 19 years of age. In K. E. Grossmann, K. Grossmann, & E. Waters (Eds.), *Attachment from infancy to adulthood: The major longitudinal studies* (pp. 245–304). New York: Guilford Press.

Main, M., Kaplan, N., & Cassidy, J. (1985). Security in infancy, childhood, and adulthood: A move to the level of representation. In I. Bretherton & E. Waters (Eds.), Growing points of attachment theory and research. *Monographs of the Society for Research in Child Development, 50*(1–2, Serial No. 209), 66–104.

Main, M., & Weston, D. (1981). The quality of the toddler's relationship to mother and to father: Related to conflict behavior and the readiness to establish new relationships. *Child Development, 52,* 932–940.

Marvin, R. S., VanDevender, T. L., Iwanaga, M. I., LeVine, S., & LeVine, R. A. (1977). Infant–caregiver attachment among the Hausa of Nigeria. In H. McGurk (Ed.), *Ecological factors in human development* (pp. 247–259). Amsterdam: North-Holland.

Mead, M. (1962). A cultural anthropologist's approach to maternal deprivation. In *Deprivation of maternal care: A reassessment of its effects* (Public Health Papers No. 14). Geneva: World Health Organization.

Miller, R., Caul, W., & Mirsky, I. (1967). Communication of affect between feral and socially isolated monkeys. *Journal of Personality and Social Psychology, 7,* 231–239.

Morgan, G. A., & Ricciuti, H. N. (1969). Infants' responses to strangers during the first year. In B. M. Foss (Ed.), *Determinants of infant behaviour* (Vol. 4, pp. 253–272). London: Methuen.

Murray, H. A. (1938). *Explorations in personality.* New York: Oxford University Press.

Passman, R. H., & Erck, T. W. (1977, March). *Visual presentation of mothers for facilitating play in childhood; The effects of silent films of mothers.* Paper presented at the biennial meeting of the Society for Research in Child Development, New Orleans, LA.

Passman, R. H., & Weisberg, P. (1975). Mothers and blankets as agents for promoting play and exploration by young children in a novel environment: The effects of social and nonsocial attachment objects. *Developmental Psychology, 11,* 170–177.

Piaget, J. (1954). *The construction of reality in the child.* New York: Basic Books.

Rheingold, H. (1969). The effect of a strange environment on the behaviour of infants. In B. M. Foss (Ed.), *Determinants of infant behaviour* (Vol. 4, pp. 137–166). London: Methuen.

Robertson, J., & Bowlby, J. (1952). Responses of young children to separation from their mothers. *Courrier du Centre International de l'Enfance, 2,* 131–142.

Rutter, M. (1981). *Maternal deprivation reassessed* (2nd ed.). New York: Penguin.

Sagi-Schwartz, A., & Aviezer, O. (2005). Correlates of attachment to multiple caregivers in kibbutz children from birth to emerging adulthood: The Haifa longitudinal study. In K. E. Grossmann, K. Grossmann, & E. Waters (Eds.), *Attachment from infancy to adulthood: The major longitudinal studies* (pp. 165–197). New York: Guilford Press.

Schaffer, H. R., & Emerson, P. E. (1964). The development of social attachments in infancy. *Monographs of the Society for Research in Child Development, 29*(3, Serial No. 94), 1–77.

Sears, R. R., Maccoby, E. E., & Levin, H. (1957). *Patterns of child rearing.* Evanston, IL: Row, Peterson.

Sorce, J., & Emde, R. (1981). Mother's presence is not enough: Effect of emotional availability on infant explorations. *Developmental Psychology, 17,* 737–745.

Solomon, J., & George, C. (1996). Defining the caregiving system: Toward a theory of caregiving. *Infant Mental Health Journal, 17,* 183–197.

Sroufe, L. A., & Waters, E. (1977). Attachment as an organizational construct. *Child Development, 48,* 1184–1199.

Steele, H., Steele, M., & Fonagy, P. (1996). Associations among attachment classifications of mothers, fathers, and their infants. *Child Development, 67,* 541–555.

Stewart, R., & Marvin, R. S. (1984). Sibling relations: The role of conceptual perspective-taking in the ontogeny of sibling caregiving. *Child Development, 55,* 1322–1332.

Teti, D., & Ablard, K. E. (1989). Security of attachment and infant–sibling relationships. *Child Development, 60,* 1519–1528.

Thompson, R. A., & Meyer, S. (2007). The socialization of emotion regulation in the family. In J. Gross (Ed.), *Handbook of emotion regulation* (pp. 249–268). New York: Guilford Press.

Trivers, R. L. (1972). Parental investment and sexual selection. In B. Campbell (Ed.), *Sexual selection and the descent of man, 1871–1971* (pp. 136–179). Chicago: Aldine-Atherton.

Trivers, R. L. (1974). Parent–offspring conflict. *American Zoologist, 14,* 249–264.

Vandell, D. L. (1980). Sociability with peer and mother during the first year. *Developmental Psychology, 16,* 355–361.

van IJzendoorn, M., & De Wolff, M. S. (1997). In search of the absent father—meta-analyses of infant–father attachment: A rejoinder to our discussants. *Child Development, 68,* 604–609.

Vaughn, B. E., Waters, H. S., Coppola, G., Cassidy, J., Bost, K. K., & Verissimo, M. (2006). Script-like attachment representations and behavior in families and across cultures: Studies of parental secure base narratives. *Attachment and Human Development, 8,* 179–184.

Weinraub, M., Brooks, J., & Lewis, M. (1977). The social network: A reconsideration of the concept of attachment. *Human Development, 20,* 31–47.

Weiss, R. S. (1982). Attachment in adult life. In C. M. Parkes & J. Stevenson-Hinde (Eds.), *The place of attachment in human behavior* (pp. 171–184). New York: Basic Books.

CHAPTER 2

Disruptions in Attachment Bonds
Implications for Theory, Research, and Clinical Intervention

ROGER KOBAK
STEPHANIE MADSEN

Young children's reactions to separations from their parents have played a central role in conceptualizing and studying the operation and regulation of the attachment system. During the 1940s and 1950s, John Bowlby and James Robertson used films of young children undergoing such separations to demonstrate the emotional significance of the attachment relationship (e.g., Bowlby, Robertson, & Rosenbluth, 1952; Robertson, 1953). It was apparent to most observers that the children experienced the separations as a fundamental threat to their well-being. The films documented how the disruptions of children's bonds with their parents resulted in expressions of fear, angry protests, and desperate efforts to find the missing parents. The more extreme emotions of fear and anger that were immediately evident following the parents' departure eventually gave way to more subtle expressions of sadness and despair. Careful observation revealed that after a prolonged period of sadness, the infants regained some composure and became detached and less emotionally expressive. Subdued activity and a notable lack of joy or enthusiasm marked this detached stance. Much of the impetus for Bowlby's (1969/1982) attachment theory came from his efforts to account for the mechanisms

and processes that organize children's reactions to separation.

Yet, despite the power of separations to illustrate the emotional significance of the attachment bond, it soon became evident that the simple presence or absence of an attachment figure was inherently limited as a means of understanding how older children and adults maintain their relationships with attachment figures. The most casual observer of children could see that by 3 or 4 years of age, physical separations no longer present as serious a threat to a child's bond with a parent, and consequently do not produce the same kinds of emotional reactions. As a result, Bowlby (1973) faced the challenge of demonstrating the continuing importance of attachment bonds "from the cradle to the grave." In the volume titled *Separation: Anxiety and Anger,* he introduced two theoretical ideas that laid the foundation for understanding attachment relationships across the lifespan. First, he emphasized that humans' capacity to forecast the future makes their expectations of caregiver availability, or "working models," increasingly important in understanding individual differences in security and anxiety. Later attachment researchers (e.g., Bretherton, 1985; Main, Kaplan, & Cassidy,

1985) substantially extended this emphasis on cognitive processes or working models of attachment figures (see Bretherton & Munholland, Chapter 5, this volume).

A second important notion has received less attention from later researchers. Bowlby stated that an individual's sense of safety and security is derived from *maintaining* a bond with an *accessible and responsive* caregiver. Several implications follow from Bowlby's definition of caregiver availability as the set goal of the attachment system. First, unchallenged maintenance of an attachment bond contributes to a feeling security. Second, when an individual perceives a threat to a caregiver's availability, he or she will feel anxious and angry. Third, a persistent disruption of an attachment bond will result in a feeling of sadness and despair. When caregiver availability is viewed as the set goal of the attachment system, physical separations in infancy and early childhood can be understood as constituting one kind of threat to a caregiver's accessibility and responsiveness (Adam, Gunnar, & Tanaka, 2004). Older children and adults are likely to perceive threats to a caregiver's availability when lines of communication are disrupted by prolonged absence, emotional disengagement, or signals of rejection or abandonment. As a result, disrupted lines of communications produce feelings of anxiety, anger, and sadness similar to those that have been documented in young children's reactions to physical separation.

In this chapter, we review the role of separations in the development of attachment theory, and highlight Bowlby's emphasis on the continuing role of caregivers' availability in shaping children's confidence and feelings of security. We suggest that although attachment researchers have made exciting advances in understanding the cognitive and personality processes involved in child and adult attachment, less attention has been directed toward the caregiving and communication processes that contribute to the formation, maintenance, and repair of attachment bonds across the lifespan. Much of Bowlby's (1973) *Separation* volume directs attention to the continuing importance of open communication in maintaining a secure attachment bond. Similarly, Mary Ainsworth's seminal study of infant attachment (Ainsworth, Blehar, Waters, & Wall, 1978) highlights the ongoing quality of mother–infant communication as the context within which working models and attachment strategies initially develop. In reviewing Bowlby's volume on separation, we highlight Bowlby's and Ainsworth's ideas about

how open communication with an attachment figure maintains feelings of security, and about how threats to the availability of an attachment figure can produce fear, anger, and sadness. This focus on communication holds considerable promise for extending attachment research and clinical practice to older children and adults.

MATERNAL DEPRIVATION AND THE ORIGINS OF ATTACHMENT THEORY

In the decade following World War II, Bowlby laid much of the foundation for attachment theory. He developed his ideas in the context of scientific and political settings that gave little recognition to the importance of a child's ties to parents. In the scientific arena, the major learning theories of child development portrayed the infant's relationship with a primary caregiver as simply a learned by-product of the drive to feed. Since the mother most often happened to be associated with feeding, the child eventually developed positive associations to her. This view implied that if a child was fed by a variety of caregivers, the relationship with mother would hold no special significance for the child. Professional child care workers of that era often maintained institutional practices that assigned little importance to a child's relationship with a parent or primary caregiver (Karen, 1994). Social workers in many industrialized countries would routinely separate young children from their mothers because the mothers were extremely poor or lacked husbands. These well-intended practices placed the physical health and well-being of the children ahead of the children's need for a primary relationship with their mothers. A similar attitude influenced hospital practice. If a young child needed to be hospitalized, it was standard to prevent or severely restrict parental visitation.

Beginning with his earliest work, Bowlby stressed the importance of maintaining a continuous relationship between child and mother. In a widely noted paper, Bowlby (1944) investigated the early home environments and parent–child relationships of 44 children who had been institutionalized for stealing. Social workers' reports indicated that in nearly all of these cases, the subjects had experienced highly deviant parenting marked by parental violence and emotional abuse. In several cases, a child had been blamed for a sibling's death. However, Bowlby found similar sorts of deviant parent–child relationships in a comparison group of other clinic children. The one factor that distinguished the thieves from the clinic children was evidence of prolonged separations from parents, and this difference was particularly striking among a subgroup of thieves Bowlby diagnosed as "affectionless." In many cases, the prolonged separations resulted from parental illness, death, or other family disruptions that resulted in placement of the children in foster care settings. Although many clinic children had experienced disruptions in parent–child relationships, Bowlby noted that the affectionless children had all experienced a prolonged separation after 6 months of age, and hence after they had begun to form a bond with their mothers.

In the late 1940s, Bowlby extended his investigation of the importance of the mother–child relationship by integrating research findings on the effects of institutionalization on young children for a report published by the World Health Organization (WHO) (Bowlby, 1951). Across a variety of studies from different countries, Bowlby found a similar pattern: Children who had been seriously deprived of maternal care tended to develop the same symptoms that Bowlby had identified in his "affectionless" young thieves. Institutionalized children developed into individuals who lacked feeling, had superficial relationships, and exhibited hostile or antisocial tendencies. Dorothy Burlingham and Anna Freud (1944) had reached similar conclusions, based on their work in a residential nursery for children whose parents had been unable to care for them as a result of World War II. Burlingham and Freud noted that despite extensive efforts by child care workers to develop relationships with the institutionalized children, some were nearly impossible to reach. Bowlby's conclusions from his review of research were clear. In a much-quoted passage, he noted that the provision of mothering is as important to a child's development as proper diet and nutrition.

The WHO report (Bowlby, 1951) signaled with unmistakable clarity the importance of the parent–child bond to the development of young children, as well as the potential emotional damage resulting from disruptions of the bond. Institutional care provided by child care experts and professionals could not substitute for the attachment bond with parents. Bowlby (cited in Karen, 1994) stated, "The services which mothers and fathers habitually render their children are so taken for granted that their magnitude is forgotten. In no other relationship do human beings place themselves so unreservedly and so continuously at the disposal of others. This holds true even for bad

parents—a fact far too easily forgotten by their critics, especially critics who have never had the care of children of their own" (p. 66). The clear emphasis on the importance of the primary parent–child relationship suggested to Bowlby that many of the assumptions underlying child care in such institutions as hospitals, foster homes, and residential nurseries were open to serious question: "The mothering of a child is not something which can be arranged by roster; it is a live human relationship which alters the characters of both partners" (cited in Karen, 1994, p. 66).

These claims concerning the emotional significance of the parent–child bond stirred a great deal of controversy among a range of human service professionals responsible for child welfare (Karen, 1994). If Bowlby's claims were correct, much of then-current policy in social work training, child care agencies, and hospitals needed to be reconsidered. For the most part, these professions stressed the physical needs of children in settings where relatively little attention was paid to the emotional significance of the parent–child relationship. In sharp contrast, Bowlby suggested that the parent–child bond provides an irreplaceable context for emotional development. Emphasizing the importance of the parent–child relationship for emotional development also stirred controversy within Bowlby's own discipline of psychiatry, where psychoanalytic theory suggested that many of children's and adults' problems are the products of internal conflicts and fantasies (Spitz, 1958). By placing so much emphasis on the adverse effects of maternal deprivation, Bowlby suggested that many childhood and adult difficulties result from a child's actual experience, as opposed to internal conflicts and fantasies. Such claims were ripe for testing and debate.

Children's Responses to Disruptions of the Attachment Bond

Notably absent from Bowlby's 1951 monograph was any theoretical understanding of the mechanisms through which maternal deprivation produces adverse effects (Bowlby, 1988). The post-World War II period proved to be a critical time for developing the theory and research that would lay the foundation for the attachment field. Bowlby was faced with a dual task: On the one hand, he needed a theory to explain the importance of the parent–child bond; on the other hand, he needed research evidence demonstrating the importance of this bond for children's adaptation.

The literature on maternal deprivation had been largely devoid of theory, and the individual studies that Bowlby reviewed were subject to alternative interpretations (Ainsworth, 1962; Rutter, 1981). Without a theory, it was difficult to conduct research that would answer critical questions about the mechanisms through which disruptions in the attachment bond adversely affect children's emotional development.

Beginning in the late 1940s, Bowlby began a research project designed to gather the critical observations needed to understand young children's responses to separation. The hospital practices in the United Kingdom at that time provided a natural opportunity to document the effects of prolonged separations on young children. During the 1940s and 1950s, parents were allowed to visit their sick children in the hospital for only 1 hour per week (Karen, 1994). For older children and their parents, this policy was manageable, but for infants, toddlers, and young children, the prolonged separation led to a substantial and largely unexplained disruption of the attachment relationship. Bowlby and Robertson spent 4 years, 1948 to 1952, documenting and filming the effects of these separations on young children (Robertson, 1962). The children that they observed ranged in age from 18 months to 4 years, and all were separated from their families in residential nurseries or hospitals for periods of a week or more. These separations consisted of removals from the primary caregiver and placements in unfamiliar environments in the care of a succession of unfamiliar figures. Following the children's stays in these institutions, Robertson and Bowlby continued to observe their adjustment upon return to their families. Although there was substantial variation among the young children, Robertson and Bowlby were able to identify three phases that the children typically passed through during separations, each characterized by a particular attitude toward the missing mother figure. These phases, labeled "protest," "despair," and "detachment," not only were descriptive of Bowlby and Robertson's subjects, but seemed to echo many of the descriptions of children's responses to separation provided by other observers (e.g., Burlingham & Freud, 1944).

Further evidence for these phases came from careful descriptions provided by Heinicke and Westheimer (1966). The initial phase, protest, typically lasted from a few hours to a week or more. It began at the moment a parent prepared to leave a child at the nursery or hospital. Crying or screaming was the rule. During this phase the child signaled separation distress in a variety of ways, such as crying loudly, showing anger, following the mother, pounding the door, or shaking his or her cot. Any sight or sound might produce a temporary respite, as the child eagerly checked to see whether it was a sign of the mother's return. The dominant attitude during this phase was hope that the mother would return, and the child actively attempted to regain contact with her. During this phase, efforts by alternative adults to comfort or soothe the child typically met with little success, and some children actively spurned potential caregivers. Although crying gradually subsided over time, it commonly recurred, especially at bedtime or during the night. Searching for the missing parent often continued on a sporadic basis over a number of days. During the protest phase, the dominant emotions were fear, anger, and distress. Fear and distress signaled a child's appraisal of danger at being separated from a primary attachment figure, and anger served to mobilize the child's efforts to reestablish contact with the mother.

The phase of despair, which succeeded protest, was marked by behavior that suggested increased hopelessness about the mother's return. Although a child might continue to cry intermittently, active physical movements diminished, and the child withdrew or disengaged from people in the environment. Bowlby (1973) interpreted this phase as similar to deep mourning, in that the child interpreted the separation as a loss of the attachment figure. He suggested that adults often misinterpreted the reduced activity and withdrawal as signs of the child's recovery from the distress of separation. Sadness accompanied this withdrawn state. Heinicke and Westheimer (1966) also noted that hostile behavior, directed toward another child or toward a favorite object brought from home, tended to increase over time. A child's active turning of attention to the environment marked the final phase, detachment. In this phase, the child no longer rejected alternative caregivers, and some children even displayed sociability toward other adults or peers. The nature of this phase became most evident during reunion with the mother.

A child who reached the phase of detachment showed a striking absence of joy at the mother's return; instead of enthusiastically greeting her, the detached child was likely to appear apathetic. In the Heinicke and Westheimer (1966) study, varying degrees of detachment were reported among 10 children following separations that lasted from 12 days to 21 weeks. On their initial reunion with their mothers, two of the children seemed not to recognize their mothers, and the other eight children either turned or walked away from their mothers. Children often alternated between crying and showing blank, expressionless faces. Some degree of detachment persisted following the reunions, with five of the mothers complaining that their children treated them like strangers. For many children, detachment and neutrality alternated with clinging and showing fear that the mother might leave again. Following the reunions, children felt frightened by home visits from observers they knew from the nursery.

These early efforts to document young children's distress and pain caused by separations were initially met with a great deal of disbelief and hostility from professional audiences (Karen, 1994). Because these children were too young to communicate their feelings effectively in words, it was easy for adults to downplay the significance of the mother–child separation, particularly as the children themselves moved beyond immediate protest to more subtle forms of despair and detachment. Furthermore, the distress reported by Bowlby and Robertson would have major implications for hospital policy regarding parental visitation and the degree to which nursing and pediatric staffs would have to adapt to the needs of young children and their families. Despite initial denial and criticism, Robertson persisted in documenting the effects of separation, and during the 1950s he produced a series of films that vividly dramatized children's emotional reactions to the disruption of the attachment bond. His work, along with Bowlby's writings, would eventually alter hospital practice and lay the foundations for attachment theory.

A Theoretical Explanation for Separation Distress

To many professionals and child care workers, young children's apparent distress at being separated from their parents in a well-managed hospital setting could easily be dismissed as unrealistic and immature. There was little in psychological theory to contradict these professionals. As noted earlier, the major theories of the parent–child relationship that were current in the 1950s viewed this relationship as a secondary by-product of the infant's more primary need for food. Such a perspective suggested that as long as a child receives adequate physical care, the relationship with a parent is relatively unimportant. Furthermore, existing theory suggested that separation from a parent and the distress this produces in a child should be

relatively short-lived disruptions with no lasting consequences.

Bowlby viewed psychology's failure to recognize children's separation distress as a fundamental anomaly in contemporary theories of human nature. In searching for an alternative paradigm, he discovered the field of ethology, with its roots in naturalistic observation and evolutionary biology; he became particularly enthusiastic about Lorenz's observations of bonding in geese. Lorenz (1957) had demonstrated that a strong bond could develop between a mother figure and her offspring, even in a species in which the young can feed themselves. Bowlby also recognized that ethology provided new and powerful tools for reconsidering the nature of the parent–child bond. Drawing on the concept of a "behavioral system," Bowlby suggested that many of the human infant's behaviors are organized around maintaining proximity to a parent (see Cassidy, Chapter 1, this volume). Viewed in its evolutionary context, the attachment behavioral system offers a distinct survival advantage in species that have a prolonged period of development before reaching reproductive maturity.

The notion of behavioral systems also provided a way of understanding fear behaviors. Bowlby (1973) posited a fear system that is activated by "natural" clues to danger, which for humans include unfamiliarity, sudden change of stimulation, rapid or looming approach, heights, and being alone. In addition to natural clues are a variety of cultural clues that are learned through observation or association. Bowlby noted that the fear system is most likely to be activated in "compound" fear situations, in which more than one clue to danger is present. Various fear behaviors, such as avoidance, withdrawal, and attack, are well known. The goal of these behaviors is to increase distance or to eliminate the feared object. Fear and proximity-seeking behaviors are often elicited together by the same set of circumstances. When a child is frightened or in pain, he or she not only wants to avoid the source of discomfort, but also actively seeks a source of protection and safety. If the attachment figure is not available, the child faces a compound fear situation: Not only is the child facing danger, but he or she is cut off from a critical source of protection. Both aspects of this situation elicit fear, though Bowlby sought to reserve the term "fear" for situations that alarm a child as a result of the presence of frightening stimuli, and the term "anxiety" for situations in which an attachment figure or trusted companion is absent.

This distinction clarifies the situation faced by the children Bowlby and Robertson observed in the residential nurseries and hospitals. Not only were the children alarmed at being placed in unfamiliar surroundings and cared for by unfamiliar adults; they were also anxious at not being able to gain ready access to their mothers.

Ainsworth and Wittig's (1969) naturalistic observations of mother–infant interaction illustrated the interplay among the attachment, exploration, and fear systems. In contrast to the fear system, the exploration system, whose primary function is learning, interlocks in a quite different fashion with the attachment system. In observing infants in naturalistic settings, Ainsworth noted that the presence of the mother often increased the quality of the child's play and exploration. In contrast, if the infant became distressed or the attachment system was activated, play and exploration rapidly diminished until the child had gained reassurance or comfort from the mother. Ainsworth described this interplay between the attachment and exploration systems in terms of the infant's using the mother as a "secure base" from which to explore. She noted that this balance between the attachment system, whose function is protection, and the exploration system, whose function is learning, provides a mechanism that allows the child to learn and develop without straying too far away or remaining away for too long (Ainsworth et al., 1978). Viewing attachment, fear, and exploration as behavioral systems allows for increased precision in understanding infants' and young children's behavior.

The development of the Strange Situation marked a significant advance in the study of separation from Bowlby's early review of the maternal deprivation literature. Ainsworth's procedure showed that a brief 20-minute laboratory paradigm using what she termed "minuscule separations" could systematically activate the attachment system and demonstrate the interrelations among the attachment, fear, and exploration behavioral systems. The interplay between attachment and exploration was strikingly supported by Ainsworth's data (Ainsworth et al., 1978). Frequency counts of exploratory locomotion, manipulation, and visual exploration during each episode of the Strange Situation showed that exploration peaked during Episode 2, when an infant was alone with the mother, and then dramatically declined. In contrast, frequency measures of separation protest that included crying and search behavior peaked in Episode 6, when the baby was alone, while attach-

ment behaviors measured by seeking proximity and contact showed a linear increase from Episode 2 through the reunion in Episode 8. Thus, as the attachment system became increasingly activated over the course of the eight episodes, the exploration system became increasingly deactivated. The importance of the attachment system was now apparent not only in the case of severe disruption, but also in much more subtle day-to-day situations experienced by all children.

REDEFINING SEPARATIONS AS THREATS TO THE AVAILABILITY OF ATTACHMENT FIGURES

Clarifying the Set Goal of the Attachment System

Observations of children's responses to separations from their parents had provided critical evidence for the emotional significance of the attachment bond. As a result, it was tempting to view the primary purpose of the attachment system as the regulation and maintenance of physical proximity to the parent. This view of attachment was enormously appealing to behavioral researchers, who could easily quantify proximity seeking. Even more appealing was the notion that attachment behavior could be turned on by the absence of the parent and turned off by the presence of the parent. Yet, by the 1970s, the limitations of using simple physical proximity or the physical presence or absence of the parent as the set goal of the attachment system were obvious to attachment theorists. Such a model did not adequately explain Ainsworth's observations of mothers and infants, and Bowlby (1973) was aware that sole reliance on physical proximity and separations would limit his efforts to extend attachment theory to older children and adults.

Ainsworth and colleagues' (1978) Baltimore study of mothers and their infants had not only documented the operation of the attachment, fear, and exploration behavioral systems; of equal significance was her discovery of important individual differences in infants' responses to separations in the Strange Situation. The identification of "secure," "avoidant," and "ambivalent" or "resistant" patterns in the Strange Situation suggested that the infants entered this standardized situation with different cognitive expectations for how their parents would respond to them in times of distress. Ainsworth's detailed observations of mother–infant interaction suggested that these different expectations resulted from the infants' actual experience with their mothers during the first year of life. These expectations or "working models" of the mothers led to observable differences in how infants responded to the stress of brief separations. Thus the simple presence or absence of a parent did not provide an adequate account of these individual differences, and it was clear to Ainsworth that cognitive processes had to be incorporated into a model of how the attachment system functions. Although Bowlby (1969/1982) initially stressed that proximity to the parent is the predictable outcome of the attachment system, he was aware that the increasing cognitive complexity that accompanies development can alter how the child maintains the attachment relationship. With the capacity to plan and to negotiate plans about separations with parents, the child can adjust his or her goals from one situation to the next. "At one moment the child is determined to sit on his mother's knee and nothing else will do; at another he is content to watch her through the doorway. In ordinary circumstances, it seems clear, whatever conditions are at any one time necessary to terminate his attachment behavior become the set-goal of whatever attachment plan he adopts" (Bowlby, 1969/1982, p. 351). The notion that distal communication can serve at times to reassure the child suggested that the set goals for the attachment system are flexible and must include more than simple proximity or physical contact with the caregiver. In the first volume of the *Attachment and Loss* trilogy, however, Bowlby was less clear about how to replace physical proximity as the set goal of the attachment system.

Ainsworth's Emphasis on Appraisals of Availability and Responsiveness

Although separations were clearly one condition activating attachment behavior and resulting in an infant's effort to gain physical proximity to the parent, Ainsworth was clearly not satisfied with the apparent implication that the set goal of the attachment system is physical proximity to the parent. Ainsworth expressed major reservations with this "simple regulator model" of the attachment system. She and her colleagues wrote: "Overemphasis on the simple model has led many to assume that Bowlby's attachment theory defines attachment behavior rigidly and exclusively in terms of seeking literal proximity—a conception that is inadequate even when describing the attachment and attachment behavior of a 1-year-old and that is clearly misleading when attempting to comprehend the behavior of the older child or

adult" (Ainsworth et al., 1978, p. 11). Ainsworth's reservations about limiting the set goal of the attachment system to physical proximity came from several sources. If proximity were indeed the set goal, even by 1 year of age most children should respond with the same level of alarm to separations. It was clear to Ainsworth, however, that infants' responses to separations in the Strange Situation were influenced by other factors. For instance, infants displayed greater separation distress in the context of a strange laboratory environment than in the familiar home environment. It was also evident that infants were more distressed in the second separation episode than they were in the first. These problems disappear when separation distress is viewed as resulting from a child's *appraisal* or evaluation of the mother's departure, and not from the actual physical absence of the parent.

The importance of cognitive processes in infants' responses to separations was further highlighted by the substantial individual differences in how infants responded to the Strange Situation. Most notable were marked differences in reunion behavior following the second separation episode. Whereas most children actively sought contact with their mothers and were soothed by such contact, others ignored or avoided their mothers, and still others mixed contact seeking with anger. To account for these differences, Ainsworth again relied on cognitive processes, suggesting that differences in infants' attachment behavior result from different *expectations* of how their mothers will respond. According to Ainsworth, an infant's model of a parent, built from previous experiences, guides the infant's expectations regarding the mother's availability and acts as an important "modifier" of the infant's set goal of proximity. Thus a child whose model includes confident expectations concerning the mother's availability and responsiveness will react to a separation and subsequent reunion with open bids for contact; a child who anticipates rejection will approach more cautiously or not at all.

Ainsworth's notion that expectations for the caregiver's availability organize the operation of the attachment system also explains why brief laboratory separations gradually cease to be stressful for older children. Marvin (1977), in a cross-sectional study of 2-, 3-, and 4-year-olds in the Strange Situation, found that whereas 2-year-olds responded to the separation episodes in much the same way as 1-year-olds, 3-year-olds showed little disturbance in the first separation episode. Although the 3-year-olds became distressed when left alone, they were more readily comforted by the stranger than were the younger children. The 4-year-olds showed even less distress, with the exception of several children who asked to go with their mothers. When the mothers, following the experimenter's instructions, refused their children's requests, the children became very distressed. These children were angry, crying, and demanding when their mothers returned. Ainsworth and colleagues (1978) suggested that it was not the physical separation that distressed the 4-year-olds, but their mothers' apparently arbitrary behavior—which violated the children's expectations of caregiver availability.

Ainsworth's observations of infants and their mothers, and her emphasis on cognitive appraisals, plans, and working models, helped Bowlby to refine his claims about the effects of separation and maternal deprivation. Just as simple proximity seeking failed to account for children's responses to the Strange Situation, the simple presence or absence of the attachment figure was proving inadequate as a defining condition for attachment security. For instance, efforts to review studies of "maternal deprivation" indicated that this term was too broad and gave the mistaken impression that separations regardless of moderating conditions could create irreversible damage to a child (Ainsworth, 1962; Rutter, 1981). Although the study of separations had proved invaluable in revealing important mechanisms and showing how children cope with disruptions of the attachment bond, it was now clear that these disruptions were moderated by an increasingly complex set of appraisals and emotional processes. Claims about the consequences of separation and the set goal of the attachment system had to be substantially refined and clarified.

Bowlby's Clarification: From Physical Proximity to Availability and Responsiveness

In the second volume of *Attachment and Loss*, Bowlby (1973) refined his definition of the set goal of the attachment system. In considering the effects of separations on children, he moved toward the notion that security derives from a child's appraisal of an attachment figure's availability. In the first chapter, Bowlby stated:

> "Presence" and "absence" are relative terms and, unless defined, can give rise to misunderstanding. By presence is meant "ready accessibility," by absence "inaccessibility." The words "separation" and "loss" as used in this work imply always that the subject's attachment figure is inaccessible, either temporarily (separation) or permanently (loss). (1973, p. 23)

However, even "ready accessibility" is not enough to establish security for the child. Bowlby presented the case of the physically accessible but "emotionally absent" parent. To address this issue, he added a second criterion for attachment security: The child needs to experience a parent who is not only accessible but also *responsive*. This aspect of security incorporated Ainsworth's findings that it is the quality of day-to-day interactions, not just major separations, that influences infants' attachment expectations. Ainsworth's ratings of mothers' sensitivity to their infants' signals in the home showed a strong association with infants' confident expectation for mothers' response in the Strange Situation. Ainsworth viewed a mother's sensitivity to infant signals as increasing her infant's confidence in her availability and responsiveness. In contrast, various nonresponsive or insensitive forms of care can undermine the infant's confidence or even lead to expectations for rejection or inconsistent response.

The set goal of maintaining the caregiver's accessibility and responsiveness also accounted for the three phases of children's responses to separation observed by Robertson and Bowlby. Different emotions accompany a child's changing appraisals of parents' availability and play a central role in organizing a child's behavioral responses. Separation distress results from the appraisal that a parent is inaccessible. This perceived threat to a parent's accessibility activates the attachment system and motivates a child to reestablish contact. Emotional reactions accompanying the appraisal of threat include fear and anger. Fear activates the attachment system and signals the child's distress. Anger results from frustrations that the child encounters in trying to regain access, and it mobilizes efforts to reestablish contact. Fear and anger are often combined in a child's protest of a parent's departure. As initial attempts to reestablish contact fail and the child's expectations for reunion are disappointed, he or she *reappraises* the situation, and frightened and angry efforts to reunite give way to sadness. Despair accompanies the recognition that protest will not succeed in reestablishing contact with the parent. Since prolonged despair and failure to reestablish contact leave the child in an intolerably painful state, the child may attempt to reduce this pain by defensively excluding thoughts, feelings, and memories about the absent parent. Defensive detachment becomes the only available means of coping with the severe distress that the child experiences.

Moreover, defining the set goal as maintaining the caregiver's accessibility and responsiveness within comfortable limits provided an explanation for the decline of separation distress during the third and fourth years of life. As a child gains the ability to talk with an attachment figure and to understand his or her goals and plans, it becomes possible to make plans for separations that reassure the child of the attachment figure's continued accessibility and responsiveness. Because separation is no longer perceived as a threat to the caregiver's availability, separation distress declines dramatically. The decline of separation distress does not mean that the importance of the attachment relationship declines. Bowlby's focus on the parent's accessibility and responsiveness raised new questions about how the maintenance of the attachment bond changes with age. As a child gains an increased capacity to maintain the relationship through distal communication and representations of the caregiver, the nature of threats to availability also changes. Consequently, attachment theory was no longer limited to an account of young children's responses to the physical absence of their parents. The new criteria of accessibility and responsiveness allowed Bowlby (1973) to make a bolder and much broader claim: "Whether a child or adult is in a state of security, anxiety, or distress is determined in large part by the accessibility and responsiveness of his principal attachment figure" (p. 23). This claim extended the scope of attachment theory well beyond early childhood. The challenge for researchers was (and indeed still is) to move beyond the Strange Situation to find alternative ways of assessing older children's and adults' appraisals of their attachment figures' availability and strategies for maintaining attachment bonds.

Although Bowlby defined the set goal of the attachment system in the first chapter of his 1973 volume, he did not address the critical role of cognitive appraisals in the operation of the attachment system until the third section of that book. The importance of cognitive appraisals became clear when Bowlby discussed individual differences in susceptibility to fear. He began by clarifying the notion of "caregiver responsiveness," or a parent's willingness to act as a comforter and protector when a child is afraid. Bowlby then provided a single term, "availability," to encompass both a caregiver's accessibility and responsiveness as the set goal of the attachment system. With the set goal defined as caregiver "availability," three critical propositions followed that provided the scaffolding for the volume on separation:

> When an individual is confident that an attachment figure will be available to him whenever he desires it, that person will be much less prone to either intense or chronic fear than will an individual who for any reason has no such confidence. Confidence in the availability of attachment, or lack of it, is built up slowly during the years of immaturity—infancy, childhood, and adolescence—and whatever expectations are developed during those years tend to persist relatively unchanged throughout the rest of life. The varied expectations of the accessibility and responsiveness of attachment figures that different individuals develop during their years of immaturity are tolerably accurate reflections of the experiences those individuals have actually had. (p. 202)

All three of these propositions depend on the expectations or forecasts that an individual makes about the availability of his or her attachment figure. These expectations or working models become a central aspect of personality and bias how an individual will respond to frightening situations and interpret a caregiver's response. Yet in spite of these individual differences in a child's expectations, the quality of caregivers' accessibility and responsiveness will continue to shape these expectancies over the course of childhood and adolescence. Because maintaining the attachment figure's availability remains the set goal of the attachment system, the caregiver's availability continues to influence the individual's feelings of security and insecurity across the lifespan.

An Alternative Definition of the Set Goal: Felt Security

In 1977, Sroufe and Waters published a seminal and very influential paper titled "Attachment as an Organizational Construct." This paper highlighted the emotional processes that organize infants' behavior in the Strange Situation, and helped to explain how a variety of locomotive and signaling behaviors can all serve the common function of gaining access to the mother. The paper also provided a compelling demonstration of how behavior needs to be interpreted according to the context and the underlying goals of the child, instead of being reduced to simple frequency counts of discrete behaviors. The emphasis on the organization of behavior in the Strange Situation further emphasized the problems with physical proximity as the set goal of the attachment system. The concerns of Sroufe and Waters were similar to those of Ainsworth. If proximity were indeed the set goal, why should an infant be any more distressed during the second separation than during the first? Furthermore, why should distal communication with the attachment figure be reassuring to the child? Sroufe and Waters believed these questions could be addressed by specifying a set goal that makes reference to internal emotional processes, as opposed to simple distance regulation. They proposed "felt security" as the set goal of the attachment system. With felt security as the set goal, a wider range of factors could be shown to influence the activation of the attachment system, including internal cues such as mood or illness, as well as external cues such as preceding events and context.

The notion of felt security provided a useful way of talking about the operation of the attachment system in older children and adults (Cicchetti, Cummings, Greenberg, & Marvin, 1990; Mikulincer & Shaver, 2007). However, this concept substituted a set goal that was too broad (felt security) for a goal that had clearly been too narrow (physical proximity). There is little reason to believe that reliance on an attachment figure is the only source of feeling secure. As Ainsworth (1990) pointed out, an individual can increase felt security simply by avoiding dangerous situations. The attachment relationship has little or nothing to do with this strategy or with many other strategies for maintaining felt security. Making felt security the set goal for attachment suggested that "the child plans how to become secure rather than planning for conditions that, as it turns out, make him secure" (Ainsworth, 1990, p. 474). Ainsworth's response to Sroufe and Waters led to further clarification of the set goal of the attachment system. After reiterating that "maintenance of proximity can still be conceived as the set-goal of the attachment system, given that the definition of closeness is extended by cognitive development" (Ainsworth, 1990, p. 474), Ainsworth cited Bowlby's statement that "availability of the attachment figure is the set-goal of the attachment system in older children and adults." Bowlby's definition of availability "turns on cognitive processes: (a) belief that lines of communication with the attachment figure are open, (b) that physical accessibility exists, and (c) that the attachment figure will respond if called upon for help" (Ainsworth, 1990, p. 474).

Bowlby's emphasis on the caregiver's availability as the set goal of the attachment system fit with his view that an individual's feelings of security are derived from successful maintenance of an attachment bond, and that anxiety accompanies perceived threats to availability. Although internal working models guide appraisals, these appraisals continue to be influenced by the actual behavior of the attachment figure. Thus older children and adults continue to monitor the physical accessibility and responsiveness of caregivers, although this monitoring may occur through distal forms of communication. Bowlby's and Ainsworth's focus on appraisals of caregiver availability suggests the continued need for the observational study of attachment *relationships* in older children and adults. This view is consistent with a transactional model of attachment, in which internalized aspects of personality interact with the quality of a current attachment relationship in a dynamic and reciprocal manner (Bowlby, 1973; Sroufe, Egeland, Carlson, & Collins, 2005).

THREATS TO THE AVAILABILITY OF ATTACHMENT FIGURES

During childhood, adolescence, and adulthood, many individuals encounter difficulties in their relationships with parents and spouses that shake their confidence in the availability of these attachment figures. Such difficulties may fundamentally disrupt attachment bonds and dramatically reduce an individual's capacity to adapt to challenges outside the family (Adam & Chase-Lansdale, 2002; Kobak, Little, Race, & Acosta, 2001). Just as prolonged separations have been shown to have dramatic effects on the emotional life of young children, a lifespan view of attachment should identify situations that produce similar reactions in older children and adults. Bowlby's and Ainsworth's criteria for the availability of attachment figures provide valuable guidelines for identifying threats to the attachment bonds of older children and adults. Disrupted communication, physical inaccessibility, and lack of responsiveness may lead to many of the emotional responses that are evident in young children's responses to physical separations. The degree of threat is likely to be greatest when beliefs in all three aspects of caregivers' availability are simultaneously challenged. Since both responsiveness and open communication are premised on the possibility that the attachment figure is physically accessible, threats of abandonment by or loss of an attachment figure may produce the most distress (Kobak, Cassidy, & Ziv, 2004). Less severe threats may result from lack of responsiveness or emotional disengagement during communication. Threats to the availability of an attachment figure are often the source of many child and family problems encountered by clinicians.

Threats to Availability in Child–Parent and Marital Relationships

Much of Bowlby's 1973 volume was devoted to the types of threats that would shake older children and adults' confidence in the availability of their attachment figures. The perception of physical accessibility remains the most fundamental appraisal of an attachment figure's availability. With age, there are dramatic advances in the cognitive mapping of the attachment figure's whereabouts, the resources for seeking proximity, and the types of distal communication with the attachment figure. Although these advances make distance less of an obstacle to maintaining an attachment bond, the notion that the individual can reunite with the attachment figure if necessary remains a fundamental aspect of availability. Furthermore, when lines of communication are closed or cut off, older children and adults can perceive physical separations as a major threat to maintaining an attachment bond. For instance, separations in which a caregiver leaves in an angry or unexplained manner may disrupt a child's ability to plan for reunion and leave the child uncertain about the parent's whereabouts. Bowlby cited a research study by Newson and Newson (1968) describing how a 4-year-old had become anxious and clingy following her father's desertion of the family 3 months earlier. The child's mother speculated that her child's difficulty with staying at day care resulted from her fear that the mother would also not come back—a speculation supported by the child's repeatedly saying to the mother, "Do you love me? You won't leave me, Mummy, will you?" (Bowlby, 1973, p. 214).

The development of verbal communication creates new possibilities for both maintaining and disrupting attachment bonds. For instance, without actually leaving, a parent can threaten to leave or to send the child away. Such behavior is likely to occur in disciplinary contexts when the parent has become angry and exasperated with the child. For instance, Bowlby (1973) quoted a mother from the Newson and Newson (1968) study:

I used to threaten him with the Hartley Road Boys' Home, which isn't a Home any more; and since then, I haven't been able to do it; but I can always say I shall go down town and see about it you know. And Ian says, "Well, if I'm going with Stuart (7) it won't matter"; so I say, "Well, you'll go to different ones— you'll go to one Home, and *you'll* go to another." But it really got him worried, you know, and I really got him ready one day and I thought I'll take him a walk round, *as if* I was going, you know, and he really *was* worried. In fact, I had to bring him home, he started to cry. He saw I was in earnest about it—he *thought* I was, anyway. And now I've only got to threaten him. I say "It won't take me long to get you ready." (pp. 227–228)

It is difficult to document the frequency of such statements, because many parents are ashamed to admit them to researchers. However, in his review of parenting studies, Bowlby reported that the incidence of such statements was as high as 27% in the Newson and Newson (1968) study of families in England, and 20% in a study of parents in the United States (Sears, Maccoby, & Levin, 1957).

Threats of suicide by a desperate parent may elicit even more anxiety about the parent's availability. In addition to the obvious threat to the parent's physical accessibility, the child is faced with the fear of violence and with the prospect of loss. These threats often occur in the context of hostile and conflictual relations, which may further create the implication for the child that his or her angry feelings toward the parent may be responsible for the parent's desperation and despair. Bowlby noted that many children not only are exposed to threats of suicide, but may actually witness suicidal attempts. A parent may also make statements that attribute responsibility for future abandonment to the child. Statements to the child such as "You will be the death of me," or threats of abandonment that follow a child's misbehavior, are likely to confound attachment-related fears with feelings of guilt. This kind of attribution not only shakes the child's confidence in the parent's availability, but also leads directly to negative perceptions of the self.

Witnessing violence between parents may also threaten a child's confidence in the parents' availability (Davies & Cummings, 1995, 1998). The child's appraisal of marital violence is likely to include the fear that harm may come to one or both of the parents. In addition, parents who are living with constant conflict and fear are likely to have reduced capacities to attend to the child. Thus, in addition to fear of harm coming to the parents, attachment anxiety is increased by uncertainty about the parents' ability to respond to the child's distress and the lack of open communication with both parents.

Even in situations with less extreme conflict, parents who become emotionally disengaged from each other and decide to separate or divorce may create fears in the child that the parents will also decide to leave the child. For the child, the notion that a parent may leave and not return creates a fundamental threat to physical accessibility. Most parents who divorce will make efforts to communicate with the child and reassure the child of their continued availability. Such efforts substantially reduce the perceived threat and restore the child's confidence in both parents' continuing availability.

Adults may experience threats to the availability of their adult attachment figures as well. Gottman (1994) observed that distressed spouses are prone to entering into negative absorption states. These states are marked by intense negative affect in both partners and by the partners' failure to find a way of exiting from this negative state. A common self-perpetuating pattern of this type occurs when one partner rigidly pursues the other in a manner that is perceived as critical or nagging, and the partner responds by emotionally disengaging. Such disengagement can take a variety of forms: contemptuous or aloof responses, silent stonewalling, or actual physical withdrawal from the partner. Although this disengagement can be seen as an effort to escape from a painful interaction, it paradoxically heightens the pursuing partner's efforts to engage the withdrawing partner. Each partner in this state perceives the other as behaving aversively, and both see their own efforts as legitimate attempts to reduce the distress in the relationship (Johnson & Greenman, 2006; see Johnson, Chapter 34, this volume).

From an attachment perspective, these negative emotional states are maintained by the perceived threat to the availability of the partner. The emotions accompanying an individual's appraisal that a partner is no longer available as an attachment figure and has emotionally abandoned the individual may fuel the rigid negative absorption states that mark distressed marriages. Unfortunately, fear of losing the partner or of being hurt is often mixed with defensive anger. As a result, attachment-related fears and vulnerabilities are often hidden behind cycles of blame and defense that dominate many of a distressed couple's interactions. Marital therapists are faced with the challenge of helping members of such couples access underlying attachment fears associated with appraisals that their partners are unavailable and unresponsive (Kobak, Hazan, & Ruckdeschel, 1994). Shifting from an externally focused attentional set in which a partner is viewed as primarily a source of danger, to a more internally focused awareness of the fear and distress caused by the threat to the attachment relationship, can be a critical step in marital therapy. When the fears that accompany perceived threats to a partner's availability are openly communicated, the high level of conflict and disengagement found in distressed marriages can be deescalated (Johnson, 1996, 2003).

Threats to Caregiver Availability, Communication, and Attachment Strategies

Stressful events that occur in the context of an attachment relationship do not necessarily result in perceived threats to the caregiver's availability. Such events as marital conflict, divorce, parental dysfunction or illness, and parent–child conflict become threats only when a child or adult *perceives* them as jeopardizing the attachment bond. A child's perception of threat to a caregiver's availability is shaped both by internal expectations and by the quality of communication between the caregiver and the child. A secure relationship, in which the child has confident expectations in the caregiver's availability and maintains open lines of communication, reduces the likelihood that stressful events will be perceived as threats to the caregiver's availability. By contrast, an anxious relationship, in which the child lacks confidence in the caregiver's availability and communication is characterized by defensively distorted signals or strategies, increases the likelihood that disruptive events will be perceived as further threats to the caregiver's availability.

Open lines of communication can increase confidence in a caregiver's availability when the child encounters a stressful challenge. As discipline becomes a focal task for caregivers of toddlers and young children, positive parenting strategies lead to more cooperative responses from the child (Kochanska, 2001). Alternatively, negative or inconsistent parenting can result in noncompliance and negative reinforcement of controlling or coercive child behaviors (Patterson, 1986). Parental discipline can be perceived by a child either as a signal that the child needs to alter his or her behavior, or as a rejection or threat of abandonment. When lines of communication is open, parental discipline is usually accompanied by an explanation that provides the child with a clear understanding of the expectations and rules. This understanding allows the child to appraise the parent's concerns and to adjust his or her behavior accordingly (van Zeijl et al., 2006). In contrast, a parent may discipline a child with hostile, critical remarks that fail to provide a clear account of the child's misbehavior. This kind of discipline can easily be perceived as a potential indicator of rejection or abandonment and as a threat to a parent's availability. Open communication continues to be an important marker of security in parent–child relationships (Adam et al., 2004), in parent–adolescent relationships (Allen et al., 2003; Kobak & Cole, 1994; Roisman, Madsen, Hennighausen, Sroufe, & Collins, 2001), and later in marriages (Crowell et al., 2002; Johnson, 1996; Kobak & Hazan, 1991; Treboux, Crowell, & Waters, 2004).

A child's appraisal of stressful events is also influenced by his or her expectations or working model of the attachment figure. This working model is built from the child's previous interactions with the parent and is a tolerably accurate representation of the child's experience. Ainsworth believed that these expectations "modified" infants' appraisals of the separations they encountered in the Strange Situation (Ainsworth et al., 1978). Infants who had confident expectations of their caregivers' availability actively sought comfort and used the parents as a safe haven following the separations. Avoidant infants, who had reason to expect rejection from their caregivers, modified their attachment behavior by avoiding their caregivers, effectively reducing anticipated conflict or rejection following the separation. Ambivalent/resistant infants, who had reason to be uncertain about their mothers' response, showed angry resistant or passive behavior that served to increase their proximity to the caregivers. Infants who lack confidence in the responsiveness of their mothers develop either avoidant or ambivalent/resistant strategies; these two types of strategies can be viewed as organized ways of maintaining proximity to unresponsive parents (Main, 1990; Main & Weston, 1982).

The interplay among attachment strategies, communication, and stressful events is likely to provide much more predictive power in considering outcomes such as social competence and psychopathology than any one of these factors in isolation. For example, an avoidant child, who lacks confidence in a parent's responsiveness, may have found ways of reducing conflict and subse-

quent anxiety about the parent's availability. However, if that child encounters a disruptive event—including an outburst of anger from a parent, or a more prolonged event such as marital conflict and divorce—he or she is more likely to interpret that event as a threat to the parent's availability. Similarly, the nature of parent–child communication will also bias that child's interpretation of subsequent disruptions in attachment relationships. When lines of parent–child communication are open, disruptive events can be discussed with parents, and perceived threats to availability can be disconfirmed. Infants and toddlers lack the ability to discuss and negotiate physical separations, and as a result are much more vulnerable to perceiving physical separations as threats to the availability of their parents.

A comprehensive account of attachment relationships requires a dual focus on *intrapersonal* processes (described with internal working models and attachment strategies) and *interpersonal* processes (described with such constructs as sensitivity/responsiveness, positive parenting, and open communication). This account should include (1) current disruptions in the attachment relationship (prolonged separations, chronic conflict, marital separation, and loss); (2) the nature of communication in the attachment relationship; and (3) the attachment strategies that the child has developed to maintain attachment bonds with insensitive or unresponsive caregivers. The risk for psychopathology is highest when multiple factors coincide to increase the child's anxiety about his or her parent's availability. The anxiety and accompanying defensive processes that are associated with threats to availability increase the risk that attachment related fear, anger, and sadness will be expressed in symptomatic forms.

The Special Case of Trauma and Loss

During the 1970s and 1980s, the increased awareness of child physical and sexual abuse and child neglect called attention to difficulties in attachment relationships that pose unique problems for children's adaptation. A traditional focus on the availability of an attachment figure assumes that the attachment relationship will serve as a source of safety; however, children exposed to abuse or extreme forms of punishment must manage a profound dilemma, as their attachment figures are potential sources of danger. Main and Hesse (1990) noted that infants who have been unpredictably frightened by their attachment figures are caught in a conflict when placed in a situation that normally elicits attachment behavior. Although these infants may display the typical secure and insecure attachment strategies, many show temporary lapses in their strategies; such lapses are marked by fear, freezing, and disorientation.

Main and Solomon (1986) developed a new classification, "disorganized/disoriented" (D), for infants showing these behaviors in the Strange Situation. Initial studies of the parents of D infants pointed to a parallel form of disorganization in their discussions of loss and trauma in the Adult Attachment Interview (AAI; see Hesse, Chapter 25, this volume). In the interview context, these adults show momentary lapses in "monitoring discourse or reason" that include disorientation as to time and space, loss of monitoring of discourse, and reports of extreme behavioral reactions. These lapses can be seen as indications that aspects of the loss or trauma remain unresolved or not fully processed at a conscious level. These parents are thought to be vulnerable to similar lapses in organized behavior with their children, causing the children to perceive their parent as "frightened or frightening" (Main & Hesse, 1990).

The infant and adult disorganized classifications have been consistently linked to a variety of adjustment difficulties and to psychopathology (Kobak, Cassidy, Lyons-Ruth, & Ziv, 2006; Lyons-Ruth & Jacobvitz, Chapter 28, this volume). During early childhood, infant D status has been associated with aggressive and externalizing symptoms (Shaw, Owens, Vondra, Keenan, & Winslow, 1996). In a 6-year longitudinal study, children who were classified as D in infancy were much more likely to develop aggressive behavior problems in preschool and elementary school (Lyons-Ruth, 1996; Lyons-Ruth, Alpern, & Repacholi, 1993; Moss, Cyr, & Dubois-Comtois, 2004; Moss et al., 2006). Longitudinal data from Sroufe and Egeland's sample of high-risk families indicate that the infant D classification predicts adjustment problems consistently from childhood and through adolescence, and that it specifically predicts dissociative symptoms (Carlson, 1998; Sroufe, 2005). Similar patterns of maladaptation have been identified in adolescents and adults who are classified as "unresolved with respect to loss or trauma" in the AAI (Allen, Hauser, & Borman-Spurrell, 1996) or as having disorganized, hostile/helpless states of mind (Lyons-Ruth, Melnick, Patrick, & Hobson, 2007; Lyons-Ruth, Yellin, Melnick, & Atwood, 2005b). Symptomatic expressions of aggression, anxiety, or sadness are likely to be most evident at times when normal coping strategies break down. Similarly, parents are likely to be most frightening to their children when their unusual behavior occurs in unpredictable ways. These sorts of events not only threaten the availability of a caregiver, but also threaten a child's safety, which is fundamental to the attachment relationship.

During the past decade, new attention has been focused on children who experience permanent disruptions in their attachment bonds with biological parents. As foster care families have replaced residential nurseries for children who have been removed from their biological parents, new questions about the effects of disruptions of bonds with biological parents and the potential formation of bonds to foster parents have begun to be investigated (Stovall-McClough & Dozier, 2004; see Dozier & Rutter, Chapter 29, this volume). These studies suggest that infants and young children in foster care will display attachment behaviors toward their new caregivers within the first few weeks of placement. In contrast to bonds to biological parents that are formed over the first 9 months of life, there is a question about whether attachment behaviors directed toward foster parents necessarily indicate that the children have formed an attachment bond. In contrast to a child's attachment behaviors, a foster parent's "commitment" to the foster child measured early in the relationship was found to be a strong predictor of the long-term stability of the placement and of adoption (Dozier & Lindhiem, 2006). These findings illustrate that assessment of the foster parent can yield a better prediction of bond formation than either home or laboratory assessments of the foster child's attachment behavior. The importance of maintaining an enduring attachment bond is further highlighted by a prospective study of foster and maltreated children: Higher rates of behavior problems were found in children who had been placed in foster care than in children who remained placed with maltreating caregivers with whom they had presumably maintained an attachment bond (Lawrence, Carlson, & Egeland, 2006).

EMOTIONAL REACTIONS TO ATTACHMENT DISRUPTIONS

When physical separations are viewed as one example of a larger class of attachment disruptions, observations of infants' and toddlers' emotional reactions to separation can be used to anticipate older children's and adults' responses to disruptive events. What constitutes a threat to an attachment figure's availability may change with age, along with the capacities to manage emotional reactions. However, the core emotional reactions that accompany threats to the maintenance of an attachment bond remain similar across the lifespan. These reactions can directly signal the individual's concerns and promote open communication, or they can be expressed in distorted forms that reduce the likelihood of eliciting an effective response from a caregiver.

Fear, Anger, and Sadness as Responses to Attachment Disruptions

From infancy through adulthood, specific emotions accompany an individual's appraisals of an attachment figure's availability. These emotions normally serve important motivational, self-monitoring, and communication functions for the individual (Bowlby, 1969/1982). For instance, when access to the attachment figure is jeopardized, fear activates the attachment system and leads to attachment behaviors that normally serve to reestablish access to the attachment figure. When communication is open and direct, fear serves as a communicative signal alerting the attachment figure to the child's or adult's distress and eliciting comforting responses. Anger also plays an important role in responding to disruptions in attachment relationships. Increased anger is often observed when children experience prolonged separations from their caregivers. In a doll-play situation, Heinicke and Westheimer (1966) reported that children in a residential nursery displayed hostile themes four times as often as children living at home did. They also noted that the hostility of the separated children was frequently directed at parent dolls. Bowlby likewise reported several studies indicating that hostile behavior often continued at increased levels following a prolonged separation. He suggested that when separations are only temporary, anger can serve to (1) motivate a child to overcome obstacles to reuniting with the attachment figure, and (2) communicate reproach to the attachment figure and discourage him or her from becoming unavailable in the future (Bowlby, 1973).

Dramatic evidence that the emotions of fear, anger, and sadness persist as responses to disruptions in adult attachment relationships comes from Weiss's (1975) study of individuals who were dissolving their marriages. In studying individuals who had separated from their partners, Weiss gathered extensive descriptive information about attachment processes, with some striking parallels to the phases of separation identified by Robertson and Bowlby in young children. Weiss discovered what he termed the "persistence of attachment" in the separated spouses, despite their decision to live separate lives and end their marital relationships. Many spouses reported that when they considered leaving their marriages, they became almost paralyzed with fear. The nature of separation distress was vividly depicted by one of Weiss's (1975, p. 49) subjects, who said, "When my husband left I had this panicky feeling which was out of proportion to what was really happening. I was afraid I was being abandoned. I couldn't shake the feeling." Many of the subjects had difficulty giving up hopes of restoring the relationship and regaining access to their former partners. Weiss also found that spouses' fears were accompanied by intense anger. As one woman described it, "In separating from someone you discover in yourself things that you had never felt before in your life. That's one of the things that really freak you out. I've always used my mind to keep down anything I didn't like. And now I discover, wow, I can hate!" (Weiss, 1975, p. 98; see also B. C. Feeney & Monin, Chapter 39, this volume).

A spouse often played on a partner's fears of separation, using threats to leave as a weapon to frighten the partner. However, as Weiss noted, such threats were double-edged swords that only increased both partners' insecurity and fear. Together, the recurrent bouts of anger and fear were reminiscent of the protest phase identified in young children. Like adolescents who were relinquishing their parents as attachment figures (but had not yet formed attachments with romantic partners), the adults in Weiss's studies gradually experienced loneliness. This phase mirrors the despair of young children who were losing hope of reuniting with their attachment figures. In many, it led to symptoms of depression and a perception that the world seemed "desolate of potential attachment … barren, silent, dead" (pp. 56–57). Similarly, feelings about the self were depleted, with many subjects describing feeling empty or hollow. Throughout the process of dissolving the marital attachment, subjects attempted to reduce the fear of separation and the despair of loneliness with defensive coping. For instance, Weiss (1975) noted:

> In most marriages headed for separation the partners seem not to relinquish their attachment for one another. It would be too painful to do so, and even if they wanted to, they cannot control their feelings.

But often for reasons of pride, because of hurt and anger, or from impulses toward self-protection, *they attempt to hide their attachment behind a mask of indifference.* (p. 45, emphasis added)

Despite trying to control the pain of separation by feigning indifference, many in Weiss's sample experienced breakdowns in their defenses that resulted in desperate efforts to reunite with their spouses. Weiss's study documented the role of fear, anger, and sadness as emotional responses to disruptions in adult attachment relationships. By considering situations that threaten the availability of adults' attachment figures, he demonstrated how attachment theory can provide a guide for understanding and normalizing many of the extreme emotions that accompany threats to the availability of attachment figures in later life. His work suggests that the availability and responsiveness of attachment figures remain critical aspects of adult security and happiness. Furthermore, threats to the availability of romantic attachment figures elicit adult emotional reactions that are strikingly similar to those observed in young children's responses to separation.

Open and Distorted Emotional Communication

When an individual maintains open lines of communication, perceptions of threat can be managed in ways that restore confidence in the caregiver. Open communication and secure working models go hand in hand (Bretherton, 1987, 1990; Kobak & Duemmler, 1994). During infancy, open communication depends on a caregiver's ability to read a child's signals accurately (Crowell & Feldman, 1988), which in turn promotes sensitive response to the infant's signals. Ainsworth and her colleagues observed that mothers of infants who would later be judged secure in the Strange Situation were able to manage feedings in a manner that responded to infant signals, at times requiring adjustments to the intake of bottled and solid foods. Feeding was responsive to infants' initiatives and never forced by the mothers of secure infants (Ainsworth & Bell, 1969). In face-to-face interactions, some mothers were able to skillfully regulate pacing to establish smooth turn taking and coordination with the children's initiatives (Blehar, Lieberman, & Ainsworth, 1977). Physical contact between secure infants and their mothers was marked by a gentle and tender style that made the contact pleasurable for both mothers and infants. By the end of infancy, infants who had experienced open communica-

tion marked by sensitive care were more effective in communicating with their mothers. Grossmann, Grossmann, and Schwan (1986) also observed that infants judged secure in the Strange Situation engaged in more "direct communication" with their mothers, as evidenced in more eye contact, facial expression, vocalization, and showing and affective sharing of objects.

Open parent–child communication allows a child to develop and maintain confident expectations for his or her caregiver's availability. These expectations result in more open and direct signaling to the parent. Secure relationships often foster a self-sustaining "circle of security" (Hoffman, Marvin, Cooper, & Powell, 2006). In a relationship marked by confident expectations for caregiver availability and open communication, perceived threats to the caregiver's availability often result in conversations that restore the child's confidence in the caregiver. The child in such a relationship is more likely to directly express the negative feelings associated with perceived threats. For instance, a child worrying about a mother who has an increased work schedule may tell the mother that he or she misses her. The mother in such a relationship is more likely to be accepting of her child's need and to be capable of acknowledging the stresses in her life in a way that reassures the child of her continued availability. Even if the child responds to perceived threats with indirect expressions of anger, fear, or sadness, a perceptive parent may recognize the connection between a child's angry oppositional behavior and his or her fears about perceived threats to the caregiver's availability. Such an understanding can in turn allow the parent to understand and respond in a more empathetic manner to the anxious child. In secure relationships, negative emotions serve as signals of the child's goals and needs, and thus facilitate open communication.

Symptomatic Expressions of Attachment Emotions and Psychopathology

States of anxiety and depression that occur during the adult years, and also psychopathic conditions, can, it is held, be linked in a systematic way to the states of anxiety, despair, and detachment described by Burlingham and Freud.

—Bowlby (1973, pp. 4–5)

Although fear, anger and sadness can serve as signals that promote open communication in secure attachment relationships, these feelings may be expressed in distorted or symptomatic forms in anxious relationships. Anger can easily become destructive and dysfunctional when the caregiver misreads the child's anger and responds with reciprocated anger or withdrawal. Sadness naturally accompanies the recognition that an attachment figure is not accessible and that efforts to reestablish contact cannot succeed. Unlike fear and anger, which are especially evident when an individual protests a threat to the attachment figure's availability, sadness tends to occur as the individual begins to accept the loss of an attachment figure. Withdrawal is the behavior that normally accompanies sadness, and this disengagement offers the individual time to accept unwelcome changes and revise working models.

When negative emotions fail to restore a child's confidence in his or her caregiver's availability, such emotions can rapidly become dysfunctional and contribute to distorted expressions that "miscue" the caregiver (Hoffman et al., 2006). One source of distorted communication can be traced to the detached phase of separation. This phase is characterized by an attempt to downplay attachment feelings. Bowlby viewed detachment as a defensive effort to deactivate the attachment system and thus to gain control over the painful emotions. Although this defensive detachment gives children a way of coping with anxious and angry feelings, it leads to difficulties when the children are reunited with their parents. Detached children show cool neutrality toward parents and an apparent apathy. In some cases, children may appear not to recognize their parents and show a striking absence of joy at the parents' return. Following reunions, children often alternate between crying and showing blank, expressionless faces. When children defensively hide or distort anxious and angry feelings, parents and other observers can easily misunderstand the children's neutrality as a rebuff or lack of concern about the attachment relationship. The blank, expressionless faces described by observers of detached children can also be interpreted as general emotional disengagement. More significantly, the fear, anger, and sadness that serve to signal parents of the children's concerns are likely to be hidden by detached children, leading their parents to ignore or misunderstand their children's concerns. If emotions associated with threats to caregiver availability are "shut away from further conscious processing," they no longer serve as signals that facilitate self-understanding and interpersonal adjustment, and instead become symptoms that appear puzzling and problematic (Kobak et al., 1994).

Under extreme stress, when the detached defense breaks down, anger, fear, and sadness may emerge in uncontrolled forms. Anger resulting from disruptions in attachment relationships is especially prone to distorted expression. Bowlby (1973, p. 249) described how anger as a signal of "hot displeasure" with a caregiver's lack of availability can become instead the "malice" of hatred. Hatred and resentment toward parents may be accompanied by thoughts of wanting to harm parents, which paradoxically increase anxiety about the parents' availability. It is not uncommon for even very young children to redirect or displace anger toward other targets, such as peers. In a study of children's behavior in a day care setting, George and Main (1979) observed that children who had been physically abused by their parents were much more likely than nonabused children to attack their peers, particularly at moments when their peers were distressed. This type of hostile behavior increases the likelihood that parents will be angry at the children's misbehavior, and in turn results in further interactions that heighten the children's anxiety about their parents' availability.

Clinicians often encounter difficulty in getting accurate information about family interaction. Bowlby (1973) called attention to parents' tendency to feel ashamed about the sorts of threats to availability that might account for their children's anxiety, anger, and sadness. This shame often results in parents' attempts to deny, hide, or distort any role that they may have played in their children's difficulties. These parents are acutely sensitive to any implication that family difficulties may be playing a role in their children's problems. As a result, parents are likely to omit information about attachment disruptions or actually to falsify their depictions of conflicted family relationships. A history of poor parent–child communication combined with a child's lack of confidence in the availability of attachment figures will exacerbate these problems. Not only does such a child receive little help in identifying threats to availability, but the child may suppress the memories of attachment disruptions in order to reduce painful feelings. Thus attachment-related feelings become cognitively disconnected from the family situations in which they originated.

Bowlby's review of the clinical treatment literature found substantial evidence for perceived threats to parents' availability and distorted communication in the families of pseudophobic children. He identified four family patterns. In one, a parent suffers from chronic anxiety and often unconsciously comes to reverse roles with a child, using him or her as a source of safety. In such a family, the parent may often keep the child at home. In another pattern, a child fears that something dreadful may happen to a parent and stays at home to maintain a vigilant watch on the parent. In such families, parental threats of suicide or abandonment are common. The child fearing for his or her own safety when he or she is away from home marks the third pattern. In yet another pattern, a parent may fear that something dreadful will happen to a child at school and may consequently work to keep the child at home. In nearly all these cases, Bowlby suggested that parents themselves may have suffered from lack of available and responsive care from their own parents. He also noted that the marital relations in the families of school-refusing children are often disturbed.

In considering agoraphobia and animal phobias in children, Bowlby was more circumspect and reported a lack of data on family interaction that made it impossible to determine the contribution of attachment fears. Although he suspected that such children may be more susceptible to fear because of anxious attachments, Bowlby left open the possibility that true phobias may develop through conditioning and avoidance learning. Failure to understand the emotional significance of the attachment relationship in the lives of young children leads many parents and child care workers to ignore the potential impact of family disturbance. Bowlby believed that a great deal of psychopathology and many later difficulties emerge from this neglected aspect of children's experience. Not only separations, but also threats to the availability of attachment figures in general, leave children vulnerable to later depression, anxiety, aggression, and defensive distortions of vulnerable feelings in close relationships.

During the past decade, simplistic models linking insecure attachment to psychopathology have given way to more complex models that take into account the dynamic transaction between personality and the caregiving environment (Sroufe et al., 2005). This toward a more sophisticated understanding of attachment and psychopathology was anticipated by Bowlby's (1973, 1988) developmental-pathways model. In the developmental-pathways framework, psychopathology is viewed as the product of complex transactions among internal aspects of the child derived from his or her developmental history, the current caregiving environment, and ongoing contextual stressors (Kobak et al., 2006). Threats

to availability not only during infancy, but also during childhood, adolescence, and adulthood, continue to play a prominent role in the quality of care available to the individual and in the emergence of psychopathology (Johnson, 1996; Klerman, Weissman, Rounsaville, & Chevron, 1984; Mufson, Moreau, Weissman, & Klerman, 1993). In addition, such contextual stressors as financial strain, residential change, and neighborhood violence reduce caregivers' capacities for providing available and responsive care. The way in which children and caregivers adapt to these stresses so as to maintain an attachment bond is an important topic for future research.

RESEARCH AND CLINICAL IMPLICATIONS

Maintaining access to an attachment figure continues to be the set goal of the attachment system from infancy through adulthood. However, the individual's cognitive appraisals of the attachment figure's availability play a pivotal role in how the individual regulates attachment behavior and maintains the attachment relationship (Ainsworth, 1990; Bowlby, 1973). Confident expectations in a caregiver's availability (physical access, responsiveness, open lines of communication) are accompanied by feelings of security. Much of attachment research has focused on *intrapersonal* processes (internal working models, attachment strategies) that shape appraisals of availability and that guide attachment behavior. These intrapersonal processes form the basis for attachment as a personality construct and have been assessed with the Strange Situation, the AAI, and measures of adult attachment styles (Mikulincer & Shaver, 2007; Shaver & Mikulincer, 2007).

Although observations of parent–infant communication were the primary focus of Ainsworth's study of infant attachment, subsequent attachment research with older children and adults has devoted much less attention to observing *interpersonal* processes (e.g., positive parenting, cooperative negotiation of goal conflicts). Bowlby and Ainsworth's theory emphasizes the need to assess security as a *transaction* between intrapersonal expectations and interpersonal communication. As a result, attachment security from childhood through adulthood remains both a relationship and a personality construct (Sroufe & Fleeson, 1986). This transactional view suggests that a person may experience variability in the security of a relationship, depending on the behavior of a current attachment partner. Furthermore, intrapersonal expectations or working models may be subject to change as the result of communication processes in attachment relationships (Bowlby, 1980). Consequently, attachment security results from a dynamic transaction between internal working models and the degree of open communication in current attachment relationships.

Research Implications

During the past 20 years, measures of attachment-related aspects of personality—the AAI (George, Kaplan, & Main, 1984, 1985, 1996) and Hazan and Shaver's (1987) self-report measure of romantic attachment styles—have led to an explosion of research on attachment as a personality construct (see Crowell, Fraley, & Shaver, Chapter 26, this volume). Both measures were designed to assess adult patterns that parallel the three patterns of infant attachment identified by Ainsworth in the Strange Situation. In her work with discourse processes in the AAI, Main has suggested that cognitive advances from infancy and adulthood allow attention, feeling, and memory to be organized in such a manner that individual states of mind are preserved (Main et al., 1985). This focus on the mental processes of adolescents and adults provides an account of how attachment strategies in infancy may become internalized aspects of an individual's personality.

Hazan and Shaver (1987) further extended the personality model to adult attachment relationships by asking subjects how they managed closeness across their romantic relationships. The personality model emphasizes continuity with infant patterns of attachment and focuses exclusively on Bowlby's construct of internal working models. Attachment research over the past two decades has largely neglected Bowlby's claim that the quality of interpersonal communication continues to be the major factor in whether a child or adult is in a secure, anxious, or distressed state. The view of attachment as a relationship construct offers an alternative to a personality model that views attachment security as largely determined in infancy. Although few attachment researchers explicitly endorse such a model, it implicitly informs many attachment studies. For instance, longitudinal prediction of adult (AAI) patterns of attachment from infant patterns with mothers in the Strange Situation is considered a criterion for "thorough" validation of Main and Goldwyn's (1984; Main, Goldwyn, & Hesse, 2003) AAI cod-

ing system (e.g., van IJzendoorn, 1995). Such an assumption is consistent with a personality model of attachment in which individual differences in infant attachment determine adolescent and adult attachment patterns.

The view of attachment as a relationship construct suggests that the validity of any measure of attachment security will depend on concurrent evidence that the individual maintains a secure attachment bond with a primary attachment figure. Bowlby's theory challenges researchers to understand the communication processes through which attachment bonds are formed, maintained, and repaired. Open communication also needs to be specified according to developmental level (Bretherton, 1990). For example, by age 4, the formation of "goal-corrected partnerships" engenders confidence in the attachment figure; this confidence is reflected in cooperative discussion of goal conflicts, negotiation of plans, and perspective-taking communication (Kobak & Duemmler, 1994), all of which results in mutually responsive communication (Askan, Kochansaka, & Ortmann, 2006). Attachment-related emotions can facilitate or undermine open communication. In a secure relationship, emotions directly signal each individual's concerns and help parent and child or romantic partners to accommodate to each other (Pietromonaco, Greenwood, & Barrett, 2004). In adolescence, security of parent–teen attachment should be reflected in both the parent's and the teen's capacity to directly assert different goals and yet to maintain a sense of closeness or relatedness (Allen, Hauser, Bell, & O'Connor, 1994; Sroufe, Egeland, Carlson, & Collins, 2005). As new attachment bonds are formed with romantic partners, confident expectations in self and others should support more open negotiation of goal conflicts and the capacity for both vulnerability and empathy (Furman & Simon, 2006; Simpson, Collins, Tran, & Haydon, 2007; Sroufe, 2005). In contrast, fear or anger that accompanies perceived lack of availability may result in critical commentary or disengagement that evokes further defensive or coercive response from a caregiver.

As measures of communication in parent–child and romantic relationships are developed and validated, Bowlby's (1973, 1988) developmental-pathways model of continuity and change can be tested. Viewing attachment as a relationship construct opens up important questions. The major longitudinal studies of attachment suggest that the influence of infant attachment security on developmental outcomes during childhood, adolescence, and adulthood is largely mediated through the subsequent quality of parent–child and peer relationships (Grossmann, Grossmann, & Kindler, 2005; Sroufe, 2005; Sroufe et al., 2005). Furthermore, specific predictions of the quality of communication in adult romantic relationships are most strongly influenced by the quality of peer relationship in childhood (Simpson et al., 2007) and the quality of parent–teen interaction in early adolescence (Roisman et al., 2001). Viewing attachment as a relationship construct also raises new questions about the way in which the quality of parent–child attachments influences the formation of pair bonds with romantic partners during adolescence and early adulthood (Connolly, Furman, & Konarski, 2000; Fraley & Davis, 1997; Furman & Wehner, 1997; Hazan & Shaver, 1994) (see Zeifman & Hazan, Chapter 20, this volume), and about how the quality of marital relationships influences the child's appraisals of parental availability (Cowan, 1997; Garcia-O'Hearn, Margolin, & John, 1997).

Clinical Implications

By studying young children's responses to separations, Bowlby (1973) gained an understanding of the emotional dynamics of the attachment system that would lead to a new understanding of clinical problems. Threats to the availability of attachment figures, in conjunction with defensive processes and distorted or miscued communication, can result in symptomatic expressions of fear, anger, and sadness. Clinical symptoms such as depression, anxiety, and aggression motivate individuals to seek help and account for many of the presenting problems found in clinic settings. Bowlby believed that careful assessments of family context often reveal that behind these presenting symptoms lie basic threats to the availability of attachment figures, disrupted attachment bonds, and subsequent defensive distortions. To understand the contribution of attachment processes to child and adult psychopathology, clinicians and researchers need to assess for events that may have shaken individuals' confidence in the availability of their attachment figures. Interviews with family members about changes in relationships, losses experienced by family members, and marital functioning can provide clinicians with valuable information about the attachment disruptions associated with child and adolescent psychopathology. Observations of family interaction may also indicate the extent to which family communica-

tion is open and the degree to which relationships have become distressed or conflicted.

Comprehensive assessments of threats to caregivers' availability, disruptions of attachment bonds, working models, and communication are needed to determine the role of attachment processes in children and adults' presenting problems. Review of the history of childhood and adolescent attachment, using a format similar to George and colleagues' (1984, 1985, 1996) AAI, can help clinicians identify the extent to which attachment disruptions have been processed and integrated into a coherent model of self and others. Recent progress in identifying disorganized attachment points to important hypotheses about how more extreme forms of attachment trauma may lead a child to respond in fear or terror to a caregiver, thus illustrating a breakdown of organized attachment strategies (Hesse & Main, 2006; Lyons-Ruth, Yellin, Melnick, & Atwood, 2005a). Initial longitudinal studies of disorganized infants suggest that these children are at particular risk for later psychopathology (Carlson, 1998). In these cases, clinicians may be presented with dissociative (Carlson, 1998) or aggressive (Lyons-Ruth, 1996) symptoms. Research and theory suggest that clinicians need to observe family interactions carefully and to review both children's and parents' attachment histories to understand how attachment traumas have created extreme emotional dilemmas in these families.

The transaction between intrapersonal processes (working models) and interpersonal processes (communication) is a focal point for defining intervention strategies in attachment-based treatments. Whereas some treatments target change in internal working models, other treatments place more emphasis on altering patterns of emotional communication in attachment relationships. Bowlby wrote most extensively about individual therapy with adults. The goal of his approach was to provide a client with a secure base from which he or she could access painful emotional experiences that had been shut away from conscious processing. This type of treatment often involves linking symptomatic expressions of fear and anger to disturbances in attachment relationships. In doing so, a clinician can help a client experience and integrate painful experiences in order to gain control over symptoms. Accessing previously avoided experiences makes it possible for the individual to update working models and reduce defensively distorted emotions that contribute to miscued communication. Although this description of adult therapy focuses on intrapersonal working models, intrapersonal change is premised on the notion that the interpersonal relationship with the therapist provides the client with a model of open communication about attachment-related experiences (see Slade, Chapter 32, this volume).

Attachment interventions with infants and young children focus extensively on altering interpersonal processes in attachment dyads. Thus, while these treatments involve some effort to change the caregivers' working models of the children, their primary goal is to improve parent–child communication and the children's perception of the caregivers' availability and responsiveness. For instance, the Circle of Security intervention provides parents with a model of open communication in secure relationships (Hoffman et al., 2006). Therapists collaborate with parents in examining video replays of parent–child interaction. This process helps parents to identify their children's miscued or defensively distorted emotional signals. By altering their interpretation of children's signals, parents can respond in new ways that increase their children's perception of their availability. Pre- and posttreatment assessment of children's attachment indicate that this intervention moved a substantial number of children from disorganized to organized attachments with their caregivers. Other attachment interventions, such as infant–parent psychotherapy with toddlers, focus more on parents' working models derived from childhood experience and the effects of these models on current parent–child interaction (Lieberman, 1992). This approach has also produced increased attachment security in a randomized trial with mothers diagnosed with major depressive disorder (Toth & Cicchetti, 2006). (See Berlin, Zeanah, & Lieberman, Chapter 31, this volume, for a review of early intervention programs designed to enhance attachment security.)

Developmental changes in the parent–child relationship create new parental tasks that include discipline and cooperative negotiation of goal conflicts. These emerging features of parent–child relationships require new definitions of caregiver availability and responsiveness. In their intervention with 1- to 3-year-old children who were at increased risk for externalizing problems, van Zeijl (2006) developed a measure of sensitive discipline. These investigators used observations and discussions of parent–child goal conflicts as a way of improving "sensitive discipline" in a randomized clinical trial. This focus on sensitivity during goal conflicts produced improved management of disciplinary interactions in the intervention group and reduced externalizing behavior in families with multiple interpersonal stressors.

Innovations in marital therapy provide a prototype for how attachment theory can be used as a basis for treatment. Beginning with the well-documented negative absorption states that characterize distressed couples (Gottman, 1994), Johnson (1996, 2003, and Chapter 34, this volume) has developed exploratory techniques that help distressed partners to access the attachment fears and vulnerabilities hidden behind angry and defensive interaction sequences. Through close observations of couples' interactions and exploration of individuals' experience of "attachment injuries," Johnson's therapy focuses on facilitating reconciliation and forgiveness in distressed couples. This approach has been found to produce increased levels of marital satisfaction in the majority of couples completing treatment (Makinen & Johnson, 2006). Extension of these techniques to the treatment of children and their parents offers a promising direction for attachment-based treatment for parent–child relationships (Kobak & Esposito, 2004).

CONCLUSION

The field of attachment research has progressed substantially beyond the early studies of young children's separations. The partnership of Ainsworth and Bowlby provided a model for how theory and research can mutually inform each other: Ainsworth was guided by Bowlby's theory in nearly every aspect of her study of mothers and their infants, and her observations forced clarification and increased precision in the theory. Initial efforts to extend attachment research to older children and adults focused on attachment as an intrapersonal process, at the expense of investigating the ongoing communication processes that mediate the formation and maintenance of attachment bonds. Following Bowlby and Ainsworth, we have argued that *intrapersonal* expectations and strategies continually influence and are shaped by the quality of *interpersonal* communication in attachment relationships. When aspects of an individual's personality are viewed as a part of ongoing transaction with a caregiver's availability, we gain a more complete understanding of how attachment bonds are maintained and repaired. Recent longitudinal studies have called attention to this complex transaction and provided a new focus on Bowlby's (1973,

1988) developmental-pathways model (Grossmann et al., 2005; Simpson et al., 2007; Sroufe, 2005; Sroufe et al., 2005). These studies illustrate the importance of repeated assessments of internal working models, the caregiving environment, and communication in attachment relationships. We believe that the true value of personality measures of attachment strategies and working models will be realized only when they are studied in conjunction with the ongoing communication processes that maintain attachment bonds.

REFERENCES

Adam, E. K., & Chase-Lansdale, P. L. (2002). Home sweet home(s): Parental separations, residential moves, and adjustment problems in low-income adolescent girls. *Developmental Psychology, 38,* 792–805.

Adam, E. K., Gunnar, M. R., & Tanaka, A. (2004). Adult attachment, parent emotion, and observed parenting behavior: mediator and moderator models. *Child Development, 75,* 110–122.

Ainsworth, M. D. S. (1962). The effects of maternal deprivation: A review of findings and controversy in the context of research strategy. In *Deprivation of maternal care: A reassessment of its effects.* Geneva: World Health Organization.

Ainsworth, M. D. S. (1990). Some considerations regarding theory and assessment relevant to attachments beyond infancy. In M. T. Greenberg, D. Cicchetti, & E. M. Cummings (Eds.), *Attachment in the preschool years* (pp. 463–488). Chicago: University of Chicago Press.

Ainsworth, M. D. S., & Bell, S. M. (1969). Some contemporary patterns in the feeding situation. In A. Ambrose (Ed.), *Stimulation in early infancy* (pp. 133–170). London: Academic Press.

Ainsworth, M. D. S., Blehar, M. C., Waters, E., & Wall, S. (1978). *Patterns of attachment: A psychological study of the Strange Situation.* Hillsdale, NJ: Erlbaum.

Ainsworth, M. D. S., & Wittig, B. A. (1969). Attachment and exploratory behaviour of one-year-olds in a strange situation. In B. M. Foss (Ed.), *Determinants of infant behaviour* (Vol. 4, pp. 111–136). London: Methuen.

Aksan, N., Kochanska, G., & Ortmann, M. R. (2006). Mutually responsive orientation between parents and their young children: Toward methodological advances in the science of relationships. *Developmental Psychology, 42,* 833–848.

Allen, J. P., Hauser, S. T., Bell, K. L., & O'Connor, T. G. (1994). Longitudinal assessment of autonomy and relatedness in adolescent–family interactions as predictors of adolescent ego development and self-esteem. *Child Development, 65,* 179–194.

Allen, J. P., Hauser, S. T., & Borman-Spurrell, E. (1996). Attachment theory as a framework for understand-

ing sequelae of severe adolescent psychopathology: An 11-year follow-up study. *Journal of Consulting and Clinical Psychology, 64,* 254–263.

Allen, J. P., McElhaney, K. B., Land, D. J., Kuperminc, G. P., Moore, C. W., O'Beirne-Kelly, H., et al. (2003). A secure base in adolescence: Markers of attachment security in the mother–adolescent relationship. *Child Development, 74,* 292–307.

Blehar, M. C., Lieberman, A. F., & Ainsworth, M. D. S. (1977). Early face-to-face interaction and its relation to later infant–mother attachment. *Child Development, 48,* 182–194.

Bowlby, J. (1944). Forty-four juvenile thieves: Their characters and home life. *International Journal of Psycho-Analysis, 25,* 19–52, 107–127.

Bowlby, J. (1951). *Maternal care and mental health* (WHO Monograph No. 2). Geneva: World Health Organization.

Bowlby, J. (1969/1982). *Attachment and loss: Vol. 1. Attachment.* New York: Basic Books.

Bowlby, J. (1973). *Attachment and loss: Vol. 2. Separation: Anxiety and anger.* New York: Basic Books.

Bowlby, J. (1980). *Attachment and loss: Vol. 3. Loss: Sadness and depression.* New York: Basic Books.

Bowlby, J. (1988). *A secure base: Parent–child attachment and healthy human development.* New York: Basic Books.

Bowlby, J., Robertson, J., & Rosenbluth, D. (1952). A two-year-old goes to hospital. *Psychoanalytic Study of the Child, 7,* 82–94.

Bretherton, I. (1985). Attachment theory: Retrospect and prospect. In I. Bretherton & E. Waters (Eds.), Growing points of attachment theory and research. *Monographs of the Society for Research in Child Development, 50*(1–2, Serial No. 209), 3–35.

Bretherton, I. (1987). New perspectives on attachment relations: Security, communication, and internal working models. In J. Osofsky (Ed.), *Handbook of infant development* (2nd ed., pp. 1061–1100). New York: Wiley.

Bretherton, I. (1990). Open communication and internal working models: Their role in the development of attachment relationships. In R. A. Thompson (Ed.), *Nebraska Symposium on Motivation: Vol. 36. Socioemotional development* (pp. 57–113). Lincoln: University of Nebraska Press.

Burlingham, D., & Freud, A. (1944). *Infants without families.* London: Allen & Unwin.

Carlson, E. A. (1998). A prospective longitudinal study of disorganized/disoriented attachment. *Child Development, 69,* 1107–1128.

Cicchetti, D., Cummings, E. M., Greenberg, M. T., & Marvin, R. S. (1990). An organizational perspective on attachment beyond infancy: Implications for theory, measurement, and research. In M. T. Greenberg, D. Cicchetti, & E. M. Cummings (Eds.), *Attachment in the preschool years* (pp. 3–50). Chicago: University of Chicago Press.

Connolly, J., Furman, W., & Konarski, R. (2000). The role of peers in the emergence of heterosexual romantic relationships in adolescence. *Child Development, 71,* 1395–1408.

Cowan, P. (1997). Beyond meta-analysis: A plea for a family systems perspective on attachment. *Child Development, 68,* 600–603.

Crowell, J., & Feldman, S. (1988). Mothers' internal models of relationships and children's behavioral and developmental status: A study of mother–child interaction. *Child Development, 59,* 1273–1285.

Crowell, J. A., Treboux, D., Gao, Y., Fyffe, C., Pan, H., & Waters, E. (2002). Assessing secure base behavior in adulthood: Development of a measure, links to adult attachment representations, and relations to couples' communication and reports of relationships. *Developmental Psychology, 38,* 679–693.

Davies, P. T., & Cummings, E. M. (1995). Marital conflict and child adjustment: An emotional security hypothesis. *Psychological Bulletin, 116,* 387–411.

Davies, P. T., & Cummings, E. M. (1998). Exploring children's emotional security as a mediator of the link between marital relations and child adjustment. *Child Development, 69,* 124–139.

Dozier, M., & Lindhiem, O. (2006). This is my child: Differences among foster parents in commitment to their young children. *Child Maltreatment, 11,* 338–345.

Fraley, C., & Davis, K. E. (1997). Attachment formation and transfer in young adults' close friendships and romantic relationships. *Personal Relationships, 4,* 131–144.

Furman, W., & Simon, V. A. (2006). Actor and partner effects of adolescents' romantic working models and styles on interactions with romantic partners. *Child Development, 77,* 588–604.

Furman, W., & Wehner, E. A. (1997). Adolescent romantic relationships: A developmental perspective. *New Directions for Child Development, 78,* 21–36.

Garcia-O'Hearn, H., Margolin, G., & John, R. (1997). Mothers' and fathers' reports of children's reactions to naturalistic marital conflict. *Journal of the American Academy of Child and Adolescent Psychiatry, 36,* 1366–1373.

George, C., Kaplan, N., & Main, M. (1984). *Adult Attachment Interview protocol.* Unpublished manuscript, University of California at Berkeley.

George, C., Kaplan, N., & Main, M. (1985). *Adult Attachment Interview protocol* (2nd ed.). Unpublished manuscript, University of California at Berkeley.

George, C., Kaplan, N., & Main, M. (1996). *Adult Attachment Interview protocol* (3rd ed.). Unpublished manuscript, University of California at Berkeley.

George, C., & Main, M. (1979). Social interactions of young abused children: Approach, avoidance, and aggression. *Child Development, 50,* 306–318.

Gottman, J. (1994). *What predicts divorce?* Hillsdale, NJ: Erlbaum.

Grossmann, K., Grossmann, K. E., & Kindler, H. (2005). Early care and the roots of attachment and partnership representations. In K. E. Grossmann, K. Grossmann, & E. Waters (Eds.), *Attachment from infancy to adulthood: The major longitudinal studies* (pp. 98–136). New York: Guilford Press.

Grossmann, K. E., Grossmann, K., & Schwan, A. (1986). Capturing the wider view of attachment: A reanalysis of Ainsworth's Strange Situation. In C. E. Izard & P. B. Read (Eds.), *Measuring emotions in infants and children* (pp. 124–171). New York: Cambridge University Press.

Hazan, C., & Shaver, P. R. (1987). Romantic love conceptualized as an attachment process. *Journal of Personality and Social Psychology, 52,* 511–524.

Hazan, C., & Shaver, P. R. (1994). Attachment as an organizational framework for research on close relationships. *Psychological Inquiry, 5,* 1–22.

Heinicke, C., & Westheimer, I. (1966). *Brief separations.* New York: International Universities Press.

Hesse, E., & Main, M. (2006). Frightened, threatening, and dissociative parental behavior in low-risk samples: Description, discussion, and interpretations. *Development and Psychopathology, 18,* 309–343.

Hoffman, K. T., Marvin, R. S., Cooper, G., & Powell, B. (2006). Changing toddlers' and preschoolers' attachment classifications: The Circle of Security intervention. *Journal of Consulting and Clinical Psychology, 74,* 1017–1026.

Johnson, S. M. (1996). *Creating connection: The practice of emotionally focused marital therapy.* New York: Brunner/Mazel.

Johnson, S. M. (2003). Attachment theory: A guide for couple therapy. In S. M. Johnson & V. E. Whiffen (Eds.), *Attachment processes in couple and family therapy* (pp. 103–123). New York: Guilford Press.

Johnson, S. M., & Greenman, P. S. (2006). The path to a secure bond: Emotionally focused couple therapy. *Journal of Clinical Psychology, 62,* 597–609.

Karen, R. (1994). *Becoming attached.* New York: Warner.

Klerman, G. L., Weissman, M. M., Rounsaville, B. J., & Chevron, E. S. (1984). *Interpersonal psychotherapy of depression.* New York: Basic Books.

Kobak, R., Cassidy, J., Lyons-Ruth, K., & Ziv, Y. (2006). Attachment, stress and psychopathology: A developmental pathways model. In D. Cicchetti & D. Cohen (Eds.), *Developmental psychopathology* (2nd ed., Vol. , pp. 333–369). Hoboken, NJ: Wiley.

Kobak, R., Cassidy, J., & Ziv, Y. (2004). Attachment-related trauma and posttraumatic stress disorder: Implications for adult adaptation. In W. S. Rholes & J. A. Simpson (Eds.), *Adult attachment: Theory, research, and clinical implications* (pp. 388–407). New York: Guilford Press.

Kobak, R., & Cole, H. (1994). Attachment and meta-monitoring: Implications for adolescent autonomy and psychopathology. In D. Cicchetti (Ed.), *Rochester Symposium on Development and Psychopathology: Vol. 5. Disorders of the self* (pp. 267–297). Rochester, NY: University of Rochester Press.

Kobak, R., & Duemmler, S. (1994). Attachment and conversation: A discourse analysis of goal-corrected partnerships. In K. Bartholomew & D. Perlman

(Eds.), *Advances in personal relationships: Vol. 5. Attachment processes in adulthood* (pp. 121–149). London: Jessica Kingsley.

Kobak, R., & Esposito, A. (2004). Levels of processing in parent–child relationships: Implications for clinical assessment and treatment. In L. Atkinson & S. Goldberg (Eds.), *Attachment issues in psychopathology and intervention* (pp. 139–166). Mahwah, NJ: Erlbaum.

Kobak, R., & Hazan, C. (1991). Attachment in marriage: The effects of security and accuracy of working models. *Journal of Personality and Social Psychology, 60,* 861–869.

Kobak, R., Hazan, C., & Ruckdeschel, K. (1994). From symptom to signal: An attachment view of emotion in marital therapy. In S. M. Johnson & L. Greenberg (Eds.), *Emotions in marital therapy* (pp. 46–71). New York: Brunner/Mazel.

Kobak, R., Little, M., Race, E., & Acosta, M. C. (2001). Attachment disruptions in seriously emotionally disturbed children: Implications for treatment. *Attachment and Human Development, 3,* 243–258.

Kochanska, G. (2001). Emotional development in children with different attachment histories: The first three years. *Child Development, 72,* 474–490.

Lawrence, C. R., Carlson, E. A., & Egeland, B. (2006). The impact of foster care on development. *Development and Psychopathology, 18,* 57–76.

Lieberman, A. (1992). Infant–parent psychotherapy with toddlers. *Development and Psychopathology, 4,* 559–574.

Lorenz, K. (1957). *Instinctive behavior.* New York: International Universities Press.

Lyons-Ruth, K. (1996). Attachment relationships among children with aggressive behavior problems: The role of disorganized early attachment patterns. *Journal of Consulting and Clinical Psychology, 64,* 64–73.

Lyons-Ruth, K., Alpern, L., & Repacholi, B. (1993). Disorganized infant attachment classification and maternal psychosocial problems as predictors for hostile-aggressive behavior in the preschool classroom. *Child Development, 64,* 572–585.

Lyons-Ruth, K., Melnick, S., Patrick, M., & Hobson, R. P. (2007). A controlled study of hostile-helpless states of mind among borderline and dysthymic women. *Attachment and Human Development, 9,* 1–16.

Lyons-Ruth, K., Yellin, C., Melnick, S., & Atwood, G. (2005a). Childhood experiences of trauma and loss have different relations to maternal unresolved and hostile-helpless states of mind on the AAI. *Attachment and Human Development, 5,* 330–352.

Lyons-Ruth, K., Yellin, C., Melnick, S., & Atwood, G. (2005b). Expanding the concept of unresolved mental states: Hostile/helpless states of mind on the Adult Attachment Interview are associated with disrupted mother–infant communication and infant disorganization. *Development and Psychopathology, 17,* 1–23.

Main, M. (1990). Cross-cultural studies of attachment organization: Recent studies, changing methodologies, and the concept of conditional strategies. *Human Development, 33,* 48–61.

Main, M., & Goldwyn, R. (1984). *Adult attachment scoring and classification system.* Unpublished manuscript, University of California at Berkeley.

Main, M., Goldwyn, R., & Hesse, E. (2003). *Adult attachment scoring and classification system.* Unpublished manuscript, University of California at Berkeley.

Main, M., & Hesse, E. (1990). Parents' unresolved traumatic experiences are related to infant disorganized attachment status: Is frightening and/or frightened parental behavior the linking mechanism? In M. T. Greenberg, D. Cicchetti, & E. M. Cummings (Eds.), *Attachment in the preschool years* (pp. 121–160). Chicago: University of Chicago Press.

Main, M., Kaplan, N., & Cassidy, J. (1985). Security in infancy, childhood and adulthood: A move to the level of representation. In I. Bretherton & E. Waters (Eds.), Growing points of attachment theory and research. *Monographs of the Society for Research in Child Development, 50*(1–2, Serial No. 209), 66–104.

Main, M., & Solomon, J. (1986). Discovery of a new, insecure disorganized/disoriented attachment pattern. In T. B. Brazelton & M. Yogman (Eds.), *Affective development in infancy* (pp. 95–124). Norwood, NJ: Ablex.

Main, M., & Weston, D. R. (1982). Avoidance of the attachment figure in infancy: Descriptions and interpretations. In C. Parkes & J. Stevenson-Hinde (Eds.), *The place of attachment in human behavior* (pp. 31–59). New York: Basic Books.

Makinen, J. A., & Johnson, S. M. (2006). Resolving attachment injuries in couples using emotionally focused therapy: Steps toward forgiveness and reconciliation. *Journal of Consulting and Clinical Psychology, 74,* 1055–1064.

Marvin, R. S. (1977). An ethological–cognitive model for the attenuation of mother–child attachment behavior. In T. M. Alloway, L. Krames, & P. Pliner (Eds.), *Advances in the study of communication and affect: Vol. 3. The development of social attachments* (pp. 25–60). New York: Plenum Press.

Mikulincer, M., & Shaver, P. R. (2007). *Attachment in adulthood: Structure, dynamics, and change.* New York: Guilford Press.

Moss, E., Cyr, C., & Dubois-Comtois, K. (2004). Attachment at early school age and developmental risk: Examining family contexts and behavior problems of controlling-caregiving, controlling-punitive, and behaviorally disorganized children. *Developmental Psychology, 40,* 519–532.

Moss, E., Smolla, N., Cyr, C., Dubois-Comtois, K., Mazzarello, T., & Berthiaume, C. (2006). Attachment and behavior problems in middle childhood as reported by adult and child informants. *Development and Psychopathology, 18,* 425–444.

Mufson, L., Moreau, D., Weissman, M., & Klerman, G.

(1993). *Interpersonal psychotherapy for depressed adolescents.* New York: Guilford Press.

Newson, J., & Newson, E. (1968). *Four years old in an urban community.* Chicago: Aldine.

Patterson, G. R. (1986). Performance models for antisocial boys. *American Psychologist, 41,* 432–444.

Pietromonaco, P. R., Greenwood, D., & Barrett, L. F. (2004). Conflict in close relationships: An attachment perspective. In W. S. Rholes & J. A. Simpson (Eds.), *Adult attachment: Theory, research, and clinical implications* (pp. 267–299). New York: Guilford Press.

Robertson, J. (Producer). (1953). *A two-year-old goes to hospital: A scientific film record* [Film]. Nacton, UK: Concord Film Council.

Robertson, J. (1962). *Hospitals and children: A parent's eye view.* New York: Gollancz.

Roisman, G. I., Madsen, S. D., Hennighausen, K. H., Sroufe, L. A., & Collins, W. A. (2001). The coherence of dyadic behavior across parent–child and romantic relationships as mediated by the internalized representation of experience. *Attachment and Human Development, 3,* 156–172.

Rutter, M. (1981). *Maternal deprivation reassessed.* Harmondsworth, UK: Penguin.

Sears, R. R., Maccoby, E., & Levin, H. (1957). *Patterns of child rearing.* Evanston, IL: Row, Peterson.

Shaver, P. R., & Mikulincer, M. (2007). Adult attachment strategies and the regulation of emotion. In J. J. Gross (Ed.), *Handbook of emotion regulation* (pp. 446–465). New York: Guilford Press.

Shaw, D. S., Owens, E. B., Vondra, J. I., Keenan, K., & Winslow, E. B. (1996). Early risk factors and pathways in the development of early disruptive behavior problems. *Development and Psychopathology, 8,* 679–699.

Simpson, J. A., Collins, W. A., Tran, S., & Haydon, K. C. (2007). Attachment and the experience and expression of emotions in romantic relationships: A developmental perspective. *Journal of Personality and Social Psychology, 92,* 355–367.

Spitz, R. (1958). Discussion of Dr. Bowlby's paper. *Psychoanalytic Study of the Child, 15,* 85–94.

Sroufe, L. A. (2005). Attachment and development: A prospective, longitudinal study from birth to adulthood. *Attachment and Human Development, 7,* 349–367.

Sroufe, L. A., Egeland, B., Carlson, E. A., & Collins, W. A. (2005). Placing attachment experience in developmental context. In K. Grossmann, K. E. Grossmann, & E. Waters (Eds.), *Attachment from infancy to adulthood: The major longitudinal studies* (pp. 48–97). New York: Guilford Press.

Sroufe, L. A., & Fleeson, J. (1986). Attachment and the construction of relationships. In W. W. Hartup & Z. Rubin (Eds.), *Relationships and development* (pp. 51–71). Hillsdale, NJ: Erlbaum.

Sroufe, L. A., & Waters, E. (1977). Attachment as an organizational construct. *Child Development, 48,* 1184–1199.

Stovall-McClough, K. C., & Dozier, M. (2004). Forming attachments in foster care: Infant attachment behaviors during the first 2 months of placement. *Development and Psychopathology, 16,* 253–271.

Toth, S. L., & Cicchetti, D. (2006). Promises and possibilities: The application of research in the area of child maltreatment to policies and practices. *Journal of Social Issues, 62,* 863–880.

Treboux, D., Crowell, J. A., & Waters, E. (2004). When "new" meets "old": Configurations of adult attachment representations and their implications for marital functioning. *Developmental Psychology, 40,* 295–314.

van IJzendoorn, M. H. (1995). Of the way we are: On temperament, attachment, and the transmission gap: A rejoinder to Fox (1995). *Psychological Bulletin, 117,* 411–415.

van Zeijl, J., Mesman, J., van IJzendoorn, M. H., Bukersmans-Kranenburg, M. J., Juffer, F. Stolk, M. N., et al. (2006). Attachment-based intervention for enhancing sensitive discipline in mothers of 1- to 3-year-old children at risk for externalizing behavior problems: A randomized controlled trial. *Journal of Consulting and Clinical Psychology, 74,* 994–1005.

Weiss, R. S. (1975). *Marital separation: Coping with the end of a marriage and the transition to being single again.* New York: Basic Books.

CHAPTER 3

Attachment, Loss, and Grief
Bowlby's Views and Current Controversies

PHILLIP R. SHAVER
R. CHRIS FRALEY

The first time the full significance of [my father, John Bowlby's] work struck me was during a family walk ... just after his paper on "The nature of the child's tie to his mother" was first published [in 1958]. He said to me, "You know how distressed small children get if they're lost and can't find their mother and how they keep searching? Well, I suspect it's the same feeling that adults have when a loved one dies, they keep on searching too. I think it's the same instinct that starts in infancy and evolves throughout life as people grow up, and becomes part of adult love." I remember thinking, well, if you're right, you're on to something really big!
—R. BOWLBY (2005, pp. vi–vii)

For most of his life, evolutionary theorist Charles Darwin—one of John Bowlby's intellectual heroes—suffered from a perplexing set of symptoms, including recurrent and persistent gastric pains, nausea, and heart palpitations. These are common symptoms of hyperventilation syndrome, a condition that can be triggered by trauma, stress, or bereavement. In Bowlby's (1990) final book, *Charles Darwin: A New Life*, he attributed Darwin's hyperventilation syndrome and related symptoms to suppressed and unresolved grief following the death of his mother when he was 8 years old. Bowlby emphasized that Darwin's father did not allow his children to speak about their deceased mother following her death, and that Darwin suffered fainting spells and other signs of hyperventilation from then on.

Bowlby believed that suppression of grief inhibits a natural sequence of painful emotional reactions that, unless allowed to run their natural course, can lead to psychological and physical ill health. Although his final book was primarily concerned with understanding Darwin's loss in particular, Bowlby had been deeply concerned with the psychological consequences of loss more

generally throughout his career. In his first empirical study (Bowlby, 1946), he argued that loss of a primary attachment figure is a predisposing factor in juvenile delinquency. Decades later, in his landmark trilogy, *Attachment and Loss*, bereavement and grief were the focus of the entire third volume, *Loss: Sadness and Depression* (Bowlby, 1980).

Although Bowlby's ideas about grief changed over the course of his career, he continued to view loss of an attachment figure as an important influence on personality development. He considered suppressed and unresolved grief to be pathogenic forces, and portrayed grief itself as a natural feature of what he called the "attachment behavioral system"—a system "designed" by natural selection to discourage prolonged separation of an individual from his or her primary attachment figures (see Cassidy, Chapter 1, this volume).

Our aims in this chapter are to summarize Bowlby's contributions to the study of bereavement, and to review recent research and controversies related to those contributions.[1] We begin with a broad overview of the volume *Loss: Sadness and Depression*. We discuss Bowlby's thoughts about the function and course of mourning, and about patterns of "disordered" mourning. We then discuss recent work that challenges some of Bowlby's claims (work reviewed, e.g., by Wortman & Boerner, 2007)—for example, his claims that grief follows identifiable stages, that suppression of grief has negative effects on mental and physical health, and that recovery from grief requires "detachment" or "reorganization." Throughout, we comment briefly on clinical applications of Bowlby's ideas and of bereavement research more generally. There is considerable disagreement about whether and when grief counseling is called for, whether it does more good than harm, and how it is best carried out (e.g., Bonanno, 2004; Jordan & Neimeyer, 2003; Larson & Hoyt, 2007).

AN ATTACHMENT PERSPECTIVE ON SEPARATION AND BEREAVEMENT

Bowlby's thoughts on loss and grief were developed over several decades, but they were expressed most completely in his 1980 volume, where he addressed a wide range of issues (e.g., whether children are capable of grieving and whether they can harbor multiple conflicting representations of loss events, such as remembering a dead father's body hanging in the closet but recalling embarrassed relatives' denials that the father killed himself). Two of Bowlby's aims are particularly relevant to the present chapter. First, he wished to show that seemingly irrational or "immature" reactions to loss, such as disbelief, anger, searching, and sensing the continued presence of a lost attachment figure, are understandable when viewed from an ethological or evolutionary perspective. Second, he wished to show that how an individual responds to loss stems partly from the way his or her attachment system became organized during childhood. He thought that people whose attachment systems are organized in such a way as to chronically anticipate rejection and loss (i.e., those who are high in attachment anxiety) or to defensively suppress attachment-related feelings (i.e., avoidant or compulsively self-reliant individuals) are likely to suffer from psychological and physical distress following bereavement.

The Function and Course of Mourning in Infancy and Adulthood

One of Bowlby's most important contributions to the literature on bereavement was his ethological perspective on attachment and loss. He observed

that infants of many species require protection and care from older individuals in order to survive. To obtain this protection, infants have evolved physical adaptations (such as large eyes and facial expressions of emotion) and behavioral adaptations (such as crying and reaching) that attract and hold the attention of potential caregivers. In addition to these more basic adaptations, however, infants possess a motivational system (the attachment system) designed by natural selection to regulate and maintain proximity between infants and their caregivers (see Cassidy, Chapter 1, this volume). When an attachment figure is judged to be sufficiently available and responsive, an infant is thought to experience what Sroufe and Waters (1977) called "felt security," and is more likely to explore the environment and engage in playful social interactions. In contrast, when the attachment figure is judged to be inaccessible or unresponsive, the infant experiences anxiety and vigorously attempts to reestablish contact by calling, searching, approaching, and clinging.

The following passage illustrates the protest of a 16-month-old girl after learning that her father would be leaving her in the nursery for an extended time.

> When Dawn sensed that her father was leaving, she again whined "Mm, mm, mm," and as he got up she broke into a loud cry and clutched him around the neck. Father became upset, put her down and tried to console her. . . . As he was departing through the door, she almost knocked her head on the floor. When the nurse picked her up, she continued to scream but later comforted herself by sucking her finger and some candy. (Heinicke & Westheimer, 1965, pp. 94–95)

According to Bowlby (1969/1982), these "protest" reactions are biologically functional because in the environment of evolutionary adaptedness they would have kept infants close to their protective attachment figures (see also Archer, 1999). This natural anxiety and yearning for an attachment figure motivate continued searching and calling until either success is attained or all efforts are exhausted. Viewed in this light, many of the seemingly perplexing reactions to separation and loss (such as continuing to yearn and search even when a lost caregiver is objectively irretrievable) appear more reasonable and, in many situations, adaptive. By doing everything possible to prevent the loss of attachment figures or by successfully reuniting with temporarily absent or distracted attachment figures, infants would have substantially increased their chances of survival, and ultimately their reproductive fitness.

The same tendency to search and reunite expresses itself strongly, and in ways that may seem irrational, when an adult loses a loved spouse. Gilbert (2006) writes in *Death's Door*, a book about grief and the autobiographical literature it has spawned:

> In an account of his 34-year-old wife's death from breast cancer, the memoirist David Collins summarizes with poignant precision the rationale underlying his feeling that "I wanted to die too—so I could be with her." Explaining "so freshly present she seemed [that] I had this thought: *I could follow her*," he adds, "I just wanted to go after her, not let her get away. I wanted to find her again. Hadn't I found her once [before]?" (p. 3; original emphasis)

Unfortunately, this natural impulse sometimes leads to suicide (e.g., Harwood, Hawton, Hope, Harriss, & Jacoby, 2006; M. Stroebe, Stroebe, & Abakoumkin, 2005).

During the protest phase of separation and loss, infants generally react very forcefully. However, the intensity of these reactions eventually wanes if the separation is extended, as is obviously the case following a caregiver's death. Anxiety, anger, and denial give way to sadness and hopelessness. This second phase, which Bowlby (1980) called "despair," is thought to be a natural result of failure to bring about the attachment figure's return. A third phase, which Bowlby at first called "detachment," marks an apparent recovery and gradual renewal of interest in other activities and social relationships. The term "detachment" is misleading, however, because Bowlby (e.g., 1973) and his coworkers provided evidence that reunion with a lost attachment figure, who may at first be treated coolly or warily, can suddenly cause a powerful upsurge in attachment behavior (e.g., crying, persistent following and clinging). The apparent "detachment," therefore, is not a simple wearing away or diminishing of the attachment bond; it is a sign of defensive suppression of attachment responses that have repeatedly failed to bring about the attachment figure's return.

Although Bowlby was primarily concerned with understanding infant–caregiver attachment, he considered adult romantic or pair-bond relationships within the same theoretical framework he used to explain infant attachment (as indicated in the quotation from his son used at the beginning of the present chapter as an epigraph). Bowlby (1969/1982, 1980) and his colleagues (e.g.,

Parkes, 2006; Parkes & Weiss, 1983; Weiss, 1975) observed that adults who lose or are separated from their romantic attachment figures (e.g., a spouse) undergo a series of reactions similar to those observed in infants. As an illustration, consider the following passage, which describes the protest reaction of a woman whose husband died after spending several months in the hospital with leukemia. Although she had anticipated the loss (and knew specifically that her husband was expected to die that evening), she still felt compelled to hold on to him and keep him from leaving.

> I went over to him. I remember my brother-in-law taking me away from him because he said I kept holding on to him and patting his head. I cried my heart out. But I remember my brother-in-law coming to me and taking me away from him. (Parkes & Weiss, 1983, p. 78)

When a separation turns into a permanent loss, the protest phase may be marked by enduring preoccupation with the missing person. It is not uncommon for even adults to experience intense yearning for a lost mate, and to continue for some time to find it surprising or disquieting when aspects of the normal routine are interrupted by the attachment figure's conspicuous absence.

> The hardest thing for me, I think, is at night. We have a neighbor [who] works the second shift and we hear his pickup truck every night. And my husband would always say something like, 'When's he going to get his brakes fixed?' And every night I'm sitting here when he comes along, and that's when I really think about my husband, because he would always say something. (Parkes & Weiss, 1983, p. 87)

Once the bereaved individual realizes that the partner will not be returning (which can sometimes occur even before the partner dies, if he or she has suffered a long and irrevocable decline because of a terminal illness; e.g., Bonanno, Moskowitz, Papa, & Folkman, 2005), some degree of sadness and of mental or physiological disorganization is likely. For both adults and children, this phase is characterized by sleeping and eating disturbances, social withdrawal, loneliness, and dysphoria. (In some cases, the stress may hasten the bereaved individual's own death; Hart, Hole, Lawlor, Smith, & Lever, 2007; see M. Stroebe, Schut, & Stroebe, 2007, for a review.) As Weiss (1973) noted, the feelings of loneliness stem specifically from the absence of the attachment figure and cannot be fully alleviated by the presence of others (see W. Stroebe, Stroebe, Abakoumkin, & Schut, 1996, for empirical evidence on this point). Although many bereaved individuals definitely derive comfort from the presence of close, supportive friends or family members, who can be viewed as parts of a hierarchy of attachment figures (Bowlby, 1969/1982), a support network does not necessarily fill the emotional gap left by a specific missing attachment figure. According to Bowlby, attachment bonds are person-specific and involve many memories and feelings unique to a history of interactions with that particular person.

For many bereaved individuals, the phase of sadness and disorganization lasts for weeks or months. In the first few months following conjugal bereavement, according to early studies, roughly 30–40% of adults could be classified as clinically depressed (Clayton, Halikas, & Maurice, 1972; Futterman, Gallagher, Thompson, Lovett, & Gilewski, 1990). In Wortman and Boerner's (2007) review of more recent studies (e.g., Bonanno et al., 2002; Bonanno, Wortman, & Nesse, 2004), the rate of depression following bereavement was observed to depend on how "depression" was measured (e.g., as mild dysphoria or as a state fitting the current clinical criteria for major depression).

During the first several months following a loss, symptoms of grief appear to decrease in a negative exponential manner. Roughly 12 months after bereavement, approximately 18–30% of bereaved adults exhibit signs of depression (Bornstein, Clayton, Halikas, Maurice, & Robins, 1973; Clayton et al., 1972; Jacobs, Hansen, Berkman, Kasl, & Ostfeld, 1989). After 24–30 months, approximately 18% of adults exhibit signs of depression (Futterman et al., 1990; Lund et al., 1985; Lund, Caserta, Dimond, & Shaffer, 1989)—a figure almost twice the base rate of depression in a nonbereaved population. In more recent reviews (e.g., Bonanno et al., 2002; Wortman & Boerner, 2007), these figures are lower, based on more recent diagnostic criteria for depression. Also, more emphasis is placed on the fact that some people show improvement rather than deterioration after a loss, especially if they were depressed before the loss because a relationship partner was suffering a painful, demoralizing decline toward death (e.g., Bonanno, Papa, Lalande, Zhang, & Noll, 2005). Especially important is the fact (discussed in a later section of this chapter) that a sizable proportion of people (the "resilient" ones; Bonanno, 2004) function well before, during, and after a loss. One of the difficulties in establishing a single, simple account of loss and grief is that so many factors

influence the course and outcome of grieving (M. Stroebe, Folkman, Hansson, & Schut, 2006): age; gender; type and quality of the relationship with the deceased; suddenness or gradualness of the death; nature of the illness that caused the death; acceptance of comforting religious beliefs about death; and so on.

Still, the impact of the loss of a loved one is likely to reverberate for months or years. In 1993, Shuchter and Zisook reported that 13 months after a spouse's death, 63% of adults sensed that their spouse was with them at times, 47% thought the spouse was watching out for them, and 34% frequently "talked" with them. In a more recent study, Carnelley, Wortman, Bolger, and Burke (2007) surveyed 768 American adults who had lost a spouse at some point, varying from a few months to 64 years before the study. These adults continued to talk, think, and have feelings about the deceased spouse. For example, 13 years after their loss, respondents reported feeling upset at times when they thought about the spouse, and even 20 years after the loss, widows and widowers thought about the spouse once every week or two and had a conversation about the spouse once a month, on average. A minority of people—those suffering from what is now called "complicated" or "prolonged" grief (e.g., Maciejewski, Zhang, Block, & Prigerson, 2007; Prigerson, Maciejewski, Newson, Reynolds, & Frank, 1995; Simon et al., 2007)—experienced intense yearning, preoccupation with the deceased, intrusive images of the dying person, and efforts to avoid painful reminders of the death many months or years after it occurred.

In Bowlby's (1980) writings about loss in adulthood, the phases of mourning based on observations of young children, who exhibited protest, despair, and defensive detachment, were supplemented by a new initial phase, "numbing." This phase was added because research and clinical observations indicated that mourners often fail to register the loss of the attachment figure at first, presumably because the event is too painful to accept or seems cognitively incomprehensible. The following example describes the initial numbing reaction of a woman whose husband died suddenly and unexpectedly.[2] At the morgue, she found it difficult to acknowledge that her husband was dead.

> I didn't believe it. I stayed there for twenty minutes. I rubbed him, I rubbed his face, I patted him, I rubbed his head. I called him, but he didn't answer. And I knew if I called him he'd answer me because he's

used to my voice. But he didn't answer me. They said he was dead, but his skin was just as warm as mine. (Parkes & Weiss, 1983, p. 84)

Importantly, on the basis of adults' ability to talk about their troubling experiences and to deal cognitively and emotionally with loss, Bowlby changed the name of the final phase of adult mourning from "detachment" to "reorganization." As we explain in detail later, this change is important because it reflects Bowlby's belief that many mourners do not, and do not wish to, "detach" defensively from their lost attachment figure; instead, they rearrange their representations of self and the lost figure so that a continuing bond *and* adjustment to postloss circumstances are both possible.

The distinction between detachment and reorganization is related to arguments in the clinical field (e.g., Klass, Silverman, & Nickman, 1996a, 1996b) concerning whether Freud (1917/1957), in his classic paper "Mourning and Melancholia," advocated complete detachment ("decathexis") from mental representations of lost loved ones or did not advocate complete detachment. Interestingly, there is evidence in Freud's personal correspondence that he did not "get over" the death of his daughter Sophie, and even years later did not wish to detach himself from his memory of her. In a letter to a professional friend whose son had recently died, Freud wrote:

Although we know that after such a loss the acute stage of mourning will subside, we also know that we shall remain inconsolable and will never find a substitute. ... Actually, this is how it should be. It is the only way of perpetuating that love which we do not wish to relinquish. (in E. L. Freud, 1960, p. 386)

Bowlby's (1980) concept of reorganization allowed for the fact that bereaved individuals usually need to do considerable cognitive and emotional work to update their working models of themselves and their attachment relationships, but this updating does not require complete "detachment." One reason for the differences between Freud's and Bowlby's models of the grieving process is that Freud conceptualized the mind as powered by psychic energy; this suggested to him that energy invested in one close relationship will have to be withdrawn when the relationship ends, so that the "energy" can be reinvested in a new relationship. Bowlby favored a cybernetic rather than an energy-based model of the mind, and he acknowledged that most people have multiple attachment figures. Neither

the cybernetic nor the hierarchy-of-attachment-figures aspects of his theory require that a person relinquish mental "bonds" to one person in order to establish bonds with other people.

As might be expected, given Bowlby's ethological perspective on separation and loss, there is considerable evidence that grief responses are characteristic of many species, not just humans (Archer, 1999). For animals born without the capacity to care for themselves, the loss of a primary attachment figure evokes intense anxiety and protest, and leads eventually to what seems to human observers to be sorrow and despair (see Bowlby, 1969/1982). For example, in one of the earliest studies on attachment in rhesus macaques, Seay, Hansen, and Harlow (1962) separated 5-month-old rhesus infants from their mothers for a 3-week period. They reacted at first with extreme signs of protest and agitation, including screeching and attempting to break the barriers separating them from their mothers. When these attempts failed to establish contact, the infants became lethargic and withdrawn.[3] Such responses are also characteristic of some nonmammalian species that exhibit attachment behavior (including elephants; e.g., Poole, 1996). Konrad Lorenz (1963), one of the ethologists whose work influenced Bowlby's ideas, provided an illustration of these emotional reactions in the greylag goose:

The first response to the disappearance of the partner consists in the anxious attempt to find him again. The goose moves about restlessly by day and night, flying great distances and visiting all places where the partner might be found, uttering all the time the penetrating trisyllabic long-distance call. ... The searching expeditions are extended farther and farther, and quite often the searcher himself gets lost, or succumbs to an accident. ... All the objectively observable characteristics of the goose's behaviour on losing its mate are roughly identical with those accompanying human grief. (Lorenz, 1963, pp. 200–201)

Cross-cultural research on humans also attests to the prevalence of these emotional and behavioral responses to loss (Rosenblatt, Walsh, & Jackson, 1976). As W. Stroebe and Stroebe (1987) observed, however, the specific ways in which grief is manifested vary substantially across cultures. Some societies are structured in ways that accentuate, and perhaps romanticize, the anxiety, anger, and yearning experienced after a loss. For example, Mathison (1970) described the rituals of certain Trobriand Islanders. As part of mourning, a widow is expected to cry for several days.

In contrast, the display of emotion is restricted to a brief period among the Navajo. After this time, a widow is expected to return to her normal everyday activities and not to speak of the deceased (Miller & Schoenfeld, 1973). Nevertheless, despite the variability in mourning rituals observed by cultural anthropologists, the loss of a loved one appears to be very distressing in every part of the world and throughout recorded history (Rosenblatt et al., 1976).[4]

A few words should be said about the fact that many professionals interpreted Bowlby (1980) as saying that a bereaved person will move through the stages of shock/numbing, protest, despair, and detachment or reorganization. This generated a large literature that we need not review, because most experts now agree that there is no rigid stage sequence (in Fraley & Shaver, 1999, we used quotations from Bowlby's writings to show that he did not argue for a rigid stage sequence in any case). Many mourners go through a range of emotional states, over and over and in no particular order, depending on what they happen to focus on (Shaver & Tancredy, 2001).

Still, it is worth noting that in the first study of its kind, Maciejewski and colleagues (2007) questioned a large sample of bereaved adults within 6 months of their loss, again 6 months later, and then 6 months after that. They used single-item measures of possible grief stages based on work by Jacobs (1993), who was influenced by Bowlby: disbelief, yearning, anger, depression, and acceptance of the death. Answers ranged from 1 ("less than once a month") to 5 ("several times a day"). The data in their raw form did not seem to support a stage model: "Disbelief was not the initial, dominant grief indicator. Acceptance was the most frequently endorsed item and yearning was the dominant negative grief indicator from 1 to 24 months post-loss" (p. 716). However, when the responses were rescaled so that all had the same range, "disbelief decreased from an initial high at 1 month post-loss, yearning peaked at 4 months post-loss, anger peaked at 5 months post-loss, and depression peaked at 6 months post-loss" (p. 716). Acceptance, which received the highest mean score to begin with, increased throughout the study period.

The authors concluded that the "five grief indicators achieved their respective maximum values in the sequence (disbelief, yearning, anger, depression, and acceptance) predicted by the stage theory of grief" (p. 716). The results are compatible with Bowlby's general ideas, especially the fact that yearning was the strongest negative feeling throughout the study period. Bowlby did not, however, lead us to expect that acceptance would be as high as it was across the grieving period. This may be due to his emphasis on clinical or other cases in which distress was severe, as it is when losses are unexpected and/or traumatic (e.g., Currier, Holland, & Neimeyer, 2006; Prigerson, Vanderwerker, & Maciejewski, in press). Whatever the reason for Bowlby's lack of emphasis on acceptance as a "stage," its presence in the study by Maciejewski and colleagues (2007) is compatible with the greater emphasis in recent research on the contribution of positive thoughts and emotional states to remaining resilient in the face of loss (e.g., Bonanno, 2004; Bonanno & Kaltman, 1999, 2001).

Bowlby's Conceptualization of Disordered Mourning

In addition to offering an explanation of normative reactions to the loss of an attachment figure, Bowlby proposed a framework for conceptualizing atypical forms of mourning. His analysis of these disordered forms suggested that they can be arrayed along a single conceptual dimension running from "chronic mourning" to "prolonged absence of conscious grieving" (Bowlby, 1980, p. 138).[5] Chronic mourning is characterized by protracted grief and prolonged difficulty in normal functioning. Individuals who suffer from chronic mourning may find themselves overly preoccupied with thoughts of their missing partners and unable to return to normal functioning for months or even years after the loss. In contrast, an absence of grief is characterized by a conspicuous lack of conscious sorrow, anger, or distress. According to Bowlby, individuals exhibiting an absence of grief may express relatively little distress following the loss, continue in their jobs or activities without any noticeable disruption, and seek little support or solace from friends and family. It was Bowlby's belief that this manner of reacting to loss can lead to difficulties in long-term adjustment if a person has lost someone to whom he or she is deeply attached. He expected the majority of people (who are likely to be fairly secure with respect to attachment) to experience and express negative feelings, revise and reorganize relevant internal working models, and establish a satisfactory way of moving on with life despite the loss.

For a while, modern clinicians agreed with Bowlby's description of these opposing patterns of grief (e.g., Middleton, Raphael, Martinek, & Misso, 1993; W. Stroebe & Stroebe, 1987). According to Middleton and colleagues (1993), most clinicians distinguished between two forms of disordered mourning: "delayed" and "chronic." Similar to Bowlby's description of a prolonged absence of conscious grieving, delayed mourning is characterized by denials of distress and a continuation of normal affairs without substantial disruption. This category of disordered mourning is similar to what Parkes (1965) referred to as "inhibited" mourning and what Deutsch (1937) called "absent" mourning. Chronic mourning, as understood by clinicians until recently, encompasses what Bowlby likewise called chronic mourning and is characterized by prolonged symptoms of depression and anxiety, possibly also with aspects of posttraumatic stress disorder (PTSD). Chronic mourning might also include what some clinicians and attachment researchers call "unresolved grief " (e.g., Ainsworth & Eichberg, 1991; Main & Hesse, 1990; Zisook & DeVaul, 1985), although the precise meaning of this term varies across theorists, as we explain later.

In recent years, at least two things have happened to change the previous conceptualization of reactions to bereavement. First, empirical studies (reviewed, e.g., by Wortman & Boerner, 2007) have suggested that there are many patterns of reactions to loss, including stable resilience; stable depression or other form of distress; a temporary rise in distress, followed by a return to normal; and even a decrease in distress (which is easy to understand in cases where the survivor was worn down by the dying process of a parent or spouse, or the survivor had been abused in some way by the relationship partner). Although these various patterns are not incompatible with Bowlby's ideas, he was clearly focused on understanding some patterns (e.g., "secure" patterns of recovery and disordered mourning) rather than others. An important goal for future research on attachment is to understand how these various patterns might result from the kinds of dynamics that Bowlby and his colleagues observed.

Second, because much of the early research on loss and grief was influenced by theories (including Bowlby's) that emphasized the pain of loss and the desirability of acknowledging and expressing negative emotions, relatively little was said about the role of positive emotions, the potential for personal growth following loss, or the adaptive potential of avoiding rumination. In the current era of "positive psychology" (Peterson, 2006),

there is greater emphasis on the role of meaning making (e.g., Gillies & Niemeyer, 2006) and positive emotions (e.g., Bonanno, Moskowitz, et al., 2005; Moskowitz, Folkman, & Acree, 2003; Ong, Bergeman, & Bisconti, 2004) in coping with bereavement.

Because the main purpose of the present chapter is to recount and reconsider Bowlby's theorizing about loss, in addition to attachment researchers' explorations of some of his ideas, we do not review all of the new findings regarding loss and recovery. However, we will mention some, both to acknowledge their existence and to provide key references for interested readers.

CURRENT RESEARCH ISSUES AND PERSPECTIVES

Complicated or Prolonged Grief

One recent trend that deserves mention, because it fits with and refines some of Bowlby's (1980) ideas about disordered mourning, is the attempt to define, measure, and treat complicated or prolonged grief. As mentioned earlier, recent research suggests that the majority of bereaved individuals experience negative emotions, physiological disorganization, and health problems to only a modest or moderate degree, and that they react with considerable acceptance and resilience (Bonanno, 2004; Bonanno, Moskowitz, Papa, & Folkman, 2005; Bonanno et al., 2002). Nevertheless, about 10–15% suffer more extreme grief reactions (Bonanno & Kaltman, 2001; Lichtenthal, Cruess, & Prigerson, 2004), and there has been disagreement about how to define and measure such reactions (M. Stroebe et al., 2000). The current edition of the *Diagnostic and Statistical Manual of Mental Disorders* (DSM-IV-TR; American Psychiatric Association, 2000) classifies negative reactions to bereavement under such rubrics as depression and PTSD or other anxiety disorders, and much recent research on loss and grief is concerned with rates of those disorders. To the extent that normal grieving does not involve reactions extreme enough to warrant a clinical label or clinical intervention (Bonanno, 2004), it seems important to distinguish normal grieving from more extreme reactions.

Some researchers (e.g., Jacobs, Mazure, & Prigerson, 2000; Lichtenthal et al., 2004) have proposed a separate clinical category, initially called "complicated grief" but more recently called "prolonged grief" (Maciejewski et al., 2007). The criteria for this classification include (1) chronic and persistent yearning for the deceased on a daily basis and in an intrusive, distressing way; (2) four or more of the following seven symptoms at least several times a day or to a degree that is distressing and disruptive: trouble accepting the death, inability to trust other people, excessive bitterness or anger related to the death, being uneasy about moving on, survivor guilt, feeling that life is empty or meaningless without the deceased, and being preoccupied with thoughts of the deceased; (3) marked and persistent dysfunction in social, occupational, or other important domains because of symptoms in categories 1 and 2; and (4) lasting for at least 6 months (which Maciejewski et al., 2007, found to be the length of time taken by most adults to experience a notable reduction in grief reactions).

As Bonanno and colleagues (2007) explain, "according to this perspective, [complicated or prolonged grief] is a syndrome with symptoms not captured by depression or PTSD. ... Advocates of [this] diagnosis also argue that existing treatments for either depression or PTSD are not efficacious in [such cases]" (e.g., Shear, Frank, Houck, & Reynolds, 2005). Factor-analytic studies have supported the claim that complicated, prolonged grief is separable from depression and anxiety (e.g., Boelen, van den Bout, & de Keijser, 2003; Ogrodniczuk et al., 2003; Prigerson et al., 1996). A few studies have shown that various indicators of adjustment—psychological, behavioral (e.g., friend or observer reports), and physiological—are predicted by measures of complicated or prolonged grief, even after scores on measures of other clinical conditions, such as depression and PTSD, are statistically controlled for (e.g., Bonanno et al., 2007; Simon et al., 2007).

For present purposes, what is most important is the existence of severe grief reactions that include the phenomena Bowlby (and his associates such as Parkes, 2006; Parkes & Weiss, 1983) emphasized, such as intense yearning, intrusive preoccupation with the lost figure, and inability to understand or accept the loss. These phenomena are not fully captured by clinical categories such as depression and PTSD.

Research on Patterns of Mourning

It is noteworthy that variants of the two major endpoints of Bowlby's (1980) continuum of patterns of grief—chronic mourning and prolonged absence of conscious grieving—have been identified in multiple ways throughout the history of attachment research. In the literatures on both infant and adult attachment relationships, researchers have focused on individuals who experience intense distress after losing attachment figures and on individuals who apparently experience little distress following loss or separation. Although this research has not focused exclusively on irretrievable losses (e.g., death of a spouse), it provides important insights into the nature of bereavement, because, according to Bowlby (1980), the same psychological mechanisms underlie reactions to both brief and permanent separations.

One of the earliest researchers to study reactions to separation from an attachment figure was Mary Ainsworth. As explained by Solomon and George (Chapter 18, this volume), Ainsworth developed the Strange Situation assessment procedure (Ainsworth, Blehar, Waters, & Wall, 1978) to investigate the interplay of attachment and exploration in a controlled laboratory setting. As most readers of this volume know, Ainsworth et al. identified three major patterns of infant–mother attachment: secure, resistant, and avoidant. Of special interest here is the fact that these patterns, like those identified by Bowlby as kinds of reactions to an irretrievable loss, can be arrayed along a dimension ranging from intense and chronic distress to an absence or suppression or avoidance of distress.[6]

Resistant infants in the Strange Situation exhibit a tendency to remain focused on their attachment figure (rather than playing wholeheartedly with attractive toys provided by the experimenter), to cry profusely during separations, *and to refuse to calm down once their attachment figure returns*. In other words, they exhibit a miniature version of grief, becoming extremely distressed by separation and then finding it impossible to "resolve" this upset when conditions seem to call for resolution. Avoidant infants in the Strange Situation are marked by a kind of cool nonchalance regarding their attachment figures' whereabouts, and—at least in some cases—an active ignoring of them when they return following a separation. This can be viewed as a small, short-term version of failure to become anxious, angry, or bereft in the face of loss. Secure infants fall somewhere in between the two major insecure groups, often reacting with distress to separations but also being quick to achieve a happy resolution once their attachment figure returns.[7]

Research on adults' reactions to separation from or loss of attachment figures also indicates that responses can be arrayed along a conceptual dimension running from absent to chronic distress. As noted above, research by Parkes and his colleagues (Parkes, 1985, 2006; Parkes & Weiss, 1983) suggested that some individuals experience chronic anxiety, whereas others report little impact of the loss on their well-being. In our own research on relationship breakups (Fraley, Davis, & Shaver, 1997) and marital separations (Fraley & Shaver, 1998), we have also identified reactions falling along this dimension. Specifically, after separation from a romantic partner or spouse, some individuals report experiencing intense anxiety and depression (see B. Feeney & Monin, Chapter 39, this volume, for a related account of attachment patterns and reactions to divorce). Moreover, naturalistic observations indicate that these anxious individuals are likely to cling to their partners and actively resist separation (Fraley & Shaver, 1998). In contrast, some individuals appear less distressed when separated from their romantic or marital partner. They are unlikely to protest separation and appear to be relatively unaffected by it.

Research on "Attachment Styles" and Reactions to Loss

Empirical tests of Bowlby's ideas in studies by personality and social psychologists, including ourselves, have focused on "attachment style"—the systematic pattern of relational expectations, emotions, and behaviors that results from internalization of a particular history of attachment experiences (Fraley & Shaver, 2000). Research, beginning with Ainsworth and colleagues (1978) and continuing through hundreds of studies by personality and social psychologists (reviewed by Mikulincer & Shaver, 2007), indicates that individual differences in attachment style can be measured with self-report measures of a person's location along two orthogonal dimensions: attachment-related anxiety and attachment-related avoidance.[8] A person's position on the avoidance dimension indicates the extent to which he or she distrusts relationship partners and strives to maintain independence and emotional distance from others. A person's position on the anxiety dimension indicates the degree to which he or she is dependent and frequently worries that a partner will not be available and supportive in times of need. People who score low on both dimensions are considered secure or securely attached. People who score high on both dimensions are said to be "fearfully avoidant" (Bartholomew & Horowitz, 1991).

Based on extensive literature reviews, we (Fraley & Shaver, 2000; Mikulincer & Shaver, 2007) proposed a three-phase model of attachment system activation and dynamics in adulthood. Following Bowlby (1969/1982), we assumed that relatively continuous monitoring of internal and external events (e.g., thoughts, worries, and external stressors) results in activation of the attachment system when a potential threat is detected. Once the attachment system is activated, an affirmative answer to the question "Is an attachment figure available and likely to be responsive to my needs?" results in a sense of security and facilitates the use of security-related affect regulation strategies. These strategies are aimed at alleviating distress, maintaining comfortable and supportive relationships, and increasing effective adjustment. They consist of optimistic beliefs about distress management, trust in others' good will, and a sense of self-efficacy about coping with threats (see Mikulincer & Shaver, Chapter 23, this volume). They also include genuinely constructive coping strategies: acknowledgment and display of distress, but without exaggeration or personal disorganization; effective support seeking; and successful problem solving. These characteristics of people who score as secure on adult attachment measures have been amply documented in hundreds of studies (Mikulincer & Shaver, 2007).

In the second step of the model, perceived unavailability or unresponsiveness of an attachment figure arouses feelings of insecurity, which forces a decision about seeking or not seeking proximity to an attachment figure. When proximity seeking is expected (or at least hoped) to be successful, a person makes energetic, insistent attempts to attain proximity, protection, and support. These efforts are called "hyperactivating strategies" (Cassidy & Berlin, 1994), because they involve strong activation of the attachment system until an attachment figure is perceived to be available and responsive. These strategies include approaching, begging, crying, clinging; being hypervigilant concerning a partner's intentions, motives, and behavior; and intense distress and protest if a partner seems insensitive or unresponsive.

In contrast, viewing proximity seeking as unlikely to achieve safety or comfort, and perhaps even as likely to elicit anger or punishment and thereby exacerbate distress, results in efforts to deactivate the attachment system and handle the problem alone. These efforts are called "deactivating strategies" (Cassidy & Kobak, 1988), because their primary goal is to keep the attachment system shut down. This involves denying or de-emphasizing attachment needs, avoiding emotional involvement in and dependence on close relationship partners, suppressing attachment-related thoughts, and remaining autonomous—a stance Bowlby (1973) called "compulsive self-reliance."

Interestingly, reorganization of attachment working models following bereavement involves some degree of both hyperactivating and deactivating strategies (Mikulincer & Shaver, in press; M. Stroebe & Schut, 1999). By causing a person to experience the pain of loss, to reactivate memories of the deceased alongside realizations that he or she is no longer present, and to yearn for the deceased's proximity and love, attachment system hyperactivation allows the mourner to explore the meaning and significance of the loss and find ways of reorganizing symbolic bonds with the lost loved one. When this form of hyperactivation is tolerable and manageable—that is, not overwhelming or disorganizing—it allows the bereaved person to incorporate the past into the present without splitting off important segments of personal history and identity.

Deactivating strategies can also contribute to postloss reorganization by enabling momentary detachment from thoughts of the deceased loved one and inhibition or suppression of painful thoughts and feelings. While using a certain degree of "avoidance" and denial (Coifman, Bonanno, Ray, & Gross, 2007), a bereaved person can manage the funeral, clean out the deceased partner's closet, begin to create and explore a new life, return to work and daily activities, and recognize that the lost relationship continues to have meaning while life presents new opportunities.

Without some degree of attachment system hyperactivation, a bereaved person could not consider and experience all aspects of his or her new situation and find constructive ways of remembering the lost attachment figure. This kind of hyperactivation is what Freud (1917/1957) meant by "hypercathexis" followed by "decathexis" of mental representations of the deceased. Moreover, without some degree of attachment system deactivation (targeted on the lost figure), the bereaved person might continue to pine, feel hopeless, and be unable to cope with new demands. In other words, the person might suffer from clinically significant complicated or prolonged grief.

Attachment reorganization requires both processes, hyper- and deactivation, acting in dynamic balance—a process M. Stroebe and Schut (1999) called "oscillation" between a "loss orientation"

and a "restoration orientation." Loss orientation is conceptually similar to attachment system hyper-activation and Freud's notion of hypercathexis; it includes yearning, ruminating, and processing the implications of the loss. Restoration orientation accomplishes the same functions as attachment system deactivation—attending to life changes, doing new things, distracting oneself from grief, denying or suppressing grief, and forming new relationships. In this model, oscillation between the two orientations brings about a gradual reorganization of life and mind, such that the deceased person's absence and the survivor's new situation are integrated into his or her identity. According to M. Stroebe, Schut, and Stroebe (2005), "oscillation occurs in the short term (transient fluctuations in the course of any particular day) as well as across time, because adaptation to bereavement is a matter of . . . exploring and discovering what has been lost and what remains: what must be avoided or relinquished versus what can be retained, created, and built on" (p. 52). With successful reorganization of the attachment system, this oscillation is reduced, and a person begins to feel comfortable with memories and images of the deceased loved one and more able to engage with life and other people.

Bonanno, Papa, Lalande, Westphal, and Coifman (2004) conducted an interesting experiment related to "oscillation," or what they called "flexible" use of the two kinds of coping strategies. Actually, the experiment did not deal with bereavement per se, but rather with a combination of adjusting to college and dealing with shock and stress following the September 11, 2001, terrorist attack in New York City. The researchers had college students who lived in the city perform a laboratory task in which they "enhanced emotional expression, suppressed emotional expression, and behaved normally on different trials" (p. 482). Their performance was used as a prospective predictor of adjustment to college during the following 2 years. The results indicated that students who were better able to enhance *and* suppress the expression of emotion in the laboratory were less distressed 2 years later. The result fits with many studies of attachment style and coping, which suggest that secure individuals are more flexible in their coping strategies, and more successful in maintaining good adjustment (see Mikulincer & Shaver, 2007, for a review).

In another study, Fraley, Fazzari, Bonanno, and Dekel (2006) assessed people who had been exposed to the September 11 attack—many of whom had lost someone as a result—7 and 18 months later, using measures of the two attachment style dimensions (anxiety and avoidance), PTSD, and depression. They also asked study participants' friends and relatives to provide reports of these people's adjustment before and after the attack. Results indicated that secure participants suffered fewer symptoms of PTSD and depression than insecure participants (as indicated by self-reports), and that the secure individuals were viewed by friends and relatives as exhibiting good adjustment before and after the attack. The least well-adjusted after the attack, according to friends and relatives, were the "preoccupied" participants (those scoring high on attachment anxiety but low on avoidance). "Dismissing" participants (those high on avoidance but low on anxiety) described themselves as distressed and were viewed by observers as less well adjusted than the secure participants 7 months after the attack, but not at 18 months after. Fearfully avoidant individuals, despite feeling distressed, were judged as about average in reactions 7 and 18 months after the attack.

Despite the logic of Bowlby's and of Stroebe and colleagues' ideas about coping with and adjusting to loss, no longitudinal study has been conducted on hyperactivation–deactivation oscillations and their implications for mental health and adjustment. Most of the research has focused on attachment style differences in coping with loss. But Schut, Stroebe, and van den Bout (1997) found that men who habitually avoided confronting their grief benefited from counseling that encouraged them to deal with neglected aspects of their loss. They also found that women who habitually dwelled on the emotional meaning and deep personal implications of the loss benefited from counseling that focused on learning how to deal with changed everyday activities.

Attachment Insecurities and Disordered Patterns of Mourning

Bowlby (1980) suggested that attachment reorganization depends on the ways a person's attachment system has become organized over the course of development, resulting in the patterns we are calling attachment styles. Attachment-anxious individuals, who find it difficult to operate autonomously and handle life tasks on their own, find it difficult to deactivate or inhibit painful feelings, thoughts, and memories related to a deceased partner; this difficulty makes the deactivation side of the oscillation between hyperactivation and deactivation

impossible. Avoidant individuals, who regularly suppress attachment-related thoughts and feelings and distance themselves mentally from sources of distress (even when they are not grieving), may be unwilling to experience thoughts, feelings, and memories related to a deceased partner. In contrast, attachment security facilitates the reorganization of working models of self and partner, and makes adjustment to loss easier (M. Stroebe, Schut, & Stroebe, 2005). Securely attached people can recall and think about a deceased partner without becoming lost in rumination or having to disengage. They can acknowledge feelings of love and grief, and discuss the loss coherently in the same way they are able, in the Adult Attachment Interview (AAI; see Hesse, Chapter 25, this volume), to discuss good and bad memories of their childhood relationships with parents, including important losses.

Anxious Attachment and Chronic Mourning

Even when their attachment figures are alive, attachment-anxious people are preoccupied with these figures' availability and responsiveness, likely to make intrusive demands for greater closeness, prone to jealousy, quick to cry, and eager for love and reassurance (Mikulincer & Shaver, 2007; Shaver, Schachner, & Mikulincer, 2005). Anxiously attached people often blame themselves for not having sufficient resources and skills to gain a partner's attention and affection, and they invest heavily in their relationships and become highly dependent on their partners (e.g., Alonso-Arbiol, Shaver, & Yárnoz, 2002). Not surprisingly, when they lose a primary attachment figure, they are likely to experience intense anxiety, anger, and sorrow; yearn persistently for the lost partner; fail to accept the loss; and have difficulty establishing a new life. These are some of the core features of what Bowlby (1980) called "chronic" mourning. Another characteristic of chronic mourning is that a bereaved person is frequently reminded of the deceased by diverse stimuli and situations that unintentionally trigger intrusive thoughts, feelings, and memories (Boelen, van den Hout, & van den Bout, 2006; Lichtenthal et al., 2004). This inability to control the flow of intrusive grief reactions can overwhelm a person and prevent calm exploration of new possibilities in life and successful reorganization of attachment working models. In many cases, these tendencies of attachment-anxious individuals were probably present in some form even before bereavement.

In an experimental study of emotional memories, Mikulincer and Orbach (1995) asked participants to recall early childhood experiences of anger, sadness, anxiety, or happiness. The researchers interpreted the memory retrieval latencies as indicators of mental accessibility or inaccessibility. Participants also rated the intensity of focal and nonfocal emotions in each recalled event (i.e., the emotion they were asked to target vs. other emotions that might also be aroused). In the memory task, attachment-anxious individuals had the readiest access to targeted memories. Moreover, whereas secure people took more time to retrieve negative than positive emotional memories, anxious people took longer to retrieve positive than negative memories. In the emotion-rating task, secure individuals rated focal emotions (e.g., sadness when they had been instructed to retrieve a sad memory) as much more intense than nonfocal emotions (e.g., anger when instructed to retrieve a sad memory). In contrast, anxious individuals reported intense focal *and* nonfocal emotions when asked to remember examples of anxiety, sadness, and anger. Negative emotional memories seemed to spread like wildfire throughout their memory systems, and this did not depend on thoughts about loss or grief in particular.

Roisman, Tsai, and Chiang (2004) reported related findings concerning people's facial expressions during the AAI. Whereas securely attached interviewees' facial expressions were congruent with the valence of the childhood events they were describing, anxiously attached individuals exhibited marked discrepancies between the quality of the childhood experiences they described and their facial expressions (e.g., facial expressions of sadness or anger were noticeable while they were speaking about neutral or positive childhood experiences). According to Roisman and colleagues, these discrepancies reflect anxious individuals' confusion and emotional dysregulation when they talk about emotional experiences. We believe that this same kind of confusion/disorganization occurs when anxiously attached mourners are bombarded with intrusive images, thoughts, feelings, and memories about the deceased. This makes them especially likely candidates for complicated or prolonged grief (see Wijngaards-de Meij et al., 2007, for suggestive evidence).

In two experiments examining the link between negative moods and cognitive processing, Pereg and Mikulincer (2004) again noticed attachment-anxious individuals' lack of control over the spread of activation from one distress-eliciting thought to another. Participants were assigned to a negative mood condition (reading an article about a car accident) or a control condition (reading about how to construct and use a hobby kit), and their incidental recall and causal attributions were assessed. Induction of a negative mood, as compared with the control condition, influenced secure participants to recall more positive information and to attribute a negative event to less global and less stable causes (findings reminiscent of the previously discussed September 11 study by Fraley et al., 2006). Participants scoring higher on attachment anxiety reacted to an induced negative mood with heightened recall of negative information and a tendency to attribute the negative event to more global and stable causes. In the case of bereaved individuals, this pattern of emotional dysregulation is likely to make it difficult to manage intrusive memories of the deceased.

Another feature of chronic mourning is the presence of negative beliefs about oneself, one's life, and the future—beliefs such as "I'm worthless without my beloved," "My life is meaningless after the loss," and "The future is hopeless" (e.g., Boelen, van den Hout, & van den Bout, 2003; Neimeyer, Prigerson, & Davies, 2002). According to Foa and Rothbaum (1998), these negative beliefs can be particularly resistant to change when the loss confirms negative views of the self, hopeless beliefs, and catastrophic cognitions that were present before the loss. As already mentioned, this is more likely to be the case when a person was already anxiously attached, possessed negative views of self, exaggerated even fairly minor threats, held pessimistic beliefs about managing distress, and attributed threatening events to uncontrollable causes and pervasive personal inadequacies (Bonanno, Wortman, et al., 2004).

Avoidant Attachment and the Absence of Grief

As we have explained, avoidant people try to deny attachment needs, suppress attachment-related thoughts and emotions, and inhibit unwanted urges to seek proximity or support (Mikulincer & Shaver, 2007). This kind of person values independence to the point of avoiding deep emotional interdependence even with a long-term mate (Edelstein & Shaver, 2004; Fraley, Davis, & Shaver, 1998). Following the loss of an attachment figure, such a person is likely to use well-established defenses to inhibit anxiety and sadness, downplay the importance of the loss, and try to steer clear of thoughts and memories focused on the deceased.

This is what Bowlby (1980) meant by the "absence of conscious grieving." He considered this to be a defensive reaction involving redirection of attention away from painful thoughts and feelings ("defensive exclusion") and the segregation or dissociation of memories of the deceased, which nevertheless continue to influence emotions and behaviors without the individual's awareness of their existence or effects.

Bowlby (1980) thought that the prolonged absence of grief can eventually lead to difficulties in mental and physical health, perhaps especially when subsequent losses are experienced. He thought that people who fail to mourn will have difficulties integrating losses meaningfully into their working models and personal narratives. (This is what leads to a person's being classified as "unresolved with respect to losses or traumas" in the AAI; see Hesse, Chapter 25, this volume.) Since a bereaved person is likely to have engaged in many daily activities with the now deceased partner, each of those activities or the places where they occurred becomes an unwanted reminder of the loss and a further source of either distress or an attempt to suppress thoughts that evoke distress. In our chapter in the first edition of this handbook, we (Fraley & Shaver, 1999) said: "Repeated activation of inexplicable and partially suppressed negative emotions may eventually have a negative impact on psychological well-being or physical health" (p. 743). As mentioned at the beginning of the present chapter, Bowlby (1990) provided a detailed example of such negative consequences in his book about Charles Darwin: Darwin's hyperventilation syndrome.

Of course, the negative emotional and physical sequelae of "absence of grieving" are most likely to emerge when a mourner was deeply attached to the lost partner and the partner was the individual's primary safe haven and secure base. If an avoidant person was able to avoid proximity seeking, deep interdependence, and extensive attachment to a partner while he or she was alive, he or she might experience less anxiety and sadness following the loss even without strenuous suppression or mental segregation. In such cases, the absence of grieving might indicate a real absence of distress (relative to that experienced by other bereaved individuals), rather than a defensive reaction to the pain of a meaningful loss. Compatible with this idea, there is evidence that many people who show few signs of grief shortly after the loss of a partner do not exhibit heightened distress or maladjustment

months or years later (see Bonanno, 2001, for a review). It may be difficult, however, to tell the difference between successful but defensive suppression on the one hand, and true absence of anything to suppress on the other. But a number of new social-cognitive and physiological methods allow this issue to be studied more carefully than was possible in the past.

Using Wegner's (1994) thought suppression paradigm, we (Fraley & Shaver, 1997) asked study participants to write about whatever thoughts and feelings they were experiencing, while being allowed to think about anything except thoughts about their mates' leaving them for someone else. (All of the participants were involved in long-term couple relationships.) In one study, the ability to suppress these thoughts was assessed by the number of times they appeared in participants' stream of consciousness following the suppression effort (during what Wegner, 1994, called the "rebound" period). In another study, this ability was assessed by the level of physiological arousal (skin conductance) during the suppression task—the lower the arousal, the greater the presumed ability to suppress the troubling thoughts. The results indicated that avoidant attachment was associated with both less frequent thoughts of loss following the suppression task and lower skin conductance during the task, suggesting that avoidant defenses block unwanted thoughts and prevent the emotional arousal they might otherwise cause. A recent functional magnetic resonance imaging study (Gillath, Bunge, Shaver, Wendelken, & Mikulincer, 2005) shows that these avoidant defenses are also evident in patterns of brain activation and deactivation when people are attempting to suppress thoughts about breakups and losses.

While probing further into the regulatory mechanisms underlying avoidant defenses, we (Fraley, Garner, & Shaver, 2000) asked whether they function in a "preemptive" manner (e.g., by directing attention away from, or encoding in a shallow way, attachment-related information) or in a "postemptive" manner (repressing material that has already been encoded). Participants listened to a genuinely emotional interview about the loss of a close relationship partner and were later asked to recall details of the interview, either soon after hearing them (Study 1) or at various delays ranging from 30 minutes to 21 days (Study 2). An analysis of forgetting curves plotted over time revealed that (1) avoidant people initially encoded less information about the interview, and (2) people with different attachment styles forgot encoded information at the same rate. Thus avoidant defenses sometimes act preemptively, by blocking threatening material from awareness before it is fully encoded.

However, although these studies imply that avoidant defenses are effective in suppressing memories and thoughts concerning separation and loss, Mikulincer, Dolev, and Shaver (2004) found that avoidant people can nevertheless be disturbed by the unwanted resurgence of suppressed thoughts (a phenomenon Freud, 1926/1959, called "the return of the repressed"). In one study, participants were asked to think about a painful relationship breakup and were either instructed or not instructed to suppress thoughts about this separation. The researchers then examined the rebound of the suppressed separation-related thoughts under conditions of low or high cognitive load, which enabled them to determine whether avoidant defenses would be capable of inhibiting the postsuppression rebound effect even when other cognitive demands drew upon limited psychological resources. The implicit activation of previously suppressed thoughts was assessed by measuring the extent to which they influenced performance on a Stroop color-naming task. Participants performed a Stroop task under low or high cognitive load (holding a one- or seven-digit number in mind), and color-naming reaction times were assessed for separation-related words. (Longer reaction times imply greater activation of the verbal content printed in color.)

In a second study, Mikulincer and colleagues (2004) examined possible consequences of failed suppression efforts on avoidant individuals' self-concepts: If a high cognitive load impairs the effectiveness of avoidant defenses, it may render avoidant persons defenseless against reactivation of doubts about their lovability and sense of personal worth (doubts resulting, according to attachment theory, from a history of relationships with unavailable and rejecting partners). So that this possibility could be examined, study participants were asked to recall either a painful breakup with a romantic partner or a more neutral experience (being at a drugstore), and to perform a 5-minute stream-of-consciousness task. In this task, participants were either instructed or not instructed to suppress thoughts about the just-recalled episode. All participants then performed the Stroop color-naming task, while at the same time carrying out a relatively easy or demanding cognitive task. The main dependent variables were color-naming

reaction times for participant-specific negative self-traits and positive self-traits taken from lists supplied by the participants in a previous research session weeks before.

The results showed, as predicted, that avoidant attachment was associated in the control condition with the prevention of unwanted reactivation of previously suppressed thoughts about a painful separation. Under a low cognitive load, avoidant people were able to suppress thoughts related to the breakup, and at the same time they activated *positive* self-representations following thought suppression. However, the effectiveness of their avoidant defenses was significantly impaired when a high cognitive load taxed the mental resources needed to maintain thought suppression. Under a high cognitive load, avoidant people exhibited greater automatic activation of thoughts of separation and *negative* self-traits following suppression. In other words, their avoidant defenses collapsed when mental resources were too scarce to maintain them, and this collapse was associated with a spread of activation from unwanted attachment-related thoughts to formerly suppressed negative self-representations. This is the kind of psychodynamic phenomenon, central to Bowlby's theory, that research psychologists have often thought could not be empirically demonstrated, but that has now been clearly demonstrated in the laboratory (Mikulincer & Shaver, Chapter 23, this volume; Shaver & Mikulincer, 2005).

Moreover, naturalistic studies (e.g., Berant, Mikulincer, & Shaver, 2008) support the idea that more avoidant individuals are sometimes unable to use avoidant disattention or suppression effectively to deal with real-world stressors that cannot be ignored. In the Berant et al. study, avoidant women who gave birth to a child with a congenital heart defect—something that cannot be ignored and requires years of adaptive coping—suffered emotionally more than less avoidant mothers in the same situation, experienced greater deterioration in their marriages, and had children who at age 7 were also poorly adjusted.

These kinds of findings seem to mesh well with the conclusion we reached in the first edition of this chapter—namely, that Bowlby was largely correct in assuming that the apparent absence of grief can sometimes be a defensive maneuver that has the potential, under certain circumstances (e.g., lack of attentional resources, additional salient losses), to give way to problems. But we wish to underscore as well that he clearly stated that some of the individuals who do not show common signs of grief are not necessarily destined to experience adverse consequences later. Some individuals may be relatively uninvested in their relationships, and as a consequence may have relatively little to grieve about when those bonds are severed. Other individuals may be quite defensive, but do not encounter anything that overloads their defenses. In our opinion, the research conducted to date has not fully mapped the reasons for absence of grieving. Some people who fail to grieve may have nothing to grieve about, may not have been deeply attached to the deceased individual, may have been worn down by caregiving before the person's death, or (a very different possibility) may be quite secure and able to deal resiliently with a loss. In most of the studies showing that a group of people were resilient following a loss and did not have a troubled or avoidant relationship with the deceased (e.g., Bonanno et al., 2002), the participants we would consider relatively secure and those we would consider relatively dismissive or avoidant were probably combined in the "resilient" group, which was then compared with a more anxious, depressed, and traumatized group. Such a one-dimensional group study design does not allow a clear distinction to be drawn between secure and avoidant individuals.

Another point to consider is that different kinds of grief processing may work for different kinds of people. Wortman and Boerner (2007, p. 300) say, "Those who have difficulty expressing their emotions seem to benefit the most from interventions such as writing about their experience (Lumley, Tojeck, & Macklem, 2002; Norman, Lumley, Dooley, & Diamond, 2004)." Interestingly, these are likely to be the more avoidant people. Recall the study we mentioned earlier by Schut and colleagues (1997), which showed that men who avoided confronting their grief benefited from counseling that encouraged "loss processing," whereas women who dwelled on the emotional meaning and personal implications of the loss benefited from counseling that encouraged "restoration processing" (focusing on ways to deal with changed everyday activities).

Empirical Evidence on Attachment Style Differences in Adjustment to Loss

Beyond experimental evidence for attachment-related differences in coping with thoughts and memories related to loss, there are now a few studies that have directly examined attachment style differences in adjustment to the loss of a close relationship partner. They generally support the hypothesis that attachment security contributes to emotional adjustment following a loss. For example, van Doorn, Kasl, Beery, Jacobs, and Prigerson (1998) interviewed adults while they were caring for their terminally ill spouses and found that attachment security in romantic relationships in general and specific attachment security in the marriage were both associated with less intense grief following the loss of a spouse. Similarly, Fraley and Bonanno (2004) found that people classified as securely attached 4 months after the loss of a spouse reported relatively low levels of bereavement-related anxiety, grief, depression, and posttraumatic distress 4 and 18 months after the loss. Conceptually similar findings were reported by Wayment and Vierthaler (2002), Waskowic and Chartier (2003), and Wijngaards-de Meij and colleagues (2007).

There is also evidence concerning anxiously attached individuals' complicated grief reactions (Field & Sundin, 2001; Fraley & Bonanno, 2004; Wayment & Vierthaler, 2002). For example, Field and Sundin (2001) found that anxious attachment, assessed 10 months after the death of a spouse, predicted higher levels of psychological distress 14, 25, and 60 months after the loss. With regard to avoidant attachment, studies have generally found no association between this dimension and depression, grief, or distress (Field & Sundin, 2001; Fraley & Bonanno, 2004; Wayment & Vierthaler, 2002; however, see Fraley et al., 2006, and Wijngaards-de Meij et al., 2007, for findings that may suggest a breakdown of avoidant defenses in some cases).

Interestingly, Wayment and Vierthaler (2002) found that avoidance was associated with somatic symptoms, implying that avoidant defenses might block conscious access to anxiety and depression without blocking more subtle and less conscious somatic reactions to loss. These results are similar to ones obtained by Berant, Mikulincer, and Florian (2001), Mikulincer, Florian, and Weller (1993), and Berant and colleagues (2008), and are compatible with studies of bereaved individuals by Bonanno, Keltner, Holen, and Horowitz (1995) and Bonanno and Field (2001), which showed that respondents with an avoidant style (measured by methods differing from the self-report scales used by attachment researchers) had more somatic symptoms 6 months after the loss. In addition, Fraley and Bonanno (2004) and Wijngaards-de Meij and colleagues (2007) found that the combination of avoidance and attachment anxiety (the pattern that Bartholomew & Horowitz, 1991, called "fearful avoidance") was associated with the highest levels of anxiety, depression, grief, trauma-related symptoms, and alcohol consumption following the death of a spouse.

There is also evidence concerning attachment style differences in continuing attachment to and detachment from a lost partner. Field and Sundin (2001), for example, found that more avoidant people reported more negative thoughts about a lost spouse 14 months after the loss, perhaps reflecting a distancing, derogating attitude toward the deceased (something commonly found in studies of avoidant attachment and relationship dissatisfaction when a partner is still alive). In contrast, attachment anxiety was associated with more positive thoughts about the lost spouse, possibly reflecting a degree of idealization. This kind of idealization was also evident in Nager and de Vries's (2004) content analysis of memorial websites created by adult daughters for their deceased mothers. Comments about intensely missing a deceased mother and providing an idealized description of her (e.g., "You were the most beautiful, strongest, most determined, smartest, fascinating woman in the world") were more frequently found on websites created by anxiously attached daughters. Using the Continuing Bonds Scale, Waskowic and Chartier (2003) found that secure individuals ruminated less about, and were less preoccupied with, a deceased spouse; the secure participants also had more positive memories and symbolic exchanges with mental representations of the lost person.

Unresolved Traumas and Losses in the AAI

As explained in detail by Hesse in Chapter 25 and by Lyons-Ruth and Jacobvitz in 28 of the present volume, the AAI and its scoring system were developed by George, Kaplan, and Main (1984, 1985, 1996; see also Main & Goldwyn, 1984; Main, Goldwyn, & Hesse, 2003) to assess an adult's "current state of mind with respect to attachment." The coding system for the interview was developed partly to identify parents whose children were likely to have one or another attachment pattern as assessed in the Strange Situation. One of the most interesting discoveries in AAI research is that children classified as disorganized/disoriented in the Strange Situation (Main & Hesse, 1990; Main & Solomon, 1990) are significantly more likely than other children to have

mothers who show signs of "unresolved loss or trauma" in the AAI.

Unresolved loss or trauma is marked by (1) lapses in metacognitive monitoring, such as indications of disbelief that a deceased person is still alive or still present, false ideas of having contributed to the death, indications of confusion between the dead person and the self, and other psychologically confused statements; (2) lapses in the metacognitive monitoring of discourse, such as prolonged, inappropriate silences, odd associations, unusual attention to detail, or poetic or eulogistic phrasing of speech; and (3) reports of extreme behavioral responses at the time of the loss or trauma, in the absence of convincing evidence that resolution has taken place (Main & Goldwyn, 1984, as summarized by Adam, Sheldon-Keller, & West, 1995, p. 318).

The unresolved designation is assigned when a person receives a high rating on the unresolved coding scale, but he or she is also assigned to a best-fitting primary AAI category (dismissing, secure-autonomous, or preoccupied) as well. In every study of which we are aware, there is an association between unresolved mourning and preoccupied (anxious) attachment. For example, Ainsworth and Eichberg (1991) reported that 50% of the mothers in their sample who received an unresolved classification were also given a secondary classification of preoccupied. In contrast, only 18% of the sample who did not experience a loss or who had resolved their loss were classified as preoccupied. In a study by Adam and colleagues (1995), 49% of an adolescent clinic sample received a classification as unresolved. Of this subsample, 48% were given a secondary classification of preoccupied, compared with 12% of those not classified as unresolved. These findings provide additional evidence that unresolved or chronic mourning is associated with preoccupied or anxious attachment.

There is also a body of research *not* rooted in the attachment perspective that links characteristics associated with anxious attachment to chronic mourning and difficulties in recovery. This research indicates that both neuroticism and low self-esteem, which are correlates of anxious attachment (e.g., Noftle & Shaver, 2006; Shaver & Brennan, 1992), are also correlates of chronic mourning in bereaved individuals. For example, Vachon and colleagues (1982), M. Stroebe and Stroebe (1993), and Wijngaards-de Meij and colleagues (2007) found that neuroticism was associated with depression in the months following bereavement. Lund and colleagues (1989) found that low self-esteem was associated with stress and depression 2 years after bereavement.

CONTINUING BONDS: A CONTROVERSY CONCERNING DETACHMENT AND RESOLUTION

A challenge to Bowlby's account of loss and grief appeared in *Continuing Bonds: New Understandings of Grief* (Klass et al., 1996a). The authors who contributed chapters to the volume portrayed Freud and Bowlby as "modernists," in contrast with the authors' "postmodernism." They claimed that the modernist emphasis on extreme individualism and mechanistic science led Freud and Bowlby mistakenly to view mourning as a biological, rigidly sequenced process with a fixed healthy endpoint: decathexis or detachment, defined by Klass and colleagues as complete severance of the emotional bond to a lost attachment figure. In the first edition of the present chapter (Fraley & Shaver, 1999), we examined the evidence and rationale for this "postmodern" position and found it wanting—partly because it unfairly caricatured Bowlby's views, partly because it ignored the possibility of unresolved grief associated with disorganized attachment. Nevertheless, we credited some of the book's insights and showed how they might be incorporated into attachment theory.

Since 1999, the discussion of *Continuing Bonds* has itself "continued," and in 2006 the journal *Death Studies* published two special issues on the topic. Here we briefly recapitulate our criticisms of *Continuing Bonds* and then consider the recent literature, some of which (as mentioned by Field, 2006) was influenced by our chapter.

Far from advocating an abrupt and complete detachment from a lost attachment figure, Bowlby (1980) reacted *against* that idea. In his opinion, it had caused psychoanalytically oriented therapists to hasten the grieving process and incorrectly to view many of its healthy manifestations as pathological. The grief reactions that many clinicians apparently viewed as immature or pathological—searching, yearning, and sometimes expressing anger or ambivalence toward the lost attachment figure—are aspects of the normal functioning of the attachment system, as explained in earlier sections of this chapter. It was part of Bowlby's general approach to attachment phenomena to be sympathetic to people of any age, and in any circumstances, whose attachment behavioral sys-

tem had been activated by distress or by unavailability or loss of an attachment figure. He strongly disapproved of characterizing such individuals' reactions as childish, irrational, or inappropriately dependent.

As mentioned earlier, even Freud, at least in his personal correspondence, did not agree with the position that subsequent writers attributed to him. In our view, the notion of decathexis from mental representations of a lost attachment figure, when stripped of its outdated theoretical language (concerning the investment and disinvestment of psychic energy), refers to a commonly experienced emotional reaction when one suddenly remembers a deceased attachment figure and realizes once again that he or she is gone. This often happens when one has a glancing thought or memory of the deceased person and is jolted by the realization that the thought or related expectation is no longer appropriate. C. S. Lewis (1961) described this experience in a book about grieving for his dead wife:

> There are moments … when something inside me tries to assure me that I don't really mind so much. … Love is not the whole of a man's life. I was happy before I ever met H. I've plenty of what are called "resources." People get over these things. Come, I shan't do so badly. One is ashamed to listen to this voice but it seems for a little to be making out a good case. *Then comes a sudden jab of red-hot memory and all this "commonsense" vanishes like an ant in the mouth of a furnace.* (pp. 5–6; emphasis added)

This kind of "jab" can occur scores or hundreds of times over many weeks or months; it is a normal part of coming to terms with a loss that is not yet fully represented in all of a bereaved person's unconscious and preconscious memories. As elements of "internal working models" of the lost attachment figure are called up unexpectedly (by situations or associations), altered to acknowledge the loved one's death, and forgotten again as one returns to current activities and concerns, the emotional charge associated with them typically decreases—partly by virtue of habituation and desensitization, partly by virtue of being reorganized into more realistic, updated working models (Shaver & Tancredy, 2001). But this does not mean that the bereaved person's attachment to the lost figure is erased from memory; far from it.

As M. Stroebe and Schut (2005) said when discussing this issue, "The process involved in the working through of grief—this need to invest energy in the struggle to 'decathect' the loved object—can be interpreted as one of emotional neutralization, not forgetting" (p. 479). Horowitz (1997) described this process of repeatedly confronting one's changed reality and outdated working models until an attachment figure's loss is fully represented in memory and integrated into updated working models. Bowlby (1980) said: "The resolution of grief is not to sever bonds but to establish a changed bond with the dead person" (p. 399). Hence Bowlby the "modernist" was talking about continuing bonds 16 years before the "postmodern" authors of *Continuing Bonds*.

Evidence for Continuing Bonds

The evidence for attachments to lost attachment figures caused the authors of *Continuing Bonds* to question their clinical training and allegiance to what they mistakenly viewed as attachment theory (Balk, 1996, p. 312):

> Hogan and DeSantis (1992) discovered that bereaved adolescents typically maintained ongoing attachments to their dead siblings. Silverman, Nickman, and Worden (1992) noted that bereaved children made conscious efforts to sustain connections to their dead parents and incorporated those attachments into their ongoing social environment. Tyson-Rawson (1993) ... reported that 14 of her 20 [college student] research participants mentioned "an ongoing attachment to [their deceased fathers]" (p. 166).

The editors of *Continuing Bonds* summarized their experiences as follows:

> We realized that *we were observing phenomena that could not be accounted for within the models of grief that most of our colleagues were using.* ... [W]hat we were observing was not a stage of disengagement, *which we were educated to expect,* but rather, we were observing people altering and then continuing their relationship to the lost or dead person. *Remaining connected seemed to facilitate both adults' and children's ability to cope with the loss and the accompanying changes in their lives. These "connections" provided solace, comfort and support, and eased the transition from the past to the future.* (Klass et al., 1996b, pp. xvii–xviii; emphases added)

The *Continuing Bond* authors' perspective was repeatedly contrasted with what they claimed to be Bowlby's position:

Bowlby continued the [Freudian] model that the purpose of grief is to sever the bond with the dead. ... He defined a distinct and unvarying sequence of behaviors that can be identified in children separated from their mothers [leading to detachment]. ... Those who follow the Bowlby/Parkes theory continue to define the resolution of grief as severing bonds rather than as establishing a changed bond with the dead person. (Silverman & Klass, 1996, pp. 9–13)

> In Bowlby's view ... the attempt to restore proximity [to the deceased attachment figure] is inappropriate or nonfunctional. ... Like psychoanalytic theory, which focuses on the importance of relinquishing ties, Bowlby's work suggests that bonds with the deceased need to be broken for the bereaved to adjust and recover. ... Those who retain ties are considered maladjusted. (Balk, 1996, p. 311)

What Bowlby Actually Said about Continuing Bonds

The comments quoted above distort Bowlby's theory. They fail to mention that when writing about permanent losses as distinct from temporary separations, Bowlby (1980) used the term "reorganization" rather than "detachment." The term "detachment" was originally coined to describe a *defensive* reaction to the *return* of a temporarily absent attachment figure. When infants are separated from their attachment figures, they protest before eventually exhibiting sadness. Eventually they seem to recover and begin to explore their environments with renewed interest; they seem once again to be interested in other people. However, if the attachment figures return, Bowlby (1969/1982) noted that many children respond with coldness and an absence of attachment behavior, as if they are punishing the attachment figures for abandoning them or are unsure how to organize their conflicting desires to seek comfort and express anger. Bowlby (1969/1982) emphasized that this defensive response is best described as "apparent" detachment, because once the children reaccept their attachment figures' care, they are particularly clingy and hypervigilant, not wanting to let the figures out of sight. The following quotations from Bowlby (1980) are illuminating:

> [There is] a bias that runs through so much of the older literature on how human beings respond to loss. ... there is a tendency to under-estimate how intensely distressing and disabling loss usually is and for how long the distress, and often the disablement, commonly lasts. Conversely, there is a tendency to suppose that a normal healthy person can and should

get over a bereavement not only fairly rapidly but also completely. (pp. 7–8)

So comforting did widows find the sense of a dead husband's presence [which Bowlby described as persisting for a long time "at its original intensity"] that some deliberately evoked it whenever they felt unsure of themselves or depressed. (pp. 96–97)

Indeed, an occasional recurrence of active grieving, especially when some event reminds the bereaved of her loss, is the rule. I emphasize these findings ... because I believe that clinicians sometimes have unrealistic expectations of the speed and completeness with which someone can be expected to get over a major bereavement. (p. 101)

There is no reason to regard any of these experiences as either unusual or unfavourable, rather the contrary. For example, in regard to the Boston widows Glick, [Weiss, and Parkes] (1974) report: "Often the widow's progress toward recovery was facilitated by inner conversations with her husband's presence ... this continued sense of attachment was not incompatible with increasing capacity for independent action" (p. 154). ... [I]t seems likely that for many widows and widowers it is precisely because they are willing for their feelings of attachment to the dead spouse to persist that their sense of identity is preserved and they become able to reorganize their lives along lines they find meaningful. (p. 98; emphasis added)

[A secure] person ... is likely to possess a representational model of attachment figure(s) as being available, responsive and helpful and a complementary model of himself as at least a potentially lovable and valuable person. ... On being confronted with the loss of someone close to him such a person will not be spared grief; on the contrary he may grieve deeply. ... [But] he is likely to be spared those experiences which lead mourning to become unbearable or unproductive or both. ... Since he will not be afraid of intense and unmet desires for love from the person lost, he will let himself be swept by pangs of grief; and tearful expression of yearning and distress will come naturally. During the months and years that follow he will probably be able to organize life afresh, fortified perhaps by an abiding sense of the lost person's continuing and benevolent presence. (pp. 242–243; emphasis added)

These quotations from Bowlby are important not only because they show that Continuing Bonds mischaracterized his views, but also because they suggest the possibility that continuing bonds might be handled in either a secure or an insecure way—a possibility that was largely missing from Continuing Bonds.

Valid Insights Regarding Continuing Bonds

Despite misrepresenting Bowlby and attachment theory, the authors of Continuing Bonds reported a number of interesting findings that extend Bowlby's analysis. For example, Silverman and Nickman (1996) found that five kinds of activities helped children maintain healthy mental connections to their deceased parents:

1. The children located the parents in a place (usually heaven) where they could imagine them continuing to observe and take an interest in the children's activities and needs.
2. They experienced the parents' continuing presence.
3. They "reached out" to the deceased parents to maintain interaction with them.
4. The children made special efforts, often augmented by family members, to remember the deceased's characteristics and love for them.
5. Many children kept objects (e.g., clothing, jewelry) that belonged to their lost parents, and contact with these objects seemed to prolong the sense of closeness and of being loved and protected.

Many of the children studied by Silverman and Nickman seemed to realize that their needs and wishes for continued contact with their parents were partly responsible for their views about their parents' continued existence in another realm. A 14-year-old boy said, "I want my father to see me perform. If I said a dead person can't see then I would not be able to have my wish that he see what I am doing" (Silverman & Nickman, 1996, p. 77). A 15-year-old girl said, "I think heaven is not a definite place. ... It's not as if I actually see him standing there, but I feel him and, like, in my mind I hear his voice" (p. 78). A majority of the studied children dreamed of their parents and experienced them, during the dream, as alive: "I dreamed he met me on the way home from school and ... he hugged me" (p. 79).

According to the authors of another chapter in Continuing Bonds (Normand, Silverman, & Nickman, 1996), this kind of coherence and balance characterizes many of the relationships children construct between themselves and their dead parents:

A sign of the mental openness and "coherence" of this [pattern] is that the positive or even idealized memories are sometimes interspersed with more negative ones. For example, a number of children reminisced about the good times they had shared with their deceased parent, but also at times recalled the pain caused by the death. Similarly, in their description of the deceased, children were more likely in the [follow-up] interview … to be willing to include a few "bad points" along with the deceased's "good points" that had been more easily shared with the interviewer. (Normand et al., 1996, p. 102)

These are also examples of the balanced, open, coherent attachment representations coded as secure in the AAI.

Distortions Encouraged by the Wish to Reject Bowlby's Analysis of Loss

Unfortunately, while providing many interesting examples of the kinds of processes that Bowlby analyzed in terms of searching and reorganizing working models, the authors of *Continuing Bonds* overlooked the implications of some of their most important findings. Because they wanted to criticize what they regarded as Bowlby's advocacy of "broken bonds," they uncritically celebrated all continuing bonds. In the process, they ignored data indicating that ambivalent or chronic grieving can be a sign of serious psychological difficulty. One of the problems with their "postmodern" perspective is that it oversimplifies the concept of dependence. Consider this passage from Silverman and Klass (1996, p. 16):

We can see the consequences of [modernism's] valuing autonomy in the criteria for what has been called pathological grief. In the dominant model of grief, dependence has often been seen as a condition for "pathological" grief. [For example], Raphael (1983) assumes that dependent personalities are more prone to pathological grief: " … it may be suggested that people with personal characteristics that lead them to form dependent, clinging, ambivalent relationships with their spouses are at greater risk of having a poor outcome" (p. 225).

In the first volume of his *Attachment and Loss* trilogy, Bowlby critically analyzed the concept of dependence (see Bowlby, 1969/1982, pp. 228–229; see also Ainsworth, 1969). He thought that psychoanalysts had failed to make an important distinction between two kinds of dependence: "secure" dependence and "anxious" dependence. In the case of secure dependence, a person is able to function in a free and autonomous manner due to the security afforded by an attachment figure, who can be

called upon when needed and who is confidently expected to be helpful. In the anxious case, however, autonomy and exploration are compromised by an attachment figure's uncertain accessibility.

Some of the examples from Rosenblatt's (1996) chapter illustrate the danger of considering all forms of dependence as adaptive. In line with the "postmodern" theme of the volume, he considers virtually any sign of prolonged grief and psychological pain healthy and common, even quotations such as the following—from an adult woman whose father died when she was an infant, decades before Rosenblatt interviewed her:

I … went through some stuff where I feel I caused the death, and that was really, really deep stuff, because I, it was, I couldn't verbalize it. It made no sense to me … but I think in searching, I had this sort of replacement idea, that once you had a birth you automatically had a death. And I got born so he died, you know. (p. 51)

This passage would probably score high on the "unresolved" AAI rating scale—a rating that has been associated with troubled childhoods, adult dissociative tendencies, and being at risk for inducing disorganized/disoriented attachment in one's children. (See Hesse, Chapter 25, and Lyons-Ruth & Jacobvitz, Chapter 28, this volume.)

In another chapter, Silverman and Nickman (1996) noted other individual differences reminiscent of the literature on disorganized attachment. They encountered bereaved children who could not answer the question "What advice would you give another child who had lost a parent?" Such children replied, "I don't know," or "I can't think of anything." The authors report that "these were the same children who did not dream about the deceased, and who did not talk to the deceased [in their minds]" (p. 80). These "I don't know" responses are similar to ones noted by Kaplan (1987; see also Slough & Greenberg, 1990) in a study of disorganized children's responses to the Separation Anxiety Test, a measure developed by Hansburg (1972) for adolescents and later modified for 4- to 7-year-old children by Klagsbrun and Bowlby (1976). (See Solomon & George, Chapter 18, this volume, for details.) In both Silverman and Nickman's (1996) study and in the studies of children classified as disorganized with respect to attachment, secure children *did* offer helpful suggestions, which reflected their ability to organize memories of their experiences and think about how they might be helpful to other children.

Normand and colleagues (1996) discuss four kinds of relationships that bereaved children constructed with their images of dead parents: "Seeing the Parent as a Visiting Ghost," "Holding on to Memories from the Past," "Maintaining an Interactive Relationship," and "Becoming a Living Legacy." The first kind, "Seeing the Parent as a Visiting Ghost," is especially interesting in light of the "unresolved trauma or loss" scale in the AAI coding system:

> [These] children conceived of their deceased parent as a ghost whose presence was frightening, unpredictable, and out of their control. . . . Most notably, [they] located the deceased as being "right beside me," unlike all the other children in the sample who located their deceased parent either in heaven or were uncertain about his/her location. Unlike any of the other children in the sample who reported feeling watched by the deceased, these children were frightened by the idea. At the 1-year interview, 12-year-old Justin explained, "Like, it's just quiet, and I think she's right there behind me and she's gonna . . . Like when I look in the mirror in the morning, like to comb my hair, I always think that she's gonna pop up behind me and scare me." . . . Children who experienced their parent as a visiting ghost did not feel sad or glad, only frightened. [They] said they "never" cried during the first year after the death. All the other children in the sample said they cried every day or at least several times a week at that time. (pp. 88–89)

Normand and colleagues found this pattern "difficult to explain," saying that the children appeared "very distraught" and had hardly changed after 2 years. "Despite the small number of indicators [collected in our study], we favor the interpretation that the parent–child relationship prior to the death must account in part for this representation" (p. 109). This conclusion is consistent with the notion that disorganized attachment results from an attachment figure's "frightened" or "frightening" behavior (e.g., Main & Hesse, 1990).

In a separate study of late-adolescent women whose fathers had died, described in a *Continuing Bonds* chapter by Tyson-Rawson (1996), 30% of the women who had some kind of continuing attachment to their fathers experienced an "intrusive presence" suggestive of insecure attachment. One woman said:

> After he died, I was so depressed that I couldn't go to school or sleep or anything. So they put me on an antidepressant. . . . Lately, I've been feeling that way again. I have these dreams, nightmares, and I can't

stop thinking about him dying. I think he's mad at me. . . . I don't know why, no, I think I feel this way because I never said good-bye to him. I knew he was dying and all that time I just stayed away, went to someone else's house. (p. 138)

Anxiety and guilt were commonly reported by such women. As Tyson-Rawson (1996) noted,

> These women's responses had a desperate, struggling quality. . . . [Their sense of intrusive presence was] typically expressed in nightmares, intrusive thoughts, and high levels of anxiety that debilitated the subject in one or more areas of functioning. . . . The common factor that united the experience of these . . . women was a sense of "unfinished business" (McGoldrick, 1991). Each reported thinking that she had not been able to effect closure in the relationship with her father. . . . [Two] had highly conflicted relationships with their fathers, characterized by cutoff from contact and minimal interaction. In comparison to those who welcomed their father's presence in their lives, *those who experienced an Intrusive Presence were unanimous in reporting no sense of having resolved their grief.* (pp. 128, 139; emphasis added)

In other words, a tendency toward preoccupied or disorganized attachment seems to have been involved in failure to resolve grief constructively, failure to view the lost attachment figure as a security provider within the realm of imagination, self-blame for the death, and failure to emphasize positive memories of interactions with the deceased while he was alive.

In the end, it is clear both that bereaved individuals do maintain mental representations of their relationships with deceased attachment figures (as Bowlby contended long before *Continuing Bonds*), and that these representations and the bonds they incorporate may partake of and contribute to either security or insecurity. Resolving grief, according to attachment theory, does not entail complete severance of affectional bonds or complete excision of mental representations of dead attachment figures.

Subsequent Writings on the Construct of Continuing Bonds

The *Continuing Bonds* book, which was based more on qualitative than on quantitative data, stimulated a flurry of more quantitative studies, many of which were reviewed by Boerner and Heckhausen (2003). They concluded, in line with our analysis (Fraley & Shaver, 1999), that "different types of connections [with the deceased] may be more or less adaptive" (p. 211). They also emphasized that when such connections were obtained in correlational studies, it was unclear which variable—grief severity or continuing bonds—was cause and which was effect, or what third factor might have caused the two variables to be related.

Subsequent studies (e.g., Field & Friedrichs, 2004; Field, Gal-Oz, & Bonanno, 2003) obtained results inconsistent with some of the earlier ones and also failed to discern causal relationships among key variables. In a review of this literature, M. Stroebe and Schut (2005) concluded that it was impossible to tell whether continuing bonds were generally beneficial or detrimental when coping with bereavement. In most studies, continuing bonds (at least as measured) were associated with grief severity, not with resolution. But this fact seemed partially attributable to content overlap in measures of grief severity and continuing-bonds (Schut, Stroebe, Boelen, & Zijerveld, 2006). In fact, most operationalizations of the continuing bonds construct seemed inadvertently to make continuing bonds a part of grieving. To make matters more confusing, Lalande and Bonanno (2007) found that the relation between continuing bonds and grief severity, assessed over time, differs between the United States and China.

Our earlier suggestion (Fraley & Shaver, 1999) that continuing bonds can take either secure or insecure forms, and in particular can be part of "unresolved" or "disorganized" attachment, has been most fully developed by Field (e.g., 2006). He points out that there is a huge difference between, on the one hand, thinking positively about a deceased attachment figure's admirable and loving qualities and incorporating some of this figure's positive qualities and goals into oneself, and, on the other hand, being haunted by the person's sudden (imagined) appearance (as in one of the examples quoted above) or being confused about whether the person is or is not still available in the physical world.[9] Viewed from this perspective, which is based on Main's (1991) conception of unresolved grief, the empirical studies conducted so far (most of which ask about concrete aspects of continuing bonds, such as keeping physical objects or clothes that belonged to the deceased or keeping the person in mind in various ways) do not seem adequate to resolve arguments about such bonds. A coded interview, based on insights from research with the AAI, might be more productive. The goal would be to determine how a

person represents, relates to, and talks about (coherently or incoherently) a particular deceased attachment figure.

Our conclusions are similar regarding therapeutic interventions based on the continuing-bonds construct. Whereas many psychotherapists were apparently taught in the past to help bereaved clients decathect and detach from mental representations of deceased attachment figures, many are now being taught to help bereaved clients continue their bonds with lost loved ones. In light of attachment theory and research, it would make more sense to help each person articulate his or her experiences and ideas about the loss, and move toward models of the lost attachment figure and the relationship that are maximally compatible with maintaining a secure stance toward the future. In cases where a person's memories and continuing bonds are positive, there is no reason to alter them (and perhaps no reason for them to be a focus of psychotherapy; Bonanno, 2004). In cases where a person's emotions and mental representations seem deeply conflicted, painful, disorganized, and incoherent, therapeutic interventions should be focused on more than continuing bonds per se. (Some examples can be found in an article by Malkinson, Rubin, & Witztum, 2006.)

Interestingly, in a commentary on the recent research articles about continuing bonds, Klass (2006), one of the authors of *Continuing Bonds*, distanced himself from the growing pro-bonds movement among bereavement counselors:

> As the idea of continuing bonds has made its way into the clinical lore, some clinicians and lay authors have mistaken a description (that survivors do maintain bonds) for a prescription (that it is helpful for survivors to do so). I have seen workshops advertised that promise techniques by which therapists and others can help the bereaved continue their bond with the deceased as if that were the sine qua non of good survivorship. My work is often cited wrongly as claiming that continuing bonds support better adjustment. If I have ever implied such a thing, I apologize. ... I did not and do not believe it is so. (p. 844)

It may require a postmodern perspective to square this quotation with one from Klass and colleagues' (1996b) preface: "Remaining connected seemed to facilitate both adults' and children's ability to cope with the loss and the accompanying changes in their lives. These "connections" provided solace, comfort and support, and eased the transition from the past to the future" (pp. xvii–xviii).

SUMMARY AND CONCLUSION

From a combination of attachment theory and numerous clinical case studies, Bowlby (1980) developed a theory of loss, grief, and mourning that remains the deepest and most comprehensive available. His theory is recognized as one of the major theories of bereavement (W. Stroebe & Stroebe, 1987), and it has generated an enormous amount of research on reactions to loss and individual differences in the way people respond to and adapt to loss. Not surprisingly, Bowlby's theory has also generated criticism and controversy. In this chapter, we have considered some of the main criticisms of the theory: (1) that grief may not follow a prescribed sequence of stages; (2) that failing to grieve intensely may be a sign of resilience and positive emotion, rather than of avoidant suppression; and (3) that "detachment" is ill advised and "continuing bonds" are more natural and desirable. In each case, we have considered the possibility that critics have mischaracterized Bowlby's views in an effort to supersede them. But we have also acknowledged that data collected and reported long after Bowlby's death make it clearer that many people weather losses without becoming disorganized, depressed, or vulnerable to later breakdown; that positive emotion plays a role in resilience; and that the stages Bowlby inferred from studies of young children's separations from and reunions with their parents may not apply directly or without modification to the course of normal grieving. We are still not sure what to think about avoidant defenses and the possibility that they hide vulnerabilities that may suddenly emerge under extreme stress. Our own experimental studies cause us to remain cautious about lumping avoidant suppression with secure resilience, but we admit that the data collected to date in studies of grief, with a few notable exceptions, do not allow us to distinguish avoidant from secure grieving. This is an important issue for future research.

The field of bereavement studies has made several advances over the studies from Bowlby's era. There are beginning to be prospective studies, which allow us to see how prebereavement experiences and mental health affect postbereavement reactions. There is a clearer distinction emerging between normal grief and complicated or prolonged grief (the latter is likely to be a consequence, in part, of anxious attachment). There is a more explicit recognition that there are continuing bonds, and that those bonds can be either adaptive or maladaptive—in the latter case, being closely associated with what AAI researchers call "unresolved loss or trauma." The clinical application of all the new and old insights will require considerable judgment and training, because it is clear that there is no one-size-fits-all form of therapy that will work or be helpful for every bereaved individual.

Bowlby was not able to answer every important question about grief and mourning. Nevertheless, having reconsidered his work in light of what came before and what has come since, we are humbled by his ability to incorporate so much of the available evidence while keeping an eye on a coherent, comprehensive, and deep theory of human attachment and loss. His work will continue to inform researchers and clinicians interested in bereavement.

ACKNOWLEDGMENTS

We would like to thank the following people for providing us with new material from their own research and writing programs: George Bonanno, Mario Mikulincer, Margaret Stroebe, and Camille Wortman. We also thank Mario Mikulincer and Jude Cassidy for commenting on previous drafts of this chapter.

NOTES

1. Following now-standard usage (see Zhang, El-Jawahri, & Prigerson, 2006), we use the term "bereavement" for the state of having lost an attachment figure or loved one to death, and the terms "grief" and "mourning" to refer to the emotional distress associated with that loss.

2. A degree of numbing, combined with other emotions, is common even when a bereaved individual has anticipated a partner's death. In a recent book written mostly by her dying husband (O'Kelly, 2006), Corinne O'Kelly describes how she felt immediately after her husband died, 3 months after learning he had an inoperable brain tumor: "Now that Gene's journey was over, I was somewhat relieved. *I felt numb the rest of the evening.* ... The next morning, I felt sublime joy and tranquility. The pain of loss would set in later. ... Gene had left in peace" (p. 172; emphasis added). (This quotation also shows how difficult it may be to get an accurate assessment of a bereaved individual's emotional state shortly after a loss.)

3. See Plimpton and Rosenblum (1987) and Laudenslager, Boccia, and Reite (1993) for reviews of additional studies of reactions to loss in nonhuman primates. See Hennessy, Deak, and Schiml-Webb (2001) and Hennessy and colleagues (2007) for recent evidence that some of the passivity is due to

stress-induced "sickness behavior," which can be counteracted with anti-inflammatory medications. This latter idea has yet to be applied in studies of humans.

4. A PsycINFO search using the keywords "grief" and "culture" turns up many interesting recent studies, but each goes into detail about a particular culture and a particular kind of loss, which is not the purpose of the present chapter.

5. Bowlby (1980) also discussed "compulsive caregiving" as a disordered form of mourning. Because of space limitations and the relative lack of research examining this pattern, we do not discuss it further in this chapter.

6. The three attachment patterns are actually locations in a two- rather than a three-dimensional space (see Crowell, Fraley, & Shaver, Chapter 26, this volume), but it is possible to draw a diagonal dimension across the space, with avoidance and resistance lying at the two ends of the dimension and attachment security located in the middle.

7. As readers of this volume know, there is a fourth infant category, disorganized/disoriented, discussed by Solomon and George (Chapter 18, this volume) and Lyons-Ruth and Jacobvitz (Chapter 28, this volume). This category, identified by Main and Solomon (1990), was added after Bowlby (1980) wrote about loss and after Ainsworth and colleagues (1978) wrote about the Strange Situation.

8. Typical measures can be found in Brennan, Clark, and Shaver (1998); Fraley, Waller, and Brennan (2000); and Chapter 4 of Mikulincer and Shaver (2007). Interesting new measures by a pioneer bereavement researcher can be found in Parkes (2006). Parkes's measures are based on questions about childhood experiences and relationships with parents rather than adolescent and adult relationship experiences. Parkes used these measures in an interesting study of normal and pathological grieving, finding much support for hypotheses based on attachment theory. His book also provides many provocative and insight-generating clinical case studies.

9. Epstein, Kalus, and Berger (2006) showed that even when specific scales were used to measure continuing bonds, bereaved individuals with similar scores could differ considerably in psychologically significant ways: "One participant, whose scores on the measures of pathological grief were elevated ... , said that she could sometimes sense the odor of her husband in the house and this would upset her. By contrast, another participant ... said, "I don't feel he has completely gone—I can feel his presence in the house, and this makes me feel good" (p. 263).

REFERENCES

Adam, K. S., Sheldon-Keller, A. E., & West, M. (1995). Attachment organization and vulnerability to loss, separation, and abuse in disturbed adolescents. In S. Goldberg, R. Muir, & J. Kerr (Eds.), *Attachment theory: Social, developmental, and clinical perspectives* (pp. 309–341). Hillsdale, NJ: Analytic Press.

Ainsworth, M. D. S. (1969). Object relations, dependency, and attachment: A theoretical review of the infant–mother relationship. *Child Development, 40,* 969–1025.

Ainsworth, M. D. S., Blehar, M. C., Waters, E., & Wall, S. (1978). *Patterns of attachment: A psychological study of the Strange Situation.* Hillsdale, NJ: Erlbaum.

Ainsworth, M. D. S., & Eichberg, C. (1991). Effects on infant–mother attachment of mother's unresolved loss of an attachment figure, or other traumatic experience. In C. M. Parkes, J. Stevenson-Hinde, & P. Marris (Eds.), *Attachment across the life cycle* (pp. 160–183). London: Routledge.

Alonso-Arbiol, I., Shaver, P. R., & Yarnoz, S. (2002). Insecure attachment, gender roles, and interpersonal dependency in the Basque country. *Personal Relationships, 9,* 479–490.

American Psychiatric Association. (2000). *Diagnostic and statistical manual of mental disorders* (4th ed., text rev.). Washington, DC: American Psychiatric Association.

Archer, J. (1999). *The nature of grief: The evolution and psychology of reactions to loss.* New York: Routledge.

Balk, D. E. (1996). Attachment and the reactions of bereaved college students: A longitudinal study. In D. Klass, P. R. Silverman, & S. L. Nickman (Eds.), *Continuing bonds: New understandings of grief* (pp. 311–328). Washington, DC: Taylor & Francis.

Bartholomew, K., & Horowitz, L. M. (1991). Attachment styles among young adults: A test of a four-category model. *Journal of Personality and Social Psychology, 61,* 226–244.

Berant, E., Mikulincer, M., & Florian, V. (2001). Attachment style and mental health: A one-year follow-up study of mothers of infants with congenital heart disease. *Personality and Social Psychology Bulletin, 8,* 956–968.

Berant, E., Mikulincer, M., & Shaver, P. R. (2008). Mothers' attachment style, their mental health, and their children's emotional vulnerabilities: A 7-year study of mothers of children with congenital heart disease. *Journal of Personality, 76,* 31–65.

Boelen, P. A., van den Bout, J., & de Keijser, J. (2003). Traumatic grief as a disorder distinct from bereavement-related depression and anxiety: A replication study with bereaved mental health care patients. *American Journal of Psychiatry, 160,* 1339–1341.

Boelen, P. A., van den Bout, J., & van den Hout, M. A. (2003). The role of cognitive variables in psychological functioning after the death of a first degree relative. *Behaviour Research and Therapy, 41,* 1123–1136.

Boelen, P. A., van den Bout, M. A., & van den Hout, J. (2006). A cognitive-behavioral conceptualization of complicated grief. *Clinical Psychology: Science and Practice, 13,* 109–128.

Boerner, K., & Heckhausen, J. (2003). To have and have not: Adaptive bereavement by transforming mental ties to the deceased. *Death Studies, 27*, 199–226.

Bonanno, G. (2001). Grief and emotion: A social-functional perspective. In M. Stroebe, W. Stroebe, R. O. Hansson, & H. A. W. Schut (Eds.), *Handbook of bereavement research: Consequences, coping, and care* (pp. 493–515). Washington, DC: American Psychological Association.

Bonanno, G. (2004). Loss, trauma, and human resilience: Have we underestimated the human capacity to thrive after extremely aversive events? *American Psychologist, 59*, 20–28.

Bonanno, G. A., & Field, N. P. (2001). Evaluating the delayed grief hypothesis across 5 years of bereavement. *American Behavioral Scientist, 44*, 798–816.

Bonanno, G. A., & Kaltman, S. (1999). Toward an integrative perspective on bereavement. *Psychological Bulletin, 125*, 760–786.

Bonanno, G. A., & Kaltman, S. (2001). The varieties of grief experience. *Clinical Psychology Review, 21*, 705–734.

Bonanno, G. A., Keltner, D., Holen, A., & Horowitz, M. J. (1995). When avoiding unpleasant emotions might not be such a bad thing: Verbal–autonomic response dissociation and midlife conjugal bereavement. *Journal of Personality and Social Psychology, 69*, 975–989.

Bonanno, G. A., Moskowitz, J. T., Papa, A., & Folkman, S. (2005). Resilience to loss in bereaved spouses, bereaved parents, and bereaved gay men. *Journal of Personality and Social Psychology, 88*, 827–843.

Bonanno, G. A., Neria, Y., Mancini, A., Coifman, K. G., Litz, B., & Insel, B. (2007). Is there more to complicated grief than depression and posttraumatic stress disorder?: A test of incremental validity. *Journal of Abnormal Psychology, 116*, 342–351.

Bonanno, G. A., Papa, A., Lalande, K., Westphal, M., & Coifman, K. (2004). The importance of being flexible: The ability to both enhance and suppress emotional expression predicts long-term adjustment. *Psychological Science, 15*, 482–487.

Bonanno, G. A., Papa, A., Lalande, K., Zhang, N., & Noll, J. G. (2005). Grief processing and deliberate grief avoidance: A prospective comparison of bereaved spouses and parents in the United States and the People's Republic of China. *Journal of Consulting and Clinical Psychology, 73*, 86–98.

Bonanno, G. A., Wortman, C. B., Lehman, D., Tweed, R., Sonnega, J., Carr, D., et al. (2002). Resilience to loss, chronic grief, and their pre-bereavement predictors. *Journal of Personality and Social Psychology, 83*, 1150–1164.

Bonanno, G. A., Wortman, C. B., & Nesse, R. M. (2004). Prospective patterns of resilience and maladjustment during widowhood. *Psychology and Aging, 19*, 260–271.

Bornstein, P. E., Clayton, P. J., Halikas, J. A., Maurice, W. L., & Robins, E. (1973). The depression of widowhood after thirteen months. *British Journal of Psychiatry, 122*, 561–566.

Bowlby, J. (1946). *Forty-four juvenile thieves: Their characters and home-life.* London: Bailliére, Tindall, & Cox.

Bowlby, J. (1969/1982). *Attachment and loss: Vol. 1. Attachment.* New York: Basic Books.

Bowlby, J. (1973). *Attachment and loss: Vol. 2. Separation: Anxiety and anger.* New York: Basic Books.

Bowlby, J. (1980). *Attachment and loss: Vol. 3. Loss: Sadness and depression.* New York: Basic Books.

Bowlby, J. (1990). *Charles Darwin: A new life.* New York: Norton.

Bowlby, R. (2005). Introduction. In J. Bowlby, *The making and breaking of affectional bonds* (Routledge Classics ed.). New York: Routledge.

Brennan, K. A., Clark, C. L., & Shaver, P. R. (1998). Self-report measurement of adult romantic attachment: An integrative overview. In J. A. Simpson & W. S. Rholes (Eds.), *Attachment theory and close relationships* (pp. 46–76). New York: Guilford Press.

Carnelley, K. B., Wortman, C. B., Bolger, N., & Burke, C. T. (2007). The time course of grief reactions to spousal loss: Evidence from a national probability sample. *Journal of Personality and Social Psychology, 91*, 476–492.

Cassidy, J., & Berlin, L. J. (1994). The insecure/ambivalent pattern of attachment: Theory and research. *Child Development, 65*, 971–991.

Cassidy, J., & Kobak, R. R. (1988). Avoidance and its relation to other defensive processes. In J. Belsky & T. Nezworski (Eds.), *Clinical implications of attachment* (pp. 300–323). Hillsdale, NJ: Erlbaum.

Clayton, P. J., Halikas, J. A., & Maurice, W. L. (1972). The depression of widowhood. *British Journal of Psychiatry, 120*, 71–76.

Coifman, K. G., Bonanno, G. A., Ray, R. D., & Gross, J. J. (2007). Does repressive coping promote resilience?: Affective–autonomic response discrepancy during bereavement. *Journal of Personality and Social Psychology, 92*, 745–758.

Currier, J. M., Holland, J. M., & Neimeyer, R. A. (2006). Sense-making, grief, and the experience of violent loss: Toward a mediational model. *Death Studies, 30*, 403–428.

Deutsch, H. (1937). Absence of grief. *Psychoanalytic Quarterly, 6*, 12–22.

Edelstein, R. S., & Shaver, P. R. (2004). Avoidant attachment: Exploration of an oxymoron. In D. Mashek & A. Aron (Eds.), *Handbook of closeness and intimacy* (pp. 397–412). Mahwah, NJ: Erlbaum.

Epstein, R., Kalus, C., & Berger, M. (2006). The continuing bonds of the bereaved towards the deceased and adjustment to loss. *Mortality, 11*, 253–269.

Field, N. P. (2006). Continuing bonds in adaptation to bereavement: Introduction. *Death Studies, 30*, 709–714.

Field, N. P., & Friedrichs, M. (2004). Continuing bonds in coping with the death of a husband. *Death Studies, 28*, 597–620.

Field, N. P., Gal-Oz, E., & Bonanno, G. A. (2003). Continuing bonds and adjustment at 5 years after the death of a spouse. *Journal of Consulting and Clinical Psychology, 71*, 110–117.

Field, N. P., & Sundin, E. C. (2001). Attachment style in adjustment to conjugal bereavement. *Journal of Social and Personal Relationships, 18*, 347–361.

Foa, E. B., & Rothbaum, B. O. (1998). *Treating the trauma of rape: Cognitive-behavioral therapy for PTSD.* New York: Guilford Press.

Fraley, R. C., & Bonanno, G. A. (2004). Attachment and loss: A test of three competing models on the association between attachment-related avoidance and adaptation to bereavement. *Personality and Social Psychology Bulletin, 30*, 878–890.

Fraley, R. C., Davis, K. E., & Shaver, P. R. (1997). *Attachment behavior and romantic relationship dissolution.* Unpublished manuscript, University of California, Davis.

Fraley, R. C., Davis, K. E., & Shaver, P. R. (1998). Dismissing-avoidance and the defensive organization of emotion, cognition, and behavior. In J. A. Simpson & W. S. Rholes (Eds.), *Attachment theory and close relationships* (pp. 249–279). New York: Guilford Press.

Fraley, R. C., Fazzari, D. A., Bonanno, G. A., & Dekel, S. (2006). Attachment and psychological adaptation in high exposure survivors of the September 11th attack on the World Trade Center. *Personality and Social Psychology Bulletin, 32*, 538–551.

Fraley, R. C., Garner, J. P., & Shaver, P. R. (2000). Adult attachment and the defensive regulation of attention and memory: Examining the role of preemptive and postemptive defensive processes. *Journal of Personality and Social Psychology, 79*, 816–826.

Fraley, R. C., & Shaver, P. R. (1997). Adult attachment and the suppression of unwanted thoughts. *Journal of Personality and Social Psychology, 73*, 1080–1091.

Fraley, R. C., & Shaver, P. R. (1998). Airport separations: A naturalistic study of adult attachment behavior and dynamics in separating couples. *Journal of Personality and Social Psychology, 75*, 1198–1212.

Fraley, R. C., & Shaver, P. R. (1999). Loss and bereavement: Attachment theory and recent controversies concerning "grief work" and the nature of detachment. In J. Cassidy & P. R. Shaver (Eds.), *Handbook of attachment: Theory, research, and clinical applications* (pp. 735–759). New York: Guilford Press.

Fraley, R. C., & Shaver, P. R. (2000). Adult romantic attachment: Theoretical developments, emerging controversies, and unanswered questions. *Review of General Psychology, 4*, 132–154.

Fraley, R. C., Waller, N. G., & Brennan, K. A. (2000). An item response theory analysis of self-report measures of adult attachment. *Journal of Personality and Social Psychology, 78*, 350–365.

Freud, E. L. (Ed.). (1960). *Letters of Sigmund Freud* (T. Strachey & J. Strachey, Trans.). New York: Basic Books.

Freud, S. (1957). Mourning and melancholia. In J. Strachey (Ed. & Trans.), *The standard edition of the complete psychological works of Sigmund Freud* (Vol. 14, pp. 237–260). New York: Basic Books. (Original work published 1917)

Freud, S. (1959). Inhibitions, symptoms, and anxiety. In J. Strachey (Ed. & Trans.), *The standard edition of the complete psychological works of Sigmund Freud* (Vol. 20, pp. 75–175). London: Hogarth Press. (Original work published 1926)

Futterman, A., Gallagher, D., Thompson, L. W., Lovett, S., & Gilewski, M. (1990). Retrospective assessment of marital adjustment and depression during the first two years of spousal bereavement. *Psychology and Aging, 5*, 277–283.

George, C., Kaplan, N., & Main, M. (1984). *Adult Attachment Interview protocol.* Unpublished manuscript, University of California, Berkeley.

George, C., Kaplan, N., & Main, M. (1985). *Adult Attachment Interview protocol* (2nd ed.). Unpublished manuscript, University of California, Berkeley.

George, C., Kaplan, N., & Main, M. (1996). *Adult Attachment Interview protocol* (3rd ed.). Unpublished manuscript, University of California, Berkeley.

Gilbert, S. M. (2006). *Death's door: Modern dying and the ways we grieve.* New York: Norton.

Gillath, O., Bunge, S. A., Shaver, P. R., Wendelken, C., & Mikulincer, M. (2005). Attachment-style differences in the ability to suppress negative thoughts: Exploring the neural correlates. *NeuroImage, 28*, 835–847.

Gillies, J., & Neimeyer, R. A. (2006). Loss, grief, and the search for significance: Toward a model of meaning reconstruction in bereavement. *Journal of Constructivist Psychology, 19*, 31–65.

Glick, I. O., Weiss, R. S., & Parkes, C. M. (1974). *The first year of bereavement.* New York: Wiley.

Hansburg, H. G. (1972). *Adolescent separation anxiety: Vol. 1. A method for the study of adolescent separation problems.* Springfield, IL: Thomas.

Hart, C. L., Hole, D. J., Lawlor, D. A., Smith, G. D., & Lever, T. F. (2007). Effect of conjugal bereavement on mortality of the bereaved spouse in participants of the Renfrew/Paisley Study. *Journal of Epidemiology and Community Health, 61*, 455–460.

Harwood, D. M. J., Hawton, K., Hope, T., Harriss, L., & Jacoby, R. (2006). Life problems and physical illness as risk factors for suicide in older people: A descriptive and case-control study. *Psychological Medicine, 36*, 1265–1274.

Heinicke, C. M., & Westheimer, I. J. (1965). *Brief separations.* New York: International Universities Press.

Hennessy, M. B., Deak, T., & Schiml-Webb, P. A. (2001). Stress-induced sickness behaviors: An alternative hypothesis for responses during maternal separation. *Developmental Psychobiology, 39*, 76–83.

Hennessy, M. B., Schiml-Webb, P. A., Miller, E. E., Maken, D. S., Bullinger, K. L., & Deak, T. (2007). Anti-inflammatory agents attenuate the passive responses of guinea pig pups: Evidence for stress-induced sickness behavior during maternal separation. *Psychoneuroendocrinology, 32*, 508–515.

Hogan, N., & DeSantis, L. (1992). Adolescent sibling

bereavement: An ongoing attachment. *Qualitative Health Research, 2*, 159–177.

Horowitz, M. (1997). *Stress response syndromes* (3rd ed.). Northvale, NJ: Aronson.

Jacobs, S. (1993). *Pathologic grief: Maladaptation to loss.* Washington, DC: American Psychiatric Press.

Jacobs, S., Hansen, F., Berkman, L., Kasl, S., & Ostfeld, A. (1989). Depressions of bereavement. *Comprehensive Psychiatry, 30*, 218–224.

Jacobs., S., Mazure, C., & Prigerson, H. (2000). Diagnostic criteria for traumatic grief. *Death Studies, 24*, 185–199.

Jordan, J. R., & Neimeyer, R. A. (2003). Does grief counseling work? *Death Studies, 27*, 763–786.

Kaplan, N. (1987). *Individual differences in six-year-olds' thoughts about separation: Predicted from attachment to mother at one year of age.* Unpublished doctoral dissertation, University of California, Berkeley.

Klagsbrun, M., & Bowlby, J. (1976). Responses to separation from parents: A clinical test for children. *British Journal of Projective Psychology, 21*, 7–21.

Klass, D. (2006). Continuing conversation about continuing bonds. *Death Studies, 30*, 843–858.

Klass, D., Silverman, P. R., & Nickman, S. L. (Eds.). (1996a). *Continuing bonds: New understandings of grief.* Washington, DC: Taylor & Francis.

Klass, D., Silverman, P. R., & Nickman, S. L. (1996b). Preface. In D. Klass, P. R. Silverman, & S. L. Nickman (Eds.), *Continuing bonds: New understandings of grief* (pp. xvii–xxi). Washington, DC: Taylor & Francis.

Lalande, K. M., & Bonanno, G. A. (2007). Culture and continuing bonds: A prospective comparison of bereavement in the United States and the People's Republic of China. *Death Studies, 30*, 303–324.

Larson, D. G., & Hoyt, W. T. (2007). What has become of grief counseling?: An evaluation of the empirical foundations of the new pessimism. *Professional Psychology: Research and Practice, 38*, 347–355.

Laudenslager, M. L., Boccia, M. L., & Reite, M. L. (1993). Biobehavioral consequences of loss in nonhuman primates: Individual differences. In M. S. Stroebe, W. Stroebe, & R. O. Hansson (Eds.), *Handbook of bereavement: Theory, research, and intervention* (pp. 129–142). New York: Cambridge University Press.

Lewis, C. S. (1961). *A grief observed.* London: Faber & Faber.

Lichtenthal, W. G., Cruess, D. G., & Prigerson, H. G. (2004). A case for establishing complicated grief as a distinct mental disorder in DSM-V. *Clinical Psychology Review, 24*, 637–662.

Lorenz, K. (1963). *On aggression.* New York: Bantam.

Lumley, M. A., Tojeck, T. M., & Macklem, D. J. (2002). The effects of written and verbal disclosure among repressive and alexithymic people. In S. J. Lepore & J. M. Smyth (Eds.), *The writing cure: How expressive writing promotes health and emotional well-being* (pp. 75–95). Washington, DC: American Psychological Association.

Lund, D. A., Caserta, M. S., Dimond, M. F., & Shaffer, S. K. (1989). Competencies, tasks of daily living, and adjustments to spousal bereavement in later life. In D. A. Lund (Ed.), *Older bereaved spouses: Research with practical applications* (pp. 135–152). Washington, DC: Taylor & Francis.

Lund, D. A., Dimond, M. F., Caserta, M. S., Johnson, R. J., Poulton, J. L., & Connelly, J. R. (1985). Identifying elderly with coping difficulties after two years of bereavement. *Omega, 16*, 213–223.

Maciejewski, P. K., Zhang, B., Block, S. D., & Prigerson, H. G. (2007). An empirical examination of the stage theory of grief. *Journal of the American Medical Association, 297*, 716–723.

Main, M. (1991). Metacognitive knowledge, metacognitive monitoring, and singular (coherent) vs. multiple (incoherent) model of attachment: Findings and directions for future research. In C. M. Parkes, J. Stevenson-Hinde, & P. Marris (Eds.), *Attachment across the life cycle* (pp. 127–159). London: Tavistock/Routledge.

Main, M., & Goldwyn, R. (1984). *Adult attachment scoring and classification system.* Unpublished manuscript, University of California, Berkeley.

Main, M., Goldwyn, R., & Hesse, E. (2003). *Adult attachment scoring and classification system.* Unpublished manuscript, University of California, Berkeley.

Main, M., & Hesse, E. (1990). Parents' unresolved traumatic experiences are related to infant disorganized attachment status: Is frightened and/or frightening parental behavior the linking mechanism? In M. T. Greenberg, D. Cicchetti, & E. M. Cummings (Eds.), *Attachment in the preschool years: Theory, research, and intervention* (pp. 161–182). Chicago: University of Chicago Press.

Main, M., & Solomon, J. (1990). Procedures for identifying infants as disorganized/disoriented during the Ainsworth Strange Situation. In M. T. Greenberg, D. Cicchetti, & M. Cummings (Eds.), *Attachment in the preschool years: Theory, research, and intervention* (pp. 121–160). Chicago: University of Chicago Press.

Malkinson, R., Rubin, S. S., & Witztum, E. (2006). Therapeutic issues and the relationship to the deceased: Working clinically with the two-track model of bereavement. *Death Studies, 30*, 797–815.

Mathison, J. (1970). A cross-cultural view of widowhood. *Omega, 1*, 201–218.

McGoldrick, M. (1991). The legacy of loss. In F. Walsh & M. McGoldrick (Eds.), *Living beyond loss: Death in the family* (pp. 104–129). New York: Norton.

Middleton, W., Raphael, B., Martinek, N., & Misso, V. (1993). Pathological grief reactions. In M. S. Stroebe, W. Stroebe, & R. O. Hansson (Eds.), *Handbook of bereavement: Theory, research, and intervention* (pp. 44–61). New York: Cambridge University Press.

Mikulincer, M., Dolev, T., & Shaver, P. R. (2004). Attachment-related strategies during thought-suppression: Ironic rebounds and vulnerable self-representations. *Journal of Personality and Social Psychology, 87,* 940–956.

Mikulincer, M., Florian, V., & Weller, A. (1993). Attachment styles, coping strategies, and posttraumatic psychological distress: The impact of the Gulf war in Israel. *Journal of Personality and Social Psychology, 64,* 817–826.

Mikulincer, M., & Orbach, I. (1995). Attachment styles and repressive defensiveness: The accessibility and architecture of affective memories. *Journal of Personality and Social Psychology, 68,* 917–925.

Mikulincer, M., & Shaver, P. R. (2007). *Attachment in adulthood: Structure, dynamics, and change.* New York: Guilford Press.

Mikulincer, M., & Shaver, P. R. (in press). An attachment perspective on bereavement. In M. S. Stroebe, R. O. Hansson, W. Stroebe, & H. A. W. Schut (Eds.), *Handbook of bereavement research and practice: 21st century perspectives.* Washington, DC: American Psychological Association.

Miller, S. I., & Schoenfeld, L. (1973). Grief in the Navajo: Psychodynamics and culture. *International Journal of Social Psychiatry, 19,* 187–191.

Moskowitz, J. T., Folkman, S., & Acree, M. (2003). Do positive psychological states shed light on recovery from bereavement?: Findings from a 3-year longitudinal study. *Death Studies, 27,* 471–500.

Nager, E. A., & de Vries, B. (2004). Memorializing on the World Wide Web: Patterns of grief and attachment in adult daughters of deceased mothers. *Omega, 49,* 43–56.

Neimeyer, R. A., Prigerson, H. G., & Davies, B. (2002). Mourning and meaning. *American Behavioral Scientist, 46,* 235–241.

Noftle, E. E., & Shaver, P. R. (2006). Attachment dimensions and the big five personality traits: Associations and comparative ability to predict relationship quality. *Journal of Research in Personality, 40,* 179–208.

Norman, S. A., Lumley, M. A., Dooley, J. A., & Diamond, M. P. (2004) For whom does it work?: Moderators of the effects of written emotional disclosure in a randomized trial among women with chronic pelvic pain. *Psychosomatic Medicine, 66,* 174–183.

Normand, C. L., Silverman, P. R., & Nickman, S. L. (1996). Bereaved children's changing relationships with the deceased. In D. Klass, P. R. Silverman, & S. L. Nickman (Eds.), *Continuing bonds: New understandings of grief* (pp. 87–111). Washington, DC: Taylor & Francis.

Ogrodniczuk, J. S., Piper, W. E., Joyce, A. S., Weideman, R., McCallum, M., Azim, H. F., et al. (2003). Differentiating symptoms of complicated grief and depression among psychiatric outpatients. *Canadian Journal of Psychiatry/Revue Canadienne de Psychiatrie, 48,* 87–93.

O'Kelly, E. (2006). *Chasing daylight: How my forthcoming death transformed my life.* New York: McGraw-Hill.

Ong, A. D., Bergeman, C. S., & Bisconti, T. L. (2004). The role of daily positive emotions during conjugal bereavement. *Journals of Gerontology: Series B. Psychological Sciences and Social Psychology, 59B,* 168–176.

Parkes, C. M. (1965). Bereavement and mental illness. *British Journal of Medical Psychology, 38,* 388–397.

Parkes, C. M. (1985). Bereavement. *British Journal of Psychiatry, 146,* 11–17.

Parkes, C. M. (2006). *Love and loss: The roots of grief and its complications.* New York: Taylor & Francis.

Parkes, C. M., & Weiss, R. S. (1983). *Recovery from bereavement.* New York: Basic Books.

Pereg, D., & Mikulincer, M. (2004). Attachment style and the regulation of negative affect: Exploring individual differences in mood congruency effects on memory and judgment. *Personality and Social Psychology Bulletin, 30,* 67–80.

Peterson, C. (2006). *A primer in positive psychology.* New York: Oxford University Press.

Plimpton, E. H., & Rosenblum, L. A. (1987). Maternal loss in nonhuman primates: Implications for human development. In J. Bloom-Feshbach & S. Bloom-Feshbach (Eds.), *The psychology of separation and loss* (pp. 63–86). San Francisco: Jossey-Bass.

Poole, J. H. (1996). *Coming of age with elephants.* New York: Hyperion.

Prigerson, H. G., Bierhals, A. J., Kasl, S. V., Reynolds, C. F., III, Shear, M. K., Newsom, J. T., et al. (1996). Complicated grief as a disorder distinct from bereavement-related depression and anxiety: A replication study. *American Journal of Psychiatry, 153,* 1484–1486.

Prigerson, H. G., Maciejewski, P. K., Newson, J., Reynolds, C. F., & Frank, E. (1995). The Inventory of Complicated Grief: A scale to measure maladaptive symptoms of loss. *Psychiatry Research, 59,* 65–79.

Prigerson, H. G., Vanderwerker, L. C., & Maciejewski, P. K. (in press). Prolonged grief disorder as a mental disorder: Inclusion in the *DSM.* In M. S. Stroebe, R. O. Hansson, W. Stroebe, & H. A. W. Schut (Eds.), *Handbook of bereavement research and practice: 21st century perspectives.* Washington, DC: American Psychological Association.

Raphael, B. (1983). *The anatomy of bereavement.* New York: Basic Books.

Reite, M., & Boccia, M. L. (1994). Physiological aspects of adult attachment. In M. B. Sperling & W. H. Berman (Eds.), *Attachment in adults* (pp. 98–127). New York: Guilford Press.

Roisman, G. I., Tsai, J. L., & Chiang, K. H. (2004). The emotional integration of childhood experience: Physiological, facial expressive, and self-reported emotional response during the Adult Attachment Interview. *Developmental Psychology, 40,* 776–789.

Rosenblatt, P. C. (1996). Grief that does not end. In D. Klass, P. R. Silverman, & S. L. Nickman (Eds.), *Continuing bonds: New understandings of grief* (pp. 45–58). Washington, DC: Taylor & Francis.

Rosenblatt, P. C., Walsh, R. P., & Jackson, D. A. (1976). *Grief and mourning in cross-cultural perspective.* New Haven, CT: Human Relations Area Files.

Schut, H. A. W., Stroebe, M. S., Boelen, P. A., & Zijerveld, A. M. (2006). Continuing relationships with the deceased: Disentangling bonds and grief. *Death Studies, 30,* 757–766.

Schut, H. A. W., Stroebe, M. S., & van den Bout, J. (1997). Intervention for the bereaved: Gender differences in the efficacy of two counselling programmes. *British Journal of Clinical Psychology, 36,* 63–72.

Seay, B., Hansen, E., & Harlow, H. F. (1962). Mother–infant separation in monkeys. *Journal of Child Psychology and Psychiatry, 3,* 123–132.

Shaver, P. R., & Brennan, K. A. (1992). Attachment styles and the "Big Five" personality traits: Their connections with each other and with romantic relationship outcomes. *Personality and Social Psychology Bulletin, 18,* 536–545.

Shaver, P. R., & Mikulincer, M. (2005). Attachment theory and research: Resurrection of the psychodynamic approach to personality. *Journal of Research in Personality, 39,* 22–45.

Shaver, P. R., Schachner, D. A., & Mikulincer, M. (2005). Attachment style, excessive reassurance seeking, relationship processes, and depression. *Personality and Social Psychology Bulletin, 31,* 1–17.

Shaver, P. R., & Tancredy, C. M. (2001). Emotion, attachment, and bereavement: A conceptual commentary. In M. S. Stroebe, W. Stroebe, R. O. Hansson, & H. Schut (Eds.), *Handbook of bereavement research: Consequences, coping, and care* (pp. 63–88). Washington, DC: American Psychological Association.

Shear, K., Frank, E., Houck, P. R., & Reynolds, C. F. (2005). Treatment of complicated grief: A randomized controlled trial. *Journal of the American Medical Association, 293,* 2601–2608.

Shuchter, S., & Zisook, S. (1993). The course of normal grief. In M. Stroebe, W. Stroebe, & R. O. Hansson (Eds.), *Handbook of bereavement: Theory, research, and intervention* (pp. 23–43). New York: Cambridge University Press.

Silverman, P. R., & Klass, D. (1996). Introduction: What's the problem? In D. Klass, P. R. Silverman, & S. L. Nickman (Eds.), *Continuing bonds: New understandings of grief* (pp. 3–25). Washington, DC: Taylor & Francis.

Silverman, P. R., & Nickman, S. L. (1996). Children's construction of their dead parents. In D. Klass, P. R. Silverman, & S. L. Nickman (Eds.), *Continuing bonds: New understandings of grief* (pp. 73–86). Washington, DC: Taylor & Francis.

Silverman, P. R., Nickman, S., & Worden, J. W. (1992). Detachment revisited: The child's reconstruction of a dead parent. *American Journal of Orthopsychiatry, 62,* 494–503.

Simon, N. M., Shear, K. M., Thompson, E. H., Zalta, A. K., Perlman, C., Reynolds, C. F., et al. (2007). The prevalence and correlates of psychiatric comorbidity in individuals with complicated grief. *Comprehensive Psychiatry, 48,* 395–399.

Slough, N. M., & Greenberg, M. T. (1990). Five-year-olds' representations of separation from parents: Responses from the perspective of self and other. *New Directions for Child Development, 48,* 67–84.

Sroufe, L. A., & Waters, E. (1977). Attachment as an organizational construct. *Child Development, 48,* 1184–1199.

Stroebe, M., Folkman, S., Hansson, R. O., & Schut, H. (2006). The prediction of bereavement outcome: Development of an integrative risk factor framework. *Social Science and Medicine, 63,* 2440–2451.

Stroebe, M., & Schut, H. (1999). The dual process model of coping with bereavement: Rationale and description. *Death Studies, 23,* 197–224.

Stroebe, M., & Schut, H. (2005). To continue or relinquish bonds: A review of consequences for the bereaved. *Death Studies, 29,* 477–494.

Stroebe, M., Schut, H., & Stroebe, W. (2005). Attachment in coping with bereavement: A theoretical integration. *Review of General Psychology, 9,* 48–66.

Stroebe, M., Schut, H., & Stroebe, W. (2007). Health outcomes in bereavement. *Lancet, 370,* 1960–1973.

Stroebe, M., & Stroebe, W. (1993). The mortality of bereavement: A review. In M. S. Stroebe, W. Stroebe, & R. O. Hansson (Eds.), *Handbook of bereavement: Theory, research, and intervention* (pp. 175–195). New York: Cambridge University Press.

Stroebe, M., Stroebe, W., & Abakoumkin, G. (2005). The broken heart: Suicidal ideation in bereavement. *American Journal of Psychiatry, 162,* 2178–2180.

Stroebe, M., van Son, M., Stroebe, W., Kleber, R., Schut, H., & van den Bout, J. (2000). On the classification and diagnosis of pathological grief. *Clinical Psychology Review, 20,* 57–75.

Stroebe, W., & Stroebe, M. (1987). *Bereavement and health: The psychological and physical consequences of partner loss.* New York: Cambridge University Press.

Stroebe, W., Stroebe, M., Abakoumkin, G., & Schut, H. (1996). The role of loneliness and social support in adjustment to loss: A test of attachment versus stress theory. *Journal of Personality and Social Psychology, 70,* 1241–1249.

Tyson-Rawson, K. (1993). *College women and bereavement: Late adolescence and father death.* Unpublished doctoral dissertation, Kansas State University.

Tyson-Rawson, K. (1996). Relationship and heritage: Manifestations of ongoing attachment following father death. In D. Klass, P. R. Silverman, & S. L. Nickman (Eds.), *Continuing bonds: New understandings of grief* (pp. 125–145). Washington, DC: Taylor & Francis.

Vachon, M. L. S., Sheldon, A. R., Lancee, W. J., Lyall, W. A. L., Rogers, J., & Freeman, S. J. J. (1982). Correlates of enduring stress patterns following bereavement: Social network, life situation and personality. *Psychological Medicine, 12,* 783–788.

van Doorn, C., Kasl, S. V., Beery, L. C., Jacobs, S. C., & Prigerson, H. G. (1998). The influence of marital quality and attachment styles on traumatic grief and depressive symptoms. *Journal of Nervous and Mental Disease, 186,* 566–573.

Waskowic, T. D., & Chartier, B. M. (2003). Attachment and the experience of grief following the loss of a spouse. *Omega, 47*, 77–91.

Wayment, H. A., & Vierthaler, J. (2002). Attachment style and bereavement reactions. *Journal of Loss and Trauma, 7*, 129–149.

Wegner, D. M. (1994). Ironic processes of mental control. *Psychological Review, 101*, 34–52.

Weiss, R. S. (1973). *Loneliness: The experience of social and emotional isolation*. Cambridge, MA: MIT Press.

Weiss, R. S. (1975). *Marital separation*. New York: Basic Books.

Wijngaards-de Meij, L., Stroebe, M., Schut, H., Stroebe, W., van den Bout, J., van der Heijden, P. G. M., et al. (2007). Patterns of attachment and parents' adjustment to the death of their child. *Personality and Social Psychology Bulletin, 33*, 537–548.

Wortman, C. B., & Boerner, K. (2007). Beyond the myths of coping with loss: Prevailing assumptions versus scientific evidence. In H. S. Friedman & R. C. Silver (Eds.), *Foundations of health psychology* (pp. 285–324). New York: Oxford University Press.

Zhang, B., El-Jawahri, A., & Prigerson, H. G. (2006). Update on bereavement research: Evidence-based guidelines for the diagnosis and treatment of complicated grief. *Journal of Palliative Medicine, 9*, 1188–1203.

Zisook, S., & DeVaul, R. A. (1985). Unresolved grief. *American Journal of Psychoanalysis, 45*, 370–379.

CHAPTER 4

Individual Differences
in Infant–Caregiver Attachment
Conceptual and Empirical Aspects of Security

NANCY S. WEINFIELD
L. ALAN SROUFE
BYRON EGELAND
ELIZABETH CARLSON

Almost every infant will develop an attachment relationship with a caregiver, and will endeavor to use that caregiver as a source of comfort and reassurance in the face of challenges or threats from the environment. The presence of attachment relationships in human infant–caregiver relationships seems to be universal. The nature of the relationship and the effectiveness with which the caregiver can be used as a source of comfort in the face of danger, however, differ across infant–caregiver dyads. These variations are individual differences in the quality of attachment relationships.

This chapter describes the nature of individual differences in infant–caregiver attachment as John Bowlby and Mary Ainsworth conceptualized it. It reviews how individual differences are described and assessed in infancy, as well as the meaning of attachment classification as an assessment of relationship history. This chapter also discusses core theoretical predictions regarding the meaning of individual differences in early attachment relationships for subsequent child adjustment and relationship functioning. Empirical findings are reviewed supporting these predictions, drawn from the findings of our own research on the Minnesota Parent–Child Project, a longitudinal study of children at high risk for poor developmental

outcomes; from a Minnesota longitudinal study of middle-class families; and from other independent longitudinal studies.

INDIVIDUAL DIFFERENCES IN ATTACHMENT: DEVELOPMENT AND DEFINITIONS

The distinction between the *presence* of an attachment relationship and the *quality* of an attachment relationship is important. According to Bowlby, a human infant will form an attachment to a caregiver as long as someone is there to interact with the infant and to serve as an attachment figure. Forming attachments is strongly built into the human repertoire through evolution. Children will be unattached only if there is no stable caregiver, such as is the case in certain kinds of institutional rearing. For all others, even those who are mistreated, attachment relationships are formed with caregivers.

Individual differences in these attachment relationships reflect differences in the history of care. They do not arise suddenly, nor are they carried solely in the traits of the infant or the caregiver (Ainsworth, Blehar, Waters, & Wall, 1978; Bowlby, 1969/1982; Sroufe & Waters, 1977). Patterns of interaction are built out of a history of bids and responses within the dyad, and these patterns of interaction, rather than individual behaviors, reveal the underlying character of the relationship.

Through repeated interactions with the same adults over time, infants begin to recognize their caregivers and to anticipate the behavior of primary caregivers. Bowlby and Ainsworth were the first to elaborate on these early relationships in terms of both survival behavior and psychological processes. They described the infant as biologically predisposed to use the caregiver, usually the mother, as a "haven of safety" and as a "secure base" while exploring the environment (Ainsworth, 1967; Ainsworth et al., 1978; Bowlby, 1969/1982). When the infant feels threatened, he or she will turn to the caregiver for protection and comfort. In fact, Bowlby and Ainsworth described a delicate balance in the infant between exploration and seeking proximity to the caregiver when exploration proves threatening. Individual differences are most easily seen in this attachment–exploration balance. From this theoretical perspective, assessments of attachment security in infancy must be related to such secure-base behavior.

When seeking comfort or reassurance, infants direct behaviors toward their caregivers such as approaching, crying, seeking contact, and maintaining that contact. These behaviors are called "attachment behaviors" (Ainsworth et al., 1978; Bowlby, 1969/1982). Attachment behaviors do not yield sufficient information, however, if one studies only the number of behaviors expressed. All infants display attachment behaviors at times, the quantity of which may vary with the degree of threat an infant perceives in the environment. In a dangerous environment, when protection is needed, it is maladaptive for an infant to refrain from expressing attachment behaviors. In an environment that poses little danger and warrants exploration, it might be maladaptive for an infant to forgo exploration in favor of seeking out the caregiver. The study of attachment behaviors becomes most meaningful when one focuses on individual differences in the patterning of attachment behavior—the timing and effectiveness of their expression. The focus in studying individual differences in attachment relationships is not the quantity of attachment behaviors expressed, but rather the organization of attachment-related behavior in the relationship—the quality of the attachment relationship (Ainsworth, 1972; Sroufe & Waters, 1977).

Individual differences in quality of attachment relationships have been broadly divided into two categories: "secure" attachment relationships and "insecure" attachment relationships (Ainsworth, 1972; Ainsworth et al., 1978; Bowlby, 1973). The terms "secure" and "insecure" do not describe simply the manifest behaviors of the infant within the attachment relationship. Rather, the terms describe an infant's apparent perception of the availability of the caregiver if a need for comfort or protection should arise, and the organization of the infant's responses to the caregiver in light of those perceptions of availability.

Security of attachment does not mean that an infant never feels fear or apprehension (Bowlby, 1973). Fear and anxiety are normal human reactions, and all infants will occasionally feel unsettled or fearful of something in the environment. Such reactions are adaptive because they prompt proximity to the protective caregiver, as well as movement away from the source of threat. Security in the attachment relationship indicates that an infant is able to rely on that caregiver as an available source of comfort and protection if the need arises. Infants with secure attachment relationships may direct few attachment behaviors toward their caregivers when there are no threats in the environment. When threat-based feelings of apprehension arise, however, infants in secure relationships are able to direct attachment behaviors to their caregivers and take comfort in the reassurance offered by them. Secure relationships promote infants' exploration of the world and expand their mastery of the environment, because experience tells such infants that if the exploration proves unsettling, they can rely on their caregivers to be there and alleviate their fears. Infants with secure attachment relationships are confident in the sensitive and responsive availability of their caregivers, and consequently these infants are confident in their own interactions with the world.

This confidence is not instilled by the experiences of infants who have insecure attachment relationships with their caregivers. Infants with insecure attachment relationships have not experienced consistent availability of and comfort from their caregivers when the environment has proven threatening. Bids for attention may have been met with indifference, with rebuffs, or with notable inconsistency (Ainsworth et al., 1978; Bowlby, 1973). The result of such histories is that these infants are anxious about the availability of their caregivers, fearing that the caregivers will be unresponsive or ineffectively responsive when needed.

They may also be angry with their caregivers for this lack of responsiveness. Anger seems to be a normative reaction to inaccessibility of caregivers, similar to that which occurs in prolonged separation (Robertson & Robertson, 1971). Bowlby (1973) speculated that angry reactions might have evolved because they punish caregivers for unresponsiveness, and may be intended to discourage caregivers from further unresponsiveness.

A history of unresponsiveness or erratic responsiveness results in infants' being unable to direct attachment behaviors at caregivers when doing so would be appropriate. When there is no apparent danger in the environment, some infants with insecure attachment relationships may still direct many attachment behaviors to their caregivers, reflecting a constant low-level anxiety about the caregivers' availability. When there is a perceived threat from the environment and anxiety is high, some infants may not be able to direct appropriate attachment behaviors to their caregivers, or may not be easily comforted by caregivers who have been unreliable in the past. Because insecurely attached infants are not free to explore the environment without worry, they cannot achieve the same confidence in themselves and mastery of their environments that securely attached infants can.

Insecure attachments are nonoptimal organizations of attachment behaviors because they can compromise exploration. At the same time, patterns of insecure attachment may be viewed as adaptations, in that they are suitable responses to the unresponsiveness of the caregivers. Main and Hesse (1990), for example, argue that establishing a low threshold for threat can be described as "maximizing" expressions of attachment even in low-threat situations. This may ensure that inconsistent caregivers will be available if genuine threat should occur. Alternatively, some infants can be described as "minimizing" expressions of attachment, even in conditions of mild threat. This may forestall alienating caregivers who are already rejecting, and it may leave open the possibility of responsiveness if a more serious threat should arise. Within the theoretical tradition of Bowlby and Ainsworth, all infants are viewed as adapting their attachment behavioral systems to the caregiving environment at the same time as the environment adapts to them. In a proximal sense, both secure and insecure attachments can be considered adaptive: They promote proximity to caregivers, and consequently promote survival past the vulnerable period of infancy and to the age of reproductive maturity. In purely evolutionary terms, secure and insecure attachments are both distally adaptive as well, in that neither pattern should compromise reproductive success (Sroufe, 1988). In nonevolutionary terms, however, there are ways in which a history of insecure attachment may compromise an individual's subsequent development.

DESCRIPTIONS AND ASSESSMENTS OF INDIVIDUAL DIFFERENCES IN ATTACHMENT SECURITY

It is not possible to observe directly the conscious and unconscious processes that guide the infant's responses within the attachment relationship. And as mentioned previously, observing the number of attachment behaviors expressed in a given situation is insufficient, because infants with insecure attachment relationships may not be making attachment-related overtures to their caregivers in an adaptive fashion. The key to assessing attachment rests in determining how an infant organizes attachment behaviors to balance the need for protection and comfort with the desire to explore the environment.

The Strange Situation (Ainsworth et al., 1978; Ainsworth & Wittig, 1969) was the method Ainsworth developed for assessing the infant–caregiver attachment relationship, and it has become the standard by which measures at later ages are judged. The Strange Situation is so named because it is intended to be a mildly to moderately stressful experience for an infant, akin to an experience in a doctor's office waiting room. It introduces several strange and therefore stressful elements to an infant—a laboratory context that is unfamiliar, an unfamiliar adult who interacts with the child, and two brief separations from the mother. The premise of the situation is that the multiple increasing stressors will activate the infant's attachment behavioral system, and that individual differences in the child's expectations about the availability of the caregiver will thus be revealed. The situation also reveals the infant's ability to balance exploration of a new environment with a need for reassurance from the caregiver (see Solomon & George, Chapter 18, this volume, for a detailed discussion of the Strange Situation).

Based on the pattern of interactive behavior across the session and especially the two reunions, each relationship is classified as "secure," "avoidant," or "resistant" (Ainsworth et al., 1978). An additional classification, "disorganized/disoriented," is now also used because some infants exhibit unusual behaviors that seem to represent breakdowns in the organization of attachment behavior, or that reflect striking episodes of disorientation (Main & Solomon, 1990; see also Solomon & George, Chapter 18, and Lyons-Ruth & Jacobvitz, Chapter 28, this volume). Such infants, like avoidant and resistant infants, are considered insecurely attached.

Infants classified as secure with their caregivers in the Strange Situation are able to use the caregivers as a secure base for exploration in the novel room. An infant may check back with a caregiver, but usually engages in exploring the toys. Upon separation the infant may be overtly distressed, and play may become impoverished. A secure infant may be friendly with the stranger, and may even be somewhat comforted by the stranger during separation, but there is a clear preference for comfort by the caregiver. Upon reunion with the caregiver, a distressed secure infant will seek proximity or contact with the caregiver, will be readily comforted by the proximity or contact, and will maintain contact as long as it is needed. Eventually, most secure infants will return to play. Even when not distressed, a secure infant is responsive to the caregiver's return, greeting with a smile or vocalization and initiating interaction.

Infants classified as avoidant with their caregivers will usually engage with the toys in the presence of their caregivers. These infants are unlikely to show affective sharing (e.g., smiling or showing toys to the caregiver) before the first separation, although they may engage the caregiver for instrumental assistance (Waters, Wippman, & Sroufe, 1979). Upon separation the infant is unlikely to be distressed, although some distress when left alone is possible. Avoidant infants tend to treat the stranger similarly to the caregiver, and in some cases the infants are actually more responsive with the stranger. Upon reunion with the caregiver, avoidant infants show signs of ignoring, looking or turning away from, or moving past the caregiver rather than approaching. If picked up, avoidant infants will make no effort to maintain the contact.

Infants classified as resistant with their caregivers are conspicuously unable to use their caregivers as a secure base for exploration of the novel setting. These infants may seek proximity and contact with the caregivers even before separation occurs, and may be quite wary of the situation and of the stranger. Upon separation resistant infants are likely to be quite distressed, and are not easily calmed by the stranger. Upon reunion they are likely to want proximity or contact with their caregivers, but not to be calmed by the contact. Some resistant infants display unusual passivity, continuing to cry but failing to seek contact actively. In most cases, however, the hallmark of this classification is seeking contact and then resisting contact angrily once it is achieved. There is a palpable ambivalence in many of these relationships.

An infant who is classified as disorganized in the Strange Situation (in addition to an alternate, best-fitting classification of secure, avoidant, or resistant) exhibits conflicted, contradictory, or disoriented behaviors that indicate an inability to maintain one coherent attachment strategy in the face of distress (Main & Solomon, 1990). Disorganization can manifest itself in a variety of ways, including, but not limited to, behaviors such as behavioral stilling, stereotypies, or direct fear of the parent.

Waters and Deane (1985) developed an Attachment Q-Sort that uses extended observations of the home behavior of children as indicators of attachment. The procedure does not result in attachment classifications, but rather a continuous score for security based on home behaviors that are relevant to attachment and that should discriminate between secure and insecure attachment. Vaughn and Waters (1990) found that infants who were secure with their mothers in the Strange Situation had significantly higher security scores on the Attachment Q-Sort when the sort was completed by observers, confirming the link between home behavior and Strange Situation classification. (The Attachment Q-Sort is addressed in greater depth by Solomon & George, Chapter 18, this volume.)

THEORETICAL PREDICTIONS REGARDING INDIVIDUAL DIFFERENCES IN ATTACHMENT

Bowlby (1969/1982, 1973) proposed two major hypotheses regarding individual differences in attachment. The first addressed antecedents of individual differences in attachment. Bowlby defined security of attachment in terms of preferential desire for contact with the caregiver under conditions of threat, and secure-base behavior more generally. He viewed both as outgrowths of a child's confidence in a caregiver's responsiveness. Through a history of responsive care, infants develop expectations (or, in Bowlby's terms, "internal working models") of their caregivers' likely responses to signs of distress or bids for contact. The specific prediction, then, is that caregiver responsiveness early in infancy is related to individual differences in attachment security later in infancy. In the simplest terms, Bowlby postulated that what infants expect is what has happened before. (See Belsky & Fearon, Chapter 13, this volume, for further discussion of the antecedents of individual differences in attachment.)

Bowlby's second hypothesis concerned the likely consequences of individual differences in attachment security for a child's development, particularly social and personality development (Bowlby, 1973). Bowlby argued that because attachment relationships are internalized or represented, attachment experiences and consequent expectations get taken forward to serve later behavioral and emotional adaptation, even in totally new contexts and with different people. In particular, internal working models are a foundation not only for expectations concerning the self, but also for later relationships with caregivers and noncaregivers alike. Caregiver responsiveness (and the ensuing confidence in that responsiveness) is more than a foundation for the developing parent–child relationship. The model of parent as responsive is inextricably associated with a complementary model of the self as effective, since the child is predictably effective at eliciting a parental response. This pattern of responsiveness also generalizes to the belief that relationships are a context in which needs are met. Thus there are implications for later efficacy, self-esteem, and social relationships. (See Thompson, Chapter 16, this volume, for further discussion of links between infant attachment and later social functioning.)

This is not meant to imply that early attachment relationships are destiny. In Bowlby's (1973) view, adaptation always depends both on the prior history of adaptation *and* on current circumstances, with established patterns influencing selection and interpretation of, and reactions to, the environment. Current experiences are capable of transforming adaptation and subsequent expectations, while not erasing the influence of history. Bowlby adapted Waddington's (1957) pathway model to argue both that change is always possible,

and that change is at the same time constrained by prior adaptation.

These issues are elaborated in the sections to follow. We then conclude with a discussion of current issues in the arena of individual differences in attachment, including when attachment-based differences are not expected.

Antecedents of Individual Differences in Attachment Security

Research on Bowlby's first hypothesis—that individual differences in attachment arise from experiences and expectations regarding the availability of caregivers—was pioneered by Ainsworth, who was the first to provide a formal description of individual differences in infants' attachment security. Inspired by Bowlby's theory and her own ethological observations of caregiving practices and infant behavior in Uganda (Ainsworth, 1967), Ainsworth and her research team began by making hours of detailed observations of exploratory behavior, crying, and other attachment-related behaviors in the home for a small sample of infants. She also developed carefully crafted, behaviorally anchored rating scales for caregiver behavior: Sensitivity to Signals, Cooperation–Interference, Acceptance–Rejection, and Availability–Unavailability. Thus Ainsworth established anchors in attachment behavior in the home, as well as in assessments of caregiver sensitivity, before developing the Strange Situation. This impressive and methodical pursuit of validation against home behavior was an essential first step in the development of the laboratory-based Strange Situation.

Ainsworth and colleagues (1978) reported extensively on the home behaviors of their participants over the first year of the infants' lives leading up to the Strange Situation. Although the full sample size used for the development of the Strange Situation coding procedures was 106 dyads, the more intensive study of home behavior was undertaken only for a subsample of 23 dyads. In general, small sample sizes reduce the likelihood of finding significant between-group differences. The fact that Ainsworth and her colleagues found group differences despite the small sample size attests to the magnitude of the differences. They found that infants who would later be classified as insecurely attached (avoidant and resistant) with their mothers in the Strange Situation were more overtly angry and noncompliant and cried more at home than infants who would later be classified as secure. Mothers of infants who would later be classified as insecure were less sensitive in interactions, more interfering with the children's behavior, and less responsive to the children's bids than mothers of infants who would later be classified as secure. In addition, mothers of infants who would later be classified as avoidant expressed an aversion to physical contact with their infants and expressed little emotion during interactions with them.

Numerous others have replicated the core findings of a relation between caregiver insensitivity and later insecure attachment (Bates, Maslin, & Frankel, 1985; Grossmann, Grossmann, Spangler, Suess, & Unzner, 1985; Isabella, 1993; Kiser, Bates, Maslin, & Bayles, 1986; National Institute of Child Health and Human Development [NICHD] Early Child Care Research Network, 1997; Pederson, Gleason, Moran, & Bento, 1998; Posada et al., 1999). In the Minnesota Parent–Child Project, Egeland and Farber (1984) found that mothers of infants who would later be classified as secure were more sensitive and expressive during a feeding situation than mothers of avoidant or resistant infants. Mothers of avoidant infants were insensitive to their infants' timing cues and seemed to dislike close physical contact with their infants. The magnitude of the relation between caregiver sensitivity and attachment security is often modest, especially when compared to the findings in Ainsworth and colleagues' (1978) original study, and there have been occasional nonreplications (e.g., Seifer, Schiller, Sameroff, Resnick, & Riordan, 1996). Some of the problems in replicating these findings may be found in the difficulty of devising a good measure of caregiver sensitivity, as well as in the different numbers of hours of home observation that form the basis for the different sensitivity measures. Despite some variability in findings, a meta-analysis did find a significant relation between sensitivity and attachment (De Wolff & van IJzendoorn, 1997). In addition, the large multisite NICHD Study of Early Child Care and Youth Development (NICHD SECCYD), although finding little impact of day care on attachment, supported the significance of caregiver sensitivity in predicting individual differences in attachment (NICHD Early Child Care Research Network, 1997).

The finding that infant home behavior during the first year of life is related to later Strange Situation classification led to the suggestion that attachment classification could be a simple manifestation of infant temperament, and not a product of the relationship. Direct comparisons of temperament and attachment, however, have suggested that there is not in fact a direct link between temperament and attachment security (Belsky & Rovine, 1987; Crockenberg, 1981; Egeland & Farber, 1984; Gunnar, Mangelsdorf, Larson, & Hertsgaard, 1989; Seifer et al., 1996; Vaughn, Lefever, Seifer, & Barglow, 1989; see Vaughn, Bost, & van IJzendoorn, Chapter 9, this volume). Research has demonstrated that what can be predicted by temperament are specific behaviors during the Strange Situation, particularly distress during separation from, but not during reunion with, the mother (Gunnar et al., 1989; Vaughn et al., 1989). These findings bolster the supposition that the attachment relationship is not reducible to infant characteristics, and that attachment and temperament represent two distinct constructs (Mangelsdorf & Frosch, 2000).

Other researchers have sought to explain the relation between temperament and attachment by looking at the interaction of maternal and infant characteristics. Although Crockenberg (1981) found no direct relation between infant temperament and attachment classification, she did find a significant interaction between maternal social support and infant temperament in predicting attachment classification. Mothers with irritable infants (as assessed shortly after birth) and poor social support were more likely to have insecurely attached infants. When social support was high, infant irritability had no impact on attachment quality. Mangelsdorf, Gunnar, Kestenbaum, Lang, and Andreas (1990) explored infant temperament and maternal personality in relation to attachment. Like previous researchers, they found no direct relations between temperament, or personality, and attachment; however, they did find a significant interaction. Infants who were highly prone to distress and had mothers who were rigid and traditional were most likely to be insecurely attached. In the Minnesota Parent–Child Project, Susman-Stillman, Kalkoske, Egeland, and Waldman (1996) found that maternal sensitivity during the first year of life predicted attachment security, that infant temperamental characteristics predicted type of insecure attachment, and that maternal sensitivity mediated the link between infant irritability and attachment security. Thus, although some of the behaviors seen in the Strange Situation may be related to temperament, security in the infant–caregiver relationship is not determined by infant temperament (see Vaughn et al., Chapter 9, this volume, for a more extensive discussion of attachment and temperament).

Predictive Meaning of Individual Differences in Attachment Security

Bowlby's second hypothesis concerns the developmental significance of individual differences in early attachment relationships. This hypothesis includes the nature of meaningful variations in infant–caregiver attachment; the aspects of development they affect; and the processes by which this effect occurs.

Bowlby described two types of variation in attachment: presence versus absence of an attachment relationship, and individual differences in organization of secure-base behavior across infant–caregiver dyads. Although absence of attachment is likely to affect survival, Bowlby did not predict that individual differences in attachment security should influence survival. Both secure and insecure patterns of attachment serve to promote survival to reproductive maturity by keeping infants in proximity to their caregivers.

Individual differences in attachment security, because of their impact on emotion regulation and exploration, are nonetheless conceptualized as important both for social and personality development and for psychopathology. Bowlby argued, as Freud had previously, that early attachment experiences are of special importance because of their implications for mastery, emotion regulation, and interpersonal closeness. Rejecting the notion of drive reduction, Bowlby expanded on Freud's original focus on the role of actual experience. Bowlby elaborated on the idea of an internal world of mental processes as central to the ongoing influence of early history (Sroufe, 1986). Expectations about oneself and the social world, according to Bowlby, are based on the quality and patterning of early care. From a history of responsive care and smooth dyadic emotion regulation come a sense of efficacy, a capacity for self-regulation, and positive expectations regarding interpersonal relationships. Within this developmental process, the individual is viewed as active—adapting, coping, and shaping his or her own experiences.

There are at least four possible explanations of why early attachment relationships influence later development. These explanations are not mutually exclusive, and it is likely that each plays a part in the continuing influence of attachment. First, it is possible that the experiences within the early attachment relationship influence the developing brain, resulting in lasting influences at a neuronal level (Schore, 1994). This possibility, though compelling and a promising area of future research, is not a focus of the present discussion (see Cicchetti & Tucker, 1994).

Second, as suggested by Isabella (1993), Cassidy (1994), and Sroufe (1979, 1996), the early attachment relationship may serve as a foundation for learning emotional self-regulation. Emotion regulation denotes the ability to control and modulate emotional responses, coping with arousal in order to maintain a motivating, but not debilitating, level of emotion (Cole, Martin, & Dennis, 2004). Infants are ill equipped to regulate their own emotions, so as they experience such emotions as distress, anger, and fear, they turn to their caregivers for assistance. Tronick (1989) detailed a process of coordination, miscoordination, repair, and recoordination of emotion that cycles within well-functioning infant–caregiver dyads. This process of miscoordination and caregiver-driven repair gives the infant guided experience with managing stressful emotions and provides a foundation for self-regulatory abilities. Individual differences in attachment relationships should give infants repeated experiences with predictable patterns of coregulation of emotion (Thompson, 1994), and these experiences should lead to predictable patterns of self-regulation. According to theory regarding organized patterns of attachment (Cassidy, 1994; Sroufe, Egeland, Carlson, & Collins, 2005a), infants in secure relationships should be flexible in their self-regulation strategies in the face of negative emotion, and their mothers should be accepting of a wide range of emotional expressions. Infants in insecure-avoidant relationships should minimize direct expressions of distress, and have poor regulation skills in the face of such emotions, due to experience with caregivers who reject such expressions. Infants in insecure-resistant relationships should maximize expressions of distress, and manage these emotions poorly, due to experiences with caregivers who respond erratically to bids and therefore respond more predictably to amplified emotions. Disorganized attachment, which represents a breakdown in attachment strategies, should predict an absence of predictable emotional strategies, and thus the most poorly managed emotions (DeOliveira, Bailey, Moran, & Pederson, 2004; Lyons-Ruth & Jacobvitz, Chapter 28, this volume). Empirical research has supported some of these propositions (Berlin & Cassidy, 2003; Denham, Blair, Schmidt, & DeMulder, 2002; Diener,

Mangelsdorf, McHale, & Frosch, 2002; NICHD Early Child Care Research Network, 2004), demonstrating overall that children who have secure attachment histories with their mothers regulate their emotions more effectively than do children with insecure histories.

A third possible avenue for attachment to influence subsequent development is through behavioral regulation and behavioral synchrony. Through observing and interacting with an attachment figure, an infant learns what it is like to behave in a relationship (Elicker, Englund, & Sroufe, 1992; Gianino & Tronick, 1988; Pastor, 1981). The sensitive, responsive behavior of the caregiver in a secure dyad teaches the secure infant that communication is contingent upon each partner's cues and responses. The insensitive, uncoordinated interactions of an insecure dyad teach the insecure infant that communication is not a responsive interaction, but a series of poorly coordinated bids and responses. All infants carry forward not only the expectations of how interactions with social partners are coordinated, but also their experiences with caregivers in succeeding or failing to construct synchronous, reciprocal social and emotional exchanges. Secure children develop such abilities as self-control and behavioral reciprocity, which result in more skilled interactions than those of insecure children. These interactional skills can then be applied to new settings and new relationships, resulting in continued differences that are reinforced and strengthened across development.

The fourth way in which individual differences in attachment influence later development is through representation. According to Bowlby (1969/1982), from the early attachment relationship the child begins to represent what to expect from the world and from other people, as well as how he or she can expect to be treated by others. These beliefs and expectations, or "internal working models," begin in the relationship with the caregiver as the infant starts to anticipate caregiver responses to the infant's signals. Infants who have secure relationships have been treated in a consistently sensitive manner. They grow to see the world as good and responsive, and the self as deserving such consideration. Infants who have insecure relationships are responded to harshly, erratically, or not at all. They grow to see the world as unpredictable and insensitive, and the self as not deserving better treatment. These internal working models are then carried forward to new relationships and new experiences, guiding chil-

dren's expectations and behavior. In Bowlby's terms (1973, 1980), the environment is engaged within the confines of models of self, other, and relationships that have been previously formulated. (See Bretherton & Munholland, Chapter 5, this volume, for a detailed discussion of internal working models.)

There are specific predictions regarding individual differences in early attachment quality and later outcomes. Particular patterns are expected to have particular correlates, in terms of social behavior, personality, and psychopathology. Moreover, not all developmental outcomes, whether of good or poor quality, are viewed as related to attachment history. As we discuss later, many outcomes are viewed as independent of the attachment system.

Theory dictates that the influence of infant attachment relationships should be principally apparent in some specific domains of adjustment. These domains include dependency, self-reliance, and efficacy; anxiety, anger, and empathy; and interpersonal competence (Ainsworth, 1972; Ainsworth & Bell, 1974; Bowlby, 1969/1982, 1973, 1988; Sroufe, 1988; Sroufe & Fleeson, 1986, 1988). These issues should be specifically related to attachment because they are intricately connected to the emotion regulation, behavioral reciprocity, and expectations and beliefs about self and other that arise from early attachment relationships. Theoretical predictions and empirical findings follow not only from individual differences in secure versus insecure attachment, but also in some cases from more specific individual differences between those with a history of avoidant attachment and those with a history of resistant attachment (and, in some cases, those with a history of disorganized attachment).

In the following section, we review empirical predictions from individual differences in infant attachment to theoretically relevant dimensions of behavior in childhood and adolescence.

EMPIRICAL STUDIES OF INFANT ATTACHMENT AND LATER ADAPTATION

Dependency, Self-Reliance, and Efficacy

Infants whose caregivers are sensitive and responsive to cues learn that they can influence the world around them, successfully getting their needs met and having an effect on the world. They acquire the experience and confidence to function autonomously. Infants whose caregivers are unresponsive or erratically responsive to cues learn that they are not able to influence the world to meet their needs. Consequently, these infants do not acquire the confidence to function autonomously (Ainsworth & Bell, 1974; Sroufe, Fox, & Pancake, 1983). This prediction regarding the development of self-reliance was a cornerstone of Bowlby's theory (Bowlby, 1973).

When the attachment construct was first introduced, it was necessary for researchers to differentiate between attachment and dependency (Ainsworth, 1969, 1972; Bowlby, 1969/1982; Sroufe et al., 1983). Because attachment behavior and signs of dependency are similar (e.g., crying, clinging, seeking proximity), attachment quality was misunderstood to be a measure of dependency (Gewirtz, 1972). Some secure infants were mistakenly thought to be dependent, whereas avoidant infants were thought to be precociously independent. In Bowlby's view, however, it is not possible for an infant to be either too dependent or truly independent. Because of their immaturity and inability to care for themselves, infants may be effectively or ineffectively dependent.

The key to the relation among infant attachment, dependency, and self-reliance has been articulated by Sroufe and colleagues (1983), who explained that infants who are effectively dependent will consequently become effectively independent. Signaling needs to sensitive and responsive caregivers and having those needs met will lead infants to develop confidence in their ability to influence the world and achieve their goals. This confidence allows children with secure histories to function autonomously and with a belief that they will be successful in their efforts. Several studies have examined the relations between attachment and dependency, and between attachment and environmental mastery.

In the Minnesota Parent–Child Project, dependency has been studied in preschool, middle childhood, and adolescence. Sroufe and colleagues (1983) and Sroufe (1983) studied dependent behavior in preschool. "Dependency" was defined primarily in terms of seeking attention and proximity to the teacher, extreme reliance on the teacher for help, and seeking teacher attention at the expense of peer relations. Data were obtained through multiple methods, including observer data and teacher rankings and Q-sorts. Children with resistant or avoidant histories, as compared to children with secure histories, had more interactions with teachers, sat next to them more often during circle time, and were judged to be more

dependent overall. Children with secure histories did seek teacher attention, but they tended to seek attention in positive ways, and not at the expense of peer relations. Dependency was later studied in this sample at age 10 in a summer camp context by Urban, Carlson, Egeland, and Sroufe (1991), who assessed dependency through camp counselor ratings and observer data on contact sought with adults. As in the preschool context, they found that children with insecure histories, both resistant and avoidant, were rated as more dependent. Children with secure histories sought less contact with adults at the camp overall.

Differences continued to be manifest at age 15, the latest age at which dependency was examined in the Minnesota Parent–Child Project (Sroufe, Carlson, & Shulman, 1993). Both those adolescents with histories of resistant attachment and those with histories of avoidant attachment continued to show more dependency on adults than those with secure histories. This finding held even when variance attributable to contemporary parenting measures was taken into account.

Confidence, belief that one can succeed, and tolerance of frustration in goal seeking have also been studied in relation to early attachment history. In the Minnesota studies, this took the form of studying ego resilience, or a child's ability to respond flexibly to the changing requirements of a situation, particularly in the face of frustration. In the Parent–Child Project, children with secure histories were rated by their preschool teachers as more ego-resilient than children with insecure attachment histories (Sroufe, 1983). Most striking was the fact that there was no overlap in ego resilience between the secure and avoidant groups.

These dimensions of efficacy were also explored in the Minnesota study of middle-class families. At 2 years old, children and their mothers were seen in a tool use situation. Matas, Arend, and Sroufe (1978) found that children with secure histories appeared more competent in the tool use tasks than those with insecure histories, showing more enthusiasm, compliance with maternal directives, and persistence. When these children were in preschool, Arend, Gove, and Sroufe (1979) found the same relation between attachment and ego resilience that would later be replicated in the Parent–Child Project: Children with secure histories were judged to be more ego-resilient than their insecure counterparts in a teacher Q-sort.

Other studies have explored these efficacy constructs as well. Frankel and Bates (1990), in a replication of Matas and colleagues (1978), found that toddlers with secure histories were more persistent in a tool use task than were children with insecure histories. In an Israeli kibbutz study of attachment between young children and their *metaplot* (the primary caregivers in a kibbutz children's house), Oppenheim, Sagi, and Lamb (1988) found that children who had secure histories with their *metaplot* were described (by their *metaplot*, in Q-sorts) as more goal-directed and achievement-oriented than children with insecure-resistant histories. In a German study of interaction with a stranger, Lütkenhaus, Grossmann, and Grossmann (1985) looked at 3-year-old children's responses to playing a competitive game with an unfamiliar experimenter. When the children saw that they might be failing, those with secure histories increased their efforts, whereas those with insecure histories decreased their efforts. This finding was interpreted as indicating that the children with secure histories believed they had more control over their environments and could succeed by using their skills if they tried.

Overall, these findings on dependency, self-reliance, and efficacy suggest that early attachment history does contribute to a child's growing effectiveness in the world. Children with secure histories seem to believe that, as was true in infancy, they can get their needs met and achieve their goals through their own efforts and bids. In contrast, children with insecure histories seem to believe that, as in their early attachment relationships, their efforts are often ineffective, and they must rely extensively on others who may or may not meet their needs. These beliefs are translated into both differences in effort and differential success in affecting the world.

Anxiety, Anger, and Empathy

Chronic rejection by and inconsistent availability of the caregiver, which are characteristic of insecure attachment, take their toll on an infant over the course of development. Unlike a secure infant, who can count on the responsiveness of the caregiver, an insecurely attached infant must deal with the constant possibility of needing an unavailable caregiver, as well as coping with the accumulating frustration and dysregulation inherent in being treated insensitively (Bowlby, 1973).

According to Bowlby (1973) and Stayton and Ainsworth (1973), insecurely attached infants must be constantly concerned about the whereabouts of their caregivers, because the caregivers cannot be relied upon to be accessible in times of

need. Because of the potential unavailability of the caregivers, these infants live with the constant fear of being left vulnerable and alone. This fear of separation or abandonment continues beyond infancy, because the fear of being alone when comfort or protection is needed continues throughout childhood and adulthood (Bowlby, 1973). Thus the anxiety associated with this fear of separation lasts beyond infancy as well. Such anxiety should be particularly characteristic of individuals with resistant attachment histories, because these relationships are characterized by an unpredictable, erratic responsiveness that can prove particularly anxiety-provoking and can give rise to a coping strategy centered on chronic vigilance (Bowlby, 1973; Cassidy & Berlin, 1994).

Another response to unavailable, rejecting caregiving is anger. Some anger is a natural response to the fear engendered by separation from an attachment figure, because it serves to express displeasure over the separation and to prevent it from recurring (Bowlby, 1973). Chronic anger as a response to chronic unavailability, however, can be highly maladaptive and manifest itself through angry, aggressive behavior toward the caregiver. When the expectation of being hurt, disappointed, and afraid is carried forward to new relationships, the insecure infant becomes an angry, aggressive child. Avoidant infants, who are chronically rejected, and disorganized infants, who are conflicted in the face of frightened or frightening caregivers, are the most likely to show these angry, aggressive responses later (Ainsworth et al., 1978; Bowlby, 1973, 1980; Lyons-Ruth, Alpern, & Repacholi, 1993; Renken, Egeland, Marvinney, Mangelsdorf, & Sroufe, 1989).

Empathy is in many ways the complement or counterpoint to aggression. Whereas aggression often reflects an alienation from others, empathy reflects an amplified connectedness, and whereas aggression reflects a breakdown or warping of dyadic regulation, empathy reflects heightened affective coordination. In fact, in many ways aggression is dependent upon a lack of empathy or emotional identification with others.

Attachment theory makes a strong prediction with regard to the development of empathic capacity. Given that not only roles but basic properties of relating are learned within the attachment relationship (Sroufe & Fleeson, 1986), the responsiveness that underlies security is also predicted to give rise to empathy. Earlier we have argued, following Bowlby, that consistently providing for infants' needs does not condemn them to perpetual dependency, but in fact serves as a springboard for self-reliance because it instills a sense of efficacy concerning the environment. Similarly, being consistently nurtured and responded to empathically leads not to a spoiled, self-indulged child, but rather to an empathic child. All children learn about the patterning of relating and dyadic emotion regulation through experience. Those whose caregivers are responsive to their needs learn that when one person is needy, the other responds with assistance; when one person is emotionally overaroused, the other provides comfort or reassurance. All that these children require are the cognitive advances necessary to play the more mature role. Recapitulating experienced patterns of dyadic interaction and regulation is a natural tendency. For some, particularly those with secure attachment histories, this gives rise to the capacity for empathy. Empirical studies on anxiety, anger, and empathy and their relation to infant attachment are reviewed below.

Both in laboratory assessments and in school settings, children with histories of resistant attachment have been found to be less forceful and confident, more hesitant in the face of novelty, and generally more anxious than those with either secure histories or avoidant histories. For example, using Banta's (1970) curiosity box situation at age 4½, Nezworski (1983) found the resistant group to be more hesitant about engaging this novel object than either the avoidant or the secure group. In elementary school, children with resistant histories were identified by their teachers as more passive and withdrawn than children with secure or avoidant histories (Renken et al., 1989). In addition, 6-year-old children with insecure attachment histories, and particularly those with resistant histories, reported higher levels of separation anxiety than did children with secure histories (Dallaire & Weinraub, 2005). Further data on more extreme anxiety symptoms are reported in the section on psychopathology.

Anger and aggression, as related to attachment history, have been examined in several samples. In the Minnesota Parent–Child Project, angry and aggressive behavior was assessed in preschool and in elementary school. During preschool, teacher Q-sorts and detailed behavioral coding by observers indicated that more negative affect, anger, and aggression were expressed by children with insecure attachment histories than by those with secure histories. Q-sort data from elementary school teachers yielded the same results

(Sroufe, 1983; Sroufe, Schork, Motti, Lawroski, & LaFreniere, 1984).

Another analysis in the same sample revealed differences between those with avoidant and resistant histories. Troy and Sroufe (1987) observed children in the preschool setting who were assigned to play pairs based on attachment history. Analysis of the interactions between the children in each pair revealed a systematic relation between victimization and attachment. Children with avoidant histories were significantly more likely than other children to victimize their play partners. Children with secure histories were never either victimizers or victims, whereas children with resistant histories were likely to be victims if they were paired with children with avoidant histories.

Research in other samples has replicated these findings on anger and aggression. In a study examining peer interaction in preschool in relation to attachment history in a German sample, Suess, Grossmann, and Sroufe (1992) found that children with avoidant attachment histories exhibited more hostility and scapegoating of other children than did children with secure histories. In the NICHD SECCYD sample, 36-month-old children with avoidant histories showed more instrumental aggression when interacting with a friend than did children with either secure or resistant histories (McElwain, Cox, Burchinal, & Macfie, 2003).

In the middle-class Minnesota sample mentioned previously, differences as a function of attachment history were found in expressions of anger and aggression toward mothers at 2 years of age (Matas et al., 1978). Matas and her colleagues found that children with insecure histories were more likely than children with secure histories to display aggressive behavior toward their mothers during a tool use task. These findings were replicated by Frankel and Bates (1990), using the same procedure in an independent sample. Interestingly, no difference in aggression was found between the groups with avoidant and resistant histories when the aggression was directed at mothers rather than peers.

A history of disorganized attachment is also related to angry and aggressive behavior during childhood. Kochanska (2001) found that in laboratory situations designed to induce anger in young children, children with disorganized attachment relationships, but not those with organized attachment classifications, showed significant longitudinal increases in levels of expressed anger. By 33 months of age, their anger levels were significantly higher than those expressed by secure or resistant infants. Disorganized attachment, particularly in high-risk samples, may also put children at risk for clinical levels of anger and aggression during childhood (Lyons-Ruth, 1996; Lyons-Ruth, Easterbrooks, & Cibelli, 1997). Such findings are addressed in the later section on psychopathology.

Empathy has also been assessed empirically in relation to attachment. In the Minnesota studies, empathic behavior was assessed in two ways. First, ratings were composited from preschool teacher Q-sort descriptions on items pertaining to empathy (e.g., "shows concern for others," "is empathic"). The ratings significantly distinguished those with secure and insecure histories, often at the item level (see also Waters et al., 1979). In the written descriptions teachers provided of individual children, those described as "empathic" in each case had secure histories, whereas those described as "mean" were always those with avoidant histories. Second, empathic behavior was assessed from videotapes of preschool interaction (Kestenbaum, Farber, & Sroufe, 1989; Sroufe, 1983). Tapes made of free play interactions were examined for instances in which a child in the frame was distressed, and children in the vicinity of the distressed child were rated for empathic responses. Results indicated that children with secure histories were more empathic than children with avoidant histories. Children with resistant histories did not differ significantly from either of the other attachment groups on these measures, although they did seem to have trouble maintaining a boundary between someone else's distress and their own; that is, they became distressed in response to witnessing distress in another. This is consistent with the idea that differences in attachment will be reflected in differences in emotion regulation.

Overall, attachment history does seem to contribute to the prediction of anxiety, anger, and empathy during childhood. Children with resistant attachment histories are more likely than children with other histories to have problems with anxiety, perhaps in response to the constant vigilance they have developed in their early attachment relationships. Children with avoidant or disorganized/disoriented histories are most likely to show angry, aggressive behavior both with parents and with peers, perhaps as a response either to chronic rejection and insensitivity from their caregivers, or to the unmanageable paradox of attachment to frightened or frightening caregivers.

In contrast, children with secure histories seem to have acquired a foundation for empathy from their early relationships; they bring to new relationships the ability to be sensitive to another's emotional cues, as well as a pattern of dyadic affect regulation in which the one who is not distressed helps to regulate the other.

Social Competence

Navigating the world of social relationships is an important task of development. Because humans are inherently social beings, social competence is an essential lifelong component of competence in school, work, and personal/family life, as well as of overall adjustment. There are two avenues through which infant–caregiver attachment relationships prepare individuals for this task: expectations about the social world, and the ability to coordinate behavior in social interactions.

One way attachment relationships contribute to social competence is by providing a foundation for a child's expectations about and approach to other relationships (Sroufe & Fleeson, 1986, 1988). Secure infants, as they develop, bring forward with them experience-based expectations that social partners will be responsive to them and that they are worthy of such positive responses. Insecure infants, as they develop, bring forward experience-based expectations that they will be treated inconsistently or rejected outright by social partners, and that they are not worthy of better treatment (Bowlby, 1969/1982). Such expectations could affect the ways in which children approach relationships, as well as the ways in which they respond to socially ambiguous cues from relational partners. Another way in which attachment relationships contribute to social competence is through teaching infants about behavioral reciprocity, synchrony, and communication (Ainsworth & Bell, 1974; Sroufe, Egeland, & Carlson, 1999).

The data on social competence illustrate particularly well the coherence between individual differences in early attachment and later social functioning, despite changes in settings and relational partners. Research both from the Minnesota studies and from other laboratories has revealed differences in orientation toward peers as early as the toddler period (Belsky & Fearon, 2002; Pastor, 1981). As children expand their social worlds, they must begin to function with some proficiency in a group, and must also engage in more extensive reciprocity with particular partners. When teacher ratings were focused on such capacities, children with secure histories were found to be dramatically more competent (Sroufe, 1983). In observational research, secure children also demonstrate more subtle skill in coordinating behavior with a play partner: Positive bids by children with secure histories are more often accepted and reciprocated by peers, whereas the less synchronous bids of children with insecure histories are more often rebuffed by playmates (Fagot, 1997; Jacobson & Wille, 1986).

By middle childhood children not only must interact with others, but must forge loyal and enduring friendships, find a place in the more organized peer group, and coordinate friendships with group functioning. In the Minnesota Parent–Child Project, global ratings by school teachers confirmed the greater interpersonal competence of those with secure histories (Sroufe et al., 1999). In other research in the school setting, children with secure histories were rated by teachers as more popular and taking more social initiative, and were rated by observers as engaging in more prosocial behavior than their insecure counterparts (Bohlin, Hagekull, & Rydell, 2000). More detailed analysis of 47 children in the Parent–Child Project summer camp revealed differences with regard to each of the age-related competence issues. Those with secure histories, compared to those with insecure histories, more often formed friendships at a summer camp (and more often with those who also had been secure), as revealed by reciprocated sociometric choices, counselor nominations, and direct observations of frequency of interaction (Elicker et al., 1992). Those with secure histories were also more accepted by the group and adhered more to group norms, such as those regarding maintenance of gender boundaries, than those with insecure histories (Sroufe, Bennett, Englund, Urban, & Shulman, 1993). Finally, those with secure histories were better able than those with insecure histories to manage complex social situations, as witnessed by the ease of incorporating others into their activities while still maintaining a reciprocated focus with their partners (Shulman, Elicker, & Sroufe, 1994).

In adolescence, at a camp reunion for the Parent–Child Project camp subsample, teens with secure histories were effective in the ways they had been at camp; they were also rated by camp counselors as more competent in general, and more effective in the mixed-gender crowd in particular (Sroufe, Bennett, et al., 1993; Weinfeld,

Ogawa, & Sroufe, 1997). In addition, ratings in group problem-solving situations revealed greater leadership abilities for those with secure histories, who were also significantly more often elected spokespersons for their groups (Englund, Levy, Hyson, & Sroufe, 2000). In an interview study of the full sample at age 16, the friendships of girls with secure histories were judged to be more intimate than those of girls with insecure histories (Ostoja, 1996). Also, again at age 16 years, competence rankings by high school teachers using the full sample favored those with secure histories (Sroufe et al., 1999).

In the Parent–Child Project, children's social competence was correlated over time. Attachment history, along with earlier social competence, did predict later social competence better than attachment alone, as developmental theory derived from Bowlby would predict. But it was also the case that attachment history accounted for additional variance in the later outcomes, even after earlier social competence was taken into account (Sroufe et al. 1999). Overall, the empirical data on social competence and attachment are strongly supportive of Bowlby's theory. (See Berlin, Cassidy, & Appleyard, Chapter 15, this volume, for additional discussion of the links between infant attachment and later relationships with friends and peers.)

INFANT ATTACHMENT AND PSYCHOPATHOLOGY

In the conceptualization presented here, adapted from Bowlby, individual differences in infant attachment quality are not viewed as inherently pathological or nonpathological. In the pathways perspective, the hypothesis is that patterns of insecure attachment represent initiations of pathways that, if pursued, will increase the likelihood of pathological conditions. Thus, although insecure attachment is considered a risk factor for pathology, not all, or even most, insecurely attached infants will develop psychopathology. Psychopathology is a developmental construction involving a myriad of influences interacting over time (Sroufe, 1997). Similarly, secure attachment is not a guarantee of mental health, but rather is viewed as a protective factor or buffer. Research has demonstrated that children with secure histories are more resistant to stress (Pianta, Egeland, & Sroufe, 1990) and more likely to rebound toward adequate functioning following a period of troubled behavior (Sroufe, Egeland, & Kreutzer, 1990). Thus resilience too is viewed as a developmental construction within this framework. Children who are resilient in the face of stress, or who recover following struggle, have been found to have had either early supportive care or increased support during the time of recovery; resilience is a process rather than a trait (Egeland, Carlson, & Sroufe, 1993; Sroufe et al., 2005a). Secure attachment appears to be part of this process. There is minimal evidence that some children simply are innately resilient (Sroufe, 1997).

There are numerous reasons why insecure attachment histories put children at risk for psychopathology. The anxiety and low frustration tolerance of individuals with resistant histories may make them vulnerable to anxiety disorders. The alienation, lack of empathy, and hostile anger of those with avoidant histories may make them vulnerable to conduct problems and certain personality disorders. Both may be vulnerable to depression, but for different reasons (passivity and helplessness on the one hand, alienation on the other). Both struggle with social relationships, which can exacerbate developmental problems through mistreatment by others or through association with deviant peer groups, and can limit social support, thus reducing an important buffer for stress. Those with histories of disorganized attachment, characterized by a failure to maintain a coherent attachment strategy and postures resembling trance-like states (Main & Hesse, 1990), are at risk for diverse forms of pathology, particularly dissociation (Liotti, 1992; Main & Morgan, 1996) and externalizing problems (Lyons-Ruth, 1996). (See also Lyons-Ruth & Jacobvitz, Chapter 28, and Dozier, Stovall-McClough, & Albus, Chapter 30, this volume, for further discussion of disorganized attachment and psychopathology.)

Data from the Minnesota Parent–Child Project provide some evidence for these predictions in a high-risk sample. From individual interviews with the Schedule for Affective Disorders and Schizophrenia for Adolescents (administered at age 17½), an overall index of psychopathology was created based on the number and severity of disorders manifested. The combination of avoidant and disorganized attachment histories across 12- to 18-month assessments accounted for more than 16% of the variance in this outcome. It was also the case, consistent with the developmental-construction view, that later assessments (including other aspects of parenting) added to the predictability of pathology, ultimately accounting

for more than 30% of the variance. Attachment history remained significant after other variables were accounted for, and early measures based on competing hypotheses (e.g., infant temperament) did not predict pathology significantly (Carlson, 1998).

As predicted by theory, a history of resistant attachment was related specifically and uniquely to anxiety disorders (Warren, Huston, Egeland, & Sroufe, 1997). Resistant attachment history did not predict externalizing disorders, and other forms of insecure attachment did not predict anxiety disorders. Some markers of infant neurological status (e.g., "slow to habituate" on the Brazelton Neonatal Behavioral Assessment Scale) also predicted anxiety disorders, although not as powerfully as resistant attachment, and resistant attachment remained significant after predictions from the Brazelton measure were taken into account.

Predicting anxiety-related symptoms was one focus of an independent study by Lewis, Feiring, McGuffog, and Jaskir (1984). In a longitudinal study extending from infancy to age 6, they examined the connection between infants' attachment history and later maternal reports of the children's psychopathological symptoms. They found that boys with resistant histories were more likely than boys with secure histories to have somatic complaints at age 6, and that boys with insecure histories (both avoidant and resistant) were more likely than boys with secure histories to be socially withdrawn.

Conduct problems have also been predicted by attachment history, both from avoidant attachment and from disorganized attachment. Renken and colleagues (1989) examined conduct problems in elementary school for children in the Parent–Child Project. Problem behaviors were assessed through ratings on the Child Behavior Checklist (Achenbach, 1978) by the children's teachers in first through third grades. Results indicated that boys with avoidant histories were rated as more aggressive by teachers than boys with secure or resistant histories were. By adolescence, a history of avoidant attachment in this same sample predicted a pattern of conduct problems that began in childhood and persisted at clinical levels to age 16 (Aguilar, Sroufe, Egeland, & Carlson, 2000).

In research from an independent laboratory, Lyons-Ruth and colleagues (1997) focused on the relation between disorganized attachment in infancy and severe externalizing behavior problems at age 7. They found that disorganized attachment significantly predicted externalizing problems, particularly when combined with mild deficits in cognitive functioning. Avoidant attachment, although not predictive of externalizing problems in their sample, was predictive of non-clinical-level internalizing symptoms.

Finally, disorganized attachment has significantly predicted dissociative symptoms. In the Parent–Child Project, disorganized attachment in infancy predicted adolescent dissociative symptoms based on the Child Behavior Checklist at age 16 and the Putnam Dissociative Experiences Scale at age 19. Dissociation was, of course, also predicted by a history of maltreatment and trauma (Carlson, 1998; Ogawa, Sroufe, Weinfield, Carlson, & Egeland, 1997), but the relation between disorganized attachment and dissociation remained after childhood trauma was partialed out (Ogawa, Egeland, & Carlson, 1998). Of particular interest is that disorganization in infancy predicted clinical levels of dissociation in each assessment from middle childhood to late adolescence, with the strength of the prediction *increasing* over time (Ogawa et al., 1997). The finding that infant disorganization predicts dissociative symptoms at age 19 was recently replicated in another sample characterized by high social risk (Dutra & Lyons-Ruth, 2005; Lyons-Ruth, Dutra, Schuder, & Bianchi, 2006), strengthening the proposition that disruptions in early attachment relationships, and caregiving interactions that underlie disorganized attachment, put children at risk for dissociative pathology years later.

CATEGORICAL VERSUS CONTINUOUS CONCEPTUALIZATIONS OF INDIVIDUAL DIFFERENCES IN ATTACHMENT

Although the Attachment Q-Sort, which yields a continuous score, has been in use for over 20 years, the majority of infant attachment research still uses the Strange Situation and thus its classifications of secure, avoidant, resistant, and disorganized attachment. This taxonomic approach was chosen by Ainsworth and colleagues to capture the patterned nature of Strange Situation behavior—multifaceted behavioral configurations that unfold as the stress of the situation increases (Ainsworth et al., 1978). As the validity of the Attachment Q-Sort demonstrates, however, the taxonomy is not the only way to describe individual differences in attachment. Nonetheless, it is one that has proven extremely fruitful in theory and research. Recently

Fraley and Spieker (2003) employed complex taxometric analyses to test whether there is evidence that the attachment classifications represent naturally occurring types (e.g., naturally differentiated groups that are fundamentally divergent), rather than empirically and conceptually constructed groups based on underlying dimensions of behaviors. Their analysis did not yield evidence for naturally occurring types, suggesting that individual differences in attachment might also be described continuously—through multivariate combinations of behaviors displayed during the Strange Situation, such as avoiding contact, resisting contact, seeking proximity to the caregiver, and maintaining contact with the caregiver. Of course, no empirical issue is ever settled by one study, and this study provided a somewhat imperfect test of this extremely complex issue (Sroufe, 2003; Waters & Beauchaine, 2003); the results are provocative nonetheless.

As attachment researchers become increasingly adept with sophisticated multivariate statistics, such techniques might help uncover new complexities in individual differences. Expansions of our exploration of individual differences, however, do not negate or even lessen the importance of the research done with the existing classifications. The taxonomy resulted in the recognition that some infants who did not fit the classifications were unified in the disorganization of their strategies (Cassidy, 2003); facilitated the search for individual differences in attachment across the lifespan (Cassidy, 2003); and made possible a plethora of research that has elucidated the differences between avoidant and resistant organizations (Sroufe, 2003). If advances in multivariate statistics result in new ways of conceptualizing individual differences, these methods are likely to supplement rather than supplant the utility of the Strange Situation classifications, much in the way that the Attachment Q-Sort has done.

A DEVELOPMENTAL PERSPECTIVE ON INDIVIDUAL DIFFERENCES IN ATTACHMENT

Bowlby proposed a very particular view of individual differences over time, based on an adaptation of Waddington's (1957) "developmental pathways" (analogous to branching tracks in a train yard; see Sroufe, 1997). In this view, early differences in attachment do not directly cause later differences in functioning; rather, they initiate pathways that are probabilistically related to certain later outcomes.

Because any outcome is always the joint product of earlier history and current circumstances, changes in patterns of adaptation always remain possible. Prior adaptation, however, constrains subsequent development: Following a particular developmental trajectory limits the degree and nature of change, both in the sense that the longer a pathway has been followed the more difficult it is to achieve substantial change in direction, and in the sense that not all patterns of subsequent adaptation are equally likely. This results in change that is lawful rather than unpredictable.

Stability of the surrounding environment is certainly a partial explanation for the stability of individual differences. There is, however, a transaction between individual history and environment. One reason why change away from maladaptive behavioral patterns is difficult is that the environment itself is influenced by the individual; it does not simply wash over the person as an independent force. Individuals interpret, select, and influence the people and circumstances surrounding them to confirm existing beliefs and adaptational pathways (Scarr & McCartney, 1983; Sroufe, 1983; Sroufe, Egeland, & Kreutzer, 1990). Patterns of maladaptation *are* maladaptive in part because they lead to environmental experiences that perpetuate them. Take, for example, the case of avoidant attachment. If such children encounter responsive peers and teachers, countering the rejection they have experienced previously, in time one would expect changes in their working models of self and relationships. Such environmental inputs become less likely, however, because children with these histories are more likely to isolate themselves (Sroufe, 1983), to interpret the ambiguous or even supportive efforts of others as hostile (Suess et al., 1992), and to be rejected by both peers (Fagot, 1997) and teachers. In the Minnesota Parent–Child Project, the children with avoidant histories were the only children in the nursery school who made teachers angry, perhaps because of their cool defiance or aggression toward vulnerable children (Sroufe & Fleeson, 1988; Troy & Sroufe, 1987). It is because children have a role in creating their own later experiences that describing individual history and stability of the environment as completely separate influences is unduly simplistic.

The patterns of adaptation reflected in early attachment are, of course, subject to change. The pathways model implies two things about change: (1) The earlier a change in circumstances is seen (the shorter the time a pathway has been pursued), the more readily change may be accom-

plished; and (2) the more sustained the forces of change, the more permanent the change will be. Attachment classification itself has been shown to change between the ages of 12 and 18 months with changes in caregiver life stress (Egeland & Farber, 1984; Vaughn, Egeland, Sroufe, & Waters, 1979). Beyond infancy, the later functioning of children who were securely (or insecurely) attached as infants is sometimes worse (or better) than would have been predicted from attachment alone. Such change is lawful, with the most potent factors identified thus far being changes in caregiver life stress, social support, and depression (Erickson, Sroufe, & Egeland, 1985; Pianta et al., 1990). Longitudinally assessed changes in attachment security between the Strange Situation in infancy and attachment state of mind on the Adult Attachment Interview in adolescence and adulthood have been lawfully predicted by divorce, life stress, family functioning, and features of the home environment during the interim years (Hamilton, 2000; Sampson, 2004; Waters, Merrick, Treboux, Crowell, & Albersheim, 2000; Weinfield, Sroufe, & Egeland, 2000; Weinfield, Whaley, & Egeland, 2004).

Current patterns of care and other environmental circumstances are clearly related to current adaptation, but this does not erase the influence of prior history. Early attachment history has been shown to add to the prediction of functioning even after the influence of contemporary experiences has been taken into account. For example, in the Parent–Child Project, peer competence and psychopathology measures obtained in adolescence were predicted by assessments of family functioning at age 13 years. Nonetheless, early history of care and adaptation still added predictive power (Englund et al., 2000). Even in the face of changes in adaptation, therefore, early experience still informs later behavior (Sroufe et al., 1990).

ON FINDING AND NOT FINDING PREDICTIONS FROM ATTACHMENT

Researchers do not always find the degree of predictability with regard to individual differences in attachment that we have reported here, both from the Minnesota studies and from other research. Indeed, the Minnesota Parent–Child Project findings with regard to attachment are often modest as well. There is some inconsistency in the literature (see Thompson, Chapter 16, this volume), with some findings being small or nonsignificant, and others being quite powerful. There are many possible reasons for these varied results.

Measurement Challenges

One issue that warrants consideration is measurement. Constructs such as secure and insecure attachment and subsequent socioemotional outcomes are extraordinarily difficult to assess. In studying such issues, investigators face not only the complexity of the constructs themselves, but also their changing manifestations across development.

Adequacy of measurement is a basic requirement for research of any type. With regard to early attachment, the only laboratory measure that is thoroughly validated against secure-base behavior at home is Ainsworth's Strange Situation coding scheme, as used for infants between 12 and 20 months old. Beyond 20 months of age, the original observational paradigm and coding scheme need to be modified or changed entirely to account for developmental changes in the child and relationship (Ainsworth et al., 1978; Marvin, 1997). Other laboratory procedures for assessing early attachment, though perhaps promising, have yet to be as thoroughly validated against home behavior (see Solomon & George, Chapter 18, this volume). Research using unvalidated measures to assess attachment relationships may be introducing as-yet-unidentified measurement error into analyses.

Single assessments of constructs can also introduce unanticipated measurement error into analyses. Multiple assessments of constructs, particularly when gleaned from multiple reporters, can capture more of the true variance associated with the construct than a single measurement, even when that single measurement is sufficiently valid and reliable.

In the Parent–Child Project, multiple measurements were administered at different times, using multiple reporters. Attachment security was assessed twice, at 12 and 18 months, and these assessments were often pooled for a more robust indicator of attachment. We also pooled outcome assessments to establish more robust variables. Although individual differences in attachment did relate to teacher appraisals of social competence and behavior problems, relations based on the report of one teacher for each participant were significant but very small. Combining the reports of multiple teachers across years increased effect sizes. Pooling the reports of four independent counselors in the

project summer camps served a similar purpose, yielding dramatically more impressive findings.

Counterintuitive research findings lead to natural questions about the psychometric properties of the measures used. Sound measurement strategies can help reduce psychometric problems, permitting confident exploration of counterintuitive results. A useful example comes from the work of the Grossmanns. They found an unusually high rate of avoidant attachment in the Strange Situation assessments of their Bielefeldt sample (Grossmann et al., 1985). Avoidant attachment in this sample, however, was related to caregiver sensitivity at 6 months and to other external correlates of avoidant attachment that had been established in previous samples, thus reducing the likelihood that the results could be attributed to measurement error. Further assessments showed this high rate of avoidant attachment to be a cohort effect, reflecting difficult societal circumstances at the time that may have influenced caregiving environments. The high rate of avoidant attachment in fact represented a coherent and informative consequence of a characteristic of the sample. Such research holds an important place in the study of attachment, because it allows us to understand more about the processes that influence individual differences.

Specificity of the Role of Attachment in Development

Beyond these measurement concerns, conceptual problems are often at issue. Not only are many aspects of early care outside of the attachment domain (e.g., the socialization of impulse control; Sroufe, 1997), but variations in quality of care, even broadly conceived, are not responsible for all aspects of development and behavior. For example, one early inconsistency in the literature concerned the relation between attachment security and the age of mirror self-recognition (Cicchetti, 1986; Lewis, Brooks-Gunn, & Jaskir, 1985; Sroufe, 1988). Such inconsistencies do not diminish the value of Bowlby and Ainsworth's elaboration of attachment theory, however, because nothing in the theory would lead to a strong prediction regarding a variable that is so heavily influenced by cognitive maturation. To the extent that such relations are found in research, they are most likely to be indirect, and are not validations of attachment theory per se. In the Parent–Child Project, there was an impressive link between infant attachment and math achievement at age 16 years (Teo, Carlson,

Mathieu, Egeland, & Sroufe, 1996). This relation certainly did not come about because attachment security has a direct influence on the brain's ability to process math problems. More likely, math achievement requires regular attendance at school and perhaps specific support at home. Adolescents with secure histories, both because their parents remain more involved and for a variety of other reasons, attend school more regularly. Relations between attachment history and reading achievement in high school are less strong, probably because reading proficiency is established early. Although this finding is interesting, it cannot be taken as a confirmation of attachment theory.

Bowlby did not conceive of the internal working model as a model for all things, but rather as a model of expectations and beliefs about oneself, other people, and relationships. Consequently, attachment should be expected to exert its influence on a child's later adaptation primarily in the context of beliefs about the self and relationships, rather than indiscriminately predicting all things, both good and bad. The emotion regulation and behavioral reciprocity learned in this early relationship should also be most influential in the realm of subsequent personality and relationship issues.

Even within the parent–child relationship, not all interactions are driven by the attachment–exploration balance. Minimally stressful free-play sessions, for example, may appear quite similar for secure and insecure dyads (Ainsworth, 1990). Other elements of parent–child relationships, and other elements of children's lives overall, predict individual differences in adaptation as well (Sroufe, Carlson, Egeland, & Collins, 2005b). It would be both naive and incorrect to suggest that infant attachment is solely and directly responsible for adaptation during childhood and adolescence. Attachment does *contribute*, however, to explaining individual differences in trajectories of adaptation during childhood, particularly when it is combined with other assessments of subsequent experience and current circumstances (Bowlby, 1973, 1980; Yates, Sroufe, & Egeland, 2003). Attachment theory is concerned with social behavior and emerging expectations of self, others, and relationships. The strong theoretical predictions relate to feelings of self-worth, expectations regarding others, and capacities for close relationships. One could argue that these areas of personality and interpersonal functioning may influence diverse aspects of life, but the core predictions of the theory are clear.

Even within the domain of psychopathology, it is not reasonable to expect individual differences in attachment to be equally predictive of all problems. In the Parent–Child Project, we deliberately singled out anxiety problems, conduct problems, and dissociation as prototypical resistant, avoidant, and disorganized outcomes, respectively. Anxiety and alienation (along with impoverished empathic capacity) are clear derivatives of the patterns of care associated with resistance and avoidance, respectively, and the disorganization and disorientation inherent in the failure to maintain an attachment orientation should have consequences for self-integration. Other kinds of problems should not be expected to be closely related to attachment history. For example, attention-deficit/hyperactivity disorder is more consistently related to early patterns of overstimulation and parent–child boundary violations than to attachment history (Carlson, Jacobvitz, & Sroufe, 1995). A full understanding of development and developmental psychopathology requires much more than knowledge of attachment history.

The Value of Studying Differing Samples

A final reason for varying results among studies might be the particular samples studied. Participants in the Parent–Child Project were at risk because of poverty and high life stress. At-risk samples tend to have higher rates of maladaptation in general and psychopathology in particular; indeed, this was the original rationale for studying this population. Certainly the increased range of outcomes might have strengthened the relation between insecure attachment and pathology, particularly as compared to smaller middle-class samples with a more restricted range of outcomes. Middle-class samples have some advantages in that they include more stable attachments and much stronger relations with certain outcomes, in part because of more stable life circumstances. Waters and colleagues (2000) found dramatic continuity between infant attachment classification and Adult Attachment Interview classification in a young adult middle-class sample. In the Parent–Child Project, a nonsignificant relation was found between organized infant attachment classifications and Adult Attachment Interview classification at age 19 (Weinfield et al., 2000, 2004), and a modest but significant relation was found between 18-month (but not 12-month) infant attachment and the Adult Attachment Interview at age 26 (Sampson, 2004). We believe that the difference in the samples is at the heart of the difference in findings. In both samples, negative attachment-related life experiences were associated with instability of attachment classifications. The middle-class sample allows us to see that attachment can be stable over a long period of time; the higher rate of discontinuity (and the higher rate of negative life events) in the Parent–Child Project, however, allows for a more in-depth examination of types of experiences related to stability and change. Both middle-class samples and samples that are more at risk for developmental difficulties are needed in continuing research. Only through research that spans geographic, socioeconomic, family structure, and cultural boundaries will we gain a full understanding of the complexities of attachment's role in development.

CONCLUSION

In general, the meaning of individual differences in attachment security, as conceptualized by Bowlby and Ainsworth, has been well substantiated by research. At times, of course, well-conceptualized, rigorous studies have failed to obtain predictive relations. Development is extraordinarily complex, and longitudinal research is very difficult to carry out. Despite these challenges, research has repeatedly confirmed core propositions of this individual-differences theory.

In this chapter, we have described Bowlby and Ainsworth's theory of attachment security with regard to the normative function of attachment relationships, antecedents and qualities of individual differences in attachment, and consequences of individual differences in attachment for social and personality development and for psychopathology. Bowlby focused on attachment because of its evolutionary value in the survival of the human infant, and because of its central role in subsequent human adaptation and development. The normative stages of attachment formation he proposed (see Marvin & Britner, Chapter 12, this volume) inspired Ainsworth's assessment procedure. The similarity of resistance and avoidance to the patterns of protest, anger, and detachment that are normal responses in the face of loss of a caregiver led Ainsworth to focus on these behaviors in ongoing infant–caregiver relationships. The advent of the Strange Situation procedure has generated 30 years of research on the meaning and consequences of individual differences in

infant attachment for development, and has been the starting point for the emergent study of attachment processes after infancy.

Bowlby's theories about the implications of individual differences in attachment for personality development remain not only testable but also critically important to our understanding of the role of early experience in socioemotional development. These ideas have guided substantial infant research, and (as the contents of this volume demonstrate) will no doubt continue to contribute to our understanding of attachment as Bowlby (1969/1982) conceptualized it, "from the cradle to the grave" (p. 208).

REFERENCES

Achenbach, T. (1978). The child behavior profile: I. Boys aged 6–11. *Journal of Consulting and Clinical Psychology, 46,* 478–488.

Aguilar, B., Sroufe, L. A., Egeland, B., & Carlson, E. (2000). Distinguishing the early-onset/persistent and adolescence-onset antisocial behavior types: From birth to 16 years. *Development and Psychopathology, 12,* 109–132.

Ainsworth, M. D. S. (1967). *Infancy in Uganda.* Baltimore: Johns Hopkins University Press.

Ainsworth, M. D. S. (1969). Object relations, dependency, and attachment: A theoretical review of the infant–mother relationship. *Child Development, 40,* 969–1025.

Ainsworth, M. D. S. (1972). Attachment and dependency: A comparison. In J. L. Gewirtz (Ed.), *Attachment and dependency* (pp. 97–137). Washington, DC: V. H. Winston.

Ainsworth, M. D. S. (1990). Epilogue: Some considerations regarding theory and assessment relevant to attachments beyond infancy. In M. T. Greenberg, D. Cicchetti, & E. M. Cummings (Eds.), *Attachment in the preschool years* (pp. 463–488). Chicago: University of Chicago Press.

Ainsworth, M. D. S., & Bell, S. M. (1974). Mother–infant interaction and the development of competence. In K. Connolly & J. Bruner (Eds.), *The growth of competence* (pp. 97–118). New York: Academic Press.

Ainsworth, M. D. S., Blehar, M., Waters, E., & Wall, S. (1978). *Patterns of attachment: A psychological study of the Strange Situation.* Hillsdale, NJ: Erlbaum.

Ainsworth, M. D. S., & Wittig, B. A. (1969). Attachment and exploratory behaviour of one-year-olds in a strange situation. In B. M. Foss (Ed.), *Determinants of infant behaviour* (Vol. 4, pp. 111–136). London: Methuen.

Arend, R., Gove, F., & Sroufe, L. A. (1979). Continuity of individual adaptation from infancy to kindergarten: A predictive study of ego-resiliency and curiosity in preschoolers. *Child Development, 50*, 950–959.

Banta, T. J. (1970). Tests for the evaluation of early childhood education: The Cincinnati Autonomy Test Battery (CATB). In J. Hellmuth (Ed.), *Cognitive studies* (pp. 424–490). New York: Brunner/Mazel.

Bates, J., Maslin, C., & Frankel, K. (1985). Attachment security, mother–child interactions, and temperament as predictors of behavior problem ratings at age three years. In I. Bretherton & E. Waters (Eds.), Growing points of attachment theory and research. *Monographs of the Society for Research in Child Development, 50*(1–2, Serial No. 209), 167–193.

Belsky, J., & Fearon, R. M. P. (2002). Early attachment security, subsequent maternal sensitivity, and later child development: Does continuity in development depend upon continuity of caregiving? *Attachment and Human Development, 4*, 361–387.

Belsky, J., & Rovine, M. (1987). Temperament and attachment security in the Strange Situation: An empirical rapprochement. *Child Development, 58*, 787–795.

Berlin, L., & Cassidy, J. (2003). Mothers' self-reported control of their preschool children's emotional expressiveness: A longitudinal study of associations with infant–mother attachment and children's emotion regulation. *Social Development, 12*, 477–495.

Bohlin, G., Hagekull, B., & Rydell, A. (2000). Attachment and social functioning: A longitudinal study from infancy to middle childhood. *Social Development, 9*, 24–39.

Bowlby, J. (1969/1982). *Attachment and loss: Vol. 1. Attachment.* New York: Basic Books.

Bowlby, J. (1973). *Attachment and loss: Vol. 2. Separation: Anxiety and anger.* New York: Basic Books.

Bowlby, J. (1980). *Attachment and loss: Vol. 3. Loss: Sadness and depression.* New York: Basic Books.

Bowlby, J. (1988). Developmental psychiatry comes of age. *American Journal of Psychiatry, 145*, 1–10.

Carlson, E. (1998). A prospective longitudinal study of attachment disorganization/disorientation. *Child Development, 69*, 1107–1128.

Carlson, E., Jacobvitz, D., & Sroufe, L. A. (1995). A developmental investigation of inattentiveness and hyperactivity. *Child Development, 66*, 37–54.

Cassidy, J. (1994). Emotion regulation: Influences of attachment relationships. In N. Fox (Ed.), The development of emotion regulation. *Monographs of the Society for Research in Child Development, 59*(2–3, Serial No. 240), 228–249.

Cassidy, J. (2003). Continuity and change in the measurement of infant attachment: Comment on Fraley and Spiker (2003). *Developmental Psychology, 39*, 409–412.

Cassidy, J., & Berlin, L. (1994). The insecure/ambivalent pattern of attachment: Theory and research. *Child Development, 65*, 971–981.

Cicchetti, D. (1986, April). *Organization of the self-system in atypical populations.* Paper presented at the biennial meeting of the International Conference on Infant Studies, Los Angeles.

Cicchetti, D., & Tucker, D. (1994). Development and self regulatory structures of the mind. *Development and Psychopathology, 4*, 533–549.

Cole, P., Martin, S., & Dennis, T. (2004). Emotion regulation as a scientific construct: Methodological challenges and directions for child development research. *Child Development, 75*, 317–333.

Crockenberg, S. (1981). Infant irritability, mother responsiveness, and social support influences on the security of infant–mother attachment. *Child Development, 52*, 857–865.

Dallaire, D. H., & Weinraub, M. (2005). Predicting children's separation anxiety at age 6: The contributions of infant–mother attachment security, maternal sensitivity, and maternal separation anxiety. *Attachment and Human Development, 7*, 393–408.

Denham, S., Blair, K., Schmidt, M., & DeMulder, E. (2002). Compromised emotional competence: Seeds of violence sown early? *American Journal of Orthopsychiatry, 72*, 70–82.

DeOliveira, C. A., Bailey, H. N., Moran, G., & Pederson, D. (2004). Emotion socialization as a framework for understanding the development of disorganized attachment. *Social Development, 13*, 437–467.

De Wolff, M., & van IJzendoorn, M. (1997). Sensitivity and attachment: A meta-analysis on parental antecedents of infant attachment. *Child Development, 68*, 571–591.

Diener, M., Mangelsdorf, S., McHale, J., & Frosch, C. (2002). Infants' behavioral strategies for emotion regulation with fathers and mothers: Associations with emotional expressions and attachment quality. *Infancy, 3*, 153–174.

Dutra, L., & Lyons-Ruth, K. (2005, April). Maltreatment, maternal and child psychopathology, and quality of early care as predictors of adolescent dissociation. In J. Borelli (Chair), *Interrelations of attachment and trauma symptoms: A developmental perspective.* Symposium conducted at the biennial meeting of the Society for Research in Child Development, Atlanta, GA.

Egeland, B., Carlson, E., & Sroufe, L. A. (1993). Resilience as process. *Development and Psychopathology, 5*, 517–528.

Egeland, B., & Farber, E. (1984). Infant–mother attachment: Factors related to its development and changes over time. *Child Development, 55*, 753–771.

Elicker, J., Englund, M., & Sroufe, L. A. (1992). Predicting peer competence and peer relationships in childhood from early parent–child relationships. In R. Parke & G. Ladd (Eds.), *Family–peer relationships: Modes of linkage* (pp. 77–106). Hillsdale, NJ: Erlbaum.

Englund, M., Levy, A., Hyson, D., & Sroufe, L. A. (2000). Adolescent social competence: Effectiveness in a group setting. *Child Development, 71*, 1049–1060.

Erickson, M. F., Sroufe, L. A., & Egeland, B. (1985).

The relationship of quality of attachment and behavior problems in preschool in a high risk sample. In I. Bretherton & E. Waters (Eds.), Growing points of attachment theory and research. *Monographs of the Society for Research in Child Development, 50*(1–2, Serial No. 209), 147–186.

Fagot, B. (1997). Attachment, parenting, and peer interactions of toddler children. *Developmental Psychology, 33,* 489–499.

Fraley, R. C., & Spieker, S. (2003). Are infant attachment patterns continuously or categorically distributed?: A taxometric analysis of strange situation behavior. *Developmental Psychology, 39,* 387–404.

Frankel, K. F., & Bates, J. E. (1990). Mother–toddler problem solving: Antecedents in attachment, home behavior, and temperament. *Child Development, 61,* 810–819.

Gewirtz, J. L. (1972). Attachment, dependence, and a distinction in terms of stimulus control. In J. L. Gewirtz (Ed.), *Attachment and dependency* (pp. 179–215). Washington, DC: V. H. Winston.

Gianino, A., & Tronick, E. Z. (1988). The mutual regulation model: The infant's self and interactive regulation coping and defensive capacities. In T. Field, P. McCabe, & N. Schneiderman (Eds.), *Stress and coping* (pp. 47–68). Hillsdale, NJ: Erlbaum.

Grossmann, K., Grossmann, K. E., Spangler, G., Suess, G., & Unzner, L. (1985). Maternal sensitivity and newborn orienting responses as related to quality of attachment in northern Germany. In I. Bretherton & E. Waters (Eds.), Growing points of attachment theory and research. *Monographs of the Society for Research in Child Development, 50*(1–2, Serial No. 209), 233–256.

Gunnar, M., Mangelsdorf, S., Larson, M., & Hertsgaard, L. (1989). Attachment, temperament, and adrenocortical activity in infancy: A study of psychoendocrine regulation. *Developmental Psychology, 25,* 355–363.

Hamilton, C. (2000). Continuity and discontinuity of attachment from infancy through adolescence. *Child Development, 71,* 690–694.

Isabella, R. (1993). Origins of attachment: Maternal interactive behavior across the first year. *Child Development, 64,* 605–621.

Jacobson, J., & Wille, D. (1986). The influence of attachment pattern on developmental changes in peer interaction from the toddler to the preschool period. *Child Development, 57,* 338–347.

Kestenbaum, R., Farber, E., & Sroufe, L. A. (1989). Individual differences in empathy among preschoolers: Relation to attachment history. *New Directions for Child Development, 44,* 51–64.

Kiser, L., Bates, J., Maslin, C., & Bayles, K. (1986). Mother–infant play at six months as a predictor of attachment security at thirteen months. *Journal of the American Academy of Child Psychiatry, 25,* 68–75.

Kochanska, G. (2001). Emotional development in children with different attachment histories: The first three years. *Child Development, 72,* 474–490.

Lewis, M., Brooks-Gunn, J., & Jaskir, J. (1985). Individual differences in visual self-recognition as a function of mother–infant attachment relationship. *Developmental Psychology, 21,* 1181–1183.

Lewis, M., Feiring, C., McGuffog, C., & Jaskir, J. (1984). Predicting psychopathology in six-year-olds from early social relations. *Child Development, 55,* 123–136.

Liotti, G. (1992). Disorganized/disoriented attachment in the etiology of the dissociative disorders. *Dissociation: Progress in the Dissociative Disorders, 5,* 196–204.

Lütkenhaus, P., Grossmann, K. E., & Grossmann, K. (1985). Infant–mother attachment at twelve months and style of interaction with a stranger at the age of three years. *Child Development, 56,* 1538–1542.

Lyons-Ruth, K. (1996). Attachment relationships among children with aggressive behavior problems: The role of early disorganized attachment patterns. *Journal of Consulting and Clinical Psychology, 64,* 64–73.

Lyons-Ruth, K., Alpern, L., & Repacholi, B. (1993). Disorganized infant attachment classification and maternal psychosocial problems as predictors of hostile-aggressive behavior in the preschool classroom. *Child Development, 64,* 572–585.

Lyons-Ruth, K., Dutra, L., Schuder, M., & Bianchi, I. (2006). From infant attachment disorganization to adult dissociation: Relational adaptations or traumatic experiences? *Psychiatric Clinics of North America, 29,* 63–86.

Lyons-Ruth, K., Easterbrooks, M. A., & Cibelli, C. D. (1997). Infant attachment strategies, infant mental lag, and maternal depressive symptoms: Predictors of internalizing and externalizing symptoms at age 7. *Developmental Psychology, 33,* 681–692.

Main, M., & Hesse, E. (1990). Parents' unresolved traumatic experiences are related to infant disorganized attachment status: Is frightened and/or frightening parental behavior the linking mechanism? In M. T. Greenberg, D. Cicchetti, & E. M. Cummings (Eds.), *Attachment in the preschool years* (pp. 161–182). Chicago: University of Chicago Press.

Main, M., & Morgan, H. (1996). Disorganization and disorientation in infant strange situation behavior: Phenotypic resemblance to dissociative states. In L. Michelson & W. Ray (Eds.), *Handbook of dissociation: Theoretical, empirical, and clinical perspectives* (pp. 107–138). New York: Plenum Press.

Main, M., & Solomon, J. (1990). Procedures for identifying infants as disorganized/disoriented during the Ainsworth Strange Situation. In M. T. Greenberg, D. Cicchetti, & E. M. Cummings (Eds.), *Attachment in the preschool years* (pp. 121–160). Chicago: University of Chicago Press.

Mangelsdorf, S., & Frosch, C. (2000). Temperament and attachment: One construct or two? In H. W. Reese (Ed.), *Advances in child development and behavior* (Vol. 27, pp. 181–220). San Diego, CA: Academic Press.

Mangelsdorf, S., Gunnar, M., Kestenbaum, R., Lang, S., & Andreas, D. (1990). Infancy proneness-to-distress temperament, maternal personality, and mother–

infant attachment: Associations and goodness of fit. *Child Development, 61,* 820–831.

Marvin, R. S. (1997). Ethological and general systems perspectives on child–parent attachment during the toddler and preschool years. In N. Segal, G. Weisfeld, & C. Weisfeld (Eds.), *Uniting psychology and biology: Integrative perspectives on human development* (pp. 189–216). Washington, DC: American Psychological Association.

Matas, L., Arend, R., & Sroufe, L. A. (1978). Continuity of adaptation in the second year: The relationship between quality of attachment and later competence. *Child Development, 49,* 547–556.

McElwain, N., Cox, M., Burchinal, M., & Macfie, J. (2003). Differentiating among insecure infant–mother classifications: A focus on child–friend interaction and exploration during solitary play at 36 months. *Attachment and Human Development, 5,* 136–164.

National Institute of Child Health and Human Development (NICHD) Early Child Care Research Network. (1997). The effects of infant child care on mother–infant attachment security. *Child Development, 68,* 860–879.

National Institute of Child Health and Human Development (NICHD) Early Child Care Research Network. (2004). Affect dysregulation in the mother–child relationship in the toddler years: Antecedents and consequences. *Development and Psychopathology, 16,* 43–68.

Nezworski, T. (1983). *Continuity in adaptation into the fourth year: Individual differences in curiosity and exploratory behavior of preschool children.* Unpublished doctoral dissertation, University of Minnesota.

Ogawa, J. R., Egeland, B., & Carlson, E. A. (1998). [The relation between disorganized attachment, childhood trauma, and psychopathological dissociation]. Unpublished raw data.

Ogawa, J. R., Sroufe, L. A., Weinfield, N. S., Carlson, E., & Egeland, B. (1997). Development and the fragmented self: A longitudinal study of dissociative symptomatology in a nonclinical sample. *Development and Psychopathology, 9,* 855–879.

Oppenheim, D., Sagi, A., & Lamb, M. (1988). Infant–adult attachments on the kibbutz and their relation to socioemotional development four years later. *Developmental Psychology, 24,* 427–433.

Ostoja, E. (1996). *Developmental antecedents of friendship competence in adolescence: The roles of early adaptational history and middle childhood peer competence.* Unpublished doctoral dissertation, University of Minnesota.

Pastor, D. (1981). The quality of mother–infant attachment and its relationship to toddlers' initial sociability with peers. *Developmental Psychology, 17,* 326–335.

Pederson, D., Gleason, K., Moran, G., & Bento, S. (1998). Maternal attachment representations, maternal sensitivity, and the infant–mother attachment relationship. *Developmental Psychology, 34,* 925–933.

Pianta, R., Egeland, B., & Sroufe, L. A. (1990). Maternal stress in children's development: Predictions of school outcomes and identification of protective factors. In J. E. Rolf, A. Masten, D. Cicchetti, K. Neuchterlen, & S. Weintraub (Eds.), *Risk and protective factors in the development of psychopathology* (pp. 215–235). New York: Cambridge University Press.

Posada, G., Jacobs, A., Carbonell, O., Alzate, G., Bustamante, M., & Arenas, A. (1999). Maternal care and attachment security in ordinary and emergency contexts. *Developmental Psychology, 35,* 1379–1388.

Renken, B., Egeland, B., Marvinney, D., Mangelsdorf, S., & Sroufe, L. A. (1989). Early childhood antecedents of aggression and passive withdrawal in early elementary school. *Journal of Personality, 57,* 257–281.

Robertson, J., & Robertson, J. (1971). Young children in brief separation: A fresh look. *Psychoanalytic Study of the Child, 26,* 264–315.

Sampson, M. (2004). *Continuity and change in patterns of attachment between infancy, adolescence, and early adulthood in a high risk sample.* Unpublished doctoral dissertation, University of Minnesota.

Scarr, S., & McCartney, K. (1983). How people make their own environments: A theory of genotype → environment effects. *Child Development, 54,* 424–435.

Schore, A. (1994). *Affect regulation and the origin of the self: The neurobiology of emotional development.* Hillsdale, NJ: Erlbaum.

Seifer, R., Schiller, M., Sameroff, A., Resnick, S., & Riordan, K. (1996). Attachment, maternal sensitivity, and infant temperament during the first year of life. *Developmental Psychology, 32,* 12–25.

Shulman, S., Elicker, J., & Sroufe, L. A. (1994). Stages of friendship growth in preadolescence as related to attachment history. *Journal of Social and Personal Relationships, 11,* 341–361.

Sroufe, L. A. (1979). The coherence of individual development. *American Psychologist, 34,* 834–841.

Sroufe, L. A. (1983). Infant–caregiver attachment and patterns of adaptation in preschool: The roots of maladaptation and competence. In M. Perlmutter (Ed.), *Minnesota Symposium on Child Psychology: Vol. 16. Development and policy concerning children with special needs* (pp. 41–83). Hillsdale, NJ: Erlbaum.

Sroufe, L. A. (1986). Bowlby's contribution to psychoanalytic theory and developmental psychopathology. *Journal of Child Psychology and Psychiatry, 27,* 841–849.

Sroufe, L. A. (1988). The role of infant–caregiver attachment in development. In J. Belsky & T. Nezworski (Eds.), *Clinical implications of attachment* (pp. 18–38). Hillsdale, NJ: Erlbaum.

Sroufe, L. A. (1996). *Emotional development: The organization of emotional life in the early years.* New York: Cambridge University Press.

Sroufe, L. A. (1997). Psychopathology as outcome of development. *Development and Psychopathology, 9,* 251–268.

Sroufe, L. A. (2003). Attachment categories as reflections of multiple dimensions: Comment on Fraley and Spieker (2003). *Developmental Psychology, 39*, 413–416.

Sroufe, L. A., Bennett, C., Englund, M., Urban, J., & Shulman, S. (1993). The significance of gender boundaries in preadolescence: Contemporary correlates and antecedents of boundary violation and maintenance. *Child Development, 64*, 455–466.

Sroufe, L. A., Carlson, E., & Shulman, S. (1993). Individuals in relationships: Development from infancy through adolescence. In D. C. Funder, R. Parke, C. Tomlinson, L. Keesey, & K. Widaman (Eds.), *Studying lives through time: Approaches to personality and development* (pp. 315–342). Washington, DC: American Psychological Association.

Sroufe, L. A., Egeland, B., & Carlson, E. A. (1999). One social world. In W. A. Collins & B. Laursen (Eds.), *Minnesota Symposium on Child Psychology: Vol. 30. Relationships as developmental context* (pp. 241–261). Mahwah, NJ: Erlbaum.

Sroufe, L. A., Egeland, B., Carlson, E. A., & Collins, W. A. (2005a). *The development of the person: The Minnesota Study of Risk and Adaptation from Birth to Adulthood.* New York: Guilford Press.

Sroufe, L. A., Egeland, B., Carlson, E. A., & Collins, W. A. (2005b). Placing early attachment experiences in developmental context: The Minnesota longitudinal study. In K. E. Grossmann, K. Grossmann, & E. Waters (Eds.), *Attachment from infancy to adulthood: The major longitudinal studies* (pp. 48–70). New York: Guilford Press.

Sroufe, L. A., Egeland, B., & Kreutzer, T. (1990). The fate of early experience following developmental change: Longitudinal approaches to individual adaptation in childhood. *Child Development, 61*, 1363–1373.

Sroufe, L. A., & Fleeson, J. (1986). Attachment and the construction of relationships. In W. Hartup & Z. Rubin (Eds.), *Relationships and development* (pp. 239–252). Hillsdale, NJ: Erlbaum.

Sroufe, L. A., & Fleeson, J. (1988). The coherence of individual relationships. In R. A. Hinde & J. Stevenson-Hinde (Eds.), *Relationships within families: Mutual influences* (pp. 27–47). Oxford, UK: Oxford University Press.

Sroufe, L. A., Fox, N., & Pancake, V. (1983). Attachment and dependency in developmental perspective. *Child Development, 54*, 1615–1627.

Sroufe, L. A., Schork, E., Motti, E., Lawroski, N., & LaFreniere, P. (1984). The role of affect in social competence. In C. Izard, J. Kagan, & R. Zajonc (Eds.), *Emotions, cognition, and behavior* (pp. 289–319). New York: Cambridge University Press.

Sroufe, L. A., & Waters, E. (1977). Attachment as an organizational construct. *Child Development, 48*, 1184–1199.

Stayton, D., & Ainsworth, M. D. S. (1973). Individual differences in infant responses to brief, everyday separations as related to other infant and maternal behaviors. *Developmental Psychology, 9*, 226–235.

Suess, G. J., Grossmann, K. E., & Sroufe, L. A. (1992). Effects of infant attachment to mother and father on quality of adaptation in preschool: From dyadic to individual organisation of self. *International Journal of Behavioral Development, 15*, 43–65.

Susman-Stillman, A., Kalkoske, M., Egeland, B., & Waldman, I. (1996). Infant temperament and maternal sensitivity as predictors of attachment security. *Infant Behavior and Development, 19*, 33–47.

Teo, A., Carlson, E., Mathieu, P., Egeland, B., & Sroufe, L. A. (1996). A prospective longitudinal study of psychosocial predictors of achievement. *Journal of School Psychology, 34*, 285–306.

Thompson, R. (1994). Emotion regulation: A theme in search of definition. In N. Fox (Ed.), The development of emotion regulation. *Monographs of the Society for Research in Child Development, 59*(2–3, Serial No. 240), 25–52.

Tronick, E. (1989). Emotions and emotional communication in infants. *American Psychologist, 44*, 112–119.

Troy, M., & Sroufe, L. A. (1987). Victimization among preschoolers: The role of attachment relationship theory. *Journal of the American Academy of Child and Adolescent Psychiatry, 26*, 166–172.

Urban, J., Carlson, E., Egeland, B., & Sroufe, L. A. (1991). Patterns of individual adaptation across childhood. *Development and Psychopathology, 3*, 445–460.

Vaughn, B. E., Egeland, B., Sroufe, L. A., & Waters, E. (1979). Individual differences in infant–mother attachment at twelve and eighteen months: Stability and change in families under stress. *Child Development, 50*, 971–975.

Vaughn, B. E., Lefever, G. B., Seifer, R., & Barglow, P. (1989). Attachment behavior, attachment security, and temperament during infancy. *Child Development, 60*, 728–737.

Vaughn, B. E., & Waters, E. (1990). Attachment behavior at home and in the laboratory: Q-sort observations and Strange Situation classifications of one-year-olds. *Child Development, 61*, 1965–1973.

Waddington, C. (1957). *The strategy of the genes.* London: Allen & Unwin.

Warren, S. L., Huston, L., Egeland, B., & Sroufe, L. A. (1997). Child and adolescent anxiety disorders and early attachment. *Journal of the American Academy of Child and Adolescent Psychiatry, 36*, 637–644.

Waters, E., & Beauchaine, T. P. (2003). Are there really patterns of attachment?: Comment on Fraley and Spieker (2003). *Developmental Psychology, 39*, 417–422.

Waters, E., & Deane, K. (1985). Defining and assessing individual differences in attachment relationships: Q-methodology and the organization of behavior in infancy and early childhood. In I. Bretherton & E. Waters (Eds.), Growing points of attachment theory and research. *Monographs of the Society for Research in Child Development, 50*(1–2, Serial No. 209), 41–65.

Waters, E., Merrick, S., Treboux, D., Crowell, J., & Albersheim, L. (2000). Attachment security in infancy and early adulthood: A twenty-year longitudinal study. *Child Development, 71*, 684–689.

Waters, E., Wippman, J., & Sroufe, L. A. (1979). Attachment, positive affect, and competence in the peer group: Two studies in construct validation. *Child Development, 50*, 821–829.

Weinfield, N. S., Ogawa, J. R., & Sroufe, L. A. (1997). Early attachment as a pathway to adolescent peer competence. *Journal of Research on Adolescence, 7*, 241–265.

Weinfield, N. S., Sroufe, L. A., & Egeland, B. (2000). Attachment from infancy to young adulthood in a high-risk sample: Continuity, discontinuity and their correlates. *Child Development, 71*, 695–702.

Weinfield, N. S., Whaley, G. J. L., & Egeland, B. (2004). Continuity, discontinuity, and coherence in attachment from infancy to late adolescence: Sequelae of organization and disorganization. *Attachment and Human Development, 6*, 73–97.

Yates, T., Sroufe, L. A., & Egeland, B. (2003). Rethinking resilience: A developmental process perspective. In S. Luthar (Ed.), *Resilience and vulnerability: Adaptation in the context of childhood adversities* (pp. 243–266). New York: Cambridge University Press.

CHAPTER 5

Internal Working Models in Attachment Relationships
Elaborating a Central Construct in Attachment Theory

INGE BRETHERTON
KRISTINE A. MUNHOLLAND

Bowlby's attachment theory (1969/1982, 1973, 1980) accorded a central role in adaptive human development to supportive interpersonal relationships. From the cradle to the grave, he argued, an individual's mental health is intimately tied to relationships with attachment figures who afford emotional support and physical protection:

> For not only young children, it is now clear, but human beings of all ages are found to be at their happiest and to be able to deploy their talents to best advantage when they are confident that, standing behind them, there are one or more trusted persons who will come to their aid should difficulties arise. The person trusted provides a secure base from which his (or her) companion can operate. (1973, p. 359)

How well attachment relationships can fulfill these safe-haven and secure-base functions, however, turns not only on attachment partners' actual behaviors, but on the translation of their interaction patterns into relationship representations—or, as Bowlby termed them, "internal working models." Internal working models of self and other in attachment relationships, Bowlby claimed, help members of an attachment dyad (parent and child, or adult couple) to anticipate, interpret, and guide interactions with partners. In

the course of development, infants' sensorimotor–affective internal working models become increasingly complex and mentally "manipulable," enabling not only simple short-term predictions but also reflection on current, past, and future relationships by means of *internal simulation* (Bowlby, 1988). We deliberately emphasize the term "internal simulation" to indicate that Bowlby employed it before it was adopted by philosophers (e.g., Goldman, 1991) and neuroscientists (e.g., Adolphs, 2006; Gallese, 2005).

Bowlby's proposals about the formation, development, function, and intergenerational transmission of internal working models of self and attachment figures are scattered across the three volumes of his seminal trilogy *Attachment and Loss* (1969/1982, 1973, 1980) and his book *A Secure Base* (1988). To make these ideas more accessible as a whole, we summarize them in the first section of this chapter. In the second section, we discuss possible elaborations and extensions of the working-model construct by drawing on the literature from neuroscience and memory development. In the third section, we turn to studies conducted by attachment researchers. Specifically, we focus on the extent to which findings obtained with representational measures of attachment suitable for adults and children support, extend, and raise new questions about Bowlby's conceptualization of working models. We conclude with suggestions for future research.

BOWLBY AND THE PSYCHOANALYTIC INNER WORLD

That Bowlby emphasized the *function* of representation in the conduct of interpersonal relationships is not surprising. As a member of the British Psycho-Analytic Society, he was familiar with Freud's (1940/1963) definition of the inner world in *An Outline of Psychoanalysis*, which uncannily prefigured his own notion about the simulation and guidance function of "internal working models":

> The yield brought to light by scientific work from our primary sense perceptions will consist of an insight into connections and dependent relations which are present in the external world, which can somehow be reliably *reproduced or reflected in the internal world of our thought and a knowledge of which enables us to 'understand' something in the external world, to foresee it and possibly to alter it.* (p. 85; emphasis added)

When Freud's comments about representation were posthumously published (he died in 1939), most mainstream academic psychologists subscribed to behaviorism and considered the study of mental processes to be "unscientific." Thirty years later, when Bowlby undertook the task of reworking Freudian theory in light of new evidence (e.g., 1969/1982, 1973), academic psychology was still largely dominated by behaviorist precepts. To garner helpful theoretical ideas and empirical findings about the role of representation in attachment relationships, Bowlby therefore cast a wider, interdisciplinary net. The result was not a fully worked-out theory, but a promising conceptual framework to be filled in by others.

Bowlby's (1969/1982) conception of representation as mental model building was inspired by the writings of an eminent biologist (Young, 1964) who had borrowed the idea from a slim volume on *The Nature of Understanding* written by Kenneth Craik (1943). Craik was a young, philosophically trained psychologist and brilliant pioneer in what would later be called "artificial intelligence." Taking an evolutionary approach, he proposed that organisms that could generate "internal working models" of the environment would considerably improve their chances of survival by using these

models to mentally "run off" alternative courses of action and evaluate their likely outcome. Unfortunately, Craik's early death cut short any further work on this topic.

Conceding that the notion of internal working models might seem fanciful to researchers "steeped in extreme behaviorism," Bowlby (1969/1982) contended: "The notion that brains do in fact provide more or less elaborate models that 'can be made to conduct, as it were, small scale experiments in the head,' is one that appeals to anyone concerned to understand the complexity of behavior, and especially human behavior" (pp. 80–81). Bowlby rejected related terms such as "cognitive map," because "the word conjures up merely a static representation of topography" (p. 80). The term "internal working model," in contrast, implies a representational system that allows us, for example, to imagine interactions and conversations with others, based on our previous experiences with them:

> Every situation we meet with in life is construed in terms of the representational models we have of the world about us and of ourselves. Information reaching us through our sense organs is selected and interpreted in terms of those models, its significance for us and those we care for is evaluated in terms of them, and plans of action executed with those models in mind. On how we interpret and evaluate each situation, moreover, turns also how we feel. (Bowlby, 1980, p. 229)

This quotation shows that Bowlby regarded internal working models as a general construct, not one limited to attachment. It was with respect to relationship representations (of self and other in attachment relationships), however, that he most extensively discussed mental model building, model use, and model revision, and it is on this aspect that we focus in this chapter.

> Starting, we may suppose, towards the end of his first year, and probably especially actively during his second and third when he acquires the powerful and extraordinary gift of language, a child is busy constructing working models of how the physical world may be expected to behave, how his mother and other significant persons may be expected to behave, how he himself may be expected to behave, and how each interacts with the other. Within the framework of these working models he evaluates his situation and makes his plans. And within the framework of the working models of his mother and himself he evaluates special aspects of his situation and makes his attachment plans. (1969/1982, p. 354)

In our review of Bowlby's notions about internal working models, we highlight several issues that have caused misunderstandings in the literature: (1) whether attachment working models are to be understood as relationship-specific representations or as general strategies of relating; (2) how to understand the stability and change of working models; (3) to what degree and under which circumstances internal working models are consciously accessible and subject to defensive processes; and (4) how to conceptualize the processes in the intergenerational transmission of attachment working models.

Relationship Specificity

Bowlby (1969/1982, 1988, p. 129) postulated that a child's attachment working models are based "on real-life experiences of day-to-day interactions with his parents," and are therefore relationship-specific. Moreover, because they are constructed in interpersonal relationships, models of self and attachment figure(s) are perforce mutually confirming (e.g., parent as loving/protective and self as loved/secure):

> In the working model of the world that anyone builds a key feature is his notion of who his attachment figures are, where they may be found, and how they may be expected to respond. Similarly, in the working model of the self that anyone builds a key feature is his notion of how acceptable or unacceptable he himself is in the eyes of his attachment figures. On the structure of these complementary models are based that person's forecasts of how accessible and responsive his attachment figures are likely to be should he turn to them for support. In terms of the theory now advanced, it is on the structure of those models that depends, also, whether he feels confident that his attachment figures are in general readily available or whether he is more or less afraid that they will not be available—occasionally, frequently or most of the time. (1973, p. 203)

In short, the complementary models of self and parents represent both sides of the relationship.

Bowlby also advanced the idea that internal working models of self with specific attachment figures in infancy and early childhood "increasingly become a property of the child himself" (1988, p. 127)—a process that would be more complex for a child with two very different relationship-specific attachment working models. Acknowledging that little is known about the relative influence on personality development of the child's relationship

with father and mother, Bowlby speculated that during the early years, the model of self interacting with mother may be more influential because the mother is likely to be the child's principal caregiver (p. 129).

Continuity of Security in the Face of Developmental Change

In the attachment literature, the label "secure" is used regardless of age to describe an individual's trust that a protective, supportive figure will be emotionally available and responsive in case of need. This general definition obscures developmental changes that take place in how individuals experience and understand security.

Bowlby (1980, 1988) repeatedly stressed that a continuously secure attachment relationship requires an infant's embryonic working models of self and attachment figure(s) to be updated in step with communicative, social, and cognitive competencies that develop in childhood and adolescence. The same holds for a parent's working models of the child and of the self as attachment figure (see George & Solomon, Chapter 35, this volume).

Bowlby drew particular attention to young children's developing understanding that their attachment figures have separate (non-child-focused) goals. This cognitive advance permits secure attachment relationships to become "goal-corrected partnerships" (1969/1982, p. 355) in which there is give-and-take on *both* sides and in which inevitable conflicts can be resolved through reciprocal adjustment of goals (hence the term "goal correction"; see Marvin & Britner, Chapter 12, this volume). Pointing to mothers' role in this development, Bowlby cited a study by Light (1979) showing that mothers who referred to feelings and intentions while discussing the mother–child relationship had children with better perspective-taking skills (Solomon & George, Chapter 18, this volume). Bowlby also speculated that 2½-year-olds' abilities to talk meaningfully of their own and others' mental states, reported by Bretherton and Beeghly (1982), might be more advanced in children "whose mothers treat them sensitively" (2nd edition of *Attachment*, 1982, p. 370).

Although working models can and must be updated as children develop, Bowlby (1969/1982) mentioned several processes that ensure their relative stability. First, habitual interaction patterns bias perceptions—an idea borrowed from Piaget's (1952) concept of "assimilation." Thus a child's confidence in an attachment figure's emotional availability is not likely to be shattered by occasional lapses in a caregiver's sensitivity. Second, *two* individuals' working models (and hence expectations) are involved in a relationship; hence when *one* partner tries out new behaviors, the other may resist, and attempt to return the relationship to the old pattern. Third, frequently repeated interaction patterns have a tendency to become increasingly "automatized," making lesser demands on attention, but hindering the conscious revision of working models.

This being said, in secure relationships these normal stabilizing processes give way to revisions of the working models as a child (or an adult) realizes that the current models no longer yield adequate predictions. In Bowlby's (1988) own words, "As a securely attached child grows older and his parents treat him differently, a gradual updating of models occurs. This means that, though there is always a time-lag, his currently operative models continue to be reasonably good simulations of himself and his parents in interaction" (p. 130).

Aside from developmental revisions of internal working models in attachment relationships, Bowlby (1973) also considered what we here call their "affective discontinuity." Relying on evidence from clinical case studies of children with severe emotional problems, Bowlby (1973, 1980, 1988) argued that defensive changes in a child's working models are likely when parental behaviors, such as threats of abandonment, undercut trust in the parent as an attachment figure. Conversely, when a family's stressful circumstances improve, or effective support by others becomes available, a previously rejecting or neglectful parent may become able to respond more sensitively to his or her child's attachment needs. However, once defensive aspects of working-model organization are established in an insecure attachment relationship, such positive reconstructions can become quite difficult. As we discuss in the next subsection, representational processes take a considerably less straightforward course when previously secure relationships become insecure.

Consciousness and Working Model Organization in Light of Defensive Processes

The advent of psychology's cognitive revolution provided Bowlby with new tools for developing an alternative theoretical approach to Freud's ideas about the "dynamic unconscious" and repression.

We stress, however, that Bowlby (1980) regarded his proposals in this area as particularly tentative, conceding that "there is clearly a long way to go before the theory sketched is within sight of doing justice to the wide range of defensive phenomena met with clinically" (p. 44).

Using as his primary sources Dixon (1971), Erdelyi (1974), and Norman (1976), Bowlby (1980, p. 65) explained repression as the systematic exclusion from further processing of "certain information of significance to the individual" for long periods or permanently. To justify this view he cites extensive evidence that incoming information is always subjected to many stages of unconscious analysis and synthesis before becoming conscious. At each stage, information most relevant to current goals is selectively retained and sharpened, whereas less salient information is discarded. What distinguishes defensive from other types of selective exclusion is the goal: to prevent an individual from becoming aware of events or thoughts that would be unbearable if they were accepted as true. Whereas "defensive exclusion" may be temporarily adaptive, however, it is likely to become maladaptive if maintained in the long run or when circumstances change.

To demonstrate the effect of defensive exclusion on attachment working models, Bowlby (1973, 1980) reanalyzed published case studies of children and adults with severe emotional problems, but contended that the proposed processes also apply in less troubled relationships. Two situations struck Bowlby as particularly likely instigators of defensive exclusion in young children: (1) intense arousal of attachment behavior that is persistently rejected, ignored, ridiculed, or punished by a parent; and (2) knowing something about the parent that the parent does not wish the child to "know about and would punish him for accepting as true" (1980, p. 73). Examples of the latter are sexual abuse by a parent who denies that such behavior occurred or witnessing a father's suicide but being told by the mother that the death was due to a heart attack. A common response by children faced with such representational conflict is to develop two conflicting sets of working models of self with parent. One set, based on the child's adverse experience with the parent, is defensively excluded, whereas the other set, reflecting what the parent wants the child to believe, remains consciously accessible.

Bowlby provided two reasons why children commonly accept the parental version of what happened. First, it may be more frightening for a child to see his or her attachment figure as non-caring than to view the self as "bad." Second, a parent may have strongly forbidden the child to question the meaning of what occurred and may have threatened severe punishment if the child divulges the parent's behavior to others. In this context, Bowlby (1973) pointed out that many emotionally troubled adults in therapy still seem to harbor defensively excluded working models that were developed "in the early years on fairly simple lines" (p. 205) and that conflict with much more sophisticated, radically different conscious models dating from a later period. Here he appeared to propose that incompatible working models can develop sequentially as well as concurrently, and that the defensively excluded model, even though it has not been updated, reveals itself in an individual's adult behavior.

Alongside defensive exclusion, Bowlby (1980, citing research on hypnosis by Hilgard, 1974) proposed a second process, termed "segregation of (principal) systems," that seems more akin to dissociation than repression. "Principal system" denotes a self capable of self-perception and agency. Segregated multiple selves are said to be cognitively "walled off" from each other, each self having its own "sectionalized memory store" (or working models). These selves can alternate in consciousness, but generally only one self is dominant at any one time whereas the other (including its working models) is in a state of complete or partial deactivation (see pp. 59–60, 345–349). Bowlby defined a deactivated principal system as "an organized one and no less self-consistent than is the system with free access to action and consciousness" (p. 347). He contended that when "it takes control of behavior the segregated system is capable of framing plans ... albeit in clumsy and ineffective ways" (p. 348). As an example, Bowlby presented the case of an adolescent who, most of the time, was fully aware that her mother had died when she was 3 years old but who had no conscious memory of grieving. Yet occasionally this girl entered fugue states during which she disappeared from her home in what appeared to be a search for her mother. Bowlby also discussed a patient with two conflicting selves that were consciously accessible at the same time. Rather than being deactivated, one of the selves was merely kept secret from other people. He likened this condition to Freud's concept of "split in the ego."

The notion of defensive exclusion involves one self that is protected from conscious conflict because one of two incompatible sets of working models (self with parent) is defensively excluded. The notion of segregated principal systems, in contrast, involves multiple dissociated selves each with access to a different organized working model. The distinction seems important, but Bowlby did not pursue it in subsequent writings. While revisiting his earlier ideas in *A Secure Base* (1988), he linked defensive exclusion to "a spectrum of related syndromes within their commoner and less severe forms tend to be diagnosed as 'narcissism' or 'false self' and in their more severe forms may be labeled a fugue, a psychosis, or a case of multiple personality" (p. 113). Likewise, he uses defensive exclusion as an explanation for personality-splitting (p. 114), but segregated principal systems are no longer mentioned.

Finally, pertaining both to defensively excluded working models and working models sequestered in segregated selves, Bowlby proposed that contradictory working models that are derived from different sources (own experience or parental input) may also be differently encoded. Drawing on Tulving's (1972) distinction between "episodic" (autobiographical) and "semantic" memory (general knowledge base), he suggested that children's conscious representations of what parents or others misleadingly told them may be stored as general propositions in the semantic memory system while the child's own (defensively excluded or segregated) memories of traumatic attachment experiences might be stored "analogically" in the episodic memory system. This, Bowlby noted, might explain why patients often give starkly conflicting accounts of their parents during therapy sessions. Some provide general descriptions of parents as highly admirable, but then supply detailed contradictory anecdotes of how the parents had actually behaved or what they had actually said. Others make "uniformly adverse" generalizations about parents, but their detailed memories portray a more favorable image (1980, p. 62).

Whereas Bowlby frequently attributed a child's construction of conscious, but highly distorted attachment working models to misleading parental input, his discussion of the consequences of persistent defensive exclusion is also pertinent to this topic. The consequences he had in mind include most of the phenomena described as defenses in the psychoanalytic literature, but Bowlby (1980, pp. 64–69) preferred to group them into two broad categories: (1) deactivation of behavioral systems and (2) cognitive disconnection.

In regard to the first category, Bowlby stressed that behavioral systems, when deprived of their required input (be the source external or internal), will become partially or completely deactivated. If the deactivated systems are those controlling attachment, attachment-related behaviors, thoughts, and feelings "will cease to occur or to be experienced" (1980, p. 66), resulting in emotional detachment. Should fragments of relevant information seep through, system deactivation will be only partial, and fragments of attachment behavior or affect may become conscious in the form of moods, memories, or dreams. The activities, feelings, and thoughts normally governed by deactivated system(s) will be replaced by other activities that tend to absorb an undue portion of a person's attention. Bowlby contended that there is virtually no activity that cannot be used for this diversionary purpose.

In regard to the second set of consequences, Bowlby proposed that systematic and persistent defensive exclusion may result in three distinct ways of cognitive disconnection between an individual's affective and behavioral responses and the otherwise anxiety-provoking interpersonal situations that caused them. When this occurs, the disconnected feelings or behaviors are likely to receive a less threatening but erroneous explanation. First, individuals may misidentify the situation that is responsible for their negative affect. For example, a child may unconsciously fear that his mother might abandon him if he does not stay home with her, but consciously he may refuse to attend school because he is afraid of his teacher's criticism. Second, individuals may direct their negative feelings away from the person who aroused them, and instead direct them toward an irrelevant person or themselves. For example, an adult or child may defensively exclude his or her own unassuaged attachment needs, and instead direct compulsive caregiving behaviors toward a rejecting or helpless attachment figure. Third, an individual may react to a painful interpersonal situation by turning away from it and instead become morbidly preoccupied with psychological and physiological aspects of his or her own suffering.

Bowlby rejected psychoanalytic labels for defense mechanisms (e.g., projection, projective identification, denial, or displacement), because he feared that their use might prevent therapists from adequately exploring patients' real-life experiences. For the same reason, he urged great caution when using terms like "fantasy" and "magical thinking":

The more details one comes to know about the events in a child's life, and about what he has been told, what he has overheard and what he has observed but is not supposed to know, the more clearly can his ideas about the world and what may happen in the future be seen as perfectly reasonable constructions. (1979, p. 23)

Communication and Intergenerational Transmission

Bowlby (1973, 1988) envisioned two processes through which internal working models of secure and insecure attachment relations may be communicated from parent to child: (1) the quality of interaction, and (2) open discussion of emotion and relationships. Like other psychoanalysts (e.g., Stern, 1985), Bowlby focused extensively on the role of deliberate parental *miscommunications* in disorganizing or confusing children's internal working models, but he also acknowledged that parents perform a positive role in helping a child construct and revise working models through emotionally open dialogue:

Thus the family experience of those who grow up anxious and fearful is found to be characterized not only by uncertainty about parental support but often also by covert yet strongly distorting parental pressures: pressure on the child, for example, to act as caregiver for a parent; *or to adopt, and thereby to confirm, a parent's false models—of self, of child and of their relationship.* Similarly the family experience of those who grow up to become relatively stable and self-reliant is characterized not only by unfailing parental support when called upon but also by a steady yet timely encouragement toward increasing autonomy, and *by the frank communication by parents of working models—of themselves, of child and of others—that are not only tolerably valid but are open to be questioned and revised.* (1973, pp. 322–323; emphasis added)

Bowlby went on to explain that the experience of open communication in the family of origin may foster parents' ability to engage in emotionally open communication with their own children:

Because in all these respects children tend unwittingly to identify with parents and therefore adopt, when they become parents, the same patterns of behavior towards their children that they themselves have experienced during their own childhood, patterns of interaction are transmitted, more or less faithfully, from one generation to another. (1973, p. 323)

These statements are noteworthy for two reasons: (1) They lay out the processes whereby attachment working models may be transmitted from parents to children through behavioral and emotional interactions; and (2) they stress that children are most likely to develop adaptive, revisable attachment working models when parents encourage exploration of the inner world by modeling emotionally open (frank) verbal communication about relationships.

Throughout his writings, Bowlby drew a sharp distinction between attachment working models as they develop in secure and insecure relationships, most likely out of a desire for clearer exposition of unfamiliar ideas. It is important to stress, however, that he saw these contrasting descriptions not as a dichotomy, but as two ends of a continuum:

> Between the groups of people with extremes of either good or bad experience lie groups of people with an almost infinite range of intermediate sorts of experience. ... For example, some may have learnt that an attachment figure responds in a comforting way only when coaxed to do so. They grow up expecting that all such figures have to be coaxed. Others may have learnt during childhood that the wished for response can be obtained only if certain rules are kept. Provided the rules and the sanctions are mild and predictable, a person can still come to believe that support will always be available. (1973, pp. 208–209)

We encourage readers to keep this point in mind throughout the remainder of this chapter.

Summary

In formulating propositions about the function of working models in attachment relationships, Bowlby systematically sought validation and support from outside the psychoanalytic domain. Before the "cognitive revolution" took hold in psychology, he adopted Craik's (1943) enormously powerful concept of representation as model building and model use in the service of predicting and guiding interpersonal behavior. He then wedded this idea to Piaget's (1951, 1952) theory of sensorimotor development, representation, and perspective taking. Based on information-processing studies, he contrasted representational processes in secure and insecure attachment relationships, but acknowledged many gradations in between. Viewing representation and interpersonal communication as mutually reinforcing, he proposed that emotionally open dialogue with responsive attachment figures facilitates an individual's construction of well-functioning, revisable internal working models, which in their turn foster the

continuation of open communication. Bowlby also argued that frank discussion of emotions and other mental states encourages the development of social cognition. In insecure relationships, he noted, clear communication becomes more difficult as partners' conscious and unconscious working models become less consistent with each other because of defensive processes.

Many of Bowlby's intuitions about working models have proven to be remarkably prophetic. Since his last publication on attachment in 1988, numerous studies of neural processes and memory development have provided findings that help to flesh out and elaborate his proposals about the working-model construct. We review a selection of these contributions in the next section.

SELECTED PERSPECTIVES FROM THE FIELDS OF NEUROSCIENCE AND MEMORY DEVELOPMENT

Internal Working Models and Meaning Making

As our quotations from Bowlby's work reveal, he did not intend the concept of working models to be construed in terms of dispassionate mappings of an "objective" reality. Rather, he regarded emotional appraisals and goal setting as integral aspects of representation—a viewpoint that has much in common with the work of social psychologists Lewin (1933) and Heider (1958), with whose theories Bowlby was apparently unfamiliar.

Influenced by Gestalt psychology and with little concern for the hegemony of behaviorism, Lewin and Heider wrote extensively about representation in terms of personal and interpersonal meaning making, proposing ideas that are useful in thinking about working models. According to Lewin (1933), humans construe their psychological environment or "life space" in terms of the actions it is seen to invite, repel, permit, or prohibit in the context of current goals and competencies. Hence an infant who is likely to perceive a staircase as an impediment to reaching his or her disappearing mother may, a year or so later, perceive the same staircase as a means of joining her. Related ideas have appeared in James and Eleanor Gibson's concept of "affordances" (see E. Gibson, 1982).

Heider (1958) extended Lewin's (1933) concept of psychological life space to the interpersonal context, stressing that when we react to others, we do not usually perceive their actions as meaningless movement patterns that have to be laboriously interpreted. Rather, we understand others' behaviors (and we construct working models) in terms of how they make us feel, and what we believe our interaction partners are intending, thinking, perceiving and feeling.

Very much in accord with Lewin's and Heider's ideas, neuroimaging studies performed during the last decade have revealed a great deal about the brain as a meaning-making organ. These discoveries provide a new understanding of the human capacity to envision others as psychological beings who can evaluate and decide on a course of action—all highly relevant to the working-model construct.

A Model in the Brain

Since Bowlby (1969/1982) incorporated Craik's term "internal working model" into attachment theory, it was independently rediscovered by cognitive scientist Johnson-Laird (1983). Through his influence, it has been adopted by neuroscientists (e.g., Adolphs, 2003; Gallese, 2005) whose work is surprisingly consistent with Bowlby's notion that the brain constructs working models of self, attachment figures, and the environment. We begin this review with macaque studies, but devote most of it to insights relevant to working models that can be gleaned from neuroimaging of human brains.

Mirror Neuron Systems

While recording from single cells in monkeys' premotor cortex, Rizzolatti, Fadiga, Gallese, and Fogassi (1996) serendipitously discovered "mirror neurons." These neurons are triggered when a monkey performs a goal-directed hand action (e.g., picking up a peanut), but also when it merely observes a conspecific or even a human perform a similar action. What matters, is whether the observed action is goal-directed, not whether a particular hand shape or hand orientation is adopted. Other neurons (termed "canonical") fire when a monkey looks at an object that requires a particular hand shape for pickup, as well as when it actually uses that same hand shape to grasp the object. One might say that the monkey's brain creates an embodied awareness of the object's "pickuppable" affordance. Based on these and related findings, Gallese (2005) proposed that premotor mirror neurons and other neurons coupling perception and action enable monkeys to understand their peers' *intentional* (meaningful) actions in space through a process of "embodied simulation."

These findings naturally raised the question whether humans, too, possess mirror systems that enable the mental simulation of others' actions, goals, and emotions. The discovery that newborns are able to imitate mouth opening, tongue protrusion, lip pursing, finger movements, and even some facial expressions (e.g., Meltzoff & Moore, 1977) had suggested that humans may begin extrauterine life with a rudimentary mirror neuron system already in place. Neuroimaging studies of human action, emotion, and other aspects of "mentalizing" (thinking about mental states) confirmed and extended Gallese's (2005) notion of embodied simulation by using such techniques as positron emission tomography (PET) and functional magnetic resonance imaging (fMRI). Results to date are largely confined to adults, because brain imaging is not appropriate for children unless medically indicated, but the findings have important developmental implications for the conceptualization of working models that we discuss later.

Specific sites in humans' premotor cortex, corresponding to the correct location in the premotor body map or "homunculus," do indeed show increased activity when study participants view video clips of other humans performing mouth, hand, foot, and face movements (Buccino et al., 2001). Moreover, imagining or recalling an action (one's own or that of another person) induces activation in the same premotor sites as action execution and observation (Decety, Chaminade, Grèzes, & Meltzoff, 2002), suggesting that "embodied" representations form the basis for simulating one's own and others' behavior.

Findings for emotions are similar. The anterior insula, which receives input from all parts of the autonomic nervous system (Damasio, 2003), responds in the same way when study participants sniff a foul-smelling substance and when they observe video clips of human faces displaying disgust expressions (Wicker et al., 2003). The authors' interpretation of the disgust findings is captured in the pithy title of their article: "Both of Us Disgusted in My Insula." Corresponding findings have been obtained for the psychological aspects of physical pain and the pain of social rejection (Eisenberger & Lieberman, 2004).

In addition, brain regions involved in the experience of personal and vicarious emotions are recruited during more complex mentalizing functions. Ruby and Decety (2004), for example, observed the same levels of amygdala activation whether participants imagined their own or their mothers' feelings in a variety of embarrassing situations. However, and possibly in the service of distinguishing the two perspectives, participants' right somatosensory cortex was engaged only when they considered their own feelings, whereas their temporoparietal junction (TPJ) responded only while they took their own mother's perspective.

Also relevant to attachment working models, several somatotopically organized face- and body-responsive sites in the temporal and prefrontal cortices are recruited when individuals interpret and imagine social interactions. The superior temporal sulcus (STS) becomes activated during the perception of biological motion (eye gaze direction; facial expressions; purposeful movement of lips and mouth during speech, as well as hands, arms, and legs; see review by Haxby, Hoffman, & Gobbini, 2000). However, the same region is also recruited during more complex mentalizing functions, as when individuals imagine *themselves* as the protagonist in a story (Vogeley et al., 2001), solve false-belief tasks and moral dilemmas (see review by Frith & Frith, 2003), or judge the intentionality of others' actions in context (Saxe, Xiao, Kovacs, Perrett, & Kanwisher, 2004). A complementary function, individual face identification, enabling differential emotional responses to attachment figures, is supported by the fusiform face area (FFA) in the inferior temporal cortex (e.g., Kanwisher & Yovel, 2006). Patients with focused lesions in the FFA cannot recognize the faces of familiar individuals or their own reflections in a mirror (prosopagnosia; Damasio, 1999).

These and other neuroimaging studies suggest that human brains are built for "intersubjectivity," or the ability to understand other people and to imagine interactions with them through embodied (and experiential) simulation. Brain systems previously believed to support self-related appraisals are also recruited when people vicariously "feel" others' actions and emotions—not only while observing or interacting with them, but while imagining interactions with them. That this capacity begins early is strongly suggested, not only by the evidence for neonatal imitation, but by Trevarthen and Hubley's (1978) studies of primary and secondary intersubjectivity, including the emergence before the end of the first year of a capacity for shared attention. Studies of intentional gestural communication at about 9 months of age likewise appear to indicate a rudimentary understanding than minds can be interfaced (Bretherton & Bates, 1979). In "good enough" attachment relationships, we argue, a child's experiential understanding of others' actions and emotions develops naturally in the

course of mutually responsive social interactions. Rather than having to explain how it is even possible for humans to comprehend others' feelings at an experiential level, the new question concerns the conditions that suppress the natural capacity for empathy and mentalizing implied in studies of embodied simulation.

The neuroimaging findings reviewed here are compatible with an emerging functional view of memory as constructive and reconstructive rather than reproductive, allowing individuals to "reexperience" past and "preexperience" future episodes (see review by Schacter & Addis, 2007). Schacter and Addis (2007) point out that because the future is rarely an exact repetition of the past, simulation of future scenarios requires a system that can draw on the past in a manner that flexibly extracts and recombines elements of previous experiences. They cite evidence of considerable overlap between the neural processes involved in recalling the past and imagining the future, as well as in adopting others' perspectives.

Neuroimaging Studies and the Mental "Operation" of Working Models

A stated function of working models is to evaluate the potential effectiveness of alternative courses of action. Neuroimaging studies are beginning to show that many sites in the prefrontal cortex (PFC) are involved in aspects of this task. These PFC sites form an interconnected network, but they also receive signals from and transmit signals to many other brain areas (particularly those reviewed above). In collaboration with other cortical and subcortical regions, they are involved in the "top-down" regulation of emotional and social responses, whereas automatic behaviors such as orienting to unexpected movement and other behaviors that have become automated through practice are no longer subject to control by the PFC (Miller & Cohen, 2001).

Demonstrating the enormous role of emotions in so-called "executive functions," the orbital (pre)frontal cortex (OFC) guides the processing of learned and unlearned sensory and psychological rewards, including the reward value of specific faces (Rolls, 1996). Relevant to attachment, Bartels and Zeki (2004) found that face-responsive OFC neurons (along with other regions related to the brain's reward circuitry) responded considerably more strongly when mothers viewed the faces of their own children as compared to faces of same-age acquainted children. At the same time, areas associated with more analytic social judgments (e.g., the STS and amygdala) were suppressed.

Important for conceptualizing working-model change and adaptive decision making, the OFC plays a vital role in overriding habitual responses, thereby facilitating adaptive new behaviors if a particular stimulus or behavioral strategy ceases to be rewarding. Patients with circumscribed OFC damage who lack this capacity for flexible evaluation (perhaps also the associated "gut feelings") tend to make poor decisions, whether in their day-to-day lives or an experimental economic game (Damasio, 1999). They make these maladaptive decisions even though they can describe the adaptive choices that they could or should make instead. Infants with this kind of prefrontal damage suffer even more severely. Not only do they fail to express (and seemingly fail to experience) social emotions of sympathy, embarrassment, or guilt; they are also unable to develop an understanding of social rules and rule violations. In such cases, the brain is not developmentally plastic enough to make up for the damage (Anderson, Bechara, Damasio, Tranel, & Damasio, 1999).

A second prefrontal region, the anterior cingulate cortex (ACC), is involved in signaling information-processing conflicts (Botvinick, Carter, Braver, Barch, & Cohen, 2001). Its activation during top-down processing of mental conflict was studied by Singer and colleagues (2006), who demonstrated that distrust affects empathic reactions. Viewing a photograph of someone in a situation likely to cause pain (a finger pinched by a closing door) normally recruits both amygdala and ACC regions, but these activations are substantially diminished if the pictured person previously behaved in a deceptive rather than a trustworthy manner toward the study participant.

A third prefrontal area with functions relevant to working model operation is the dorsolateral prefrontal cortex (DLPFC), which has been identified as important for working memory. This region contains neurons that can remain activated, or hold representations "online" for tens of seconds after a stimulus has been removed (Fuster, 1997). A review by Miller and Cohen (2001) suggests that this region, as part of working memory function, is involved in the comparison, manipulation, and integration of rules for goal or task achievement, rather than the recall of unique episodes. In another review, Krawczyk (2002) argued that the DLFPC is critical for making decisions under conditions of uncertainty that require evaluation of multiple sources of information. Also,

perhaps in the service of comparative appraisal before engaging in impulsive action, the output of the OFC reward network is transmitted to the primary motor cortex only indirectly via the DLPFC (Rolls, 1996).

In short, neuroimaging studies shed new light on the proposed capacity to "run off" aspects of working models to generate and evaluate alternative plans of action. This capacity involves the simultaneous activation and collaboration of many specialized brain sites, and is consistent with a view of memory that includes emotion as an integral and necessary aspect of meaning making, representation, and adaptive decisions. That many of the cortical sites involved in guiding, planning, and imagining individual behavior and social interactions are organized in terms of body maps (i.e., somatotopically) is presumably not a coincidence, and may facilitate the integration of related information via a mysterious process neuroscientists call "binding." Not only are these neuroimaging findings consonant with Bowlby's thinking about the function of working models in planning, and with the approaches to memory reviewed by Schacter and Addis (2007); they also accord well with Nelson's (1996) theoretical reformulation of memory development, to which we turn next.

Developmental Memory Research

As mentioned, Bowlby proposed that "the generalizations of mother, father, and self enshrined in what I am terming working models or representational models will be stored semantically" (1980, p. 62). However, Bretherton (1985) contended that studies of adults' memory for scripts (Schank & Abelson, 1977) and children's event representations (e.g., Nelson & Gruendel, 1981) provide a better fit with Bowlby's view that working models of specific attachment figures allow an individual to mentally simulate habitual interaction patterns with these figures, and thus to anticipate the likely course of ongoing and future interactions with them. Nelson's (1996, 2005) revised conceptualization of experiential event memory makes this fit even clearer.

For Nelson (1996), as for Bowlby (1969/1982, 1980), the everyday function of representation is to guide actions in the present and anticipate future events in light of what has generally happened in the past. Based on infant research, Nelson posited that (nonverbal) event memory is the basic experiential memory system that develops first, and that generic event representations (GERs) provide the initial building blocks for a child's "world model." Events are defined as "whole scenes unfolding over time that involve people and/or other animates acting over time and in particular places" (Nelson, 2005, p. 360).

Nelson (1996) considered event memory to be primary, in contrast to Schacter and Tulving (1994), who subsumed event memory under the semantic memory system. Nelson (p. 154) argued that semantic memory ("general knowledge, undated and unlocalized") is constructed by reprocessing the constituents of generic event memory. For example, children may group particular food items into one semantic category because the items fit the same "slot" in a generic event, such as "lunch at the day care center." Nelson also proposed that GERs help to organize autobiographical memories. Finally, she explained that GERs are not to be confused with procedural memory, at least as defined by Sherry and Schacter (1987). Procedural memory is said to operate outside awareness, whereas event memory "is a form of representation that involves a degree of conscious awareness" (Nelson, 1996, p. 62).

Although Nelson initially assumed that early (experiential, nonverbal) event memory is always GER- or script-like, she changed her mind after studies documented that very young children can display memory for unique events through external *reenactments* weeks to months later (e.g., Bauer & Wewerka, 1995), which Nelson (1996, following Donald, 1991), called "mimetic." However, as they approach the end of their second year and if their efforts are supported by caregivers, many children already begin to translate experiential event representations into language and gain a rudimentary ability to translate *others'* verbal narratives back into their own meaningful event representations, or—as Damasio (1999) termed them—"nonverbal narratives." Fuller mastery of these processes extends over the preschool years and beyond (Nelson, 1996). A fascinating account of a young child's solitary verbal rehearsal of daily routines before falling asleep was published by Nelson in 1989.

Nelson's (1996) theory is highly consonant with the notion of attachment working models, once a few assumptions are added. First, even though children's nonverbal and verbal event knowledge has most often been studied in relation to emotionally neutral scripts (e.g., "lunch at the day care center"), Nelson's definition of GERs can easily be extended to include affects and intentions of agents and recipients (e.g., Bretherton, 1990, 1991, 2005), especially in light of neuroscience findings on embodied simulation. Second, whereas the event schemas proposed by Nelson may allow more than one person to fill the agent and recipient "slots" in an event representation, a child's generic representation of, say, "self with father" would be specific to the father and would not allow other caregivers or other adults as substitutes. Third, an internal working model of self with a specific other would be unworkable if conceptualized as a mere collection of GERs. A better approach would be to regard working models as an organized, multilayered, hierarchical network or web of GERs with different levels of generality (Bretherton, 1985, 1991). In such a network, habitual, experience-near, relationship-specific scenarios would serve as inputs to higher-order general event categories.

Elaborating on these ideas in terms of attachment theory, we propose that an infant's repeated experience-near attachment scenario with his or her father could consist of feeling and expressing distress, being picked up and cuddled against the father's chest, and being soothed by comforting sounds, followed by feelings of relaxation (see Stern, 1985). Such a nonverbal, experiential GER would be relationship-specific because of the particular way in which the father has cuddled or comforted the child, and therefore might allow the infant to mentally "simulate" the father's anticipated behavior in similar contexts. In addition, such a script, along with other father scenarios, could form the basis of a more general but still relationship-specific (nonverbal) event category, verbally expressed as "When I feel bad/sad, Dad helps me feel better." This in turn might be embedded in (or nested under) what H. S. Waters and Waters (2006) have called a "secure-base script" in relation to the father, verbally abbreviated as "When I need help, Dad is usually there for me." It would represent basic trust not only in the father's ability to provide emotional support and protection, but also in his willingness and availability to do so. As noted above, it is at this general level that Bowlby most often wrote about working models, but without access to underlying experience-near GERs, such trust could not, in our view, come into being or be sustained. Trait adjectives such as "trustworthy" or "loving" are but stand-ins for general event categories that are meaningful only because of underlying experience-near GERs (see also E. Waters, Crowell, Elliott, Corcoran, & Treboux, 2002). The developmental process whereby relationship-specific working models of self with several attachment figures and of other familial and extrafamilial relationships become integrated into a reasonably coherent general model of the self is only beginning to become a focus of attachment research, although the social-cognitive literature provides guiding ideas (see Bretherton, 1990; Mikulincer & Shaver, 2004; Thompson, Laible, & Ontai, 2003).

Space limitations preclude a detailed discussion of experiential (verbal and nonverbal) event memory in relation to defensive processes (for an attempt, see Bretherton, 1991), but we briefly alert readers to the usefulness of attribution theory in this regard. Given that information in everyday life (as opposed to experimental situations) is usually incomplete and interpretable in multiple ways, *defensive manipulation* of causal information could be highly effective in working-model change. A switch of causal attributions from external and transient (an individual behaves in a certain way because of situational factors) to internal and stable (the individual's behavior is caused by his or her personality) is likely to have drastic relationship consequences when it concerns an attachment figure's unreliable behavior (see Collins, 1996, for an example based on a study of young adults).

Parent–Child Memory Talk

Bowlby's (1973) proposition that working models of self develop as a result of interactions and dialogues with attachment figures was shared by psychoanalysts in the object relations tradition, but it also parallels Mead's (1934) and other symbolic interactionists' notions about the social self. According to Mead, children learn the meaning of their gestures through the responses others make to them, but Bowlby's claims are somewhat different. Because evolutionary processes are believed to have prepared infants to *expect* appropriate and caring parental responses to attachment signals, parental ignoring or deliberate misinterpretation of emotional signals would not render an infant's communication meaningless, but rather would convey rejection. If pervasive and consistent, such rejection is likely to lead to an internal working model of self stated verbally as "My needs [or I myself] don't count" (Bretherton, 1990). Seen in this way, meanings derived from attachment interactions hold tremendous emotional significance for the child's developing model of self. We surmise that the adaptive development of neural mirror systems that underlie experiential understanding

of others' emotions and intentions is fostered by parental responses conveying to the infant that he or she has been understood. Independently, psychoanalysts have claimed that appropriate parental "mirroring" of infants' emotions enables the development of a reflective/reflected understanding that is likely the foundation for a secure sense of self (e.g., Fonagy, Gergely, & Target, Chapter 33, this volume).

Also relevant is Mead's work on the social origins of thought, conceptualized as inner conversations with imagined others or the self. For young children, Mead suggested, these inner conversations should be viewed as "dramatic," involving mental reenactments of conversations between child and parent. Later, "the inner stage changes into the forum and workshop of thought. The features and intonations of the dramatis personae fade out and the emphasis falls upon inner speech, though thought can always return to the personal mode" (Mead, 1913, p. 377). Applied to attachment, these ideas suggest that young children's thoughts may in some instances consist of holding inner conversations with parents. For example, to allay fears, they may repeat to themselves remembered parental reassurances that the monster under the bed is only a shadow. However, "outer" reassuring conversations must precede the ability to conduct them internally.

Despite Bowlby's (1973) proposals about the importance of parent–child dialogue in the co-construction of attachment working models, Mead's (1934) and Vygotsky's (1978) theories about the social self were what inspired the pioneering research. Studies of conversations about past and future events by parents and their young children (e.g., Fivush & Fromhoff, 1988) revealed that some mothers (termed "elaborative") welcomed their children's additions to the dialogue, even if minimal, and expanded on their children's contributions through affirmations and questions. Other mothers, with a "low-elaborative" or "repetitive" style, tended to brush aside what their children had to say if it seemed irrelevant to the conversational topic and to reiterate the same question without waiting for an answer. Overall, they seemed more interested in obtaining what they regarded as the correct answer than in co-constructing a collaborative account.

These descriptions reminded Bretherton (1993) strongly of Ainsworth, Bell, and Stayton's (1974) definitions of the sensitive and insensitive maternal behaviors during nonverbal interactions at home that predict infant–mother attachment security. Correlations between assessments of child–mother attachment and maternal reminiscing style have indeed emerged (e.g., Fivush & Vasudeva, 2002; Laible & Thompson, 2000). Particularly revealing were findings from a longitudinal study of mother–child memory talk at 19, 25, 32, 40, and 51 months (Newcombe & Reese, 2004). Attachment security at 19 months was assessed by mothers with the E. Waters (1995) Attachment Q-Set (AQS), and AQS scores were dichotomized to form two groups of children. Mothers of the secure group used more evaluative language (internal-state words, intensifiers, affect modifiers, and emphasis) at each successive age, whereas the opposite held for mothers of the insecure group. Furthermore, during all five sessions, children in the secure group used more evaluative language than their insecure peers, and maternal and child evaluative language scores in secure (but not insecure) dyads became correlated, beginning at 25 months. In a related study of short-term reminiscing, Etzion-Carasso and Oppenheim (2000) found that mothers of boys who had been secure as infants engaged in open and responsive communication after a brief separation, and that their children reciprocated with free expression of their needs and concerns.

In summary, Nelson's (1996) theory of experiential and verbal event representation not only fits well with the neuroimaging studies of embodied simulation, but is also highly consonant with the notion that attachment working models are based on experiential memories of repeated interpersonal experiences in the context of specific attachment relationships. With a few additional assumptions, Nelson's theory allows us to conceptualize how a child's working models of specific relationships might also come to serve as input for more general attachment representations and even worldviews. Studies of memory talk additionally indicate that children in more secure dyads tend to adopt their mothers' mentalizing reminiscing style—not only affecting how the children remember specific experiences, but helping them to incorporate an understanding of mental states into their conscious, verbally articulable working models of self with mother and others.

The findings on embodied simulation, experiential event memory, and mentalizing parent–child conversations discussed in this section are beginning to make limited inroads into representational attachment research, but as the next section demonstrates, their influence is still quite small. The major emphasis has been on the development and validation of representational attachment measures.

ATTACHMENT RESEARCH RELEVANT TO WORKING MODELS

Until the mid-1980s, attachment researchers focused almost exclusively on the quality of infant–parent attachment patterns in the Strange Situation (Ainsworth, Blehar, Waters, & Wall, 1978)—either to predict developmental outcomes, or to examine precursors of secure and insecure attachment classifications. Bowlby's (1969/1982, 1973, 1980) notions about attachment working models were largely ignored. This changed after Main, Kaplan, and Cassidy (1985) introduced several instruments for evaluating attachment at the level of representation.

Most influential among these was the Adult Attachment Interview (AAI; George, Kaplan, & Main, 1984, 1996), an hour-long, semistructured interview about adults' childhood attachment experiences and their impact on personality development (see Hesse, Chapter 25, this volume). Also important was Kaplan's (see Main et al., 1985) revised version of Klagsbrun and Bowlby's (1976) Separation Anxiety Test (SAT), a semiprojective instrument for eliciting attachment narratives from young children.

That this work had an almost immediate impact on developmental and clinical attachment research is attributable to two findings. First, representational features of parents' AAIs seemed to parallel their infants' behavioral attachment patterns in the Strange Situation, suggesting intergenerational transmission. Second, Strange Situation classifications in infancy predicted "mental aspects of security" assessed with the SAT at age 6, revealing developmental continuity in attachment patterns from the behavioral-experiential to the verbal-representational level.

Several replication studies and the creation of additional instruments by other researchers quickly followed, including at least four AAI-like interviews about the current parent–child attachment relationship, adaptations of the AAI to younger ages, and several projective attachment measures for children and adults (see the review by Solomon & George, Chapter 18, this volume). During this period, a methodological tradition evolved within the field whereby new representational attachment measures were recognized only if they were successfully validated against classifications or scales used to code the Strange Situation and the AAI. Although enormously fruitful in many ways, this emphasis on refining assessment and coding methods had the somewhat unfortunate side effect that theoretical links with Bowlby's notions about attachment working models were often overlooked or not clearly drawn. Our goal in this section is to make up for this neglect by examining research conducted with the AAI in light of relationship-specific and generalized attachment working models, their intergenerational transmission, and longitudinal consistency. Next, we consider further insights offered by the SAT and a selection of other semiprojective attachment measures for children and adults. With apologies to colleagues, our review must often refer to other chapters for specific citations and related findings.

Not included, although important to the conceptualization of attachment working models, are findings based on paper-and-pencil self-report measures of attachment styles pioneered by Hazan and Shaver (1987) and used in hundreds of studies conducted primarily by personality and social psychologists. As elucidated by Crowell, Fraley, and Shaver (Chapter 26, this volume), these measures seem to tap somewhat different constructs than the narrative assessments created by developmental psychologists do. For a detailed consideration of the large literature on attachment styles and their correlates, see J. Feeney (Chapter 21, this volume) and Mikulincer and Shaver (Chapter 23, this volume).

The AAI in Working-Model Perspective

Although the AAI focuses on an interviewee's family-of-origin attachment experiences, the AAI classification procedures developed by Main and Goldwyn (1984; Main, Goldwyn, & Hesse, 2003) do not purport to assess working models of an interviewee's past or ongoing attachment relationships. Main and colleagues (1985) initially attempted an explanation of these classifications in terms of working models, but Main (1995, 1999) later explicitly distanced herself from this approach. Instead, she proposed the term "state of mind with respect to attachment" to denote an individual's habitual or "organized" manner of attention regulation when confronted with attachment cues, whether in the course of interviews, interpersonal interactions, or intrapersonal reflection. Thus AAI classifications represent a single predominant state of mind ("secure-autonomous," "dismissing," or "preoccupied") that pervades the discussion of

several possibly quite different attachment relationships and topics. The additional "unresolved/disorganized" AAI designation applies only to portions of the interview that concern experiences of loss and abuse (see Hesse, Chapter 25, this volume), whereas the remainder of the transcript can generally be assigned to one of the three organized classifications. Elaborating on previous work (e.g., Bretherton, 1985, 2005; Bretherton & Munholland, 1999), we argue for a *complementary* interpretation of AAI classifications in terms of general and relationship-specific attachment working models as affected by defensive processes (Bowlby, 1980).

The hallmarks of secure-autonomous AAI transcripts are coherence, emotional openness, and valuing of attachment relationships, but coherence is not restricted to positive depictions of an interviewee's childhood attachments. That some secure-autonomous adults described very difficult relationships with their own parents led Bowlby (1988, p. 135) to suggest that they had achieved a freely accessible and coherent organization of attachment-relevant information (working models) by reprocessing, and thus coming to terms with, their unhappy childhood memories. The term "earned-secure," coined for these parents, was based on the unstated assumption that AAI coherence reflects the reworking of formerly incoherent attachment working models.

Questions about this interpretation arose from findings of the Minnesota Study of Risk and Adaptation from Birth to Adulthood. In that study, about half of the young adult participants with AAIs considered earned-secure were found, on consultation of earlier records, to have received supportive caregiving as toddlers and children (Roisman, Padrón, Sroufe, & Egeland, 2002). The ensuing debate about a more stringent definition and meaning of "earned security" has not yet been resolved. Whatever its outcome, parents' AAI coherence remains the best predictor of their infants' attachment security. AAI coherence is also strongly correlated with the security of young adults' current relationships with close friends or romantic partners, whether assessed observationally or with AAI-like interviews (e.g., Grossmann, Grossmann, & Kindler, 2005). AAI evaluations even forecast an individual's cooperative behavior in a laboratory task with strangers (Roisman, 2006).

Given consistent evidence that secure-autonomous AAI classifications predict an adult's supportive and quite stable behavior within attachment relationships, as well as the concomitant ability to discuss these relationships coherently and openly (see Hesse, Chapter 25, this volume), we interpret the secure-autonomous AAI status as an *indicator* that a person has developed a general working model of a secure self in close relationships. Drawing on our earlier discussion of event memories and scripts, we contend that such a generalized model of the relational self must be rooted in past working models of at least some specific attachment relationships within which an individual has learned to communicate attachment feelings, thoughts, and behaviors with relative openness and honesty. Research suggests that secure parent–child relationships play the most influential role, but that the quality of subsequent close relationships (including those with peers, teachers, and friends) is also important (e.g., Simpson, Collins, Tran, & Haydon, 2007; Sroufe, Egeland, Carlson, & Collins, 2005). In at least some cases, a secure relational self may develop despite early attachment insecurity, as long as the individual has had an opportunity to learn that experiences of rejecting or inconsistent caregiving do not define his or her self-worth. We note, however, that the psychological pathway whereby an individual can develop a secure relational self in the context of both secure and insecure, or consistently insecure, early relationships is at present not well understood. Moreover, as shown by Sroufe and colleagues (2005), early attachment experiences are never fully erased.

We further propose that a general model of the relational self does not replace existing relationship-specific working models or preclude the development of specific working models in new relationships at any age. For example, secure-autonomous parents are likely to construct a coherent, well-organized, relationship-specific working models of their infant and of themselves as caregivers to this infant. Without relationship-specific working models, a person could neither reflect on past nor imagine future interactions with a particular attachment partner, except in the most general way. In line with the "embodied simulations" described in our review of neuroimaging studies, we argue that individuals who recall or imagine relationships with particular others engage in mental enactments of emotional experiences drawn or inferred from relationship-specific working models.

In this context, we wish to dispute the oft-stated notion that working models are invariably unconscious or rely entirely on procedural or implicit memories. During live interactions, individuals will not usually be aware that their relationship-specific working models are activated (operating) unless their partners behave in completely unexpected ways. This does not mean, however, that individuals cannot recall valid aspects of these models when reflecting on close relationships. In clinical practice, Bowlby (1988, p. 149) suggested that "whenever plenty of consistent detail is given," individuals' memories of childhood should be considered as "reasonable approximations of the truth." We contend that this is also a fair provisional assumption for secure-autonomous AAIs, although the word "truth" should be understood to refer an adult's current constructions (see also Main, 1991).

The proposed generalized working model of a confident relational self as a property of the person (to use Bowlby's [1988] phrase) should not be regarded as a trait, however, because its operation in a developing attachment relationship depends on how and whether trust and commitment are reciprocated (see also Sroufe et al., 2005). Some individuals with secure-autonomous AAIs respond with low coherence to an AAI-like interview about their relationship to a romantic partner to whom they are engaged, but these individuals tend to leave the relationship rather than marrying the partner (Crowell & Waters, 2005). A *capacity* for secure relationships indicated by the AAI, it appears, affects the likelihood but does not guarantee that attempted attachment relationships will be secure or coherently represented.

Secure-autonomous interviewees not only provide coherent and emotionally open AAI narratives, but also tend to discuss relationships reflectively and empathically. Both during the AAI itself (Fonagy, Steele, Moran, Steele, & Higgitt, 1993) and during an AAI-like interview about the parent–toddler relationship (Slade, Grienenberger, Bernbach, Levy, & Locker, 2005), adults with secure-autonomous AAI status often describe themselves and close others (parents or children) in terms of needs, wishes, beliefs, regrets, and values. Fonagy and Target (1997, p. 683) hypothesized that such "mentalizing" also enables parents to empathize with their infant as a mental being with feelings and needs, and thus to appropriately mirror (reflect back) the infant's internal states so that "he now knows what he is feeling." Revealing this mentalizing tendency in their speech before their infants are verbal, mothers of secure, but not insecure, infants appropriately label and comment on their infants' emotions during observed interactions (Meins et al., 2002). Moreover, once able to participate in verbal dialogue, a secure child tends to acquire from the mother a mentalizing reminiscing style (see the earlier review) that may help him or her construct a verbalizable model of the mother as an individual with her own goals, emotions, and intentions; such a model is important for a goal-corrected partnership (Bowlby, 1969/1982). An understanding of others in mental terms, accompanied by emotional openness and considerateness, is also useful in repairing the unavoidable conflicts and misunderstandings that arise between parents and children or adolescents and later between adult mates (see integrative reviews by Cassidy, 2001; Kobak & Duemmler, 1994; and Fonagy et al., Chapter 33, this volume).

In contrast to the coherent, fresh, lively, and believable accounts of childhood attachments that characterize secure-autonomous AAIs, narratives classified into one of the three insecure statuses (dismissing, preoccupied, and unresolved/disorganized) exhibit various inconsistencies and confusions. The evaluation of these transcripts requires close analysis of the interview content in terms of its relative consistency, relevance, and connotative meanings, supporting Bowlby's proposal that working models acquired in insecure relationships develop in a less straightforward manner than those indicative of security.

Although the intergenerational match between specific subtypes of parental AAI insecurity and infant Strange Situation classifications is lower for insecurity than for security (van IJzendoorn, 1995), the number of parents with dismissing AAI status whose infants are classified as avoidant is substantial. Main (1999, p. 862) explained this intergenerational link in terms of a parent's *singular* overall classifiable "state of mind," held in place by minimizing attention to attachment cues. The adult's implicit goal is to maintain a *false* sense of felt security, whether by evading AAI questions or by rejecting a distressed infant's bids for physical contact (Main, Hesse, & Kaplan, 2005, p. 282). Although we consider this emphasis on regulatory processes valuable, we suggest that processes beyond attention regulation should be probed. A working-model perspective on dismissing AAIs emphasizes defensive exclusion and conflicting working models.

Two somewhat different defensive strategies (idealization and dismissiveness) characterize most dismissing AAIs. Idealization is coded when respondents provide glowing adjectives about their relationships with parents in childhood, but are unable or unwilling to recall relevant memories. This is consistent with Bowlby's (1980) notion that defensive exclusion, followed by partial or complete deactivation of the systems mediating attachment, results in conflicting conscious and unconscious working models of self with attachment figures. Dismissiveness is coded when the respondents recall negative attachment episodes while answering direct questions about separation, rejection, and other untoward situations, but render them emotionally "harmless" by discounting their affective importance and influence. We hypothesize that what are being regulated or suppressed in such cases are affective components of otherwise relatively accessible working models that might create anxiety if they became fully conscious. We return to this issue in our discussion of semiprojective measures.

Regarding physiological aspects of such representational conflict, Dozier and Kobak (1992) discovered that AAI dismissiveness (but not idealization) was accompanied by significantly elevated electrodermal responses, usually considered indicative of emotional inhibition, conflict, and deception. Roisman (2007) observed similar autonomic reactivity in married adults with high AAI deactivating scores (related to dismissiveness) who were engaged in problem-solving discussions with their spouses, suggesting that these adults have developed a defensively excluded working model of self with spouse that conflicts with their conscious models. We suspect that autonomic inhibition may also be demonstrated in parents who ignore their infant's distress and reject bids for close bodily contact. By contrast, avoidant infants, who turn or move away from their parents on reunion in the Strange Situation, exhibit physiological *arousal* (elevated heart rate) rather than inhibition (Spangler & Grossmann, 1993). Although behaviorally avoidant, such infants may not yet have learned to inhibit physiological arousal when expecting that the desired parental reassurance will not forthcoming.

Because of space limitations, we omit discussion of the preoccupied AAI designation, but recommend more attention to its disproportionate co-occurrence with the unresolved classification (see below). As a consequence, "purely" preoccupied AAI transcripts are rare (Main et al., 2005). They are also not systematically associated with infant–parent ambivalence in the Strange Situation (van IJzendoorn, 1995).

The third insecure AAI classification (unresolved/disorganized) is given when discussions of loss or abuse contain subtle cognitive and discourse lapses (e.g., inappropriately detailed narratives, use of inappropriate speech registers, and irrational thinking). Regardless of secondary AAI status (based on the overall transcript), a substantial number of parents with these classifications tend to have infants who exhibit behavioral disorganization in the Strange Situation (see Weinfield, Sroufe, Egeland, & Carlson, Chapter 4, this volume).

AAI lapses associated with discussions of unresolved trauma remind us of dissociative phenomena that Bowlby (1980) conceptualized as "segregated selves" (or "principal systems"), capable of alternation in consciousness without possibility of intercommunication, and therefore liable to cause inexplicable, erratic behavior. Note, however, that Bowlby's examples concerned very severe disorders (e.g., fugues) and that he did not clarify specific triggers for the proposed alternations. Main (1999) has explained the unresolved state of mind in terms of the temporary collapse or disorganization of attention when confronted with reminders of traumatic attachment experiences, whether during the AAI or while interacting with an infant. Again, deeper probing for explanations beyond attention regulation seems necessary, but given the subtle and temporary nature of AAI disorganization, we also do not find an explanation in terms of segregated principal systems or selves and their working models fully satisfactory.

In their work with clinical and high-risk groups, Lyons-Ruth, Yellin, Melnick, and Atwood (2005) felt the need for a disorganized AAI category that, unlike the unresolved status, could be assessed on an *interview-wide* basis. Foremost among indicators of a "pervasively unintegrated state of mind" was frank discussion of a helpless and/or hostile primary caregiver in childhood with whom the interviewee currently identified, implicitly or explicitly. Associated indicators were frequent laughter following descriptions of highly negative childhood events; numerous references to fear, but not in relation to trauma; and reports of severe abuse (resolved or unresolved). After independent reconsideration with this new coding system, many AAI transcripts of high-risk women were reclassified with the new designation "hostile-helpless," including half of those previously deemed secure-autonomous in view of the openness and coherence with which these mothers had discussed highly negative family-of-origin experiences. Lyons-Ruth and colleagues interpret the reclassified hostile-helpless AAI status in terms of alternating "split" (or segregated) work-

ing models of self as good and bad, arguing that that the negative episodes in these AAIs were "too encompassing to be dealt with by lack of memory … so the difficulties are presented as matter of fact or even as having a certain entertainment or shock value" (p. 20). Supporting the validity of the hostile-helpless status were findings of its strong associations with infant disorganization at 18 months.

Overall, AAI findings suggest that parents induct their infants into a way of relating that is consistent with their own secure or conflicted/defensive models of self in relationships. Developmental continuity from nonverbal behavioral and emotional attachment patterns with mother in infancy to adult representational AAI status has been established in several longitudinal studies of middle-class families, but is greater for security than for specific subtypes of insecurity (e.g., Main et al., 2005; Waters, Merrick, Treboux, Crowell, & Albersheim, 2000). In particular, infants classified as disorganized with their mothers in infancy frequently produce dismissing rather than unresolved AAIs in adulthood (e.g., Main et al., 2005). However, in a German longitudinal study, later AAI status was not predictable from infant Strange Situations, but was correlated with attachment measures in childhood (Grossmann et al., 2005).

Concerning which of several caregivers' AAI status is more influential in a child's general model of the relational self, Main and colleagues (2005) reported longitudinal links of infant–mother, but not infant–father, attachment with later AAI status. Grossmann, Grossmann, Kindler, and Zimmermann (see Chapter 36, this volume), on the other hand, have found that both mother- and father-related attachment-relevant assessments beyond infancy contribute unique and joint variance to the prediction of young adult AAIs.

Finally, in a study of disadvantaged families exposed to numerous life stresses, many individuals who were *secure* with their mothers as infants produced *insecure* (usually dismissing) AAIs as young adults. However, in that study relationship quality with peers and teachers added considerable additional variance to the prediction of young adult AAI status, as did the mother–child relationship quality at age 13 (Sroufe et al., 2005). An important next step will be to go beyond correlational explanations to gain an expanded understanding of why specific relational patterns (underpinned by coherent or conflicting working models) are intergenerationally transmitted in many dyads but not in others, and why some remain stable in unstable circumstances whereas others undergo gradual or sudden longitudinal "affective change" from security to insecurity, or from one pattern of insecurity to another.

OTHER REPRESENTATIONAL ATTACHMENT MEASURES IN WORKING MODEL PERSPECTIVE

Semiprojective Measures for Young Children

We now consider additional insights that semiprojective measures may contribute to the working-model perspective on attachment. We focus first on two child assessments, the SAT (Main et al., 1985) and the Attachment Story Completion Task (ASCT; Bretherton & Ridgeway, 1990).

Following Bowlby's (1973) precept that attachment working models are rooted in real-life experiences, researchers assume that young children draw on aspects of these models when responding to semiprojective attachment tasks. In the SAT, children are shown six pictures of parent–child separations, both mild (saying goodnight) and severe (leaving for 2 weeks). They are then asked what the pictured child would feel and do in each situation. In the ASCT, an interviewer invites children to "show me and tell me what happens next" after enacting and narrating a variety of attachment-related story beginnings or stems with small family figures and simple props (an accidental mishap, a painful fall, a monster in the bedroom, a parent–child separation and reunion). Whereas the SAT was intended for somewhat older preschoolers, the enactive format of the ASCT was designed for children as young as 3 years. However, with minor adaptations, both instruments have been effectively used with children up to 8 or 9 years of age.

The semiprojective format enables children to create imaginary responses not available during interviews about everyday life. Even though real-life events are sometimes incorporated, story content cannot be assumed to represent literal replays of reality, and attachment narratives could easily be written off as "pure fantasy." However, a (by now considerable) number of studies in the United States and elsewhere have documented significant longitudinal and concurrent correlations of SAT and ASCT evaluations with earlier and concurrent attachment measures (e.g., the Strange Situation, the AQS, naturalistic home observations). One study (Main et al., 2005) also reported significant longitudinal correlations of the SAT with the AAI in terms of the secure–insecure dichotomy.

Young children's responses to attachment issues presented in SAT pictures and ASCT stems are taken as indicators of security if they are resolved constructively and coherently. Coherent stories about noncaring parents are very rare.

Avoidance of attachment topics in both the SAT and ASCT can be conveyed by refusing to acknowledge the attachment issue presented in the picture or story stem (claiming that a troublesome event, such as a fall, did not take place). Alternatively, children may completely sidestep attachment topics (by talking about the protagonist's appearance) or generate attachment-avoidant story content, wherein child protagonists do not seek, and their parents do not provide, comfort in distressing situations.

Most striking are highly unusual, if not bizarre, stories told by some children in response to SAT pictures (the child figure is locked in a closet) and ASCT stems (the family car drives off a cliff and everyone dies). During the SAT, such stories were produced by kindergarten children who, as infants, had been disorganized with their mothers in the Strange Situation (e.g., Main et al., 2005). Upon reunion with their mothers after a 1-hour separation at age 6, these children exhibited not disorganized but controlling behavior. Reminiscent of a defensive response that Bowlby (1980, p. 223) called "inverting the parent–child relationship," they either issued peremptory commands or acted toward their mothers in an oversolicitous fashion. Here, behavioral (organized) and representational (disorganized) assessments reflected different facets of attachment working models that together provide a more comprehensive, but not fully understood, picture.

Following Bowlby's (1980) contention that unrealistic "fantasies" may become comprehensible when viewed in context, we suggest closer examination of seemingly bizarre attachment narratives. Examples from an ASCT study of preschoolers from postdivorce families (Bretherton & Page, 2004) appeared very meaningful when construed as metaphorical portrayals of overwhelming emotions about family situations (e.g., a child protagonist becomes a ghost who is trapped under furniture by a parent, or a family is uncontrollably battered and tossed about by a tornado). These children also enacted stories that appeared to portray a hoped-for future (e.g., "Daddy will live with us now") or a feared future (e.g., the children are abandoned and have to take care of themselves). Their narratives recall proposals by Parkes (1971) that relinquishing working models of an anticipated future is a difficult aspect of all loss experiences—a topic that calls for more systematic investigation in adults as well. In our study, the loss concerned parents no longer living together. Many children tried to undo this fact in their narratives, while some focused more on a feared future.

Not yet sufficiently understood within these assessments are gender differences in children's responses—especially evident in the ASCT, with boys often portraying more aggression and less prosocial behavior than girls (e.g., Page & Bretherton, 2003)—although the main results in most studies have held even when child gender was statistically controlled for. In addition, story completions become more coherent with age, making assessment potentially problematic if the same coherence criteria are applied to groups with a wide age range (for a more detailed consideration of the validity and limitations of these and other semiprojective attachment instruments for children, see Solomon & George, Chapter 18, this volume). Finally, we note that only *one* representational classification or rating is given to each child's narratives, even though the pictures and stories include two parents, and the observational attachment measures with the two parents may differ in security. For this reason, we would not call a child who produces "secure" stories "securely attached."

Two Semiprojective Measures for Adults

Both of the instruments we consider here were developed after the semiprojective child measures and were, in part, inspired by them. Whereas the first measure provides ratings of security, the second is based on classifications and places stress on defensive processes.

The Secure Base Scriptedness measure (H. S. Waters & Rodrigues-Doolabh, 2004) emerged from the idea that children's ASCT narratives could be rated in terms of their resemblance to a secure-base script (see reanalysis by H. S. Waters, Rodrigues, & Ridgeway [1998] of transcripts from the Bretherton et al. [1990] study). Adults are not asked to complete attachment stories, but to generate narratives by using words from carefully constructed prompt lists. The words can be used in any order, but each list, if read in sequence, suggests a specific instantiation of a more general or prototypical secure-base script (i.e., pleasant interaction interrupted by a troublesome event that is resolved by appeal to and effective intervention by an attachment figure).

The assumption underlying this task is that individuals who have acquired generalized secure-base beliefs or working models in past relationships will "see" the secure base script in the word list. In contrast, adults who "do not know" or do not have access to this script will produce narratives that only partially conform or do not conform to a secure-base script (H. S. Waters & Waters, 2005, p. 190), because of inconsistent or insufficient attachment support in the past. This seemingly simple idea has been remarkably productive.

Secure-base ratings of narratives created in response to the (usually) four prompt lists were very highly intercorrelated. Because some lists included words suggesting parent–child dyads while others referred to couples, these findings support the hypothesis that the task reflects a generalized working model. Test–retest correlations over approximately 1 year were highly significant (r's above .50), suggesting considerable stability (Vaughn et al., 2006). Significant associations between mothers' secure-base script ratings and AAI coherence scales have already been reported in several U.S. and international studies (e.g., Vaughn et al., 2007), showing that this working-model-based approach is compatible with AAI security. We suggest, however, that the Secure Base Scriptedness instrument, because it does not assess types of insecurity, is most likely to be useful in nonclinical groups.

The Adult Attachment Projective (AAP; George & West, 2004) was influenced by the SAT and a coding system that Solomon, George, and De Jong (1995) developed for their adaptation of the original ASCT. In contrast to the Secure Base Scriptedness task, the AAP was specifically created to line up with the Main and Goldwyn (1984; Main et al., 2003) AAI categories (secure, dismissing, preoccupied, and unresolved). However, unlike that of the AAI, the AAP coding system is closely tied to Bowlby's (1980) theory of defensive processes. Another difference is that the AAP requires the participant to tell stories about pictured scenarios, whereas the AAI asks for childhood memories. Nevertheless, the developers of the measure found, in a sample of 144 adults of diverse ages and backgrounds, substantial AAP–AAI concordance (kappa = .84; C. George, personal communication, January 7, 2007).

Participants are asked to tell stories about eight somewhat ambiguous line drawings that depict adult–child dyads, adult couples, and solitary figures in a variety of situations likely to elicit attachment distress (e.g., separation, solitude, fear, injury, and death). A secure stance is indicated by coherent and constructively resolved narratives in which the distressed protagonists either receive care or (in response to "alone" pictures) rely on inner resources, such as reflecting on and exploring feelings. The latter responses are coded as indicative of an "internalized secure base." Dismissing AAP narratives emphasize relational disconnection and avoidance of attachment topics, interpreted in terms of Bowlby's (1980) notion of attachment system deactivation. Preoccupied AAP stories also focus on relational disconnection, but the protagonists are more passive, and their wavering story lines are very hard to follow. In line with Bowlby, George and West view preoccupied stories as evidence for cognitive disconnection of affect from its source. Finally, plots of unresolved AAP narratives contain themes of helplessness, loss of control, violence, or isolation; the authors ascribe these to the breakdown of severe repression, referring to Bowlby's (1980) notion of segregated (principal) systems, but not the link to dissociation. We suspect that the AAP may be particularly suitable for use with clinical groups, as shown in a neuroimaging AAP study of women with borderline personality disorder by Buchheim and colleagues (in press).

Summary and Comments

Aware that our selective review cannot comprehensively cover (or even touch on) all important theoretical issues and empirical work on attachment at the representational level, we conclude this section by contrasting and comparing the findings obtained with the AAI and semiprojective measures. This comparison has yielded an interesting set of similarities and differences relevant to, but also raising questions about, the conceptualization of attachment working models.

First, whether produced in response to questions about childhood experiences or hypothetical attachment situations, coherent narratives about attachment relationships by children and adults are indicators of attachment-related security assessed with observational attachment measures). However, coherent narratives about lived experiences in the AAI describe both positive and negative attachment relationships, whereas coherence and constructive content usually go hand in hand in children's and adults' narratives about hypothetical situations. We expected this link in children's stories, because "earned security" seems improbable when children are still living with parents to whom they are insecurely attached. Given that the same result was obtained for adults, a preferable explanation may be that individuals who have experienced or are experiencing secure relationships will create positive hypothetical attachment scenarios based on their *generalized* expectations or working models, even though their actual relationships are likely to be uncaring from time to time.

Second, we consider the notion of an "internalized secure base," proposed by George and West (2004) in conjunction with AAP narratives to "alone" pictures. In explaining this construct, George and West argue that maintenance of proximity to attachment figures in adulthood becomes an almost exclusively internal process related to "internalized attachment figures." They do not specify whether they are referring to representations of caregiving figures from childhood, current attachment figures, or generalized working models not linked to a specific figure. Their construct resembles, but is not equivalent to, Main's (1999, p. 862) statement that secure-autonomous adults "feel secure in themselves." Elaborating on this explanation, Main and colleagues (2005, p. 268) posited that "in theory, an adult with all attachment figures deceased and no close relationship available could still be secure-autonomous and raise secure offspring." Although we recognize the value of an "internalized secure base" and of autonomy (and similar proposals by Mikulincer & Shaver, 2004), we believe that Bowlby would not accord this much power to "states of mind" or generalized attachment working models in the complete absence of actual support. Moreover, children, by Main and colleagues' definition, cannot be autonomous, because they need the physical presence of an attachment figure. This obscures the fact that even young children can express a degree of autonomy in their attachment relationships as they gain the ability to take their parents' perspective in goal-corrected partnerships, and as they become able to spend more time apart from their attachment figures, trusting that these figures will be available when needed.

Third, with respect to attachment avoidance, the AAI and the semiprojective measures for children and adults elicit both dissimilar and similar defensive strategies. Idealization of attachment figures, considered one of the hallmarks of dismissing AAIs, is not seen during the SAT, ASCT, or AAP. This raises the possibility that AAI idealization may be due to dismissing individuals' concerns about self-presentation or self-disclosure in a face-to-face interview about their own experiences—perhaps indicating a form of self-deception, an attempt at positive self-presentation, or merely a way of trying to head off further inquiries. Main and colleagues (2005) have suggested that the validity of the AAI does not depend on how the reasons underlying the idealization strategy are explained, but an examination of this issue is important for theory. In contrast, devaluation and discounting of attachment feelings are common to the AAI, ASCT, and AAP; during the SAT, however, children who were avoidant with their mothers in infancy labeled the pictured child as sad about the separation, but unable to act.

Fourth, the plots of disorganized SAT and ASCT narratives and unresolved AAP narratives contain many portrayals of helplessness, loss of control, violence, or abandonment. The readiness with which some children and adults produce such narratives raises the question of why indices of disorganization during the AAI are more subtle and fleeting, yet are so striking in projective assessments for children and adults. These findings make us wonder whether individuals who tell these narratives also have daydreams that are pervasively filled with chaotic fantasies, possibly surfacing from dissociated working models. This would make their inner lives much more disturbing than is apparent from the more fleeting indicators of attachment disorganization seen during the AAI.

More generally, we conclude that assessments of specific attachment relationships or sets of relationships by means of interviews, projective tests, or observations never yield "pure" insights about specific and general working models because of bidirectional influences between them (see also Sroufe et al., 2005). Despite strong evidence that the AAI *reflects* a general stance (and associated working models), the inferences about this stance must rely on descriptions of specific relationships and may provide insights into these particular relationships as well. In addition, the developmental phase at which it becomes appropriate to speak of a generalized attachment working model, and ways to conceptualize the complexity of such a model at different stages of development, are not settled. Even by the end of early childhood, security ratings of attachment stories predict higher ratings for general self-worth and the quality of relations with peers and teachers in preschool (e.g., Cassidy, 1988; Gullon-Rivera, 2008). At that age, children's attachment stories may already be related to a general view of peers as more or less trustworthy (e.g., Suess, Grossmann, & Sroufe, 1992). On the other hand, why one approach (trusting,

avoidant, ambivalent, or disorganized) becomes most predominant in early childhood, even when an individual is exposed to both secure and insecure attachment relationships at home, remains to be clarified. In addition, it is evident that different methods of assessment reveal different aspects of an individual's attachment working models, especially with respect to dismissiveness and disorganization. These findings require integration into a complete and coherent picture.

Finally, our review suggests that the narrative assessments reviewed here may be effective as indicators of general working models because they elicit descriptions of attachment interactions in specific relationship contexts rather than asking individuals to rate general statements such as "my mother loves me." Perhaps one can most fully access information about differences in the organization of participants' attachment working models by asking them to describe remembered or imagined (embodied and felt) interactions in specific attachment relationships.

CONCLUDING STATEMENT

To make further progress in elaborating and clarifying the working-model construct and to foster new discoveries in representational attachment research, we strongly urge close collaboration with cutting-edge researchers who study memory, narratives, and storytelling in adults and children. We need to gain a deeper understanding of the development and operation of the collaborating brain systems that Bowlby (1969/1982) subsumed under the label "attachment behavioral system," and to which he later referred as "systems-mediating attachment" (1980). These systems influence representational and experiential processes, and are in turn influenced by them. In addition, new developments in clinical and social psychology as well as neuroscience may offer useful constructs and findings to expand and refine ideas about the operation of defensive processes, as urged by Bowlby (1980); they may also help us discover more about the many factors that make for working-model change, whether in a secure or insecure direction, and whether gradual or abrupt (see Mikulincer & Shaver, Chapter 23, this volume). Mining the rich AAI texts for the specific adaptive or maladaptive ways in which interviewees process relationship information may be helpful as well.

Finally, we feel compelled to voice concerns about what may be becoming an excessively monadic (one-person) emphasis on the role of attachment representations, whether these are conceptualized as working models or as states of mind. Evaluations of interview-based and semiprojective attachment measures are currently used to explain an individual's mental health, emotion regulation, and other desirable and important outcomes. Even when interactions between both members of a dyad are observed or both members are interviewed, researchers most often evaluate the responses of each separately, rather than examining relationship functioning when partners' attachment working models mesh well or diverge. Similarly, proposals that secure-autonomous individuals are "secure within themselves" (Main et al., 2005) or rely most of the time on an "internalized secure base" (George & West, 2004) may lead to an exaggerated notion about the extent to which attachment representations per se, in the absence of actual supportive relationships, enable self-reliance.

We recommend an increased focus on dyadic (two-person) approaches. The incoherent, conflicted representational processes observed in insecure relationships can be characterized as self-protective and therefore adaptive from a monadic point of view (e.g., defensive exclusion of anxiety-provoking attachment-related thoughts and feelings). However, the associated behaviors turn out to be maladaptive for constructive communication in ongoing attachment relationships. By contrast, coherent and open representational processes in secure relationships not only encourage self-reliance and autonomy, but also foster relationships that are likely to be more satisfying to both members of an attachment dyad.

ACKNOWLEDGMENTS

We thank the following colleagues with whom we engaged in stimulating exchanges of ideas during the writing of this chapter (in alphabetical order): Carol George, Roger Kobak, Karlen Lyons-Ruth, Glenn Roisman, L. Alan Sroufe, and Everett Waters. We are also grateful for the enormously helpful feedback we received from Jude Cassidy and Phillip Shaver. Finally, Inge Bretherton wishes to convey her appreciation to Stein Bråten for inspiring her to link John Bowlby's ideas about internal working models with insights from neuroscience at the 2004 Theory Forum Symposium of the Norwegian Academy of Science and Letters, Oslo.

REFERENCES

Adolphs, R. (2003). Cognitive neuroscience of human social behavior. *Nature Reviews, Neuroscience, 4*, 165–177.

Adolphs, R. (2006). How do we know the minds of others?: Domain-specificity, simulation, and enactive social cognition. *Brain Research, 1079*, 25–35.

Ainsworth, M. D. S., Bell, S. M., & Stayton, D. (1974). Infant–mother attachment and social development: "Socialization" as a product of reciprocal responsiveness to signals. In P. M. Richards (Ed.), *The integration of a child into a social world* (pp. 99–135). Cambridge, UK: Cambridge University Press.

Ainsworth, M. D. S., Blehar, M. C., Waters, E., & Wall, S. (1978). *Patterns of attachment: A psychological study of the Strange Situation.* Hillsdale, NJ: Erlbaum.

Anderson, S., Bechara, A., Damasio, H., Tranel, D., & Damasio, A. (1999). Impairment of social and moral behavior related to early damage in the prefrontal cortex. *Nature Neuroscience, 2*, 1032–1037.

Bartels, A., & Zeki, S. (2004).The neural correlates of maternal and romantic love. *NeuroImage, 21*, 1155–1166.

Bauer, P. J., & Wewerka, S. S. (1995). One- to two-year-olds' recall of events: The more impressed, the more expressed. *Journal of Experimental Child Psychology, 59*, 475–496.

Botvinick, M. M., Carter, C. S., Braver, T. S., Barch, D. M., & Cohen, J. D. (2001). Conflict monitoring and cognitive control. *Psychological Review, 108*, 624–652.

Bowlby, J. (1969/1982). *Attachment and loss: Vol. 1. Attachment.* New York: Basic Books.

Bowlby, J. (1973). *Attachment and loss: Vol. 2. Separation: Anxiety and anger.* New York: Basic Books.

Bowlby, J. (1979). *The making and breaking of affectional bonds.* London: Tavistock/Routledge.

Bowlby, J. (1980). *Attachment and loss: Vol. 3. Loss: Sadness and depression.* New York: Basic Books.

Bowlby, J. (1988). *A secure base.* New York: Basic Books.

Bretherton, I. (1985). Attachment theory: Retrospect and prospect. In I. Bretherton & E. Waters (Eds.), Growing points of attachment theory and research. *Monographs of the Society for Research in Child Development, 50*(1–2), Serial No. 209, 3–35.

Bretherton, I. (1990). Open communication and internal working models: Their role in the development of attachment relationships. In R. A. Thompson (Ed.), *Nebraska Symposium on Motivation: Vol. 36. Socioemotional development* (pp. 59–113). Lincoln: University of Nebraska Press.

Bretherton, I. (1991). Pouring new wine into old bottles: The social self as internal working model. In M. Gunnar & L. A. Sroufe (Eds.), *Minnesota Symposia on Child Psychology: Vol. 23. Self processes in development* (pp. 1–41). Hillsdale, NJ: Erlbaum.

Bretherton, I. (1993). From dialogue to representation: The intergenerational construction of self in relationships. In C. A. Nelson (Ed.), *Minnesota Symposia on Child Development: Vol. 26. Memory and affect in development* (pp. 237–263). Hillsdale, NJ: Erlbaum.

Bretherton, I. (2005). In pursuit of the internal working model construct and its relevance to attachment relationships. In K. E. Grossmann, K. Grossmann, & E. Waters (Eds.), *Attachment from infancy to adulthood: The major longitudinal studies* (pp. 13–47). New York: Guilford Press.

Bretherton, I., & Bates, E. (1979). The emergence of intentional communication. In I. C. Užgiris (Ed.), *Social interaction and communication during infancy* (pp. 81–100). San Francisco: Jossey-Bass.

Bretherton, I., & Beeghly, M. (1982). Talking about internal states: The acquisition of an explicit theory of mind. *Developmental Psychology, 18,* 906–921.

Bretherton, I., & Munholland, K. A. (1999). Internal working models in attachment relationships: A construct revisited. In J. Cassidy & P. R. Shaver (Eds.), *Handbook of attachment: Theory, research, and clinical applications* (pp. 89–111). New York: Guilford Press.

Bretherton, I., & Page, T. (2004). Shared or conflicting working models?: Relationships in postdivorce families seen through the eyes of mothers and their preschool children. *Development and Psychopathology, 16,* 551–575.

Bretherton, I., & Ridgeway, D. (1990). An Attachment Story Completion Task to assess young children's internal working models of child and parents in the attachment relationship. In M. T. Greenberg, D. Cicchetti, & E. M. Cummings (Eds.), *Attachment in the preschool years: Theory, research, and intervention* (pp. 300–308). Chicago: University of Chicago Press.

Bretherton, I., Ridgeway, D., & Cassidy, J. (1990). Assessing internal working models of the attachment relationship: An Attachment Story Completion Task for 3-year-olds. In D. Cicchetti, M. Greenberg, & E. M. Cummings (Eds.), *Attachment in the preschool years: Theory, research, and intervention* (pp. 272–308). Chicago: University of Chicago Press.

Buccino, G., Binkofski, F., Fink, G. R., Fadiga, L., Fogassi, L., Gallese, V., et al. (2001). Action observation activates premotor and parietal areas in a somatotopic manner: An fMRI study. *European Journal of Neuroscience, 13,* 400–404.

Buchheim, A., Erk, S., George, C., Kächele, H., Kircher, T., Martius, P., et al. (in press). Neural correlates of attachment trauma in borderline personality disorder: A functional magnetic resonance imaging study. *Psychiatry Research.*

Cassidy, J. (1988). Child–mother attachment and the self in six-year-olds. *Child Development, 59,* 121–134.

Cassidy, J. (2001). Truth, lies, and intimacy: An attachment perspective. *Attachment and Human Development, 3,* 121–155.

Collins, N. L. (1996). Working models of attachment: Implications for explanation, emotion, and behavior. *Journal of Personality and Social Psychology, 71,* 810–832.

Craik, K. (1943). *The nature of explanation.* Cambridge, UK: Cambridge University Press.

Crowell, J., & Waters, H. (2005). Attachment representations, secure-base behavior, and the evolution of adult relationships. In K. E. Grossmann, K. Gross-

mann, & E. Waters (Eds.), *Attachment from infancy to adulthood: The major longitudinal studies* (pp. 223–244). New York: Guilford Press.

Damasio, A. R. (1999). *The feeling of what happens.* New York: Harcourt Brace.

Damasio, A. R. (2003). *Looking for Spinoza: Joy, sorrow, and the feeling brain.* Orlando, FL: Harcourt.

Decety, J., Chaminade, T., Grèzes, J., & Meltzoff, A. N. (2002). A PET exploration of the neural mechanisms involved in reciprocal imitation. *NeuroImage, 15,* 265–272.

Dixon, N. F. (1971). *Subliminal perception: The nature of a controversy.* London: McGraw-Hill.

Donald, M. (1991). *Origins of the modern mind.* Cambridge, MA: Harvard University Press.

Dozier, M., & Kobak, R. R. (1992). Psychophysiology in Adult Attachment Interviews: Converging evidence for de-activating strategies. *Child Development, 63,* 1473–1480.

Eisenberger, N. E., & Lieberman, M. D. (2004). Why rejection hurts: A common neural alarm system for physical and social pain. *Trends in Cognitive Sciences, 8,* 294–300.

Erdelyi, M. H. (1974). A new Look at the New Look: Perceptual defense and vigilance. *Psychological Review, 81,* 1–25.

Etzion-Carasso, A., & Oppenheim, D. (2000). Open mother–preschooler communication: Relations with early secure attachment. *Attachment and Human Development, 2,* 347–370.

Fivush, R., & Fromhoff, F. (1988). Style and structure in mother–child conversations about the past. *Discourse Processes, 11,* 337–355.

Fivush, R., & Vasudeva, A. (2002). Remembering to relate: Socioemotional correlates of mother–child reminiscing. *Journal of Cognition and Development, 3,* 73–90.

Fonagy, P., Steele, M., Moran, G., Steele, H., & Higgitt, M. D. (1993). Measuring the ghost in the nursery: An empirical study of the relation between parents' mental representation of childhood experiences and their infants' security of attachment. *Journal of the American Psychoanalytic Association, 41,* 957–989.

Fonagy, P., & Target, M. (1997). Attachment and reflective function: Their role in self-organization. *Development and Psychopathology, 9,* 679–700.

Freud, S. (1963). *An outline of psychoanalysis* (J. Strachey, Trans). New York: Norton. (Original work published 1940)

Frith, U., & Frith, C. D. (2003). Development and the neurophysiology of mentalizing. *Philosophical Transactions of the Royal Society of London, Series B, 358,* 459–473.

Fuster, J. M. (1997). *The prefrontal cortex: Anatomy, physiology, and neuropsychology of the frontal lobe.* New York: Raven Press.

Gallese, V. (2005). Embodied simulation: From neurons to phenomenal experience. *Phenomenology and the Cognitive Sciences, 4,* 23–48.

George, C., Kaplan, N., & Main, M. (1984). *Adult Attachment Interview protocol*. Unpublished manuscript, University of California at Berkeley.

George, C., Kaplan, N., & Main, M. (1985). *Adult Attachment Interview protocol* (2nd ed.). Unpublished manuscript, University of California at Berkeley.

George, C., Kaplan, N., & Main, M. (1996). *Adult Attachment Interview protocol* (3rd ed.). Unpublished manuscript, University of California at Berkeley.

George, C., & West, M. (2004). The Adult Attachment Projective: Measuring individual differences in attachment security using projective methodology. In M. Hersen (Series Ed.) & M. Hilsenroth & D. Segal (Vol. Eds.), *Comprehensive handbook of psychological assessment: Vol. 2. Personality assessment* (pp. 431–447). Hoboken, NJ: Wiley.

Gibson, E. J. (1982). The concept of affordances in development: The renascence of functionalism. In W. A. Collins (Ed.), *Minnesota Symposia on Child Psychology: Vol. 15. The concept of development* (pp. 55–81). Hillsdale, NJ: Erlbaum.

Goldman, A. I. (1991). In defense of simulation. *Mind and Language, 7*, 104–119.

Grossmann, K., Grossmann, K. E., & Kindler, H. (2005). Early care and the roots of attachment and partnership representations. In K. E. Grossmann, K. Grossmann, & E. Waters (Eds.), *Attachment from infancy to adulthood: The major longitudinal studies* (pp. 98–136). New York: Guilford Press.

Gullon-Rivera, A. (2008). *Examining Puerto Rican children's self-representation as reflected in the Attachment Story Completion Task: Linkages with global self-worth, mother–child relationship, and social competence.* Unpublished doctoral dissertation, University of Wisconsin–Madison.

Haxby, J. V., Hoffman, E. A., & Gobbini, M. I. (2000). The distributed human neural system for face perception. *Trends in Cognitive Sciences, 4*, 223–233.

Hazan, C., & Shaver, P. R. (1987). Romantic love conceptualized as an attachment process. *Journal of Personality and Social Psychology, 52*, 511–524.

Heider, F. (1958). *The psychology of interpersonal relations.* New York: Wiley.

Hilgard, E. (1974). Toward a neo-dissociation theory: Multiple cognitive controls in human functioning. *Perspectives in Biology and Medicine, 17*, 301–316.

Johnson-Laird, P. N. (1983). *Mental models.* Cambridge, MA: Harvard University Press.

Kanwisher, N., & Yovel, G. (2006). The fusiform face area: A cortical region specialized for the perception of faces. *Philosophical Transactions of the Royal Society of Long, Series B, 361*, 2109–2128.

Klagsbrun, M., & Bowlby, J. (1976). Responses to separation from parents: A clinical test for young children. *British Journal of Projective Psychology, 21*, 7–21.

Kobak, R., & Duemmler, S. (1994). Attachment and conversation: A discourse analysis of goal-directed partnerships. In K. Bartholomew & D. Perlman (Eds.), *Advances in personal relationships: Vol. 5. Attachment processes in adulthood* (pp. 121–149). London: Jessica Kingsley.

Krawczyk, D. C. (2002). Contributions of the prefrontal cortex to the neural basis of human decision making. *Neuroscience and Biobehavioral Reviews, 26*, 631–664.

Laible, D. J., & Thompson, R. (2000). Mother–child discourse, attachment security, shared positive affect and early conscience development. *Child Development, 71*, 1424–1440.

Lewin, K. (1933). Environmental forces. In C. Murchison (Ed.), *A handbook of child psychology* (2nd ed., pp. 590–625). Worcester, MA: Clark University Press.

Light, P. (1979). *The development of social sensitivity.* Cambridge, UK: Cambridge University Press.

Lyons-Ruth, K., Yellin, C., Melnick, S., & Atwood, G. (2005). Expanding the concept of unresolved mental states: Hostile-helpless states of mind on the Adult Attachment Interview are associated with disrupted mother–infant communication and infant disorganization. *Development and Psychopathology, 17*, 1–23.

Main, M. (1991). Metacognitive knowledge, metacognitive monitoring, and singular (coherent) versus multiple (incoherent) models of attachment. In C. M. Parkes, J. Stevenson-Hinde, & P. Marris (Eds.), *Attachment across the life cycle* (pp. 127–159). London: Routledge.

Main, M. (1995). Recent studies in attachment. In S. Goldberg, R. Muir, & J. Kerr (Eds.), *Attachment theory: Social, developmental, and clinical perspectives* (pp. 407–474). Hillsdale, NJ: Analytic Press.

Main, M. (1999). Epilogue. Attachment theory: Eighteen points with suggestions for future studies. In J. Cassidy & P. R. Shaver (Eds.), *Handbook of attachment: Theory, research, and clinical applications* (pp. 845–887). New York: Guilford Press.

Main, M., & Goldwyn, R. (1984). *Adult attachment scoring and classification system.* Unpublished manuscript, University of California at Berkeley.

Main, M., Goldwyn, R., & Hesse, E. (2003). *Adult attachment scoring and classification system.* Unpublished manuscript, University of California at Berkeley.

Main, M., Hesse, E., & Kaplan, N. (2005). Predictability of attachment behavior and representational processes at 1, 6 and 19 years of age. In K. E. Grossmann, K. Grossmann, & E. Waters (Eds.), *Attachment from infancy to adulthood: The major longitudinal studies* (pp. 245–304). New York: Guilford Press.

Main, M., Kaplan, K., & Cassidy, J. (1985). Security in infancy, childhood, and adulthood: A move to the level of representation. In I. Bretherton & E. Waters (Eds.), Growing points of attachment theory and research. *Monographs of the Society for Research in Child Development, 50*(1–2, Serial No. 209), 66–104.

Mead, G. H. (1913). The social self. *Journal of Philosophy, Psychology and Scientific Methods, 10*, 374–380.

Mead, G. H. (1934). *Mind, self, and society.* Chicago: University of Chicago Press.

Meins, E., Fernyhough, C., Wainwright, R., Gupta, M. D., Fradley, E., & Tuckey, M. (2002). Maternal mind-mindedness and attachment security as predictors of theory of mind understanding. *Child Development, 73,* 1715–1726.

Meltzoff, A. N., & Moore, M. K. (1977). Imitation of facial and manual gestures by human neonates. *Science, 198,* 75–98.

Mikulincer, M., & Shaver, P. R. (2004). Security-based self-representations in adulthood: Contents and processes. In W. S. Rholes & J. A. Simpson (Eds.), *Adult attachment: Theory, research, and clinical implications* (pp. 159–195). New York: Guilford Press.

Miller, E. K., & Cohen, J. D. (2001). An integrative theory of prefrontal cortex function. *Annual Review of Neuroscience, 24,* 167–202.

Nelson, K. (1989). *Narratives from the crib.* Cambridge, MA: Harvard University Press.

Nelson, K. (1996). *Language in cognitive development: Emergence of the mediated mind.* New York: Cambridge University Press.

Nelson, K. (2005). Evolution and the development of human memory systems. In S. Ellis & D. Bjorklund (Eds.), *Origins of the social mind: Evolutionary psychology and child development* (pp. 319–345). New York: Guilford Press.

Nelson, K., & Gruendel, J. (1981). Generalized event representations: Basic building blocks of cognitive development. In M. E. Lamb & A. Brown (Eds.), *Advances in developmental psychology* (Vol. 1, pp. 131–158). Hillsdale, NJ: Erlbaum.

Newcombe, R., & Reese, E. (2004). Evaluations and orientations in mother–child narratives as a function of attachment security: A longitudinal investigation. *International Journal of Behavioral Development, 28,* 230–245.

Norman, D. A. (1976). *Memory and attention: Introduction to human information processing* (2nd ed.). New York: Wiley.

Page, T., & Bretherton, I. (2003). Gender differences in stories of violence and caring by preschool children in post-divorce families: Implications for social competence. *Child and Adolescent Social Work Journal, 20,* 485–504.

Parkes, C. M. (1971). Psychosocial transitions: A field for study. *Social Sciences and Medicine, 5,* 1110–1115.

Piaget, J. (1951). *Play, dreams, and imitation.* New York: Norton.

Piaget, J. (1952). *The origins of intelligence in children.* New York: Norton.

Rizzolatti, G., Fadiga, L., Gallese, V., & Fogassi, L. (1996). Premotor cortex and the recognition of motor actions. *Brain Research: Cognitive Brain Research, 3,* 131–141.

Roisman, G. (2006). The role of adult attachment security in non-romantic, non-attachment-related first interactions between same-sex strangers. *Attachment and Human Development, 8,* 341–352.

Roisman, G. (2007). The psychophysiology of adult attachment relationships: Autonomic reactivity in marital and premarital interactions. *Developmental Psychology, 43,* 39–53.

Roisman, G., Padrón, E., Sroufe, L. A., & Egeland, B. (2002). Earned attachment status in retrospect and prospect. *Child Development, 73,* 1204–1219.

Rolls, E. T. (1996). The orbitofrontal cortex. *Philosophic Transactions of the Royal Society of London, Series B, 351,* 1433–1444.

Ruby, P., & Decety, J. (2004). How would *you* feel versus how do you think *she* would feel?: A neuroimaging study of perspective-taking with social emotions. *Journal of Cognitive Neuroscience, 16,* 988–999.

Saxe, R., Xiao, D.-K., Kovacs, G., Perrett, D. I., & Kanwisher, N. (2004). A region of right posterior superior temporal sulcus responds to observed intentional actions. *Neuropsychologia, 42,* 1435–1446.

Schacter, D. L., & Addis, D. R. (2007). The cognitive neuroscience of constructive memory: Remembering the past and imagining the future. *Philosophical Transactions of the Royal Society of London, Series B, 362,* 773–786.

Schacter, D. L., & Tulving, E. (1994). What are the memory systems of 1994? In D. Schachter & E. Tulving (Eds.), *Memory systems* (pp. 1–38). Cambridge, MA: MIT Press.

Schank, R. C., & Abelson, R. P. (1977). *Scripts, plans, goals, and understanding.* Hillsdale, NJ: Erlbaum.

Sherry, D. F., & Schacter, D. L. (1987). The evolution of multiple memory systems. *Psychological Review, 94,* 439–454.

Simpson, J. A., Collins, W. A., Tran, S., & Haydon, K. C. (2007). Attachment and the experience and expression of emotions in romantic relationships: A developmental perspective. *Journal of Personality and Social Psychology, 92,* 355–367.

Singer, T., Seymour, B., O'Doherty, J., Stephan, K. E., Dolan, R. J., & Frith, C. D. (2006). Empathic neural responses are modulated by the perceived fairness of others. *Nature, 439,* 466–469.

Slade, A., Grienenberger, J., Bernbach, E., Levy, D., & Locker, A. (2005). Maternal reflective functioning, attachment, and the transmission gap: A preliminary study. *Attachment and Human Development, 7,* 283–298.

Solomon, J., George, C., & De Jong, A. (1995). Children classified as controlling at age six: Evidence of disorganized representational strategies at home and school. *Development and Psychopathology, 7,* 447–464.

Spangler, G., & Grossmann, K. E. (1993). Biobehavioral organization in securely and insecurely attached infants. *Child Development, 64,* 1439–1450.

Sroufe, L. A., Egeland, B., Carlson, E., & Collins, W. A. (2005). *The development of the person: The Minnesota Study of Risk and Adaptation from Birth to Adulthood.* New York: Guilford Press.

Stern, D. N. (1985). *The interpersonal world of the infant.* New York: Basic Books.

Suess, G., Grossmann, K. E., & Sroufe, L. A. (1992). Effects of infant attachment to mother and father on quality of adaptation in preschool: From dyadic to individual organization of self. *International Journal of Behavioural Development, 15,* 43–65.

Thompson, R. A., Laible, D. J., & Ontai, L. L. (2003). Early understanding of emotion, morality, and the self: Developing a working model. In R. V. Kail (Ed.), *Advances in child development and behavior* (Vol. 31, pp. 137–171). San Diego, CA: Academic Press.

Trevarthen, C., & Hubley, P. (1978). Secondary inter-subjectivity: Confidence, confiding, and acts of meaning in the first year. In A. Lock (Ed.), *Action, gesture, and symbol* (pp. 183–229). London: Academic Press.

Tulving, E. (1972). Episodic and semantic memory. In E. Tulving & W. Donaldson (Eds.), *Organization of memory* (pp. 381–403). New York: Academic Press.

van IJzendoorn, M. H. (1995). Adult attachment representations, parental responsiveness, and infant attachment: A meta-analysis on the predictive validity of the Adult Attachment Interview. *Psychological Bulletin, 117,* 387–403.

Vaughn, B., Coppola, G., Veríssimo, M., Monteiro, L., Santos, A. J., Posada, G., et al. (2007). The quality of maternal secure base scripts predicts children's secure base behavior at home in three socio-cultural groups. *International Journal of Behavioral Development, 31,* 65–76.

Vaughn, B. E., Veríssimo, M., Coppola, G., Bost, K. K., Shin, N., McBridge, B., et al. (2006). Maternal attachment script representations: Longitudinal stability and associations with stylistic features of maternal narratives. *Attachment and Human Development, 8,* 199–208.

Vogeley, K., Bussfeld, P., Newen, A., Herrmann, S., Happe, F., Falkai, P., et al. (2001). Mind reading: Neural mechanisms of theory of mind and self-perspective. *NeuroImage, 14,* 170–181.

Vygotsky, L. S. (1978). *Mind in society.* Cambridge, MA: Harvard University Press.

Waters, E. (1995). The Attachment Q-Set (Version 3.0). In E. Waters, B. E. Vaughn, G. Posada, & K. Kondo-Ikemura (Eds.), Caregiving, cultural and cognitive perspectives on secure base behavior and working models: New growing points of attachment theory and research. *Monographs of the Society for Research in Child Development, 60*(2–3, Serial No. 244), 234–246.

Waters, E., Crowell, J., Elliott, M., Corcoran, D., & Treboux, D. (2002). Bowlby's secure base theory and the social/personality psychology of attachment styles: Work(s) in progress. *Attachment and Human Development, 4,* 230–242.

Waters, E., Merrick, S., Treboux, D., Crowell, J., & Albersheim, L. (2000). Attachment security in infancy and early adulthood: A 20-year longitudinal study. *Child Development, 71,* 684–689.

Waters, H. S., Rodrigues, L. M., & Ridgeway, D. (1998). Cognitive underpinnings of narrative attachment assessment. *Journal of Experimental Child Psychology, 71,* 211–234.

Waters, H. S., & Rodrigues-Doolabh, L. (2004). *Manual for decoding secure base narratives.* Unpublished manuscript, State University of New York at Stony Brook.

Waters, H. S., & Waters, E. (2006). The attachment working models concept: Among other things, we build script-like representations of secure base experiences. *Attachment and Human Development, 8,* 185–197.

Wicker, B., Keysers, C., Plailly, J., Royet, J.-P., Gallese, V., & Rizzolatti, G. (2003). Both of us disgusted in my insula: The common neural basis of seeing and feeling disgust, *Neuron, 3,* 655–664.

Young, J. Z. (1964). *A model for the brain.* London: Oxford University Press.

PART II

BIOLOGICAL PERSPECTIVES

CHAPTER 6

Attachment Theory
within a Modern Evolutionary Framework

JEFFRY A. SIMPSON
JAY BELSKY

It has often been assumed that animals were in the first place rendered social, and that they feel as a consequence uncomfortable when separated from each other, and comfortable whilst together; but it is a more probable view that these sensations were first developed, in order that those animals which would profit by living in society, should be induced to live together, ... for with those animals which were benefited by living in close association, the individuals which took the greatest pleasure in society would best escape various dangers; whilst those that cared least for their comrades and lived solitary would perish in greater numbers.
—Darwin (1871/1981, Vol. 1, p. 80)

As this quotation suggests, Charles Darwin may have been the first attachment theorist. Although he focused on "society" (instead of significant persons in an individual's life) and "comrades" (instead of attachment figures), Darwin was perhaps the first scientist to appreciate the deep degree to which human social nature is a product of selection pressures. John Bowlby, who admired Darwin's theoretical vision and was one of his biographers (see Bowlby, 1991), spent most of his brilliant career treading the intellectual path that Darwin began paving. Integrating ideas from Darwin's theory of evolution by natural selection, object relations theory, control systems theory, evolutionary biology, and the fields of ethology and cognitive psychology, Bowlby (1969/1982, 1973, 1980) developed a grand synthesis of social and personality development across the lifespan—attachment theory. Among the reasons why attachment theory is so unique, generative, and prominent today are its deep intellectual ties to fundamental principles of evolution.

Indeed, attachment theory is one of a handful of major middle-level evolutionary theories. Bowlby's interest in the cognitive, emotional,

and behavioral ties that bind humans to one another began with an astute observation. Across all human cultures and most primate species, young and vulnerable infants display a specific sequence of reactions following separation from their stronger, older, and wiser caregivers. Immediately following separation, most infants protest vehemently, typically crying, screaming, and throwing temper tantrums as they search for their caregivers. Bowlby surmised that vigorous protest during the early phases of caregiver absence is a good initial strategy to promote survival, particularly in species born in a developmentally immature and highly dependent state. Intense protests usually draw the attention of caregivers to their infants, who during evolutionary history would have been susceptible to injury or predation if left unattended.

If loud and persistent protests fail to retrieve the caregiver, infants enter a second stage—despair, during which their motor activity declines and they fall silent. From an evolutionary standpoint, Bowlby realized that despondency is a good "second" strategy to promote survival. Excessive movement may result in accident or injury, and loud protests combined with movement may

131

draw predators. Thus, if protests fail to retrieve the caregiver, the next best survival strategy is to avoid actions that may increase the risks of self-inflicted harm or predation.

Bowlby observed that after a period of despair, infants who are not reunited with their caregivers enter a third and final stage—detachment. During this phase, an infant begins to resume normal activity without the caregiver, learning to behave in an independent and self-reliant manner. Bowlby (1969/1982) conjectured that the function of detachment is to permit the formation of emotional bonds with new caregivers. He reasoned that emotional ties with previous caregivers must be partially if not fully relinquished before new bonds can be formed. From the standpoint of evolution, detachment allows infants to cast off old ties and begin the process of forming new ones with caregivers who may be willing to provide the resources necessary for survival.

Bowlby believed that the cognitive, emotional, and behavioral reactions characterizing each stage reveal the operation of an innate attachment system. The reason why the attachment system evolved and remains so deeply ingrained in human nature is that it provided a good solution to one of the most daunting adaptive problems our ancestors faced: how to increase the probability of survival through the most perilous years of social and physical development. Guided by Darwin, Bowlby believed that the attachment system was genetically "wired" into many species through intense directional selection during evolutionary history.

There were, of course, limitations to Bowlby's and other early attachment theorists' understanding and application of evolutionary thinking, many of which Bowlby corrected during the development of attachment theory (see Belsky, 1999; Bowlby, 1969/1982; Simpson, 1999). One shortcoming was Bowlby's initial focus on the differential survival of species rather than of individuals. Another shortcoming was his nearly exclusive focus on the survival function of attachment rather than its implications for differential reproduction. To enhance reproductive fitness, individuals must not only survive to reproductive age; once there, they must successfully mate and raise children, who in turn must mate and raise their own children, and so on. Fortunately, as we shall see, contemporary attachment theorists have shifted attention to how attachment phenomena and processes in childhood may be systematically linked to the enactment of different reproductive strategies in adulthood (Belsky, 2007; Belsky, Steinberg, & Draper, 1991; Chisholm, 1996, 1999). Nevertheless, because in-

dividuals cannot reproduce without first surviving to reproductive age, Bowlby was wise to build the foundation of attachment theory on this vital prerequisite to ultimate reproductive fitness.

Early attachment theorists also harbored the erroneous view that most rearing environments in the "environment of evolutionary adaptedness" (EEA) were benign, resulting in the secure attachment pattern being "species-typical" (see Ainsworth, 1979; Main, 1981). The EEA, however, was probably not nearly as uniform, resource-rich, or benign as many early attachment theorists envisioned (Edgarton, 1992; Foley, 1992), meaning that no single attachment pattern should have been primary or species-typical. In fact, as we shall see, the adoption of different attachment patterns (in children) or orientations (in adults) may actually reflect evolved, unpremeditated tactics designed to improve reproductive fitness in response to the specific environments in which individuals grow and develop. "Reproductive fitness" reflects the extent to which an individual's genes are present in his or her descendants. The concept of "inclusive fitness" (see below) highlights the important distinction between genes present in direct descendants (i.e., children) and those present in indirect descendants (e.g., grandchildren, nieces, nephews). From an evolutionary standpoint, the maximization of reproductive or inclusive fitness is the goal of all living organisms, including humans.

Perhaps the biggest impediment to Bowlby's understanding of evolution, however, was the nascent state of evolutionary thinking when he began formulating attachment theory in the 1950s and 1960s. The foundation of attachment theory was well established long before several important "middle-level" theories of evolution—theories addressing the major adaptive problems that humans probably confronted at different life stages during evolutionary history—were introduced in the early to mid-1970s. As a result, Bowlby was not privy to much of what is now known as the "modern" evolutionary perspective when he began erecting the tenets of attachment theory. Until recently, few of the modern middle-level evolutionary theories have been systematically linked with mainstream attachment theory and research. We hope to facilitate this process.

The overarching goal of this chapter is to place attachment theory in a modern (neo-Darwinian) evolutionary perspective. As will become apparent, the modern evolutionary perspective includes an array of theories, principles, and assumptions, all of which share a central premise: that much of the human mind and human social behavior reflect adaptations to the major obstacles to inclusive fitness that humans repeatedly faced throughout evolutionary history.

The chapter is divided into seven sections. The first section briefly reviews theoretical developments that have transformed Darwin's (1859, 1871/1981) original theory of natural selection into the modern evolutionary perspective. We also discuss where attachment theory fits within the hierarchy of evolutionary principles and middle-level theories. The second section describes the major adaptive problems that our ancestors had to overcome, given the probable nature of the environments they most likely inhabited in the past 100,000 years. Highlighting anthropological evidence from hunter–gatherer tribes, we identify the most stable features of the social EEAs that humans probably inhabited.

The third section focuses on how the two major components of attachment theory—the normative component and the individual-difference component—fit within a modern evolutionary view of human behavior. In discussing normative attachment, we briefly review the species-typical course through which attachment bonds develop and unfold across the lifespan. Different patterns or styles of attachment are construed as adaptive, ecologically contingent behavioral strategies that could have facilitated reproduction in adulthood, given the probable environments that individuals would inhabit as adults.

The fourth section reveals how another major middle-level theory of evolution—Trivers's (1974) theory of parent–offspring conflict—sheds new light on several attachment-related phenomena, including how and why parents and children negotiate issues of weaning, parental investment, and the children's eventual independence. In the fifth section, we review and evaluate several attachment/life history models, most of which articulate how and why different attachment patterns in childhood may affect the trajectory of social and personality development, culminating in divergent reproductive strategies in adulthood. In the final two sections, we highlight some important unresolved issues and promising new directions for research, and offer concluding comments.

THE PLACE OF ATTACHMENT THEORY IN MODERN EVOLUTIONARY THINKING

Though it remains one of the greatest intellectual accomplishments in the history of science, Darwin's (1859) original theory of evolution was incomplete and imprecise, especially in view of recent theoretical advances that have shaped the modern evolutionary perspective. Darwin's thinking was constrained by several factors. First, his theory predated our understanding of genes and patterns of inheritance. Mendel's pioneering research on heritable traits in plants, though initially published in 1866, was neither understood nor appreciated until well after the turn of the 20th century. Second, because Darwin did not focus on genes as the principal units on which natural selection operates, he could not explain why some organisms engage in self-sacrificial or nonreproductive behavior. This enigma was not solved until Hamilton (1964) introduced and provided compelling empirical evidence for the concept of inclusive fitness (i.e., the notion that differential gene replication really drives evolution). Third, Darwin had only a faint understanding of how sexual recombination and genetic mutations provide the variation from which better adaptations and new species are selected. Fourth, Darwin did not fully appreciate the extent to which specific adaptations are associated with both benefits and costs. Similar to many theorists of his time, he focused more on the benefits bestowed by certain adaptations and did not fully consider potential costs (see Cronin, 1991). Darwin's brilliance allowed him to sketch the ways in which natural selection might operate, *without* the benefits of all this knowledge.

The Rise of Modern Evolutionary Theories

Few theoretical advances occurred in the evolutionary sciences for almost a century after Darwin published his second landmark book, *The Descent of Man*, in 1871. This state of affairs changed in the mid-1960s. With the development of inclusive fitness theory, Hamilton (1964) introduced the notion of kin selection. By focusing on the gene rather than the individual organism as the primary unit on which selection operates, Hamilton solved the biggest paradox that Darwin never unraveled: Namely, in the evolutionary struggle for reproductive fitness, why do some organisms forgo reproduction to assist the reproductive efforts of their biological relatives?

Hamilton solved this riddle by realizing that an individual's total (inclusive) fitness should depend on his or her own reproductive output, plus the total reproductive output of all kin who share some portion of the individual's genes. If genes are the units on which selection operates, and if individuals can facilitate the reproductive output of their biological relatives, there may be situations in which it would pay to sacrifice one's own reproductive output, including one's life, in order to facilitate the reproduction of close relatives. Unlike Darwin, Hamilton could calculate the degree to which pairs of individuals are likely to share novel genes. On average, parents share half of their genes with their children; full siblings share half of their genes with each other; grandparents share one-quarter of their genes with their grandchildren; aunts and uncles share one-quarter of their genes with their nieces and nephews; and first cousins share one-eighth of their genes.

Armed with this knowledge, Hamilton confirmed that self-sacrificial behavior could have been selected in situations where the costs of engaging in an act were less than the benefits to be gained times the degree to which individuals were biologically related (i.e., altruistic behavior should occur when $C < Br$, where C = costs, B = benefits, and r = the degree of relatedness; see Simpson, 1999). For example, although it would make sense to sacrifice one's own life to save at least two biological children (each of whom shares 50% of a parent's genes), one would have to save many more nieces or nephews (who carry fewer genes) to achieve the same fitness benefits. Hamilton's intellectual breakthrough marked the dawn of the modern evolutionary perspective. Indeed, inclusive fitness theory is the overarching theory of natural selection from which virtually all middle-level evolutionary theories are derived. Although Hamilton's research was not cited by Bowlby (1969/1982), Bowlby's first major statement on attachment proved to be one of the first middle-level evolutionary theories. In developing attachment theory, Bowlby sought to understand and explain how our ancestors successfully "solved" the first critical barrier to inclusive fitness—how to survive the many perils and dangers of infancy.

Several important theoretical advances followed in the early 1970s, many of which were spearheaded by Robert Trivers. In 1971, he introduced the theory of reciprocal altruism, which explains why organisms who have inherently "selfish" genes should at times behave in a cooperative manner with non-kin. Trivers outlined some of the specific conditions under which selective reciprocal altruism could enhance an individual's inclusive fitness. Axelrod (1984) then demonstrated how a quid pro quo strategy of helping others (i.e., a tit-for-tat strategy) could evolve and become stable amid alternate competing strategies.

In 1972, Trivers unveiled the theory of parental investment and sexual selection. According to this theory, different amounts of parental investment in children govern sexual selection, which explains why females and males in many species differ on certain physical attributes (e.g., relative body size) and behavioral characteristics (e.g., aggressiveness). Trivers (1972) argued that in species where one sex *initially* invests more time, effort, resources, and energy in producing and raising offspring (usually women, in the case of humans), the other sex (usually men) should compete to mate with the higher-investing sex. The intense intrasexual competition that results should have produced some of the modal physical, behavioral, and emotional differences witnessed between the sexes.

In 1974, Trivers introduced the theory of parent–offspring conflict. This theory explains why parents and their children—individuals who share half their genes, and thus should be jointly invested in passing them on to future generations—experience conflict: Their individual self-interests are not identical. Because the theory of parent–offspring conflict has several fascinating implications for how patterns of attachment between children and their caregivers can be understood, we discuss it in greater detail below.

In recent years, life history theory (LHT; Charnov, 1993; Clutton-Brock, 1991; Stearns, 1976, 1992; Williams, 1966) has become a prominent, unifying perspective within the evolutionary sciences. In order to leave descendants, individuals must solve multiple problems tied to survival, growth, development, and reproduction across the lifespan. Depending on life circumstances, the time, effort, and energy that an individual has can be allotted to somatic effort (i.e., investing in growth and development of one's body to facilitate survival en route to later reproduction) and reproductive effort (i.e., funneling effort toward progeny). Reproductive effort, in turn, has two components: mating effort (i.e., locating, courting, and retaining suitable mates) and parenting effort (i.e., gestating, giving birth, postnatal child care, and teaching/socialization). LHT addresses how individuals should best allocate somatic versus reproductive effort, given their past, current, and anticipated (future) life circumstances.

Attachment Theory in the Hierarchy of Evolutionary Theories

Inclusive fitness theory, which encompasses Darwin's concept of fitness due to one's own reproduction (i.e., direct descendants—children) as well as Hamilton's notion of fitness due to the reproduction of one's biological relatives (i.e., indirect descendants—grandchildren, nieces, etc.), is the superordinate theory of evolution from which nearly all middle-level evolutionary theories flow. The middle-level theories, each of which addresses special adaptive problems that humans faced during evolutionary history, reside one level below inclusive fitness theory, being more specific and less general. As discussed above, some of the major middle-level theories are reciprocal altruism theory (Trivers, 1971), sexual selection and parental investment theory (Trivers, 1972), parent–offspring conflict theory (Trivers, 1974), and attachment theory (Bowlby, 1969/1982).[1] Because it addresses how individuals should allocate their finite resources across the entire lifespan, LHT (Charnov, 1993; Stearns, 1992) intersects with and interconnects many of the other middle-level theories. Each middle-level theory contains a small set of basic principles that reside at the next level down (see Simpson, 1999). Most evolutionary hypotheses and predictions are derived from these basic principles.

Sexual selection and parental investment theory, for instance, contains two major principles relevant to mate selection. The theory suggests that the search for mates is governed by the extent to which prospective mates (1) are likely to be good investors in and providers for future offspring, and (2) possess desirable attributes (e.g., physical attractiveness or other mate-attracting features) that can be passed on genetically to offspring (Gangestad & Simpson, 2000). Specific predictions and hypotheses are then derived from each of these principles. Attachment theory also has two primary theoretical components. The normative component of attachment theory makes predictions about relatively universal, stable patterns of behavior, particularly in response to situations in which individuals feel ill, fatigued, afraid, or upset (Bowlby, 1969/1982). The individual-difference component offers predictions about the ontogenic origins and developmental sequelae of different patterns or orientations (styles) of attachment, including why each pattern or style should be "adaptive" in certain environments.

Even though each middle-level evolutionary theory was formulated to address a specific adaptive problem, many of them have overlapping implications for social behavior. The theory of kin selection, for example, also stipulates when conflict ought to arise between parents and their children; the theory of parent–offspring conflict specifies

when reciprocal altruism should emerge between different sets of parents; and the theory of reciprocal altruism addresses when men and women may strive to attain status and ascend social hierarchies in local groups (see Simpson, 1999). Moreover, in some cases, middle-level theories generate different hypotheses and predictions about a given outcome. This highlights a critical point: For some phenomena, there is no single evolutionary prediction, particularly if competing middle-level theories are involved (see Buss, 1995).

STABLE FEATURES OF THE SOCIAL EEA

To gain a clearer understanding of the context in which the attachment system evolved and the problems it was designed to "solve," one must consider the physical and social environments that humans probably inhabited in evolutionary history. Although attachment theorists have speculated some about what the EEA might have been like (especially the physical EEA; see Bowlby, 1969/1982), less consideration has been given to the *social* EEA (for an exception, see Brewer & Caporael, 1990, 2006). Unfortunately, we do not know many concrete details about the environments in which our ancestors lived. What we do know is that, given their diverse migration patterns, humans inhabited a wide array of geographical and climatic environments, ranging from arid and barren deserts to lush tropical jungles. Thus there was no single EEA, particularly no monolithic physical environment. The social environments in which most humans evolved, however, may have had some reasonably consistent and stable features (see Simpson, 1999).

During much of human evolutionary history, for example, people were hunters and gatherers (Cronk, 1999; Kelly, 1995). Anthropological observations of contemporary hunter–gatherer tribes, such as the !Kung San of Africa, the Inuit of the Arctic, the Ache of Paraguay, and the Aborigines of Australia, provide perhaps the best views of what ancient tribal life might have been like. For thousands of generations, our ancestors lived in small, cooperative groups (Brewer & Caporael, 1990; Eibl-Eibesfeldt, 1989). Most people within a tribe were biologically related to one another, and strangers were encountered rather infrequently, probably during intertribal trading or war (Wright, 1994). Though people occasionally migrated in and out of their natal groups, most remained in the same tribe their entire lives.

Most men and women formed long-term pair bonds (Cronk, 1999), but serial monogamy was probably the norm (Fisher, 1992). Children were typically born approximately 4 years apart and were raised with considerable help from extended family and perhaps non-kin (Wright, 1994); few children were raised exclusively by their biological parents. In fact, humans were probably "cooperative breeders" who shared childrearing with their kin (Hrdy, 1999, 2005). In all likelihood, younger children spent considerable time being socialized by older children (Eibl-Eibesfeldt, 1989). Both men and women were involved in securing food, with men doing most of the hunting and women doing most of the gathering (Wood & Eagly, 2002). Whereas some of these inferences are more speculative than others, the human mind probably evolved to deal with problems arising in social environments that had these features. Indeed, participation in the daily functioning of small, cooperative groups may have been the predominant survival strategy of early humans (Brewer & Caporael, 1990). These likely features of the social EEA must be considered when attachment theory is conceptualized within an evolutionary framework.

NORMATIVE AND INDIVIDUAL-DIFFERENCE COMPONENTS OF ATTACHMENT

As mentioned earlier, attachment theory has two primary components: (1) a normative component, which seeks to explain modal or species-typical patterns and stages of attachment in humans (e.g., "How and why are attachment bonds formed?"); and (2) an individual-difference component, which attempts to explain deviations from modal or normative patterns and stages (e.g., "How and why do different patterns of attachment exist?"). The attempt to explain both species-typical patterns of behavior and predictable individual differences is a hallmark of most major middle-level evolutionary theories (Simpson, 1999). Bowlby and Ainsworth were, in fact, among the first middle-level evolutionary theorists to recognize the need to explain not only normative behavior, but systematic individual differences as well.

Normative Features of Attachment

There are several normative features of attachment, three of which have especially important ties to evolutionary principles: the apparent "synchronization" of infant–parent responses/behav-

iors in the opening months of life; young children's need to maintain contact with and seek proximity to their caregivers; and basic stages through which attachment propensities develop.

Synchronized Capabilities

Compared to other species, human infants are born in an underdeveloped and premature state (Kaplan, Lancaster, & Hurtado, 2000). From the moment of birth, however, human infants are prepared to bond with their caregivers (see Simpson, 1999). In addition, several postpartum reactions of mothers seem to operate in synchrony with those of their newborns, facilitating the early formation of infant–caregiver bonds. Systems that operate in a synchronous, lock-and-key fashion between codependent individuals are often telltale signs of evolved adaptations (Andrews, Gangestad, & Matthews, 2002).

Immediately after delivery, for example, mothers experience a rush of hormones that make them feel euphoric and receptive to emotional bonding, despite the fact that they are exhausted from giving birth (Eibl-Eibesfeldt, 1989). Without instruction, mothers in all cultures place themselves about 30 centimeters from their young infants, which happens to be an optimal distance for young infants to see faces clearly (Eibl-Eibesfeldt, 1989). Mothers also work hard to establish eye contact with their infants (Klaus & Kennell, 1976), and when infants reciprocate eye contact, mothers become livelier, speak with greater voice inflections, and approach their infants more closely (Grossmann, 1978, cited in Eibl-Eibesfeldt, 1989). Eye contact and smiling by infants are extremely rewarding to new mothers, who interpret such cues as signs of genuine affection (Eibl-Eibesfeldt, 1989). When interacting with their infants, mothers typically exaggerate their facial expressions, change them more slowly, and maintain visual contact for longer periods of time (Eibl-Eibesfeldt, 1989), all of which are ideally suited to an infant's developing visual system. When talking to their infants, mothers intentionally slow their speech, accentuate certain syllables, and talk one octave above normal speech (Anderson & Jaffe, 1972; Grieser & Kuhl, 1988). This pattern of speech, termed "motherese," is preferred by most young infants (Fernald, 1985) and is well suited to infants' developing auditory capacities. It is simply implausible that such well-coordinated and interconnected behaviors and proclivities did not coevolve. The evolutionary hypothesis is that by tying mother to baby and baby to mother, these coordinated responses, skills, and inclinations promoted the survival and probably the reproductive fitness of mothers and their children.

Contact Maintenance and Proximity Seeking

According to Bowlby (1980), attachment behaviors include actions that promote proximity between children and their attachment figures. Young children engage in three classes of behavior that establish or maintain proximity to their caregivers (Belsky & Cassidy, 1994). Signaling behaviors (e.g., vocalizing, smiling) tend to draw caregivers toward children, usually for positive interactions. Aversive behaviors (e.g., crying, screaming) bring caregivers to children, typically to terminate the aversive reactions. Active behaviors (e.g., approaching, following) move children toward caregivers. Though different phenotypically, these behaviors all serve the same biological function: to keep vulnerable infants in close physical proximity to their caregivers, thereby increasing their chances of survival. Given that death prior to reproduction was the first major threat to inclusive fitness, Bowlby reasoned that directional selection shaped the attachment system in humans, setting the foundation of our social nature.

Phases of Development

According to Bowlby (1969/1982; see Marvin & Britner, Chapter 12, this volume), attachment propensities develop through four phases in humans. In the first phase, which takes place between birth and 2–3 months, infants respond to a variety of social stimuli and people, not exhibiting strong preferences for one attachment figure. Although Bowlby may have overestimated how open very young infants are to contact comfort from multiple caregivers (see above), he was correct in believing that infants are malleable in terms of whom they can bond with in the opening months of life. During the second phase, which runs from 2–3 months to about 7 months, infants display greater discrimination in social responsiveness. They begin, for instance, to distinguish caregivers and family members from strangers, to selectively prefer certain persons, and to direct their attachment behaviors toward specific attachment figures.

In the third phase, which extends from 7 months to roughly 3 years, children learn to play a more active role in seeking proximity and initiating social contact. During this phase, they start to develop "internal working models" (i.e., beliefs,

expectancies, and attitudes about relationships based on experiences with attachment figures) of the self and significant others (Bowlby, 1973). This is also the phase during which the three primary functions of attachment are first seen in the child's behavior: proximity maintenance (staying near to, and resisting separations from, the attachment figure), safe haven (turning to the attachment figure for comfort and support), and secure base (using the attachment figure as a base from which to engage in nonattachment behaviors). If children in this phase have prolonged separations from their attachment figures, they experience the three stages of response to separation: protest, despair, and detachment. The fourth phase, which begins at about age 3, marks the beginning of behaviors that signal the development of a "goal-corrected partnership" with attachment figures. That is, given the further development of language skills and theory-of-mind capabilities, children begin to see the world from the perspective of their interaction partners. This allows them to incorporate the goals, plans, and desires of their interaction partners into their decision making, resulting in the negotiation of joint plans and activities.

As children move through the toddler years, their desire for physical proximity is gradually replaced by a desire to maintain psychological proximity (i.e., felt security; Sroufe & Waters, 1977). Early in adolescence, overt manifestations of attachment bonds with parents start to subside (Hinde, 1976). The three functions of attachment—proximity maintenance, safe haven, and secure base—are slowly transferred from parents to peers and romantic partners as adolescents enter adulthood (see Furman & Simon, 1999; Hazan & Shaver, 1994).

In summary, each of these normative capabilities and proclivities was probably shaped by selection pressures. Infants (and mothers) who forged stronger emotional bonds had, on average, higher reproductive fitness. Young children who were motivated to maintain closer contact to their parents (and parents who encouraged such tendencies) achieved greater fitness, as did individuals who successfully moved through each attachment stage and were able to transfer critical attachment functions from their parents to adult romantic partners.

Individual Differences in Attachment

Although infants are biologically predisposed to form attachment bonds with their caregivers, the type of bonds they form ought to depend on the conditions in which they are raised, just as Bowlby (1969/1982) and Ainsworth (1979) argued. Perceptions of environmental conditions, in turn, are likely to be filtered through evolved psychological mechanisms. Psychological mechanisms are typically activated by specific environmental cues, resulting in "optimal" ecologically contingent strategies that evolved to solve specific adaptive problems posed by different kinds of environments (see Buss, 1995; Tooby & Cosmides, 1992). The term "strategy" refers to a set of coevolved anatomical, physiological, psychological, and/or behavioral traits designed by natural selection to increase inclusive fitness. Use of this term does not imply foresight, conscious awareness, or premeditation. In addition, the term "optimal" does not imply that natural selection is geared to produce a single, perfect phenotype. Optimal strategies are sets of coevolved traits that are best suited to increasing inclusive fitness in specific environments, given various tradeoffs.

Infants, of course, do not have the cognitive ability to appraise the quality of local environmental conditions (e.g., whether the environment is safe, plentiful, and rich in resources vs. threatening, harsh, and impoverished). However, they do have the ability to determine whether their caregivers are sensitive, responsive, and attentive to their biological needs. Such information ought to provide clues about the nature and quality of current—and perhaps future—environmental conditions (Belsky, 1997; Belsky et al., 1991; Chisholm, 1996). If caregivers in evolutionary history were able to devote the time, effort, and energy necessary to be sensitive, responsive, and attentive to the needs of their children, the local environment was probably safe and sufficiently rich in resources (broadly defined). If caregivers were insensitive, nonresponsive, and devoted less attention to their children, the local environment was probably less resource-rich and perhaps even dangerous.

Ainsworth's Strange Situation is well suited to detect different patterns of attachment because it presents infants with two common cues to danger in the EEA: being left alone, and being left with a stranger. Examining reunions between mothers and their 12- to 18-month-old infants, Ainsworth, Blehar, Waters, and Wall (1978) identified three primary attachment patterns in young children: "secure," "anxious-ambivalent," and "anxious-avoidant."[2] Upon reunion, securely attached children use their caregivers to regulate and attenuate their distress, usually resuming other activities (e.g., exploration, play) quickly

after calming down. Anxious-avoidant children retract from their caregivers upon reunion, opting to control and dissipate their negative affect in an independent, self-reliant manner. Anxious-ambivalent children make inconsistent and conflicted attempts to derive comfort and support from their caregivers, often intermingling clinginess with outbursts of anger (what Bowlby [1973] termed the "anger of hope").

Each attachment pattern reflects a different "strategy" that could have solved adaptive problems presented by different kinds of rearing environments (see Belsky, 1997; Chisholm, 1996; Main, 1981). Mothers of securely attached infants tend to be available and responsive to the needs and signals of their infants (Ainsworth et al., 1978; De Wolff & van IJzendoorn, 1997). In particular, they are attuned to signs that their infants are distressed (Del Carmen, Pedersen, Huffman, & Bryan, 1993); provide moderate and appropriate levels of stimulation (Belsky, Rovine, & Taylor, 1984; Feldstein, Crown, Beebe, & Jaffe, 1995); engage in synchronous interactions with their infants (Isabella & Belsky, 1990; Isabella, Belsky, & von Eye, 1989; Leyendecker, Lamb, & Scholmerich, in press); and behave in a warm, involved, and contingently responsive manner (Braungart-Rieker, Garwood, Powers, & Wang, 2001; National Institute of Child Health and Human Development [NICHD] Early Child Care Network, 1997). Partly because their caregivers are sensitive and responsive, secure children need not worry about the availability and responsiveness of their caregivers, which permits them to concentrate on other life tasks.

Anxious-ambivalent children, in contrast, have caregivers who behave inconsistently toward them (Ainsworth et al., 1978), sometimes because of poor or deficient parenting skills. Mothers of such infants tend to respond erratically to their infants' needs and signals, sometimes appearing to be underinvolved parents (Belsky et al., 1984; Isabella et al., 1989; Lewis & Feiring, 1989; Scholmerich, Fracasso, Lamb, & Broberg, 1995; Smith & Pedersen, 1988; Vondra, Shaw, & Kevinides, 1995). Among children who are maltreated, anxious-ambivalent children are more likely to have been victims of parental neglect (Youngblade & Belsky, 1989). Thus the demanding nature of ambivalent children might reflect an ecologically contingent strategy designed to obtain, retain, or improve greater parental attention and care (Cassidy & Berlin, 1994; Main & Solomon, 1986). More specifically, the constellation of behaviors characteristic of ambivalent children—including hypervigilance and rumination about potential relationship loss (Cassidy & Berlin, 1994)—could have evolved to counteract deficiencies in caregiving by young, naive, overburdened, or underinvolved parents. For children who had such parents, this behavioral strategy would have increased proximity to caregivers, solicited better care, and improved their chances of survival. In view of cross-cultural evidence indicating that insecure infants in Israel are disproportionately likely to develop anxious-ambivalent attachments (van IJzendoorn & Sagi-Schwartz, Chapter 37, this volume), this pattern might also have been an evolved strategy for inducing helpless dependency in order to keep children excessively close in a world filled not only with strangers, but with people who had actually harmed biological relatives in the past.

Anxious-avoidant children usually have caregivers who are cold and rejecting (Ainsworth et al., 1978). Indeed, mothers of avoidant children are less responsive to their infants' distress (Crockenberg, 1981), use overly stimulating styles of interaction (Belsky et al., 1984; Scholmerich et al., 1995; Vondra et al., 1995), and dislike close body contact (Ainsworth et al., 1978). Among maltreated children, avoidant children are more likely to have suffered physical or emotional abuse from their parents (Youngblade & Belsky, 1989). The evolutionary origins of anxious avoidance, however, may be more complex and multifaceted than the origins of anxious ambivalence. Bowlby (1980) conjectured that avoidance allows infants to disregard cues that may activate the attachment system. If such cues were fully processed, avoidant infants might recognize the true inaccessibility and rejecting demeanor of their primary caregivers, which could be incapacitating.

Two further evolutionary explanations for avoidance in childhood have been developed. Main (1981) suggests that the distant, self-reliant behavior characteristic of avoidant infants permits them to maintain reasonably close proximity to belligerent or overwhelmed caregivers without driving them away. Avoidance, in other words, might have evolved to overcome deficiencies in caregiving provided by highly distressed, hostile, or unmotivated parents. During evolutionary history, this behavioral strategy would have increased survival among infants who, if they placed too many demands on their parents, might have been abandoned. Alternately, earlier reproduction might have facilitated inclusive fitness in some circumstances, especially in harsh environments with few resources (Trivers, 1985). If maternal rejection served as a proximal cue of the severity of future environments, avoidant tendencies might have allowed children not only to move away from their parents earlier, but to become more opportunistic and advantage-taking, thereby facilitating survival and early reproduction in such arduous environments (Belsky, 1997; Belsky et al., 1991).

Given the complex neural foundations of the attachment system (see Simpson, Beckes, & Weisberg, 2007), the basic functions of the attachment system ought to be fairly consistent across the lifespan. As children enter adolescence, however, cumulative experiences in relationships should be assimilated into internal working models, which are continually being updated and revised. These models reflect the degree to which individuals (1) believe they are worthy of love and affection, and (2) view significant others as loving and affectionate (Bartholomew & Horowitz, 1991; Collins & Read, 1994). Unlike the attachment system in childhood, in adulthood the system becomes integrated with the mating and caregiving systems (Kirkpatrick, 1998; Shaver, Hazan, & Bradshaw, 1988; Zeifman & Hazan, 1997). The infusion of these other systems makes adult attachment orientations (styles) more challenging to interpret than attachment patterns in children.

ATTACHMENT THEORY AND PARENT–OFFSPRING CONFLICT THEORY

One middle-level evolutionary theory that has considerable relevance to attachment theory is parent–offspring conflict theory (Trivers, 1974). According to this theory, children (who share 50% of their genes with parents and full siblings) should desire greater investment from their parents than their parents have been selected to provide. As a result, parents and offspring ought to have slightly divergent reproductive interests, resulting in bouts of conflict that climax during the final stages of weaning.

Parent–Offspring Conflict Theory and Parental Investment

According to Trivers (1972), parental investment includes any actions performed by a parent for his or her offspring that increase the offspring's chances of survival while reducing the parent's ability to invest in other offspring (including current or future children). The level of investment is a function of the costs and benefits associated with a given parental act or behavior. "Costs" are defined as units of foregone reproductive success by any other current or future offspring, and "benefits" are defined as units of reproductive success of the current offspring (Trivers, 1974). In humans, acts of investment include allocating time, effort, energy, or resources to children through such activities as feeding, protecting, sheltering, and teaching. The amount of investment that children seek and parents offer should depend on how both parties view the costs and benefits of different forms of parental investment. Hamilton (1964), for example, has shown that altruistic behaviors (i.e., acts that lower an individual's future reproductive success while raising the recipient's success) could have evolved if beneficiaries were biological relatives who carried the same altruistic genes. When $1 < r(b/c)$ (where r = the degree of relatedness [.5 between parents and their offspring], b = benefits of an altruistic act, and c = costs of the act), altruism would have increased inclusive fitness and been selected.

When infants are young and highly dependent on their parents for care and resources, the costs of investment to parents are low and the benefits to infants are high from the reproductive standpoint of each party. During the early stages of childrearing, therefore, the reproductive interests of parents and their offspring coincide. However, as infants grow, consume more resources, and become more self-sufficient, the reproductive interests of parents and offspring diverge. From a parent's perspective, the costs of investment continue to rise over time, while the benefits an infant derives from additional investment reach an asymptote. During this phase, directing investment to new offspring may enhance parents' reproductive success more than continuing to invest in an increasingly autonomous, self-sufficient child. This is the point at which weaning takes place in many cultures.

Because children share only half of their genes with their parents and full siblings, two of an infant's siblings must survive and successfully reproduce to fully propagate the infant's genes to future generations. Accordingly, infants should devalue the costs of investment incurred by their parents by 50%, expecting twice as many benefits as their parents have been selected to provide. A child and parent, therefore, should experience conflict until, from the perspective of the parent, the cost of parental investment is more than twice the benefit to the infant (or, from the perspective of the child, the cost of parental investment exceeds self-benefit). When this point is reached, the child's inclusive fitness will be reduced if he or she continues to demand additional investment. Conflict should then

subside as the child accepts the diversion of parental investment to other siblings.

Trivers (1974) hypothesized that the intensity and duration of parent–offspring conflict should also depend on factors that affect the cost–benefit ratio over time. Several novel predictions flow from the theory. For instance, conflict should be greater when there are stepsiblings in families. Because stepsiblings share only 25% of their genes, four stepsiblings must survive and reproduce to fully propagate a child's genes. Within "pure" stepfamilies, therefore, offspring should demand approximately four times as much investment as their parents are willing to grant, resulting in unusually long and intense periods of parent–offspring conflict. Conflict should also be more pronounced in families with very young mothers. Because younger mothers have more reproductive years ahead of them (and therefore more and possibly better reproductive opportunities in the future) than older mothers do, younger mothers should be less tolerant of high-cost infants.

Attachment theory does not fully recognize and account for the slightly different reproductive interests of infants and their caregivers (see Main, 1990). Indeed, many attachment theorists assume that the evolutionary interests of parents and their children are equivalent, and that (barring significant abnormalities) each child should be of equal "reproductive value" to its parents. Both of these assumptions are questionable. The reproductive value of a child should depend on several factors (Daly & Wilson, 1981; Trivers, 1974), including attributes of (1) the infant (e.g., his or her health, normality); (2) the mother (e.g., her health, age, ability to provide for the infant); (3) the father (e.g., the certainty of his paternity, his resources, his willingness to invest in the infant); (4) the nuclear family (e.g., the number of existing children, their birth spacing); and (5) the local environment (e.g., whether or not resources are available to minimize the costs and maximize the benefits of further parental investment). When the costs of investing in a given child are disproportionately high relative to the benefits, parents should display discriminative parental solicitude (i.e., preferential investment in certain children; Daly & Wilson, 1981). In some instances, attachment insecurity may arise from conditions that lower parental investment. Lower investment should be revealed by inadequate or poor caregiving behaviors, including parental inattentiveness, neglect, rejection, abuse, and even infanticide in extreme cases.[3]

Cross-cultural research indicates that parental investment is in fact lower when a family contains at least one stepparent; when fathers question their paternity; when infants are ill, weak, or deformed; during periods of famine; when families are poor or lack social support; when mothers are very young; when families have too many children; and when birth spacing is too short (see Daly & Wilson, 1984, 1988; Dickemann, 1975; Hrdy, 1999; Minturn & Stashak, 1982, for reviews). The incidence of parental neglect, abuse, and occasional infanticide increases sharply when certain conditions are present. For example, when adjustments are made for the prevalence of stepfamilies, the probability of child abuse is up to 100 times greater in households containing at least one stepparent than in households that have two biological parents (Daly & Wilson, 1985). Stepparents, especially stepfathers, are many times more likely to kill their biologically unrelated stepchildren than biological parents are to kill their children (Daly & Wilson, 1988). If biological parents maltreat their children, they typically engage in neglect rather than more active abuse, and usually for reasons associated with poverty (Daly & Wilson, 1981). Moreover, even when financial resources and marital status are statistically controlled for, younger mothers are more likely to kill their infants than are older mothers (Daly & Wilson, 1988), and older mothers are much less likely to abuse or harm their infants (Daly & Wilson, 1985).

From an evolutionary perspective, each of the precipitating conditions listed above should have incrementally deleterious effects on the quality and/or quantity of parent–infant interactions, setting the stage for insecure attachment patterns. For children who have congenital disabilities (e.g., blindness, mental retardation, severe emotional disturbances), or for mothers who feel overburdened (due to youth, depression, lack of paternal investment, or inadequate social support), neonatal emotional bonding may be disrupted by limited mother–infant postpartum contact or the inability of mothers and their infants to communicate in ways that facilitate early bonding (Daly & Wilson, 1981). Some evidence suggests that mothers deprived of postpartum interaction sometimes report feeling emotionally detached from their infants (Kennell, Trause, & Klaus, 1975). Infants separated from their mothers during the first few days of life may be slightly more likely to be abused as toddlers (Klaus & Kennell, 1976; Lynch, 1975; O'Connor, Vietze, Hopkins, & Altemeier, 1977) and both disabled children and overburdened mothers are more likely to have experienced early separations (Irvin, Kennell, & Klaus, 1976; Sugarman, 1977). If these precipitating conditions persist over time, this may reinforce poor, insensitive, or noncontingent caregiving.

Parental Investment and Attachment

Relatively little is known about whether the conditions that should reduce parental investment *cause* insecure attachment in children. Certain contextual factors, however, predict the development of insecure patterns (see Belsky & Fearon, Chapter 13, this volume). For example, parents who have better psychological health and well-being typically provide their offspring with higher-quality care (Belsky, 1984; Gelfand & Teti, 1990), and their children tend to be securely attached (Belsky & Isabella, 1988; Benn, 1986; NICHD Early Child Care Network, 1997; O'Connor, 1997). And clinically depressed mothers, who tend to display intrusive/hostile or detached/unresponsive styles of caregiving (Belsky & Jaffee, 2006), are more likely to have insecurely attached infants (for a meta-analysis, see Atkinson et al., 2000).

In addition, spouses involved in happier and more supportive marriages when their children are infants and toddlers exhibit better and more sensitive parenting skills (for reviews, see Belsky & Jaffee, 2006; Krishnakumar & Buehler, 2000), and as a result have securely attached infants (Goldberg & Easterbrooks, 1984; Howes & Markman, 1989; Teti, Gelfand, Messinger, & Isabella, 1995). Spouses who display the lowest levels of parental support are more likely to have infants with the most severe form of insecurity—the disorganized/disoriented (D) attachment pattern (Spieker, 1988; Spieker & Booth, 1988). Isabella (1994) has found that the relation between marital quality and infant attachment is mediated by maternal role satisfaction and maternal sensitivity to the child's needs.

External social support also has a positive impact on both parenting behavior and attachment security in infants and young children. Mothers who perceive more support from the community interact with their infants more positively (for a meta-analysis, see Andersen & Telleen, 1992), whereas those who perceive less support provide less sensitive care (Smith, Landry, & Swank, 2000). Poor mothers given material resources are more likely to hold, touch, kiss, and vocalize with their young infants (Feiring, Fox, Jaskir, & Lewis, 1987). Indeed, in samples of high-risk infants, the level of social support that mothers receive correlates positively with the long-term attachment security of their children (Crnic, Greenberg, & Slough, 1986), which is mediated by the quality of mothers' daily care (Crittenden, 1985). Although some studies have found no connection between social support and attachment security (e.g., Zeanah et al., 1993), several experimental studies have confirmed this link (e.g., Jacobson & Frye, 1991; Lieberman, Weston, & Pawl, 1991; Lyons-Ruth, Connell, & Grunebaum, 1990).

In summary, parent–offspring conflict theory offers novel insights into the conditions that should, from an evolutionary perspective, reduce parental investment. Attachment theorists have not taken full advantage of these and other insights (see Belsky, 1999; Simpson, 1999). Although the level of caregiver sensitivity appears to be one of the proximal causes of secure versus insecure attachment in infants and young children (van IJzendoorn, 1995b), attachment theorists need to consider the full range of contextual factors that, from the vantage point of ultimate causation, should govern caregiver sensitivity.

EVOLUTIONARY MODELS OF SOCIAL DEVELOPMENT ACROSS THE LIFESPAN

Attachment theory addresses social and personality development "from the cradle to the grave" (Bowlby, 1979, p. 129). Most early attachment research, however, investigated certain barriers to inclusive fitness (e.g., problems associated with infant survival), to the relative exclusion of other barriers (e.g., problems related to mating and reproduction). Even though some early attachment theorists (e.g., Main, 1981) conjectured that different attachment patterns observed in children might reflect different evolution-based strategies for promoting survival under certain rearing conditions, childhood attachment patterns were not systematically tied to the development of different adult romantic attachment styles and mating orientations until the early 1990s, when Belsky and his colleagues (1991) published an influential paper on human social development from an evolutionary/attachment perspective.

Life History Theory

More recent theoretical developments have been guided by ideas from LHT (Charnov, 1993; Stearns, 1992). LHT (see Kaplan & Gangestad, 2005, for a recent review) addresses how and why individuals allocate time, energy, and resources to different traits, behaviors, and life tasks when they make tradeoff decisions that could influence their

reproductive fitness. In particular, LHT models the selection pressures in our ancestral past that should have determined when, and the conditions under which, individuals allocated time, energy, and resources to physical development, growth, reproduction, body repair, or aging.

According to most life history models, individuals can increase their reproductive fitness in two general ways (Parker & Maynard Smith, 1991). First, they can "invest" in traits or attributes that will affect the timing of their mortality (i.e., the age at which they deteriorate and die). Second, they can "invest" in traits or attributes that influence the timing of their fertility (i.e., the age and rate at which they reproduce). Many life history traits/attributes, however, have countervailing effects on mortality and fertility (Kaplan & Gangestad, 2005). Traits or attributes that improve fertility through more frequent or more intense mating effort, for example, usually shorten survival, because many of the traits that make people (particularly men) more attractive to the opposite sex may compromise the immune system (Grafen, 1990). Moreover, the allocation of energy and resources to growth during development tends to retard fertility when individuals are young, but enhances it once individuals mature sexually (Stearns, 1992). And the allocation of time, energy, and resources needed to ensure that one's children grow to be strong and healthy typically undermines one's own future fertility and survival.

Individuals must negotiate three fundamental tradeoffs during their lives: (1) whether to invest in present (immediate) reproduction or future (delayed) reproduction; (2) whether to invest in higher-quantity or higher-quality offspring; and (3) whether to invest in mating effort or parenting effort. How each tradeoff is resolved should depend on several factors, including the demands of the local environment (e.g., how taxing it is, the amount of pathogens it contains, whether biparental care is required); the skills, abilities, and resources available to an individual at that time; the skills, abilities, and resources possessed by others (e.g., kin, potential mates, competitors); and so on.

The Belsky, Steinberg, and Draper Model

Inspired by LHT and earlier research on father absence during childhood (Draper & Harpending, 1982), Belsky and colleagues (1991) developed the first major evolution-based lifespan model of human social development. According to this model, the main evolutionary function of early social experience is to prepare children for the social and physical environments they are likely to inhabit during their lifetime. The model focuses primarily on offspring quantity versus quality tradeoffs. Certain information gleaned from the early environment should allow individuals to adopt an appropriate reproductive strategy—one that, on average, best increases inclusive fitness—in future environments. Hinde (1986), for example, proposed that if maternal rejection is induced by harsh environments in which competition for limited resources is intense, offspring who are aggressive and noncooperative should have higher reproductive fitness as adults than those who fail to display these attributes. Conversely, offspring raised in environments with abundant resources could increase their fitness by adopting a more cooperative and communal orientation toward others in adulthood.

The Belsky and colleagues (1991) model includes five stages. It proposes that (1) early contextual factors in the family of origin (e.g., level of stress, spousal harmony, financial resources) affect (2) early childrearing experiences (e.g., level of sensitive, supportive, and responsive caregiving). These experiences then affect (3) psychological and behavioral development (e.g., attachment patterns, internal working models), which in turn influences (4) somatic development (how quickly sexual maturation is reached) and eventually (5) the adoption of specific reproductive strategies. Although Belsky and colleagues suggested that these stages are linked sequentially, they also suggested that earlier stages may statistically interact to predict later outcomes (see Belsky, 2007). Early contextual factors in the family of origin, for example, may interact with early childrearing experiences to forecast the rate of somatic development.

Belsky and colleagues (1991) hypothesized that two developmental trajectories culminate in two distinct reproductive strategies in adulthood (although they also entertained the possibility that these may be opposite ends of a single continuum rather than alternate types). One strategy entails a short-term, opportunistic orientation toward close relationships (especially those pertaining to mating and parenting), in which sexual intercourse occurs earlier in life, romantic pair bonds are short-lived and less stable, and parental investment is lower. This orientation is geared toward increasing the *quantity* of offspring. The second strategy entails a long-term, investing orientation toward mating relationships, in which sexual intercourse occurs

later in life, romantic pair bonds are enduring, and parental investment is greater. This orientation focuses on maximizing offspring *quality*. A critical prediction derived from the model—one that distinguishes it from all other nonevolutionary theories of psychological and behavioral development—is that early rearing experiences should influence the timing of puberty. In particular, puberty should occur earlier for individuals who develop along the "quantity trajectory" than for those who develop along the "quality trajectory." According to classical philosophy of science, a theory that explains what competing theories can explain, but also makes original predictions that other theories do not make, should supplant competing theories if its novel predictions prove accurate (see Ketelaar & Ellis, 2000).

A growing body of evidence supports the Belsky et al. model (for recent reviews, see Belsky, 2007; Ellis, 2004). For example, in accord with nonevolutionary perspectives, greater socioemotional stress in families is related to more insensitive, harsh, rejecting, inconsistent, and/or unpredictable parenting practices. Economic hardship (Burgess & Draper, 1989; McLoyd, 1990), occupational stress (Bronfenbrenner & Crouter, 1982), marital discord (Belsky, 1981; Emery, 1988), and psychological distress (McLoyd, 1990) are all precursors of more hostile and/or detached parenting styles. Conversely, greater social support and more economic resources seem to facilitate warmer and more sensitive childrearing practices (Belsky, 2007; Lempers, Clark-Lempers, & Simons, 1989), perhaps because less taxed parents are more patient with or tolerant of their young children (Belsky, 1984).

The link between parental sensitivity and the psychological and behavioral development of children is also well established, in line with predictions from many theories, including classical attachment theory. During the first year of life, insensitive and unresponsive caregiving predicts the development of insecure attachments (see De Wolff & van IJzendoorn, 1997), which in turn predict assorted behavior problems later in development. Insecurely attached 2-year-olds, for instance, are less tolerant of frustration (Matas, Arend, & Sroufe, 1978). Insecurely attached preschoolers are more socially withdrawn (Waters, Wippman, & Sroufe, 1979), less likely to display sympathy to distressed peers (Waters et al., 1979), less willing to interact with friendly adults (Lütkenhaus, Grossmann, & Grossman, 1985), and less well liked by their classmates (LaFreniere &

Sroufe, 1985). During elementary school, insecure children display more severe behavior problems, especially aggression and disobedience (Erickson, Sroufe, & Egeland, 1985; Lewis, Feiring, McGuffog, & Jaskir, 1984). According to Belsky and colleagues (1991), these behaviors are governed by insecure working models, which "prepare" the child for negative, noncommunal relationships later in life. (For more recent evidence supporting the model, see Amato, 2001; Belsky & Fearon, 2002 and Chapter 13, this volume; Buehler & Gerard, 2002; Parke et al., 2004; Seccombe, 2000.)

As already noted, the most novel part of the model is the factors that predict the rate of somatic development. Belsky and colleagues (1991) claimed that children exposed to higher levels of socioemotional stress develop insecure attachments, exhibit behavior disorders, and should reach puberty—and therefore reproductive capacity—earlier than children without these attributes. According to LHT logic (Chisholm, 1993, 1999; Promislow & Harvey, 1990), environments in which resources are scarce and relationship ties are tenuous should cause more energy and effort to be allocated to rapid physical development, early mating, and short-term romantic pair bonds. Delayed maturation and reproduction in such arduous environments may cost individuals dearly, especially if they die before reproducing. On the other hand, environments in which resources are plentiful and relationship ties are reciprocal and enduring should result in efforts being channeled to additional somatic development, later sexual maturity, delayed mating, and longer-term romantic pair bonds that contribute to greater parental investment. In more benign environments, reproductive fitness could be enhanced by deferring reproduction until (1) individuals have acquired the skills and resources needed to maximize the quality of each offspring, and (2) offspring can benefit from all of the embodied capital that humans need to reproduce successfully.

Three strands of evidence support this novel feature of the Belsky and colleagues (1991) model. First, greater parent–child warmth, cohesion, and positivity predict delayed pubertal development in both prospective longitudinal studies (Ellis, McFadyen-Ketchum, Dodge, Pettit, & Bates, 1999; Graber, Brooks-Gunn, & Warren, 1995; Steinberg, 1988) and retrospective or concurrent ones (Kim & Smith, 1998a; Kim, Smith, & Palermiti, 1997; Miller & Pasta, 2000; Romans, Martin, Gendall, & Herbison, 2003; Rowe, 2000). Second, greater parent–child conflict and coercion predict earlier

pubertal timing in both prospective longitudinal studies (Moffitt, Caspi, Belsky, & Silva, 1992) and retrospective or concurrent ones (Jorm, Christensen, Rodgers, Jacomb, & Easteal, 2004; Kim & Smith, 1998a, 1998b; Kim et al., 1997; Mezzich et al., 1997; Wierson, Long, & Forehand, 1993). Third, the happier and/or less conflict-ridden the parental relationship, the later pubertal maturation occurs in girls, both in prospective longitudinal studies (Ellis et al., 1999; Ellis & Garber, 2000) and in those employing less rigorous research designs (Kim et al., 1997; Romans et al., 2003).

Virtually all of these findings are based on studies of girls, because of the difficulties associated with measuring pubertal development in boys. In the few studies that have examined boys, parallel pubertal timing effects have not been found (Ellis, 2004). Moreover, some studies have not found certain hypothesized links for girls. Ellis and colleagues (1999), Miller and Pasta (2000), and Steinberg (1988), for instance, did not find associations between the amount of family conflict/coercion and pubertal timing in girls. Nevertheless, in an outstanding comprehensive review of this literature, Ellis (2004, pp. 935–936) concluded that "empirical research has provided reasonable, though incomplete" support for the Belsky and colleagues model.

Evidence relevant to the final stages of the Belsky and colleagues (1991) model (i.e., the mating strategies that individuals adopt in adulthood) comes from two sources: (1) research tying adult attachment styles to mating and romantic relationship functioning, and (2) research bridging adult attachment and parenting practices. Individuals who report being more securely attached to their romantic partners are less likely to have promiscuous sexual attitudes or to engage in sex with other partners (Brennan & Shaver, 1995; Simpson & Gangestad, 1991). Indeed, more securely attached adults claim that they would ideally desire only one sexual partner (mate) during the next 30 years (Miller & Fishkin, 1997), and more secure women tend to have first sexual intercourse at a later age than do insecure women (Bogaert & Sadava, 2002).

Satisfaction is also higher in the romantic relationships of more securely attached adults (J. Feeney, Chapter 21, this volume; Rholes, Simpson, Campbell, & Grich, 2001; Simpson, 1990), and observational research confirms that more secure adults display less negative affect and more constructive conflict resolution tactics when interacting with their romantic partners (J. Feeney,

Chapter 21, this volume; Simpson, Rholes, & Phillips, 1996). Greater attachment security is also related to better communication in romantic relationships, including greater self-disclosure and responsivity to self-disclosures by partners (Kobak & Hazan, 1991; Mikulincer & Nachson, 1991). In addition, more secure adults are less likely to divorce or separate from their partners (Kirkpatrick & Hazan, 1994; see B. Feeney & Monin, Chapter 39, this volume); they have longer-lasting romantic relationships (Hazan & Shaver, 1987; Kirkpatrick & Davis, 1994); and they report greater commitment to and trust in their dating partners (Brennan & Shaver, 1995; Simpson, 1990) and their spouses (Feeney, 1994; Fuller & Fincham, 1995; Kobak & Hazan, 1991).

In line with the Belsky and colleagues (1991) model, adult attachment is also associated with differential expectations about children and parenting even before individuals have children. Rholes, Simpson, Blakely, Lanigan, and Allen (1997), for instance, have found that less securely attached college students anticipate being more easily aggravated by their young children if/when they become parents, expect to be more strict disciplinarians, believe they will express less warmth toward their children, and are less confident about their ability to relate well to them. In addition, more avoidant college students believe they will derive less satisfaction from caring for their young children and express less interest in having them. Once they have children, more avoidant parents report feeling less emotionally close to their first newborn child merely 2 weeks after birth (Wilson, Rholes, Simpson, & Tran, 2007), and more avoidant mothers are less emotionally supportive of their preschooler children, adopting a more detached, controlling, or instrumentally focused mode of relating to them (Crowell & Feldman, 1988, 1991; Rholes, Simpson, & Blakely, 1995).

Furthermore, mothers classified as secure on the Adult Attachment Interview (who probably received greater warmth and contingent care from their own parents) are more sensitive to the needs of their children and are more supportive of them (see Belsky, 2005a; Hesse, Chapter 25, this volume; van IJzendoorn, 1995b). Specifically, greater attachment security is associated with more warmth and appropriate structuring of learning tasks by both fathers and mothers (Adam, Gunnar, & Tanaka, 2004; Cohn, Cowan, Cowan, & Pearson, 1992), greater emotional support in different situations (Crowell & Feldman, 1998, 1991), less negativity (Adam et al., 2004; Slade, Belsky, Aber,

& Phelps, 1999), and greater awareness of children's needs (Das Eiden, Teti, & Corns, 1995).

The Chisholm Model

Chisholm (1993, 1996, 1999) has proposed a slightly revised and expanded model of alternate reproductive strategies—one that addresses the life history tradeoff of immediate versus delayed reproduction. Chisholm (1993) claims that local mortality rates are one of the critical environmental cues that shunt people down different developmental and reproductive pathways. According to bet-hedging theory (Horn & Rubenstein, 1984; Promislow & Harvey, 1990), when mortality rates are high in a local area, the optimal reproductive strategy is to mate early so that current fertility is maximized. When mortality rates are low, the best strategy may be deferred, long-term reproduction in which fewer progeny are given more intensive care. In abundant and safe environments that signal longer life expectancies, therefore, a delayed/high-investment reproductive strategy should increase the total number of descendants over multiple generations by minimizing the *variance* of surviving offspring within each generation. This, in turn, should decrease the likelihood that an entire generation will fail to reproduce.

High mortality rates, which should have been a barometer of the difficulty of local environments, typically should have been associated with poorer caregiving in the EEA. Chisholm (1993, 1996) claims that parental indifference or insensitivity should have been a valid cue of local mortality rates, motivating children to develop avoidant working models and behaviors that would have been better suited to increasing fitness in such arduous environments. Low mortality rates, which should have signaled more hospitable environments, should have been associated with better, more attentive caregiving. Sensitive parenting, in other words, should have conveyed to children that premature death was less likely, resulting in more secure working models and behaviors that might have enhanced fitness in benign environments.

In addition, Chisholm (1999) proposes another psychological mediator linking childhood experience and reproductive strategies: time preference. Time preference, which is associated with delay-of-gratification tendencies, reflects the degree to which individuals prefer to—or believe they will—achieve—their desires now (immediately) versus later (in the future). Individuals raised in dangerous or uncertain environments in which waiting for rewards may result in leaving no descendants should prefer immediate payoffs, even if delayed ones may be superior (Wilson & Daly, 2005).

Chisholm (1996) proposes that there were two parent-based threats to the survival and growth of children in the EEA: (1) parents' *inability* to invest in offspring, and (2) their *unwillingness* to do so. He contends that children and adolescents have evolved psychological mechanisms to detect and respond to these different forms of threat. Young infants are in fact fairly skilled observers of their parents' moods and motivations (Cohn & Tronick, 1983), and they are aware of others' intentions early in life (Woodward, Sommerville, & Guajardo, 2001). According to Chisholm's model and also in line with Belsky and colleagues' (1991) theorizing, the secure attachment pattern is a facultative adaptation to parents' psychological and parenting orientations, particularly to their ability *and* willingness to provide high investment. The anxious-avoidant attachment pattern, on the other hand, is an adaptation to parents' unwillingness to invest (regardless of their ability), whereas the anxious-ambivalent pattern is an adaptation to parents' inability to invest. The model proposes that warm/sensitive caregiving is a good indicator of parents' ability and willingness to invest, that cold/rejecting caregiving signals parents' unwillingness to invest, and that inconsistent/unpredictable caregiving conveys parents' inability to invest.

Building on the Belsky and colleagues model, Chisholm (1996) suggests how each of the three attachment patterns in children should map on to distinct reproductive strategies—something that Belsky and colleagues (1991) did vis-à-vis the secure versus insecure attachment distinction, and that Belsky (1997, 1999) did vis-à-vis all three primary attachment patterns. During childhood, secure individuals should maximize long-term learning to enhance their overall developmental quality, which explains why securely attached children typically grow faster than do insecure children in high-risk samples (Valenzuela, 1990) and why they display more advanced cognitive-perceptual and socioemotional skills earlier in development (Belsky & Cassidy, 1994; Sroufe, 1988). When parents are both able and willing to invest, and rearing environments are nonthreatening, greater effort can be allocated to long-term developmental quality and hence to future reproductive potential. Therefore, consistent with Belsky and colleagues' quality trajectory framework, more secure adults seek long-term mates, are able and willing parents, invest heavily in their children, and provide more sensitive and responsive care, all in the service of enhancing the phenotypic quality of their children.

Because avoidantly attached children have harsh and rejecting parents who force them to become independent at an early age, avoidant children must allocate resources differently. When parents are unwilling to invest and local environments are threatening, less effort and fewer resources can be devoted to physical growth. Effort and resources must be funneled to immediate reproduction, which accelerates sexual maturation. Consequently, more avoidant adults have shorter romantic relationships, are less willing to invest in children, allot more time and energy to mating effort, and feel less close to their children, all of which should increase offspring quantity.

Whereas Belsky and colleagues (1991) linked unsupportive rearing and insecure attachment patterns in general to accelerated pubertal development, Chisholm (1996) developed intriguing ideas about anxious-ambivalent individuals (see also Belsky, 1997, 1999). Chisholm believes that anxious-ambivalent children should channel more effort toward early sexual maturity (see also Belsky et al., 1991) while attempting to extract greater investment from their negligent or underinvolved caregivers (see also Cassidy & Berlin, 1994). According to Chisholm's LHT, when parents are willing but unable to invest, children should try to obtain as many resources as they can, funneling most of them to earlier reproduction. This helps to explain why anxious-ambivalent individuals are so irritable, demanding, and hypervigilant about gaining and maintaining time and attention from their caregivers, including their romantic partners (Cassidy & Berlin, 1994; Kunce & Shaver, 1994). It might also explain why more ambivalently attached adults experience rapid and extreme sexual attraction to prospective mates (Hazan & Shaver, 1987). According to both Chisholm (1996) and Belsky and colleagues (1991), such adults should engage in short-term mating, want to but perhaps not be fully able to invest in children, and hence behave inconsistently toward them. Belsky (1997, 1999), on the other hand, has proposed that anxious ambivalence may reflect an evolved "helper-at-the-nest" reproductive strategy in which parenting effort is directed toward kin (siblings), particularly when local conditions demand more caregiving than parents can provide. However, no evidence consistent with such thinking has emerged to date.

Several additional findings are consistent with Chisholm's (1996, 1999) theorizing. As life expectancy declines in a local area, the probability that women will reproduce by age 30 increases (Wilson & Daly, 1997). Similarly, teen mothers who expect to die at a younger age are more likely to become mothers at an earlier age (Johns, 2003). These findings are consistent with Geronimus's (1996) "weathering hypothesis," which proposes that early birth is a strategic response to the rapid decline in health among women in their 30s and 40s. In addition, meta-analytic research has revealed that when a mother experiences the loss of a loved one through death and the loss remains emotionally "unresolved," the probability of her offspring developing a disorganized attachment pattern increases (van IJzendoorn, 1995a). These findings highlight the value of treating local mortality rates as a powerful cue in the development of alternate reproductive strategies.

The Belsky et al. and Chisholm models have both played important roles in getting scholars to think more deeply about how and why early experiences shape subsequent development—something that had been taken for granted by many developmental psychologists. Both models, however, could be expanded and further refined by the infusion of additional evolutionary considerations. First, neither model addresses all of the factors that, from an evolutionary standpoint, should govern the adoption of specific reproductive strategies in adulthood. Mate selection is contingent on a multitude of factors, ranging from a potential mate's genetic quality, to his or her ability to accrue and share resources, to his or her capacity to impart knowledge and information to offspring (see Gangestad & Simpson, 2000). Many of these factors have not been incorporated into current lifespan attachment models. One might pose the question, for example, whether secure individuals are better able than insecure individuals to attract partners who have higher mate value. Second, current models are not sufficiently sensitive to the different roles that men and women assume in reproduction (Buss & Schmitt, 1993; Geary, 2005; Hinde, 1991). The fact that women must make greater *initial* investments in their offspring than men do should influence how each gender makes reproductive decisions and the mating strategies they ultimately adopt (Hinde, 1984; Trivers, 1972). Sex-differentiating factors are not addressed by current lifespan attachment models. For example, relative to males, do females require stronger "doses" of poor or noncontingent early

care to launch them down short-term, quantity-focused reproductive pathways? Third, evidence of pubertal timing effects in boys is absent. If future well-conducted studies fail to find theoretically meaningful pubertal timing effects for boys, the Belsky and colleagues and Chisholm models will obviously require revision. It is possible that the reproductive strategies of human females may be more sensitive to environmental inputs than those of human males are (cf. Gangestad & Simpson, 2000). Despite these limitations, the Belsky and colleagues and Chisholm models represent important advances in our understanding of attachment and social development across the lifespan.

The Ellis Model

Melding ideas from Belsky and colleagues (1991), Draper and Harpending (1982), and parental investment theory (Trivers, 1972), Ellis and colleagues (1999; Ellis & Garber, 2000) hypothesize that fathers may assume a special role in the development of girls' reproductive strategies. Belsky and colleagues viewed early father absence as a marker of stress in the family of origin and appreciated the influence of the quality of mothering and fathering. Ellis (2004), on the other hand, claims that father absence or stepfather presence may serve as a particularly important paternal investment cue signaling low, unpredictable, or changing levels of paternal investment within families.

Father absence does in fact predict accelerated pubertal development among girls, both in prospective studies in which girls are followed from childhood into adolescence (Campbell & Udry, 1995; Ellis & Garber, 2000; Ellis et al., 1999; Hetherington & Kelly, 2002; Moffitt et al., 1992; Rowe, 2000; Wierson et al., 1993) and in retrospective studies of adults (Doughty & Rodgers, 2000; Hoier, 2003; Jones, Leeton, McLeod, & Wood, 1972; Jorm et al., 2004; Kiernan & Hobcraft, 1997; Quinlan, 2003; Romans et al., 2003; Surbey, 1990). Similar effects, however, have not been found in African American samples (Campbell & Udry, 1995; Rowe, 2000).

Additional work has shown that the earlier father absence occurs in a child's life (especially within the first 5 years), the greater effect it has on the speed of female pubertal development (Ellis & Garber, 2000; Jones et al., 1972; Quinlan, 2003; Surbey, 1990). Stepfather presence may also affect pubertal timing, perhaps even accounting for some of the father absence effects (see Ellis, 2004). Supporting this view is the observation that greater conflict between the mother and stepfather, combined with earlier stepfather presence in the home, seems to be particularly influential in accelerating pubertal development in girls (Ellis & Garber, 2000). Consistent with Belsky and colleagues' (1991) emphasis on the quality of parent–child relationships, Ellis and colleagues (1999) also found that girls' pubertal development is delayed the more time fathers spend caring for their daughters in the first 5 years of life and the more fathers have positive/affectionate interactions with their daughters at age 5.

Thus there are good empirical and theoretical grounds for *not* treating mothers and fathers as interchangeable agents of influence in understanding how childhood experiences shape reproductive strategies. Greater attention may need to be paid to the presence of biologically unrelated male figures in the home during development, as well as to the differential influence of maternal and paternal investment (i.e., quality of parenting).

The Hazan/Zeifman and Kirkpatrick Models

Scholars have also sought to explain the nature and strength of adult romantic pair bonds from a life history/attachment perspective. Hazan and Zeifman (1999; Zeifman & Hazan, 1997; see also Zeifman & Hazan, Chapter 20, this volume), for example, suggest that adult romantic relationships are an instantiation of attachment relationships formed earlier in life. They note numerous similarities between childhood attachment to caregivers and adult attachment to close peers and romantic partners (see also Shaver et al., 1988). For example, infants and adults display very similar reactions to separation from or loss of their attachment figures. In addition, people value qualities in prospective mates that parallel those they valued in their caregivers, and children and adults behave quite similarly when seeking close contact, physical intimacy, and affection from their attachment figures. Parent–child and adult–adult attachment relationships also pass through similar sets of developmental stages.

Hazan and Zeifman (1999) suggest that the primary evolutionary function of secure attachment in adult relationships is to increase the likelihood of stable and enduring pair bonds so that mates can provide better mutual support. Pair bonding is thus believed to enhance the reproductive fitness of both parents and their offspring. Adult mating strategies are in fact related to the pair-bond status of one's parents, with father ab-

sence and greater marital discord in the family of origin predicting earlier sexual maturation, short-term mating strategies in adulthood, and less stable marriages (Belsky, 1999). Children who have more pair-bonded parents, by comparison, should adopt long-term mating strategies and emphasize quality rather than quantity of investment when they have their own children (Hazan & Zeifman, 1999). More pair-bonded partners should also contribute to their own reproductive success by providing one another with greater support, which tends to be associated with better long-term physical and mental health and more regular ovulation patterns (see Zeifman & Hazan, 1997).

Partially in response to this model, Kirkpatrick (1998) claims that adult attachment styles evolved to enhance reproductive fitness in light of early childhood experiences, but he questions whether security and protection are the *primary* functions of adult attachment. Instead, Kirkpatrick suggests that components of the caregiving system (e.g., love) may have been coopted during evolutionary history to cement romantic pair bonds in adulthood, and that (similar to the Belsky and colleagues and Chisholm models) adult attachment styles primarily reflect evolved reproductive strategies.

One of the principal life history tradeoffs involves allocating time and energy to mating effort more or less than to parenting effort. Kirkpatrick (1998) argues that it was not always adaptive or advantageous for women and men to enact long-term, monogamous mating strategies (see also Gangestad & Simpson, 2000). Consequently, adult attachment styles may be "mechanisms" for choosing the best mating strategy, given the nature of early childhood experiences and the quality of early parental investment as discussed by Belsky and colleagues (1991). Individuals who receive consistently sensitive and responsive parenting should develop secure working models and thus should adopt long-term, committed mating strategies. These individuals should also develop greater trust and intimacy in their relationships (Simpson, 1990) and should fall in love rather easily with partners who tend to have higher mate value (Hazan & Shaver, 1987), which they do. More avoidant individuals, in contrast, should be involved in less committed relationships, should pursue short-term mating strategies, and should have more unrestricted sociosexual orientations, which they do (see Simpson, Wilson, & Winterheld, 2004). And more anxious-ambivalent persons should desire and want to pursue long-term mating strategies, but their strong desire to be attractive to and merge with their romantic partners may result in short-term sexual relationships in which they eventually drive partners away (see Kirkpatrick, 1998). For these reasons, Kirkpatrick believes that features of the caregiving system—especially love operating as a "commitment device" (Frank, 1988)—could have been coopted to bind and stabilize long-term romantic pair bonds.

UNRESOLVED ISSUES AND PROMISING DIRECTIONS

Several unresolved issues and promising directions for future research exist, only a few of which can be covered here to complement some of the questions and hypotheses raised in this chapter. Two of the most perplexing questions in the attachment field center on (1) why maternal sensitivity accounts for only a portion of the variance in children's attachment status, and (2) why the intergenerational transmission of attachment patterns is not stronger than it is (see also van IJzendoorn & Bakermans-Kranenburg, 1997). Possible solutions to these puzzles might be achieved through applications of LHT. Applying bet-hedging logic, Belsky (1997, 2000, 2005b) has theorized that children should differ in their susceptibility to parental influence (see also Boyce & Ellis, 2005). Experimental evidence relevant to this prediction focusing on the influence of maternal sensitivity on attachment security has recently been reported (Velderman, Bakermans-Kranenburg, Juffer, & van IJzendoorn, 2006). Also relevant are twin studies showing that nonshared environmental influences explain much more of the variation underlying most traits and behaviors than shared environmental influences do (Bouchard, 2004; Turkheimer & Waldron, 2000), and that attachment security is not heritable (Bokhorst et al., 2003). Belsky (2000, 2005b) suggests that differential susceptibility *might* be adaptive for parents, children, and their siblings if a parent's attempt to "prepare" his or her children for the future environment could be mistaken, due to the inherent unpredictability of future conditions. This would explain why, from an evolutionary standpoint, differential susceptibility to parental influence is witnessed within families. It would also explain why intergenerational transmission effects are weaker than initially expected (Belsky, 2005a).

Less-than-perfect intergenerational transmission rates also raise intriguing questions about the possible "time span of influence" on present and future decision making. To date, transmission has been assumed to be a single-generation process (e.g., a mother's attachment status shapes her child's attachment status, with little consideration of the possible impact of grandparents, great-grandparents, etc.). The concept of "intergenerational phenotypic inertia" (see Kuzawa, 2005), however, suggests that some forms of influence may endure over multiple generations, even when the most proximate generational experiences are at odds with the modal family trajectory. In particular, this model proposes that individuals should typically place greater diagnostic weight on conditions in the current (immediate) environment when allocating life history resources than on cues signaling the environments in which their parents, their grandparents, or more distant relatives lived, even if past environments were stable over multiple generations. There may be cases, however, when looking back only one generation may not be the best way to interpret or model intergenerational transmission processes, particularly when environments are very stable across several generations.

This raises another critical set of issues. Although evolutionary forces should have shaped developmental trajectories, organisms also evolved to respond adaptively to rapid changes in local environments. The field of behavioral ecology in fact models such adaptive behaviors (see Gangestad & Simpson, 2007). Indeed, the strategic pluralism model (Gangestad & Simpson, 2000) proposes that human females may have evolved to base mating decisions (including decisions about parenting qualities in mates) on two dimensions: the extent to which prospective mates display evidence of (1) viability (i.e., good health or other desirable mate-attracting attributes that could be passed on genetically to offspring) and (2) investment potential (in both the romantic relationship and any resulting offspring). In pathogen-prevalent environments, which still characterize the current world and perhaps characterized the EEA, women should place more weight on men's viability attributes so that the "good genes" of such mates may be passed on to their children. In environments that demand heavy investment in children or biparental care, women should place greater importance on men's investment potential to enhance the likelihood of offspring survival. Given their different life experiences, adults with different attachment histories and styles may evaluate, calibrate, or apply each mate dimension somewhat differently. This returns us to an issue raised earlier about the mate value of relationship partners. Highly avoidant women, for instance, may expect and require less paternal investment in light of their independence and self-reliance, and due to their mistrust of others, they may want less. Highly anxious women, in contrast, may expect and demand greater investment, given their chronic concerns about relationship loss and abandonment.

Finally, epigenetics research holds the promise of advancing our understanding of intergenerational attachment issues in major ways. Recent animal work, for example, has shown that maternal grooming of newborn female rat pups not only calibrates their stress response system when they are adults and raise their own offspring. Through nongenetic mechanisms, such care also influences the development of the *grandoffspring* of the original grooming mother (see Cameron et al., 2005). These findings are important because they partially complete the attachment/mothering intergenerational cycle. This research calls attention to the fact that rearing experiences stimulate gene action, which launches a cascade of developmental processes and outcomes leading to different reproductive strategies in adulthood, which are then transmitted intergenerationally via nongenetic means. This evidence raises additional intriguing questions about recent research on gene–environment interactions (see Caspi et al., 2002). This work, which supports the notion of differential susceptibility to parental influence, shows that the impact of rearing effects (e.g., child maltreatment) on the development of antisocial behavior varies as a function of genotype. What remains unclear, however, is whether individuals who possess genetic vulnerabilities succumb to environmental risks, or whether early rearing experiences activate certain genes that then facilitate the development of antisocial behavior.

CONCLUSIONS

At its (secure) base, attachment theory is an evolutionary theory of human social behavior "from the cradle to the grave" (Bowlby, 1979, p. 129). Although the theory's initial ties to evolution focused on how the normative and individual difference components of attachment should have promoted infant survival, recent work has shed light on how attachment patterns across the lifespan—including adult romantic attachment styles—may have evolved to increase reproductive fitness. These new theoretical advances are

important for several reasons. Until recently, attachment theorists have not addressed *why* early developmental experiences should be systematically related to later life outcomes, *why* intergenerational transmission of attachment should exist, or *why* maternal sensitivity plays perhaps the leading role in shaping attachment security in children (Belsky, 2007). Traditionally, attachment theorists and researchers have focused on *how* these processes work. Recent applications of LHT within attachment theory have begun to rectify this deficiency in the original theory, directing attention to questions concerning both ultimate *and* proximate causation. These recent theoretical advances are also important because they suggest that adult attachment styles may *not* be inconsequential evolutionary "artifacts" of the attachment system in children. According to life history accounts, the attachment system in young children should have facilitated survival and development through the perilous years of early childhood, not just psychological health and well-being. In adulthood, the attachment system may further enhance inclusive fitness via the adoption of environmentally contingent, alternate reproductive strategies, not just satisfaction and happiness in close relationships.

In the future, attachment scholars would be well advised to base more of their thinking on a modern evolutionary framework. As Dobzhansky (1973) once exclaimed, "Nothing in biology makes sense except in the light of evolution" (p. 125). The same claim applies to much of psychology in general and much of developmental and social psychology in particular, especially those fields that focus on close interpersonal relationships. We strongly advocate treading the intellectual path first paved by Darwin and then extended by Bowlby and other modern evolutionary theorists. Various middle-level evolutionary theories—especially parent–offspring conflict theory, parental investment and sexual selection theory, and LHT—have a tremendous amount to offer scholars interested in attachment phenomena across the lifespan. Future advances in attachment theory and research are likely to rest on the successful and complete integration of attachment theory into a modern evolutionary perspective.

NOTES

1. These are only some of the major middle-level evolutionary theories that have been developed. Others include host–parasite coevolution theory (Hamilton & Zuk, 1982; Tooby, 1982) and intragenomic conflict theory (Trivers, 1997).

2. Main and Solomon (1990) identified a fourth attachment pattern in children, labeled "disorganized/disoriented." These children do not have a clear, coherent strategy for managing negative affect, frequently intermixing anxious-avoidant and anxious-ambivalent behavioral tactics with bizarre ones. This pattern, which has the lowest base rate, tends to be witnessed when caregivers are abusive, depressed, or emotionally disturbed (see Lyons-Ruth & Jacobvitz, Chapter 28, this volume).

3. These precipitating conditions may interact in interesting ways. For example, males in most polygynous species have more variable reproductive success than females do (Trivers, 1985). In our ancestral past, nearly all fertile females reproduced and had approximately the same number of children, whereas some males had large numbers of children and others failed to reproduce. Trivers and Willard (1973) have proposed that when environmental resources are limited, daughters should receive more parental investment than sons. Most daughters will eventually bear children if environmental conditions are not too severe, whereas sons who cannot amass resources or display evidence of their fitness may never attract mates. When environmental conditions are better, however, sons should receive greater investment than daughters, because the most reproductively successful males should, on average, propagate their parents' genes more extensively than should daughters. This reasoning suggests that when environmental conditions are harsh, the pattern of parental investment may lead to more daughters than sons being securely attached, whereas the reverse may be true when environmental conditions are favorable.

REFERENCES

Adam, E., Gunnar, M., & Tanaka, A. (2004). Adult attachment, parent emotion, and observed parenting behavior. *Child Development, 75,* 110–122.

Ainsworth, M. D. S. (1979). Infant–mother attachment. *American Psychologist, 34,* 932–937.

Ainsworth, M. D. S., Blehar, M. C., Waters, E., & Wall, S. (1978). *Patterns of attachment: A psychological study of the Strange Situation.* Hillsdale, NJ: Erlbaum.

Amato, P. (2001). Children of divorce in the 1990s. *Journal of Family Psychology, 15,* 355–370.

Andersen, P., & Telleen, S. (1992). The relationship between social support and maternal behavior and attitudes: A meta-analytic review. *American Journal of Community Psychology, 20,* 753–774.

Anderson, S. W., & Jaffe, J. (1972). *The definition, detection and timing of vocalic syllables in speech signals* (Scientific Report No. 12). New York: Department of Communication Sciences, New York State Psychiatric Institute.

Andrews, P. W., Gangestad, S. W., & Matthews, D. (2002). Adaptationism—how to carry out an exaptationist program. *Behavioral and Brain Sciences, 25,* 489–504.

Atkinson, L., Paglia, A., Coolbear, J., Niccols, A., Parker, K. C. H., & Guger, S. (2000). Attachment security: A meta-analysis of maternal mental health correlates. *Clinical Psychology Review, 20,* 1019–1040.

Axelrod, R. (1984). *The evolution of cooperation.* New York: Basic Books.

Bartholomew, K., & Horowitz, L. M. (1991). Attachment styles among young adults: A test of a four-category model. *Journal of Personality and Social Psychology, 61,* 226–244.

Belsky, J. (1981). Early human experience: A family perspective. *Developmental Psychology, 17,* 3–23.

Belsky, J. (1984). The determinants of parenting: A process model. *Child Development, 55,* 83–96.

Belsky, J. (1997). Attachment, mating, and parenting: An evolutionary interpretation. *Human Nature, 8,* 361–381.

Belsky, J. (1999). Modern evolutionary theory and patterns of attachment. In J. Cassidy & P. R. Shaver (Eds.), *Handbook of attachment: Theory, research, and clinical applications* (pp. 141–161). New York: Guilford Press.

Belsky, J. (2000). Conditional and alternative reproductive strategies. In J. L. Rodgers, D. C. Rowe, & W. B. Miller (Eds.), *Genetic influences on human fertility and sexuality: Theoretical and empirical contributions from the biological and behavioral sciences* (pp. 127–145). Boston: Kluwer.

Belsky, J. (2005a). The developmental and evolutionary psychology of intergenerational transmission of attachment. In C. S. Carter, L. Ahnert, K. Grossmann, S. Hrdy, M. Lamb, S. Porges, et al. (Eds.), *Attachment and bonding: A new synthesis* (pp. 169–198). Cambridge, MA: MIT Press.

Belsky, J. (2005b). Differential susceptibility to rearing influence. In B. J. Ellis & D. F. Bjorklund (Eds.), *Origins of the social mind: Evolutionary psychology and child development* (pp. 139–163). New York: Guilford Press.

Belsky, J. (2007). Childhood experiences and reproductive strategies. In R. Dunbar & L. Barrett (Eds.), *Oxford handbook of evolutionary psychology* (pp. 237–254). Oxford, UK: Oxford University Press.

Belsky, J., & Cassidy, J. (1994). Attachment: Theory and evidence. In M. Rutter & D. Hay (Eds.), *Development through life: A handbook for clinicians* (pp. 373–402). Oxford, UK: Blackwell.

Belsky, J., & Fearon, R. M. P. (2002). Infant–mother attachment security, contextual risk, and early development. *Development and Psychopathology, 14,* 293–310.

Belsky, J., & Isabella, R. (1988). Maternal, infant, and social-contextual determinants of attachment security. In J. Belsky & T. Nezworski (Eds.), *Clinical implications of attachment* (pp. 41–94). Hillsdale, NJ: Erlbaum.

Belsky, J., & Jaffee, S. (2006). The multiple determinants of parenting. In D. Cicchetti & D. Cohen (Eds.), *Developmental psychopathology: Vol. 3. Risk, disorder, and adaptation* (2nd ed., pp. 38–85). Hoboken, NJ: Wiley.

Belsky, J., Rovine, M., & Taylor, D. G. (1984). The Pennsylvania Infant and Family Development Project: III. The origins of individual differences in infant–mother attachment: Maternal and infant contributions. *Child Development, 55*, 718–728.

Belsky, J., Steinberg, L., & Draper, P. (1991). Childhood experience, interpersonal development, and reproductive strategy: An evolutionary theory of socialization. *Child Development, 62*, 647–670.

Benn, R. K. (1986). Factors promoting secure attachment relationships between employed mothers and their sons. *Child Development, 57*, 1224–1231.

Bogaert, A. F., & Sadava, S. (2002). Adult attachment and sexual behavior. *Personal Relationships, 9*, 191–204.

Bokhorst, C., Bakermans-Kranenburg, J., Fearon, R. M. P., van IJzendoorn, M., Fonagy, P., & Schuengel, C. (2003). The importance of shared environment in mother–infant attachment security: A behavioral genetic study. *Child Development, 74*, 1769–1782.

Bouchard, T. (2004). Genetic influence on human psychological traits. *Current Directions in Psychological Science, 13*, 148–151.

Bowlby, J. (1969/1982). *Attachment and loss: Vol. 1. Attachment.* New York: Basic Books.

Bowlby, J. (1973). *Attachment and loss: Vol. 2. Separation: Anxiety and anger.* New York: Basic Books.

Bowlby, J. (1979). *The making and breaking of affectional bonds.* London: Tavistock.

Bowlby, J. (1980). *Attachment and loss: Vol. 3. Loss: Sadness and depression.* New York: Basic Books.

Bowlby, J. (1991). *Charles Darwin: A new life.* New York: Norton.

Boyce, W. T., & Ellis, B. J. (2005). Biological sensitivity to context. *Development and Psychopathology, 17*, 271–301.

Braungart-Rieker, J. M., Garwood, M. M., Powers, B. P., & Wang, X. (2001). Parental sensitivity, infant affect, and affect regulation: Predictors of later attachment. *Child Development, 72*, 252–270.

Brennan, K. A., & Shaver, P. R. (1995). Dimensions of adult attachment, affect regulation, and romantic relationship functioning. *Personality and Social Psychology Bulletin, 21*, 267–283.

Brewer, M. B., & Caporael, L. R. (1990). Selfish genes versus selfish people: Sociobiology as origin myth. *Motivation and Emotion, 14*, 237–243.

Brewer, M. B., & Caporael, L. R. (2006). An evolutionary perspective of social identity: Revisiting groups. In M. Schaller, J. A. Simpson, & D. T. Kenrick (Eds.), *Evolution and social psychology* (pp. 143–161). New York: Psychology Press.

Bronfenbrenner, U., & Crouter, A. (1982). Work and family through time and space. In S. Kamerman & C. Hayes (Eds.), *Families that work* (pp. 39–83). Washington, DC: National Academy Press.

Buehler, C., & Gerard, J. (2002). Marital conflict, ineffective parenting, and children's and adolescents' adjustment. *Journal of Marriage and the Family, 64*, 78–92.

Burgess, R., & Draper, P. (1989). The explanation of family violence: The role of biological behavioral and cultural selection. In L. Ohlin & M. Tonry (Eds.), *Family violence* (pp. 59–116). Chicago: University of Chicago Press.

Buss, D. M. (1995). Evolutionary psychology: A new paradigm for psychological science. *Psychological Inquiry, 6*, 1–30.

Buss, D. M., & Schmitt, D. P. (1993). Sexual strategies theory: A contextual evolutionary analysis of human mating. *Psychological Review, 100*, 204–232.

Cameron, N. M., Champagne, F. A., Parent, C., Fish, E. W., Ozaki-Kuroda, K., & Meaney, M. (2005). The programming of individual differences in defensive responses and reproductive strategies in the rat through variations in maternal care. *Neuroscience and Biobehavioral Reviews, 29*, 843–865.

Campbell, B. C., & Udry, J. R. (1995). Stress and age at menarche of mothers and daughters. *Journal of Biosocial Science, 27*, 127–134.

Caspi, A., McClay, J., Moffitt, T. E., Mill, J., Martin, J., Craig, I. W., et al. (2002). Role of genotype in the cycle of violence in maltreated children. *Science, 297*, 851–854.

Cassidy, J., & Berlin, L. J. (1994). The insecure/ambivalent pattern of attachment: Theory and research. *Child Development, 65*, 971–991.

Charnov, E. L. (1993). *Life history invariants.* Oxford, UK: Oxford University Press.

Chisholm, J. S. (1993). Death, hope, and sex: Life-history theory and the development of reproductive strategies. *Current Anthropology, 34*, 1–24.

Chisholm, J. S. (1996). The evolutionary ecology of attachment organization. *Human Nature, 7*, 1–38.

Chisholm, J. S. (1999). *Death, hope, and sex.* New York: Cambridge University Press.

Clutton-Brock, T. (1991). *The evolution of parental care.* Princeton, NJ: Princeton University Press.

Cohn, D., Cowan, P., Cowan, C., & Pearson, J. (1992). Mothers' and fathers' working models of childhood attachment relationships, parenting style, and child behavior. *Development and Psychopathology, 4*, 417–431.

Cohn, J., & Tronick, E. (1983). Three-month-old infants' reactions to simulated depression. *Child Development, 54*, 185–193.

Collins, N. L., & Read, S. J. (1994). Cognitive representations of attachment: The structure and function of working models. In K. Bartholomew & D. Perlman (Eds.), *Attachment processes in adulthood* (pp. 53–90). London: Kingsley.

Crittenden, P. M. (1985). Social networks, quality of child rearing, and child development. *Child Development, 56*, 1299–1313.

Crnic, K. A., Greenberg, M. T., & Slough, N. M. (1986). Early stress and social support influences on mothers' and high-risk infants' functioning in late infancy. *Infant Mental Health Journal, 7*, 19–33.

Cronin, H. (1991). *The ant and the peacock*. Cambridge, UK: Cambridge University Press.

Cronk, L. (1999). *That complex whole: Culture and the evolution of human behavior*. Boulder, CO: Westview Press.

Crowell, J., & Feldman, S. (1988). Mothers' internal models of relationships and children's behavioral and developmental status: A study of mother–child interaction. *Child Development, 59*, 1273–1285.

Crowell, J., & Feldman, S. (1991). Mothers' working models of attachment relationships and mother and child behavior during separation and reunion. *Developmental Psychology, 27*, 597–605.

Daly, M., & Wilson, M. I. (1981). Abuse and neglect of children in evolutionary perspective. In R. D. Alexander & D. W. Tinkle (Eds.), *Natural selection and social behavior: Recent research and new theory* (pp. 405–416). Oxford, UK: Blackwell.

Daly, M., & Wilson, M. (1984). A sociobiological analysis of human infanticide. In G. Hausfater & S. B. Hrdy (Eds.), *Infanticide* (pp. 487–502). New York: Aldine de Gruyter.

Daly, M., & Wilson, M. (1985). Child abuse and other risks of not living with both parents. *Ethology and Sociobiology, 6*, 197–210.

Daly, M., & Wilson, M. (1988). *Homicide*. New York: Aldine de Gruyter.

Darwin, C. (1859). *On the origins of species*. London: John Murray.

Darwin, C. (1981). *The descent of man, and selection in relation to sex*. Princeton, NJ: Princeton University Press. (Original work published 1871)

Das Eiden, R., Teti, D. M., & Corns, K. M. (1995). Maternal working models of attachment, marital adjustment, and the parent–child relationship. *Child Development, 66*, 1504–1518.

Del Carmen, R., Pedersen, F., Huffman, L., & Bryan, Y. (1993). Dyadic distress management predicts security of attachment. *Infant Behavior and Development, 16*, 131–147.

De Wolff, M., & van IJzendoorn, M. (1997). Sensitivity and attachment: A meta-analysis on parental antecedents of infant attachment. *Child Development, 68*, 571–591.

Dickemann, M. (1975). Demographic consequences of infanticide in man. *Annual Review of Ecology and Systematics, 7*, 107–137.

Dobzhansky, T. (1973). Nothing in biology makes sense except in the light of evolution. *American Biological Teacher, 35*, 125–129.

Doughty, D., & Rodgers, J. L. (2000). Behavior genetic modeling of menarche in US females. In J. L. Rodgers, D. C. Rowe, & W. B. Miller (Eds.), *Genetic influences on human fertility and sexuality* (pp. 169–181). Boston: Kluwer.

Draper, P., & Harpending, H. (1982). Father absence and reproductive strategy: An evolutionary perspective. *Journal of Anthropological Research, 38*, 255–273.

Edgarton, R. (1992). *Sick societies: Challenging the myth of primitive harmony*. New York: Free Press.

Eibl-Eibesfeldt, I. (1989). *Human ethology*. New York: Aldine de Gruyter.

Ellis, B. J. (2004). Timing of pubertal maturation in girls. *Psychological Bulletin, 130*, 920–958.

Ellis, B. J., & Garber, J. (2000). Psychosocial antecedents of variation in girls' pubertal timing. *Child Development, 71*, 485–501.

Ellis, B. J., McFadyen-Ketchum, S., Dodge, K. A., Pettit, G. S., & Bates, J. E. (1999). Quality of early family relationships and individual differences in the timing of pubertal maturation in girls. *Journal of Personality and Social Psychology, 77*, 387–401.

Emery, R. (1988). *Marriage, divorce, and children's adjustment*. Beverly Hills, CA: Sage.

Erickson, M. F., Sroufe, L. A., & Egeland, B. (1985). The relationship between quality of attachment and behavior problems in preschool in a high risk sample. In I. Bretherton & E. Waters (Eds.), Growing points of attachment theory and research. *Monographs of the Society for Research in Child Development, 50*(1–2, Serial No. 209), 147–193.

Feeney, J. A. (1994). Attachment style, communication patterns and satisfaction across the life cycle of marriage. *Personal Relationships, 1*, 333–348.

Feiring, C., Fox, N. A., Jaskir, J., & Lewis, M. (1987). The relation between social support, infant risk status and mother–infant interaction. *Developmental Psychology, 23*, 400–405.

Feldstein, S., Crown, C., Beebe, B., & Jaffe, J. (1995, April). *Temporal coordination and the prediction of mother–infant attachment*. Paper presented at the biennial meeting of the Society for Research in Child Development, Indianapolis, IN.

Fernald, A. (1985). Four-month-old infants prefer to listen to motherese. *Infant Behavior and Development, 8*, 181–195.

Fisher, H. E. (1992). *Anatomy of love: The natural history of monogamy, adultery, and divorce*. New York: Norton.

Foley, R. (1992). Evolutionary ecology and fossil hominids. In E. Smith & B. Winterholder (Eds.), *Evolutionary ecology and human behavior* (pp. 29–64). New York: Aldine de Gruyter.

Frank, R. H. (1988). *Passions within reason: The strategic role of the emotions*. New York: Norton.

Fuller, T. L., & Fincham, F. D. (1995). Attachment style in married couples: Relation to current marital functioning, stability over time, and method of assessment. *Personal Relationships, 2*, 17–34.

Furman, W., & Simon, V. A. (1999). Cognitive representations of adolescent relationships. In W. Furman, B. B. Brown, & C. Feiring (Eds.), *The development of romantic relationships in adolescence* (pp. 75–98). New York: Cambridge University Press.

Gangestad, S. W., & Simpson, J. A. (2000). The evolution of human mating: Trade-offs and strategic pluralism. *Behavioral and Brain Sciences, 23*, 573–587.

Gangestad, S. W., & Simpson, J. A. (Eds.). (2007). *The evolution of mind: Fundamental questions and controversies*. New York: Guilford Press.

Geary, D. C. (2005). Evolution of paternal investment. In D. M. Buss (Ed.), *The handbook of evolutionary psychology* (pp. 483–505). Hoboken, NJ: Wiley.

Gelfand, D., & Teti, D. (1990). The effects of maternal depression on children. *Clinical Psychology Review, 10*, 329–353.

Geronimus, A. T. (1996). What teen mothers know. *Human Nature, 7*, 323–352.

Goldberg, W. A., & Easterbrooks, M. A. (1984). The role of marital quality in toddler development. *Developmental Psychology, 20*, 504–514.

Graber, J., Brooks-Gunn, J., & Warren, M. (1995). The antecedents of menarcheal age. *Child Development, 66*, 346–359.

Grafen, A. (1990). Biological signals as handicaps. *Journal of Theoretical Biology, 144*, 517–546.

Grieser, D. L., & Kuhl, P. K. (1988). Maternal speech to infants in a tonal language: Support for universal prosodic features in motherese. *Developmental Psychology, 24*, 14–20.

Hamilton, W. D. (1964). The genetical evolution of social behaviour. *Journal of Theoretical Biology, 7*, 1–52.

Hamilton, W. D., & Zuk, M. (1982). Heritable true fitness and bright birds: A role for parasites? *Science, 218*, 384–387.

Hazan, C., & Shaver, P. R. (1987). Romantic love conceptualized as an attachment process. *Journal of Personality and Social Psychology, 52*, 511–524.

Hazan, C., & Shaver, P. R. (1994). Attachment as an organizational framework for research on close relationships. *Psychological Inquiry, 5*, 1–22.

Hazan, C., & Zeifman, D. (1999). Pair bonds as attachments: Evaluating the evidence. In J. Cassidy & P. R. Shaver (Eds.), *Handbook of attachment: Theory, research, and clinical applications* (pp. 336–354). New York: Guilford Press.

Hetherington, E. M., & Kelly, J. (2002). *For better or for worse*. New York: Norton.

Hinde, R. A. (1976). On describing relationships. *Journal of Child Psychology, 17*, 1–19.

Hinde, R. A. (1984). Why do the sexes behave differently in close relationships? *Journal of Social and Personal Relationships, 1*, 471–501.

Hinde, R. A. (1986). Some implications of evolutionary theory and comparative data for the study of human prosocial and aggressive behaviour. In D. Olweus, J. Block, & M. Radke-Yarrow (Eds.), *Development of anti-social and prosocial behaviour* (pp. 13–32). Orlando, FL: Academic Press.

Hinde, R. A. (1991). When is an evolutionary approach useful? *Child Development, 62*, 671–675.

Hoier, S. (2003). Father absence and age at menarche. *Human Nature, 14*, 209–233.

Horn, H., & Rubenstein, D. (1984). Behavioural adaptations and life history. In J. R. Krebs & N. B. Davies (Eds.), *Behavioural ecology: An evolutionary approach* (2nd ed., pp. 279–300). Oxford, UK: Blackwell.

Howes, P., & Markman, H. J. (1989). Marital quality and child functioning: A longitudinal investigation. *Child Development, 60*, 1044–1051.

Hrdy, S. B. (1999). *Mother nature*. New York: Ballantine.

Hrdy, S. B. (2005). Evolutionary context of human development: The cooperative breeding model. In C. S. Carter, L. Ahnert, K. Grossmann, S. Hryd, M. Lamb, S. Porges, et al. (Eds.), *Attachment and bonding: A new synthesis* (pp. 9–32). Cambridge, MA: MIT Press.

Irvin, N. A., Kennell, J. H., & Klaus, M. H. (1976). Caring for parents of an infant with a congenital malformation. In M. H. Klaus & J. H. Kennell (Eds.), *Maternal–infant bonding* (pp. 167–208). St. Louis, MO: Mosby.

Isabella, R. (1994). Origins of maternal role satisfaction and its influences upon maternal interactive behavior and infant–mother attachment. *Infant Behavior and Development, 17*, 381–387.

Isabella, R., & Belsky, J. (1990). Interactional synchrony and the origins of infant–mother attachment: A replication study. *Child Development, 62*, 373–384.

Isabella, R., Belsky, J., & von Eye, A. (1989). Origins of infant–mother attachment: An examination of interactional synchrony during the infant's first year. *Developmental Psychology, 25*, 12–21.

Jacobson, S. W., & Frye, K. F. (1991). Effect of maternal social support on attachment: Experimental evidence. *Child Development, 62*, 572–582.

Johns, S. E. (2003). *Environmental risk and the evolutionary psychology of teenage motherhood.* Unpublished doctoral dissertation, University of Bristol, Bristol, UK.

Jones, B., Leeton, J., McLeod, I., & Wood, C. (1972). Factors influencing the age of menarche in a lower socio-economic group in Melbourne. *Medical Journal of Australia, 21*, 533–535.

Jorm, A. F., Christensen, H., Rodgers, B., Jacomb, P. A., & Easteal, S. (2004). Association of adverse childhood experiences, age of menarche and adult reproductive behavior: Does the androgen receptor gene play a role? *American Journal of Medical Genetics: Part B. Neuropsychiatric Genetics, 125*, 105–111.

Kaplan, H. S., & Gangestad, S. W. (2005). Life history theory and evolutionary psychology. In D. M. Buss (Ed.), *The handbook of evolutionary psychology* (pp. 68–95). Hoboken, NJ: Wiley.

Kaplan, H. S., Lancaster, J., & Hurtado, A. M. (2000). A theory of human life history evolution. *Evolutionary Anthropology, 9*, 156–185.

Kelly, R. L. (1995). *The foraging spectrum: Diversity in hunter–gatherer lifeways*. Washington, DC: Smithsonian Institution Press.

Kennell, J. H., Trause, M. A., & Klaus, M. H. (1975). Evidence for a sensitive period in the human mother. In T. Brazelton, E. Tronick, L. Adamson, H. Als, & S. Wise (Eds.), *Parent–infant interaction* (pp. 87–101). New York: Elsevier/Excerpta Medica/North Holland.

Ketelaar, T., & Ellis, B. J. (2000). Are evolutionary explanations falsifiable?: Evolutionary psychology and Lakatosian philosophy of science. *Psychological Inquiry, 11*, 1–21.

Kiernan, K. E., & Hobcraft, J. (1997). Parental divorce during childhood. *Population Studies, 51,* 41–55.

Kim, K., & Smith, P. K. (1998a). Childhood stress, behavioral symptoms and mother–daughter pubertal development. *Journal of Adolescence, 21,* 231–240.

Kim, K., & Smith, P. K. (1998b). Retrospective survey of parental marital relations and child reproductive development. *International Journal of Behavioral Development, 22,* 729–751.

Kim, K., Smith, P. K., & Palermiti, A. L. (1997). Conflict in childhood and reproductive development. *Evolution and Human Behavior, 18,* 109–142.

Kirkpatrick, L. A. (1998). Evolution, pair-bonding, and reproductive strategies. In J. A. Simpson & W. S. Rholes (Eds.), *Attachment theory and close relationships* (pp. 353–393). New York: Guilford Press.

Kirkpatrick, L. A., & Davis, K. E. (1994). Attachment style, gender and relationship stability. *Journal of Personality and Social Psychology, 66,* 502–512.

Kirkpatrick, L. A., & Hazan, C. (1994). Attachment styles and close relationships. *Personal Relationships, 1,* 123–142.

Klaus, M., & Kennell, J. (1976). Parent-to-infant attachment. In D. Hull (Ed.), *Recent advances in pediatrics* (pp. 129–152). New York: Churchill Livingstone.

Kobak, R. R., & Hazan, C. (1991). Attachment in marriage. *Journal of Personality and Social Psychology, 60,* 861–869.

Krishnakumar, A., & Buehler, C. (2000). Interparental conflict and parenting behaviors: A meta-analytic review. *Family Relations, 49,* 25–44.

Kunce, L. J., & Shaver, P. R. (1994). An attachment-theoretical approach to caregiving in romantic relationships. In K. Bartholomew & D. Perlman (Eds.), *Attachment processes in adulthood* (pp. 205–237). London: Kingsley.

Kuzawa, C. W. (2005). Fetal origins of developmental plasticity: Are fetal cues reliable predictors of future nutritional environments? *American Journal of Human Biology, 17,* 5–21.

LaFreniere, P. J., & Sroufe, L. A. (1985). Profiles of peer competence in the preschool: Interrelations between measures, influence of social ecology, and relation to attachment history. *Developmental Psychology, 21,* 56–69.

Lempers, J., Clark-Lempers, D., & Simons, R. (1989). Economic hardship, parenting, and distress in adolescence. *Child Development, 60,* 25–49.

Lewis, M., & Feiring, C. (1989). Infant, mother, and mother–infant interaction behavior and subsequent attachment. *Child Development, 60,* 831–837.

Lewis, M., Feiring, C., McGuffog, C., & Jaskir, J. (1984). Predicting psychopathology in six-year-olds from early social relations. *Child Development, 55,* 123–136.

Leyendecker, B., Lamb, M., & Scholmerich, A. (in press). Studying mother–infant interaction: Effects of context and length of observation in two cultural groups. *Infant Behavior and Development.*

Lieberman, A. F., Weston, D. R., & Pawl, J. H. (1991). Preventative intervention and outcome with anxiously attached dyads. *Child Development, 62,* 199–209.

Lütkenhaus, P., Grossmann, K. E., & Grossmann, K. (1985). Infant–mother attachment at twelve months and style of interaction with a stranger at the age of three years. *Child Development, 56,* 1538–1542.

Lynch, M. A. (1975). Ill-health and child abuse. *Lancet, 2,* 317–319.

Lyons-Ruth, K., Connell, D. B., & Grunebaum, H. U. (1990). Infants at social risk: Maternal depression and family support services as mediators of infant development and security of attachment. *Child Development, 61,* 85–98.

Main, M. (1981). Avoidance in the service of attachment: A working paper. In K. Immelmann, G. Barlow, M. Main, & L. Petrinovich (Eds.), *Behavioral development: The Bielefeld Interdisciplinary Project* (pp. 651–693). New York: Cambridge University Press.

Main, M. (1990). Cross-cultural studies of attachment organization: Recent studies, changing methodologies, and the concept of conditional strategies. *Human Development, 33,* 48–61.

Main, M., & Solomon, J. (1986). Discovery of an insecure-disorganized/disoriented attachment pattern: Procedures, findings, and implications for the classification of behavior. In T. B. Brazelton & M. Yogman (Eds.), *Affective development in infancy* (pp. 95–124). Norwood, NJ: Ablex.

Main, M., & Solomon, J. (1990). Procedures for identifying disorganized/disoriented infants in the Ainsworth Strange Situation. In M. T. Greenberg, D. Cicchetti, & E. M. Cummings (Eds.), *Attachment in the preschool years: Theory, research, and intervention* (pp. 121–160). Chicago: University of Chicago Press.

Matas, L., Arend, R., & Sroufe, L. A. (1978). Continuity in adaptation in the second year: The relationship between quality of attachment and later competence. *Child Development, 49,* 547–556.

McLoyd, V. (1990). The declining fortunes of black children: Psychological distress, parenting, and socioemotional development in the context of economic hardship. *Child Development, 61,* 311–346.

Mezzich, A. C., Tarter, R. E., Giancola, P. R., Lu, S., Kirisci, L., & Parks, S. (1997). Substance use and risky sexual behavior in female adolescents. *Drug and Alcohol Dependence, 44,* 157–166.

Mikulincer, M., & Nachshon, O. (1991). Attachment styles and patterns of self-disclosure. *Journal of Personality and Social Psychology, 61,* 321–331.

Miller, C., & Fishkin, S. A. (1997). On the dynamics of human bonding and reproductive success. In J. A. Simpson & D. T. Kenrick (Eds.), *Evolutionary social psychology* (pp. 197–235). Mahwah, NJ: Erlbaum.

Miller, W. B., & Pasta, D. J. (2000). Early family environment, reproductive strategy and contraceptive behavior. In J. L. Rodgers, D. C. Rowe, & W. B. Miller (Eds.), *Genetic influences on human fertility and sexuality* (pp. 183–230). Boston: Kluwer.

Minturn, L., & Stashak, J. (1982). Infanticide as a terminal abortion procedure. *Behavior Science Research*, *17*, 70–90.

Moffitt, T. E., Caspi, A., Belsky, J., & Silva, P. A. (1992). Childhood experience and the onset of menarche: A test of a sociobiological model. *Child Development, 63*, 47–58.

National Institute of Child Health and Human Development (NICHD) Early Child Care Network. (1997). The effects of infant child care on infant–mother attachment security: Results of the NICHD Study of Early Child Care. *Child Development, 68*, 860–879.

O'Connor, M. (1997, March). *Maternal personality characteristics on the MMPI and infant attachment*. Paper presented at the biennial meeting of the Society for Research in Child Development, Washington, DC.

O'Connor, S. M., Vietze, P. M., Hopkins, J. B., & Altemeier, W. A. (1977). Postpartum extended maternal–infant contact: Subsequent mothering and child health. *Pediatric Research, 11*, 380.

Parke, R., Coltrane, S., Duffy, S., Buriel, R., Dennis, J., Powers, J., et al. (2004). Economic stress, parenting, and child adjustment in Mexican American and European families. *Child Development, 75*, 1632–1656.

Parker, G. A., & Maynard Smith, J. (1991). Optimality theory in evolutionary biology. *Nature, 348*, 27–33.

Promislow, D., & Harvey, P. (1990). Living fast and dying young: A comparative analysis of life-history variation among mammals. *Journal of the Zoological Society of London, 220*, 417–437.

Quinlan, R. J. (2003). Father absence, parental care, and female reproductive development. *Evolution and Human Behavior, 24*, 376–390.

Rholes, W. S., Simpson, J. A., & Blakely, B. S. (1995). Adult attachment styles and mothers' relationships with their young children. *Personal Relationships, 2*, 35–54.

Rholes, W. S., Simpson, J. A., Blakely, B. S., Lanigan, L., & Allen, E. A. (1997). Adult attachment styles, the desire to have children, and working models of parenthood. *Journal of Personality, 65*, 357–385.

Rholes, W. S., Simpson, J. A., Campbell, L., & Grich, J. (2001). Adult attachment and the transition to parenthood. *Journal of Personality and Social Psychology, 81*, 421–435.

Romans, S. E., Martin, M., Gendall, K., & Herbison, G. P. (2003). Age of menarche: The role of some psychosocial factors. *Psychological Medicine, 33*, 933–939.

Rowe, D. C. (2000). Environmental and genetic influences on pubertal development. In J. L. Rodgers, D. C. Rowe, & W. B. Miller (Eds.), *Genetic influences on human fertility and sexuality* (pp. 147–168). Boston: Kluwer.

Scholmerich, A., Fracasso, M., Lamb, M., & Broberg, A. (1995). Interactional harmony at 7 and 10 months of age predicts security of attachment as measured by Q-sort ratings. *Social Development, 34*, 62–74.

Seccombe, K. (2000). Families in poverty in the 1990s. *Journal of Marriage and the Family, 62*, 1094–1113.

Shaver, P. R., Hazan, C., & Bradshaw, D. (1988). Love as attachment: The integration of three behavioral systems. In R. J. Sternberg & M. L. Barnes (Eds.), *The psychology of love* (pp. 68–99). New Haven, CT: Yale University Press.

Simpson, J. A. (1990). Influence of attachment styles on romantic relationships. *Journal of Personality and Social Psychology, 59*, 971–980.

Simpson, J. A. (1999). Attachment theory in modern evolutionary perspective. In J. Cassidy & P. R. Shaver (Eds.), *Handbook of attachment: Theory, research, and clinical applications* (pp. 115–140). New York: Guilford Press.

Simpson, J. A., Beckes, L., & Weisberg, Y. J. (2007). Evolutionary accounts of individual differences in adult attachment orientations. In J. V. Wood, A. Tesser, & J. G. Holmes (Eds.), *The self and relationships* (pp. 183–206). New York: Psychology Press.

Simpson, J. A., & Gangestad, S. (1991). Individual differences in sociosexuality: Evidence for convergent and discriminant validity. *Journal of Personality and Social Psychology, 60*, 870–883.

Simpson, J. A., Rholes, W. S., & Phillips, D. (1996). Conflict in close relationships: An attachment perspective. *Journal of Personality and Social Psychology, 71*, 899–914.

Simpson, J. A., Wilson, C. L., & Winterheld, H. A. (2004). Sociosexuality and romantic relationships. In J. H. Harvey, A. Wenzel, & S. Sprecher (Eds.), *Handbook of sexuality in close relationships* (pp. 87–112). Mahwah, NJ: Erlbaum.

Slade, A., Belsky, J., Aber, J. L., & Phelps, J. L. (1999). Maternal representations of their relationship with their toddlers. *Developmental Psychology, 35*, 611–619.

Smith, K. E., Landry, S. H., & Swank, P. R. (2000). The influence of early patterns of positive parenting on children's preschool outcomes. *Early Education and Development, 11*, 147–169.

Smith, P. B., & Pederson, D. R. (1988). Maternal sensitivity and patterns of infant–mother attachment. *Child Development, 59*, 1097–1101.

Spieker, S. J. (1988). Patterns of very insecure attachment forward in samples of high-risk infants and toddlers. *Topics in Early Childhood Special Education, 6*, 37–53.

Spieker, S. J., & Booth, C. (1988). Maternal antecedents of attachment quality. In J. Belsky & T. Nezworski (Eds.), *Clinical implications of attachment* (pp. 95–135). Hillsdale, NJ: Erlbaum.

Sroufe, L. A. (1988). The role of infant–caregiver attachment in development. In J. Belsky & T. Nezworski (Eds.), *Clinical implications of attachment* (pp. 18–38). Hillsdale, NJ: Erlbaum.

Sroufe, L. A., & Waters, E. (1977). Attachment as an organizational construct. *Child Development, 48*, 1184–1199.

Stearns, S. (1976). Life-history tactics: A review of the ideas. *Quarterly Review of Biology, 51*, 3–47.

Stearns, S. (1992). *The evolution of life histories*. New York: Oxford University Press.

Steinberg, L. (1988). Reciprocal relation between parent–child distance and pubertal maturation. *Developmental Psychology, 24,* 122–128.

Sugarman, M. (1977). Parental influences of maternal–infant attachment. *American Journal of Orthopsychiatry, 47,* 407–421.

Surbey, M. (1990). Family composition, stress, and human menarche. In F. Bercovitch & T. Zeigler (Eds.), *The socioendocrinology of primate reproduction* (pp. 71–97). New York: Liss.

Teti, D., Gelfand, D., Messinger, D., & Isabella, R. (1995). Maternal depression and the quality of early attachment. *Developmental Psychology, 31,* 364–376.

Tooby, J. (1982). Pathogens, polymorphism, and the evolution of sex. *Journal of Theoretical Biology, 97,* 557–576.

Tooby, J., & Cosmides, L. (1992). Psychological foundations of culture. In J. Barkow, L. Cosmides, & J. Tooby (Eds.), *The adapted mind* (pp. 19–136). New York: Oxford University Press.

Turkheimer, E., & Waldron, M. (2000). Non-shared environment. *Psychological Bulletin, 126,* 78–108.

Trivers, R. L. (1971). The evolution of reciprocal altruism. *Quarterly Review of Biology, 46,* 35–57.

Trivers, R. L. (1972). Parental investment and sexual selection. In B. Campbell (Ed.), *Sexual selection and the descent of man, 1871–1971* (pp. 136–179). Chicago: Aldine-Atherton.

Trivers, R. L. (1974). Parent–offspring conflict. *American Zoologist, 14,* 249–264.

Trivers, R. L. (1985). *Social evolution.* Menlo Park, CA: Benjamin/Cummings.

Trivers, R. L. (1997). Genetic basis of intrapsychic conflict. In N. L. Segal, G. E. Weisfeld, & C. C. Weisfeld (Eds.), *Uniting psychology and biology: Integrative perspectives on human development* (pp. 385–395). Washington, DC: American Psychological Association.

Trivers, R. L., & Willard, D. E. (1973). Natural selection of parental ability to vary the sex ratio of offspring. *Science, 179,* 90–92.

Valenzuela, M. (1990). Attachment in chronically underweight young children. *Child Development, 61,* 1984–1996.

van IJzendoorn, M. H. (1995a). Adult attachment representations, parental responsiveness, and infant attachment. *Child Development, 68,* 604–609.

van IJzendoorn, M. H. (1995b). Adult attachment representations, parental responsiveness, and infant attachment: A meta-analysis on the predictive validity of the Adult Attachment Interview. *Psychological Bulletin, 117,* 387–403.

van IJzendoorn, M. H., & Bakermans-Kranenburg, M. J. (1997). Intergenerational transmission of attachment: A move to the contextual level. In L. Atkinson & K. J. Zucker (Eds.), *Attachment and psychopathology* (pp. 135–170). New York: Guilford Press.

Velderman, M. K., Bakermans-Kranenburg, M. J., Juffer, F., & van IJzendoorn, M. H. (2006). Effects of attachment-based interventions on maternal sensitivity and infant attachment: Differential susceptibility of highly reactive infants. *Journal of Family Psychology, 20,* 266–274.

Vondra, J., Shaw, D., & Kevinides, M. (1995). Predicting infant attachment classification from multiple, contemporaneous measures of maternal care. *Infant Behavior and Development, 18,* 415–425.

Waters, E., Wippman, J., & Sroufe, L. A. (1979). Attachment, positive affect, and competence in the peer group: Two studies in construct validation. *Child Development, 50,* 821–829.

Wierson, M., Long, P. J., & Forehand, R. L. (1993). Toward a new understanding of early menarche. *Adolescence, 28,* 913–924.

Williams, G. (1966). *Adaptation and natural selection.* Princeton, NJ: Princeton University Press.

Wilson, C. L., Rholes, W. S., Simpson, J. A., & Tran, S. (2007). Labor, delivery, and early parenthood: An attachment theory perspective. *Personality and Social Psychology Bulletin, 33,* 505–518.

Wilson, M., & Daly, M. (1997). Life expectancy, economic inequality, homicide and reproductive timing in Chicago neighbourhoods. *British Medical Journal, 314,* 1271–1274.

Wilson, M., & Daly, M. (2005). Carpe diem: Adaptation and devaluing the future. *Quarterly Review of Biology, 80,* 55–60.

Wood, W., & Eagly, A. H. (2002). A cross-cultural analysis of the behavior of men and women: Implications for the origins of sex differences. *Psychological Bulletin, 128,* 699–727.

Woodward, A. L., Sommerville, J. A., & Guajardo, J. J. (2001). How infants make sense of intentional action. In B. F. Malle, L. J. Moses, & D. A. Baldwin (Eds.), *Intentions and intentionality: Foundations of social cognition* (pp. 149–169). Cambridge, MA: MIT Press.

Wright, R. (1994). *The moral animal.* New York: Vintage.

Youngblade, L. M., & Belsky, J. (1989). Child maltreatment, infant–parent attachment security, and dysfunctional peer relationships in toddlerhood. *Topics in Early Childhood Special Education, 9,* 1–15.

Zeanah, C., Benoit, D., Barton, M., Regan, C., Hirshberg, L., & Lipsett, L. (1993). Representations of attachment in mothers and their one-year-old infants. *Journal of the American Academy of Child and Adolescent Psychiatry, 32,* 278–286.

Zeifman, D., & Hazan, C. (1997). Attachment: The bond in pair-bonds. In J. A. Simpson & D. T. Kenrick (Eds.), *Evolutionary social psychology* (pp. 237–263). Mahwah, NJ: Erlbaum.

CHAPTER 7

Psychobiological Origins of Infant Attachment and Its Role in Development

H. JONATHAN POLAN
MYRON A. HOFER

John Bowlby (1969/1982) was the first to give the psychological concept of human attachment a strong base in evolutionary theory. He was convinced that early attachment was evidence of a previously unrecognized motivational system present in both mammals and birds, which had been selected during evolution for the survival value of the protection it afforded offspring through the emotional bond that developed between infant and mother. The strong tendency for young to stay close to their mothers, and their prolonged emotional distress upon separation, were the core behavioral indicators of what Bowlby viewed as a basic instinct organized according to the principle of goal-corrected feedback—a concept borrowed from engineering, which had proved useful in understanding physiological adaptation and homeostasis.

With the discovery of qualitatively different patterns of attachment in children and of mental representations (internal working models) in mothers, attachment research moved quickly in these new directions, as if the nature of the "bond" and the separation response were well understood. But for many behavioral scientists who were studying early development experimentally, evidence from their research did not fit Bowlby's concept

of a *unitary* attachment system at work within the mother–infant interaction. Instead, they found a number of relatively independent systems (e.g., for orientation, for early learning and memory, for thermal regulation, or for early affect expression), each with its own organizing principles. In addition, Bowlby's concept did not generate research questions, but rather seemed to answer questions with a frustrating form of circular reasoning. For example, an infant's attachment bond was inferred from the infant's response to separation (Bowlby, 1973), which itself was explained as a consequence of disruption of the attachment bond.

Evolutionary principles give us a conceptual common ground that can be shared by neuroscience, psychology, and psychoanalysis, providing answers to questions about how the human mind and brain have come into being and why they have their present form. The historical nature of both development and evolution bridges the gap between the "reductionist" emphasis of the molecular/cellular neurosciences and the "holistic" emphasis on meaning that is the central focus of psychoanalytically oriented clinicians. Early human development traverses a series of levels of scale and organization—from the multicellular interactions of the embryo, to the integrated systems and behavior of the fetus, to the emerging cognitive and affective capacities of the child. The biological, behavioral, and psychological processes at work at those levels of organization seem very different. But the new properties that emerge at each level arise from the combined operation of simpler processes taking place at the previous level. Understanding those transitions, and the emergence of new properties at higher levels, is one of the central issues for research in early human development as well as for attempts to integrate neuroscience, psychology, and psychoanalysis.

In the first edition of this handbook, Simpson (1999) and Belsky (1999) contributed chapters that extended the evolutionary theoretical approach, begun by Bowlby, to the possible long-term developmental effects of early attachment patterns and the transmission of these patterns across generations. (See also Simpson & Belsky, Chapter 6, this volume.) Drawing on recent advances in evolutionary theory, they described the contribution of different developmental attachment patterns for enhancing reproductive fitness as well as simple survival in the next generation. For example, a secure attachment pattern may prepare offspring best in a predictable, secure environment where prolonged parental investment in offspring is possible; however, the insecure patterns may be more adaptive in chaotic, dangerous, and depriving environments where fearful responses maximize short-term survival, and where early sexual maturation maximizes the number of offspring produced.

New discoveries in the genetic mechanisms of early development in the past several years have provided the basis for an integration of the fields of evolutionary and developmental biology (for a review, see Carroll, 2005). In this view, development can be viewed as a major source of potentially adaptive variation for selection to act upon in the course of evolution. We have learned that genes are not only instruments of inheritance in evolution, but also targets of molecular signals originating both within the organism and in the environment outside it. These signals regulate development. Rapid progress in understanding these molecular genetic mechanisms has revealed an unexpected potential for plasticity, which can enable a relatively few evolutionarily conserved cellular processes to be linked together by differential gene expression into a variety of adaptive patterns that respond to environmental changes as well as to genetic mutations. The resulting plasticity allows a variety of developmental pathways, evident

in both behavior and physiology, to be generated from the same genome. This discovery of a central role for the regulation of gene expression in development has at last provided a specific mechanism for the frustratingly vague and much-debated concept of gene–environment interaction.

These advances in our understanding of both development and evolution have important implications for the study of attachment, including our understanding of the environment provided by a mother–infant relationship. They have given us a new way to understand recent studies of the biological processes that underlie the psychological constructs and life history consequences of early attachment. In this chapter, we outline how the strategy of uncovering the component processes underlying the psychological constructs created in the study of early human attachment, and the new perspective of evolutionary developmental biology, offer new and potentially useful ways of thinking about attachment and creating new ways to help patients.

The term "early attachment" has a number of different meanings in the psychological literature. In its most general sense, the term refers to a set of behaviors we observe in infants and to the feelings and thought processes (conscious and/or unconscious) we suppose infants to have, based on our own experiences and the psychological concepts we have formed ourselves or learned from others. Within this range of usage of the word "attachment," several different schools of thought have emerged—some within psychoanalysis, and others within different schools of psychodynamic psychotherapy. Common to all, however, are three themes: (1) some sort of emotional tie or bond that is inferred to develop between an infant and its caretaker, and that keeps the infant physically close; (2) a series of responses to separation that constitute the infant's emotional reaction to interruption or rupture of that bond; and (3) the existence of different patterns or qualities of interaction between infants and mothers that have important long-term effects on the infants' subsequent development, and that lead to a repetition of particular patterns of mothering by daughters in the next generation. These three central concepts of attachment theory have been extremely useful clinically, but they leave a number of observations unexplained and questions unanswered, as we explain below.

We use recent psychobiological research to provide answers to questions left open by attachment theory, and we organize the answers by the three concepts just outlined. The answers emerging from our laboratory research with animals, and from research by others, have tended to support clinical observations, but they have also extended them in unexpected ways. We cannot settle questions of human nature by studying other animals, but we can generate new hypotheses, concepts, and ways of thinking that ultimately may apply to our clinical work with patients.

DEVELOPMENT OF THE BOND

Exclusive, or preferential, orienting and proximity seeking by offspring directed toward their mothers are defining behaviors of a filial attachment system. To perform them, offspring must be able to recognize their mothers and to distinguish between maternal and nonmaternal stimuli. Although rat pups are unable to see or hear until at least 11 days of age, their sense of smell, on the way to becoming far more sensitive and discriminating than a human's, is quite competent at birth. A number of studies showed that rat pups discriminate familiar from unfamiliar odors, beginning immediately after birth based on odors learned *in utero* (Hepper, 1987) and extending to postnatally encountered odors (Gregory & Pfaff, 1971; Johanson, Turkewitz, & Hamburgh, 1980; Leon, 1974; Nyakas & Endroczi, 1970). We asked whether pups could also discriminate *among the familiar odors* in their environment—specifically, between those of their mothers and their home shavings. That ability would be evidence of *filial* attraction, not simply a nonspecific orienting toward *any* familiar cues, and its onset would mark an important developmental milestone for the infant.

We tested 1- to 10-day-old pups in a two-choice test chamber, comparing proximity seeking toward the mothers with proximity seeking toward the home nest. Pups as young as 4–5 days crawled closer to their mothers' odor than to that of their home nest shavings, and they performed certain other behaviors, such as probing with their snouts into the test platform, more often when responding to their mothers' odor. Furthermore, pups increased both maternal preference and differential responding to maternal scent after overnight isolation, demonstrating early development of a motivational component. We also found that if we supplied as little as 0.5° C of additional warmth over the mothers' side of the test chamber, even 2-day-old pups would express a preference for maternal odor (Polan & Hofer, 1998), whereas

1-day-old pups in our test paradigm did not yet show a preference for maternal odor over that of equally familiar home nest shavings. These results suggested that preference for the odor of mothers over home shavings may be acquired between 1 and 2 days of age, and that the earliest distinction between mothers and home shavings may require the convergence in time and space of both olfactory and thermal cues.

Although it had long been suspected that infant rats *learned* their olfactory preferences, we found some rather surprising reinforcers of that learning. During the first 9 postnatal days of a rat pup's life, in classical conditioning experiments using novel odors as the conditioned stimulus, we found reinforcers that neither satisfy an obvious physiological need state (unlike such reinforcers as milk or warmth) nor are themselves attractive (Sullivan, Hofer, & Brake, 1986). Examples of these reinforcers include pinching the tail, vigorous repetitive stroking with a soft brush (Sullivan & Hall, 1988), and mild foot shock (Camp & Rudy, 1988). Each of these artificial reinforcers is thought to imitate something that a mother does to her pups in the normal course of returning to the nest and initiating a nursing bout. When she returns to the nest, she often steps on the pups, then picks them up with her teeth one by one, carries them, and then begins to lick them rapidly and vigorously before replacing them in the litter pile. Thus tail pinching may mimic the sensation of being stepped on, and stroking may mimic the sensation of being licked; perhaps mild shock mimics the sensation of teeth gripping the skin. What these and the other primary reinforcers in neonates (even milk ingestion) have in common is that they are vigorously behaviorally arousing to pups.

These classical conditioning experiments (reviewed in Sullivan & Hall, 1988; Wilson & Sullivan, 1994) showed that a wide variety of stimuli that seem to mimic specific maternal behaviors toward the pups, and that all vigorously activate pups, also support the learning of a preference for a novel odor with which they are paired. It is now known that norepinephrine plays a key role in mediating these events. Thus it is theorized that during a sensitive period extending through the first week and a half of life, associative preference learning depends on an activated norepinephrinergic state induced by the reinforcer.

What advantage might there be in newborn rats' predisposition to learn approach responses to a wide range of unconditioned stimuli—some of which might seem to us noxious at worst, or not very maternal at best, but which nevertheless get their attention and activate them? We believe that this ability was selected in evolution precisely because it enables pups to learn from the widest range of maternal interactions and cues. Thus they begin to learn about their mother from the moment she reenters the nest and activates them by her movements. They are not limited to the cues that accompany the rewarming of the litter pile after she settles over it, nor to just the sensations of milk letdown. Because the mother activates her young pups repeatedly—up to 20 times a day at each return to the nest—we can see how by stepping on, retrieving, licking, crouching over, and providing milk to them, she powerfully conditions an attraction in them to her own odor and tactile cues (e.g., fur texture). In essence, these findings substantiate Bowlby's (1969/1982) positing of an imprinting-like basis for the formation of mammalian attachment. We can see that this process of approach behavior conditioning by a broad range of activating stimuli during the 9-day sensitive period, and its continuance beyond 9 days for cues originally conditioned during the sensitive period (Sullivan, 1996), is the *functional equivalent* of imprinting in an altricial mammalian species.

We recognized that although the study of olfactory preference behavior—measuring orienting responses to odors presented on one side or the other—provided important insights into the psychobiological basis of filial attachment, more complex aspects of the infants' environment had to be modeled to further our understanding of the emergence of attachment. The next set of studies in our laboratory modeled the pups' entire three-dimensional world and revealed an unexpected complexity to pups' maternally directed behaviors, and to the range of the mother's sensory cues that guide those behaviors.

A rat pup is born into a "sandwich" world, consisting of the substrate of its nest materials beneath it and the canopy of its mother's belly looming above as she hovers over the litter. In this environment, the newborn pup must (1) burrow under the mother's abdominal surface and (2) orient and maintain itself in relation to her ventrum so that (3) contact with her body will permit heat transfer, protection, nipple grasp, and access to ongoing maternal cues that regulate the pup's endocrinological, physiological, and behavioral processes. In this sandwich world, the mother's body is both the *source* of stimuli to which the pups are responding and the *superstructure* upon which the pups organize their responses.

We conducted a series of experiments to determine precisely what maternal stimuli guided the entire complex repertoire. We modeled the mother's ventral body surface with overhead "roof" surfaces featuring increasingly dam-like tactile and olfactory cues. Under even the least mother-like roof, a wire mesh, pups became aroused, crawled, turned supine onto their backs, and audibly barked. Once supine, some pups planted their feet against the overlying mesh and crawled on their backs. Thus an overhead mesh roof evokes behaviors that appear identical in form to those we observed in the nest, and by which pups orient toward and seek proximity to the maternal ventrum. When they found themselves under roof surfaces that featured increasingly mother-like cues, 2- to 3-day-olds engaged in correspondingly higher frequencies of the behaviors (Polan & Hofer, 1999a). These experiments showed that early maternally directed proximity-seeking behaviors are not simple reflexes stimulated by nonspecific inputs, but are graded responses to specific maternal features.

We next asked whether that system might be responsive to changes in the pups' motivational state. Operationally, we asked whether a period of acute deprivation was necessary for the expression of the maternally directed orienting and proximity-seeking behaviors. Therefore, we compared the behaviors of pups that had received acute overnight deprivation with nondeprived pups. We found that although maternal deprivation was not *necessary* to the performance of the behaviors, it did significantly *enhance* responding to sufficiently motherlike surfaces, but did not affect behavior in the absence of maternal stimuli. These findings suggested that the motivational component of the system specifically modulates maternally directed orienting behaviors, but not undirected behaviors performed in isolation.

Finally, we asked how early in development the entire repertoire of behaviors is present and when they come under the sensory guidance of maternal features. We tested newborn pups that were deprived just before and after their very first nursing bout. We found that after the first nursing experience, the behaviors were already subject to sensory guidance by maternal features, whereas before any nursing occurred, pups performed the behaviors vigorously but independently of the type of stimulus encountered (Polan, Milano, Eljuga, & Hofer, 2002). Thus the first experience of nursing organizes an important transition in the control of these orienting behaviors from reflex-like action patterns to responsiveness to specific maternal features.

NEW VIEWS OF SENSITIVE PERIODS

Since the original descriptions of avian imprinting by Lorenz and Tinbergen, the concept of, and search for, sensitive periods have occupied attachment researchers. The identification of maternal licking and grooming as the stimulus that promotes long-term programming of the hypothalamic–pituitary–adrenocortical (HPA) axis led to the finding of an apparent sensitive period in the development of attachment in an altricial mammal. "Handling," or brief daily maternal separation during infancy, which evidently promotes extra maternal licking and grooming upon reunion, causes permanent down-regulation of the HPA axis and a high tolerance for stress in adulthood. But to be effective, handling has to be initiated within the first week of postnatal life (Meaney & Aitken, 1985).

This sensitive period for HPA axis programming by the mother's behavior coincides with a sensitive period for early olfactory learning, which also depends on maternal behavior. Olfactory preference learning is our best current model for how learned preferences for maternal cues begin to establish mother-seeking attachment behaviors in the infant. There is a sensitive period for this kind of learning, which extends through postnatal day (PND) 9. Learning of maternal odor cues depends on behavioral stimulation, which serves as the unconditioned stimulus (US) that is paired with the odor. Up through PND 9, all sufficiently arousing stimuli—whether presumed pleasant ones, such as stroking with a soft brush to mimic the mother's licking, or ostensibly aversive ones, such as a tail pinch or foot shock that mimic rough handling by the mother—cause pups to seek proximity with and prefer the odor with which they are paired (Camp & Rudy, 1988; Sullivan, Hofer, & Brake, 1986). During this sensitive period, it is difficult to condition *avoidance* behavior to an odor paired with any exteroceptive US. This strong predominance of preference learning over avoidance learning can be seen as an evolutionarily determined developmental adaptation that serves an infant's need to form a bond to its mother.

Abruptly at PND 10, however, the behavior learned from odor–shock pairings reverses to become the more adult-like response, avoidance. Furthermore, from PND 10 on, stroking no longer conditions proximity seeking or preference behavior to a new odor. Sullivan, Landers, Yeaman, and Wilson (2000) determined that the brain uses a special mechanism for preference learning during this pre-PND 10 sensitive period. It consists of an overactive locus ceruleus, a midbrain nucleus that mediates attention and arousal while releasing very large amounts of the neuromodulator norepinephrine at its synapses in the olfactory bulb. When stroking is paired with a new odor, the olfactory nerve action potentials reaching the bulb converge with the strong norepinephrinergic arousal signals arriving from the midbrain. These combined signals are transduced into a new response pattern—namely, approach behavior—the next time the odor is encountered. This simple learning circuit omits several brain regions involved in adult learning. A particular region that is bypassed is the amygdala, which later plays a crucial role in fear conditioning. During the sensitive period for olfactory preference learning, the amygdala is kept "offline" even during aversive stimulation (Moriceau & Sullivan, 2005). This special early learning process, which strongly favors preference learning and inhibits avoidance learning, may well be the basis by which infant mammals, from puppies to humans, form strong attachments to even abusive caregivers (Scott, 1963).

Although the amygdala is kept "offline" from the olfactory learning circuit, it is by no means inactive during the sensitive period. Rather, during this time it initiates the long-term processes of HPA axis programming by maternal licking and grooming. Adults that, as infants, experienced high levels of licking and grooming have a "toned-down" stress axis, which has an attenuated "on" switch in the form of decreased secretion of corticotropin-releasing hormone by the hypothalamus and an augmented "off" switch in the form of extra corticosterone receptors in the hippocampus. The amygdala is the first brain locus to register added daily maternal care. As early as PND 6, after just 4 days of augmented maternal care, there are changes in two elements of the stress response system—namely, increased production of corticotropin-releasing factor, a hormone that induces the production of the stress hormone corticosterone, and, by PND 9, decreased glucocorticoid receptors (GRs) (Fenoglio, Chen, & Baram, 2006), which detect corticosterone in the brain and provide feedback to its production mechanisms. These changes occur well in advance of the permanent increase in GR expression in the hippocampus, which appears after PND 23 and, although transient, may be part of the cascade of events that establishes the permanent changes in HPA axis regulation in the hypothalamus and hippocampus. These early changes in elements of the corticosterone response system in the amygdala also have a surprising immediate influence on the circuits for olfactory learning. An early boost in corticosterone levels hastens the end of the sensitive period, turning off preference learning and ushering in precocious avoidance learning (Moriceau, Wilson, Levine, & Sullivan, 2006).

Thus the period from birth through PND 9 harbors at least two sensitive periods: one for the emergence of the attachment relationship itself, which equips the pup to survive the immediately demanding transition to postnatal life; and one that is, in a sense, banked for the pup's later benefit, the emotional tuning of its adult life, as a legacy of its rearing, but that under emergency conditions even alters the duration of the first sensitive period. Through evolution's conservative economy of form and function, the pup's nervous system is equipped to generate both kinds of behavioral plasticity from the same maternal care behaviors, licking and grooming.

RESPONSES TO SEPARATION

Up to this point, we have explored new views of the processes by which approach and proximity-seeking behaviors develop in infant rats. But behavioral systems that maintain an infant in close proximity to the mother and promote physical attachment to the nipple do not fulfill our criteria for a fully developed attachment system. Another essential component is a particular set of responses to maternal separation. In fact, Bowlby's attachment theory was developed to explain the separation responses that became all too evident during the societal devastations of World War II (Bowlby, 1969/1982). It was maternal separation that revealed the existence of a deeper layer of processes beneath the apparently simple interactions of mother and infant. Bowlby viewed these processes as primarily psychological. The behavioral and physiological responses of the infant to separation, in Bowlby's conception, were consequences of "rupture" of a psychological "bond" formed as part of an integrated psychophysiological organization that Bowlby called "the attachment system." More recent research, however, has revealed a network of simple behavioral and biological processes underlying this and other psychological constructs used to define and understand early human social relationships.

Experiments in our laboratory have shown that infant rats have complex and lasting responses to maternal separation similar to those of primates,

and that these responses occur in a number of different physiological and behavioral systems. Years ago we found that the slower developing components (Bowlby's "despair" phase) were *not* an integrated psychophysiological response, as had been supposed, but were the results of a novel mechanism (reviewed in Hofer, 1994). As separation continued, each individual system of the infant rat responded to the loss of one or another of the components of the infant's previous interactions with its mother. Providing one of these components to a separated pup (e.g., maternal warmth) maintained the level of brain biogenic amine function underlying the pup's general activity level, but it had no effect on other systems. For example, the pup's cardiac rate continued to fall, regardless of whether supplemental heat was provided. The heart rate, normally maintained by sympathetic autonomic tone, we found was regulated by provision of milk to neural receptors in the lining of the pup's stomach. With loss of the maternal milk supply, sympathetic tone fell and cardiac rate was reduced by 40% in 12–18 hours.

By studying a number of additional systems, such as those controlling sleep–wake states, activity level, sucking pattern and blood pressure, we found different components of the mother–infant interaction (such as olfaction, taste, touch, warmth, and texture) that either up-regulated or down-regulated each of these functions. We therefore concluded that in maternal separation, all these regulatory components of the mother–infant interaction are withdrawn at once. This widespread loss creates a pattern of increases or decreases in level of function of the infant's systems, depending on whether the particular system was up- or down-regulated previously by specific components of mother–infant interactions. We called these "hidden regulators," because they were not evident from simply observing the ongoing mother–infant relationship.

One of the best-known responses to maternal separation is the infant's separation cry, a behavior that occurs in a wide variety of species, including humans. In the rat, this call is in the ultrasonic range and appears on PND 1 or 2. Pharmacological studies by Susan Carden in our laboratory and by a number of others showed that the ultrasonic vocalization (USV) response to isolation is attenuated or blocked in a dose-dependent manner by clinically effective anxiolytic drugs that act at benzodiazepine and serotonin receptors (reviewed in Hofer, 1996). Conversely, USV rates are increased by compounds known to be anxiogenic in humans.

This evidence strongly suggests that separation produces an early affective state in rat pups that is expressed by the rate of infant calling. This calling behavior (and its inferred underlying affective state) develops as a communication system between mother and pup. Infant rat USVs are a powerful stimulus for the lactating rat, capable of causing her to interrupt an ongoing nursing bout, initiate searching outside the nest, and direct her search toward the source of the calls. The mother's retrieval response to the pup's vocal signals then results in renewed contact between pup and mother. This contact in turn quiets or comforts the pup.

The separation and comfort responses in attachment theory are described as expressions of interruption and reestablishment of a social bond. Such a formulation would predict that since a rat pup recognizes its own mother by her scent, pups deprived of their sense of smell (anosmic) would fail to show a comfort response. But we discovered that anosmic pups showed comfort responses that were virtually unaffected by loss of their capacity to recognize their mother by smell (Hofer & Shair, 1991). Instead, we found multiple regulators of infant USV within the contact between mother and pup: warmth, tactile stimuli, and milk, as well as the mother's scent (Hofer, 1996). The full "comfort" quieting response was elicited only when all modalities were presented together, and maximum calling rates occurred when all were withdrawn at once. In essence, we found parallel regulatory systems involving different sensory modalities. These functioned as a pattern across sensory modalities, with the rate of infant calling reflecting the sum total of effective maternal regulatory stimuli present at any given time.

In the case of sleep–wake state organization, a *temporal* patterning of stimulation is necessary, based on the timing of the mother's periodic nursing bouts and absences. For older human infants, more complex interactions such as attunement, imitation, and play are likely to have regulatory effects on developing infant cognitive and affective systems. It seems likely that these form the early building blocks of mental representations.

HIDDEN REGULATORS OF EARLY DEVELOPMENT

The regulatory effects described thus far were observed to be acting over periods of 24 hours, but it seemed likely that regulatory effects that were "hidden" within the mother–infant interaction would normally act over longer periods of time during development. This was soon found to be true.

Kuhn and Schanberg (1998) have published a series of studies in which they found that removal of the mother from rat pups produced a rapid (30-minute) fall in the pups' growth hormone (GH) levels, and that vigorous tactile stroking of maternally separated pups (mimicking maternal licking) prevented this fall in GH. There are several biological similarities between this maternal deprivation effect in rats and the growth retardation that occurs in some variants of human reactive attachment disorders of infancy. Applying this new knowledge about the regulation of GH to low-birthweight, prematurely born babies, Field and coworkers joined the Schanberg group (Field et al., 1986). They used a combination of stroking and limb movement, administered 3 times a day for 15 minutes each time and continued through the infants' 2 weeks of hospitalization. This intervention increased weight gain, head circumference, and behavioral development test scores in relation to those of a randomly chosen control group, with enhanced maturational effects discernible many months later. Clearly, early regulators are effective in humans, and over time periods as long as several weeks to months.

As we began to understand the infants' separation response as one of loss—loss of a number of individual regulatory processes that were hidden within the interactions of the previous relationship—an important implication of this finding emerged: These ongoing regulatory interactions can shape the development of an infant's brain and behavior throughout the preweaning period, when mother and infant remain in close proximity. We could now think of mother–infant interactions as regulators of normal infant development, with variations in the intensity and patterning of these interactions gradually shaping infant behavior and physiology. These processes go beyond the adaptive evolutionary role of the attachment "bond" as a protection against predators, as proposed by Bowlby (1969/1982). The rapid onset and prolonged duration of processes keeping infants close to their mothers described above provide the necessary conditions for the regulatory effects of early mother–infant interactions. The two are likely to have evolved together, because they provide a developmental mechanism through which an infant's novel adaptive capabilities can be created and shaped by variations in maternal behavior.

LASTING EFFECTS OF EARLY RELATIONSHIPS

One of the major tenets of attachment theory is the idea that an infant's early attachment pattern can have long-term developmental effects—on the internal working models that later close relationships will be built upon (the attachment pattern in the next generation in particular), but also on broader aspects of behavior, such as levels of anxiety, aggression, and later social interactions. As described in the introduction to this chapter, such a developmental system may have evolved as a result of the competitive advantages to be gained by young who are shaped by their parents, in advance, to deal most effectively with the kind of environment they are likely to face as adolescents and adults. Furthermore, we can surmise that this "predictive" role of parenting in development will be most effective if it allows for "corrective" effects of later developmental interactions, such as those with peers and with the broader social system, if these are of a different quality from that predicted by the earlier interactions. This is the evolutionary basis for the effects of social support interventions, such as those found to be effective in reducing the risk for depression conveyed by both the short variant of the serotonin transporter gene and early maltreatment in 5- to 15-year-old children (Kaufman et al., 2004).

What basis do we have for this new evolutionary interpretation? The evidence in humans is suggestive (Simpson & Belsky, Chapter 6, this volume), but not conclusive. By observing naturally occurring variations in mother–infant interactions in strains of genetically identical rats, we were able to identify three behaviors in the first 2 weeks of life that were correlated significantly with the severity of hypertension in adults of this susceptible strain (Myers, Brunelli, Shair, Squire, & Hofer, 1989). We were able to replicate the finding in another genetic strain, and because the animals in each strain were genetically identical, the differences in adulthood could be attributed to the early mother–infant interactions—in particular, the time spent in contact, the amount of maternal licking and grooming, and the time mothers spent in a highly stimulating high-arched resting position. This effect was also observed in cross-fostering studies. Thus we were able to conclude that early differences in the pattern of early maternal regulating interactions could initiate long-term developmental effects lasting into adulthood. But the evolutionary advantages for maternal regulation of offspring's blood pressure were not clear, and we had no clue as to how the biological effects of such early experiences were represented in a way that could be maintained into adulthood.

The work of Meaney and his colleagues over the past decade has greatly enlarged our understanding of the biological processes at work in these lasting effects of early relationships (reviewed in Cameron et al., 2005). They discovered that normal variation in two of the same mother–infant behaviors observed in our studies (maternal licking of pups and high-arched maternal nursing position) systematically modified the development of the adrenocortical stress response and the behavioral fear response to open spaces in adult offspring, with low levels of those maternal behaviors leading to greater adrenocortical and fear responses. In a remarkable series of cell biological studies, Meaney and his colleagues were able, first, to trace the effects of maternal behaviors to the hippocampal cell membrane receptors that sense the level of adrenocortical hormone and inhibit the hormonal response to stress in the adult—a form of feedback inhibition, as in a thermostat. Next, they found that the genes responsible for the synthesis of these receptors in the infant offspring of the high- or low-licking/grooming mothers were differently regulated by their specific transcription factors, and that the rates of genetic expression of these transcription molecules were in turn modified by a process of methylation within the chromatin layer that surrounds and controls which genes will be available for activation (Weaver et al., 2004). These findings link variation within normally occurring levels of mother–infant interactions to molecular processes regulating gene expression in the developing young.

But how are the behavioral interactions translated into changes in the brain of the infant and how are the changes maintained into adulthood? The question of how early attachment patterns in humans are established and maintained was posed by Main (1999) in an epilogue to the first edition of this handbook as an area in our understanding of attachment suffering from an "embarrassing poverty of information" (p. 849). This gap was equally present in the animal work until 2006, when two important discoveries were made.

Fenoglio, Chen, and Baram (2006) reported that the changes in brain systems known to be primarily involved in the integration of adrenocortical and behavioral stress responses (central nucleus of the amygdala, thalamic paraventricular area, and bed nucleus of the stria terminalis) were specifically activated in pups by high levels of maternal grooming that took place when pups were returned to their mothers after handling. One grooming bout produced minor changes, but after recurrent daily handling during the first 9 postnatal days, there was activation in cell signaling pathways known to be involved in learning and memory storage. At PND 9, only the first steps in the pathway were involved; by PND 23, areas regulating corticosterone production showed persistent reduction in gene activation in the hypothalamic paraventricular nucleus; and by PND 45, the stress-related brain regions described above were found to show enduring changes in the activation levels of key regulatory factors and gene functions that are responsible for the full range of adrenocortical and behavioral fear responses. What these studies indicate is that an activity-dependent process, based on known mechanisms of learning, underlies the long-term developmental regulatory effects of different levels of mother–infant interaction during the early postnatal period.

Second, Meaney's research group found that differences between the two mothering types were associated with changes in a newly recognized system of gene regulation called "epigenetics" (Weaver et al., 2004). Chromatin, the complex molecular structure that supports and surrounds the long, thin DNA strands, includes several mechanisms for silencing some genes and opening others to activation (gene transcription) in response to outside signals. Two known genes in the brain cell regions known to be involved in adrenocortical responses showed evidence of modification (methylation and deacetylation) in their epigenetic regulation. And the adrenocortical changes could be reversed by specifically blocking these epigenetic modifications.

Most recently, Weaver, Meaney, and Szyf (2006) carried out a massive analysis of all the changes in gene activation in adults of the two early-experience groups. They used a new technique, the gene "chip," that allows simultaneous assessment of the activation state of all the roughly 30,000 genes in a piece of brain tissue—in this case, the hippocampus. Of the 300 genes that were differently activated in the two mothering groups, about 100 are known to be involved in cell-to-cell signaling in pathways of brain formation and function. A few are known to regulate cell metabolism and energy expenditure, and about 50% have unknown functions.

Can the cellular memory mechanism of the Baram group (Fenoglio et al., 2006) be integrated with the epigenetic changes described by the Meaney group? In the process of answering these questions in the next few years, we will learn a great deal more about the long-range developmental effects of different early mother–infant interaction patterns. What these studies have done for us is to uncover some of the component processes through which different patterns of early mother–infant interactions regulate the long-term development of physiological and behavioral systems into adulthood. Given that the number of genes involved in this long-term regulation apparently number in the hundreds, it seems likely that the effects of different early mother–infant interaction patterns are more extensive and may well involve more systems than those already identified.

We can speculate from clinical observations of humans that attachment patterns tend to be repeated by daughters in the next generation—an effect thought to be mediated by processes of psychological representation (Bowlby's "internal working model"). Now we have good evidence for underlying biological processes in this transgenerational process as well. Meaney's group (Cameron et al., 2005) has gone on to find that mothers with high and low interaction levels pass these different maternal behavior patterns on to their daughters, along with the different levels of adult adrenocortical and fear responses. This transgenerational effect on maternal behavior is beginning to be linked to the effects of maternal interaction patterns on 1-week-old pups' developing brain systems (estrogen-induced oxytocin receptors) in the area most central to later maternal behavior, the preoptic area (Champagne, Diorio, Sharma, & Meaney, 2001).

How do these widespread biological effects fit into the evolutionary perspective on attachment described at the beginning of this section? The changes in offspring physiology and behavior generated by the two different mother–infant interaction types showed widespread, recognizable "preadaptations" to two different kinds of environments. Low levels of maternal interaction resulted in more fearful adult offspring with heightened startle responses and intense adrenocortical responses to stress. Their capacity for avoidance learning was enhanced, whereas their spatial learning and memory were relatively impaired, as reflected in slower hippocampal synapse growth. In addition to transmitting their own low-level maternal behavior pattern to their offspring, young adults in this group also showed more rapid sexual maturation (vaginal opening), greater sexual receptivity, more rapidly repeated sexual encounters, and a higher rate of pregnancy following mating than offspring of high-interaction-level mothers. These differences appear to be suited to a harsh, unpredictable, and threatening environment with few resources—an environment in which intense defensive responses, fearful avoidance of threats, and early, increased sexual activity will be likely to result in maximal survival and more offspring born in the next generation. In this way, the developmental mechanisms, previously described, that support this form of "soft" inheritance will have been selected during evolution.

High levels of mother–infant interaction in turn lead to a pattern of slower sexual development, more exploration than fear of novelty, a predisposition to learn spatial maps rather than avoidance responses, and lower levels of adrenocortical responses—traits that would be liabilities in very harsh environments, but that allow optimal adaptation to a stable, supportive environment with abundant new opportunities and resources.

This remarkable research is revealing a network of biological processes—extending down to the regulatory mechanisms within the genome—that appear to be developmental and evolutionary precursors of the psychological processes, such as enduring mental representations, that are fundamental to concepts of human attachment. From an evolutionary perspective, maternal behavior not only prepares an infant for its likely adult environment, but can exert a transgenerational propagation of maternal behavior, extending effects into a third generation. These developmental mechanisms of inheritance are not "Lamarckian" because they do not involve the germline genes, and, unlike that of genetic mutations, their inheritance does not depend on more permanent changes in DNA. They provide a more limited but also more flexible way of passing biological information from one generation to the next, resembling the cultural inheritance of ideas, beliefs, and psychological predispositions. They fit remarkably well with previous human studies of transgenerational continuity in attachment patterns (e.g., Main, Kaplan, & Cassidy, 1985).

APPLYING THE NEW TOOLS OF MOLECULAR BIOLOGY

As discussed above, the tools of molecular biology have opened up an entirely new route of approach to the biology of attachment. Now it is even pos-

sible to manipulate the genes themselves that are thought to regulate the biology and behavioral processes of attachment and separation. The basic approach is to manipulate the genetic instructions of those genes whose products are thought by prior research to be mediators of attachment behaviors. One of the major insights of molecular biology is that genes—once viewed as static repositories of the information contained in the organism's basic plan, akin to a house's blueprint that is rolled up and stored away after construction—are now known to be active participants in all cellular processes throughout life, whose ongoing contributions are regulated from moment to moment. The regulated activity of genes directs everything from cell and tissue differentiation to organogenesis and neurogenesis, and after birth it modulates all ongoing behavior, responding to changes in the organism's entire environment and in each cell's unique local environment. The environment signals the genes through numerous chemical messengers that make their way to the nucleus and its DNA.

Through molecular engineering, we can manipulate the information contained in the genes in several ways. We can delete a gene (i.e., knock it out) and infer directly the function of that gene on attachment or any other behavior by seeing what behaviors are then dysfunctional or absent. We can add a gene to the animal's DNA (a "transgene"), so that the animal makes extra amounts of the gene product; we can thereby infer the gene's function by seeing what behaviors are enhanced, or potentially diminished, by the molecular superabundance. Finally, we can add copies of a gene that makes a nonfunctional product, which dominates the endogenous gene's normal product and thereby disables the system for which the gene is responsible (a "transdominant negative").

However, straightforward genetic manipulations like these are limited, because they may give "false-negative" results. Developmental compensation mechanisms may be activated in response to the mutation, or "false-positive" results may be due to the mutation occurring in brain regions responsible for nonspecific behavioral disruptions. To overcome these problems, we have at hand two techniques that are tremendously useful for studying precisely how the brain influences behavioral development. First, we can target our genetic manipulations to specific parts of the brain, and we can turn the gene's activity on or off by throwing molecular switches to start or stop its transcription into messenger RNA—the secondary instructions that are then translated into the protein product.

These spatial and temporal controls over transcription of the mutation are accomplished by exploiting the specificity of "promoter regions" on genes. These are noncoding regions of the DNA lying upstream of the coding regions, which serve as sites for the DNA to receive specific chemical messengers. When a messenger molecule makes contact with a specific promoter region that is sensitive to it, it binds to the DNA at this point, thereby instigating the RNA polymerase to start transcribing the downstream coding regions of the DNA. By engineering our knockouts and transgenic mice with specific promoters, which respond only to chemical messengers found in specific brain regions, we can control where in the brain the genetic mutation will be expressed. Likewise, by spiking the animals' food or water with a bit of the molecular switch that represses or derepresses the gene's promoter, we can start or stop transcription of a genetically modified gene at will.

The application of these powerful techniques has only just begun. The following are the few cases in which a candidate gene has been studied for its role in filial attachment behaviors by using one of these methods. There are other cases—a few examples of which are also described below—in which gene candidates for behaviors related to attachment, such as fear, anxiety, and learned safety, have been studied by these methods, and in particular in which candidate genes for the development of emotional behavior have been expressed in specific brain regions of interest and at specific times during development. We discuss these examples, and then consider the implications of these early studies for the future of the field.

Although these kinds of studies are exciting, they mark the start of an investigation, not the end. Linking genes directly to attachment-related behaviors through genetic manipulation can tell us what molecules a young mammal needs to set up a fully functional filial attachment system. It cannot tell us *how* these molecules are used in making the system or *what* they do for the system. This matter is much more complex and sets the molecular biologist on a path that can involve many experiments to discover the role of the molecule of interest in the development of attachment behavior.

These new methods are so powerful that they illustrate how methodological advances can change fundamental concepts (Shair, Barr, & Hofer, 1991). There has been lingering doubt as to how good a model the rat is for infant–mother attachment, because the pups and dams readily accept same-age or same-lactating age pup and mother substitutes from the same colony. Thus rat filial attachment was thought by some not to exist, because the behaviors lack the high degree of specificity for *individuals* seen in humans (Gubernick, 1981). But the ability to model many fundamental aspects of filial attachment—such as the mosaic of behavioral, physiological, and endocrine separation responses; the formation of attachment in terms of its earliest manifestations of maternally directed orienting behaviors and maternal preference learning; and the brain substrates of these—has proven the rat to be an extremely informative animal model. Of course, there are *aspects* of attachment that can be modeled only in primates, and some that are uniquely human. However, the fundamental aspects of attachment common to all or most mammals, illustrated by the rat, can serve as the foundation for a basic biology of attachment.

Now, with the advent of molecular biology, the mouse genome, and the technology to introduce very precise mutations into the mouse oocyte's DNA, the mouse is beginning to take the stage in the study of filial attachment. Like the rat, the mouse may evoke objections that its social behavior lacks the nuances of primates, thereby limiting its use as a model of filial attachment; some may perhaps even argue that it is a step back from the rat. However, what clearly happened in the case of the rat is also happening in the case of the mouse: Powerful new methods are reshaping old concepts. In some respects, the mouse may or may not be as behaviorally sophisticated as the rat with respect to attachment. This question calls for additional basic behavioral research. At the same time, what is already known about the mouse's behavioral repertoire is that it is sufficiently sophisticated to provide a treasure trove of information about attachment if we use the techniques of molecular biology.

Only a few genetic models of the impact of filial behavior of infants and juvenile mice have so far been studied. Two are described here. In one, our collaborators knocked out the gene for glutaminase type 1 (GLS1), which is the enzyme responsible for most of the brain's main excitatory neurotransmitter, glutamate (Masson et al., 2006). Newborns that lack both copies of the gene (also called "null" or "knockout" mice) die within a day or two after birth, lacking milk in the stomach, whereas their siblings that have one copy of the gene (i.e., the heterozygotes) survive and develop, on gross inspection, normally.

Our studies of maternally directed orienting behaviors in the GLS1 animals shed light on the mechanism of death in the nulls and suggested a more complex view of the heterozygotes. We found that the nulls' failure to obtain milk was not due simply to behavioral debilitation. They were as active as their heterozygote and wild-type littermates, but the nulls' maternally directed orienting behaviors were disorganized. Specifically, after supinating under the mother's ventrum, the nulls failed to maintain the supine orientation. They also emitted far too little audible calling (barking) when encountering the mother, whereas they engaged in undirected and inappropriately high frequencies of mouthing and licking, even when not in the mother's presence. All of these behavioral anomalies suggest either that the nulls fail to recognize the mother or cannot organize an appropriate response to her.

Furthermore, the nulls' sleep–wake states were dysregulated. The wild-type littermates slept twice as much in the control test condition without the mother as they did when under the mother's ventrum, indicating that they were appropriately stimulated to wakefulness when encountering the mother. By contrast, the nulls slept less than the wild types and their sleep was unaffected by the presence of the mother. Thus the nulls' deficiency of the excitatory transmitter glutamate did not result in a simple generalized deficiency of maternally directed behaviors or wakefulness. Rather, it caused dysregulated expressions of these behaviors, which may be evidence of deficits in sensory processing or in central integration, severe enough to prevent nursing and contribute to neonatal mortality.

The heterozygotes had a behavioral phenotype intermediate between the nulls and wild types on all measures, demonstrating that they were not in fact "normal." Their mild deficit of glutamate neurotransmission caused them to hold the supine orientation under the mother's belly for less than half the amount of time typical of the wild types. This particular maternally directed orienting behavior—which brings the pup into ventrum-to-ventrum contact with the dam and is critical for the pup to be able to locate a nipple and nurse, and the absence of which is devastating for the null mouse—is evidently effective even in lesser amounts than normal, enabling the heterozygote pups to compete well enough for nipples and maternal contact with their wild-type siblings to survive and grow. New evidence indicates that as adults, the heterozygotes have deficient baseline activity in the hippocampus (a brain region needed for spatial learning and explicit memory), as measured by functional magnetic resonance imaging. Likewise, they fail to properly activate their frontal cortex (a brain region needed for attention, working memory, and cognitive flexibility) when pharmacologically challenged with a glutamate receptor antagonist. The causal chain of events leading to these adult deficits are unknown, but searching for the mechanisms is typical of the research that will increasingly occupy us as we pursue genetic models of attachment. We will want to know whether the adult deficits are direct effects of the glutamate deficiency or are caused by the relative deficiency of filial interaction with the mother.

Another study examined the effects of the gene for the mu opioid receptor on the infant mouse's isolation-induced USV. As described earlier, USV is a behavior that is functionally and pharmacologically analogous to the human infant's separation call and is regarded as a necessary indicator of the establishment of a filial attachment relationship (Hofer, 1996). A large pharmacological literature shows that the mu receptor mediates the behavioral and physiological effects of many natural rewards. On the basis of some pharmacological studies, the mu receptor has been hypothesized also to mediate the infant's response to social isolation. However, the pharmacological evidence is controversial; thus the genetic model was investigated as an important alternative perspective. Isolation-induced USV was recorded for knockout infant mice lacking both copies of the mu receptor gene and for wild-type controls (Moles, Kieffer, & D'Amato, 2004). The knockouts exhibited significantly less USV during the first 2 postnatal weeks of life, and they failed to "potentiate" their calling rates after being reexposed briefly to their mothers and then isolated again. However, the knockouts' sensitivity to physically or socially threatening stimuli was not impaired: They responded to isolation in a cold environment and to isolation in the presence of the odor of a strange male with robust USVs, as did the wild types. Nor were the knockouts grossly deficient in olfactory competence. Thus this study of the mu receptor knockout mouse lends support to the hypothesis that the mu opioid receptor in the infant plays a specific role in pathways that mediate the reinforcing properties of maternal stimuli. Neither of these knockout studies is definitive; as with all methods, replications and convergent evidence are required. However, these studies represent the leading edge of a barrage of emerging work on the effects of specific candidate genes on the formation and competence of filial behaviors.

A third study illustrates two other approaches taken in molecular studies to shed light on attachment (Gross et al., 2002). The investigators used a genetic model to examine the development of an emotion, anxiety, that figures critically in the development of attachment. In this study, the investigators knocked out the gene for one of the receptors for serotonin—a neurotransmitter that is central to the maintenance of normal mood and affect and, when dysfunctional, permits pathological states of anxiety and depression. The particular receptor knocked out was the serotonin 1A receptor, whose action has anxiolytic properties. The knockout mouse was demonstrably more anxious than the wild type (normal), as measured on behavioral tests of anxiety; these tests included exploration versus wall hugging in a novel open and therefore anxiety-provoking field, and willingness to sample food placed in the center of the open field. The researchers used a molecular rescue strategy to turn the knocked-out gene's expression back on in the mouse's forebrain, and were able to control the timing of this rescue. They found that expression of this gene (and hence production of serotonin 1A receptors) in the forebrain, during just the first 2 weeks of the mouse's postnatal life, was sufficient to restore normal emotional responsiveness in adulthood. This postnatal window is equivalent neurodevelopmentally and experientially to the human third trimester and infancy.

The potential implications of this finding for filial attachment are clear. First, the work urges a reexamination in new ways of old questions about sensitive periods. The new research tools permit us to determine, at the molecular level, the quality, quantity, and timing of developmental provisions that support the emergence of normal emotional capacities. In addition, because anxiety is the affect most closely connected to separation, and because this work shows that anxiety's neural substrate forms when filial attachment is the infant's main environmental experience, we must ask whether attachment experiences shape the nascent brain substrates for anxiety. We know that experiences of maternal separation or variations in maternal behavior in infant rodents reprogram the stress axis, leading to altered levels of anxiety and stress responsiveness in adulthood (Cameron et al., 2005; Meaney et al., 1996). Meaney and others have hypothesized that maternal separation, and the altered patterns of maternal behavior that occur with reunion, are transduced in part by the

pups' serotonin systems. The serotonin 1A receptor knockout mouse provides evidence that serotonin is indeed a key player in the mechanism by which altered separation and attachment experiences in infancy can reprogram the stress axis and its affective manifestation, anxiety.

PERSPECTIVES FOR FUTURE RESEARCH

We concluded our chapter in the first edition of this handbook (Polan & Hofer, 1999b) with a set of questions for future investigation. Some of these have been partially answered as explained above. We now propose a new set of questions, arising in part from the answers to the old ones and in part from the new perspectives that the molecular methods have opened up.

• Are the processes of olfactory learning and stress axis programming during the sensitive period reversible? If so, what implications might this have for the treatment of abuse, neglect, and early abandonment?

• What is the precise relation between the development of proximity seeking and separation or loss responses? Is the achievement of one necessary for the emergence of the other? If so, what mechanisms link them?

• Are there genetically based differences in the neural and endocrine substrates for attachment and separation processes? How might these interact with the environmental and genetic mechanisms described above? Does such genetically based variation in the population confer an evolutionary advantage on the species by producing individuals suited to environments that change unpredictably?

• What is the relation of later-differentiated affects to early primitive affective states, such as norepinephrine-mediated activation, benzodiazepine-receptor-mediated separation and comfort responses, and serotonin-mediated anxiety?

• What is the relation between filial preferences and other social attachments through the life cycle, such as mate selection ("sexual imprinting") and parental behavior? Do early experiential and/or biological substrate characteristics influence the quality (security) of attachment in infancy and adulthood?

• Are there commonalities between the known biological substrates of attachment and the neurodevelopmental disorders that have long been thought to involve deficits in attachment, such as autism and schizophrenia? If so, will knowledge of these lead to advances in treatment or prevention of these often devastating disorders?

Clinical research on human infant attachment is coming of age. Attachment has already acquired status as a causal agent; its disturbances are often hypothesized to contribute to social and psychological pathologies of childhood (DeKlyen & Greenberg, Chapter 27, this volume; Lyons-Ruth & Jacobvitz, Chapter 28, this volume; Main, 1996). At this juncture, it is critical for basic researchers to provide clinical researchers and clinicians with clarity concerning the biobehavioral origins of attachment. In the first edition, we argued that the concept of filial attachment in infant rats has come of age. We now advance the view that the mouse model must be embraced for its provision of previously unimagined molecular and evolutionary insights.

REFERENCES

Belsky, J. (1999). Modern evolutionary theory and patterns of attachment. In J. Cassidy & P. R. Shaver (Eds.), *Handbook of attachment: Theory, research, and clinical applications* (pp. 141–161). New York: Guilford Press.

Bowlby, J. (1969/1982). *Attachment and loss: Vol. 1. Attachment* (2nd ed.). New York: Basic Books.

Bowlby, J. (1973). *Attachment and loss: Vol. 2. Separation: Anxiety and anger.* New York: Basic Books.

Cameron, N. M., Champagne, F. A., Carine, P., Fish, E. W., Ozaki-Kuroda, K., & Meaney, M. J. (2005). The programming of individual differences in defensive responses and reproductive strategies in the rat through variations in maternal care. *Neuroscience and Biobehavioral Reviews, 29,* 843–865.

Camp, L. L., & Rudy, J. W. (1988). Changes in the categorization of appetitive and aversive events during postnatal development of the rat. *Developmental Psychobiology, 21,* 25–42.

Carroll, S. B. (2005). *Endless forms most beautiful: The new science of evo devo and the making of the animal kingdom.* New York: Norton.

Champagne, F., Diorio, J., Sharma, S., & Meaney, M. J. (2001). Variations in maternal care in the rat are associated with differences in estrogen-rated changes in oxytocin receptor levels. *Proceedings of the National Academy of Sciences USA, 98,* 12736–12741.

Fenoglio, K. A., Chen, Y., & Baram, T. Z. (2006). Neuroplasticity of the hypothalamic–pituitary–adrenal axis early in life requires recurrent recruitments of stress-regulating brain regions. *Journal of Neuroscience, 26,* 2434–2442.

Field, T. M., Schanberg, S. M., Scafidi, F., Bauer, C. R., Vega-Lahr, N., Garcia, R., et al. (1986). Tactile/kinesthetic stimulation effects on preterm neonates. *Pediatrics, 77,* 654–658.

Gregory, E. H., & Pfaff, D. W. (1971). Development of olfactory guided behavior in infant rats. *Physiology and Behavior, 6,* 573–576.

Gross, C., Zhuang, X., Stark, K., Ramboz, S., Oosting, R., Kirby, K., et al. (2002). Serotonin 1A receptor acts during development to establish normal anxiety-like behaviour in the adult. *Nature, 416,* 396–400.

Gubernick, D. J. (1981). Parent and infant attachment in mammals. In D. J. Gubernick & P. H. Klopfer (Eds.), *Parental care in mammals* (pp. 272–273). New York: Plenum Press.

Hepper, P. G. (1987). The amniotic fluid: An important priming role in kin recognition. *Animal Behaviour, 35,* 1343–1346.

Hofer, M. A. (1994). Early relationships as regulators of infant physiology and behavior. *Acta Paediatrica Supplement, 397*(Suppl.), 9–18.

Hofer, M. A. (1996). Multiple regulators of ultrasonic vocalization in the infant rat. *Psychoneuroendocrinology, 21,* 203–217.

Hofer, M. A., & Shair, H. N. (1991). Trigeminal and olfactory pathways mediating isolation distress and companion comfort responses in rat pups. *Behavioral Neuroscience, 105,* 699–706.

Johanson, I. B., Turkewitz, G., & Hamburgh, M. (1980). Development of home orientation in hypothyroid and hyperthyroid rat pups. *Developmental Psychobiology, 13,* 331–342.

Kaufman, J., Yang, B.-Z., Douglas-Palumberi, H., Houshyar, S., Lipschitz, D., Krystal, J. H., et al. (2004). Social supports and serotonin transporter gene moderate depression in maltreated children. *Proceedings of the National Academy of Sciences USA, 101,* 17316–17321.

Kuhn, C. M., & Schanberg, S. M. (1998). Responses to maternal separation: Mechanisms and mediators. *International Journal of Developmental Neuroscience, 16,* 261–270.

Leon, M. (1992). The neurobiology of filial learning. *Annual Review of Psychology, 43,* 377–398.

Main, M. (1996). Introduction to the special section on attachment and psychopathology: 2. Overview of the field of attachment. *Journal of Consulting and Clinical Psychology, 64,* 237–243.

Main, M. (1999). Epilogue: Attachment theory: Eighteen points with suggestions for further studies. In J. Cassidy & P. R. Shaver (Eds.), *Handbook of attachment: Theory, research, and clinical applications* (pp. 845–887). New York: Guilford Press.

Main, M., Kaplan, N., & Cassidy, J. (1985). Security in infancy, childhood, and adulthood: A move to the level of representation. In I. Bretherton & E. Waters (Eds.), Growing points of attachment theory and research. *Monographs of the Society for Research in Child Development, 50*(1–2, Serial No. 209), 66–104.

Masson, J., Darmon, M., Conjard, A., Chuhma, N., Ropert, N., Thoby-Brisson, M., et al. (2006). Mice lacking brain/kidney phosphate-activated glutaminase have impaired glutamatergic synaptic transmission, altered breathing, disorganized goal-directed behavior and die shortly after birth. *Journal of Neuroscience, 26*, 4660–4671.

Meaney, M. J., & Aitken, D. H. (1985). The effects of early postnatal handling on hippocampal glucocorticoid receptor concentrations: Temporal parameters. *Brain Research, 354*, 301–304.

Meaney, M. J., Diorio, J., Francis, D., Widdowson, J., LaPlante, P., Caldji, C., et al. (1996). Early environmental regulation of forebrain glucocorticoid receptor gene expression: Implications for adrenocortical responses to stress. *Developmental Neuroscience, 18*, 49–72.

Moles, A., Kieffer, B. L., & D'Amato, F. R. (2004). Deficit in attachment behavior in mice lacking the mu-opioid receptor gene. *Science, 304*, 1983–1986.

Moriceau, S., & Sullivan, R. M. (2005). Neurobiology of infant attachment. *Developmental Psychobiology, 47*, 230–242.

Moriceau, S., Wilson, D. A., Levine, S., & Sullivan, R. M. (2006). Dual circuitry for odor–shock conditioning during infancy: Corticosterone switches between fear and attraction via amygdala. *Journal of Neuroscience, 26*, 6737–6748.

Myers, M. M., Brunelli, S. A., Shair, H. N., Squire, J. M., & Hofer, M. A. (1989). Relationships between maternal behavior of SHR and WKY dams and adult blood pressures of cross-fostered F1 pups. *Developmental Psychobiology, 22*, 55–67.

Nyakas, C., & Endroczi, E. (1970). Olfaction guided approaching behaviour of infantile rats to the mother in maze box. *Acta Physiologica Academiae Scientiarum Hungaricae, 38*, 59–65.

Polan, H. J., & Hofer, M. A. (1998). Olfactory preference for mother over home nest shavings by newborn rats. *Developmental Psychobiology, 33*, 5–20.

Polan, H. J., & Hofer, M. A. (1999a). Maternally-directed orienting behaviors of newborn rats. *Developmental Psychobiology, 34*, 269–279.

Polan, H. J., & Hofer, M. A. (1999b). Psychobiological origins of infant attachment and separation responses. In J. Cassidy & P. R. Shaver (Eds.), *Handbook of attachment: Theory, research, and clinical applications* (pp. 162–180). New York: Guilford Press.

Polan, H. J., Milano, D., Eljuga, L., & Hofer, M. A. (2002). Development of rats' maternally-directed orienting from birth to day 2. *Developmental Psychobiology, 40*, 81–103.

Scott, J. P. (1963). Process of primary socialization in canine and human infants. *Monographs of the Society for Research in Child Development, 28*(1, Serial No. 85), 1–47.

Shair, H. N., Barr, G. A., & Hofer, M. A. (Eds.). (1991). *Developmental psychobiology: New methods and changing concepts.* New York: Oxford University Press.

Simpson, J. A. (1999). Attachment theory in modern evolutionary perspective. In J. Cassidy & P. R. Shaver (Eds.), *Handbook of attachment: Theory, research, and clinical applications* (pp. 115–140). New York: Guilford Press.

Sullivan, R. M. (1996, November). *Neural correlates of neonatal olfactory learning.* Paper presented at the meeting of the International Society for Developmental Psychobiology, Washington, DC.

Sullivan, R. M., & Hall, W. G. (1988). Reinforcers in infancy: Classical conditioning using stroking or intra-oral infusions of milk as UCS. *Developmental Psychobiology, 21*, 215–223.

Sullivan, R. M., Hofer, M. A., & Brake, S. (1986). Olfactory-guided orientation in neonatal rats is enhanced by a conditioned change in behavioral state. *Developmental Psychobiology, 19*, 615–623.

Sullivan, R. M., Landers, M., Yeaman, B., & Wilson, D. A. (2000). Good memories of bad events in infancy. *Nature, 407*, 38–39.

Weaver, I. C., Cervoni, N., Champagne, F. A., D'Alessio, A. C., Sharma, S., Seckl, J. R., et al. (2004). Epigenetic programming by maternal behavior. *Nature Neuroscience, 7*, 847–854.

Weaver, I. C., Meaney, M. J., & Szyf, M. (2006). Maternal care effects on the hippocampal transcriptome and anxiety-mediated behaviors in the offspring that are reversible in adulthood. *Proceedings of the National Academy of Sciences USA, 103*, 3480–3486.

Wilson, D. A., & Sullivan, R. M. (1994). Neurobiology of associative learning in the neonate: Early olfactory learning. *Behavioral and Neural Biology, 61*, 1–18.

CHAPTER 8

Attachment in Rhesus Monkeys

STEPHEN J. SUOMI

Attachment is not an exclusively human phenomenon. Although the theory that John Bowlby developed during the 1950s and 1960s and refined during the 1970s reflected his clinical observations of infants and young children, it also had a strong biological foundation that stemmed in large part from his long-standing interest in ethological studies of developmental phenomena in animals, especially nonhuman primates (van der Horst, van der Veer, & van IJzendoorn, 2007). Indeed, it can be argued that Bowlby (1969/1982) specifically tailored the basic biological features of his attachment theory to account for clear-cut commonalities in the strong behavioral and emotional ties that infants typically develop with their mothers—not only across virtually all of humanity, but also among our closest evolutionary relatives.

At about the time that Bowlby published, with James Robertson, his seminal studies of mother–infant separation via hospitalization (Robertson & Bowlby, 1952), he was also becoming familiar with the classic ethological studies of filial imprinting in precocial birds. During this period, he developed a close friendship with Cambridge University ethologist Robert Hinde, who at that time was in the process of shifting his own basic research interests from song learning in birds

to mother–infant interactions in rhesus monkeys. Hinde soon had rhesus monkey mothers raising babies in small captive social groups (e.g., Hinde, Rowell, & Spencer-Booth, 1964), and Bowlby came to recognize patterns of behavior shown by the infant monkeys toward their mothers—but not toward other adult females in the group—that strikingly resembled recurrent response patterns of human infants and young children he had observed over years of clinical practice (van der Horst et al., 2007). These common patterns provided Bowlby with powerful evidence supporting his basic assumption that attachment has its foundation in biology.

Indeed, virtually all of the classic features of human infant behavior that Bowlby's attachment theory specifically ascribed to our evolutionary history could be clearly observed in the patterns of mother-directed activity exhibited by rhesus monkey infants, as described by Hinde and other primate researchers. For Bowlby (1958, 1969/1982), the fact that rhesus monkey infants and human babies share unique physical features, behavioral propensities, and emotional labilities linked to highly specific social situations was consistent with the view that they also share significant parts of their respective evolutionary histories. He argued that these features, present in newborns of each species but often largely absent (or at least largely obscured) in older individuals, reflect successful adaptations to selective pressures over millions of years. To Bowlby, those characteristics common to both human and monkey infants represent evolutionary success stories and should be viewed as beneficial, if not essential, for promoting the survival of both the individual infant and the species.

What are those common characteristics, and what is their relevance for attachment theory? This chapter begins by describing how attachment relationships between rhesus monkey infants and their mothers are typically established and maintained throughout development. Next, those features that are unique to attachment relationships are examined, as is conflict within these relationships. Attachment relationships in rhesus monkeys and other primates are subject to influence from a variety of sources, and some of these influences are reviewed next. Some long-term behavioral and biological consequences of different early attachment experiences are then examined in detail. Finally, the implications for attachment theory of recent findings regarding cross-generational transmission of specific attachment patterns in rhesus monkey families are discussed.

NORMATIVE PATTERNS OF INFANT–MOTHER ATTACHMENT IN RHESUS MONKEYS

The first detailed longitudinal studies of species-normative attachment relationships in rhesus monkeys were carried out over 40 years ago (e.g., Hansen, 1966; Harlow, Harlow, & Hansen, 1963; Hinde & Spencer-Booth, 1967). These seminal investigations provided descriptions of infant behavioral development and emerging social relationships that not only appear remarkably accurate today, but also have repeatedly been shown to generalize to other rhesus monkey infants growing up across a variety of naturalistic settings, as well as to infants of other Old World monkey and ape species (see Higley & Suomi, 1986, for one of many comprehensive reviews). Virtually all infants in these species spend their initial days, weeks, and (for infant apes) months of life in near-continuous physical contact with their biological mothers, typically clinging to their mothers' ventral surface for most of their waking (and virtually all of their sleeping) hours each day.

Newborn rhesus monkeys clearly and consistently display four of the five "component instinctual responses" that Bowlby (1958) listed as universal human attachment behaviors in his initial monograph on attachment: sucking, clinging, crying, and following (the fifth, smiling, is seen in chimpanzee but not monkey infants). Rhesus monkey infants, like human infants, are also able to imitate specific facial expressions of their mothers shortly after birth (Ferrari et al., 2006). All of these response patterns reflect efforts on the part of an infant to obtain and maintain physical contact with or proximity to its mother.

Rhesus monkey mothers, in turn, provide their newborns with essential nourishment; physical and psychological warmth (e.g., Harlow, 1958); and protection from the elements, potential predators, and even other members of the infants' immediate families (e.g., jealous older siblings). During this time a strong and enduring social bond inevitably develops between a mother and infant—a bond that is unique in terms of its exclusivity, constituent behavioral features, and ultimate duration. The attachment bond that a rhesus monkey infant typically develops with its mother is like no other social relationship it will ever experience during the rest of its life, except (in reciprocal form) for a female when she grows up to have infants of her own. For a male infant this bond will last at least until puberty, whereas for a female it will be maintained as long as mother and daughter are both alive (Suomi, 1995).

In their second month of life, most rhesus monkey infants start using their mothers as a "secure base" from which to begin exploring their immediate physical and social environment. At this age monkey infants are inherently curious (Harlow, 1953), and most attempt to leave their mothers for brief periods as soon as they become physically capable of doing so. Mothers typically monitor these attempts quite closely, and they often physically restrain their infants' efforts—or retrieve them if they have wandered beyond arm's length—at the slightest sign of potential danger. Several studies (e.g., Hinde & White, 1974) have demonstrated that at this stage of an infant's development, the mother is primarily responsible for maintaining mutual contact and/or proximity. With the emergence of social fear in the infant's emotional repertoire between 2 and 3 months of age—functionally and developmentally equivalent to the emergence of "stranger anxiety" in 8- to 12-month-old human infants (Sackett, 1966; Suomi & Harlow, 1976)—this pattern reverses, and thereafter the infant is primarily responsible for maintaining proximity and initiating physical contact with its mother. Once an infant monkey has become securely attached to its mother and begins to use her as an established base from which to make exploratory ventures toward stimuli that have caught its interest, it soon learns that if it becomes frightened or is otherwise threatened by the stimuli it has sought out, it can always run back to its mother, who usually is able to provide immediate safety and comfort via mutual ventral contact. Initiation of ventral contact with the mother has been shown to promote rapid decreases in the infant's hypothalamic–pituitary–adrenocortical (HPA) activity (as indexed by lowered plasma cortisol concentrations) and in sympathetic nervous system arousal (as indexed by reductions in heart rate), along with other physiological changes commonly associated with soothing (e.g., Gunnar, Gonzalez, Goodlin, & Levine, 1981; Mendoza, Smotherman, Miner, Kaplan, & Levine, 1978; Reite, Short, Seiler, & Pauley, 1981; see Cassidy, Chapter 1, this volume, for discussion of Bowlby's concept of the secure base in humans).

As they grow older, most monkey infants voluntarily spend increasing amounts of time at increasing distances from their mothers, apparently confident that they can return to their mothers' protective care without interruption or delay should circumstances so warrant. The presence of their mothers as a secure base clearly promotes exploration of their ever-expanding physical and social world (Dienske & Metz, 1977; Harlow et al., 1963; Simpson, 1979). On the other hand, when rhesus monkey infants develop less than optimal attachment relationships with their mothers, their exploratory behavior is inevitably compromised (e.g., Arling & Harlow, 1967; McCormack, Sanchez, Bardi, & Maestripieri, 2006); this is consistent with Bowlby's observations regarding human attachment relationships (e.g., Bowlby, 1969/1982, 1988), as will be discussed later.

At approximately 3 months of age, monkey infants start developing distinctive social relationships with other members of their social group. Increasingly, these come to involve their peers—other infants of similar age and comparable physical, cognitive, and socioemotional capabilities. After weaning (usually in the fourth and fifth months) and essentially until puberty (during the third or fourth year), play with peers represents the predominant social activity for young monkeys (Ruppenthal, Harlow, Eisele, Harlow, & Suomi, 1974). During this time, social play becomes increasingly gender-specific and sex-segregated; that is, males tend to play more with males, and females with females (Harlow & Lauersdorf, 1974). Play interactions with peers also become more and more behaviorally and socially complex, such that

by the third year the play bouts typically involve patterns of behavior that appear to simulate almost the entire range of adult social activity (e.g., Suomi & Harlow, 1975). By the time they reach puberty, most rhesus monkey juveniles have had ample opportunity to develop, practice, and perfect behavioral routines that will become crucial for normal functioning in adult life, especially patterns involved in reproduction and in dominance/aggressive interactions (Suomi, 1979b). Virtually all of them will also have maintained close ties with their mothers throughout their juvenile years (e.g., Berman, 1982).

The onset of puberty is associated with major life transitions for both male and female rhesus monkeys. Adolescence is associated not only with major hormonal alterations, pronounced growth spurts, and other obvious physical changes, but also with major social changes for both sexes (Suomi, Rasmussen, & Higley, 1992). Males experience the most dramatic and serious social disruption: They typically leave their natal troop, severing all social ties not only with their mothers and other kin, but also with all others in that troop. Virtually all of these adolescent males soon join all-male "gangs," and after several months most of them then attempt to enter a different troop, typically composed entirely of individuals largely unfamiliar to the adolescent males. Field studies have revealed substantial individual differences among these males in the timing of their emigration, in the basic strategies they follow in attempting to join other established social groups, and in their ultimate success or failure in these efforts (Howell et al., 2007; Mehlman et al., 1995). Adolescent females, by contrast, almost never leave their maternal family or natal social group (Lindburg, 1971). Puberty for them is instead associated with increases in social activities directed toward maternal kin, typically at the expense of interactions with unrelated peers. Rhesus monkey females continue to be involved in family social affairs for the rest of their lives, even after they cease having infants of their own. Thus their experiences with specific attachment relationships tend to be lifelong (Suomi, 1998).

UNIQUE ASPECTS OF PRIMATE INFANT–MOTHER ATTACHMENT RELATIONSHIPS

Is infant–mother attachment fundamentally different from the other social relationships a young rhesus monkey (or, for that matter, a human infant) will establish during its lifetime? Clearly, some aspects of the attachment relationship are exclusive to the mother–infant dyad, because the mother is the exclusive source not only for all that passes through the placenta but also for a prenatal environment uniquely attuned to her own circadian and other biological rhythms. In addition, there is increasing evidence of predictable fetal reactions that can be traced to specific activities (including vocalizations) of the mother, perhaps providing the basis for exclusive multimodal proto-communication between mother and fetus (e.g., Busnell & Granier-Deferre, 1981; DeCasper & Fifer, 1980; Fifer, 1987; Novak, 2006; Schneider, 1992). Such types of prenatal stimulation are, of course, routinely (and exclusively) provided by pregnant females in all placental mammalian species.

Some of these unique aspects of maternal support and stimulation are basically continued into an infant's initial postnatal weeks and months, including obviously the mother's status as the primary (if not sole) source of its nutrition. Mothers also keep sharing their own specific antibodies with their infants postnatally via the nursing process. Moreover, the essentially continuous contact or proximity between a mother and her newborn provides the infant with extended exposure to its mother's odor, taste (of milk, at least), relative warmth, sound, and sight, representing a range and intensity of social stimulation seldom if ever provided by any other family or group members. In addition, rhesus monkey mothers continue to communicate their internal circadian and other biological rhythms to their offspring via extended ventral–ventral contact, and there is some evidence that their offspring typically develop synchronous parallel rhythms during their initial weeks of life (Boyce, Champoux, Suomi, & Gunnar, 1995). As before, these maternally specific postnatal aspects of infant support and stimulation are not limited to primates, but instead are characteristic of mothers of many other mammalian species, at least until the time of weaning (e.g., Hofer, 1995; see also Polan & Hofer, Chapter 7, this volume). But other aspects of a rhesus monkey mother's relationship with her infant are not shared by all mammalian mothers, not even by mothers of some other primate species.

What are these unique features of a rhesus monkey (and human) mother's relationship with her infant? It turns out that they are the very characteristics that Bowlby made the defining features of maternal attachment: (1) the mother's ability to reduce fear in her infant via direct social contact

and other soothing behavior, and (2) the mother's capacity to provide a secure base to support her infant's exploration of the environment. Numerous longitudinal studies of rhesus monkey social ontogeny, carried out in both laboratory and field environments, have consistently found that mothers have a virtual monopoly on these capabilities—or at least on the opportunity to express them with their infants (e.g., Berman, 1982; Harlow & Harlow, 1965). Thus rhesus monkey infants rarely if ever use other group members (even close relatives) as secure bases, or even as reliable sources of ventral contact (Suomi, 1979a). Moreover, on those occasions when they "mistakenly" seek the company of someone other than their own mothers, they are unlikely to experience decreases in physiological arousal comparable to those resulting from contact with their mothers; instead, they are likely to experience *increases* in arousal. (See Coan, Chapter 11, this volume, for a discussion of a study of humans in which a woman's having her hand held by her husband reduced activation in brain regions related to autonomic arousal. The benefits were greatly reduced when her hand was held by a male experimenter rather than her husband.)

The attachment relationship a rhesus monkey infant establishes with its mother differs in additional fundamental ways from all other social relationships it will ever develop during its lifetime. As previously noted, rhesus monkeys routinely establish a host of distinctive relationships with different siblings, peers, and adults of both sexes throughout development; however, each is strikingly different from the initial attachment they establish with their mothers in terms of primacy, constituent behaviors, reciprocity, and course of developmental change (Suomi, 1979b, 2002). Given these findings, perhaps Bowlby was not entirely correct when he argued that the infant's attachment to the mother provides the *prototype* for all of its subsequent social relationships (Bowlby, 1969/1982), because (at least for rhesus monkeys) the relationship an infant establishes with its mother is like no other. On the other hand, Bowlby was absolutely correct (at least for rhesus monkeys) when he argued that the nature of the specific attachment relationship an infant develops with its mother can profoundly affect both concurrent and future relationships the infant may develop with others in its social sphere, as will be discussed in detail later.

A somewhat different issue concerns the question of whether attachment phenomena as originally defined by Bowlby generalize to other species, including other primates. As outlined above, Bowlby clearly believed that basic features of attachment phenomena are essentially homologous in rhesus monkey infants and human babies, but are these characteristic features of attachment seen in other mammalian species as well? It all depends on how one defines "attachment," or related terms such as "partner preference" or "imprinting."

Without question, infant preference for the mother (and vice versa) represents an exceedingly widespread phenomenon across most mammalian and avian species, as well as in numerous other taxa (Wilson, 1975). One specific (and, for Bowlby, a particularly relevant) form of partner preference involves "imprinting." According to Lorenz's (1937) classical definition, imprinting is restricted to those partner preferences that are (1) acquired during a critical period, (2) irreversible, (3) generally species-specific, and (4) typically established prior to any behavioral manifestation of the preference. According to a slightly broadened version of this definition, imprinting-like phenomena can be observed in numerous insect, fish, avian, and mammalian species, including most if not all primates (Immelmann & Suomi, 1981).

On the other hand, it can be argued that infant–mother attachment as originally defined by Bowlby (1958, 1969/1982) represents a special case of imprinting that may itself be limited largely to Old World monkeys, apes, and humans (Suomi, 1995). To be sure, infants of all the other primate species (i.e., prosimians and New World monkeys) are initially at least as dependent on their mothers for survival, and spend at least as much time in physical contact with them, as do rhesus monkey (and human) infants (Higley & Suomi, 1986). In these other primate species, however, the predominant form of mother–infant physical contact is usually different (dorsal–ventral vs. ventral–ventral); the frequency and diversity of mother–infant interactions are generally reduced; the patterns of developmental change are also different (often dramatically so); and, most importantly, the specific defining features of attachment are largely absent.

Consider the case of capuchin monkeys (*Cebus apella*), a highly successful New World species whose natural habitat covers much of South America, including both Amazonian and Andean regions. These primates are remarkable in many respects, not the least of which is an amazing capability for manufacturing and using tools to ma-nipulate their physical environment both in captivity and in their natural habitats (Darwin, 1794; Visalberghi, 1990; Visalberghi et al., 2007). In this respect, they are probably superior to rhesus monkeys and, for that matter, all other primates except humans and perhaps chimpanzees. On the other hand, capuchin mother–infant relationships seem somewhat primitive by rhesus monkey standards.

A capuchin monkey infant spends virtually all of its first 3 months of life clinging to its mother's back, moving ventrally only during nursing bouts (Welker, Becker, Hohman, & Schafer-Witt, 1987). During this time, there is very little visual, vocal, or grooming interaction between mother and infant—in marked contrast to rhesus monkey infants, who by 1 month of age are already actively interacting with their mothers in extensive one-on-one bouts involving a wealth of visual, auditory, olfactory, tactile, and vestibular stimulation, and who typically are already beginning to use their mothers as a secure base. When capuchin monkeys finally get off their mothers' backs in their fourth month, they seem to be surprisingly independent and can spend long periods away from their mothers without getting visibly upset. If frightened, they are almost as likely to seek protective contact from other group members as from their mothers (Byrne & Suomi, 1995). At this age and thereafter, capuchin monkey youngsters spend only about one-third as much time grooming their mothers as do young rhesus monkeys, and their other activities with their mothers are not markedly different from their activities with siblings, peers, or unrelated adults (Byrne & Suomi, 1995; Welker, Becker, & Schafer-Witt, 1990), in sharp contrast to rhesus monkeys of comparable age. All in all, capuchin monkey infants seem far less attached to their biological mothers in terms of the prominence of the relationship, the relative uniqueness of constituent behaviors, and the nature and degree of secure-base-mediated exploration. One wonders how Bowlby's attachment theory might have looked if Hinde had been studying capuchin rather than rhesus monkeys!

Comparative studies of infant–mother relationships in other New World monkey and prosimian species have found that in most cases, the relationships more closely resemble those of capuchin monkeys than those of rhesus monkeys (e.g., Fragaszy, Baer, & Adams-Curtis, 1991); in a few species (e.g., some marmosets and tamarins), the mother is not even an infant's primary caregiver (Higley & Suomi, 1986). To be sure, infants in all these primate species appear to be "imprinted" on their mothers, according to Lorenz's (1937) definition. However, attachment involves considerably more developmental complexity and reciprocity, especially with respect to secure-base phenomena, than do classical notions of imprinting. It can therefore be argued that, strictly speaking, attachment represents a special, *restricted* case of imprinting. Moreover, because infant–mother attachment is most apparent in humans and their closest phylogenetic kin, it may also represent a relatively recent evolutionary adaptation among primates (Suomi, 1995).

CONFLICT IN RHESUS MONKEY INFANT–MOTHER RELATIONSHIPS

The relationships that rhesus monkeys develop with their mothers over time involve many behavioral patterns that go beyond attachment phenomena per se (Hinde, 1976). Indeed, a rhesus monkey female is extensively involved in a wide variety of interactions with her mother virtually every day that both are alive (and a male is thus involved every day until adolescence). However, this does not mean that all of these interactions are uniformly positive and pleasant. To the contrary, conflicts between mothers and offspring are frequent and often predictable, if not inevitable, occurrences in everyday rhesus monkey social life.

Sociobiologists have long argued that although mothers and infants share many genes and (therefore) many long-term goals, their short-term interests are not always mutual, and hence periodic conflict is inevitable (Trivers, 1974). Regardless of the validity of this view, an obvious instance of parent–offspring conflict occurs for virtually every rhesus monkey infant at approximately 20 weeks of age, when its mother begins to wean it from her own milk to solid food. Whether this process begins because the mother "wants" her infant to cease nursing (so she can stop lactating, begin cycling, and be able to produce another offspring, as the sociobiologists propose); because she "knows" that she cannot continue to produce enough milk to sustain her infant's rapidly growing energy requirements; or because her infant's erupting teeth make nursing increasingly uncomfortable is certainly open to question. What *is* clear is that weaning is almost always associated with significant changes in the basic nature of the infant's relationship with its mother, and those changes are seldom placid (e.g., Hinde & White, 1974).

Mothers, for their part, make increasingly frequent efforts to deny their infants access to their nipples—albeit with considerable variation in the precise form, timing, and intensity of their weaning behavior, ranging from the exquisitely subtle to what borders on abuse. Infants, on the other hand, dramatically increase their efforts to obtain and maintain physical contact with their mothers, even when nipple contact is not attainable. As with mothers, there is substantial variation in the nature, intensity, and persistence of the infants' efforts to prevent or at least delay the weaning process (Berman, Rasmussen, & Suomi, 1993). In virtually all cases, an infant's newfound preoccupation with maintaining maternal contact clearly inhibits its exploratory behavior, and noticeably alters and diminishes its interactions with peers (and often other kin) as well. Indeed, it usually takes a month or more (if at all) before those interaction patterns return to some semblance of normality (Hinde & White, 1974; Ruppenthal et al., 1974). Weaning therefore appears to undermine basic attachment security for the infant, perhaps permanently in some cases.

Postweaning "normality" for a young rhesus monkey seldom lasts for more than a few additional weeks before a second form of conflict with its mother typically arises. Most mothers return to reproductive receptivity at about the time their infants are 6–7 months old, at which point they begin actively soliciting selected adult males for the next 2 or 3 months (rhesus monkeys are seasonal breeders in nature). Throughout this period they may enter into consort relationships with several different males, typically lasting 1–3 days each. During this time a female and her chosen partner usually leave the main body of the monkey troop for most (if not all) of the time they are together, often seeking relative seclusion to avoid harassment or other interruptions from other troop members (Manson & Perry, 1993). At the same time, the offspring from the previous year's consort tends to be ignored, actively avoided, or even physically rejected by both the mother and her current mate (Berman, Rasmussen, & Suomi, 1994).

Not surprisingly, most rhesus monkey yearlings become quite upset in the face of such functional maternal separations; indeed, a few actually develop dramatic behavioral and physiological symptoms that parallel Bowlby's (1960, 1973) descriptions of separation-induced depression in human infants and young children (Suomi, 1995). Most of their cohorts likewise exhibit an initial period of intense protest following loss of access to their mothers, but soon begin directing their attention elsewhere. Interestingly, female offspring "left behind" by their mothers during consorts tend to seek out other family members during their mothers' absence, whereas young males are more likely to increase interactions with peers while their mothers are away (Berman et al., 1994). These gender differences in the prototypical response to maternal separation at 6–7 months of age thus appear to presage the much more dramatic gender differences in life course that emerge during adolescence and continue throughout adulthood.

It would seem that a rhesus monkey mother would always have the upper hand in conflicts with her offspring during both weaning and breeding periods, given her great size and strength advantage over even the most persistent 5- to 7-month-old infant. A number of research findings, however, suggest that infants bring resources of their own into these conflicts. For example, Simpson, Simpson, Hooley, and Zunz (1981) reported that infants who remained in physical contact with their mothers more and explored less during the preweaning months were more likely to delay the onset of weaning by several weeks, and in some cases even to preempt their mothers' cycling during the normal breeding season; this pattern was especially clear for male infants. More recently, Berman and colleagues (1993) found that infants who achieved the most frequent nipple contacts with their mothers during the breeding season had mothers who were least likely to conceive, even if they entered into relationships with multiple consorts during that period. The end result in both cases was that these infants could, by their own actions, "postpone" their mothers' next pregnancy for another year, thus gaining additional opportunities for unfettered access to her not shared by agemates whose mothers had become pregnant during the same period. In the process, such an infant was also able to postpone by at least a year the appearance of a new source of conflict—that of "rivalry" with the mother's next infant.

The birth of a new sibling has major consequences for a yearling rhesus monkey. From that moment on, the yearling's relationship with the mother is altered dramatically, especially with respect to attachment-related activities. No longer is a yearling the primary focus of its mother's attention. Instead, many of its attempts to use her as a source of security and comfort are often ignored or rebuffed, especially when its newborn sibling is nursing or merely clinging to the mother's ventrum (Suomi, 1982). Moreover, whenever the yearling tries to push its younger sibling off the mother, to obstruct its access to her, or to disrupt its activity when it moves away from her, the mother's most likely response is to physically punish the yearling quickly, without warning, and often with considerable severity. In contrast, the mother seldom if ever punishes the younger sibling when it interrupts the yearling's attempts to interact with her or otherwise disrupts the yearling's activities (Berman, 1992).

Thus the arrival of a younger sibling inevitably alters the yearling's attachment relationship with its mother. This relationship generally continues to wane (i.e., proximity seeking and secure-base exploratory behavior both diminish) throughout the rest of the childhood years, especially after the birth of each succeeding sibling. For males, the waning process continues into puberty—eventually culminating with their natal troop emigration, which effectively terminates any remnant of their relationship with their mothers. Although attachment-related activities likewise decline throughout childhood for females, the daughters tend to increase other forms of affiliative interaction with their mothers (e.g., mutual grooming bouts), most notably after they start having offspring of their own. Coincidentally, episodes involving obvious conflict with their mothers become increasingly frequent for both male and female offspring as they approach puberty; thereafter, any semblance of attachment-like behavior directed toward mothers is infrequent at best among daughters and, of course, impossible for sons once they have left their natal troop (Suomi, 1998).

FACTORS INFLUENCING ATTACHMENT RELATIONSHIPS IN RHESUS MONKEYS

Although Bowlby (1969/1982) believed that attachment has a strong biological basis and represents the product of evolutionary processes, he also observed that there is substantial variation among mother–infant dyads in fundamental aspects of their attachment relationships, and he recognized the potential developmental significance of such variation. Indeed, he lived to see his collaborator Mary Ainsworth's Strange Situation assessment paradigm become almost reified in its identification and characterization of different "types" (groups A, B, C, and [more recently] D) and even "subtypes" of human infant–mother attachment relationships (e.g., Goldberg, 1995; see Solomon & George, Chapter 18, this volume). Perhaps not surprisingly, there appears to be comparable variation in the attachment relationships formed by different rhesus monkey mother–infant dyads. Indeed, there exist compelling parallel examples in rhesus monkey attachment relationships to each of the major human attachment types, if not at least some of the subtypes (Higley & Suomi, 1989). Moreover, a substantial body of research has identified numerous factors that can significantly influence the nature and ultimate developmental trajectory of these different attachment relationships. Some of these influences derive from factors external to the mother–infant dyad, and others appear to be derived from specific behavioral and biological features of the mother and the infant.

With respect to external factors, numerous studies carried out over the past 30 years have demonstrated that most rhesus monkey mothers are usually highly sensitive to those aspects of their immediate physical and social environment that pose a potential threat to their infants' well-being, and they appear to adjust their maternal behavior accordingly. Both laboratory and field studies have consistently shown that mothers from low-ranking families typically are much more restrictive of their infants' exploratory efforts than are mothers from high-ranking matrilines, whose maternal style tends to be more "laissez-faire" (e.g., Fairbanks, 1996). The standard interpretation of these findings has been that low-ranking mothers risk reprisal from others if they try to intervene whenever their infants are threatened, so they minimize such risk by restricting their infants' exploration. High-ranking mothers usually have no such problem and hence can afford to let their infants explore as they please (Suomi, 1998). Other studies have found that mothers generally become more restrictive and increase their levels of infant monitoring when their immediate social environment becomes less stable, such as when major changes in dominance hierarchies take place or when a new male joins the social group (Fairbanks et al., 2001). They also tend to monitor their infants' social activities with peers more closely and become more restrictive about the range of social partners with whom they allow their infants to interact as the size of their troop increases (Berman, Rasmussen, & Suomi, 1997). For those infants whose opportunities to explore and to interact with peers are chronically limited during their first few months of life, their ability to develop species-normative relationships with others in their social group (especially peers) can be compromised, often with long-term consequences for both the infants and the troop itself (Suomi, 1999).

Changes in various aspects of the physical environment, such as the food supply becoming less predictable, have also been associated with al-

terations in the day-to-day relationships between monkey mothers and their infants, with significant short-term and surprising long-term consequences for the infants as they mature. In a series of landmark studies, Rosenblum and his colleagues (e.g., Rosenblum & Paulley, 1984) developed a laboratory procedure that permitted experimental manipulation of the amount of time and effort a mother had to spend to obtain the nutrition to satisfy her own and her infant's daily needs. Specifically, they created a low-foraging-demand (LFD) condition in which food was available *ad libitum*, and a high-foraging-demand (HFD) condition in which the mother had to spend several hours each day to obtain equivalent nutrition for both her infant and herself, but in which there was no food deprivation per se. These researchers found that although there were no major differences among bonnet macaque infants reared under either condition, there were profound consequences for infants whose mothers experienced a *shift* in foraging conditions (e.g., from LFD to HFD and back) every 2 weeks—a situation termed the variable-foraging-demand (VFD) condition—even if this condition was in place for only a period of 12 weeks. They observed major changes in the amount of time and the manner in which the mothers interacted with their infants during VFD periods, largely due to changes in the way the mothers were interacting with each other within their social group (Andrews & Rosenblum, 1991). The end result was that the attachment relationships of VFD mothers and infants became less secure (Andrews & Rosenblum, 1993).

Offspring raised by VFD mothers exhibited persistent effects of this experience when compared with those raised in either the LFD or the HFD condition only. As juveniles, they showed less social affiliation, greater affective withdrawal, and more subordinate behavior toward others in their social group (Andrews & Rosenblum, 1994; Rosenblum, Forger, Noland, Trost, & Coplan, 2001). They also exhibited a different profile of HPA activity—with higher cerebrospinal fluid (CSF) concentrations of corticotropin-releasing factor (CRF), but, interestingly, lower CRF concentrations of cortisol than in non-VFD subjects—not only as infants immediately following the VFD manipulation (as did their mothers), but actually continuing well into adulthood (Coplan et al., 1996; Matthew et al., 2002). Interestingly, these VFD effects on offspring HPA activity patterns were significantly less pronounced for offspring of socially dominant mothers. Moreover, these effects were not limited to the HPA system: Infants whose mothers experienced the VFD condition also had significantly higher CSF levels of 5-hydroxyindoleacetic acid (5-HIAA, the primary central serotonin metabolite), somastatin, and homovanillic acid (HVA, the primary central dopamine metabolite) than did those whose mothers experienced only the LFD condition (Coplan et al., 1998). Significant VFD–LFD differences were also found in growth hormone levels and in several measures of immune response, and these differences also persisted into adulthood (Coplan et al., 2000). In sum, these findings clearly indicate that environmental factors falling short of what might be characterized as truly traumatic in nature, but sufficient to alter attachment relationships between a mother monkey and her infant, can have profound and long-lasting consequences not only for the infant's subsequent behavioral and emotional development, but also for the functioning of various biological systems throughout its ontogeny.

Numerous other studies have shown that differences among monkey mothers in their characteristic maternal "style" can also affect the types of attachment relationships they develop with their offspring, even when they are living in the same physical and social environmental settings. Although a comprehensive review of the relevant literature is beyond the scope of this chapter, it is worth noting that most primate females tend to be remarkably consistent in the specific manner in which they rear their infants, at least after their initial pregnancy (Higley & Suomi, 1986; Suomi, 1987). It is also worth noting that some of the differences one can observe among monkey mothers in their respective maternal styles can be related to specific temperamental characteristics they displayed as infants, as well as to the nature of the attachment relationship they formed with their own mothers (e.g., Champoux, Byrne, Delizio, & Suomi, 1992; Suomi, 1995, 1999; Suomi & Ripp, 1983).

It is now apparent that differences in maternal style can have major and lasting consequences not only for the attachment relationships that mothers develop with their offspring, but also, as in the case of external environmental influences described above, for their offspring's behavioral and biological functioning throughout life. One of the most dramatic examples of the effects of differential maternal style comes from the work of Maestripieri and his colleagues at the Yerkes National Primate Research Center field facility near Atlan-

ta, Georgia, where large breeding groups of rhesus monkeys are maintained in outdoor corrals. These investigators observed that successive generations of females in several long-standing matrilines maintained in this setting physically abuse most of their offspring to a degree not seen in other families. Most of the abuse occurs during their infants' first month of life and is rarely seen after the third month (Maestripieri, McCormack, Higley, Lindell, & Sanchez, 2006). In addition, these abusive mothers tend to exhibit unusually high levels of infant rejection (i.e., preventing their infants from obtaining ventral or nipple contact, or pushing them away if such contact has already been established), and these high rates of rejection continue long after all incidents of abuse have ceased (McCormack et al., 2006). Thus, for females living in these families, high levels of infant neglect and abuse appear to be the norm rather than the exception across successive generations of mothers.

Such extreme styles of maternal care are not without behavioral and biological consequences for infants growing up in these matrilines. The maternally abused and neglected infants exhibit much higher rates of screams, tantrums, and other behavioral indices of obvious distress throughout their first 6 months of life—long after they are no longer being physically abused—than do offspring of nonabusive mothers. They also appear to become much more emotionally reactive than their nonabused agemates, including delayed independence from their mothers, less environmental exploration, and much lower levels of social play during this same developmental period (McCormack et al., 2006). In addition, as was the case for monkey infants whose mothers were exposed to VFD conditions during their initial 6 months, physically abused infants exhibit deviations from the normative pattern of HPA activity and central serotonin metabolism shown by nonabused infants, and these aberrant patterns continue well into the juvenile years, if not beyond. However, it appears that the nature of these deviations is quite different from that seen in VFD infants: Abused infants exhibit unusually high levels of HPA reactivity in their first month, but thereafter HPA reactivity appears to be blunted relative to that of nonabused infants, and abused infants have significantly *lower* CSF concentrations of 5-HIAA—exactly the opposite of infants growing up under VFD conditions (Maestripieri et al., 2006; Sanchez, 2006). Moreover, it has now been well documented that a high proportion of females who experienced such abuse and rejection by their mothers early in life grow up to be abusive mothers themselves (Maestripieri & Carroll, 1998).

These and other findings clearly support the proposition that individual differences in maternal style, including attachment-related activities, among rhesus monkey mothers can have profound consequences for the behavioral and biological functioning of their offspring throughout development, especially when the differences are extreme. (See Hesse, Chapter 25, and George & Solomon, Chapter 35, this volume, for discussions of how maternal attachment relates to maternal caregiving behavior in humans.)

Finally, variance in rhesus monkey attachment relationships may stem in part from differences among infant monkeys in their temperamental characteristics and the physiological processes that underlie their behavioral expression early in life. Researchers studying rhesus and other monkey species in both laboratory and field settings have long recognized developmentally stable individual differences along certain temperamental dimensions. One dimension involves relative fearfulness, as reflected by individual differences in prototypical behavioral and biological responses to environmental novelty and/or challenge. Some monkey infants consistently respond to such mildly stressful situations with obvious behavioral expressions of fear and anxiety, as well as significant (and often prolonged) cortisol elevations, unusually high and stable heart rates, and dramatic increases in norepinephrine metabolism (e.g., Capitanio, Rasmussen, Snyder, Laudenslager, & Reite, 1986; Clarke & Boinski, 1995; Kalin & Shelton, 1989; Suomi, 1981, 1991; Suomi, Kraemer, Baysinger, & Delizio, 1981). These distinctive behavioral and physiological features appear early in infancy; they show remarkable interindividual stability throughout development; and there is increasing evidence that they are highly heritable (Higley et al., 1993; Williamson et al., 2003).

One consequence of these behavioral and biological proclivities is that such "high-reactive" infants tend to spend more time with their mothers and less time with peers during their initial weeks and months of life. High-reactive young monkeys are also more likely to exhibit depressive-like reactions to functional maternal separations during the breeding season, as described above, than the rest of their birth cohort (Berman et al., 1994; Suomi, 1995). On the other hand, a high-reactive infant may ultimately be more "successful" than others in its peer group in postponing its mother's next pregnancy and, eventually, a new sibling rival

for her attention (Berman et al., 1993; Simpson et al., 1981; Suomi, 1998). These and other findings provide impressive evidence that an infant's temperamental reactivity can influence, if not substantially alter, fundamental aspects of its relationship with its mother throughout development. (See Vaughn, Bost, & van IJzendoorn, Chapter 9, this volume, for discussion of temperament and attachment in humans.)

Another temperamental dimension on which there are obvious individual differences among rhesus monkey infants is relative impulsivity, especially in social settings (where inappropriately impulsive behavior often leads to aggressive exchanges). This temperamental pattern is most readily apparent in peer play interactions. Impulsive males in particular seem unable to moderate their behavioral responses to rough-and-tumble play initiations from peers, instead escalating initially benign play bouts into full-blown, tissue-damaging aggressive exchanges, disproportionately at their own expense (Higley, Suomi, & Linnoila, 1996). Prospective longitudinal studies have shown that individuals who develop such response patterns typically exhibit poor state control and significant deficits in visual orienting capabilities during their first month of life (Champoux, Suomi, & Schneider, 1994). They also tend to exhibit chronically low rates of central metabolism of serotonin, a prominent inhibitory neurotransmitter implicated in ubiquitous aspects of metabolic, regulatory, and emotional functioning (Coccaro & Murphy, 1990). In particular, impulsive and aggressive monkeys consistently have lower CSF 5-HIAA than their peers throughout development (e.g., Champoux, Higley, & Suomi, 1997; Higley, King, et al., 1996; Higley & Suomi, 1996; Mehlman et al., 1994; Shannon et al., 2005). As is the case for high reactivity, these behavioral and biological characteristics of impulsive aggression are remarkably stable throughout development, and they appear to be highly heritable (Higley et al., 1993; Higley & Suomi, 1996).

Highly impulsive rhesus monkeys typically develop difficult attachment relationships with their mothers. They seem to be unusually fussy in their initial weeks (reflecting their generally poor state control; cf. Champoux et al., 1994), and their conflicts with their mothers intensify substantially during and shortly after the time of weaning (Suomi, 1998). As they grow older, highly impulsive youngsters usually continue to exhibit difficulties in their social interactions with their mothers, with peers, and with others in their social group; these social problems generally carry over into adolescence and adulthood—and sometimes into the next generation (Higley & Suomi, 1996; Suomi, 2006).

EFFECTS OF DIFFERENTIAL ATTACHMENT RELATIONSHIPS ON LONG-TERM DEVELOPMENTAL TRAJECTORIES

Although considerable evidence from both field and laboratory studies has shown that individual differences among rhesus monkeys in certain temperamental characteristics tend to be quite stable from infancy to adulthood and are at least in part heritable, this does not mean that these behavioral and physiological features are necessarily fixed at birth or are immune to subsequent environmental influence. On the contrary, an increasing body of evidence from laboratory studies has demonstrated that prototypical behavioral and biological response patterns can be modified substantially by certain early experiences, especially those involving attachment relationships. This is perhaps most clearly illustrated by the results of experimental studies in which monkey infants have been separated from their biological mothers at or shortly after birth and reared in the presence of other monkeys, other species, or a variety of animate or inanimate objects. In most of these circumstances, rhesus monkey infants readily develop Bowlby-like attachments with whatever mother substitutes might be available, although some potential attachment objects are clearly preferred to others. The classic case is Harlow's research involving cloth- and wire-covered surrogates (Harlow, 1958), which Bowlby found so compelling (e.g., Bowlby, 1969/1982), but there have been many others. Over the years, rhesus monkey infants have been reported to become attached to unrelated adult female conspecifics, adult male conspecifics, adult females from other primate species, dogs, cats, hobby horses, and a range of variations on the original Harlow cloth surrogates (e.g., Dettmer, Novak, Meyer, Ruggiero, & Suomi, 2008; Mason & Berkson, 1975; Mason & Kenney, 1974; Redican & Mitchell, 1973). It is clearly in their nature to become attached, but attachments with these different classes of individuals and objects often have vastly different consequences, especially for different infants.

One extensive set of studies has focused on rhesus monkey infants raised with peers instead of their biological mothers. Infants in these studies were permanently separated from their biological mothers at birth; hand-reared in a neonatal nursery for their first month of life; housed with same-age, like-reared peers for the rest of their first 6 months; and then moved into larger social groups containing both peer-reared and mother-reared agemates. During their initial months, these infants readily developed strong social attachment bonds to each other, much as mother-reared infants develop attachments to their own mothers (Harlow, 1969). However, perhaps because peers are not nearly as effective as typical monkey mothers in reducing fear in the face of novelty, or in providing a secure base for exploration, the attachment relationships that these peer-reared infants developed were almost always dysfunctional in nature (Suomi, 1995). As a result, although peer-reared monkeys showed completely normal physical and motor development, their early exploratory behavior was somewhat limited: They seemed reluctant to approach novel objects, and they tended to be shy in initial encounters with unfamiliar peers (Suomi, 2006).

Even when peer-reared youngsters interacted with their same-age cagemates in familiar settings, their emerging social play repertoires were usually retarded in both frequency and complexity. One explanation for their relatively poor play performance is that their cagemates had to serve as both attachment figures and playmates—a dual role that neither mothers nor mother-reared peers have to fulfill. Another explanation is that they faced difficulties in developing sophisticated play repertoires with basically incompetent play partners. Perhaps as a result of either or both of these factors, peer-reared youngsters typically dropped to the bottom of their respective dominance hierarchies when they were grouped with mother-reared monkeys their own age (Higley, King, et al., 1996).

Several prospective longitudinal studies have found that peer-reared monkeys consistently exhibit more extreme behavioral, HPA, and neurochemical reactions to social separations than do their mother-reared cohorts, even after they have been living in the same social groups for extended periods (Higley & Suomi, 1989; Shannon, Champoux, & Suomi, 1998). Such differences in prototypical behavioral reactions to separation persist from infancy to adolescence, if not beyond. Interestingly, the general nature of the separation reactions of peer-reared monkeys seems to mirror that of the naturally occurring reactions in high-reactive mother-reared subjects. In this sense, early rearing by peers appears to have the effect of making rhesus monkey infants generally more high-reactive than they might have been if reared by their biological mothers (Suomi, 1997).

Early peer rearing has another long-term developmental consequence for rhesus monkeys: It tends to make them more impulsive, especially if they are males. Peer-reared males initially exhibit aggressive tendencies in the context of juvenile play; as they approach puberty, the frequency and severity of their aggressive episodes typically exceed those of mother-reared group members of similar age. Peer-reared females tend to groom (and be groomed by) others in their social group less frequently and for shorter durations than their mother-reared counterparts, and (as noted above) they usually stay at the bottom of their respective dominance hierarchies (Higley, King, et al., 1996). These differences between peer-reared and mother-reared agemates in aggression, grooming, and dominance remain relatively robust throughout the preadolescent and adolescent years (Higley, Suomi, & Linnoila, 1996). Peer-reared monkeys also consistently show lower CSF concentrations of 5-HIAA than their mother-reared counterparts. These group differences in 5-HIAA concentrations appear well before 6 months of age, and they remain stable at least throughout adolescence and into early adulthood (Higley & Suomi, 1996; Shannon et al., 2005). Thus peer-reared monkeys as a group resemble the impulsive subgroup of wild-living (and mother-reared) monkeys, not only behaviorally but also in terms of decreased serotonergic functioning (Suomi, 1997).

Other laboratory studies of peer-reared monkeys have disclosed additional differences from their mother-reared counterparts—differences that are not readily apparent in free-ranging populations of rhesus monkeys. Peer-reared adolescent monkeys consistently consume larger amounts of alcohol under comparable *ad lib.* conditions than their mother-reared agemates do (Higley, Hasert, Suomi, & Linnoila, 1991; see Mikulincer & Shaver, 2007, for a review of studies linking substance abuse and attachment in humans). Recent follow-up studies have demonstrated that the peer-reared subjects quickly develop a greater tolerance for alcohol; this can be predicted by their central nervous system serotonin turnover rates, which in turn appear to be associated with differential serotonin transporter availability (Heinz et al., 1998). Peer-reared adolescent and adult males require larger doses of the anesthetic ketamine to reach a comparable state of sedation. They also exhibit significantly higher rates of whole-brain glucose metabolism under mild isoflurane anesthesia, as determined by positron emission tomography (PET) imaging, than mother-reared controls do (Doudet et al., 1995). Additional studies involving PET imaging have reported that peer-reared juveniles have significantly lower levers of serotonin-binding potential and cerebral blood flow in multiple brain regions than do their mother-reared counterparts (Ichise et al., 2006). Thus the development of early attachments to peers in the absence of mothers can have significant long-term consequences for monkeys not only at the levels of behavioral expression and emotional regulation, but also at the levels of hormonal output, neurotransmitter metabolism, drug sensitivity, and even brain structure and function.

Clearly, a range of adverse early experiences— be they exposure to a mother dealing with the demands of a VFD environment, experience with an abusive and rejecting mother, or peer rearing in the absence of attachment opportunities with any adult—can have significant developmental consequences for individuals at multiple levels of analysis. It also seems apparent that heritable factors may influence individual developmental trajectories at one or more levels of analysis. But do these genetic and environmental factors operate separately, or do they interact in some fashion? Recent research has demonstrated several significant interactions between specific genetic and experiential factors in shaping developmental trajectories for rhesus monkeys.

For example, the serotonin transporter gene (5-HTT), a candidate gene for impaired serotonergic function (Heils et al., 1996), has length variation in its promoter region that results in allelic variation in 5-HTT expression. A heterozygous short allele (LS) confers low transcriptional efficiency to the 5-HTT promoter relative to the homozygous long allele (LL), raising the possibility that low 5-HTT expression may result in decreased serotonergic function (Lesch et al., 1996, 1997).

Several studies have now demonstrated that the consequences of having the LS allele differ dramatically for peer-reared monkeys and their mother-reared counterparts. For example, Champoux and colleagues (2002) examined the relation between early rearing history and 5-HTT polymorphic status on measures of neonatal neurobehavioral development during the first month of life, and found further evidence of maternal buffering. Specifically, infants possessing the LS allele who were being reared in the laboratory neonatal nursery showed significant deficits in measures of attention, activity, and motor maturity relative to nursery-reared infants possessing the LL allele, whereas both LS and LL infants who were being reared by competent mothers exhibited normal values for each of these measures. One interpretation of this interaction is that effective maternal rearing, including the development of secure attachment relationships, appeared to buffer any potentially deleterious effects of the LS allele on these measures.

In a similar vein, Bennett and colleagues (2002) found that CSF 5-HIAA concentrations did not differ as a function of 5-HTT status for securely attached mother-reared subjects, whereas among peer-reared monkeys, individuals with the LS allele had significantly lower CSF 5-HIAA concentrations than those with the LL allele. Once again, maternal rearing appeared to buffer any potentially deleterious effects of the LS allele on serotonin metabolism. A similar pattern appeared with respect to aggression: High levels of aggression were shown by peer-reared monkeys with the LS allele, whereas mother-reared LS monkeys exhibited low levels comparable to those of both mother-reared and peer-reared LL monkeys, again suggesting a buffering effect of maternal rearing (Barr et al., 2003).

An even more dramatic pattern of gene–environment interaction was revealed by an analysis of alcohol consumption data: Whereas peer-reared monkeys with the LS allele consumed more alcohol than peer-reared monkeys with the LL allele, the reverse was true for mother-reared subjects, with individuals possessing the LS allele actually showing relatively low levels of alcohol consumption (Barr et al., 2004). In other words, the LS allele appeared to represent a significant *risk* factor for excessive alcohol consumption among monkeys with adverse early attachment experiences, but a significant *protective* factor for mother-reared subjects, most of whom had experienced positive attachment experiences with their mothers.

In sum, peer-reared monkeys with the LS allele displayed deficits in measures of neurobehavioral development during their initial weeks of life, and reduced serotonin metabolism and excessive alcohol consumption as adolescents, compared with those possessing the LL allele. In contrast, mother-reared subjects with the LS allele were characterized by normal early neurobehavioral development and serotonin metabolism, as well as reduced risk for excessive alcohol consump-

tion later in life, compared with their mother-reared counterparts with the LL allele. It could be argued on the basis of these findings that having the LS allele of the 5-HTT gene may well lead to psychopathology among monkeys with poor early rearing histories, but may actually be adaptive for monkeys who develop a secure early attachment to their mothers. (See Simpson & Belsky, Chapter 6, this volume, for discussion of the evolutionary advantages of such differential susceptibility to environmental influence. See also Vaughn et al., Chapter 9, this volume, for a review of behavior genetic and molecular studies of attachment in humans.)

The implications of these recent findings may be considerable with respect to the cross-generational transmission of these behavioral and biological characteristics, in that (as mentioned above) the attachment style of a monkey mother tends to be mirrored by her daughters when they grow up and become mothers themselves (Fairbanks, 1989; Maestripieri, 2005). If similar buffering is indeed experienced by the next generation of infants carrying the LS 5-HTT polymorphism, then having had their mothers develop a secure attachment relationship with their own mothers may well provide the basis for a nongenetic means of transmitting its apparently adaptive consequences to that new generation. On the other hand, if contextual factors (e.g., changes in dominance rank, instability within the troop, or changes in the availability of food) were to alter young mothers' care of their infants in ways that compromised such buffering, one might expect any offspring carrying the LS polymorphism to develop some if not all of the problems described above.

CROSS-GENERATIONAL CONSEQUENCES OF EARLY ATTACHMENT RELATIONSHIPS: IMPLICATIONS FOR HUMAN ATTACHMENT THEORY

One of the most intriguing aspects of the long-term consequences of different early attachment experiences, especially in light of the speculation outlined above, is the apparent transfer of specific features of maternal behavior across successive generations. Several studies of rhesus monkeys and other Old World monkey species have demonstrated strong continuities between the type of attachment relationship a female infant develops with her mother and the type of attachment relationship she develops with her own infant(s) when she becomes a mother herself. In particular, the pattern of ventral contact a female infant has with her mother (or mother substitute) during her initial months of life is a powerful predictor of the pattern of ventral contact she will have with her own infants during their first 6 months of life (Champoux et al., 1992; Fairbanks, 1989, 1996). This predictive cross-generational relationship appears to be as strong in females who were foster-reared from birth by unrelated multiparous females as it is for females reared by their biological mothers. An even more impressive demonstration of cross-generational transmission of maternal characteristics comes from a study by Maestripieri (2005), who cross-fostered female infants of abusive mothers to nonabusive multiparous mothers—and also cross-fostered offspring of nonabusive mothers to unrelated females with a prior history of abuse. Maestripieri found that whereas approximately half of the female offspring of nonabusive mothers who were reared by abusive foster mothers grew up to be abusive toward their own offspring, *none* of the female offspring of abusive mothers who had nonabusive foster mothers subsequently abused their own infants! These findings clearly demonstrate that cross-generational transmission of at least some aspects of mother–infant attachment necessarily involves nongenetic mechanisms (cf. Suomi & Levine, 1998). What those nongenetic mechanisms may be, and through what developmental processes they may act, are questions at the heart of ongoing investigations. (See Dozier & Rutter, Chapter 29, this volume, for discussion of attachment and foster care in humans.)

Contemporary attachment theorists considering the long-term consequences of differential early attachment relationships in humans have also focused on possible cross-generational continuities in attachment styles. Some authors have posited the likely existence of strong cross-generational continuities, such that mothers who experienced secure attachments when they were infants may tend to raise infants who are securely attached to them, whereas those who experienced avoidant or ambivalent attachments with their own mothers may tend to promote avoidant or ambivalent attachments as mothers themselves (e.g., Berlin & Cassidy, 1999; Main, 1995). Moreover, current attachment theorists attribute these postulated infancy-to-parenthood continuities in attachment type to "internal working models" initially based on early memories and periodically transformed by more recent experiences (see Bretherton & Munholland, Chapter 5, this volume). Most of the empirical findings that have led to these hypoth-

eses have come from comprehensive interviews of adults (e.g., with the Adult Attachment Interview; see Hesse, Chapter 25, this volume) retrospectively probing memories of events and experiences. On the other hand, the most powerful empirical support for apparently parallel long-term continuities in attachment behavior from the nonhuman primate literature comes from prospective longitudinal observations and physiological recordings, both in controlled experimental settings and in naturalistic habitats, as reviewed above.

One insight that the nonhuman primate data bring to discussions *in the absence of language or complex imagery* about long-term consequences of early experiences is that strong developmental continuities can unfold. It is difficult to argue that rhesus monkeys, for example, possess sufficient cognitive capabilities to develop internal working models requiring considerable self-reflection, given that they are probably not capable of self-awareness or self-recognition (e.g., Gallup, 1977; Povinelli, Parks, & Novak, 1992). What cognitive, emotional, and mnemonic processes may underlie these continuities, and do they have parallels in human nonverbal mental processes?

Alternatively, one might argue that working models are exclusively human constructions that are built upon a basic foundation that is essentially biological in nature and universal among the more advanced primate species. According to this view, cognitive constructions per se may not be necessary for long-term developmental or cross-generational continuities in attachment phenomena to transpire. That is, such continuities are essentially "programmed" to occur in the absence of major environmental disruption and are in fact the product of strictly biological processes that reflect the natural evolutionary history of advanced primate species, human and nonhuman alike (for discussion of attachment and evolutionary processes, see Simpson & Belsky, Chapter 6, this volume). If this is the case, then working models (or other comparable cognitive processes) may represent a luxury for humans that enables individuals to cognitively reinforce the postulated underlying biological foundation, in which case the predicted developmental continuity may actually be strengthened.

On the other hand, the existence of a working model that has the potential to be *altered* by specific experiences (and/or insights) in late childhood, adolescence, or adulthood may provide a basis for breaking an otherwise likely continuity between one's early attachment experiences and subsequent performance as a parent. These important issues deserve not only further theoretical consideration, but empirical investigation as well. As Bowlby (1988) himself said, "All of us, from cradle to the grave, are happiest when life is organized as a series of excursions, long or short, from the secure base provided by our attachment figure(s)" (p. 62). Research with nonhuman primates has clearly provided compelling evidence in support of a strong biological foundation for attachment phenomena. Indeed, such a foundation may well serve as a secure base for future research excursions in the realm of attachment phenomena.

REFERENCES

Andrews, M. W., & Rosenblum, L. A. (1991). Security of attachment in infants raised in variable- or low-demand environments. *Child Development, 62,* 686–693.

Andrews, M. W., & Rosenblum, L. A. (1993). Assessment of attachment in differentially reared infant monkeys (*Macaca radiata*). *Journal of Comparative Psychology, 107,* 84–90.

Andrews, M. W., & Rosenblum, L. A. (1994). The development of affiliative and agonistic patterns in differentially reared monkeys. *Child Development, 65,* 1398–1404.

Arling, G. L., & Harlow, H. F. (1967). Effects of social deprivation on maternal behavior of rhesus monkeys. *Journal of Comparative and Physiological Psychology, 64,* 371–377.

Barr, C. S., Newman, T. K., Becker, M. L., Parker, C. C., Champoux, M., Lesch, K. P., et al. (2003). The utility of the non-human primate model for studying gene by environment interactions in behavioral research. *Genes, Brain and Behavior, 2,* 336–340.

Barr, C. S., Newman, T. K., Lindell, S. G., Shannon, C., Champoux, M., Lesch, K. P., et al. (2004). Interaction between serotonin transporter gene variation and rearing condition in alcohol preference and consumption in female primates. *Archives of General Psychiatry, 61,* 1146–1152.

Bennett, A. J., Lesch, K. P., Heils, A., Long, J. C., Lorenz, J. G., Shoaf, S. E., et al. (2002). Early experience and serotonin transporter gene variation interact to influence primate CNS function. *Molecular Psychiatry, 7,* 118–122.

Berlin, L. J., & Cassidy, J. (1999). Relations among relationships: Contributions from attachment theory and research. In J. Cassidy & P. R. Shaver (Eds.), *Handbook of attachment: Theory, research, and clinical applications* (pp. 688–712). New York: Guilford Press.

Berman, C. M. (1982). The ontogeny of social relationships with group companions among free-ranging rhesus monkeys: I. Social networks and differentiation. *Animal Behavior, 30,* 149–162.

Berman, C. M. (1992). Immature siblings and mother–infant relationships among free-ranging rhesus monkeys on Cayo Santiago. *Animal Behavior, 44,* 247–258.

Berman, C. M., Rasmussen, K. L. R., & Suomi, S. J. (1993). Reproductive consequences of maternal care patterns during estrus among free-ranging rhesus monkeys. *Behavioral Ecology and Sociobiology, 32,* 391–399.

Berman, C. M., Rasmussen, K. L. R., & Suomi, S. J. (1994). Responses of free-ranging rhesus monkeys to a natural form of maternal separation: I. Parallels with mother–infant separation in captivity. *Child Development, 65,* 1028–1041.

Berman, C. M., Rasmussen, K. L. R., & Suomi, S. J. (1997). Group size, infant development, and social networks: A natural experiment with free-ranging rhesus monkeys. *Animal Behavior, 53,* 405–421.

Bowlby, J. (1958). The nature of the child's tie to his mother. *International Journal of Psycho-Analysis, 39,* 1–24.

Bowlby, J. (1960). Separation anxiety. *International Journal of Psycho-Analysis, 51,* 1–25.

Bowlby, J. (1969/1982). *Attachment and loss: Vol. 1. Attachment.* New York: Basic Books.

Bowlby, J. (1973). *Attachment and loss: Vol. 2. Separation: Anxiety and anger.* New York: Basic Books.

Bowlby, J. (1988). *A secure base.* New York: Basic Books.

Boyce, W. T., Champoux, M., Suomi, S. J., & Gunnar, M. R. (1995). Salivary cortisol in nursery-reared rhesus monkeys: Interindividual stability, reactions to peer interactions, and altered circadian rhythmicity. *Developmental Psychobiology, 28,* 257–267.

Busnell, M.-C., & Granier-Deferre, C. (1983). And what of fetal audition? In A. Oliverio & M. Zappella (Eds.), *The behavior of human infants* (pp. 93–126). New York: Plenum Press.

Byrne, G. D., & Suomi, S. J. (1995). Activity patterns, social interaction, and exploratory behavior in *Cebus apella* infants from birth to 1 year of age. *American Journal of Primatology, 35,* 255–270.

Capitanio, J. P., Rasmussen, K. L. R., Snyder, D. S., Laudenslager, M. L., & Reite, M. (1986). Long-term follow-up of previously separated pigtail macaques: Group and individual differences in response to unfamiliar situations. *Journal of Child Psychology and Psychiatry, 27,* 531–538.

Champoux, M., Bennett, A. J., Shannon, C., Higley, J. D., Lesch, K. P., & Suomi, S. J. (2002). Serotonin transporter gene polymorphism, differential early rearing, and behavior in rhesus monkey neonates. *Molecular Psychiatry, 7,* 1058–1063.

Champoux, M., Byrne, E., Delizio, R. D., & Suomi, S. J. (1992). Motherless mothers revisited: Rhesus maternal behavior and rearing history. *Primates, 33,* 251–255.

Champoux, M., Higley, J. D., & Suomi, S. J. (1997). Behavioral and physiological characteristics of Indian and Chinese–Indian hybrid rhesus macaque infants. *Developmental Psychobiology, 31,* 49–63.

Champoux, M., Suomi, S. J., & Schneider, M. L. (1994). Temperamental differences between captive Indian and Chinese–Indian hybrid rhesus macaque infants. *Laboratory Animal Science, 44*, 351–357.

Clarke, A. S., & Boinski, S. (1995). Temperament in nonhuman primates. *American Journal of Primatology, 37*, 103–125.

Coccaro, E. F., & Murphy, D. L. (1990). *Serotonin in major psychiatric disorders.* Washington, DC: American Psychiatric Press.

Coplan, J. D., Andrews, M. W., Rosenblum, L. A., Owens, M. J., Friedman, S., Gorman, J. M., et al. Persistent elevations of cerebrospinal fluid concentrations of corticotrophin-releasing factor in adult nonhuman primates exposed to early-life stressors: Implications for the pathophysiology of mood and anxiety disorders. *Proceedings of the National Academy of Sciences USA, 93*, 1619–1623.

Coplan, J. D., Trost, R. C., Owens, M. J., Cooper, T. B., Gorman, J. M., Nemeroff, C. B., et al. (1998). Cerebrospinal fluid concentrations of somatostatin and biogenic amines in grown primates reared by mothers exposed to manipulated foraging conditions. *Archives of General Psychiatry, 55*, 473–477.

Coplan, J. H., Smith, E. L., Trost, R. E., Scharf, B. A., Altemus, M., Bjornson, J., et al. (2000). Growth hormone response to clonidine in adversely reared young adult primates: Relationship to serial cerebrospinal fluid corticotropin-releasing factor concentrations. *Psychiatry Research, 95*, 93–102.

Darwin, E. (1794). *Zoonomia, or the laws of organic life.* London: Johnson.

DeCasper, A. J., & Fifer, W. P. (1980). Of human bonding: Newborns prefer their mothers' voices. *Science, 208*, 1174–1176.

Dettmer, A. M., Novak, M. A., Meyer, J. S., Ruggiero, A. M., & Suomi, S. J. (2008). Surrogate mobility and orientation affect the early neurobehavioral development of infant rhesus macaques (Macaca mulatta). *Developmental Psychobiology, 50*, 218–222.

Dienske, H., & Metz, J. A. J. (1977). Mother–infant body contact in macaques: A time interval analysis. *Biology of Behaviour, 2*, 3–21.

Doudet, D., Hommer, D., Higley, J. D., Andreason, P. J., Moneman, R., Suomi, S. J., et al. (1995). Cerebral glucose metabolism, CSF 5-HIAA, and aggressive behavior in rhesus monkeys. *American Journal of Psychiatry, 152*, 1782–1787.

Fairbanks, L. A. (1989). Early experience and cross-generational continuity of mother–infant contact in vervet monkeys. *Developmental Psychobiology, 22*, 669–681.

Fairbanks, L. A. (1996). Individual differences in maternal style: Causes and consequences for mothers and offspring. *Advances in the Study of Behavior, 25*, 59–61.

Ferrari, P. F., Visalberghi, E., Paukner, A., Fogassi, L., Ruggiero, A., & Suomi, S. J. (2006). Neonatal imitation in infant macaques. *PLoS Biology, 4*, 1501–1508.

Fifer, W. P. (1987). Neonatal preference for mother's voice. In N. A. Krasnagor, E. M. Blass, M. A. Hofer, & W. P. Smotherman (Eds.), *Perinatal development: A psychobiological perspective* (pp. 39–60). New York: Academic Press.

Fragaszy, D. M., Baer, J., & Adams-Curtis, L. (1991). Behavioral development and maternal care in tufted capuchins (*Cebus apella*) and squirrel monkeys (*Saimiri sciureus*) from birth through seven months. *Developmental Psychobiology, 24*, 375–393.

Gallup, G. G. (1977). Self-recognition in primates: A comparative approach to the bidirectional properties of consciousness. *American Psychologist, 32*, 329–338.

Goldberg, S. (1995). Introduction. In S. Goldberg, R. Muir, & J. Kerr (Eds.), *Attachment theory: Social, developmental, and clinical perspectives* (pp. 1–15). Hillsdale, NJ: Analytic Press.

Gunnar, M. R., Gonzalez, C. A., Goodlin, B. L., & Levine, S. (1981). Behavioral and pituitary–adrenal responses during a prolonged separation period in rhesus monkeys. *Psychoneuroendocrinology, 6*, 65–75.

Hansen, E. W. (1966). The development of maternal and infant behavior in the rhesus monkey. *Behaviour, 27*, 109–149.

Harlow, H. F. (1953). Mice, monkeys, men, and motives. *Psychological Review, 60*, 23–35.

Harlow, H. F. (1958). The nature of love. *American Psychologist, 13*, 673–685.

Harlow, H. F. (1969). Age-mate or peer affectional system. *Advances in the Study of Behavior, 2*, 333–383.

Harlow, H. F., & Harlow, M. K. (1965). The affectional systems. In A. M. Schrier, H. F. Harlow, & F. Stollnitz (Eds.), *Behavior of nonhuman primates* (Vol. 2, pp. 287–334). New York: Academic Press.

Harlow, H. F., Harlow, M. K., & Hansen, E. W. (1963). The maternal affectional system of rhesus monkeys. In H. L. Rheingold (Ed.), *Maternal behavior in mammals* (pp. 254–281). New York: Wiley.

Harlow, H. F., & Lauersdorf, H. E. (1974). Sex differences in passions and play. *Perspectives in Biology and Medicine, 17*, 348–360.

Heils, A., Teufel, A., Petri, S., Stober, G., Riederer, P., Bengel, B., et al. (1996). Allelic variation of human serotonin transporter gene expression. *Journal of Neurochemistry, 6*, 2621–2624.

Heinz, A., Higley, J. D., Gorey, J. G., Saunders, R. C., Jones, D. W., Hommer, D., et al. (1998). In vivo association between alcohol intoxication, aggression, and serotonin transporter availability in nonhuman primates. *American Journal of Psychiatry, 155*, 1023–1028.

Higley, J. D., Hasert, M. L., Suomi, S. J., & Linnoila, M. (1991). A new nonhuman primate model of alcohol abuse: Effects of early experience, personality, and stress on alcohol consumption. *Proceedings of the National Academy of Sciences USA, 88*, 7261–7265.

Higley, J. D., King, S. T., Hasert, M. F., Champoux, M., Suomi, S. J., & Linnoila, M. (1996). Stability of individual differences in serotonin function and its relationship to severe aggression and competent social behavior in rhesus macaque females. *Neuropsychopharmacology, 14,* 67–76.

Higley, J. D., & Suomi, S. J. (1986). Parental behaviour in primates. In W. Sluckin & M. Herbert (Eds.), *Parental behaviour in mammals* (pp. 152–207). Oxford, UK: Blackwell.

Higley, J. D., & Suomi, S. J. (1989). Temperamental reactivity in nonhuman primates. In G. A. Kohnstamm, J. E. Bates, & M. K. Rothbart (Eds.), *Temperament in childhood* (pp. 153–167). New York: Wiley.

Higley, J. D., & Suomi, S. J. (1996). Reactivity and social competence affect individual differences in reaction to severe stress in children: Investigations using nonhuman primates. In C. R. Pfeffer (Ed.), *Intense stress and mental disturbance in children* (pp. 3–58). Washington, DC: American Psychiatric Press.

Higley, J. D., Suomi, S. J., & Linnoila, M. (1996). A nonhuman primate model of Type II alcoholism?: Part 2. Diminished social competence and excessive aggression correlates with low CSF 5-HIAA concentrations. *Alcoholism: Clinical and Experimental Research, 20,* 643–650.

Higley, J. D., Thompson, W. T., Champoux, M., Goldman, D., Hasert, M. F., Kraemer, G. W., et al. (1993). Paternal and maternal genetic and environmental contributions to CSF monoamine metabolites in rhesus monkeys (*Macaca mulatta*). *Archives of General Psychiatry, 50,* 615–623.

Hinde, R. A. (1976). On describing relationships. *Journal of Child Psychology and Psychiatry, 17,* 1–19.

Hinde, R. A., Rowell, T. E., & Spencer-Booth, Y. (1964). Behavior of socially living monkeys in their first six months. *Proceedings of the Zoological Society of London, 143,* 609–649.

Hinde, R. A., & Spencer-Booth, Y. (1967). The behaviour of socially living rhesus monkeys in their first two and a half years. *Animal Behaviour, 15,* 169–176.

Hinde, R. A., & White, L. E. (1974). Dynamics of a relationship: Rhesus mother–infant ventro–ventro contact. *Journal of Comparative and Physiological Psychology, 86,* 8–23.

Hofer, M. A. (1995). Hidden regulators: Implications for a new understanding of attachment, separation, and loss. In S. Goldberg, R. Muir, & J. Kerr (Eds.), *Attachment theory: Social, developmental, and clinical perspectives* (pp. 203–230). Hillsdale, NJ: Analytic Press.

Howell, S., Westergaard, G. C., Hoos, B., Chavanne, T. J., Shoaf, S. E., Cleveland, A., et al. (2007). Serotonergic influences on life-history outcomes in free-ranging male rhesus macaques. *American Journal of Primatology, 69,* 851–865.

Ichise, M., Vines, D. C., Gura, T., Anderson, G. M., Suomi, S. J., Higley, J. D., et al. (2006). Effects of early life stress on [11C] DABS PET imaging of serotonin transporters in adolescent peer- and mother-reared rhesus monkeys. *Journal of Neuroscience, 26,* 4638–4643.

Immelmann, K., & Suomi, S. J. (1981). Sensitive phases in development. In K. Immelmann, G. W. Barlow, L. Petrinovich, & M. Main (Eds.), *Behavioral development: The Bielefeld Project* (pp. 395–431). New York: Cambridge University Press.

Kalin, N. H., & Shelton, S. E. (1989). Defensive behaviors in infant rhesus monkeys: Environmental cues and neurochemical regulation. *Science, 243,* 1718–1721.

Lesch, K. P., Bengel, D., Heils, A., Sabol, S. Z., Greenberg, B. D., Petri, S., et al. (1996). Association of anxiety-related traits with a polymorphism in the serotonin transporter gene regulatory region. *Science, 274,* 1527–1531.

Lesch, L. P., Meyer, J., Glatz, K., Flugge, G., Hinney, A., Hebebrand, J., et al. (1997). The 5-HT transporter gene-linked polymorphic region (5-HTTLPR) in evolutionary perspective: Alternative biallelic variation in rhesus monkeys. *Journal of Neural Transmission, 104,* 1259–1266.

Lindburg, D. G. (1971). The rhesus monkey in north India: An ecological and behavioral study. In L. A. Rosenblum (Ed.), *Primate behavior: Developments in field and laboratory research* (Vol. 2, pp. 1–106). New York: Academic Press.

Lorenz, K. (1937). Der Kumpan in der Umwelt des Vogels. *Journal für Ornithologie, 83,* 137–213, 289–413.

Maestripieri, D. (2005). Early experience affects the intergenerational transmission of infant abuse in rhesus monkeys. *Proceedings of the National Academy of Sciences USA, 102,* 9726–9729.

Maestripieri, D., & Carroll, K. A. (1998). Risk factors for infant neglect and abuse in group-living rhesus monkeys. *Psychological Science, 9,* 143–145.

Maestripieri, D., McCormack, K. M., Higley, J. D., Lindell, S. G., & Sanchez, M. M. (2006). Influence of parenting style and offspring behavior and CSF monoamine metabolites in cross-fostered and non-crossfostered rhesus macaques. *Brain and Behavioral Research, 175,* 90–95.

Main, M. (1995). Recent studies in attachment: Overview, with selected implications for clinical work. In S. Goldberg, R. Muir, & J. Kerr (Eds.), *Attachment theory: Social, developmental, and clinical perspectives* (pp. 407–474). Hillsdale, NJ: Analytic Press.

Manson, J. H., & Perry, S. E. (1993). Inbreeding avoidance in rhesus macaques: Whose choice? *American Journal of Physical Anthropology, 90,* 335–344.

Mason, W. A., & Berkson, G. (1975). Effects of maternal mobility on the development of rocking and other behaviors in rhesus monkeys: A study with artificial mothers. *Developmental Psychobiology, 8,* 213–221.

Mason, W. A., & Kenney, M. D. (1974). Re-direction of filial attachments in rhesus monkeys: Dogs as mother surrogates. *Science, 183,* 1209–1211.

Matthew, S. J., Coplan, J. H., Smith, E. L., Scharf, B. A., Owens, M. J., Nemeroff, C. B., et al. (2002). Cerebrospinal fluid concentrations of biogenic amines and corticotrophin-releasing factor in adolescent nonhuman primates as a function of the timing of adverse early rearing experiences. *Stress, 5,* 185–193.

McCormack, K. M., Sanchez, M. M., Bardi, M., & Maestripieri, D. (2006). Maternal care patterns and behavioral development of rhesus macaque abused infants in the first 6 months of life. *Developmental Psychobiology, 48*, 537–550.

Mehlman, P. T., Higley, J. D., Faucher, I., Lilly, A. A., Taub, D. M., Vickers, J., et al. (1994). Low cerebrospinal fluid 5-hydroxyindoleacetic acid concentrations are correlated with severe aggression and reduced impulse control in free-ranging nonhuman primates (*Macaca mulatta*). *American Journal of Psychiatry, 151*, 1485–1491.

Mehlman, P. T., Higley, J. D., Faucher, I., Lilly, A. A., Taub, D. M., Vickers, J. M., et al. (1995). CSF 5-HIAA concentrations are correlated with sociality and the timing of emigration in free-ranging primates. *American Journal of Psychiatry, 152*, 907–913.

Mendoza, S. P., Smotherman, W. P., Miner, M., Kaplan, J., & Levine, S. (1978). Pituitary–adrenal response to separation in mother and infant squirrel monkeys. *Developmental Psychobiology, 11*, 169–175.

Mikulincer, M., & Shaver, P. R. (2007). *Attachment in adulthood: Structure, dynamics, and change.* New York: Guilford Press.

Novak, M. F. (2006). Tethering with maternal and fetal catheterization as a model for studying pre-to postnatal continuities. In G. P. Sackett, G. C. Ruppenthal, & K. Elias (Eds.), *Nursery rearing of nonhuman primates in the 21st century* (pp. 513–536). New York: Springer.

Povinelli, D. J., Parks, K. A., & Novak, M. A. (1992). Role reversal by rhesus monkeys, but no evidence of empathy. *Animal Behavior, 43*, 269–281.

Redican, W., & Mitchell, G. D. (1973). A longitudinal study of paternal behavior in adult male rhesus monkeys: I. Observations on the first dyad. *Developmental Psychology, 8*, 135–136.

Reite, M., Short, R., Selier, C., & Pauley, J. D. (1981). Attachment, loss, and depression. *Journal of Child Psychology and Psychiatry, 22*, 141–169.

Robertson, J., & Bowlby, J. (1952). Responses of young children to separation from their mothers. *Cours du Centre International de l'Enfance, 2*, 131–142.

Rosenblum, L. A., Forger, C., Noland, S., Trost, R. C., & Coplan, J. D. (2001). Response of adolescent bonnet macaques to an acute fear stimulus as a function of early rearing conditions. *Developmental Psychobiology, 39*, 40–45.

Rosenblum, L. A., & Paulley, G. S. (1984). The effects of varying demands on maternal and infant behavior. *Child Development, 55*, 305–314.

Ruppenthal, G. C., Harlow, M. K., Eisele, C. D., Harlow, H. F., & Suomi, S. J. (1974). Development of peer interactions of monkeys reared in a nuclear family environment. *Child Development, 45*, 670–682.

Sackett, G. P. (1966). Monkeys reared in isolation with pictures as visual input: Evidence for an innate releasing mechanism. *Science, 154*, 1468–1472.

Sanchez, M. M. (2006). The impact of early adverse care on HPA development: Nonhuman primate models. *Hormones and Behavior, 50*, 623–631.

Schneider, M. L. (1992). Delayed object permanence in prenatally stressed rhesus monkey infants. *Occupational Therapy Journal of Research, 12*, 96–110.

Shannon, C., Champoux, M., & Suomi, S. J. (1998). Rearing condition and plasma cortisol in rhesus monkey infants. *American Journal of Primatology, 46*, 311–321.

Shannon, C., Schwandt, M. L., Champoux, M., Shoaf, S. E., Suomi, S. J., Linnoila, M., et al. (2005). Maternal absence and stability of individual differences in CSF 5-HIAA concentrations in rhesus monkey infants. *American Journal of Psychiatry, 162*, 1658–1664.

Simpson, M. J. A. (1979). Daytime rest and activity in socially living rhesus monkey infants. *Animal Behaviour, 27*, 602–612.

Simpson, M. J. A., Simpson, A. E., Hooley, J., & Zunz, M. (1981). Infant-related influences on birth intervals in rhesus monkeys, *Nature, 290*, 49–51.

Suomi, S. J. (1979a). Differential development of various social relationships by rhesus monkey infants. In M. Lewis & L. A. Rosenblum (Eds.), *Genesis of behavior: Vol. 2. The child and its family* (pp. 219–244). New York: Plenum Press.

Suomi, S. J. (1979b). Peers, play, and primary prevention in primates. In M. Kent & J. Rolf (Eds.), *Primary prevention in psychopathology: Vol. 3. Social competence in children* (pp. 127–149). Hanover, NH: University Press of New England.

Suomi, S. J. (1981). Genetic, maternal, and environmental influences on social development in rhesus monkeys. In A. B. Chiarelli & R. S. Corruccini (Eds.), *Primate behavior and sociobiology: Selected papers (Part B) of the VIII Congress of the International Primatological Society, 1980* (pp. 81–87). New York: Springer-Verlag.

Suomi, S. J. (1982). Sibling relationships in nonhuman primates. In M. E. Lamb & B. Sutton-Smith (Eds.), *Sibling relationships: Their development and significance* (pp. 284–309). Hillsdale, NJ: Erlbaum.

Suomi, S. J. (1987). Genetic and maternal contributions to individual differences in rhesus monkey biobehavioral development. In N. A. Krasnagor, E. M. Blass, M. A. Hofer, & W. P. Smotherman (Eds.), *Perinatal development: A psychobiological perspective* (pp. 397–420). New York: Academic Press.

Suomi, S. J. (1991). Up-tight and laid-back monkeys: Individual differences in the response to social challenges. In S. Brauth, W. Hall, & R. Dooling (Eds.), *Plasticity of development* (pp. 27–56). Cambridge, MA: MIT Press.

Suomi, S. J. (1995). Influence of Bowlby's attachment theory on research on nonhuman primate biobehavioral development. In S. Goldberg, R. Muir, & J. Kerr (Eds.), *Attachment theory: Social, developmental, and clinical perspectives* (pp. 185–201). Hillsdale, NJ: Analytic Press.

Suomi, S. J. (1997). Early determinants of behaviour: Evidence from primate studies. *British Medical Bulletin, 53*, 170–184.

Suomi, S. J. (1998). Conflict and cohesion in rhesus monkey family life. In M. Cox & J. Brooks-Gunn

(Eds.), *Conflict and cohesion in families* (pp. 283–296). Mahwah, NJ: Erlbaum.

Suomi, S. J. (1999). Developmental trajectories, early experiences, and community consequences: Lessons from studies with rhesus monkeys. In D. Keating & C. Hertzman (Eds.), *Developmental health and the wealth of nations: Social, biological, and educational dynamics* (pp. 185–200). New York: Guilford Press.

Suomi, S. J. (2002). Parents, peers, and the process of socialization in primates. In J. G. Borkowski, S. L. Ramey, & M. Bristol-Power (Eds.), *Parenting and the child's world: Influences on academic, intellectual, and social-emotional development* (pp. 265–279). Mahwah, NJ: Erlbaum.

Suomi, S. J. (2006). Risk, resilience, and gene × environment interactions in rhesus monkeys. *Annals of the New York Academy of Sciences, 1094*, 52–62.

Suomi, S. J., & Harlow, H. F. (1975). The role and reason of peer friendships. In M. Lewis & L. A. Rosenblum (Eds.), *Friendships and peer relations* (pp. 310–334). New York: Basic Books.

Suomi, S. J., & Harlow, H. F. (1976). The facts and functions of fear. In M. Zuckerman & C. D. Spielberger (Eds.), *Emotions and anxiety: New concepts, methods, and applications* (pp. 3–34). Hillsdale, NJ: Erlbaum.

Suomi, S. J., Kraemer, G. W., Baysinger, C. M., & Delizio, R. D. (1981). Inherited and experiential factors associated with individual differences in anxious behavior displayed by rhesus monkeys. In D. G. Klein & J. Rabkin (Eds.), *Anxiety: New research and changing concepts* (pp. 179–200). New York: Raven Press.

Suomi, S. J., & Levine, S. (1998). Psychobiology of intergenerational effects of trauma: Evidence from animal studies. In Y. Danieli (Ed.), *International handbook of multigenerational legacies of trauma* (pp. 623–637). New York: Plenum Press.

Suomi, S. J., Rasmussen, K. L. R., & Higley, J. D. (1992). Primate models of behavioral and physiological change in adolescence. In E. R. McAnarney, R. E. Kriepe, D. P. Orr, & G. D. Comerci (Eds.), *Textbook of adolescent medicine* (pp. 135–139). Philadelphia: Saunders.

Suomi, S. J., & Ripp, C. (1983). A history of motherless mother monkey mothering at the University of Wisconsin Primate Laboratory. In M. Reite & N. Caine (Eds.), *Child abuse: The nonhuman primate data* (pp. 49–77). New York: Liss.

Trivers, R. L. (1974). Parent–offspring conflicts. *American Zoologist, 14*, 249–264.

van der Horst, F. C. P., van der Veer, R., & van IJzendoorn, M. H. (2007). John Bowlby and ethology: An annotated interview with Robert Hinde. *Attachment and Human Development, 9*, 1–15.

Visalberghi, E. (1990). Tool use in *Cebus*. *Folia Primatologica, 54*, 146–154.

Visalberghi, E., Frazasgy, D., Ottoni, E., Izar, P., de Oliveria, M. G., & Andrade, F. R. D. (2007). Characteristics of hammer stones and anvils used by wild bearded capuchin monkeys (*Cebus libidinosus*) to crack open palm nuts. *American Journal of Physical Anthropology, 132*, 426–444.

Welker, C., Becker, P., Hohman, H., & Schafer-Witt, C. (1987). Social relations in groups of the black-capped capuchin *Cebus apella* in captivity: Interactions of group-born infants during their first 6 months of life. *Folia Primatologica, 49*, 33–47.

Welker, C., Becker, P., & Schafer-Witt, C. (1990). Social relations in groups of the black-capped capuchin (*Cebus apella*) in captivity: Interactions of group-born infants during their second half-year of life. *Folia Primatologica, 54*, 16–33.

Williamson, D. E., Coleman, K., Bacanu, S. A., Devlin, B. J., Rogers, J., Ryan, N. D., et al. (2003). Heritability of fearful-anxious endophenotypes in infant rhesus macaques: a preliminary study. *Biological Psychiatry, 53*, 284–291.

Wilson, E. O. (1975). *Sociobiology*. New York: Cambridge University Press.

CHAPTER 9

Attachment and Temperament
Additive and Interactive Influences on Behavior, Affect, and Cognition during Infancy and Childhood

BRIAN E. VAUGHN
KELLY K. BOST
MARINUS H. VAN IJZENDOORN

When planning this chapter, we intended to pick up the discussion of relations between attachment and temperament at the point where our review of the literature left off in the first edition of this handbook (Vaughn & Bost, 1999), and to add a review of recent twin studies of attachment being reported by developmental scientists with interests in behavior genetics (e.g., O'Connor & Croft, 2001). In 1999 we concluded that attachment and temperament domains might overlap, insofar as constructs from both domains refer to the expression of affect in social contexts, but that neither domain of constructs could be reduced to the other. We further suggested that both attachment and temperament constructs should be assessed in studies of the development of individual behavioral and personality traits. This conclusion was echoed in a second major review of the literature published the same year (Mangelsdorf & Frosch, 1999).

We rather expected that investigators committed to more biologically based interpretations of social behavior, interactions, and relationships during infancy and childhood would challenge the conclusions of these two reviews. To our surprise, computer searches (from PsycLIT, PsycARTI-CLES, and Google Scholar) for published articles

and chapters focusing on the prediction of attachment security from temperament (or temperament from attachment) returned remarkably few "hits" in the years since 1997. Moreover, in a number of these (e.g., Marshall & Fox, 2005), relations between temperament and attachment security per se were not the central focus; rather, the authors explored tendencies to seek (or not to seek) proximity to a caregiver across episodes of the Strange Situation. Apparently, developmental scientists, with perhaps the exception of some old-guard holdouts (e.g., Kagan, 1995, 2003), have accepted our earlier conclusions and now study the complementary and interactive effects of both attachment and temperament as domains of influence on a range of social and developmental outcomes.

This shift in the focus of developmental studies of attachment and temperament prompted us to revise our orientation to this chapter. On the one hand, several points that concerned us in the first edition seem worth restating, including the scope and claims of attachment theory, the conceptual connections between attachment and temperament theories, and an updated account of studies examining empirical relations between measures of temperament and attachment. On the other hand, temperament theories and measures have shifted considerably since the early 1990s (e.g., compare Rothbart & Bates, 1998, with Rothbart & Bates, 2006)—from an emphasis on behavioral style measured largely by parental reports, to an emphasis on neurologically based action or reactivity tendencies in the domains of attention, affect, and motor behavior. Temperament is being measured with both objective, standardized tests (e.g., the Laboratory Temperament Assessment Battery; Goldsmith, Reilly, Lemery, Longley, & Prescott, 1999) and more refined and precise adult reports (by parents and others). Consequently, the detailed exposition of different temperament theories required in 1999 is no longer necessary.

Our goals in this chapter, then, are to describe briefly the conceptual and empirical domains covered and the claims about socioemotional development advanced from attachment theory and from the neural theories of temperament; to review new studies directly relating attachment and temperament constructs; to review the behavior genetic studies addressing genetic and shared or nonshared environmental influences on attachment; and to devote the bulk of the chapter to reviewing studies that have used both attachment and temperament concepts and measures as "levers" to help understand the construction of personality and social functioning during development.

CONTENT DOMAINS AND CLAIMS OF ATTACHMENT AND TEMPERAMENT THEORIES REDUX

Bowlby and Ainsworth's attachment theory takes as its *explicanda* the co-construction of parent–child bonds in the early years of life and the ways in which shared experiences in attachment relationship(s) direct a child's developmental trajectories with regard to the assembly of subsequent interpersonal relationships, especially intimate relationships. The theory contains both explicit and implicit implications for individual personality and emotional development and functioning across the lifespan; nevertheless, attachment relationships themselves are obviously social, and the central premises of the theory concern the making, maintenance, breaking, and subjective meaning of those relationships. By way of comparison, both archaic and modern temperament theories have been proposed as explanations for endogenously organized individual differences in action styles, reactivity, and regulation. Modern theories emphasize the grounding of these differences in the neurophysiological mechanisms underlying activ-

ity, affect, attention, and the regulation of these domains (Rothbart & Bates, 2006). Dimensions of temperament are often (but not always) explicitly discussed as "core" aspects of personality (Rothbart & Bates, 2006), and some theorists (e.g., Buss & Plomin, 1984) view temperament traits as maturing into personality traits. The individual-difference dimensions referenced in temperament theories carry substantial implications for the quality and adaptiveness of personality and social behavior throughout the life course, although the routes of temperamental influences can be both direct and indirect (e.g., Rothbart, Posner, & Hershey, 1995). Unlike attachments, however, temperamental traits usually are not construed as products of social interactions or relationships.

Attachment Theory

Bowlby (1969/1982, 1973, 1980) grounded attachment theory in concepts, insights, and empirical findings from several intellectual traditions. Psychoanalytic/object relations theory was a source of insights concerning the nature of the infant–caregiver relationship. For example, the infant–caregiver relationship was viewed as a true love relationship, with all of the emotional implications of a love relationship, and dissolution of the child–caregiver bond through prolonged separations was thought to cause a full-fledged grief reaction in the child; the early child–caregiver relationship was viewed as serving as a model that can influence the ways in which the child co-constructs future intimate relationships with new partners; and social and psychological adjustment was conceptualized in terms of the capacities to work, love, affiliate, and play. To the extent that the early love relationship constructed in the context of caregiver–infant interactions constituted the foundation for learning to "love well," the child–caregiver attachment could be construed as a cornerstone for inter- and intrapersonal adjustment across a lifetime. Findings from ethology and research on animal behavior provided Bowlby with the motivational constructs (e.g., the attachment behavioral system) and empirical data (e.g., Harlow's studies of "motherless" monkeys) needed to explain the child's tendency to seek and maintain proximity to caregivers. Bowlby (1969/1982) suggested that the human infant comes equipped with a rudimentary attachment behavioral system, organized to maintain proximity to the caregiver in the first years of life, and that this behavioral system governs the expression of attachment behavior on a moment-to-moment basis. Bowlby explained the presence of this behavioral system in terms of evolution by natural selection (see Cassidy, Chapter 1, this volume).

Properties of the attachment behavioral system were characterized in terms of control systems concepts (e.g., the attachment system has proximity to the caregiver as its "set goal," and the degree of proximity is dynamically adjusted through "goal-corrected behavior" informed by "feedback" from sensory inputs to the system). Bowlby also coordinated his developmental schedule for the emerging attachment relationship with Piaget's periods of sensorimotor and preoperational intelligence (see Marvin & Britner, Chapter 12, this volume). Like Piaget, Bowlby believed that infants and young children actively participate in their own development, and he saw this as a defining distinction between attachment theory and both classical psychoanalytic and behaviorist explanations of the child–caregiver bond.

However, Piaget was not the primary cognitive-psychological influence on attachment theory. Bowlby based his concept of "internal working models" (e.g., Bowlby, 1973, 1980) on the ideas of Craik (1943), who had suggested that people construct mental models for all kinds of physical and social phenomena as heuristics for explanation of the operation and functioning of those phenomena (see also Johnson-Laird, 1989; Bretherton & Munholland, Chapter 5, this volume). Bowlby found the concept attractive because it suggested both a process and a structure for preserving the child's attachment relationship in the absence of overt attachment behavior, and indeed in the absence of the caregiver altogether.

Normative Claims

From an attachment theory perspective, the child's tie to the caregiver is assumed to constitute a special sort of relationship (i.e., a love relationship, as already mentioned), arising from the operation of a behavioral system designed by natural selection to promote proximity and contact with the primary caregiver in the service of survival. As the system is activated in both normal and emergency situations (i.e., when the infant is stressed by internal or by external inputs), and as the set goal is repeatedly attained (i.e., contact or proximity is achieved), the pattern of individual interactions becomes organized as a recognizable and unique relationship characterizing the child–caregiver dyad (for discussions of connections between interac-

tions and relationships, see Hinde, 1987; Hinde & Stevenson-Hinde, 1987). This relationship is co-constructed with the caregiver over ontogenetic time in a regular, expectable sequence that parallels the growth of sensorimotor intelligence during the first years of life.

Further activity of the behavioral system in the context of the attachment relationship provides input for the assembly of an internal working model of the relationship, and of collateral models of the attachment figure and of the self. Because these models take their initial forms from interactions and associated emotions experienced prior to the onset of verbal representation, Bowlby (1980) argued that core aspects of internal working models are sometimes difficult to bring into conscious awareness. These assumptions constitute the normative, species-specific claims for attachment theory (see also Waters, Kondo-Ikemura, Posada, & Richters, 1991).

Individual-Difference Claims

Yet another influence on Bowlby's thinking about attachment arose from his association with Mary Ainsworth. Ainsworth's work focused on the construct of "security" (i.e., the feeling of safety and comfort arising from the satisfaction of basic physical and psychological needs, and from knowledge that future satisfaction of needs is not at risk). She met Bowlby in the early 1950s (see Ainsworth & Marvin, 1995) and recognized that the attachment relationship should be the primary source of security for a young child. That this relationship is indeed a source of security can be inferred from the organization of the child's behavior with reference to the caregiver. As Ainsworth observed, the child uses the caregiver as a base for exploring the surrounding environment in both familiar and unfamiliar settings. Furthermore, when the child is distressed, threatened, or simply bored, proximity and contact with the caregiver generally return the "system" to its prior state, allowing the child to continue exploration. Ainsworth referred to the balance of attachment and exploratory behavior organized around a specific caregiver as the "secure-base" and "haven-of-safety" phenomena (see Weinfield, Sroufe, Egeland, & Carlson, Chapter 4, this volume).

Although attachment theory provides a normative account of when, how, and why child–caregiver bonds emerge and are maintained, it is both explicit and implicit in the theory that attachments have individual-difference implications in the domains of personality and interpersonal adaptation. Security theory provided a venue for exploring those implications. Fieldwork convinced Ainsworth (e.g., Ainsworth, 1967; Ainsworth, Blehar, Waters, & Wall, 1978) that differences in the patterns of secure-base behavior characterizing different child–mother pairs reflect differences in the effectiveness of the attachment relationship as a source of security. Although differences in the organization of secure-base behavior were apparent in home observations (e.g., Ainsworth et al., 1978; Vaughn & Waters, 1990; Waters & Deane, 1985; Waters et al., 1991), they were distinguished by qualitatively distinct responses of the child to separation and reunion events in Ainsworth's Strange Situation procedure. In most nonclinical samples, from 50% to 70% of cases are assigned to the "secure" (Group B) classification, whereas the remaining cases are assigned to one of three "insecure" (Groups A, C, D) classifications. Secure as well as "insecure-avoidant" (A) or "insecure-ambivalent" (C) attachment relationships are considered to involve organized strategies, adaptive to a child's environment (e.g., Main, 1990). However, some insecure attachment relationships are best characterized by the absence or breakdown of an organized strategy, and hence are defined as "disorganized" (D—Main & Solomon, 1990; see Solomon & George, Chapter 18, this volume).

Drawing on her naturalistic observations of child–mother interactions at home, Ainsworth argued that the differences in secure-base behavior seen in the Strange Situation could be predicted from qualities of interaction over the first year of life (Ainsworth et al., 1978). Other researchers (e.g., Grossmann, Grossmann, Spangler, Suess, & Unzner, 1985; Pederson & Moran, 1995) have also distinguished securely from insecurely attached infants on the basis of home observations in the first year. In general, caregivers who typically respond sensitively to their child's communicative signals have securely attached children (De Wolff & van IJzendoorn, 1997; van IJzendoorn & De Wolff, 1997; see Belsky & Fearon, Chapter 13, this volume).

Attachment theory assumes that individual differences in the organization of secure-base behavior, and associated differences in the experience and expression of affects, arise as a consequence of quantitative and qualitative differences in the patterns of interactions over the first years of life. Individual differences in the organization of attachment behavior observed in infancy and childhood (Ainsworth et al., 1978) reflect accommodations of the child's attachment behavioral system to characteristic qualities of the interactive environment provided by the attachment figure. Differences in experienced attachment relationships (and the resulting internal working models) influence personality development and psychosocial adjustment by virtue of their influences on beliefs and expectations concerning the self and the self in relation to others (see Waters, Vaughn, Posada, & Kondo-Ikemura, 1995, for examples; see also Thompson, Chapter 16, this volume).

Temperament Theory

Diverse theories of temperament have been unified within the psychobiological theory and empirical achievements of Mary Rothbart, Hill Goldsmith, and their associates over the past 20 years (Kagan, 2003, offers a similar appraisal). Derryberry and Rothbart (1997) have defined "temperament" as affective, motivational, and cognitive (attentional) adaptations that are constitutional (i.e., grounded in neuroanatomical and physiological structures that are inherited), but also are shaped by experience. Constitutionally based individual differences in reactivity and regulation in the domains of attention, emotionality, and motor activity are the phenotypic expressions of temperament (Rothbart & Derryberry, 1981). Temperament theorists have defined "reactivity" as a person's characteristic mode of responding to changes in stimulation, including responses at behavioral, autonomic, and neuroendocrine levels. "Self-regulation" has been defined as those processes operating to adjust the person's characteristic level of reactivity across the several domains (i.e., affect, cognition, motor activity) and levels in response to variations in environmental demands (see Block & Block, 1980, for a similar characterization of broad personality constructs).

Biological mechanisms associated with individual differences in reactivity are thought to be present in the earliest period of life, although reactivity is expressed within motivational systems that develop as individual modules (e.g., individual differences in appetitive motivation may be present by 6 months, but individual differences in fear are not reliable until 9+ months of age; Rothbart, 1988, 1989). Regulatory processes depend on central nervous system maturation, and these processes also develop on an uneven schedule over the first several years of life (e.g., regulatory mechanisms controlling autonomic and neuroendocrine functions mature earlier than conscious regulatory processes such as "effortful control," which modulate reactivity for motor behavior, thought, and emotions) (e.g., Jones, Rothbart, & Posner, 2003; Rothbart, Ellis, Rueda, & Posner, 2003; Rothbart & Rueda, 2005). Importantly, Rothbart and Bates (2006) suggested that the consolidation of regulatory capacity may change the child's characteristic levels of reactivity between 3 and 6 years of age. As a consequence, rank-order stability of temperament may be expected to be modest in the first years, with increases after 3 years of age (Roberts & DelVecchio, 2000; Rothbart et al., 1995).

Rothbart and Bates (2006) review an extensive literature concerning some of the molecular (genetic) and neuroanatomical structures that support both the reactive and the regulatory facets of temperament. Much of this research is recent, and relatively few of the molecular results have been replicated; nevertheless, it seems that alleles contributing to differences in serotonin transport and dopamine reception are implicated in both appetitive and fear systems of human children and adults, as well as of other primates. Various brain structures and asymmetries of brain activation have also been identified in support of both approach and inhibitory aspects of temperament (e.g., Calkins, Fox, & Marshall, 1996; Fox, Calkins, & Bell, 1994). Autonomic indicators (both sympathetic and parasympathetic) have been implicated in individual differences with respect to both appetitive and inhibitory motivational systems. To give some examples, skin conductance (considered a sympathetic nervous system indicator) may prove to be as valid a measure of fear as parent report or laboratory test (e.g., Fowles & Kochanska, 2000); hypothalamic–pituitary–adrenocortical (HPA) axis reactivity may be predicted by the combination of high negative emotionality and low self-regulation (e.g., Dettling, Parker, Lane, Sebanc, & Gunnar, 2000); and heart rate variability and respiratory sinus arrhythmia (RSA) (both considered parasympathetic nervous system indicators) have been implicated in the development of attention regulation (Katz & Gottman, 1995; Porges, Doussard-Roosevelt, Portales, & Suess, 1995) and generally better-adapted functioning (Beauchaine, 2001).

These kinds of results provide compelling evidence that variations in human action, cognition, and emotion (and those of other animals) have a material basis, and that the central nervous system participates in these functions in a complex, transactional manner. Moreover, the results of psychobiological and molecular genetic studies clearly support the notion that virtually every "structure" associated with temperamental variability has multiple functions in both development and adaptation, and that these functions may become reorganized as the environments to which the child must adapt change over ontogenetic time. Finally, the results of these studies highlight the interactive nature of this underlying material participation in behavior, cognition, and emotion, insofar as "effects" of temperament and the functioning of physical structures underlying temperament are generally moderated or mediated by aspects of the environment (both internal to the individual and external/social).

Normative Claims

Although it may seem paradoxical to suggest that structures underlying *differences* between persons with respect to characteristic levels of reactivity and regulation show species-specific patterns of growth, Rothbart (e.g., 1989, 2004) has argued that the underlying neural and physiological structures governing motivation (e.g., approach vs. withdrawal and/or avoidance), emotion (e.g., fear, anger, joy), and their regulation (e.g., inhibition and effortful control) are shared (i.e., normative) features of our species, and that these structures are assembled according to species-specific developmental schedules over the first several years of life. Importantly, these structures have functions that are intimately connected to viability and survival of the infant or child, suggesting that the structures are adaptations in the evolutionary sense. For example, emotions or affects convey information to the experiencing child concerning the salience and valence of the immediate environment, in terms of that environment's support (or threat) to the experiencing infant or child's current well-being (e.g., Campos, Frankel, & Camras, 2004; Campos, Mumme, Kermoian, & Campos, 1994; Campos, Thein, & Owen, 2003), and the behavioral expression of affect serves to regulate behavior of both self and others (Campos et al., 2003). Likewise, mechanisms and processes regulating the experience of emotions or affects (as well as thought and action)—both in terms of the intensity and duration of the experience, and in terms of the frequency with which specific states are entered—have important adaptive consequences for the developing person (Diamond & Aspinwall, 2003; Fox, Henderson, Marshall, Nichols, & Ghera, 2005). Normatively, then, temperament is the nexus of linkages among neuroanatomical, neuroendocrine, and physiological systems that controls the phenotypic expression of system functions at the behavioral, feeling, and mental levels.

Individual-Difference Claims

Of course, the concept of temperament refers to differences among individuals within a population, and it is the variability of phenotypic expression that gives rise to notions of temperamental reactivity *dimensions* (e.g., negative and positive reactivity, activity level, impulsivity) and their regulation (e.g., behavioral inhibition, effortful control). As noted above, Rothbart and Bates (2006) argue that these differences arise as a consequence of constitutional differences among individuals that are inherited. An individual infant's temperament is construed as a biological "given" or a primitive trait (in the sense of being at least potentially present from birth or even before) that defines the mode(s) of adaptation possible for a given child in the face of a variable environment.

Because temperament constitutes a biological primitive, Rothbart and Bates (2006) argue that temperamental variability necessarily contributes to later variability along dimensions of personality (e.g., Caspi, 2000; Caspi et al., 2003; Rothbart, Ahadi, & Evans, 2000). Moreover, temperament is linked, both directly and indirectly (i.e., it interacts with the social or physical environments), with adjustment during childhood, adolescence, and even young adulthood (e.g., Bates, 1989; Belsky, Friedman, & Hsieh, 2001; Eisenberg, Guthrie, et al., 2000; Lonigan, Vasey, Phillips, & Hazen, 2004; Rubin, Burgess, Dwyer, & Hastings, 2003; Sanson, Hemphill, & Smart, 2004). Interestingly, with respect to adjustment, it is suboptimal adaptation (usually defined in terms of internalizing or externalizing problem behaviors and troubled peer relationships) that is predictable from temperament measures, rather than optimal functioning (Rothbart & Bates, 2006).

CONCEPTUAL AND EMPIRICAL OVERLAP BETWEEN ATTACHMENT AND TEMPERAMENT

Conceptual Overlap and Distinctions

Bowlby and Ainsworth's attachment theory and the psychobiological theory of temperament proposed by Rothbart, Goldsmith, and their associates are similar in a number of respects. In both theories, the expression of action, affect, and thought in relevant domains is grounded in neu-

roanatomical and physiological structures whose functions promote the immediate survival of the individual, and these structures orient the individual's trajectory of future growth and adaptation within particular domains. Likewise, both theories emphasize regulatory mechanisms and processes within the domains of action, affect, and thought relevant to the theories. In each theoretical framework, the underlying processes related to the phenotypic expression of system function and system regulation are assumed to develop during the early years of life. Finally, both theories propose that aspects of personality growth and intra- and interpersonal adjustment are influenced by the quality of adaptation within those domains. Given these metatheoretical similarities and the overlap in content between the two theories, perhaps especially with respect to affect or emotions, it is not surprising that earlier research focused on contests over that content at both conceptual and empirical levels (for reviews and discussions, see Mangelsdorf & Frosch, 1999; Vaughn & Bost, 1999).

Despite these metatheoretical similarities, attachment and temperament theories are meant to explain very different phenomena. Attachment theory is centered on the construction and maintenance of interpersonal relationships and their consequences for the developing child. As such, attachment is a social and psychological phenomenon that cannot depend solely on material structures in the central and peripheral nervous systems that govern the expression of proximity and contact seeking. The infant–caregiver attachment relationship is co-constructed and exists *between* dyadic partners, as well as *within* each one. The function of the attachment behavioral system, in Bowlby's (e.g., 1969/1982) theory, is to promote the proximity and contact between the child and caregiver that result in the assembly of this relationship. The child's internal states are relevant to the frequency and intensity of attachment behavioral system activation, but a social process involving the child and attachment figure is what determines the outcome of this activation. Attachment exists between persons first, and within the child only at a much later point in development. The psychobiological temperament theory, on the other hand, assumes that reactivity and regulation of affect, attention, and motor activity are determined primarily by the "set points" for neuroanatomical and physiological structures that are internal to the child and variable across children. Rothbart and Bates (2006) acknowledge the possibility that a child's characteristic degree of reactivity may be modified internally, as regulatory mechanisms and processes mature, or externally, as a consequence of experience (e.g., Blair, Granger, Willoughby, Kivlighan, & the Family Life Project Investigators, 2006). Nevertheless, temperament remains an attribute of the child and is not situated *between* the child and salient others at any developmental period.

The developmental aspects of temperament theory address questions concerning the sources of variation among individuals with respect to reactivity and regulation of affect, behavior, and attention, whereas the developmental aspects of attachment theory address questions concerning the gradual assembly of the attachment relationship between the child and caregiver(s) over the early years of life. As a result, normative questions arising from several of the assumptions of attachment theory (e.g., Bowlby's arguments concerning attachments as love relationships, and his assumption that establishing a primary attachment relationship is a normative developmental accomplishment in the first year of life) do not seem to carry implications for temperament theory. However, Rothbart (e.g., 1989, 2004) and others have drawn attention to the developmental/organizational aspects of temperamental reactivity and the (potentially) reorganizing effects of emergent regulatory mechanisms that mature according to different timetables, as well as the potential effects of external regulators of reactivity, which may include attachment.

Empirical Overlap

Recent research examining both attachment and temperament domains has suggested that the caregiving environment supporting the formation of attachment relationships also serves to regulate infant reactivity. For example, Blair and colleagues (2006) found that mothers who were sensitive to their 6-month-olds' communicative signals had babies with a more typical pattern of cortisol reactivity in response to a challenge than did mothers where were less sensitive (whose infants showed a blunted cortisol reactivity response). Similarly, Jahromi, Putnam, and Stifter (2004) reported that maternal interventions served to regulate distress reactivity in 2- and 6-month-olds, and that multiple modes of intervention were more effective than any single intervention strategy. In a different study, Crockenberg and Leerkes (2006) found that maternal engagement or sensitivity at 6 months of age moderated the interaction of regula-

tory and reactive temperamental attributes in the prediction of anxious behavior 2 years later (i.e., moderating effects of regulation were observed only when mothers were less engaged and/or less sensitive). Haley and Stansbury (2003) found that parental responsiveness in a modified still-face reunion sequence was associated with both physiological reactivity and regulation. Lastly, Hane and Fox (2006) studied neural indicators (electroencephalographic asymmetries in the frontal cortex) of stress reactivity and emotionality in relation to maternal care behavior, and reported elevated indicators of stress reactivity for infants of mothers who provided low-quality care. Furthermore, in that study temperament had been assessed independently of the neural data, and temperament did not account for the elevated levels of stress indicators.

None of these studies can speak to causal ordering of infant reactivity and maternal regulation, because temperament assessments and maternal regulatory activities were assessed simultaneously. Nevertheless, the findings suggest that reactivity of (at least some) physiological and psychological systems underlying temperament is relatively labile during the early years of life (see also Schore, 2000, 2005, for a discussion of social tuning of regulatory circuits connecting the limbic system and frontal cortex). This conclusion is consistent with the observation that rank-order stability of temperamental reactivity over the first 3 years is modest (Roberts & DelVecchio, 2000), and with Rothbart and Bates's (2006) suggestion that social forces can modify initial levels of reactivity. Further research on the normative growth of the structures underlying both temperament and attachment relationships (and the context each provides for the other) should prove fruitful.

Individual Differences in Attachment and Temperament

As noted above, the central question addressed in our earlier chapter on temperament and attachment (Vaughn & Bost, 1999) was whether temperament and attachment theories are redundant construct systems with respect to explanations of individual differences in the organization of attachment behavior. We reviewed data from over 50 published studies including over 60 nonclinical samples of children and covering all of the major temperament theories. The results of these studies were inconsistent and occasionally contradictory (as when one investigator reported that children classified in one Strange Situation category had high scores for some temperament dimension, and another reported that children with the same classification were low on the same temperament dimension). We concluded that the fundamental individual-differences distinction in attachment theory (i.e., security vs. insecurity) could not be explained by temperament constructs derived from any of the major temperament approaches, although we recognized that modest to moderate correlations might be found for measures from the two domains that emphasize the expression of affect. We also concluded that attachment constructs were not sufficient to explain individual differences in temperament identified by the major theories. For the most part, these conclusions have been sustained in the handful of studies testing relations between attachment and temperament over the intervening decade. Indeed, for most of the studies reviewed below, the test of attachment–temperament relations was peripheral to the main interests of the investigators.

Marshall and Fox (2005) tested the relation between emotional reactivity and motor activity (assessed with laboratory tests and observer ratings) at 4 months of age and attachment security (Strange Situation classifications) at 14 months. Pearson chi-square tests indicated that neither the two-way (i.e., secure vs. insecure) nor the three-way (i.e., A vs. B vs. C) associations with 4-month reactivity were significant. However, when Ainsworth subgroup classifications were taken into account and the B1 + B2 cases were grouped with the A cases and the B3 + B4 cases were grouped with the C cases, the resulting chi-square did reach significance (see also Belsky & Rovine, 1987). Stevenson-Hinde and Marshall (1999) examined relations among attachment security, behavioral inhibition, heart period (considered as a reactivity indicator), and RSA (considered as a regulation indicator) in a sample of 4½-year-olds. Attachment security moderated relations between behavioral inhibition and both heart period and RSA (predicted associations were found for secure cases only). Again, no main effects of security were obtained (although complex interactions between the physiological measures were moderated by attachment status). Burgess, Marshall, Rubin, and Fox (2003) examined relations between attachment security–insecurity (A, B, and C in the Strange Situation) and behavioral inhibition (assessed with laboratory tests) at 24 months of age. The overall F-test did not reach significance, but post hoc tests showed that avoidant (Group A in the Strange Situation) cases showed significantly less behavioral inhibition than the secure (Group B) cases, and that resistant (Group C) cases did not differ from either of the other groups. Analyses testing the Belsky–Rovine split (i.e., A, B1, B2 vs. B3, B4, C cases) did not reach significance.

Pauli-Pott, Haverkock, Pott, and Beckmann (2007) compared laboratory assessments of negative emotionality completed at 4, 8, and 12 months against Strange Situation classifications and found no significant associations. Kochanska, Aksan, and Carlson (2005) used a different measure of negative reactivity (proneness to anger from laboratory tasks) at 7 months as one predictor (along with three additional nontemperament predictors) of Strange Situation classifications with both mothers and fathers at 15 months. Temperamental proneness to anger was not a significant predictor of attachment behavior with either mothers or fathers.

In a number of other studies, investigators have examined parent reports of temperament as predictors of attachment classifications (e.g., Rydell, Bohlin, & Thorell, 2005; Shamir-Essakow, Ungerer, & Rapee, 2005; Stams, Juffer, & van IJzendoorn, 2002). As with the studies using laboratory tasks to assess temperament, these studies have failed to yield significant associations between attachment classifications (using the secure vs. insecure split) and measures of temperament. In one additional study, parent-rated negative emotionality during infancy was not a significant correlate of attachment security in the Strange Situation, but attachment security did predict parent ratings of negative emotionality for the same children at preschool ages (r = –.23; Hagekull & Bohlin, 2004). Taken together, these studies are consistent with our initial conclusions (Vaughn & Bost, 1999) that attachment security and temperament domains are at best only partially, and rarely consistently, overlapping. This conclusion also holds for disorganized attachment (see Lyons-Ruth & Jacobvitz, Chapter 28, this volume). Based on a meta-analysis of 12 samples including 1,877 participants, van IJzendoorn, Schuengel, and Bakermans-Kranenburg (1999) found no association between disorganized attachment behavior in infancy and constitutional and temperamental variables (r = .003). In the eight studies (N = 1,639) that assessed difficult temperament, again no association was found with disorganized attachment.

A somewhat different pattern of results is found when attachment security is assessed with the Attachment Q-Sort (AQS; Waters et al., 1995). As noted in our earlier review, Bowlby (1969/1982) recognized that affect expression and regulation are central features of attachment relationships. He believed that the presence (or return after separation) of the attachment figure is an occasion for joy and pleasure, whereas the loss or threat of loss of this figure arouses sadness and anger or fear in the attached child. Consistent with Bowlby's argument, securely attached children are often described as expressing more positive affect in the context of interactions with their attachment figures than are insecure children (e.g., Waters, Wippman, & Sroufe, 1979). The AQS includes items descriptive of a child's expression of positive and negative affect in the context of interaction and in the context of impending or realized separations, which reflect Bowlby's emphasis on the attachment figure's regulation of the child's affect experience. Consequently, the AQS and measures of negative emotionality are usually somewhat negatively correlated in published reports. Several studies have appeared since our earlier review that support this conclusion.

Two studies reported by van Bakel and Riksen-Walraven (2004a, 2004b) found modest associations (−.15 to −.29) between the AQS security score and anger proneness (scored from maternal ratings) and social fearfulness (scored from a laboratory task) in a sample of 15-month-olds. A third study (Szewczyk-Sokolowski, Bost, & Wainwright, 2005) also yielded a moderate association ($r = -.33$) between the AQS security score and mother-rated temperamental difficulty (for preschool-age children). In each of these studies, observers completed the AQS after one or more home visits. In four additional studies, mothers served as the AQS informants *and* provided temperament ratings. Diener, Nievar, and Wright (2003) found an association ($r = -.33$) between the AQS security score and temperamental difficulty. Ispa, Fine, and Thornburg (2002) reported correlations of −.44 between the AQS security score and both fearfulness and distress to limitations. Laible (2004) reported correlations of −.35 and .41 with temperament measures of negative reactivity and effortful control. Finally, Nair and Murray (2005) reported a correlation of −.62 between temperamental difficulty (rated from a behavioral style questionnaire and scored as "difficult" or "not difficult") and the AQS security score.

The ranges of correlations between temperament scores and observer versus maternal AQS security scores show almost no overlap. Several re-

viewers have identified a range of concerns about maternal AQS scores (see Moss, Bureau, Cyr, & Dubois-Comtois, 2006; van IJzendoorn, Vereijken, Bakermans-Kranenburg, & Riksen-Walraven, 2004), and it seems likely that the elevated correlations reviewed above were obtained because the attachment and temperament data came from a common source. van IJzendoorn and colleagues (2004) have speculated that mothers of insecure children may lack the observational skills necessary for a balanced registration of secure-base behaviors in their children. They have argued that the maternal AQS may suffer from the paradox of self-diagnosis, because the observer is an active part of the observed dyadic system. Mothers of secure children may be less defensive in their perception of (negative) attachment behavior (Main, 1990; Zeijlmans van Emmichhoven, van IJzendoorn, de Ruiter, & Brosschot, 2003).

Nevertheless, the overall pattern of results when observers complete the AQS suggests that aspects of negative emotionality overlap with AQS security scores, but only to a small degree. For example, across 10 studies including 831 children, the relation between observer AQS scores and temperamental reactivity yielded an average effect size of 0.16 (van IJzendoorn et al., 2004). More secure children tend to show less negative affect. These findings are consistent with Bowlby's characterization of the affective experiences of secure children, but they also leave open questions about causality: Do secure children express less negative emotion in the presence of their mothers *because* they are secure and/or have a history of sensitive and cooperative interactions that supports optimal secure-base behavior, or are constitutionally less negatively reactive children *predisposed* to use their mothers as a secure base for exploration and a haven of safety when distressed? Careful and nuanced longitudinal studies will be required to address these issues.

Although temperamental reactivity and regulation do not seem to influence attachment security per se, it may be that specific organizations of secure-base behavior (as characterized by the avoidant vs. resistant/ambivalent vs. disorganized classifications based on child behavior in the Strange Situation) may reflect underlying differences along temperament dimensions. This speculative hypothesis—namely, that negative reactivity (alternatively, negative emotionality) distinguishes children classified as B2, B1, and A in the Strange Situation from children classified as B3, B4, and C—was first proposed by Thompson (e.g., Thompson & Lamb, 1984) and tested by Belsky and Rovine (1987). In our earlier review, we reported that subsequent tests of that hypothesis were largely negative (i.e., differences between the two groups were not significant). Several investigators have reported analyses testing the hypothesis since 1996, and the results remain mixed (see our discussion of the studies by Marshall & Fox, 2005, and Burgess et al., 2003, above). Braungart-Rieker, Garwood, Powers, and Wang (2001) did find significant relations between infant affect and regulatory activity at 4 months of age and attachment (using the A to B2 vs. C to B3 split), and they found that infant regulatory activity mediated the relation between sensitivity and attachment outcome (i.e., the Belsky–Rovine split). However, infant regulation did not mediate relations between sensitivity and security versus insecurity (i.e., B vs. all others) in their sample.

Overall, the more recent data suggest the possibility that temperamental differences may bias an insecure infant in the direction of avoidance or resistance as a strategy for proximity maintenance to the attachment figure, but that the caregiving environment is what determines security (vs. insecurity). It is not clear from existing studies whether reactivity/behavioral inhibition (e.g., Marshall & Fox, 2005) or regulatory aspects of temperament (Braungart-Rieker et al., 2001) underlie these differences. Furthermore, to the extent that aspects of stress reactivity are tuned by experience as well as by constitutional factors (e.g., Hane & Fox, 2006), it is difficult to maintain strong distinctions between "constitutional" and "socialization" influences on stress reactivity, especially insofar as stress reactivity contributes to the formation of attachment relationships. Future studies that focus more on differences among the A, C, and D classifications from the Strange Situation, rather than combining the insecure and secure cases in contrast groups, may lead to greater understanding of the etiology of specific categories of insecure attachments. Similar analyses among the secure subgroups (B1, B2, B3, B4) may also prove informative regarding the origins of subgroup differences.

Genetic Studies of Temperament and Attachment

The nature of relations between attachment and temperament may also be clarified through (behavioral and molecular) genetic studies. In the Rothbart and Goldsmith psychobiological temperament models, differences between children are rooted, at least in part, in genetic variability. Certainly, for temperamental traits like reactivity and behavioral inhibition, a rather large role of genetic influences has been confirmed (Bouchard & Loehlin, 2001; Emde et al., 1992; Goldsmith, Lemery, Buss, & Campos, 1999; O'Connor & Croft, 2001). In contrast, attachment theory proposes that although every human infant is born with an innate bias to become attached, individual differences in attachment security are explained by parental caregiving rather than by genes (O'Connor & Croft, 2001; O'Connor, Croft, & Steele, 2000; van IJzendoorn et al., 2000). Estimates of concordance between non-twin siblings assessed with the same parent are substantially greater than would be expected on the basis of genetic similarity alone and are similar to concordance rates for monozygotic twins (e.g., van IJzendoorn et al., 2000). These findings are consistent with the conclusion that temperamental influences on *security* of attachment are at best modest, even if we do find that differences along dimensions of reactivity/inhibition or regulation do help explain differences between categories of insecurity or differences among the secure subgroups.

Twin studies also show the minor role of temperament and other constitutional factors in the development of attachment. Of the four twin studies on child–mother attachment security that have been published thus far, three document a minor role for genetic influences on differences in attachment security and a rather substantial role for shared environment (making siblings within the same family more similar to each other and less similar to children in other families) (Bokhorst et al., 2003; O'Connor & Croft, 2001; Ricciuti, 1992). The fourth study, the Louisville Twin Study (Finkel & Matheny, 2000), investigated the quality of attachment in twin pairs with an adapted separation–reunion procedure originally designed for assessing temperament, which might have increased the estimate of heritability of attachment (25%).

In the Bokhorst and colleagues (2003) study, the heritability of temperament was large, in contrast to the large role of shared environment (and not heritable factors) in attachment. Genetic factors explained 77% of the variance in temperamental reactivity, and measurement error and unique environmental factors (making siblings within the same family different from each other) 23%. The study also showed that temperamental reactivity of twins who were similar in their attachment security was not more similar than the reactivity of twins with divergent attachment classifications. Thus differences or similarities in temperamental reactivity were not associated with attachment concordance within twin pairs. In the same sample, Fearon and colleagues (2006) found no evidence for a contribution of genetic factors residing in the infants to differences in maternal sensitivity. Correlations for sensitivity as rated from 1½ hours of home observations by independent coders for each of the twin siblings were high in both monozygotic and dizygotic twins (between .64 and .69). Genetic modeling indicated that shared environmental factors explained 66% of the variance in sensitivity as experienced by the children, and nonshared environmental factors explained 34%. Thus parents interact with twins in a similar sensitive or insensitive way, but it does not matter whether the twins are more or less alike genetically—or, for that matter, temperamentally.

A behavior genetic study of infant–father attachment security suggests that genetic differences do not play a role in the development of attachment to fathers, either (Bakermans-Kranenburg, van IJzendoorn, Bokhorst, & Schuengel, 2004). Again, infant–father attachment appeared to be determined by shared environment to a substantial degree (59%). In contrast, temperamental dependency was found to be largely (66%) genetically determined. Dependency was indexed by behaviors such as excessive distress before and after separation at home, clinging, and fussy or demanding behaviors. Security and dependency were assessed in the same context and with the same Q-sort measure (the AQS; Vaughn & Waters, 1990). Therefore, procedural differences cannot explain the contrasting behavior genetic outcomes for attachment and dependency. Moreover, concordance of attachment to father within twin pairs was not associated with greater twin similarity in temperament.

Recently, the first behavior genetic study with the Adult Attachment Interview (AAI) measuring current adult representations of childhood attachment experiences (see Hesse, Chapter 25, this volume) has been reported (Caspers, Yucuis, Troutman, Arndt, & Langbehn, 2007). Interestingly, Caspers et al. found in a sample of genetically unrelated (adopted) adult sibling pairs (mean age of 39 years) 61% concordance of AAI attachment security, suggesting that shared environment influences sibling similarities in adult attachment.

Molecular genetic studies on attachment have focused on the dopamine D4 receptor

(DRD4) 7-repeat allele. The dopaminergic system is engaged in attentional, motivational, and reward mechanisms (Robbins & Everitt, 1999), and the 7-repeat allele has been linked to lower dopamine reception efficiency. In the first molecular genetic study on attachment, Lakatos and colleagues (2000) found an estimated relative risk of 4.15 for disorganized attachment among children carrying the 7-repeat allele. There was no association between the 7-repeat allele and the three organized attachment classifications. The appealing link between the DRD4 7-repeat allele and disorganized attachment has now been tested in six samples with a combined sample size of 542 infant–mother dyads, but no association between DRD4 and disorganized attachment or attachment security has been found (Bakermans-Kranenburg & van IJzendoorn, 2007; see also Lyons-Ruth & Jacobvitz, Chapter 28, this volume).

In the absence of main genetic effects, gene–environment interactions shaping the development of attachment and other developmental outcomes have been proposed (e.g., Rutter, 2006; Rutter, Moffitt, & Caspi, 2006). For disorganized attachment, the crucial question may be whether infants with the DRD4 7-repeat allele are more susceptible to parental unresolved loss or trauma (see Hesse, Chapter 25, this volume) than infants without this allele. In a sample of 63 mothers who had experienced at least one important loss, a moderating role of the DRD4 gene was indeed found: Maternal unresolved loss or trauma was associated with infant disorganization, but only in the presence of the DRD4 7-repeat allele. Children with the shorter DRD4 variants did not show higher scores for disorganized attachment when their mothers had unresolved loss (van IJzendoorn & Bakermans-Kranenburg, 2006). In a sample of 138 mother–infant dyads (including the Lakatos et al., 2000, sample), Gervai and colleagues (2005) found that the short DRD4 allele led to a strong relation between quality of maternal communication and infant disorganization. Among infants with the long allele, however, the relation between anomalous maternal communication and infant disorganization was not significant. These contrasting findings require replication in independent studies with larger samples (see Lyons-Ruth & Jacobvitz, Chapter 28, this volume, for a similar call for replication).

In sum, both molecular (i.e., single-gene effects) and twin studies document the crucial role of shared environmental factors in attachment, contrasting with the large role of genetic influences in temperament. Twins are not similar with respect to attachment security because of similarity in their temperamental profiles, but rather because they are treated more similarly by their parents. Nevertheless, the available evidence from behavior genetic studies does not exclude the possibility that temperamental differences affect the type of attachment insecurity (avoidance vs. resistance) a child co-constructs when the parental environment provided by the caregiver fosters attachment insecurity. Finally, molecular genetic studies leave open the possibility that attachment disorganization may result when a genetic vulnerability is coupled with a caregiving environment containing the necessary elements for intergenerational transmission of trauma (although these studies will be more compelling if it is discovered that children with the DRD4 7-repeat allele are at increased risk for attachment disorganization with multiple attachment figures). Genetic differences may therefore play an indirect role in the processes leading to the co-construction of attachment relationships.

ATTACHMENT AND TEMPERAMENT AS INTERACTING INFLUENCES ON BEHAVIOR, COGNITION, AND AFFECT

It is clear from the discussion above that attachment and temperament constructs are at most obliquely related; nevertheless, theorists and investigators from both construct domains make legitimate claims that attachment security or temperament dimensions are antecedent to and underlie individual differences in behavior, cognition, and affect that together characterize personality and adjustment. Both conceptual frameworks assume that the phenomena explained by their respective theories are grounded in material systems of the body and brain, and that development of these material systems influences the development in both attachment and temperament domains (e.g., Hofer, 2006; Oosterman & Schuengel, 2007; Rueda, Posner, & Rothbart, 2005). But the two frameworks differ in terms of when, how, and why individual differences arising from the respective domains affect personality and adjustment at later ages. In this section, we consider the kinds of claims made about specific aspects of behavior, cognition, and affect, and we review studies employing constructs and measures from both attachment and temperament that may relate to those claims.

According to Bowlby and Ainsworth, the attachment *system* regulates proximity and contact with the caregiver, whereas the secure-base *relationship* supports the child's exploration of the immediate and far environments by regulating his or her experience of security in the context of novelty and challenge (see Sroufe, 1996; Sroufe, Egeland, Carlson, & Collins, 2005). The secure-base relationship also supports construction of mental representations of the self and others, especially others with whom a close relationship has been co-constructed. Thus, while the attachment system functions autonomously (i.e., in a manner analogous to autonomic nervous system functioning) most of the time, internal working models are at least potentially accessible to conscious contemplation (although preverbal children's mental representations are believed to be sensorimotor rather than cognitive). They are also susceptible to instruction from the social environment. This leads us to suggest that consequences of attachment in personality and adjustment domains should be most apparent when interpersonal outcomes in these domains are considered. This may be especially true when personality and adjustment outcomes are contingent on socializing transactions between the child and attachment figure. Furthermore, the patterns of caregiving associated with the different forms of organization of attachment behaviors among insecurely attached children should be related to specific adjustment outcomes (e.g., Jacobvitz & Sroufe, 1987). Conversely, we may expect to find that influences of attachment security or type of insecurity are less evident (although not absent) in broad aspects of personality (e.g., extraversion or conscientiousness), cognitive functioning (e.g., IQ), and other outcomes that are largely heritable. Likewise, it seems probable that attachment-related variables are less strongly associated with aspects of adjustment (e.g., measures of problem behaviors or criminality or achievement in academic and work settings), which, although often explicit targets of parental and other socialization efforts, may be more directly associated with contextual factors (e.g., socioeconomic status, ethnicity/race, immigrant status, neighborhood quality, behavioral profiles of peers) and with the heritable attributes identified above than with attachment relationships per se.

In contrast with outcomes contingent on attachment security, the emphasis in psychobiological theories of temperament on constitutionally based reactivity and regulation in relation to activity, attention, and affect (e.g., Buss, Davidson,

Kalin, & Goldsmith, 2004; Gunnar, Porter, Wolf, Rigatuso, & Larson, 1995; Kagan, 1994; Rothbart, 2004; Rothbart et al., 2004) implies significant associations with heritable dimensions of personality (e.g., Halverson, Kohnstamm, & Martin, 1994; McCrae et al., 2000; Rothbart et al., 2000). Furthermore, to the extent that temperament is defined as *regulation* of motor activity, attention, and affect, individual differences in regulatory capacity and motivation should be causal antecedents to a range of outcomes—such as externalizing problem behaviors, including attention-deficit/hyperactivity disorder and conduct disorder (e.g., Nigg, Goldsmith, & Sachek, 2004; Rettew, Copeland, Stanger, & Hudziak, 2004); anxiety disorders (e.g., Kagan, Snidman, Zentner, & Peterson, 1999; Prior, Smart, Sanson, & Oberklaid, 2000); and adjustment in settings such as schools (e.g., Eisenberg et al., 2004; Nelson, Martin, Hodge, Havill, & Kamphaus, 1999). We would also expect that associations between temperament and relational outcomes (e.g., friendship quality, teacher–child relationships) would be less prominent (but not necessarily absent) than associations between aspects of temperament and heritable aspects of personality and cognitive functioning. Of course, these broad dimensions of adjustment, personality, and cognition overlap to an extent with the kinds of outcomes we suggest are consequences of attachment, so interactions across these domains should be expected, even though the nature of those interactions (e.g., mediating, moderating) may not be readily derivable from either attachment or temperament theories.

Interactions between Attachment and Temperament: Interpersonal Outcomes

That attachment security is a significant predictor of parent–child interaction and relationship quality, and of aspects of peer interaction throughout the childhood years, has been well documented by Sroufe and associates (e.g., Arend, Gove, & Sroufe, 1979; Matas, Arend, & Sroufe, 1978; Waters & Sroufe, 1983; Waters et al., 1979) as well as many others. Secure attachments in infancy predict smoother and more harmonious parent–child interactions during the toddler period, perhaps especially in the context of developmentally challenging tasks (Matas et al., 1978; Waters et al., 1979), and specific patterns of positive peer interactions in preschoolers (e.g., LaFreniere & Sroufe, 1985). However, the early studies did not

consider the possibility that a child's temperamental characteristics may also contribute to these interactions and the relationships they reflect (see Chess & Thomas, 1982, for a discussion). Our earlier chapter (Vaughn & Bost, 1999) documented the exchanges between attachment and temperament approaches to this question, but it was not until the 1990s that investigators tested interactions between construct domains in predicting interpersonal outcomes. Kochanska's studies (e.g., Kochanska, 1995) are exemplars of this approach to parent–child interactions and relationships, and we review representative studies from her research program (and qualifications on her conclusions suggested by other research teams) below.

Compliance, Cooperation, and Conscience

Kochanska has tested several temperament dimensions, especially fearfulness/anxiety proneness, as mediators of relations among attachment security, maternal discipline, and behavioral and cognitive indicators of children's developing conscience across the toddler and early childhood periods (e.g., Kochanska, 1995, 1997, 2001). In her earlier studies, Kochanska (e.g., Fowles & Kochanska, 2000; Kochanska, 1995, 1997) reported that different aspects of parent–infant (and parent–toddler) interactions and relationships contributed to conscience development in children with lower versus higher levels of temperamental fearfulness. For fearless children, attachment security was the primary predictor of internalization (of maternal directives/prohibitions); for more fearful children, maternal gentle discipline was the primary predictor. In a subsequent report (Kochanska, Askan, & Carlson, 2005), children's temperamental proneness to anger and their attachment security were examined as predictors of receptive cooperation with their mothers at 15 months of age. Security, but not anger proneness, significantly predicted later receptive cooperation. Anger proneness did not interact with attachment security in predicting later receptive cooperation in mother–child interactions (although a significant interaction between temperamental anger proneness and maternal responsiveness was observed). For the father–child data, however, a significant interaction was obtained. Attachment security moderated the relation between children's anger proneness and receptive cooperation; the association between anger proneness and receptive cooperation was significant only for insecure dyads. Furthermore, maternal responsiveness had a positive, significant association with children's receptive cooperation with their fathers (but the reverse relation was not significant).

Schieche and Spangler (2005) tested the predictive utility of behavioral inhibition (a presumed component of fearfulness/anxiety proneness), adrenocortical reactivity (assessed in the problem-solving task context), and attachment security for toddlers' behavior in a problem-solving assessment (analogous to assessments reported by Matas et al., 1978). Attachment security in infancy predicted toddler task orientation, help seeking, and the balance of attachment and exploratory behaviors in the problem-solving tasks, whereas behavioral inhibition predicted aspects of a child's approach to the task. For insecure children, high behavioral inhibition predicted elevated adrenocortical reactivity, but this relation was not found in the group of secure children. Furthermore, physiological reactivity showed different patterns of relations with toddler behavior in the problem-solving tasks for secure and insecure children (with significant relations found only for insecure cases). Thus, in contrast with Kochanska's (1995, 1997) findings, attachment security moderated the potential influences of behavioral inhibition and physiological reactivity on child behavior.

van der Mark, Bakermans-Kranenburg, and van IJzendoorn (2002) also examined relations among fearfulness, attachment security, and compliance with maternal directives ("Do X" vs. "Don't do X") in a longitudinal study of girls from 16 to 22 months of age. Fearfulness was unrelated to attachment security at both ages (although at 22 months, avoidant children had significantly lower fearfulness scores than did infants in the resistant category). In this study, neither attachment, fearfulness, nor their interaction had consistent significant relations with children's committed compliance; rather, compliance was related to the quality of maternal behavior (as sensitive or intrusive). In addition, developmental level (i.e., the Bayley Mental Development Index [MDI]) was also uniquely predictive of compliance, but only in the prohibition tasks. These findings are consistent with more recent findings from Kochanska's team (e.g., Kochanska, Forman, Aksan, & Dunbar, 2005; Kochanska & Murray, 2000) suggesting that qualities of parental behavior (which are themselves presumed to be antecedents of a child's attachment security), rather than security per se, affect various aspects of conscience development.

Even so, Kochanska, Aksan, Knaack, and Rhines (2004) suggested that the efficacy of parental socialization is contingent on attachment security. That is, securely attached toddlers were more readily influenced by parental socialization attempts than were insecurely attached children.

Relationships with Teachers and Peer Social Competence

Both attachment security and temperamental reactivity and regulation have been identified as critical antecedents to peer social competence and to relationships with peers and teachers (e.g., Arend et al., 1979; Bost, Vaughn, Washington, Cielinski, & Bradbard, 1998; Eisenberg, Fabes, Guthrie, & Reiser, 2000; Fabes, Shepard, Guthrie, & Martin, 1997; Park & Waters, 1989; Rubin, Coplan, Fox, & Calkins, 1995; Suess, Grossmann, & Sroufe, 1992). There are, however, fewer reports concerning joint relations between attachment and temperament as predictors of aspects of teacher and peer relationships or peer social competence, and a number of the reports (e.g., Denham et al., 2001) did not report tests of interactions between the attachment and temperament measures.

Szewczyk-Sokolowski and colleagues (2005) assessed attachment security (i.e., AQS security score), temperamental difficulty (from maternal report), and children's sociometric acceptance (vs. rejection) concurrently for a sample of preschool-age children. They reported that both attachment security and child difficult temperament were significant correlates (positive for attachment, negative for temperamental difficulty) of peer sociometric acceptance (based on a nomination task), whereas only difficult temperament was significantly (positively) associated with peer rejection. The interaction of attachment security and difficult temperament did not add significantly to the overall R^2 in the regression analyses for either peer acceptance or peer rejection. Rydell and colleagues (2005) tested joint relations of attachment representation (assessed with a story completion task), shyness, and peer competence as well as teacher–child relationships in a preschool sample. As in the Szewczyk-Sokolowski and colleagues' report, there were main effects of both attachment and shyness measures, but the interaction of these dimensions did not add to the predicted variance in any outcome. Attachment security positively predicted peer competence outcomes and teacher–child relationship patterns, with avoidant and resistant representations having somewhat different patterns of (negative) correlates. Shy children tended to have fewer conflicts with peers than more uninhibited children did, but they also had less optimal relationships with teachers than their more uninhibited peers did.

Bohlin, Hagekull, and Andersson (2005) tested relations among attachment, temperament, and peer social competence at early school age. Attachment assessed at 15 months was a significant positive correlate of social competence at 8 years (measures included parent and teacher ratings as well as direct observations). Behavioral inhibition assessed during infancy (at 13 and 15 months) did not predict social competence measures; however, behavioral inhibition assessed at 4 years was a significant negative predictor of social competence at 8 years. These latter results were qualified by an interaction with attachment. For securely attached cases, high behavioral inhibition showed a significant positive association with social competence at 8 years, whereas for insecure cases high behavioral inhibition was significantly negatively associated with social competence.

In a longitudinal study of children adopted as infants, Juffer and associates (e.g., Jaffari-Bimmel, Juffer, van IJzendoorn, Bakermans-Kranenburg, & Mooijaart, 2006; Stams et al., 2002) have examined relations among attachment, temperament, and social adaptation from infancy to adolescence. Attachment security (Strange Situation classifications converted to a 6-point continuous scale) assessed during infancy, as well as easy temperament (from the Dutch Temperament Questionnaire; Kohnstamm, 1984) predicted prosocial development at age 7 years (based on parent and teacher ratings and Q-sorts; see Stams et al., 2002). Effects of attachment during infancy on positive social development at age 14 (from parent and teacher Q-sort data) were mediated by childhood (age 7) positive social development and by a social development (age 7) to maternal sensitivity (age 14) pathway. Effects of infant and childhood temperament were also mediated by positive social development at age 7 and by temperament and maternal sensitivity at age 14. Temperament explained a substantially larger portion of the variance in social development than did either attachment security or parental sensitivity. The interaction of attachment and temperament in infancy did not have a significant pathway in the overall model (Jaffari-Bimmel et al., 2006). This is a complicated study, but it is exemplary in that the investigators attempted to assess common constructs across the infancy, childhood, and adolescence periods (although attach-

ment security was not explicitly assessed beyond infancy). The results suggest that both attachment and temperament constructs contribute to subsequent positive social development, albeit through different and noninteracting pathways.

Considered together, the results from parent–child interaction studies and from studies of peer competence are consistent with our suggestion that attachment security should be a significant predictor of outcomes in socially relevant domains. Temperamental qualities, perhaps especially behavioral inhibition/fear/anxiety, also show significant relations with social outcomes measured later in childhood, and these may moderate relations between attachment and certain social outcomes. However, results from Kochanska's research program suggest that parental socialization practices are the proximal causal factors leading to variations in social outcomes (at least with respect to compliance and conscience), and that these may be moderated by attachment quality, so that securely attached children are more easily socialized by parents than are insecure children (a conclusion anticipated by Stayton, Hogan, & Ainsworth, 1971). Social outcomes assessed outside the family tend to be predictable from both attachment and temperament measures. There is only modest evidence of interaction between attachment security and temperament domains in the predictions to outcomes in the peer group, and the available data suggest that when an interaction is observed, attachment security moderates relations between temperament and peer competence outcomes.

Interactions between Temperament and Attachment: Intrapersonal Outcomes

Although Bowlby believed that attachment (or attachment-related phenomena) should be causal antecedents to aspects of personality and psychopathology (e.g., Bowlby, 1980), and although temperament has been linked explicitly with somatic reactivity and regulation as well as with personality and psychopathology, only a handful of studies have attempted to assess both attachment and temperament constructs as predictors of outcomes in these domains, and older or nonstandard temperament models were used in some studies. We review representative studies for each of three outcome domains (physiological reactivity and regulation; personality and cognition; and problem behaviors), but none of these offer the breadth of programmatic research available for the interpersonal outcome domains discussed above.

Biobehavioral Response Systems

Both attachment theory and neurophysiological temperament theories posit associations between their constitutive construct domains and adaptive responses to stress/distress. Whereas temperament approaches tend to treat reactivity and regulation of affect and behavior as broad trait-like aspects of a person (i.e., reactivity and regulation are not context-specific), attachment theory assumes that arousal and regulation of affect, cognition, and behavior in the context of the threat of loss or separation from an attachment figure are governed by the attachment behavioral system, and that with the assembly of internal working models, these adaptive processes may generalize to other social contexts (see Sroufe et al., 2005, for an extended treatment of these ideas). Furthermore, attachment theory suggests that the attachment figure plays an important role in regulating arousal during infancy, toddlerhood, and beyond; this is not solely the child's responsibility (e.g., Spangler, Schieche, Ilg, Maier, & Ackermann, 1994). Given the relevance of arousal and regulation in both attachment and temperament domains, it is not surprising that many studies have related temperament and/or attachment to the physiological systems governing the production and breakdown of cortisol (a major stress hormone), especially the HPA axis (e.g., Gunnar, Larson, Hertsgaard, Harris, & Brodersen, 1992; McEwen, 2001; Spangler, Fremmer-Bombik, & Grossmann, 1996). Of significance here, several of these studies included measures of both attachment and temperament as correlates of cortisol reactivity in response to stress.

Gunnar and associates (e.g., Gunnar, Brodersen, Nachmias, Buss, & Rigatuso, 1996) were among the first to systematically examine relations among attachment security, fearful temperament, and cortisol reactivity. In their study, attachment security (based on Strange Situation classifications) was related to *baseline* cortisol levels (taken during medical checkups and inoculations at 2, 4, and 6 months of age) and to maternal responsiveness. Neither cortisol *reactivity* nor behavioral *reactivity* at the clinic visits predicted attachment classifications, but attachment security moderated relations between fearfulness and cortisol reactivity: A positive relation between the two was observed only for insecurely attached children. This suggests that attachment security was a protective factor buffering the effects of high fearfulness on cortisol reactivity. Schieche and Spangler (2005; see discussion above) reached a similar conclu-

sion concerning protective effects of attachment security, although they used a different assessment context and different indices of temperamental reactivity. Schieche and Spangler also noted that security moderated relations between behavioral inhibition and task behavior in a problem-solving task. Whereas insecure inhibited children decreased task involvement and sought proximity to their mothers as the tasks became more difficult, secure inhibited children increased task-related help seeking in the difficult tasks. For the insecure inhibited children, proximity seeking was associated with increasing cortisol reactivity, but for the secure inhibited youngsters, seeking task-relevant instrumental assistance was negatively associated with cortisol reactivity.

van Bakel and Riksen-Walraven (2004a, 2004b) used both the Strange Situation and the AQS as attachment security indicators in a study of temperament (based on parent reports using the Toddler Behavior Assessment Questionnaire [TBAQ]), parent–child interaction in the context of a teaching task, and cortisol reactivity in a task testing both social (stranger) and nonsocial (toy robot) fearfulness. Strange Situation classifications were unrelated to the temperament measures and the measure of cortisol reactivity, but the AQS security score had significant associations with anger proneness (negative) and pleasure (positive) from the TBAQ, task orientation (in the parent–child teaching task), and social fear (in the stranger interaction task). Cortisol reactivity was positively associated with AQS security, whereas anger proneness and social fear (from the TBAQ) were negatively associated with attachment security. However, AQS security was not related significantly to either observed social or nonsocial fear in this study, although cortisol reactivity predicted nonsocial fear, and anger proneness predicted social fear. Interactions of the attachment and temperament measures did not yield significant effects. Thus, in contrast to the other studies reviewed in this section, no special protective effect of attachment security (assessed by either the Strange Situation or the AQS) was observed in the relation between cortisol reactivity and fearfulness/inhibition.

In addition to cortisol activation, researchers have examined cardiac reactivity in relation to child temperament and attachment security. In general, these studies are based on the theoretical notion that individual differences in autonomic nervous system responses related to arousal may influence social engagement behaviors. In particular, the vagal system is proposed to regulate vagal input to the heart and facilitate changes in heart rate required to promote social communication when there are challenges to homeostasis; when this regulatory mechanism is not applied, the sympathetic nervous system is recruited, and more defensive behavior may be exhibited (e.g., Porges, Doussard-Roosevelt, Portales, & Greenspan, 1996).

Stevenson-Hinde and Marshall (1999) examined heart period (the interval between heartbeats) and RSA during a modified Strange Situation in relation to children's attachment security and behavioral inhibition in a sample of preschool children (4½ years old). They reported that for secure and for temperamentally less inhibited children, heart period significantly increased upon reunion with the caregiver, but this increase was not evident for highly inhibited or insecure children. RSA was also found to increase upon reunion, except for those children who were highly inhibited. Thus, in general, separation from caregivers tended to be associated with increases in heart rate, whereas reunion tended to be associated with decreasing heart rate (with the exceptions noted), and these physiological changes were affected by both attachment quality and temperament. Oosterman and Schuengel (2007) extended the Stevenson-Hinde and Marshall (1999) study to include continuous ambulatory recordings of changes in heart rate, RSA (parasympathetic activity or withdrawal), and preejection period (PEP; sympathetic activity or withdrawal) in a sample of 50 children ages 3–6 years who participated in a separation–reunion episode with their mothers and a stranger. The AQS served as the measure of attachment security (observer sort), and inhibition to the stranger was assessed with a composite of selected items from the AQS (e.g., "child laughs and smiles easily with a lot of different people"). The inhibition-to-stranger score was found to be unrelated to security ($r = .09$), but was significantly associated with the Shyness scale of the Child Behavior Questionnaire completed by a subsample of mothers ($r = .37, p < .05$). Results indicated an overall decrease in RSA over the separation–reunion episodes and a decrease at separation from mothers (but not the stranger), but no significant PEP effects were reported even for insecure and inhibited children.

A recent example of the moderating role of attachment in buffering the influences of temperamental reactivity is the research by Gilissen and colleagues (Gilissen, Bakermans-Kranenburg, van IJzendoorn, Van der Veer, in press; Gilissen, Koolstra, van IJzendoorn, Bakermans-Kranenburg, & Van der Veer, 2007) on physiological stress responses to fear-inducing film clips. In these two studies, 4- and 7-year-old children were shown fear-inducing film clips; during the film clips, their skin conductance and heart rate variability were measured. Both 4- and 7-year-olds responded to the fear-inducing film clips with increases in skin conductance and decreases in heart rate variability. A secure relationship (as assessed by the Emotional Availability Scales and the Attachment Story Completion Task; see Solomon & George, Chapter 18, this volume) affected the physiological reactivity to the film clips in temperamentally reactive children but not in less reactive children, regardless of age. Temperamentally reactive children with less secure relationships showed the highest skin conductance responses to the film clips, whereas reactive children with more secure relationships showed the lowest skin conductance responses. These findings indicate that attachment may be more important for temperamentally reactive children, for the better *and* for the worse, supporting the differential-susceptibility hypothesis (Bakermans-Kranenburg & van IJzendoorn, 2007; Belsky, 2005).

Although the results of these studies are not consistent, the many procedural differences between them (e.g., age ranges, measures of behavioral inhibition, length of separation from mother) make any strong interpretation difficult. Additional studies will be needed to clarify relations between these sympathetic and parasympathetic nervous system indicators and both attachment and temperament domains.

Personality and Cognitive Outcomes

Hagekull and Bohlin (2003) reported a study examining both attachment security and temperament (assessed with the Colorado Childhood Temperament Inventory; Rowe & Plomin, 1977) during toddlerhood as predictors of the "Big Five" personality traits at 8 to 9 years of age. The temperament variables were not associated with attachment security. Attachment security predicted extraversion, openness (positively), and neuroticism (negatively) (3 of 5 correlations were significant). The temperament dimensions yielded only 2 (of 15) significant associations, both with extraversion. One interaction (out of 15 tested) between attachment security and the three temperament scores was significant. Although secure children had lower scores on neuroticism than insecure children at both high and low levels of emotionality, secure children with high emotionality scores had higher neuroticism scores at age 8–9 than did secure children with low emotionality scores.

Although attachment theory does not address questions concerning individual differences in cognitive development, some studies have shown that infant developmental tests (e.g., the Bayley MDI) favor secure babies (especially as compared to insecure-resistant babies; Egeland & Farber, 1984). Karrass and Braungart-Reiker (2004) tested effects of attachment (Strange Situation classifications at 12 months) and temperament (distress to novelty, distress to limitations) on IQ (Stanford–Binet) at preschool age. Neither attachment security nor distress to limitations yielded significant, unique effects on IQ; however, distress to novelty did show a significant positive relation to IQ. This relation was partially moderated by attachment, such that distress to novelty predicted higher preschool IQs only for insecure children, $r(14) = .73$, $p < .01$, versus $r(47) = .03$ for secure children. The van Bakel and Riksen-Walraven (2004a) study also included the Bayley MDI, and it yielded a significant association with the AQS. Furthermore, developmental status (MDI) interacted with attachment security with regard to cortisol reactivity, so that for insecure (but not secure) children, cortisol reactivity was positively associated with cognitive competence.

Problem Behaviors

Although both attachment and temperament frameworks have been invoked by investigators studying problem behaviors (e.g., Eisenberg, Fabes, Nyman, Bernzweig, & Pineulas, 1994; Kobak, Sudler, & Gamble, 1991), only a few reports include measures from both domains. McCartney, Tresch Owen, Booth, Clarke-Stewart, and Vandell (2004) used data from the National Institute of Child Health and Human Development Study of Early Child Care and Youth Development data set to examine attachment (assessed with the Strange Situation at 15 and 36 months, and with the AQS at 24 months) as a predictor of externalizing problems. A temperament measure based on a subset of items from the Infant Temperament Questionnaire (Carey & McDevitt, 1978) was completed by each mother at the 6-month home visit and was used to index temperamental difficulty. Problem behaviors were rated by mothers and by teachers at 36 months. Small but significant associations between attachment security and maternal ratings

of both internalizing and externalizing behavior problems were found. Difficult temperament also predicted maternal ratings of behavior problems. The interaction of temperament and attachment did not yield any significant effects. Attachment security also had modest but significant predictive associations with caregiver-rated internalizing and externalizing behaviors; however, there was no significant predictive association between teacher-rated problems and temperamental difficulty. Adding the attachment × difficulty interaction term did not add significant variance to the regression equation.

Burgess and colleagues (2003) also reported direct effects of infant behavioral inhibition (vs. uninhibited temperament) and attachment on mother-reported externalizing behaviors at 4 years of age. In this study, however, it was only the insecure-avoidant infants who had elevated externalizing scores, and the interaction of avoidance and uninhibited temperament produced the highest externalizing scores. A similar finding was reported by Pierrehumbert, Miljkovitch, Planherel, Halfon, and Ansermet (2000): Insecure-avoidant children (Strange Situation classification, 21 months) had higher scores on ratings of externalizing behavior (mothers completed a checklist when their children were 5 years of age). Curiously, although temperament assessments were available in this study (based on a Thomas and Chess measure), those data were not analyzed with reference to problem behaviors. However, Pierrehumbert et al. treated the Belsky–Rovine split as a dichotomous temperamental reactivity variable and did find some associations with both externalizing and internalizing problem ratings. No interaction analyses were reported.

A few studies have examined the role of both attachment and temperament in the development of anxiety disorders. Manassis, Bradley, Goldberg, Hood, and Swinson (1995) examined these relations in a clinical sample of preschool-age children of anxious mothers. Insecure attachment was found to be significantly associated with internalizing problems and indicators of childhood anxiety, whereas behavioral inhibition was significantly associated with somatic difficulties. In addition, Warren, Huston, Egeland, and Sroufe (1997) followed up 172 adolescents who had been observed in the Strange Situation with their mothers at age 1 and found that insecure-resistant attachment predicted anxiety disorders in adolescence, over and beyond maternal anxiety and maternal reports of child temperament. More recently,

Shamir-Essakow and colleagues (2005) examined relations between insecure attachment (preschool version of the Strange Situation; Cassidy & Marvin, 1992), behavioral inhibition (maternal report and lab procedure), and anxiety disorders (criteria from the *Diagnostic and Statistical Manual of Mental Disorders*, fourth edition) in an at-risk sample of preschool-age children. Both behavioral inhibition and insecure attachment were unique and significant predictors of child anxiety even after maternal anxiety was controlled for. Children who were inhibited and insecure, and whose mothers were anxious, tended to have the highest anxiety levels.

The results reported in this section are quite mixed and difficult to reconcile. In most of the studies, results run contrary to our expectations that temperament rather than attachment would be the primary predictor of outcomes in developmental domains with high heritability (e.g., physiological reactivity, personality, IQ). When interactions were significant, it was typically the attachment variable that moderated effects of temperament on a given outcome rather than the reverse, and this held across all areas we reviewed.

CONCLUSION

We have begun this chapter with the assumptions that attachment and temperament constitute separate domains of development, and that constructs from one domain do not explain individual differences in the other. The bulk of the recent literature is consistent with these assumptions. Nevertheless, aspects of both domains contribute meaningfully to a broad range of interpersonal and intrapersonal developmental outcomes, both as direct effects and as products of their interaction. Given the breadth of the areas in which moderating interactions involving attachment and temperament measures have been documented, it would seem prudent to recommend that measures from both domains be included in all future studies of the "consequences" of either attachment or temperament. Although we had anticipated that attachment and temperament variables would each have a suite of "principal" correlates (attachment in the interpersonal domain, temperament in the intrapersonal), this proved not to be the case. Both attachment and temperament were important in the decomposition of variance for both inter- and intrapersonal outcomes. Interestingly, in several studies, attachment effects were obtained

for specific categories of insecurity (i.e., avoidant, resistant, disorganized), so future research might profit by exploring these specific attachment consequences more thoroughly. Finally, evidence is accumulating that both attachment and the physiological mechanisms underlying temperamental differences are tuned by the social environment associated with the behavior patterns of significant caregivers (with the qualification that the focus has been on mothers, which reflects the common practice in the developmental sciences of letting "someone else" do the father–child work). We also suspect that aspects of the *physical* environment act to tune mechanisms underlying both temperament and attachment. Further exploration of the contextual parameters that tune attachment and temperament systems will be important over the next decade.

ACKNOWLEDGMENTS

Preparation of this chapter has been supported in part by National Science Foundation Grant Nos. BCS 0126163 and BCS 0623019. We gratefully acknowledge the tolerance and encouragement of the volume editors, and the invaluable contributions of Marian J. Bakermans-Kranenburg to the preparation of this chapter. Errors of commission or omission are our responsibility.

REFERENCES

Ainsworth, M. D. S. (1967). *Infancy in Uganda: Infant care and the growth of love*. Baltimore: Johns Hopkins University Press.

Ainsworth, M. D. S., Blehar, M. C., Waters, E., & Wall, S. (1978). *Patterns of attachment: A psychological study of the Strange Situation*. Hillsdale, NJ: Erlbaum.

Ainsworth, M. D. S., & Marvin, R. (1995). On the shaping of attachment theory and research: An interview with Mary D. S. Ainsworth. In E. Waters, B. E. Vaughn, G. Posada, & K. Kondo-Ikemura (Eds.), Caregiving, cultural, and cognitive perspectives on secure-base behavior and working models: New growing points of attachment theory and research. *Monographs of the Society for Research in Child Development*, 60(2–3, Serial No. 244, pp. 3–21).

Arend, R., Gove, F. L., & Sroufe, L. A. (1979). Continuity of individual adaptation from infancy to kindergarten: A predictive study of ego resiliency and curiosity in preschoolers. *Child Development, 50*, 950–959.

Bakermans-Kranenburg, M. J., & van IJzendoorn, M. H. (2007). Genetic vulnerability or differential susceptibility in child development?: The case of attachment. *Journal of Child Psychology and Psychiatry, 48*, 1160–1173.

Bakermans-Kranenburg, M. J., van IJzendoorn, M. H., Bokhorst, C. L., & Schuengel, C. (2004). The importance of shared environment in infant–father attachment: A behavioral genetic study of the Attachment Q-Sort. *Journal of Family Psychology, 18*, 545–549.

Bates, J. E. (1989). Applications of temperament concepts. In G. A. Kohnstamm, J. E. Bates, & M. K. Rothbart (Eds.), *Temperament in childhood* (pp. 321–355). Chichester, UK: Wiley.

Beauchaine, T. (2001). Vagal tone, development, and Gray's motivational theory: Toward an integrated model of autonomic nervous system functioning in psychopathology. *Development and Psychopathology, 13*, 183–214.

Belsky, J. (2005). Differential susceptibility to rearing influence: An evolutionary hypothesis and some evidence. In B. Ellis & D. Bjorklund (Eds.), *Origins of the social mind: Evolutionary psychology and child development* (pp. 139–163). New York: Guilford Press.

Belsky, J., Friedman, S., & Hsieh, K. (2003). Testing a core emotion-regulation prediction: Does early attentional persistence moderate the effect of infant negative emotionality on later development? *Child Development, 72*, 123–133.

Belsky, J., & Rovine, M. (1987). Temperament and attachment security in the Strange Situation: An empirical rapprochement. *Child Development, 58*, 787–795.

Blair, C., Granger, D., Willoughby, M., Kivlighan, K., & the Family Life Project Investigators. (2006). Maternal sensitivity is related to hypothalamic–pituitary–adrenal axis stress reactivity and regulation in response to emotion challenge in 6-month-old infants. *Annals of the New York Academy of Sciences, 1094*, 263–267.

Block, J. H., & Block, J. (1980). The role of ego-control and ego-resiliency in the organization of behavior. In W. A. Collins (Ed.), *Minnesota Symposium on Child Psychology: Vol. 13. Development of cognition, affect, and social relations* (pp. 39–101). Hillsdale, NJ: Erlbaum.

Bohlin, G., Hagekull, B., & Andersson, K. (2005). Behavioral inhibition as a precursor of peer social competence in early school age: The interplay with attachment and nonparental care. *Merrill–Palmer Quarterly, 51*, 1–19.

Bokhorst, C. L., Bakermans-Kranenburg, M. J., Fearon, R. M. P., van IJzendoorn, M. H., Fonagy, P., & Schuengel, C. (2003). The importance of shared environment in mother–infant attachment security: A behavioral genetic study. *Child Development, 74*, 1769–1782.

Bost, K. K., Vaughn, B. E., Washington, W. N., Cielinski, K. L., & Bradbard, M. R. (1998). Social competence, social support, and attachment: Demarcation of construct domains, measurement, and paths of influence for preschool children attending Head Start. *Child Development, 69*, 192–218.

Bouchard, T., & Loehlin, J. C. (2001). Genes, evolution, and personality. *Behavior Genetics, 31*, 243–273.

Bowlby, J. (1969/1982). *Attachment and loss: Vol. 1. Attachment.* New York: Basic Books.

Bowlby, J. (1973). *Attachment and loss: Vol. 2. Separation: Anxiety and anger.* New York: Basic Books.

Bowlby, J. (1980). *Attachment and loss: Vol. 3. Loss: Sadness and depression.* New York: Basic Books.

Braungart-Rieker, J. M., Garwood, M. M., Powers, B. P., & Wang, X. (2001). Parental sensitivity, infant affect, and affect regulation: Predictors of later attachment. *Child Development, 72*, 252–270.

Burgess, K. B., Marshall, P. J., Rubin, K. H., & Fox, N. A. (2003). Infant attachment and temperament as predictors of subsequent externalizing problems and cardiac physiology. *Journal of Child Psychology and Psychiatry, 44*, 819–831.

Buss, A., & Plomin, R. (1984). *Temperament: Early developing personality traits.* Hillsdale, NJ: Erlbaum.

Buss, K. A., Davidson, R. J., Kalin, N. H., & Goldsmith, H. H. (2004). Context-specific freezing and associated physiological reactivity as dysregulated fear response. *Developmental Psychology, 40*, 583–594.

Calkins, S. D., Fox, N. A., & Marshall, T. R. (1996). Behavioral and psychological antecedents of inhibition in infancy. *Child Development, 67*, 523–540.

Campos, J. J., Frankel, C. B., & Camras, L. (2004). On the nature of emotion regulation. *Child Development, 75*, 377–394.

Campos, J. J., Mumme, D. L., Kermoian, R., & Campos, R. G. (1994). A functionalist perspective on the nature of emotion. In N. A. Fox (Ed.), The development of emotion regulation: Biological and behavioral considerations. *Monographs of the Society for Research in Child Development, 59*(2–3, Serial No. 240), 284–303.

Campos, J. J., Thein, S., & Owen, D. (2003). A Darwinian legacy to understanding human infancy: Emotional expressions as behavior regulators. *Annals of the New York Academy of Sciences, 1000*, 110–134.

Carey, W. B., & McDevitt, S. C. (1978). Revision of the Infant Temperament Questionnaire. *Pediatrics, 61*, 735–739.

Caspers, K., Yucuis, R., Troutman, B., Arndt, S., & Langbehn, D. (2007). A sibling adoption study of adult attachment: The influence of shared environment on attachment states of mind. *Attachment and Human Development, 9*, 375–392.

Caspi, A. (2000). The child is father of the man: Personality continuities from childhood to adulthood. *Journal of Personality and Social Psychology, 78*, 158–172.

Caspi, A., Harrington, H. L., Milne, B., Amell, J. W., Theodore, R. F., & Moffitt, T. E. (2003). Children's behavioral styles at age 3 are linked to their adult personality traits at age 26. *Journal of Personality, 71*, 495–513.

Cassidy, J., & Marvin, R. S. (1992). *Attachment organization in preschool children: Procedures and coding manual.* Unpublished manuscript, MacArthur Group on Attachment, Seattle, WA.

Chess, S., & Thomas, A. (1982). Infant bonding: Mystique and reality. *American Journal of Orthopsychiatry*, 52, 213–222.

Craik, K. (1943). *The nature of exploration*. Cambridge, UK: Cambridge University Press.

Crockenberg, S. B., & Leerkes, E. M. (2006). Infant and maternal behavior moderate reactivity to novelty to predict anxious behavior at 2.5 years. *Development and Psychopathology*, 18, 17–34.

De Wolff, M. S., & van IJzendoorn, M. H. (1997). Sensitivity and attachment: A meta-analysis on parental antecedents of infant attachment. *Child Development*, 68, 571–591.

Denham, S., Mason, T., Caverly, S., Schmidt, M., Hackney, R., Caswell, C., et al. (2001). Preschoolers at play: Co-socializers of emotional and social competence. *International Journal of Behavioral Development*, 25, 290–301.

Derryberry, D., & Rothbart, M. K. (1997). Reactive and effortful processes in the organization of temperament. *Development and Psychopathology*, 9, 633–652.

Dettling, A. C., Parker, S., Lane, S. K., Sebanc, A. M., & Gunnar, M. R. (2000). Quality of care and temperament determine whether cortisol levels rise over the day for children in full-day childcare. *Psychoneuroendocrinology*, 25, 819–836.

Diamond, L. A., & Aspinwall, L. G. (2003). Emotion regulation across the life span: An integrative perspective emphasizing self-regulation, positive affect, and dyadic processes. *Motivation and Emotion*, 27, 125–156.

Diener, M. L., Nievar, M. A., & Wright, C. (2003). Attachment security among mothers and their young children living in poverty: Associations with maternal, child, and contextual characteristics. *Merrill–Palmer Quarterly*, 49, 154–182.

Egeland, B., & Farber, E. A., (1984). Infant–mother attachment: Factors related to its development and changes over time. *Child Development*, 55, 753–771.

Eisenberg, N., Fabes, R. A., Guthrie, I. K., & Reiser, M. (2000). Dispositional emotionality and regulation: Their role in predicting quality of social functioning. *Journal of Personality and Social Psychology*, 78, 136–157.

Eisenberg, N., Fabes, R. A., Nyman, M., Bernzweig, J., & Pinuelas, A. (1994). The relations of emotionality and regulation to children's anger-related reactions. *Child Development*, 65, 109–128.

Eisenberg, N., Guthrie, I. K., Fabes, R. A., Shepard, S., Losoya, S., & Murphy, B. C. (2000). Prediction of elementary school children's externalizing problem behaviors from attentional and behavioral regulation and negative emotionality. *Child Development*, 71, 1367–1382.

Eisenberg, N., Spinrad, T. L., Fabes, R. A., Reiser, M., Cumberland, A., Shepard, S. A., et al. (2004). The relations of effortful control and impulsivity to children's resiliency and adjustment. *Child Development*, 75, 25–46.

Emde, R. N., Plomin, R., Robinson, J., Corley, R., DeFries, J., Fulker, D. W., et al. (1992). Temperament, emotion, and cognition at fourteen months: The MacArthur Longitudinal Twin Study. *Child Development*, 63, 1437–1455.

Fabes, R. A., Shepard, S. A., Guthrie, I. K., & Martin, C. L. (1997). Roles of temperamental arousal and gender-segregated play in young children's social adjustment. *Developmental Psychology*, 33, 693–702.

Fearon, R. M., van IJzendoorn, M. H., Fonagy, P., Bakermans-Kranenburg, M. J., Schuengel, C., & Bokhorst, C. L. (2006). In search of shared and nonshared environmental factors in security of attachment: A behavior-genetic study of the association between sensitivity and attachment security. *Developmental Psychology*, 42, 1026–1040.

Finkel, D., & Matheny, A. P. (2000). Genetic and environmental influences on a measure of infant attachment security. *Twin Research*, 3, 242–250.

Fowles, D. C., & Kochanska, G. (2000). Temperament as a moderator of pathways to conscience in children: The contribution of electrodermal activity. *Psychophysiology*, 37, 788–795.

Fox, N. A., Calkins, S. D., & Bell, M. A. (1994). Neural plasticity and development in the first two years of life: Evidence from cognitive and socioemotional domains of research. *Development and Psychopathology*, 6, 667–696.

Fox, N. A., Henderson, H. A., Marshall, P. J., Nichols, K. E., & Ghera, M. M. (2005). Behavioral inhibition: Linking biology and behavior within a developmental framework. *Annual Review of Psychology*, 56, 235–262.

Gervai, J., Nemoda, Z., Lakatos, K., Ronai, Z., Toth, I., Ney, K., et al. (2005). Transmission disequilibrium tests confirm the link between DRD4 gene polymorphism and infant attachment. *American Journal of Medical Genetics. Part B, Neuropsychiatric Genetics*, 132, 126–130.

Gilissen, R., Bakermans-Kranenburg, M. J., van IJzendoorn, M. H., & Van der Veer, R. (in press). Parent–child relationship, temperament, and physiological reactions to fear-inducing film clips: Further evidence for differential susceptibility. *Journal of Experimental Child Psychology*.

Gilissen, R., Koolstra, C. M., van IJzendoorn, M. H., Bakermans-Kranenburg, M. J., & Van der Veer, R. (2007). Physiological reactions of preschoolers to fear-inducing film clips: Effects of temperamental fearfulness and quality of the parent–child relationship. *Developmental Psychobiology*, 49, 187–195.

Goldsmith, H. H., Lemery, K. S., Buss, K. A., & Campos, J. J. (1999). Genetic analyses of focal aspects of infant temperament. *Developmental Psychology*, 35, 972–985.

Goldsmith, H. H., Reilly, J., Lemery, K. S., Longley, S., & Prescott, A. (1999). *The Laboratory Temperament Assessment Battery*. Unpublished manuscript, University of Wisconsin, Madison.

Grossmann, K., Grossmann, K. E., Spangler, G., Suess, G., & Unzner, L. (1985). Maternal sensitivity and newborns' orientation responses as related to quality of attachment in northern Germany. In I. Bretherton & E. Waters (Eds.), Growing points of attachment theory and research. *Monographs of the Society for Research in Child Development, 50*(1–2, Serial No. 209), 233–256.

Gunnar, M. R., Brodersen, L., Nachmias, M., Buss, K., & Rigatuso, J. (1996). Stress reactivity and attachment security. *Developmental Psychobiology, 29,* 191–204.

Gunnar, M. R., Larson, M. C., Hertsgaard, L., Harris, M., & Brodersen, L. (1992). The stressfulness of separation among 9-month-old infants: Effects of social context variables and infant temperament. *Child Development, 63,* 290–303.

Gunnar, M. R., Porter, F. L., Wolf, C. M., Rigatuso, J., & Larson, M. C. (1995). Neonatal stress reactivity: Predictions to later emotional temperament. *Child Development, 66,* 1–13.

Hagekull, B., & Bohlin, G. (2003). Early temperament and attachment as predictors of the five factor model of personality. *Attachment and Human Development, 5,* 2–18.

Haley, D. W., & Stansbury, K. (2003). Infant stress and parent responsiveness: Regulation of physiology and behavior during still-face and reunion. *Child Development, 74,* 1534–1546.

Halverson, C. F., Kohnstamm, G. A., & Martin, R. (1994). *The developing structure of temperament and personality from infancy to adulthood.* Hillsdale, NJ: Erlbaum.

Hane, A. A., & Fox, N. A. (2006). Ordinary variations in maternal caregiving influence human infants' stress reactivity. *Psychological Science, 17,* 550–556.

Hinde, R. A. (1987). *Individuals, relationships, and culture.* Cambridge, UK: Cambridge University Press.

Hinde, R. A., & Stevenson-Hinde, J. (1987). Interpersonal relationships and child development. *Developmental Review, 7,* 1–21.

Hofer, M. A. (2006). Psychobiological roots of early attachment. *Current Directions in Psychological Science, 15,* 84–88.

Ispa, J. M., Fine, M. A., & Thornburg, K. R. (2002). Maternal personality as a moderator of relations between difficult infant temperament and attachment security in low-income families. *Infant Mental Health Journal, 23,* 130–144.

Jacobvitz, D., & Sroufe, L. A. (1987). The early caregiver–child relationship and attention deficit disorder with hyperactivity in kindergarten: A prospective study. *Child Development, 58,* 1496–1504.

Jaffari-Bimmel, N., Juffer, F., van IJzendoorn, M. H., Bakermans-Kranenburg, M. J., & Mooijaart, A. (2006). Social development from infancy to adolescence: Longitudinal and concurrent factors in an adoption sample. *Developmental Psychology,* 1143–1153.

Jahromi, L. B., Putnam, S. P., & Stifter, C. A. (2004). Maternal regulation of infant reactivity from 2 to 6 months. *Developmental Psychology, 40,* 477–487.

Johnson-Laird, P. N. (1989). Mental models. In M.

I. Posner (Ed.), *Foundations of cognitive science* (pp. 125–156). Cambridge, MA: MIT Press.

Jones, L. B., Rothbart, M. K., & Posner, M. I. (2003). Development of executive attention in preschool children. *Developmental Science, 6,* 498–504.

Kagan, J. (1995). On attachment. *Harvard Review of Psychiatry, 3,* 104–106.

Kagan, J. (1994). *Galen's prophecy: Temperament and human nature.* New York: Basic Books.

Kagan, J. (2003). Biology, context, and developmental inquiry. *Annual Review of Psychology, 54,* 1–23.

Kagan, J., Snidman, N., Zentner, M., & Peterson, E. (1999). Infant temperament and anxious symptoms in school age children. *Development and Psychopathology, 11,* 209–224.

Karrass, J., & Braungart-Reiker, J. M. (2004). Infant negative emotionality and attachment: Implications for preschool intelligence. *International Journal of Behavioral Development, 28,* 221–229.

Katz, L. F., & Gottman, J. M. (1995). Vagal tone protects children from marital conflict. *Development and Psychopathology, 7,* 83–92.

Kobak, R. R., Sudler, N., & Gamble, W. (1991). Attachment and depressive symptoms during adolescence: A developmental pathways analysis. *Development and Psychopathology, 3,* 461–474.

Kochanska, G. (1995). Children's temperament, mothers' discipline, and security of attachment: Multiple pathways to emerging internalization. *Child Development, 66,* 597–615.

Kochanska, G. (1997). Multiple pathways to conscience for children with different temperaments: From toddlerhood to age 5. *Developmental Psychology, 33,* 228–240.

Kochanska, G. (2001). Emotional development in children with different attachment histories: The first three years. *Child Development, 72,* 474–490.

Kochanska, G., Aksan, N., & Carlson, J. J. (2005). Temperament, relationships, and young children's receptive cooperation with their parents. *Developmental Psychology, 41,* 648–660.

Kochanska, G., Askan, N., Knaack, A., & Rhines, H. M. (2004). Maternal parenting and children's conscience: Early security as a moderator. *Child Development, 75,* 1229–1242.

Kochanska, G., Forman, D. R., Aksan, N., & Dunbar, S. B. (2005). Pathways to conscience: Early mother–child mutually responsive orientation and children's moral emotion, conduct, and cognition. *Journal of Child Psychology and Psychiatry, 46,* 19–34.

Kochanska, G., & Murray, K. T. (2000). Mother–child mutually responsive orientation and conscience development: From toddler to school age. *Child Development, 71,* 417–431.

Kohnstamm, G. A. (1984, April). *Bates' Infant Characteristics Questionnaire (ICQ) in the Netherlands.* Paper presented at the fourth biennial International Conference on Infant Studies, New York.

LaFreniere, P. J., & Sroufe, L. A. (1985). Profiles of peer competence in the preschool: Interrelations among measures, influence of social ecology, and relation to attachment history. *Developmental Psychology, 21,* 56–66.

Laible, D. (2004). Maternal emotional expressiveness and attachment security: Links to representations of relationships and social behavior. *Merrill–Palmer Quarterly, 52,* 645–670.

Lakatos, K., Toth, I., Nemoda, Z., Ney, K., Sasvari-Szekely, M., & Gervai, J. (2000). Dopamine D4 receptor (DRD4) gene polymorphism is associated with attachment disorganization in infants. *Molecular Psychiatry, 5,* 633–637.

Lonigan, C. J., Vasey, M. W., Phillips, B. M., & Hazen, R. A. (2004). Temperament, anxiety, and the processing of threat-relevant stimuli. *Journal of Clinical Child and Adolescent Psychology, 33,* 8–20.

Main, M. (1990). Cross-cultural studies of attachment organization: Recent studies, changing methodologies, and the concept of conditional strategies. *Human Development, 33,* 48–61.

Main, M., & Solomon, J. (1990). Procedures for identifying infants as disorganized/disoriented during the Ainsworth Strange Situation. In M. T. Greenberg, D. Cicchetti, & E. M. Cummings (Eds.), *Attachment in the preschool years: Theory, research, and intervention* (pp. 121–160). Chicago: University of Chicago Press.

Manassis, K., Bradley, S., Goldberg, S., Hood, J., & Swinson, R. (1995). Behavioural inhibition, attachment, and anxiety in children of mothers with anxiety disorders. *Canadian Journal of Psychiatry, 40,* 87–92.

Mangelsdorf, S. C., & Frosch, C. A. (1999). Temperament and attachment: One construct or two? *Advances in Child Development and Behavior, 27,* 181–220.

Marshall, P. J., & Fox, N. A. (2005). Relations between behavioral reactivity at 4 months and attachment classification at 14 months in a selected sample. *Infant Behavior and Development, 28,* 492–502.

Matas, L., Arend, R. A., & Sroufe, L. A. (1978). Continuity of adaptation in the second year: The relationship between quality of attachment and later competence. *Child Development, 49,* 547–556.

McCartney, K., Tresch Owen, M., Booth, C. L., Clarke-Stewart, A., & Vandell, D. L. (2004). Testing a maternal attachment model of behavior problems in early childhood. *Journal of Child Psychology and Psychiatry, 45,* 765–778.

McCrae, R. R., Costa, P. T., Jr., Ostendorf, F., Angleitner, A., Hrebickova, M., Avia, M. D., et al. (2000). Nature over nurture: Temperament, personality, and life span development. *Journal of Personality and Social Psychology, 78,* 173–186.

McEwen, B. S. (2001). From molecules to mind: Stress, individual differences, and the social environment. *Annals of the New York Academy of Sciences, 935,* 42–49.

Moss, E., Bureau, J.-F., Cyr, C., & Dubois-Comtois, K. (2006). Is the maternal Q-set a valid measure of preschool child attachment behavior? *International Journal of Behavioral Development, 30,* 488–497.

Nair, H., & Murray, A. D. (2005). Predictors of attachment security in preschool children from intact and divorced families. *Journal of Genetic Psychology, 166,* 245–263.

Nelson, B., Martin, R. P., Hodge, S., Havill, V., & Kamphaus, R. (1999). Modeling the prediction of elementary school adjustment from preschool temperament. *Personality and Individual Differences, 26,* 687–700.

Nigg, J. T., Goldsmith, H. H., & Sachek, J. (2004). Temperament and attention deficit hyperactivity disorder: The development of a multiple pathway model. *Journal of Clinical Child and Adolescent Psychology, 33,* 42–53.

O'Connor, T. G., & Croft, C. M. (2001). A twin study of attachment in preschool children. *Child Development, 72,* 1501–1511.

O'Connor, T. G., Croft, C. M., & Steele, H. (2000). The contributions of behavioral genetic studies to attachment theory. *Attachment and Human Development, 2,* 107–122.

Oosterman, M., & Schuengel, C. (2007). Physiological effects of separation and reunion in relation to attachment and temperament in young children. *Developmental Psychobiology, 49,* 119–128.

Park, K. A., & Waters, E. (1989). Security of attachment and preschool friendships. *Child Development, 60,* 1076–1081.

Pauli-Pott, U., Haverkock, A., Pott, W., & Beckmann, D. (2007). Negative emotionality, attachment quality, and behavior problems in early childhood. *Infant Mental Health Journal, 28,* 39–53.

Pederson, D. R., & Moran, G. (1995). A categorical description of infant–mother relationships in the home and its relation to Q-sort measures of infant–mother interaction. In E. Waters, B. E. Vaughn, G. Posada, & K. Kondo-Ikemura (Eds.), Caregiving, cultural, and cognitive perspectives on secure-base behavior and working models: New growing points of attachment theory and research. *Monographs of the Society for Research in Child Development, 60*(2–3, Serial No. 244), 111–132.

Pierrehumbert, B., Miljkovitch, R., Plancherel, B., Halfon, D., & Ansermet, F. (2000). Attachment and temperament in early childhood: Implications for later behavior problems. *Infant and Child Development, 9,* 17–32.

Porges, S. W., Doussard-Roosevelt, J. A., Portales, A. L., & Greenspan, S. I. (1996). Infant regulation of the vagal "brake" predicts child behavior problems: A psychobiological model of social behavior. *Developmental Psychobiology, 29,* 697–712.

Porges, S. W., Doussard-Roosevelt, J. A., Portales, A. L., & Suess, P. E. (1995). Cardiac vagal tone: Stability and relation to difficultness in infants and 3-year-olds. *Developmental Psychobiology, 27,* 289–300.

Prior, M., Smart, D., Sanson, A., & Oberklaid, F. (2000). Does shy-inhibited temperament in childhood lead to anxiety problems in adolescence? *Journal of the American Academy of Child and Adolescent Psychiatry, 39,* 461–468.

Rettew, D. C., Copeland, W., Stanger, C., & Hudziak, J. J. (2004). Associations between temperament and DSM-IV externalizing disorders in children and adolescents. *Journal of Developmental and Behavioral Pediatrics, 25*, 383–391.

Ricciuti, A. E. (1992). Child–mother attachment: A twin study. *Dissertation Abstracts International, 54*, 3364B. (UMI No. 9324873)

Robbins, T. W., & Everitt, B. J. (1999). Motivation and reward. In M. J. Zigmond (Ed.), *Fundamental neuroscience* (pp. 1246–1260). San Diego, CA: Academic Press.

Roberts, B. W., & DelVecchio, W. F. (2000). The rank-order consistency of personality traits from childhood to old age: A quantitative review of longitudinal studies. *Psychological Bulletin, 126*, 3–25.

Rothbart, M. K. (1988). Temperament and the development of inhibited approach. *Child Development, 59*, 1241–1250.

Rothbart, M. K. (1989). Temperament and development. In G. Kohnstamm, J. Bates, & M. K. Rothbart (Eds.), *Temperament in childhood* (pp. 26–64). Chichester, UK: Wiley.

Rothbart, M. K. (2004). Temperament and the pursuit of an integrated developmental psychology. *Merrill–Palmer Quarterly, 50*, 492–405.

Rothbart, M. K., Ahadi, S. A., & Evans, D. E. (2000). Temperament and personality: Origins and outcomes. *Journal of Personality and Social Psychology, 78*, 122–135.

Rothbart, M. K., & Bates, J. E. (1998). Temperament. In W. Damon & R. M. Lerner (Series Eds.) & N. Eisenberg (Vol. Ed.), *Handbook of child psychology: Vol. 3. Social, emotional, and personality development* (4th ed., pp. 105–176). New York: Wiley.

Rothbart, M. K., & Bates, J. E. (2006). Temperament. In W. Damon & R. M. Lerner (Series Eds.) & N. Eisenberg (Vol. Ed.), *Handbook of child psychology: Vol. 3. Social, emotional, and personality development* (5th ed., pp. 99–166). New York: Wiley.

Rothbart, M. K., & Derryberry, D. (1981). Development of individual differences in temperament. In M. E. Lamb & A. L. Brown (Eds.), *Advances in developmental psychology* (Vol. 1, pp. 37–86). Hillsdale, NJ: Erlbaum.

Rothbart, M. K., Ellis, L. K., & Posner, M. I. (2004). Temperament and self-regulation. In R. F. Baumeister & K. D. Vohs (Eds.), *Handbook of self-regulation: Research, theory, and applications* (pp. 357–370). New York: Guilford Press.

Rothbart, M. K., Ellis, L. K., Rueda, M. R., & Posner, M. I. (2003). Developing mechanisms of temperamental effortful control. *Journal of Personality, 71*, 1113–1143.

Rothbart, M. K., Posner, M. I., & Hershey, K. (1995). Temperament, attention, and developmental psychopathology. In D. Cicchetti & J. D. Cohen (Eds.), *Developmental psychopathology* (Vol. 1, pp. 315–340). New York: Wiley.

Rothbart, M. K., & Rueda, M. R. (2005). The development of effortful control. In U. Mayr, E. Awh, & S. Keele (Eds.), *Developing individuality in the human brain: A tribute to Michael I. Posner* (pp. 167–188). Washington, DC: American Psychological Association.

Rowe, D. C., & Plomin, R. (1977). Temperament in early childhood. *Journal of Personality Assessment, 41*, 150–156.

Rubin, K. H., Burgess, K. B., Dwyer, K. M., & Hastings, P. D. (2003). Predicting preschoolers' externalizing behaviors from toddler temperament, conflict, and maternal negativity. *Developmental Psychology, 39*, 164–176.

Rubin, K. H., Coplan, R. J., Fox, N. A., & Calkins, S. D. (1995). Emotionality, emotion regulation, and preschoolers' social adaptation. *Development and Psychopathology, 7*, 49–62.

Rueda, M. R., Posner, M. I., & Rothbart, M. K. (2005). The development of executive attention: Contributions to the emergence of self-regulation. *Developmental Neuropsychology, 28*, 573–594.

Rutter, M. (2006). *Genes and behavior: Nature–nurture interplay explained.* Oxford, UK: Blackwell.

Rutter, M., Moffitt, T. E., & Caspi, A. (2006). Gene–environment interplay and psychopathology: Multiple varieties but real effects. *Journal of Child Psychology and Psychiatry, 47*, 226–261.

Rydell, A.-M., Bohlin, B., & Thorell, L. B. (2005). Representations of attachment to parents and shyness as predictors of children's relationships with teachers and peer competence in preschool. *Attachment and Human Development, 7*, 187–204.

Sanson, A., Hemphill, S. A., & Smart, D. (2004). Connections between temperament and social development: A review. *Social Development, 13*, 142–170.

Schieche, M., & Spangler, G. (2005). Individual differences in biobehavioral organization during problem-solving in toddlers: The influence of maternal behavior, infant–mother attachment, and behavioral inhibition on the attachment–exploration balance. *Developmental Psychobiology, 46*, 293–306.

Schore, A. N. (2000). Attachment and the regulation of the right brain. *Attachment and Human Development, 2*, 23–47.

Schore, A. N. (2005). Attachment, affect regulation, and the developing right brain: Linking developmental neuroscience to pediatrics. *Pediatrics Review, 26*, 204–217.

Shamir-Essakow, G., Ungerer, J. A., & Rapee, R. M. (2005). Attachment, behavioral inhibition, and anxiety in preschool children. *Journal of Abnormal Child Psychology, 33*, 131–143.

Spangler, G., Fremmer-Bombik, E., & Grossmann, K. (1996). Social and individual determinants of attachment security and disorganization during the first year. *Infant Mental Health Journal, 17*, 127–139.

Spangler, G., Schieche, M., Ilg, U., Maier, U., & Ackermann, C. (1994). Maternal sensitivity as an external organizer for biobehavioral regulation in infancy. *Developmental Psychobiology, 27*, 425–437.

Sroufe, L. A. (1996). *Emotional development: The organization of emotional life in the early years.* New York: Cambridge University Press.

Sroufe, L. A., Egeland, B., Carlson, E. A., & Collins, W. A. (2005). *The development of the person: The Minnesota Study of Risk and Adaptation from Birth to Adulthood.* New York: Guilford Press.

Stams, G. J., Juffer, F., & van IJzendoorn, M. H. (2002). Maternal sensitivity, infant attachment, and temperament in early childhood predict adjustment in middle childhood: The case of adopted children and their biologically unrelated parents. *Developmental Psychology, 38,* 806–821.

Stayton, D. J., Hogan, R., & Ainsworth, M. D. S. (1971). Infant obedience and maternal behavior: The origins of socialization reconsidered. *Child Development, 42,* 1057–1069.

Stevenson-Hinde, J., & Marshall, P. J. (1999). Behavioral inhibition, heart period, and respiratory sinus arrhythmia: An attachment perspective. *Child Development, 70,* 805–816.

Suess, G. J., Grossmann, K., & Sroufe, L. A. (1992). Effects of infant attachment to mother and father on quality of adaptation in preschool: From dyadic to individual organization of self. *International Journal of Behavioral Development, 15,* 43–65.

Szewczyk-Sokolowski, M., Bost, K. K., & Wainright, A. B. (2005). Attachment, temperament, and preschool children's peer acceptance. *Social Development, 14,* 379–397.

Thompson, R. A., & Lamb, M. (1984). Assessing qualitative dimensions of emotional responsiveness in infants: Separation reactions in the Strange Situation. *Infant Behavior and Development, 7,* 423–445.

van Bakel, H. J. A., & Riksen-Walraven, J. M. (2004a). AQS security scores: What do they represent? A study in construct validation. *Infant Mental Health Journal, 25,* 175–193.

van Bakel, H. J. A., & Riksen-Walraven, J. M. (2004b). Stress reactivity in 15-month-old infants: Links with infant temperament, cognitive competence, and attachment security. *Developmental Psychobiology, 44,* 157–167.

van der Mark, I. L., Bakermans-Kranenburg, M. J., & van IJzendoorn, M. H. (2002). The role of parenting, attachment, and temperamental fearfulness in the prediction of compliance in toddler girls. *British Journal of Developmental Psychology, 20,* 361–378.

van IJzendoorn, M. H., & Bakermans-Kranenburg, M. J. (2006). DRD4 7-repeat polymorphism moderates the association between maternal unresolved loss or trauma and infant disorganization. *Attachment and Human Development, 8,* 291–307.

van IJzendoorn, M. H., & De Wolff, M. S. (1997). In search of the absent father: Meta-analyses of infant–father attachment: A rejoinder to our discussants. *Child Development, 68,* 604–609.

van IJzendoorn, M. H., Moran, G., Belsky, J., Pederson, D., Bakermans-Kranenburg, M. J., & Kneppers, K.

(2000). The similarity of siblings' attachments to their mothers. *Child Development, 71,* 1086–1098.

van IJzendoorn, M. H., Schuengel, C., & Bakermans-Kranenburg, M. J. (1999). Disorganized attachment in early childhood: Meta-analysis of precursors, concomitants, and sequelae. *Development and Psychopathology, 11,* 225–249.

van IJzendoorn, M. H., Vereijken, C. M. J. L., Bakermans-Kranenburg, M. J., & Riksen-Walraven, J. M. (2004). Assessing attachment security with the Attachment Q Sort: Meta-analytic evidence for the validity of the observer AQS. *Child Development, 75,* 1188–1213.

Vaughn, B. E., & Bost, K. K. (1999). Attachment and temperament: Redundant, independent, or interacting influences on interpersonal adaptation and personality development? In J. Cassidy & P. R. Shaver (Eds.), *Handbook of attachment: Theory, research, and clinical applications* (pp. 198–225). New York: Guilford Press.

Vaughn, B. E., & Waters, E. (1990). Attachment behavior at home and in the laboratory: Q-sort observations and Strange Situation classifications of one-year-olds. *Child Development, 61,* 1965–1973.

Warren, S., Huston, L., Egeland, B., & Sroufe, L. A. (1997). Child and adolescent anxiety disorders and early attachment. *Journal of the American Academy of Child and Adolescent Psychiatry, 36,* 637–644.

Waters, E., & Deane, K. (1985). Defining and assessing individual differences in attachment relationships: Q-methodology and the organization of behavior in infancy and early childhood. In I. Bretherton & E. Waters (Eds.), Growing points of attachment theory and research. *Monographs of the Society for Research in Child Development, 50*(1–2, Serial No. 209), 41–65.

Waters, E., Kondo-Ikemura, K., Posada, G., & Richters, J. (1991). Learning to love: Mechanisms and milestones. In M. Gunnar & L. A. Sroufe (Eds.), *Minnesota Symposium on Child Psychology: Vol. 23. Self processes in early development* (pp. 217–255). Hillsdale, NJ: Erlbaum.

Waters, E., & Sroufe, L. A. (1983). Social competence as a developmental construct. *Developmental Review, 3,* 79–97.

Waters, E., Vaughn, B. E., Posada, G., & Kondo-Ikemura, K. (Eds.). (1995). Caregiving, cultural, and cognitive perspectives on secure-base behavior and working models: New growing points of attachment theory and research. *Monographs of the Society for Research in Child Development, 60*(2–3, Serial No. 244).

Waters, E., Wippman, J., & Sroufe, L. A. (1979). Attachment, positive affect, and competence in the peer group: Two studies in construct validation. *Child Development, 50,* 821–829.

Zeijlmans van Emmichhoven, I. A., van IJzendoorn, M. H., de Ruiter, C., & Brosschot, J. F. (2003). Selective processing of threatening information: Effects of attachment representation and anxiety disorder on attention and memory. *Development and Psychopathology, 15,* 219–237.

CHAPTER 10

Studying the Biology of Human Attachment

NATHAN A. FOX
AMIE ASHLEY HANE

There has always been great interest in research that illuminates the brain circuitry underlying human behavior. This interest has increased recently because of innovative technologies that cognitive and social psychologists can use to study brain activation while eliciting specific psychological states. One technology that is prevalent in the literature is functional magnetic resonance imaging (fMRI), which involves presenting people with stimuli in either a task or a passive viewing design while measuring their brain activity. In the field of cognitive neuroscience, there are now multiple studies examining brain activation during standard cognitive tasks that elicit states of attention, perception, or memory. In the field of social and affective neuroscience, similar approaches have examined brain activation during tasks designed to elicit different emotions.

In both areas of imaging, it has been assumed that a specific psychological state can be elicited by a particular experimental manipulation. For example, studies of working memory have involved presenting a series of stimuli to people and asking them to remember the stimulus that was one, two, or three back from a particular target stimulus (called an "N-back" task; e.g., Ciesielski, Lesnik, Savoy, Grant, & Ahlfors, 2006). This task

robustly activates the dorsolateral prefrontal cortex. Designers of other studies have attempted to elicit feelings of social rejection in subjects by having them participate in tasks in which they rate their willingness to interact with another person, only to receive feedback that the person is not interested in interacting with them (Somerville, Heatherton, & Kelley, 2006). Such tasks appear to activate an area of the brain called the anterior cingulate, which is known for its role in conflict detection. In both of these examples and in most fMRI studies, tasks are designed to elicit specific psychological states whose brain correlates can then be measured. We contrast this approach, often thought of as defining cognitive, social, and affective neuroscience, with an approach known as *psychophysiology*.[1]

Psychophysiology is the study of how physiological processes intersect with and influence psychological processes and behavior. Psychophysiological research includes measurement of physiological systems that are correlated with observed behavioral responses, as well as the manner in which individual differences in the level of a physiological response predispose people to certain kinds of behavior. Two examples of this approach are studies measuring task-elicited autonomic activity and research measuring the activity of the hypothalamic–pituitary–adrenocortical (HPA) axis during tasks designed to provoke stress.

In studies assessing autonomic activity, the measures are generally thought to provide an index of physiological arousal. Increased heart rate (HR), respiration, or skin conductance is often viewed as reflecting enhanced sympathetic or parasympathetic activity in response to a task demand (e.g., Phillips, Carroll, Hunt, & Der, 2006). Autonomic measures have also been used to detect different states of attention. For example, HR change has been measured in response to visual or auditory stimuli in preverbal infants. Sustained HR deceleration is viewed as indicating sustained attention (Courage, Reynolds, & Richars, 2006). In the case of research measuring HPA axis activity, the assumption is that changes in the level of activation of the HPA axis reflect the individual's response to stress (Gunnar & Donzella, 2002). Psychologists measure cortisol change as an index of HPA activity and interpret it as an indirect measure of an individual's stress reactivity.

Measuring either of these physiological systems provides a window into the ways body and mind respond together to meet environmental task demands. But a psychophysiological approach may be thought to differ from a neuroscientific approach in several important ways. First, unlike techniques that image or measure brain activity, measures of autonomic or HPA axis activity are necessarily indirect assessments of brain–behavior links. A second, and related, difference is that imaging techniques—and here we include electroencephalography (EEG) and measures of evoked response potentials (ERPs) from stimulus-locked EEG—are attempts to localize or identify brain–behavior links by providing information about the neural circuitry involved in certain behaviors. As such, these approaches, particularly fMRI, provide better spatial resolution for identifying underlying structural features of brain activity than measures of other physiological systems do. Third, the time course of autonomic or HPA axis activity is generally much slower than the time course of brain activity. Methods such as ERP provide greater temporal resolution for neural events than the activity of other physiological systems.

Both approaches have their benefits. The psychophysiological approach has been especially useful for studies of infants and young children, because it is difficult to apply brain imaging technologies to them. Both neuroscience and psychophysiology have been used to study the psychological states involved in attachment. In the past, most

attachment research was conducted with infants and young children, and most studies involving physiological measures assessed autonomic and HPA reactivity. The development of conceptual and methodological approaches for measuring and understanding adult attachment has provided an opportunity to use brain imaging measures. In this chapter, although we focus especially on psychophyiological measures, we review both approaches to the study of psychological states associated with attachment. And we comment on possible new approaches to thinking about studies of both infants and adults.

Attachment has long been viewed as a biobehavioral state in which multiple physiological and behavioral systems are organized to provide an individual with a sense of security (i.e., safety within an environment) and intimacy with significant others (Bowlby, 1969/1982). Individual differences in the organization of certain behaviors have been well characterized as reflecting different attachment classifications based on experiences in attachment relationships (Ainsworth, Blehar, Waters, & Wall, 1978). And there is growing empirical evidence that individual differences in attachment are associated with differences in the processing of perceptual information (e.g., Cohen & Shaver, 2004; Mikulincer & Shaver, 2007, Ch. 6). Thus the study of attachment can be approached from a physiological perspective by examining either (1) individual differences in arousal or stress reactivity as a function of differences in attachment classification, or (2) individual differences in cognitive and affective brain circuitry associated with attachment classifications.

PSYCHOPHYSIOLOGY AND ATTACHMENT

In this section, we review studies of infant attachment that have included measures of either autonomic activity or activity of the HPA axis. These studies can be grouped into two categories: those examining physiological responses of human infants in Ainsworth's Strange Situation (Ainsworth & Wittig, 1969), and those in which infant physiological responses have been assessed as correlates of behavior in the Strange Situation. The former kinds of studies focus on individual differences in physiological reactivity that may be related to attachment classification or to infant behavior in the Strange Situation.

We next review animal and human research demonstrating that the quality of early caregiving environments shapes individual differences in physiological and behavioral responses to stress. We then turn to the physiological effects of caregiver variables and review studies that have included psychophysiological measures in conjunction with measures of caregiver sensitivity and responsiveness. Next, we review recent studies that have used psychophysiological responses during the Adult Attachment Interview (AAI) or in conjunction with self-report measures of "attachment style." We end the chapter with a review of studies that have applied a neuroscientific (i.e., imaging) approach to the study of adult attachment and to the assessment of behaviors relevant to the development of the attachment system. Throughout these reviews, we hope to inform the reader about both the problems and the benefits of using psychophysiological and imaging methods to study different aspects of attachment behavior.

Before reviewing particular studies, it is important to raise a number of caveats concerning psychophysiological studies, particularly those measuring autonomic or HPA axis activity. The first caveat concerns the multidetermined nature of the response. Despite its simplicity of measurement, HR, for example, is complexly determined; there are both neural and extraneural influences on it. Extraneural influences include hormonal effects that are the result of sympathetic activity or metabolic effects that may be a function of somatic activity ranging from digestion to muscle movement. There are also mechanical influences on HR, including changes in respiratory activity that affect HR via the stretch receptors in the lungs (Porges & Byrne, 1992). There are intrinsic influences on HR as well; the heart beats at a particular rate as a function of electrical discharge via pacemaker cells at the sinoatrial node. HR responds to changes in other systems, such as fluctuations in blood pressure. Most neural influence on the heart is via the vagus or 10th cranial nerve (Katona & Jih, 1985). The vagus nerve, which originates in the brain stem, has complex interconnections with neural centers regulating respiration and is linked with both afferent and efferent connections to the midbrain and cortical regions of the brain (Porges, 1995). Thus HR (and HR change) may be the result of multiple physiological factors, only some of which may directly affect or reflect psychological state.

Changes in cortisol level are also multidetermined. Cortisol is a hormone secreted by the actions of the HPA axis. It is the hormone of energy and hence is released as a result of many aspects of an organism's interaction with its environment, including responses to novelty, appetitive behavior, sexual stimulation, and injury or illness, as well as psychological stressors (Adam, Klimes-Dougan, & Gunnar, 2007). The secretion of cortisol within the HPA system has its own circadian rhythm, and the adrenocortical system is slow to respond; thus it may take 25–30 minutes before a change in cortisol levels can be detected.

The multidetermined nature of psychophysiological responses requires, at the very least, careful methodological consideration. The measurement of HR has sometimes been supplemented with measures of somatic activity, to rule out these influences on rate. Attempts have also been made to extract from the HR signal the portion of variance that can be exclusively related to neural influence (e.g., Porges & Bohrer, 1991). Studies of cortisol response should take into account time of day for sample collection, because of changes due to circadian rhythms. These precautions and concerns are critical in allowing inferences about psychophysiological responses to be made.

A second caveat regarding the measurement and interpretation of physiological responses such as autonomic and HPA axis activity is the issue of individual differences in the initial level of response. The "law of initial values" states that the initial baseline level of a physiological system will affect the degree to which that system responds to stimulus presentation. For example, people with high levels of basal cortisol and those with more normative levels may respond differently to a stressor. The notion is that there is a ceiling level above which the system usually does not operate. It is important, therefore, that individual differences in baseline level be incorporated into any analysis of phasic responses. The usual approaches include computing change scores between baseline and phasic responses, or using analysis of covariance with baseline level as the covariate.

The issue of baseline level is complicated when researchers are assessing infants and young children. Because these research participants cannot be instructed to sit quietly for a baseline recording, researchers have attempted to devise methods for recording physiological responses when infants are not responding to a strong stimulus challenge. The key is to record "baseline" in a noninvasive experimental condition that may be replicated across children. It is often necessary to record behavior during such "baseline" physiological assessments, to ensure that all children are in the same state.

Baseline differences may also speak to the underlying physiological mechanisms that affect magnitude of response. Porges, Stamps, and Walter (1974) noted, for example, that some infants do not display HR deceleration in response to a visual stimulus. These infants have relatively high HRs. When studying this issue, Porges and colleagues found that the same high-HR group also displayed low HR variability. When subjects were grouped into those displaying high versus low resting HR variability, those with high resting variability were more likely to show the supposedly normative decelerative pattern. In his subsequent work, Porges (1991, 1996; Porges, Doussard-Roosevelt, Portales, & Suess, 1994) argued that initial baseline differences in HR are due to vagal control of the heart, and that differences in the degree of this control predict HR responsivity.

Psychophysiology within the Strange Situation

Heart Rate

The Strange Situation (Ainsworth & Wittig, 1969) was designed to assess the quality of an infant's attachment to a primary caregiver. The Strange Situation includes a series of conditions beginning with the infant and caregiver being together in an unfamiliar playroom, followed by the introduction of an unfamiliar adult, separation from the caregiver, and the infant's being left alone in the playroom. There are two conditions of reunion between caregiver and infant, and it is principally on the basis of the infant's behavior during these reunion episodes that he or she is classified as being "securely" or "insecurely" attached to that caregiver. There are four subtypes of secure infants, ranging from those who show little proximity seeking during reunion to those who seek a good deal of contact and comfort. Securely attached infants may cry and become distressed in response to separation from their caregivers, although such distress is not a prerequisite behavior for a secure attachment.

There are three insecure classifications: "avoidant," "resistant," and "disorganized." Avoidant infants ignore their caregivers' return and may actively avoid proximity and contact. Resistant infants display proximity- and contact-seeking behaviors, while at the same time displaying resistance to caregiver attempts to soothe distress. Disorganized infants are likely to display contradictory emotions; to appear confused, apprehensive, and hypervigilant; to make incomplete or undirected movements; and to show depressed affect and possibly behavioral stilling. Unlike the disorganized infants, the secure, avoidant, and resistant infants are viewed as having a coherent

strategy for coping with separation, although the secure infants are viewed as having the most adaptive strategy. (See Solomon & George, Chapter 18, this volume, for a detailed description of the Strange Situation.)

Within the confines of the Strange Situation paradigm, infants may locomote where they please in the unfamiliar playroom. Some infants run to the door after their caregiver leaves. Some move close to their caregiver when the unfamiliar adult enters, whereas others play with toys and explore the room. The high mobility within the confines of the experimental setting places limits on the ability to measure ongoing physiological activity. Nevertheless, there have been a number of attempts to assess psychophysiological reactions during the Strange Situation.

One of the first attempts to record HR during the Strange Situation was reported by Sroufe and Waters (1977). They described individual case studies of infant HR response during preseparation, separation, and reunion episodes. Infant HR was recorded via telemetry: Each infant wore a small transmitter that sent an FM radio signal containing the electrocardiogram (EKG) to a receiver—a procedure that allowed the infant complete mobility within the playroom. The researchers were primarily interested in the HR responses of insecure infants. Avoidant infants, who usually appear undisturbed by the separation, seem to exhibit "displacement behavior" during reunion, in which they continue to play with toys in a rigid or uninspired way. Sroufe and Waters hypothesized that these infants, although showing no overt behavioral distress at reunion, are in fact upset and should therefore show elevations in HR during reunion, in contrast to the decelerative HR responses shown by most infants during object play prior to separation. Similarly, Sroufe and Waters were interested in the HR patterns of resistant infants, who appear highly distressed during separation and have difficulty being soothed by their caregivers during reunion. Resistant infants, they thought, should continue to show elevated HR during the reunion episodes, reflecting their inability to regulate their heightened arousal.

Sroufe and Waters (1977) reported that secure, avoidant, and resistant infants all showed increased HR upon separation, which remained elevated during reunion. Secure infants' HR recovered on average after less than 1 minute of contact with their mothers. After the secure infants were put down, they showed HR deceleration when they returned to play and attended to objects. Resistant infants, in contrast, requested to be put down before their HR recovered to the preseparation level; then, after being put down, with their HR still elevated, they reached up to be held again. Avoidant infants showed an increase in HR from the beginning of separation until long into the reunion session, even though they outwardly appeared to be unaffected by the separation. These case studies demonstrated not only that HR could be recorded from infants in the Strange Situation, but that changes in HR were helpful in interpreting the behavior of different categories of infants. Donovan and Leavitt (1985a) also examined HR response in infants during the Strange Situation. Using telemetry, they recorded EKG synchronized to the ongoing sequence of behavioral episodes in the Strange Situation. Thirty-seven infants were tested, 29 of whom provided usable EKG data. Of the 29 infants, 22 were classified as securely attached, 4 as avoidant, and 3 as resistant. Because of the low number of infants in the insecure categories, most of the statistical analyses were computed only on the subcategories (B1 through B4) of the secure infants.

The data suggested that in response to the entrance and approach of the unfamiliar adult, secure infants displayed HR deceleration, relative to a preentrance baseline. In addition, in response to impending separation (when their mothers said goodbye), secure infants displayed acceleratory trends in their HR. Although no inferential statistical comparisons were reported, Donovan and Leavitt (1985a) presented the mean HR data for the combined avoidant and resistant infants during these same situations. These insecure infants did not appear to display HR deceleration to either stranger entrance or approach; they did, however, display HR acceleration to the impending separation. Donovan and Leavitt interpreted the deceleratory responses of secure infants as indexing attention and orienting to the stranger, whereas they viewed the acceleratory responses to impending separation as a defensive response. Unfortunately, the small number of insecure infants, and the need to combine avoidant and resistant infants, precluded any assessment of the hypotheses proposed by Sroufe and Waters (1977) regarding the utility of HR in distinguishing the behaviors of avoidant and resistant infants.

In this same study, Donovan and Leavitt (1985a) also examined the HR changes of the mothers and their infants. The HR data for the 22 securely attached infants and their mothers paralleled each other, whereas the HR data for the combined insecurely attached infants and their mothers did not. Securely attached infants and their mothers both displayed HR decreases as the stranger entered the room and approached the infant. Donovan and Leavitt suggested that this concordance between the secure infants and their mothers reflects the mothers' involvement in their infants' behavior. Specifically, by responding to an infant's gaze and/or events surrounding her infant, a mother displays a sensitivity that contributes to the development of a secure attachment. The mothers of insecurely attached infants failed to show consistency to the stranger's entrance and approach. The authors suggested that this inconsistency reflected lower involvement on the part of such a mother in an infant's behavior.

A later attempt to examine HR responses of infants during the Strange Situation provided little support for differentiating between avoidant and secure attachment classifications. Spangler and Grossmann (1993) observed 41 infants in the Strange Situation, recording EKG via telemetry. Although no description was provided of how behavior and physiology were synchronized, the authors reported usable HR data for 18 secure, 6 avoidant, and 6 disorganized infants. The analyses revealed no group differences in infant HR change during any of the reunion episodes. The one episode in which significant group differences in HR change appeared was Episode 6, when the infant was alone in the room. In this episode, disorganized infants displayed greater HR acceleration than did the other two groups (avoidant and secure). Interestingly, the secure and disorganized infants displayed similar levels of negative vocalizations during this episode, whereas only the disorganized infants displayed the elevated HR pattern. Willemsen-Swinkels and her colleagues (Willemsen-Swinkels, Bakermans-Kranenburg, Buitelaar, van IJzendoorn, & van Engeland, 2000) noted a similar HR acceleration-upon-separation effect when assessing attachment security in a sample of children with pervasive developmental disorder who were classified as having disorganized attachments. Such evidence supports Spangler and Grossmann's (1993) contention that disorganized infants may be intensely alarmed by separation in the Strange Situation, to the point that activation of their attachment behavior cannot be systematically controlled.

Spangler and Grossmann (1993) also examined the HR of attachment-classified infants during object manipulation and play with their mothers. They found that the avoidant infants did not display HR acceleration when looking at their mothers, whereas the secure and disorganized infants did. The avoidant infants did, however, display acceleration while looking at objects or during object manipulation, whereas the disorganized and secure infants displayed HR deceleration. It appears that these behavior–EKG links were aggregates of data from across the different episodes of the Strange Situation; this makes their interpretation difficult.

Similarly, it is unclear why secure and disorganized infants displayed similar HR patterns while the HR patterns of avoidant infants differed, particularly during visual regard of their mothers. Spangler and Grossmann (1993) stated that "the heightened heart rate when looking to the mother [of secure infants] indicates that visual contact with mother was initiated specifically during episodes of physiological arousal" (p. 1447). In the absence of a precise linkage between measures of visual regard and specification of when these behaviors were coded, however, such an explanation seems post hoc at best.

Bono and Stifter (1995) examined the relations between measures of HR and HR variability assessed immediately before and after the Strange Situation as a function of infant attachment classification at 18 months of age. The authors reported that infants categorized as resistant displayed faster HR and less variability in heart period (HP, the interval between heart beats, which is inversely related to HR) than secure infants did after the Strange Situation. These differences, however, may be due to the extreme degree of upset displayed by resistant infants and their inability to be soothed during reunion. To the extent that resistant infants display behavioral problems in regulating their affect in the Strange Situation and immediately thereafter, autonomic activity will mimic those patterns of dysregulation.

Another, more recent study examined the degree of physiological attunement between mothers and infants in a sample of low-socioeconomic-status young women (age 20 or under, M = 17.8) (Zelenko et al., 2005). In this report, mean HR was recorded by Mini-Logger monitors that collected and stored HR signals every 10 seconds from mothers and infants as they underwent the Strange Situation procedure. Forty-one mother–infant dyads participated, of which 23 were classified as securely attached, 6 as insecure-avoidant, and 12 as insecure-resistant. No mean attachment group differences in HR were detected from the infants at baseline; nor were there significant differences in HR change across separation and reunion episodes between the attachment groups. All infants showed a pattern of HR acceleration during separations and deceleration upon reunion. Mothers showed no significant differences in baseline HR across the groups. However, the pattern of mean HR change for mothers of resistant infants differed significantly from the secure and avoidant groups. For mothers of secure and avoidant infants, HR followed a pattern consistent with that of their infants—acceleration during separation, and deceleration upon reunion. However, mothers of resistant infants showed HR acceleration during reunion episodes. For securely attached infants, maternal HR slowed after the successful calming of the infant, whereas the HR of mothers of resistant infants remained elevated. This inability of mothers of resistant infants to recover from the stress of separation may be a function of maternal dysregulation that contributed to the insecure attachment of the infant, a by-product of the stress associated with soothing a distress-prone infant, or a combination of these states. Although not statistically significant, the descriptive findings obtained from calculating dyadic consistency (a crude index of physiological attunement) in HR revealed that mothers and their resistant infants scored lower in dyadic consistency than securely attached dyads—an effect necessarily driven by the discrepant profile of the mothers of resistant infants, given the lack of significant HR differences among the infants across attachment groups.

Zelenko and her colleagues (2005) also assessed frequency and intensity of infant crying during the Strange Situation, and noted descriptively that resistant infants cried more than the other two attachment groups. Hence resistant infants themselves showed a discordance between behavioral distress and physiological arousal; this is reminiscent of the discordance between physiological and behavioral distress of the avoidant infants studied by Spangler and Grossmann (1993), but it is discrepant from Bono and Stifter's (1995) findings regarding increased physiological arousal in resistant infants. It is important to note that Zelenko et al.'s sample consisted of young, poor mothers and their infants, who were probably at increased risk for poor developmental outcomes. It is unclear whether similar effects would be obtained from a more normative sample. As well, Bono and Stifter measured cardiac functioning before and after but not during the Strange Situation, whereas Zelenko and colleagues' effects were driven by changes in cardiac functioning during the procedure.

Stevenson-Hinde and Marshall (1999) examined the role of attachment security in the relation between behavioral inhibition and cardiac reactivity. Using an extreme-groups approach, they selected 126 children (age 4½ years), based on level of behavioral inhibition (high, medium, or low). Behavioral inhibition was assessed via maternal report and behavioral observation in the laboratory, and children underwent the Strange Situation procedure to have their attachment security assessed while cardiac data were recorded from both the mother and the infant via telemetry. HP and HR variability (respiratory sinus arrhythmia, or RSA) were noted during four specific periods in the Strange Situation paradigm: after Episode 3 with the stranger reading a story; at the start of Episode 7, with the examiner playing a recorded story; following a structured self-esteem interview (Harter & Pike, 1984), while another excerpt from the story was played from an audiocassette; and at the end of Episode 9, as mother and child sat quietly alone. Of the children with usable cardiac data, 38 were classified as securely attached, 6 as insecure-avoidant, and 8 as insecure-resistant. No significant inhibition group or attachment group differences were found in child mean HP or RSA (aggregated across all four assessment points). A significant interaction effect indicated that children low in behavioral inhibition who were securely attached had significantly higher mean HP than securely attached children who were high in behavioral inhibition and insecurely attached children who were low in inhibition did. A similar effect was found for RSA (itself highly correlated with mean HP in this sample, $r = .80$), with low-inhibition, securely attached children showing the highest degree of RSA, although the interaction effect was not significant. Securely attached children who were not highly inhibited showed significant increase in HP upon reunion with their mothers. Highly inhibited children, regardless of attachment status, showed no such increase, indicating that attachment security and the absence of behavioral inhibition are requisite for a significant increase in HP upon reunion. Hence this study provides additional support for the notion that insecurely attached children and inhibited children manifest disorganization in psychophysiological responses to the challenges of the Strange Situation. Notably, this study also provides evidence for the benefit of considering temperament, attachment, and physiological reactivity in concert, because there was no relation between attachment status and cardiac reactivity when inhibition was not considered.

Cortisol

A number of researchers have measured the cortisol levels of infants assessed in the Strange Situation. The cortisol response takes place over a much longer time course than other physiological systems do. Thus measuring cortisol in saliva or plasma 15–30 minutes after completion of the Strange Situation may accurately capture an infant's HPA response during the testing procedure. Gunnar, Mangelsdorf, Larson, and Hertsgaard (1989) observed 66 infants in the Strange Situation at 13 months of age. Saliva was obtained from them, first at home prior to coming to the lab, then immediately before and immediately after the Strange Situation procedure. Of the 66 infants, 37 were classified as secure, 10 as avoidant, 16 as resistant, and 3 as disorganized. There were no differences among attachment groups in either cortisol level or the degree of cortisol change. In a follow-up, Gunnar, Colton, and Stansbury (1992) examined differences in salivary cortisol between 47 securely attached infants and 24 insecurely attached infants. Again, saliva was collected immediately prior to and immediately after the Strange Situation. No differences in salivary cortisol reactivity were found among infants classified as avoidant, resistant, and secure.

Spangler and Grossmann (1993), on the other hand, reported finding differences in salivary cortisol reactivity between their infant attachment groups. In their study of 41 infants, saliva was collected immediately prior to the Strange Situation and then 15 and 30 minutes afterward. They found significant cortisol increases in infants categorized as disorganized compared to secure infants 15 minutes after the Strange Situation, as well as significant secure–insecure differences 30 minutes after the Strange Situation. Spangler and Grossmann argued that these data support a cortisol–coping hypothesis, with secure infants being better able than insecure infants to cope with the stress of separation in the Strange Situation. Spangler and Grossmann also commented on the differences between their findings and those of the two studies conducted by Gunnar's group (Gunnar et al., 1989, 1992). They noted that these differences could have resulted from variation in the length of time after the session before saliva was collected. In the Gunnar and colleagues (1989, 1992) studies, saliva was collected 5–10 minutes after the session; in the Spangler and Grossmann study, it was collected at 15 and then again at 30 minutes after the Strange Situation. Given the slow response time of cortisol, the Gunnar and colleagues data may not have reflected the full effect of the Strange Situation upon the insecure infants.

In a subsequent study, Hertsgaard, Gunnar, Erickson, and Nachmias (1995) examined 38 infants from a high-risk population. Unlike other studies, this one did not control for time of day at which saliva was obtained; nor was there any pretest cortisol measurement. Of the 34 subjects with usable data, 17 were classified as secure, 5 as avoidant, 1 as resistant, and 11 as disorganized. Results of the analyses revealed, first, that the infants with disorganized classifications had elevated cortisol levels compared to all of the other infants combined. Further inspection of the data revealed that the main difference in level was between the avoidant and disorganized infants. That is, avoidant infants displayed the lowest cortisol values, and disorganized infants displayed the highest. The authors argued that these data support the notion that infants categorized as disorganized may have greater vulnerability to stressful situations. It is, of course, also interesting that the infants classified as avoidant did not show elevated cortisol levels. If in fact avoidant infants are physiologically stressed during the Strange Situation, one would expect their cortisol levels to be higher than those of secure infants. It is also important to note that the initial level of cortisol was not assessed; therefore, it is unclear whether the cortisol levels represent different responses to the Strange Situation or initial differences between groups in levels of cortisol.

In a subsequent study, Nachmias, Gunnar, Mangelsdorf, Parritz, and Buss (1996) examined 73 children at 18 months of age in the Strange Situation. There were 13 children classified as avoidant, 12 classified as resistant, and 48 classified as secure. Salivary samples were collected immediately prior to the Strange Situation and 45 minutes after the onset of the testing session. The children had also been observed on a previous occasion responding to several novel events presented as part of assessing behavioral inhibition. "Behavioral inhibition" was defined as the tendency to restrain or restrict one's approach to new people, places, events, and/or objects (Kagan & Snidman, 1991). Although the authors did not find a relation between inhibition and security of attachment, they did find that children with higher behavioral inhibition had higher postsession cortisol levels if they

were also insecure. Secure inhibited children did not exhibit significant cortisol reactivity; nor, for that matter, did insecure infants who were low in inhibition. Thus the degree of cortisol reactivity to the Strange Situation in insecure children was heightened among those with higher behavioral inhibition. These results nicely illustrate Gunnar's stress model, in which the security of attachment is viewed as a buffer against stress; in this model, infants who are securely attached should exhibit a reduced stress response. In fact, inhibited infants who were securely attached did show lower cortisol responses.

In sum, the results of studies conducted to examine the physiological correlates of attachment classification during the Strange Situation have been mixed. Few studies have measured HR responses of infants in the Strange Situation, despite the technical feasibility of doing so. Those studies that have measured HR responses in the Strange Situation contain small numbers of subjects in different attachment categories, so that interpretation of the HR data is problematic. Greater success has been found in studies utilizing cortisol in the Strange Situation. The results indicate that infants who appear stressed during the Strange Situation are more likely to exhibit increases in cortisol levels.

Individual Differences in Physiology and Behavior in the Strange Situation

Heart Rate

Although attachment theorists for the longest time believed that an infant's temperament is orthogonal to the quality of the child's attachment to the caregiver (Sroufe, Egeland, Carlson, & Collins, 2005), there have been attempts to reconcile temperament and attachment positions (see Vaughn, Bost, & van IJzendoorn, Chapter 9, this volume). Belsky and Rovine (1987), for example, argued that temperament may play a role in the manner in which behaviors are expressed within the Strange Situation, regardless of attachment classification. That is, temperamentally reactive and fearful infants may be more likely to cry during separation and may have more difficulty in being soothed during reunion. Belsky and Rovine suggested that instead of comparing secure (B), avoidant (A), and resistant groups, researchers should compare A1-through-B2 infants with B3-through-C2 infants (the former group is relatively avoidant, whereas the latter group is relatively resistant). Organizing attachment classifications in this manner may assist in conceptualizing the influence of temperament on behavior in the Strange Situation. One might expect infants in the A1-through-B2 range not to react as intensely to separation as infants in the B3-through-C2 range.

Several researchers interested in the psychophysiological correlates of temperament have examined the physiological correlates of reactivity and regulation in infants (e.g., Fox, 1989; Stifter & Fox, 1990). Some have attempted to relate their findings to subsequent attachment behavior or status (Izard et al., 1991). For example, Porges and colleagues (1994) conceptualized their measure of vagal tone as reflecting the degree to which infants will be reactive and able to self-regulate. Infants with high vagal tone are thought to display more mature autonomic regulation and thus may exhibit both greater reactivity and superior self-regulatory strategies. Izard and colleagues (1991) examined the relation between vagal tone measured at 3, 4½, 6, and 9 months and attachment status at 13 months of age in 54 infants. Forty infants were classified as securely attached, 8 as avoidant, and 6 as resistant. Measures of vagal tone, HR, and HR variance were collected at each age assessed during the first year of life. A continuous measure of security was used as the dependent measure, and vagal tone scores were computed for each of the different assessment points on that score.

Izard and colleagues (1991) reported that measures of vagal tone at the earliest months significantly predicted attachment insecurity at 13 months. Specifically, infants with high vagal tone at 3 months and high HR variance at 4½ months were more likely to be classified as insecure at 13 months, although there were no differences between avoidant and resistant infants. Izard and colleagues' findings seem contrary to Porges's (1991) prediction regarding the role of vagal tone in emotion regulation. Porges argues that high vagal tone should reflect more mature autonomic regulation and greater regulatory capacity. It is unclear why these autonomic measures at this young age differed in the direction that they did; nor is it clear why there was a lack of differentiation at each of the other ages assessed.

Fox and colleagues conducted a series of studies aimed at examining relations among individual differences in emotion expression and emotion regulation and measures of autonomic activity (Fox, 1989; Fox & Gelles, 1984; Stifter & Fox, 1990). Fox and Gelles (1984) found that 3-month-old infants who displayed high HR vari-

ability and low HR were more likely to express positive emotions in response to maternal bids than were infants with high HR and low HR variability. "HR variability" was defined in this study as the mean of the successive differences in HR over the recording epoch. HR variability (particularly of the mean successive differences) is highly correlated with measures of RSA such as vagal tone. The authors reasoned that high HR variability, like vagal tone, should reflect an infant's ability to mount an organized behavioral response. This was confirmed when they found that infants with high HR variability displayed more positive interactive behavior. In subsequent studies, Fox (e.g., Fox, 1985) found that infants with high vagal tone were more reactive as young infants and also more likely to display positive social behaviors as toddlers. In contrast to Izard and colleagues' (1991) findings, but consistent with Porges's prediction, these data suggest that high vagal tone is associated with more organized social responsivity. Porges has argued that the level of vagal tone reflects the degree to which the organism will exhibit an organized response to stimulus challenge. The manner of autonomic response is reflected in organized overt behavior. Thus infants with high vagal tone should display less dysregulated and more organized behavioral responses to novelty and challenge; infants with low vagal tone should display less organized behavioral responses to stimulation.

Fox (1985) related individual differences in HR variability to attachment status within a high-risk (premature) infant sample. In a sample of 60 infants, Fox reported relations among measures of HR variability at 3 months of age and attachment status at 12 months of age. Of the 60 infants in the sample, 43 were classified at 12 months of age as secure, 16 as avoidant, and only 1 as resistant. Although there were no differences between attachment classification groups (avoidant vs. secure) on any of the autonomic measures, individual differences in behavior in the Strange Situation were related to 3-month HR variability. Specifically, infants who cried during the Strange Situation at 12 months had higher HR variability at 3 months. In addition, infants with high HR variability at 3 months displayed greater regulation at reunion during the Strange Situation; that is, they resumed playing in a shorter period of time. Fox argued that high HR variability, like vagal tone, reflects better physiological organization, such that children with high variability are more reactive but are also better able to self-regulate than infants with low variability.

More recent evidence suggests that attachment security predicts cardiac reactivity in early childhood (Burgess, Marshall, Rubin, & Fox, 2003). In their study of 172 families, Burgess et al. examined relations between attachment classification at 14 months, behavioral inhibition at 24 months, social behavior at 4 years, and cardiac functioning (HP and RSA) at 14 and 24 months and at 4 years. Cardiac assessments at each age were made during 3 minutes in which the child quietly attended to a video monitor. No significant group differences were yielded for attachment group on HP or RSA at 14 or 24 months. Also, no significant group differences for inhibition (low, medium, and high) on HP or RSA at 14 or 24 months were found. However, attachment security (and not behavioral inhibition) predicted HP and RSA at 4 years. Specifically, avoidant infants showed significantly higher HP and RSA than secure and resistant infants did.

The association between 14-month attachment status and cardiac reactivity some 3 years thereafter is an impressive demonstration of the potential evocative effects of attachment security on physiological arousal. The predictive association between 14-month attachment and 4-year cardiac reactivity, and the lack of association with contemporaneous (or more proximal) assessment of cardiac reactivity and attachment security, suggest that the avoidant pattern of attachment acquired in infancy may have influenced the development of physiological reactivity. That is, infants who employed a coping strategy characterized by avoidance, or seeming indifference to maternal separation and reunion, may have acquired a generalized pattern of underarousal that continued to develop across late infancy and was not salient until early childhood. In the same study, Burgess and colleagues (2003) revealed that children who were classified as avoidant in infancy and who were low in inhibition at 24 months scored significantly higher than all other attachment–inhibition groups on externalizing behavior problems on the Child Behavior Checklist (CBCL; Achenbach & Edelbrock, 1991), and that this effect was largely carried by high scores on the aggression narrow band of the CBCL.

Raine (1996) has proposed a model of physiological underarousal in the development of antisocial behavior, which has been met with empirical validation (e.g., Raine, Venables, & Williams, 1990). Although three-way interactions involving attachment security, behavioral inhibition, and cardiac reactivity as determinants of childhood behavior problems were not examined in the Burgess and colleagues (2003) report, it seems plausible that avoidant infants who are also uninhibited and who acquire a cardiac profile characterized by underarousal may be at considerable risk for the development of antisocial behavior in early childhood and beyond. Such a proposal awaits substantiation from future research.

Cortisol

Emergent evidence suggests that attachment security foretells subsequent physiological regulation as assessed via salivary cortisol. In a comprehensive examination of biobehavioral organization, attachment security, and behavioral inhibition, Schieche and Spangler (2004) assessed 76 toddlers in the Strange Situation at 12 months; inhibited temperament at 22 months via maternal report; maternal and child behavior during a challenge task (i.e., a series of structured tasks of progressive difficulty, which culminated in the necessary involvement of the mother for successful completion) at 22 months; and salivary cortisol in infants before and 15 and 30 minutes following the challenge paradigm. Nineteen infants were classified as insecure-avoidant, 23 as secure, 11 as insecure-resistant, and 23 as disorganized.

Contemporaneous associations between behavior during the challenge task and cortisol showed that elevated cortisol was associated with low task orientation and exploration in the infants, which were in turn associated with low supportive maternal presence and reduced quality of maternal assistance during the challenge task (although no significant relations between cortisol and maternal behavior during the task were revealed). Across the sample, infants showed a decline in cortisol during the challenge task, and this was particularly evident for infants who were reported by their mothers as low on behavioral inhibition. However, differential levels of cortisol were revealed for highly inhibited children depending on attachment status, with securely attached inhibited infants showing the expected decrease in cortisol from task onset to 30 minutes after the task. Avoidant infants in contrast showed a decrease from task onset to 15 minutes after the task, but a modest (and nonsignificant) increase in cortisol 30 minutes after the task, suggesting a delayed activation of the HPA axis. This finding was complemented by behavioral findings indicating that avoidant infants manifested less effective coping and an inability to use their mothers as a source of support during the challenge task. Within-group analyses revealed that elevated cortisol was associated with low task orientation and exploration, low help-seeking behavior, and high proximity seeking for the insecure group (A, C, and D combined). No significant correlations involving cortisol within the secure group were obtained.

Taken together, these findings suggest that the association between early attachment, stress reactivity, and social behavior later in infancy is dependent upon an infant's temperamental disposition, and that for an insecurely attached infant, physiological reactivity is associated with a corresponding behavioral profile characterized by an inability to use the mother effectively as a source of support in the face of environmental challenge.

EEG Asymmetry

Various data from a number of different sources have implicated the anterior regions of the left and right cerebral hemispheres as being involved in the expression and/or experience of different emotions (Davidson & Fox, 1982; Fox, 1991; Fox & Davidson, 1984). In an initial study, Davidson and Fox (1982) found that 10-month-old infants viewing a videotape of an actress portraying either positive affect (smiling and laughter) or negative affect (sad expression and crying) exhibited asymmetric activation in frontal scalp leads, depending on the valence of the video stimulus. While viewing the positive segment, infants exhibited left frontal EEG asymmetry (relatively greater activation in the left frontal region). Follow-up studies found this asymmetry in frontal EEG activity to be present also in infants' responses to sweet and sour tastes (Fox & Davidson, 1986), as well as to the approach of the infants' mothers or a stranger (Fox & Davidson, 1988). Infants exhibited left frontal EEG asymmetry during the expression of positive affect and right frontal EEG asymmetry during the expression of negative affect (Fox & Davidson, 1984).

Fox and Davidson (1984) argued that the functional significance of frontal asymmetry with regard to emotion may be conceptualized in terms of the motivational systems of approach and withdrawal. The right frontal region may be specialized for behaviors associated with withdrawal, whereas the left may be specialized for behaviors associated with approach. Subsequently, Fox (1991, 1994) speculated that activity in the frontal region may also be involved in the regulation of approach or withdrawal behaviors. He based this position partly on studies of the behavioral effects of unilateral frontal brain damage. Patients with either left or right frontal lesions often report an inability to control or regulate the expression of negative or positive affects; these same patients can, if requested, produce facial expressions of either positive or negative affect. Their deficit thus appears to be in the control of emotion expression, rather than in the ability to produce the expressions themselves.

Fox therefore argued that both left and right frontal activation may be associated with the ability to modulate approach or withdrawal behaviors. Left frontal activation may be associated with the ability to control approach behavior and the expression of positive affect. A decrement in left frontal activation may be associated with the absence of the expression of positive affect. Pizzagalli, Sherwood, Henriques, and Davidson (2005) suggest that resting left prefrontal EEG asymmetry is associated with the propensity to develop approach-related tendencies. Right frontal activation may be associated with the ability to control withdrawal behaviors and the expression of negative affect. A decrement in right frontal activation may be associated with the absence of the expression of negative affect.

There is some evidence for this model. Henriques and Davidson (1990) found that depressed individuals (even those who had previously been depressed and were currently in remission) exhibited right frontal EEG asymmetry. Inspection of the EEG power values revealed that the asymmetry in these individuals was a function of less activity in the left frontal region. The authors argued that some depression may be characterized by an absence of positive affect rather than the presence of extreme negative affect. On the other hand, Davidson and Fox (1988) found that infants with right frontal EEG asymmetry were more likely to cry at maternal separation than were those displaying left frontal EEG asymmetry. Fox, Bell, and Jones (1992) replicated this finding and reported that the locus of the effect was in the right hemisphere: Infants most likely to cry were those displaying less power in the right frontal region (e.g., right frontal asymmetry). In addition, Calkins, Fox, and Marshall (1996) found that inhibited infants displayed right frontal EEG asymmetry, which was a function of right frontal activation. Finally, Schmidt, Shahinfar, and Fox (1996) reported that toddlers selected for externalizing behaviors exhibited left frontal EEG asymmetry, which was a function of high right frontal power (less right activation).

They speculated that this pattern may reflect a decreased ability to experience punishment among aggressive children.

Dawson and her colleagues (2001) examined the associations of maternal depression and attachment security with frontal EEG asymmetry in 13- to 15-month-old infants. Mothers were sorted into groups based on depression status as follows: no depression ($n = 69$), subthreshold depression ($n = 63$), and depression ($n = 27$). Infants and their mothers underwent the Strange Situation procedure, and 20 infants were classified as insecure-avoidant, 54 as secure, 23 as insecure-resistant, and 35 as disorganized. EEG data were collected independently of the Strange Situation and included recordings at baseline, during mother play, and during experimenter play.

Results revealed that infants of depressed mothers and insecurely attached infants (types A, C, and D combined) exhibited a pattern of reduced right frontal EEG activity relative to infants of subthreshold depressed and nondepressed mothers. Also, a trend for a significant depression–attachment interaction indicated that within the sample of insecurely attached infants, infants of mothers with major depression showed significantly greater attenuated left frontal activity than infants of mothers with no or subthreshold depression. Hence infants of depressed mothers and insecurely attached infants, and particularly insecurely attached infants of depressed mothers, showed a physiological bias toward withdrawal motivation that is consistent with theoretical and empirical evidence regarding the heightened levels of emotion dysregulation of infants of depressed mothers (Murray & Cooper, 1997) and insecurely attached infants (Calkins & Fox, 1992; Kochanska, 1998).

Although there are no data directly assessing EEG differences in the prediction of attachment classification, there is indirect evidence of a relation between dispositional patterns of frontal EEG asymmetry and attachment classification. In a series of studies, Fox and colleagues (Calkins & Fox, 1992; Calkins et al., 1996; Fox, Calkins, & Bell, 1994) examined the pattern of EEG asymmetry in temperamentally inhibited infants. These infants displayed a pattern of right frontal EEG asymmetry as early as 9 months of age. Indeed, infants displaying stable right frontal EEG asymmetry across the first 2 years of life were more likely to display reticence and social withdrawal at age 4 than were infants whose pattern was unstable or who showed a stable pattern of left frontal EEG asymmetry over that period of time (Fox et al., 1994). In a parallel

study, Calkins and Fox (1992) reported that inhibited infants were more likely to be categorized as resistant than were uninhibited infants. Fifty infants were seen at both 14 and 24 months of age. At 14 months of age, the infants were videotaped in the Strange Situation, and later 34 were classified as secure, 7 as avoidant, and 9 as resistant. At 24 months of age, these same infants were seen in the laboratory and assessed for behavioral inhibition. The pattern of cross-age findings revealed that at 24 months avoidant infants were likely to be assessed as uninhibited, resistant infants were likely to be assessed as highly inhibited, and secure infants were likely to display behaviors around the mean. The temperamentally inhibited infants displayed right frontal EEG asymmetry, suggesting an underlying predisposition toward withdrawal. Inhibited infants displaying right frontal EEG asymmetry were most likely to be categorized as resistant in their attachment, due to their disposition to express negative affect in response to mild stress and their inability to modulate that affective response.

Similar findings were obtained in a study examining the influence of maternal depression on attachment security in both clinical and nonclinical populations (Dawson, Klinger, Panagiotides, Spieker, & Frey, 1992). These researchers reported that secure infants of symptomatic mothers displayed reduced left frontal EEG activity in response to a positive affect elicitor, compared to securely attached infants of nonsymptomatic mothers. They argued that the infants of symptomatic mothers may have had more difficulty expressing positive affect, as indexed by the reduced left frontal EEG activity. The small number of subjects and lack of comparisons with insecure infants, however, do not allow for a generalization about EEG as indicative of affect expression in attachment.

Although the influence of individual differences in temperament on attachment security remains a point of discussion and dissension among researchers, there appears to be evidence for physiological markers of certain infant dispositions. In particular, proneness to distress and negative affect seem to have distinct physiological markers. These dispositions most certainly have some influence on behavior in the Strange Situation and perhaps on attachment classification as well. More importantly, the manner in which caregiving styles interact with such dispositions to produce attachment classification and social competencies should be a productive avenue of future research.

QUALITY OF CAREGIVING
AND PHYSIOLOGICAL AROUSAL

Quality of maternal caregiving, particularly caregiving that is sensitive (i.e., involving prompt, contingent, and appropriate responsiveness to infant cues and signals; Ainsworth et al., 1978), is the key theoretical antecedent to attachment security. An exciting emergent body of research involving both animals and humans is revealing that natural (in the case of animals) or ordinary (for humans) variations in the quality of maternal caregiving shape the neurological systems that regulate stress reactions.

Meaney and his colleagues (Caldji et al., 1998; Francis, Diorio, Liu, & Meaney, 1999; Liu & Diorio, 1997) have shown that naturally occurring variations in quality of maternal caregiving behavior (MCB) among rat dams shapes the development of the neural substrates that underlie the phenotypic behavioral and endocrine responses to stress in offspring. These researchers noted that the MCB of rat dams in the postnatal period—specifically, in terms of nursing posture (arch-backed vs. lying) and frequency of licking and grooming behavior—is normally distributed. They created extreme groups of pups based on the quality of MCB received (low vs. high levels of licking/grooming and arch-backed nursing), and followed these offspring into adulthood. Compared with adult offspring that received high degrees of maternal licking/grooming and arch-backed nursing in the postnatal period, the adult offspring of dams that provided low degrees of maternal licking/grooming and arch-backed nursing showed a behavioral response reflective of heightened levels of stress reactivity, including higher frequencies of startle responses, less open-field exploration, and elongated latencies to eat food presented in a novel environment (Caldji et al., 1998; Francis et al., 1999). These differences in behavior were accompanied by a corresponding neuroendocrine profile characteristic of heightened fearfulness (Caldji et al., 1998), such as increased plasma adrenocorticotropic hormone and corticosterone responses to restraint stress, and decreased sensitivity to the inhibitory effects of glucocorticoids during acute stress (Liu & Diorio, 1997). The behavioral differences were also associated with decreased central benzodiazepine receptor density in the central, lateral, and basolateral nuclei of the amygdala and locus ceruleus (Caldji et al., 1998).

In a study based on retrospective self-report, Pruessner, Champagne, Meaney, and Dagher (2004) found that human adults who reported extremely low-quality relationships with their parents evidenced significantly more release of dopamine in the ventral striatum and a higher increase in salivary cortisol during a stressful event than individuals who reported extremely high-quality parental relations. Such an effect suggests that early human caregiving may similarly affect the development of the systems that underlie stress reactivity. In an effort to extend this provocative set of findings to human infants, we (Hane & Fox, 2006) examined the relation between quality of MCB and behavioral and physiological indices of stress reactivity in 9-month-old infants. The quality of MCB during routine activities in the home (e.g., feeding and changing) was assessed with Ainsworth's original global scales for rating degree of maternal sensitivity, which included ratings for acceptance, availability, appropriateness of interaction, and delight in the infant, as well as with an intrusiveness scale developed by Park, Belsky, Putnam, and Crnic (1997).

We then compared the infants who received low-quality MCB to those who experienced high-quality MCB on indices of stress reactivity also assessed at age 9 months, and found that infants who experienced low-quality MCB displayed significantly more fearfulness during the presentation of novel stimuli and less sociability with an experimenter. In addition, the infants receiving low-quality MCB showed a pattern of right frontal EEG asymmetry. These infants were not found to differ in terms of earlier temperament from the infants who received high-quality MCB, based on degree of positive and negative reactivity to novelty assessed at age 4 months. However, infants who received low-quality MCB were more likely to express higher levels of negative affect during interactions with their mothers than infants in the high-quality MCB group, suggesting that the infants' negativity may have influenced the quality of mother–infant interactions.

The work described above (Caldji et al., 1998; Francis et al., 1999; Hane & Fox, 2006; Liu & Diorio, 1997) breaks new ground in demonstrating that the quality of maternal caregiving, not just extreme instances of maternal deprivation, influence neurological development. The infants in our (Hane & Fox, 2006) sample came from a middle-class, low-risk demographic group, and the measure of MCB, which assessed degree of maternal sensitivity and intrusiveness, captured typical variations in MCB seen in previous research on attachment. Also, the research examining the biobehavioral concomitants and sequelae of MCB provides the first evidence that early relationships may affect both behavioral and health outcomes. Meaney (2001) has noted that exposure to early and pronounced stressors that cause dysregulation of the HPA axis predisposes individuals to further problems in dealing with environmental stressors, and persistent difficulty in coping with stress exacerbates risk for behavioral and health problems. The neuroendocrine changes associated with dysregulation of the HPA axis alter the organism's availability and distribution of energy and increases of cardiovascular tone, which over time may predispose individuals to steroid-induced diabetes, hypertension, and other risk factors for heart disease (Brindley & Rolland, 1989).

Indeed, Bowlby, Ainsworth, and others have contended that the importance of the quality of the mother–infant relationship is far-reaching. Emergent evidence indicates that attachment quality predicts general health outcomes, including well-being (Konstantinos & Sideridis, 2006), symptom perception and health care utilization (Ciechanowski, Walker, Katon, & Russo, 2002), and severity of disability associated with migraine (Rossi et al., 2005).

Most importantly, this emergent evidence showing that quality of caregiving shapes the development of the neurological systems that regulate reactions to stress provides the first suggestion of a mechanism of influence by which early caregiving environments shape behavior, including sociability with unfamiliar adults (Hane & Fox, 2006). We have suggested elsewhere (Hane & Fox, 2007) that the process by which early experience shapes developmental outcomes may be a function of phenotypic plasticity, whereby early caregiving shapes the expression of innate temperamental tendencies by yielding phenotypic changes to the neurological systems that regulate reactivity to stress and novelty. Those changes in stress reactivity may then elicit changes in the environment by altering the quality of maternal behavior. Certain features of the early caregiving environment may yield contemporaneous phenotypic changes to the systems involved in regulation of stress, and also to the organism's propensity to manifest similar phenotypic changes in the future—a phenomenon documented by evolutionary biologists and referred to as "phenotypic plasticity" (Hane & Fox, 2007).

Bowlby (1969/1982) and Main, Kaplan, and Cassidy (1985) contended that security of mother–infant attachment influences the quality of an individual's future social relationships via the formation of "internal working models," or cognitive representations that are based on early attachment experiences; these models set the rules and expectations for, and ultimately influence the quality of, future attachment relationships. According to this notion, an insecure attachment relationship with one's primary caregiver should lead to future difficulties in intimate relationships. This has been supported empirically by studies showing that adult attachment representations (Treboux, Crowell, & Waters, 2004) and attachment style (Volling, Notaro, & Larsen, 1998) are related to the quality of marital relationships.

Phenotypic plasticity in the development of stress reactivity vis-à-vis quality of MCB may offer a complementary biological model for the mechanism of influence of early attachment security throughout the lifespan. In this model, quality of MCB shapes the development of the neurological systems that regulate stress responses and social behavior, and this effect is apparent in the social behavior of adults as a function of phenotypic plasticity, which increases an individual's vulnerability to react physiologically and behaviorally to future relationship stressors (see Mikulincer & Shaver, Chapter 23, this volume, for examples).

PHYSIOLOGICAL RESPONSES OF CAREGIVERS AND ATTACHMENT

The development of the attachment relationship is thought to be based on the manner in which a caregiver responds to an infant's signals. A mother who is insensitive and ignores her infant's needs contributes to the development of an avoidant attachment; a mother who is inconsistent in her responses contributes to the development of a resistant attachment; and a mother who is sensitive and responsive to the infant contributes to the development of a secure attachment (Ainsworth, 1973). It is for this reason that a good deal of research has examined the parameters of sensitivity and responsiveness in maternal behavior during the first year of life, and its association with the subsequent quality of attachment (Ainsworth, 1973; Ainsworth, Bell, & Stayton, 1971; Ainsworth et al., 1978; Bell & Ainsworth, 1972; Belsky & Isabella, 1987; Egeland & Farber, 1984; see Belsky & Fearon, Chapter 13, this volume).

Among studies assessing these parameters and subsequent quality of attachment are those that have used psychophysiological measures to examine maternal sensitivity to infant signals, as well as the underlying aspects of sensitive MCB (e.g., Donovan & Leavitt, 1985a, 1985b, 1989; Frodi, Lamb, Leavitt, Donovan, Neff, et al., 1978). For example, in a study assessing the behavioral sensitivity of mothers to their infants during a feeding session, Donovan and Leavitt (1978) showed that physiological reactivity (the degree of a mother's HR deceleration) to an infant's signals predicted the mother's behavioral sensitivity when feeding the infant. HR deceleration was interpreted as reflecting maternal attention. The authors suggested that mothers showing the HR deceleration pattern were more attentive to their infants' needs than were mothers who did not show this pattern of HR deceleration.

Researchers have argued that the quality of maternal responsiveness is in part influenced by the infant's behavior. In order to examine this, researchers have presented adult participants with audiotapes or videotapes of different types of cries of familiar and unfamiliar infants, and measured the autonomic responses to these cries. Frodi, Lamb, Leavitt, and Donovan (1978) presented 48 mother–father pairs with a 6-minute videotape showing either a smiling infant or a crying infant. The infant in the videotape was randomly labeled prior to presentation as either "normal," "difficult," or "premature." Blood pressure and skin conductance were recorded while each participant watched the tape. Results revealed little autonomic change in response to the smiling infant, but significant increases in blood pressure (interpreted as reflecting an "aversive state" or a "disposition to aggress") and skin conductance (interpreted as an index of autonomic arousal to "aggress") in response to the crying infant, with the highest increases in parents who were told that the infant was premature. The authors speculated that perception of an infant's difficultness may lead some individuals to respond aversively to that infant's signals. In a follow-up study, these same authors (Frodi, Lamb, Leavitt, Donovan, Neff, et al., 1978) examined 64 parents who were presented with a videotape of either a full-term or a premature infant and heard, paired with it, either a full-term or a premature infant's cry. HR and skin conductance were measured and found to be significantly elevated when subjects heard the cry of a premature infant, particularly when this cry was paired with the video of the premature infant.

The increases in HR and skin conductance were interpreted within a general model of arousal as reflecting aversiveness. The authors speculated

that "high-risk" infants may emit cries that are more aversive and thus more likely to reduce caregivers' responsiveness. Several other studies have employed variants of the paradigm described above to examine factors that might influence parental response to infant cries (these data are reviewed extensively in Donovan & Leavitt, 1985b). For example, Boukydis and Burgess (1982) examined the effects of parity on a parent's response to infant crying, finding that primiparous parents showed higher levels of skin potential response. Wiesenfeld, Malatesta, and DeLoach (1981) reported that both mothers and fathers responded with HR deceleration to unfamiliar infant cries, although mothers were better able than fathers to discriminate between their own infants' cries and those of an unfamiliar infant. In most of these studies, HR deceleration has been interpreted as reflecting attention to the stimulus, whereas HR acceleration has been considered evidence of an aversive or defensive response. Such correspondence may not always be evident, however. For example, Wiesenfeld and Klorman (1978) found that mothers responded with HR acceleration to videotapes of their own infants' smiles. Similarly, Donovan, Leavitt, and Balling (1978) found an initial HR acceleration in mothers in response to their smiling 3-month-old infants. The acceleration of HR found in such studies does not easily fit a model of linking acceleration and defensive response. Nevertheless, the finding of HR deceleration across studies in response to "normal" infant cries does seem to reflect an early component of the attention system and may play a role in directing maternal responses to a distressed infant.

In a series of innovative studies, Donovan and Leavitt studied factors that may elicit an attentional response in mothers of young infants (Donovan & Leavitt, 1989; Donovan, Leavitt, & Walsh, 1990, 1997). They examined the degree to which mothers felt they had control over the termination of an infant's cry. Their task—a modification of the illusion-of-control paradigm (Alloy & Abramson, 1979)—consisted of having each mother make one of two responses, with the goal of terminating an infant's cry, after which the mother was asked to estimate her perceived control over the event. On each of 42 trials, a red light was followed by cry onset. Subjects had the option of either pressing or not pressing a button. Responses were followed by a fixed schedule of cry termination in half the trials and cry continuation in the other half. On trial 41, the cry stimulus was omitted. After the trials, mothers of 5-month-old infants were asked to rate the degree to which they felt they had control over cry termination during the task. HR was monitored continuously during the task, and change scores were computed between prestimulus HR level and levels during (1) the 10-second interval prior to onset of the cry, (2) the initial 5 seconds of the cry, (3) the 20-second interval during omission of the cry on trial 41, and (4) the 10-second period on trial 42. Mothers were grouped into those who reported either a high illusion of control, a midlevel illusion of control, or a low illusion of control during the task.

Mothers in the high-illusion group displayed an augmented HR acceleration in anticipation of the impending cry, which habituated rapidly and remained low during the middle of the task, and displayed increasing acceleration toward the final trials. Mothers in the high-illusion group did not show the same pattern of deceleration to the omitted cry that mothers in the middle- and low-illusion groups did. Thus maternal HR reflected attentional processes in a mother's response to her perception of control over an infant's cries. Mothers with a high illusion of control displayed more aversive responses, coped less well over time (as reflected in their pattern over trials), and were not as attentive to the omitted cry. Donovan and Leavitt (1989) claimed that this pattern of HR findings reflects a degree of insensitivity to infant signals.

In this same study, Donovan and Leavitt (1989) assessed the mothers and infants in the Strange Situation when the infants were 15 months of age. Infants were classified as either secure or insecure, and comparisons were made with the 5-month sensitivity ratings. Four insecurely attached infants had mothers in the low- or middle-illusion groups, and three had mothers in the high-illusion group. These small group sizes precluded any direct test of the relations between illusion group and attachment security. Donovan and Leavitt also reported that mothers of insecurely attached infants were more depressed at 5 (but not at 16) months than were mothers of securely attached infants. And mothers of insecurely attached infants exhibited cardiac acceleration to the impending cry.

In two follow-up studies, Donovan and Leavitt (Donovan et al., 1990, 1997) further refined their model of illusion of control in relation to sensitive caregiving. Donovan and colleagues (1990) presented mothers of 5-month-olds with the illusion-of-control task. A week later, the mothers participated in a learned helplessness paradigm, in which they were presented with an infant cry and told to try to terminate it by pressing a button. For all mothers, pushing the button had no effect on the cry. Mothers were then given a second task consisting of a shuttle box with a movable handle. Again, they were asked to attempt to terminate the cry by moving the handle. HR was recorded throughout the session. As in the earlier study, mothers were categorized as having a high, middle, or low illusion of control. In addition, mothers completed a temperament questionnaire designed to assess their own infants' behavior; based on their responses, their infants were categorized as either "easy" or "difficult."

The HR data revealed an interaction between illusion group and infant temperament. Mothers in the high-illusion group who rated their infants as difficult responded with cardiac acceleration in the learned helplessness task. Only mothers in the middle-illusion group displayed significant cardiac deceleration to the impending cry as they completed the task. Donovan and colleagues (1990) argued that mothers who had a high illusion of control were less attentive and more "defensive" in response to infant signals than were mothers in the other two groups.

In a subsequent study, Donovan and colleagues (1997) assessed mothers of 4- to 6-month-olds in their lab twice—once with the illusion-of-control task, and a second time with a signal detection task in which they were asked to differentiate infant cries that varied in frequency. HR was monitored throughout the illusion-of-control task. Mothers were divided into three groups based on sensitivity scores collected during the signal detection task. Analysis of the HR data revealed that only the most sensitive mothers exhibited a smooth pattern of habituation over trials in HR; mothers in the latter two groups failed to habituate across trials. Thus greater sensitivity of mothers to infant cries was associated with habituation of the HR response during the illusion-of-control task. In addition, mothers' perception of their ability to control terminating an infant cry was related to their sensitivity to discriminate between different infant cry patterns.

The Donovan and Leavitt work has systematically addressed factors that may be associated with maternal sensitivity to infant cries, and possibly to a secure pattern of attachment. They reported across studies that maternal sensitivity was related to the degree to which mothers realistically estimated the control they had over terminating an infant's cry, as well as the degree to which they were susceptible to learned helplessness. The picture emerging from this body of work is one in which particular maternal personality characteristics contribute to a mother's lack of sensitivity toward her infant's signals. This apparent insensitivity is further supported by the absence of clear deceleratory HR patterns in the data. The links among this apparent insensitivity, maternal personality characteristics, and associated HR response have not yet been fully explored, however. In only one study (Donovan & Leavitt, 1989) did these investigators follow up the mothers and children to age 15 months and assess them in the Strange Situation. As in many studies of this type, the number of insecure children who had mothers in the high-illusion group was too small to permit any definite conclusions to be drawn. Nevertheless, the work represents the best available attempt to integrate physiological indices of attention with cognitive and personality attributes of caregiving, in order to clarify the factors involved in maternal sensitivity.

PSYCHOPHYSIOLOGY AND MEASURES OF ADULT ATTACHMENT

Conceptual advances in the study of attachment have led to the development of an instrument for assessing an adult's current state of mind regarding attachment to his or her parents. Researchers administering the AAI (George, Kaplan, & Main, 1984, 1985, 1996) ask subjects to describe experiences they may have had as children interacting with their parents. Particular emphasis is placed on themes of separation and loss. Subjects are asked to generate memories regarding their parents' caregiving and to characterize the relationships they had with their parents. Interviews are recorded on audiotape and then scored from verbatim transcripts. Important elements in the scoring are a subject's coherence and nature of discourse. That is, an interview is scored for the degree to which there is consistency across responses and the extent to which a coherent story is generated. On the basis of these scores, subjects are classified into one of four attachment groups: "secure-autonomous," "dismissing," "preoccupied," or "unresolved" (see Hesse, Chapter 25, and Crowell, Fraley, & Shaver, Chapter 26, this volume).

An excellent review paper by Diamond (2001) presented a number of approaches for studying individual differences in adult attachment organization, including both the AAI and questionnaire measures. Not surprisingly, her review focused on the use of either autonomic activity or measurement of the HPA axis in the study of such individual differences. Diamond's paper makes two conceptual points that are important guides to research in this area. First, she frames the study of adults who vary in classification on the AAI or in scores on attachment style questionnaires clearly within the tradition of individual differences and personality. Thus, as they do in other personality characteristics (such as neuroticism or the "Big Five" typology), individuals may vary in their attachment organization. Identifying differences in autonomic reactivity among adults differing in attachment classification or style is one means of validating these categories. Second, Diamond frames individual differences in adult attachment within an emotion regulation framework. That is, individuals who differ in their attachment classification will display differences in reactions to stress and different patterns of emotion regulation, which can be measured in part by autonomic and HPA reactivity.

Relatively few studies to date have utilized this approach for studying individual differences in adult attachment. Diamond (2001) cites a number of papers that examined adults' responses to stressors when the presence of significant others was manipulated. For example, Spitzer, Llabre, Ironson, and Gellman (1992) found that individuals had lower blood pressure when their family members were present than when they were in the presence of strangers. In a study with a similar approach, Kirkpatrick and colleagues (Carpenter & Kirkpatrick, 1996; Feeney & Kirkpatrick, 1996) examined college-age women's responses to stress once in the presence of a romantic partner and once by themselves. They found that women who were insecure in their attachment styles (measured with a questionnaire) exhibited greater blood pressure and HR changes when their romantic partners were present than when they were alone. Interestingly, securely attached women showed no differences in reactivity with or without their romantic partners. Diamond writes that this pattern of data may reflect the greater internalization of an attachment figure's stress-buffering capacities. Thus securely attached individuals don't "need" their attachment figures present to regulate their emotional reactions to a stressor.

In one of the only studies that has directly examined adults' autonomic responses during the AAI, Dozier and Kobak (1992) measured skin conductance while adults were questioned about their recall of experiences of separation, rejection, and threat from their parents. They reported that subjects employing "deactivating" strategies showed marked increases in skin conductance, compared to those who were securely attached. The authors relate their findings to emotion regulation strategies used during the AAI interview. These studies varied in the manner in which subjects were characterized as having different attachment styles. For example, the Kirkpatrick studies used questionnaire methods, whereas the Dozier study used AAI responses. Although interesting differences between subjects with different styles of attachment were found, it would be helpful to examine the possible underlying latent trait or traits that are measured with these various approaches to individual differences in attachment style.

Recently a number of studies have begun to examine physiological and behavioral differences among adults who have different AAI classifications. In one study, Roisman, Tsai, and Chiang (2004) measured skin conductance, HR, and facial expression in adults while they reported on their experiences during the AAI. The study was framed around the issue of individual differences in emotion regulation strategies as they are related to differences in AAI organization. Roisman and colleagues reported that their results replicated those of Dozier and Kobak (1992): Adults who were dismissing about their early attachment experiences displayed enhanced electrodermal activity. Roisman and colleagues found that these differences were not present for HR measures, but were true for both men and women of two different ethnic groups. According to the authors, their data support the notion that attachment organization as assessed by the AAI is associated with distinct emotion regulation patterns measured both physiologically and behaviorally.

A recent study by Powers, Pietromonaco, Gunlicks, and Sayer (2006) examined HPA axis activity (via measurement of cortisol) in dating couples. Cortisol was measured before and after a stressful procedure (a conflict negotiation task). And each of the individuals in the couple was categorized via questionnaire as fearfully avoidant, dismissing, preoccupied, or secure. Results revealed differences between those adults categorized as securely versus insecurely attached, with the latter displaying greater physiological reactivity, although there were differences between men and women in the pattern of responses.

A recent study by Diamond, Hicks, and Otter-Henderson (2006) of 74 cohabitating heterosexual couples examined the relation between autonomic reactivity (via skin conductance) during administration of various laboratory-based psychological stressors (math, speech, and anger tasks) and attachment-related tasks, and self-reported attachment anxiety and avoidance. To evoke reactivity to attachment-related issues, participants were asked to describe their thoughts and feelings regarding their current relationships and any anticipated or hypothetical separations from their partners. Results indicated that avoidance was associated with greater autonomic reactivity across all tasks, with this trend growing more robust across tasks, despite self-reported level of decreased distress across these same tasks. In contrast, attachment anxiety was not associated with sympathetic reactivity across the sample, and for women, attachment anxiety was associated with a decrease in sympathetic reactivity across tasks. According to Diamond and her colleagues, such evidence supports the notion that avoidant adults employ a repressive coping style, which is ineffective in regulating their heightened levels of physiological arousal.

In sum, a growing number of studies now take a traditional individual-differences approach to the study of variations in attachment organization among adults. The investigators have framed their approach, for the most part, around the study of emotion regulation or responses to stress, and have made specific predictions about the nature of physiological responses to stress among different attachment categories. It appears that the different AAI categories and questionnaire-based assessments of attachment style do tap individual differences that are related to adaptive coping with stress, although the relations are complex. In particular, gender differences appear to be found in many of the studies. Further research on the physiological correlates of individual differences assessed with the AAI and with attachment style questionnaires will elucidate these issues.

NEUROSCIENTIFIC APPROACHES TO STUDYING DIFFERENCES IN ADULT ATTACHMENT

There are at least two approaches to the study of attachment that involve neuroscience—specifically, imaging of brain activity. The first involves assessment of behaviors thought to be important in the support of attachment. The second involves imaging of individuals who differ in their attachment styles or adult attachment classifications. There are numerous studies in the imaging literature that have examined individuals' responses to pictures of faces.

Often researchers who conduct these studies are interested in whether pictures of faces with different emotion expressions elicit or activate different regions of the brain. For example, several studies have found that individuals display heightened amygdala activation in response to faces displaying fear or anger (Whalen, 1999; Whalen et al., 1998). More recently, a number of studies have examined patterns of neural activation to familiar versus unfamiliar faces, and in some instances have examined differences in women's responses to faces of their own children versus faces of unfamiliar children.

For example, Nitschke and colleagues (2004) showed women photographs of their own infants, unfamiliar infants, and unfamiliar adults. Women also rated their hedonic responses to each of the photographs. Results revealed strong bilateral activation of orbitofrontal cortex when women viewed pictures of their own infants, compared to either unfamiliar infants or unfamiliar adults. Women's ratings of their hedonic response to the pictures revealed heightened positive affect to pictures of their own children versus other children. Interestingly, the brain response to own versus unfamiliar infants diminished over time. That is, in a second block of exposures, the difference in brain response (but not in the hedonic rating) between own and unfamiliar infants decreased. The orbitofrontal cortex is a region of the prefrontal cortex that has been implicated in the decoding of affective valence of a stimulus. It has been implicated in rodent and human work as a brain region important for reward processing (Knutson, Westdorp, Kaiser, & Hommer, 2000; Schoenbaum, Chiba, & Gallagher, 1998). Nitschke and colleagues suggest that it may also be involved in attachment-related behaviors, particularly those involved in positive affect toward an attachment figure.

In similar work, Leibenluft, Gobbini, Harrison, and Haxby (2004) examined women's neural activation while each woman was viewing pictures of her own child, a friend's child, an unfamiliar child, or an unfamiliar adult. The design of their study allowed comparison of familiar versus unfamiliar children and own children versus familiar children to determine the neural specificity of each comparison. Results revealed that a complex set of brain networks was activated for each of the different types of stimuli. Viewing one's own child vs. viewing a familiar child activated amygdala, insula, anterior paracingulate cortex, and superior temporal sulcus. Viewing familiar versus unfamiliar children activated regions similar to those seen in prior studies in which familiar versus unfamiliar adults were viewed. The authors suggested that viewing one's own child (vs. another familiar child) activates emotion responses and cognitions that may reflect attachment, protection, and empathy. Although subjects were asked prior to scanning to rate the stimuli, the questions did not cover the psychological states that are proposed to underlie activation of these different neural structures.

The two studies just described represent the possibility of an approach to studying psychological and brain processes that should be related to attachment. That is, to the extent that viewing the face of one's own infant, or the face of one's own caregiver, elicits positive emotion, this state should be distinct (and so far does appear to be distinct) from that elicited by viewing either familiar or unfamiliar infants or adults. The emotions and social cognitions, and the underlying neural circuitry involved in identifying attachment figures, could be probed in this manner.

A second brain imaging approach to attachment is similar to that described earlier with regard to physiological measures such as HR or cortisol. Individuals who vary in attachment style or AAI classification are probed with an attachment-relevant task, and patterns of neural activity that differ between attachment groups are explored. For example, Gillath, Bunge, Shaver, Wendelken, and Mikulincer (2005) examined the pattern of neural activity in women while they were told to think about various relationship scenarios. The researchers found that when women thought about negative scenarios, dispositional attachment anxiety was correlated with activation in brain regions thought to subsume the control of negative emotion (anterior temporal pole) and inversely correlated with activation in brain regions associated with emotion regulation (orbitofrontal cortex). This study is notable for its attempt to combine the individual-difference approach with a neurological assessment of emotion regulation. On the other hand, asking participants to imagine certain scenarios runs the risk of having to speculate about what the participants are doing (or how engaged they are) during the scan.

In another recent study, Lemche and colleagues (2006) examined adults performing a stressful task while in the scanner. The task consisted of two series of 32 statements describing self or other, and participants were asked to push one of two buttons ("agree" or "disagree"). Prior to sentence presentation, individuals were primed subliminally with either nonsense information or descriptions of unpleasant attachment experiences (e.g., "My mom rejects me"). On the basis of performance on the behavioral task, the researchers classified adult participants as secure or insecure in their attachment organization. The study revealed heightened amygdala activation during the stress condition, as well as a significant correlation between attachment insecurity and amygdala activation (the more insecure, the more heightened the amygdala activation). The study is complex, but again noteworthy for attempting to identify relations between individual differences in attachment organization and cognitive and neural processing. The complicated design and use of nonstandard methods for identifying differences in attachment security make generalization difficult, however.

In sum, with the advent of innovative imaging techniques, it is now possible to examine the neural circuitry underlying information processing and emotion regulation among individuals who differ in attachment organization. These studies are new, and the methods are not as clear and crisp as they could be to allow definitive examination of these individual differences. But methodological advances will occur and allow attachment researchers to further probe the neural circuitry underlying differences in adult attachment organization. (See also Coan, Chapter 11, this volume.)

CONCLUSIONS

The use of psychophysiological and neuroscientific (brain imaging) approaches to studying attachment involves complex technologies, each with its own set of methodological issues and problems. If such approaches are to be informative, they should be used in studies asking questions that cannot easily be answered without the addition of psychophysiological or imaging data. One example is the question of reactivity of avoidant infants. For quite some time, attachment researchers have been interested in whether infants who are classified as avoidant undergo stress during the Strange Situation. Research utilizing HR or cortisol has attempted to answer this question, albeit with limited success. Physiological approaches have been more successful in describing individual differences in infant disposition, including reactivity to stress. Using measures of cortisol response or EEG asymmetry, studies have identified physiological

markers of infant temperament that influence infant behavior toward caregivers and behavior in the Strange Situation. These measures have also aided our understanding of the manner in which attachment may act as a buffer or moderator of initial physiological disposition, and they point to the possibility that the early caregiving environment influences the physiological processes that underlie individual differences in reactivity. Future studies should examine whether these initial physiological dispositions change as a function of such moderators. Such work holds great promise for understanding the interplay of biology and environment as they shape personality.

NOTE

1. We realize that this distinction may be viewed as artificial. Studies of brain imaging have long been included within the realm of psychophysiology. Nevertheless, distinguishing between studies directly examining brain activity during psychological states and studies measuring other physiological systems that support or are connected with such states is helpful for our review of the attachment literature. See Coan (Chapter 11, this volume) for a review of brain imaging studies.

REFERENCES

Achenbach, T., & Edelbrock, C. (1991). *Manual for the Child Behavior Checklist and Revised Child Behavior Profile*. Burlington: University of Vermont, Department of Psychiatry.

Adam, E. K., Klimes-Dougan, B., & Gunnar, M. (2007). Social regulation of stress physiology in infancy, childhood, and adolescence: Implications for mental health and education. In D. Coch, G. Dawson, & K. Fischer (Eds.), *Human behavior, learning, and the developing brain: Atypical development* (pp. 264–304). New York: Guilford Press.

Ainsworth, M. D. S. (1973). The development of infant–mother attachment. In B. M. Caldwell & H. N. Ricciuti (Eds.), *Review of child development research* (Vol. 3, pp. 1–94). Chicago: University of Chicago Press.

Ainsworth, M. D. S., Bell, S. M., & Stayton, D. J. (1971). Individual differences in Strange-Situation behavior of one year olds. In H. R. Schaffer (Ed.), *The origins of human social relations* (pp. 17–58). New York: Academic Press.

Ainsworth, M. D. S., Blehar, M. C., Waters, E., & Wall, S. (1978). *Patterns of attachment: A psychological study of the Strange Situation*. Hillsdale, NJ: Erlbaum.

Ainsworth, M. D. S., & Wittig, B. A. (1969). Attachment and exploratory behaviour of one-year-olds in a strange situation. In B. M. Foss (Ed.), *Determinants of infant behaviour* (Vol. 4, pp. 113–136). London: Methuen.

Alloy, L. B., & Abramson, L. Y. (1979). Judgment of contingency in depressed and nondepressed students: Sadder but wiser? *Journal of Experimental Psychology: General, 108,* 441–487.

Bell, S. M., & Ainsworth, M. D. S. (1972). Infant crying and maternal responsiveness. *Child Development, 43,* 1171–1190.

Belsky, J., & Isabella, R. (1987). Maternal, infant, and social contextual determinants of attachment security: A process analysis. In J. Belsky & T. Nezworski (Eds.), *Clinical implications of attachment* (pp. 40–94). Hillsdale, NJ: Erlbaum.

Belsky, J., & Rovine, M. (1987). Temperament and attachment security in the Strange Situation: An empirical rapprochement. *Child Development, 58,* 787–795.

Bono, M., & Stifter, C. A. (1995, April). Changes in infant cardiac activity elicited by the Strange Situation and its relation to attachment status. In C. A. Brownell (Chair), *Early development of self-regulation in the context of the mother–child relationship.* Symposium conducted at the biennial meeting of the Society for Research in Child Development, Indianapolis, IN.

Boukydis, C. F. Z., & Burgess, R. (1982). Adult physiological response to infant cries: Effects of temperament, parental status, and gender. *Child Development, 53,* 704–713.

Bowlby, J. (1969/1982). *Attachment and loss: Vol. 1. Attachment.* New York: Basic Books.

Brindley, D. N., & Rolland, Y. (1989). Possible connections between stress, diabetes, obesity, hypertension, and altered lipoprotein metabolism that may result in atheroselerosis. *Clinical Science, 77,* 453–461.

Burgess, K. B., Marshall, P. J., Rubin, K. H., & Fox, N. A. (2003). Infant attachment and temperament as predictors of subsequent externalizing problems and cardiac physiology. *Journal of Child Psychology and Psychiatry, 6,* 819–831.

Caldji, C., Tannenbaum, B., Sharma, S., Francis, D., Plotsky, P. M., & Meaney, M. J. (1998). Maternal care during infancy regulates the development of neural systems mediating the expression of fearfulness in the rat. *Proceedings of the National Academy of Sciences USA, 95,* 5335–5340.

Calkins, S. D., & Fox, N. A. (1992). The relations among infant temperament, security of attachment, and behavioral inhibition at twenty-four months. *Child Development, 63,* 1456–1472.

Calkins, S. D., Fox, N. A., & Marshall, T. R. (1996). Behavioral and physiological antecedents of inhibition in infancy. *Child Development, 67,* 523–540.

Carpenter, E. M., & Kirkpatrick, L. A. (1996). Attachment style and presence of a romantic partner as moderators of psychophysiological responses to a stressful laboratory situation. *Personal Relationships, 3,* 351–367.

Ciechanowski, P. S., Walker, E. A., Katon, W. J., &

Russo, J. E. (2002). Attachment theory: A model for health care utilization and somatization. *Psychosomatic Medicine, 64,* 660–667.

Ciesielski, K. T., Lesnik, P. G., Savoy, R. L., Grant, E. P., & Ahlfors, S. P. (2006). Developmental neural networks in children performing a categorical *N*-back task. *NeuroImage, 33,* 980–990.

Cohen, M. X., & Shaver, P. R. (2004). Avoidant attachment and hemispheric lateralisation of the processing of attachment- and emotion-related words. *Cognition and Emotion, 18,* 799–813.

Courage, M. L., Reynolds, G. D., & Richars, J. E. (2006). Infants' attention to patterned stimuli: Developmental change from 3 to 12 months of age. *Child Development, 77,* 680–695.

Davidson, R. J., & Fox, N. A. (1982). Asymmetrical brain activity discriminates between positive and negative affective stimuli in human infants. *Science, 218,* 1235–1237.

Davidson, R. J., & Fox, N. A. (1988). Frontal brain asymmetry predicts infants' response to maternal separation. *Journal of Abnormal Psychology, 98,* 127–131.

Dawson, G., Ashman, S. B., Hessl, D., Spieker, S., Frey, K., Panagiotides, H., et al. (2001). Autonomic and brain electrical activity in securely—and insecurely—attached infants of depressed mothers. *Infant Behavior and Development, 24,* 135–149.

Dawson, G., Klinger, L. G., Panagiotides, H., Spieker, S., & Frey, K. (1992). Infants of mothers with depressive symptoms: Electroencephalographic and behavioral findings related to attachment status. *Development and Psychopathology, 4,* 67–80.

Diamond, L. M. (2001). Contributions of psychophysiology to research on adult attachment: Review and recommendations. *Personality and Social Psychology Review, 5,* 276–295.

Diamond, L. M., Hicks, A. M., & Otter-Henderson, K. (2006). Physiological evidence for repressive coping among avoidantly attached adults. *Journal of Social and Personal Relationships, 23,* 205–229.

Donovan, W. L., & Leavitt, L. A. (1978). Early cognitive development and its relation to maternal physiologic responsiveness. *Child Development, 49,* 1251–1254.

Donovan, W. L., & Leavitt, L. A. (1985a). Physiological assessment of mother–infant attachment. *Journal of the American Academy of Child Psychiatry, 24,* 65–70.

Donovan, W. L., & Leavitt, L. A. (1985b). Physiology and behavior: Parents' response to the infant cry. In B. Lester & C. F. Z. Boukydis (Eds.), *Infant crying: Theoretical and research perspectives* (pp. 241–261). New York: Plenum Press.

Donovan, W. L., & Leavitt, L. A. (1989). Maternal self-efficacy and infant attachment: Integrating physiology, perceptions, and behavior. *Child Development, 60,* 460–472.

Donovan, W. L., Leavitt, L. A., & Balling, J. D. (1978). Maternal physiological response to infant signals. *Psychophysiology, 15,* 68–74.

Donovan, W. L., Leavitt, L. A., & Walsh, R. O. (1990). Maternal self-efficacy: Illusory control and its effect on susceptibility to learned helplessness. *Child Development, 61,* 1637–1647.

Donovan, W. L., Leavitt, L. A., & Walsh, R. O. (1997). Cognitive set and coping strategy affect mothers' sensitivity to infant cries: A signal detection approach. *Child Development, 5,* 760–772.

Dozier, M., & Kobak, R. R. (1992). Psychophysiology in attachment interviews: Converging evidence for deactivating strategies. *Child Development, 63,* 1473–1480.

Egeland, B., & Farber, E. A. (1984). Infant–toddler attachment: Factors related to its development and changes over time. *Child Development, 55,* 753–771.

Feeney, B. C., & Kirkpatrick, L. A. (1996). Effects of adult attachment and presence of romantic partners on physiological responses to stress. *Journal of Personality and Social Psychology, 70,* 255–270.

Fox, N. A. (1985). Behavioral and autonomic antecedents of attachment in high-risk infants. In M. Reite & T. Field (Eds.), *The psychobiology of attachment and separation* (pp. 389–414). Orlando, FL: Academic Press.

Fox, N. A. (1989). Psychophysiological correlates of emotional reactivity during the first year of life. *Developmental Psychology, 25,* 364–372.

Fox, N. A. (1991). If it's not left, it's right: Electroencephalogram asymmetry and the development of emotion. *American Psychologist, 46,* 863–872.

Fox, N. A. (1994). Dynamic cerebral processes underlying emotion regulation. In N. A. Fox (Ed.), The development of emotion regulation: Biological and behavioral considerations. *Monographs of the Society for Research in Child Development, 59*(2–3, Serial No. 240), 152–166.

Fox, N. A., Bell, M. A., & Jones, N. A. (1992). Individual differences in response to stress and cerebral asymmetry. *Developmental Neuropsychology, 8,* 161–184.

Fox, N. A., Calkins, S. D., & Bell, M. A. (1994). Neural plasticity and development in the first year of life: Evidence from cognitive and socio-emotional domains of research. *Development and Psychopathology, 6,* 677–696.

Fox, N. A., & Davidson, R. J. (1984). Hemispheric substrates of affect: A development model. In N. A. Fox & R. J. Davidson (Eds.), *The psychobiology of affective development* (pp. 353–382). Hillsdale, NJ: Erlbaum.

Fox, N. A., & Davidson, R. J. (1986). Taste-elicited changes in facial signs of emotion and the asymmetry of brain electrical activity in human newborns. *Neuropsychologia, 24,* 417–422.

Fox, N. A., & Davidson, R. J. (1988). Patterns of brain electrical activity during the expression of discrete emotions in ten-month-old infants. *Developmental Psychology, 24,* 230–236.

Fox, N. A., & Gelles, M. (1984). Face-to-face interaction in term and preterm infants. *Infant Mental Health Journal, 5,* 192–205.

Francis, D. D., Diorio, J., Liu, D., & Meaney, M. J. (1999). Nongenomic transmission across generations of maternal behavior and stress response in the rat. *Science, 286,* 1155–1158.

Frodi, A., Lamb, M. E., Leavitt, L., & Donovan, W. (1978). Fathers' and mothers' responses to infant smiles and cries. *Infant Behavior and Development, 1,* 187–198.

Frodi, A., Lamb, M. E., Leavitt, L., Donovan, W., Neff, C., & Sherry, D. (1978). Fathers' and mothers' responses to the appearance and cries of premature and normal infants. *Developmental Psychology, 14,* 490–498.

George, C., Kaplan, N., & Main, M. (1984). *Adult Attachment Interview protocol.* Unpublished manuscript, University of California at Berkeley.

George, C., Kaplan, N., & Main, M. (1985). *Adult Attachment Interview protocol* (2nd ed.). Unpublished manuscript, University of California at Berkeley.

George, C., Kaplan, N., & Main, M. (1996). *Adult Attachment Interview protocol* (3rd ed.). Unpublished manuscript, University of California at Berkeley.

Gillath, O., Bunge, S. A., Shaver, P. R., Wendelken, C., & Mikulincer, M. (2005). Attachment-style differences in the ability to suppress negative thoughts: Exploring the neural correlates. *NeuroImage, 28,* 835–847.

Gunnar, M. R., Colton, M., & Stansbury, K. (1992, May). *Studies of emotional behavior, temperament, and adrenocortical activity in human infants.* Paper presented at the Eighth International Conference on Infant Studies, Miami, FL.

Gunnar, M. R., & Donzella, B. (2002). Social regulation of the cortisol levels in early human development, *Psychoneuroendocrinology, 27,* 199–220.

Gunnar, M. R., Mangelsdorf, S., Larson, M., & Hertsgaard, L. (1989). Attachment, temperament, and adrenocortical activity in infancy: A study of psychoendocrine regulation. *Developmental Psychology, 25,* 355–363.

Hane, A. A., & Fox, N. A. (2006). Ordinary variations in maternal caregiving of human infants influence stress reactivity. *Psychological Science, 17,* 550–556.

Hane, A. A., & Fox, N. A. (2007). A closer look at the transactional nature of early social development: The relations among early caregiving environments, temperament, and early social development and the case for phenotypic plasticity. In F. Santoianni & C. Sabatano (Eds.), *Brain development in learning environments: Embodied and perceptual advancements* (pp. 1–15). Newcastle, UK: Cambridge Scholars Publishing.

Harter, S., & Pike, R. (1984). The Pictorial Scale of Perceived Competence and Acceptance in Young Children. *Child Development, 55,* 1969–1982.

Henriques, J. B., & Davidson, R. J. (1990). Regional brain electrical asymmetries discriminate between previously depressed and healthy control subjects. *Journal of Abnormal Psychology, 99,* 22–31.

Hertsgaard, L., Gunnar, M., Erickson, M. F., & Nachmias, M. (1995). Adrenocortical responses to the Strange Situation in infants with disorganized/disoriented attachment relationships. *Child Development*, 66, 1100–1106.

Izard, C. E., Porges, S. W., Simons, R. F., Haynes, O. M., Hyde, C., Parisi, M., et al. (1991). Infant cardiac activity: Developmental changes and relations with attachment. *Developmental Psychology, 27*, 432–439.

Kagan, J., & Snidman, N. (1991). Infant predictors of inhibited and uninhibited profiles. *Psychological Science, 2*, 40–44.

Katona, P. G., & Jih, F. (1985). Respiratory sinus arrhythmia: A noninvasive measure of parasympathetic cardiac control. *Journal of Applied Physiology, 39*, 801–805.

Knutson, B., Westdorp, A., Kaiser, G., & Hommer, D. (2000). fMRI visualization of brain activity during a monetary incentive delay task. *NeuroImage, 12*, 20–27.

Kochanska, G. (1998). Mother–child relationship, child fearfulness, and emerging attachment: A longitudinal study. *Developmental Psychology, 34*, 480–490.

Konstantinos, K., & Sideridis, G. D. (2006). Attachment, social support, and well being in young and older adults. *Journal of Health Psychology, 11*, 863–876.

Leibenluft, E., Gobbini, M. I., Harrison, T., & Haxby, J. V. (2004). Mothers' neural activation in response to pictures of their children and other children. *Biological Psychiatry, 56*, 225–232.

Lemche, E., Giampietro, V. P., Surguladze, S. A., Amaro, E. J., Andrew, C. M., Williams, S. C. R., et al. (2006). Human attachment security is mediated by the amygdala: Evidence from combined fMRI and psychophysiological measures. *Human Brain Mapping, 27*, 623–635.

Liu, D., & Diorio, J. (1997). Maternal care, hippocampal glucocorticoid receptors, and hypothalmic–pituitary–adrenal responses to stress. *Science, 277*, 1659–1663.

Main, M., Kaplan, N., & Cassidy, J. (1985). Security in infancy, childhood, and adulthood: A move to the level of representation. In I. Bretherton & E. Waters (Eds.), Growing points of attachment theory and research. *Monographs of the Society for Research in Child Development, 50*(1–2, Serial No. 209), 66–104.

Meaney, M. J. (2001). Maternal care, gene expression, and the transmission of individual differences in stress reactivity across generations. *Annual Review of Neuroscience, 24*, 1161–1192.

Mikulincer, M., & Shaver, P. R. (2007). *Attachment in adulthood: Structure, dynamics, and change.* New York: Guilford Press.

Murray, L., & Cooper, P. J. (1997). The impact of physiological treatments if postpartum depression on maternal mood and infant development. In L. Murray & P. J. Cooper (Eds.), *Postpartum depression and child development* (pp. 201–220). New York: Guilford Press.

Nachmias, M., Gunnar, M., Mangelsdorf, S., Parritz, R., & Buss, K. (1996). Behavioral inhibition and stress reactivity: The moderating role of attachment security. *Child Development, 67*, 508–522.

Nitschke, J. B., Nelson, E. E., Rusch, B. D., Fox, A. S., Oakes, T. R., & Davidson, R. J. (2004). Orbitofrontal cortex tracks positive mood in mothers viewing pictures of their newborn infants. *NeuroImage, 21*, 583–592.

Park, S., Belsky, J., Putnam, S., & Crnic, K. (1997). Infant emotionality, parenting, and 3-year inhibition: Exploring stability and lawful discontinuity in a male sample. *Developmental Psychology, 32*, 218–227.

Phillips, A. C., Carroll, D., Hunt, K., & Der, G. (2006). The effects of the spontaneous presence of a spouse/partner and others on cardiovascular reactions to an acute psychological challenge. *Psychophysiology, 43*, 633–640.

Pizzagalli, D. A., Sherwood, R., Henriques, J. B., & Davidson, R. J. (2005). Frontal brain asymmetry and reward responsiveness. *Psychological Science, 16*, 805–813.

Porges, S. W. (1991). Vagal tone: An autonomic mediator of affect. In J. A. Garber & K. A. Dodge (Eds.), *The development of affect regulation and dysregulation* (pp. 111–128). New York: Cambridge University Press.

Porges, S. W. (1995). Orienting in a defensive world: Mammalian modifications of our evolutionary heritage. A polyvagal theory (Presidential address, 1994). *Psychophysiology, 32*, 301–318.

Porges, S. W. (1996). Physiological regulation in high-risk infants: A model for assessment and potential intervention. *Development and Psychopathology, 8*, 43–58.

Porges, S. W., & Bohrer, R. E. (1991). The analysis of periodic processes in psychophysiological research. In J. T. Cacioppo & L. G. Tassinary (Eds.), *Principles of psychophysiology: Physical, social, and inferential elements* (pp. 708–753). New York: Cambridge University Press.

Porges, S. W., & Byrne, E. A. (1992). Research methods for measurement of heart rate and respiration. *Biological Psychology, 34*, 93–130.

Porges, S. W., Doussard-Roosevelt, J. A., Portales, A. L., & Suess, P. E. (1994). Cardiac vagal tone: Stability and relation to difficultness in infants and 3-year-olds. *Developmental Psychology, 27*, 289–300.

Porges, S. W., Stamps, L. E., & Walter, G. F. (1974). Heartrate variability and newborn heart-rate responses to illumination changes. *Developmental Psychology, 10*, 507–513.

Powers, S. I., Pietromonaco, P. R., Gunlicks, M., & Sayer, A. (2006). Dating couples' attachment styles and patterns of cortisol reactivity and recovery in response to a relationship conflict. *Journal of Personality and Social Psychology, 90*, 613–628.

Pruessner, J. C., Champagne, F., Meaney, M. J., & Dagher, A. (2004). Dopamine release in response to a psychological stress in humans and its relationship to early maternal care: A positron emission tomography study using [C]raclopride. *Journal of Neuroscience, 24*, 2825–2831.

Raine, A. (1996). Autonomic nervous system activity and violence. In D. M. Stoff & R. B. Cairns (Eds.), *Neurobiological approaches to clinical aggression research* (pp. 145–168). Mahwah, NJ: Erlbaum.

Raine, A., Venables, P. H., & Williams, M. (1990). Relationships between central and autonomic measures of arousal at age 15 years and criminality at age 24 years. *Archives of General Psychiatry, 47,* 1003–1007.

Roisman, G. I., Tsai, J. L., & Chiang, K. S. (2004). The emotional integration of childhood experience: Physiological, facial expressive, and self-reported emotional response during the Adult Attachment Interview. *Developmental Psychology, 40,* 776–789.

Rossi, P., Di Lorenzo, G., Malpezzi, M. G., Di Lorenzo, C., Cesarino, F., Faroni, J., et al. (2005). Depressive symptoms and insecure attachment as predictors of disability in a clinical population of patients with episodic and chronic migraine. *Headache: The Journal of Head and Face Pain, 45,* 561–570.

Schieche, M., & Spangler, G. (2005). Individual differences in biobehavioral organization during problem solving in toddlers: The influence of maternal behavior, infant–mother attachment, and behavioral inhibition on the attachment–exploration balance. *Developmental Psychobiology, 46,* 293–306.

Schmidt, L. A., Shahinfar, A., & Fox, N. A. (1996). Individual differences in temperament. In V. S. Ramachandran (Ed.), *Encyclopedia of human behavior* (Vol. 2, pp. 621–629). San Diego, CA: Academic Press.

Schoenbaum, G., Chiba, A. A., & Gallagher, M. (1998). Orbitofrontal cortex and basolateral amygdale encode expected outcomes during learning. *Nature Neuroscience, 1,* 155–159.

Somerville, L. H., Heatherton, T. F., & Kelley, W. M. (2006). Anterior cingulate cortex responds differentially to expectancy violation and social rejection. *Nature Neuroscience, 9,* 1007–1008.

Spangler, G., & Grossmann, K. E. (1993). Biobehavioral organization in securely and insecurely attached infants. *Child Development, 64,* 1439–1450.

Spitzer, S. B., Llabre, M. M., Ironson, G. H., & Gellman, M. D. (1992). The influence of social situations on ambulatory blood pressure. *Psychosomatic Medicine, 54,* 79–86.

Sroufe, L. A., Egeland, B., Carlson, E., & Collins, W. A. (2005) *The development of the person: The Minnesota Study of Risk and Adaptation from Birth to Adulthood.* New York: Guilford Press.

Sroufe, L. A., & Waters, E. (1977). Heart rate as a convergent measure in clinical and developmental research. *Merrill–Palmer Quarterly, 23,* 3–27.

Stevenson-Hinde, J., & Marshall, P. J. (1999). Behavioral inhibition: Heart period, respiratory sinus arrhythmia: An attachment perspective. *Child Development, 70,* 805–832.

Stifter, C. A., & Fox, N. A. (1990). Infant reactivity: Physiological correlates of newborn and 5-month temperament. *Developmental Psychology, 26,* 582–588.

Treboux, D., Crowell, J. A., & Waters, E. (2004). When "new" meets "old": Configurations of adult attachment representation and their implications for marital functioning. *Developmental Psychology, 40,* 295–314.

Volling, B. L., Notaro, P. C., & Larsen, J. (1998). Adult attachment styles: Relations with emotional well-being, marriage, and parenting. *Family Relations, 47,* 355–367.

Whalen, P. (1999). Fear, vigilance and ambiguity: Initial neuroimaging studies of the human amygdala. *Current Directions in Psychological Science, 7,* 177–188.

Whalen, P. J., Rauch, S. L., Etcoff, N. L., McInerney, S. C., Lee, M. B., & Jenike, M. A. (1998). Masked presentations of emotional facial expressions modulate amygdala activity without explicit knowledge. *Journal of Neuroscience, 18,* 411–418.

Wiesenfeld, A. R., & Klorman, R. (1978). The mother's psychophysiological reactions to contrasting expressions by her own and unfamiliar infant. *Developmental Psychology, 14,* 294–304.

Wiesenfeld, A. R., Malatesta, C. Z., & DeLoach, L. L. (1981). Differential parental response to familiar and unfamiliar infant distress signals. *Infant Behavior and Development, 4,* 281–295.

Willemsen-Swinkels, S. H., Bakermans-Kranenburg, M. J., Buitelaar, J. K., van IJzendoorn, M. H., & van Engeland, H. (2000). Insecure and disorganized attachment in children with pervasive developmental disorder: Relationship with social interaction and heart rate. *Journal of Child Psychology and Psychiatry, 41,* 759–767.

Zelenko, M., Kraemer, H., Huffman, L., Gschwendt, M., Pageler, N., & Steiner, H. (2005). Heart rate correlates of attachment status in young mothers and their infants. *Journal of the American Academy of Child and Adolescent Psychiatry, 44,* 470–476.

CHAPTER 11

Toward a Neuroscience of Attachment

JAMES A. COAN

Neurobiological studies of attachment are either abundant or scarce, depending on one's research tradition and one's scientific understanding of the term "attachment." On the one hand, the past two decades have seen a great deal of non-human animal work detailing the various neural manifestations of social bonding, familiarity, affiliation, caregiving, and other behaviors that can (and often do) fall under the general rubric of "attachment." On the other hand, neuroscientific investigations of normative attachment in *humans* have been limited and slow to develop, and similar investigations of the neural circuits supporting, or even associated with, individual differences in attachment (e.g., secure, anxious or ambivalent, and avoidant, in the social psychology tradition; autonomous, preoccupied, and dismissing, in the clinical and developmental tradition; see Crowell, Fraley, & Shaver, Chapter 26, this volume) are exceedingly rare. These facts (and a cursory glance at the table of contents for this volume) underscore the complexity of attachment as a domain of inquiry, and suggest that at present any neuroscience of attachment is likely to strike some as limited in both empirical foundation and theoretical scope.

Nevertheless, it is important to make a beginning somewhere, and a neuroscience of attach-

ment has much to gain from the integration of multiple research perspectives. Following Bowlby (1969/1982) and Ainsworth (1989), I consider attachment bonds in the present chapter to be those characterized by a high frequency of close proximity to the putative "attachment figure," especially during times of emotional stress. Moreover, attachment relationships are considered in this chapter to serve regulatory functions, often in relation to basic physiological needs, but also with respect to many forms of emotional responding. These regulatory functions are *social*, insofar as they result from interaction with "conspecifics" (other members of the same species). Some of the regulatory functions of attachment relationships are obvious and fundamental. For example, human infants literally cannot survive without the assistance of an adult caregiver. In later childhood, however, and in adult attachment relationships, emotion becomes the primary target of social regulation (Mikulincer & Shaver, Chapter 23, this volume). A major source of interest here is that the likely mechanism underlying the well-known link between social contact and health is the social regulation of emotion, particularly the social regulation of threat responding. The social regulation of threat responding is itself a major feature of attachment (Carter & DeVries, 1999; Edens, Larkin, & Abel, 1992; Hofer, 1995).

A large literature now suggests that a range of interactive social behaviors target physiological systems, temperamental dispositions, and overt behaviors associated with the stress response (Berscheid, 2003; Diamond, 2001; Sapolsky, 1998; Uchino, Cacioppo, & Kiecolt-Glaser, 1996). For example, supportive social behaviors are known to attenuate stress-related activity in the autonomic nervous system (ANS) and the hypothalamic–pituitary–adrenocortical (HPA) axis (Boccia, Reite, & Laudenslager, 1989; Flinn & England, 1997; Lewis & Ramsay, 1999; Weiss, 1990; Wiedenmayer, Magarinos, McEwen, & Barr, 2003). Maternal grooming behaviors affect glucocorticoid receptor gene expression underlying hippocampal and HPA axis stress reactivity in rat pups (Weaver et al., 2004). In the context of a novel, mildly stressful environment, rats in the company of a familiar companion engage in more exploration and play-soliciting behavior than rats in the company of an unfamiliar companion do (Terranova, Cirulli, & Laviola, 1999).

Theorists have long argued that social bonding serves the regulatory functions of security provision and distress alleviation with respect to negative affect and arousal (Bowlby, 1973; Mikulincer, Shaver, & Pereg, 2003). Prominent evolutionary theorists dating to Darwin have even argued that because mammalian emotional responding evolved in a social context, emotional behavior is virtually inextricable from social behavior (Brewer & Caporael, 1990; Buss & Kenrick, 1998; Darwin, 1872/1998). These diverse perspectives and literatures suggest that any robust conception of attachment will include multiple, distributed subsystems, including (but probably not limited to) those devoted to emotion, motivation, emotion regulation, and social affiliation.

The promise of the emerging field of what we can here consider to be "attachment neuroscience" is at once to provide critical information about how the brain supports attachment behaviors and to forge links among research traditions as diverse as the basic neurosciences, behavioral ecology, and various subdomains of psychology (e.g., developmental, social, and clinical), as well as affective science. In this chapter, the neural systems supporting emotion, motivation, emotion regulation, and social behavior are first reviewed. Following this, the social regulation of emotion and individual differences in attachment behavior are considered from the perspective of behavioral neuroscience. Based on these reviews, the "social baseline model" of social affect regulation is proposed. The social baseline model uses a neuroscientific framework to integrate models of attachment with a neuroscientific principle—"economy of action" in the management of metabolic resources devoted to emotional and social behavior. Finally, recommendations are made for the development of a robust future neuroscience of attachment.

ATTACHMENT AS A NEURAL CONSTRUCT

Although attachment bonds are widely believed to result from a universal, innate "attachment behavioral system," attempts to locate a single, dedicated attachment circuit is likely to be (to paraphrase Wittgenstein) a bit like trying to find the real artichoke by peeling away all its leaves. Almost any interpretation of the attachment behavioral system reveals it to be a higher-order construct constituted of behaviors about which a great deal is known, even at the neural level (Fox & Hane, Chapter 10, and Polan & Hofer, Chapter 7, this volume). For example, many studies have addressed the neurobiology of such social behaviors as recognition and familiarity, proximity seeking, separation distress, soothing behaviors, and maternal caregiving. Thus, one of the goals of this chapter is to introduce the neuroscientific study of attachment from the perspective of what is currently known about its social and emotional *constituents*.

A corollary goal is to move toward bridging two broad, rigorous, productive, and unfortunately disparate literatures. One is a thriving animal literature dedicated to what is variously termed "social bonding," "pair bonding," and "attachment bonding." The other contains a vast body of research on human attachment behavior, including studies of individual differences in internal working models of attachment (reviewed in Mikulincer & Shaver, 2007, and in J. Feeney, Chapter 21, this volume). Traditionally, these two worlds have had little to say to each other—a reflection of their starkly different research strategies as much as their different subject populations. Animal models, partly by virtue of what is ethically permissible with the population, often emphasize the study of social processes in terms of specific causal neural structures, circuits, neurotransmitters, neuropeptides, pheromones, or hormones. Attachment relationships are defined observationally, by the presence of separation distress or physiological soothing (or both) as a function of close proximity. By contrast, social, clinical, and developmental psychologists often focus their efforts on "behavioral systems," seeking to understand how humans behave in—and, importantly, what they have to *say* about—relational contexts.

This is not to say that research on attachment in humans has not utilized physiological measurement. On the contrary, psychologists have used measures of ANS physiology, electroencephalography (EEG), glucocorticoid levels, and more recently functional magnetic resonance imaging (fMRI). These measures have provided valuable insights into human social behavior, but they are rarely capable of identifying causal brain–behavior relationships (Norris, Coan, & Johnstone, 2007), and their frequent dependence on self-report measures (including coded interviews) may result in neurobiological correlates that are quite distinct from those of behaviorally defined animal models (cf. Williamson, 2006).

Yet another difficulty presents itself in bridging these literatures. Even if the definitions of attachment were perfectly matched, and if the neural measures applied to humans and nonhuman animals were identical, the neural processes associated with attachment behaviors in nonhuman animals may not generalize perfectly to those in humans. Work on the social communication value of pheromones provides an excellent example of this point. Pheromones are chemical substances that convey information between members of the same species (Insel & Fernald, 2004). It is certain that nearly all animals, including humans, show at least some evidence of two distinct olfactory systems. The "primary olfactory system" is dedicated to the detection of odors that convey information about food or the presence or predators, and this system is most commonly associated with the sense of smell. By contrast, the "accessory olfactory system" is, in many species, dedicated to the detection of specific pheromonal information. This accessory olfactory system consists of the vomeronasal organ (VNO) and the accessory olfactory bulb (AOB). Pheromones make contact with the VNO, exciting pheromone-specific sensory neurons projecting to the AOB.

In a wide variety of species, this system is capable of providing rapid and powerful information about sex, reproductive capacity, mate location, territorial boundaries, and even social status (Insel & Fernald, 2004). Nevertheless, the strongest of these findings derive exclusively from studies of animal populations. After a great deal of initial excitement about the possibility of a human pheromone system, enthusiasm has waned significantly amid evidence that although there does appear to be a human VNO, (1) there is no obvious pheromone-specific sensory neuron associated with it; (2) vomeronasal receptor genes present in the human genome appear to be "pseudogenes" (genes that have lost their protein-coding ability); and (3) the AOB does not appear to exist at all in the brains of adult humans (Meredith, 2001). In other words, the VNO—the primary and best-understood mechanism of socially critical pheromonal communication in animals—appears to be vestigial in humans.

Interestingly, evidence does suggest that chemical communication between humans can occur (e.g., Jacob & McClintock, 2000). However, unlike what we know about so many social species, the extent to which such effects are pheromonal, and whether they have anything whatever to do with the VNO, are uncertain at best. It is more likely that odors can moderate social information in humans, and that they do so through a distinct mechanism that is as yet poorly defined and understood (Meredith, 2001).

Despite all of these cautions, it is clear that research on animals has yielded invaluable information about the neurobiology of attachment, without which any understanding of human attachment would, at the neural level, be severely impoverished. Moreover, advanced neuroimaging techniques such as high-density EEG, positron emission tomography (PET), transcranial magnetic stimulation (TMS), and fMRI promise access to human neural processes at a level of detail undreamed of until the very end of the 20th century. Hence the potential for building bridges between the animal and human attachment literatures is higher than it has ever been. fMRI studies in particular are, by virtue of their rapid proliferation and relative lack of invasiveness, beginning to supply pieces of the human social bonding puzzle that will complement anatomical and molecular work in animals. Such advances promise the formation of a more comprehensive neuroscience of attachment.

THE NEURAL CONSTITUENTS OF ATTACHMENT

Neural systems supporting attachment are likely to include, at a minimum, those underlying incentive motivation; certain forms of emotional responding; emotion regulation; and such discrete social behaviors as the establishment of familiarity and preference, proximity seeking, separation distress, and social affect regulation. This chapter is not intended to provide an exhaustive treatment of all possible constituent systems underlying attachment. In truth, because so many neural structures are involved one way or another in attachment behavior, it is possible to think of the entire human brain as a neural attachment system. Auditory, olfactory, and visual sensory systems are heavily implicated for obvious reasons. Memory processes—involving, for example, long-term memory consolidation and retrieval in the hippocampus—underlie familiarity, recognition, and the maintenance of shared histories. Many different regulatory needs affected by attachment relationships are likely to be related to activity in the hypothalamus. Conflict-monitoring demands will be made on the anterior cingulate cortex (ACC). Each of these systems and more contribute to attachment in a variety of ways. In this chapter, however, I review a smaller number of putatively basic elements.

Preliminary Considerations

Behavioral versus Neural Systems

I should first distinguish between what ethologists have long referred to as "behavioral systems" and what neuroscientists refer to as "neural systems." In ethology, a behavioral system is a set of behaviors associated with a common causal antecedent and resulting, once activated, in a common consequence, which in turn deactivates the system. Drawing on an ethological approach, Bowlby (1969/1982) described several behavioral systems associated with attachment. When we are discussing behavioral systems such as these, there is a great temptation to view the behavioral system as having a one-to-one relationship with some underlying neural system. But such tidy correspondences are rare. The term "neural system" describes coordinated neural inputs and signaling targets among a population of neurons that form a circuit. Neural systems can be tightly organized in close physical proximity or distributed throughout the brain. Highly similar or even identical behaviors may, across individuals, result from different combinations of activity in dissimilar neural systems. Moreover, similar neural activations can result in quite distinct behaviors. Thus the search for specific neural circuits associated with time-honored, observationally defined behavioral systems is fraught with theoretical and empirical difficulty.

Bottom-Up versus Top-Down Processing

Although the terms "bottom-up" and "top-down" processing are frequently used in the cognitive neurosciences (and throughout the remainder of this chapter), their meanings may not be immediately obvious. Bottom-up processes are thought to begin, more or less, with sensory information or with more evolutionarily "primitive" brain structures, working "up" to more integrative and evolutionarily modern areas such as the cortex. The process of receiving sensory inputs from the environment and converting those inputs into neural pulses that are relayed to cortical structures as consciously perceived information about one's surroundings would be an example of this. Top-down processes are essentially the opposite. In this case, integrative and evolutionarily "new" structures pass neural information "down" to more sensory-oriented and evolutionarily old structures, often to suit some regulatory purpose. One example of a top-down process might be the brain's tendency to impute information from memory and experience into stimuli in the periphery of the visual field, thereby imposing "best guesses" on ambiguous visual information.

Emotional and Motivational Elements

Incentive Motivation, Reward, and the Dopamine System

Incentive motivation involves the acquisition of rewarding stimuli. The intensity of incentive motivation varies as a function of the state of the individual and the magnitude of the reward. For example, if a typical Westerner is mildly hungry and is offered a kind of food that is normally undesirable to him or her—uni (raw sea urchin), for example—there will be little incentive motivation to eat the food. If the individual is extremely hungry, however, the incentive motivation to eat the uni will be high. Similarly, if the same individual is again only mildly hungry, but is given a food item that is deemed highly desirable—say, a piece of chocolate cake—the incentive motivation to eat the cake will be high.

Incentive motivation plays a key role in a number of attachment-related processes (e.g., proximity seeking) and is tightly linked to the dopamine projection system of the ventral tegmental area (VTA). Dopamine is produced in the VTA and substantia nigra, and is projected to as many as 30 distinct networks (Le Moal & Simon, 1991). It has long been held that dopaminergic activity represents a neural substrate for the facilitation of goal-directed behavior (Berridge, 2007; Depue & Collins, 1999). Strongly implicated in this function is the nucleus accumbens, which is a major terminal area of dopaminergic projections from the VTA (Tzschentke & Schmidt, 2000). Dopaminergic activity within the VTA and nucleus accumbens has been repeatedly associated with reinforcing stimuli and the experience of pleasure. For example, rats capable of directly stimulating these circuits with a lever press will repeatedly do so, even in lieu of access to food, water, and sex. This preference for lever pressing over food and water will continue even to the point of death (Bozarth & Wise, 1996).

Dopaminergic cells in the VTA are also highly responsive to conditioning (Depue & Collins, 1999), especially to cues that predict the receipt of reward (Schultz, Dayan, & Montague, 1997). Importantly, the VTA is also responsive to stimuli that are *unconditioned*. Unconditioned stimuli are those that naturally, automatically, and unconditionally trigger a response in an organism. Positive unconditioned stimuli act as reinforcers, and include certain flavors, water, sleep, touch, and the presence of a variety of social cues. Negative unconditioned stimuli act as punishers or negative reinforcers, and include pain, social deprivation, and putrefying odors (Rolls, 2007a). With repeated exposure to unconditionally reinforcing stimuli, dopaminergic neurons in the VTA become sensitive to cues associated with those stimuli. In this way, the VTA begins to activate the nucleus accumbens earlier and earlier in a "chain of cues" that increase the probability of coming into contact with the original unconditioned reinforcer (e.g., an attractive potential mate). Put another way, conditioned associations between cues related to desirable unconditioned stimuli and dopaminergic activity in the VTA increase the predictability of those unconditioned stimuli, and hence the opportunities for obtaining them (Depue & Collins, 1999).

The Amygdala and Hippocampus in Affect and Memory

The amygdala is now one of the most widely recognized brain structures associated with emotion (Phelps & LeDoux, 2005). Far from a unitary structure, the amygdala contains many subnuclei, accounting for its involvement in a vast array of emotional responses. A large body of research now supports the notion that the amygdala is sensitive to both conditioned and unconditioned signs of threat. Moreover, at least two pathways to amygdala activation associated with visual stimuli

exist, both of which can mediate fear learning. One is a very rapid and direct route through the thalamus (the thalamoamygdala pathway) that processes obvious or highly specific sensory information (e.g., the shape of a snake) (LeDoux, 2000; Öhman, 2005). Another pathway processes slower and more complex information in the visual cortex before activating the amygdala. When paired with unconditioned aversive stimuli (e.g., a loud noise, pain), otherwise meaningless stimuli quickly come to be associated with the presence of a threat, and this conditioning appears to be dependent to a large degree on amygdala functioning in humans as well as animals. Importantly, although it at first appears as if threat responding in the amygdala is an entirely bottom-up phenomenon, there is evidence that amygdala activity is modulated by top-down processes related to attention (Pessoa, Kastnerb, & Ungerleider, 2002).

Interestingly, the amygdala is exquisitely sensitive to social signals expressed on the face (Benuzzi et al., 2007; Rolls, 2007b). Human patients with impaired amygdala functioning have difficulty processing emotional facial expressions, especially those communicating social emotions (Adolphs, Baron-Cohen, & Tranel, 2002; Adolphs & Tranel, 2003; Adolphs, Tranel, & Damasio, 1998). Fearful faces in particular reliably activate the amygdala in normal human subjects (Thomas et al., 2001; Whalen, 2007), even when the presentation of faces is so rapid that subjects have no conscious memory of them (Whalen et al., 1998), or when the faces are reduced to "essential elements" (e.g., when no cue but the raised upper eyelid is shown) (Whalen et al., 2004).

As we bear all of this in mind, it is noteworthy that the amygdala also plays a major role in the consolidation of both positive and negative long-term memories. Amygdala activity during memory encoding is associated with the recall of emotionally salient information even weeks after testing (Hamann, Ely, Grafton, & Kilts, 1999). Beta-adrenergic blockade of amygdala function appears to impair these effects (Cahill, Prins, Weber, & McGaugh, 1994). These findings suggest that the amygdala "tags" sensory experiences as significant or salient, and that this tagging is prominently represented in long-term memory consolidation. Importantly, the hippocampus appears to support the formation, storage, and consolidation of associations between internal states and spatial or contextual environmental stimuli (Brasted, Bussey, Murray, & Wise, 2003; Kennedy & Shapiro, 2004).

Ultimately, both the amygdala and the hippocampus are likely to underlie the identification and consolidation of significant interactions between attachment figures and emotionally salient situations. The amygdala will tag emotionally salient stimuli and will participate, along with the hippocampus, in the consolidation of contextual cues associated with those stimuli in long-term memory. Among those contextual cues will be the behavior of attachment figures.

Threat Responding, Social Soothing, and the Hypothalamus

The hypothalamus regulates a variety of metabolic and autonomic processes, as well as linking the central nervous system to the endocrine system, most famously in the case of cortisol release via the HPA axis (Kemeny, 2003). The hypothalamus receives inputs from a wide variety of structures implicated in social behavior, emotion, stress, and attachment, including the amygdala, prefrontal cortex (PFC), and hippocampus (McEwen, 2007). The periventricular nucleus of the hypothalamus is capable of synthesizing corticotropin-releasing hormone (CRH; Gainer & Wray, 1994). In threat responding, CRH released by the hypothalamus stimulates the release of adrenocorticotropic hormone (ACTH) in the pituitary gland. ACTH causes increased production of cortisol and catecholamines (e.g., epinephrine and norepinephrine) in the adrenal cortex. This cortisol is circulated throughout the body, including the brain. Critically, circulating cortisol in the brain is capable of activating glucocorticoid receptors in the hippocampus that feed back to inhibit the HPA axis (Kemeny, 2003).

Importantly, the hypothalamus is one of the key structures implicated in the regulatory effects of social soothing on neural threat responding, including interactions with attachment figures (Carter, 2003; Coan, Schaefer, & Davidson, 2006). The precise mechanisms by which social soothing down-regulates HPA axis activity are currently unknown (Coan, Schaefer, et al., 2006), but the hypothalamus is known to coordinate the activity of many behavioral and physiological systems, including those involved in maternal behavior and pair bonding. Moreover, maternal and pair-bonding behaviors are strongly associated with oxytocin and vasopressin—neuropeptides (reviewed below) that the hypothalamus is capable of synthesizing in abundance (Carter, 2003; Gainer & Wray, 1994).

The PFC, Emotion, and Emotion Regulation

Many regions of the PFC are implicated in emotion, motivation, and emotion regulation (Coan & Allen, 2004; Coan, Allen, & McKnight, 2006). Indeed, portions of the PFC are strongly connected to the dopaminergic projection system (e.g., nucleus accumbens and VTA), and the PFC shares numerous connections with the amygdala, hippocampus, and hypothalamus. For example, the orbitofrontal region of the PFC assists the amygdala and hippocampus in linking the emotional value of secondary sensory information (e.g., place cues) to primary reinforcers, such as food, water, and social contact (Rolls, 2007a).

One of the major functions of the PFC is the regulation of emotion. Prefrontal regions may bias brain circuits responsible for appraising the emotional content of sensory stimuli and instantiating behavior directed toward approach- or avoidance-related goals (e.g., via amygdala or nucleus accumbens; Davidson & Irwin, 1999). Different portions of the PFC underlie different emotion regulation strategies (see Ochsner & Gross, 2005, for a review). These can include "automatic" forms of emotion regulation, as well as effortful forms related to the cognitive control of attention or stimulus appraisal (Ellenbogen, Schwartzman, Stewart, & Walker, 2006). Some automatic forms of emotion regulation are conditioning and extinction learning, including instrumental avoidance. These rapid and automatic regulatory functions (especially extinction learning) have been associated with the ventromedial and medial orbital PFC (Milad et al., 2005; Quirk & Beer, 2006; Sierra-Mercado, Corcoran, Lebrón-Milad, & Quirk, 2006). More "effortful" forms of regulation require attention, working memory, and other cognitive operations (Ochsner, Bunge, Gross, & Gabrieli, 2002). For example, cognitive reappraisals have been used to alter the meaning of a stimulus, and attentional practices (e.g., meditation) have been used to alter attentional foci associated with affective stimuli. These processes have been associated with more lateral, especially dorsolateral, portions of the PFC—regions also known to support working memory, language, and action planning operations (Ochsner et al., 2002).

Thus the PFC may be associated with attachment processes in at least two ways. First, over time, medial orbital circuits may encode conditioned or "automatic" responses to attachment figures related to excitatory or inhibitory responses to threat cues. Second, dorsolateral circuits may modulate cognitive operations associated with attachment figures in reflective, working memory. In truth, these distinctions are not likely to be as discrete as the formulation above suggests, but the distinction between medial orbital and dorsolateral circuits of the PFC offers a useful neural heuristic for thinking about the regulatory influences of attachment figures in automatic versus explicit terms, respectively.

Emotional Constituents in Combination

Because all of the constituent systems described above are linked, it is possible for them to coordinate in important ways. For example, dopaminergic neurons in the VTA share connections with many regions other than the nucleus accumbens, including the amygdala (in various nuclei as well as the extended amygdala), the hippocampus, the hypothalamus, and the PFC (Depue & Collins, 1999). In this way, these structures form their own distributed networks of often reciprocal influence. To understand how such a network may function, consider the distribution of activity following an encounter with an unconditionally rewarding stimulus. Dopamine is released from the VTA, which stimulates dopaminergic activity in the nucleus accumbens associated with pleasure. The amygdala "tags" sensory properties of the stimulus as affectively salient or significant, placing special emphasis on those properties during the process of long-term memory consolidation via the hippocampus, which also encodes contextual information as part of the consolidation process. The PFC uses this information to effect action plans and regulate subsequent behavior—both automatic and effortful—relevant to the stimulus. As experience with the rewarding stimulus increases in frequency (partly as a function of successful regulation and action planning activity in the PFC), the affective "tagging" of cues associated with it proceeds down a "chain of cues," increasing the probability that the rewarding stimulus will be accessed (or avoided in the case of unconditionally negative reinforcers).

For a more concrete example, consider an encounter with an attractive potential mate. In many species, including humans, such an encounter is unconditionally reinforcing. The encounter initially elicits pleasurable feelings and an increase in incentive motivation associated with the partner. The amygdala tags sensory features of the encounter as salient during the process of memory consolidation, in cooperation with the hippocampus; the

VTA becomes conditioned to cues associated with (and predictive of) the potential mate, thereby activating incentive motivation circuits early in the "chain of cues" that will increase the likelihood of encountering the potential mate again. With repeated exposures, and perhaps a bit of luck, the potential mate may even respond in kind. With this, the foundation of pair-bond attachment has been set, and the complex process of attachment bonding has begun (see Zeifman & Hazan, Chapter 20, this volume). During the attachment bonding process, the PFC utilizes information about the potential mate to adjust its emotion regulation activities, opting in many cases to cede some level of regulatory effort to the potential mate, as discussed below.

Social Elements

Familiarity and Preference

One of the bedrock features of any species deemed "social" (as well as any conception of attachment) is the ability to distinguish individuals who are familiar from those who are not—an ability that in turn is yoked to a preference for the familiar. Indeed, the establishment and maintenance of preferences for familiar others (caregivers, peers, one's mate, etc.) form the first necessary condition of attachment bonds. Through evolutionary time, familiarity was probably a matter of survival, and so it remains in the case of infants and their caregivers. One of the striking things about humans (and many other mammals) is how well *designed* we are for affiliation (Depue & Morrone-Strupinsky, 2005). Many stereotyped behaviors, including facial expressions, vocalization, bodily gestures, and so forth, are calibrated to signal social closeness and/or discomfort. These signals are readily recognized by most humans, and may in many cases be innate (Laird & Strout, 2007; Rolls, 2007a).

Nearly 40 years ago, Bowlby (1969/1982) suggested that infant–mother bonds, characterized by both the ability to distinguish the caregiver from others and a strong preference for the caregiver, formed very rapidly; this appears to be true in many species. Most researchers who study infants agree that the development of attachment bonds is critical, because infants often must survive long periods of early development totally dependent upon their caregivers, even when those caregivers are neglectful or abusive (Simpson & Belsky, Chapter 6, this volume). The formation of such bonds appears mainly among birds and mammals, and is thought to have been present in their common ancestors, the therapsids (Insel & Winslow, 1998).

Among social species, the most common manifestation of the attachment bond—indeed, its commonest exemplar—is, as Bowlby suggested, the bond between an infant and its mother (Insel & Fernald, 2004). Human infants have the capacity to distinguish their mothers from others within hours after birth (DeCasper & Fifer, 1980). Most researchers agree, however, that in many species attachment bonding represents a more generalized capacity—one that is only *very frequently* applied to the actual mother. Indeed, many birds become bonded within hours to the first moving object they encounter. Interestingly, Lorenz (1935) discovered that geese reared by him not only bonded to him (and followed him) as if he was the parent, but also that they "courted" him upon reaching sexual maturity, preferring him to other geese. These observations raise important questions for a neuroscience of attachment, concerning the degree to which early sensory objects associated with a caregiver are rapidly and permanently "etched" into the developing brain, how such a thing can occur, and whether a critical period of bonding formation exists in early development.

Filial Bonding, the Locus Coeruleus, and the Amygdala

Filial affiliations are those concerning an offspring relating to a parent. In humans, strong attachment to the caregiver usually develops at 6 months of age, but filial bonds resembling this process appear from birth. Filial bonds may, however, differ from adult affiliation behaviors in important ways, due to the dependent nature of the offspring–parent relationship. Many offspring of social species are totally dependent upon a caregiver for survival, and attachments are imperative regardless of the quality of the care (Hofer & Sullivan, 2001). Indeed, nonhuman primates have been observed to exhibit strong attachments to their mothers even when the mothers are abusive, and this pattern extends to human children (Moriceau & Sullivan, 2005). Rat pups have been observed to form preferences even to stimuli paired with electric shock. This seemingly paradoxical effect is thought to have developed as a means of preventing pups from aversion learning while being handled roughly by the mother (Hofer, 2006)—an unfortunate predicament, but generally not as unfavorable as being abandoned. Ultimately, filial bonds need to be understood in the context of this high level of dependence, at least early in development.

It is largely for this reason that at least some of the neural circuitry associated with attachment in infants is likely to be different from that in adults. This may explain why filial bonds occur so rapidly and unconditionally by comparison with attachment formation in adulthood. In fact, filial bonding may precede birth, where learning about the mother's voice and odor may occur. In many species, odor is thought to play a significant role in the identification of the primary caregiver soon after birth and thereafter, even among human infants (Insel & Fernald, 2002). For example, maternal odor has been observed to elicit orienting responses in infants, as well as having soothing effects on human infant crying (Marlier & Schaal, 2005; Schaal, Marlier, & Soussignan, 1998).

Filial bonding also occurs in a context of significant neural development. The human brain grows exponentially during the first year of life and continues to develop rapidly into the second year (Franceschini et al., 2007). Glucose metabolism rises gradually until about the fourth year, and on average the level of brain glucose metabolism is more than double that of adults until about age 10 (Chugani, 1998). The production of neurotrophins (proteins that aid in neuron survival) are dependent upon neuronal activity and, by extension, environmental stimuli (Berardi & Maffei, 1999; Cancedda et al., 2004). Within the first 2 years of development in humans, the brain's production of axons, dendrites, and synapses far exceeds its needs. Synaptic connections are then "pruned" throughout childhood by lack of use; that is, synaptic connections that go unused are discarded (Reichardt, 2006). In this way, the environment exerts its influence on the otherwise genetically determined neural development of the brain. At a systems level, neural organization tends to follow functioning—repetitive and patterned activation—during development (Hebb, 1949; Posner & Rothbart, 2007).

Throughout the earliest stages of this process, at least two brain structures, the locus coeruleus and the amygdala, interact to facilitate the familiarity and reinforcement associated with the caregiver in filial bonding. Although in adults norepinephrine *moderates* memory consolidation and learning (Cahill et al., 1994), norepinephrine from the locus coeruleus appears to be both necessary and sufficient for learning in human and animal neonates (Sullivan, 2003). And the neonate locus coeruleus releases large amounts of norepinephrine early in development (Nakamura & Sak-aguchi, 1990). When it is combined with sensory information, such as the look, sound, and smell of a caregiver, that sensory information is likely to be learned rapidly. Importantly, this learning is occurring alongside a neonatal amygdala that is not yet fully functional, making it difficult or impossible for aversive conditioning to occur (Sullivan, 2003). In other words, the amygdala, being immature during early neonatal development, may not be capable of associating aversive stimuli with alarm or avoidance behavior; this may leave virtually all stimuli to be simply encoded as "familiar," which is, for many intents and purposes at this stage, unconditionally reinforcing.

During this developmental period, neural pathways linking amygdala to hippocampus are similarly underdeveloped, as are many regions within the PFC (Herschkowitz, 2000). This suggests that learning in neonates may not involve the PFC, or may do so only in limited ways. In either case, these systems begin to develop rapidly in infancy, leading many to refer to this developmental time as a "critical" or "sensitive" period for neural development. Sensitive periods have been studied extensively in terms of the brain's sensory systems. For example, Hubel and Wiesel (1970) observed that a temporary blockage of visual input to one eye in cats during early development caused irreversible impairment in the visual cortex. Similarly, children born deaf have been observed to cease vocalizations in late infancy, probably due to a lack of auditory stimuli (Schauwers et al., 2004). Interestingly, research on the social complexity of rearing environments in rats suggests that environments rich in social and cognitive complexity are associated with significantly more synapses per neuron throughout the visual cortex than are simple socially paired housing and individual housing (Briones, Klintsova, & Greenough, 2004). These effects remain even after later environments are changed or reversed, suggesting that plastic changes associated with early experiences are persistent.

In combination, these findings suggest that filial bonding occurs rapidly and unconditionally. Moreover, the filial bond develops in a context of rapid neural development, during what appears to be a sensitive period of learning. As discussed in greater detail below, this process (especially to the extent that it involves developing links between the PFC and affective structures like the amygdala and nucleus accumbens) may result in the development of different reflexive "assumptions" about the nature of the social world, including that world as it will be encountered in the future. This may set the stage for different broad strategies for engaging (or avoiding) social stimuli, perhaps especially during emotional situations. Indeed, conditions under which the filial bond forms and develops may constitute a kind of rudimentary "preworking model" of interdependence and affect regulation—of attachment—that is either altered or reinforced during the course of development throughout childhood.

Adult Affiliation, Nucleus Accumbens, and the Social Neuropeptides

Of course, attachment bonds characterized by interdependence and affect regulation extend far beyond the prototypic mother–infant relationship. Adult attachments occur in the context of romantic relationships, especially monogamous ones—but adult attachment is probably not restricted to this. Indeed, relationships that meet attachment criteria have by now been documented between pairs of individuals as diverse as adult romantic partners (Fraley & Shaver, 2000), captive chimpanzee cagemates (Bard, 1983; Miller, Bard, Juno, & Nadler, 1986), chimpanzees and their human caretakers (Miller, Bard, Juno, & Nadler, 1990), and domesticated dogs and their owners (Topal, Miklosi, Csanyi, & Doka, 1998). Aspects of attachment seem to occur even between organization members and their leaders (Davidovitz, Mikulincer, Shaver, Ijzak, & Popper, 2007).

Of interest here are neural circuits that support the establishment and maintenance of attachment bonds in later childhood and adulthood. How does the brain facilitate movement from close proximity to familiarity to attachment? To start, positive, possibly unconditioned social affiliation behaviors (e.g., eye gaze, soothing vocalizations, nonthreatening facial and bodily behaviors) increase proximity between conspecifics, setting the stage for motivated attachment bonding. It is clear that some social cues are unconditionally capable of activating neural structures supporting incentive or reward motivation, especially the nucleus accumbens and the VTA (Allen et al., 2003). For example, passively viewed images of female faces have been observed to activate the VTA and nucleus accumbens unconditionally in heterosexual men (Aharon et al., 2001). In rats, maternal females show an increase in dopamine release in the nucleus accumbens when exposed to pups (Hansen, Bergvall, & Nyiredi, 1993). Depletion of dopamine in the VTA and nucleus accumbens via lesions or dopamine antagonists virtually eliminates rat maternal behavior (Hansen, Harthon, Wallin, Löfberg, & Svensson, 1991). Interestingly, maternal behaviors not directly associated with caregiving, such as nest building, passive nursing, and aggression, are virtually unaffected by these manipulations. Other studies have linked dopamine release in the nucleus accumbens and VTA to the spontaneous establishment of partner preferences (Aragona et al., 2006).

Mating behavior in the absence of partner preference is also associated with dopamine in the nucleus accumbens (Balfour, Yu, & Coolen, 2004; Pfaus, Kippin, & Centeno, 2001), however, suggesting that dopaminergic activity in the nucleus accumbens is insufficient for the establishment of partner preferences. This raises the question of how the establishment of partner preferences is "linked up" to the dopaminergic incentive motivation system. Here the neuropeptides oxytocin and vasopressin appear to play major roles (Depue & Morrone-Strupinsky, 2005; Young & Wang, 2004). Both have been associated with the formation of partner preferences regardless of mating behavior, and both, especially oxytocin, are elicited by positive social behaviors (Uvnaes-Moberg, 1998).

Perhaps the most celebrated example of the function of these neuropeptides derives from work on pair bonding within monogamous prairie voles (Borman-Spurrell, Allen, Hauser, Carter, & Cole-Detke, 1995; Carter, 2003; Insel & Fernald, 2004; Young & Wang, 2004). When these animals forge a pair bond, they mate, share nests and territory, cooperate in the care of their young, and forcefully reject intruders of either sex (Borman-Spurrell et al., 1995). Unlike in nonmonogamous animals— including other variants of voles—the nucleus accumbens in these animals is rich in oxytocin receptors. Moreover, structures like the VTA and ventral palladium are rich in receptors for vasopressin (Lim, Hammock, & Young, 2004; Lim & Young, 2006).

Findings such as these provide clues as to how social cues activate incentive motives associated with dopaminergic activity and in turn the formation of partner preferences and proximity-seeking behavior. Socially sensitive oxytocin and vasopressin circuits in the VTA, nucleus accumbens, and ventral palladium probably stimulate dopaminergic activity linked to incentive motivation. Because activation of this dopaminergic system is frequently associated with positive affect and reward, the degree of oxytocin and vasopressin activity may determine the degree to which a social experience is rewarding, by virtue of the dopaminergic cascade that follows it.

Proximity Seeking, the Dopamine System, and Endogenous Opiates

One of the natural consequences of familiarity, preference, and bonding is proximity seeking, a characteristic of social behavior strongly associated with attachment. Proximity seeking is likely to be an extension of motivational circuits associated with reward and partner preference. Of course, individuals can seek close proximity as a function of positive affect and reward, or in response to cues of punishment where the goal is the provision of safety (Depue & Morrone-Strupinsky, 2005). In the case of positive affect, proximity is sought because the attachment figure has become associated with rewarding feelings of pleasure, and close proximity increases the frequency or intensity of these feelings. In the case of negative affect, the attachment figure may serve as a safety cue, eliciting approach behaviors oriented toward the acquisition of security. In this way, proximity seeking can involve both reward-related approach behaviors and approach behaviors associated with active avoidance.

Behaviorally, these motivations may appear to be identical, but they are likely to involve both shared and distinct neural circuits. Moreover, although attachment theory emphasizes the emotion regulation function of proximity seeking due to the need for security, it may be counterproductive to downplay the role of proximity seeking due to reward processes. It may be the case, for example, that at the neural level reward-related proximity conditioning is tightly bound to the provision of security by the attachment figure in other contexts. From the perspective of the VTA and nucleus accumbens, there may be little difference, because they become in either case sensitized to the presence of the attachment figure as a positive outcome.

In addition to the reinforcing nature of dopaminergic activation, consummatory pleasure may play a role in rewarding social interaction. After all, positive social experiences are characterized in everything from semistructured scientific interviews to ancient literature as involving feelings of warmth, closeness, love, affection, and pleasure. Depue and Morrone-Strupinsky (2005) have argued that feelings of consummatory pleasure promote the development of contextual associative memory networks that help both to establish and to maintain social bonds, and that are ultimately responsible for many of the *regulatory* effects associated with the soothing and security provided by attachment relationships. The critical substrate for these feelings, and perhaps for the socioaffective regulatory effects that accompany them, may be the release of opiates that often follows activation of oxytocin receptors—also in structures like the nucleus accumbens and VTA.

There is abundant evidence for the role of endogenous opiates in a wide variety of social behaviors. In humans and other animals, these opiates are released during childbirth, nursing, maternal caregiving, sexual activity, and many modes of tactile stimulation, including grooming and play behavior (Carter & Keverne, 2002; Keverne, Martensz, & Tuite, 1989). This release may mediate the reward associations that are forged between infants and mothers, as well as between romantic partners and even platonic friends. For example, morphine, an opiate receptor agonist, increases the reinforcing effects of a host of maternal behaviors, mother–infant bonding, time spent by juveniles (rats) with their mothers after a brief separation, grooming, and juvenile play behavior (Agmo, Barreau, & Lemaire, 1997; Niesink, Vanderschuren, & van Ree, 1996; Nocjar & Panksepp, 2007; Panksepp, Nelson, & Siviy, 1994). By contrast, opiate receptor antagonists such as naltrexone reduce the reward-conditioning effects associated with each of these forms of social contact (Graves, Wallen, & Maestripieri, 2002; Holloway, Cornil, & Balthazart, 2004). In humans, the administration of the opiate antagonist naltrexone was associated with increased voluntary isolation from friends, as well as decreased levels of enjoyment in the company of others (Jamner & Leigh, 1999).

Importantly, tactile stimulation appears to play a particularly powerful role in the activation of affiliative reward conditioning (Burgdorf & Panksepp, 2001; Melo et al., 2006). In some animals, the affiliative conditioning associated with maternal behavior is attenuated in the absence of tactile stimulation (Melo et al., 2006).

ATTACHMENT AND THE SOCIAL REGULATION OF EMOTION

Many evolutionary accounts of the reproductive advantages of infant–caregiver bonds have been proposed, but similar accounts of adult attachment bonds are relatively recent (Simpson & Belsky, Chapter 6, and Zeifman & Hazan, Chapter 20, this volume). Fraley and Shaver (2000) have proposed that adult attachments represent homologies of the infant–caregiver bond coopted by natural selection to facilitate pair bonding. By this account, adult and infant–caregiver attachment systems entail similar goals (the survival of offspring) and operate according to similar conditions of activation (e.g., presence of a threat) and termination (e.g., regulation of threat responding by the attachment figure). Evolutionary perspectives like these address *ultimate* functions, in the sense of explaining why attachment bonds and capabilities persist among so many species.

Function can be considered in a more proximal, ontogenetic sense as well, and it is at this level that the regulation of affect may take center stage. Proximal functions of the attachment system are, following basic survival during infancy (Hofer, 2006), primarily concerned with the social regulation of emotional responding. Bowlby (1969/1982), following along with Ainsworth and her colleagues (e.g., Ainsworth, Blehar, Waters, & Wall, 1978), argued that a critical function of attachment figures is the provision of a "secure base" from which infants can explore their worlds relatively free of anxiety, and a "safe haven" to which the infants can return when distressed. It was proposed, for example, that the base from which an infant can explore his or her world is secure to the extent that the caregiver is responsive to the infant's distress. Many have since proposed that the quality of the caregiver–infant attachment bond—especially of the caregiver's status as a secure base—holds consequences for child and adult emotional functioning, including styles of interpersonal relating and emotion regulation capabilities. A very large behavioral database now supports this notion with respect to both childhood and adulthood (for reviews, see Thompson, Chapter 16, and Mikulincer & Shaver, Chapter 23, this volume).

Throughout childhood, and certainly by adulthood, the regulatory effects of attachment relationships are likely to be felt in two broad ways. The first is immediate, as when the attachment figure is present and regulating emotional responding "online." An example of this may be when a caregiver holds a child's hand during a blood draw at the doctor's office, thus actively soothing the child's anxiety as it occurs. The second is generalized, where the attachment figure is present only in the form of a mental representation. These representations may in theory be manifested either as internal working models based on procedural and semantic memory, or as declarative, explicitly recalled mental images. Indeed, online regulation experiences are likely to condition mental representations in both implicit and declarative memory. In the sections that follow, immediate, online regulation is considered in contrast to mental representations of the attachment figure, often referred to as "internal working models," that may serve to preempt the level of distress an individual experiences in the face of a potential threat.

The Online Social Regulation of Emotion

Many researchers have observed the stress-buffering effects of social contact on behaviors and physiological systems related to emotional responding. This social buffering occurs at all levels (e.g., group, caregiver, familiar conspecific), but familiarity and attachment are associated with the strength of social regulation effects. Even in rats, the presence of familiar conspecifics ("buddy" rats) increases exploration and attenuates HPA axis activity under conditions of threat (Kiyokawa, Kikusui, Takeuchi, & Mori, 2004; Ruis et al., 1999; Terranova et al., 1999). Familiar conspecifics attenuate emotional stress responding in nonhuman primates during new social group formation and social conflict (Gust, Gordon, Brodie, & McClure, 1996; Weaver & de Waal, 2003). As reviewed above, these effects are widely believed to derive from social cues that activate the release of oxytocin and vasopressin in the VTA, ventral palladium, and nucleus accumbens (Carter & DeVries, 1999; Heinrichs et al., 2001; Izzo et al., 1999; Uvnaes-Moberg, 1998; Windle, Shanks, Lightman, & Ingram, 1997). This release in turn is thought to activate dopaminergic and endogenous opiate activity associated with incentive motivation, consummatory pleasure, and physiological soothing.

In humans, very little work to date has actually sought to identify how neural circuits associated with social affiliation and emotion function in a context that combines social interaction with externally generated emotional stress. Recently my colleagues and I (Coan, Schaefer, et al., 2006) collected functional brain images from 16 married women as they were subjected to the threat of mild electric shock while either holding their husbands' hands, holding the hand of an anonymous male experimenter, or holding no hand at all. Our results suggested that physical contact from both attachment figures and strangers attenuated threat-responsive neural activity in affect-related action and bodily arousal circuits (e.g., in the ventral ACC), but also that down-regulation of such structures as the nucleus accumbens, dorsolateral prefrontal cortex, and superior colliculus was achieved only via holding hands with the attachment figure. Moreover, we (Coan, Schaefer, et al., 2006) observed that some of the regulatory effects of soothing physical contact varied as a function of relationship quality, with higher quality predicting yet greater attenuation of threat-related neural activation in the right anterior insula, superior frontal gyrus, and hypothalamus during spousal, but not stranger, hand holding. These findings suggest that social proximity in general, and the presence of an attachment figure in particular, exert bottom-up regulatory influences on the perception of threat in the brain. Moreover, the fact that holding a stranger's hand conferred regulatory benefits at all suggests that the human brain is unconditionally soothed to some extent by social proximity, which may lay the groundwork for the additional regulatory benefits associated with attachment figures.

Internal Working Models and Individual Differences

Thus far, we have primarily considered basic systems supporting "normative" manifestations of attachment behavior, as well as a concrete example of how the emotion regulation functions of the attachment system occur "online" in real time. However, the emotion regulation effects of caregiving experiences such as those between infants and caregivers, or even between romantic partners, are likely to extend far beyond online moments of soothing and security provision. Bowlby (1979) considered many facets of early attachment experiences to hold implications for interpersonal and emotional functioning "from the cradle to the grave" (p. 129), and in the past several decades many researchers have adopted this idea as one way to understand adult interpersonal functioning and emotion regulation capabilities.

Unfortunately, a large portion of what is known about links among early social experience, neural development, and subsequent emotional behavior has been derived from studies of abuse and neglect. For example, neglect and abuse (both physical and verbal aggression) are associated with risks for heightened stress reactivity, anxiety, depression, and social deviance that extend well into adulthood (Teicher, Samson, Polcari, & McGreenery, 2006). In one recent study, children who had experienced social deprivation and neglect in Romanian orphanages were observed to have lower overall levels of vasopressin, as well as blunted oxytocin responses to physical contact with their caregivers, relative to normally family-reared children (Wismer-Fries, Ziegler, Kurian, Jacoris, & Pollak, 2005). This is consistent with findings regarding social isolation as a well-known risk factor for a number of neurodevelopmental and psychosocial problems, ranging from anxiety and depression to increased risk of suicide, family problems, and even stress-related dwarfism (Barber, Eccles, & Stone, 2001; Kawachi & Berkman, 2001; Newcomb & Bentler, 1988; Skuse, Albanese, Stanhope, Gilmour, & Voss, 1996). In nonhuman primates, frequent or prolonged separation of offspring from caregivers (primarily mothers) can result in socially deviant behavior and physiology later in life (Mineka & Suomi, 1978). Among brown capuchin monkeys, patterns of mother–offspring behavior partially determine the postconflict reconciliation styles of offspring during later interactions with nonfamilial conspecifics (Weaver & de Waal, 2003).

Neural Mechanisms

Neural mechanisms linking early parental care to trait-like individual differences in threat responding over the lifespan have been expertly described by Meaney and colleagues (Weaver et al., 2004). This work suggests that in rats, grooming behavior by the mother "sets" or "programs" the degree to which her offspring react to threat cues throughout their lives. This modulation of threat reactivity has been observed both in behavior and in HPA axis activity. Moreover, associations between maternal grooming and offspring threat reactivity have been linked to the expression of specific genes that moderate HPA axis functioning. As reviewed earlier, the HPA axis has its own built-in regulatory mechanism in the hippocampus, whereby circulating cortisol activates hippocampal glucocorticoid receptors, which in turn down-regulate the production of CRH in the hypothalamus. Grooming induces the expression of genes that encode for glucocorticoid receptors in the hippocampus, thus making the hippocampus more sensitive to circulating cortisol and hence more susceptible to down-regulation during stress. Cross-fostering studies by Meaney and colleagues strongly suggest that lifelong stress reactivity, and even the subsequent maternal behavior of female rat pups, is largely attributable to the degree of postnatal maternal grooming and not to genetic inheritance (Weaver et al., 2004).

Attachment and Internal Working Models

According to attachment theory (Bowlby, 1969/1982, 1973; Mikulincer & Shaver, 2007 and Chapter 23, this volume), threat detection capabilities evolved in part to activate the attachment behavioral system, thus increasing the likelihood that humans would seek out and maintain proximity to attachment figures from infancy onward. Moderating the degree to which proximity to attachment figures is sought in the context of a threat is "attachment security," which is itself the product of many attachment-related experiences involving both threats and attachment figures. These experiences shape "internal working models" of attachment that guide emotion regulation throughout life (see Bretherton & Munholland, Chapter 5, this volume). According to Bowlby (1969/1982), internal working models are mental representations of the availability and practical utility of attachment figures when threats arise, and of the self in relationship with these figures.

Recently, Hofer (2006) described a process by which very early developmental experiences in interactions with a caregiver may plausibly proceed from the online regulation of fundamental neural systems supporting sensorimotor, thermal, and nutrient functions to the shaping of internal working models of attachment security. In this model, access to primary reinforcers (e.g., food, water, warmth, touch) is dependent in early development on (1) caregiver support and (2) affective brain circuitry used to solicit caregiver support via expressed affect. Over the course of development, what begins as the regulation of physiological needs via affect becomes the regulation of affect per se (Hofer, 2006). Throughout this process, the regulatory behavior of the attachment figure (e.g., the provision of security, the alleviation of distress) is likely to set expectations about the availability of attachment figures during times of stress—the internal working models reflecting attachment security.

Thus, internal working models are likely to reflect conditioned associations between proximity to attachment figures and both internal needs and external signs of threat, mediated through the amygdala, nucleus accumbens, and hippocampus, as well as portions of the PFC. These conditioned associations may remain stable for long periods of time, especially to the extent that they continue to be reinforced by internal feelings of security, prevailing social contingencies, or both.

This process probably allows individuals to adapt themselves to a variety of environmental conditions (e.g., security-restoring or security-enhancing experiences with attachment figures, frequent or lengthy absence of the caregiver, abuse by the caregiver, excessive caregiving). Such adaptations are referred to in various research traditions as "attachment patterns," "attachment styles," or "attachment states of mind" (e.g., secure, anxious or ambivalent, avoidant, preoccupied). These adaptations are thought to be relatively stable when the individual remains in a stable environment, and can be measured by observations, self-report questionnaires, and structured interviews (e.g., Crowell et al., Chapter 26; Kerns, Chapter 17; and Solomon & George, Chapter 18, this volume).

Behavioral research on the effects of different adult attachment styles suggests the presence of two relatively independent axes regarding attachment insecurity—anxiety and avoidance—along which individuals can vary (J. Feeney, Chapter 21, this volume; Mikulincer & Shaver, 2007). Moreover, different combinations of scores along these dimensions can result in particular styles of interpersonal relating. For example, individuals low in attachment anxiety and low in attachment avoidance are considered generally secure in their attachments to others. Individuals high in both avoidance and anxiety are thought to avoid attachment relationships out of fear, while those high in avoidance but low in anxiety are thought to be dismissing of attachments, compulsively self-reliant, and unlikely to seek proximity to attachment figures under stress (Bartholomew & Horowitz, 1991; Brennan, Clark, & Shaver, 1998). Finally, individuals low on avoidance but high on anxiety are thought to be preoccupied with attachment relationships.

Few studies to date have investigated individual differences in attachment styles using measures of neural activity, and some of the work that has been done serves only as an approximation. Indeed, attachment styles may, at a neural level, manifest as little more than individual differences in response capabilities among neural circuits supporting emotion, emotion regulation, and social behavior. Interestingly, Dawson and colleagues (2001) observed that insecurely attached infants of depressed mothers were more likely to show PFC asymmetries lateralized to the right. By this metric, asymmetries in EEG activity in the alpha (8–13 Hz) range (Coan & Allen, 2003, 2004) correspond with emotion regulation capabilities (Coan, Allen, et al., 2006), with relatively greater left PFC activity indexing an increased probability of approach behavior (e.g., anger, joy), and

relatively greater right PFC activity indexing an increased probability of withdrawal behavior (e.g., sadness, fear). Thus, according to Dawson and colleagues insecurely attached infants of depressed mothers have a trait-like propensity to engage in withdrawal behavior.

A very few studies have begun using functional neuroimaging technology to associate adult attachment styles with brain function. Recently, we (Coan, Schaefer, & Davidson, 2005) reported a variety of interaction effects between self-reported attachment scores and hand-holding condition (spouse, stranger, alone) on threat-related neural activity throughout the brain. For example, under threat of mild electric shock, secure attachment scores were negatively associated with activity in the ventral ACC during spouse hand holding, and positively correlated with activity in the same region during stranger hand holding. The ventral ACC is implicated in the modulation of affect-related arousal. Avoidance scores corresponded with increased activation during spouse hand holding, and decreased activation during stranger hand holding, in the right ventromedial PFC—a region commonly associated with the regulation of negative affect.

In another recent fMRI study, 20 women were asked to think about—and then to stop thinking about—various relationship scenarios (Gillath, Bunge, Shaver, Wendelken, & Mikulincer, 2005). Attachment anxiety was positively associated with activity in the dorsal ACC, and anxiety scores were positively correlated with brain activity in the temporal pole, but negatively with brain activity in the orbitofrontal cortex, during thoughts about negative relationship scenarios. This suggests that attachment-anxious individuals are not engaging neural systems that would help to regulate their emotional responses during negative relationship thoughts.

More recently, Buchheim and colleagues (2006) collected functional images of the brain while subjects told "attachment stories" in response to images from the Adult Attachment Projective (Lorberbaum et al., 1999) intended to activate the attachment behavioral system. These attachment stories were used to classify individuals as either "organized" or "disorganized." Individuals classified as disorganized were more likely to show amygdala and hippocampal activation when shown pictures portraying traumatic as opposed to neutral attachment situations.

Although findings from each of the studies described above should be considered preliminary, they do contribute to our understanding of how attachment styles and internal working models may moderate neural processes associated with the regulation of emotion. They are the initial steps in what is likely to be an increasing effort to use brain imaging techniques to study the neural correlates and underpinnings of processes studied previously only through verbal and behavioral reactions to laboratory procedures.

THE SOCIAL BASELINE MODEL

Social influences on the regulation of affect are sufficiently powerful and unconditioned to suggest that the brain's first and most powerful approach to affect regulation is via social proximity and interaction. This is most obvious in infancy, where very basic physiological needs are regulated first via affect expression, leading to a dynamic of regulating affect per se, where caregivers become the primary agent through which infants regulate affective responding (Hofer, 2006). For the infant, this is occurring in a context of rapid and expansive neural development—possibly a "critical period" during which a number of expectations about the nature of the infant's future environment are being formed. A great deal of this development is occurring in the PFC, a region of the brain powerfully implicated in self-regulation of affect. Because the PFC is underdeveloped in infancy, the caregiver effectively serves as a kind of "surrogate PFC"— a function that attachment figures probably continue to serve for each other to varying degrees throughout life.

What I call the "social baseline model" suggests that social affect regulation was long ago adopted as an efficient and cost-effective means of regulating affect. It draws on the principle of "economy of action," which states that organisms must, over time, consume more energy than they expend if they are to survive to reproduce (Proffitt, 2006). Because all bodily activities (including neural activities) expend energy, energy expenditure must be managed. Proffitt (2006) has proposed that one of the ways in which the brain manages energy expenditure is via alterations in sensory perception that aid in decision making about the deployment of an organism's resources. For example, Proffitt has observed that donning a heavy backpack causes hills to appear steeper and objects to appear farther away, thus discouraging individuals from using their resources to climb those hills or approach those objects. In this way, the brain

can be thought of as a "Bayesian machine," making "bets" at any given time about what resources to deploy and at what level of effort (Addis, Wong, & Schacter, 2007; Bar, 2007).

The social baseline model proposes that social species are hard-wired to *assume* relatively close proximity to conspecifics, because they have adopted social proximity and interaction as a strategy for reducing energy expenditure relative to energy consumption. This implies that the *absence* of conspecifics, in defying this baseline assumption, functionally adds to the perceived cost of interacting with the environment—especially in threatening contexts (an implication discussed explicitly by Bowlby, 1969/1982). In other words, the social baseline model proposes that social isolation is, for a social organism, akin to donning a heavy backpack: It alters the real and perceived demands associated with its environment. There are at least two ways in which the presence of conspecifics may reduce, for social organisms, the actual and perceived cost of engagement with the environment. I call these strategies "risk distribution" and "load sharing."

Risk Distribution

The first way in which social species, including humans, benefit from close social proximity is via the simple distribution of risk in the environment. Many species benefit from living in groups, and simple risk distribution strategies are likely to be "plesiomorphic," or relatively ancient in evolutionary terms. Although group living comes at a cost at the level of resource consumption, the benefits may outweigh those costs sufficiently to create conditions under which group cohesion ultimately promotes the survival of each individual in the group. Risk distribution speaks to the amount of risk a given individual carries as a function of the degree to which he or she is alone, and it can manifest in many ways (Krebs & Davies, 1993). For example, the larger the group, the more individuals there are to scan for possible signs of danger. Similarly, a given individual is at substantially reduced risk of personal danger (e.g., predation) when group size increases. A similar example among warm-blooded species may be the thermal advantage of huddling together. Some social species utilize group size to maximize their performance as predators; this too can be a form of risk distribution, for if predation (especially of large target animals) is maximized in groups of predators, the risk that any one predator will perish from starvation is minimized.

From the perspective of the social baseline model, it is important that the brains of social species appear to be capable of assessing the distribution of risk and making Bayesian decisions about the cost-effectiveness of affective behavior at any given time. Practically speaking, the presence or absence of conspecifics provides, at the lowest level of social proximity, a heuristic for deploying potentially costly resources. For example, in the presence of others, individuals may work less hard at being vigilant for—or even fleeing—predators. These activities, which may be yoked to perceived bodily resources (Proffitt, 2006), are deployed only as needed. The resources that are saved by close social proximity are either simply conserved or used for other valuable purposes.

Load Sharing

Risk distribution processes are not likely to have strong effects on processing at the cortical level, especially in the prefrontal regions supporting attention, working memory, and the self-regulation of affect. Interestingly, such prefrontally mediated activities are thought to be particularly costly to deploy (Galliot & Baumeister, 2007). Evidence for this derives from studies of cognitive depletion as a consequence of effortful attention and self-control. In this work, individuals who are asked to engage in tasks requiring self-regulation are subsequently less capable of similar tasks. Moreover, engaging in these tasks has been observed to result in temporary depletions in blood glucose concentration (Galliot & Baumeister, 2007).

The social baseline model predicts that the PFC and many of the regulatory processes it supports may be particularly affected by the presence of an attachment figure, especially in the context of a threat. Here the advantage of close proximity extends far beyond simple models of risk distribution: Over and above the dilution of risk via large numbers, a trusted and interdependent associate can be counted on to engage in a number of health- and safety-enhancing behaviors on one's behalf. Such behaviors may include the identification and acquisition of resources, vigilance for environmental threats, caring for one's needs, and nurturing of one's offspring. These allegiances—these attachments—serve to distribute the cost of many of life's metabolically expensive activities, not least being the regulation of one's own negative affect. Simply put, affect regulation is possible, but more difficult, in isolation. I refer to this second level of social regulation as "load sharing," and I believe it is an essential component of attachment relationships throughout the lifespan. Load sharing is likely to be "apomorphic," or relatively advanced in evolutionary terms, having arisen as a strategy relatively recently. Human brains are highly sensitive to the load-sharing significance of close attachment bonds, and adjust their efforts accordingly. For example, individuals in close, trusted relationships will invest less effort in down-regulating their negative affect, leaving them less responsive to threat cues and other signs of possible harm (Coan, Schaefer, et al., 2006; Edens et al., 1992; Mikulincer & Florian, 1998; Robles & Kiecolt-Glaser, 2003). Thus the social brain is designed in part to distribute affect regulation activities to attachment figures. As with the metabolic benefits of risk distribution, this should produce major metabolic resource savings.

Unlike risk distribution strategies, which are primarily sensitive to numbers alone, load sharing, especially in adult attachment relationships, is likely to develop as the brains of individuals in a relationship become conditioned to one another, especially in the context of coping with threats. Over time, individuals in attachment relationships literally become part of each other's emotion regulation strategy. This is not metaphorical, but literal, even at the neural level. For example, a man who has been alone for a long period of time may have learned to exercise his PFC in the service of regulating his threat responses. The social baseline model predicts that upon his establishing an attachment relationship, this man's perception of the degree to which his environment is threatening or dangerous will change, decreasing the frequency with which he exercises his PFC in the service of emotion regulation. Note that this is because his brain assumes a decrease in the need for emotion regulation. With sufficient experience in the relationship, the level of interdependence associated with emotion regulation needs can become strong. Indeed, a grim reminder of this occurs when one or the other member of an attached pair is suddenly absent due to death or divorce, leaving the partner severely dysregulated (Bowlby, 1980; Sbarra, 2006; see Shaver & Fraley, Chapter 3, this volume).

An example of this dynamic of increasing need for self-regulation as a function of distance from an attachment figure can be found in our previously mentioned study (Coan, Schaefer, et al., 2006), in which married women in an MRI scanner were confronted with the threat of a mild electric shock under each of three conditions: while alone, while holding a stranger's hand, and while holding their spouses' hands. Women in the highest-quality relationships showed the lowest degree of threat-related brain activation, limiting their response to relatively automatic regulation of threat perception via structures such as the ventromedial PFC. When a marital relationship was of relatively poor quality, however, the number of problems confronting a woman's brain under threat increased to include attention to bodily sensory afferents, presumably related to the threat of shock (right anterior insula), task salience (superior frontal gyrus), and release of regulatory stress hormones (hypothalamus).

Presumably the regulatory benefits associated with attachment figures in both the higher- and lower-quality relationships reflected the load-sharing function of attachment relationships. As the nature of the hand-holding partner switched from attachment figure to stranger, however, yet more problems presented themselves, with additional threat-related brain activations triggered to solve them. For example, threat-related vigilance increased (e.g., via the superior colliculus); effortful emotion regulation strategies were employed (e.g., via the right dorsolateral PFC); and areas were recruited that indicated increased threat-related avoidance motivation (e.g., the caudate and nucleus accumbens).

Still, a woman's brain was less active while she was holding the hand of a stranger than while she was alone, presumably reflecting the effects of risk distribution via fairly minimal social proximity. In the alone condition, the brain appeared to get busy solving yet more perceived problems, adding—to the already enumerated somatic preparations for threat responding—increasing bodily arousal (e.g., through the ventral ACC) and coordinating visceral and musculoskeletal responses (e.g., via the posterior cingulate, supramarginal gyrus, and postcentral gyrus).

It is important to emphasize that social affect regulation appears to be a relatively bottom-up process, as opposed to one's solo affect regulation, which is more top-down. When engaging in self-regulation, a person is likely to need to engage in costly, effortful cognitive and attentional strategies in the service of inhibiting either somatic responses or structures supporting the identification of threat cues. This effortful regulation of affect relies to a great degree on the PFC. In this way, self-regulation frequently occurs in the context of an affective response that has already transpired.

By contrast, social affect regulation may often affect the perception of threat in the first place, thereby decreasing the need for threat responding and leaving the PFC with relatively little or nothing to regulate. Thus social affect regulation could be said to be more efficient, or less costly, than self-regulation strategies, such as the suppression of emotional responses, the cognitive reappraisal of threatening situations, and even popular strategies such as meditation. The extent to which this is true awaits further investigation.

Attachment Styles as Bayesian Priors

Of course, the preceding discussion offers only a simplified, idealized model of social affect regulation, and one highly dependent on situational contingencies. It is likely that superimposed on all of the processes described above are trait-like assumptions about the function and metabolic cost of social factors in regulating the perception of threat cues, and hence of affect. Accordingly, one way to conceptualize attachment styles and internal working models is as prior probabilities in a Bayesian decision-making process, where the goal is to predict the regulatory cost-effectiveness of attachment figures. In this way, attachment styles come to represent strategies, based on prior experience, for making decisions about how to utilize one's own neural resources in the presence or absence of strangers and attachment figures. A secure attachment style presumably disposes a person to make bets closely in accordance with the idealized picture described above. By contrast, avoidant and anxious strategies may encourage individuals to make greater use of their own resources even in the presence of social support, or to place themselves outside the reach of social support in the hopes of avoiding additional costs (e.g., having to regulate others as well as self), thus again requiring them to rely on their own emotion regulation strategies.

At present, the social baseline model, as well as this Bayesian conceptualization of attachment style, is predominantly a matter of conjecture. As I have stated at the outset of this chapter, however, we have to begin somewhetre in the move from evolutionary, behavioral-observational, self-report, and interview-based analyses of attachment processes to analyses based on the methods provided by rapidly developing neuroscience. I expect that future neuroscientific studies of attachment will provide additional clues to the nature of social affect regulation in the brain.

RECOMMENDATIONS AND CONCLUSIONS

In this chapter, I have sought (1) to synthesize a broad array of studies in the service of introducing the reader to the current state of the neurosciences as they pertain to research on attachment, and (2) to propose a plausible model of how what is known about the social brain and affect regulation may eventually be combined with attachment theory. This effort has necessarily included discussions of the neural constituents of attachment, from neural systems supporting emotion and motivation to those supporting emotion regulation, filial bonding, familiarity, proximity seeking, and individual differences in attachment style. What follows is a partial list of recommendations for researchers excited about pursuing the neuroscience of attachment. (Other models and suggestions can be found in other chapters in the present volume, especially Simpson & Belsky, Chapter 6; Fox & Hane, Chapter 10; and Polan & Hofer, Chapter 7.)

- *Use designs that combine social contact with emotional provocations.* Studies of the neural systems underlying attachment should combine the presence or absence of attachment cues (e.g., proximity to attachment figures) with laboratory situations that elicit emotional responses, including threats either to the participant's attachment system or to the participant directly. Many theorists have proposed that the attachment behavioral system is activated during threats to the individual or to the individual's attachment bond, but few studies of attachment processes at the neural level have actually designed studies with this in mind. Moreover, no work to date has sought to identify how social contact influences neural responses to positive affect elicitations.
- *Be sensitive to sex differences.* Little is known about how the sex of an individual under study affects activity in the attachment behavioral system, or the neural constituents of attachment. Self-reported sex differences have been noted in behavioral studies, however. For example, women are more likely to endorse items indicating a preoccupied attachment strategy (characterized by worry that their partners will leave them), whereas men are more likely to endorse a dismissive or avoidant strategy (characterized by discomfort with interpersonal closeness) (Bartholomew & Horowitz, 1991). And many studies have found that women are most bothered by their male partners' avoidance, whereas men are most bothered by their female partners' anxiety (Mikulincer &

Shaver, 2007). Others have reported sex differences in relationship stability as a function of attachment styles, suggesting that attachment styles may interact in important ways with gender roles (Kirkpatrick & Davis, 1994). Our own work on the normative regulation of affect via social channels was done only with women, and it may not generalize to men.

- *Pursue animal models of attachment style.* To date, virtually no studies exist of attachment styles in nonhuman animals, despite growing evidence that other personality dimensions are evident in nonhuman animals (Gosling & John, 1999). For example, King and Figueredo (1997) provided strong evidence that the "Big Five" personality structure and its distribution are very similar in humans and chimpanzees, and the anxiety and avoidance dimensions of attachment style are somewhat related to the Big Five traits of neuroticism and agreeableness, respectively (Noftle & Shaver, 2006). Other personality traits shared to one degree or another with humans have been observed in species as diverse as gorillas, hyenas, domesticated dogs, cats, donkeys, pigs, rats, octopi, and even guppies (Gosling & John, 1999). Attempts to study attachment styles in nonhuman animals would constitute a badly needed step toward bridging the gaps between the human and animal literatures addressing attachment behavior.
- *Allow for systemic effects in research designs.* Most attachment style research identifies effects of a given participant's attachment style on that person's own attachment behavior. One question of great interest is the degree to which the attachment style of one member of a dyad effects the behavior of the other member. (See J. Feeney, Chapter 21, this volume, for examples.) For instance, we (Coan et al., 2005) presented evidence that a husband's preoccupation score corresponded with increased neural threat reactivity throughout his wife's brain *if* she was holding the hand of a stranger (while her possibly jealous husband looked on). These sorts of effects are likely to be numerous and are of great interest to any neuroscience of attachment. (Such findings also suggest that the effects of context are likely to be profound.)
- *Seek to understand contextual and situational influences.* Nearly a half-century of research makes clear that personality is most stable within classes of situations as opposed to across situations (Mischel, Shoda, & Mendoza-Denton, 2002). Such questions as these can reasonably be asked: Is a given woman secure in her relationship with her spouse to the same degree as she is in her relation-

ship with her best friend, mother, or sister? Moreover, does her attachment style manifest itself in the same way to a threat to her relationship as it does to her personal sense of bodily harm? Would she have endorsed the same level of security during a previous relationship as she does in her current one? Some studies suggest that within-person variation in attachment style across different relationships is substantial (La Guardia, Ryan, Couchman, & Deci, 2000). This is likely to be especially true at the neural level, where measures can be very sensitive to small changes in context.

• *Implement longitudinal designs.* One extremely important problem for the neuroscience of attachment is delineating the process by which two individuals progress from not being attached to being attached. (See Zeifman & Hazan, Chapter 20, this volume, for a discussion of this issue.) What is the rate at which this typically occurs? How is this affected by attachment style? With special relevance to the present chapter, which neural structures associated with emotional responding, motivation, and emotion regulation are particularly sensitive to this process? For example, at what point, or with what kinds of interpersonal experiences, does a stranger who regulates the brain's autonomic and musculoskeletal response to threat become a partner who regulates additional neural processes related to effortful affect regulation and threat vigilance? Longitudinal studies may also address questions of within-subject variation in attachment style over both time and relationships.

• *Pursue clinical implications.* As reviewed briefly above, and by scores of other scholars in recent decades (Cacioppo et al., 2002; Coyne et al., 2001; Flinn & England, 1997; Harrison, Williams, Berbaum, Stem, & Leeper, 2000; House, Landis, & Umberson, 1988; Kawachi & Berkman, 2001; Kim & McKenry, 2002; Robles & Kiecolt-Glaser, 2003; Uchino et al., 1996; Uvnaes-Moberg, 1998), social relationships hold major implications for health and well-being. As the neural mechanisms supporting these effects become better known, it may be possible to implement clinical interventions that not only emphasize the forging and maintenance of close relationships, but also focus on the use of social affect regulation for clinical purposes.

For example, it may be possible to use certain relationship interventions (see Johnson, Chapter 33, this volume) to transform couples that do not show a strong social regulation effect on neural threat responding into those that do. Johnson (2002) has already used attachment-related mari-

tal interventions to help with the treatment of posttraumatic stress disorder.

It warrants emphasis here that most stress reduction techniques involve highly individualized activities (e.g., cognitive-behavioral therapy, mindfulness meditation) that may be less efficient or more costly than using social networks or attachment relationships in the implementation of affect regulation strategies. Few or no interventions are designed with this specifically in mind, and even those that are rarely if ever offer training in how to allow oneself to be soothed by another person.

Finally, the careful delineation of neural systems underlying attachment can expand our basic understanding of a wide variety of disorders that implicate social processes. The potential exists for this work to inform research on disorders ranging from autism to fragile X syndrome, Williams syndrome, depression, social anxiety, schizophrenia, and virtually all of the personality disorders (most or all of which are more or less defined in terms of social behaviors).

• *Differentiate behavioral from neural systems.* A major challenge to future neuroscientists interested in the study of attachment will be the temptation to think of the attachment behavioral system as a unitary neural construct, which it almost certainly is not. Numerous neural processes, each with its own unique problems to solve, contribute to what we have come to call the "attachment behavioral system"; indeed, this system may be little more than a convenient rubric for describing the collective social activities of social bonding and social affect regulation. On the other hand, the attachment behavioral system may represent an emergent property of its constituent neural components that is, under some conditions and in some situations, relatively irreducible.

• *Collaborate.* The neuroscience of attachment represents uncommonly fertile ground for a wide variety of researchers, from neuroscientists to psychologists, biologists, physicians, epidemiologists, and others. Individuals from diverse scientific traditions can contribute many essential pieces to this fundamentally important puzzle. Because this area is so necessarily multidisciplinary, researchers interested in these and related questions will do well to explore contacts in related disciplines as their particular research questions call for it (Cacioppo et al., 2007). It is for precisely this reason that collaborations are increasingly the norm among the social, cognitive, and affective neurosciences. Such collaborations enrich the science, and often richly reward the scientists who take part. When such efforts are focused on a question as fundamentally important as the neuroscience of attachment, it is expected that collaborative efforts will be embraced with great enthusiasm.

ACKNOWLEDGMENTS

I would like to thank Jude Cassidy, Jennifer La Guardia, and Philip R. Shaver for their helpful comments on early drafts of this chapter.

REFERENCES

Addis, D. R., Wong, A. T., & Schacter, D. L. (2007). Remembering the past and imagining the future: Common and distinct neural substrates during event construction and elaboration. Neuropsychologia, 45, 1363–1377.

Adolphs, R., Baron-Cohen, S., & Tranel, D. (2002). Impaired recognition of social emotions following amygdala damage. Journal of Cognitive Neuroscience, 14, 1264–1274.

Adolphs, R., & Tranel, D. (2003). Amygdala damage impairs emotion recognition from scenes only when they contain facial expressions. Neuropsychologia, 41, 1281–1289.

Adolphs, R., Tranel, D., & Damasio, A. R. (1998). The human amygdala in social judgment. Nature, 393, 470–474.

Agmo, A., Barreau, S., & Lemaire, V. (1997). Social motivation in recently weaned rats is modified by opiates. Developmental Neuroscience, 19, 505–520.

Aharon, I., Etcoff, N., Ariely, D., Chabris, C. F., O'Connor, E., & Breiter, H. C. (2001). Beautiful faces have variable reward value: fMRI and behavioral evidence. Neuron, 32, 537–551.

Ainsworth, M. D. S. (1989). Attachments beyond infancy. American Psychologist, 44, 709–716.

Ainsworth, M. D. S., Blehar, M. C., Waters, E., & Wall, S. (1978). Patterns of attachment: A psychological study of the Strange Situation. Hillsdale, NJ: Erlbaum.

Allen, J. P., McElhaney, K. B., Land, D. J., Kuperminc, G. P., Moore, C. M., O'Beirne-Kelley, H., et al. (2003). A secure base in adolescence: Markers of attachment security in the mother–adolescent relationship. Child Development, 74, 292–307.

Aragona, D. J., Liu, Y., Yu, Y. J., Curtis, J. T., Detwiler, J. M., Insel, T. R., et al. (2006). Nucleus accumbens dopamine differentially mediates the formation and maintenance of monogamous pair bonds. Nature Neuroscience, 9, 134–139.

Balfour, M. E., Yu, L., & Coolen, L. M. (2004). Sexual behavior and sex-associated environmental cues activate the mesolimbic system in male rats. Neuropsychopharmacology, 29, 718–730.

Bar, M. (2007). The proactive brain: Using analogies and associations to generate predictions. Trends in Cognitive Sciences, 11, 280–289.

Barber, B. L., Eccles, J. S., & Stone, M. R. (2001). Whatever happened to the jock, the brain, and the princess?: Young adult pathways linked to adolescent activity involvement and social identity. Journal of Adolescent Research, 16(5), 429–455.

Bard, K. A. (1983). The effect of peer separation in young chimpanzees (Pan troglodytes). American Journal of Primatology, 5, 25–37.

Bartholomew, K., & Horowitz, L. M. (1991). Attachment styles among young adults: A test of a four-category model. Journal of Personality and Social Psychology, 61, 226–244.

Benuzzi, F., Pugnaghi, M., Meletti, S., Lui, F., Serafini, M., Baraldi, P., et al. (2007). Processing the socially relevant parts of faces. Brain Research Bulletin, 74, 344–356.

Berardi, N., & Maffei, L. (1999). From visual experience to visual function: Roles of neurotrophins. Journal of Neurobiology, 41, 119–126.

Berridge, K. C. (2007). The debate over dopamine's role in reward: The case for incentive salience. Psychopharmacology, 191, 391–431.

Berscheid, E. (2003). The human's greatest strength: Other humans. In U. M. Staudinger (Ed.), A psychology of human strengths: Fundamental questions and future directions for a positive psychology (pp. 37–47). Washington, DC: American Psychological Association.

Boccia, M. L., Reite, M., & Laudenslager, M. (1989). On the physiology of grooming in a pigtail macaque. Physiology and Behavior, 45, 667–670.

Borman-Spurrell, E., Allen, J. P., Hauser, S. T., Carter, A., & Cole-Detke, H. C. (1995). Assessing adult attachment: A comparison of interview-based and self-report methods. Unpublished manuscript, Yale University, New Haven, CT.

Bowlby, J. (1969/1982). Attachment and loss: Vol. 1. Attachment. New York: Basic Books.

Bowlby, J. (1973). Attachment and loss: Vol. 2. Separation: Anxiety and anger. New York: Basic Books.

Bowlby, J. (1979). The making and breaking of affectional bonds. London: Tavistock/Routledge.

Bowlby, J. (1980). Attachment and loss: Vol. 3. Loss: Sadness and depression. New York: Basic Books.

Bozarth, M. A., & Wise, R. A. (1996). Toxicity associated with long-term intravenous heroin and cocaine self-administration in the rat. Journal of the American Medical Association, 254, 81–83.

Brasted, P. J., Bussey, T. J., Murray, E. A., & Wise, S. P. (2003). Role of the hippocampal system in associative learning beyond the spatial domain. Brain, 126, 1202–1223.

Brennan, K. A., Clark, C. L., & Shaver, P. R. (1998). Self-report measurement of adult attachment: An integrative overview. In J. A. Simpson & W. S. Rholes (Eds.), Attachment theory and close relationships (pp. 46–76). New York: Guilford Press.

Brewer, M. B., & Caporael, L. R. (1990). Selfish genes

vs. selfish people: Sociobiology as origin myth. *Motivation and Emotion, 14*, 237–243.

Briones, T. L., Klintsova, A. Y., & Greenough, W. T. (2004). Stability of synaptic plasticity in the adult rat visual cortex induced by complex environment exposure. *Brain Research, 1018*, 130–135.

Buchheim, A., Erk, S., George, C., Kächele, H., Ruchsow, M., Spitzer, M., et al. (2006). Measuring attachment representation in an fMRI environment: A pilot study. *Psychopathology, 39*, 144–152.

Burgdorf, J., & Panksepp, J. (2001). Tickling induces reward in adolescent rats. *Physiology and Behavior, 72*, 167–173.

Buss, D. M., & Kenrick, D. T. (1998). Evolutionary social psychology. In D. T. Gilbert, S. T. Fiske, & G. Lindzey (Eds.), *The handbook of social psychology* (4th ed., pp. 982–1026). New York: McGraw-Hill.

Cacioppo, J. T., Amaral, D. G., Blanchard, J. J., Cameron, J. L., Carter, C. S., Crews, D., et al. (2007). Social neuroscience: Progress and implications for mental health. *Perspectives on Psychological Science, 2*, 99–123.

Cacioppo, J. T., Hawkley, L. C., Crawford, L. E., Ernst, J. M., Burleson, M. H., Kowalewski, R. B., et al. (2002). Loneliness and health: Potential mechanisms. *Psychosomatic Medicine, 64*(3), 407–417.

Cahill, L., Prins, B., Weber, M., & McGaugh, J. L. (1994). Beta-adrenergic activation and memory for emotional events. *Nature, 371*, 702–704.

Cancedda, L., Putignano, E., Sale, A., Viegi, A., Berardi, N., & Maffei, L. (2004). Acceleration of visual system development by environmental enrichment. *Journal of Neuroscience, 24*, 4840–4848.

Carter, C. S. (2003). Developmental consequences of oxytocin. *Physiology and Behavior, 79*, 383–397.

Carter, C. S., & DeVries, A. C. (1999). Stress and soothing: An endocrine perspective. In M. Lewis & D. Ramsay (Eds.), *Soothing and stress* (pp. 3–18). Mahwah, NJ: Erlbaum.

Carter, C. S., & Keverne, E. B. (2002). The neurobiology of social affiliation and pair bonding. *Hormones, Brain and Behavior, 1*, 299–337.

Chugani, H. T. (1998). A critical period of brain development: Studies of cerebral glucose utilization with PET. *Preventive Medicine, 27*, 184–188.

Coan, J. A., & Allen, J. J. B. (2003). The state and trait nature of frontal EEG asymmetry in emotion. In K. Hugdahl & R. J. Davidson (Eds.), *The asymmetrical brain* (pp. 565–615). Cambridge, MA: MIT Press.

Coan, J. A., & Allen, J. J. B. (2004). Frontal EEG asymmetry as a moderator and mediator of emotion. *Biological Psychology, 67*, 7–49.

Coan, J. A., Allen, J. J. B., & McKnight, P. E. (2006). A capability model of individual differences in frontal EEG asymmetry. *Biological Psychology, 72*, 198–207.

Coan, J. A., Schaefer, H. S., & Davidson, R. J. (2005). Marital adjustment and interpersonal styles moderate the effects of spouse and stranger hand holding on activation of neural systems underlying response to threat. *Psychophysiology, 42*, S44.

Coan, J. A., Schaefer, H. S., & Davidson, R. J. (2006). Lending a hand: Social regulation of the neural response to threat. *Psychological Science, 17*, 1032–1039.

Coyne, J. C., Rohrbaugh, M. J., Shoham, V., Sonnega, J. S., Nicklas, J. M., & Cranford, J. A. (2001). Prognostic importance of marital quality for survival of congestive heart failure. *American Journal of Cardiology, 88*, 526–529.

Darwin, C. (1998). *The expression of the emotions in man and animals.* Oxford, UK: Oxford University Press. (Original work published 1872)

Davidovitz, R., Mikulincer, M., Shaver, P. R., Ijzak, R., & Popper, M. (2007). Leaders as attachment figures: Their attachment orientations predict leadership-related mental representations and followers' performance and mental health. *Journal of Personality and Social Psychology, 93*, 632–650.

Davidson, R. J., & Irwin, W. (1999). The functional neuroanatomy of emotion and affective style. *Trends in Cognitive Sciences, 3*, 11–21.

Dawson, G., Ashman, S. B., Hessl, D., Spieker, S., Frey, K., Panagiotides, H., et al. (2001). Autonomic and brain electrical activity in securely- and insecurely-attached infants of depressed mothers. *Infant Behavior and Development, 24*, 135–149.

DeCasper, A. J., & Fifer, W. P. (1980). Of human bonding: Newborns prefer their mothers' voices. *Science, 208*, 1174–1176.

Depue, R. A., & Collins, P. F. (1999). Neurobiology of the structure of personality: Dopamine, facilitation of incentive motivation, and extraversion. *Behavioral and Brain Sciences, 22*, 491–517.

Depue, R. A., & Morrone-Strupinsky, J. V. (2005). A neurobehavioral model of affiliative bonding: Implications for conceptualizing a human trait of affiliation. *Behavioral and Brain Sciences, 28*, 313–395.

Diamond, L. M. (2001). Contributions of psychophysiology to research on adult attachment: Review and recommendations. *Personality and Social Psychology Review, 5*, 276–296.

Edens, J. L., Larkin, K. T., & Abel, J. L. (1992). The effect of social support and physical touch on cardiovascular reactions to mental stress. *Journal of Psychosomatic Research, 36*, 371–382.

Ellenbogen, M. A., Schwartzman, A. E., Stewart, J., & Walker, C. D. (2006). Automatic and effortful emotional information processing regulates different aspects of the stress response. *Psychoneuroendocrinology, 31*, 373–387.

Flinn, M. V., & England, B. G. (1997). Social economics of childhood glucocorticoid stress response and health. *American Journal of Physical Anthropology, 102*, 33–53.

Fraley, R. C., & Shaver, P. R. (2000). Adult romantic attachment: Theoretical developments, emerging controversies, and unanswered questions. *Review of General Psychology, 4*, 132–154.

Franceschini, M. A., Thaker, S., Themelis, G., Krishnamoorthy, K. K., Bortfeld, H., Diamond, S. G.,

Boas, D. A., et al. (2007). Assessment of infant brain development with frequency-domain near-infrared spectroscopy. *Pediatric Research*, *61*, 546–551.

Gainer, H., & Wray, S. (1994). Cellular and molecular biology of oxytocin and vasopressin. In E. Knobil & J. Neill (Eds.), *The physiology of reproduction* (pp. 1099–1129). New York: Raven Press.

Galliot, M. T., & Baumeister, R. F. (2007). The physiology of willpower: Linking blood glucose to self-control. *Personality and Social Psychology Review*, *11*, 303–327.

Gillath, O., Bunge, S. A., Shaver, P. R., Wendelken, C., & Mikulincer, M. (2005). Attachment-style differences and ability to suppress negative thoughts: Exploring the neural correlates. *NeuroImage*, *28*, 835–847.

Gosling, S. D., & John, O. P. (1999). Personality dimensions in non-human animals: A cross-species review. *Current Directions in Psychological Science*, *8*, 69–75.

Graves, F. C., Wallen, K., & Maestripieri, D. (2002). Opioids and attachment in rhesus macaque (*Macaca mulatta*) abusive mothers. *Behavioral Neuroscience*, *116*, 489–493.

Gust, D. A., Gordon, T. P., Brodie, A. R., & McClure, H. M. (1996). Effect of companions in modulating stress associated with new group formation in juvenile rhesus macaques. *Physiology and Behavior*, *59*, 941–945.

Hamann, S. B., Ely, T. D., Grafton, S. T., & Kilts, C. D. (1999). Amygdala activity related to enhanced memory for pleasant and aversive stimuli. *Nature Neuroscience*, *2*, 289–293.

Hansen, S., Bergvall, A. H., & Nyiredi, S. (1993). Interaction with pups enhances dopamine release in the ventral striatum of maternal rats: A microdialysis study. *Pharmacology, Biochemistry and Behavior*, *45*, 673–676.

Hansen, S., Harthon, C., Wallin, E., Löfberg, L., & Svensson, K. (1991). The effects of 6-OHDA-induced dopamine depletions in the ventral or dorsal striatum on maternal and sexual behavior in the female rat. *Pharmacology, Biochemistry and Behavior*, *39*, 71–77.

Harrison, L. L., Williams, A. K., Berbaum, M. L., Stem, J. T., & Leeper, J. (2000). Physiologic and behavioral effects of gentle human touch on preterm infants. *Research in Nursing and Health*, *23*(6), 435–446.

Hebb, D. O. (1949). *The organization of behavior*. New York: Wiley.

Heinrichs, M., Meinlschmidt, G., Neumann, I., Wagner, S., Kirschbaum, C., Ehlert, U., et al. (2001). Effects of suckling on hypothalamic–pituitary–adrenal axis responses to psychosocial stress in postpartum lactating women. *Journal of Clinical Endocrinology and Metabolism*, *86*, 4798–4804.

Herschkowitz, N. (2000). Neurological bases of behavioral development in infancy. *Brain and Development*, *22*, 411–416.

Hofer, M. A. (1995). Hidden regulators: Implications for a new understanding of attachment, separation, and loss. In S. Goldberg, R. Muir, & J. Kerr (Eds.), *Attachment theory: Social, developmental, and clinical perspectives* (pp. 203–232). Hillsdale, NJ: Analytic Press.

Hofer, M. A. (2006). Psychobiological roots of early attachment. *Current Directions in Psychological Science*, *15*, 84–88.

Hofer, M. A., & Sullivan, R. M. (2001). Toward a neurobiology of attachment. In C. A. Nelson & M. Luciana (Eds.), *Handbook of developmental cognitive neuroscience* (pp. 599–616). Cambridge, MA: MIT Press.

Holloway, K. S., Cornil, C. A., & Balthazart, J. (2004). Effects of central administration of naloxone during the extinction of appetitive sexual responses. *Behavioural Brain Research*, *153*, 567–572.

House, J. S., Landis, K. R., & Umberson, D. (1988). Social relationships and health. *Science*, *241*, 540–545.

Hubel, D. H., & Wiesel, T. N. (1970). The period of susceptibility to the physiological effects of unilateral eye closure in kittens. *Journal of Physiology*, *206*, 419–436.

Insel, T. R., & Fernald, R. D. (2004). How the brain processes social information: Searching for the social brain. *Annual Review of Neuroscience*, *27*, 697–722.

Insel, T. R., & Winslow, J. T. (1998). Serotonin and neuropeptides in affiliative behaviors. *Biological Psychiatry*, *44*, 207–219.

Izzo, A., Rotondi, M., Perone, C., Lauro, C., Manzo, E., Casilli, B., et al. (1999). Inhibitory effect of exogenous oxytocin on ACTH and cortisol secretion during labour. *Clinical and Experimental Obstetrics and Gynecology*, *26*, 221–224.

Jacob, S., & McClintock, M. K. (2000). Psychological state mood effects of steroidal chemosignals in women and men. *Hormones and Behavior*, *37*, 57–78.

Jamner, L. D., & Leigh, H. (1999). Repressive/defensive coping, endogenous opioids and health: How a life so perfect can make you sick. *Psychiatry Research*, *85*, 17–31.

Johnson, S. M. (2002). *Emotionally focused couple therapy with trauma survivors: Strengthening attachment bonds*. New York: Guilford Press.

Kawachi, I. B., & Berkman, L. F. (2001). Social ties and mental health. *Journal of Urban Health*, *78*(3), 458–467.

Kemeny, M. E. (2003). The psychobiology of stress. *Current Directions in Psychological Science*, *12*, 124–129.

Kennedy, P. J., & Shapiro, M. L. (2004). Retrieving memories via internal context requires the hippocampus. *Journal of Neuroscience*, *24*, 6979–6985.

Keverne, E. B., Martensz, N. D., & Tuite, B. (1989). Beta-endorphin concentrations in cerebrospinal fluid of monkeys are influenced by grooming relationships. *Psychoneuroendocrinology*, *14*, 155–161.

Kim, H. K., & McKenry, P. C. (2002). The relationship between marriage and psychological well-being: A longitudinal analysis. *Journal of Family Issues*, *23*(8), 885–911.

King, J. E., & Figueredo, A. J. (1997). The five-factor model plus dominance in chimpanzee personality. *Journal of Research in Personality*, *31*, 271–271.

Kirkpatrick, L. A., & Davis, K. E. (1994). Attachment style, gender, and relationship stability: A longitudinal analysis. *Journal of Personality and Social Psychology, 66,* 502–512.

Kiyokawa, Y., Kikusui, T., Takeuchi, Y., & Mori, Y. (2004). Partner's stress status influences social buffering effects in rats. *Behavioral Neuroscience, 118,* 798–804.

Krebs, J. R., & Davies, N. B. (1993). *An introduction to behavioural ecology* (3rd ed.). Oxford, UK: Blackwell.

La Guardia, J. G., Ryan, R. M., Couchman, C. E., & Deci, E. L. (2000). Within-person variation in security of attachment: A self-determination theory perspective on attachment, need fulfillment, and well-being. *Journal of Personality and Social Psychology, 79,* 367–384.

Laird, J. D., & Strout, S. (2007). Emotional behaviors as emotional stimuli. In J. A. Coan & J. J. B. Allen (Eds.), *The handbook of emotion elicitation and assessment* (pp. 54–64). New York: Oxford University Press.

LeDoux, J. E. (2000). Emotion circuits in the brain. *Annual Review of Neuroscience, 23,* 155–184.

Le Moal, M., & Simon, H. (1991). Mesocorticolimbic dopaminergic network: Functional and regulatory roles. *Physiological Reviews, 71,* 155–234.

Lewis, M., & Ramsay, D. S. (1999). Effect of maternal soothing on infant stress response. *Child Development, 70*(1), 11–20.

Lim, M. M., Hammock, E. A., & Young, L. J. (2004). The role of vasopressin in the genetic and neural regulation of monogamy. *Journal of Neuroendocrinology, 16,* 325–332.

Lim, M. M., & Young, L. J. (2006). Neuropeptidergic regulation of affiliative behavior and social bonding in animals. *Hormones and Behavior, 50,* 506–517.

Lorberbaum, J., Newman, J., Dubno, J., Horwitz, A., Nahas, Z., Teneback, C., et al. (1999). Feasibility of using fMRI to study mothers responding to infant cries. *Depression and Anxiety, 10,* 99–104.

Lorenz, K. (1935). Der kumpan in der umwelt des vogels. *Journal of Ornithology, 83,* 137–413.

Marlier, L., & Schaal, B. (2005). Human newborns prefer human milk: Conspecific milk odor is attractive without postnatal exposure. *Child Development, 76,* 155–168.

McEwen, B. S. (2007). Physiology and neurobiology of stress and adaptation: Central role of the brain. *Physiological Reviews, 87,* 873–904.

Melo, A. I., Lovic, V., Gonzalez, A., Madden, M., Sinopoli, K., & Fleming, A. S. (2006). Maternal and littermate deprivation disrupts maternal behavior and social-learning of food preference in adulthood: Tactile stimulation, nest odor, and social rearing prevent these effects. *Developmental Psychobiology, 48,* 209–219.

Meredith, M. (2001). Human vomeronasal organ function: A critical review of best and worst cases. *Chemical Senses, 26,* 433–445.

Mikulincer, M., & Florian, V. (1998). The relationship between adult attachment styles and emotional and cognitive reactions to stressful events. In J. A. Simpson & W. S. Rholes (Eds.), *Attachment theory and close relationships* (pp. 143–165). New York: Guilford Press.

Mikulincer, M., & Shaver, P. R. (2007). *Attachment in adulthood: Structure, dynamics, and change.* New York: Guilford Press.

Mikulincer, M., Shaver, P. R., & Pereg, D. (2003). Attachment theory and affect regulation: The dynamics, development, and cognitive consequences of attachment-related strategies. *Motivation and Emotion, 27,* 77–102.

Milad, M. R., Quinn, B. T., Pitman, R. K., Orr, S. P., Fischl, B., & Rauch, S. L. (2005). Thickness of ventromedial prefrontal cortex in humans is correlated with extinction memory. *Proceedings of the National Academy of Sciences USA, 102,* 10706–10711.

Miller, L. C., Bard, K. A., Juno, C. J., & Nadler, R. D. (1986). Behavioral responsiveness of young chimpanzees (*Pan troglodytes*) to a novel environment. *Folia Primatologica, 47,* 128–142.

Miller, L. C., Bard, K. A., Juno, C. J., & Nadler, R. D. (1990). Behavioral responsiveness to strangers in young chimpanzees (*Pan troglodytes*). *Folia Primatologica, 55,* 142–155.

Mineka, S., & Suomi, S. J. (1978). Social separation in monkeys. *Psychological Bulletin, 85,* 1376–1400.

Mischel, W., Shoda, Y., & Mendoza-Denton, R. (2002). Situation–behavior profiles as a locus of consistency in personality. *Current Directions in Psychological Science, 11,* 50–54.

Moriceau, S., & Sullivan, R. M. (2005). Neurobiology of infant attachment. *Developmental Psychobiology, 47,* 230–242.

Nakamura, S., & Sakaguchi, T. (1990). Development and plasticity of the locus coeruleus: A review of recent physiological and pharmacological experimentation. *Progress in Neurobiology, 34,* 505–526.

Newcomb, M. D., & Bentler, P. M. (1988). Impact of adolescent drug use and social support on problems of young adults: A longitudinal study. *Journal of Abnormal Psychology, 97*(1), 64–75.

Niesink, R. J., Vanderschuren, L. J., & van Ree, J. M. (1996). Social play in juvenile rats after *in utero* exposure to morphine. *Neurotoxicology, 17,* 905–912.

Nocjar, C., & Panksepp, J. (2007). Prior morphine experience induces long-term increases in social interest and in appetitive behavior for natural reward. *Behavioural Brain Research, 181,* 191–199.

Noftle, E. E., & Shaver, P. R. (2006). Attachment dimensions and the Big Five personality traits: Associations and comparative ability to predict relationship quality. *Journal of Research in Personality, 40,* 179–208.

Norris, C. J., Coan, J. A., & Johnstone, I. T. (2007). Functional magnetic resonance imaging and the study of emotion. In J. A. Coan & J. J. B. Allen (Eds.), *The handbook of emotion elicitation and assessment* (pp. 440–459). New York: Oxford University Press.

Ochsner, K. N., Bunge, S. A., Gross, J. J., & Gabrieli, J. D. (2002). Rethinking feelings: An fMRI study of the cognitive regulation of emotion. *Journal of Cognitive Neuroscience, 14,* 1215–1229.

Ochsner, K. N., & Gross, J. J. (2005). The cognitive control of emotion. *Trends in Cognitive Sciences, 9,* 242–249.

Öhman, A. (2005). The role of the amygdala in human fear: Automatic detection of threat. *Psychoneuroendocrinology, 30,* 953–958.

Panksepp, J., Nelson, E., & Siviy, S. (1994). Brain opioids and mother–infant social motivation. *Acta Paediatrica, 397,* 40–46.

Pessoa, L., Kastnerb, S., & Ungerleider, L. G. (2002). Attentional control of the processing of neutral and emotional stimuli. *Cognitive Brain Research, 15,* 31–45.

Pfaus, J. G., Kippin, T. E., & Centeno, S. (2001). Conditioning and sexual behavior: A review. *Hormones and Behavior, 40,* 291–321.

Phelps, E. A., & LeDoux, J. E. (2005). Contributions of the amygdala to emotion processing: From animal models to human behavior. *Neuron, 48,* 175–187.

Posner, M. I., & Rothbart, M. K. (2007). Research on attention networks as a model for the integration of psychological science. *Annual Review of Psychology, 58,* 1–23.

Proffitt, D. R. (2006). Embodied perception and the economy of action. *Perspectives on Psychological Science, 1,* 110–122.

Quirk, G. J., & Beer, J. S. (2006). Prefrontal involvement in the regulation of emotion: Convergence of rat and human studies. *Current Opinion in Neurobiology, 16,* 723–727.

Reichardt, L. F. (2006). Neurotrophin-regulated signalling pathways. *Philosophical Transactions of the Royal Society of London, 361,* 1545–1564.

Robles, T. F., & Kiecolt-Glaser, J. K. (2003). The physiology of marriage: Pathways to health. *Physiology and Behavior, 79,* 409–416.

Rolls, E. T. (2007a). Emotion elicited by primary reinforcers and following stimulus-reinforcement association learning. In J. A. Coan & J. J. B. Allen (Eds.), *The handbook of emotion elicitation and assessment* (pp. 137–157). New York: Oxford University Press.

Rolls, E. T. (2007b). The representation of information about faces in the temporal and frontal lobes. *Neuropsychologia, 45,* 124–143.

Ruis, M. A. W., te Brake, J. H. A., Buwalda, B., De Boer, S. F., Meerlo, P., Korte, S. M., et al. (1999). Housing familiar male wildtype rats together reduces the long-term adverse behavioural and physiological effects of social defeat. *Psychoneuroendocrinology,* 285–300.

Sapolsky, R. M. (1998). *Why zebras don't get ulcers.* New York: Holt.

Sbarra, D. A. (2006). Predicting the onset of emotional recovery following nonmarital relationship dissolution: Survival analyses of sadness and anger. *Personality and Social Psychology Bulletin, 32,* 298–312.

Schaal, B., Marlier, L., & Soussignan, R. (1998). Olfactory function in the human fetus: Evidence from selective neonatal responsiveness to the odor of amniotic fluid. *Behavioral Neuroscience, 112,* 1438–1449.

Schauwers, K., Gillis, S., Daemers, K., De Beukelaer, C., De Ceulaer, G., Yperman, M., et al. (2004). Normal hearing and language development in a deaf-born child. *Otology and Neurotology, 25,* 924–929.

Schultz, W., Dayan, P., & Montague, P. R. (1997). A neural substrate of prediction and reward. *Science, 275,* 1593–1599.

Sierra-Mercado, D. J., Corcoran, K. A., Lebrón-Milad, K., & Quirk, G. J. (2006). Inactivation of the ventromedial prefrontal cortex reduces expression of conditioned fear and impairs subsequent recall of extinction. *European Journal of Neuroscience, 24,* 1751–1758.

Skuse, D., Albanese, A., Stanhope, R., Gilmour, J., & Voss, L. (1996). A new stress-related syndrome of growth failure and hyperphagia in children, associated with reversibility of growth-hormone insufficiency. *Lancet, 348,* 353–358.

Sullivan, R. M. (2003). Developing a sense of safety: The neurobiology of neonatal attachment. *Annals of the New York Academy of Sciences, 1008,* 122–131.

Teicher, M. H., Samson, J. A., Polcari, A., & McGreenery, C. E. (2006). Sticks, stones, and hurtful words: Relative effects of various forms of childhood maltreatment. *American Journal of Psychiatry, 163,* 993–1000.

Terranova, M. L., Cirulli, F., & Laviola, G. (1999). Behavioral and hormonal effects of partner familiarity in periadolescent rat pairs upon novelty exposure. *Psychoneuroendocrinology, 24,* 639–656.

Thomas, K. M., Drevets, W. C., Whalen, P. J., Eccard, C. H., Dahl, R. E., Ryan, N. D., et al. (2001). Amygdala response to facial expressions in children and adults. *Biological Psychiatry, 49,* 309–316.

Topal, J., Miklosi, A., Csanyi, V., & Doka, A. (1998). Attachment behavior in dogs (*Canis familiaris*): A new application of Ainsworth's (1969) Strange Situation test. *Journal of Comparative Psychology, 112,* 219–229.

Tzschentke, T. M., & Schmidt, W. J. (2000). Functional relationship among medial prefrontal cortex, nucleus accumbens, and ventral tegmental area in locomotion and reward. *Critical Reviews in Neurobiology, 14,* 131–142.

Uchino, B. N., Cacioppo, J. T., & Kiecolt-Glaser, J. K. (1996). The relationship between social support and physiological processes: A review with emphasis on underlying mechanisms and implications for health. *Psychological Bulletin, 119,* 488–531.

Uvnaes-Moberg, K. (1998). Oxytocin may mediate the benefits of positive social interaction and emotions. *Psychoneuroendocrinology, 23*(8), 819–835.

Weaver, A., & de Waal, F. B. M. (2003). The mother–offspring relationship as a template in social development: Reconciliation in captive brown capuchins (*Cebus apella*). *Journal of Comparative Psychology, 117,* 101–110.

Weaver, I. C. G., Cervoni, N., Champagne, F. A., D'Alessio, A. C., Sharma, S., Seckl, J. R., et al. (2004). Epigenetic programming by maternal behavior. *Nature Neuroscience, 7,* 847–854.

Weiss, S. J. (1990). Effects of differential touch on nervous system arousal of patients recovering from cardiac disease. *Heart and Lung, 19,* 474–480.

Whalen, P. J. (2007). The uncertainty of it all. *Trends in Cognitive Sciences, 11,* 499–500.

Whalen, P. J., Kagan, J., Cook, R. G., Davis, F. C., Kim, H., Polis, S., et al. (2004). Human amygdala responsivity to masked fearful eye whites. *Science, 306,* 2061.

Whalen, P. J., Rauch, S. L., Etcoff, N. L., McInerney, S. C., Lee, M. B., & Jenike, M. A. (1998). Masked presentations of emotional facial expressions modulate amygdala activity without explicit knowledge. *Journal of Neuroscience, 18,* 411–418.

Wiedenmayer, C. P., Magarinos, A. M., McEwen, B. S., & Barr, G. A. (2003). Mother lowers glucocorticoid levels of preweaning rats after acute threat. *Annals of the New York Academy of Sciences, 1008,* 304–307.

Williamson, A. (2006). Using self-report measures in neurobehavioral toxicology: Can they be trusted? *Neurotoxicology, 28,* 227–234.

Windle, R. J., Shanks, N., Lightman, S. L., & Ingram, C. D. (1997). Central oxytocin administration reduces stress-induced corticosterone release and anxiety behavior in rats. *Endocrinology, 138,* 2829–2834.

Wismer-Fries, A. B., Ziegler, T. E., Kurian, J. R., Jacoris, S., & Pollak, S. D. (2005). Early experience in humans is associated with changes in neuropeptides critical for regulating social behavior. *Proceedings of the National Academy of Sciences USA, 102,* 17237–17240.

Young, L. J., & Wang, Z. (2004). The neurobiology of pair bonding. *Nature Neuroscience, 7,* 1048–1054.

PART III

ATTACHMENT IN INFANCY AND CHILDHOOD

CHAPTER 12

Normative Development
The Ontogeny of Attachment

ROBERT S. MARVIN
PRESTON A. BRITNER

Whilst especially evident during early childhood, attachment behavior is held to characterize human beings from the cradle to the grave.

—BOWLBY (1979, p. 129)

During the 1940s and 1950s, a number of studies emerged suggesting that very young children, when separated from their mothers for a considerable period of time, proceed through a series of reactions that have become known as "protest," "despair," and "detachment" (e.g., Burlingham & Freud, 1942; Heinicke & Westheimer, 1966; Robertson, 1953). These or similar reactions were so common, despite variations in familiarity of the setting or quality of care received by a youngster, that John Bowlby (as well as others) departed from the contemporary scientific and clinical consensus and decided that the loss of the *specific mother figure* was the most important factor in these reactions. It was from this beginning that Bowlby went on to develop his "ethological–control systems" theory of the infant's tie, or attachment, to his or her mother or primary caregiver (Bowlby, 1958, 1969/1982, 1973, 1980). In a partnership that went on to span nearly 40 years, Bowlby and Mary Ainsworth (e.g., Ainsworth, 1967; Ainsworth, Blehar, Waters, & Wall, 1978), among others, decided to embark on a quest to answer questions such as these: Why does a young child become so distressed by the loss of his or her mother? What processes account for each of the three phases of loss? What *is* the bond that ties the child to the mother? What are

its forms, and how do they emerge? What happens to these forms as the child matures? Do such bonds exist in the adult, and if so, in what form? And ultimately, how do we understand form and functioning "when things go wrong"?

At that point, Bowlby and his colleagues decided that answering those questions required a shift to the study of the early development of this bond in normally developing children and their families. They were convinced that only by understanding the normal formation and functioning of an attachment would we be able to understand its malfunctioning. This decision led to Ainsworth's naturalistic observational studies in Uganda and Baltimore, and to the first volume of Bowlby's trilogy on attachment. These efforts resulted in some of the most significant, and empirically and theoretically coherent, contributions to the study of children's development in the second half of the 20th century. The theory that emerged was consistent with then-current theories of biology, embryology, cognitive science, and general systems theory. It was at the same time specific enough to incorporate species and cultural differences, and general enough to incorporate species and cultural similarity. It came closer than any other theory to being equally applicable to questions of normative

269

development and of individual differences and maladaptive developmental pathways. The chapters in this volume are a tribute to the power of the theory and the methods that have both evolved from and been informed by the theory.

Through the mid-1970s, Bowlby's theory of the ontogeny of attachment generated much excitement and controversy. However, by 1980 the field of attachment research had undergone a significant change: The study of individual differences had come to occupy so much of the focus that exploration of the *ontogeny* of attachment had nearly been abandoned. Ainsworth's identification of three "primary" strategies of attachment (e.g., Ainsworth et al., 1978), Main and Solomon's (1990) discovery of a "disorganized" pattern of attachment, and Main and colleagues' research on adults' attachment strategies (e.g., Main & Goldwyn, 1984; Main, Goldwyn, & Hesse, 2003) have contributed enormously to our understanding of differential strategies within intimate relationships, as well as of child and adult psychopathology. The history of biology, however, demonstrates that despite some analogical similarities between immature and mature forms of an organism, any attempt to understand adaptive or maladaptive versions of the mature form without constant reference to structural transformations throughout ontogeny is doomed to failure (e.g., Bateson, 1976; Waddington, 1957). Ethological studies of behavioral development also point to the obvious but often ignored importance of survival of the individual at each developmental point. This will certainly be no less the case in the study of human attachment. Only by studying individual pathways *through the course of development* will we truly understand the origins, nature, and sequelae of the attachment bond.

So the question becomes this: Do we already know enough about the form of the attachment behavioral system at different points in development to move so exclusively to the study of individual differences? And if not, what are the risks of failing to study those changing forms? If the goal of developmental research in this area is to discover reliable and valid measures of infant behavior that predict concurrent and future outcomes, then the answer to the first question is a qualified "yes." Or if attachment behavior, and a secure attachment, are assumed to be developmental tasks only of infancy, to be superseded by such later tasks as internal control and self-reliance (Freud, 1965), individuation (Mahler, Pine, & Bergman, 1975), autonomy (Erikson, 1950), or independent and

socialized behavior (Bandura, 1978; Baumrind, 1980), it is again tempting to answer "yes." There are, however, theoretical and empirical reasons for rejecting a strong developmental-task position (Ainsworth, 1990; Cicchetti, Cummings, Greenberg, & Marvin, 1990).

Perhaps the most important reason for studying the developing forms of attachment behavior is related to common experience and to one of Bowlby's most fundamental theoretical claims: that the biological function of attachment behavior is protection of the youngster from a variety of dangers. Preschool and even older children, in our present environment and in our "environment of evolutionary adaptedness" (Bowlby, 1969/1982), are vulnerable to a wide range of dangers. How children and their caregivers organize protective proximity and contact, and how they continue to use their caregivers as a secure base for exploration, remain as important during later periods of development as during the first year of life. Although the frequency of attachment behavior may wane across development, it remains as important when activated in a 4- or 8-year-old as it is during infancy. And how the attachment behavioral system is organized with other behavioral systems in an individual (and the caregivers), so that the person is protected while engaging in developmentally appropriate exploration or other activities, becomes a crucial question in understanding many developmental domains across the entire lifespan.

Bowlby (1969/1982) placed his theory of the development of attachment squarely within the biological, general systems, and cognitive sciences. The theory is actually an integration and elaboration of several conceptual schemes: general systems theory, including especially communication and control systems theory; cognitive science, much of which itself can be considered part of systems theory; evolutionary theory; ethology and the study of primate behavior; and descriptive studies of human infants and young children interacting with their caregivers. The description of the development of attachment across the lifespan presented in this chapter combines Bowlby's theory, as originally presented; the elaboration provided by Marvin and his colleagues regarding developmental changes during the preschool years; and a brief review of contributions by others regarding possible further changes during later childhood, adolescence, and adulthood. More detailed descriptions of attachment theory as applied to adolescence and adulthood are presented in the chapters in Part IV of this volume. Reviews of the nonhuman primate literature on the bond between parent(s) and offspring, of the crucial role played by that literature in the development of Bowlby's theory, and of the usefulness of that literature, are available in Bowlby (1969/1982), Hinde (1982), Marvin (1977, 1997), Maestripieri (2005), and Suomi (1995 and Chapter 8, this volume).

GENERAL SYSTEMS PERSPECTIVE

At an abstract information-theoretic level, if a system is to survive, there must be certain invariants both among its constituent elements and in its relationship with its environment (Ashby, 1952, 1956). In certain essential respects, variety must be kept within certain limits, or the system will not survive. In human development, the best-known examples are our many physiological invariants. Furthermore, if a system does not have the ability to control input from the environment in a manner that keeps these essential variables within the limits required for survival, then it must be "coupled" with another system that does have the ability to keep the variety in the first system within such limits. In other words, there must be a close coupling, bond, or attachment between the two systems that serves to protect the less "self-reliant" system. This is a formal statement of Bowlby's basic thesis regarding the biological function of child–parent attachment: It protects the child from a wide range of dangers—from either internal changes or environmental inputs—that would push some essential variable(s) beyond the system's (i.e., the child's) limits of survival.

In a system that develops toward increasing self-reliance over time, this coupling can have another aspect. In many biological organisms, the protective bond has a component that facilitates the youngster's tendency to explore and learn— that is, to develop the skills necessary to protect itself through its autonomous integration in the larger group. Within this protective relationship, the developing organism thus becomes progressively less and less dependent on the bond with its parent (i.e., the system with more variety) to provide that protection. Eventually, the developing organism contains the necessary variety or skills within itself, and within its coupling with its larger social network, to control internal change and environmental input in ways that maintain its essential variables within the limits necessary for survival. This compound, and very complex, developmental pattern constitutes the crux of Ainsworth's

(1967) concept of the child's use of its mother as a haven of safety and secure base for exploration. It emphasizes that at each point in development, the attachment–caregiving interactions between the youngster and its attachment figure(s) compensate for and complement the lack of motor, communication, and social skills on the youngster's part, so that the youngster is always protected while being afforded as much independence as possible within which to learn those skills. Finally, it suggests that at any given point in development, skills or behavior systems across developmental domains will fit together in a manner that makes adaptive sense in terms of survival at that point.

BOWLBY'S CONTROL SYSTEMS MODEL OF DEVELOPMENT

Much research on both primates and humans indicates that this developmental pattern takes place in the context of a complex network of "affectional bonds," of which the close attachment of infant to mother is one. Ainsworth (1967) defines an affectional bond as a relatively long-enduring tie in which the partner is important as a unique individual, and non-interchangeable. Harlow was one of the first to propose distinct affectional systems or bonds (Harlow & Harlow, 1965), with the explicit connotation that different bonds function to achieve different outcomes. Bowlby took this a step further in distinguishing among a number of behavioral systems, each with its own predictable outcome and biological function (see Cassidy, Chapter 1, this volume). Following on Harlow's early work, a number of distinct affectional bonds have been identified, including the attachment bond, the parent's complementary caregiving bond, the sexual pair bond, sibling/kinship bonds, and friendship bonds (Ainsworth, 1990; George & Solomon, Chapter 35, this volume; Zeifman & Hazan, Chapter 20, this volume).

In our opinion, the essential contribution of Bowlby's theory is the way in which Bowlby explained these bonds in terms of the behavioral systems underlying them, and the developmental changes in those behavioral systems. Specific criticisms over the years have challenged some of Bowlby's propositions. For example, Hrdy (2005) has argued that common allomothering practices necessitate the need to study nonmothers, and Porges (2005) has contended that traditional attachment theory has failed to articulate the mechanisms mediating engagement between bonding individuals. Nonetheless, it is striking how pre-scient Bowlby's systems theory was in light of more recent scientific evidence from neuroscientific and psychobiological studies of attachment and bonding (Hofer, 2006; Miller & Rodgers, 2001; Polan & Hofer, Chapter 7, this volume; Schore, 2000).

Behavioral Systems

Attachment theory proposes a number of behavioral systems that are species-universal, although there may be (subtle) differences across both individuals and breeding populations (e.g., Freedman & Gorman, 1993). Each behavioral system consists of a set of interchangeable, functionally equivalent behaviors—in other words, behaviors that have the same predictable effect or outcome (Bowlby, 1969/1982). At the same time, each behavior serves more than one behavioral system. For example, locomotion serves, among others, the attachment, exploration, and wariness behavioral systems. It is for this reason that Sroufe and Waters (1977) insisted that the infant's attachment behavior can be fully understood only from an organizational perspective.

A nonexhaustive list of behavioral systems would include those related to feeding, reproduction, caregiving, attachment, exploration, sociability, and fear/wariness. Following ethological theory, Bowlby proposed that the behavior patterns associated with each of these behavioral systems have been selected through evolution because they fulfill a biological function: They help ensure the survival and reproductive success of the individual and his or her genes. The biological function of attachment behavior, as well as of wary behavior, is protection of the youngster from a wide range of dangers. The biological function of exploratory and sociable behavior is that of learning the skills necessary for more self-reliant survival, in terms of both individual skills and smooth integration into the social group.

Behavioral systems[1] include rules that govern the selection, activation, and termination of the behaviors as a specifiable function of the individual's internal state and the environmental context. As implied above, attachment researchers have focused on three specific behavioral systems: attachment, fear/wariness, and exploration. Ainsworth (1990) and Marvin (1997) have suggested that it is useful to think of a fourth, the sociability behavioral system, which is related to children's friendly interactions.

Attachment theory proposes that in normal development, the operation of these four behavioral systems is affected not only by specific environmental and organismic events. They also exhibit a complex dynamic balance among themselves (Ainsworth, 1967), which has the predictable outcome of ensuring that the youngster develops more sophisticated coping skills, but does so within the protective bond to the attachment figure(s). Specifically, when the youngster's attachment and/or wariness behavior systems are minimally activated, its exploration and/or sociability behavior systems can easily be activated. Activation of the wariness system serves as a terminating condition for the exploration and/or sociability systems, and at the same time as an activating condition for the attachment behavior system. Proximity or contact with the attachment figure then often serves to minimize activation of the attachment and wariness behavioral systems, which in turn can reactivate the exploration and/or sociability systems. This is part of the underlying control system for what Ainsworth (1967, pp. 345–346) described as "using the mother as a secure base for exploration." Finally, as many mothers, fathers, babysitters, and child care providers know, a strongly activated exploration system can reduce activation of the attachment system.

One can see a delightful, if somewhat disjointed, illustration of this equilibration process in a child between the ages of 18 and 30 months who is greeted by a friendly adult stranger in the presence of the attachment figure. The child will sometimes retreat warily to the attachment figure, and from the security of that position become interested in the stranger, make a partial approach to the stranger, retreat again to the attachment figure in wariness, and then repeat the process a number of times. Repeated oscillation through this equilibration process is analogous, in control theory terms, to having separate thermostatically controlled heating and cooling systems in a single room, with slightly different settings on their separate thermostats. There is some evidence that as the youngster develops through the preschool years, the organization among these four behavior systems changes and becomes more elaborate (e.g., Greenberg & Marvin, 1982). There is also some evidence that in young children raised in environments extremely dissimilar from the "environment of evolutionary adaptedness" (e.g., in a maltreating or institutional setting without consistent caregivers), these four behavior systems often do not exhibit this equilibrated organization, leading to what could appropriately be called a developmental disorder (e.g., Goldberg, Marvin, & Sabbagh, 1996; O'Connor et al., 2003; see review by Dozier & Rutter, Chapter 29, this volume).

Complexity of Behavioral Systems

Drawing from ethology, Bowlby (1969/1982) proposed that behavioral systems differ not only in function but also in their structural complexity. The simplest is a reflex—a highly stereotyped behavior activated by a stimulus at a specific threshold and carried to completion. A more complex behavior, called a "fixed action pattern" by ethologists, is also a highly stereotyped behavior activated and terminated by specific stimuli, but its threshold for activation varies according to the state of the organism, and it often makes use of some feedback from the environment during its execution. Several social displays of birds and fish are of this type. Many of the basic attachment behaviors that Ainsworth (1967) identified, such as grasping, crying, and smiling, might also be considered fixed action patterns.

Although quite primitive when considered in isolation, these simple behavior patterns can assume an elegant complexity when placed in the context in which they evolved. In the case of attachment behavior, the context is one of close proximity to a caregiver who responds with specific behaviors that complement the infant's behavior. The immediate effect of many behaviors is to bring about a change in the environment, which itself serves as an activating condition for another behavior, often forming a lengthy sequence with an eventual outcome that is necessary for the individual's survival. For example, when a hungry neonate cries, that behavior *predictably* activates the maternal behavior of picking the infant up and placing him or her at the breast. The picking up, or at least the stimulus of the breast or nipple on the infant's face, terminates the cry and activates rooting. This predictably brings the infant's mouth in contact with the nipple, which serves as a terminating condition for rooting and an activating condition for grasping the nipple with the lips. The stimulus of the nipple in the mouth in turn activates sucking, and finally liquid in the mouth stimulates swallowing. Although the complexity and predictability of this sequence might appear purposeful, goal-directed, or (in Bowlby's terms) "goal-corrected" on the part of the infant, in fact

it is not. Interruption of the sequence at any point will lead to failure of the overall sequence, unless the probable cry causes the caregiver to reactivate and correct the sequence. Instead, Bowlby referred to these behaviors as having a specified "predictable outcome," as long as the behavior is executed in an environment similar to the one in which the behavior evolved. In the case of rooting, for example, the predictable outcome is food intake. The predictable outcome of attachment behaviors more generally is proximity and/or contact with a caregiver/attachment figure. This construct of a predictable outcome is especially important for at least two reasons. First, it allows us to understand relatively simple forms of behavior as achieving an important outcome without our inferring that the youngster executed the behavior intentionally, despite the fact that the behavior sequence occurs in a predictable way. Second, it forces us to view these simple behavior patterns as taking place in a dyadic or larger context: They have little meaning if they are not described and understood in the relationship context in which they evolved.

A yet more complicated pattern of behavior is a goal-corrected pattern. Like the simpler forms of behavior, goal-corrected behaviors have activating and terminating conditions, as well as predictable outcomes, but they achieve the outcome through a more sophisticated process. The process is one of choosing, from a repertoire of behaviors, specific ones that progressively bring the individual closer to achieving the goal state or "set goal." Since Bowlby first published *Attachment* in 1969, this construct of purposeful behavior has become commonplace in the study of motor and cognitive development, and is implicit in much research on social development.

In order to engage in goal-corrected behavior, an organism must have an especially complex, dynamic, internal representation of relevant aspects of self, his or her behavior, the environment, and the object or person toward whom the behavior is directed. Bowlby used the term "internal working model" (IWM) for these representations, but he also referred to them as "representational models," which are loosely equivalent to Piagetian "schemes." IWMs are not static images, but flexible models that are used to understand and predict one's relations with the environment, and to construct complex sequences of behavior based on plans that can achieve specific, internally represented outcomes from a variety of starting points. When a goal-corrected behavior sequence, such as moving toward the caregiver in order to make physical contact, is activated, the child continuously orients its behavior and selects alternative behaviors, based in part on the feedback received from the effects of the behavior. When the set goal is achieved, the perceived discrepancy between the set goal and the organism's state is reduced to zero, and the behavioral plan terminates. The theory posits that there is a logical parallel between the organization of behavior and that of the IWM. The structure of IWMs therefore can be inferred from observing the organization of behavior across situations. Although the operation of IWMs often takes place within awareness, for reasons of information-processing efficiency much takes place outside of awareness, especially as the operation becomes more automatic (see Bretherton & Munholland, Chapter 5, this volume).

Drawing again from the work of the ethologists, Bowlby (1969/1982) proposed that there are variations in how behaviors, and behavior systems, are coordinated into more complex wholes. Among them are the following:

1. Very simple behaviors can be coordinated in chain-linked sequences, with the terminating condition for one behavior serving as the activating condition for the next. This is the context for many of the complex sequences of interaction that take place between mother and infant during the first months of life.

2. There can be chains with alternative links. In this case, when one link in the chain fails to achieve an outcome that activates the next link in the chain, some other link is activated in a non-goal-corrected manner. For example, Ainsworth (1967) described how an infant of 3 months or so may look at the caregiver and smile and babble, and if that behavior does not result in contact, it is terminated and crying is activated.

3. Complex, goal-corrected behavior patterns can themselves be organized together in chain-linked sequences, with the terminating condition for the first goal-corrected pattern serving as the activating condition for the second.

4. An action based on one behavior system alternates with an action based on another system. Ethologists have found that these complex sequences, derived from two or more conflicting behavior systems, often form the basis for important social interactions and communicative signals.

5. Partially executed behaviors from one behavior system can occur simultaneously with partially executed behaviors from another, conflicting

behavior system. Sensitive parents and clinicians frequently use these cues in making inferences about a child's emotional state, and again these behaviors have been found by ethologists to form the basis for many important communicative displays.

An example specifically relevant to this chapter is that of coy expressions in older preschool children (see Marvin, 1997). Whether displayed in an alternating or a simultaneous manner, conflicting behavioral tendencies have long been of interest to ethologists and clinicians as cues to behavior and internal events occurring under stress. As will be discussed below, however, they are also important for studying the elaboration of behavior systems through ontogeny.

Ontogeny of Behavioral Systems

The final step in laying the groundwork for Bowlby's model of the ontogeny of attachment is to outline the three processes that he proposed as basic to development in general. First, in their early forms, behaviors are sometimes directed toward objects in the environment that differ from those to which they are directed in their mature form. Usually the range of stimuli that elicit a particular behavior becomes restricted over the course of development. Second, behavior systems that are functional early in development are often of a very simple type. Over the course of development, these simpler systems tend to become superseded by more complex, sophisticated ones. This often involves a simpler system becoming incorporated into a more complex system of goal-corrected behaviors organized into plan hierarchies, with their correspondingly complex IWMs. Third, whereas some behavior systems are functional in simple form early in development, others start out being executed only partially, in a nonfunctional way, or in an inappropriate place in a behavioral sequence. In this case, the important developmental process is the integration of these nonfunctional components into functional wholes at an appropriate point in development.

Among the most important implications of this third process is that once a behavior system has become organized, it assumes some inherent stability, like other open systems (Ashby, 1956; Thelen & Ulrich, 1991). It may maintain the same organization even if it has developed along nonfunctional lines, and may persist even in the absence of the external and internal conditions in which it developed. This part of the developmental model has clear implications for the study of developmental psychopathology. However, it also has important implications for more adaptive development: It suggests both that there may be systemic, structurally based sensitive periods in development, and that beyond a certain point in development, it may be especially difficult (albeit not impossible) for a developmental process or outcome to take shape in a "normal" fashion.

From the perspective of further advances in attachment theory and general developmental theories, an especially exciting body of current research is that stemming from the "natural experiment" involving children adopted from Eastern European orphanages (e.g., O'Connor et al., 2003; Rutter et al., 2007; Zeanah, Smyke, Koga, & Carlson, 2005). Although perhaps even more complex than Bowlby anticipated, the results and theoretical implications of this research suggest that he was correct in attempting to focus researchers and clinicians on three developmental processes: changes and restriction of range of activating conditions; simpler systems becoming incorporated into more complex systems; and the limitations associated with the increased stability of behavior systems as they become integrated into more complex wholes.

THE ONTOGENY OF ATTACHMENT

Development of Attachment during the First Year of Life

Bowlby proposed four phases in the development of the attachment behavioral system—the first three occurring during the first year of life, and the fourth beginning sometime around the child's third birthday.

Phase I: Orientation and Signals without Discrimination of Figure

Consistent with much new research of the 1960s was Bowlby's proposal that immediately or very soon after birth, babies respond to stimuli in a manner that increases the likelihood of continued contact with other humans. In a complementary way, a baby's signal and motor systems are especially adept at eliciting interest and caregiving from other humans, so that proximity, physical contact, nutrition, and warmth are the predictable outcomes. In this sense, the development of the infant's attachment behavior cannot be fully understood except as taking place in the context of

the complementary behavior, and changes in the behavior, of his or her caregivers. Although extensive consideration of these caregiving behaviors and their developmental changes is beyond the scope of this chapter (but see, e.g., Britner, Marvin, & Pianta, 2005; George & Solomon, 1996 and Chapter 35, this volume; Marvin & Britner, 1996), they are assumed at all times.

During this first phase, a baby and a caregiver engage in much interaction, and from the perspective of the caregiver's behavior, many of these interactions are goal-corrected. From the perspective of the baby's own behavioral organization and control, there are *predictable outcomes* of the behaviors, rather than set goals. Thus, during Phase I, the infant's IWMs are present but primitive, and are probably limited to internal "on-again, off-again" experiences associated with the activation and termination of individual behaviors. In this sense, the functioning of the young infant's IWMs are no more separate from actual behaviors than in Stage I of Piaget's (1952) theory of the sensorimotor period.

At birth or very soon thereafter, every sensory system in the infant is working, and these systems continue to improve in functioning. Discrimination is relatively poor in some of them; yet there is much evidence that the sensory systems are structured so that the baby is particularly likely to respond to behavior from humans in general (Bowlby, 1969/1982).

Among the sensory systems especially important in the development of attachment behavior are the auditory and visual systems. At or soon after birth, most infants are capable of visual orientation and tracking, and are especially responsive to contour and pattern, especially if the stimulus is moving slowly. By no later than 4 weeks of age, most infants exhibit a preference for looking at the human face compared to other objects (McGraw, 1943; Wolff, 1969). And very soon after birth, infants tend to quiet and attend to soft auditory stimuli, and appear especially responsive to the human voice. Infants, and even full-term fetuses, recognize and prefer their own mothers' voices to that of a stranger (Kisilevsky et al., 2003). During this first phase, each of these systems has its own activating and terminating conditions, and there is as yet no "internal" connection between the systems. For example, hearing a human voice does not yet activate visual search behavior. Reaching, grasping, and clinging are also crucial attachment behaviors in all primates, and they develop relatively late in humans. It is not until after about 2 months of age that the human infant's grasp is highly developed and controlled by anything other than a reflex-like process of activation by stimulation of the palm region of the hand. It is at about this same time that the visual system becomes chain-linked with the motor system in a manner allowing the infant to make ballistic-like movements toward an object in the visual field. Finally, smiling and crying are additional important attachment behaviors displaying a similar developmental course. Smiling tends to be activated, and crying terminated, in a relatively automatic way by a range of specific conditions. These conditions become increasingly selective and integrated within more complex behavior systems over the first 6 months.

Thus at first it is largely the caregiver who maintains proximity and protects the infant, despite the fact that the newborn is equipped to be especially responsive to other humans, and to elicit caregiving and affection from them. Over the course of the first weeks of life, these patterns of infant–caregiver interaction are repeated frequently. If the caregiver's initiations and responses are well attuned to the infant's behaviors (i.e., if the baby's attachment behaviors are predictably terminated by the caregiver's behavior), then stable patterns of interaction are established. These reciprocal patterns of caregiver–infant behaviors ultimately minimize the frequency and intensity of such attachment behaviors as crying, and more readily elicit other behaviors, such as visual orientation and smiling. In this context the infant is seen as establishing its own behavioral and autoregulatory rhythms (e.g., Stern, 1985), so that stable internal and dyadic rhythms are becoming established at the same time.

Bowlby (1969/1982) proposed that in the environment of evolutionary adaptedness, Phase I lasts from birth to sometime between 8 and 12 weeks of age. He suggested, however, that under unfavorable conditions this phase can last much longer.

Phase II: Orientation and Signals Directed toward One or More Discriminated Figures

The shift from Phase I to Phase II is gradual, and it takes place earlier with some attachment behaviors and complex attachment behavior patterns than with others (Ainsworth, 1967; Bowlby, 1969/1982). Three related issues are important in defining this transition.

First, during Phase II, there is an elaboration of simple behavior systems into more complex ones. The simple behavior systems characteristic of the Phase I infant become integrated within the infant into complex, chain-linked behavior systems. The primary focus here is on the *control* of the individual systems. Whereas in Phase I the caregiver provides the conditions for terminating one behavioral link in a chain and activating the next, during Phase II the infant assumes much of this control. Many of the sensorimotor advances of the 3- to 6-month-old infant illustrate this shift in behavioral control. For example, as early as 3 months of age, perception of the bottle or breast itself serves as an activating stimulus for opening the mouth, and often for bringing the hand(s) toward the mouth (Hetzer & Ripin, 1930, cited in Bowlby, 1969/1982). By 4 months the infant's visual system begins to activate the motor behavior of reaching for an object. Through a reciprocal feedback process, the infant alternates its gaze between hand and the object, and then grasps the object. By 5 months the infant is so adept at this that he or she is able to reach out and grasp parts of the mother's body and clothing while being held by her, or as she is leaning over the infant. By the end of the first year of life, infants clearly understand the causal mechanism of reaching, grasping, and attaining an object (Sommerville & Woodward, 2005). Other researchers have studied related developmental elaborations, using other theoretical models positing self-organization from multiple components (e.g., Hsu & Fogel, 2003; Piaget, 1952; Thelen & Ulrich, 1991).

The second defining issue for Phase II is the restriction of range of effective activating and terminating conditions. Bowlby proposed that as infant and caregiver repeat these sequences of interaction, and as the sequences come increasingly under the infant's control in this chain-linked fashion, there is a tendency for the activating and terminating conditions to become restricted to those that are most commonly part of the behavioral sequence (cf. Thelen & Ulrich's, 1991, notion of "attractor states"). Specifically, Phase II is operationally defined in terms of the infant differentiating between the most familiar caregivers and others in directing his or her attachment behavior.

Drawing from Ainsworth (1967), Bowlby (1969/1982) identified 13 relatively complex patterns of behavior that are differentially displayed toward one figure, usually the mother. At least seven of these differential attachment patterns develop during Phase II, while the remainder probably emerge during Phase III. Each of the patterns can be described in terms of relatively complex, chain-linked systems of behavior, now directed primarily toward one or a few principal caregivers. The behavior patterns that develop during Phase II are differential: termination of crying; crying when the caregiver leaves; smiling; vocalization; visual–motor orientation; greeting; and climbing and exploring.

A third and equally important component of Phase II is the infant's increasing tendency to initiate attachment–caregiving and sociable interactions with the principal caregiver(s). Ainsworth (1967) observed that as early as 2 months of age, and increasingly thereafter, infants are active in seeking interaction rather than passively responding to it. Thus, in at least two ways, the infant of Phase II is assuming increasing responsibility for gaining and maintaining contact and interaction with attachment figure(s): initiating more of the interaction, and being able to exert more control over the interaction through the use of increasingly complex chain-linked behaviors.

The elaboration of chain-linked behavior systems, and the infant's increasingly differential attachment and sociable behavior, may also have important implications for describing the distinct developmental pathways toward the individual differences in patterns of attachment discovered by Ainsworth (e.g., Ainsworth et al., 1978; see Weinfield, Sroufe, Egeland, & Carlson, Chapter 4, this volume), and found to be applicable to preschoolers (Cassidy & Marvin, 1992), young school-age children (Main & Cassidy, 1988), and adults (Main, Kaplan, & Cassidy, 1985). There is substantial evidence that the pathways to differential strategies of attachment begin in the first quarter of the first year of life. For example, parents of infants who are later "avoidant" tend to terminate their infants' cries less often and hold them less during the first months of life (Ainsworth et al., 1978). In such a case, an infant is left in a "painful" state for considerable periods of time. The context is then ripe for the infant eventually to develop alternative links in its behavioral chains, in which some behavior on the part of the infant terminates its distress (e.g., turning its focus in a rather forced manner to exploration). The patterns of infant–parent interaction along this developmental pathway can become stabilized through the same processes at work in the normative, eventually "secure" infant, leading to an avoidant strategy and a tendency for the infant to contribute to the perpetuation of the pattern. The divergent developmental pathway of the "resistant" infant develops

according to an analogous process (Ainsworth, 1967; Cassidy & Berlin, 1994).

Finally, these characteristics of Phase II have implications for describing the nature of the infant's IWMs. Most importantly, the infant can increasingly differentiate his or her primary caregiver(s) from others, and in that sense "know" who the caregiver or caregivers are. However, the infant cannot yet conceive of an attachment figure as someone with a separate existence from his or her own experience. Consistent with Piaget's (1952) theory of Stages II and III of the sensorimotor period, Bowlby's theory also implies that this infant's IWMs parallel its chain-linked sequences of behavior: The infant's awareness has expanded to encompass the continuity represented by these relatively complex sequences, but not yet to the point where he or she can use internal experimentation or manipulation of images, goals, and intentions to devise a plan for achieving a set goal.

Phase III: Maintenance of Proximity to a Discriminated Figure by Locomotion and Signals

Phase III, beginning sometime between 6 and 9 months of age, is the phase during which the infant is thought to consolidate attachment to its caregiver(s). It is characterized by a number of important motor, cognitive, and communicative changes, as well as changes in the organization among behavioral systems. Although some would consider an infant in Phase II to be attached because his or her attachment behavior is differential toward one or a few adults, it is during Phase III that most experts would consider the infant to be "really" attached, due to the organizational changes in behavior.

New Attachment Behaviors. The most notable change is the onset of locomotion. As an addition to the behaviors available to the attachment system, locomotion provides the infant with a vastly increased ability to control proximity to the attachment figure, and to move off to explore, to expand his or her horizons in innumerable ways, but also to place him- or herself in significant danger. In fact, four of the six additional attachment behaviors that Ainsworth (1967) identified are based on this newly developed motor skill. These behaviors, and the earliest ages at which Ainsworth observed them, are as follows: differential approach to mother, especially on reunion or when distressed, 28 weeks; differential following of mother when she leaves the room, 24 weeks; use of mother as a secure base for exploration (making exploratory excursions from mother, returning to her from time to time, and terminating exploratory behavior and attempting to regain proximity if she moves off), 28 weeks; and flight to mother as a haven of safety when alarmed, 34 weeks. Two other attachment behaviors to emerge during this same period depend less directly on locomotion, although they are often organized together with it (Ainsworth, 1967). These are differential burying of face (while climbing on the mother; or after an excursion away from her, baby buries face in mother's lap), 28 weeks; and differential clinging to the mother when alarmed, ill, or distressed, 43 weeks. By 6–8 months, the baby is able to cling to the caregiver in a rather automatic way as the infant's attention is directed elsewhere.

Information Processing and IWMs. A second and equally revolutionary change associated with the shift to Phase III is an elaboration of the infant's cognitive skills. Some of the systems mediating a child's attachment behavior and many of the earlier, chain-linked behaviors become organized under the infant's intentional control. Bowlby suggested that the Phase III infant has an internal image of an end state or "set goal" that he or she would like to achieve (e.g., physical contact with the attachment figure). The infant can now operate internally on available behaviors (i.e., a plan) and select behaviors that are likely to achieve this set goal (e.g., crawl around the sofa to mother); execute the plan; alter it as a function of feedback; and then terminate the plan when the discrepancy between the set goal and the infant's perception of his or her position is reduced to zero.

This describes, in control systems terminology, what traditional cognitive theorists have referred to as the infant's newly emerging ability to differentiate means from ends. The ability to organize attachment behavior on a goal-corrected basis also implies that the infant now has an internal image of the attachment figure that is independent of perception (object permanence). In a rather elegant longitudinal study, Bell (1970) demonstrated the parallel (in Piaget's terms, the "horizontal decalage") between the development of object permanence, person (mother) permanence, and the onset of goal-corrected proximity seeking. Consistent with the proposition that children will develop such a general-purpose skill first in relationship-based and emotionally salient contexts, Bell found that most infants developed person permanence before object permanence.

The baby's set goal in interactions with the attachment figure will vary from time to time. Sometimes the set goal will be maintaining some distance from the attachment figure while exploring the social and physical world. At other times it will be mere proximity, or nothing short of close physical contact. What "setting" a goal takes at any given time is the result of many factors, including physiological state (e.g., hunger, fatigue); the presence or absence of an alarming event in the environment; assessment of the caregiver's attention to the infant; and whether the caregiver is present, departing/absent, or returning from an absence (Bowlby, 1969/1982). It will also depend on the dyad's history of relatively stable patterns (i.e., individual differences) of attachment–caregiving interactions.

Communication Skills. Concurrent with these locomotor and cognitive changes are those in the infant's communication skills, both nonverbal and language-based. During Phase II the infant displays increased visual and vocal engagement with others, and much of his or her interaction is of a turn-taking, prelanguage format, to which caregivers tend to respond as if it were intentional (Bates, O'Connell, & Shore, 1987; Bruner, 1981). During Phase III the infant uses communicative signals in a goal-corrected manner, as part of a repertoire of plans for achieving a set goal that often involves regulating the behavior of others for purposes of requesting or rejecting actions or objects; attracting or maintaining another's attention; and/or establishing/maintaining joint attention for purposes of sharing an experience (Bruner, 1981). At first through the infant's display and understanding of nonverbal utterances and signals, later through single-word utterances, and still later (at 18–36 months of age) complex verbal communication, youngster and caregiver(s) are now able to alter each other's behavior indirectly by directly altering each other's set goals (Marvin, 1977).

All these changes have important implications for the Phase III baby's IWMs. At this point the baby has separate models of caregiver(s) and of self. These consist of images and plans ordered in some form of a hierarchy—or event schemas or scripts (Nelson & Gruendel, 1981; Stern, 1985)—of self and other, based on the newly developed ability to operate internally on the images and likely behaviors that were chain-linked during Phase II. The content of the infant's IWMs are probably derived from some combination of the stable, chain-linked sequences of interaction already developed in interaction with the caregiver(s) and the newly stabilizing patterns that emerge with the motor, cognitive, and communication skills developing during Phase III.

Although they are much more sophisticated than in Phase II, even in Phase III the infant's IWMs remain primitive in at least two ways. First, the infant is limited, at least early in this phase, to thinking about caregiver and self only in terms of their behaviors. The infant has yet to comprehend that the attachment figure has unique perceptions and goals, and that these can differ from his or her own. Second, early in this phase the infant is unable to think about behaviors in terms of long sequences. The early Phase III infant's ability to operate in this internal fashion is limited to individual goal–plan hierarchies or event schemas, with each thought activated and terminated by specific stimuli.

The Exploration System. The fourth important change that takes place during Phase III is especially related to the changes in the infant's locomotor and cognitive changes—namely, the elaboration of his exploration behavior system. The development of locomotion and of object permanence, the more sophisticated understanding of mean–ends relations, the ability increasingly to organize exploration on the basis of goal-corrected behavior, and emerging imitation and conversational skills (e.g., Piaget, 1952) all enhance the infant's ability to learn about and interact with the physical and social environment, to test and learn the "rules" that govern those interactions, and to categorize those interactions symbolically and linguistically.

The Sociability System. Closely related to the exploration system is the infant's sociability system. Phase III infants are particularly likely to display wariness toward other conspecifics, yet tend at the same time to be attracted to them. Although there appear to be individual differences related to both temperament and relationship history, infants in this phase are likely to stop exploration when confronted by a strange person, to remain wary (or even fearful) for some moments, and either to remain stationary or to move away from the stranger and toward the attachment figure. After some few moments, if the stranger displays positive affect, is not intrusive, and matches his or her responses to the infant's behavior, the infant is likely to interact sociably, with rapidly decreasing wariness (e.g., Bretherton & Ainsworth, 1974).

The Wariness System. The fifth and final major Phase III change to be considered involves the infant's wariness behavior system. Wariness toward novel, and especially sudden, nonhuman events has obvious survival value. Less obvious are the nature, developmental course, and role played by wariness toward unfamiliar *humans*. Despite the earlier bias toward responding to human stimuli, during the last quarter of the first year infants increasingly are more wary of unfamiliar adults than they are of unfamiliar nonhuman objects (Bretherton & Ainsworth, 1974). Although there may be individual and reproductive gene pool differences in temperamental reactivity to strangers (e.g., Kagan, 1989), this developmental shift appears to exist whether the infant is raised in a culture in which the norm is single or multiple caregivers (cf. Ainsworth, 1967).

Reciprocal linkages among the older infant's wariness, sociability, and attachment behavior systems are more obvious and predictable than they had been earlier. If the wariness system is highly activated, the infant tends to retreat to the parent as a haven of safety; if it is not, the infant may continue to stare at a nonintrusive stranger, or may initiate sociable behavior or respond sociably. In many cases, one can see a cycling of conflicting behavior systems, with the infant moving back and forth from parent to stranger as the distance from each tends to activate one system and terminate the other.

Sensitive Periods. That infants become more, rather than less, wary toward unfamiliar humans over the period from 6 to 18–24 months of age is important for at least two reasons. First, infants *are* vulnerable to danger from other humans, and until they are more able to predict which individuals are dangerous, it is adaptive that their initial reaction be wariness. Second, one of the developmental mechanisms involved in the consolidation of the infant's attachment is the reduction in the range of individuals able to activate and terminate his or her attachment behavior (Bowlby, 1969/1982). The infant comes more and more to approach familiar caregiver(s) and to retreat from unfamiliar individuals of the same species. In its general form, this phenomenon is characteristic of many species, and is common in the study of "sensitive periods" in development (see Bateson, 1976).

There are many examples of sensitive periods in nonhuman and human ontogeny, from the extreme of imprinting in many avian species to that of language development in humans. Bowlby

(1969/1982) proposed that the consolidation of infant–caregiver attachment during Phase III is one such period. The reorganization of the infant's increasingly active attachment behavior along goal-corrected lines, combined with heightened wariness of the unfamiliar and the strong emotions associated with the activation of attachment and wariness behavioral systems, results in this being a period during which the infant is particularly ready to focus attachment behavior and IWMs of attachment on one or a few familiar figures. Presumably, parallel neurological changes take place as well. It is after these changes have stabilized that disruption of the bond is so likely to lead to the short- and sometimes long-term effects that led Bowlby to the study of this early tie.

Bowlby (1969/1982) suggested that the readiness to become quickly attached remains intact at least through the end of the first year. This does not imply that the specific attachment, a more versus less adaptive *form* of attachment, or the lack of an attachment is completely irreversible after this sensitive period. Nor, it is important to note, does it invoke the construct of "critical periods" (see Bateson, 1976). The results from studies of infants placed in foster care or raised in East European orphanages and adopted into low-risk homes suggest that children *can* form discriminating or selective attachments for the first time well after 1 year of age. However, infants placed in foster care after 12 months of age have been found to be more rejecting toward their new caregivers than infants placed at younger ages are (see Dozier & Rutter, Chapter 29, this volume). And contemporary studies of children adopted from orphanages (e.g., Chisholm, Carter, Ames, & Morison, 1995; Goldberg et al., 1996; O'Connor et al., 2003; Rutter et al., 2007) are increasingly indicating that these children form attachments, but that these attachments are at increased risk of being organized in a significantly less adaptive manner than would be expected, given that they are being raised in low-risk homes. One example of organizational anomaly is the surprisingly high incidence of children adopted after 6 months of age who, at 4 and 6 years of age, are classified as securely attached but continue to exhibit disinhibited or indiscriminate attachment and sociable behavior toward strangers and other nonattachment figures.

Organization among Behavioral Systems. It is during Phase III that the dynamic balance described earlier among the four behavioral systems fully emerges (Ainsworth et al., 1978). For most infants, this balance culminates in organizing essentially all the new developments of this phase into what Ainsworth (1990) referred to as the "hallmark" of an attachment—the infant's use of the attachment figure as a secure base for exploration. Stable *variations* in this organization are evident in the different insecure strategies of attachment (Ainsworth et al., 1978; Main & Solomon, 1990). In the "avoidant" strategy, the infant tends, when the attachment system is highly activated, to inhibit attachment behavior and (often) to activate the exploration system. In the "resistant" strategy, the infant tends to overamplify the attachment and wariness systems. In the case of an infant classified as having a "disorganized" attachment, the simultaneous and/or sequential activation and termination of behavior systems are especially contradictory and take a form that puts the infant at risk of not being protected (e.g., activation of the attachment system also serves to activate wary behavior toward the caregiver).

Subordinate Attachment Figures and Types of Relationships. It is apparent that throughout human evolution children have been raised in families, which themselves are part of larger groups of varied size and composition. Most children have experienced multiple caregivers, giving them the opportunity to form specific attachments to a number of figures. Even in his early writings, Bowlby (e.g., 1958) proposed that infants tend to become attached to a number of caregivers, and that "for a child of 18 months to have only one attachment figure is quite exceptional" (Bowlby, 1969/1982, p. 304).

Several studies across many cultures have suggested that a minority of infants select more than one attachment figure almost as soon as they begin to show any differential attachment behavior, whereas a majority do so by 18 months (e.g., Ainsworth, 1967; Konner, 1976; Marvin, Van Devender, Iwanaga, LeVine, & LeVine, 1977; Schaffer & Emerson, 1964). These and other studies (e.g., Myers, Jarvis, & Creasey, 1987), however, suggest that not all attachment figures are treated by the infant as equivalent. Infants are attached to a range of caregivers; however, attachment behavior tends, especially when an infant is distressed, hungry, tired, or ill, to be focused on a particular person when both that person and other attachment figures are available. Thus most infants seem to have a network of attachment figures, but the available data suggest that they may tend to choose one figure as the "primary" attachment figure. Importantly, others may be chosen as the primary figure for play or other types of interactions (see van IJzendoorn & Sagi-Schwartz, Chapter 37, this volume).

Development of Attachment during the Toddler and Preschool Years

Most research on social and emotional development during the postinfancy preschool period has focused on issues other than attachment—for example, autonomy, self-control, independence, and socialization. These issues imply a decline in attachment behavior, as the youngster deals with these later "developmental tasks." Although the framework of developmental tasks can be helpful in guiding our research, it can also lead us astray by restricting the focus to single issues. A full understanding requires viewing development across multiple domains. In fact, while the child *is* becoming more autonomous and self-reliant during the preschool years, he or she remains vulnerable to a range of dangers. The child makes increasingly distant forays from the attachment figure while exploring the environment, but is still at an early point in developing the skills needed for self-protection. The close attachment to the caregiver thus remains crucially important to the child's survival and socialization. It is adaptive, rather than "regressive," that attachment behavior remains easily activated.

The general systems model outlined at the beginning of this chapter suggests a focus on the functional relations among various behavior systems in the child, and between the child's organization and that of caregivers and larger social context, so that (1) the child will be protected from danger; (2) he or she will take increased responsibility in self-protection and the integration of behavior with others; and (3) changes across multiple developmental domains will tend to occur simultaneously.

As we move to the study of attachment in the postinfancy years, we must also be careful not to lose the focus on *behavior* as the child's representational and communicative abilities become increasingly noticeable. Because infants' mental models of attachment cannot possibly be symbolic (i.e., language-based), it must be assumed that those cognitive structures that relate to attachment *behavior* in infancy constitute the mental model (Bretherton, 1993). There is a natural shift in research on attachment past infancy to move more and more to the level of cognitive–

emotional representation. The trap is to move to the cognitive level, to the relative exclusion of behavior. This would be a terrible error. Bowlby's whole theory—or the cognitive-behavioral part of it—is based on the important linkage between IWMs and behavior. The point is that older children do not move from the level of behavior to the level of internal representation; they become able to process and manipulate plans and goals at that internal level, and increasingly to control behavior with that internal processing. We must remember that the function of an IWM is to organize behavior in more flexible ways.

Changes in Attachment Behavior during the Toddler/Preschool Years

Although most of our knowledge about the ontogeny of attachment behavior is restricted to the first 12–15 months of life, a few naturalistic studies (e.g., Blurton-Jones, 1972; Konner, 1976) and a number of laboratory-based studies (e.g., Main & Cassidy, 1988; Marvin, 1977; Marvin & Greenberg, 1982) provide a general outline of the normative course of attachment behavior over the preschool and early school years. In reviewing the literature, Bowlby (1969/1982) suggested that during the second year and most of the third year of life, attachment behavior is shown at neither less intensity nor less frequency than at the first birthday. In fact, use of attachment figures as a secure base is a critical component of the child's rapidly expanding physical and social world, and attachment behavior therefore remains a major part of his or her behavioral organization.

Overall, 2-year-olds tend to maintain as much (or more) proximity to their mothers as do 1-year-olds. At the same time, they also make more extensive excursions away in order to explore with their more elaborate cognitive and motor abilities. Several studies (e.g., Schaffer & Emerson, 1964) have found that a toddler tends actively to monitor not only the mother's movements, but also her attention. When she is not attending to him or her, the child often executes attachment behavior with the set goal of regaining her attention. This adaptive behavior pattern is unappreciated in Western cultures, in which it is commonly seen as regressive or controlling "attention seeking," and as such is frustrating to parents.

Before the third birthday, a child is not very adept at maintaining proximity to the attachment figure when the figure is moving. The perception of the caregiver moving off is typically a condition that terminates the toddler's exploratory behavior and activates attachment behavior. At this younger age, a child can follow the caregiver around the familiar home, but finds it difficult to follow if he or she is moving steadily off. In this situation, one or both members of the dyad initiate physical contact, and the toddler is carried. After the third birthday, with much improved locomotor skills, the child is much less likely to be carried under relaxed circumstances. In fact, in his study of the Zhuntwa hunter–gatherers, Konner (1976) found that in day-to-day living, children in that culture maintain very close physical ties with their mothers until sometime between 3 and 4 years of age, after which ties to the multiage peer group become increasingly important.

When undergoing a separation from their mothers that is not of their own initiative, 2-year-olds tend to be as distressed as 1-year-olds, although they are more able to rely on calling and active search behaviors rather than crying. Many 3- and 4-year-olds also become mildly upset by such brief separations, but they are less so than 2-year-olds, and they are more willing than younger children to be left for brief periods in the company of friendly adults. By the third birthday, it appears that it is being left *alone* that is especially upsetting and likely to elicit strong attachment behavior. If briefly left alone, or if mildly distressed by being left with a friendly adult, most 3- and 4-year-olds are able to wait for the attachment figure's return before executing attachment behavior (Marvin, 1977).

When the caregiver returns after a brief, laboratory separation, 2-year-olds tend to seek proximity and contact in much the same way as 1-year-olds, albeit with much more locomotor efficiency. They also tend to require a short period of physical contact with the caregiver before being able to move off again to explore, and display the same secure, avoidant, resistant/ambivalent, and disorganized strategies in forms so similar to those of 1-year-olds that the same attachment classification procedure (Ainsworth et al., 1978) can be used, with only minor changes and extrapolation.

By the third birthday things have changed. At least partially because they are less distressed by brief separations, most children 3 years of age and older seem to require less physical contact with the attachment figure on reunion before returning to exploration. In one study, however, most 3-year-olds did seek brief proximity to their mothers before returning to exploration, in spite of the fact that they were less distressed by the separation than 2-year-olds were (Marvin, 1977). Four-year-olds, especially boys, were less likely to seek physical proximity or contact on reunion than the 1- to 3-year-olds.

Whereas there is clearly a decrease in physical proximity and contact across the preschool period, it is not the case that an older child is any less attached than an infant is to the caregiver(s). In addition to the obvious fact that older children continue to retreat to their attachment figures when distressed or frightened, at least two lines of research suggest that the *organization* of the attachment system changes significantly between the ages of 3 and 5 years. First, Marvin (1977) and Marvin and Greenberg (1982) found that 4-year-olds, but not 3-year-olds, tended not to be distressed by brief separations if they and their mothers had negotiated or agreed upon a shared plan regarding the separation and reunion prior to the mothers' departure. The 3-year-olds tended to accept or protest the impending departure, but did not negotiate a shared plan. Second, Cassidy and Marvin (1992) and Main and Cassidy (1988) found physical proximity and contact to be less important in distinguishing among strategies of attachment in preschool and early school-age children than in infants and toddlers. These older children increasingly organized their intimate interactions with their attachment figures on the basis of physical orientation, eye contact, nonverbal expressions, and affect, as well as conversations about personal matters (e.g., the separation and reunion, feelings, and shared activities and plans).

These two lines of research suggest the importance of Bowlby's (1969/1982) proposed final phase in the development of attachment, the "goal-corrected partnership." They are also congruent with earlier research suggesting that sometime around age 4, children are much less dependent on physical proximity and contact with their attachment figure(s) to maintain a sense of security, and are increasingly comfortable spending appreciable periods of time in the company of nonfamilial peers and adults (Blurton-Jones, 1972; Konner, 1976). In the following sections, we briefly review literature on other developmental domains relevant to the changes in attachment behavior outlined above, and then review the theoretical and empirical work on the goal-corrected partnership.

Developmental Changes in Relations among Behavior Systems

Ainsworth and colleagues (1978) showed how, in 1-year-olds, the attachment, exploration, wariness, and sociability systems function in the dynamic equilibrium described earlier. Observation of young children's behavior when the children are introduced to a friendly adult stranger presents an excellent opportunity to study this dynamic balance, and it has yielded some evidence that this organization changes over the preschool years in a way consistent with a youngster's gradually increased responsibility for protecting him- or herself through increasingly sophisticated behavioral organization.

Greenberg and Marvin (1982) studied young children's initial reactions to a friendly stranger. The most common response among 3- and 4-year-olds was to (apparently) ignore the stranger and continue exploring without activation of either the wariness or attachment behavior systems. The next most common response was the *simultaneous* activation of the wariness and sociability systems (usually in the form of coy expressions) and coincidental activation of the attachment system. No 2-year-olds displayed this more complex pattern. Most children of all three ages eventually played sociably with the stranger. Whereas a few of the younger children remained fearful of the stranger throughout the situation, none of the older children did so. Finally, all 2-year-olds (but none of the 3- or 4-year-olds) who displayed wariness toward the stranger while their mothers were gone also displayed attachment behavior toward the mothers when they returned. Greenberg and Marvin suggested that this decreased developmental coupling of the wariness and attachment behavior systems, and the increased developmental coupling of the wariness and sociability systems, may have important implications for children's increasing ability to cope with strangers on their own. The careful approach implied by the coincidental activation of the wariness and sociability systems, whether in the form of coy expressions or shy conversation, may provide the basis for strategies of social interaction that could fulfill the same protective function earlier fulfilled by the close physical bond between a child and his or her attachment figure(s).

Changes in Locomotor and Self-Care Skills

Humans exhibit a developmental organization during the preschool years similar to that of nonhuman primates during their late infancy—one that suggests the crucial importance of a continuing protective attachment, while at the same time providing a young child with the independence necessary to learn the skills that will be required during the following phase. The emergence of

milk teeth is complete between 2 and 3 years, and by 3 years children are quite independent in feeding themselves. Although Western cultures are now clearly different, in less industrialized cultures breast feeding tapers off between 3 and 4 years of age. By age 3, a child's locomotor skills have developed to the point where he or she can assume much of the responsibility for gaining and maintaining proximity to the attachment figure under most conditions, as well as engage in vigorous play with other children and practice many of the social skills he or she will use in a more stable fashion during the juvenile (school-age) period. By the beginning of the juvenile period, the child is capable of most of the motor skills of older children, although strength, endurance, coordination, and so forth continue to improve.

Changes in Communication Skills

Consistent with studies of nonhuman primates, it is during the preschool period that children develop most of the communication skills that will later be required for stable integration into their social groups, independent of the close physical tie to their attachment figures. By 30 months, children increasingly communicate about past and future events and emotional states, and connected narrative discourse emerges as children begin to relate logical sequences of events across many utterances (e.g., Bretherton, 1993; Dunn, 1994). Dunn (1994) found that during the second and third years children were increasingly able to recognize, understand, and converse about the feelings and behaviors of other family members; they comforted, teased, argued, joked, and blamed. She has concluded that by 3 years of age, which is much younger than previously thought, children understand surprisingly complex rules for social interaction, interpret others' feelings and goals, and use such rules to manipulate others' internal states. It now seems clear that by age 4, most children are becoming competent at one of our species' most sophisticated communication skills: thinking and conversing about the feelings, goals, and plans of others with whom they are interacting (see Lewis & Mitchell, 1994). As Bowlby (1969/1982) and Marvin (1977) have suggested, this skill should have important implications for the organization of attachment interactions.

Although there has been little recent research on the ontogeny of nonverbal expressions in preschool children, some of the early work in human ethology (Blurton-Jones, 1972; Hinde, 1976) suggests that many of the expressions used to regulate interactions during childhood and adolescence develop, and are employed with increasing effectiveness, during the preschool years. Furthermore, studies of coy expressions (Marvin, 1997) and of posed expressions of happiness, surprise, anger, fear, sadness, and disgust (Lewis, Sullivan, & Vasen, 1987) again suggest that the period between the third and fourth birthdays is especially important in the developmental elaboration and understanding of a range of complex expressions used to regulate interactions.

Changes in Information-Processing Skills and IWMs

Extensive research—including the work of Bretherton (1993), Cassidy and Marvin (1992), Dunn (1994), Main and colleagues (1985), Marvin and Greenberg (1982), Miljkovitch, Pierrehumbert, Bretherton, and Halfon (2004), Nelson and Gruendel (1981), Slough and Greenberg (1990), Stern (1985), and Waters and Waters (2006)—suggests that during the second through sixth years of life, children are elaborating more and more sophisticated and accurate (in the sense of nonegocentric) IWMs of both their own and others' behavior and internal experiences. At the same time, they are developing surprisingly sophisticated IWMs of implicit and explicit rules for social behavior and interaction. The reader is referred to the studies listed above and to other chapters in this volume for information about the *content* of, and individual differences in, these IWMs; in this section we focus on developmental changes in their underlying *form*.

This work was not available at the time Bowlby (1969/1982) first developed his model or when Marvin (1977) expanded it. Bowlby's model of information processing during the preschool years relied predominantly on Piaget's (e.g., 1952) theory of the preoperational stage, and the role played by the child's emerging ability to make accurate inferences about others' goals. Although not contradictory to Piaget's theory, Bowlby's model is actually more consistent with contemporary work on cognition and with script and event representation theories (see Bretherton & Munholland, Chapter 5, this volume; Nelson & Gruendel, 1981).

Drawing on Bowlby's general model of the organization and ontogeny of behavioral systems, Marvin (1977) proposed that the developmental changes in IWMs during the preschool years should demonstrate a formal parallel to the changes Bowlby had earlier identified with respect to behavioral organization and development in general. Specifi-

cally, the early Phase III IWM has developed to the point where the toddler is able to represent individual goal-corrected image–plan hierarchies. At that point, the internal "experiments" the child conducts take place as image sequences, in which images serve as activating and terminating conditions for other images. These schemas or action representations can also be activated or terminated by conditions or events in the child's environment. As Phase III progresses, the toddler establishes a growing number of increasingly complex, internal, "chain-linked" action images (or "event representations"). Consistent with more recent work (see Bretherton, 1993), these links may actually take the form of a network rather than a linear chain. It is these structures that the preschool child is so curious and energetic in building, as to be constantly asking, "Why?" in an attempt to establish more links in the network. It is also in the context of conversations between the youngster and caregivers that so many of these links are established (Bretherton, 1993; Dunn, 1994).

Marvin (1977) proposed that one important component of this elaboration is the child's eventual ability to inhibit the execution of a plan in order to formulate a more complex IWM of the situation, devise a more complex plan for achieving a given set goal, or postpone execution of some step in a plan until an anticipated and appropriate link in the chain exists. With the concurrent elaboration of conversational skills, this ability to inhibit ongoing thought and behavior sets the stage for the child to "insert" one of the caregiver's plans or goals into his or her own action plan. Thus the child and caregiver are able to interact under a shared goal plan hierarchy, or a partnership (Bowlby, 1969/1982).

There is, however, an additional parallel (in Piagetian terms, a "vertical decalage") between the operation of the Phase II infant's behavior and that of the older child in this partnership. At first, the partnership between child and attachment figure is a predictable outcome of their interaction, and is not (yet) goal-corrected on the child's part. This youngster cannot alter the goals or plans of self or other *in order* to achieve a shared goal or plan. That is, the youngster cannot internally *operate on* this emerging network of event representations; he or she can only *operate behaviorally in terms of* them. In order for these internal events themselves to operate in a goal-corrected manner, they need the input (increased "variety," in the terms of Ashby, 1956) of another person who already has that ability.

Later in this phase (sometime between 3½ and 5 years of age, the child's information processing skills undergo a further hierarchical reorganization (Marvin, 1977), in line with Piaget's theory of the shift to the intuitive period, followed soon by concrete operations. This reorganization is essentially a "second-order" abstraction, through which the child is now able internally to operate in a goal-corrected manner on an already existing network of event representations. No longer limited to sequential processing through a chain-linked network of thoughts–images–plans, this older preschooler can now comprehend two or more of these images as component parts of a yet higher-order image–goal–plan. This is consistent with what Piaget (1952) termed "operational reversibility." One type of this higher-order image or schema is a representation of the coordination of the child's own plans with those of another with whom he or she is interacting. Whereas the younger preschool child is able to think of and converse about the goals and plans of self and others, he or she is unable to operate on them simultaneously. Although the child will often refer to others' internal events, and will often do so "correctly," Marvin (1977) suggested that this limitation should often result in the child confusing his or her own perspective with that of the other.

Once the child's IWMs have achieved this later hierarchical reorganization, however, the child should be able internally to operate on his or her own perspective and representation of the caregiver's perspective simultaneously; this enables the child to keep them distinct, to recognize when they are shared or in conflict, and to organize a plan to construct a *shared* perspective. If this shared perspective becomes a new set goal in the child's relationship with the caregiver, then the child should (1) become disequilibrated or distressed when that set goal of a shared set of plans is unattainable; and (2) execute plans to establish that shared perspective, usually by attempting to change the caregiver's goals.

There remains some controversy regarding the age by which a young child is able to make such complex inferences about others' internal events and their relations to his or her own (see Lewis & Mitchell, 1994). There is ample evidence that between the second and third birthdays children come to realize that others have their own feelings, goals, and plans, and that their IWMs are significantly influenced by that realization. There is also evidence that by the fourth birthday most children are able accurately to distinguish between

their own and others' perspectives, and simultaneously maintain both perspectives in awareness while assessing whether or not they match (Marvin, Greenberg, & Mossler, 1976). By this same age, most children are able to reason in a nonegocentric manner about the causal relations between others' goals and plans and the others' behavior (Greenberg, Marvin, & Mossler, 1977). These are all component skills that allow a child and caregiver *both* to take responsibility, when their goals or plans conflict, in negotiating in a goal-corrected way toward a shared set of plans.

Over the last two decades, there has been an explosion of research on children's "theory of mind," or their ability to recognize and infer their own and others' mental states. A review is beyond the scope of this chapter, but studies of theory of mind have both supported the developmental timetables outlined in attachment research and advanced our understanding of the ontogenetic processes by which social perspective taking and interpersonal relations are elaborated. See, for example, recent research by Sabbagh, Xu, Carlson, Moses, and Lee (2006) on the development of executive functioning and preschoolers' theory of mind across cultures; Pears and Moses (2003) on parenting strategies and preschoolers' theory of mind; and Cahill, Deater-Deckard, Pike, and Hughes (2007) on how mother–child warmth and responsiveness (cornerstones of attachment research) moderate the relation between preschoolers' theory of mind and self-worth.

Phase IV: Implications of the Partnership for the Organization of Attachment Behavior during the Preschool Years

Although the partnership is certainly a general-purpose skill used in interactions with family members, other adults, and peers, it is likely that it will first be applied in emotionally powerful interactions, such as attachment–caregiving interactions. Marvin (1977) and Marvin and Greenberg (1982) studied its application to this type of interaction and suggested two important organizational changes. The first is related to a young preschooler's ability to inhibit attachment behavior and insert the caregiver's plans into the child's own plan for proximity, resulting in what might be called the "emergent partnership." The second is related to the older preschooler's ability to operate internally on the goals and plans of self and other simultaneously; to understand objectively (i.e., nonegocentrically) the causal relations between the caregiver's goals/plans and behavior; and to engage in goal-corrected negotiations with the caregiver regarding a shared plan for proximity, forming a goal-corrected partnership.

With regard to the first organizational change, Bowlby (1969/1982) proposed that a toddler's attachment plans vary in the extent to which they are designed to influence the behavior of the attachment figure. He suggested that the earliest goal-corrected plans for changing the caregiver's behavior are primitive (e.g., pushing the caregiver in certain directions, knocking a book off his or her lap, throwing a tantrum). These early attempts are based on changing the caregiver's behavior either directly through physical means or indirectly through crying and anger. During this same period, parents rely largely on techniques such as distracting the toddler to influence his or her behavior.

However, the changes associated with the early form of the partnership already outlined offer the dyad a new opportunity. As the dyad's conversational skills become elaborated, and as the child becomes more able to inhibit his or her ongoing behavior, it should become increasingly the case that child and caregiver are able to change each other's behavior indirectly by inserting one of each other's goals or plans into the goal or plan structure of the other through linguistic communication. Although the child cannot yet negotiate a shared plan with the caregiver in a goal-corrected manner, the child *can* attempt to change the caregiver's goal or plan, inhibit ongoing behavior, insert one of the caregiver's goals into his or her own plan for action, and thus function in an interaction that has the "predictable outcome" of shared goals.

Marvin (1977) provided an initial test for this hypothesis by administering two analogous procedures to a sample of 2-, 3-, and 4-year-old children, one relevant to interaction in a nonattachment context (a waiting task), and the other in an attachment–caregiving context (the Strange Situation). The results of both procedures suggest that by 3 years of age a child is usually able to inhibit ongoing, goal-corrected behavior across at least two types of interactions, to insert one of the mother's communicated goals into his or her own plan, and to wait until the circumstances are appropriate for both mother and child before executing the plan. These findings are consistent with Bowlby's (1969/1982) suggestion that by the third birthday children are more able to feel secure in the presence of alternative (even unfamiliar) caregivers, and that the frequency and intensity

of attachment behavior are likely to diminish because of developmental changes in the processes that control its activation and termination. The results are also consistent with the conclusion that the 3-year-old's attachment set goal continues to be represented in physical–spatial–temporal terms, and that separations that are not directly under his or her own control continue to disturb or disequilibrate that set goal.

The results also suggest a further change in the organization of attachment behavior sometime around the fourth birthday. As implied earlier, the hierarchical reorganization of the older preschooler's IWMs and information-processing skills that enables the child to operate in a nonegocentric fashion *simultaneously* on the perspectives of self and others, and to construct shared plans with the caregiver in a goal-corrected manner, should have important implications for the organization of attachment behavior. Marvin (1977) suggested that at least five component skills are involved: (1) the ability to recognize that the attachment figure possesses internal events (including thoughts, goals, plans, feelings, etc.); (2) the ability to distinguish between the caregiver's point of view and the child's own, especially when they differ; (3) the ability to infer, from logic and/or experience, what factors control the caregiver's goals and plans; (4) the ability to assess the degree of coordination, or match, between their respective points of view; and (5) the ability to influence the caregiver's goals and plans in a goal-corrected manner. On the basis of much research over the past 30 years (see Bretherton, 1993; Dunn, 1994; Greenberg et al., 1977), it seems possible that by 3 years of age and certainly by 4, children possess the first two component skills. In a series of studies, Marvin and his colleagues (e.g., Greenberg et al., 1977; Marvin, 1977; Marvin & Greenberg, 1982; Marvin et al., 1976; Stewart & Marvin, 1984) studied these five components and how they are associated with the organization of the child's attachment behavior in 2- to 6-year-old children. The results of these studies suggest that by their fourth birthdays, most children raised in low-risk settings have all five skills.

Marvin and Greenberg (1982) examined the behavior patterns of young children during leave-taking, separation, and reunion events. The purpose was to see whether those children who demonstrated the communication and perspective-taking components required for a goal-corrected partnership in fact behaved during the Strange Situation in a manner consistent with such developmental reorganization. Simply stated, the model suggests that the set goal for these children should no longer be mere physical proximity or contact; rather, it should be a *shared plan for that proximity*. Using specific behavioral criteria based on this model, Marvin and Greenberg found that most of the 3-year-olds conformed to the separation and reunion pattern consistent with the emergent partnership (i.e., the set goal was still structured in terms of physical proximity and contact), whereas most of the 4-year-olds conformed to the pattern consistent with the goal-corrected partnership. The expected association between level of partnership and ability to reason objectively about the mother's perspective and behavior also emerged. Stewart and Marvin (1984) found essentially the same within-child association between accurate perspective-taking components and separation–reunion behavior patterns that reflected a goal-corrected partnership.

These studies of developmental changes in attachment during the preschool years thus suggest, consistent with Bowlby's (1969/1982) theory, that from 1 until about 3 years of age the organization of the youngster's attachment to the caregiver remains relatively unchanged. Toward the third birthday, significant elaboration of the child's IWMs is exemplified by a more complex network of event schemas, and by an increased ability to inhibit ongoing behavior in a way that allows the child increasingly to integrate his or her goals, plans, and behavior with those of the attachment figure. By this point, the child's attachment behavior has become organized in terms of an emergent partnership, and the amount and intensity of attachment behavior become somewhat attenuated. However, the set goal in the attachment–caregiving component of the relationship with the caregiver continues to be structured in terms of physical proximity.

By the fourth birthday, with the newly developed internal ability to operate simultaneously on both his or her own perspective and that of the caregiver, the child is now able to function within a relationship that is no longer so dependent on physical proximity and contact. The child's IWMs of caregiver and self have developed to the point where he or she can conceive of, and maintain in a goal-corrected way, a relationship that is based on shared goals, plans, and feelings. To the extent that child and caregiver are able to maintain this goal-corrected partnership, the child's set goal with respect to attachment–caregiving interactions should shift from some specifiable degree of

physical proximity and contact to some specifiable degree of availability in case of need (Bowlby, personal communication, cited in Ainsworth, 1990). To the same extent, attachment behavior should be further attenuated.

This is not meant to imply that children 4 years or older do not want, need, or enjoy physical proximity and contact with their attachment figures. Under conditions of distress, illness, and fear, children—even much older children—continue to retreat to their attachment figures as a haven of safety. As suggested by the attachment classification systems developed by Cassidy and Marvin (1992) and Main and Cassidy (1988), preschool and young school-age children also continue to maintain and enjoy this close tie through a range of intimate behaviors. What is implied by the model is that an older preschooler has come to organize attachment behavior in a new way—one that enables the child to realize that he or she and the attachment figure have a continuing relationship, whether or not they are in close proximity. This new organization is one in which the child is increasingly responsible for maintaining whatever protective proximity is necessary. In conjunction with the other recently developed locomotor, communication, and information-processing skills, this organization allows the child entering the juvenile phase of development to maintain a close tie to the attachment figure(s) while increasingly moving off from them and spending more time with a peer group, teachers, and other conspecifics.

Changes in Attachment Behavior beyond the Preschool Years

Bowlby (1969/1982) suggested that the goal-corrected partnership is probably the last phase in the ontogeny of attachment. By this he seems to have meant that there are no further "stage" changes in this behavioral system. The attachment behavioral system, however, remains important throughout the lifespan and does continue to undergo significant changes. These probably include further elaborations at the same "level," as well as changes in the relations between the attachment and other behavioral systems (the higher-order control structures), activating and terminating conditions, and IWMs. Certainly there are also many instances in which children form new attachments. One clear implication is that attachment becomes increasingly difficult to measure as it becomes more sophisticated, more abstract, and less dependent on proximity and contact, as the behavioral systems become elaborated into more and more complex systems (Bowlby, 1969/1982).

During middle childhood, or the juvenile period in primate terminology, children continue to be vulnerable to a wide range of dangers, and continue to use their attachment figures as secure bases from which to explore. Increasingly, however, they use other adults and groups of specific peers in the same manner. With their much more sophisticated communication skills and IWMs, they become able to assume primary responsibility for their own protection through their integration into the larger social structure for longer periods of time and under conditions of greater physical separation from their parents.

The child–parent relationship, however, remains a close one, and attachment–caregiving interactions remain organized according to an increasingly sophisticated goal-corrected partnership. The attachment behavioral system is no less important than earlier, in that school-age children still do not have the wisdom or knowledge to make decisions completely on their own regarding their activities, their supervision, or their protection while away from their parents. Not only is it important for a child to know where the parents are and to have a secure sense of the parents' accessibility, but the parents themselves must know where the child is and who is responsible for the child's protection. For this to function well, an effective goal-corrected partnership is necessary.

Bowlby anticipated this complex state of affairs when he proposed that *availability* of the attachment figure, rather than physical proximity, becomes the set goal of the attachment system in older children and adults. This he says, "turns on cognitive processes: (a) belief that lines of communication with the attachment figure are open, (b) that physical accessibility is possible, and (c) that the attachment figure will respond if called upon for help" (Bowlby, 1987, cited as personal communication by Ainsworth, 1990, p. 474). The work of Marvin (1977) and Marvin and Greenberg (1982) suggests that this shift begins to take place during the late preschool years. Certainly it continues to develop and elaborate through the remainder of childhood, and enables children to maintain their attachment to their parents while increasingly separated from them.

The goal-corrected partnership needs much research. Very little is known except for the general construct, its early development, some implications regarding its relations with self-concept and academic performance during middle childhood (e.g., Kerns, Chapter 17, this volume; Kerns, Schlegelmilch, Morgan, & Abraham, 2005; Mayseless, 2005; Moss, St.-Laurent, & Parent, 1999), and its importance for the relationship between adolescents and their parents (e.g., Allen, Chapter 19, this volume; Kobak, 1994). In this context it will be important to remember that the goal-corrected partnership is, in Bowlby's terms, a general-purpose skill—one that is used in much wider contexts than attachment–caregiving interactions, despite the suggestion that attachment interactions may be the first in which it is used. What is needed is continued development of standardized procedures for studying attachment during the juvenile years. These procedures would include observations of interactions between children and attachment figures in situations designed to mildly activate attachment–caregiving interactions, as well as interview and projective techniques designed to access children's IWMs regarding this part of the relationship (see Kerns, Chapter 17, this volume). It will also be important to include procedures for gathering information about children's attachments to nonparental figures, including both adults and other children.

Observations and shared experiences regarding relationships during the school-age period suggest that most children develop other close, helping relationships with a range of other children and adults. Older siblings, specific teachers, adult members of the extended family, older neighbors, and coaches all become important people in the lives of school-age children and adolescents. Are these affectional bonds? And are they attachment bonds, or other types of bonds? Given the specificity and strong emotional component of many of these relationships, some certainly qualify as bonds, despite the fact that many of them are relatively short-lived (Ainsworth, 1990). Many of them, however, fall under the category of "peer affectional bonds," whose similarities to and differences from attachment bonds need much research. Others (e.g., relationships with some teachers and older neighbors) can be helping and/or protective relationships without constituting actual bonds as defined earlier. It is likely that some of these relationships actually reflect coordinations of the attachment behavioral system with other behavioral systems, and will not be fully understood outside that context. Although we already know something about the relations between individual differences in early attachment–caregiving bonds and the quality of other, later bonds (see Berlin,

Cassidy, & Appleyard, Chapter 15, this volume), there has been almost no research on the normative developmental course involved.

Child–parent attachment interactions organized in terms of a goal-corrected partnership also continue through adolescence, as these older children continue to use their parents as a secure base for expanding their increasing "autonomy" (Allen, Chapter 19, this volume). As throughout life, attachment behaviors are especially evident when an adolescent is distressed, ill, afraid, or reunited with an attachment figure after a long absence (Ainsworth, 1990; Bowlby, 1979). The degree, however, to which adolescents' movements away from parental proximity and control are interspersed with adaptive, temporary returns to that safe haven is greatly underestimated in the developmental literature. The developmental course of these cycles, the complex combinations of attachment behavior with patterns from other behavioral systems, and the parental caregiving behaviors that terminate or continually activate those cycles constitute much of the core of adolescent and family therapy (e.g., Haley, 1977), and will be some of the most important topics for the study of attachment during adolescence.

During adolescence and young adulthood, another developmental change takes place that is precipitated by hormonal changes. During these years the adolescent or young adult begins to search for a permanent, goal-corrected partnership with an agemate, usually of the opposite sex. The biological function of this relationship is to produce offspring and raise them to reproductive age. This reproductive partnership, or adult pair bond (see Zeifman & Hazan, Chapter 20, this volume), does not imply the cessation of attachments to parents. In fact, knowledge of most cultures, as well as the recent shift in Western culture toward more adult offspring living with their own parents in two- and three-generation homes, suggests that adult offspring–parent attachment–caregiving relationships often actively continue while the offspring are forming their own "nuclear" families. As Ainsworth (1990) suggested, what it does imply is that these earlier attachments no longer penetrate as many aspects of an adult child's life as they did before.

For understandable reasons there is a tendency, in lifespan developmental, social, and clinical psychology, to base research on the assumption that this adult pair bond is a homologue to, or at least a direct outgrowth of, the earlier child–parent attachment–caregiving bond. In the field

of attachment research specifically, Hazan and Shaver (1987, 1994; see also J. Feeney, Chapter 21, this volume, and Mikulincer & Shaver, 2007) argue that there is a correspondence between adult pair bonds and individuals' earlier attachment styles. That is, the history of interactions with one's primary attachment figures is hypothesized to produce a trait-like "style" for involvement in close relationships.

Bowlby (1956), like psychoanalysts before him, noted the important parallels between child–parent and adult pair bonds: "Indeed, this profound attachment to a particular person is both as strong as, and often as irrational as, falling in love, and the very similarity of these two processes suggest strongly that they may have something in common" (p. 63). Bowlby argued strongly, however, for shifting the emphasis from taking for granted the similarities to taking for granted the *differences* between the two behavioral systems. Attachment–caregiving relationships and adult pair bond relationships need to be distinguished from one another because the two systems are activated and terminated by different conditions, because they are directed toward different objects, and because they have different sensitive phases in their development (Bowlby, 1969/1982). At the same time, like so many adult behavior patterns and relationships, they do appear to share some components.

Bowlby (1969/1982) and Ainsworth (e.g., 1990; see also Mikulincer & Goodman, 2006; Shaver, Hazan, & Bradshaw, 1988) proposed that at least three basic behavioral systems are involved in sexual pair bonds: the reproductive, attachment, and caregiving systems. We suspect that the sociability behavior system (or some component reflecting close friendship) is an equally important component in many pair bonds (see also Furman, Simon, Shaffer, & Bouchey, 2002). In most pair bonds, each partner displays each of these components toward the other, sometimes simultaneously and at other times in a complementary manner. There may also be individual and cultural differences in the overall, stable balance among these components. As an example specifically related to attachment research, in some couples the attachment and caregiving components may predictably be *symmetrical* and *reciprocal* (i.e., the partners share/alternate equally in taking each role). In others, there may be a relatively stable and *complementary* organization (cf., Hinde, 1976), with one partner usually seeking protection and care from the other, who is viewed as stronger and wiser. As

Ainsworth (1990) suggested, the latter relationship may not be ideally secure, but it may be nonetheless enduring.

This complex adult bond does not develop directly out of the individual's earlier attachment behavioral system. If the underlying principles of Bowlby's theory of development presented earlier in this chapter are correct, it develops instead through a complex systemic process involving the coordination and organization of multiple behavioral systems, with changes in activating and terminating conditions, into a more complex, functional whole. We are convinced that the application of these principles of development will serve to enrich our understanding of adult pair bonds.

In order to be successful, a theory of adult pair bonds will have to include attachment and caregiving components—but, just as importantly, sexual and friendship components. It will also require much descriptive research on the entire developmental pathway from the early attachment–caregiving bond, through peer affectional bonds, to the adult pair bond itself (see Furman et al., 2002; Roisman, Collins, Sroufe, & Egeland, 2005). It will require explicit recognition that characteristics of later-developing components along this pathway may exacerbate or attenuate the effects of earlier components. For example, a young child who has a very insecure goal-corrected attachment partnership with his or her parent may develop an intimate and smoothly functioning peer bond—a bond that may constitute a branch along the developmental pathway and provide increased likelihood of a secure adult pair bond. To understand this complex development fully, we need to know more than the fact that the secure peer bond is a predictor of a secure adult pair bond: We need to know as well *how* the secure peer bond component is structurally and developmentally *organized* within the later pair bond.

Finally, Ainsworth (1990) proposed that attachment behavior remains especially important throughout the period of aging. It is usually considered dysfunctional for a parent and young child to reverse roles, so that the child is the one providing care, support, and security. However, in the case of an aging or ill parent of an adult offspring, this role reversal may be both appropriate and functional. As the aging or illness begins to make the parent less able to protect him- or herself, that individual tends to seek an attachment–caregiving relationship with a younger, stronger adult (see Antonucci, Akiyama, & Takahashi, 2004; Magai,

Chapter 24, this volume; Mikulincer & Shaver, 2007; Shaver & Mikulincer, 2004). Traditionally this new attachment figure is the adult offspring, with the aging parent now functioning as the less autonomous member of the partnership. The changes over this period—including possible "uncoupling" of some of the systems that had become progressively coupled earlier in development; individual differences in attachment patterns among aging persons; and the conflict that aging people must experience between wanting to be protected and still wanting control over their own lives—will all be important research questions reflecting Bowlby's belief that attachment behavior functions "from the cradle to the grave."

CONCLUSION

Attachment theory began with Bowlby's (e.g., 1958) attempt to understand the psychopathological effects of maternal deprivation by studying the normative course of the ontogeny of this earliest relationship. Bowlby's hope was that if we better understood this normative course, we would be in an improved position to understand disruption. We are convinced that Bowlby's attempt to integrate the study of individual differences with that of normative development is as important today as it was 50 years ago.

Whether the issue is the consolidation of the infant's attachment late in the first year of life (e.g., Ainsworth, 1967), identification of patterns of caregiving associated with secure vs. insecure attachments during the preschool period (e.g., Britner et al., 2005; Stevenson-Hinde & Shouldice, 1995), increased numbers of children in foster care (Rutter, Chapter 40, this volume), children's relationships with peers (e.g., Berlin et al., Chapter 15, this volume; Cassidy, Kirsh, Scolton, & Parke, 1996), or adult intimate relationships in this time of high divorce rates (B. Feeney & Monin, Chapter 39, this volume), a full understanding of the isolated issue will not be possible without considering the organization of the individual's attachment behavioral system in the period under study. In fact, the most powerful design would be to *integrate* normative and differential approaches through the use of the developmental-pathway models first discussed by Bowlby (1969/1982; based on Waddington, 1957) and supplemented by our growing understanding of the different kinds of relationships that emerge in different periods of development.

NOTE

1. In order to avoid confusion between the organization of observable behaviors, and the cognitive or emotional organization that governs the behaviors, we adopt Greenberg and Marvin's (1982) use of the terms "behavior system" to refer to the organization of observable behaviors, and "behavioral system" to refer to the entire system, consisting of both behaviors *and* their corresponding cognitive or emotional components.

REFERENCES

Ainsworth, M. D. S. (1967). *Infancy in Uganda: Infant care and the growth of love*. Baltimore: Johns Hopkins University Press.

Ainsworth, M. D. S. (1990). Some considerations regarding theory and assessment relevant to attachments beyond infancy. In M. T. Greenberg, D. Cicchetti, & E. M. Cummings (Eds.), *Attachment in the preschool years: Theory, research, and intervention* (pp. 463–488). Chicago: University of Chicago Press.

Ainsworth, M. D. S., Blehar, M. C., Waters, E., & Wall, S. (1978). *Patterns of attachment: A psychological study of the Strange Situation*. Hillsdale, NJ: Erlbaum.

Antonucci, T. C., Akiyama, H., & Takahashi, K. (2004). Attachment and close relationships across the life span. *Attachment and Human Development, 6*, 353–370.

Ashby, W. R. (1952). *Design for a brain*. New York: Wiley.

Ashby, W. R. (1956). *An introduction to cybernetics*. New York: Wiley.

Bandura, A. (1978). Social learning theory of aggression. *Journal of Communication, 28*, 12–29.

Bates, E., O'Connell, B., & Shore, C. (1987). Language and communication in infancy. In J. D. Osofsky (Ed.), *Handbook of infant development* (2nd ed., pp. 149–203). New York: Wiley.

Bateson, P. P. G. (1976). Rules and reciprocity in behavioural development. In P. P. G. Bateson & R. A. Hinde (Eds.), *Growing points in ethology* (pp. 401–421). Cambridge, UK: Cambridge University Press.

Baumrind, D. (1980). New directions in socialization research. *American Psychologist, 35*, 639–652.

Bell, S. M. V. (1970). The development of the concept of the object as related to infant–mother attachment. *Child Development, 40*, 291–311.

Blurton-Jones, N. (1972). *Ethological studies of child behaviour*. Cambridge, UK: Cambridge University Press.

Bowlby, J. (1956). The growth of the independent child. *Royal Society of Health Journal, 76*, 587–591.

Bowlby, J. (1958). The nature of the child's tie to his mother. *International Journal of Psycho-Analysis, 39*, 350–373.

Bowlby, J. (1969/1982). *Attachment and loss: Vol. 1. Attachment*. New York: Basic Books.

Bowlby, J. (1973). *Attachment and loss: Vol. II. Separation: Anxiety and anger*. New York: Basic Books.

Bowlby, J. (1979). *The making and breaking of affectional bonds*. London: Tavistock.

Bowlby, J. (1980). *Attachment and loss: Vol. III. Loss: Sadness and depression*. New York: Basic Books.

Bretherton, I. (1993). From dialogue to internal working models: The co-construction of self in relationships. In C. A. Nelson (Ed.), *Minnesota Symposium on Child Psychology: Vol. 26. Memory and affect in development* (pp. 237–263). Hillsdale, NJ: Erlbaum.

Bretherton, I., & Ainsworth, M. D. S. (1974). Responses of 1-year-olds to a stranger in a strange situation. In M. Lewis & L. A. Rosenblum (Eds.), *The origins of fear* (pp. 131–164). New York: Wiley.

Britner, P. A., Marvin, R. S., & Pianta, R. C. (2005). Development and preliminary validation of the Caregiving Behavior System: Association with child attachment classification in the preschool Strange Situation. *Attachment and Human Development, 7*, 83–102.

Bruner, J. (1981). The social context of language acquisition. *Language and Communication, 1*, 155–178.

Burlingham, D., & Freud, A. (1942). *Young children in war-time*. London: Allen & Unwin.

Cahill, K. R., Deater-Deckard, K., Pike, A., & Hughes, C. (2007). Theory of mind, self-worth, and the mother–child relationship. *Social Development, 16*, 45–56.

Cassidy, J., & Berlin, L. (1994). The insecure/ambivalent pattern of attachment: Theory and research. *Child Development, 65*, 971–991.

Cassidy, J., Kirsh, S., Scolton, K. L., & Parke, R. D. (1996). Attachment and representations of peers. *Developmental Psychology, 32*, 892–904.

Cassidy, J., & Marvin, R. S., with the MacArthur Attachment Working Group. (1992). *Attachment organization in preschool children: Coding guidelines* (4th ed.). Unpublished manuscript, University of Virginia.

Chisholm, K. M., Carter, M. C., Ames, E. W., & Morison, S. M. (1995). Attachment security and indiscriminately friendly behavior in children adopted from Romanian orphanages. *Development and Psychopathology, 3*, 397–411.

Cicchetti, D., Cummings, E. M., Greenberg, M. T., & Marvin, R. S. (1990). An organizational perspective on attachment beyond infancy. In M. T. Greenberg, D. Cicchetti, & E. M. Cummings (Eds.), *Attachment in the preschool years: Theory, research and intervention* (pp. 3–49). Chicago: University of Chicago Press.

Dunn, J. (1994). Changing minds and changing relationships. In C. Lewis & P. Mitchell (Eds.), *Children's early understanding of mind: Origins and development* (pp. 297–310). Hillsdale, NJ: Erlbaum.

Erikson, E. H. (1950). *Childhood and society*. New York: Norton.

Freedman, D. G., & Gorman, J. (1993). Attachment and the transmission of culture: An evolutionary perspective. *Journal of Social and Evolutionary Systems, 16*, 297–329.

Freud, A. (1965). *Normality and pathology in childhood:*

Assessments of development. New York: International Universities Press.

Furman, W., Simon, V. A., Shaffer, L., & Bouchey, H. A. (2002). Adolescents' working models and styles for relationships with parents, friends, and romantic partners. *Child Development, 73,* 241–255.

George, C., & Solomon, J. (1996). Representations of relationships: Links between caregiving and attachment. *Infant Mental Health Journal, 17,* 198–216.

Goldberg, S., Marvin, R., & Sabbagh, V. (1996). *Child–parent attachment and indiscriminately friendly behavior toward strangers in Romanian orphans adopted into Canadian families.* Paper presented at the biennial meeting of the International Society for Infant Studies, Providence, RI.

Greenberg, M. T., & Marvin, R. S. (1982). Reactions of preschool children to an adult stranger: A behavioral systems approach. *Child Development, 53,* 481–490.

Greenberg, M. T., Marvin, R. S., & Mossler, D. G. (1977). The development of conditional reasoning skills. *Developmental Psychology, 13,* 527–528.

Haley, J. (1977). *Problem solving therapy.* San Francisco: Jossey-Bass.

Harlow, H. F., & Harlow, M. K. (1965). The affectional systems. In A. M. Schrier, H. F. Harlow, & F. Stollnitz (Eds.), *Behavior of nonhuman primates* (Vol. 2, pp. 287–334). New York: Academic Press.

Hazan, C., & Shaver, P. R. (1987). Romantic love conceptualized as an attachment process. *Journal of Personality and Social Psychology, 52,* 511–524.

Hazan, C., & Shaver, P. R. (1994). Deeper into attachment theory: Authors' response. *Psychological Inquiry, 5,* 68–79.

Heinicke, C., & Westheimer, I. (1966). *Brief separations.* New York: International Universities Press.

Hinde, R. A. (1976). On describing relationships. *Journal of Child Psychology and Psychiatry, 17,* 1–19.

Hinde, R. A. (1982). The uses and limitations of studies of nonhuman primates for the understanding of human social development. In L. W. Hoffman, R. Gandelman, & H. R. Schiffman (Eds.), *Parenting: Its causes and consequences* (pp. 5–17). Hillsdale, NJ: Erlbaum.

Hofer, M. A. (2006). Psychobiological roots of early attachment. *Current Directions in Psychological Science, 15,* 84–88.

Hrdy, S. B. (2005). Evolutionary context of human development: The cooperative breeding model. In C. S. Carter, L. Ahnert, K. Grossmann, S. Hrdy, M. Lamb, S. Porges, et al. (Eds.), *Attachment and bonding: A new synthesis* (pp. 9–32). Cambridge, MA: MIT Press.

Hsu, H.-C., & Fogel, A. (2003). Stability and transitions in mother–infant face-to-face communication during the first 6 months: A microhistorical approach. *Developmental Psychology, 39,* 1061–1082.

Kagan, J. (1989). *Unstable ideas: Temperament, cognition, and self.* Cambridge, MA: Harvard University Press.

Kerns, K. A., Schlegelmilch, A., Morgan, T. A., & Abraham, M. M. (2005). Assessing attachment in middle childhood. In K. A. Kerns & R. A. Richardson (Eds.), *Attachment in middle childhood* (pp. 46–70). New York: Guilford Press.

Kisilevsky, B. S., Hains, S. M., Lee, K., Xie, X., Huang, H., Ye, H. H., et al. (2003). Effects of experience on fetal voice recognition. *Psychological Science, 14,* 220–224.

Kobak, R. (1994). Adult attachment: A personality or relationship construct? *Psychological Inquiry, 5,* 42–44.

Konner, M. (1976). Maternal care, infant behavior and development among the !Kung. In R. Lee & I. DeVore (Eds.), *Kalahari hunter gatherers: Studies of the !Kung San and their neighbors* (pp. 377–394). Cambridge, MA: Harvard University Press.

Lewis, C., & Mitchell, P. (Eds.). (1994). *Children's early understanding of the mind: Origins and development.* Hillsdale, NJ: Erlbaum.

Lewis, M., Sullivan, M. W., & Vasen, A. (1987). Making faces: Age and emotion differences in the posing of emotional expressions. *Developmental Psychology, 23,* 690–697.

Maestripieri, D. (2005). On the importance of comparative research for the understanding of human behavior and development: A reply to Gottlieb & Lickliter (2004). *Social Development, 14,* 181–186.

Mahler, M., Pine, F., & Bergman, A. (1975). *The psychological birth of the human infant.* New York: Basic Books.

Main, M., & Cassidy, J. (1988). Categories of response to reunion with the parent at age six: Predictable from infant attachment classifications and stable over a one-month period. *Developmental Psychology, 24,* 415–426.

Main, M., & Goldwyn, R. (1984). *Adult attachment scoring and classification system.* Unpublished manuscript, University of California at Berkeley.

Main, M., Goldwyn, R., & Hesse, E. (2003). *Adult attachment scoring and classification system.* Unpublished manuscript, University of California at Berkeley.

Main, M., Kaplan, N., & Cassidy, J. (1985). Security in infancy, childhood, and adulthood: A move to the level of representation. In I. Bretherton & E. Waters (Eds.), Growing points of attachment theory and research. *Monographs of the Society for Research in Child Development, 50*(1–2), 66–104.

Main, M., & Solomon, J. (1990). Procedures for identifying infants and disorganized/disoriented during the Ainsworth Strange Situation. In M. T. Greenberg, D. Cicchetti, & E. M. Cummings (Eds.), *Attachment in the preschool years: Theory, research, and intervention* (pp. 134–146). Chicago: University of Chicago Press.

Marvin, R. S. (1977). An ethological–cognitive model for the attenuation of mother–child attachment behavior. In T. M. Alloway, L. Krames, & P. Pliner (Eds.), *Advances in the study of communication and affect: Vol. 3. Attachment behavior* (pp. 25–60). New York: Plenum Press.

Marvin, R. S. (1997). Ethological and general systems perspectives on child–parent attachment during the toddler and preschool years. In N. Segal, G. We-isfeld, & C. Weisfeld (Eds.), *Genetic, ethological, and evolutionary perspectives on human development* (pp. 189–216). Washington, DC: American Psychological Association.

Marvin, R. S., & Britner, P. A. (1996). *Classification system for parental caregiving patterns in the preschool Strange Situation.* Unpublished manuscript, University of Virginia.

Marvin, R. S., & Greenberg, M. T. (1982). Preschoolers' changing conceptions of their mothers: A social-cognitive study of mother–child attachment. *New Directions for Child Development, 18,* 47–60.

Marvin, R. S., Greenberg, M. T., & Mossler, D. G. (1976). The early development of conceptual perspective taking: Distinguishing among multiple perspectives. *Child Development, 47,* 511–514.

Marvin, R. S., Van Devender, T. L., Iwanaga, M., LeVine, S., & LeVine, R. A. (1977). Infant–caregiver attachment among the Hausa of Nigeria. In H. M. McGurk (Ed.), *Ecological factors in human development* (pp. 247–260). Amsterdam: North Holland.

Mayseless, O. (2005). Ontogeny of attachment in middle childhood: Conceptualization of normative changes. In K. A. Kerns & R. A. Richardson (Eds.), *Attachment in middle childhood* (pp. 1–23). New York: Guilford Press.

McGraw, M. B. (1943). *The neuromuscular maturation of the human infant.* New York: Columbia University Press.

Mikulincer, M., & Goodman, G. S. (Eds.). (2006). *Dynamics of romantic love: Attachment, caregiving, and sex.* New York: Guilford Press.

Mikulincer, M., & Shaver, P. R. (2007). *Attachment in adulthood: Structure, dynamics, and change.* New York: Guilford Press.

Miljkovitch, R., Pierrehumbert, B., Bretherton, I., & Halfon, O. (2004). Associations between parental and child attachment representations. *Attachment and Human Development, 6,* 305–325.

Miller, W. B., & Rodgers, J. L. (2001). *The ontogeny of human bonding systems: Evolutionary origins, neural bases, and psychological manifestations.* Boston: Kluwer.

Moss, E., St.-Laurent, D., & Parent, S. (1999). Disorganized attachment and developmental risk at school age. In J. Solomon & C. George (Eds.), *Attachment disorganization* (pp. 160–186). New York: Guilford Press.

Myers, B. J., Jarvis, P. A., & Creasey, G. L. (1987). Infants' behavior with their mothers and grandmothers. *Infant Behavior and Development, 10,* 245–259.

Nelson, K., & Gruendel, J. (1981). Generalized event representations: Basic building blocks of cognitive development. In M. E. Lamb & A. Brown (Eds.), *Advances in developmental psychology* (Vol. 1, pp. 131–158). Hillsdale, NJ: Erlbaum.

O'Connor, T. G., Marvin, R. S., Rutter, M., Olrick, J., Britner, P. A., & The English and Romanian Adoptees Study Team. (2003). Child–parent attachment following early severe institutional deprivation. *Development and Psychopathology, 15,* 19–38.

Pears, K. C., & Moses, L. J. (2003). Demographics, parenting, and theory of mind in preschool children. *Social Development, 12,* 1–20.

Piaget, J. (1952). *The origins of intelligence in children.* New York: International Universities Press.

Porges, S. W. (2005). The role of social engagement in attachment and bonding: A phylogenetic perspective. In C. S. Carter, L. Ahnert, K. Grossmann, S. Hrdy, M. Lamb, S. Porges, et al. (Eds.), *Attachment and bonding: A new synthesis* (pp. 33–54). Cambridge, MA: MIT Press.

Robertson, J. (Producer). (1953). *A two-year-old goes to hospital* [Film]. London: Tavistock Child Development Research Unit.

Roisman, G. I., Collins, W. A., Sroufe, L. A., & Egeland, B. (2005). Predictors of young adults' representations of and behavior in their current romantic relationship: Prospective test of the prototype hypothesis. *Attachment and Human Development, 7,* 105–121.

Rutter, M., Colvert, E., Kreppner, J., Beckett, C., Castle, J., Groothues, C., et al. (2007). Early adolescent outcomes for institutionally deprived and non-deprived adoptees: I. Disinhibited attachment. *Journal of Child Psychology and Psychiatry, 48,* 17–30.

Sabbagh, M. A., Xu, F., Carlson, S. M., Moses, L. J., & Lee, K. (2006). The development of executive functioning and theory of mind: A comparison of Chinese and U.S. preschoolers. *Psychological Science, 17,* 74–81.

Schaffer, H. R., & Emerson, P. E. (1964). The developments of social attachments in infancy. *Monographs of the Society for Research in Child Development, 29*(3, Serial No. 94).

Schore, A. N. (2000). Attachment and the regulation of the right brain. *Attachment and Human Development, 2,* 23–47.

Shaver, P. R., Hazan, C., & Bradshaw, D. (1988). Love as attachment: The integration of three behavioral systems. In R. J. Sternberg & M. Barnes (Eds.), *The psychology of love* (pp. 68–99). New Haven, CT: Yale University Press.

Shaver, P. R., & Mikulincer, M. (2004). Attachment in the later years: A commentary. *Attachment and Human Development, 6,* 451–464.

Slough, N. M., & Greenberg, M. T. (1990). Five-year-olds' representations of separation from parents: Responses from the perspective of self and other. *New Directions for Child Development, 48,* 67–84.

Sommerville, J. A., & Woodward, A. L. (2005). Pulling out the intentional structure of action: The relation between action processing and action production in infancy. *Cognition, 95,* 1–30.

Sroufe, L. A., & Waters, E. (1977). Attachment as an organizational construct. *Child Development, 48,* 1184–1199.

Stern, D. (1985). *The interpersonal world of the infant.* New York: Basic Books.

Stevenson-Hinde, J., & Shouldice, A. (1995). Maternal

interactions and self-reports related to attachment classifications at 4.5 years. *Child Development, 66,* 583–596.

Stewart, R. B., & Marvin, R. S. (1984). Sibling relations: The role of conceptual perspective taking in the ontogeny of sibling caregiving. *Child Development, 55,* 1322–1332.

Suomi, S. J. (1995). Influence of attachment theory on ethological studies of biobehavioral development in non-human primates. In S. Goldberg, R. Muir, & J. Kerr (Eds.), *Attachment theory: Social, developmental, and clinical perspectives* (pp. 185–201). Hillsdale, NJ: Analytic Press.

Thelen, E., & Ulrich, B. D. (1991). Hidden skills: A dynamic systems analysis of treadmill stepping during the first year of life. *Monographs of the Society for Research in Child Development, 56*(1, Serial No. 223).

Waddington, C. H. (1957). *The strategy of the genes.* London: Allen & Unwin.

Waters, H. S., & Waters, E. (2006). The attachment working models concept: Among other things, we build script-like representations of secure base experiences. *Attachment and Human Development, 8,* 185–197.

Wolff, P. H. (1969). The natural history of crying and other vocalizations in early infancy. In B. M. Foss (Ed.), *Determinants of infant behavior* (Vol. 4, pp. 81–109). New York: Barnes & Noble.

Zeanah, C., Smyke, A., Koga, S., & Carlson, E. (2005). Attachments in institutionalized and community children in Romania. *Child Development, 76,* 1015–1028.

CHAPTER 13

Precursors of Attachment Security

JAY BELSKY
R. M. PASCO FEARON

Why do some infants develop secure attachments to their primary caregivers, whereas others establish insecure relationships? That is the central question to be addressed in this chapter. In certain respects, one might regard such a question as more American than British. This is because even though John Bowlby, a British psychiatrist, was concerned with the consequences of variation in the quality of early attachment, it was his American colleague, psychologist Mary Ainsworth, who brought the topic of the origins of individual differences in infant–parent attachment security to center stage. Whereas Bowlby's (1944, 1958) original thinking on the roots of security–insecurity was organized around the development of disorders (e.g., juvenile delinquency) and led to a focus on major separations from parents early in life, Ainsworth (1973) was the first to devote considerable empirical and theoretical energies to consideration of the determinants of secure and insecure infant–mother attachments in the normal, nonclinical population.

At the core of Ainsworth's extension of Bowlby's attachment theory was the contention that a sensitive, responsive caregiver is of fundamental importance to the development of a secure as opposed to an insecure attachment bond during the opening years of life. According to Ainsworth, a caregiver capable of providing security-inducing, sensitive, responsive care understands the child's individual attributes; accepts the child's behavioral proclivities; and is thus capable of consistently orchestrating harmonious interactions between self and child, especially those in which the soothing of distress is involved. In elaborating on and thereby further developing Bowlby's theory, Ainsworth never expressed the belief that the development of the relationship between infant and mother was determined entirely by the mother. Nevertheless, she was convinced that the developing relationship between child and adult was not shaped equally by the two participants. Recognizing the greater maturity and power of the mother, Ainsworth attributed disproportionate influence to her rather than to the child.

Nonetheless, the notion of maternal sensitivity championed by Ainsworth in her efforts to account for individual differences in attachment security was defined in terms of what the child brought to the relationship and, more specifically, how the child behaved at a particular time. By definition, then, care that is sensitive and theorized to promote security in the child does not take exactly the same form for all children. Nor does

295

it take the same form across all situations in the case of a particular child. This is why Ainsworth (1973) adopted the methodology of rating maternal behavior after extensive observation, rather than microcoding interactions on a moment-by-moment basis.

The first part of this chapter contains a summary of research on the effects of mothering and mother–infant interaction on attachment security—the issues raised most directly by Ainsworth. Related evidence pertaining to the effects of the quality of fathering and of nonparental caregivers' care on attachment to father and to caregiver, respectively, is also considered. Attention is devoted to the origins of security in these nonmaternal infant–adult relationships, because they too underscore the role of sensitive care in promoting attachment security. In addition, the issue of whether effects of sensitive care on attachment security are evident outside the Western world is considered, as this is important for understanding how universal or general these developmental processes are.

In the second part of the chapter, the broader social context of attachment is considered. At approximately the same time that interest in the interactional origins of attachment security was growing in the field of developmental psychology, Bronfenbrenner (1979) advanced an ecological perspective, drawing attention to the broader context of human development beyond the confines of the mother–child relationship. Even though some (including Bronfenbrenner) regarded his framework as a challenge to a developmental psychology that seemed to be excessively concerned with the mother–child relationship, those who were already intrigued by Ainsworth's ideas saw Bronfenbrenner's ecological framework as providing a means for expanding the attachment research agenda (Belsky, 2005a). This was because it drew attention to issues that were not explicitly emphasized in attachment theory, but that seemed latent in the theory.

Whereas caregiver sensitivity is regarded within attachment theory as the principal determinant of whether an infant develops a secure or insecure relationship with the caregiver, from an ecological perspective the psychological attributes of the mother, her relations with her partner, and the degree to which she has access to other social agents who provide instrumental and emotional support should also be associated with the security of the infant–mother relationship. This is because these factors are theorized to affect the quality of care that a mother (or other caregiver)

provides (for a review, see Belsky & Jaffee, 2006). Thus, whereas attachment theory is essentially a theory of the microprocesses of development, emphasizing the daily interactional exchanges between parent and child and the developing internal working model of the child, the ecological/social-contextual perspective draws attention to the contextual factors and processes likely to influence these microdevelopmental processes.

THE QUALITY OF MATERNAL AND NONMATERNAL CARE

Not long after Ainsworth first advanced her ideas and evidence regarding the role of maternal sensitivity in fostering the development of a secure attachment relationship (Ainsworth, 1973; Ainsworth, Blehar, Waters, & Wall, 1978), what might be regarded as a "cottage industry" developed within the field of developmental psychology seeking to replicate—or refute—her findings. Child temperament was the major focus of those seeking to disconfirm Ainsworth's theory and evidence, and it is thus difficult to consider the role of maternal sensitivity and the quality of maternal care more generally without devoting some attention to what might be regarded as a competing theoretical perspective.

The Role of Temperament

According to a variety of classical temperament theorists, the source of security and insecurity lie not in the caregiver's ministrations, but in the constitutional attributes of the child. Those like the child psychiatrist Stella Chess regarded the Ainsworth–Bowlby view as little more than refurbished psychoanalytic theory, attributing far too much influence to parents and "blaming" them for difficulties inherent in the child (Chess & Thomas, 1982). Two basic views regarding the role temperament plays in the development and assessment of individual differences in infant–mother attachment relationships merit discussion here. One, embraced principally by students of attachment theory, is that temperament does not directly influence the quality of attachment that develops between infant and mother, because even a difficult infant, given sensitive care, can become secure (Sroufe, 1985). Thus no main effect of temperament on attachment security is expected.

The second school of thought contends that an infant's temperament (particularly his or her child's susceptibility to distress) directly affects attachment security via its impact upon mother–infant interaction, *and* is the principal determinant of behavior observed in the Strange Situation (Chess & Thomas, 1982; Kagan, 1982). The claim has been advanced, moreover, that infants classified as securely attached are simply less upset by separation in the Strange Situation, whereas those infants classified as insecurely attached are simply more distressed, despite the fact that both secure *and* insecure infants display the same kinds of discrete behaviors (e.g., crying) in the Strange Situation. These arguments can be broken down into two different elements. The first is the broad issue of whether attachment security reflects genetically based characteristics of the child. The second concerns a related but more narrowly defined question about the role of specific dimensions of temperament in the development of attachment security.

Genetics and Attachment

In recent years, knowledge about genetic contributions to variation in infant attachment organization has increased significantly. The first line of evidence on this topic comes from studies of concordance rates of attachment security in individuals who vary in their degree of biological relatedness (twins, siblings, unrelated infants). In the earliest sibling study, Ward, Vaughn, and Robb (1988) found significant correspondence (63%; $N = 65$) between siblings in attachment security measured from 1 to 4½ years apart. Teti and Ablard (1989) found converging evidence in a concurrent design with 50 sibling pairs; they measured attachment with the Strange Situation for younger siblings, and with the Attachment Q-Sort (AQS; Waters & Deane, 1985) for the older ones. After the older siblings were divided into secure and insecure groups on the basis of their AQS scores, concordance for attachment between siblings was 64%. In a larger sibling sample of 138 pooled from three studies, van IJzendoorn and colleagues (2000) found a concordance rate remarkably consistent with those reported above (62%).

Sibling concordances themselves cannot differentiate between similarities broadly attributable to common environmental factors and those associated with genetics. Four studies have conducted infant–mother attachment assessments on samples of monozygotic (MZ) and dizygotic (DZ) twins. In a sample of 157 MZ and DZ twins seen in the Strange Situation at 12 months, Bokhorst and colleagues (2003) found 60% correspondence in MZ twins and 57% in DZ twins. In genetic modeling, 52% of the variance in attachment security within

the organized categories was attributable to shared environmental effects, whereas the remainder was estimated to be due to nonshared environment and measurement error. When disorganization was considered, no genetic or shared environmental effects were detected, and all of the variance was attributable to nonshared environment and measurement error. Broadly convergent results have been reported by O'Connor and Croft (2001) in an older sample of preschoolers with the MacArthur modified Strange Situation, although rather different degrees of twin similarity emerged in a relatively large sample by Finkel, Wille, and Matheny (1998): substantial genetic effects (72%) and no shared environmental effects. This result appeared to derive primarily from the low DZ correspondence (compared to other DZ samples or fraternal siblings) of 44%, rather than a high correspondence among MZ twins (which was 63%).

Despite the modest sample sizes of all the aforementioned studies, the cumulative picture is quite consistent, suggesting a significant role for shared and nonshared environmental effects and apparently little role for genetics, at least within the range of low-risk samples studied. This conclusion is substantiated by results from the only genetic study of infant–*father* attachment, which relied on AQS security scores derived from mother sorts of infant behavior vis-à-vis the father (Bakermans-Kranenburg, van IJzendoorn, Bokhorst, & Schuengel, 2004): Genetic modeling showed that attachment was explained virtually exclusively by shared environmental (59%) and unique environmental (41%) factors.

Molecular genetic studies of attachment have advanced the field beyond estimates of heritability. Lakatos and colleagues (2000, 2002) reported an association between disorganized attachment and a polymorphism of the DRD4 dopamine receptor gene (Exon III 48-bp VNTR). Of 17 disorganized infants, 12 had the 7-repeat allele of this gene (which has been found to confer lower dopamine neurotransmission than the more common 4-repeat allele), compared to 21 of 73 nondisorganized infants. These investigators also attempted to rule out a range of confounds (e.g., population stratification) by testing whether disorganized infants showed higher transmission of the 7-repeat allele from their parents (Gervai et al., 2005). Because this transmission test requires a sample of heterozygous parents, the n for this analysis was small, and differential transmission in the disorganized group was only at a trend level (Gervai et al., 2005). However, significant nontransmission of the 7-repeat allele emerged in the group of secure infants (which had a larger *n*). Further analyses using the same sample suggested that a single nucleotide substitution in the promoter region of the DRD4 gene amplified the effect of the 7-repeat allele on disorganization.

   Bakermans-Kranenburg, van IJzendoorn, and Juffer (2005) recently failed to replicate these molecular genetic effects in an independent sample of twins. Such cross-study inconsistency, not unusual in molecular genetic research on behavior (Rutter, 2006), suggests that there is not a strong "main effect" of genetics on attachment. If there is a role for genetics considered broadly, and for dopaminergic genes more narrowly, it may be dependent upon a variety of poorly understood contingencies with proximal and contextual factors.

Temperament and Attachment

A meta-analysis of some 18 studies carried out two decades ago provides some support for the assertion that insecurity is a direct function of an infant's proneness to distress (Goldsmith & Alansky, 1987). Resistant behavior in the Strange Situation (e.g., kicking legs, pushing away upon reunion) proved to be reliably, though weakly, associated with proneness to distress. Notably, however, more recent work has failed to consistently support the view that attachment *security* is influenced by temperament. As Vaughn, Bost, and van IJzendoorn (Chapter 9, this volume) explain, whereas some recent studies have found negative correlations between indices of negative emotionality and attachment security—typically when the caregiver provides reports of both, though sometimes even when observers provide AQS security evaluations—many have not (for a meta-analysis, see van IJzendoorn, Vereijken, Bakermans-Kranenburg, & Riksen-Walraven, 2004). The latter appears to be especially true when attachment security is evaluated by means of the Strange Situation (e.g., Kochanska, Aksan, & Carlson, 2005; Marshall & Fox, 2005).

   Nevertheless, several studies that have examined associations between temperament and avoidant or resistant *behavior* in the Strange Situation, rather than between temperament and *security* per se, have found evidence for such associations (though see Vaughn et al., Chapter 9, this volume, for a somewhat different view). In fact, evidence continues to be reported—as Belsky and Rovine (1987) contended—that temperament *may* play some role in the ways in which insecurity is expressed, but not in whether a child is secure or insecure. Kochanska (1998) found, for

example, that fearful temperament in the first year predicted *type of insecurity* at 13–15 months, with A (avoidant) babies manifesting lower distress or fearfulness than other insecure types (and no significant association between temperament and attachment security; see also Kochanska & Coy, 2002). Moreover, Braungart-Rieker, Garwood, Powers, and Wang (2001) reported that the Belsky and Rovine "temperamental split" of Strange Situation attachment classifications—A1-B2 versus B3-C2—proved related to infant affect and regulatory activity measured at 4 months of age. Especially noteworthy is Marshall and Fox's (2005) related finding that 4-month-olds who manifested elevated distress and motor activity were more likely to be classified A1-B2 rather than B3-C2 in the Strange Situation at 14 months. (And, once again, early temperament did not distinguish security from insecurity.) It would be a mistake, however, to leave the impression that all efforts to use this split to account for the effects of early temperament on affective behavior measured in the Strange Situation have provided positive evidence (see Vaughn et al., Chapter 9, this volume). Nevertheless, it is difficult to avoid the conclusion that fearfulness and other manifestations of negativity *may* predispose a child to express resistant behavior when reunited with the parent following separation (see Kochanska & Coy, 2002), whereas low levels of negativity *may* predispose a child to exhibit avoidant behavior. Critical to note here is that the discussion is about resistant and avoidant *behavior*, not about insecure-resistant or insecure-avoidant attachments.

   Thus evidence repeatedly, even if not universally, shows that temperamental negative emotionality correlates with separation distress, with variations in Strange Situation subclassifications along the A1-C2 dimension and with avoidance versus resistance. This evidence, in conjunction with unpublished results from the Bokhorst and colleagues (2003) twin study documenting strong genetic influence on the A1-C2 dimension, raises questions about what to make of apparent differences in parenting associated with avoidance versus resistance (see below). Although the theoretical distinction between rejection/intrusiveness (as a cause of avoidance) and inconsistency/unavailability (as a cause of resistance) is appealing, the possibility cannot be ignored that these stylistic differences in parenting associated with types of insecurity may at least partially be parental adaptations to differences in infant behavioral dispositions (i.e., gene–environment correlations). Seemingly inconsistent with this argument, however, is evidence reported by Dozier, Stovall, Albus, and Bates (2001) that the quality of the attachment an infant establishes with a foster mother is systematically and significantly related to the foster mother's state of mind regarding attachment. Nevertheless, the possibility that infant behavioral dispositions can influence attachment security, even if only indirectly, is underscored by the collection of (not entirely replicated) findings linking temperament and maternal sensitivity (Vaughn et al., Chapter 9, this volume).

To our minds, the somewhat dated findings of van den Boom (1990, 1994) are particularly important to consider with regard to the issue of the role of temperament in the development of attachment security. In a sample of economically at-risk families in the Netherlands, van den Boom longitudinally followed 100 infants who scored very high on irritability on two separate neonatal examinations. Contrary to the Goldsmith and Alansky (1987) meta-analytic findings, as well as to the preceding review suggesting that negative emotionality may predispose an infant to develop an insecure-resistant attachment if sensitive caregiving is not experienced, more than three of every four distress-prone infants whose mothers received no intervention services (*n* = 50) and who were classified as insecure were categorized as insecure-avoidant, not insecure-resistant. As van den Boom (1990) noted, these data directly challenge the contention of Chess and Thomas (1982) and Kagan (1982) that variation in security of attachment is reducible to temperamental differences among babies. As just implied, these findings are also inconsistent with the Belsky–Rovine "temperamental split" perspective suggesting that negatively emotional infants, when they develop insecure attachments, will be predisposed to develop insecure-resistant ones. After all, how does a temperament theory of attachment account for the fact that highly irritable newborns express limited negative affect in the Strange Situation? Furthermore, the fact that another Dutch parenting-focused intervention effort (to be described below) proved highly effective in shaping the attachment security of infants with high negative emotionality documents a strong causal role of sensitivity in moderating associations between temperament and attachment insecurity (Velderman, Bakermans-Kranenburg, Juffer, & van IJzendoorn, 2006).

In addition to the Dutch findings and the more extensive evidentiary base considered by Vaughn and colleagues (Chapter 9, this volume), one final consideration should be raised in any discussion of attachment and temperament. Throughout much of the temperament–attachment debate over the past 25 years, temperament has been treated more or less as a fixed trait. Yet there is not only evidence that temperament can and does change (Rothbart & Bates, 1998), but that features of families, including the quality of care that parents provide, contribute to changes in temperament (e.g., Belsky, Fish, & Isabella, 1991). The most important implication of this latter fact is that even when temperament, especially measured late in the first year (or thereafter), covaries with attachment security, it cannot be presumed—as it often is—that such a finding reflects an effect of temperament on attachment, rather than an effect of parental care on both temperament and attachment.

Maternal Care

There can be little doubt that, in accord with Ainsworth's (1973) original theorizing and her intensive research on just 26 mother–infant dyads, variation in rated maternal sensitivity in the first year is linked to security in the Strange Situation. This is revealed in studies of middle-class U.S. (Ainsworth et al., 1978; Braungart-Reiker et al., 2001; Cox, Owen, Henderson, & Margand, 1992; Fish & Stifter, 1995 [girls only]; Isabella, 1993; Kochanska, 1998; Teti, Gelfand, Messinger, & Isabella, 1995), Canadian (Pederson & Moran, 1996), and German (Grossmann, Grossmann, Spangler, Suess, & Unzner, 1985) families, as well as economically disadvantaged, often single-parent families (Egeland & Farber, 1984; Krupka, Moran, & Pederson, 1996; Susman-Stillman, Kalkoske, Egeland, & Waldman, 1996). Furthermore, security is associated with prompt responsiveness to distress (Crockenberg, 1981; Del Carmen, Pedersen, Huffman, & Bryan, 1993), moderate, appropriate stimulation (Belsky, Rovine, & Taylor, 1984; Feldstein, Crown, Beebe, & Jaffe, 1995), and interactional synchrony (Isabella & Belsky, 1991; Isabella, Belsky, & von Eye, 1989), as well as with warmth, involvement, and responsiveness (Bates, Maslin, & Frankel, 1985; Leyendecker, Lamb, Fracasso, Scholmerich, & Larson, 1997; National Institute of Child Health and Human Development [NICHD] Early Child Care Network, 1997; O'Connor, Sigman, & Kasasi, 1992). In contrast, insecure-avoidant attachments are related to intrusive, excessively stimulating, controlling interactional styles, and insecure-resistant attachments to an unresponsive, underinvolved approach to caregiving (Belsky et al., 1984; Isabella et al., 1989; Lewis & Fiering, 1989; Malatesta,

Grigoryev, Lamb, Albin, & Culver, 1986; Smith & Pederson, 1988; Vondra, Shaw, & Kevinides, 1995).

In addition to such associations from studies using the Strange Situation procedure, similar contemporaneous and time-lagged relations have emerged in North American research using the AQS to assess attachment security (Krupka et al., 1996; Moran, Pederson, Pettit, & Krupka, 1992; Pederson et al., 1990; Scholmerich, Fracasso, Lamb, & Broberg, 1995) and in related research conducted in Japan (Vereijken, Riksen-Walraven, & Kondo-Ikemura, 1997). All this is not to say that there have been no failures to replicate such theoretically anticipated results (Murray, Fiori-Cowley, Hooper, & Cooper, 1996; Notaro & Volling, 1999; Schneider-Rosen & Rothbaum, 1993; Seifer, Schiller, Sameroff, Resnick, & Riordan, 1996), but rather that there are many consistent findings in the literature.

It must be noted, however, that the strength of the discerned association between quality of rearing (e.g., sensitivity) and attachment security is not large. As Goldsmith and Alansky (1987) observed in their meta-analysis of 15 studies carried out between 1978 and 1987, "the effect [of maternal interactive behavior on attachment security] that has enjoyed the confidence of most attachment researchers is not as strong as was once believed" (p. 811). A decade ago, De Wolff and van IJzendoorn (1997) reexamined relations between parenting and attachment security by means of meta-analysis. Drawing upon data from 66 investigations involving some 4,176 infant–mother dyads, they discerned an overall effect size of 0.17 between attachment security and various measures of mothering and of mother–child interaction (e.g., sensitivity, contiguity of maternal response, physical contact, cooperation). When the meta-analysis was restricted to only the subset of 30 investigations that measured sensitivity ($n = 1,666$), the effect size was somewhat larger (0.22). And when the 16 studies ($n = 837$) that relied on Ainsworth's original sensitivity rating scales were considered, the effect size was larger still (0.24). Nevertheless, effect sizes across investigations that relied upon different operationalizations of mothering and mother–infant interaction were more similar than different. And, moreover, the magnitude of the discerned effects was not influenced (i.e., moderated) by the length of observations of mother–child interaction, or by whether security was assessed with the Strange Situation or the AQS. Worth noting as well is that De Wolff and van IJzendoorn did not include the findings of the

original Ainsworth and colleagues (1978) study in their meta-analyses because its results, like those more recent (null) ones of Seifer and colleagues (1996) (which were included), were regarded as outliers relative to the entire corpus of findings.

Whether one regards the magnitude of the effect of maternal care as weak or moderate, it is indisputable that Ainsworth's core theoretical proposition linking maternal sensitivity with attachment security has been empirically confirmed (Belsky, 1997). Four possibilities might account for why attachment security is less well accounted for by maternal sensitivity than many expected. The first is a "technological" gap, in that the quality, intensity, or context of measurement of sensitivity is suboptimal. The fact that several recent studies, using arguably improved measurement methods, have repeatedly found substantially higher associations between sensitivity and attachment than the earlier meta-analytic average lends some credence to this first argument (Pederson, Gleason, Moran, & Bento, 1998; Raval et al., 2001; Tarabulsy et al., 2005; see also Atkinson et al., 2005).

The second possibility—of a "moderator" gap—concerns the fact that unidentified variables may moderate the sensitivity–attachment link, thereby diminishing the overall meta-analytic average when studies fail to consider potential moderating factors. This gap is addressed later in this chapter, when the proposition of differential susceptibility to rearing influences is discussed. The third and fourth possibilities for why effects of sensitivity are at best modest in magnitude are that the most predictive elements of parenting behavior have perhaps not been identified and fall outside of the definition of sensitivity (i.e., a "domain" gap), and that other factors unrelated to parental behavior contribute to attachment security and mediate the association (a "third-variable" gap) (Belsky, 2005b). Such possibilities are considered later in this chapter, in the discussion of broader ecological influences on attachment security when personal/psychological resources of mothers are examined—particularly the constructs of "mindmindedness" and "reflective functioning." What should be clear at this juncture is that the modest variance in attachment accounted for by sensitivity clearly indicates that the quest to elucidate the causal antecedents of attachment is far from over (De Wolff & van IJzendoorn, 1997).

From Correlational to Experimental Evidence

The modesty of the meta-analytically derived correlation between maternal behavior and attachment security, coupled with the logical possibility that this reliably discerned association could be a product of the effect of infant characteristics (especially temperament) on maternal interactive style, provides a basis for questioning the causal role of maternal care in fostering security or insecurity. Fortunately, van den Boom's (1990) aforementioned investigation of 100 irritable Dutch infants from economically at-risk families put the issue to rest, especially the argument that insecurity reflects negative emotionality or difficult temperament. This is because her study design included an experimental manipulation to foster maternal sensitivity: Three home visits designed to foster mothers' "contingent, consistent, and appropriate responses to both positive and negative infant signals" were administered to 50 mothers randomly assigned to an experimental group. The home visitor/intervenor "aimed to enhance mothers' observational skills … [and] assisted mothers to adjust their behaviors to their infant's [sic] unique cries" (p. 208). Control group mothers were simply observed in interaction with their babies. Importantly, the two groups of mothers were equivalent in terms of maternal behavior prior to the implementation of the intervention.

Impressively, not only did postintervention observations reveal that maternal sensitivity was greater in the experimental group, but results of Strange Situation evaluations 4 months after the termination of the intervention were strongly consistent with predictions derived from attachment theory: Whereas a full 68% (34 of 50) of the infants in the control group were classified as insecure, this was true of only 28% (14 of 50) of the experimental subjects! No doubt these findings resulted from the fact that "experimental mothers respond[ed] to the whole range of infant signals (during post-intervention home observation), whereas control mothers mainly focus[ed] on very negative infant signals" (van den Boom, 1990, p. 236). More specifically, in the insecurity-producing control group,

> mildly negative infant behaviors like fussing are ignored for most of the time or are responded to ineffectively. Positively toned attachment behaviors, on the contrary, are ignored for the most part. And infant exploration is either ignored or interfered with. The program mothers' infants' negative actions boost maternal positive actions. Maternal anger is not observed. … Positive social infant behaviors are also responded to in a positive fashion. And program mothers are attentive to the infant's exploration, but they do not interfere in the process. (van den Boom, 1990, p. 236)

These findings chronicling a causal—not just correlational—impact of the quality of maternal care on attachment security are, in the main, in accord with those emanating from other experimental investigations. In both an original (van IJzendoorn, Juffer, & Duyvesteyn, 1995) and a more recently updated (Bakermans-Kranenburg, van IJzendoorn, & Juffer, 2003) meta-analysis of intervention studies, van IJzendoorn and colleagues showed that interventions are effective in enhancing maternal sensitivity, and that in particular, short-term interventions (like van den Boom's) can therefore increase the probability of an infant developing a secure attachment to its mother. Indeed, the combined effect size for 10 studies that sought to promote security by enhancing sensitivity was 0.39 (Bakermans-Kranenburg et al., 2003). These results extend those from correlational studies in documenting a truly causal effect of maternal care on attachment security.

The Case of Disorganization

Studies documenting links between child maltreatment and disorganized attachment gave birth to Main and Hesse's (1990) hypothesis that fear in the attachment relationship serves as the driving force behind disorganization. Research testing this proposition provides the clearest example of the need to move beyond sensitivity in seeking to understand the interactional determinants of attachment. This is because at least six independent studies have found that disorganized attachment is associated with disturbances in parenting behavior that could be considered frightening to the infant (rather than insensitive) (Abrams, Rifkin, & Hesse, 2006; Goldberg, Benoit, Blokland, & Madigan, 2003; Lyons-Ruth, Bronfman, & Parsons, 1999; Madigan, Moran, & Pederson, 2006; Schuengel, Bakermans-Kranenburg, & van IJzendoorn, 1999; True, Pisani, & Oumar, 2001). Maternal sensitivity, in contrast, appears to be only very weakly associated with disorganized attachment when subjected to meta-analysis (van IJzendoorn, Schuengel, & Bakermans-Kranenburg, 1999). Furthermore, two studies chronicle the effect of frightening behavior on disorganization even when maternal sensitivity is controlled for (Schuengel et al., 1999; True et al., 2001).

A recent series of studies has broadened the domain of inquiry from an emphasis on frightening/frightened/dissociative (FR) behavior to disturbances in parental affective communication (Lyons-Ruth et al., 1999). The latter category subsumes FR behavior but also includes less obviously frightening atypical maternal behavior, such as affective communication errors (e.g., contradictory cues), role confusion (e.g., role reversal or sexualized behavior), and withdrawal (creating physical or verbal distance from the infant; see Lyons-Ruth et al., 1999). Empirically, this broader set of maternal behaviors has been found to correlate quite consistently with disorganized attachment (Abrams et al., 2006; Goldberg et al., 2003; Lyons-Ruth et al., 1999 [see also Lyons-Ruth, Yellin, Melnick, & Atwood, 2005, on the same sample]; Madigan et al., 2006; see Lyons-Ruth & Jacobvitz, Chapter 28, this volume, for a review).

What currently cannot be discerned from these studies is the extent to which disrupted affective communication contributes additional predictive power over and above that accounted for by FR behavior. No research has tested this; nor, indeed, has there been any examination of whether there is variable discriminative power within the domains of FR behavior itself. Although one study found that dissociative behavior predicted infant disorganization independently of other FR elements (Abrams et al., 2006), this work was based on an analysis of the sample from which the original FR coding system was developed and hence may have partially capitalized on chance. Schuengel and colleagues (1999) and Madigan and colleagues (2006) also found stronger associations between dissociative behavior and infant disorganization than the other FR scales, but did not test whether the effect size was significantly different from or independent of the other scales. In three studies, the preeminence of dissociative behavior was not found (Goldberg et al., 2003; Lyons-Ruth et al., 1999) or was not examined (True et al., 2001).

Quite apart from whether available measures of maternal behavior have greater or lesser predictive power, a critical question that no correlational study has been in a position to address directly is whether any of the associations detected are truly causal, though one recent study has linked *change* in atypical maternal behavior with *change* in attachment disorganization from 12 to 24 months (Forbes, Evans, Moran, & Pederson, 2007). Interestingly, Juffer, Bakermans-Kranenburg, and van IJzendoorn (2005) reported a reanalysis of data from their earlier sensitivity-based intervention study, discovering that the intervention had reduced disorganized attachment. Intriguingly, despite the focus of the intervention, the positive impact on disorganization was not mediated by changes in sensitivity. The authors speculate that the intervention may have indirectly reduced FR

behavior, perhaps by increasing parents' attention to and awareness of their child's behavior and the impact of their own behavior on the child. The positive impact of sensitivity-based interventions on disorganized attachment has been confirmed in a recent meta-analysis of 15 intervention studies (that were also not designed to reduce FR behavior) (Bakermans-Kranenburg et al., 2005). Collectively, these results indicate that disorganization is susceptible to environmental remediation, but how these changes take place is an important question for clinicians and scientists alike.

Cultural Variation

Cross-cultural variation in parenting can shed further light on the nature of the interactional antecedents of attachment security (see also van IJzendoorn & Sagi-Schwartz, Chapter 37, this volume). One might wonder, for example, whether the association between sensitivity and attachment emerges in non-U.S. or non-European samples, where cultural norms for raising infants may be quite different. Posada, Carbonell, Alzate, and Plata (2004) conducted an intensive investigation of patterns of parenting behavior in 30 Colombian families to address this very issue. Data were gathered via standardized assessments of maternal sensitivity (using the Maternal Behavior Q-Sort [MBQS]) and open-ended ethnographic transcripts of parenting behavior. There was considerable correspondence between the domains of parenting behavior identified through ethnographical analysis and those originally developed by Ainsworth and refined by Pederson and colleagues. Furthermore, both maternal sensitivity identified by the MBQS and the ethnographically derived parenting parallel to sensitivity correlated significantly with infant attachment security as measured with the AQS. Similar results were obtained by Zevalkink, Riksen-Walraven, and Van Lieshout (1999) with a Sudanese–Indonesian sample, and by Peterson, Drotar, Olness, Guay, and Kiziri-Mayengo (2001) in a study of Ugandan mothers and infants. Tomlinson and colleagues (2005) also detected robust associations between attachment and various indices of parenting quality (sensitivity, intrusiveness, coerciveness, remoteness) in a sample of extremely impoverished black South African mother–infant dyads. They were also able to show that disorganized attachment was associated with a modified measure of maternal FR behavior administered when the infants were 2 months of age. True and colleagues (2001) also found infant disorganization to be correlated with observed maternal FR behavior in a sample of Malian infants and mothers, whereas broader measures of sensitivity were only marginally correlated with security. Using data from the NICHD Study of Early Child Care, Bakermans-Kranenburg, van IJzendoorn, and Kroonenburg (2004) recently examined whether patterns of association between attachment and sensitivity were similar between European American and African American families. The associations proved to be highly consistent across groups, and the significantly lower mean attachment security score (measured via the AQS) in the African American group was fully accounted for by differences in socioeconomic status (SES).

There is thus reasonably consistent evidence that the overall direction of findings relating security to parenting sensitivity is relatively preserved across a range of cultural contexts. Despite this, some evidence suggests caveats that may be required for such a conclusion. Carlson and Harwood (2003) found, for example, that Puerto Rican mothers used more physically controlling tactics in caregiving than European American mothers did, and that higher physically controlling parenting was associated with secure attachment in the Puerto Rican group but not in the European American mothers, where it was associated with infant avoidance. Although the small sample and imperfect matching of the two groups limit interpretation of this finding, it does indicate that further research is warranted on potentially important culture-specific associations between parenting and attachment.

Nonmaternal Care

Even though attachment theory is often cast as a theory of the infant–*mother* relationship, most attachment scholars consider attachment to be involved in emotionally close child–*adult* relationships more generally. Indeed, Bowlby made it clear that in writing about the mother, he was assuming that mothers are usually the primary caregivers. If, as is now widely recognized, infants and young children can establish relationships with more than a single individual (neither Bowlby nor Ainsworth argued otherwise), a theoretically important question is whether the interactional processes highlighted as important to the development of secure relationships with mothers also operate with other adults. The few available studies of fathers and of nonparental caregivers indicate that this is indeed the case.

Infant–Father Attachment

In fact, even though the majority of investigations that have examined the relation between quality of paternal care and infant–father attachment security have individually failed to document a significant effect of fathering on attachment security (Belsky, 1983; Braungart-Reiker et al., 2001; Caldera, Huston, & O'Brien, 1995; Easterbrooks & Goldberg, 1984; Grossmann & Grossmann, 1992; Schneider-Rosen & Rothbaum, 1993; Volling & Belsky, 1992), a different picture emerges when the results of these and two other studies showing a significant relation (Cox et al., 1992; Goossens & van IJzendoorn, 1990) are combined and subjected to meta-analysis. When data from the eight investigations are considered together, a significant ($p < .001$), even if small (0.13), effect size emerges ($N = 546$) (van IJzendoorn & De Wolff, 1997). This is smaller than the 0.24 figure for infant–mother attachment relationships. As the meta-analysts point out, however, the small effect size represents the lower boundary of the association between paternal sensitivity and infant–father attachment: Nonsignificant findings that were insufficiently specified in the original research reports had to be replaced with zero correlations (or probability values of .50) in the analysis, when they might actually have been higher.

Infant–Caregiver Attachment

Ahnert, Pinquart, and Lamb's (2006) recent meta-analysis of 40 investigations involving almost 3,000 children (average age = 29.6 months) reveals a great deal about the security of children's relationships with nonparental caregivers. First, attachments to nonparental providers were less likely to be secure than attachments to parents (in studies that measured both) when assessed by means of the Strange Situation, but equally secure attachments were more likely when Q-sort methods were used. Second, the security of children's relationships with their mothers and fathers was significantly related to the security of their attachment to their care providers. Third, secure attachment to caregivers was more likely in home-based than in center-based care, more likely for girls than for boys, and more likely when children had been with particular caregivers for longer periods. The fact that secure attachments to caregivers were more likely to be detected in older than in newer studies across the quarter century of research covered by the meta-analysis suggests that this trend may be the result of the ever-increasing emphasis on education (i.e., literacy, numeracy) in child care, at the expense of emotional development.

Most important from the standpoint of the current chapter was evidence addressing the influence of caregiver sensitivity on security of attachment to caregiver. Making a distinction between sensitivity to individual children (as always investigated in the case of parents) and sensitivity to a group of children, Ahnert and colleagues (2006) found that setting mattered: Whereas care providers' sensitivity to individual children predicted attachment security in the small groups that characterize home-based settings (and more so when the number of children being cared for was smaller), sensitivity to the group as a whole best predicted security of attachment to caregivers in larger groups (i.e., centers), though individual sensitivity was also related to security.

Evidence from an intervention study suggests, at least in the case of home-based care, that the relations detected in the meta-analysis are causal. When Galinsky, Howes, and Kontos (1995) improved the care of home-based caregivers via a training program, security of infant–provider attachments improved. Unfortunately, no such research has been carried out in groups to document either indisputably causal relations or differential effects of individual versus group sensitivity in the development of secure attachment to care provider. These comments notwithstanding, the evidence reviewed suggests that relationship processes somewhat similar to those delineated in studies of mothering appear relevant to the development of secure relationships with others with whom a child is expected to develop a close, affectional bond.

Summary of the Evidence

When considered in its entirety, the evidence summarized in this section pertaining to mothering, fathering, and the care provided by some other consistent caregiver offers support for Ainsworth's (1973) extension of Bowlby's theory of attachment. Individual differences in attachment security, whether measured with the laboratory-based Strange Situation or the home-based AQS procedure, are systematically related to the quality of the care that an infant or toddler experiences with a particular caregiver; this is true of both the role of sensitivity in fostering security and of FR behavior in fostering disorganization. What makes the former (and some of the latter) evidence par-

ticularly convincing is that it is both correlational and experimental in nature; longitudinal as well as cross-sectional; apparently cross-culturally generalizable; and derived from studies of fathers and child care providers as well as of mothers. Finally, even though infant temperamental characteristics may contribute to the quality of interaction between caregiver and child, the evidence that such attributes are the primary determinants of attachment security is especially limited.

Differential Susceptibility

However theoretically important the data linking adult–infant interaction to attachment security may be, the fact remains that associations between rearing and attachment are only modest in magnitude. Recent evolutionary theorizing highlights one reason—referred to above as a "moderator" gap—for this less than strong association. Moreover, intriguing evidence is offered that temperament may be important to attachment in ways that have not heretofore been appreciated.

Elsewhere, Belsky (1997, 2005c) notes that because the future is uncertain, it makes biological sense for children to vary, particularly within a family, in their susceptibility to rearing influence (see also Boyce & Ellis, 2005). If all children are equally influenced by parental care, then there may be—or would have been in the environment of evolutionary adaptedness—the risk that when the future does not prove consistent with parents' (not necessarily conscious) expectations, presumed to guide (often in unconscious ways) their rearing practices, then all children within a family may be led into a literal or at least a reproductive dead end. That is, they may fail to succeed in the biologically fundamental task of surviving to reproductive age and passing on genes to future generations.

Perhaps one way that natural selection has reduced the likelihood of this pitfall in the course of shaping human development is by increasing the probability that parents will conceive children who vary in their tendencies to be influenced by their rearing experiences, with some being more and others less susceptible. "Fixed strategists" may develop along lines established principally by their biological makeup, whereas "plastic strategists" may navigate the ship of development according to prevailing (rearing) winds. In line with general evolutionary terminology, the term "strategist" in no way implies conscious intent on the part of a child, any more than the terminology of "difficult" temperament implies deliberate effort on the child's part to make rearing especially challenging for parents.

If differential susceptibility to rearing represents an evolved characteristic of our species, then all research efforts failing to distinguish infants/children along these lines may both over- and underestimate effects of rearing, including studies of rearing influences on attachment security. Research may overestimate rearing influences for fixed strategists and underestimate them for plastic ones. Not only does some evidence (both correlational and experimental) suggest that highly negatively emotional infants/toddlers may be especially susceptible to rearing influence, especially with regard to developmental outcomes related to self-control and socioemotional development (for a review, see Belsky, 2005c); this is also true in the case of studies of mothering and attachment security. Consider first the fact that the intervention study documenting perhaps the largest indisputably causal effect of rearing on attachment was carried out on a sample preselected for being highly negatively emotional (van den Boom, 1994). Consider next the fact that when Velderman and colleagues (2006) formally tested Belsky's (1997) differential-susceptibility hypothesis by means of an experimental intervention, they found support for it: Attachment security proved most susceptible to intervention-induced changes in maternal sensitivity among infants who were highly negative.

Further evidence that the influence of the quality of maternal care on attachment security is not the same for all children comes from two recent molecular-genetic studies investigating the existence of gene × environment interactions in the case of attachment security. In one study, Gervai and colleagues (2007) found that a dopamine receptor gene—*DRD4*—interacted with a measure of disrupted forms of maternal communication in the prediction of attachment organization. More specifically, the anticipated adverse effect of such disrupted communication on the development of disorganized attachment held only for those infants who had the short form of the *DRD4* allele, with no relation between mothering and disorganization emerging in the case of those with the 7-repeat *DRD4* allele (but see van IJzendoorn & Bakermans-Kranenburg, 2006, for failure to replicate this result when "frightening" maternal behavior was used to index disrupted mothering). In the second study, the outcome to be explained was security of attachment and evidence indicated

the maternal sensitive responsiveness predicted attachment security only in the case of infants carrying one or two short alleles of a serotonin transporter gene—*5HTTLPR*—and thus no apparent influence of sensitive responsiveness on infants carrying two long versions of the *5HTTLPR* allele (Barry, Kochanska, & Philibert, in press). Of particular interest given the previous discussion of the role of infant negative emotionality in moderating the effect of rearing experience on attachment security is further molecular-genetic evidence indicating that the short version of the *5HTTLPR* polymorphism is itself related to infant negativity (e.g., Auerbach et al., 1999). This raises the possibility, of course, that the reason why studies considered in the preceding paragraph by van den Boom (1994) and Velderman and colleagues (2006) may have generated the results that they did showing that highly negative infants were more susceptible to the effects of rearing on attachment was because they, too, were carriers of the short *5HTTLPR* allele. Further consideration of the contribution that evolutionary theory can make to thinking about attachment and human development can be found in Simpson and Belsky's (Chapter 6) contribution to this volume.

PSYCHOLOGICAL AND SOCIAL-CONTEXTUAL DETERMINANTS

Having considered the interactional determinants of attachment security, we now turn our attention to the role of more "distal" factors implicated by an ecological perspective and likely to impact the quality of care that mothers (and other caregivers) provide. First to be considered are parental personality and related psychological attributes. The influence of parental state of mind regarding attachment is not considered, however, because Hesse (Chapter 25, this volume) addresses that topic. After considering parental psychological makeup, we consider the broader context of child–parent attachment relationships, including the social-contextual sources of stress and support—specifically, the marital/couple relationship and social support from associates other than spouses or partners.

Parental Psychological Resources and Personality

Because the provision of security-inducing sensitive care requires the accurate reading of, and timely and empathic responding to, a child's affective and behavioral cues, there are theoretical grounds for expecting the caregiver's psychological attributes to be related to the security of attachment that the child develops. Moreover, much theory and evidence having little to do with attachment indicate that both mothers' and fathers' psychological health and well-being affect the quality of care that parents provide (for a review, see Belsky & Jaffee, 2006). Evidence from both normal and clinical samples underscores the importance of parental psychological makeup vis-à-vis infant attachment security.

Normal Samples

Cross-sectional studies (Benn, 1986; Ricks, 1985) and longitudinal ones (in which personality is measured prior to attachment security) indicate that in nondisturbed populations, secure attachment relationships are more likely to develop when mothers are psychologically healthy. Maslin and Bates (1983) found, for example, that mothers of secure infants scored higher than mothers of insecure infants on a series of personality subscales measuring nurturance, understanding, autonomy, inquisitiveness, and dependence, and lower on a subscale assessing aggressiveness. Subsequently, Del Carmen and colleagues (1993) reported that mothers who scored higher on prenatal anxiety were more likely than those scoring lower on anxiety to have insecure 1-year-olds; and O'Connor (1997) observed that mothers of secure infants were likely to describe themselves as self-confident, independent, cheerful, adaptable, and affectionate. In the largest study to date, involving more than 1,100 infants, maternal personality was assessed when infants were 1 month of age, and it was found that mothers of infants classified as secure at 15 months of age scored higher on a composite index of psychological adjustment (agreeableness + extraversion – neuroticism – depression) than mothers of insecure infants (NICHD Early Child Care Network, 1997). Atkinson and colleagues' (2000) meta-analysis revealed, moreover, that across 13 studies maternal stress was significantly associated with attachment insecurity (mean effect size = 0.19). It is notable that findings like these are not restricted to economically advantaged families, but also emerge in research on high-risk, low-SES households (Jacobson & Frye, 1991; Sims, Hans, & Cox, 1996), as well as in countries outside North America (Scher & Mayseless, 2000).

Not all relevant investigations, however, provide evidence of statistically significant associations between parental personality and attachment security (Barnett, Blignault, Holmes, Payne, & Parker, 1987; Belsky, Rosenberger, & Crnic, 1995; Levitt, Weber, & Clark, 1986; Zeanah et al., 1993). Perhaps more noteworthy, though, is the lack of any evidence indicating that parents of secure infants are *less* psychologically healthy than other parents.

In addition to focusing upon maternal personality and psychological distress, research on attachment has considered other aspects of maternal psychological functioning in an effort to better understand what van IJzendoorn (1995) has labeled the "transmission gap"—a reference to the fact that measured sensitivity does not fully account for the link, as some anticipated it might, between a mother's own state of mind regarding attachment and infant attachment security. Meins, Fernyhough, Fradley, and Tuckey (2001, p. 638) have focused on "mind-mindedness," which they define as a mother's readiness "to treat her infant as an individual with a mind, rather than merely as a creature with needs that must be satisfied." Support for the Meins and colleagues hypothesis that mind-mindedness contributes to attachment security comes from work showing that mothers of secure infants are more likely than mothers of insecure infants to make appropriate mind-minded comments when interacting with their infants. Meins and colleagues also found that the effect of mind-mindedness was independent of the significant contribution of maternal sensitivity to the prediction of attachment security, though it has not yet been reported that it helps fill the "transmission gap." Slade, Grienenberger, Bernbach, Levy, and Locker (2005) have reported similar results upon measuring a construct seemingly related to "mind-mindedness" labeled "reflective functioning" (Fonagy, Steele, Moran, Steele, & Higgitt, 1991), even showing in a pilot study that it mediates some of the effect of adult attachment on infant attachment. Exactly how parental thought processes and related comments come to influence the organization of the infant's attachment behavior remains unclear, though (see Fonagy, Gergely, & Target, Chapter 33, this volume).

Clinical Samples

Depression in its various manifestations—unipolar and bipolar—is the clinical disorder most often studied in relation to attachment security. On the basis of evidence linking both unresponsive/detached and intrusive/rejecting mothering with maternal depression (see Belsky & Jaffee, 2006, for a review), there are strong grounds for expecting children of depressed mothers to be at heightened risk of insecure attachment. Perusal of the available evidence reveals seemingly inconsistent findings, however. Whereas some research fails to find the expected significant association between maternal psychological disorder and elevated rates of insecurity (Frankel, Maslin-Cole, & Harmon, 1991; Lyons-Ruth, Zoll, Connell, & Grunebaum, 1986 [12-month data]; Sameroff, Seifer, & Zax, 1982), other investigations do document such a linkage (Campbell, Cohn, Meyers, Ross, & Flanagan, 1993; D'Angelo, 1986; Das Eiden & Leonard, 1996; DeMulder & Radke-Yarrow, 1991; Gaensbauer, Harmon, Cytryn, & McKnew, 1984; Lyons-Ruth, 1988 [18-month data]; Murray et al., 1996; Radke-Yarrow, 1991; Radke-Yarrow, Cummings, Kuczynski, & Chapman, 1985; Spieker & Booth, 1988; Teti et al., 1995; Tomlinson, Cooper, & Murray, 2005).

Martins and Gaffan (2000) conducted a meta-analysis of 7 studies that compared rates of attachment insecurity in samples of mothers with a clinical diagnosis of unipolar depression versus nondepressed controls. They statistically documented significant variability across studies in the rates of insecurity associated with depression. When one study outlier was removed, significantly higher levels of insecurity emerged in depressed samples than controls—although when another outlying sample was removed, this effect was diminished to nonsignificance. For a homogeneous set of studies that broadly found an association with attachment, rates of infant disorganization and avoidance were significantly elevated in depressed populations, but rates of resistance were not.

In a broader meta-analysis of depression and attachment that included 15 studies of clinical and nonclinical samples, Atkinson and colleagues (2000) discerned a significant overall association between depression and attachment (effect size r = 0.18), with clinical samples yielding a stronger effect size than nonclinical ones (0.27 vs. 0.09). Like Martins and Gaffan (2000), Atkinson and colleagues also noted significant variability within the group of clinical samples, but they could detect no reliable predictor of effect size.

In sum, the relation between depression and insecurity or disorganization emerges repeatedly, though not in every study, suggesting that it is likely to be dependent upon a variety of factors. Some work raises the prospect that in addition to

whether a sample comprises clinical or nonclinical cases, degree of exposure may matter (i.e., chronicity of depression), though this prospect was not substantiated in the Atkinson and colleagues (2000) meta-analysis. In any event, evidence linking depression with insecurity and/or disorganization is likely to be driven by the actual effect of depression on the quality of care that mothers provide, as it is presumably when sensitive behavior is disrupted or FR behavior is manifested that links would emerge. This analysis is consistent with the mediational thinking informing this entire chapter, which stipulates that even though maternal psychological well-being, as well as a mother's marital/couple relationship and social support, may directly affect attachment insecurity (through some unspecified process), most of the effect of such distal factors will flow through their impact on the quality of care the mother actually provides.

Perhaps the best evidence of such a mediational process involving maternal psychological well-being comes from a study of nondisordered women, which serves as a useful conclusion to this section. Benn (1986) found that when a composite index of psychological well-being—labeled "emotional integration" and drawn from clinical interview ratings of competence, emotional responsivity, warmth, and acceptance of motherhood—was statistically controlled, a previously obtained and significant association between maternal sensitivity and attachment security was substantially attenuated. Such results are clearly in accord with the mediational view, which links distal factors with attachment security via more proximal processes of parenting.

The Marital/Couple Relationship

An abundance of evidence indicates that a supportive relationship with a spouse or partner during the infancy and toddler years is correlated with the very kinds of parenting theorized (and found) to predict attachment security (e.g., Tarabulsy et al., 2005; Tomlinson et al., 2005; for narrative reviews, see Belsky & Jaffee, 2006, and Grych, 2002; for a meta-analytic review, see Krishnakumar & Buehler, 2000). Given data linking relationship quality with many of the aspects of parenting found to be predictive of attachment security (De Wolff & van IJzendoorn, 1997), there are strong grounds to expect a relation between marital/couple functioning and infant–parent attachment security. The fact that a mediational perspective leads to such a prediction does not preclude the possibility that relationship quality may affect attachment security directly, rather than exclusively via parenting-mediated processes. Not only does Davies and Cummings's (1994) emotional security hypothesis lead to such a prediction, but Owen and Cox's (1997) failure to find evidence of a parent-mediated linkage is consistent with it. Especially in the case of overt conflict, it is not difficult to imagine how exposure to such aversive interactions between mother and father could foster insecurity directly.

Available evidence is consistent with both mediational and direct-effect theorizing. That is, children growing up with parents who have better-functioning couple relationships are more likely to develop secure attachments than those growing up in households where parents are less happy in their relationships. Such results emerge from cross-sectional studies carried out in the United States (Crnic, Greenberg, & Slough, 1986; Goldberg & Easterbrooks, 1984; Howes & Markman, 1989; Jacobson & Frye, 1991) and in Japan (Durrett, Otaki, & Richards, 1984). Moreover, in work on poor African American mothers and infants, Sims and colleagues (1996) found that when fathers were physically violent with mothers, infants were more likely to be insecurely attached to their mothers.

More important than these results from cross-sectional research are those from several longitudinal studies. In one such investigation, Howes and Markman (1989) found that wives who prenatally reported higher levels of marital satisfaction and lower levels of spousal conflict had children who scored higher on the AQS 1–3 years later. Tracking similar middle-class families across a somewhat shorter time period, Lewis, Owen, and Cox (1988) reported that 1-year-old daughters (but not sons) were more likely to be securely attached to their mothers when marriages were more harmonious during pregnancy. Subsequently, Teti and colleagues (1995) showed that greater marital harmony before a second child was born predicted greater security (via the AQS) on the part of the firstborn both in the last trimester of the mother's pregnancy and up to 2 months following the birth of the younger sibling. In a related study, Owen and Cox (1997) found that more marital conflict (observed prenatally and at 3 months postpartum) predicted less secure infant–father attachments and greater disorganization in infant–mother relationships (assessed at 12 months), even after each parent's psychological maturity was controlled for.

Such findings would seem consistent with those reported by Belsky and Isabella (1988) indicating that relationship quality declines more precipitously across the transition to parenthood in the case of infants subsequently classified as insecurely rather than securely attached to their mothers. Also noteworthy is Spieker's (1988; Spieker & Booth, 1988) research on high-risk mother–infant dyads showing that the lowest levels of spousal support measured prenatally and at 3 months postpartum characterize the marriages in families in which infants develop disorganized attachments.

Despite the seeming persuasiveness of the cross-sectional and longitudinal data, it would be a mistake to selectively cite only the aforementioned research and leave the impression that all studies of marital/couple relationships and attachment present such positive and statistically significant results. Not only have a number of investigations failed to find a significant association between some index of relationship quality and infant–parent attachment security (Belsky, 1996; Belsky et al., 1995; Das Eiden & Leonard, 1996; Harrison & Ungerer, 2002; Levitt et al., 1986; Teti, Nakasawa, Das, & Wirth, 1991; Zeanah et al., 1993); one study of an unusual sample—Japanese mothers living in the United States due to their husbands' employment—actually produced results showing higher levels of marital quality to be associated with less AQS-rated security (Nakasawa, Teti, & Lamb, 1992). Two studies draw attention to the possibility that the multiple null findings just cited may reflect the limits of inquiring into direct effects, rather than the absence of a relation between relationship quality and attachment security. In one illuminating piece of work, Isabella (1994) found that even though no direct relation between marital quality (measured prenatally) and attachment security (at one year) could be discerned, an indirect pathway of influence did appear to exist, mediated by maternal role satisfaction.

Whereas the work of Isabella (1994) underscores an indirect (and not typically studied) process by which relationship quality might affect the infant–mother attachment bond, work by Das Eiden, Teti, and Corns (1993) draws attention to the need to study relationship quality in context. Although Das Eiden and colleagues found that higher levels of marital quality were related to higher levels of security as measured via the AQS, further analyses revealed that this relation was restricted to families in which mothers were classified as insecure on the Adult Attachment Interview. What is fascinating about these data is not only that they are consistent with other research showing that a mother with a risky developmental history is less likely to mother poorly if she has a supportive relationship (see Belsky & Jaffee, 2006, for a review); they also suggest that in order for a full understanding of the relationship's impact on the development of secure or insecure attachment bonds, additional information about the family is useful.

We return to this theme of multiple determinants in the concluding section of this chapter. For now, it suffices to say that accepting null findings as conclusive may be premature when only direct effects are examined. Developmental influences do not operate in isolation, so there is a need to take into consideration not only mediational processes (e.g., via role satisfaction and mothering), but moderational ones (e.g., interactions with maternal state of mind) when considering linkages between marital/couple relationships and attachment.

Social Support from Others

It is not just relations with spouse or partner that are systematically related to what transpires between parents and their children (Belsky, 1984). Consistent with the theorizing of Cochran and colleagues (Cochran & Brassard, 1979; Cochran & Niego, 2002), numerous investigations now provide evidence that the amount and nature of contact and support that parents, especially mothers, experience from significant others in their lives affects the way they interact with their infants (for a meta-analysis, see Andersen & Telleen, 1992). For example, middle-class European American mothers with more prenatal social support were more sensitive when interacting with their 3-month-olds (Goldstein, Diener, & Mangelsdorf, 1996). Low-income African American mothers with larger social networks tended to be more responsive when interacting with their infants (Burchinal, Follmer, & Bryand, 1996). Poor Hispanic women who received more material resources from friends and relatives engaged in more proximal (touching, kissing, holding) and distal (vocalizing, looking) interactions with their 3-month-old premature infants (Feiring, Fox, Jaskir, & Lewis, 1987). And mothers of preterm infants who had the highest level of social support exhibited the most favorable patterns of parenting (Smith, Landry, & Swank, 2000). Given the mediational thinking central to this chapter, such findings lead to the expectation that nonspousal social support should be positively associated with infant attachment security.

Ten studies pertaining to the relation between social support from others and infant–mother attachment security have been reported and most failed to yield the expected association (Belsky et al., 1995; Belsky & Isabella, 1988; Crnic et al., 1986; Levitt et al., 1986; Spieker, 1988; Spieker & Booth, 1988; Zeanah et al., 1993). Notably, three efforts providing support for the hypotheses that more social support would significantly predict attachment security focus on samples at risk for insensitive maternal care or insecure attachment. Thus Crockenberg (1981) found that the absence of social support predicted insecure attachment, but only in the case of highly irritable infants. Crnic and colleagues (1986) reported that an index of total community support was positively correlated with attachment security in a sample of premature infants. And Crittenden (1985) showed that in a group of infants with abusive or neglectful mothers, low social support predicted insecurity. Perhaps more interesting and theoretically significant, however, is that this effect of social support in the Crittenden investigation disappeared once quality of maternal care (i.e., abuse or neglect) was controlled for, consistent with the mediational arguments advanced throughout this chapter. It is also interesting that a fourth study that revealed a significant association between social support and attachment did so in an Australian sample where resistant attachments were the largest insecure category by some margin (Harrison & Ungerer, 2002).

Once again, Isabella's (1994) research cautions against concluding that attachment security is not affected by social support, even when direct effects of social support do not emerge as expected. This is because he found (as was the case with marital/couple relationship quality) that high social support significantly predicted high maternal role satisfaction, and thereby quality of maternal care and attachment security. Thus, even though the contribution of social support to attachment security was neither overwhelming nor direct, a process of influence postulated by Isabella—and consistent with the mediational argument developed throughout this chapter—was confirmed. Given the conflicting results across correlational studies, as well as the fact that mediational processes may be a more appropriate venue for understanding the effects of social support on attachment security, it seems misguided to embrace the null hypothesis of no relation between social support and infant–mother attachment.

INTEGRATION AND CONCLUSIONS

Evidence considered in the first part of this chapter has documented the role played by the quality of maternal and nonmaternal care in fostering secure and insecure attachments to mothers and fathers/other caregivers, respectively, as well as the apparent influence of FR maternal behavior on attachment disorganization in both Western and non-Western cultural contexts. Importantly, the evidence pertaining to infant–mother attachment security is experimental—and thereby causal—as well as correlational in nature. Also considered is the possibility that effect sizes may be modest because children may vary (for reasons based in evolutionary biology) in their susceptibility to rearing influence, with high levels of negative emotionality perhaps demarcating infants maximally susceptible to such influence.

In the second half of this chapter, the focus has been on determinants of attachment suggested by an ecological perspective. Central to the discussion of psychological and contextual factors is the assumption that so-called "distal" influences—be they less distant, like personality, or more distant, like social support—exert most of their effects by influencing more proximal processes of parent–child interaction. Although ample evidence provides grounds for concluding that all of the factors we have considered play a role in shaping the development of a secure or insecure attachment bond, inconsistency in the evidence has been repeatedly and purposefully highlighted. Up to this point, however, these factors have themselves not been placed "in context." By organizing the second part of the chapter around various factors, even while emphasizing mediational processes of influence, we have run the risk of leaving the impression that these sources of influence on the parent–child relationship, and thus on the child's attachment to his or her parent, operate in isolation. Nothing could be further from the truth.

Theory and research draw attention to the need to consider stresses and supports (Belsky, 1984; Belsky & Isabella, 1988; Belsky & Jaffee, 2006)—or, in the terms of developmental psychopathology, risk and protective factors (Cicchetti, 1983; Sroufe & Rutter, 1984)—simultaneously. Central to both of these theoretical orientations are the postulates (1) that risks can be balanced by strengths; and (2) that risks of problematical developmental outcomes, including attachment insecurity, are more likely to be realized as risk factors accumulate and are not balanced by sup-

ports or compensatory factors. Consider in this regard Das Eiden and Leonard's (1996) finding that heavy paternal alcohol consumption amplified the adverse effect of maternal depression on attachment insecurity.

Related findings have emerged in a series of studies by Belsky and colleagues concerning the effect of the accumulation of risks on attachment security. Perhaps most notable are data showing that even though not a single one of the distal psychological and social-contextual factors considered in the second part of this chapter individually distinguished secure and insecure attachments (to mothers or to fathers), a decidedly different result emerged when indices of personality, marital/couple relationship quality, social support, infant temperament, occupational stressors, and SES were considered collectively. When risk scores on these factors were composited, a clear and significant relation with attachment emerged, replicating earlier findings reported by Belsky and Isabella (1988): The more indications there were that a family and a specific infant–parent relationship were "at risk"—due to lower levels of parental psychological adjustment, poorer marital/couple relationship quality, more negative and less positive infant temperament, less social support, more work–family stress, and lower SES—the more likely infant–mother and infant–father relationships were to be insecure (Belsky, 1996; Belsky et al., 1995). More recently, Scher and Mayseless (2000), working in Israel, reported that an index of cumulative risk (e.g., maternal stress, separation anxiety, group day care) predicted attachment insecurity.

These results underscore the final point to be made in this chapter: To understand how psychological and social contexts influence the development of the child–parent attachment relationship, we must consider multiple factors simultaneously. Having a mother who is depressed is likely to have a dramatically different effect when the parents' relationship is also conflicted and the infant is temperamentally difficult than when the relationship is supportive and the infant is easy to care for. Thus not only do processes of mediation need to be central to our understanding of the origins of individual differences in attachment (distal factors → parent–child interaction → attachment security), but so too do moderational ones, because the impact of one source of influence is highly likely to be contingent on another. As Bronfenbrenner (1979, p. 38) so astutely noted in regard to the ecology of human development, and thus with respect to the etiology of secure and insecure infant–parent attachment bonds, "the principal main effects are likely to be interactions."

REFERENCES

Abrams, K. Y., Rifkin, A., & Hesse, E. (2006). Examining the role of parental frightened/frightening subtypes in predicting disorganized attachment within a brief observational procedure. *Development and Psychopathology, 18*, 345–361.

Ahnert, L., Pinquart, M., & Lamb, M. E. (2006). Security of children's relationships with nonparental care providers: A meta-analysis. *Child Development, 74*, 664–679.

Ainsworth, M. D. S. (1973). The development of infant–mother attachment. In B. M. Caldwell & H. N. Ricciuti (Eds.), *Review of child development research* (Vol. 3, pp. 1–94). Chicago: University of Chicago Press.

Ainsworth, M. D. S., Blehar, M. C., Waters, E., & Wall, S. (1978). *Patterns of attachment: A psychological study of the Strange Situation*. Hillsdale, NJ: Erlbaum.

Andersen, P., & Telleen, S. (1992). The relationship between social support and maternal behavior and attitudes: A meta-analytic review. *American Journal of Community Psychology, 20*, 753–774.

Atkinson, L., Goldberg, S., Raval, V., Pederson, D., Benoit, D., Moran, G., et al. (2005). On the relation between maternal state of mind and sensitivity in the prediction of infant attachment security. *Developmental Psychology, 41*, 42–53.

Atkinson, L., Paglia, A., Coolbear, J., Niccols, A., Parker, K. C. H., & Guger, S. (2000). Attachment security: A meta-analysis of maternal mental health correlates. *Clinical Psychology Review, 20*, 1019–1040.

Auerbach, J., Geller, V., Lezer, S., Shinwell, E., Belmaker, R. H., Levine, J., et al. (1999). Dopamine D4 receptor (D4DR) and serotonin transporter promoter (5-HTTLPR) polymorphisms in the determination of temperament in 2-month-old infants. *Molecular Psychiatry, 4*, 369–373.

Bakermans-Kranenburg, M. J., van IJzendoorn, M. H., Bokhorst, C. L., & Schuengel, C. (2004). The importance of shared environment in infant–father attachment: A behavioral genetic study of the Attachment Q-Sort. *Journal of Family Psychology, 18*, 545–549.

Bakermans-Kranenburg, M. J., van IJzendoorn, M. H., & Juffer, F. (2003). Less is more: Meta-analysis of sensitivity and attachment interventions in early childhood. *Psychological Bulletin, 129*, 195–215.

Bakermans-Kranenburg, M. J., van IJzendoorn, M. H., & Juffer, F. (2005). Disorganized infant attachment and preventive interventions: A review and meta-analysis. *Infant Mental Health Journal, 26*, 191–216.

Bakermans-Kranenburg, M. J., van IJzendoorn, M. H., & Kroonenberg, P. M. (2004). Differences in attachment security between African-American and white

children: Ethnicity or socio-economic status? *Infant Behavior and Development, 27*, 417–433.

Barnett, B., Blignault, I., Holmes, S., Payne, A., & Parker, G. (1987). Quality of attachment in a sample of 1-year-old Australian children. *Journal of the American Academy of Child and Adolescent Psychiatry, 26*, 303–307.

Barry, R. A., Kochanska, G., & Philibert, R. A. (in press). G × E interactions in the organization of attachment. *Developmental Psychology*.

Bates, J. E., Maslin, C. A., & Frankel, K. A. (1985). Attachment security, mother–child interaction, and temperament as predictors of behavior-problem ratings at age three years. In I. Bretherton & E. Waters (Eds.), Growing points of attachment theory and research. *Monographs of the Society for Research in Child Development, 50*(1–2, Serial No. 209), 167–193.

Belsky, J. (1983). *Father–infant interaction and security of attachment: No relationship*. Unpublished manuscript, Pennsylvania State University.

Belsky, J. (1984). The determinants of parenting: A process model. *Child Development, 55*, 83–96.

Belsky, J. (1996). Parent, infant, and social-contextual determinants of attachment security. *Developmental Psychology, 32*, 905–914.

Belsky, J. (1997). Theory testing, effect-size evaluation, and differential susceptibility to rearing influence: The case of mothering and attachment. *Child Development, 64*, 598–600.

Belsky, J. (2005a). Attachment theory and research in ecological perspective. In K. E. Grossmann, K. Grossmann, & E. Waters (Eds.), *Attachment from infancy to adulthood: The major longitudinal studies* (pp. 71–97). New York: Guilford Press.

Belsky, J. (2005b). The developmental and evolutionary psychology of intergenerational transmission of attachment. In C. S. Carter, L. Ahnert, K. Grossmann, S. Hrdy, M. Lamb, S. Porges, et al. (Eds.), *Attachment and bonding: A new synthesis* (pp. 169–198). Cambridge, MA: MIT Press.

Belsky, J. (2005c). Differential susceptibility to rearing influence: An evolutionary hypothesis and some evidence. In B. Ellis & D. Bjorklund (Eds.), *Origins of the social mind: Evolutionary psychology and child development* (pp. 139–163). New York: Guilford Press.

Belsky, J., Fish, M., & Isabella, R. (1991). Continuity and discontinuity in infant negative and positive emotionality: Family antecedents and attachment consequences. *Developmental Psychology, 27*, 421–431.

Belsky, J., & Isabella, R. (1988). Maternal, infant, and social-contextual determinants of attachment security. In J. Belsky & T. Nezworski (Eds.), *Clinical implications of attachment* (pp. 41–94). Hillsdale, NJ: Erlbaum.

Belsky, J., & Jaffee, S. (2006). The multiple determinants of parenting. In D. Cicchetti & D. Cohen (Eds.), *Developmental psychopathology: Vol. 3. Risk, disorder, and adaptation* (2nd ed., pp. 38–85). Hoboken, NJ: Wiley.

Belsky, J., Rosenberger, K., & Crnic, K. (1995). Maternal personality, marital quality, social support and infant temperament: Their significance for infant–mother attachment in human families. In C. Pryce, R. Martin, & D. Skuse (Eds.), *Motherhood in human and nonhuman primates* (pp. 115–124). Basel, Switzerland: Karger.

Belsky, J., & Rovine, M. (1987). Temperament and attachment security in the Strange Situation: An empirical rapprochement. *Child Development, 58,* 787–795.

Belsky, J., Rovine, M., & Taylor, D. G. (1984). The Pennsylvania Infant and Family Development Project: III. The origins of individual differences in infant–mother attachment: Maternal and infant contributions. *Child Development, 55,* 718–728.

Benn, R. K. (1986). Factors promoting secure attachment relationships between employed mothers and their sons. *Child Development, 57,* 1224–1231.

Bokhorst, C. L., Bakermans-Kranenburg, M. J., Fearon, R. M. P., van IJzendoorn, M. H., Fonagy, P., & Schuengel, C. (2003). The importance of shared environment in mother–infant attachment security: A behavioral genetic study. *Child Development, 74,* 1769–1782.

Bowlby, J. (1944). Forty-four juvenile thieves: Their characters and home life. *International Journal of Psycho-Analysis, 25,* 19–52.

Bowlby, J. (1958). The nature of the child's tie to his mother. *International Journal of Psycho-Analysis, 39,* 350–373.

Bowlby, J. (1969/1982). *Attachment and loss: Vol. 1. Attachment.* New York: Basic Books.

Boyce, W. T., & Ellis, B. J. (2005). Biological sensitivity to context. *Development and Psychopathology, 17,* 271–301.

Braungart-Rieker, J. M., Garwood, M. M., Powers, B. P., & Wang, X. (2001). Parental sensitivity, infant affect, and affect regulation: Predictors of later attachment. *Child Development, 72,* 252–270.

Bronfenbrenner, U. (1979). *The ecology of human development.* Cambridge, MA: Harvard University Press.

Burchinal, M., Follmer, A., & Bryand, D. (1996). The relations of maternal social support and family structure with maternal responsiveness and child outcomes among African American families. *Developmental Psychology, 6,* 1073–1083

Caldera, Y. M., Huston, A., & O'Brien, M. (1995, April). *Antecedents of father–infant attachment: A longitudinal study.* Paper presented at the biennial meeting of the Society for Research in Child Development, Indianapolis, IN.

Campbell, S. B., Cohn, J. F., Meyers, T. A., Ross, S., & Flanagan, C. (1993, April). Chronicity of maternal depression and mother–infant interaction. In D. Teti (Chair), *Depressed mothers and their children: Individual differences in mother–child outcome.* Symposium conducted at the biennial meeting of the Society for Research in Child Development, New Orleans, LA.

Carlson, V. J., & Harwood, R. L. (2003). Attachment, culture, and the caregiving system: The cultural patterning of everyday experiences among Anglo and Puerto Rican mother–infant pairs. *Infant Mental Health Journal, 24,* 53–73.

Chess, S., & Thomas, A. (1982). Infant bonding: Mystique and reality. *American Journal of Orthopsychiatry, 5,* 213–222.

Cicchetti, D. (1983). The emergence of developmental psychopathology. *Child Development, 55,* 1–7.

Cochran, M., & Brassard, J. (1979). Child development and personal social networks. *Child Development, 50,* 601–616.

Cochran, M., & Niego, S. (2002). Parenting and social networks. In M. Bornstein (Ed.), *Handbook of parenting: Vol. 4. Social conditions and applied parenting* (2nd ed., pp. 123–148). Mahwah, NJ: Erlbaum.

Cox, M., Owen, M. T., Henderson, V. K., & Margand, N. A. (1992). Prediction of infant–father and infant–mother attachment. *Developmental Psychology, 28,* 474–483.

Crittenden, P. M. (1985). Social networks, quality of child rearing, and child development. *Child Development, 56,* 1299–1313.

Crnic, K. A., Greenberg, M. T., & Slough, N. M. (1986). Early stress and social support influences on mothers' and high-risk infants' functioning in late infancy. *Infant Mental Health Journal, 7,* 19–33.

Crockenberg, S. B. (1981). Infant irritability, mother responsiveness, and social support influences on the security of infant–mother attachment. *Child Developmental, 52,* 857–869.

D'Angelo, E. J. (1986). Security of attachment in infants with schizophrenic, depressed, and unaffected mothers. *Journal of Genetic Psychology, 147,* 421–422.

Das Eiden, R., & Leonard, K. (1996). Paternal alcohol use and the mother–infant relationship. *Development and Psychopathology, 8,* 307–323.

Das Eiden, R., Teti, D., & Corns, K. (1993, April). *Maternal working models of attachment, marital adjustment, and the parent–child relationship.* Paper presented at the biennial meeting of the Society for Research in Child Development, New Orleans, LA.

Davies, P., & Cummings, E. M. (1994). Marital conflict and child adjustment: An emotional security hypothesis. *Psychological Bulletin, 116,* 387–411.

Del Carmen, R., Pedersen, F., Huffman, L., & Bryan, Y. (1993). Dyadic distress management predicts security of attachment. *Infant Behavior and Development, 16,* 131–147.

DeMulder, E. K., & Radke-Yarrow, M. (1991). Attachment with affectively ill and well mothers: Current behavioral correlates. *Developmental Psychopathology, 3,* 227–242.

De Wolff, M., & van IJzendoorn, M. (1997). Sensitivity and attachment: A meta-analysis on parental antecedents of infant attachment. *Child Development, 68,* 571–591.

Dozier, M., Stovall, K. C., Albus, K., & Bates, B. (2001). Attachment for infants in foster care: The role of caregiver state of mind. *Child Development, 72,* 1467–1477.

Durrett, M. E., Otaki, M., & Richards, P. (1984). Attachment and the mother's perception of support from the father. *International Journal Behavior Development, 7*, 167–176.

Easterbrooks, M. A., & Goldberg, W. A. (1984). Toddler development in the family: Impact of father involvement and parenting characteristics. *Child Development, 55*, 744–752.

Egeland, B., & Farber, E. A. (1984). Infant–mother attachment: Factors related to its development and changes over time. *Child Development, 55*, 753–771.

Feiring, C., Fox, N. A., Jaskir, J., & Lewis, M. (1987). The relation between social support, infant risk status, and mother–infant interaction. *Developmental Psychology, 23*, 400–405.

Feldstein, S., Crown, C., Beebe, B., & Jaffe, J. (1995, April). *Temporal coordination and the prediction of mother–infant attachment.* Paper presented at the biennial meeting of the Society for Research in Child Development, Indianapolis, IN.

Finkel, D., Wille, D. E., & Matheny, A. P., Jr. (1998). Preliminary results from a twin study of infant–caregiver attachment. *Behavior Genetics, 28*, 1–8.

Fish, M., & Stifter, C. (1995). Patterns of mother–infant interaction and attachment. *Infant Behavior and Development, 18*, 435–446.

Fonagy, P., Steele, M., Moran, G., Steele, H., & Higgitt, A. (1991). The capacity for understanding mental states: The reflective self in parent and child and its significance for security of attachment. *Infant Mental Health Journal, 13*, 200–216.

Forbes, L. M., Evans, E. M., Moran, G., & Pederson, D. R. (2007). Change in atypical maternal behavior predicts change in attachment disorganization from 12 to 24 months in a high-risk sample. *Child Development, 78*, 955–971.

Frankel, K., Maslin-Cole, C., & Harmon, R. (1991, April). *Depressed mothers of preschoolers.* Paper presented at the biennial meeting of the Society for Research in Child Development, Seattle, WA.

Gaensbauer, T. J., Harmon, R. J., Cytryn, L., & McKnew, D. H. (1984). Social and affective development in infants with a manic–depressive parent. *American Journal of Psychiatry, 141*, 223–229.

Galinsky, E., Howes, C., & Kontos, S. (1995). *The family child care training study.* New York: Families and Work Institute.

Gervai, G., Nemoda, Z., Lakatos, K., Ronai, Z., Toth, I., Ney, K., et al. (2005). Transmission disequilibrium tests confirm the link between DRD4 gene polymorphism and infant attachment. *American Journal of Medical Genetics, Part B (Neuropsychiatric Genetics), 132B*, 126–130.

Gervai, J., Novak, A., Lakatos, K., Toth, I., Danis, I., Zsolt, R., et al. (2007). Infant genotype may moderate sensitivity to maternal affective communications: Attachment disorganization, quality of care, and the DRD4 polymorphism. *Social Neuroscience, 2*, 307–319.

Goldberg, S., Benoit, D., Blokland, K., & Madigan, S. (2003). Atypical maternal behavior, maternal representations, and infant disorganized attachment. *Development and Psychopathology, 15*, 239–257.

Goldberg, W. A., & Easterbrooks, M. A. (1984). The role of marital quality in toddler development. *Developmental Psychology, 20*, 504–514.

Goldsmith, H. H., & Alansky, J. A. (1987). Maternal and infant temperamental predictors of attachment: A meta-analytic review. *Journal of Consulting and Clinical Psychology, 55*, 805–816.

Goldstein, L., Diener, M., & Mangelsdorf, S. (1996). Maternal characteristics and social support across the transition to motherhood: Associations with maternal behavior. *Journal of Family Psychology, 10*, 60–71.

Goossens, F., & van IJzendoorn, M. (1990). Quality of infants' attachment to professional caregivers. *Child Development, 61*, 832–837.

Grossmann, K., & Grossmann, K. E. (1992). Newborn behavior, the quality of early parenting, and later toddler–parent relationships in a group of German infants. In J. K. Nugent, B. M. Lester, & T. B. Brazelton (Eds.), *The cultural context of infancy* (Vol. 2, pp. 3–38). Norwood, NJ: Ablex.

Grossmann, K., Grossmann, K. E., Spangler, G., Suess, G., & Unzner, L. (1985). Maternal sensitivity and newborns' orientation responses as related to quality of attachment in northern Germany. In I. Bretherton & E. Waters (Eds.), Growing points of attachment theory and research. *Monographs of the Society for Research in Child Development, 50*(1–2, Serial No. 209), 233–257.

Grych, J. (2002). Marital relationships and parenting. In M. Bornstein (Ed.), *Handbook of parenting: Vol. 4. Social conditions and applied parenting* (2nd ed., pp. 203–225). Mahwah, NJ: Erlbaum.

Harrison, L. J., & Ungerer, J. A. (2002). Maternal employment and infant–mother attachment security at 12 months postpartum. *Developmental Psychology, 38*, 758–773.

Howes, C., & Markman, H. J. (1989). Marital quality and child functioning: A longitudinal investigation. *Child Development, 60*, 1044–1051.

Isabella, R., & Belsky, J. (1991). Interactional synchrony and the origins of infant–mother attachment: A replication study. *Child Development, 62*, 373–384.

Isabella, R., Belsky, J., & von Eye, A. (1989). Origins of infant–mother attachment: An examination of interactional synchrony during the infant's first year. *Developmental Psychology, 25*, 12–21.

Isabella, R. A. (1993). Origins of attachment: Maternal interactive behavior across the first year. *Child Development, 64*, 605–621.

Isabella, R. A. (1994). Origins of maternal role satisfaction and its influences upon maternal interactive behavior and infant–mother attachment. *Infant Behavior and Development, 17*, 381–388.

Jacobson, S. W., & Frye, K. F. (1991). Effect of maternal social support on attachment: Experimental evidence. *Child Development, 62*, 572–582.

Juffer, F., Bakermans-Kranenburg, M. J., & van IJzendoorn, M. H. (2005). The importance of parenting in the development of disorganized attachment: Evidence from a preventive intervention study in adoptive families. *Journal of Child Psychology and Psychiatry, 46,* 263–274.

Kagan, J. (1982). *Psychological research on the human infant: An evaluative summary.* New York: W. T. Grant Foundation.

Kochanska, G. (1998). Mother–child relationship, child fearfulness, and emerging attachment: A short-term longitudinal study. *Developmental Psychology, 34,* 480–490.

Kochanska, G., Aksan, N., & Carlson, J. J. (2005). Temperament, relationships, and young children's receptive cooperation with their parents. *Developmental Psychology, 41,* 648–660.

Kochanska, G., & Coy, K. C. (2002). Child emotionality and maternal responsiveness as predictors of reunion behaviors in the Strange Situation: Links mediated and unmediated by separation distress. *Child Development, 73,* 228–240.

Krishnakumar, A., & Buehler, C. (2000). Interparental conflict and parenting behaviors: A meta-analytic review. *Family Relations, 49,* 25–44.

Krupka, A., Moran, G., & Pederson, D. (1996, April). *The quality of mother–infant interactions in families at risk for maladaptive behavior: A window on the process of attachment.* Paper presented at the International Conference on Infant Studies, Providence, RI.

Lakatos, K., Nemoda, Z., Toth, I., Ronai, Z., Ney, K., Sasvari-Szekely, M., et al. (2002). Further evidence for the role of the dopamine D4 receptor (DRD4) gene in attachment disorganization: Interaction of the exon III 48-BP repeat and the -521 C/T promoter polymorphisms. *Molecular Psychiatry, 7,* 27–31.

Lakatos, K., Toth, I., Nemoda, Z., Ney, K., Sasvari-Szekely, M., & Gervai, J. (2000). Dopamine D4 receptor (DRD4) gene polymorphism is associated with attachment disorganization in infants. *Molecular Psychiatry, 5,* 633–637.

Levitt, M., Weber, R., & Clark, M. (1986). Social network relationships as sources of maternal support and well-being. *Developmental Psychology, 22,* 310–316.

Lewis, M., & Feiring, C. (1989). Infant, mother, and mother–infant interaction behavior and subsequent attachment. *Child Development, 60,* 831–837.

Lewis, M., Owen, M. T., & Cox, M. J. (1988). The transition to parenthood: III. Incorporation of the child into the family. *Family Press, 27,* 411–421.

Leyendecker, B., Lamb, M., Fracasso, M., Scholmerich, A., & Larson, C. (1997). Playful interaction and the antecedents of attachment. *Merrill–Palmer Quarterly, 43,* 24–47.

Lyons-Ruth, K. (1988, April). *Maternal depression and infant disturbance.* Paper presented at the International Conference on Infant Studies, Washington, DC.

Lyons-Ruth, K., Bronfman, E., & Parsons, E. (1999). Maternal frightened, frightening, or atypical behavior and disorganized infant attachment patterns. *Mono-*

graphs of the Society for Research in Child Development, 64 (3, Serial No. 258), 67–96.

Lyons-Ruth, K., Yellin, C., Melnick, S., & Atwood, G. (2005). Expanding the concept of unresolved mental states: Hostile/helpless states of mind on the Adult Attachment Interview are associated with disrupted mother–infant communication and infant disorganization. *Development and Psychopathology, 17,* 1–23.

Lyons-Ruth, K., Zoll, D., Connell, D. B., & Grunebaum, H. U. (1986). The depressed mother and her one-year-old infant: Environmental context, mother–infant interaction and attachment. In E. Tronick & T. Field (Eds.), *Maternal depression and infant disturbance* (pp. 61–82). San Francisco: Jossey-Bass.

Madigan, S., Moran, G., & Pederson, D. R. (2006). Unresolved states of mind, disorganized attachment relationships, and disrupted interactions of adolescent mothers and their infants. *Developmental Psychology, 42,* 293–304.

Main, M., & Hesse, E. (1990). Parents' unresolved traumatic experiences are related to infant disorganized attachment status: Is frightened and/or frightening parental behavior the linking mechanism? In M. T. Greenberg, D. Cicchetti, & E. M. Cummings (Eds.), *Attachment in the preschool years: Theory, research, and intervention* (pp. 161–182). Chicago: University of Chicago Press.

Malatesta, C. Z., Grigoryev, P., Lamb, C., Albin, M., & Culver, C. (1986). Emotion socialization and expressive development in preterm and full-term infants. *Child Development, 57,* 316–330.

Marshall, P. J., & Fox, N. A. (2005). Relations between behavioral reactivity at 4 months and attachment classification at 14 months in a selected sample. *Infant Behavior and Development, 28,* 492–502.

Martins, C., & Gaffan, E. A. (2000). Effects of early maternal depression on patterns of infant–mother attachment: A meta-analytic investigation. *Journal of Child Psychology and Psychiatry, 41,* 737–746.

Maslin, C. A., & Bates, J. E. (1983, April). *Precursors of anxious and secure attachments: A multivariant model at age 6 months.* Paper presented at the biennial meeting of the Society for Research in Child Development, Detroit, MI.

Meins, E., Fernyhough, C., Fradley, E., & Tuckey, M. (2001). Rethinking maternal sensitivity: Mothers' comments on infants' mental processes predict security of attachment at 12 months. *Journal of Child Psychology and Psychiatry, 42,* 637–648.

Moran, G., Pederson, D., Pettit, P., & Krupka, A. (1992). Maternal sensitivity and infant–mother attachment in a developmentally delayed sample. *Infant Behavior and Development, 15,* 427–442.

Murray, L., Fiori-Cowley, A., Hooper, R., & Cooper, P. (1996). The impact of postnatal depression and associated adversity on early mother–infant interactions and later infant outcome. *Child Development, 67,* 2512–2526.

Nakasawa, M., Teti, D. M., & Lamb, M. E. (1992). An ecological study of child–mother attachments among

Japanese sojourners in the United States. *Developmental Psychology, 28,* 584–592.

National Institute of Child Health and Human Development (NICHD) Early Child Care Network. (1997). The effects of infant child care on infant–mother attachment security: Results of the NICHD Study of Early Child Care. *Child Development, 68,* 860–879.

Notaro, P. C., & Volling, B. L. (1999). Parental responsiveness and infant–parent attachment: A replication study with fathers and mothers. *Infant Behavior and Development, 22,* 345–352.

O'Connor, M. (1997, March). *Maternal personality characteristics on the MMPI and infant attachment.* Paper presented at the biennial meeting of the Society for Research in Child Development, Washington, DC.

O'Connor, M., Sigman, M., & Kasasi, C. (1992). Attachment behavior of infants exposed prenatally to alcohol. *Developmental Psychopathology, 4,* 243–256.

O'Connor, T. G., & Croft, C. M. (2001). A twin study of attachment in preschool children. *Child Development, 72,* 1501–1511.

Owen, M., & Cox, M. (1997). Marital conflict and the development of infant–parent attachment relationships. *Journal of Family Psychology, 11,* 152–164.

Pederson, D., Gleason, K. E., Moran, G., & Bento, S. (1998). Maternal attachment representations, maternal sensitivity, and the infant–mother attachment relationship. *Developmental Psychology, 34,* 925–933.

Pederson, D., & Moran, G. (1996). Expressions of the attachment relationship outside of the Strange Situation. *Child Development, 67,* 915–927.

Pederson, D., Moran, G., Sitko, C., Campbell, K., Ghesqure, K., & Acton, H. (1990). Maternal sensitivity and the security of infant–mother attachment. *Child Development, 61,* 1974–1983.

Peterson, N. J., Drotar, D., Olness, K., Guay, L., & Kiziri-Mayengo, R. (2001). The relationship of maternal and child HIV infection to security of attachment among Ugandan infants. *Child Psychiatry and Human Development, 32,* 3–17.

Posada, G., Carbonell, O. A., Alzate, G., & Plata, S. J. (2004). Through Colombian lenses: Ethnographic and conventional analyses of maternal care and their associations with secure base behavior. *Developmental Psychology, 40,* 508–518.

Radke-Yarrow, M. (1991). Attachment patterns in children of depressed mothers. In C. M. Parkes, J. Stevenson-Hinde, & P. Maras (Eds.), *Attachment across the life cycle* (pp. 115–126). London: Tavistock/Routledge.

Radke-Yarrow, M., Cummings, M. E., Kuczynski, L., & Chapman, M. (1985). Patterns of attachment in two- and three-year olds in normal families and families with parental depression. *Child Development, 56,* 884–893.

Raval, V., Goldberg, S., Atkinson, L., Benoit, D., Myhal, N., Poulton, L., et al. (2001). Maternal attachment, maternal responsiveness and infant attachment. *Infant Behavior and Development, 24,* 281–304.

Ricks, M. H. (1985). The social transmission of parental behavior: Attachment across generations. In I. Bretherton & E. Waters (Eds.), Growing points of attachment theory and research. *Monographs of the Society for Research in Child Development, 50*(1–2, Serial No. 209), 211–227.

Rothbart, M., & Bates, J. (1998). Temperament. In W. Damon (Series Ed.) & N. Eisenberg (Vol. Ed.), *Handbook of child psychology: Vol. 3. Social, emotional, and personality development* (5th ed., pp. 308–418). New York: Wiley.

Rutter, M. (2006). *Genes and behavior: Nature–nurture interplay explained.* Oxford, UK: Blackwell.

Sameroff, A. J., Seifer, R., & Zax, M. (1982). Early development of children at risk for emotional disorder. *Monographs of the Society for Research in Child Development, 47*(7, Serial No. 199), 1–82.

Scher, A., & Mayseless, O. (2000). Mothers of anxious/ambivalent infants: Maternal characteristics and childcare context. *Child Development, 71,* 1629–1639.

Schneider-Rosen, K., & Rothbaum, F. (1993). Quality of parental caregiving and security of attachment. *Developmental Psychology, 29,* 358–367.

Scholmerich, A., Fracasso, M., Lamb, M., & Broberg, A. (1995). Interactional harmony at 7 and 10 months of age predicts security of attachment as measured by Q-sort ratings. *Social Development, 34,* 62–74.

Schuengel, C., Bakermans-Kranenburg, M. J., & van IJzendoorn, M. H. (1999). Frightening maternal behavior linking unresolved loss and disorganized infant attachment. *Journal of Consulting and Clinical Psychology, 67,* 54–63.

Seifer, R., Schiller, M., Sameroff, A., Resnick, S., & Riordan, K. (1996). Attachment, maternal sensitivity, and infant temperament during the first year of life. *Developmental Psychology, 32,* 12–25.

Sims, B., Hans, S., & Cox, S. (1996, April). *Raising children in high-risk environments: Mothers' experience of stress and distress related to attachment security.* Poster presented at the biennial meeting of the International Conference on Infant Studies, Providence, RI.

Slade, A., Grienenberger, J., Bernbach, E., Levy, D., & Locker, A. (2005). Maternal reflective functioning, attachment, and the transmission gap: A preliminary study. *Attachment and Human Development, 7,* 283–298.

Smith, K. E., Landry, S. H., & Swank, P. R. (2000). The influence of early patterns of positive parenting on children's preschool outcomes. *Early Education and Development, 11,* 147–169.

Smith, P. B., & Pederson, D. R. (1988). Maternal sensitivity and patterns of infant–mother attachment. *Child Development, 59,* 1097–1101.

Spieker, S. J. (1988). Patterns of very insecure attachment forward in samples of high-risk infants and toddlers. *Topics in Early Childhood Special Education, 6,* 37–53.

Spieker, S. J., & Booth, C. (1988). Maternal antecedents of attachment quality. In J. Belsky & T. Nezworski (Eds.), *Clinical implications of attachment* (pp. 95–176). Hillsdale, NJ: Erlbaum.

Sroufe, L. A. (1985). Attachment classification from the perspective of infant–caregiver relationships and infant temperament. *Child Development, 56*, 1–14.

Sroufe, L. A., & Rutter, M. (1984). The domain of developmental psychopathology. *Child Development, 55*, 17–29.

Susman-Stillman, A., Kalkoske, M., Egeland, B., & Waldman, I. (1996). Infant temperament and maternal sensitivity as predictors of attachment security. *Infant Behavior and Development, 19*, 33–47.

Tarabulsy, G. M., Bernier, A., Provost, M. A., Maranda, J., Larose, S., Moss, E., et al. (2005). Another look inside the gap: Ecological contributions to the transmission of attachment in a sample of adolescent mother–infant dyads. *Developmental Psychology, 41*, 212–224.

Teti, D., & Ablard, K. E. (1989). Security of attachment and infant–sibling relationships: A laboratory study. *Child Development, 60*, 1519–1528.

Teti, D., Gelfand, D., Messinger, D., & Isabella, R. (1995). Maternal depression and the quality of early attachment. *Developmental Psychology, 31*, 364–376.

Teti, D., Nakasawa, M., Das, R., & Wirth, O. (1991). Security of attachment between preschoolers and their mothers: Relations among social interaction, parenting stress, and mothers' sorts of the attachment Q-set. *Developmental Psychology, 27*, 440–447.

Tomlinson, M., Cooper, P., & Murray, L. (2005). The mother–infant relationship and infant attachment in a South African peri-urban settlement. *Child Development, 76*, 1044–1054.

True, M. M., Pisani, L., & Oumar, F. (2001). Infant–mother attachment among the Dogon of Mali. *Child Development, 72*, 1451–1466.

van den Boom, D. (1990). Preventive intervention and the quality of mother–infant interaction and infant exploration in irritable infants. In W. Koops, H. J. G. Soppe, J. L. van der Linden, OP. C. M. Molenaar, & J. J. F. Schroots (Eds.), *Developmental psychology behind the dikes* (pp. 249–270). Amsterdam: Eburon.

van den Boom, D. (1994). The influence of temperament and mothering on attachment and exploration. *Child Development, 65*, 1457–1477.

van IJzendoorn, M. (1995). Adult attachment representations, parental responsiveness, and infant attachment: A meta-analysis on the predictive validity of the Adult Attachment Interview. *Psychological Bulletin, 117*, 387–403.

van IJzendoorn, M. H., & Bakermans-Kranenburg, M. J. (2006). DRD4 7-repeat polymorphism moderates the association between maternal unresolved loss or trauma and infant disorganization. *Attachment and Human Development, 8*, 291–307.

van IJzendoorn, M., & De Wolff, M. (1997). In search of the absent father: Meta-analysis of infant–father attachment. *Child Development, 68*, 604–609.

van IJzendoorn, M., Juffer, F., & Duyvesteyn, M. (1995).

Breaking the intergenerational cycle of insecure attachment: A review of the effects of attachment-based interventions on maternal sensitivity and infant security. *Journal of Child Psychology and Psychiatry, 36*, 225–248.

van IJzendoorn, M. H., Moran, G., Belsky, J., Pederson, D., Bakermans-Kranenburg, M. J., & Kneppers, K. (2000). The similarity of siblings' attachments to their mother. *Child Development, 71*, 1086–1098.

van IJzendoorn, M. H., Schuengel, C., & Bakermans-Kranenburg, M. J. (1999). Disorganized attachment in early childhood: Meta-analysis of precursors, concomitants, and sequelae. *Development and Psychopathology, 11*, 225–249.

van IJzendoorn, M. H., Vereijken, M., Bakermans-Kranenburg, M. J., & Riksen-Walraven, J. M. (2004). Assessing attachment security with the Attachment Q-Sort: Meta-analytic evidence for the validity of the observer AQS. *Child Development, 75*, 1188–1213.

Velderman, M. K., Bakermans-Kranenburg, M. J., Juffer, F., & van IJzendoorn, M. H. (2006). Effects of attachment-based interventions on maternal sensitivity and infant attachment: Differential susceptibility of highly reactive infants. *Journal of Family Psychology, 20*, 266–274.

Vereijken, C., Riksen-Walraven, J., & Kondo-Ikemura, K. (1997). Maternal sensitivity and infant attachment security in Japan: A longitudinal study. *International Journal of Behavioral Development, 21*, 35–49.

Volling, B. L., & Belsky, J. (1992). Infant, father, and marital antecedents of infant–father attachment security in dual-earner and single-earner families. *International Journal of Behavioral Development, 15*, 83–100.

Vondra, J., Shaw, D., & Kevinides, M. (1995). Predicting infant attachment classification from multiple, contemporaneous measures of maternal care. *Infant Behavior and Development, 18*, 415–425.

Ward, M. J., Vaughn, B. E., & Robb, M. D. (1988). Social-emotional adaptation and infant–mother attachment in siblings: Role of the mother in cross-sibling consistency. *Child Development, 59*, 643–651.

Waters, E., & Deane, K. E. (1985). Defining and assessing individual differences in attachment relationships: Q-methodology and the organization of behavior in infancy and early childhood. In I. Bretherton & E. Waters (Eds.), Growing points of attachment theory and research. *Monographs of the Society for Research in Child Development, 50*(1–2, Serial No. 209), 41–65.

Zeanah, C., Benoit, D., Barton, M., Regan, C., Hirshberg, L., & Lipsett, L. (1993). Representations of attachment in mothers and their one-year-old infants. *Journal of the American Academy of Child and Adolescent Psychiatry, 32*, 278–286.

Zevalkink, J., Riksen-Walraven, J. M., & Van Lieshout, C. F. M. (1999). Attachment in the Indonesian caregiving context. *Social Development, 8*, 21–40.

CHAPTER 14

Attachment Relationships in the Context of Multiple Caregivers

CAROLLEE HOWES
SUSAN SPIEKER

In his early writings, Bowlby (1969/1982) proposed that a child develops a hierarchy of attachment relationships—first with the mother as the primary caregiver. In 1967, Ainsworth wrote that "nearly all the babies in this sample who became attached to their mothers during the period spanned by our observations became attached also to some other familiar figure—father, grandmother, or other adult in the household, or to an older sibling" (p. 315). The Ainsworth sample was composed of Ghanda infants in East Africa. Ainsworth's next major work was the Baltimore study of child–mother attachment (Ainsworth, Blehar, Waters, & Wall, 1978). Although this work was concerned with patterns of infant–mother attachment relationships, Ainsworth still acknowledged the possibility of other attachment figures: "The mother figure is, however, the principal caregiver, whether the natural mother or someone else plays that role" (Ainsworth et al., 1978, p. 5).

Although, as these quotations show, recognition of alternative attachment figures has been part of attachment theory since its development, attachment research has largely been conducted on the child–mother attachment relationship. There are practical reasons to consider children as having a network of attachment figures. In the United States, families outside the dominant culture (par-

ticularly people of color, immigrant families, and families living in or close to poverty) have historically used a variety of childrearing configurations involving networks of caregiving adults rather than a single caregiver (Jackson, 1993). As the roles of women and men in family life have changed, and as the two-income family has become an economic necessity, most children are now regularly cared for by more than one adult. Some children who are adopted, and children in foster care, experience multiple attachment relationships not only simultaneously but also sequentially. As research on multiple attachment relationships has become more common, there is little dispute that children form attachment relationships with child care providers, and that child–mother and child–other attachments are independent in antecedents and quality (Ahnert, Pinquart, & Lamb, 2006).

Considering multiple attachment figures raises theoretical issues for attachment theory. Central to the theory is a set of propositions about how attachments are formed and about the influence of attachment relationships on subsequent development. Because alternative attachment relationships are formed in different contexts, and often in different developmental periods (i.e., subsequent to maternal attachments), examining antecedents of alternative attachment relationships can inform and expand the theory. Similarly, examining the predictive power of attachment quality with alternative attachment figures for children's development can expand our understanding of relationships in development. Moreover, including multiple caregivers as part of a network of attachment figures may expand our understanding of the organization of internal working models of attachment.

In this chapter, we first consider children's attachments to other-than-mother caregivers (alternative caregivers); we then describe, in some detail, child–mother attachment relationship quality when children attend child care and may also develop attachment relationships with nonparental caregivers.

ATTACHMENT TO NONPARENTAL CAREGIVERS

Developmental Issues

Attachment theory assumes that a mother and infant will begin to construct their relationship from the moment of birth. Children's repertoire of social signals and their capacities for memory, internal representation, and affective knowledge develop at the same time as the child–mother attachment. Children encounter alternative attachment figures at varying points in their development. We can assume that the course of attachment relationship construction is similar from a developmental point of view to that of child–mother attachment relationship construction for some alternative caregivers—fathers; grandparents and other relatives; adoptive and foster parents when a child is placed at birth; and infant child care providers. Other relationships between the child and care providers begin later in the child's life. For these relationships, both developmental considerations and previous relationship history may have shaping influences.

Simultaneously Formed Attachment Relationships

In two-parent families, children simultaneously, and from birth onward, are assumed to construct attachment relationships with their mothers and their fathers (Easterbrooks & Goldberg, 1987). Infant–mother and infant–father attachment relationships are constructed within the same developmental period and the same household. However, even though the two sets of relationships develop interdependently, attachment security with the two parents often differs, suggesting

that each attachment relationship is shaped by specific interactions (Fox, Kimmerly, & Shafer, 1991; Grossmann et al., 2002; van IJzendoorn & De Wolff, 1997).

Families vary considerably in the organization of caregiving responsibilities and caregiving behaviors that are linked to attachment relationship formation. A large literature suggests that when fathers engage in caregiving activities, there are few differences between child–mother and child–father relationships (Parke & Asher, 1983). An early study by Lamb (1977b) is illustrative, in that when mothers, fathers, and infants were all present for evening observations, infants directed attachment behaviors to both mothers and fathers. By age 2 the children showed no preference for one parent over the other in the shared caregiving context (Lamb, 1977b).

When caregiving is not shared between parents, relationships between the caregivers appear to influence the construction of alternative caregiver attachment relationships. Steele, Steele, and Fonagy (1995) examined associations among mothers' and fathers' Adult Attachment Interview (AAI; George, Kaplan, & Main, 1984, 1985, 1996; see Hesse, Chapter 25, this volume) classifications and the attachment classifications of their infants in traditional families where mothers served as primary caregivers. They found that mothers' own attachment security constrained and shaped father–infant relationship formation. Whereas mothers' own attachment security was linked to child–mother attachment quality, child–father attachment security was linked to mothers' attachment security and not fathers' own attachment security. Recent longitudinal findings from families participating in this study suggest that fathers' prebirth AAI security scores predicted their children's preteen self-reported mental health, but only when mediated by the mothers' reports of prebirth marital satisfaction (Steele & Steele, 2005).

Even when caregiving is shared, the nature of the relationship between the parents influences child–parent attachment quality. Solomon and George (1999) found that not all infants who experienced overnight visitation with their divorced fathers constructed organized (secure or insecure) attachment relationships with their parents. Instead when infants experienced high parental conflict and poor communication, whether or not the parents were divorced, they were more likely to construct disorganized attachment relationships. Disorganized child–mother attachments were associated with overnight visitation only in the context of parental conflict.

There is almost no literature on grandparent–child attachment relationships constructed concurrently with child–parent relationships. There is a small literature on adolescent parents that includes the parents of the adolescents, who are, of course, the grandparents of the infants. Under some conditions, support from a grandmother appears to enhance attachment security between an adolescent mother and her child. High grandmother support was associated with more secure infant attachment only for adolescents living with partners (Spieker & Bensley, 1994). Perhaps, through processes similar to those identified by Steele and colleagues (1995) for mothers and fathers, grandmothers' representations of attachment influence adolescent mothers' caregiving and attachment relationships with their children (Ward, Carlson, Plunket, & Kessler, 1991). Although significant life events, including having a baby, appear to be catalysts for positive change in adults' representations of attachment (Ward & Carlson, 1995), Benoit and Parker (1994) observed continuity of attachment representations between grandmothers and mothers and between these representations and child–mother attachment security.

There is also little research on attachment relationships between children and child care providers in cases where a child is enrolled in child care prior to the formation of an attachment relationship with one or both parents or parental figures. For example, the youngest children in the large ($N = 2,867$) sample used in the Ahnert and colleagues (2006) meta-analysis were toddlers and therefore enrolled in child care after establishing parental attachments. Subsequent to the meta-analysis, Howes (2006) followed a sample of 88 children born to low-income Mexican immigrant parents—24 children who were cared for by child care providers, primarily kith and kin, by 2 months of age. At 14 months of age, half of these children had secure attachments with both their mothers and their child care providers. Children who were not secure with both types of caregivers were equally likely to be secure with only their mothers or only their child care providers, suggesting an independence of the two relationships.

Sequentially Formed Attachment Relationships

Most toddlers or older children who encounter alternative attachment figures already have at least one internal working model (IWM) of an attachment relationship. In sequentially formed attachments, both the developmental context and the relationship history are different from those affecting infant–mother attachments. In this section of the chapter, we review literature on the construction of attachment relationships with sequential nonparental caregivers. When we describe the construction of sequential attachment relationships with child care providers, we are concerned with whether or not these relationships are constructed according to developmental processes similar to those seen in child–mother attachment relationships. When we describe the construction of sequential attachment relationships to foster and adoptive parents, we are concerned not only with developmental processes, but also with the issue of prior difficult relationships.

Forming New Relationships with Child Care Providers

The formation of infant–mother attachment relationships can be observed as children track or follow their mothers, cry to alert the mothers to their distress, or maintain social contact through smiles and vocalizations. Do children use these same behaviors when they are left in the care of a child care provider or a teacher, or is there another developmental process? Three studies have explicitly examined this question for toddlers. Raikes (1993) had center-based providers complete Attachment Q-Sorts (Waters, 1987) for the children in their care. Security scores increased as the toddlers spent more time with the providers, indicating relationship formation. Barnas and Cummings (1997) compared toddlers' attachment behaviors with long-term staff members (3 months or more in the center) and short-term staff members. Children directed more attachment behaviors to the long-term staffers, and long-term staffers were more successful than short-term staffers in soothing distressed children. Howes and Oldham (2001) observed toddlers daily and then weekly during their first 6 months in child care. The frequency of attachment behavior decreased over the children's first 2 months in child care. However, the initial frequency of attachment behaviors and their rate of decrease over time were unrelated to the children's attachment security by the end of 6 months in child care. Thus the formation of toddler–child care provider attachment relationships appears to be similar to infant–mother attachment formation. When toddlers begin child care, they direct attachment behaviors to the caregivers; with time in the setting, children's experiences of interacting with the caregivers become more organized. Toddlers respond differently to providers who are present for longer periods of time and are therefore more predictable, regardless of whether the relationship is more or less secure.

Forming New Relationships with Adoptive or Foster Parents

Classic studies of adoptive children indicated that children adopted after the beginnings of attachment relationship formation (6–8 months) had difficulty forming positive, trusting relationships with their adoptive parents (Tizard & Rees, 1975; Yarrow, Goodwin, Manheimer, & Milowe, 1973). More recent studies of children adopted before, during, and after the developmental period of attachment formation suggest that attachment formation in infants adopted during their first year is similar to child–mother attachment formation and does not have a critical period (Dontas, Maratos, Fafoutis, & Karangelis, 1985; Marcovitch et al., 1997; Singer, Brodzinsky, Ramsay, Steir, & Waters, 1985). (See Dozier & Rutter, Chapter 29, this volume, for further discussion of issues concerning adoption.)

Describing attachment formation in foster care children and children adopted from institutions with severe caregiving deprivation policies is a stringent test of the dual influences of developmental period and prior relationship history on the process of constructing an attachment relationship. Most foster care children have experienced difficult relationships, but not necessarily severe deprivation. Researchers question both whether these children can form secure attachments with alternative caregivers, and whether the process of attachment formation is similar to attachment formation in typical children. In an early study (Howes & Segal, 1993), almost half of the children (47%) removed from their homes because of maternal abuse or neglect and placed in high-quality shelter care were able to develop secure attachment relationships with shelter caregivers within 2 months of placement. Foster children placed in therapeutic preschool programs are also able to form secure attachments to their providers (Howes & Ritchie, 1999).

Other studies have directly examined the behaviors foster care infants initially direct to their foster parents and found high incidences of pushing caregivers away, appearing inconsolable, and engaging in emotionally dysregulated and disorganized behavior (Dozier, Lindhiem, & Ackerman, 2005; Stovall & Dozier, 2000; Stovall-McClough

& Dozier, 2004; Zeanah & Smyke, 2005). Foster parents often react to these behaviors by concluding that the children do not need or cannot benefit from warm or responsive caregiving (Dozier, Stovall, Albus, & Bates, 2001; Milam & Pinderhughes, 2000). When foster parents are helped to understand this process and to respond to children as if they needed and were signaling for a warm, organized, and nurturing environment, positive attachment formation is possible (Dozier, Albus, Fischer, & Sepulveda, 2002; Dozier et al., 2001). Recent studies of children adopted from Romanian orphanages suggest a similar pattern of behaviors toward caregivers in children with little or no experiences of trusting caregivers (Maclean, 2003; O'Conner et al., 2003). These children tend to approach strangers with disinhibited behaviors, failing to seek proximity to or engage in organized help seeking with attachment figures. Attachments to adoptive parents in these children are slow to develop, but the proportion of children who do construct secure attachments may be similar to that of nonadopted children. In summary, children who construct mother–child attachments subsequent to prior difficult caregiving relationships appear to use a different repertoire of attachment behaviors from that originally described for mother–child attachment; however, these children appear to be able to form attachments with parental and nonparental caregivers. (See Dozier & Rutter, Chapter 29, this volume, for a more detailed discussion of foster care.)

Pathways to Secure Attachment Relationships with Alternative Caregivers

An important premise of attachment theory and research is that caregiver behavior, specifically sensitive and responsive behavior, and caregiver attachment representations are important in the construction of secure attachment relationships (Ainsworth et al., 1978; Cassidy et al., 2005; van IJzendoorn, 1995). Not surprisingly, sensitive and responsive behaviors—and, to a lesser extent, caregiver "states of mind with respect to attachment" assessed in the AAI—have been the topics of research on the antecedents of secure attachments with nonparental caregivers.

Sensitive and Responsive Caregiver Behaviors

Early studies on child–father and child–caregiver attachments (with the term "caregiver" referring to a nonparental child care provider) found that more sensitive previous or current caregiving was linked to more secure attachment relationships (Anderson, Nagel, Roberts, & Smith, 1981; Cox, Owen, Henderson, & Margand, 1992; Easterbrooks & Goldberg, 1987; Goossens & van IJzendoorn, 1990; Howes & Hamilton, 1992a; Howes & Ritchie, 1998; Howes, Rodning, Galluzzo, & Myers, 1988; Howes & Smith, 1995). Recent meta-analytic work suggests that for child–caregiver attachment relationships, the form of child care may influence caregiver sensitivity (Ahnert et al., 2006). Security in child–caregiver relationships in child care centers was best predicted by warm and sensitive care that monitored both individual children's needs and the needs of the entire group of children. Caregivers were, not surprisingly, more successful at this dual focus when the groups of children were smaller. In family-based child care, with smaller groups of children, dyadic responsivity predicted attachment security.

Caregiver States of Mind

When children in the meta-analysis (Ahnert et al., 2006) had experienced discontinuous care, and perhaps were less trusting of child care providers (see Howes & Hamilton, 1993), they were less likely to be secure. This suggests that the average professional caregiver's level of sensitivity may not be sufficient to produce secure attachment relationships with children whose relationship histories have predisposed them to consider adult caregivers unavailable and untrustworthy (Howes & Ritchie, 2002).

What characteristics of caregivers cause or allow them to deal successfully with difficult child behaviors? We know of no studies directly addressing associations between professional caregivers' states of mind with respect to attachment and children's attachment security. However, recent work suggests that caregivers' perceptions of children can influence attachment security, particularly if the children are different from them in ethnic background. In one recent study of children entering center-based child care programs, caregivers were rated, on average, as very low in warmth and sensitivity (Howes & Shivers, 2006). Not surprisingly, 6 months after entering child care, fewer than half of the children had constructed secure attachment relationships with these caregivers. Child–caregiver insecurity was best predicted by mismatches in ethnic heritage and difficult interactions at entry. Children who were ethnic matches with caregivers and who had difficult

child–caregiver interactions at entry were no more likely than children who entered child care with no child–caregiver conflict to be insecure. When teachers were asked to describe their relationships with the children, the pattern of findings was similar. If children were ethnically mismatched with teachers and if the children evoked negative emotions from these teachers, the teachers were more likely to report conflictual child–teacher relationships (Rudasill, Rimm-Kaufman, Justice, & Pence, 2006; Saft & Pianta, 2001; Stuhlman & Pianta, 2002).

More is known about how adoptive and foster parents' states of mind about attachment influence attachment security than about how professional care providers' states of mind influence child security. These findings are parallel to those for mothers: Parents with more secure states of mind are more likely to construct secure attachment relationships with foster or adopted children (Dozier et al., 2001; Zeanah & Smyke, 2005; see Dozier & Rutter, Chapter 29, this volume).

Organization of IWMs in Multiple-Caregiver Contexts

Examining attachment in the context of multiple caregivers requires that we consider how representations of multiple attachment relationships are organized in a child's IWMs. According to attachment theory, the child forms internal representations of self and relationships with others based on repeated interactions with attachment figures (Bowlby, 1969/1982). Several different possibilities for the organization of IWMs of multiple attachment relationships have been suggested: "hierarchical," where the child's representation of the most salient caregiver, most often the mother, is the most influential (Bretherton, 1985); "integrative," where the child integrates all of his or her attachment relationships into a single representation (van IJzendoorn, Sagi, & Lambermon, 1992); and "independent," where the different representations are independent both in quality and in their influence on development (Howes, 1999). To evaluate the empirical support for a model of organization of IWMs, two bodies of literature must be considered. In one body of literature, researchers have examined the concordance in the quality of children's attachments to more than one caregiver. In the second body of literature, researchers have compared the predictability of children's developmental outcomes from their attachment security with different caregivers.

Concordance of Attachment Quality

There have been two major meta-analyses examining concordance of attachment relationship quality across caregivers. Fox and colleagues (1991) conducted a meta-analysis examining the concordance of infant–mother and infant–father attachment security. They concluded that mother and father relationships were modestly concordant; that is, they were not independent. This is consistent with the literature discussed earlier in this chapter suggesting that the mother shapes the father–child relationship (Steele et al., 1995), and it supports a hierarchical model of organization.

Ahnert and colleagues (2006) examined the concordance of child–mother and child–caregiver attachment security. Children were less likely to be secure with their professional care providers than with their mothers. The degree of concordance between the two relationships suggests independent yet related relationships—inconclusive evidence for any of the proposed conceptions of the organization of IWMs.

Prediction of Developmental Outcomes

Relatively few studies have examined the differential prediction of developmental outcomes from attachment quality of relationships with more than one caregiver. As might be expected from the greater amount of time mothers, as compared with fathers, spend with their children, child–mother attachment quality is generally (but not always) more predictive of child outcomes than child–father attachment quality is (Main, Hesse, & Kaplan, 2005; Main, Kaplan, & Cassidy, 1985; Suess, Grossmann, & Sroufe, 1992; Volling & Belsky, 1992; but see also Easterbrooks & Goldberg, 1985; Grossmann et al., 2002; Lamb, Hwang, Frodi, & Frodi, 1982; Main & Weston, 1981; Steele & Steele, 2005). Two longitudinal studies have examined children's developmental outcomes, using child–mother and child–caregiver relationships as predictors of children's outcomes. The Haifa longitudinal study examines prediction from quality of child–mother, child–father, and child–*metapelet* relationship in infancy to social and emotional outcomes in early childhood, early and late adolescence, and early adulthood (Sagi-Schwartz & Avierzer, 2005). In early childhood, previous child–*metapelet* attachment security predicted preschool children's social competence with peers better than child–parent attachment security did (Oppenheim, Sagi, & Lamb, 1988). Furthermore, scores based on a network of caregivers (mother,

father, *metapelet*) better predicted general social competence in early childhood than did child–mother attachment security (van IJzendoorn et al., 1992). Network security in early childhood was also most predictive of child competence with peers in a Dutch sample of children, mothers, and child care providers (van IJzendoorn et al., 1992). These findings support an independent or integrative model of IWM organization. By adolescence and adulthood, results from the Haifa study were less conclusive with regard to the organization of IWMs. Beyond early childhood, networks of attachment relationships were not as predictive of outcomes as was early attachment security with mother and father (Sagi-Schwartz & Avierzer, 2005).

The Howes longitudinal study examined the ability of child–mother, child–caregiver, and child–teacher relationships from infancy through middle childhood to predict concurrent and early and late adolescent social and emotional outcomes. In the toddler period, attachment relationships with mother and child care providers predicted behavior with peers, supporting an integrative organization of IWMs (Howes et al., 1988). At preschool, the findings suggested an independent organization, with early security of attachment to a child care provider predicting preschool children's social competence with peers (Howes, Matheson, & Hamilton, 1994). At age 9 (Howes, Hamilton, & Phillipsen, 1998) and at age 14 (Howes & Tonyan, 2000), early attachment security with mother was the best predictor of child–mother relationship quality, and early attachment security with child care providers was the best predictor of child–teacher attachment security. These results argue for an independent organization. However, peer friendships in these last two developmental periods were best predicted by preschool friendship quality, suggesting that whereas early attachment security with child care providers predicted early friendship with peers, peer relationship quality in later developmental periods was independent of early attachments to adults. By late adolescence (Howes & Aikens, 2002) the pattern of relations between early attachments to mothers and caregivers on the one hand, and social and emotional competence on the other, did not fit any of the proposed models of IWM organization. Complex relations were found among adolescent functioning, gender, and early emotion regulation in child care and early relationships with adults.

Far more research than two longitudinal studies is needed to support any of the proposed conceptions of IWM organization resulting from multiple attachment relationships (see Kobak, Rosenthal, & Serwik, 2005, and Thompson & Raikes, 2003, for further discussion of these issues). As more and more children develop social and emotional competence through attachment relationships with mothers and other salient caregivers, researchers should consider planning studies that describe relationships with multiple attachment figures.

RELATIONS BETWEEN CHILD CARE AND MATERNAL ATTACHMENT

A dramatic demographic shift in the rearing experiences of infants in the United States occurred in the closing decades of the 20th century. By the mid-1980s, the number of mothers with infants under 1 year of age who were in the paid labor force reached 50%. Social scientists began to ask whether the experience of repeated separations from mother, and time away from mother during the development of a child's primary attachments, had adverse consequences for the quality of infant–mother attachment.

Concern That Child Care Was a Risk for Insecure Infant–Mother Attachment

During the 1980s, two multistudy analyses converged on the conclusion that more that 20 hours/week of child care in the first year of life was associated with elevated rates of insecure infant–mother attachment, as measured by the Strange Situation (Ainsworth & Wittig, 1969; see Solomon & George, Chapter 18, this volume). Belsky and Rovine (1988) and Clarke-Stewart (1989) reported insecurity rates for infants with extensive child care to be 43% and 36%, respectively, compared with rates of 26% and 29% for groups with no or limited early child care experience. These differences were particularly marked for insecure-avoidant classifications. Lamb, Sternberg, and Prodromidis (1992) reanalyzed data from 13 studies and also found that children in exclusive maternal care had higher rates of security than other infants. In contrast to the studies above, however, Lamb and colleagues found elevated insecurity and avoidance for infants in any child care exceeding a mere 5 hours/week, and insecurity and avoidance rates for infants receiving this low level of child care were not different from those receiving extensive care of more than 20 hours/week.

The explanation of these effects was a matter of controversy. Barglow, Vaughn, and Molitor (1987) hypothesized that the elevation in the rate of insecure-avoidant attachment indicated that these infants experienced repeated separations from their mothers as rejection. Others wondered whether time away from each other might disrupt the proximal processes of mother–child interaction, affecting a mother's ability to respond to her infant with sensitivity (Brazelton, 1985; Jaeger & Weinraub, 1990; Owen & Cox, 1988) or the infant's expectation of an available and responsive parent (Sroufe, 1988).

Eventually, two interpretations of the data became common in the developmental and popular literature. One was that the experience of extensive child care in the first year of life was indeed a risk factor for the development of insecure infant–mother attachment (Belsky, 1990), although the majority of infants with this early experience did develop secure attachments. The second interpretation was focused on the measurement of attachment insecurity itself. Clarke-Stewart (1989) suggested that the two brief separations in the Strange Situation procedure were not stressful enough for infants with extensive child care experience, and that the autonomy and independence displayed by these less distressed infants upon reunion with their mothers was in fact misinterpreted as avoidance. Clarke-Stewart asserted that the Strange Situation may not be a valid measure of attachment for infants with extensive child care experience.

The evidence relevant to these two interpretations was mixed. The results of the 1980s studies were consistent, but Roggmann, Langlois, Hubbs-Tait, and Rieser-Danner (1994), studying a small but later-born cohort, found no association between child care experience and infant–mother attachment security. Other studies found no differences in distress or exploration in the Strange Situation for infants with insecure-avoidant classifications and varying amounts of child care experience (Belsky & Braungart, 1991; McCartney & Galanopoulos, 1988), and Berger, Levy, and Compaan (1995) supplied evidence that the Strange Situation was equally valid for infants with and without extensive child care in the first year. Thus the "infant day care controversy" (Westman, 1988) was in full swing when the National Institute of Child Health and Human Development (NICHD) initiated the Study of Early Child Care to address these and other questions about the effects of early child care on children's social, emotional, cognitive, and language development.

The NICHD Study of Early Child Care

The 1,364 participants in the NICHD Study of Early Child Care and Youth Development (NICHD SECCYD; "Youth Development" was added to the title of the study when it was extended in its third phase to follow participants through sixth grade) were recruited throughout 1991 from 31 hospitals in 10 sites across the United States, in accordance with a conditionally random sampling plan designed to ensure that participant families reflected the educational, economic, and ethnic diversity of their respective sites. The corporate author, the NICHD Early Child Care Research Network (NICHD ECCRN), published two articles (1997, 2001) on the effects of early child care on attachment as assessed by the Strange Situation at 15 and 36 months. Subsequent named-author papers (e.g., Booth, Clarke-Stewart, Vandell, McCartney, & Owen, 2002; Huston & Rosenkrantz Aronson, 2005; Tran & Weinraub, 2006), using the same data set, also addressed this question; many others have used the data to examine predictors of attachment security (e.g., Campbell et al., 2004; McElwain & Booth-LaForce, 2006) or the influence of attachment security on child development (e.g., Belsky & Fearon, 2002a, 2002b; McCartney, Owen, Booth, Clarke-Stewart, & Vandell, 2004), regardless of child care experience. And, as the title of the study suggests, the ECCRN has published extensively on the influences of early child care experiences on a wide range of developmental outcomes, including language, cognition, and achievement, peer relationships, problem behavior, and school adjustment. Other analyses focus on topics that are not related to early child care, such as the influence on developmental outcomes of variations in after school experience, physical activity, family processes, and school environments. Currently, the fourth phase of the study is following its youthful participants through middle adolescence.

The NICHD SECCYD has considerable methodological strength. The sample size has been nearly as large as the largest of the 1980s multistudy analyses (Clarke-Stewart, 1989). The study has been prospective and longitudinal, following children identified at birth, and thus reducing selection biases. Parents determined the timing, type, and amount of child care, and presumably considered quality in their choices; the researchers recorded this information regularly and observed the quality of the major arrangements during the first phase of the study at child ages 6, 15, 24, and 36 months. The design of the study used a broad multivariate framework, permitting the effects of child care on infant–mother attachment security to be studied "in context." The examination of effects in context was important, because none of the previous studies had indicated that insecurity was inevitable for children with extensive early child care experience—only that rates of insecurity were elevated. Characteristics of the child (e.g., sex, temperament), child care experience (type, amount, age of entry, stability, and quality) and characteristics of the family (including socioemotional processes and economic resources) could all interact with each other to influence child outcomes, including attachment security. Children were not randomly assigned to child care, and complex family selection factors influenced family decisions about the type of child care children would experience. The basic analytic approach of the NICHD ECCRN was to assess the amount of variance of any outcome explained by child-care-related variables that was over and above that explained by selection, family, and child factors. The major child care associations with attachment reported in the ECCRN papers are reviewed below.

The NICHD Study of Early Child Care and Infant–Mother Attachment

The NICHD ECCRN (1997) analyses had two purposes. The first was to explore the validity of the Strange Situation for assessing attachment security of infants with extensive experience in child care by comparing a subsample of infants who experienced more than 30 hours/week of child care from 4 to 15 months ($n = 263$) with infants who had fewer than 10 hours/week of child care during this period ($n = 251$). The validation measures included 5-point ratings of the infants' distress during the separation episodes of the Strange Situation, and the coders' self-rated confidence (5-point scale) with which they assigned the various secure or insecure major classifications. In these validity analyses, the five-category attachment classification (A, B, C, D, U) was used. Results of 2 (high vs. low child care intensity) × 5 (attachment classification) analyses of variance for the distress and confidence ratings provided no support for the hypothesis that the Strange Situation was a less valid measure of attachment for children with extensive child care experience. There was no main effect of child care intensity on either of these ratings. Thus there was no evidence for differential internal validity of the Strange Situation as a function of child care experience.

The second purpose of the 1997 analyses was to examine the main effects of age of entry and child care quantity, stability, and quality on infant attachment security, as well as the interaction of these features of child care with aspects of the family and/or child. Two kinds of interactions were tested. The first set addressed the "dual-risk" hypothesis: namely, that large amounts of child care, poor-quality child care, or frequent changes in care over time would promote insecure infant–mother attachment in the context of other risks, such as difficult temperament, being a male, or residing with a mother who had poor psychological adjustment or was less sensitive and responsive to the infant. A "compensatory" hypothesis was also tested: namely, that when family or child risks were high, child care that began early in life and was stable, extensive, or of high quality would foster the formation of a more secure infant–mother attachment. In a series of logistic regression analyses, the dichotomous dependent attachment variable (secure–insecure or secure–avoidant) was predicted from one of five characteristics of the mother or the child, one of five characteristics of child care, and the interaction between the two selected (mother–child and child care) variables, entered one at a time.

The "main effects" hypotheses for child care received no support. None of the five child care variables (two measures of observed quality of care, the amount of care, the age of entry, and the frequency of care starts), entered after the selection and family–child variables, significantly predicted attachment security. Six of the 25 interaction terms included in the logistic regression analyses were significant predictors of attachment security. A consistent pattern observed across five of the six significant interactions was that the highest rates of insecurity occurred under dual-risk conditions. Infants were less likely to be secure when low maternal sensitivity/responsiveness was combined with poor-quality child care, more than minimal amounts of child care, or more than one care arrangement. In addition, boys experiencing many hours in care were somewhat less likely to be securely attached (and girls experiencing more hours in care were somewhat more likely to be secure). The interaction analyses also provided evidence for compensatory effects. The proportion of attachment security among children with the least sensitive and responsive mothers was higher in high-quality child care than in low-quality care.

Additional detailed analyses of the NICHD SECCYD data set likewise found no evidence of main effects. Booth and colleagues (2002) and Huston and Rosenkrantz Aronson (2005), analyzing detailed data, examined amount of maternal time with their infants in the first year of life and found no associations with attachment security at 15 or 36 months. Thus one of the hypothesized mechanisms for earlier findings on attachment security—that extensive child care did not give mothers and children sufficient time to get to know one another—was not supported. Nevertheless, another paper by the NICHD ECCRN (1999), based on longitudinal analyses that controlled for selection, child, and family predictors, reported that more hours of child care predicted less maternal sensitivity and less positive child engagement with the mother. Apparently the effect of hours in child care does not overlap completely with the effect of time with mother. Another failure to replicate prior results completely, using different analyses from the data set, was reported by Tran and Weinraub (2006), who did not find an interaction between maternal sensitivity and stability of child care predicting infant attachment. Tran and Weinraub used a slightly different measure of stability and a somewhat different subset of participants. These instances of lack of replication highlight the relatively small effect sizes of the significant interactions in the 1997 paper.

In comparing the results of the NICHD SECCYD with those of earlier studies, considerable weight should be given to the NICHD study because of its size and the quality of the data. But the possibility of cohort effects is real and may be responsible for some of the differences in findings between this and earlier studies. Families in the 1990s that used child care may have been different in important ways from their earlier counterparts. Maternal employment during a child's infancy became an increasingly "mainstream" practice; also, families and child care providers may have been more aware of the child care controversy than were families in the 1970s and 1980s, and so may have worked harder to support the infant–parent relationship.

The limitations of the NICHD SECCYD should not be ignored. The highest-risk families, including those with adolescent mothers or families with vulnerable ill or premature newborns were not included in the sample. Although nearly a quarter of the sample was low-income, low income was almost completely confounded with racial minority status (specifically, African American), making it impossible to examine these factors independently. Finally, the researchers were less likely to be permitted to observe child care arrangements presumed to be of low quality. All of these limitations affect the generalizability of conclusions from the seminal 1997 study about the main and interactive effects of family–child characteristics and child care quality on infant attachment and other outcomes.

The Haifa Study of Early Child Care and Infant–Mother Attachment

A later Israeli study modeled on the NICHD SEC-CYD was designed to address some of these issues. The Haifa Study of Early Child Care (Sagi, Koren-Karie, Gini, Ziv, & Joels, 2002), also funded by the NICHD, "was designed to shed further light on issues pertaining to the effects of early child care on the development of the infant–mother attachment relationship in general, and on the published data from the NICHD Early Child Care Research Network in particular" (Sagi et al., 2002, p. 1167). Because in Israel child care centers are part of a nationwide network, the quality is relatively homogeneous and not confounded with socioeconomic status (SES), as infants from families of all income and education levels are placed in the same centers. The researchers used a randomized stratified sampling strategy for all healthy, singleton births in the greater Haifa metropolitan area in a 1-year period. The final sample consisted of 758 families at all SES levels. The analytic approach closely followed that reported by the NICHD ECCRN (1997). Like the NICHD SECCYD researchers, the Haifa researchers controlled for selection, family, and child characteristics before testing for main and interaction effects involving features of child care. Sagi et al. found that infants who experienced center care in the first year of life (46% insecure), as compared to those who experienced no child care or care by relatives, paid individuals, or family day care (26% insecure overall), were more likely to be insecurely attached to their mothers. Further analyses implicated the high infant–caregiver ratio ($M = 8.01$, $SD = 1.69$) in Israeli centers. Among infants cared for by professional caregivers, those experiencing infant–caregiver ratios of 3:1 or less had a security rate of 72%, compared to 57% for infants experiencing higher infant–caregiver ratios. The researchers also demonstrated that infant–caregiver ratios, not amount of care, were what predicted infant attachment security. When only infants cared for in centers were considered, there was no difference in amount of care experienced by infants who were secure or

insecure with their mothers. Finally, 8 of 24 interaction terms were significant, most supporting a dual-risk interpretation. Low maternal sensitivity combined with an indicator of low-quality child care always yielded the lowest proportion of securely attached infants. Three interactions with child gender indicated that boys were particularly vulnerable to center care, unstable care, and high infant–caregiver ratios.

Most of the insecure Israeli infants were ambivalent; very few were avoidant, consistent with previous studies of infant attachment in Israel (Scher & Mayseless, 2000; van IJzendoorn & Sagi, 1999). In contrast, many of the child care studies in the United States found that most of the infants in child care classified as insecure with their mothers were avoidant, and this difference underscores the cultural context in which these studies were conducted. Both the NICHD ECCRN (1997) study and the Haifa study found small effect sizes for child care variables. The results of the two studies are similar and complementary. The Haifa study compensates for one of the limitations of the NICHD SECCYD, which was that observations of quality in the lowest-quality settings were frequently denied. In Israel, the centers were of uniformly very poor quality, and access was readily available. The Haifa study's inclusion of very low-quality center care for infants from a range of SES groups expands the continuum of quality under which the effects of child care have been studied, and has important policy implications for the well-being of infants placed in center care.

In summary, the NICHD SECCYD and the Haifa infant study examined effects of child care experience during the development of primary attachments in infancy on the security of the infant–mother attachment relationship. The 2001 report of the NICHD ECCRN extended the approach of the 1997 paper to examine the continued effects of this early experience, and also examined the effects of child care that began after the formation of the infant–mother attachment relationship on children's preschool Strange Situation classifications with mothers at 36 months. Because the 1999 NICHD ECCRN report found that more hours/week in child care was associated with lower maternal sensitivity and less positive engagement of child with mother over the first 3 years of life, main effects of child care on attachment security that were not noted at 15 months might have emerged by 36 months. The 2001 analyses addressed whether child care experience (amount, number of arrangements, age of entry, and quality), alone or in combination with family, maternal, or child factors, was associated with attachment security at 36 months. In addition, analyses examined child, family, and child care correlates of stability–instability of Strange Situation attachment classifications from 15 to 36 months.

Child Care and Infant–Mother Attachment Stability

Several authors have reported links between early child care experience and attachment stability from infancy to preschool. In a low-risk sample, Howes and Hamilton (1992b) found significant stability in attachment from infancy to the preschool period. In addition, they found instability to be associated with hours/week in child care. Children who entered part-time child care as infants or 3-year-olds had more stable maternal attachment classifications, regardless of quality of attachment, than children who entered full-time care as infants or 3-year-olds. The stability described by Howes and Hamilton (1992b) is interesting in light of a report by Egeland and Heister (1995). In their high-risk sample from the 1970s, early and extensive child care beginning in the first year seemed to have a negative effect on children who were secure as infants, but a positive effect on those who were insecure. Furthermore, infant attachment security predicted later outcomes only for children who were not in early and extensive child care before 18 months of age. Egeland and Heister speculated that these relations may be mediated by a change in attachment security from infancy to preschool for children in child care, with greater stability of attachment to mother for children who did not experience child care. Egeland and Heister did not, however, actually assess preschool security in their study. In contrast, Rauh, Ziegenhain, Muller, and Wijnroks (2000), following a German sample, found that attachment stability in the first 2 years of life was related to maternal sensitivity, but not to variations in child care experience across that time period.

Unlike the 1997 NICHD ECCRN study, the NICHD ECCRN (2001) analyses considered all four attachment classifications (A, B, C, D) using multinomial logistic regression. Results revealed that mothers who exhibited more sensitivity and responsiveness across play assessments between 6 and 36 months were more likely to have children with secure rather than insecure-controlling classifications, and marginally more likely to have children with insecure-avoidant versus insecure-

controlling, insecure-ambivalent versus insecure-controlling, and secure versus insecure-ambivalent classifications. None of the three child care predictors available for the whole sample significantly predicted any attachment classification. That is, variations in the amount of care, the frequency of care arrangements, or age of entry did not increase or decrease a child's chances of being assigned a particular attachment classification, after controls for all selection and mother–family–child variables. As a direct follow-up of the 15-month interaction findings, four interactions (sensitivity × quality, sensitivity × hours, sensitivity × number of arrangements, and hours × child gender) at 36 months were tested, one at a time, in the multinomial logistic regression models. One interaction term was significant, suggesting that as hours in care increased, children with more sensitive parents were more likely to be classified as secure, and children with less sensitive parents were more likely to be classified as insecure-ambivalent. Thus, overall, findings concerning the follow-up effects of child care experience were congruent with the findings on earlier effects, and they support the conclusion that the effects of child care experience that begins during the development of primary attachments persist into the preschool years.

The ECCRN (2001) also reported logistic regression analyses predicting security vs. insecurity at 36 months within both the initially secure and initially insecure groups. These analyses determined whether child care experience could explain why some children who were initially secure remained that way over time whereas others did not, and why some children who were initially insecure remained that way whereas others did not. There was one effect of child care experience for children who were classified as secure at 15 months: Those whose classification changed from secure to insecure were more likely to have initiated at least 10 hours/week of child care during the interval between 15 and 35 months, compared with children whose classification remained secure. This was a small effect ($r_\phi = .09$). These new results for sequential effects of child care after the formation of primary attachments are in contrast to the results for simultaneous child care experiences, described earlier.

In summary, analyses from the NICHD SEC-CYD have consistently found that family influences are stronger than child care effects in determining the quality of child–mother attachment as measured by the Strange Situation at 15 and 36 months. However, some evidence for dual-risk effects has been found at both ages. It seems that long daily separations from mothers, for children whose interactions with their mothers are already distressed, increase the likelihood of insecure attachment. Entry into child care after developing a primary attachment also appears to elevate risk for insecurity somewhat. A similar finding was reported by Lamb and colleagues (1992), who found that insecure infant–mother attachments were significantly more common among infants assessed after 15 months of age, and among those who entered care between 7 and 12 months of age rather than earlier.

In both the NICHD SECCYD and the Haifa study, any adverse effects of child care on child–mother attachment were observed more in groups at risk because the quality of maternal care was less sensitive and responsive—that is, because the relationship was already troubled. As an extreme example of this phenomenon, Crittenden (1983) reported on the effects of mandatory protective day care (respite care) for young children of maltreating and neglecting mothers. After 4 years the outcomes for the two groups were similar, except that those placed in day care had earlier removals for foster care than comparable children who could not be placed in day care. Crittenden concluded that mandatory protective day care had hastened, but not caused, the removal of the children. She explained this surprising outcome in terms of attachment theory, citing evidence that both maltreating mothers and their infants could be considered anxiously attached, and that as such they would be more vulnerable to experiences of separation. Both mothers and infants reacted to the day care placement with a combination of direct and repressed anger, which exacerbated their already strained relationship and accelerated infants' removal from the home.

The Haifa study complements the NICHD SECCYD by including a range of child care quality that was not confounded by family SES. Together, these studies add to the literature on child–mother attachment in the context of multiple caregiving. Much of child care (especially in infancy, and for some cultural groups more than others) is provided by fathers, grandparents, relatives, friends, and neighbors. The literature suggests little or no impact of these caregiving arrangements on the primary infant–mother attachment relationship. However, there appears to be a threshold effect that is illustrated by results from the Haifa study: More formal group care, with large number of chil-

dren and large child–caregiver ratios, may make the formation of *any* secure attachment—whether to the mother or an alternative caregiver—less likely. This conclusion is supported by the Ahnert and colleagues (2006) meta-analysis, which found that children's attachments to caregivers in child care were observed to be less secure when group size and child–caregiver ratios were large. It may be that children under these adverse circumstances develop strategies with all of their caregivers that are adapted to increase the probability of protection and survival under threatening conditions, which after all is the evolutionary purpose of attachment.

SUMMARY AND CONCLUSIONS

Most children grow and develop within a changing network of attachment relationships, which includes some enduring attachment figures and some that change with time and circumstances. The child is a co-constructor of all of these relationships. Children construct relationships with mothers and residential fathers within the same family. Children come and go between home and child care facilities; the adult caregivers communicate with each other or do not; they collaborate in caring for the child or they do not. However, child–parent and child–caregiver attachment relationships are largely independent in quality and may have different antecedents. The process of forming attachment relationships is similar for parents and alternative caregivers for typical children, particularly children who are very young and/or experiencing positive parental relationships. The construction of secure attachments appears more dependent on particularly skilled and sensitive adult behaviors when children have experienced prior difficult relationships. As with parents, the quality of caregiving may influence attachment formation, but other attributions of the children by the caregivers may also be important.

We know less about the role of alternative caregivers in terms of children's long-term development. Parents, particularly mothers, are undoubtedly the emotionally salient and sustaining attachment figures in most cases. Child care providers are not long-term participants in the social networks of most children. In general, we can draw few conclusions about the importance of early versus later or sustained experiences with alternative attachment figures. We could find no longitudinal studies of long-term alternative attachment relationships—for example, those with grandparents. Far more research than currently exists is needed to support any of the proposed conceptions of the organization of IWMs based on multiple attachment relationships.

ACKNOWLEDGMENT

Susan Spieker's work on this chapter was facilitated by Grant Nos. U10 HD025447 and P30 HD02274 from the National Institute of Child Health and Human Development.

REFERENCES

Ahnert, L., Pinquart, M., & Lamb, M. E. (2006). Security of children's relationships with nonparental care providers: A meta-analysis. *Child Development, 77,* 664–679.

Ainsworth, M. D. S. (1967). *Infancy in Uganda: Infant care and the growth of love.* Baltimore: Johns Hopkins University Press.

Ainsworth, M. D. S., Blehar, M., Waters, E., & Wall, S. (1978). *Patterns of attachment: A psychological study of the Strange Situation.* Hillsdale, NJ: Erlbaum.

Ainsworth, M. D. S., & Wittig, B. (1969). Attachment and exploratory behaviour of one-year-olds in a strange situation. In B. Foss (Ed.), *Determinants of infant behaviour* (Vol. 4, pp. 111–173). London: Methuen.

Anderson, C. W., Nagel, P., Roberts, M., & Smith, K. (1981). Attachment in substitute caregivers as a function of center quality and caregiver involvement. *Child Development, 52,* 53–51.

Barglow, P., Vaughn, B. E., & Molitor, N. (1987). Effects of maternal absence due to employment on the quality of infant–mother attachment in a low-risk sample. *Child Development, 58,* 945–954.

Barnas, M. V., & Cummings, E. M. (1997). Caregiver stability and toddlers' attachment-related behaviors towards caregivers in day care. *Infant Behavior and Development, 17,* 171–177.

Belsky, J. (1990). Developmental risks associated with infant day care: Attachment insecurity, noncompliance, and aggression? In S. S. Chehrazi (Ed.), *Psychosocial issues in day care* (pp. 37–68). Washington, DC: American Psychiatric Association.

Belsky, J., & Braungart, J. M. (1991). Are insecure-avoidant infants with extensive day-care experience less stressed by and more independent in the Strange Situation? *Child Development, 62,* 567–571.

Belsky, J., & Fearon, R. (2002a). Early attachment security, subsequent maternal sensitivity, and later child development: Does continuity in development depend upon continuity of caregiving? *Attachment and Human Development, 4,* 361–387.

Belsky, J., & Fearon, R. (2002b). Infant–mother attachment security, contextual risk, and early development: A moderational analysis. *Development and Psychopathology, 14,* 293–310.

Belsky, J., & Rovine, M. J. (1988). Nonmaternal care in the first year of life and the security of infant–parent attachment. *Child Development, 59,* 157–167.

Benoit, D., & Parker, K. C. H. (1994). Stability and transmission of attachment across three generations. *Child Development, 65,* 1444–1456.

Berger, S., Levy, A., & Compaan, K. (1995, March). *Infant attachment outside the laboratory.* Paper presented at the biennial meeting of the Society for Research in Child Development, Indianapolis, IN.

Booth, C. L., Clarke-Stewart, K. A., Vandell, D. L., McCartney, K., & Owen, M. T. (2002). Childcare usage and mother–infant "quality time." *Journal of Marriage and the Family, 64,* 16–26.

Bowlby, J. (1969/1982). *Attachment and loss: Vol. 1. Attachment.* New York: Basic Books.

Brazelton, T. B. (1985). *Working and caring.* New York: Basic Books.

Bretherton, I. (1985). Attachment theory: Retrospect and prospect. In I. Bretherton & E. Waters (Eds.), Growing points of attachment theory and research. *Monographs of the Society for Research in Child Development, 50*(1–2, Serial No. 209), 3–35.

Campbell, S. B., Brownell, C. A., Hungerford, A., Spieker, S. I., Mohan, R., & Blessing, J. S. (2004). The course of maternal depressive symptoms and maternal sensitivity as predictors of attachment security at 36 months. *Development and Psychopathology, 16,* 231–252.

Cassidy, J., Woodhouse, S. S., Cooper, G., Hoffman, K., Powell, B., & Rodenberg, M. (2005). Examining the precursors of infant attachment security: Implications for early intervention and intervention research. In L. J. Berlin, Y. Ziv, L. Amaya-Jackson, & M. T. Greenberg (Eds.), *Enhancing early attachments: Theory, research, intervention, and policy* (pp. 34–60). New York: Guilford Press.

Clarke-Stewart, K. A. (1989). Infant day care: Maligned or malignant? *American Psychologist, 44,* 266–273.

Cox, M. J., Owen, M., Henderson, V. K., & Margand, N. A. (1992). Prediction of infant–father and infant–mother attachment. *Developmental Psychology, 28,* 777–783.

Crittenden, P. M. (1983). The effect of mandatory protective daycare on mutual attachment in maltreating mother–infant dyads. *Child Abuse and Neglect, 7,* 297–300.

Dontas, C., Maratos, O., Fafoutis, M., & Karangelis, A. (1985). Early social development in institutionally reared Greek infants: Attachment and peer interaction. In I. Bretherton & E. Waters (Eds.), Growing points of attachment theory and research. *Monographs of the Society for Research in Child Development, 50*(1–2, Serial No. 209), 135–175.

Dozier, M., Albus, K., Fisher, P. A., & Sepulveda, S. (2002). Interventions for foster parents: Implications for developmental theory. *Development and Psychopathology, 14,* 843–860.

Dozier, M., Lindhiem, O., & Ackerman, J. P. (2005). Attachment and biobehavioral catchup. In L. J. Berlin, Y. Ziv, L. Amaya-Jackson, & M. T. Greenberg (Eds.), *Enhancing early attachments: Theory, research, intervention, and policy* (pp. 178–194). New York: Guilford Press.

Dozier, M., Stovall, K. C., Albus, K., & Bates, B. (2001). Attachments for infants in foster care: The role of the caregiver state of mind. *Child Development, 72,* 1467–1477.

Easterbrooks, M. A., & Goldberg, W. (1987). Toddler development in the family: Impact of father involvement and parenting characteristics. *Child Development, 55,* 770–752.

Egeland, B., & Heister, M. (1995). The long-term consequences of infant day-care and mother–infant attachment. *Child Development, 66,* 474–485.

Fox, N. A., Kimmerly, N. L., & Schafer, W. D. (1991). Attachment to mother/attachment to father: A meta-analysis. *Child Development, 52,* 210–225.

George, C., Kaplan, N., & Main, M. (1984). *Adult Attachment Interview protocol.* Unpublished manuscript, University of California at Berkeley.

George, C., Kaplan, N., & Main, M. (1985). *Adult Attachment Interview protocol* (2nd ed.). Unpublished manuscript, University of California at Berkeley.

George, C., Kaplan, N., & Main, M. (1996). *Adult Attachment Interview protocol* (3rd ed.). Unpublished manuscript, University of California at Berkeley.

Goossens, F. A., & van IJzendoorn, M. H. (1990). Quality of infants' attachment to professional caregivers: Relation to infant–parent attachment and daycare characteristics. *Child Development, 51,* 832–837.

Grossmann, K., Grossmann, K. E., Fremmer-Bombik, E., Kindler, H., Scheuerer-Englisch, H., & Zimmermann, P. (2002). The uniqueness of the child–father attachment relationship: Fathers' sensitive and challenging play as a pivotal variable in a 16-year longitudinal study. *Social Development, 11,* 307–331.

Howes, C. (1999). Attachment relationships in the context of multiple caregivers. In J. Cassidy & P. R. Shaver (Eds.), *Handbook of attachment: Theory, research, and clinical applications* (pp. 671–687). New York: Guilford Press.

Howes, C. (2006). [Attachment security scores at 14 months]. Unpublished raw data.

Howes, C., & Aikens, J. W. (2002). Peer relations in the transition to adolescence. In H. W. Reese & R. Kail (Eds.), *Advances in child development and behavior* (Vol. 30, pp. 195–230). San Diego, CA: Academic Press.

Howes, C., & Hamilton, C. E. (1992a). Children's relationships with caregivers: Mothers and child care teachers. *Child Development, 63,* 859–866.

Howes, C., & Hamilton, C. E. (1992b). Children's relationships with child care teachers: Stability and concordance with parental attachments. *Child Development, 63,* 867–878.

Howes, C., & Hamilton, C. E. (1993). The changing experience of child care: Changes in teachers and in teacher–child relationships and children's social

competence with peers. *Early Childhood Research Quarterly, 8,* 15–32.

Howes, C., Hamilton, C. E., & Phillipsen, L. C. (1998). Stability and continuity of child–caregiver relationships. *Child Development, 69,* 418–426.

Howes, C., Matheson, C. C., & Hamilton, C. E. (1994). Maternal, teacher, and child care history correlates of children's relationships with peers. *Child Development, 55,* 257–273.

Howes, C., & Oldham, E. (2001). Attachment formation in child care: Processes in the formation of attachment relationships with alternative caregivers. In A. Göncü & E. Klein (Eds.), *Children in play, story, and school* (pp. 267–287). New York: Guilford Press.

Howes, C., & Ritchie, S. (1998). Changes in child–teacher relationships in a therapeutic preschool program. *Early Education and Development, 4,* 411–422.

Howes, C., & Ritchie, S. (1999). Attachment organizations in children with difficult life circumstances. *Development and Psychopathology, 11,* 254–268.

Howes, C., & Ritchie, S. (2002). *A matter of trust: Connecting teachers and learners in the early childhood classroom.* New York: Teachers College Press.

Howes, C., Rodning, C., Galluzzo, D. C., & Myers, L. (1988). Attachment and child care: Relationships with mother and caregiver. *Early Childhood Research Quarterly, 3,* 703–715.

Howes, C., & Segal, J. (1993). Children's relationships with alternative caregivers: The special case of maltreated children removed from their homes. *Journal of Applied Developmental Psychology, 17,* 71–81.

Howes, C., & Shivers, E. M. (2006). New child–caregiver attachment relationships: Entering child care when the caregiver is and is not an ethnic match. *Social Development, 15,* 574–590.

Howes, C., & Smith, E. W. (1995). Children and their child care caregivers: Profiles of relationships. *Social Development, 4,* 44–61.

Howes, C., & Tonyan, H. A. (2000). Links between adult and peer relations across four developmental periods. In K. A. Kerns, J. Contreras, & A. Neal-Barnett (Eds.), *Examining associations between parent–child and peer relationships* (pp. 85–114). New York: Greenwood.

Huston, A. C., & Rosenkrantz Aronson, S. (2005). Mothers' time with infant and time in employment as predictors of mother–child relationships and children's early development. *Child Development, 76,* 467–482.

Jackson, J. F. (1993). Multiple caregiving among African Americans and infant attachment: The need for an emic approach. *Human Development, 35,* 87–102.

Jaeger, E., & Weinraub, M. (1990). Early maternal care and infant attachment: In search of process. In K. McCartney (Ed.), *Child care and maternal employment: A social ecology* (pp. 71–90). San Francisco: Jossey-Bass.

Kobak, R., Rosenthal, N., & Serwik, A. (2005). The attachment hierarchy in middle childhood: Conceptual and methodological issues. In K. A. Kerns & R.

A. Richardson (Eds.), *Attachment in middle childhood* (pp. 71–88). New York: Guilford Press.

Lamb, M. E. (1977a). The development of infant–mother and father–infant attachments in the second year of life. *Developmental Psychology, 13,* 637–648.

Lamb, M. E. (1977b). Father–infant and mother–infant interaction in the first year of life. *Child Development, 48,* 167–181.

Lamb, M. E., Hwang, C. P., Frodi, A., & Frodi, M. (1982). Security of mother- and father-attachment and its relation to sociability with strangers in nontraditional Swedish families. *Infant Behavior and Development, 5,* 355–367.

Lamb, M. E., Sternberg, K. J., & Prodromidis, M. (1992). Nonmaternal care and the security of infant–mother attachment: A reanalysis of the data. *Infant Behavior and Development, 15,* 71–83.

Maclean, K. (2003). The impact of institutionalization on child development. *Development and Psychopathology, 15,* 853–884.

Main, M., Hesse, E., & Kaplan, N. (2005). Predictability of attachment behavior and representational processes at 1, 6, and 19 years of age: The Berkeley longitudinal study. In K. E. Grossmann, K. Grossmann, & E. Waters (Eds.), *Attachment from infancy to adulthood: The major longitudinal studies* (pp. 245–304). New York: Guilford Press.

Main, M., Kaplan, N., & Cassidy, J. (1985). Security in infancy, childhood, and adulthood: A move to the level of representation. In I. Bretherton & E. Waters (Eds.), Growing points of attachment theory and research. *Monographs of the Society for Research in Child Development, 50*(1–2, Serial No. 209), 66–104.

Main, M., & Weston, D. R. (1981). The quality of toddlers' relationships to mother and to father: Related to conflict and the readiness to establish new relationships. *Child Development, 52,* 932–970.

Marcovitch, S., Goldberg, S., Gold, A., Washington, J., Wasson, C., Krekewich, K., et al. (1997). Determinants of behavioral problems in Romanian children adopted in Ontario. *International Journal of Behavioral Development, 20,* 17–31.

McCartney, K., & Galanopoulos, A. (1988). Child care and attachment: A new frontier the second time around. *American Journal of Orthopsychiatry, 58,* 17–24.

McCartney, K., Owen, M. T., Booth, C. L., Clarke-Stewart, A., & Vandell, D. L. (2004). Testing a maternal attachment model of behavior problems in early childhood. *Journal of Child Psychology and Psychiatry, 45,* 765–778.

McElwain, N. L., & Booth-LaForce, C. (2006). Maternal sensitivity to infant distress and nondistress as predictors of infant–mother attachment security. *Journal of Family Psychology, 20,* 247–255.

Milam, S., & Pinderhughes, E. E. (2000). Factors influencing maltreated children's early adjustment in foster care. *Development and Psychopathology, 12,* 63–81.

National Institute of Child Health and Human Development (NICHD) Early Child Care Research Network (ECCRN). (1997). The effects of infant child care on infant–mother attachment security: Results of the NICHD Study of Early Child Care. *Child Development, 68,* 860–879.

National Institute of Child Health and Human Development (NICHD) Early Child Care Research Network (ECCRN). (2001). Child-care and family predictors of preschool attachment and stability from infancy. *Developmental Psychology, 37,* 847–862.

National Institute of Child Health and Human Development (NICHD) Early Child Care Research Network (ECCRN). (1999). Child care and mother–child interaction in the first 3 years of life. *Developmental Psychology, 35,* 1399–1413.

O'Conner, T. G., Marvin, R. S., Rutter, M., Olrick, J. T., Britner, P. A., & The English and Romanian Adoptees Study Team. (2003). Child–parent attachment following early institutional deprivation. *Development and Psychopathology, 15,* 19–38.

Oppenheim, D., Sagi, A., & Lamb, M. E. (1988). Infant–adult attachments on the kibbutz and their relation to socio-emotional development four years later. *Developmental Psychology, 27,* 727–733.

Owen, M., & Cox, M. (1988). Maternal employment and the transition to parenthood: Family functioning and child development. In A. Gottfried & A. Gottfried (Eds.), *Maternal employment and children's development: Longitudinal research* (pp. 85–119). New York: Plenum Press.

Parke, R. D., & Asher, S. R. (1983). Social and personality development. *Annual Review of Psychology, 37,* 755–509.

Raikes, H. A. (1993). Relationship duration in infant care: Time with a high ability teacher and infant–teacher attachment. *Early Childhood Research Quarterly, 8,* 309–325.

Rauh, H., Ziegenhain, U., Muller, B., & Wijnroks, L. (2000). Stability and change in infant–mother attachment in the second year of life: Relations to parenting quality and varying degrees of day-care experience. In P. M. Crittenden & A. H. Claussen (Eds.), *The organization of attachment relationships: Maturation, culture, and context* (pp. 251–276). New York: Cambridge University Press.

Roggmann, L. A., Langlois, J. H., Hubbs-Tait, L., & Rieser-Danner, L. A. (1994). Infant day-care, attachment, and the "file drawer problem." *Child Development, 65,* 1429–1443.

Rudasill, K. M., Rimm-Kaufman, S. E., Justice, L. M., & Pence, K. (2006). Temperament and language skills as predictors of teacher–child relationship quality in preschool. *Early Education and Development, 17,* 271–291.

Saft, E., & Pianta, R. C. (2001). Teacher perceptions of their relationships with students: Effects of child age, gender, and ethnicity of teachers and children. *School Psychology Quarterly, 16,* 125–141.

Sagi, A., Koren-Karie, N., Gini, M., Ziv, Y., & Joels, T. (2002). Shedding further light on the effects of various types and quality of early child care on infant–

mother attachment relationship: The Haifa Study of Early Child Care. *Child Development, 73*, 1166–1186.

Sagi-Schwartz, A., & Aviezer, O. (2005). Correlates of attachment to multiple caregivers in kibbutz children from birth to emerging adulthood: The Haifa longitudinal study. In K. E. Grossmann, K. Grossmann, & E. Waters (Eds.), *Attachment from infancy to adulthood: The major longitudinal studies* (pp. 165–197). New York: Guilford Press.

Scher, A., & Mayseless, O. (2000). Mothers of anxious/ambivalent infants: Maternal characteristics and child-care context. *Child Development, 71*, 1629–1639.

Singer, L. M., Brodzinsky, D. M., Ramsay, D., Steir, M., & Waters, E. (1985). Infant–mother attachment in adoptive families. *Child Development, 55*, 1573–1551.

Solomon, J., & George, C. (1999). The development of attachment in separated and divorced families: Effects of overnight visitation, parent and couple variables. *Attachment and Human Development, 1*, 2–33.

Spieker, S. J., & Bensley, L. (1994). Roles of living arrangements and grandmother social support in adolescent mothering and infant attachment. *Developmental Psychology, 30*, 102–111.

Sroufe, L. A. (1988). A developmental perspective on day care. *Early Childhood Research Quarterly, 3*, 51–50.

Steele, H., & Steele, M. (2005). Understanding and resolving emotional conflict: The London Parent Child Project. In K. E. Grossmann, K. Grossmann, & E. Waters (Eds.), *Attachment from infancy to adulthood: The major longitudinal studies* (pp. 137–164). New York: Guilford Press.

Steele, H., Steele, M., & Fonagy, P. (1995). Associations among attachment classifications of mothers, fathers, and their infants. *Child Development, 57*, 571–555.

Stovall, K. C., & Dozier, M. (2000). The development of attachment in new relationships: Single subject analyses for ten foster infants. *Development and Psychopathology, 12*, 133–156.

Stovall-McClough, K. C., & Dozier, M. (2004). Forming attachments in foster care: Infant attachment during the first two months in placement. *Development and Psychopathology, 16*, 253–271.

Stuhlman, M., & Pianta, R. C. (2002). Teachers' narratives about their relationships with children: Associations with behaviors in the classroom. *School Psychology Review, 31*, 148–163.

Suess, G. J., Grossmann, K. E., & Sroufe, L. A. (1992). Effects of infant attachment to mother and father on quality of adaptation in preschool: From dyadic to individual organization of self. *International Journal of Behavioral Development, 15*, 73–55.

Thompson, R., & Raikes, H. A. (2003). Towards the next quarter century: Conceptual and methodological challenges for attachment theory. *Development and Psychopathology, 15*, 691–718.

Tizard, B., & Rees, J. (1975). The effect of early institutional rearing on the behavior problems and affectional relationships of four-year-old children. *Journal of Child Psychology and Psychiatry, 15*, 51–77.

Tran, H., & Weinraub, M. (2006). Child care effects in context: quality, stability, and multiplicity in non-maternal child care arrangements during the first 15 months of life. *Developmental Psychology, 42*, 566–582.

van IJzendoorn, M. H. (1995). Adult attachment representations, parental responsiveness and infant attachment: A meta-analysis on the predictive validity of the Adult Attachment Interview. *Psychological Bulletin, 117*, 387–403.

van IJzendoorn, M. H., & De Wolff, M. S. (1997). In search of the absent father: Meta-analysis of infant–father attachment. A rejoinder to our discussants. *Child Development, 60*, 71–91.

van IJzendoorn, M. H., & Sagi, A. (1999). Cross-cultural patterns of attachment: Universal and contextual dimensions. In J. Cassidy & P. R. Shaver (Eds.), *Handbook of attachment: Theory, research, and clinical applications* (pp. 713–734). New York: Guilford Press.

van IJzendoorn, M. H., Sagi, A., & Lambermon, M. W. E. (1992). The multiple caregiver paradox: Data from Holland and Israel. *New Directions for Child Development, 57*, 5–27.

Volling, B., & Belsky, J. (1992). The contribution of child–mother and father–child relationships to the quality of sibling interaction: A longitudinal study. *Child Development, 53*, 1209–1222.

Ward, M. J., & Carlson, E. A. (1995). Associations among adult attachment representations, maternal sensitivity, and infant–mother attachment in a sample of adolescent mothers. *Child Development, 55*, 59–79.

Ward, M. J., Carlson, E. A., Plunket, S. W., & Kessler, D. B. (1991). *Adolescent infant–mother attachment: Interactions, relationships, and working models.* Unpublished manuscript, Cornell Medical College.

Waters, E. (1987). *Attachment Behavior Q-Set (Revision 3.0).* Stony Brook: State University of New York at Stony Brook, Department of Psychology.

Westman, J. C. (1988). The infant day care controversy. *American Journal of Psychiatry, 145*, 1177–1178.

Yarrow, L. J., Goodwin, M. S., Manheimer, H., & Milowe, I. D. (1973). Infancy experiences and cognitive and personality development at 10 years. In L. J. Stone, H. T. Smith, & L. B. Murphy (Eds.), *The competent infant: Research and commentary* (pp. 1277–1281). New York: Basic Books.

Zeanah, C., & Smyke, A. T. (2005). Building attachment relationships following maltreatment and severe deprivation. In L. J. Berlin, Y. Ziv, L. Amaya-Jackson, & M. T. Greenberg (Eds.), *Enhancing early attachments: Theory, research, intervention, and policy* (pp. 195–216). New York: Guilford Press.

CHAPTER 15

The Influence of Early Attachments on Other Relationships

LISA J. BERLIN
JUDE CASSIDY
KAREN APPLEYARD

Questions about the influence of early attachments on other relationships cut to the heart of attachment theory and research. According to Bowlby (1979), "there is a strong causal relationship between an individual's experiences with his parents [attachments] and his later capacity to make affectional bonds" (p. 135). By "affectional bonds," Bowlby was referring to particularly close ties "in which the partner is important as a unique individual and interchangeable with none other" (Ainsworth, 1989, p. 711). An attachment is a specific type of affectional bond that a person has to another from whom he or she attempts to derive security, as with an infant to a parent or an adult to a romantic partner. Affectional bonds that do not contain an attachment component typically include bonds to one's children, and, during childhood, most relationships with siblings and friends. Bowlby (1969/1982, 1973) also specified that the mechanisms underlying the "causal relationship" between early child–parent attachment and later affectional bonds are "internal working models"—mental representations based on early interactions between infants and their parents that tend to stabilize over time.

In this chapter, we discuss attachment theory and research concerning the influence of early attachments on other relationships. We consider the influence of early attachments on several kinds of affectional bonds: those with siblings, friends, romantic partners, and children. We also consider the large body of research on the influence of early attachments on children's most important relationships that typically do not meet Bowlby's criteria for classification as affectional bonds: relationships with peers (as opposed to relationships with friends). Throughout this review, we examine not only the extent to which there are associations between early attachments and other relationships, but also what is known about the mechanisms underlying these associations.

THE INFLUENCE OF EARLY ATTACHMENTS ON OTHER RELATIONSHIPS: THEORETICAL CONSIDERATIONS

According to attachment theory, the infant–parent attachment relationship is an evolutionarily adaptive relationship, a key function of which is to protect the child (Bowlby, 1969/1982). Bowlby (1969/1982) maintained that the "attachment behavioral system" is one of several species-specific "control systems" that have evolved to facilitate survival and reproductive fitness. According to Bowlby (1969/1982, 1973), individuals develop internal working models that guide the attachment behavioral system (see Bretherton & Munholland, Chapter 5, this volume). Bowlby (1973) asserted that repeated daily transactions between the infant and parent lead the infant to develop expectations about the parent's caregiving that are gradually organized into internal working models of the caregiver, of the self in relation to this caregiver, and of the attachment relationship as a whole. Sensitive caregiving potentiates a secure attachment and the development of internal working models of the caregiver as trustworthy and supportive, of the self as worthy of the caregiver's support, and of the relationship as a nurturing "safe haven." Conversely, insensitive caregiving leads to an insecure attachment, and to working models of the caregiver as unavailable and untrustworthy, of the self as unworthy of the caregiver's support, and of the attachment relationship as fundamentally unreliable.

According to Bowlby, it is individuals' internal working models derived from their earliest attachments that guide the development of other relationships. This influence occurs initially through an individual's expectations about others' emotional availability: " ... the kinds of experiences a person has, especially during childhood, greatly affect ... whether he expects later to find a secure personal base, or not" (Bowlby, 1979, p. 104). Thus a securely attached child will expect others to be sensitive and supportive. An insecure child will expect others to be insensitive and not consistently supportive, or directly rejecting. It is important to note that internal working models are not viewed as immutable. Major changes in the environment and/or in the person require the reformulation of internal working models. Such experiences as traumas, losses, and new attachments are the most likely to alter internal working models. Understanding the conditions under which internal working models about relationships change is especially important for understanding the influence of early attachments on other relationships, and especially the *limits* of this influence—an issue that we address throughout this chapter.

During the past 20 years, attachment scholars have elaborated on Bowlby's propositions, bringing greater specificity to both theory and research. Sroufe and Fleeson (1986, 1988) have elaborated on the concept of working models of relationships, arguing that it is the working model of the attachment relationship as a coherent whole—the

model of how a close relationship should be—that is carried forward from early attachments to other relationships. This model then guides not only expectations of others, but also behavior toward others, behavior elicited from others, and the selection of relationship partners. From early interactions with caregivers during infancy, therefore, the child learns fundamental rules of relating to others, especially in terms of reciprocity, synchrony, and communication (Weinfield, Sroufe, Egeland, & Carlson, Chapter 4, this volume). Sroufe and his colleagues also have argued that a secure attachment fosters such intrapersonal qualities as confidence, self-efficacy, self-esteem, social skills, and the ability to explore the environment competently, which in turn foster mutually satisfying interpersonal interactions and relationships (Sroufe, Egeland, & Carlson, 1999; Sroufe, Egeland, Carlson, & Collins, 2005).

Cassidy and Berlin (1999) have proposed several ways in which parents of secure children may directly facilitate their children's positive relationships with others: (1) by providing their children with more social experiences, which in turn may increase opportunities for practicing social skills and making friends; (2) by directing and advising their children in ways that help them develop and maintain positive relationships; and (3) by serving as role models of sensitive and supportive behavior toward others. Similarly, Thompson and his colleagues have recently emphasized the ways in which mothers discuss emotions with their young children as an important component of early attachments and of children's developing social competence, including their relationships with others. (See Thompson, Chapter 16, this volume, for a review and further discussion.)

Main (1990) and other scholars have expanded on Bowlby's ideas concerning the evolutionary function of early attachments (Belsky, 1999, 2005; Simpson, 1999; Simpson & Belsky, Chapter 6, this volume). In particular, according to Main's (1990) concept of "conditional behavioral strategies," infants have the biologically based ability to tailor the output of their attachment behavioral systems (i.e., their attachment-seeking behaviors) to particular caregiving environments in order to elicit as much parental investment and protection as possible. In a *sensitive* caregiving environment, when an infant's attachment system is activated, he or she seeks protection from the caregiver. In an *insensitive* caregiving environment, the infant must manipulate attachment-seeking behaviors to fit the particular (implicit or explicit) demands of the caregiver. Main proposed that each of the three principal attachment patterns (secure, insecure-avoidant, and insecure-ambivalent) reflects a particular attachment strategy. The strategy of a secure infant is to seek support from attachment figures. In mildly threatening situations, the strategy of an insecure-avoidant infant is to minimize dependence on attachment figures (see also Cassidy & Kobak, 1988). The strategy of an insecure-ambivalent infant is to emphasize or maximize dependence on attachment figures (see also Cassidy & Berlin, 1994).

Conditional behavioral strategies can be viewed as unconscious plans, guided by internal working models of attachment, which influence cognition and behavior. To the extent that these conditional behavioral strategies guide infants' behaviors toward their parents, these strategies may also be carried forward to guide behavior toward other attachment figures or potential relationship partners. In fact, although not directly derived from Main's concept of conditional behavioral strategies, social-psychological research on adult attachment "styles" (e.g., J. Feeney, Chapter 21, this volume; Hazan & Shaver, 1987; Mikulincer & Shaver, 2007) can be viewed as categorizing adults' proclivities in romantic relationships according to Main's three attachment strategies of support seeking, minimizing, or maximizing (see also Kobak & Sceery, 1988; Mikulincer & Shaver, 2004 and Chapter 23, this volume). Consistent with Main's (1990) arguments, Belsky and his colleagues have argued that individuals' earliest experiences with caregivers lead not only to strategic care-eliciting behaviors during infancy, but also to variation in other behavioral and biological processes (such as pubertal timing, mate selection, and parenting), in order to maximize the individual's reproductive fitness (Belsky, Steinberg, & Draper, 1991; Simpson & Belsky, Chapter 6, this volume).

In sum, Bowlby's original writings emphasized a strong influence of early attachments on other relationships characterized by affectional bonds, operating largely through internal working models. Contemporary attachment theorists have elaborated on Bowlby's hypotheses, especially in terms of possible mediators and moderators of the associations between early attachments and other relationships. In the literature review that follows, we examine empirical evidence of associations between early attachments and other relationships; the extent to which these associations support Bowlby's hypothesis of a causal influence of early attachment on later relationships; and especially the processes and mechanisms underlying both continuities and discontinuities between early attachments and other relationships.

THE INFLUENCE OF EARLY ATTACHMENTS ON OTHER RELATIONSHIPS: RESEARCH EVIDENCE

We begin this section by examining affectional bonds within families: first, the concordance of an infant's multiple attachments; and second, the associations between early attachments and sibling relationships. We next discuss the associations between early attachments and relationships with childhood friends and peers. Last, we examine associations between early attachments and subsequent relationships with romantic partners and children. In light of the vast number of studies examining the influence of early attachments on other relationships, we intend this literature review to be representative, not exhaustive. In addition, our review highlights findings from studies that can best address the question of the influence of early attachment on other relationships: prospective, longitudinal studies.

Associations among Early Attachments: The Concordance of Infant–Caregiver Attachments

Bowlby and other theorists have clearly stated that an infant can form an attachment to more than one caregiver at a time. Observational studies support this claim (e.g., Ainsworth, 1967). Associations among infants' multiple attachments are less clear, however. If, as attachment theory and research suggest, the quality of an infant's attachment to the parent reflects the quality of interaction with that parent, then the infant's attachments across parents would be similar only to the extent that the two sets of interactions were similar, and neither attachment relationship would influence the formation of the other. Yet according to Bowlby's (1958, 1969/1982) concept of "monotropy," infants tend to have a principal attachment figure who is sought preferentially as a secure base in times of trouble (even above other attachment figures). It may be that the infant's attachment to the principal attachment figure influences the formation of the infant's attachments to other caregivers. Ainsworth noted that infant–mother and infant–father attachments may be particularly likely to reflect unique and specific relationship histories because they are simultaneously formed initial attachments; in contrast, attachments formed later (e.g., a relationship with a nanny formed later in infancy), may be more likely to be influenced by the earlier attachment(s) (M. D. S. Ainsworth, personal communication to J. Cassidy, August 1988). Another important question, about which little is known, concerns concordance across parents: If the infant has formed different-quality attachments to different parents, which of these early attachments is more likely to influence (which) other relationships?

Numerous studies have examined the associations among infants' attachments to different caregivers, including mothers, fathers, and kibbutz *metaplot* (Belsky & Rovine, 1987; Easterbrooks, 1989; Fox, Kimmerly, & Schafer, 1991; Grossmann, Grossmann, Huber, & Wartner, 1981; Main & Weston, 1981; Sagi et al., 1985; Steele, Steele, & Fonagy, 1996). Although some studies have indicated that an infant can form different types of attachments to different caregivers (e.g., Belsky & Rovine, 1987; Grossmann et al., 1981; Main & Weston, 1981), there is stronger evidence of concordance, especially between parents, as demonstrated by two meta-analyses (Fox et al., 1991; van IJzendoorn & De Wolff, 1997). What needs to be better understood, however, is what accounts for this concordance. In reflecting on their findings, Fox and his colleagues highlighted the possibilities of (1) caregivers' shared childrearing values and practices and (2) infant temperament as contributors to concordant attachment classifications. Because some studies of adult romantic or marital attachment relationships find concordance of partners on attachment "style" (reviewed by Mikulincer & Shaver, 2007), it is also important to consider that concordant security of attachment between two parents and their children may be attributable in part to similarities in attachment and caregiving styles between the parents. These various possibilities remain to be rigorously tested.

Surprisingly, in one study of infant–parent and adult attachment, when parents had similar Adult Attachment Interview (AAI; George, Kaplan, & Main, 1984, 1985, 1996) classifications— classifications that should overlap at least partially with their childrearing values and practices—there was not also greater concordance between infant–mother and infant–father attachment (Steele et al., 1996). One post hoc explanation that received some support from the data was that infant–mother attachment was influencing infant–father attachment. The data also suggested that infant characteristics could be contributing to the finding of concordance, however.

Further study of the associations among early attachments is required. In addition, the large majority of the research on the associations between early attachments and other relationships has focused exclusively on child–mother attachment. In the sections that follow, we include findings, when available, about child–father attachment and about the ways in which attachments to mother and father compare.

Associations between Early Attachments and Relationships with Siblings

Sibling relationships are frequently people's longest-lasting close relationships. They are especially interesting from an attachment perspective, because they usually develop in the context of each sibling's attachment to the same set of parents. Two studies have examined the associations between infant–parent attachment and sibling interaction. One study found that infant–mother, but not infant–father, attachment security was associated with less sibling conflict observed in the home approximately 5 years later (Volling & Belsky, 1992). A second sibling study found that infant–mother attachment security was related to positive treatment of and from an older sibling (Teti & Ablard, 1989; see also Booth, Rubin, & Rose-Krasnor, 1998). In addition, 70% of the secure infants had siblings classified as "more secure" according to mothers' ratings on the Attachment Q-Sort (AQS; Waters & Deane, 1985). Thus, consistent with attachment theory, the quality of sibling relationships appears to derive primarily from each sibling's attachment to the mother. The associations between infant–father attachment and sibling interaction is an area that requires further investigation.

Associations between Early Attachments and Relationships with Childhood Friends and Peers

Attachment theory's predictions of causal links between early attachments and other relationships have galvanized multiple investigations of these associations. Researchers have examined the qualities of children's established and "best" friendships, as well as children's interactions with less intimate peers. Supporting attachment theory, studies generally have revealed positive associations between early attachment security and childhood friendship and peer relationships. Moreover, supporting Main's (1990) concept of conditional behavioral strategies, the attachment group differences in children's relationships with friends and peers appear consistent with distinct attachment-based strategies. Further supporting the theory, studies have provided some evidence of children's representational processes mediating the associations between early attachments and peer relationships. Most recently, researchers have begun to examine child–parent attachment, children's friendships, and peer interactions simultaneously and over long time periods (i.e., from infancy to adolescence), offering greater specificity about each of these factors and the relations among them.

Associations between Early Attachments and Children's Friendships

Numerous inquiries have addressed the associations between infant– or child–parent attachment and the qualities of established friendships in children as young as 2 and as old as 12. Findings from both home- and lab-based studies using a variety of measures are generally quite consistent in illustrating associations between early child–mother attachment and friendship quality, in terms of greater responsiveness toward toddler "best playmates" (Pierrehumbert, Ianotti, Cummings, & Zahn-Waxler, 1989); more positive interaction between 4-year-old best friends (Kerns, 1994; Park & Waters, 1989; although see Booth et al., 1998, for differing longitudinal findings); and less negative interaction between 6-year-old best friends (although positive behavior was, surprisingly, *less* evident in children who had been securely attached to their fathers; Youngblade & Belsky, 1992; Youngblade, Park, & Belsky, 1993). In addition, in the longitudinal Minnesota Study of Risk and Adaptation from Birth to Adulthood of approximately 180 low-income mothers and their children, a subset of approximately 40 children was assessed over the course of a 1-month summer camp at age 10 (Elicker, Englund, & Sroufe, 1992; Shulman, Elicker, & Sroufe, 1994; Sroufe et al., 1999). Children classified as secure with their mothers at both 12 and 18 months were more likely to make friends with other children with secure attachment histories. Similarly, in a longitudinal inquiry of north German families, infant–mother (but not infant–father) attachment predicted interviewer ratings of children's "competence in establishing close friendships" at age 10 (Freitag, Belsky, Grossmann, Grossmann, & Scheuerer-Englisch, 1996).

Children's attachments to their parents may influence not only the quality but also the quan-

tity of children's friendships. In three longitudinal studies, children who had been securely attached as infants were judged to have made more friends in middle childhood than children who had been insecurely attached (Elicker et al., 1992; Grossmann & Grossmann, 1991; Lewis & Feiring, 1989).

Associations between Early Attachments and Children's Peer Relationships

Despite Bowlby's emphasis on the influence of early attachments on later affectional bonds, a large body of attachment research addresses the connections between child–parent attachment and children's peer relationships—relationships typically *not* characterized by affectional bonds. Although this emphasis may seem misplaced, Sroufe and his colleagues (1999, 2005) have argued persuasively that, especially during toddlerhood and the preschool years, relating to one's agemates is a key developmental task—important in and of itself and because it paves the way for subsequent tasks, including the development of close friendships and intimate partnerships. Based on this rationale, a multifaceted literature has developed, including contemporaneous and longitudinal investigations of toddlers, preschoolers, school-age children, and adolescents from different socioeconomic strata, with data provided by mothers, teachers, independent observers, and peers on children's behavior *toward* others as well as treatment received and elicited *from* others. Although findings are not completely uniform, they are strikingly consistent in illustrating a relation between a secure child–mother attachment and more harmonious interactions with peers, higher regard from peers, and fewer behavior problems in preschool and elementary school classrooms (see Berlin & Cassidy, 1999, for a review; see also Booth-LaForce & Kerns, in press; Thompson, Chapter 16, this volume). Moreover, in the Minnesota study, infant–mother attachment predicted peer competence 15 years later as observed in small-group interactions during a summer camp reunion (Englund, Levy, Hyson, & Sroufe, 2000), as well as parent- and teacher-rated social competence at age 16 (Sroufe et al., 1999).

The overwhelming majority of these studies examine child–mother attachment and thus cannot offer definitive findings about the role of child–father attachment in children's developing peer relationships—a conclusion also drawn by the authors of a recent meta-analysis on attachment and peer relationships (Schneider, Atkinson, & Tardif, 2001). It is interesting to note, however, that two studies examining multiple child–caregiver attachments, one longitudinal and one cross-sectional, have revealed an advantage of multiple secure attachments for a child's social competence (including competence with classmates) (Sagi-Schwartz & Aviezer, 2005; Verschueren & Marcoen, 1999).

Early Attachments and Relationships with Childhood Friends and Peers: Minimizing and Maximizing Strategies

The research on the associations between early attachment and childhood relationships with friends and peers not only provides consistent evidence of these associations, but also begins to suggest that children's minimizing and maximizing "strategies" (Main, 1990), developed in response to their caregivers' particular attachment-related demands, affect relationships with peers and friends. These suggestions come from the relatively few studies in which the principal insecure groups of children (avoidant and ambivalent) are examined as separate groups. Taken as a whole, the peer studies portray both avoidant and ambivalent children as followers—not leaders—of their peers and as overly dependent on their classroom teachers. Yet, whereas the ambivalent children appear tentative, inhibited, and anxiously (if unsuccessfully) seeking positive peer interaction, the avoidant children appear aggressive, hostile, and actively repudiating positive peer interaction (Cassidy & Berlin, 1994; Sroufe et al., 2005).

The insecure-ambivalent profile of an inhibited, anxious child is consistent with a strategy of maximizing child–caregiver attachment because it emphasizes the child's needs for extra attention and care. This pattern of behavior also communicates the child's vulnerability and neediness to his or her peers and potential friends, which in turn may elicit further peer rejection or neglect. The avoidant profile of an aggressive and rejecting child is consistent with a strategy of minimizing child–caregiver attachment, because it emphasizes the child's power and "independence." This pattern of behavior also repels and alienates peers.

These characterizations are also reflected in a study of infant–mother attachment and friendship in 3-year-olds, involving 1,060 participants from the prospective, longitudinal National Institute of Child Health and Human Development (NICHD) Study of Early Child Care (McElwain, Cox, Burchinal, & Macfie, 2003). In observational assessments of each target child and a same-sex friend, target children who at age 15 months were classified as ambivalent were significantly less self-assertive or controlling than children

who had been classified avoidant. Avoidant children demonstrated more instrumental aggression (defined as unprovoked physical attempts to take a toy from the friend) than secure or ambivalent children. In addition, the friends of disorganized children (those children without an organized attachment strategy; see Lyons-Ruth & Jacobvitz, Chapter 28, this volume), perhaps responding to these children's *lack* of a strategy, were more self-assertive or controlling than the friends of secure, avoidant, or ambivalent children. These associations held even when attachment classifications at 3 years and maternal sensitivity at both 15 months and 3 years were controlled.

These profiles are further reflected in children's self-reports about their relationships with friends and peers. For example, two longitudinal studies of attachment and loneliness have linked the ambivalent pattern to greater self-reported loneliness in children as young as 5 (Berlin, Cassidy, & Belsky, 1995; Raikes & Thompson, 2007). In addition, in the Grossmann and Grossmann (1991) study of 10-year-old German children's friendships described earlier, children who had been secure could identify a number of friends by name, whereas the children who had been insecure (83% avoidant) professed to have many friends but could not name any of them.

The discrepancy between the avoidant children's positive general claims and the lack of specific support for their assertions is reminiscent of the idealizing discourse of some adults classified as dismissing (avoidant) in the AAI. These adults describe their experiences in positive generalities, yet fail to substantiate their descriptions with specific examples and often provide directly contradictory examples. In the AAI, this type of idealizing is considered to reflect defensive exclusion of painful memories—a form of information processing that is consistent with minimizing attachment (i.e., not acknowledging emotional pain precludes the need for comfort and nurturance). In the Grossmann and Grossmann (1991) study, therefore, the inability of the German avoidant children to name their friends also may reflect defensive exclusion in the service of minimizing attachment. These processes require and merit further research.

These broad profiles provided by studies of childhood friendship and peer relationships are also reflected in studies focusing on attachment and early psychopathology, often measured in terms of ratings of classroom behavior problems (i.e., peer group behavior). Specifically, there is some indication that ambivalent children are at elevated risk for internalizing disorders and avoidant children are at elevated risk for externalizing disorders, although as DeKlyen and Greenberg (Chapter 27, this volume) point out in their review of this literature, these connections are "suggestive but inconclusive." As the authors note, the associations appear more pronounced in high-risk than in low-risk samples (see also Belsky & Fearon, 2002b, and Sroufe et al., 2005). Disorganized children are also at elevated risk for externalizing disorders (Lyons-Ruth & Jacobvitz, Chapter 28, this volume; see also van IJzendoorn, Schuengel, & Bakermans-Kranenburg, 1999).

Early Attachments and Relationships with Childhood Friends and Peers: Mediating Mechanisms

As described earlier, Bowlby emphasized the role of individuals' internal working models in mediating the associations between early attachments and other relationships. The most precise test of Bowlby's hypothesis would come from a mediational analysis of longitudinal data focusing on infant–parent attachment as the (sole) predictor and later representations of peer or friend relationships. Although to our knowledge this particular test has not been conducted, several studies have begun to examine this issue. All find evidence consistent with a mediational model. First, numerous studies have found associations between attachment quality and representations of self, others, and attachment in general (e.g., Booth et al., 1998; Cassidy, 1988; Colman & Thompson, 2002; Ziv, Oppenheim, & Sagi-Schwartz, 2004). Several studies have also linked attachment quality and cognitive processes theorized to reflect internal working models, such as attributional biases and memory for affectively charged information (Belsky, Spritz, & Crnic, 1996; Kirsh & Cassidy, 1997). Second, one investigation found longitudinal and contemporaneous associations between child–mother attachment and children's peer relationships *and* representations of peers (Suess, Grossmann, & Sroufe, 1992; Wartner, Grossmann, Fremmer-Bombik, & Suess, 1994). Finally, in another study, kindergarten and first-grade children's peer-related representations (i.e., interpretations of whether a hypothetical peer acted with hostile intent) partially mediated the association between the children's attachments to their mothers and their actual relationships with their peers, assessed concurrently (Cassidy, Kirsh, Scolton, & Parke, 1996). Similar findings come from a cross-sectional study of preschoolers in which children's perceptions of social support (a form of peer rep-

resentations) mediated the association between child–mother attachment, assessed according to an observer's ratings on the Attachment Q-Sort (Waters, 1987; Waters, Vaughn, Posada, & Kondo-Ikemura, 1995), and a composite measure of children's social competence that included peer relationships (Bost, Vaughn, Newell Washington, Cielinski, & Bradbard, 1998; see also Anan & Barnett, 1999).

Relevant findings also come from a structural equation analysis of data from the Minnesota study (Carlson, Sroufe, & Egeland, 2004). This analysis tested the associations among "early experience" (including infant–mother attachment security and child–mother relationship quality at age 2), representations of self and relationships, "social behavior" from age 4 to age 12, and adolescent "social functioning" (including functioning in friendships and romantic partnerships) at age 19. No direct association emerged between early experience and a comprehensive measure of social functioning at age 19. Early experience, however, significantly predicted early childhood representations, which then predicted later self- and relationship representations and later social behavior. Early experience also significantly predicted early childhood social behavior, which then predicted later social behavior and later self- and relationship representations.

In addition to representational processes, it is important to consider other possible mechanisms linking early attachments and subsequent relationships. As described earlier, parents of secure children may directly facilitate their children's positive relationships with others in several ways, such as by providing their children with more social experiences (Cassidy & Berlin, 1999). Some evidence for this supposition comes from an early study of attachment security and peer interaction, in which attachment security was positively related to the extent of children's contacts with peers (Lieberman, 1977). These and other nonrepresentational mediators require further investigation.

Associations among Early Attachments, Children's Friendships, and Children's Peer Interactions: Increased Specificity

Given Bowlby's emphasis on the influence of early attachments on later affectional bonds, Berlin and Cassidy (1999) have highlighted the need for research to specify the extent to which early attachments more strongly influence affectional bonds versus relationships that are not characterized by affectional bonds (see also Belsky &

Cassidy, 1994). A valuable step in this direction was taken in a 2001 meta-analysis of 63 studies of child–parent attachment and children's peer relationships, including friendships (Schneider et al., 2001). Although this meta-analysis did not speak exclusively to the prediction of peer relationships from *early* attachment per se (it also included studies of concurrent associations between adolescent attachment and friendship quality), its findings are nonetheless relevant. Specifically, Schneider and his colleagues reported a small to moderate effect (an effect size of 0.20) of child–parent (predominantly child–mother) attachment security on children's peer relationships in general. When the studies of children's close friendships were examined as a separate subgroup, the effect size of 0.24 was significantly stronger than the effect for the studies of children's peer relationships (0.14). This finding supports Bowlby's claims and provides important specificity to the understanding of the influence of early attachments on other relationships, suggesting that early attachment in fact does exert a stronger influence on relationships characterized by affectional bonds than on relationships that are not characterized by affectional bonds.

Increased specificity about the associations among early attachments, children's friendships, and children's peer relationships also comes from the Minnesota study (Sroufe et al., 2005) and the NICHD study (NICHD Early Child Care Research Network [ECCRN], 2005). Each of these studies includes multiple measures of the early child–parent relationship and of children's relationships with both friends and peers. Both studies provide careful examinations of the processes underlying continuity and discontinuity in the quality of children's relationships. In addition, some comparison of the prediction from early attachment to friend versus peer relationships is possible.

For example, in the Minnesota study, infant–mother attachment security was more consistently related to the quality of children's friendships than to preschool or elementary school teachers' ratings of peer competence (Sroufe et al., 1999). Associations with a composite measure of "early care" (quality of attachment and parenting from 12 to 42 months), however, were consistently significant for both friendships and peer relationships, illustrating the value of considering the quality of the child–parent relationship beyond infant–parent attachment per se. Consistent with Sroufe and colleagues' (1999) predictions about the importance of early peer relationships for later friendship quality, early peer relationships consistently predicted later peer competence and friendship quality. Moreover, factoring in earlier measures of friendship quality or peer competence typically improved the prediction to later friendship quality and peer competence (over attachment quality alone; Sroufe et al., 1999; see Jaffari-Bimmel, Juffer, van IJzendoorn, Bakermans-Kranenburg, & Mooijaart, 2006, for similar findings). Interestingly, as children aged, intermediate measures of friendship or peer competence appeared increasingly less likely to add incrementally to the prediction of social competence by earlier measures (measures of child–parent relationship quality and peer competence), leading Sroufe and colleagues to conclude that "by age 5, much of the variance in [later] adolescent social competence can be accounted for" (p. 256).

Findings from the NICHD study of approximately 1,000 families have illustrated the importance of early attachment for other relationships, as well as the value of factoring in (1) subsequent parenting quality and (2) the family's broader ecological conditions. Specifically, in addition to the associations between infant–mother attachment and friendship quality discussed earlier (McElwain et al., 2003), there were direct associations between infant–mother attachment and mother-rated social competence (in terms of children's sociability, empathy, and prosocial engagement) at age 3 (Belsky & Fearon, 2002b); mothers' ratings of children's social skills from ages 4½ through 6; and teachers' ratings of children's internalizing and externalizing behavior problems during kindergarten and first grade (NICHD ECCRN, 2006). At the same time, at age 3, the associations between attachment and social competence were moderated by a composite measure of family risk (including family income, maternal education, maternal depression, and parenting stress) (Belsky & Fearon, 2002b). Specifically, for all attachment groups, as family risk increased, social competence declined linearly; at the highest level of risk, there were no attachment group differences in social competence. The avoidant children appeared especially vulnerable to family risk. For these children, social competence dropped markedly in response to midlevel family risk. A similar pattern of findings was reported for age 3 behavior problems.

In addition, at age 3, the associations between infant–mother attachment and social competence depended on maternal sensitivity at age 2 (Belsky & Fearon, 2002a). Specifically, the most socially competent children were those who were securely attached infants and who experienced relatively more maternal sensitivity at age 2. The least socially competent children were those who were insecurely attached as infants and who experienced relatively less maternal sensitivity at age 2. Of the two intermediate groups, the more socially competent children were those who were insecurely attached infants and who experienced relatively more maternal sensitivity at age 2. These findings highlight the importance of more recent parenting behavior for social competence, at least as reported by mothers. The pattern was different for observed friendship, however: Although concurrent attachment security and maternal sensitivity added incrementally to the prediction of friendship quality, the significant associations between infant–mother attachment and friendship remained for all attachment groups.

As these children aged, main effects of earlier attachment on aspects of social competence (i.e., mother-rated social skills and teacher-rated behavior problems) remained. Moreover, between the ages of 4½ and 6, evidence emerged that these links were mediated by intermediate measures of parenting quality (according to maternal sensitivity and Home Observation for Measurement of the Environment scores from infancy through age 4½; NICHD ECCRN, 2006). Interesting moderated effects also emerged. Specifically, for children who had been insecurely attached, when parenting quality between infancy and age 4½ declined, children's teacher-rated externalizing problems increased. When parenting quality between infancy and age 4½ increased, these children's behavior problems declined. These behavior changes were not observed in children who had been securely attached. Thus the findings suggest that insecure attachment was malleable and open to change, whereas a secure infant–mother attachment may have served a lasting protective function.

Summary and Suggestions for Future Research

The many studies of the associations between early attachments and children's relationships with friends and peers have generally supported Bowlby's theory by illustrating more harmonious friendships and peer relationships for children who were (and/or are) securely attached to their mothers. Moreover, supporting Main's (1990) concept of conditional behavioral strategies, the less harmonious relationships of avoidant and ambivalent children appear consistent with distinct attachment-based strategies. In addition, the literature provides some evidence that children's representa-

tional processes mediate the associations between early attachments and peer relationships. More recently, as researchers have looked simultaneously at attachment, friendships, and peer relationships (especially in the context of prospective longitudinal studies), an increasingly nuanced view has begun to emerge. Early attachment appears to be an important predictor of children's relationships with peers and friends—and, as Bowlby claimed, a stronger predictor of close relationships than of less intimate ones. The newer view includes the discovery that the prediction from attachment to children's relationships can be moderated by the degree of risk in the family environment and can be mediated by subsequent parenting quality, sometimes more for some children than others. For longer-term outcomes, the associations with early attachment appear increasingly less likely to be direct and more likely to operate through other relationships and representations.

As we acknowledge the considerable progress made by the field of attachment theory and research in explicating the associations between attachment and children's relationships with friends and peers, we also offer two suggestions for further illuminating these associations. The first suggestion is for researchers to analyze infants and children classified as insecure-avoidant, insecure-ambivalent, and disorganized as separate groups, to allow for better understanding of each insecure pattern and for further scrutiny of minimizing and maximizing strategies. The friendships and peer relationships of disorganized children, in particular, require further study in both high- and low-risk samples (Belsky & Fearon, 2002b).

The second suggestion is for more research on child–father attachment and its role in the development of children's friendships and peer relationships. It may be that the child–father attachment (or another attachment) contributes less to these other relationships than the child–mother attachment does. It may also be that child–father relationships affect the child's other relationships quite differently than do child–mother relationships. Other elements of the child–father relationship, such as the father's behavior in play, may overshadow or interact with the influences of the child–father attachment (see, e.g., Parke, 1995, and Grossmann, Grossmann, Kindler, & Zimmermann, Chapter 36, this volume). Furthermore, these effects may differ by the sex of the child. Chodorow (1978, 1989) argued that child–mother relationships exert quite different influences on the future relational tendencies of males and females (see also Gilligan, 1982). We suggest further inquiry into (1) attachment to male caregivers versus attachment to female caregivers; (2) attachments of male children versus those of female children; and (3) the interaction between the two (e.g., what are the implications for other relationships of father–son attachment vs. father–daughter attachment?).

Early Attachments and Adult Relationships with Romantic Partners and Children

Bowlby (1979) highlighted marriage and child-rearing relationships as the subsequent relationships in which the influence of early attachments is likely to be strongest. Fully understanding the influence of early attachments on romantic and childrearing relationships, however, requires prospective data on infant–parent attachment and the infant's later (adult) romantic relationships and parenting. For romantic relationships, these data are just beginning to emerge, principally from the Minnesota study (Sroufe et al., 2005). For childrearing relationships, no prospective studies are available as yet.

As is the case for the research on associations between early attachments and children's relationships with peers and friends, the Minnesota study (Sroufe et al., 2005) serves as a key source for understanding the associations between early attachments and romantic relationships. Drawing on a subsample of 78 Minnesota study participants between the ages of 20 and 23 and their romantic partners of at least 4 months, one study focused on self-reported and observed emotional experiences as a barometer of relationship quality (Simpson, Collins, Tran, & Haydon, 2007). Structural equation modeling revealed indirect associations between infant–mother attachment at 12 months and relationship quality via double mediation. Specifically, infant–mother attachment predicted teacher-rated peer competence during early elementary school (first through third grade). Peer competence in turn predicted participants' secure representations of close friendships assessed at age 16 (based on a comprehensive interview tapping such issues as trust, disclosure, and authenticity). Secure representations then predicted target participants' and their partners' reports of positive feelings in the relationship, as well as ratings of more supportive and less negative behavior coded from videotaped interactions.

In another analysis of the same Minnesota subsample, infant–mother attachment security

(according to a composite of 12- and 18-month classifications) predicted relationship security at age 20–21 according to the Current Relationship Interview (Crowell, 1990), a coder-rated measure of adults' state of mind with respect to experiences with their romantic partners (Roisman, Collins, Sroufe, & Egeland, 2005). These associations held even when observed relationship quality and duration were controlled (see also Collins & van Dulmen, 2006). Somewhat similar findings have emerged from a subsample of 38 participants from the Grossmanns' longitudinal studies. To date, initial correlational analyses indicate associations between infant–mother attachment security and children's responses to the Separation Anxiety Test of attachment representations at age 6, as well as correlations between these representations at age 6 and the security of partnership representations according to a modified version of the Current Relationship Interview at age 22 (Grossmann, Grossmann, Winter, & Zimmermann, 2002; see also Grossmann, Grossmann, & Kindler, 2005, for related findings).

Further insight into the links between early attachment and later relationship quality comes from yet another analysis of Minnesota study participants—this time providing data about when infant–mother attachment does and does not predict functioning in romantic relationships during young adulthood. Participants with secure AAI classifications at age 19 exhibited significantly more positive "relationship processes" (including support, autonomy promotion, shared affect, and secure-base provision) with their romantic partner during videotaped interactions at age 20–21 than individuals with insecure AAI classifications, *regardless of whether those in the secure group had been securely or insecurely attached to their mothers as infants* (Roisman, Padrón, Sroufe, & Egeland, 2002). These findings, while awaiting necessary replication, highlight the limits of the influence of early attachments on later romantic relationships—or at least the limits of the influence of early insecure attachments. These findings are also consistent with Bowlby's arguments that although working models created within early attachment relationships are expected to have far-reaching effects, changes in working models can occur and can disrupt the influence of early experiences. Consistent findings have emerged from three other studies—one focusing on marital quality (Paley, Cox, Burchinal, & Payne, 1999), and two focusing on parenting (Pearson, Cohn, Cowan, & Cowan, 1994; Phelps, Belsky, & Crnic, 1998). These three studies, however, must be interpreted with caution, as they drew exclusively on AAI coder assessments of "probable childhood experience" rather than on observations made during infancy. (See Hesse, Chapter 25, this volume, and Roisman, Fortuna, & Holland, 2006, for further discussion of adult reports of childhood experiences within the AAI.)

In sum, the literature on the associations between early attachments and later relationships with romantic partners and children is young, but beginning to provide insight. Just as early attachments are associated with relationships with peers and friends, early attachments also predict later romantic relationships. At the same time, associations are often indirect, operating through intermediate relationships and representations. Moreover, the research conducted by Roisman and his colleagues (2002) highlights discontinuities and the possible influence of current relationship representations on adults' romantic relationships. As the work of Carlson and her colleagues (2004) and Simpson and his colleagues (2007) has elegantly demonstrated, the Minnesota study illustrates that "adult social competence emerges from the continuous interplay between cognitive representations of earlier relationships and current social experiences" (Simpson et al., 2007, p. 365).

CONCLUSIONS AND SUGGESTIONS FOR FUTURE RESEARCH

Our review of the literature has provided ample evidence of associations between early attachments and other relationships. Especially compelling evidence of these associations has come from two major prospective, longitudinal studies: the Minnesota Study of Risk and Adaptation from Birth to Adulthood (Sroufe et al., 2005), a 30-year study of approximately 180 high-risk families; and the NICHD Study of Early Child Care (NICHD ECCRN, 2005), a 10-year study of approximately 1,000 low-risk families. These and other studies, despite considerable variability in participants, methods, and measures, are remarkably consistent in illustrating that individuals with secure attachments to their mothers during infancy also have more harmonious and mutually supportive relationships with siblings, friends, peers, and romantic partners, even 20 years later. Moreover, as findings from prospective longitudinal studies accumulate, they support Bowlby's initial hypothesis regarding a causal influence from early attachment quality to the "later capacity to make affectional

bonds." And in keeping with the theory, the literature suggests that early attachments exert a stronger influence on relationships characterized by affectional bonds than on relationships that are not characterized by affectional bonds, even though the latter are also affected.

The research literature has also begun to provide insight into the processes and mechanisms underlying both continuities and discontinuities between early attachment relationships and other relationships. For example, continuity in parenting quality appears to be an important moderator and mediator of the associations between early attachment quality and later relationships (Belsky & Fearon, 2002b; NICHD ECCRN, 2006; Sroufe et al., 1999). A decline in parenting quality after infancy, however, may bode worse for children who were insecurely attached as infants than for children who were securely attached as infants (NICHD ECCRN, 2006). At the same time, the influence of an insecure infant–mother attachment appears to be modifiable. In the NICHD study, children who were insecurely attached as infants and who experienced improved parenting quality after infancy were rated by their elementary school teachers as having fewer externalizing behavior problems (NICHD ECCRN, 2006). Similarly, even if a 20-year-old adult had an insecure attachment to his or her mother, if the adult's *current* state of mind with respect to attachment is secure, then his or her romantic relationship quality appears to reflect current—not early—internal working models of attachment (e.g., Roisman et al., 2002).

Elucidating the conditions under which internal working models of attachment can change remains an important task for future research. Bowlby argued that although the opportunities for individual change decrease over time, individual functioning is always a product of early and current environments, especially in terms of the quality of intimate relationships in these environments. These arguments and the research that supports them offer promise to prevention and intervention programs for supporting early attachments. Recent studies in fact have suggested that careful attachment-based treatment can change an infant–parent classification from insecure to secure (Cicchetti, Rogosch, & Toth, 2006; Hoffman, Marvin, Cooper, & Powell, 2006; see Berlin, Zeanah, & Lieberman, Chapter 31, this volume, for a review).

In addition, theory and research point to the value of considering stress as an activator of both early and later internal working models of attachment. Bowlby (1979) wrote that "the stronger the emotions ... the more likely are the earlier and less conscious models to become dominant" (p. 142). Several recent studies have in fact confirmed the importance of stress or emotional arousal in determining when an individual's functioning most reflects his or her working models of attachment. For example, in one study, when mothers' self-reported daily parenting stress was high, those classified as secure on the AAI were observed to be more positive with their toddlers than mothers classified as insecure were (Phelps et al., 1998). There were, however, no such attachment group differences under conditions of low stress. Similar findings have come from a recent study in which mothers' self-reported romantic attachment styles predicted observed "positive engagement" with their infants only when self-reported psychological distress was relatively high (Mills-Koonce et al., 2007).

Another, related question for future research concerns the relative influence of an infant's multiple attachments when they are discordant. That is, if the infant has formed different-quality attachments to different caregivers (including parents and even siblings), which attachments are more likely to influence (which) other relationships? It will also be important to discover whether people with discordant working models of attachment are more susceptible to the influence of new relationships than people with concordant working models are.

A third set of questions for future research concerns the influence of nonattachment factors—either alone or in concert with early attachments—on other relationships. For example, Belsky and Fearon (2002b) found that family risk moderated the association between infant–mother attachment quality and social competence at age 3. It will be interesting to see whether this finding is replicated in other studies and, if so, for what outcomes. Belsky, Bakermans-Kranenburg, and van IJzendoorn (in press) have also argued convincingly that developmental scholars should focus less on the main effects of attachment and other rearing influences, and instead should consider children's differential susceptibility to rearing influences, including parenting quality; parenting quality in turn affects the development of attachments and the influence of early attachments on other relationships. We hope that scholars will take up these and other questions raised in this chapter, to advance the broader understanding of the influence of early attachments on other relationships.

ACKNOWLEDGMENTS

Portions of this chapter are based on Berlin and Cassidy (1999). Copyright 1999 by The Guilford Press. We thank Katherine Ehrlich for helpful comments on a previous draft, Naomi Jean-Baptiste for research assistance, and Ellen Lockwood and Jamilah Taylor for assistance with manuscript preparation. Lisa Berlin's work was supported by National Institute of Mental Health Grant No. K01MH 70378.

REFERENCES

Ainsworth, M. D. S. (1967). *Infancy in Uganda: Infant care and the growth of love*. Baltimore: Johns Hopkins University Press.

Ainsworth, M. D. S. (1989). Attachments beyond infancy. *American Psychologist, 44*, 709–716.

Anan, R., & Barnett, D. (1999). Perceived social support mediates between prior attachment and subsequent adjustment: A study of urban African American children. *Developmental Psychology, 35*, 1210–1222.

Belsky, J. (1999). Modern evolutionary theory and patterns of attachment. In J. Cassidy & P. R. Shaver (Eds.), *Handbook of attachment: Theory, research, and clinical applications* (pp. 141–161). New York: Guilford Press.

Belsky, J. (2005). Differential susceptibility to rearing influence: An evolutionary hypothesis and some evidence. In B. Ellis & D. Bjorklund (Eds.), *Origins of the social mind: Evolutionary psychology and child development* (pp. 139–163). New York: Guilford Press.

Belsky, J., Bakermans-Kranenburg, M. J., & van IJzendoorn, M. H. (in press). For better and for worse: Differential susceptibility to environmental influences. *Current Directions in Psychological Science*.

Belsky, J., & Cassidy, J. (1994). Attachment: Theory and evidence. In M. Rutter & D. Hay (Eds.), *Developmental through life* (pp. 373–402). London: Blackwell.

Belsky, J., & Fearon, R. M. (2002a). Early attachment security, subsequent maternal sensitivity, and later child development: Does continuity in development depend upon continuity of caregiving? *Attachment and Human Development, 3*, 361–387.

Belsky, J., & Fearon, R. M. (2002b). Infant–mother attachment security, contextual risk, and early development: A moderational analysis. *Development and Psychopathology, 14*, 293–310.

Belsky, J., & Rovine, M. (1987). Temperament and attachment security in the Strange Situation: An empirical rapprochement. *Child Development, 58*, 787–795.

Belsky, J., Spritz, B., & Crnic, K. (1996). Infant attachment security and affective–cognitive information processing at age 3. *Psychological Science, 7*, 111–114.

Belsky, J., Steinberg, L., & Draper, P. (1991). Childhood experience, interpersonal development, and reproductive strategy: An evolutionary theory of socialization. *Child Development, 62*, 647–670.

Berlin, L. J., & Cassidy, J. (1999). Relations among relationships: Contributions from attachment theory and research. In J. Cassidy & P. R. Shaver (Eds.), *Handbook of attachment: Theory, research, and clinical applications* (pp. 688–712). New York: Guilford Press.

Berlin, L. J., Cassidy, J., & Belsky, J. (1995). Loneliness in young children and infant–mother attachment: A longitudinal study. *Merrill–Palmer Quarterly, 41,* 91–103.

Booth, C. L., Rubin, K. H., & Rose-Krasnor, L. (1998). Perceptions of emotional support from mother and friend in middle childhood: Links with social-emotional adaptation and preschool attachment security. *Child Development, 69,* 427–442.

Booth-LaForce, C., & Kerns, K. A. (in press). Child–parent attachment relationships, peer relationships, and peer group functioning. In K. H. Rubin, W. Bukowski, & B. Laursen (Eds.), *Peer interactions, relationships, and groups.* New York: Guilford Press.

Bost, K. K., Vaughn, B. E., Newell Washington, W., Cielinski, K. L., & Bradbard, M. R. (1998). Social competence, social support, and attachment: Demarcation of construct domains, measurement, and paths of influence for preschool children attending Head Start. *Child Development, 69,* 192–218.

Bowlby, J. (1958). The nature of the child's tie to his mother. *International Journal of Psycho-Analysis, 39,* 350–373.

Bowlby, J. (1969/1982). *Attachment and loss: Vol. 1. Attachment.* New York: Basic Books.

Bowlby, J. (1973). *Attachment and loss: Vol. 2. Separation: Anxiety and anger.* New York: Basic Books.

Bowlby, J. (1979). *The making and breaking of affectional bonds.* London: Tavistock/Routledge.

Carlson, E. A., Sroufe, L. A., & Egeland, B. (2004). The construction of experience: A longitudinal study of representation and behavior. *Child Development, 75,* 66–83.

Cassidy, J. (1988). Child–mother attachment and the self in six-year-olds. *Child Development, 59,* 121–134.

Cassidy, J., & Berlin, L. J. (1994). The insecure-ambivalent pattern of attachment: Theory and research. *Child Development, 65,* 971–991.

Cassidy, J., & Berlin, L. J. (1999). Understanding the origins of childhood loneliness: Contributions of attachment theory. In K. J. Rotenberg & S. Hymel (Eds.), *Loneliness in childhood and adolescence* (pp. 34–55). New York: Cambridge University Press.

Cassidy, J., Kirsh, S., Scolton, K. L., & Parke, R. D. (1996). Attachment and representations of peers. *Developmental Psychology, 32,* 892–904.

Cassidy, J., & Kobak, R. R. (1988). Avoidance and its relation to other defensive processes. In J. Belsky & T. Nezworski (Eds.), *Clinical implications of attachment* (pp. 300–323). Hillsdale, NJ: Erlbaum.

Chodorow, N. (1978). *The reproduction of mothering.* Berkeley: University of California Press.

Chodorow, N. (1989). *Feminism and psychoanalytic theory.* New Haven, CT: Yale University Press.

Cicchetti, D., Rogosch, F. A., & Toth, S. L. (2006). Fostering secure attachment in infants in maltreating families through preventive interventions. *Development and Psychopathology, 18,* 623–649.

Collins, W. A., & van Dulmen, M. H. M. (2006). "The course of true love(s) … ": Origins and pathways in the development of romantic relationships. In A. Booth & A. Crouter (Eds.), *Romance and sex in adolescence and emerging adulthood: Risks and opportunities* (pp. 63–86). Mahwah, NJ: Erlbaum.

Colman, R. A., & Thompson, R. A. (2002). Attachment security and the problem-solving behaviors of mothers and children. *Merrill–Palmer Quarterly, 48,* 337–359.

Crowell, J. A. (1990). *Current Relationship Interview.* Unpublished manuscript, State University of New York at Stony Brook.

Easterbrooks, M. A. (1989). Quality of attachment to mother and to father: Effects of perinatal risk status. *Child Development, 60,* 825–830.

Elicker, J., Englund, M., & Sroufe, L. A. (1992). Predicting peer competence and peer relationships in childhood from early parent–child relationships. In R. D. Parke & G. W. Ladd (Eds.), *Family–peer relationships: Modes of linkages* (pp. 77–106). Hillsdale, NJ: Erlbaum.

Englund, M., Levy, A., Hyson, D., & Sroufe, L. A. (2000). Adolescent social competence: Effectiveness in a group setting. *Child Development, 71,* 1049–1060.

Fox, N. A., Kimmerly, N. L., & Schafer, W. D. (1991). Attachment to mother/attachment to father: A meta-analysis. *Child Development, 62,* 210–225.

Freitag, M., Belsky, J., Grossmann, K., Grossmann, K. E., & Scheuerer-Englisch, H. (1996). Continuity in parent–child relationships from infancy to middle childhood and relations with friendship competence. *Child Development, 67,* 1437–1454.

George, C., Kaplan, N., & Main, M. (1984). *Adult Attachment Interview protocol.* Unpublished manuscript, University of California at Berkeley.

George, C., Kaplan, N., & Main, M. (1985). *Adult Attachment Interview protocol* (2nd ed.). Unpublished manuscript, University of California at Berkeley.

George, C., Kaplan, N., & Main, M. (1996). *Adult Attachment Interview protocol* (3rd ed.). Unpublished manuscript, University of California at Berkeley.

Gilligan, C. (1982). *In a different voice.* Cambridge, MA: Harvard University Press.

Grossmann, K. E., & Grossmann, K. (1991). Attachment quality as an organizer of emotional and behavioral responses in a longitudinal perspective. In C. M. Parkes, J. Stevenson-Hinde, & P. Marris (Eds.), *Attachment across the life cycle* (pp. 93–114). New York: Routledge.

Grossmann, K. E., Grossmann, K., Huber, F., & Wartner, U. (1981). German children's behavior towards their mothers at 12 months and their fathers at 18 months in Ainsworth's Strange Situation. *International Journal of Behavioral Development, 4,* 157–181.

Grossmann, K. E., Grossmann, K., & Kindler, H. (2005). Early care and the roots of attachment and partnership representations: The Bielefeld and Regensburg longitudinal studies. In K. E. Grossmann, K. Grossmann, & E. Waters (Eds.), *Attachment from infancy to adulthood: The major longitudinal studies* (pp. 98–136). New York: Guilford Press.

Grossmann, K. E., Grossmann, K., Winter, M., & Zimmermann, P. (2002). Attachment relationships and appraisal of partnership: From early experience of sensitive support to later relationship representation. In L. Pulkkinen & A. Caspi (Eds.), *Paths to successful development: Personality in the life course* (pp. 73–105). New York: Cambridge University Press.

Hazan, C., & Shaver, P. (1987). Romantic love conceptualized as an attachment process. *Journal of Personality and Social Psychology, 52,* 511–524.

Hoffman, K. T., Marvin, R. S., Cooper, G., & Powell, B. (2006). Changing toddlers' and preschoolers' attachment classifications: The Circle of Security intervention. *Journal of Consulting and Clinical Psychology, 74,* 1017–1026.

Jaffari-Bimmel, N., Juffer, F., van IJzendoorn, M. H., Bakermans-Kranenburg, M. J., & Mooijaart, A. (2006). Social development from infancy to adolescence: Longitudinal and concurrent factors in an adoption sample. *Developmental Psychology, 42,* 1143–1153.

Kerns, K. (1994). A longitudinal examination of links between mother–child attachment and children's friendships in early childhood. *Journal of Social and Personal Relationships, 11,* 379–381.

Kirsh, S., & Cassidy, J. (1997). Preschoolers' attention to and memory for attachment relevant information. *Child Development, 68,* 1143–1153.

Kobak, R. R., & Sceery, A. (1988). Attachment in late adolescence: Working models, affect regulation, and representations of self and others. *Child Development, 59,* 135–146.

Lewis, M., & Feiring, C. (1989). Early predictors of children's friendships. In T. J. Berndt & G. W. Ladd (Eds.), *Peer relationships in child development* (pp. 246–273). New York: Wiley.

Lieberman, A. F. (1977). Preschoolers' competence with a peer: Relations with attachment and peer experience. *Child Development, 48,* 1277–1287.

Main, M. (1990). Cross-cultural studies of attachment organization: Recent studies, changing methodologies, and the concept of conditional strategies. *Human Development, 33,* 48–61.

Main, M., & Weston, D. (1981). The quality of the toddler's relationship to mother and to father: Related to conflict behavior and the readiness to establish new relationships. *Child Development, 52,* 932–940.

McElwain, N. L., Cox, M. J., Burchinal, M. R., & Macfie, J. (2003). Differentiating among insecure mother–infant attachment classifications: A focus on child–friend interaction and exploration during solitary play at 36 months. *Attachment and Human Development, 5,* 136–164.

Mikulincer, M. & Shaver, P. R. (2004). Security-based self-representations in adulthood: Contents and pro-

cesses. In W. S. Rholes & J. A. Simpson (Eds.), *Adult attachment: Theory, research, and clinical implications* (pp. 159–195). New York: Guilford Press.

Mikulincer, M., & Shaver, P. R. (2007). *Attachment in adulthood: Structure, dynamics, and change.* New York: Guilford Press.

Mills-Koonce, W. R., Appleyard, K., Barnett, M., Deng, M., Putallaz, M., & Cox, M. (2007). *Diathesis–stress model for parenting during infancy: Analysis of adult attachment styles and psychological risk.* Manuscript submitted for publication.

National Institute of Child Health and Human Development (NICHD) Early Child Care Research Network (ECCRN). (2005). *Child care and child development: Results from the NICHD Study of Early Child Care and Youth Development.* New York: Guilford Press.

National Institute of Child Health and Human Development (NICHD) Early Child Care Research Network (ECCRN). (2006). Infant–mother attachment classification: Risk and protection in relation to changing maternal caregiving quality. *Developmental Psychology, 42,* 38–58.

Paley, B., Cox, M. J., Burchinal, M. R., & Payne, C. C. (1999). Attachment and marital functioning: Comparison of spouses with continuous-secure, earned-secure, dismissing, and preoccupied attachment stances. *Journal of Family Psychology, 13,* 580–597.

Park, K., & Waters, E. (1989). Security of attachment and preschool friendships. *Child Development, 60,* 1076–1081.

Parke, R. D. (1995). Fathers and families. In M. Bornstein (Ed.), *Handbook of parenting: Vol. 3. Status and social conditions of parenting* (pp. 27–63). Mahwah, NJ: Erlbaum.

Pearson, J., Cohn, D. A., Cowan, P. A., & Cowan, C. P. (1994). Earned- and continuous-security in adult attachment: Relation to depressive symptomatology and parenting style. *Development and Psychopathology, 6,* 359–373.

Phelps, J. L., Belsky, J., & Crnic, K. (1998). Earned-security, daily stress, and parenting: A comparison of five alternative models. *Development and Psychopathology, 10,* 21–38.

Pierrehumbert, B., Iannotti, R. J., Cummings, E. M., & Zahn-Waxler, C. (1989). Social functioning with mother and peers at 2 and 5 years: The influence of attachment. *International Journal of Behavioral Development, 12,* 85–100.

Raikes, H. A., & Thompson, R. A. (2007). *Attachment and parenting quality as predictors of early social cognition.* Manuscript submitted for publication.

Roisman, G. I., Collins, W. A., Sroufe, L. A., & Egeland, B. (2005). Predictors of young adults' representations of and behavior in their current romantic relationship: Prospective tests of the prototype hypothesis. *Attachment and Human Development, 7,* 105–121.

Roisman, G. I., Fortuna, K., & Holland, A. (2006). An experimental manipulation of retrospectively defined earned and continuous attachment security. *Child Development, 77,* 59–71.

Roisman, G. I., Padrón, E., Sroufe, L. A., & Egeland, B. (2002). Earned-secure attachment status in retrospect and prospect. *Child Development, 73*, 1204–1219.

Sagi, A., Lamb, M. E., Lewkowicz, K. S., Shoham, R., Dvir, R., & Estes, D. (1985). Security of infant–mother, –father, and –*metapelet* attachments among kibbutz-reared Israeli children. In I. Bretherton & E. Waters (Eds.), Growing points of attachment theory and research. *Monographs of the Society for Research in Child Development, 50*(1–2, Serial No. 209), 257–275.

Sagi-Schwartz, A., & Aviezer, O. (2005). Correlates of attachment to multiple caregivers in kibbutz children from birth to emerging adulthood: The Haifa longitudinal study. In K. E. Grossmann, K. Grossmann, & E. Waters (Eds.), *Attachment from infancy to adulthood: The major longitudinal studies* (pp. 165–197). New York: Guilford Press.

Schneider, B. H., Atkinson, L., & Tardif, C. (2001). Child–parent attachment and children's peer relations: A quantitative review. *Developmental Psychology, 37*, 86–100.

Shulman, S., Elicker, J., & Sroufe, L. A. (1994). Stages of friendship growth in preadolescence as related to attachment history. *Journal of Social and Personal Relationships, 11*, 341–361.

Simpson, J. A. (1999). Attachment theory in modern evolutionary perspective. In J. Cassidy & P. R. Shaver (Eds.), *Handbook of attachment: Theory, research, and clinical applications* (pp. 115–140). New York: Guilford Press.

Simpson, J. A., Collins, W. A., Tran, S., & Haydon, K. C. (2007). Attachment and the experience and expression of emotions in romantic relationships: A developmental perspective. *Journal of Personality and Social Psychology, 92*, 355–367.

Sroufe, L. A., Egeland, B., & Carlson, E. A. (1999). One social world: The integrated development of parent–child and peer relationships. In W. A. Collins & B. Laursen (Eds.), *Minnesota Symposium on Child Psychology: Vol. 30. Relationships as developmental contexts* (pp. 241–262). Mahwah, NJ: Erlbaum.

Sroufe, L. A., Egeland, B., Carlson, E. A., & Collins, W. A. (2005). *The development of the person: The Minnesota Study of Risk and Adaptation from Birth to Adulthood.* New York: Guilford Press.

Sroufe, L. A., & Fleeson, J. (1986). Attachment and the construction of relationships. In W. W. Hartup & Z. Rubin (Eds.), *Relationships and development* (pp. 51–71). Hillsdale, NJ: Erlbaum.

Sroufe, L. A., & Fleeson, J. (1988). The coherence of family relationships. In R. A. Hinde & J. Stevenson-Hinde (Eds.), *Relationships within families: Mutual influences* (pp. 27–47). Oxford, UK: Clarendon Press.

Steele, H., Steele, M., & Fonagy, P. (1996). Associations among attachment classifications of mothers, fathers, and their infants. *Child Development, 67*, 541–555.

Suess, G. J., Grossmann, K. E., & Sroufe, L. A. (1992). Effects of infant attachment to mother and father on

quality of adaptation in preschool: From dyadic to individual organization of self. *International Journal of Behavioral Development, 15*, 43–65.

Teti, D. M., & Ablard, K. E. (1989). Security of attachment and infant–sibling relationships. *Child Development, 60*, 1519–1528.

van IJzendoorn, M. H., & De Wolff, M. S. (1997). In search of the absent father—Meta-analysis of infant–father attachment: A rejoinder to our discussants. *Child Development, 68*, 604–609.

van IJzendoorn, M. H., Schuengel, C., & Bakermans-Kranenburg, M. J. (1999). Disorganized attachment in early childhood: A meta-analysis of precursors, concomitants, and sequelae. *Development and Psychopathology, 11*, 225–249.

Verschueren, K., & Marcoen, A. (1999). Representation of self and socioemotional competence in kindergarteners: Differential and combined effects of attachment to mother and father. *Child Development, 70*, 183–201.

Volling, B., & Belsky, J. (1992). The contribution of mother–child and father–child relationships to the quality of sibling interaction: A longitudinal study. *Child Development, 63*, 1209–1222.

Wartner, U., Grossmann, K., Fremmer-Bombik, E., & Suess, G. (1994). Attachment patterns at age six in South Germany: Predictability from infancy and implications for preschool behavior. *Child Development, 65*, 1014–1027.

Waters, E. (1987). *Attachment behavior Q-set* (Revision 3.0). Unpublished manuscript, State University of New York at Stony Brook.

Waters, E., & Deane, K. E. (1985). Defining and assessing individual differences in attachment relationships: Q-methodology and the organization of behavior in infancy and early childhood. In I. Bretherton & E. Waters (Eds.), Growing points of attachment theory and research. *Monographs of the Society for Research in Child Development, 50*(1–2, Serial No. 209), 41–65.

Waters, E., Vaughn, B. E., Posada, G., & Kondo-Ikemura, K. (Eds.). (1995). Caregiving, cultural, and cognitive perspectives on secure-base behavior and working models: New growing points of attachment theory and research. *Monographs of the Society for Research in Child Development, 60*(2–3, Serial No. 244).

Youngblade, L. M., & Belsky, J. (1992). Parent–child antecedents of 5-year-olds' close friendships: A longitudinal analysis. *Developmental Psychology, 28*, 700–713.

Youngblade, L. M., Park, K., & Belsky, J. (1993). Measurement of young children's close friendships: A comparison of two independent assessment systems and their associations with attachment security. *International Journal of Behavioral Development, 16*, 563–587.

Ziv, Y., Oppenheim, D., & Sagi-Schwartz, A. (2004). Social information processing in middle childhood: Relations to infant–mother attachment. *Attachment and Human Development, 6*, 327–348.

CHAPTER 16

Early Attachment and Later Development
Familiar Questions, New Answers

ROSS A. THOMPSON

How does the child foreshadow the adult-to-be? Philosophers, spiritualists, playwrights, and most recently behavioral scientists have sought to understand how early dispositions and influences provide a foundation for adult personality. Among the answers they have offered is the influence of early, close relationships. This view was eventually crystallized in Freud's (1940/1963, p. 45) famous dictum that the infant–mother relationship is "unique, without parallel, established unalterably for a whole lifetime as the first and strongest love-object and as the prototype of all later love-relations." Drawing on this psychoanalytic heritage, Bowlby (1969/1982, 1973, 1980) also enlisted formulations from evolutionary biology, developmental psychology, and control systems theory to argue that a warm and continuous relationship with a caregiver promotes psychological health and well-being throughout life in a manner that accords with the adaptive requirements of the human species. In collaboration with Ainsworth (1967, 1973), he proposed that differences in the security of infant–mother attachment have significant long-term implications for later intimate relationships, self-understanding, and even risk for psychopathology.

Bowlby's conceptual integration was provocative, and with the validation of reliable methods for assessing the security of attachment for infants and young children, an enormous research literature emerged concerning the origins, correlates, and consequences of secure and insecure relationships. Guided by a general expectation that a secure attachment would predict better later functioning, developmental researchers have explored the association between early security and later relations with parents, peers, friends, and other social partners, as well as with self-concept, competence in preschool and kindergarten, personality development, social cognition, behavior problems, and indicators of emergent psychopathology. But researchers have also broadened their inquiry to explore how security predicts later cognitive and language development, exploration and play, curiosity, ego resiliency, math achievement, and even political ideology, extending the range of predictive correlates far beyond what Bowlby originally envisioned. As Belsky and Cassidy (1994) mused, one might wonder whether there is anything with which attachment security is *not* associated. Comprehending this research literature thus requires reconsidering how and why early attachment security should be associated with later development, as well as alternative models for why security might predict later functioning in direct and indirect ways. Doing so is important for interpreting research findings in a theoretically coherent manner—and equally important for highlighting the research designs that are likely to be most informative for future studies of early attachment and its sequelae.

This chapter begins, therefore, with consideration of alternative explanations for why a secure attachment should be associated with later behavior, with a focus on attachment security in the early years. Following this is a review of the research examining these associations in the developmental domains that have been best studied: parent–child relationships, close relationships with peers and other partners, personality, emotion regulation, self-concept, emotion understanding, social cognition, memory, and conscience. In a final section, these results are discussed in light of what we can conclude about how attachment security influences later developmental functioning, and which research approaches are most likely to elucidate this association in future studies.

CONCEPTUAL PERSPECTIVES

To an observer, it might appear surprising that it would be necessary to begin this discussion by sorting through the various conceptual explanations in the literature for why early attachment security should be associated with later development. After all, wasn't Bowlby's theory clear on this issue?

The challenge facing contemporary attachment researchers is not only Bowlby's theory, but also its generativity. Attachment theory was formulated decades ago, at a time when scientific understanding of infancy and early childhood underestimated the cognitive and behavioral sophistication of the child and the dynamics of early parent–child relationships. There have also been significant advances in behavioral ecology and evolutionary biology. It is natural that in efforts to keep the theory current with advancing knowledge, Bowlby's heirs would expand, elucidate, and update his formulations in ways that he could not anticipate. Furthermore, as would be expected of a conceptually innovative approach, Bowlby's theory provides a conceptual umbrella for broad and narrow constructions of the developmental impact of attachment relationships. Grossmann (1999), for example, has identified at least two different conceptualizations of "internal working models" in Bowlby's theory, and the breadth of the theory offers explanations for developmental influences related to the biologically adaptive qualities of

attachment relationships, continuity and change in parent–child interaction, and the dynamics of personality growth. Beyond theoretical breadth, of course, is the fact that subsequent attachment researchers have had their own ideas about the influence of early attachment security, which they have sought to harmonize with Bowlby's formulations.

These are all signs of a vibrant, generative theory. Indeed, it can be argued that today the proper role of Bowlby's theory is not as a source of orthodoxy for attachment theorists (much as Freud's theory was treated in the early decades of psychoanalysis), but rather as a foundation for new thinking about early parent–child relationships. The problem this presents for contemporary researchers, however, is the proliferation of conceptual explanations for why early attachment should (and sometimes should not) be associated with later development. Beyond the casual post hoc explanations offered by researchers for unexpected empirical findings, in other words, there have grown from the foundation of Bowlby's theory various attachment minitheories, with somewhat different views of the nature of the developmental influences arising from secure or insecure early relationships.

In this section, therefore, the goal is to summarize and evaluate several alternative views of the developmental influence of attachment that have become significant in contemporary attachment research. These approaches are discussed with respect to certain key conceptual questions. For which developmental domains is early security likely to be most important, and at what ages? How much should the effects of early attachment be expected to endure, and what mediators might affect its continuing influence? What are the conditions in which attachment should most influence later development? Although most of these attachment minitheories do not provide clear answers to all of these conceptual questions, the purpose in posing them is to clarify our thinking about why early attachment should be developmentally provocative.

Internal Working Models

One of Bowlby's most heuristically powerful formulations is the view that attachment security influences psychological growth through children's developing mental representations, or "internal working models" (IWMs), of the social world. IWMs are based on infants' expectations for the accessibility and responsiveness of their caregivers; these expectations develop into broader representations of themselves, their attachment figures, interpretations of their relational experiences, and decision rules about how to interact with others. These mental representations not only enable immediate forecasts of the caregiver's responsiveness, but develop into interpretive filters through which children (and adults) reconstruct their understanding of new relationships and experiences in ways that are consistent with past experiences and expectations arising from secure or insecure attachments. As a consequence, children choose new partners and behave with them in ways that are consistent with, and thus help to confirm, the expectations created from earlier attachments. IWMs thus constitute the bridge between an infant's experience of sensitive or insensitive care and the development of beliefs and expectations that affect subsequent experience in close relationships. Young children also internalize conceptions of themselves from early relational experience that form the basis for developing self-concept and other self-referential beliefs. This concept has been theoretically generative: Bretherton and Munholland (1999 and Chapter 5, this volume), Crittenden (1990), Main (1991), Sroufe and Fleeson (1988), and I (Thompson, 2006) have each offered contemporary extensions of Bowlby's concept of IWMs.

In this formulation, therefore, IWMs would be expected to be most directly associated with the child's capacities to create and maintain successful close relationships (with parents, peers, teachers, and others), establish a positive self-image, and perhaps also develop constructive social representations of people and of relationships. However, because of the imprecision of Bowlby's portrayal of IWMs (which is a conceptual metaphor rather than a well-defined theoretical construct), this concept has assumed far greater explanatory breadth in attachment research to account for a widening array of developmental outcomes, such as proneness to stress, theory of mind, and ideological values. Its use by the field has caused some to question whether IWMs constitute a "catch-all, post-hoc explanation" for almost anything to which a secure attachment is found to be associated (Belsky & Cassidy, 1994, p. 384). The inclusiveness of the contemporary IWM construct has tended to expand with every new empirical finding that is "explained" with reference to it, which is a problem for attachment theory and the discriminant validity of the attachment construct (Thompson & Raikes, 2003).

One solution to this problem of underspecificity is to understand IWMs as developing rep-

resentations that change over time with a child's conceptual growth. Thus our knowledge of young children's developing conceptual skills could establish parameters for what we would expect to be true of their IWMs of self and relationships, especially early in life. Bretherton (1993; Bretherton & Munholland, 1999 and Chapter 5, this volume) pioneered this developmental approach by conceptualizing IWMs in relation to mental schemas and constructive memory processes, underscoring that regardless of their unconscious influences, IWMs are based on consciously accessible cognitive processes that change with development. Elsewhere (Thompson, 2000, 2006), I have built on this formulation by offering a developmental account that associates the growth of IWMs with allied conceptual advances in early childhood—such as implicit memory and social expectations in infancy, the development of event representation and episodic memory in early childhood, the emergence of theory of mind and autobiographical memory in the preschool years, and the development of specific social-cognitive skills later in childhood. Each of these well-understood conceptual advances contributes to the representational capacities of Bowlby's IWM construct: understanding other people (including attachment figures), representing experience (especially in close relationships), self-concept, and understanding how to relate socially to others. When a developmental understanding of IWMs is linked to these conceptual advances in the encoding, representation, and memory of social experience, the growth of attachment-related working models can be conceptualized more precisely and studied in relation to current understanding of children's cognitive growth.

There are several other implications of this developmental formulation (Thompson, 2000, 2006). First, IWMs are likely to change in response to new relational experiences and also during periods of representational advance, such as in the transition to the symbolic representational capacities of early childhood and the emergence of abstract thought in adolescence. These transitions render IWMs more susceptible to revision, as new modes of understanding can alter earlier representations of relational experience. Second, the security or insecurity incorporated into IWMs may have their greatest influence on social and personality capacities during those periods when these capacities are maturing most significantly. The IWMs associated with a secure attachment are likely to influence self-concept or emotion understanding most strongly in early childhood, for example, when children's conceptions of themselves and others' feelings develop significantly. In this regard, contrary to the traditional research strategy of using infant Strange Situation classifications to predict later psychological functioning, the IWMs associated with attachment security may be found to be developmentally most influential when assessed during the preschool years or later, depending on the developmental outcome of interest.

Finally, especially in early childhood, IWMs are shaped not only by direct experience of sensitive care, but also by the secondary representations of experience mediated by language—particularly in parent–child conversation. This is consistent with the research literatures on constructive memory, event representation, autobiographical memory, and even theory of mind, which together document the great narrative influence of parent–child conversation (for a review, see Thompson, 2006). These literatures attest to the powerful influence of language in providing young children with insight into shared experiences, others' feelings and thoughts, and even the self. In this respect, responsive care and thoughtful, rich, accessible conversation may each be age-appropriate manifestations of parental sensitivity, once young children become capable of representing and sharing experience through language (see Wareham & Salmon, 2006). As we shall see, a growing body of research documents the different qualities of parent–child conversation of secure and insecure dyads in the preschool years.

Taken together, Bowlby's IWM construct and the extensions it has generated predicts that early security should influence a child's capacity to form close, satisfying relationships; create a positive self-concept; and develop constructive, insightful understanding of other people. More expansive views of the influence of IWMs exist, however. In some formulations, IWMs develop with a child's conceptual advances, and their influence is most significant when young children are at the vanguard of new advances in social understanding and personality development. Virtually all theorists agree that IWMs change with further experience and conceptual growth (although disagreement exists over how readily they change), suggesting that the influences of early attachment relationships may not be enduring unless the IWMs with which they are associated are maintained.

Emergent Personality Organization

Another conceptualization of the influence of early attachment on later development is that attachment security shapes emergent personality processes in infancy, which, as they mature and become consolidated, exert a continuing influence on subsequent personality growth. Early attachment is important because it inaugurates adaptive or maladaptive organizational processes in personality that render young children more or less competent in facing subsequent challenges in personality growth.

This view is best articulated in the "organizational perspective" that has been advanced by Sroufe (2005; Sroufe, Egeland, Carlson, & Collins, 2005; Weinfield, Sroufe, Egeland, & Carlson, Chapter 4, this volume) and others (e.g., Cicchetti, 2006). This neo-Eriksonian perspective portrays personality growth as a succession of age-salient developmental challenges around which critical aspects of personality development are organized. During the first year, of course, the development of a secure attachment is central. In successive years, relevant developmental issues include the growth of an autonomous self in toddlerhood, the acquisition of effective peer relationships in preschool, successful adaptation to school, coordinating friendship and group membership in middle childhood, and identity and self-reflection in adolescence. The successful mastery of earlier developmental challenges is believed to provide a stronger psychological foundation for subsequent challenges, because of the internal resources in personality organization that have developed and the supportive relationships on which the child can rely. However, even though the child builds on prior developmental accomplishments when facing new challenges for personality organization, the possibility for change in adaptation remains.

From this perspective, therefore, the developmental processes that are affected by early attachment vary, depending on the age-relevant challenges faced by the child with growing maturity. Proponents of the organizational perspective anticipate continuity over time in the adaptive success with which children address these challenges, while allowing for change in personality organization as well.

Consistency and Change in Parent–Child Relationships

In infancy and early childhood, parent–child relationships are described as secure or insecure. By adulthood, security is viewed as a characteristic of the person. Attachment theory thus seeks to explain how characteristics of relationships become incorporated into personality. In the developmental transition from attachment-as-relationship to attachment-as-personal-characteristic, the consistency of relational quality in the early years may be a foundation for the enduring significance of early attachment for later development. Quite simply, an early secure attachment provides a stronger foundation for subsequent psychosocial achievements if the sensitive, supportive parental care initially contributing to attachment security is maintained over time (Lamb, Thompson, Gardner, & Charnov, 1985). In that ongoing relationship of parental support, young children continue to enjoy the benefits of the sensitive care that they experienced in infancy; moreover, they become increasingly receptive to their parents' influences and socialization incentives as they identify with the adults' goals and behavior (Kochanska, 2002; Waters, Kondo-Ikemura, Posada, & Richters, 1991). However, if the earlier sensitive care that initially inspired a secure attachment is not maintained, there would be less reason to anticipate that early attachment security would have enduring effects on a child. In this view, therefore, the significance of early attachment for later development is contingent on the continuing sensitivity of parental care, especially in a child's early years.

In an empirical assessment of this formulation, Belsky and Fearon (2002a) analyzed data from the National Institute of Child Health and Human Development (NICHD) Study of Early Child Care, a national sample of more than 1,000 mothers and their children studied from birth. Analyzing attachment classifications in the Strange Situation at 15 months and subsequent measures of maternal sensitivity at 24 months, they reported that the children who obtained the highest scores on a broad range of social and cognitive measures at 36 months were those who were securely attached and who subsequently experienced sensitive care. Those performing most poorly at 36 months were insecurely attached in infancy and experienced later insensitive care. Of the two intermediate groups, children who were initially insecurely attached but subsequently experienced sensitive care scored higher on all outcome measures than did children who were initially secure but later experienced insensitive care. These researchers also found that maternal report measures of life stress, depression, social support, and family resources at 24 months helped to explain why some securely attached infants subsequently experienced insensitive maternal care, and why some initially insecure infants later experienced sensitive care. In each case, declines in maternal sensi-

tivity were associated with the number of negative life events and lack of support that mothers experienced when children were age 2, which were likely to affect children as well as their mothers. In a corollary report from the same NICHD study, Belsky and Fearon (2002b) reported that a cumulative measure of contextual risk during a child's first 3 years moderated some of the associations between early attachment and later behavior.

These findings are consistent with those reported by other researchers (e.g., Egeland, Kalkoske, Gottesman, & Ericson, 1990; Sroufe, Egeland, & Kreutzer, 1990), and with the literature concerning the causes of stability and change in the security of attachment (see Thompson, 2006, for a review). Taken together, they indicate that early security of attachment interacts with the quality of subsequent experience (particularly sensitive parental care and broader life stresses) in predicting developmental outcomes. Indeed, these findings suggest that later quality of care may be at least as important as early security in predicting later development. The continuing sensitivity of parental care may be especially important in the early years, when IWMs are still rudimentary. In this respect, the continuing harmony of the parent–child relationship may constitute a bridge between a secure attachment in infancy and the development of more sophisticated later IWMs of the reliability of parental care and of one's deservingness of love, which influence later personality growth.

Biological Adaptations

Bowlby (1969/1982) and his followers have portrayed attachment as a function of an evolved behavioral system to promote the inclusive fitness of the human species. More specifically, the attachment behavioral system is viewed as motivating infants to seek the protective proximity of adults, especially when offspring are distressed, alarmed, or in danger, and as organizing the behavioral competencies to maintain proximity. Attachment theorists initially viewed the secure behavioral pattern as biologically adaptive because, by contrast with the insecure behavioral patterns, it is well organized to accomplish and maintain protective proximity to a caregiver (see, e.g., Ainsworth, 1979, 1984). However, with advances in behavioral ecology and life history theory, it became apparent that the different behavioral patterns of security and insecurity can be regarded as biologically adaptive responses to different qualities of parental care (e.g., Chisholm, 1996, 1999). In this view, sensitively responsive parental care leading to a secure attachment derives from the adult's ability and willingness to provide for the child, enabling the child's confident exploration, play, and other activities that also prepare the child for maturity. By contrast, unresponsive or insensitive parental care reflects either the adult's unwillingness to invest resources in the child (leading to avoidant insecurity in offspring) or the adult's inability to do so (leading to resistant insecurity), with each insecure behavioral pattern representing a necessary means of obtaining needed resources in alternative ways. Viewed in this light, early attachment patterns can be regarded as "juvenile adaptations" that function to aid individuals through their immaturity, but have no necessarily enduring significance.

Life history theory also highlights, however, how variations in the quality of early care sensitize offspring to broader characteristics of environmental provision or deprivation that are relevant to survival and reproductive strategies beyond infancy. An influential evolutionary theory of socialization that reflects this approach was proposed by Belsky, Steinberg, and Draper (1991; see also Simpson & Belsky, Chapter 6, this volume). They argued that owing to the sensitivity of offspring to variations in parental care and the meaning of this care for long-term reproductive success, early attachment patterns are likely to be related to the later timing of pubertal maturation, the onset of sexual activity, preferences in pair bonding, and eventual parental investment. In essence, children whose family experiences are characterized by high stress (and consequent insecurity) are likely to develop reproductive strategies that are low-investment and opportunistic, with children in low-stress, secure families developing in the opposite manner. This approach portrays early attachment patterns not as juvenile adaptations, but rather as "ontogenetic adaptations" that are significant early in life, but also become incorporated into later behavioral patterns that have lifelong adaptational value (see also Chisholm, 1996, 1999, for another example of this approach).

Thus whether early attachment is viewed biologically as a juvenile or an ontogenetic adaptation is relevant to the nature of the developmental outcomes expected of early security or insecurity, as well as their long-term consequences. Research relating to the evolutionary model of Belsky and his colleagues has received considerable but not unequivocal research support, with some arguing that early family stress may be more significantly associated with the duration of childhood immaturity than with pubertal maturation and reproductive strategy (Ellis, 2004). Much more work remains to characterize the place of early attachment in the biologically adaptive processes of the human species.

Other Considerations

There are other formulations about how early attachment is associated with later development. To Weinfield, Sroufe, Egeland, and Carlson (1999 and Chapter 4, this volume), early attachment is important because of its influence on developmental functions that have long-term consequences for brain development, affect regulation, relational synchrony, and early representations of relationships. They argue that early attachment relationships should be most strongly related to later interpersonal competence, psychological adjustment, and self-understanding, but there is room for a far broader range of sequelae from the early developmental functions they identify. In a similar vein, we (Thompson & Lamb, 1983) have argued that attachments in infancy foster the development of social skills and social dispositions that, as they are generalized to other social partners, elicit complementary responses from partners and contribute to the development of relationships.

It is apparent, therefore, that attachment researchers have a variety of theoretical approaches to guide their inquiry into the developmental outcomes of early security. Moreover, these formulations differ in important and meaningful ways. They emphasize different outcomes, for example: Some highlight the relational consequences of early secure or insecure relationships, others the representational sequelae of attachment security, and still others its influence on stages of personality growth, while some evolutionary theories focus on reproductively adaptive strategies. Although some formulations view the continuing influence of parenting practices in childhood as a mediator of the enduring effects of early security, others make no such claim. In several approaches, the consequences of attachment security are developmentally graded—that is, the effects of attachment depend on when security is assessed and when outcomes are evaluated—but others offer more general predictions. Most of these approaches also expect stronger associations between attachment security and its contemporaneous correlates than in long-term predictive relations, but they differ in the reasons why.

These conceptual differences are important because they have implications for research design. If, for example, researchers expect that later behavior arises from an interaction between early security and the continuing quality of parental care, it is important to measure each of these factors in follow-up studies. Likewise, other potential moderators of this association should also be assessed, such as family stress. Moreover, the analyses of large-scale follow-up studies with many outcome measures should be guided by theoretically derived expectations concerning the behaviors that attachment security should predict and other behaviors that it should *not* predict, in order to document the discriminant validity of the attachment construct. When unexpected associations emerge (such as between early attachment security and math achievement), researchers should measure and examine whether these might arise from theoretically predicted mediators (such as parental involvement in school), rather than creating new extensions of attachment theory to explain these findings (Thompson & Raikes, 2003). Unfortunately, the research reviewed below was rarely designed with these considerations in mind, and the large majority of studies used simple pre–post designs. This is unfortunate, because in the context of a variety of minitheories to explain the association between early attachment and later behavior, it is often difficult to determine whether empirical associations confirm, disconfirm, or have no theoretical relevance at all. The needs for greater theoretical clarity concerning the sequelae of early attachment, and for research designed with direct, mediated, moderated, and nonlinear associations between attachment and later behavior in mind, are two of the greatest challenges for attachment theory and research in the 21st century.

EMPIRICAL PERSPECTIVES

Consistent with these conceptual perspectives, this review of research is organized according to the various outcome domains to which attachment security has been empirically associated. The review begins with the relational outcomes anticipated from a secure attachment (warmer subsequent parent–child relationships, closer relationships with peers and other partners); then moves on to personality outcomes and emotion regulation; and then examines more recent work on the representational correlates and outcomes of a secure attachment—self-concept, emotion

understanding, social cognition, conscience, and finally memory. The prediction of early attachment to risk for psychopathology is also an important outcome domain, but is not considered in this chapter because it is discussed extensively elsewhere in this handbook (see especially DeKlyen & Greenberg, Chapter 27, and Lyons-Ruth & Jacobvitz, Chapter 28). In light of the enormous empirical literature in this area, this review should be viewed as a representative, not an exhaustive, overview of the major findings and important new directions for research.

Parent–Child Relationship

The strongest and most direct outcome of a secure attachment should be more positive parent–child interaction in follow-up assessments. This expectation is confirmed in short-term longitudinal studies during the second year, in which securely attached children (assessed in the Strange Situation) showed greater enthusiasm, compliance, and positive affect—and less frustration and aggression—during shared tasks with their mothers (e.g., Frankel & Bates, 1990; Matas, Arend, & Sroufe, 1978; Slade, 1987). In short, securely attached infants tend to maintain more harmonious relations with their mothers in the second year.

Consistent with the view of early attachment as a relationship, however, in each of these studies the mothers of securely attached children were also more sensitive and helpful toward their offspring in follow-up assessments, and their behavior supported the positive behavior of their children. In the words of one researcher, "secure dyads 'work' better" together (Slade, 1987, p. 83), suggesting that the consistency between attachment security and later parent–child interaction is dyadic. This is a nontrivial conclusion, because it suggests that one of the benefits of a secure attachment is that it inaugurates what Maccoby (1984) called a "mutual interpersonal orientation of positive reciprocity" between parent and child; this is the foundation for cooperation, values acquisition, and the child's enthusiastic responsiveness to the parent's socialization incentives (see also Kochanska, 2002). If this relational harmony is not maintained, however, the benefits to the parent–child relationship of early security may not endure.

Over longer periods of time, evidence for the enduring benefits of early security for the parent–child relationship is mixed. On one hand, researchers have not found longer-term associations between a secure attachment in the Strange

Situation and parent–child interaction at ages 3 (Youngblade & Belsky, 1992) and 5 (van IJzendoorn, van der Verr, & van Vliet-Visser, 1987). On the other hand, some research groups have found significant associations between different measures of parent–child attachment over even longer periods (e.g., Main & Cassidy, 1988). This mixed pattern of results mirrors the inconsistent findings concerning the stability of the security of attachment over time, with some researchers finding long-term stability of security over several years, and others finding little consistency between repeated attachment assessments over as little as 6–7 months (see Thompson, 2006, for a review). Consistency in the quality of parent–child interaction over time is often mediated by intervening events, such as family stress, significant changes in family circumstances, or other conditions affecting relational harmony (Thompson, 2006). Consequently, although early attachment security may inaugurate short-term consistency in the harmony of parent–child relations, the likelihood of longer-term consistency is more contingent on other events in family life.

Other Close Relationships

One of the most important alternative relational contexts in which the benefits of early security might be observed is that of peer relationships. A meta-analysis by Schneider, Atkinson, and Tardif (2001) found a modest association between parent–child attachment security and children's peer relationships (combined effect size = 0.20), and noted that this association is stronger for studies of children's close friendships (effect size = 0.24) than for relationships with other peers (effect size = 0.14), consistent with the view that attachment security is more important for establishing and maintaining relational closeness. Attachment was assessed with the Strange Situation, Attachment Q-Sort (AQS), and self-report measures for older children (e.g., Kerns, Klepac, & Cole, 1996), and the findings for each method were consistent with these conclusions. Schneider and colleagues also concluded that the association with attachment is stronger for peer relations in middle childhood and adolescence than for those in early childhood; they suggested that this derives from the consolidation and sophistication of children's friendship representations and attachment IWMs with increasing age. The strength of this association was not affected by the amount of time between assessments of attachment and peer relationships. In a study

applying growth curve modeling to data from the NICHD Study of Early Child Care, we (Raikes, Virmani, Thompson, & Pong, 2007) found that securely attached children (assessed at 24 months via the AQS) showed lower rates of peer conflict in preschool and first grade, as well as greater declines in peer conflict from 54 to 84 months.

Differences in peer relationships by attachment security are also revealed in children's self-perceptions of their peer relationships. We (Raikes & Thompson, in press-a) analyzed data from the NICHD Study of Early Child Care and reported that AQS security scores at 24 months were negatively associated with children's self-reported loneliness in first grade, and that children deemed resistant in a modified Strange Situation procedure at 36 months were significantly higher in self-reported loneliness than children in the other attachment groups (see also Berlin, Cassidy, & Belsky, 1995). These findings are important in suggesting that securely attached children benefit not only from their enhanced social skills in developing friendships, but also from self-perceptions as fitting well into the peer group. (See Berlin, Cassidy, & Appleyard, Chapter 15, this volume, for further discussion of the links between infant attachment and children's current and subsequent relationships with peers.)

Other studies support the conclusion that attachment security is associated with children's functioning in close relationships. Bost, Vaughn, Washington, Cielinski, and Bradbard (1998) found that secure preschoolers (assessed via AQS scores) had more extensive and supportive social networks and were also higher on sociometric assessments of peer competence (similar conclusions have been reported by Booth, Rubin, and Rose-Krasnor, 1998, and DeMulder, Denham, Schmidt, & Mitchell, 2000). Anan and Barnett (1999) found in a sample of lower-income African American 6½-year-olds that secure attachment (assessed 2 years earlier) was associated with children's perceptions of greater social support, and that social support mediated the association between secure attachment and lower scores on externalizing and internalizing problems. These results underscore the importance of children's perceptions of social support, and show how social cognitions like these can mediate between attachment security and its psychosocial outcomes.

Some studies have found that securely attached infants are also more sociable with unfamiliar adults in follow-up studies (e.g., Thompson & Lamb, 1983). However, mothers were present during assessments of stranger reactions, and each study in which concurrent maternal behavior was evaluated yielded differences indicating that the mothers of secure children were more supportive of their offspring. Thus early differences in responses to unfamiliar adults appear to be reliant on maternal support. The association between attachment security and children's capacities to develop close relationships with peers and adults, by contrast, appears to be more clearly a result of the skills and predispositions that children bring to these relationships.

Personality

The largest and most comprehensive study of early attachment and its developmental consequences is the Minnesota Study of Risk and Adaptation from Birth to Adulthood (Sroufe, 2005; Sroufe et al., 2005). This prospective longitudinal study of children and families in poverty focused on the association between attachment and personality, and thus enlisted the "organizational perspective" described earlier. In this study, children were recruited with their families in infancy and followed through age 28. Strange Situation observations were conducted at 12 and 18 months; in the years that followed, personality characteristics were assessed regularly through behavioral observations, interviews, observer ratings, self-reports, and semiprojective instruments.

The reports based on this study revealed significant associations between early attachment security and personality characteristics throughout childhood and adolescence, including relations with measures of emotional health, self-esteem, agency and self-confidence, positive affect, ego resiliency, and social competence in interactions with peers, teachers, camp counselors, romantic partners, and others (see Sroufe et al., 2005, for a detailed discussion, which also includes a list of citations to specific research reports). In infancy, the researchers concluded, the association between attachment security and emergent personality owed primarily to the continuing quality of care—or, in the authors' words, "continuity at this age is still primarily at the level of the relationship" (Sroufe et al., 2005, p. 110).

As children matured, moreover, the continuing importance of early attachment was in the context of subsequent developmental influences. Sroufe and his colleagues found that the prediction of later personality was enhanced when early attachment measures were supplemented by other indicators of the quality of subsequent care, which could transform as well as sustain the effects of early security (see Carlson, Sroufe, & Egeland, 2004). Moreover, as time progressed between Strange Situation assessments and later personality outcomes, the effects of early security were more likely to be indirect—mediated and/or moderated by subsequent relational influences. In recognizing that personality outcomes are multidetermined and that attachment security is only one of many constituent influences, in other words, these researchers emphasized that both developmental history and current experience are important in shaping personality growth.

The Minnesota study has been an important and provocative contribution to the research on the sequelae of early attachment, and is one of the few studies to document long-term associations between attachment security and later personality outcomes. Few other studies have sought to replicate the findings reported from this study, however, and in view of some nonreplications (e.g., Bates, Maslin, & Frankel, 1985; Easterbrooks & Goldberg, 1990), continued efforts to confirm and extend these important findings are warranted. Equally important are future studies that are designed, as was the Minnesota study, to view the significance of early attachment security in the context of subsequent developmental influences on multidetermined personality outcomes.

Emotion Regulation

One of the functions of attachment relationships is to assist in regulating the emotional arousal of offspring, especially emotions that are potentially disturbing or overwhelming (Cassidy, 1994; Thompson, 1994). This is most evident when parents respond sensitively to the distress of their infants, but remains an ongoing feature of secure relationships even as children mature and become more capable of emotion self-regulation. Moreover, through the parents' acceptance of children's feelings and willingness to communicate openly about them, especially those that are disturbing or threatening, parents in secure relationships foster the children's developing emotional self-awareness and scaffold the growth of competent, flexible skills in emotion self-regulation. Thus children in secure relationships are likely to be stronger in emotion regulation than are children in insecure relationships, where parents may be more dismissive, punitive, or critical of the children's emotional expressions (Thompson & Meyer, 2007).

The relevance of a secure attachment to emotion regulation is apparent in infancy (see NICHD Early Child Care Research Network, 2004). In a study of the responses of 18-month-olds to moderate stressors, for example, Nachmias, Gunnar, Mangelsdorf, Parritz, and Buss (1996) reported that postsession cortisol elevations were found only for temperamentally inhibited toddlers who were in insecure relationships with their mothers. For inhibited toddlers in secure relationships, their mothers' presence helped to buffer the physiological effects of challenging events. Gilliom, Shaw, Beck, Schonberg, and Lukon (2002) reported that boys who were securely attached at age 1½ were observed to use more constructive anger management strategies at age 3½. The securely attached boys were more likely to use distraction, ask questions about the frustration task, and wait quietly than the insecurely attached boys were. These findings may help to explain the emotional behaviors that also distinguish securely attached from insecure children from early in life. In a longitudinal study over the first 3 years, Kochanska (2001) reported that over time, insecurely attached children exhibited progressively greater fear and/or anger, and diminished joy, in standardized assessments compared with secure children.

The importance of secure attachments for emotion regulation does not end with early childhood, however. Using the self-report index of attachment security developed by Kerns and colleagues (1996), Contreras, Kerns, Weimer, Gentzler, and Tomich (2000) found that security in middle childhood was significantly associated with children's constructive coping with stress, and that the measure of coping mediated the association between attachment and children's peer competence. Similar findings have been reported by Kerns, Abraham, Schlegelmilch, and Morgan (2007), using multiple measures of middle adolescent attachment (see Kerns, Chapter 17, this volume). As discussed below, preschoolers and older children engage in rich conversations about daily experiences with their parents; these provide a forum for discussion of feelings and their management, as well as a context for growth in emotion regulation skills (Wareham & Salmon, 2006). Research in our laboratory is currently devoted to exploring these influences further.

Self-Concept

Bowlby's (1969/1982, 1973, 1980) argument that attachment security influences young chil-

dren's self-concept, particularly their conceptions of themselves as loved and lovable, has guided several research inquiries into attachment and self-concept. Cassidy (1988) found that securely attached 6-year-olds described themselves in generally positive terms in a puppet interview, but were capable of admitting that they were imperfect (i.e., they were flexible or "open"). Insecurely attached children either revealed a more negative self-image or resisted admitting flaws (similar results were reported by Verschueren, Marcoen, & Schoefs, 1996). In addition, secure children were significantly more likely to exhibit globally positive self-esteem on Harter and Pike's (1984) measure. Clark and Symons (2000) also found that attachment at age 5 (on the AQS) was significantly associated with the positivity and openness of children's responses to the contemporaneous puppet task, but not with self-esteem on the Harter and Pike measure. However, attachment at age 2 (also on the AQS) for this sample was not significantly associated with either measure of self-concept at age 5. Goodvin, Meyer, Thompson, and Hayes (in press) found that AQS attachment assessments at age 4 predicted the positivity of young children's self-concept at age 5 even when contemporaneous attachment security was controlled for. Secure children also viewed themselves as more agreeable and as expressing less negative affect, and these self-concept dimensions were more stable between ages 4 and 5 for secure children. In this sample, a composite measure of maternal emotional stresses was negatively correlated with positive self-concept. Attachment security has also been associated with positive self-concept in older children (Doyle, Markiewicz, Brendgen, Lieberman, & Voss, 2000).

Each of these studies measured explicit self-concept in young children. Only two studies have measured implicit self-concept. One was by Colman and Thompson (2002), who presented 5-year-olds with both manageable and difficult puzzle tasks. Children with lower AQS security scores spontaneously expressed more self-doubt about their abilities or negative self-appraisals during *both* tasks, such as saying, "This is too hard for me" (mothers were present but otherwise occupied as children worked on the puzzles). The second study was by Cassidy, Ziv, Mehta, and Feeney (2003), who used the self-report measure of middle childhood attachment by Kerns and colleagues (1996) in a study of the association between security and children's preferences for receiving positive or negative feedback about the self. They found that a more secure attachment was associated with seeking more positive feedback about the self, and that this association was mediated by global self-worth. Thus research on implicit self-concept is consistent with the findings of explicit self-descriptions by young children in highlighting the more positive self-representations of securely attached children.

Emotion Understanding

Several attachment researchers have proposed and tested the view that owing to the greater psychological intimacy they share with the attachment figure and other partners, securely attached children should have greater understanding of emotions than insecure children. Several studies have now confirmed this to be true in contemporaneous associations with preschoolers using the AQS (Laible & Thompson, 1998; Ontai & Thompson, 2002), and in predictive associations with infant Strange Situation classifications (Steele, Steele, Croft, & Fonagy, 1999) or early childhood AQS ratings (Raikes & Thompson, 2006). Secure children are indeed more proficient at identifying emotions in others. These studies also indicate that securely attached children are especially skilled at understanding negative emotions and mixed feelings, which are conceptually more complex than are positive emotions.

Several studies have sought to understand the relational catalysts of this enhanced understanding. They have drawn on Bretherton's (1993) portrayal of the more "open, fluid communication" between securely attached children and their caregivers that enables emotional sharing and discussion—particularly of negative emotions, which may be more troubling, disturbing, or confusing to young children. We (Ontai & Thompson, 2002) found that more secure 5-year-olds had mothers who, in discussions with them of recent past events and in storybook reading, used a more descriptively rich, elaborative style of conversation about emotion (see Laible, 2004, for similar findings). A number of studies have found that the mothers of secure children are more elaborative in their style of conversation with offspring (see Reese, 2002, for a review); this finding is important, because such a conversational style has been found by other researchers to enhance young children's memory representations and contribute to the construction of autobiographical recall (Nelson & Fivush, 2004), and it is consistent with Bretherton's (1993) description of the communicative style of secure dyads. In reciprocal fashion, preschool children in secure relationships spontaneously talk about emotions more

often in their everyday conversations with their mothers (Raikes & Thompson, in press-b).

In talking about shared events in a rich, interactive, elaborative manner, the mothers of securely attached young children are likely to provide them with enhanced understanding of the psychological dimensions of human interaction, since an appreciation of the influence of emotions (and of other mental phenomena) in everyday events would naturally become incorporated into their shared recounting (Thompson, Laible, & Ontai, 2003). Indeed, Raikes and Thompson (2006) found that the quality of mother–child conversations about emotion mediated the association between attachment security and emotion understanding in 3-year-olds. Thus the association between the security of attachment and emotion understanding may have origins in the relational processes by which mothers and their preschool offspring co-construct an understanding of the psychological world through shared conversation—a view meriting further research exploration. The need for further study of this collaborative construction of psychological understanding is especially important, because of its potential connection to the capacity for mentalization that is, to researchers like Fonagy and Slade, at the heart of security and the development of secure parent–child relationships (see Fonagy, Gergely, & Target, Chapter 33, this volume, and Slade, Chapter 32, this volume).

Social Cognition

Enhanced understanding of emotions may contribute to the greater social competence of secure children. In a study by Denham, Blair, Schmidt, and DeMulder (2002), multiple measures of attachment security (including the AQS) were obtained when children were age 3, along with several measures of emotional competence, including assessments of emotion understanding, emotion regulation, and anger expression. Children were subsequently studied in their kindergarten classrooms to assess peer competence through sociometric ratings and teacher-rated social competence measures. Through latent-variable path-analytic procedures, these researchers confirmed two pathways from preschool attachment security to kindergarten social competence. The first was a direct pathway, consistent with the results of research reviewed above. The second was an indirect pathway, with attachment security at age 3 having an indirect effect on social functioning through emotional competence (see also Denham et al., 2001). The emotion understanding of secure children appears to be an important contributor to their greater social competence with peers.

Other social-cognitive contributors to children's peer relationships are also likely to be influenced by attachment security. In three studies, Cassidy, Kirsh, Scolton, and Parke (1996) examined the association between attachment and children's attributions concerning peer motivations. Infant attachment classifications were not strongly predictive of preschoolers' responses to story questions concerning the motivations of peer story characters when their negative behavior had ambiguous intent. But when attachment and attributional probes were assessed contemporaneously, securely attached kindergartners and first-graders responded as predicted: Secure children were more likely to attribute benign motives to, and insecure children to infer hostile intent in, the story characters. Moreover, these attributions concerning peer motivations were found to mediate the association between attachment security and peer friendship nominations in a sociometric procedure.

Ziv, Oppenheim, and Sagi-Schwartz (2004) examined differences in social information processing in Israeli middle schoolers on the basis of infant attachment classifications. Based on children's responses to interview questions after watching a filmed series of peer interaction vignettes, the researchers found that there were no differences by security on questions concerning the encoding or interpretation of social behavior or generation of alternative responses, but securely attached youth were more likely to believe that peers would respond positively and constructively to competent social initiatives.

Analyzing data from the NICHD Study of Early Child Care, we (Raikes & Thompson, in press-a) examined the association between early attachment security (at 15 months in the Strange Situation, 24 months in the AQS, and 36 months in the modified Strange Situation for preschoolers) and several measures of social cognition when children were 54 months and in first grade. Replicating the results of Cassidy and colleagues (1996), we found that children deemed resistantly attached at 36 months were more likely to make negative motivational attributions to peers as first graders than were secure children (although there were no differences on this measure by attachment security at 54 months). Securely attached children at 24 and 36 months were more likely to identify socially competent and relevant solutions to social problem-solving tasks than were insecure children, but there were no group differences in children's identification of aggressive solutions.

Several things make this study noteworthy. First, each of these predictive outcomes from the security of attachment controlled for the influence of later measures of parenting (including maternal sensitivity), to ensure that these were outcomes of early security rather than of continuity in parenting practices. Second, the prediction of these social-cognitive variables was especially strong when children were securely attached at more than one assessment. Finally, Strange Situation classifications never predicted later social cognition, perhaps because of the more rudimentary IWMs underlying infant attachments compared to attachments at 24 and 36 months of age.

Taken together, these findings suggest that the enhanced capacities of secure children to create and maintain more intimate, close relationships with peers and other partners may derive at least in part from aspects of their social-cognitive skills (including emotion understanding) and representations of relationships, consistent with Bowlby's IWM construct. Securely attached children have been found in these studies to exhibit greater emotion understanding and greater social problem-solving competence than insecurely attached children, to be less lonely, and to create more benign attributions for peers' motivations in ambiguous situations. The relevance of each of these social-cognitive capacities to successful peer interaction in childhood is also empirically supported, and suggests that greater inquiry into how the security of attachment is associated with social information processing is warranted.

Conscience

Kochanska (2002) has argued that one of the motivators of early conscience development is the young child's commitment to maintaining a relationship of mutual harmony with the caregiver. In this respect, a secure attachment may be associated with greater compliance and cooperation, and this association has been confirmed (Laible & Thompson, 2000). Kochanska's (1991, 1995) research has also shown that a secure attachment is especially influential for children who are temperamentally relatively fearless; for these children, the emotional incentives of the mother–child relationship (rather than the anxiety provoked by discipline practices) are motivational.

As in research on emotion understanding, attachment researchers have also sought to understand in more detail the relational catalysts to early conscience development in the context of attachment. Laible and Thompson (2000) reported an interaction between attachment security and the way in which mothers talked about prior instances of child misbehavior (and good behavior) with their children. Mothers who spoke more about people's feelings and used moral evaluatives (e.g., "That was a nice thing to do") in their recounting of past events contributed to conscience development especially for children who were less secure, suggesting that when a secure relationship does not exist, emotion-based references in discussions of misbehavior may stimulate conscience development (see also Laible & Thompson, 2002). In another study, Laible, Panfile, and Makariev (2008) reported an association between AQS attachment security and mothers' conflict resolution strategies in disputes with their children at 30 and 36 months. Mothers of secure children were more likely to use justifications and compromises with their children and were less likely to aggravate conflict, even though the frequency of mother–toddler conflict did not differ from that of insecure dyads.

Further evidence for the relational catalysts to early conscience development comes from findings of Kochanska, Aksan, Knaack, and Rhines (2004). In their longitudinal analysis, they found that for securely attached children (assessed in the Strange Situation at 14 months), the parents' responsiveness and use of gentle discipline (from 14 to 45 months) predicted later conscience (assessed at 56 months), but that for insecure children there was no such association. These findings add to other studies by Kochanska suggesting that an adult's disciplinary practices have differential emotional impact, depending on the broader quality of the parent–child relationship. But this is one of the first studies documenting that the security of attachment moderates the influence of other relational influences on early socialization—an idea that merits further study.

Memory

Why would memory be associated with the security of attachment? Considering this question requires proceeding from the well-studied *content* of IWMs to the *process* (i.e., information-processing) characteristics of IWMs, which have been much less systematically examined. Bowlby's (1980) portrayal of the functioning of IWMs included his view that IWMs guide the analysis of new information in light of previously established expectations or schemas. Attachment theory is not entirely consistent, however, in its view of how IWMs are so

influential—sometimes indicating that attention and memory will be directed *toward* information that is consistent with prior expectations and prior schemas (see below), and on other occasions (particularly in discussions of defensive processing; see also Main, Kaplan, & Cassidy, 1985) indicating that attention and memory will be directed *away* from expectation-consistent information, especially if it is painful or disturbing. Nevertheless, these theoretical views have generated several efforts to examine the hypothesized influence of attachment security on memory.

Belsky, Spritz, and Crnic (1996) hypothesized that differential processing of schema-consistent information, owing to the influences of IWMs, would cause securely attached children to remember positive events more accurately than would insecure children. In a study in which 3-year-old boys' delayed recognition memory for positive and negative events during a previously viewed puppet show was assessed, this expectation was confirmed. Children who were securely attached (assessed in infancy) remembered the positive events more accurately than the negative events; the reverse was true for those earlier deemed insecurely attached, even though there were no group differences in initial attention to the positive or negative events in the puppet show.

Kirsh and Cassidy (1997) also studied the relevance of infant attachment status for 3½-year-olds' memory for stories depicting maternal responsiveness, rejection, and exaggerated distress-related responding. Consistent with the findings of Belsky and colleagues (1996), securely attached preschoolers remembered the stories describing responsive mothers better than insecure children did. Contrary to expectations, however, secure children also better remembered rejecting and exaggerated stories, significantly better than insecure-resistant children in the case of stories describing maternal rejection. Although the authors interpreted these findings as indicating that secure children are open to a range of emotions in their processing of attachment-related information, these findings underscore the need for greater theoretical clarity concerning the relevance of attachment security for memory of certain events. It is possible (indeed, likely) that several different processes may be relevant to the association between attachment and memory for attachment-relevant events (see Alexander, Quas, & Goodman, 2002, for a thoughtful review of potential processes mediating the association between attachment and children's memory for traumatic events).

CONCLUSION

This review does not exhaust the range of correlates and outcomes of early attachment security that have been studied. Associations with theory of mind, mastery motivation, academic achievement, cognitive and linguistic functioning, and many other sequelae have also been empirically examined. The reason for focusing on outcomes related to children's functioning in relationships, personality, emotion regulation and understanding, social-cognitive capabilities, conscience, and memory is that these are the most direct derivatives from Bowlby's theory and (perhaps as a consequence) have been best studied.

In the broadest sense, the picture yielded by this vast empirical literature is both encouraging and daunting. On the one hand, there is a broader, more coherent network of correlates and outcomes of early attachment security than has ever before been revealed. This literature indicates, usually in replicated findings, that children with a secure attachment history are capable of developing and maintaining more successful close relationships, especially with their parents and with peers, than are insecure children; they develop a variety of desirable personality qualities in childhood and adolescence; they are more likely to exhibit constructive forms of emotionality and emotion self-regulation; and they exhibit more positive self-regard in both explicit and implicit assessments of self-concept. Some of the more exciting recent findings come from studies of the representational correlates and outcomes of attachment security. Securely attached children exhibit greater emotion understanding, demonstrate more competent social problem-solving skills, assume more benign attributions for peers' motivations in ambiguous situations, are more advanced in conscience development, and are less lonely than are insecurely attached children. There is also evidence for the advantages of a secure attachment for memory, especially of attachment-related events, although elucidation of this awaits greater conceptual clarity and research exploration.

Early security clearly makes a significant difference for psychological development, but the empirical yield of this literature is not as generous with respect to the reasons why. As earlier noted, the various attachment minitheories provide somewhat different explanations for why a secure attachment should be developmentally provocative; most of the studies in this literature are agnostic concerning why attachment is related to later outcomes, because the research is seldom designed to discriminate among different potential explanations. Of those that are more informatively designed, the literature yields some important and interesting clues. Early security is more strongly associated with psychological sequelae when children continue to experience sensitive parental care and security is maintained (Belsky & Fearon, 2002a, 2002b; Raikes & Thompson, in press-a). The content and quality of mother–child conversation may be part of that sensitivity, with the mothers of secure children conversing with their offspring in more elaborative and psychologically more informative ways (Raikes & Thompson, 2006; Thompson et al., 2003). Attachment security may also mediate the effects of other parenting practices on early psychological development (Kochanska et al., 2004). Early secure or insecure attachment may be especially predictive of later psychological outcomes when it is considered in the context of subsequent developmental influences, especially the continuing quality of parental care (Sroufe et al., 2005). The social-cognitive advantages of children with a secure attachment history may be an important mediator of their social competence, especially with peers and other close relational partners (Cassidy et al., 1996; Denham et al., 2002). In particular, how secure and insecure children perceive themselves and their own characteristics may be an especially significant contributor to their better psychological functioning (Cassidy et al., 2003). Attachment security may be important not only for how young children think, but for how they attend to, process, and remember events related to their relational experiences (Belsky et al., 1996).

These are important clues to how early attachment influences later psychological functioning, and constitute an agenda for future study. One of the central conclusions of this chapter, therefore, is that there will be further advances in our understanding of the association between early attachment and psychological growth when future studies are designed more incisively to examine the intervening processes that connect them. Carefully designed longitudinal research studies, together with analytical designs that enable the detection of direct and indirect associations between attachment and later outcomes, are likely to be important contributions to that productive future research literature. In addition, consistent with some of the more exciting research insights of this field, exploration of continuing parental influences (e.g., conversational fluency, discipline practices), contextual demands (e.g., family stress and disruption) and representational processes (e.g., self-referential beliefs, self-regulatory capacities, motivational influences) mediating attachment and its outcomes will be especially informative.

Another challenge facing attachment researchers in the future is that of narrowing and specifying the range of expectable correlates of a secure attachment. "All good things go together" is not a sophisticated developmental theory, but the current literature increasingly suggests that a secure attachment is associated with an ever-widening variety of good outcomes. If attachment theory does not have a coherent explanation for this variety of outcomes, the integrity of the attachment construct is in doubt (a problem currently confronting the literature on adult attachment styles), because theory development cannot be bootstrapped by findings of empirical research alone without potentially holding attachment theory accountable for formulations it should not and perhaps cannot embrace (Sroufe, 1988). Therefore, future research must be designed to examine both the convergent and the discriminant validity of the attachment construct, to determine the extent to which the associations between attachment and other behaviors derives from theoretically predicted mediators, and to facilitate further work on theory development (particularly concerning the representational dimensions of attachment security).

One manner of addressing these conceptual and empirical challenges is for attachment researchers to integrate the scholarship of contemporary developmental science more fully into their thinking about the impact of early close relationships, just as Bowlby did several decades ago. For Bowlby, new insights into children's thinking inspired by Piagetian theory were significant catalysts to his conceptualization of stages of attachment formation and the developmental outcomes of early security. For current attachment scholars, the equally profound insights deriving from literatures on implicit knowledge, theory of mind, autobiographical memory, social representation, and many other areas of contemporary scholarship have comparable potential to reinvigorate thinking about the development of attachment and its psychological outcomes. Because scientists are all studying the same developing child, there is every reason to expect that contemporary research insights into conceptual and behavioral development should inform attachment theorists' understanding of IWMs, the psychological meaning of

secure relationships, and the influence of these relationships on specific developmental outcomes at particular periods of growth. Drawing on allied developmental literatures outside of the attachment field will add greater clarity, specificity, and precision to attachment theory.

One of the reasons why attachment theory has remained vigorous over the years is that researchers have found new areas to pioneer. The "move to the level of representation" (Main et al., 1985), the exploration of adult attachment representations, and the connections between disorganized attachment and emergent risk for psychopathology are some of the ways that new research directions have reinvigorated attachment theory in the past. For the future, understanding the reasons for the psychological outcomes of attachment security in a theoretically rigorous, developmentally informed manner promises to yield equally vigorous new energy for this field of study.

ACKNOWLEDGMENT

I am grateful for the comments of Miranda Goodman-Wilson on an earlier version of this chapter.

REFERENCES

Ainsworth, M. D. S. (1967). *Infancy in Uganda: Infant care and the growth of love.* Baltimore: Johns Hopkins University Press.

Ainsworth, M. D. S. (1973). The development of infant–mother attachment. In B. Caldwell & H. Ricciuti (Eds.), *Review of child development research* (Vol. 3, pp. 1–94). Chicago: University of Chicago Press.

Ainsworth, M. D. S. (1979). Attachment as related to mother–infant interaction. In J. S. Rosenblatt, R. A. Hinde, C. Beer, & M.-C. Busnel (Eds.), *Advances in the study of behavior* (Vol. 9, pp. 1–51). New York: Academic Press.

Ainsworth, M. D. S. (1984, April). *Adaptation and attachment.* Paper presented at the meeting of the International Conference on Infant Studies, New York.

Alexander, K. W., Quas, J. A., & Goodman, G. S. (2002). Theoretical advances in understanding children's memory for distressing events: The role of attachment. *Developmental Review, 22,* 490–519.

Anan, R., & Barnett, D. (1999). Perceived social support mediates between prior attachment and subsequent adjustment: A study of urban African American children. *Developmental Psychology, 35,* 1210–1222.

Bates, J. E., Maslin, C. A., & Frankel, K. A. (1985). Attachment security, mother–child interaction, and temperament as predictors of behavior-problem ratings at age three years. In I. Bretherton & E. Waters

(Eds.), Growing points of attachment theory and re-search. *Monographs of the Society for Research in Child Development, 50*(Serial No. 209), 167–193.

Belsky, J., & Cassidy, J. (1994). Attachment: Theory and evidence. In M. Rutter & D. Hay (Eds.), *Development through life* (pp. 373–402). Oxford, UK: Blackwell.

Belsky, J., & Fearon, R. M. (2002a). Early attachment security, subsequent maternal sensitivity, and later child development: Does continuity in development depend upon continuity of caregiving? *Attachment and Human Development, 4*, 361–387.

Belsky, J., & Fearon, R. P. (2002b). Infant–mother attachment security, contextual risk, and early development: A moderational analysis. *Development and Psychopathology, 14*, 293–310.

Belsky, J., Spritz, B., & Crnic, K. (1996). Infant attachment security and affective–cognitive information processing at age 3. *Psychological Science, 7*, 111–114.

Belsky, J., Steinberg, L., & Draper, P. (1991). Childhood experience, interpersonal development, and reproductive strategy: An evolutionary theory of socialization. *Child Development, 62*, 647–670.

Berlin, L. J., Cassidy, J., & Belsky, J. (1995). Loneliness in young children and infant–mother attachment: A longitudinal study. *Merrill–Palmer Quarterly, 41*, 91–103.

Booth, C., Rubin, K., & Rose-Krasnor, L. (1998). Perceptions of emotional support from mother and friend in middle childhood: Links with social-emotional adaptation and preschool attachment security. *Child Development, 69*, 427–442.

Bost, K., Vaughn, B., Washington, W., Cielinski, K. L., & Bradbard, M. (1998). Social competence, social support, and attachment: Demarcation of construct domains, measurement, and paths of influence for preschool children attending Head Start. *Child Development, 69*, 192–218.

Bowlby, J. (1969/1982). *Attachment and loss: Vol. 1. Attachment.* New York: Basic Books.

Bowlby, J. (1973). *Attachment and loss: Vol. 2. Separation: Anxiety and anger.* New York: Basic Books.

Bowlby, J. (1980). *Attachment and loss: Vol. 3. Loss: Sadness and depression.* New York: Basic Books.

Bretherton, I. (1993). From dialogue to internal working models: The co-construction of self in relationships. In C. A. Nelson (Ed.), *Minnesota Symposium on Child Psychology: Vol. 26. Memory and affect in development* (pp. 237–263). Hillsdale, NJ: Erlbaum.

Bretherton, I., & Munholland, K. A. (1999). Internal working models in attachment relationships: A construct revisited. In J. Cassidy & P. R. Shaver (Eds.), *Handbook of attachment: Theory, research, and clinical applications* (pp. 89–111). New York: Guilford Press.

Carlson, E., Sroufe, L., & Egeland, B. (2004). The construction of experience: A longitudinal study of representation and behavior. *Child Development, 75*, 66–83.

Cassidy, J. (1988). Child–mother attachment and the self in six-year-olds. *Child Development, 59*, 121–134.

Cassidy, J. (1994). Emotion regulation: Influences of attachment relationships. In N. A. Fox (Ed.), The development of emotion regulation and dysregulation: Biological and behavioral aspects. *Monographs of the Society for Research in Child Development, 59*(2–3, Serial No. 240), 228–249.

Cassidy, J., Kirsh, S., Scolton, K., & Parke, R. (1996). Attachment and representations of peer relationships. *Developmental Psychology, 32*, 892–904.

Cassidy, J., Ziv, Y., Mehta, T. G., & Feeney, B. C. (2003). Feedback seeking in children and adolescents: Associations with self-perceptions, attachment representations, and depression. *Child Development, 74*, 612–628.

Chisholm, J. S. (1996). The evolutionary ecology of attachment organization. *Human Nature, 1*, 1–37.

Chisholm, J. S. (1999). *Death, hope and sex: Steps to an evolutionary ecology of mind and morality.* New York: Cambridge University Press.

Cicchetti, D. (2006). Development and psychopathology. In D. Cicchetti & D. J. Cohen (Eds.), *Developmental psychopathology: Vol. 1. Theory and method* (2nd ed., pp. 1–23). Hoboken, NJ: Wiley.

Clark, S., & Symons, D. (2000). A longitudinal study of Q-sort attachment security and self-processes at age 5. *Infant and Child Development, 9*, 91–104.

Colman, R. A., & Thompson, R. A. (2002). Attachment security and the problem-solving behaviors of mothers and children. *Merrill–Palmer Quarterly, 48*, 337–359.

Contreras, J. M., Kerns, K. A., Weimer, B. L., Gentzler, A. L., & Tomich, P. L. (2000). Emotion regulation as a mediator of associations between mother–child attachment and peer relationships in middle childhood. *Journal of Family Psychology, 14*, 111–124.

Crittenden, P. M. (1990). Internal representational models of attachment relationships. *Infant Mental Health Journal, 11*, 259–277.

DeMulder, E., Denham, S., Schmidt, M., & Mitchell, J. (2000). Q-sort assessment of attachment security during the preschool years: Links from home to school. *Developmental Psychology, 36*, 274–282.

Denham, S., Blair, K., Schmidt, M., & DeMulder, E. (2002). Compromised emotional competence: Seeds of violence sown early? *American Journal of Orthopsychiatry, 72*, 70–82.

Denham, S., Mason, T., Caverly, S., Schmidt, M., Hackney, R., Caswell, C., et al. (2001). Preschoolers at play: Co-socialisers of emotional and social competence. *International Journal of Behavioral Development, 25*, 290–301.

Doyle, A. B., Markiewicz, D., Brendgen, M., Lieberman, M., & Voss, K. (2000). Child attachment security and self-concept: Associations with mother and father attachment style and marital quality. *Merrill–Palmer Quarterly, 46*, 514–539.

Easterbrooks, M., & Goldberg, W. (1990). Security of toddler–parent attachment: Relation to children's sociopersonality functioning during kindergarten. In M. Greenberg, D. Cicchetti, & E. Cummings (Eds.),

Attachment in the preschool years (pp. 221–244). Chicago: University of Chicago Press.

Egeland, B., Kalkoske, M., Gottesman, N., & Erickson, M. (1990). Preschool behavior problems: Stability and factors accounting for change. *Journal of Child Psychology and Psychiatry, 31,* 891–909.

Ellis, B. J. (2004). Timing of pubertal maturation in girls: An integrated life history approach. *Psychological Bulletin, 130,* 920–958.

Frankel, K., & Bates, J. (1990). Mother–toddler problem solving: Antecedents in attachment, home behavior, and temperament. *Child Development, 61,* 810–819.

Freud, S. (1963). *An outline of psychoanalysis* (J. Strachey, Trans.). New York: Norton. (Original work published 1940)

Gilliom, M., Shaw, D. S., Beck, J. E., Schonberg, M. A., & Lukon, J. L. (2002). Anger regulation in disadvantaged preschool boys: Strategies, antecedents, and the development of self-control. *Developmental Psychology, 38,* 222–235.

Goodvin, R., Meyer, S., Thompson, R. A., & Hayes, R. (in press). Self-understanding in early childhood: Associations with attachment security, maternal perceptions of the child, and maternal emotional risk. *Attachment and Human Development.*

Grossmann, K. E. (1999). Old and new internal working models of attachment: The organization of feelings and language. *Attachment and Human Development, 1,* 253–269.

Harter, S., & Pike, R. (1984). The Pictorial Scale of Perceived Competence and Social Acceptance for Young Children. *Child Development, 55,* 1969–1982.

Kerns, K. A., Abraham, M. M., Schlegelmilch, A., & Morgan, T. A. (2007). Mother–child attachment in later middle childhood: Assessment approaches and associations with mood and emotion regulation. *Attachment and Human Development, 9,* 33–53.

Kerns, K. A., Klepac, L., & Cole, A. (1996). Peer relationships and preadolescents' perceptions of security in the child–mother relationship. *Developmental Psychology, 32,* 457–466.

Kirsh, S. J., & Cassidy, J. (1997). Preschoolers' attention to and memory for attachment-relevant information. *Child Development, 68,* 1143–1153.

Kochanska, G. (1991). Socialization and temperament in the development of guilt and conscience. *Child Development, 62,* 1379–1392.

Kochanska, G. (1995). Children's temperament, mothers' discipline, and security of attachment: Multiple pathways to emerging internalization. *Child Development, 66,* 597–615.

Kochanska, G. (2001). Emotional development in children with different attachment histories: The first three years. *Child Development, 72,* 474–490.

Kochanska, G. (2002). Mutually responsive orientation between mothers and their young children: A context for the early development of conscience. *Current Directions in Psychological Science, 11,* 191–195.

Kochanska, G., Aksan, N., Knaack, A., & Rhines, H. (2004). Maternal parenting and children's con-

science: Early security as a moderator. *Child Development, 75,* 1229–1242.

Laible, D. (2004). Mother–child discourse surrounding a child's past behavior at 30 months: Links to emotional understanding and early conscience development at 36 months. *Merrill–Palmer Quarterly, 50,* 159–180.

Laible, D., Panfile, T., & Makariev, D. (2008). The quality and frequency of mother–toddler conflict: Links with attachment and temperament. *Child Development, 79,* 426–443.

Laible, D., & Thompson, R. A. (1998). Attachment and emotional understanding in preschool children. *Developmental Psychology, 34,* 1038–1045.

Laible, D., & Thompson, R. A. (2000). Mother–child discourse, attachment security, shared positive affect, and early conscience development. *Child Development, 71,* 1424–1440.

Laible, D., & Thompson, R. A. (2002). Mother–child conflict in the toddler years: Lessons in emotion, morality, and relationships. *Child Development, 73,* 1187–1203.

Lamb, M. E., Thompson, R. A., Gardner, W., & Charnov, E. L. (1985). *Infant–mother attachment.* Hillsdale, NJ: Erlbaum.

Maccoby, E. E. (1984). Socialization and developmental change. *Child Development, 55,* 317–328.

Main, M. (1991). Metacognitive knowledge, metacognitive monitoring, and singular (coherent) versus multiple (incoherent) models of attachment: Findings and directions for future research. In C. M. Parkes, J. Stevenson-Hinde, & P. Marris (Eds.), *Attachment across the life cycle* (pp. 127–159). London: Routledge.

Main, M., & Cassidy, J. (1988). Categories of response to reunion with the parent at age 6: Predictable from infant attachment classifications and stable over a 1-month period. *Developmental Psychology, 24,* 415–426.

Main, M., Kaplan, N., & Cassidy, J. (1985). Security in infancy, childhood, and adulthood: A move to the level of representation. In I. Bretherton & E. Waters (Eds.), Growing points of attachment theory and research. *Monographs of the Society for Research in Child Development, 50*(1–2, Serial No. 209), 66–104.

Matas, L., Arend, R., & Sroufe, L. (1978). Continuity of adaptation in the second year: The relationship between quality of attachment and later competence. *Child Development, 49,* 547–556.

Nachmias, M., Gunnar, M., Mangelsdorf, S., Parritz, R. H., & Buss, K. (1996). Behavioral inhibition and stress reactivity: The moderating role of attachment security. *Child Development, 67,* 508–522.

National Institute of Child Health and Human Development (NICHD) Early Child Care Research Network. (2004). Affect dysregulation in the mother–child relationship in the toddler years: Antecedents and consequences. *Development and Psychopathology, 16,* 43–68.

Nelson, K., & Fivush, R. (2004). The emergence of autobiographical memory: A social-cultural developmental theory. *Psychological Review, 111,* 486–511.

Ontai, L., & Thompson, R. A. (2002). Patterns of attachment and maternal discourse effects on children's emotion understanding from 3 to 5 years of age. *Social Development, 11*, 433–450.

Raikes, H. A., & Thompson, R. A. (2006). Family emotional climate, attachment security, and young children's emotion understanding in a high-risk sample. *British Journal of Developmental Psychology, 24*, 89–104.

Raikes, H. A., & Thompson, R. A. (in press-a). Attachment and parenting quality as predictors of early social cognition. *Attachment and Human Development.*

Raikes, H. A., & Thompson, R. A. (in press-b). Conversations about emotions in high-risk dyads. *Attachment and Human Development.*

Raikes, H. A., Virmani, E. A., Thompson, R. A., & Pong, H. (2007). *Declines in peer conflict from preschool through first grade: The importance of social cognitive representations.* Manuscript submitted for publication.

Reese, E. (2002). Social factors in the development of autobiographical memory: The state of the art. *Social Development, 11*, 124–142.

Schneider, B., Atkinson, L., & Tardif, C. (2001). Child–parent attachment and children's peer relations: A quantitative review. *Developmental Psychology, 37*, 86–100.

Slade, A. (1987). Quality of attachment and early symbolic play. *Developmental Psychology, 23*, 78–85.

Sroufe, L. A. (1988). The role of infant–caregiver attachment in development. In J. Belsky & T. Nezworski (Eds.), *Clinical implications of attachment* (pp. 18–38). Hillsdale, NJ: Erlbaum.

Sroufe, L. A. (2005). Attachment and development: A prospective, longitudinal study from birth to adulthood. *Attachment and Human Development, 7*, 349–367.

Sroufe, L. A., Egeland, B., Carlson, E., & Collins, W. (2005). *The development of the person: The Minnesota Study of Risk and Adaptation from Birth to Adulthood.* New York: Guilford Press.

Sroufe, L. A., Egeland, B., & Kreutzer, T. (1990). The fate of early experience following developmental change: Longitudinal approaches to individual adaptation in childhood. *Child Development, 61*, 1363–1373.

Sroufe, L. A., & Fleeson, J. (1988). The coherence of family relationships. In R. A. Hinde & J. Stevenson-Hinde (Eds.), *Relationships within families* (pp. 27–47). Oxford, UK: Clarendon Press.

Steele, H., Steele, M., Croft, C., & Fonagy, P. (1999). Infant–mother attachment at one year predicts children's understanding of mixed emotions at six years. *Social Development, 8*, 161–178.

Thompson, R. A. (1994). Emotion regulation: A theme in search of definition. In N. Fox (Ed.), The development of emotion regulation and dysregulation: Biological and behavioral aspects. *Monographs of the Society for Research in Child Development, 59*(2–3, Serial No. 240), 25–52.

Thompson, R. A. (2000). The legacy of early attachments. *Child Development, 71*, 145–152.

Thompson, R. A. (2006). The development of the person: Social understanding, relationships, self, conscience. In W. Damon & R. M. Lerner (Series Eds.) & N. Eisenberg (Vol. Ed.), *Handbook of child psychology: Vol. 3. Social, emotional, and personality development* (6th ed., pp. 24–98). Hoboken, NJ: Wiley.

Thompson, R. A., Laible, D., & Ontai, L. (2003). Early understanding of emotion, morality, and the self: Developing a working model. In R. Kail (Ed.), *Advances in child development and behavior* (Vol. 31, pp. 137–171). San Diego, CA: Academic Press.

Thompson, R. A., & Lamb, M. E. (1983). Security of attachment and stranger sociability in infancy. *Developmental Psychology, 19*, 184–191.

Thompson, R. A., & Meyer, S. (2007). The socialization of emotion regulation in the family. In J. Gross (Ed.), *Handbook of emotion regulation* (pp. 249–268). New York: Guilford Press.

Thompson, R. A., & Raikes, H. A. (2003). Toward the next quarter-century: Conceptual and methodological challenges for attachment theory. *Development and Psychopathology, 15*, 691–718.

van IJzendoorn, M., van der Veer, R., & van Vliet-Visser, S. (1987). Attachment three years later: Relationships between quality of mother–infant attachment and emotional/cognitive development in kindergarten. In L. Tavecchio & M. van IJzendoorn (Eds.), *Attachment in social networks* (pp. 185–224). Amsterdam: Elsevier.

Verschueren, K., Marcoen, A., & Schoefs, V. (1996). The internal working model of the self, attachment, and competence in five-year-olds. *Child Development, 67*, 2493–2511.

Wareham, P., & Salmon, K. (2006). Mother–child reminiscing about everyday experiences: Implications for psychological interventions in the preschool years. *Clinical Psychology Review, 26*, 535–554.

Waters, E., Kondo-Ikemura, K., Posada, G., & Richters, J. E. (1991). Learning to love: Mechanisms and milestones. In M. R. Gunnar & L. A. Sroufe (Eds.), *Minnesota Symposium on Child Psychology: Vol. 23. Self processes and development* (pp. 217–255). Hillsdale, NJ: Erlbaum.

Weinfield, N., Sroufe, L. A., Egeland, B., & Carlson, E. (1999). The nature of individual differences in infant–caregiver attachment. In J. Cassidy & P. R. Shaver (Eds.), *Handbook of attachment: Theory, research, and clinical applications* (pp. 68–88). New York: Guilford Press.

Youngblade, L., & Belsky, J. (1992). Parent–child antecedents of 5-year-olds' close friendships: A longitudinal analysis. *Developmental Psychology, 28*, 700–713.

Ziv, Y., Oppenheim, D., & Sagi-Schwartz, A. (2004). Social information processing in middle childhood: Relations to infant–mother attachment. *Attachment and Human Development, 6*, 327–348.

CHAPTER 17

Attachment in Middle Childhood

KATHRYN A. KERNS

This is a new chapter in the *Handbook of Attachment*. It would have been difficult to write in the 1990s, when the first edition of the volume appeared. At that time, there was a well-established literature on attachment in young children and a rapidly developing literature on attachment in adolescence and adulthood, but middle childhood had been largely ignored by attachment researchers. Now, however, the situation has changed. In the last few years there has been rapid growth in the study of attachment in the middle childhood years, and it is worthwhile to examine and evaluate the emerging literature.

The goals of this chapter are to outline what we know about attachment in middle childhood and to highlight areas in need of further study. The chapter focuses on children 7–12 years of age, and several themes are highlighted. First, middle childhood is an important period of development in its own right, and attachment during this period is likely to be influenced by the broader developmental context. Second, there are clear differences in opinion regarding how to conceptualize and measure attachment at this age, and the lack of a common approach poses challenges for researchers. Third, there are important limitations in our knowledge of developmental change and mechanisms of continuity of attachment during this age

period. Fourth, the empirical literature demonstrates the continued salience and importance of children's attachments to parents in middle childhood. Following the elaboration of these themes, I conclude with several recommendations for future research.

THE NATURE OF ATTACHMENT IN MIDDLE CHILDHOOD

The period of middle childhood can be distinguished from both early childhood and adolescence. In early childhood, children's social worlds are largely oriented around and shaped by family members. Even if young children spend substantial time outside the home (e.g., in day care), parents have a great deal of control over the children's environments and the people with whom the children have social contact. Parents are clearly the primary social figures in children's lives, and they often function not only as attachment figures and teachers, but also as playmates. In middle childhood, children's social worlds expand: They may spend substantial time away from parents, and parents may have less control and influence over the environments and social contacts children experience. Entrance to formal schooling places new demands on children and provides an important context for mastery or failure experiences. Peers take on greater salience, and by middle childhood children have a clear preference for peers rather than parents as playmates (Kerns, Tomich, & Kim, 2006). There are important changes in parental supervision, with a shift in middle childhood from parental control to parent and child co-regulation (Maccoby, 1984). Children become more self-reliant and assume greater responsibility for their behavior both at home and at school. There are also important changes in children's cognitive development (including social cognition). For example, there are advances in metacognition, memory, and cognitive flexibility; greater self-awareness, more consideration of psychological traits, and enhanced understanding of others; and a greater capacity to regulate emotions (Raikes & Thompson, 2005). Physical changes at puberty may also affect attachment relationships (Richardson, 2005). Given the large number of changes occurring, it would be surprising if there were *not* also changes in parent–child attachments between early and middle childhood.

One change may be in the regulation of the attachment behavioral system. Bowlby (1987; cited in Ainsworth, 1990) suggested that the goal of the attachment system changes from *proximity* of the attachment figure in early childhood to the *availability* of the attachment figure in middle childhood. Compared with an infant, a child is content with longer separations and increased distance from the attachment figure, as long as the child knows it is possible to make contact with the figure (e.g., by telephone) and to reunite with the figure if needed (e.g., following an injury to the child). In addition, there is a decline in the frequency and intensity of specific attachment behaviors, such as clinging and following (Bowlby, 1969/1982). There may also be a decline in the range of conditions that elicit a need for the attachment figure, and an increase in the range of actions that can be undertaken to terminate attachment behavior (Bowlby, 1969/1982). These changes probably occur partly because of a child's increased self-reliance, and partly because of parents' and children's expectations regarding greater child autonomy (Kerns et al., 2006; Marvin & Britner, 1999). And these expectations may in turn be influenced by requirements for children to spend more time away from parents (e.g., because of school attendance and other formal activities, such as clubs and sports).

There are also likely to be changes in how parents and children assume responsibility for regulation of secure-base contact. Bowlby (1973) proposed that a fourth phase of attachment, the goal-corrected partnership, emerges sometime after age 3. At this point, a child is better able to understand a parent's desires, communications, and decisions, and is able to take these into consideration when developing plans and goals. Waters, Kondo-Ikemura, Posada, and Richters (1991) have suggested that this shift in attachment may emerge later, during middle childhood. Prior to this age, parents may assume responsibility for maintaining contact with the child. But in middle childhood there may be a change to mutual co-regulation, with the child increasingly taking responsibility for communicating with the attachment figure (e.g., informing him or her of the child's whereabouts and changes in plans). These ideas are consistent with Maccoby's (1984) proposal that a shift toward parent–child co-regulation is the key change in parent–child relationships in the middle childhood years. Children may also be able to develop more sophisticated plans that include alternative ways to achieve the set goal, and be able to evaluate and change plans as needed (Mayseless, 2005; see also Marvin & Britner, Chapter 12, this volume).

Children also develop cognitive models of themselves in relation to their attachment figures, which Bowlby (1969/1982) viewed as part of the children's attachment working models (see Bretherton & Munholland, Chapter 5, this volume). Changes in working models (also referred to as "attachment representations") are likely to occur in middle childhood, due to the changes in cognitive development noted earlier (e.g., greater self-awareness and flexibility in thinking). Children's representations may become more elaborated and organized in middle childhood (Mayseless, 2005). An important question is whether children have the capacity in middle childhood to develop a general model of attachment relationships, which has been referred to as "state of mind with respect to attachment" (Main, Kaplan, & Cassidy, 1985). Younger children's attachment representations are typically assessed in relation to particular figures (e.g., mother and father as distinct figures). By contrast, the assessment of attachment state of mind in adolescence and adulthood is usually focused on an individual's generalized model of attachment relationships, which is thought to develop in addition to (rather than in place of) representations of specific attachment relationships. Although children's cognitive processes in middle childhood are typically more abstract than they were earlier, there are nevertheless limitations on children's thinking that may limit their ability to integrate relationship experiences into a single general model. It may be that by the end of middle childhood, some children have developed a general, internally consistent representation of attachment relationships, particularly if their experiences with different attachment figures are consistent (Kerns, Schlegelmilch, Morgan, & Abraham, 2005). On the other hand, this achievement may not occur until adolescence for children who have the difficult task of integrating very different experiences with different attachment figures.

Another difference between middle childhood and adolescence is the typical constellation of attachment figures. In early childhood, parents and other adults (e.g., day care providers, grandparents) serve as attachment figures, and in some cases older siblings may also function as attachment figures for younger children (see Howes & Spieker, Chapter 14, this volume). Parents continue to function as attachment figures for children, at least through adolescence, and there is also speculation that attachments to peers may emerge in adolescence (see Allen, Chapter 19, this volume). Are peers attachment figures in middle childhood? The available evidence suggests that the answer is no. By the end of middle childhood, children do spend substantial time with peers and will sometimes seek them out for support. Nevertheless, when asked about situations likely to invoke the need for an attachment figure (e.g., times when a child is afraid or sad), even 11- to 12-year-old children show a strong preference for parents over peers (Kerns et al., 2006; Kobak, Rosenthal, & Serwik, 2005). Although peers may not function as full-fledged attachment figures, children may sometimes direct attachment behaviors to peers, particularly if parents are unavailable. Mayseless (2005) has proposed that this may serve an important evolutionary function in middle childhood, by facilitating the transition to investment in peer relationships that is likely to occur in adolescence. Although parents are clearly still children's primary attachment figures, an interesting hypothesis is that there may be greater diversification of attachment in middle childhood, with children utilizing different attachment figures in different situations (Mayseless, 2005). This may include seeking out secondary attachment figures such as grandparents or siblings in some situations. We currently know very little about the role and function of secondary attachment figures in middle childhood.

It should be noted that the developmental outline presented here is largely speculative. The empirical literature at present is limited to studies of whom children prefer in attachment situations (reviewed above) and studies of age-related changes in perceptions of attachment (to be described later). Normative studies of attachment processes are needed to document age-related changes in attachment during middle childhood.

MEASURING ATTACHMENT IN MIDDLE CHILDHOOD

Due to space limitations, this chapter does not present a thorough review of measurement issues and specific measures designed to assess attachment in middle childhood. Nevertheless, the topic deserves comment, to aid readers in evaluating the literature discussed here. There is currently no dominant conceptual or methodological approach. Rather, a wide range of techniques and specific measures have been used to assess attachment in middle childhood. The measurement approaches include questionnaires completed by a child (e.g., Finnegan, Hodges, & Perry, 1996; Kerns, Aspelmeier, Gentzler, & Grabill, 2001); child interviews based on prompted storytelling (e.g., Granot & Mayseless, 2001; Jacobsen, Edelstein, & Hofmann, 1994) or narrations of autobiographical events (e.g., Ammaniti, van IJzendoorn, Speranza, & Tambelli, 2000; Target, Fonagy, & Shmueli-Goetz, 2003); analysis of family drawings (e.g., Fury, Carlson, & Sroufe, 1997; Madigan, Ladd, & Goldberg, 2003); and observations of secure-base behavior in a separation–reunion paradigm (e.g., Easterbrooks, Davidson, & Chazan, 1993). For some methods (questionnaires and interviews), multiple measures are available.

The measures also differ in how they conceptualize attachment, and thus they are not equivalent. Measures vary by whether they are designed to assess perceptions of attachment, attachment representations, or secure-base behavior. Some measures are relationship-specific (e.g., focused on the mother–child or father–child relationship), whereas others assess a child's general orientation or state of mind in regard to attachment relationships. Some measures assess variations in security, whereas others are designed to assess specific patterns of attachment, including kinds of insecure attachment (i.e., avoidant, ambivalent, and disorganized attachment patterns). Just about every possible combination of these features is represented in the literature. Most measures are closely tied to the secure-base and safe-haven constructs, but in a few cases assessments of "attachment" appear to tap other aspects of parent–child relationships (e.g., alienation or social support).

The creation of several different kinds of measures may be due partly to the nature of middle childhood. As already noted, this is an age period during which there are a number of important changes in children's cognitive and social-cognitive abilities. One consequence is that measures thought to be appropriate during the latter half of middle childhood may not be equally sensitive and valid at younger ages, and vice versa. The diversity is probably due also to the relatively late emergence of studies on middle childhood, which allowed investigators to draw upon techniques first developed for other age periods. In developing new measures, investigators have sometimes adapted approaches first developed for early childhood (e.g., story stem narratives, observations of secure-base behavior), whereas in other cases they have adapted approaches first used in adolescence (e.g., questionnaires, autobiographical interviews).

The diversity of measures, and of the conceptualizations of attachment inherent in the measures, can be viewed as both a strength and a weakness. On the positive side, multiple measures can be advantageous: With a single measure, there is always a concern that one is studying the measure rather than the underlying construct. The use of multiple measures allows for more thorough assessment of a construct by more broadly sampling the relevant domain. In a new field, it can be helpful to have more than one approach, because some may ultimately prove to have greater validity than others. By using different measures, the field avoids prematurely relying on a single approach.

Unfortunately, several problems can arise when investigators adopt a wide range of approaches. Often the conceptual rationale for a particular measure is not developed in sufficient detail, making it unclear how authors are conceptualizing attachment. Bretherton (1985) argued for applying a narrow rather than a broad definition of attachment, which would allow researchers to distinguish attachment from other aspects of the parent–child relationship. A measure of attachment based on the secure-base concept seems closely tied to most definitions of attachment, whereas a measure that assesses social support or alienation seems less so. In addition, measures that assess global qualities such as social support may fail to be context-sensitive. Although conceptually one would expect the mother of a securely at-

tached child to be more sensitive than a mother of an avoidantly attached child to a child's distress cues, there may not be differences between the two in all contexts. For example, there is no theoretical reason to expect that a mother of an avoidantly attached child would be unsupportive of her child's academic goals or shared interests (in fact, nonsocial activities might be a focus of interaction and could function to allow maintenance of the relationship without emotional engagement).

Lack of clarity and specificity in conceptualization creates problems when a "box score" approach is taken to evaluating a particular claim of the theory, because failures to replicate may be a product of investigators studying only partially overlapping conceptualizations of attachment. This problem would be less of a concern if every study included multiple measures of attachment, so that different measures could be evaluated empirically. Unfortunately, most studies of attachment in middle childhood include only one measure of the construct. This relates to another concern—namely, that only very limited validity data are currently available for most of the measures developed for assessing attachment in middle childhood (for reviews, see Dwyer, 2005; Kerns et al., 2005; Kerns & Seibert, 2008). Even fewer studies test the discriminant validity of the measures. Thus the current situation is that many measures are available, but there may be only one or two studies evaluating the validity of some of them. In a few studies, questionnaire measures of attachment are related only to other self-reports from children. The limitations of self-report questionnaires are well known, and studies that rely entirely on child questionnaire data offer weaker tests of the theory, the results of which are subject to uninteresting alternative interpretations (e.g., that obtained correlations reflect halo effects or response bias).

There is clearly a need for additional studies that test the validity of middle childhood attachment measures. One need is for studies that include multiple measures of attachment, so that overlap among different conceptualizations and types of measures can be assessed. Most of the measures developed are reliable, as indicated by measures of internal consistency, test–retest stability, or observer agreement (Kerns & Seibert, 2008). Yet, because validity data are rare, it is less clear what interpretations these measures can bear. There needs to be more rigorous testing of the measures' validity, with special attention to tests that are theoretically derived and allow for ruling out alternative interpretations of the measures.

In reviewing the literature for the present chapter, I have included only studies in which attachment constructs were clearly what was measured; studies that employed questionnaire measures of perceived parenting (e.g., social support, parental acceptance, alienation) are not included in this review. I have included studies that used questionnaire, interview, family drawing, or observational measures to assess attachment in middle childhood. Also, some studies involved follow-up assessment of children for whom attachment was assessed in infancy or preschool with observational or narrative attachment assessments. Space limitations and limited data for any single measure preclude separating descriptions by measure. The reader should therefore keep in mind that the chapter reviews a diversity of measures.

CONTINUITY AND CHANGE IN ATTACHMENT IN MIDDLE CHILDHOOD

Although relatively little attention has been paid to normative issues, a few studies have examined whether there are age-related changes in attachment in middle childhood. These studies provide evidence that between later middle childhood and early adolescence, there may be a normative shift toward greater avoidance or a more dismissing attitude toward parental attachments; this change is found for both interview (Ammaniti et al., 2000) and questionnaire (Kerns et al., 2006) measures. During this age period, children also report relying less on attachment figures as they get older (Kerns et al., 2006; Lieberman, Doyle, & Markiewicz, 1999). The change may be partly due to increases in self-reliance. By contrast, there are no age differences in perceptions of caregiver availability (Kerns et al., 2006, Study 1; Lieberman et al., 1999), and two longitudinal studies actually suggest that there are increases in children's perceptions of caregiver availability and security within the middle childhood years (Kerns et al., 2006, Study 2; Verscheueren & Marcoen, 2005). Thus children in middle childhood do still want to have attachment figures available, although they may rely on them less frequently as they get older.

More commonly, the focus has been on the degree of continuity in individual differences in attachment over time. In the absence of disruptions in the quality of caregiving or the loss of attachment figures, one would expect at least moderate continuity over time (see Thompson, Chapter 16, and Weinfield, Sroufe, Egeland, & Carlson,

Chapter 4, this volume). Several studies have evaluated the test–retest stability of attachment within middle childhood, administering the same measure of attachment on two occasions separated by 1–3 months. Wright, Binney, and Smith (1995) did not find evidence of test–retest reliability over a 1-month interval in a small clinical sample. In three other studies (Granot & Mayseless, 2001; Kerns et al., 2005; Target et al., 2003), interview measures of attachment were administered twice with a 3-month separation; all found evidence of test–retest reliability, although the proportion of children receiving the same classification at the two time points was variable across studies (ranging from 50% to 94%). Other research has investigated the stability of attachment over a 1- to 4-year interval. Target and colleagues (2003) found significant levels of stability when a subsample of children was reassessed after 1 year. Ammaniti and colleagues (2000) administered the Attachment Interview for Childhood and Adolescence to a sample of children at ages 10 and 14 years, and found a 71% stability rate with a four-way classification system. Two studies examined stability in children's perceptions of security of attachment. Both studies first assessed children at age 8, with a follow-up assessment either 2 years (Kerns, Tomich, Aspelmeier, & Contreras, 2000) or 3 years (Verschueren & Marcoen, 2005) later. There was evidence of stability in both studies, although correlations for mother–child attachment were not significant in one study (Kerns et al., 2000), and significant correlations in both studies were of only moderate magnitude (ranging from .28 to .37).

Other published studies examined whether attachment assessed in infancy or early childhood predicted attachment in middle childhood. In two studies, children were seen in the Strange Situation at 1 year of age and then were administered a family drawing measure between 7 and 9 years of age (Fury et al., 1997; Madigan et al., 2003). In both studies, a secure classification in infancy predicted classifications and ratings of attachment representations from the later family drawing measure. Bohlin, Hagekull, and Rydell (2000) found no association between mother–child attachment assessed at age 1 in the Strange Situation and secure or avoidant attachment as assessed with an interview at age 8 years. Two other studies found that mother–infant, but not father–infant, attachment predicted children's attachment at ages 10–12 years as assessed with an interview (Aviezier, Sagi, Resnick, & Gini, 2002; Grossmann et al., 2002), although in the Aviezier and colleagues

(2002) study secure attachment in infancy predicted insecure attachment at age 11 years. Ammaniti, Speranza, and Fedele (2005) assessed attachment at age 1 year (Strange Situation), 5 years (behavioral observation, story stem), and 11 years (Attachment Interview for Childhood and Adolescence). Although stability rates from ages 1 and 5 years to age 11 years ranged from 50% to 68%, the stability was not statistically significant in this small sample (21 children).

Collectively, the studies provide mixed evidence for continuity between early attachment and attachment in middle childhood, and modest to high stability within the middle childhood years. The substantial variation in stability estimates suggests that change is also occurring for many children during these years, and studies examining factors that may account for both continuity and change are needed. Questionnaire measures yielded low estimates of stability over a 2- to 3-year period, suggesting a need to investigate further why children's perceptions of attachment relationships change in middle childhood. The available studies examined perceptions of attachment from age 8 to age 10 or 11. Although it is possible that the low stability is due to the modest reliability of these measures for younger children, a more interesting possibility is that the 8–10 age period is a time of reorganization in children's models of relationships (e.g., advances in social comparison abilities may lead children to change their evaluations of their attachment figures). If so, this might also account for the low stability between infant attachment and assessments of attachment made when children were 10–12 years of age. Multimethod stability studies within middle childhood are needed to test this hypothesis. It should also be noted that some studies of stability have related early relationship-specific measures (e.g., the Strange Situation) to later measures of general attachment representations. Weak associations may be found if the latter are based on experiences in multiple attachment relationships. In general, there is a need for additional studies examining how the attachment behavioral system changes in middle childhood, with attention also to factors that can explain continuity and change.

ASSOCIATIONS WITH PARENTING, PARENTS' WORKING MODELS, AND THE FAMILY SYSTEM

One of the strong claims derived from attachment theory is that the quality of the attachment relationship is related to the quality of caregiving provided by an attachment figure. A child who experiences sensitive and responsive care is expected to form a secure relationship with a caregiver, in which the child is able to use the parent as a secure base from which to explore and a haven of safety during times of stress (see Weinfield et al., Chapter 4, this volume). Studies of young children have documented an association between maternal sensitivity and a child's secure attachment to the mother (De Wolff & van IJzendoorn, 1997). There is also an expectation of continuity in attachment across generations; that is, parents who themselves have a secure state of mind in regard to attachment are expected to have children who form secure attachments to them (see Hesse, Chapter 25, this volume). The available data do show an association between parents' states of mind regarding attachment and the security of infants' attachment to those parents (van IJzendoorn, 1995). Finally, it may be that children's attachments to particular caregivers influence and are influenced by the broader family context, including the marital/couple relationship and sibling relationships.

A few studies have examined how attachment is related to parenting style or specific parenting practices in middle childhood. Although not studies of middle childhood attachment per se, several studies have found that secure attachment in infancy or early childhood is associated with parental sensitivity and open parent–child communication in middle childhood (Booth, Rubin, & Rose-Krasnor, 1998; Easterbrooks, Biesecker, & Lyons-Ruth, 2000; Freitag, Belsky, Grossmann, Grossmann, & Scheuerer-Englisch, 1996; Grossmann & Grossmann, 1991; Oppenheim, Koren-Karie, & Sagi-Schwartz, 2006). Other studies have examined concurrent associations between attachment and parenting in children ages 8–12 years. Children who report a more secure attachment to their parents have parents who report a greater willingness to serve as a secure base (Kerns, Klepac, & Cole, 1996, Study 2; Kerns et al., 2000). In addition, more securely attached children were more cooperative in monitoring situations and had parents who were more knowledgeable about their activities in sixth grade, but not third grade (Kerns et al., 2001). Some studies have examined associations with specific forms of insecurity. Children who reported more avoidant coping with mothers perceived their parents to exhibit lower levels of involvement, support, and monitoring of their activities (Karavasilis, Doyle, & Markiewicz, 2003; Yunger, Corby, & Perry, 2005). In another study, avoidant coping was associated negatively with mothers' and fathers' reports of willingness to serve as a secure base (Kerns et al., 2000). Children who scored higher on preoccupied coping also reported higher levels of psychological control from their mothers in one study (Yunger et al., 2005), but not another (Karavasilis et al., 2003); in a third study, preoccupation was not consistently related to measures of parenting (Kerns et al., 2000).

Another set of studies examined whether a secure attachment in middle childhood is associated with parents' models of relationships (i.e., do children form secure attachments to parents who are themselves secure?). Steele and Steele (2005) found that a parent's attachment state of mind, assessed with the Adult Attachment Interview (AAI; George, Kaplan, & Main, 1984, 1985, 1996) prior to a child's birth, predicted the coherence and quality of child attachment representations at age 11. Ammaniti and colleagues (2005) and Target and colleagues (2003) also found concordance between mothers' AAIs and children's attachment (assessed with a child version of the AAI). In a study using questionnaire assessment of child and parent attachment (Doyle, Markiewicz, Brendgen, Lieberman, & Voss, 2000), child security was related negatively to mothers' reports of anxious-ambivalent attachment, but was not related to fathers' reports of anxious-ambivalent attachment or to either mothers' or fathers' reports of avoidant attachment.

The parent–child relationship is typically embedded within a larger family system that may include more than one parent, siblings, and other relatives (e.g., grandparents). The question of how attachment influences and is influenced by the family system has not been explored in depth. Children's security of attachment is linked to the family environment, in that children from disengaged or enmeshed families report lower security in parent–child relationships compared to children from cohesive or adequate families (Davies, Cummings, & Winter, 2004). In addition, higher levels of marital or couple conflict have been related to lower security in parent–child relationships (Harold, Shelton, Goeke-Morey, & Cummings, 2004). Children who are securely attached to their parents are also less likely to be emotionally insecure in the presence of marital/couple conflict (Davies et al., 2004; Harold et al., 2004). No studies have examined the role, quality, and correlates of sibling attachments in middle childhood.

In summary, although the data are limited in comparison with data for younger age periods,

they indicate that secure attachment in middle childhood is related to sensitive, responsive, and accepting parenting, to a parent's secure state of mind, and to features of the family environment—all of which would be expected from theory. It should be noted that relatively few studies have included observational assessments of parenting. As De Wolff and van IJzendoorn (1997) found in reviewing studies of infancy and early childhood, most studies of attachment and parenting have focused on sensitivity or responsiveness rather than other aspects of parenting. Parents of children in middle childhood face many important tasks other than fostering security (e.g., encouraging independence, mastery, politeness, and conformity to rules), but these aspects of socialization have rarely been studied in relation to attachment. As a result, we lack an understanding of the broader parenting context in which attachment develops and is sustained. In addition, there has also been little consideration of how different aspects of parenting may mediate or moderate the influence of attachment. Important tasks for future research will include investigating these questions, as well as considering how the broader family system interfaces with parent–child attachments. Finally, virtually no attention has been paid to the possibility that siblings may be important attachment figures in middle childhood.

ASSOCIATIONS WITH COGNITIVE, SOCIAL, AND EMOTIONAL DEVELOPMENT

An important finding at younger ages is that the formation of a secure attachment to a parent is associated with greater cognitive, emotional, and social competence (see Thompson, Chapter 16, this volume). Studies have also investigated whether these links are found in middle childhood (ages 7–12 years). In one kind of study, assessments of attachment made when children were in infancy or preschool have been used to predict developmental outcomes for children in middle childhood. These studies show that earlier attachment predicts several indicators of competence in middle childhood, including school adaptation and cognitive competence (Aviezer, Resnick, Sagi, & Gini, 2002; Sroufe, Egeland, & Kreutzer, 1990; Stams, Juffer, & van IJzendoorn, 2002), emotion regulation and personality (Grossmann & Grossmann, 1991; Hagekull & Bohlin, 2003; Stams et al., 2002), peer relationships (Aviezer et al., 2002; Booth et al., 1998; Booth, Rose-Krasnor,

McKinnon, & Rubin, 1994; Lewis & Feiring, 1989; Shulman, Elicker, & Sroufe, 1994; Sroufe, Bennett, Englund, Urban, & Shulman, 1993; Sroufe, Egeland, Carlson, & Collins, 2005; Stams et al., 2005), and clinical symptoms (Booth et al., 1994; Carlson, 1998; Lyons-Ruth, Easterbrooks, & Cibelli, 1997; Renken, Egeland, Marvinney, Mangelsdorf, & Sroufe, 1989; Stams et al., 2002). In all of these studies, attachment was not assessed in middle childhood, and it is therefore unclear whether the effects are mediated by middle childhood attachment.

The following literature review focuses on studies in which both attachment and individual adaptation were assessed within middle childhood. As will be seen, these studies suggest that in middle childhood attachment is related in theoretically meaningful ways to indices of children's cognitive, social, and emotional adjustment. Measures of child functioning have included observations of child behavior, maternal reports, teacher reports, and child self-reports. Very few studies relied solely on child questionnaires to measure both attachment and child functioning. Studies of associations between attachment and self-concept or behavior problems were those most likely to include only child questionnaire data.

Associations with Cognitive Development and School Adaptation

Does the quality of attachment have implications for a child's cognitive competence and cognitive performance? Sroufe (1988) predicted that securely attached children may not outperform insecurely attached children on performance measures such as IQ, but that nevertheless they may show superior school adaptation, due to their sense of competence and self-efficacy. Thus it could be predicted that securely attached children will differ from insecurely attached children on indices of school adaptation that include assessments of work habits, attitude, persistence, and the like. It is also well known in the literature on cognitive development that responsive and engaged parenting is associated, in some cases, with children's cognitive development. For example, responsive parenting is related to language development, presumably because responsive caregivers provide a rich language environment in which they elaborate on and encourage their children's verbalizations; and in the toddler years secure attachment is related to children's language development (van IJzendoorn, Dijkstra, & Bus, 1995). Given these considerations, although attachment may have implications for school adaptation, it is less clear whether attachment (theoretically) would be related to cognitive performance.

The available data provide strong evidence for a link between secure attachment to the mother and a child's school attitudes and classroom behaviors. Studies show that more securely attached children report greater perceived academic competence and mastery motivation (Kerns et al., 1996, Study 1; Moss & St.-Laurent, 2001), and are rated by teachers as showing better classroom adjustment in such areas as participation, academic skills, and emotional health (Easterbrooks & Abeles, 2000; Easterbrooks et al., 1993; Granot & Mayseless, 2001; Jacobsen & Hofmann, 1997; Kerns et al., 2000). These links have been documented in both longitudinal and cross-sectional studies, using a variety of measures of attachment.

Other studies have examined how attachment is related to measures of cognitive performance, such as formal tests of reasoning, achievement test scores, and IQ tests. Here the data are more mixed. Some studies have found that secure attachment—assessed with interviews, questionnaires, or behavioral observations—is not related to IQ scores, grade point averages, or achievement test performance (Granot & Mayseless, 2001; Kerns et al., 1996, Study 1; Moss & St.-Laurent, 2001; Target et al., 2003). However, other studies have found secure attachment to be associated with higher scores on IQ or logic tests (Easterbrooks et al., 1993; Jacobsen et al., 1994; Jacobsen & Hofmann, 1997). In some samples, insecure-controlling or disorganized children have been found to have the lowest school grades or performance on tests of cognitive skills (Jacobsen et al., 1994; Moss & St.-Laurent, 2001), suggesting that this group may be especially at risk for problems in cognitive development.

Adapting to the demands of the school environment is an important challenge for children in middle childhood. Studies suggest that secure attachment is related to better adaptation to school, as manifested in children's attitudes, work habits, and persistence. Attachment has been less consistently linked to performance measures, such as IQ or the acquisition of specific cognitive skills. We especially need studies that can explain these effects. It is possible that the presence of a secure base directly fosters enthusiasm and exploration of the school environment, by providing children with the support and self-confidence needed to tackle challenges. It is also possible that associations between attachment and school outcomes are mediated by (and best explained by) correlated parenting practices or the quality of the home environment. For example, Moss, St.-Laurent, Dubois-Comtois, and Cyr (2005) found that the link between disorganized attachment and school performance could be explained by the quality of children's collaborative interactions with their caregivers. Thus specific parenting practices may play a role in explaining why attachment is sometimes related to indicators of cognitive development.

Associations with Self-Concept and Social Information Processing

Bowlby (1973) proposed that the development of a secure attachment relationship has implications for a child's self-view, in that children who experience responsive and sensitive care are likely to view themselves as worthy of others' affection. In addition, children who form secure attachments are thought to possess a balanced self-view, being able to acknowledge personal limitations (Cassidy, 1988). This leads to the expectation that securely attached children will hold positive but realistic and balanced views of themselves.

In several studies of 8- to 12-year-olds, children who reported more secure attachments to parents also reported higher self-esteem (Cassidy, Ziv, Mehta, & Feeney, 2003; Doyle et al., 2000; Kerns, Klepac, & Cole, 1996, Study 1; Sharpe et al., 1998; Verschueren & Marcoen, 2002, 2005; Yunger et al., 2005). In addition, secure attachment has been related to social self-efficacy (Coleman, 2003, for father–child but not mother–child attachment) and fewer weight concerns (Sharpe et al., 1998). These studies are limited in that both attachment and self-concept were measured with self-report questionnaires, which may overestimate the link between the two. In addition, these studies all tested the hypothesis that secure attachment would be related to higher self-esteem. However, research with 6-year-olds suggests that children with an avoidant attachment may tend to provide overly positive reports about themselves (Cassidy, 1988). Consequently, single-dimension measures that assess self-worth on a positivity dimension may not be adequate for testing the link between attachment and self-worth. That is, these measures may not be well suited to testing the hypothesis that securely attached children have a positive but *balanced* view of the self.

These problems can be reduced by employing independent assessments of attachment and self-

concept. Jacobsen and Hofmann (1997) found that children who were classified as secure based on an interview were rated by teachers as higher in self-confidence. Easterbrooks and Abeles (2000) found that children classified as secure based on an interview showed greater access to self-evaluations (i.e., they discussed the self spontaneously and easily, without tension or resistance), but did not report higher global self-esteem. Bohlin and colleagues (2000) found that interview and observational assessments of attachment were not consistently related to measures of social self-esteem. Thus, when methods other than child questionnaires are used, attachment has not been related consistently to higher self-esteem. The lack of consistent evidence for an association is curious, given Bowlby's (1973) argument that models of self and others (relationships) are mutually confirming.

One reason why more securely attached children are hypothesized to maintain positive self-views is that they are thought to process social information in a positively biased way. Two studies have directly examined this mechanism. Ziv, Oppenheim, and Sagi-Schwartz (2004) found that children classified as secure in infancy were more likely at age 7 to hold positive expectations of others, and Cassidy and colleagues (2003) found that more secure 11- to 14-year-olds were more likely to attend selectively to positive information about themselves. Thus there is some initial evidence that more securely attached children may process social information in ways that enhance their views of themselves and others.

As can be seen from this review, there are relatively few studies of attachment and self-concept, especially if one excludes studies that are based entirely on questionnaire measures of the two. The lack of attention to self-concept and social-cognitive processes is surprising, given the central role in attachment theory of working models of self and others. Middle childhood may be an interesting age period in which to study these questions, given the developmental changes at this time in the complexity and sophistication in children's self-understanding and gains in cognitive processing. Given the theory's emphasis on the explanatory role of cognitive models, this is an area where more research is needed. In addition to studies of self-esteem, further research is needed on how attachment is related to information processing. For example, in adolescence attachment is associated with memory biases for interpersonal events (Feeney & Cassidy, 2003; Gentzler & Kerns, 2006), and these biases may emerge earlier.

Associations with Emotion Regulation and Personality

Emotion regulation is an integral aspect of attachment. By definition, a securely attached child is able to use the parent as a safe haven when distressed. Emotional distress is addressed effectively in the secure parent–child dyad, which leads to the mitigation of distress (i.e., return of positive mood), and the child is then able to return to exploration of the environment. Furthermore, it is hypothesized that securely attached children internalize effective ways to cope with stress and are consequently resilient when coping with problems, even in the absence of the caregiver (Contreras & Kerns, 2000; Sroufe, 1983). By contrast, security of attachment is not hypothesized to be associated strongly with measures of temperament, such as emotionality (Vaughn, Bost, & van IJzendoorn, Chapter 9, this volume).

Relatively few studies have assessed attachment and emotion in middle childhood. There is some evidence that attachment is related to patterns of emotion regulation, with more securely attached children using more constructive coping strategies, such as seeking support from others or problem solving (Contreras, Kerns, Weimer, Gentzler, & Tomich, 2000; Kerns, Abraham, Schlegelmilch, & Morgan, 2007). Secure attachment has been related to more positive and less negative mood in daily interactions (Kerns et al., 2007). Three studies have examined whether attachment is related to homesickness at summer camp (Kerns, Brumariu, & Abraham, in press; Thurber & Sigman, 1998; Thurber, Sigman, Weisz, & Schmidt, 1999). Although there was some evidence for a link between the two, the association was small in magnitude, and attachment was less predictive of homesickness than were other factors (such as a homesickness disposition or peer relationships).

Other studies have examined how attachment is related to personality or temperament. Surprisingly, one study found that secure attachment was not related in middle childhood to global measures of ego resilience (Easterbrooks & Abeles, 2000). In addition, two other studies found no association between attachment and temperament when the latter was measured as extraversion (Jacobsen & Hofmann, 1997) or difficult temperament (Contreras et al., 2000).

The lack of research on attachment and emotional development is somewhat surprising, given the central role of emotion in attachment. This is another area where more study is needed, with attention to aspects of emotion that are not related to attachment (i.e., aspects that establish discriminant validity), as well as additional studies of emotion profiles associated with attachment. Especially needed are studies that determine whether specific forms of insecure attachment (e.g., avoidance) are associated with distinct emotion profiles, as Cassidy (1994) and Sroufe (1983) have suggested.

Associations with Peer Relationships and Peer Competence

One of the most extensively investigated questions in middle childhood is whether attachment predicts the quality of children's relationships with peers. There are several reasons for expecting an association between the two. The development of a secure attachment may foster greater exploration, including exploration of peer relationships (Kerns, 1996). In addition, children who form secure attachments to caregivers may show greater interest in and motivation for engaging with other social partners (Sroufe, Egeland, & Carlson, 1999), and may learn socially competent interaction styles from responsive caregivers (Kerns et al., 1996). Also, more securely attached children may develop more adaptive emotion regulation capacities, which are especially important for peer relationships in middle childhood when there is an emphasis on controlling one's emotions with peers (Contreras & Kerns, 2000). A meta-analysis, based mostly on studies with younger children, showed that attachment was related to both friendship and social behavior or popularity with peers, with stronger effects for friendship (Schneider, Atkinson, & Tardif, 2001). In the review below, studies are organized into three areas: friendship, peer popularity, and peer competence.

In the friendship domain, investigators have examined whether attachment is related to the quantity and quality of children's friendships in studies of 8- to 12-year-old children. Evidence for a link between attachment and the number of children's friendships is mixed. Attachment was related concurrently to the number of reciprocated friendships in one study (Kerns et al., 1996, Study 1) but not another (Lieberman et al., 1999). Consistent evidence for a link between attachment and number of friends may be lacking because most children in middle childhood have at least one friend, and numerical indices do not capture information about the quality of a friendship. By contrast, studies consistently find that attachment is related to the quality of children's friendships, as indexed by measures of support, companionship, responsiveness, and conflict (Howes & Tonyan, 2000; Kerns et al., 1996, Study 2; Lieberman et al., 1999). Thus attachment is related to friendship when the quality of children's friendships is considered.

A second group of studies, all with children 8–11 years of age, have examined whether children who form secure attachments to caregivers are more popular (more highly accepted) by their peers. Three studies found that children more securely attached to their mothers were better liked and less likely to be rejected by their peers (Bohlin et al., 2000; Granot & Mayseless, 2001; Kerns et al., 1996, Study 1). However, two studies found an association between secure attachment and peer popularity for father–child, but not mother–child, attachment (Verschueren & Marcoen, 2002, 2005); another study did not find an association between peer popularity and attachment to mothers or to fathers (Lieberman et al., 1999). Bully–victim status also was not related to attachment (Bowers, Smith, & Binney, 1994). Thus, in keeping with Schneider and colleagues' (2001) earlier review, attachment appears to be related more consistently to friendship quality than to peer sociometric status.

A final group of studies examined the association between secure mother–child attachment and global ratings of peer competence or observational measures of competent peer interactions. Securely attached children showed greater social engagement and participation with peers (Bohlin et al., 2000; Yunger et al., 2005). Secure attachment was also related to higher peer competence as rated by teachers (Contreras et al., 2000; but see Easterbrooks & Abeles, 2000, for contrary evidence). Thus most studies find attachment to be related to peer competence.

In summary, there is substantial evidence for an association between attachment and peer relationships, especially when the *quality* of children's relationships and social behavior is the focus. These associations have been found in studies using a variety of measures of both attachment and peer relationships. In their review of the link between attachment and peer relationships, Schneider and colleagues (2001) concluded that there is not a strong need for additional studies documenting an association between the two. This conclusion also seems to apply to the study of attachment and peer relationships in middle childhood. Rather, we need more studies aimed at explaining this link (e.g., Contreras et al., 2000), as well as studies that consider how attachment and peer relationships jointly influence children's social development (e.g., Sroufe et al., 2005).

Associations with Behavior Problems and Clinical Symptoms

Bowlby's interest in attachment grew out of his clinical work with children (Bretherton, 1992). He (1979, 1989) speculated that a secure attachment provides a healthy foundation for development, whereas an insecure attachment to one's primary attachment figures is likely to be associated with difficulties in personality development and in some cases clinical symptoms (see DeKlyen & Greenberg, Chapter 27, this volume). It is therefore not surprising that one of the most frequently investigated topics in middle childhood is whether attachment is related to signs of psychopathology. It should be noted that almost all of the studies measured clinical symptoms (e.g., externalizing problems) rather than assigning clinical diagnoses. In addition, many of the studies employed a developmental-psychopathology perspective, in which multiple aspects of parent–child relationships and family functioning were examined as predictors of adjustment. The review below highlights the specific findings for attachment. Readers should keep in mind, however, that attachment was often not the strongest predictor of adjustment, and that multiple measures of family functioning were usually more strongly related to adjustment than were measures of attachment examined in isolation.

Several studies have evaluated whether children who form insecure attachments to caregivers are likely to show externalizing behavior problems in middle childhood. Some studies have found that avoidant attachment is related to teacher or peer reports of more externalizing behavior problems (Easterbrooks & Abeles, 2000; Easterbrooks et al., 1993; Finnegan et al., 1996; Granot & Mayseless, 2001; Yunger et al., 2005). In addition, attachment security has been linked to lower levels of externalizing problems (Davies et al., 2004; El-Sheikh & Buckhalt, 2003; Harold et al., 2004). Lyons-Ruth (1996) proposed that disorganized attachment might be most clearly related to externalizing problems, but disorganized attachment has not been associated consistently with externalizing problems in middle childhood (Granot & Mayseless, 2001; Jacobsen & Hofmann, 1997).

Several studies have supported the hypothesis that securely attached children will experience lower levels of internalizing problems (Bohlin et al., 2000; Davies, Harold, Goeke-Morey, & Cummings, 2002; Easterbrooks & Abeles, 2000; Easterbrooks et al., 1993; Graham & Easterbrooks, 2000; Granot & Mayseless, 2001; Harold et al., 2004; Muris, Mayer, & Meesters, 2000; for an exception, see El-Sheikh & Buckhalt, 2003). Other studies have examined how internalizing problems are related to specific forms of insecurity. Although there has been speculation that internalizing problems are most likely to be related to ambivalent or preoccupied attachment (Finnegan et al., 1996; Renken et al., 1989), studies have shown measures of internalizing problems to correlate with avoidance (Finnegan et al., 1996; Yunger et al., 2005), ambivalent/preoccupied attachment (Finnegan et al., 1996; Yunger et al., 2005), and attachment disorganization (Graham & Easterbrooks, 2000). The lack of specificity in the associations with different insecure patterns is difficult to evaluate, given that the few studies available have used different measures of internalizing problems (e.g., depression, anxiety, social withdrawal, aggregate measures) and different measures of attachment (observations and questionnaires), and that only a few studies have examined attachment disorganization.

Finally, two studies have examined attachment in middle childhood in clinical populations. Wright and colleagues (1995) found that children recruited from a clinic were less secure and more avoidant in their attachments than children from a community sample were. Another study (Clarke, Ungerer, Chahoud, Johnson, & Stiefel, 2002) found that children with attention-deficit/hyperactivity disorder were more likely than those in a control group to have insecure attachment representations.

In summary, the evidence suggests that children who form a secure attachment to their mothers are less likely to experience clinical symptoms in middle childhood. There are virtually no data on father–child attachment and children's adjustment. In addition, there is currently no clear evidence that specific forms of insecurity are linked to specific clinical symptoms; however, the question has not been explored extensively, and the lack of consistency in the findings may be due to the use of different methods to assess attachment and the measurement of different symptoms across studies. Finally, it is worth reiterating that attachment is likely to be only one of many factors that influence the development of psychopathology in children (see DeKlyen & Greenberg, Chapter 27, this volume), and thus it may not be surprising that when considered in isolation attachment is not strongly related to signs of psychopathology. When attachment has been linked empirically with later psychopathology, it is possible that other factors (such as genes, poverty, abuse, and peer relationships) were also involved.

CONCLUSIONS AND FUTURE DIRECTIONS

This is an interesting time for research on attachment in middle childhood. An overview volume has been published on the topic (Kerns & Richardson, 2005), and several authors have proposed hypotheses regarding normative changes that may occur during this age period. Progress has been made in the development of new measures that now need to be validated. There appears to be an acceleration of empirical research on the topic. The extension of attachment research to middle childhood fills an important gap in our knowledge and allows for further study of how changes in attachment trajectories may predict later development.

A limitation in the literature is that research often seems driven mainly by a desire to retest old findings and questions in a new age period, rather than to take the developmental context of middle childhood into account. Certainly it is important to learn that basic tenets of attachment theory are confirmed in middle childhood (e.g., secure attachment is associated with responsive parenting). Nevertheless, it would be even more interesting if there were further consideration of how the nature of middle childhood might affect the study of attachment at this age. For example, if shifts in parental supervision are the most prominent change in parent–child relationships during this time period, it is important to consider how attachment is related not just to responsive parenting, but also to the ways in which parents and children negotiate greater child autonomy. In studies of how attachment might be related to peer relationships, it is important to consider the key features of peer relationships during middle childhood (Kerns, 1994). More broadly, an important goal for future research is to understand how attachment is influenced by intraindividual development and features of the social context in middle childhood (Richardson, 2005).

There are a number of thorny problems with the current theoretical and methodological approaches to attachment in middle childhood. Researchers have adopted several different theoretical conceptualizations that are not equivalent. This is not always made clear in research reports, where important distinctions are often blurred by the use of the same term "attachment." At a minimum, it is important to pay careful attention to defining the term "attachment," making clear how it is conceptualized in a particular study. Even when investigators share a similar orientation, they often employ different measures. Although at one time there was a lack of attachment measures for middle childhood, the current problem is that there are many measures, most of which have not been fully validated. More attention needs to be paid to validation of measures, and studies are needed to explore the overlap among different measures and approaches. Investigators need to consider their choice of measures carefully, making sure that the chosen measure captures the construct of interest. Self-report questionnaires have been used to assess children's perceptions of attachment, which is one specific way of conceptualizing attachment. Although their use should not be ruled out a priori, it is important to recognize their limitations. Studies in which questionnaire measures of attachment are correlated only with other questionnaires completed by children are methodologically quite weak and are best avoided.

The empirical literature has shown that, as found at other ages, parent–child attachment is related to individual differences in children's social, emotional, and cognitive development. For example, there is substantial evidence that mother–child attachment is related to children's school adaptation and peer relationships, and there is not a strong need for additional studies documenting these associations. There are still important gaps in our knowledge. Relatively few studies have examined specific mechanisms that might account for the documented associations. In addition, relatively few studies have explored how attachment is related to emotional development and self-concept. There has been very little study of factors that might account for both continuity and normative changes in attachment at this age period. Another limitation is that most studies have focused exclusively on mother–child attachment, without considering the possible importance of children's attachments to fathers or siblings.

In some ways, this chapter provides a narrow and perhaps somewhat misleading view of development, in that it focuses exclusively on attachment. In infancy, parents clearly have a dominant role in socialization, acting as gatekeepers as well as directly influencing their children. Although parents continue in these roles at older ages, the expansion of children's social world and changes in the developmental tasks they face mean that attachment is likely to be only one of many important influences on development. Thus a challenge for the field is to understand how attachment and other aspects of social experience operate together to influence children's social development. We need more studies that place attachment within a broader context, considering multiple influences (see Sroufe et al., 2005, for an illustration and elaboration of this point). This would also allow researchers to determine whether and how attachment mediates or moderates the influence of other variables. In conclusion, the field is poised for additional research on the topic of attachment in middle childhood. There are many opportunities for investigators to address key questions regarding the nature and significance of attachment in middle childhood.

REFERENCES

Ainsworth, M. D. S. (1990). Epilogue: Some considerations regarding theory and assessment relevant to attachments beyond infancy. In M. T. Greenberg, D. Cicchetti, & E. M. Cummings (Eds.), *Attachment in the preschool years* (pp. 463–488). Chicago: University of Chicago Press.

Ammaniti, M., Speranza, A. M., & Fedele, S. (2005). Attachment in infancy and in early and late childhood: A longitudinal study. In K. A. Kerns & R. A. Richardson (Eds.), *Attachment in middle childhood* (pp. 115–136). New York: Guilford Press.

Ammaniti, M., van IJzendoorn, M. H., Speranza, A. M., & Tambelli, R. (2000). Internal working models of attachment during late childhood and early adolescence: An exploration of stability and change. *Attachment and Human Development, 2,* 328–346.

Aviezer, O., Resnick, G., Sagi, A., & Gini, M. (2002). School competence in young adolescence: Links to early attachment relationships beyond concurrent self-perceived competence and representations of relationships. *International Journal of Behavioral Development, 26,* 397–409.

Bohlin, G., Hagekull, B., & Rydell, A. (2000). Attachment and social functioning: A longitudinal study from infancy to middle childhood. *Social Development, 9,* 24–39.

Booth, C. L., Rose-Krasnor, L., McKinnon, J., & Rubin, K. H. (1994). Predicting social adjustment in middle childhood: The role of preschool attachment security and maternal style. *Social Development, 3,* 189–204.

Booth, C. L., Rubin, K. H., & Rose-Krasnor, L. (1998). Perceptions of emotional support from mother and friend in middle childhood: Links with social-emotional adaptation and preschool attachment security. *Child Development, 69,* 427–442.

Bowers, L., Smith, P. K., & Binney, V. (1994). Perceived family relationships of bullies, victims, and bully/victims in middle childhood. *Journal of Social and Personal Relationships, 11*, 215–232.

Bowlby, J. (1969/1982). *Attachment and loss: Vol. 1. Attachment.* New York: Basic Books.

Bowlby, J. (1973). *Attachment and loss: Vol. 2. Separation: Anxiety and anger.* New York: Basic Books.

Bowlby, J. (1979). *The making and breaking of affectional bonds.* London: Tavistock.

Bowlby, J. (1989). The role of attachment in personality development and psychopathology. In S. I. Greenspan & G. H. Pollock (Eds.), *The course of life: Vol. 1. Infancy* (pp. 229–270). Madison, CT: International Universities Press.

Bretherton, I. (1985). Attachment theory: Retrospect and prospect. In I. Bretherton & E. Waters (Eds.), Growing points of attachment theory and research. *Monographs of the Society for Research in Child Development, 50*(1–2, Serial No. 209), 3–35.

Bretherton, I. (1992). The origins of attachment theory: John Bowlby and Mary Ainsworth. *Developmental Psychology, 28*, 759–775.

Carlson, E. A. (1998). A prospective longitudinal study of attachment disorganization/disorientation. *Child Development, 69*, 1107–1128.

Cassidy, J. (1988). Child–mother attachment and the self in six-year-olds. *Child Development, 59*, 121–134.

Cassidy, J. (1994). Emotion regulation: Influences of attachment relationships. In N. A. Fox (Ed.), The development of emotion regulation: Biological and behavioral considerations. *Monographs of the Society for Research in Child Development, 59*(2–3, Serial No. 240), 228–249.

Cassidy, J., Ziv, Y., Mehta, T. G., & Feeney, B. C. (2003). Feedback seeking in children and adolescents: Associations with self-perceptions, attachment representations, and depression. *Child Development, 74*, 612–628.

Clarke, L., Ungerer, J., Chahoud, K., Johnson, S., & Stiefel, I. (2002). Attention deficit hyperactivity disorder is associated with attachment insecurity. *Clinical Child Psychology and Psychiatry, 7*, 179–198.

Coleman, P. K. (2003). Perceptions of parent–child attachment, social self-efficacy, and peer relationships in middle childhood. *Infant and Child Development, 12*, 351–368.

Contreras, J. M., & Kerns, K. A. (2000). Emotion regulation processes: Explaining links between parent–child attachment and peer relationships. In K. A. Kerns, J. M. Contreras, & A. M. Neal-Barnett (Eds.), *Family and peers: Linking two social worlds* (pp. 1–25). Westport, CT: Praeger.

Contreras, J. M., Kerns, K. A., Weimer, B. L., Gentzler, A. L., & Tomich, P. L. (2000). Emotion regulation as a mediator of associations between mother–child attachment and peer relationships in middle childhood. *Journal of Family Psychology, 14*, 111–124.

Davies, P. T., Cummings, E. M., & Winter, M. A. (2004). Pathways between profiles of family functioning, child security in the interparental subsystem, and child psychological problems. *Development and Psychopathology, 16*, 525–550.

Davies, P. T., Harold, G. T., Goeke-Morey, M. C., & Cummings, E. M. (2002). Child emotional security and interparental conflict. *Monographs of the Society for Research in Child Development, 67*(3, Serial No. 270).

De Wolff, M. S., & van IJzendoorn, M. H. (1997). Sensitivity and attachment: A meta-analysis on parental antecedents of infant attachment. *Child Development, 68*, 571–591.

Doyle, A. B., Markiewicz, D., Brendgen, M., Lieberman, M., & Voss, K. (2000). Child attachment security and self-concept: Associations with mother and father attachment style and marital quality. *Merrill–Palmer Quarterly, 46*, 514–539.

Dwyer, K. M. (2005). The meaning and measurement of attachment in middle and late childhood. *Human Development, 48*, 155–182.

Easterbrooks, M. A., & Abeles, R. (2000). Windows to the self in 8-year-olds: Bridges to attachment representation and behavioral adjustment. *Attachment and Human Development, 2*, 85–106.

Easterbrooks, M. A., Biesecker, G., & Lyons-Ruth, K. (2000). Infancy predictors of emotional availability in middle childhood: The roles of attachment security and maternal depressive symptomatology. *Attachment and Human Development, 2*, 170–187.

Easterbrooks, M. A., Davidson, C. E., & Chazan, R. (1993). Psychosocial risk, attachment, and behavior problems among school-aged children. *Development and Psychopathology, 5*, 389–402.

El-Sheikh, M., & Buckhalt, J. A. (2003). Parental problem drinking and children's adjustment: Attachment and family functioning as moderators and mediators of risk. *Journal of Family Psychology, 17*, 510–520.

Feeney, B. C., & Cassidy, J. (2003). Reconstructive memory related to adolescent–parent conflict interactions: The influence of attachment-related representation on immediate perceptions and changes in perception over time. *Journal of Personality and Social Psychology, 85*, 944–955.

Finnegan, R. A., Hodges, E. V. E., & Perry, D. G. (1996). Preoccupied and avoidant coping during middle childhood. *Child Development, 67*, 1318–1328.

Freitag, M. K., Belsky, J., Grossmann, K., Grossmann, K., & Scheuerer-Englisch, H. (1996). Continuity in parent–child relationships from infancy to middle childhood and relations with friendship competence. *Child Development, 67*, 1437–1454.

Fury, G., Carlson, E. A., & Sroufe, L. A. (1997). Children's representations of attachment relationships in family drawings. *Child Development, 68*, 1154–1164.

Gentzler, A. L., & Kerns, K. A. (2006). Adult attachment and memory of emotional reactions to negative and positive events. *Cognition and Emotion, 20*, 20–42.

George, C., Kaplan, N., & Main, M. (1984). *Adult At-*

tachment Interview protocol. Unpublished manuscript, University of California at Berkeley.

George, C., Kaplan, N., & Main, M. (1985). Adult Attachment Interview protocol (2nd ed.). Unpublished manuscript, University of California at Berkeley.

George, C., Kaplan, N., & Main, M. (1996). Adult Attachment Interview protocol (3rd ed.). Unpublished manuscript, University of California at Berkeley.

Graham, C. A., & Easterbrooks, M. A. (2000). School-aged children's vulnerability to depressive symptomatology: The role of attachment security, maternal depressive symptomatology, and economic risk. Development and Psychopathology, 12, 201–213.

Granot, D., & Mayseless, O. (2001). Attachment security and adjustment to school in middle childhood. International Journal of Behavioral Development, 25, 530–541.

Grossmann, K., Grossmann, K. E., Fremmer-Bombik, E., Kindler, H., Scheuerer-Englisch, H., & Zimmermann, P. (2002). The uniqueness of the child–father attachment relationship: Fathers' sensitive and challenging play as a pivotal variable in a 16-year longitudinal study. Social Development, 11, 307–331.

Grossmann, K. E., & Grossmann, K. (1991). Attachment quality as an organizer of emotional and behavioral responses. In P. Marris, J. Stevenson-Hinde, & C. Parkes (Eds.), Attachment across the life cycle (pp. 93–114). New York: Routledge.

Hagekull, B., & Bohlin, G. (2003). Early temperament and attachment as predictors of the five factor model of personality. Attachment and Human Development, 5, 2–18.

Harold, G., T., Shelton, K. H., Goeke-Morey, M. C., & Cummings, E. M. (2004). Marital conflict, child emotional security about family relationships, and child adjustment. Social Development, 13, 350–376.

Howes, C., & Tonyan, H. (2000). Links between adult and peer relations across four developmental periods. In K. A. Kerns, J. M. Contreras, & A. M. Neal-Barnett (Eds.), Family and peers: Linking two social worlds (pp. 85–113). Westport, CT: Praeger.

Jacobsen, T., Edelstein, W., & Hofmann, V. (1994). A longitudinal study of the relation between representations of attachment in childhood and cognitive functioning in childhood and adolescence. Developmental Psychology, 30, 112–124.

Jacobsen, T., & Hofmann, V. (1997). Children's attachment representations: Longitudinal relations to school behavior and academic competency in middle childhood and adolescence. Developmental Psychology, 33, 703–710.

Karavasilis, L., Doyle, A. B., & Markiewicz, D. (2003). Associations between parenting style and attachment to mother in middle childhood and adolescence. International Journal of Behavioral Development, 27, 153–164.

Kerns, K. A. (1994). A developmental model of the relations between mother–child attachment and friendship. In R. Erber & R. Gilmour (Eds.), Theoretical

frameworks for personal relationships (pp. 129–156). Hillsdale, NJ: Erlbaum.

Kerns, K. A. (1996). Individual differences in friendship quality: Links to child–mother attachment. In W. M. Bukowski, A. F. Newcomb, & W. W. Hartup (Eds.), The company they keep: Friendship in childhood and adolescence (pp. 137–157). New York: Cambridge University Press.

Kerns, K. A., Abraham, M. M., Schlegelmilch, A., & Morgan, T. A. (2007). Mother–child attachment in later middle childhood: Assessment approaches and associations with mood and emotion regulation. Attachment and Human Development, 9, 33–53.

Kerns, K. A., Aspelmeier, J. E., Gentzler, A. L., & Grabill, C. M. (2001). Parent–child attachment and monitoring in middle childhood. Journal of Family Psychology, 15, 69–81.

Kerns, K. A., Brumariu, L. E., & Abraham, M. M. (in press). Homesickness at summer camp: Associations with the mother–child relationship, social self-concept, and peer relationships in middle childhood. Merrill–Palmer Quarterly.

Kerns, K. A., Klepac, L., & Cole, A. (1996). Peer relationships and preadolescents' perceptions of security in the child–mother relationship. Developmental Psychology, 32, 457–466.

Kerns, K. A., & Richardson, R. A. (Eds.). (2005). Attachment in middle childhood. New York: Guilford Press.

Kerns, K. A., Schlegelmilch, A., Morgan, T. A., & Abraham, M. M. (2005). Assessing attachment in middle childhood. In K. A. Kerns & R. A. Richardson (Eds.), Attachment in middle childhood (pp. 46–70). New York: Guilford Press.

Kerns, K. A., & Seibert, A. C. (2008). Finding your way through the thicket: Promising approaches to assessing attachment in middle childhood. Manuscript submitted for publication.

Kerns, K. A., Tomich, P. L., Aspelmeier, J. E., & Contreras, J. M. (2000). Attachment-based assessments of parent–child relationships in middle childhood. Developmental Psychology, 36, 614–626.

Kerns, K. A., Tomich, P. L., & Kim, P. (2006). Normative trends in children's perceptions of availability and utilization of attachment figures in middle childhood. Social Development, 15, 1–22.

Kobak, R., Rosenthal, N., & Serwik, A. (2005). The attachment hierarchy in middle childhood: Conceptual and methodological issues. In K. A. Kerns & R. A. Richardson (Eds.), Attachment in middle childhood (pp. 71–88). New York: Guilford Press.

Lewis, M., & Feiring, C. (1989). Early predictors of childhood friendship. In T. J. Berndt & G. W. Ladd (Eds.), Peer relationships in child development (pp. 246–273). New York: Wiley.

Lieberman, M., Doyle, A., & Markiewicz, D. (1999). Developmental patterns in security of attachment to mother and father in late childhood and early adolescence: Associations with peer relations. Child Development, 70, 202–213.

Lyons-Ruth, K. (1996). Attachment relationships among

children with aggressive behavior problems: The role of disorganized early attachment patterns. *Journal of Consulting and Clinical Psychology, 64,* 64–73.

Lyons-Ruth, K., Easterbrooks, M. A., & Cibelli, C. D. (1997). Infant attachment strategies, infant mental lag, and maternal depressive symptoms: Predictors of internalizing and externalizing problems at age 7. *Developmental Psychology, 33,* 681–692.

Maccoby, E. (1984). Middle childhood in the context of the family. In W. A. Collins (Ed.), *Development during middle childhood* (pp. 184–239). Washington, DC: National Academy Press.

Madigan, S., Ladd, M., & Goldberg, S. (2003). A picture is worth a thousand words: Children's representations of family as indicators of early attachment. *Attachment and Human Development, 5,* 19–37.

Main, M., Kaplan, N., & Cassidy, J. (1985). Security of infancy, childhood, and adulthood: A move to the level of representation. In I. Bretherton & E. Waters (Eds.), Growing points of attachment theory and research. *Monographs of the Society for Research in Child Development, 50*(1–2, Serial No. 209), 66–104.

Marvin, R. S., & Britner, P. A. (1999). Normative development: The ontogeny of attachment. In J. Cassidy & P. R. Shaver (Eds.), *Handbook of attachment: Theory, research, and clinical applications* (pp. 44–67). New York: Guilford Press.

Mayseless, O. (2005). Ontogeny of attachment in middle childhood: Conceptualization of normative changes. In K. A. Kerns & R. A. Richardson (Eds.), *Attachment in middle childhood* (pp. 1–23). New York: Guilford Press.

Moss, E., & St.-Laurent, D. (2001). Attachment at school age and academic performance. *Developmental Psychology, 37,* 863–874.

Moss, E., St.-Laurent, D., Dubois-Comtois, K., & Cyr, C. (2005). Quality of attachment at school age: Relations between child attachment behavior, psychosocial functioning, and school performance. In K. A. Kerns & R. A. Richardson (Eds.), *Attachment in middle childhood* (pp. 189–211). New York: Guilford Press.

Muris, P., Mayer, B., & Meesters, C. (2000). Self-reported attachment style, anxiety, and depression in children. *Social Behavior and Personality, 28,* 157–162.

Oppenheim, D., Koren-Karie, N., & Sagi-Schwartz, A. (2006). Emotion dialogues between mothers and children at 4.5 years and 7.5 years: Relations with children's attachment at 1 year. *Child Development, 78,* 38–52.

Raikes, H. A., & Thompson, R. A. (2005). Relationships past, present, and future: Reflections on attachment in middle childhood. In K. A. Kerns & R. A. Richardson (Eds.), *Attachment in middle childhood* (pp. 255–282). New York: Guilford Press.

Renken, B., Egeland, B., Marvinney, D., Mangelsdorf, S., & Sroufe, L. A. (1989). Early childhood antecedents of aggression and passive-withdrawal in early elementary school. *Journal of Personality, 57,* 257–281.

Richardson, R. A. (2005). Developmental contextual considerations of parent–child attachment in the later middle childhood years. In K. A. Kerns & R. A. Richardson (Eds.), *Attachment in middle childhood* (pp. 24–45). New York: Guilford Press.

Schneider, B. H., Atkinson, L., & Tardif, C. (2001). Child–parent attachment and children's peer relations: A quantitative review. *Developmental Psychology, 37,* 86–100.

Sharpe, T. M., Killen, J. D., Bryson, S. W., Shisslak, C. M., Estes, L. S., Gray, N., et al. (1998). Attachment style and weight concerns in preadolescent and adolescent girls. *International Journal of Eating Disorders, 23,* 39–44.

Shulman, S., Elicker, J., & Sroufe, L. A. (1994). Stages of friendship growth in preadolescence as related to attachment history. *Journal of Social and Personal Relationships, 11,* 341–361.

Sroufe, L. A. (1983). Infant–caregiver attachment and patterns of adaptation in preschool: The roots of maladaptation and competence. In M. Perlmutter (Ed.), *Minnesota Symposium on Child Psychology: Vol. 16. Development and policy concerning children with special needs* (pp. 41–83). Hillsdale, NJ: Erlbaum.

Sroufe, L. A. (1988). The role of infant–caregiver attachment in development. In J. Belsky & T. Nezworski (Eds.), *Clinical implications of attachment* (pp. 18–38). Hillsdale, NJ: Erlbaum.

Sroufe, L. A., Bennett, C., Englund, M., Urban, J., & Shulman, S. (1993). The significance of gender boundaries in preadolescence: Contemporary correlates and antecedents of boundary violation and maintenance. *Child Development, 64,* 455–466.

Sroufe, L. A., Egeland, B., & Carlson, E. A. (1999). One social world: The integrated development of parent–child and peer relationships. In W. A. Collins & B. Laursen (Eds.), *Relationships as developmental contexts* (pp. 241–261). Hillsdale, NJ: Erlbaum.

Sroufe, L. A., Egeland, B., Carlson, E. A., & Collins, W. A. (2005). *The development of the person: The Minnesota Study of Risk and Adaptation from Birth to Adulthood.* New York: Guilford Press.

Sroufe, L. A., Egeland, B., & Kreutzer, T. (1990). The fate of early experience following developmental change: Longitudinal approaches to individual adaptation in childhood. *Child Development, 61,* 1363–1373.

Stams, G. J., Juffer, F., & van IJzendoorn, M. H. (2002). Maternal sensitivity, infant attachment, and temperament in early childhood predict adjustment in middle childhood: The case of adopted children and their biologically unrelated parents. *Developmental Psychology, 38,* 806–821.

Steele, H., & Steele, M. (2005). The construct of coherence as an indicator of attachment security in middle childhood: The friends and family interview. In K. A. Kerns & R. A. Richardson (Eds.), *Attachment in middle childhood* (pp. 137–160). New York: Guilford Press.

Target, M., Fonagy, P., & Shmueli-Goetz, Y. (2003). Attachment representations in school-age children:

The development of the Child Attachment Interview (CAI). *Journal of Child Psychotherapy, 29,* 171–186.

Thurber, C. A., & Sigman, M. D. (1998). Preliminary models of risk and protective factors for childhood homesickness: Review and empirical synthesis. *Child Development, 69,* 903–934.

Thurber, C. A., Sigman, M. D., Weisz, J. R., & Schmidt, C. K. (1999). Homesickness in preadolescent and adolescent girls: Risk factors, behavioral correlates, and sequelae. *Journal of Clinical Child Psychology, 28,* 185–196.

van IJzendoorn, M. H. (1995). Adult attachment representations, parental responsiveness, and infant attachment: A meta-analysis on the predictive validity of the Adult Attachment Interview. *Psychological Bulletin, 117,* 387–403.

van IJzendoorn, M. H., Dijkstra, J., & Bus, A. G. (1995). Attachment, intelligence, and language: A meta-analysis. *Social Development, 4,* 115–128.

Verschueren, K., & Marcoen, A. (2002). Perceptions of self and relationship with parents in aggressive and nonaggressive rejected children. *Journal of School Psychology, 40,* 501–522.

Verschueren, K., & Marcoen, A. (2005). Perceived security of attachment to mother and father: Developmental differences and relations to self-worth and peer relationships at school. In K. A. Kerns & R. A. Richardson (Eds.), *Attachment in middle childhood* (pp. 212–230). New York: Guilford Press.

Waters, E., Kondo-Ikemura, K., Posada, G., & Richters, J. E. (1991). Learning to love: Mechanisms and milestones. In M. Gunnar & L. A. Sroufe (Eds.), *Minnesota Symposium on Child Psychology: Vol. 23. Self processes in early development* (pp. 217–255). Hillsdale, NJ: Erlbaum.

Wright, J. C., Binney, V., & Smith, P. K. (1995). Security of attachment in 8–12-year-olds: A revised version of the Separation Anxiety Test, its psychometric properties, and clinical interpretation. *Journal of Child Psychology and Psychiatry, 36,* 757–774.

Yunger, J. L., Corby, B. C., & Perry, D. G. (2005). Dimensions of attachment in middle childhood. In K. A. Kerns & R. A. Richardson (Eds.), *Attachment in middle childhood* (pp. 89–114). New York: Guilford Press.

Ziv, Y., Oppenheim, D., & Sagi-Schwartz, A. (2004). Social information processing in middle childhood: Relations to infant–mother attachment. *Attachment and Human Development, 6,* 327–348.

CHAPTER 18

The Measurement of Attachment Security and Related Constructs in Infancy and Early Childhood

JUDITH SOLOMON
CAROL GEORGE

In this chapter we examine the methods of assessing attachment security in infancy and early childhood, at both the level of behavior and the level of representation. Our first goal is to provide the reader with an overview and summary of available measures, including new or lesser-known measures, along with information about their psychometric properties and the ways in which they have been used in research. Our second goal is to evaluate the current state of measurement in the field of attachment. How well do the available instruments and protocols actually reflect the construct of attachment security? How useful are these measures for testing core predictions in attachment theory?

This chapter can be used in several ways. Some readers, especially those new to research in this area, can use the chapter as a source of information to help select measures appropriate to their research. For readers who are familiar with childhood attachment assessment and well grounded in attachment theory, this is an opportunity to examine all of the measures together. This kind of overview is important for understanding the development of the field and providing a sense of new directions and opportunities for theory and research.

THE DOMAIN OF ATTACHMENT SECURITY

"Attachment security" is defined by Ainsworth, Blehar, Waters, and Wall (1978) as the state of being secure or untroubled about the availability of the attachment figure. As a construct, security can never be directly observed, but must be inferred from what is observable. Furthermore, a construct is "evidenced in a variety of forms of behavior and not perfectly so in any one of them" (Nunnally, 1978, p. 84). How, then, do we determine whether a particular measure of attachment security is a "good" or valid measure of the construct?[1]

In practice, psychologists typically follow a three-step process. First, they operationalize the construct, either intuitively or with respect to theory or prior research. Second, they establish the basic reliability of the measure, asking themselves, "Can it be replicated over time [test–retest or short-term stability of scores or categories], and, to the extent that the measure is tester-derived and thus requires some judgment, can scores, codes, and so forth be agreed upon?" Finally, they evaluate how well the measure predicts (in the broadest sense) other theoretically important variables (convergent validity) or is uncorrelated with theoretically unrelated variables (discriminant validity) (Campbell & Fiske, 1959).

Although this approach is well accepted, Nunnally (1978) has pointed out that it is based on an inherent circularity in logic. We predict a relation between constructs, we "find" it using measures of the constructs at hand, and we thereby infer that our measures are valid. Optimally, construct validation requires three somewhat different steps (Nunnally, 1978): (1) The domain of relevant indices or variables ("observables") must be specified, indicating which variables are indicative of security and which are not; (2) the intercorrelations among multiple concurrent measures of the construct must be ascertained; and (3) each measure must be cross-validated with respect to a network of other theoretically important constructs that have been similarly validated. Rather than being sequential, these three steps constitute a reflective process, in which knowledge gained from one step transforms our understanding of the others.

For attachment researchers, the domain of "observables," at least for infancy and toddlerhood (12–20 months), is currently drawn from Bowlby's (1969/1982, 1973, 1980) ethological attachment theory. "Attachment behaviors" are those that increase proximity to or maintain contact with a particular attachment figure. They are understood to be organized with respect to an internal control system (the attachment system) that has the adaptive function of protection and the set goal of physical proximity or felt security (Sroufe, 1979). A critical feature of this model, with important implications for measurement, must be emphasized: The type of attachment behavior observed depends on the degree to which the attachment system is activated. When a young child is alarmed, he or she can be expected to signal clearly for proximity to and contact with the attachment figure (e.g., crying, approaching, reaching, clinging). Once these goals are achieved, and in the absence of further disturbance, the child can be expected to accept some distance from the attachment figure and return to exploration. Attachment behavior under conditions of low activation, often referred to as "secure-base behavior," can be difficult to distinguish from friendly, affiliative behavior and can be very much influenced by features of the external environment (e.g., how far away the child can wander, how visible the mother is) (Carr, Dabbs, & Carr, 1975; Rheingold & Eckerman, 1970).

Ainsworth and colleagues (1978) have argued that this basic pattern (a shift from exploration to attachment behaviors and back) will appear disturbed or distorted to the extent that the infant perceives the attachment figure to be inaccessible or unresponsive. Thus Ainsworth's classic measure of attachments in infancy (the Strange Situation), and the more recent Waters and Deane Attachment Q-Sort measure (AQS; Waters, 1995; Waters & Deane, 1985), which are described more fully later, focus on deviations from this basic pattern as a measure of insecurity in infant–parent attachment.

Attachment theory is less specific regarding appropriate measures of security in the third and fourth years of life and beyond. The attachment system is believed to function throughout this period, and indeed throughout the lifespan, but with diminishing sensitivity. Fewer situations are perceived as threatening, and knowledge of the parent's accessibility (rather than actual proximity or contact) is increasingly effective in terminating attachment behavior. In addition, the broader and more flexible behavioral repertoire of the older child, as well as the child's capacity to comprehend cognitively and therefore to anticipate and coordinate with the parent's behavior, can make it more difficult for scientific observers to perceive the underlying organization of attachment behavior. At the same time, the achievement of language and symbolic operations during this period begins to make it feasible to assess attachment security at the representational level.

CORE THEORETICAL PREDICTIONS

Whether one is following Nunnally's model of optimal construct validation or the commonly accepted but more approximate procedures of most investigators, the predictive (retrodictive, concurrent, predictive) validity of a measure is a fundamental concern. There are probably as many theoretically interesting relations among constructs in the field of attachment as there are researchers to propose them. Attachment theory as articulated by Bowlby and Ainsworth, however, provides certain key predictions regarding the relation between security and other variables that are core to the theory itself. The validity of any particular measure of security should be assessed at a minimum with respect to these. Acknowledging that there may be some dispute in the boundary areas, we propose the following core predictions:

1. *Attachment security should be positively related to the caregiver's accessibility and responsiveness to the child.* This prediction is implicit in the definition of security itself—that is, the state of being untroubled (confident) that the attachment figure will be available and will permit proximity and contact to the extent needed. An important corollary to this prediction is that attachment security with one caregiver should be independent of security with the other, insofar as the sensitivity of the two caregivers can be shown to differ. This follows from the definition of attachment security as a reflection of a particular relationship (Ainsworth et al., 1978) and not (entirely) a property of the child (i.e., not a function of temperament or some other quality).

Beginning with Ainsworth's pioneering work, which we describe more fully below, maternal responsiveness and accessibility are typically assessed through variables reflecting the mother's prompt and appropriate response to the infant's attachment signals—that is, at the behavioral level. In the last 10–15 years, the field has shown increasing interest in the representational aspects of parental (especially maternal) sensitivity, and in the maternal qualities that permit or support sensitivity. By extension, such variables ought to be related to attachment security in a similar fashion to behavioral sensitivity, and in turn can provide validity information for attachment measures. (Although discussion of this broad array of variables is beyond the scope of this chapter, further information about them and about their links to attachment measures is provided in George & Solomon, Chapter 35, and Hesse, Chapter 25, this volume.)

2. *Attachment security in a particular caregiver–child relationship should tend to remain stable over time (continuity).* Although Bowlby (1973, 1980) was well aware of destabilizing influences on infant–caregiver attachment (e.g., repeated separation, life stress) and avoided the doctrine of critical periods, he proposed that the quality of attachment should become increasingly stable and resistant to change as a function of mutual adaptation in interaction patterns and in each party's expectations about the other and the relationship. Sroufe and Waters (1977) emphasized the organizational quality of attachment; that is, although particular attachment behaviors may show little stability (due to the situation or the child's development), the underlying quality or organization of the relationship is expected to remain stable.

3. *Attachment security should predict other important aspects of development.* Related to the notion of continuity, but distinct from it, is the general hypothesis argued by Bowlby (1973) and elaborated both theoretically and empirically by Sroufe (1979) that attachment security should predict other key aspects of development. Bowlby emphasized the effects of insecurity arising from separation and loss on the development of psychopathology. In contrast, Sroufe articulated the more normative construct of "coherence" in development; that is, successes or failures in one developmental task (such as attachment in infancy) should predispose the child (and the caregiver–child dyad) to success or failure in subsequent developmental tasks (e.g., autonomy, social competence). Sroufe's notion, though perhaps less central to attachment theory proper, parallels in many respects Erikson's (1950) classic formulation of developmental stages and has captured the attention of many researchers. It is important to note that it implies prediction to constructs other than attachment security, either concurrently or from one developmental period to another. In contrast, continuity implies prediction from an attachment security measure at one time to the same or a different measure of attachment security at another. Demonstration of *coherence* across time does not necessarily establish stability in the attachment relationship.

4. *Attachment security can be assessed by using similar or parallel measures cross-culturally and across attachment figures.* In the first two volumes of his *Attachment and Loss* trilogy, Bowlby (1969/1982, 1973, 1980) painstakingly built a case for the species-specific and therefore universal nature of attachment behavior in the young child. To the degree that a measure is based upon ethological attachment theory, it should function similarly across cultures; that is, it should be as effective in describing the range of attachment relationships found in one culture (society, ethnic group, socioeconomic status [SES]) as it is in any other. In addition, it should be expected to be correlated in similar ways to measures of other theoretically important constructs, particularly to caregiver behavior. By virtue of the same reasoning, the effectiveness of security measures and the pattern of correlations to caregiver behavior should be similar for all attachment figures (e.g., mother, father, other caregivers).

ORGANIZATION OF THIS CHAPTER

For the period of infancy through early childhood (ages 12 to approximately 72 months), measures of attachment security are based on observation of behavior of one type or another. These measures can be further divided according to whether they focus on the organization of attachment behavior directed toward the caregiver or on the child's linguistic or play behavior (representational measures of attachment). Although the field of attachment has its theoretical origins in Bowlby's ethological theory of attachment, its empirical origins and the foundation of almost all subsequent efforts at assessment lie in the classification approach to attachment relationships pioneered by Ainsworth and colleagues (1978). This system of multidimensional categories of relationship, assessed on the basis of the infant's behavior in a laboratory separation and reunion context, has been both intuitively and theoretically compelling. The majority of measures for the period beyond early toddlerhood have been designed deliberately to capture these same or similar qualitative differences in child–caregiver attachment at both the behavioral and representational levels. A second strand of development is represented by Waters's (1995) AQS method, which is designed to permit observers (either trained observers or caregivers) to describe infant or child attachment behavior in the home.

We begin by describing Ainsworth's classification system and a subsequent modification of it (specifically, the inclusion of the disorganized/disoriented category). This is followed by a description and discussion of classification systems for reunion behavior and mental representation of preschool and kindergarten-age children, and then by information on the AQS approach. Each section includes a brief discussion of unresolved issues in the construct validation of the measure(s) in question. We conclude with a general discussion of measurement in the field.[2]

ATTACHMENT CLASSIFICATION IN INFANCY: THE STRANGE SITUATION

Attachment classification is based on the behavior of the young toddler (12–20 months of age) in the Strange Situation. This is a laboratory procedure that was designed to capture the balance of attachment and exploratory behavior under conditions of increasing though moderate stress (Ainsworth et al., 1978). Full directions for running the session and for classification are presented in Ainsworth and colleagues (1978). An outline of the episodes that make up the Strange Situation is shown in Table 18.1. Ainsworth's system provides instructions for classifying the infant's attachment relationship into one of three main groups: a "secure" group (B) and two "insecure" groups, "avoidant" (A) and "resistant" or "ambivalent" (C). Table 18.2 provides a brief description of classification criteria. Instructions are also available for designating eight subgroups, but the subgroups are rarely examined separately (due to limited sample sizes) and are not considered further here. Classification is based on the infant's behavior toward the caregiver during the two reunion episodes, viewed in the context of behavior in the preceding and intervening episodes and in response to the caregiver's current behavior. The infant's behavior during reunions can also be rated with respect to four scales of infant–caregiver interactive behavior that are used in the process of classification: proximity seeking, contact seeking, avoidance, and resistance to contact and interaction.

About 15% of attachments in normative samples, and much higher percentages in high-risk samples, are difficult to classify with the original

TABLE 18.1. Episodes of the Strange Situation

Episode	Duration	Description
1	1 minute	*Parent, infant:* Dyad introduced to room.
2	3 minutes	*Parent, infant:* Infant settles in, explores. Parent assists only if necessary.
3	3 minutes	*Parent, infant, stranger:* Introduction of a stranger. Stranger plays with infant during final minute.
4	3 minutes	*Infant, stranger:* Parent leaves infant with stranger. *First separation.*
5	3 minutes	*Parent, infant:* Parent returns. Stranger leaves quietly. *First reunion.*
6	3 minutes	*Infant:* Parent leaves infant alone in room. *Second separation.*
7	3 minutes	*Infant, stranger:* Stranger enters room and stays with infant, interacting as necessary.
8	3 minutes	*Parent, infant:* Parent returns. Stranger leaves quietly. *Second reunion.*

TABLE 18.2. Strange Situation Classification Groups

Group	Brief description
Secure (B) (Ainsworth et al., 1978)	Uses mother as secure base for exploration. Separation: Signs of missing parent, especially during the second separation. Reunion: Actively greets parent with smile, vocalization, or gesture. If upset, signals or seeks contact with parent. Once comforted, returns to exploration.
Avoidant (A) (Ainsworth et al., 1978)	Explores readily, little display of affect or secure-base behavior. Separation: Responds minimally, little visible distress when left alone. Reunion: Looks away from, actively avoids parent; often focuses on toys. If picked up, may stiffen, lean away. Seeks distance from parent, often interested instead in toys.
Ambivalent or resistant (C) (Ainsworth et al., 1978)	Visibly distressed upon entering room, often fretful or passive; fails to engage in exploration. Separation: Unsettled, distressed. Reunion: May alternate bids for contact with signs of angry rejection, tantrums; or may appear passive or too upset to signal, make contact. Fails to find comfort in parent.
Disorganized/disoriented (D) (Main & Solomon, 1990)	Behavior appears to lack observable goal, intention, or explanation—for example, contradictory sequences or simultaneous behavioral displays; incomplete, interrupted movement; stereotypies; freezing/stilling; direct indications of fear/apprehension of parent; confusion, disorientation. Most characteristic is lack of a coherent attachment strategy, despite the fact that the baby may reveal the underlying patterns of organized attachment (A, B, C).

Note. Descriptions in Groups A, B, and C are based on Ainsworth et al. (1978). Descriptions in Group D are based on Main and Solomon (1990).

A-B-C criteria (see Main & Solomon, 1986, 1990, for a complete discussion). Main and Solomon described the range of behaviors found in such unclassifiable infants, and developed guidelines for classification of most of these insecure infants into a fourth classification group termed "disorganized/disoriented" (D). Infants classified into Group D show a diverse set of behaviors that are characterized by a lack of observable goal, purpose, or explanation in the immediate situation; at a higher level of explanation, these behaviors suggest that the child lacks a coherent attachment strategy with respect to the parent. (Further information about this category can be found in Lyons-Ruth & Jacobvitz, Chapter 28, this volume.)

Validation of the Measure

Beginning with Ainsworth's seminal work, validation of the infant classification system has been an ongoing priority. Many chapters in this volume summarize this progress. In what follows, we briefly summarize the literature with respect to the construct validity criteria established earlier (we refer readers to other chapters in this volume, as relevant). We begin with a lengthy discussion of reliability issues because the methodology departs substantially from what researchers in other areas of psychology may be familiar with, but touch on these matters more briefly when discussing other measures later in the chapter.

Reliability

Intercoder Agreement. The Ainsworth system and other classification measures that we describe elsewhere in this chapter require extensive training. Some systems require certification or proof that the researcher can meet a minimum reliability standard (usually 80% or higher). Unlike event coding, which involves tallies of relevant, precisely defined acts, the classification process requires matching a particular case to a multidimensional, categorical template or prototype. Manuals for classification are composed mainly of written descriptions of these templates. These written descriptions cannot capture, however, the range and nuance of behavior and context that determine placement in a particular group. Only in training, where a student can see many cases of a particular type, can the student develop the expertise that will permit evaluation of new cases in terms of their fit to a particular attachment category.

Within-laboratory agreement for trained coders tends to be very high, ranging from 100% in the original Ainsworth and Bell study (Ainsworth et al., 1978) to 85–95% for researchers who were trained by Ainsworth or her students (Main

& Weston, 1981; Waters, 1978). In the one published study that examined the important question of interlaboratory agreement on A-B-C classification, five expert coders and Ainsworth independently coded all or a subset of 37 cases (videotapes), several of which were chosen because of the classification difficulties that they presented (Carlson & Sroufe, 1993). Agreement percentages ranged from 50% to 100%, with the highest agreement (86%) found between Ainsworth and others. The fact that not all coders were trained to identify the disorganized/disoriented group may have influenced average reliability. The overall level of agreement is reassuring, especially considering the difficulty of the cases. The wide range of intercoder agreement, however, raises a question about what level would have been achieved with a more diverse and less experienced group of coders. In studies that made use of coders trained to identify the disorganized/disoriented group, across- and within-laboratory agreement ranged from 80% to 88% (Carlson, 1998; Lyons-Ruth, Repacholi, McLeod, & Silva, 1991).

When classification groups are disproportionately represented in a sample, high overall agreement (between judges or between classifications in stability assessments) may mask poor concordance for one or several of the (less common) groups. This is a particular problem in attachment research, because secure classifications usually account for at least 50% of cases in nonclinical samples. Indeed, several investigators have noted that high stability in classification is actually disproportionately due to stability (continuity) in the secure group, but not in the insecure groups (Belsky, Campbell, Cohn, & Moore, 1996; Solomon & George, 1996; van IJzendoorn, Juffer, & Duyvesteyn, 1995; Waters, Merrick, Treboux, Crowell, & Albersheim, 2000). It is recommended that researchers report kappa statistics, which are adjusted for the relative frequencies of categories, along with raw reliability/stability figures. A large discrepancy between the raw (unweighted) concordance statistic and kappa indicates that agreement, stability, and so on are unevenly distributed in the sample.

Test–Retest (Short-Term) Stability. Ainsworth repeated assessments of the Strange Situation over a very short term (i.e., 2 weeks) and found low stability of classification, presumably reflecting sensitization of infants to the separation procedure (Ainsworth et al., 1978). Ainsworth was especially struck with the collapse of avoidant strategies in the second assessment; a number of previously

avoidant infants on retest showed behavior patterns that we might now classify as disorganized. Thus, where research designs require repeated testing (within or across caregivers), researchers should avoid close spacing of assessments. Separation of assessments by a month or more is recommended (Main & Cassidy, 1988; Main & Weston, 1981).

Relation to Other Measures of Security

One of the most compelling aspects of Ainsworth's original work was the exceptional effort she and her colleagues made to validate the classification groups with respect to infant behavior toward the mother in the home. Home observation data for the original sample of 23 babies was based on detailed narrative records of monthly visits over the course of the first year of life. Drawing on this work, Ainsworth was able to develop a rich and complex portrait of each relationship. Well-known findings from the study link classification in the Strange Situation to a set of variables reflecting the frequency and quality of infant attachment behavior in the home. Attachment classifications have also been assessed against home-based measures of attachment security—both a category system developed by Ainsworth and the AQS, which yields a summary security score reflecting the quality of an infant's secure-base behavior in the home. Broadly speaking, the results of using all three approaches have been consistent: Secure versus insecure laboratory attachment classifications were related to different patterns of infant behavior in the home in ways predicted by theory. The two main insecure groups (A and C), however, were generally less well discriminated from each other in the home (Ainsworth et al., 1978; Vaughn & Waters, 1990). Studies using the AQS method have shown moderate relations between AQS security scores and attachment classification, with the clearest distinctions between the secure and disorganized groups. (See the upcoming section on the AQS; see also van IJzendoorn, Vereijken, Bakermans-Kranenburg, & Riksen-Walraven, 2004.)

Prediction to Core Variables

Mother–Child Interaction. Ainsworth's original home observations established key differences among mothers of secure, avoidant, and ambivalent infants with respect to four highly intercorrelated variables: sensitivity (defined as prompt and appropriate responsiveness to the infant's signals), acceptance (vs. rejection), cooperation, and psychological accessibility. Mothers of secure infants were high on all four dimensions; mothers of avoidant infants provided the infants with little positive experience with physical proximity and were rejecting; and mothers of ambivalent infants were inconsistent or unresponsive to infant distress and other signals. These findings have been replicated in several studies in both naturalistic and structured situations, although the associations have been weaker in the replications. In an important meta-analysis, De Wolff and van IJzendoorn (1997) concluded that parental sensitivity, although clearly important, does not appear to be the exclusive factor in the development of secure attachment. Given the centrality of the sensitivity construct in contemporary attachment theory, this is a radical notion. Failure to replicate Ainsworth's original findings may reflect various kinds of measurement error—for example, reliance on limited samples of interaction, and/or shifts in the operational definition of sensitivity away from Ainsworth's original emphasis on appraisal of signals and appropriate responding toward an emphasis on such theoretically distinct constructs as warmth, acceptance, and emotional availability (Biringen et al., 2000; Bretherton, 2000; Seifer & Schiller, 1995). Recently, some researchers have focused on components of maternal sensitivity, such as sensitivity to distress versus nondistress signals (Fish, 2001; McElwain & Booth-LaForce, 2006) and contingency to affective signals (Völker, Keller, Lohaus, Cappenberg, & Chasiotis, 1999). More refined analyses such as these may contribute to an understanding of the aspects of maternal sensitivity most relevant to promoting secure infant attachment.

The identification of the disorganized/disoriented category exerts another influence on the strength of the association found between sensitivity and attachment security. Children classified into this group usually receive an alternate classification corresponding to the Ainsworth category they most nearly resemble. The alternate classification may correspond to the level of maternal sensitivity, whereas disorganization of the attachment strategy may reflect other experiences with the mother. Although no study of disorganized infants has approached the level of detail provided by Ainsworth's original home study, researchers have identified two dimensions of maternal behavior that are reliably linked to this classification—frightening or frightened/dissociative behavior, and various kinds of atypical, disrupted communication (Hesse &

Main, 2006; Lyons-Ruth, Bronfman, & Parsons, 1999; Solomon & George, 2006, in press). In addition, a number of investigators have reported links between attachment disorganization and such child characteristics as gender and neurological vulnerability (Braungart-Rieker, Garwood, Powers, & Wang, 2001; Fish, 2001; Gervai et al., 2005). (For alternative views, see Bakermans-Kranenburg & van IJzendoorn, 2004, and Lyons-Ruth & Jacobvitz, Chapter 28, this volume.)

The notion that attachment classifications reflect infant temperament or shared genetic inheritance between mother and child, rather than the history of mother–child interaction and maternal sensitivity, has a long and contentious place in the study of attachment. (For a full discussion of attachment and temperament, see Vaughn, Bost, & van IJzendoorn, Chapter 9, this volume.) Here we note merely that a growing body of research indicates that temperamental and other biologically based characteristics influence an infant's emotional reactivity to separation and capacity to read maternal signals, as well as challenge a mother's capacity to provide sensitive care (van IJzendoorn et al., 2007). Variation in infant security of attachment, however—especially the variation reflected in the standard Ainsworth A-B-C categories—is better explained by the history of mother–child interaction than by the direct effect of biological variables (Fearon et al., 2006; Fox, Susman, Feagans, & Ray, 1992).

Continuity. Studies of long-term stability or continuity of classification can be separated into those that examine stability within the toddler period (from 12 to 18 or 24 months), within early childhood (between 12 and 60 months), or across several developmental transitions (i.e., from infancy to adolescence or early adulthood). (See Weinfield, Sroufe, Egeland, & Carlson, Chapter 4, and Thompson, Chapter 16, this volume, for fuller discussions of stability.) Estimates of continuity depend on the validity of the measures involved, and, as we discuss later, this has been problematic for assessments after about age 20 months. Even without this difficulty, the empirical findings have been mixed. Findings of very high stability of classification (over 70%) have been reported across each of these time periods (e.g., Hamilton, 2000; Main & Cassidy, 1988; Waters, 1978; Waters et al., 2000). On the other hand, substantially less stability of classification or nonsignificant levels have also been reported across all three durations (e.g., Belsky et al., 1996; Cassidy, Berlin, & Belsky, 1990; Zimmermann et al., 2000). Stability of the D attachment classification over the course of the second year of life may be lower than that of the standard A-B-C classifications, due to an increase in numbers of disorganized/disoriented infants between 12 and 18 months (Lyons-Ruth, Yellin, Melnick, & Atwood, 2003; Vondra, Shaw, Swearingen, Cohen, & Owens, 2001). In a meta-analysis of nine samples ($N = 840$), however, in which the time lag between assessments ranged from 2 to 60 months, van IJzendoorn, Schuengel, and Bakermans-Kranenburg (1999) estimated the stability of the D classification as modest at best ($r = .34$).

Researchers have been at great pains to explain low stability, because this construct is so central both to attachment theory and the validation of attachment measures. Several investigators have demonstrated, however, that changes in classification are systematically related to chronic or major shifts in maternal sensitivity, or to such family events as loss, divorce, major illness, and poverty (on the negative side) and marriage or new relationships (on the positive side). Thus, while findings of low stability have been surprising, they currently are not seen as challenging the major assumptions of attachment theory, and perhaps should be given less weight overall in the evaluation of the validation of measures.

Coherence. Inspired by Sroufe's (1979) early articulation of the coherence of development across developmental tasks, the field has continued to generate a large body of research on the links between early attachment security and later functioning with parents, peers, in school, and in romantic relationships as well as psychopathology. (It is not possible to do justice to this literature here, but the reader is referred to Thompson, Chapter 16, and Weinfield et al., Chapter 4, this volume.) It should also be noted that Bowlby's seminal predictions about the links between early parent–child attachment and later psychopathology have mainly borne fruit in the study of the sequelae to disorganized attachment (summarized in Lyons-Ruth & Jacobvitz, Chapter 28, this volume; see also DeKlyen & Greenberg, Chapter 27, this volume). Evidence for links between the avoidant and resistant categories and later psychopathology are mixed, with clearest predictions from resistant classifications to anxiety disorders.

Cross-Cultural Predictions and Predictions to Other Caregivers. Studies of infants from cultures beyond North America in the Strange Situation have mainly been limited to Western Europe, but researchers have also examined infants and their mothers in Israel, Japan, China, Indonesia, Puerto Rico, Mexico, and two sites in Africa (see van IJzendoorn & Sagi-Schwartz, Chapter 37, this volume). Although secure classifications appear to be normative (modal) cross-culturally, cultural differences have emerged in the proportions of attachment groups, and debate continues regarding the cross-cultural interpretation of Strange Situation classifications (e.g., Levine & Miller, 1990). Corresponding observations of maternal behavior in the home suggest that differences in the distribution of the insecure classifications reflect systematic cultural differences in maternal sensitivity to infant signals. They may also reflect differences in the frequency with which infants in different cultures and subcultures experience even brief separations from their mothers.

Investigators have reported no difficulty in classifying infant–father attachment relationships from the Strange Situation. In several but not all studies, the modal classification category is secure (Cox, Owen, Henderson, & Margand, 1992; Easterbrooks & Goldberg, 1984; Main & Weston, 1981; Schneider-Rosen & Rothbaum, 1993). Nevertheless, at least in conventional two-parent families, infants seem to prefer their mothers as a haven of safety when they are distressed (Lamb, 1976). Measures of paternal sensitivity to infant signals in various contexts (paralleling Ainsworth's scales for maternal behavior) have not been found to predict secure infant–father attachment as they do for infants and mothers. In addition, in a middle-class sample in which child–mother attachment was very stable over time, child–father attachment was not stable, with a net movement toward greater security (Main, Kaplan, & Cassidy, 1985). Measures of reciprocity during play and a father's sensitive support of a child's exploration have emerged as the strongest predictors of secure classifications, suggesting that fathers promote their infants' security in different ways and in different contexts than do mothers (see Grossmann, Grossmann, Kindler, & Zimmerman, Chapter 36, this volume). Studies of fathers and infant attachment suggest that in comparison to mothers, fathers' behavior is more closely linked to marital conditions and to infant temperament and gender (Belsky, 1996; Schoppe-Sullivan et al., 2006). This highlights the fact that the early infant–father relationship is subject in many respects to the mother–father relationship, which influences whether the father chooses and/or is permitted to enter the "circle" of the infant–mother bond (see George & Solomon, Chapter 35, this volume, and Solomon & George, 2000). The manner in which these complex family relationships come to influence the security of the infant's attachment to the father remains unknown. Furthermore, the mechanisms by which infants arrive at qualitatively similar attachment strategies, given large culture- and parent-related differences in patterns of interaction, also need further investigation.

Discussion

There can be little doubt that attachment classification by highly trained judges captures fundamental and far-reaching qualities of the infant–mother relationship. The reliability, stability, and predictive validity of Ainsworth's classification measure are well established in U.S. and Western European populations. However, important questions still remain about the psychometric properties and meaning of the measure for infant–father relationships, relationships with other caregivers, and attachment relationships in non-Western societies. One of the most significant contributions of the method stems from its recognition of attachment relationship patterns or types, which has permitted researchers to describe and explicate individual differences in early relationships in a simple way that predicts significant developmental outcomes years later (see Weinfield et al., Chapter 4, this volume).

Ainsworth's observational and coding skills remain unsurpassed. Indeed in a meta-analysis of over 65 studies, van IJzendoorn noted that the magnitudes of the associations between theoretically important variables reported by Ainsworth have yet to be matched by other researchers (De Wolff & van IJzendoorn, 1997; van IJzendoorn et al., 2004). It should not be forgotten, however, that the A-B-C groups were based on the study of a middle-class sample of only 23 mothers and infants, observed four decades ago. As researchers have investigated larger samples and high-risk groups, inconsistencies and gaps as well as new research opportunities have emerged. For example, as described above, studies using much larger samples have revealed lower levels of stability of attachment between 12 and 18 months than were suggested by earlier, smaller studies (e.g., Waters, 1978). Mothers' work patterns, the degree of fathers' involvement in the lives of very young children, and economic conditions also have changed considerably since the early work was undertaken. Research with larger, more diverse, and more representative samples may therefore compel us to revisit and perhaps revise earlier assumptions.

Certainly the most consequential addition to the original Ainsworth system, the disorganized/disoriented group, would not have been identified had researchers not attempted to replicate early findings in larger and atypical populations, and had they not been open to unexpected variations in behavior (Main & Solomon, 1990). Systematic research following on that original work has revealed the importance of this category for understanding variation at the more insecure and even clinical end of the spectrum. This body of studies strongly suggests that the explanatory power of Ainsworth's methodology is increased when this category is included in the study.

We would also like to draw attention to an important methodological implication of Ainsworth's reliance on a categorical approach to qualitative differences in attachment. This approach reflected her background in clinical assessment, as well as her conviction that the patterns of behavioral constellations, rather than individual differences in particular behaviors, distinguish types of attachment (Ainsworth & Marvin, 1995). Statistically less sensitive than dimensional measures, categorical systems require larger samples to establish reliable group differences. Many researchers who make use of Ainsworth's classification system (or other systems derived from it) are forced to reduce variability to a simple secure–insecure dimension because of inadequate sample size, usually in the insecure groups. As a result, these studies are unable to provide complete validation of the three- and four-group classification systems. When the literature is based on small samples, researchers are also at risk of deriving false conclusions from inconsistencies in results that arise simply from sampling error.

The interactive scales that form a part of the classification procedure, along with measures of other aspects of infant behavior in the Strange Situation, have been used to derive two discriminant functions, broadly representing avoidance and resistance (Richters, Waters, & Vaughn, 1988). These can be used to produce "classifications" with high correspondence to classification by trained judges. Only a few researchers have made use of this empirical approach to classification (see Ainsworth et al., 1978; Belsky et al., 1996). Individual differences in scores on these two functions theoretically could be used to provide more sensitive, dimensional data in attachment studies. More recently, Fraley and Spieker (2003) tested the taxonomic structure of the standard Ainsworth categories, using the interactive scales and analytic procedures first developed to test the single-gene theory of schizophrenia (Meehl, 1973). They argued that a very large portion of the variance associated with the A-B-C classifications could be summarized by two dimensions broadly representing "approach–avoidance" and "resistance–emotional confidence." Researchers interested in avoiding some of the well-known methodological pitfalls of categorical analysis could also make use of this approach to dimensional scaling. Neither of the approaches described above taps aspects of behavior relevant to attachment disorganization, however, and in their present state of development they are not appropriate for studies in which attachment disorganization is a focus of interest. We return to the question of categorical versus dimensional approaches at the end of the chapter.

Finally, we call attention to the fact that infant classification procedures have become so closely identified with the construct of security that it is difficult for either new or established attachment researchers to conceive that different or additional measures may be necessary or feasible. In part, this state of affairs reflects the simple brilliance of the Strange Situation procedure: It is hard to imagine another situation that can as reliably and ethically activate attachment behavior in the second year of life. The procedure makes use of a "natural cue to danger" (Bowlby, 1973)—separation from the attachment figure—to activate the attachment system. The use of distinct episodes allows the coder to observe the infant's immediate response to particular events and the coherence of behavior across episodes. Furthermore, the situation appears to provide the "right" amount of stress. Too little stress does not activate the attachment system adequately, judging by the results of home observations (e.g., Ainsworth et al., 1978; Vaughn & Waters, 1990), and therefore may not allow critical distinctions among insecure groups to be revealed. Very high stress, such as that provided by repeating the procedure twice in 2 weeks, appears to result in a breakdown of defensive strategies, again obscuring important differences among groups. Finally, given that the primary threat to the child in the Strange Situation is a (transitory) threat to the relationship, the inferential leap from an observed pattern of attachment behavior to the infant's confidence regarding the psychological

responsiveness of the caregiver seems to be a relatively modest one.

Whatever its appeal, from a technical standpoint the validity of the security construct as measured by the Strange Situation requires its cross-validation with one or more other measures of security. Since the validation of the single alternative measure of security in early toddlerhood, the AQS, does not permit distinctions between the avoidant and resistant groups, it is still fair to conclude that construct validation for attachment classifications is technically incomplete. We hope that this rather unsettling realization will inspire researchers to devise alternative measurement approaches.

CLASSIFICATION OF ATTACHMENT RELATIONSHIPS IN THE PRESCHOOL AND KINDERGARTEN PERIOD

Investigators have followed two approaches to developing classification systems for children's attachment behavior beyond infancy. The dominant approach is based on an assumption of continuity between infancy and older ages, with allowances for developmental changes in the actual behaviors indicative of one or another type of relationship. Beginning with the challenges of interpreting the Strange Situation behavior of children older than 18 months, Marvin (1977) and later Schneider-Rosen (1990) developed general guidelines to identify the traditional Ainsworth classification groups among toddlers. These researchers modified assessment criteria developmentally; for example, the timing and quality of distance interaction (including talking) were used as indices of security, instead of the proximity seeking and contact maintenance of very young children. Marvin also emphasized the importance of considering additional aspects of parent–child interaction, such as the quality of parent–child negotiations around departures and reunions, as an index of the quality of the goal-corrected partnership that begins to emerge in an older toddler (Bowlby, 1969/1982, 1973, 1980).

The first major effort along these lines was that of Main and Cassidy (1988), who attempted to apply the continuity framework to developing a set of classification criteria for 6-year-olds. This system was developed with children whose infant attachment classifications were known. This effort was followed by the work of Cassidy, Marvin, and the MacArthur Attachment Working Group (see Cassidy & Marvin, 1992), who attempted to adjust the kindergarten system downward to develop a classification system for the preschool-age child (from 2½ to 4½ years old). Both systems can therefore be said to be founded on a priori notions of developmental transformation in the early years of life, as informed by careful and extensive observations of reunion behavior.

The second approach, called by Crittenden (1992a, 1992b, 1994) the "dynamic-maturational approach," emphasizes dynamic changes in the quality of attachment that arise from the interaction between maturation and current experience. Based on the concept of developmental pathways, this approach emphasizes more strongly than the continuity approach the possibilities for changes in quality of the attachment relationship over time. In addition, greater emphasis is placed in this system on inferences regarding the function of the child's behavior toward the parent. There are strong similarities between Crittenden's Preschool Assessment of Attachment (PAA) system and the Cassidy–Marvin system, as well as subtle but significant differences. In both systems, attachment groups are distinguished by identifying the communicative or defensive goals that underlie attachment patterns. In both, the avoidant pattern is viewed as a defensive behavioral strategy organized around the goal of decreasing the probability of emotional involvement or confrontation. In Crittenden's PAA, however, this defensive strategy includes both cool or neutral avoidance of the parent (as in the Main–Cassidy and Cassidy–Marvin systems) and behavior that might be seen as somewhat role-reversed. Manifestations of this latter pattern are termed "controlling-caregiving" in the Cassidy–Marvin and Main–Cassidy systems (i.e., placating, guiding, or acting solicitously toward the parent). The latter, according to Crittenden, is linked to cool neutrality by the fact that in both strategies, the child takes the major initiative in regulating proximity and communication with the parent.

Both approaches to preschool attachment use the Strange Situation procedure, especially the two separations and reunions of the original. Some investigators have introduced variations to accommodate the older age of the children, such as slightly longer separations, changes in the role and/or gender of the stranger, changes in the instructions to the caregiver, and blending with other laboratory tasks and procedures. A common approach in recent studies, and one that is recommended in the most recent manual (Cassidy & Marvin, 1992), is to omit the stranger episodes entirely and thus leave the child alone in the room during both separations. The manual also finds acceptable the use of the stranger as it is done for infants. Unfortunately, there has been no systematic determination of whether these variations materially affect the reunion behavior of the children.

A description of the categories used in all three systems is provided in Table 18.3. Although the Main and Cassidy system for 6-year-olds was developed earlier, we present information about the Cassidy–Marvin system first because it applies to chronologically younger children. We next consider the Main–Cassidy system. Crittenden's PAA system has been used by relatively few investigators in recent years. It is with reluctance that due to space limitations, we do not include an updated section on its use and validity in the current chapter. Interested readers are referred to the pertinent sections of the corresponding chapter in the first edition of this handbook (Solomon & George, 1999d), and to chapters by Crittenden and others in Crittenden and Claussen (2000).

The Cassidy–Marvin Assessment of Attachment in Preschoolers

The Cassidy–Marvin system for preschool-age children provides guidelines for a "secure" group (B) and four "insecure" groups as follows: "avoidant" (A), "ambivalent" (C), "controlling/disorganized" (D), and "insecure/other" (IO). Each classification group includes a set of subgroups, including types that expand upon the infant subgroups. As with the Strange Situation, classifications are based primarily on the child's behavior toward the mother during both reunions.

Reliability

Intercoder Agreement. The majority of researchers using the Cassidy–Marvin system participated in the MacArthur Working Group on Attachment (a collection of attachment researchers who collaborated to create the system), reported being trained by Cassidy or Marvin, and/or brought in a classification judge who established reliability on the system. The MacArthur Group requires a minimum of 75% agreement for certification. The range of training reliability scores reported in published studies includes percentages a bit lower (e.g., 72%), but most report reliabilities of 85% or higher.

TABLE 18.3. Early Childhood Laboratory Separation–Reunion Classification Systems: Major Classification Groups

Group	Cassidy–Marvin	PAA	Main–Cassidy
B	*Secure:* Uses parent as secure base for exploration. Reunion behavior is smooth, open, warm, positive.	*Secure/balanced:* Relaxed, intimate, direct expression of feelings, desires. Able to negotiate conflict or disagreement.	*Secure:* Reunion behavior is confident, relaxed, open. Positive, reciprocal interaction or conversation.
A	*Avoidant:* Detached, neutral nonchalance, but does not avoid interaction altogether. Avoids physical or psychological intimacy.	*Defended:* Acts to reduce emotional involvement or confrontation. Focuses on play and exploration at expense of interaction.	*Avoidant:* Maintains affective neutrality; subtly minimizes and limits opportunities for interaction.
C	*Ambivalent:* Protests separation strongly. Reunion characterized by strong proximity-seeking, babyish, coy behavior.	*Coercive:* Maximizes psychological involvement with parent; exaggerates problems and conflict. Is coercive, for example, threatening (resistant, punitive) and/or disarming (innocent, coy).	*Ambivalent:* Heightened intimacy and dependency on parent. Reunion characterized by ambivalence, subtle hostility, exaggerated cute or babyish behavior.
D	*Controlling/disorganized:* Characterized by controlling behavior (punitive, caregiving) or behaviors associated with infant disorganization.		*Controlling:* Signs of role reversal: punitive (rejecting, humiliating) or caregiving (cheering, reassuring, falsely positive).
A/C		*Defended/coercive:* Child shows both defended and coercive behaviors, appearing together or in alternation.	
AD		*Anxious/depressed:* Sad/depressed; stares, extreme distress/panic.	
IO or U	*Insecure/other:* Mixtures of insecure indices that do not fit into any of the other groups.	*Insecure/other:* Acts incoherently in relation to parent.	*Unclassifiable:* Mixture of insecure indices that do not fit into any of the other groups including behaviors associated with infant disorganization.

Note. Cassidy–Marvin, Main–Cassidy: Organized groups = A, B, C. PAA: Organized groups = A, B, C, A/C.

Short-Term Stability. There are no published studies of short-term stability.

Relation to Other Measures of Attachment Security

In a recent meta-analysis of 137 published and unpublished studies (through 2004) involving the AQS (Waters & Deane, 1985), secure classification in the Cassidy–Marvin system was significantly related to preschoolers' attachment security in the home, but at a more modest level compared to findings for infants (combined $r = .26$ for children 30 months or older; $r = .31$ for children ages 12–18 months) (van IJzendoorn et al., 2004). Since this meta-analysis, Posada (2006) reported no significant difference among attachment classification groups in either the overall AQS security or scales that tapped particular aspects of mother–child interaction in the home. Moss, Bureau, Cyr, and Dubois-Comtois (2006), however, found significant differences in AQS security overall among children classified according to the Cassidy–Marvin system. AQS scores differentiated inconsistently among the classification groups, with higher AQS security for children classified as secure than for those classified as ambivalent or disorganized (but not controlling) yet no reliable differences between the secure and avoidant or controlling groups. This partial correspondence (as well as the overall lower association between measures reported by van IJzendoorn et al., 2004) may be due to the fact that since attachment behavior is rarely elicited in the home at this age, only distinctions between preschoolers who are secure and those who are either highly dependent (and susceptible to exaggerated displays; Main, 1990) or without minimally adaptive attachment-related defenses (Solomon & George, 1999b; Solomon, George, & De Jong, 1995) are readily apparent.

Three studies have shown links between Cassidy–Marvin classifications and a representational measure of attachment security (Bretherton, Oppenheim, Buchsbaum, Emde, & the MacArthur Narrative Group, 1990; Bretherton, Ridgeway, & Cassidy, 1990; Shouldice & Stevenson-Hinde, 1992). Preschoolers classified as secure, compared to those classified as insecure, received higher scores for representational security (i.e., they were judged as more open to negative feelings and better able to tolerate attachment fears).

Prediction to Core Variables

Mother–Child Interaction. Detailed descriptive research on mother–child relationships in naturalistic situations, paralleling Ainsworth's original studies in the home as related to infant classification, has not yet been reported. In the first study of mother–child interaction in the home and laboratory as related to Cassidy–Marvin classifications, however, Stevenson-Hinde and Shouldice (1995) found predicted differences between the secure and insecure groups in measures of mothers' sensitivity, socialization, positive involvement, and scaffolding of tasks. Differences between the secure and the various insecure groups were revealed in one type of situation or the other, depending upon the group. Crittenden and Claussen (1994) found no relation between Cassidy–Marvin classifications and ratings of maternal sensitivity in a brief play situation, but did find a difference between mothers of secure and insecure children in maternal involvement and positive affect during laboratory cleanup. More recently, the National Institute of Child Health and Human Development (NICHD) Early Child Care Research Network (2001) reported a low but significant correlation between maternal sensitivity in the home and secure versus insecure attachment classifications in their large, heterogeneous U.S. sample. Significant differences between attachment groups were restricted

to the contrast between the controlling/disorganized and secure classifications. Studying a large French Canadian sample, Moss and her colleagues (Humber & Moss, 2005; Moss, Bureau, Cyr, Mongeau, & St.-Laurent, 2004; Moss, Cyr, & Dubois-Comtois, 2004) found overall smoother and more positive interaction during a brief "snacktime" between mothers and secure 3- to 5-year-olds and 5- to 7-year-olds, in comparison to dyads in which the children were judged insecure (note that the Main–Cassidy system was used for classifications for children 6 years of age and older). The clearest differences in both age periods were between dyads with children judged disorganized/controlling and secure dyads. Indeed, the former were characterized by the poorest mother–child coordination, communication, and enjoyment of all groups. A distinct pattern of significant differences among mothers of secure, avoidant, and ambivalent children, overall or with respect to other descriptive scales, was not found at the older age. A somewhat clearer pattern emerged, however, in the younger age group, with secure dyads superior to insecure ones and avoidant and dependent dyads superior to controlling/disorganized dyads. In a sample of low-income African American preschoolers, Barnett, Kidwell, and Leung (1998) reported that mothers of insecure (mainly avoidant) children were more likely than mothers of secure children to be rated as low in warmth and high in control. Britner, Marvin, and Pianta (2005) developed a classification system and rating scales to differentiate the behavior of mothers corresponding to the Cassidy–Marvin child attachment groups. In this system, a mother's behavior is classified on the basis of her behavior in the Strange Situation. Classification criteria reflect qualities captured from Ainsworth's original studies of mothers of infants and studies of adult attachment representation. Agreement between mother and child classifications was high, though not exact (kappa = .57), with many of the disagreements occurring in dyads with a disabled child. Though this system seems to provide strong evidence that distinctions exist in maternal behavior corresponding to all of the child classifications, the fact that mother and child categories are based on the same sample of behavior is problematic.

Studies in non-normative samples provide indirect evidence to suggest that classification reflects differences in maternal behavior. In a series of studies involving, variously, maltreated children; dyads with anxiety-disordered, adolescent, or impoverished mothers; mothers with depression; or mothers who were unresolved with respect to a child's disability diagnosis, the children were less likely to be classified as secure and more likely to be classified into one of the "atypical" classifications (e.g., disorganized, controlling, or insecure/other) than comparison children (Barnett et al., 2006; Campbell et al., 2004; Cicchetti & Barnett, 1991; Fish, 2004; Hoffman, Marvin, Cooper, & Powell, 2006; Lounds, Borkowski, Whitman, Maxwell, & Weed, 2005; Manassis, Bradley, Goldberg, Hood, & Swinson, 1994; Marvin & Pianta, 1996; Toth, Rogosch, Manly, & Cicchetti, 2006). Finally, Marcovitch and colleagues (1997) found that the distribution of attachment classifications among Romanian adoptees differed significantly from that of a normal comparison sample, with the disorganized classification being the most common.

Continuity. A number of studies have provided data on continuity of classification from toddlerhood. Two of the largest such studies (NICHD Network, 2001; Seifer et al., 2004) reported significant but very low stability in classifications over time, and two studies with somewhat smaller samples reported no significant stability over the early childhood period (Bar-Haim, Sutton, Fox, & Marvin, 2000; Fish, 2004). Significant but moderate continuity of classification (kappa = approximately .40) has been reported in others (Cassidy, Berlin, & Belsky, 1990; Cicchetti & Barnett, 1991; Lounds et al., 2005; Shouldice & Stevenson-Hinde, 1992; Stevenson-Hinde & Shouldice, 1995). In these studies, the secure pattern showed the highest consistency over time (though the insecure pattern showing the most change differed from study to study). In other words, a substantial portion of insecure infants appear to become secure in the preschool period. (For an exception, see Rauh, Ziegenhain, Muller, & Wijroks, 2000.) In the only study to date of stability of the Cassidy–Marvin classifications *within* the preschool period, Moss, Cyr, Bureau, Tarabulsy, and Dubois-Combois (2005) found moderate stability (kappa = .47) between 3½ and 5½ years in a sample that was heterogeneous with respect to SES (note that the Main–Cassidy system was used for 6-year-olds). Stability of group assignments was over 60% for all groups except the avoidant, which shifted considerably (44% concordant). An interesting additional finding in this study is that 70% of controlling/disorganized preschoolers shifted into the controlling category within this time period, suggesting that this is the point at which disorganized children develop their secondary controlling strategies.

The level of instability in classification might in itself raise questions about the validity of the Cassidy–Marvin system. Although lack of continuity of infant classification is more common in low-SES samples in general (see Weinfield et al., Chapter 4, this volume), this distinction does not appear to have been a key factor in the foregoing studies, which reflect the full range on this variable. Investigators in each of these studies established, however, that shifts between the secure and insecure classification(s) were related to corresponding changes in mother–child interaction and/or other key factors (e.g., marital distress and separation, losses, and other positive or negative life events that reasonably would be expected to have an impact on the mother–child relationship).

Coherence. A few studies have reported differences between secure and insecure children in other developmental domains. Secure children have been reported to be more cooperative with their mothers in brief laboratory tasks (Cassidy & Marvin, 1992), less gender-stereotyped (Turner, 1991), and less anxious (Shamir-Essakow, Ungerer, & Rapee, 2005). Fish (2004) found in a low-SES rural sample, however, that infant security classifications but not preschool ones were linked to cognitive and socioemotional competence, raising some question about the validity of the classifications for older children.

Differences in the level of behavior problems between secure and controlling/disorganized classifications are consistent with findings at later ages. Based on teacher reports, secure children were less likely than controlling/disorganized children to show externalizing and internalizing behavioral problems (Moss, Cyr, et al., 2004). In a clinical population, children classified as controlling/disorganized were more likely to be diagnosed with conduct disorder (Greenberg, Speltz, DeKlyen, & Endriga, 1991; Speltz, Greenberg, & DeKlyen, 1990).

Cross-Cultural Studies and Other Relationships. The Cassidy–Marvin system has been used to study attachment in the United States, England, Canada, and Romania. There is no published information on preschool attachment in countries or cultures other than these, or on father–child relationships.

The Main–Cassidy Attachment Classification for Kindergarten-Age Children

The Main and Cassidy (1988) attachment classification system for kindergarten-age children was developed on a sample of 33 children whose infant attachment classifications in the Strange Situation (A, B, and D) were known and who had experienced no major change in caretaking relationships. The system was further tested and extended on a new sample of 50 children that afforded enough C children to establish classification guidelines for this group. Classification is based on a child's behavior during the first 3 or 5 minutes of reunion with the parent following a 1-hour separation, rather than on the episodes and timing of the Strange Situation. Guidelines are provided for five major classification groups: "secure" (B), "avoidant" (A), "ambivalent" (C), "controlling" (D), and "unclassifiable" (U). Criteria for subgroup classifications are also provided. Rating scales for security and avoidance have been developed as well. The major criteria for classification are shown in Table 18.3.

Reliability

Intercoder Agreement. In the majority of studies, intercoder reliability between Main or Cassidy and other investigators ranged from 70% to 88%.

Short-Term Stability. Stability of classification over a 1-month period in Main and Cassidy's (1988) sample of 50 was 62%. Instability was largely due to change involving the controlling group. The authors suggest that instability in part reflects sensitization to the test situation.

Relation to Other Measures of Security

Main–Cassidy classifications have been shown to be related to secure versus insecure classifications based on three different procedures for classifying children's representations of attachments (Cassidy, 1988; Gloger-Tippelt, Gomille, Koenig, & Vetter, 2002; Solomon et al., 1995). Solomon and George's system has been shown to differentiate reliably among all of the A-B-C-D groups in both a U.S. and a Japanese sample (Kayoko, 2006). Concordance between Main–Cassidy classifications and ratings or classifications of children's responses to pictures of attachment-related events has also been reported (Jacobsen, Edelstein, & Hofmann, 1994; Jacobsen & Hofmann, 1997; Slough & Greenberg, 1990).

Prediction to Core Variables

Mother–Child Interaction. Solomon, George, and Silverman (1990) found significant correlations between ratings based on Main–Cassidy classifications and observer sorts of maternal behavior in the home (Maternal Caretaking Q-Sort). Security was related to age-appropriate maternal involvement and support; avoidance to rejection and affective distance; and ambivalence to indulgent and infantilizing behavior. Based on their studies of a French Canadian sample, Moss and colleagues reported that mother–child interaction in secure dyads was more harmonious than within insecure dyads, with the lowest scores received by mothers of controlling, disorganized, or unclassifiable children of all subtypes (Humber & Moss, 2005; Moss, Gosselin, Parent, Rousseau, & Dumont, 1997; Moss, Rousseau, Parent, St.-Laurent, & Saintonge, 1998).

Continuity. Main and Cassidy (1988) reported a very high stability (kappa = .76) between 12-month and 6-year A-B-C-D classifications with mothers. Wartner, Grossmann, Fremmer-Bombik, and Suess (1994) reported a similar level of stability over the same period in their independent German sample. As described previously, Moss and colleagues (2005) recently demonstrated moderate continuity over a 2-year period between Marvin–Cassidy preschool classifications and Main–Cassidy classifications at age 6.

Coherence. Cohn (1990) and Wartner and colleagues (1994) investigated the links between classifications at age 6 and social competence and peer acceptance in school. In both studies, the securely attached children were judged to be more socially competent and accepted than the insecurely attached children, although the studies differed as to which insecure group showed the greatest deficit (C or A, respectively). Insecure classification, especially in the D group, has been linked to behavioral problems in high- and low-risk samples (Easterbrooks, Biesecker, & Lyons-Ruth, 2000; Easterbrooks, Davidson, & Chazan, 1993; Solomon et al., 1995). Paralleling these findings, Cassidy, Kirsh, Scolton, and Parke (1996, Study 2) found at the representational level of assessment that secure children had more positive representations of peers' intentions and feelings, as assessed from social problem-solving vignettes, than did insecure children. Secure versus insecure Main–Cassidy classifications have also been found to be related to representational measures of self-esteem and attachment, with secure children judged to be more open about themselves and about feelings of vulnerability than insecure children (Cassidy, 1988; Slough & Greenberg, 1990). More recently, Bureau, Buliveau, Moss, & Lépine (2006) found that 6-year-old controlling children depicted more themes of conflict in response to the Bretherton, Oppenheim, and colleagues (1990) stories, and that secure children produced more discipline themes than avoidant children and displayed higher coherence than ambivalent children.

Cross-Cultural Studies. The Main–Cassidy system has been used in the United States, Canada, Iceland, Germany, Italy, Australia, and Japan.

Discussion

Based on widespread use and the corresponding state of validation overall, the Cassidy–Marvin system must now be considered the preferred measure for assessment of attachment of 3- and 4-year-olds and the Main–Cassidy system the preferred measure for 5- to 7-year-olds, especially for researchers who are interested in differences among the four classification groups. Both measures have been investigated with respect to all of the validation criteria described earlier and appear to be related both to other relationship measures and to the core variables in ways that broadly parallel research on infant classifications. The Main–Cassidy system appears to function as it was intended, yielding coherent and predicted differences not only between the secure and insecure groups, but among the A-B-C-D groups as well. It should be borne in mind, however, that it has been employed in relatively few studies and mainly with normative, middle-class samples. Extending its application to high-risk or more recent cohorts might yield more complex results.

The validation results for the Cassidy–Marvin system, indeed, are more complex, and at this time it is not clear why. The key problematic findings, repeated across a variety of samples and investigators, are (1) relatively low continuity between infant and preschool-age classifications, usually attributable to a shift from the insecure groups (usually A, sometimes C) to the secure group; and, (2) failure consistently to find distinctive differences in mother–child interaction associated with the avoidant and ambivalent groups. Clear distinctions usually emerge between children classified as secure and those classified as disorganized or con-

trolling. (Note that in most samples, the numbers of children in the insecure groups [A, C, or D], though relatively small, are usually comparable.)

It may indeed be the case that some attachments undergo major change between the third and fifth years of life, reflecting expectable shifts in parent–child relationships. In what follows we discuss some reasons for this; these same arguments may also apply to consideration of AQS validity, which we discuss later in the chapter. The period from infancy to preschool is one of considerable change in a child's capacity for language, goal-corrected behavior, and self-control. Parental expectations, the child's role in the family, and family life in general may shift considerably in this period as a consequence. If so, instability in classification may be a poor marker of the validity of the measure in this age range.

The failure to find strong differences in mother–child interaction also may reflect developmental shifts in relationships. As children become more mature and as fewer situations activate the attachment system, some mothers may become better able to cope with their children's needs, leading to actual improvements both in their mutual perception of their relationship and their interaction. It is also possible that researchers have simply chosen less differentiating contexts in which to observe interaction. The most salient issue for preschool parent–child dyads is the development of self-control and socialization. Indeed, the studies that have shown the clearest differences in mother–child interaction associated with Cassidy–Marvin classifications have focused on interaction in cleanup tasks (Achermann, Dinneen, & Stevenson-Hinde, 1991; Crittenden & Claussen, 1994, 2000).

Low stability may also reflect various kinds of measurement error. The procedure may not be sufficiently stressful to reliably activate the attachment system of some preschoolers. This might result in false positives for the secure group for children who are (or were) avoidant; some secure children might also be misclassified as avoidant if they are a bit "too casual" in the procedure. This interpretation is supported by a recent study by Oosterman and Schuengel (2007), which found that for preschoolers, brief laboratory separations from parents were insufficient to activate the sympathetic nervous system even if children were insecure or temperamentally inhibited.

Somewhat disconcertingly, just how distressing a child will find the separation may be a function of his or her particular "underlying" attachment strategy (ambivalent/dependent, controlling, or disorganized children might be most susceptible). The protocol advises encouraging parents to give reasons for their departure and be prepared to "negotiate." This is developmentally appropriate and yet quite different from the instructions given to parents of infants. It reflects the fact that some preschoolers can be more disturbed by the parents' departure from expectation than by the parents' *actual* departure. Thus maladroitly handled separations or other unusual features of parental behavior may have unexpectedly large consequences for preschoolers. From the perspective of evaluating stability from infancy or other important variables, then, short-separation procedures may provide a more "accurate" picture of the state of some relationships than of others. Research should focus systematically on optimal separation times and observation contexts for this age, perhaps also adding physiological measures, in order that procedural variables neither create nor mask what may be very interesting new findings about the development of mother–child attachments.

ATTACHMENT SECURITY MEASURES BASED ON SYMBOLIC REPRESENTATION

It is generally believed that infants and toddlers encode knowledge, including knowledge about their relationships with attachment figures, in terms of enactive or sensorimotor representation. Early in the preschool years, children begin to use symbolic forms of mental representation and to organize knowledge conceptually (Bretherton, Grossmann, Grossmann, & Waters, 2005). These conceptual structures and processes can be observed in contexts in which a child is asked to develop scripts for actions and events. As a result of this developmental achievement, the child is ripe for assessments that tap internal working models of attachment. Internal representational models of relationships are believed to arise from actual experiences in a relationship. They have been conceptualized as consisting of both specific content, including affect, and information-processing rules that integrate and determine perception and memory (Bowlby, 1969/1982; Bretherton et al., 2005; Main et al., 1985). Recent research has emphasized the script-like nature of what is encoded as part of repeated experiences within a relationship (Waters & Waters, 2006). Because of their link to experience, individual differences in rep-

resentational models can be expected to parallel individual differences in a child's actual behavior with an attachment figure; that is, they should be systematically related to measures of attachment security based on reunion and/or secure-base behavior in early childhood and thereafter. (The reader is referred to Bretherton & Munholland, Chapter 5, this volume, for a full discussion of internal representational models in children and adults.)

The measures that have been developed are of two kinds—those based on children's responses to pictured situations, and those based on children's doll-play narratives and enactment of attachment-related scenarios. Some researchers have attempted to develop classification schemes to parallel the Ainsworth system. Other researchers have developed scales to reflect aspects of attachment security or related constructs, but have not attempted to understand patterning of responses in such a way as to derive classifications. There is not a complete body of validation information for any of the measures developed to date. Below we describe what is known about the most influential of measures; several others, unfortunately, have been omitted due to space limitations.

Picture Response Procedures

Three interrelated measures have been developed to assess internal representations of attachment on the basis of children's responses to projective pictures or stories. Two measures (Kaplan, 1987; Slough & Greenberg, 1990) incorporate the procedures of the Separation Anxiety Test (SAT), a picture response protocol that was first developed for adolescents by Hansburg (1972) and later modified for children ages 4–7 by Klagsbrun and Bowlby (1976). The procedure consists of a set of six photographs depicting attachment-related scenes ranging from mild (a parent says goodnight to a child in bed) to stressful (a child watches a parent leave). Each picture is introduced by an adult, and the child is asked to describe how the child in the picture feels and what that child will do. The coding schemes are mainly dependent on children's verbal responses as the basis for inferring representational models.

Kaplan (1987) developed a classification system for children's responses to the pictures that differentiates attachment groups on the basis of children's emotional openness and ability to envision constructive solutions to feelings engendered by separation. The system was developed on a small sample of middle-class 6-year-olds whose attachment classifications with their mothers at 12 months were known. Children classified as "resourceful" (B) were able to discuss coping with separation in constructive ways. There was no evidence that they denied feelings of vulnerability, and no evidence that they became disorganized or disoriented. Children were classified as "inactive" (A) when they offered responses indicating feelings of vulnerability or distress at separation, but were at a loss to suggest ways in which the child in each picture might cope. Children classified as "ambivalent" (C) typically demonstrated a contradictory mixture of responses; for example, a child might seem angry toward the parent, but would shift to wanting to please the parent. Children were classified as "fearful" (D) on the basis of several types of responses: inexplicable fear, lack of constructive strategies for coping with separation, or disorganized or disoriented thought processes.

Although Kaplan's classification system has been very influential in the design of other representational measures, information regarding its reliability and validity when used with the SAT pictures is limited to Kaplan's original study. She reached 76% reliability with a second trained judge on her sample of 38 children. Correspondence between SAT responses and infant classifications was 68% for the four groups (kappa = .55). Kaplan's coding system has been used in a handful of additional studies. SAT responses were significantly related to ratings of the ease of access to self-evaluations of 8-year-olds, as well as to behavior problems at home and school (Easterbrooks & Abeles, 2000). Ackerman and Dozier (2005) found that ratings of foster children's adaptive coping responses to the SAT, but not their emotional security (openness), were related to foster mothers' acceptance of the children and to the children's self-esteem (assessed with the Puppet Interview; Cassidy, 1988). Clarke, Ungerer, Chahoud, Johnson, and Stiefel (2002), using the SAT among other representational measures, found that 5- to 10-year-old boys diagnosed with attention-deficit/ hyperactivity disorder (ADHD) gave responses most consistent with ambivalent or disorganized classifications.

Jacobsen and her colleagues (Jacobsen et al., 1994; Jacobsen & Hofmann, 1997) adapted Kaplan's classification system for use with a series of pictures depicting a long separation from parents (Chandler, 1973). These investigators were unusually thorough in establishing the validity of the measure. The Icelandic children were 7 years old

when assessed. Judges were trained by Kaplan and established excellent within-laboratory agreement (kappa = .80–.87). Stability over the following year was substantial (kappa = .78), and concordance with both infant classifications and concurrent reunion classifications based on the Main and Cassidy system was equally high. Secure versus insecure representational classification (especially the D pattern) successfully predicted several theoretically related variables for children between the ages of 7 and 15, including performance on cognitive-developmental tasks, self-esteem, teacher-reported attention and participation in class, insecurity about self, and grade point average.

Slough and Greenberg (1990) used the SAT pictures and developed four scales, apparently adapted from Kaplan's early classification criteria, to rate attachment security. The attachment scales (acknowledgment of separation-related affect in stressful separations; statements of well-being in mild separations) were positively related to security ratings (Main & Cassidy, 1988) of 5-year-olds upon reunion with their mothers following a 3-minute separation, and negatively related to ratings of avoidance. Representation ratings were unrelated, however, to reunion behavior following a second, longer (90-minute) separation. Since the Main–Cassidy ratings were based on this nonstandard separation–reunion procedure, the interpretation of these findings is open to question. No information is available regarding intercoder reliability or test–retest stability of the Slough and Greenberg measure.

Doll Play

A second approach to developing representational attachment security measures is founded on observation of children's doll play centering on attachment-relevant themes. Many different (yet overlapping) protocols have been developed, as well as major variants in approaches to classification and rating. Here we focus on three systems: the Bretherton doll-play procedure (the Attachment Story Completion Task, or ASCT; Bretherton, Ridgeway, et al., 1990); Cassidy's (1988) Incomplete Stories with Doll Family; and the Attachment Doll Play Assessment (ADPA; George & Solomon, 1990/1996/2000).

The Bretherton, Ridgeway, and colleagues (1990) doll-play procedure was originally designed to assess attachment security in 4-year-olds. This procedure involves a set of five stories, only the last four of which are involved in rating and classification (child spills juice, child hurts her knee, child "discovers" a monster in the bedroom, parents depart, and parents return). The Bretherton stories are a subset of the MacArthur Story Stem Battery, a group of 10 stories reflecting a variety of parent–child interactions, which were developed in collaboration between Bretherton and other members of the MacArthur team (Bretherton, Oppenheim, et al., 1990). In Bretherton's procedure, an adult introduces each story with a story stem that describes what has happened, and a child is asked to enact what happens next. Bretherton developed a classification system that identifies the four main attachment groups (A-B-C-D). Detailed transcripts are made of children's verbal behavior and enactment of each story, and classifications are based on children's predominant responses to the stories. Separate criteria for each story were established on a priori grounds or based on Kaplan's (SAT) findings. The system was designed with the goal of detecting parallels between the action described by a child and what might be expected of children in each of the Ainsworth groups based on what is known about their reunion behavior, what might be inferred from the various insecure attachment strategies, and Kaplan's early descriptions of SAT responses. "Secure" (B) children demonstrate coping behavior in relation to the attachment themes. For example, upon separation from parents, a secure child spontaneously (without prompting from the administrator) plays with the grandmother doll. "Avoidant" (A) children appear to avoid responding; for example, they request another story or say, "I don't know." No consistent patterns are identified for "ambivalent" (C) children. Children are classified as "disorganized" (D) if they give odd or disorganized responses—for example, throwing the child doll on the floor.

No intercoder or test–retest reliability figures are available. However, Bretherton, Ridgeway, and colleagues (1990) examined the concordance between secure and insecure doll-play classifications and corresponding classifications of children with the Cassidy–Marvin preschool system. A secure–insecure match was found for 75% of the 28 children. There was no match, however, for type of insecurity (A, C, D) across the two measures. Doll-play classifications were converted to security scores and were found to be highly correlated with AQS security scores at 25 months and marginally correlated with (concurrent) AQS security scores at 47 months. Representation security scores also showed significant though moderate relations with marital satisfaction, family adaptation and cohe-

siveness, child temperament (sociability, shyness), and language and cognition as assessed by the Bayley Scales of Infant Development. This broad network of correlations raises some question regarding the discriminant validity of the system.

Cassidy (1988) also created a set of six stories (e.g., the child gives the parent a present; the child does not like what is served for dinner; the child is awakened by a loud noise) for use with kindergartners, and devised a rating and classification scheme intended to differentiate among the secure and two of the insecure classifications (A, D). High scores and the secure classification reflected qualitative judgments that the relationship depicted between mother and child was open, warm, and trusting, and that the protagonist was depicted as valuable and worthy. Average interrater reliability on both measures was above .85, and test–retest stability (one story only) was .63 on the scale and .73 on story classification. The security scale showed a moderate, positive correlation with children's reunion security scores and reunion attachment classifications were also significantly, but moderately, associated with representational classifications. The closest correspondence between reunion and doll-play classifications appeared to be for the secure and controlling reunion groups, with most of the controlling children depicting quite negative mother–child interactions in doll play.

Verschueren, Marcoen, and Schoefs (1996), using a combination of stories from Bretherton, Ridgeway, and colleagues (1990) and Cassidy (1988), applied Cassidy's rating and classification scheme to the doll play of Belgian kindergartners in order to explore the children's self-representations and social competence and success. They reported levels of interrater agreement similar to Cassidy's, and found that both the Cassidy security score and classification scheme were moderately positively associated with representations of the self. Children also completed a second doll-play assessment with a father rather than a mother doll. Mother and father stories tended to be rated and classified similarly, and security scores from father assessments were positively associated with teacher ratings of social competence, anxious/withdrawn behavior, and school adjustment (Verschueren & Marcoen, 1999).

George and Solomon (1990/1996/2000; Solomon & George, 2002; Solomon et al., 1995) developed the ADPA, an alternative approach to deriving classifications based on doll-play responses to the ASCT (Bretherton) story stems that has been quite successful in differentiating among Main–Cassidy reunion classification groups. We introduced some changes to the Bretherton, Ridgeway, and colleagues (1990) procedures to facilitate symbolic play and enhance involvement. The system identifies four attachment groups. In our initial version of the system, we differentiated responses to the combined separation–reunion stories on the basis of narrative structure as well as content, resulting in four groups descriptively termed "confident" (B), "casual" (A), "busy" (C), and "frightened" (D).

Subsequently we reworked our classification scheme (Solomon & George, 2002) in light of our further examination of children's separation–reunion narratives, our research with maternal caregiving interviews (George & Solomon, 1996b; Solomon & George, 1996, 1999a), and the Adult Attachment Projective (George, West, Hilsenroth, & Segal, 2004). The organizing framework is derived from Bowlby's (1973, 1980) articulation of the defensive processes related to separation and loss (George & West, 1999; Solomon & George, 1999b). To summarize briefly, although security can be expected to reflect a flexible integration of attachment-related thoughts and feelings, strategies of defensive exclusion of information can be systematically brought into play as responses to anxiety and fear regarding attachment figures. These processes include "deactivation" (prevention of attachment-related thoughts and feelings) and "cognitive disconnection" (disconnection from awareness of the links between affect and thought). When attachment-related distress cannot be contained (assuaged), "dysregulation" of the attachment system (or, in Bowlby's terms, "segregated systems") is likely to be the result. Uncontained frightening and catastrophic events, as well as persistent constriction (refusal to play), are seen as evidence of dysregulation. The updated coding system, which is applied to the separation–reunion stories and two others, reflects this theoretical underpinning. Criteria for the A-B-C-D classification groups are based on features of story content and structure reflecting these processes, with indices of flexible integration corresponding to secure patterns, indices of deactivation corresponding to avoidant patterns, indices of cognitive disconnection corresponding to ambivalent patterns, and indices of dysregulation corresponding to controlling and unclassifiable patterns.

A supplementary coding system that captures specific markers for disorganization in the stories and in the child's behavior toward the story administrator is also available. Markers of one or another defensive process can be subtle. For example, in the "monster in the bedroom" story, where the child calls out to the parent in the night, having the parents give the child a rational explanation such as "Don't worry, that's just your teddy bear on the chair," would be a marker of deactivating processes. Having the parents say something such as "Don't worry, it's just a dream," would be taken as a marker of cognitive disconnection, the hallmark of which is a state of uncertainty: It provides neither a satisfying solution nor a rational explanation, but rather leaves the child with a vague feeling of unease that cannot be definitely addressed. Both the original and the revised systems were tested on a sample of 52 middle-class kindergartners (ages 5–7). Coders were required to reach 85% agreement. The concordance between the revised representation classifications and attachment classifications based on reunion behavior (Main & Cassidy, 1988) was 79% (kappa = .70), which is just slightly higher than what was achieved with the original classification procedure.

Three investigators have published applications of this updated system to high-risk populations. Venet, Bureau, Gosselin, and Capuano (2007) found that neglected children were more likely to be classified in the avoidant (deactivating) representational group and were likely to receive high scores on indices of disorganization. Katsurada (2007) found that the controlling (dysregulated) representation group was most common among Japanese children in group foster care, and that no children were judged secure (flexible). Webster and Hackett (in press) found no secure attachments in their sample of clinically referred maltreated children, but found that the presence of indices of security was negatively correlated with parent and teacher ratings of aggression and conduct disorder.

Family Drawing Measure

Several investigators have presented preliminary findings for another promising approach to representational security based on family drawing. Kaplan and Main (1986) developed a preliminary classification system for use with kindergarten-age children's drawings of their families. Some investigators, including Kaplan, have reported concordance between this system (or modifications of it) and reunion behavior classifications (Fury, Carlson, & Sroufe, 1997; Main et al., 1985); however, this finding has not been replicated in all studies

(M. Main, personal communication, 1998). Clarke and colleagues (2002) reported links among picture drawing classifications, SAT classifications, and Cassidy Puppet Interview classifications (designed to tap self-esteem) for a small group of boys with ADHD.

Discussion

A review of the available literature on measures of young children's representations of attachment reveals a wealth of efforts to capture variation related to security. Although validation of these measures is incomplete, their potential is twofold. First, the variety of children's symbolic behavior permits the development and comparison of different measures, which are necessary to establish construct validity. This has been an elusive goal for measures based on interaction. We continue to encourage researchers to undertake the systematic cross-validation of these measures, especially with respect to the four core hypotheses we have outlined earlier in this chapter. Second, investigators who have used representational materials in work with young children find them to be a rich source of information and a fruitful base for hypothesis generation. At their best, representational data reveal both the content and the structure of young children's thought, or, in Main's (2000) terms, "state of mind" regarding attachment. They may make it possible to explore psychologically important regulatory processes in young children, such as fantasy and defense, and to trace the links between children's and adults' construction of representational models. For this promise to be realized, investigators should take care to establish the congruence of new measures with interaction-based measures of attachment security. This continues to be necessary because a high level of abstraction is inherent in the construct of an attachment representation, and children's cognitive and language development can influence the quality of their responses to representational stimuli.

Much of the research on children's internal representation of attachment was inspired by work in Main's laboratory in the mid-1980s, which led to the development of the Adult Attachment Interview (AAI; George, Kaplan, & Main, 1984, 1985, 1996), Kaplan's first attempts to capture representational processes in the drawing and SAT responses of kindergartners (Kaplan, 1987), and Cassidy's self-esteem and family stories (Cassidy, 1988). Many more investigators than we have summarized here have attempted to study children's symbolic representation, leading to an almost dizzying array of instruments from which to choose. This collective effort has resulted overall in the demonstration of direct analogues to well-established qualitative differences in parent–infant and parent–child interaction, as well as to representational processes already identified in secure adults. For example, the behavior of the secure infant and kindergartner is characterized by open and direct communication of affect and by active, persistent, and unambivalent expression of attachment behavior. Criteria for representational security in several systems also include direct acknowledgment of affect (sadness, longing, anger) and a clear sense that reassurance or relief is forthcoming. In our own doll-play classification system, secure children symbolically depict separation anxiety as well as confidence in the favorable resolution to these fears and concerns. Furthermore, the cognitive complexity and narrative structure of their play clearly parallel the coherence and integration of thought characteristic of the attachment representations of secure adults (Main, 2000).

Despite these strengths, several systems have failed to differentiate completely among the various insecure representations. In our view, this is because they have focused too broadly on the surface content of children's narratives, rather than on detecting age-specific manifestations of defensive processes. This is clearest, perhaps, with respect to the avoidant group. One of the key features of the dismissing group on the AAI, linked empirically as well as theoretically to avoidant infant attachment (Main et al., 1985; van IJzendoorn et al., 1995), is the adult's tendency to idealize the self and others (see also Cassidy & Kobak, 1988). Idealization is also shown in Cassidy's (1988) study of responses to representations of the self in the Puppet Interview, where avoidant children are most likely to describe themselves as "perfect." Verscheuren and colleagues' (1996) analyses of children's representations of the family in doll play indicate that many of the children classified as "secure" in the Cassidy system also describe themselves as "perfect" in the Puppet Interview. This suggests that the attachment classification criteria fail to differentiate evidence of real confidence in the relationship from defensively asserted (portrayed) confidence, which is most likely to be shown by children with avoidant (or, as we have termed it, deactivating) defenses.

We briefly note two areas that need special attention as measures continue to be refined. First, we encourage investigators to develop measures directly from the representational material produced by a particular procedure, instead of relying on a priori considerations alone or "borrowing" criteria from one measure and applying them to another. For example, it appears that in response to SAT stimuli, avoidant children will often say, "I don't know." We find that this response is not characteristic of avoidant children when they are responding to doll-play scenarios; when it is repeated or mixed with other "response-avoidant" tactics, it is instead characteristic of some controlling/disorganized children. Transfer of Kaplan's picture-based system to doll-play materials may be one reason why several doll-play-based systems have failed to distinguish among insecure classification groups. Verbal responses to pictures and doll play may well draw on different memory processes (e.g., explicit vs. implicit memory).

Second, researchers should also consider the degree to which representational procedures activate the attachment system; this may differ depending on the age of the child being tested. Our experience in comparing the responses of children ages 3 through 7 to the Bretherton, Ridgeway, and colleagues (1990) procedure (George & Solomon, 1996a), suggests that different stories result in better discrimination between classification groups at different ages. In the stories of 3-year-olds, we see clearer distinctions in response to the "monster in the bedroom" story than to any of the other stories, including the separation–reunion scenario. In older children, we see clearer distinctions among the classification groups in response to the "hurt knee" and separation–reunion story stems. These differences may reflect an interaction between the attachment system and cognitive development (e.g., differences between preoperational and concrete operational information processing).

THE AQS: INFANCY THROUGH 5 YEARS

In contrast to systems of classifying child behavior and representation, the AQS assesses the quality of a child's secure-base behavior in the home. The system was developed by Waters to provide a practical alternative to the Ainsworth home observation narratives. Within the AQS system, "secure-base behavior" is defined as the smooth organization of and appropriate balance between proximity seeking and exploration (Posada, Waters, Crowell, & Lay, 1995). The Q-set for the AQS consists of 90 items designed to tap a range

of dimensions believed to reflect either the secure-base phenomenon itself or behavior associated with it in children ages 1–5. These items are sorted into one of nine piles, according to whether the item is considered characteristic or uncharacteristic of a child's behavior. Sorts can be completed by trained observers or by parents. Waters (1995) recommends that sorts by observers should be based on two to three visits for a total of 2–6 hours of observation in the home, with additional observations if observers fail to agree. The AQS permits the salience of a behavior in a child's repertoire to be distinguished from the frequency with which the behavior occurs. In addition, it helps to prevent observer biases and lends itself to an array of qualitative and quantitative analyses. AQS data can be analyzed in terms of individual items or summary scales, or they permit a comparison of the child's Q-sort profile to a criterion sort. Waters has developed criterion sorts for the construct of attachment security and for several other constructs (social desirability, dependence, sociability) by collecting and averaging the sorts of experts in the field. The child's security score is the correlation coefficient between the observer's sort and the criterion sort, and it represents the child's placement on a linear continuum with respect to security. Although some researchers have used different criterion sorts for the second and fourth years of life, E. Waters (personal communication, 1997) now recommends the use of a single criterion across this age range (12–60 months). Validated sorts for the A, C, or D insecure attachment groups defined by the Strange Situation are not available, although some researchers have developed classifications on a priori grounds for particular purposes (e.g., Howes & Hamilton, 1992; Kirkland, Bimler, Drawneek, McKim, & Scholmerich, 2004).

van IJzendoorn and colleagues (2004) recently undertook a meta-analysis of 139 AQS studies (N = 13,835 children ages 12–70 months) for the purpose of establishing the validity of this measure that was based on the same conceptual approach developed here. Below, for summary purposes, we rely on their findings and refer to specific studies in this area when specific points require a more fine-grained approach.

Validation of the Measure

Reliability

Intercoder Agreement. In comparison to classification systems, reliability on the AQS does not require extensive training or certification of reliability. Studies report interobserver reliability (correlations between sorts) ranging from .72 to .95. The correlation between mothers' and trained observers' sorts tends to be moderate in small to medium-size samples (approximately 35–60 subjects); however, it improves considerably as a function of training and supervision of mothers, as well as the degree to which observers are trained and have opportunity to see a sufficient range of child behavior (Teti & McGourty, 1996). We return to this issue at the conclusion of this section.

Short-Term Stability. Short-term stability data, representing repeated sorts in close succession, are not reported in the literature.

Relation to Other Measures of Attachment

AQS security scores have been found to differentiate 12- to 18-month-old infants classified as secure or insecure in the Strange Situation in several but not all published studies. Average AQS security scores for the secure group in the Strange Situation tend to be about .50, and average security scores for the insecure groups tend to be about .25 (Waters & Deane, 1985). van IJzendoorn and colleagues (2004) found a combined effect size of 0.23, indicating a moderate association between the measures. They noted that the correlation for observer-generated sorts was significantly higher than for caregiver-generated ones, and concluded that there are substantial problems with Q-sort data generated by caregivers. Paralleling Ainsworth's original finding that insecure groups were difficult to distinguish on the basis of their behavior in the home, distinctive differences between 12- to 18-month-olds classified as A or C in the Strange Situation do not emerge clearly in the AQS data. It appears to be the case, however, that infants classified as disorganized in the Strange Situation are characterized by very low AQS scores.

In the preschool period, the relation between the AQS and other security measures is less certain. van IJzendoorn and colleagues' (2004) meta-analysis revealed significantly lower correlations between reunion-based attachment measures for preschoolers and observer-generated AQS security than for younger children. The weaker relation may be accounted for at least in part by the relative paucity of validity studies existing for this age range, and the failure to explore effects of the disorganized classifications (see also Posada, 2006). Moss and colleagues (2006), in an effort

to address these gaps, compared Cassidy–Marvin classifications to AQS security (trained mothers completed the sorts) in a middle-class French Canadian sample of preschoolers. They found the two measures to be significantly associated overall; the secure group was differentiated in AQS security from the disorganized and ambivalent classifications, but not from avoidant or controlling ones. Somewhat more consistent links have been shown between AQS security in preschool and child representational measures of attachment. Bretherton, Ridgeway, and colleagues (1990) reported a strong correlation between maternal sorts completed at age 25 months and Bretherton's representational measure of attachment, but the relation between measures was considerably weaker when concurrent 37-month maternal sorts were used. Waters, Rodrigues, and Ridgeway (1998), using a script analysis approach on the Bretherton data set at 37 months, were also able to show a positive correlation to AQS security. However, Oppenheim (1997) did not find a significant relationship between AQS security and his doll-play measure of attachment.

Prediction to Core Variables

Mother–Child Interaction. Across both the infancy and preschool periods, scores or ratings of maternal sensitivity based on brief home visits were significantly related to AQS security. Meta-analysis also revealed that this relation was significantly higher for observer-generated sorts than for mother-generated ones. In contrast to what has been found for Strange Situation classifications, assessments of temperament, especially negative reactivity, have shown moderate correlations with AQS security. However, van IJzendoorn and colleagues (2004) reported that observer-generated sorts were significantly more independent of temperament measures than caregiver-generated ones (see also Vaughn et al., Chapter 9, this volume). In what may be a related set of findings, several studies report moderate concordance between mothers' and fathers' AQS security scores, which might also reflect the effect of temperament, among other factors (Bakermans-Kranenburg, van IJzendoorn, Bokhorst, & Schuengel, 2004; Caldera, 2004). Taken together, these findings suggest some limitation in the discriminant validity of AQS security, although the shared variance is not great. van IJzendoorn and colleagues found no relation between security with father and AQS scores, or between paternal sensitivity and AQS security. Since there is also a great deal of uncertainty about the meaning of father–infant security as assessed in the Strange Situation, the lack of relation between measures in the case of fathers is not surprising.

Continuity. Continuity of AQS scores appears to be low to moderate over a period of 2 or more years, similar to what has been found for the preschool-age reunion-based assessments. Using caregiver sorts, Belsky and Rovine (1990) reported low to moderate long-term stability between ages 1 and 3 (mothers, $r = .23$; fathers, $r = .53$; social desirability partialed out). Teti, Sakin, Kucera, Corns, and Das Eiden (1996), who trained mothers thoroughly on the sorting procedure, reported correlations between (approximately) .40 and .60 2 or more years later, after the birth of a sibling. Observer-generated reports appear to be variable, but potentially of comparable strength: van IJzendoorn and colleagues (2004) report that the combined stability correlation was .28. Clark and Symons (2000) found a moderate but significant positive correlation in AQS security between ages 2 and (approximately) 5, based on observer sorts. (See also Bretherton, Ridgeway, et al., 1990.)

Coherence. Using a sample of 33 studies, van IJzendoorn and colleagues (2004) found AQS security to be significantly related to measures of social competence with peers and siblings and to fewer child problem behaviors, although the correlations tended to be small. In contrast to the meta-analytic findings regarding parent and child behavior in the home, observer sorts were not superior to those of caregivers (parents or teachers). A variety of parental and marital/couple variables (e.g., marital/couple relationship quality, social support, parenting stress, SES) have also been shown to be related to AQS security (Howes & Markman, 1989; Moss et al., 2006; Nakasawa, Teti, & Lamb, 1992).

Cross-Cultural Studies. In a major study on the cross-cultural validity of the AQS, researchers determined that mothers and experts could discriminate attachment security from the constructs of dependency and social desirability in a range of countries (China, Japan, Israel, Columbia, Germany, Norway, United States) (Posada, Gao, et al., 1995). Although the structure of the data was broadly similar cross-culturally, the correlations of maternal sorts across cultures tended to be low (ranges = .15–.32) (Strayer, Verissimo, Vaughn,

& Howes, 1995; Vaughn, Strayer, Jacques, Trudel, & Seifer, 1991). This suggests that ecological factors may have a powerful effect on the patterning of young children's secure-base behavior in the home. More recently, studies bearing on the validity of the AQS have been reported for samples from Thailand (Chaimongkol & Flick, 2006), Portugal (Vaughn et al., 2007), and South Africa (Minde, Minde, & Vogel, 2006).

Discussion

The great promise of the AQS lies in its emphasis on naturalistic observation in ecologically valid contexts. Researchers have demonstrated that the procedure can be used reliably and with adequate validity across a variety of national and cultural groups. As a practical matter, this measurement approach permits researchers to estimate attachment security without the laboratory space and equipment or extensive training required for the Strange Situation procedure. For the infancy period (ages 12–18 months), there is now a substantial literature demonstrating the validity of the AQS according to the criteria we have established earlier. AQS security shows a reliable correspondence to security or insecurity in the Strange Situation, as well as to maternal sensitivity. Thus there is reason to be confident that the AQS taps a significant portion of the variance associated with the construct of attachment security. Even for infants, however, the strength of relationship among these variables is moderate or low. The AQS procedure also does not allow reliable distinctions to be made among the insecure groups, although, as would be predicted theoretically, infants and children classified as disorganized are characterized by the lowest security scores.

It is not to be expected—indeed, it may not even be desirable—for any two measures of a construct to be perfectly correlated. Nonetheless, it is helpful to explore the sources of nonconvergence, in order to better estimate and understand the underlying construct of security. A besetting question for this method has been whether mothers or trained observers are the more appropriate sources of secure-base data. Based on their meta-analytic findings, van IJzendoorn and colleagues (2004) stated definitively that observer sorts are reliable while caregiver (self-)reports are not. Indeed, there is empirical evidence that the same maternal information-processing biases that are believed to be causal factors in the development of the different types of attachment relationships come into play when mothers complete their sorts (Cassidy & Kobak, 1988; Main, 2000; Solomon & George, 1999b; Stevenson-Hinde & Shouldice, 1995). (See also George & Solomon, 1996b and Chapter 35, this volume.) Observers, on the other hand, may be susceptible to different sorts of bias or error. In contrast to the Strange Situation, a mother's behavior is not constrained in the home, and it is quite likely that an observer's impression of one interaction partner influences his or her impression of the other. In Waters and Deane's (1985) original Q-sort study, and in Teti and McGourty's (1996) more recent effort, maternal and observer agreement was moderate to very strong (.50–.80) when observers had sufficient opportunity to see relevant child behavior (see also Moss et al., 2006). Thus either caregivers or outside observers can provide reliable sorts under the proper conditions.

In our view, the most important limitation of the AQS data (which unfortunately is also its most important advantage) is that the AQS and Strange Situation classifications are rooted in the different contexts of the home and of the laboratory. In the placid and relatively safe environment of the middle-class home, there is little to activate the attachment system. That is why AQS researchers have emphasized their instrument as a measure of "secure-base" behavior, as opposed to attachment behavior in "emergency" situations, which the Strange Situation measures. Of course, observers see many kinds of behaviors in the home, many of which pertain to behavioral systems other than exploration or attachment. A consequence of this difference is not only that different behaviors are likely to be observed in the home as compared to the laboratory playroom, but that a certain amount of mother–child interaction in the home is quite likely to be a function of child temperament (including sociability), the immediate physical and social environment, the family milieu (e.g., marital/couple harmony), and more transitory influences (e.g., the health, mood, and current activities of the participants). That is, the AQS as generally employed will necessarily be imprecise with respect to a child's generalized expectations regarding parental availability and responsiveness when the child is in real need of a parent. The context of observation can be expected to be increasingly important past infancy, since situations that strongly activate attachment are very rarely observed in the home as children mature. Observations of mothers and children under more stressful or threatening conditions (e.g., busy parks, stores, doctors' offices, airports) might increase the convergence of AQS scores with reunion-based classifications and allow the quality of the attachment relationship to be disentangled from other influences in the home.

The effect of context on measures of attachment security may be even more complex. Ainsworth and colleagues (1978) noted that discrepancies between patterns of secure-base behavior in the home and attachment classifications could often be explained by recent changes in maternal sensitivity. Thus home observations may reflect the current state of a mother–child relationship rather accurately, but the child's expectations regarding the mother's responsiveness (as assessed in the Strange Situation) may lag behind. A final possibility is that the young child's attachment working model of the relationship is more heavily influenced by some experiences than by others. This would be consistent with the nature of more mature relationships. We are unlikely to hold it against those we depend on if they snub us mildly in everyday life, as long as they are truly there for us when we feel we *really* need them. The inverse should also be true: We may dismiss, discount, or at least hesitate to put faith in the sensitive responsiveness of others if we still cannot forgive them for the times they failed or disappointed us.[3]

Finally, questions may be asked about the validity of the expert (criterion) sorts themselves. AQS researchers have emphasized that the organization of secure-base relevant behaviors (i.e., the child's profile relative to the expert Q-sort of the security construct) is the best measure of security (Posada, Gao, et al., 1995). Experts may agree, and yet the criterion sort may still require some revision.[4] The validity of the criterion sort for 3-year-olds is especially problematic: It continues to be true that there is not a sufficient descriptive base from which to derive a sound criterion. A general concern is that expert sorts may confound core attachment phenomena with other behaviors that are correlated with attachment patterns under some circumstances but not others (e.g., Carlson & Harwood, 2003). The only way to determine whether the current weighting of items is appropriate is to continue to test and refine the criterion sorts themselves against classifications and other attachment measures cross-culturally.

SUMMARY AND CONCLUSIONS

In the first edition of the *Handbook of Attachment* (Solomon & George, 1999d) we described attachment research as "a robust field in a period of active expansion and experimentation" (p. 310). Our current overview of attachment security measures shows the field to be at a mature stage, with several reasonably well-validated measures available that are appropriate for children across the span of early childhood. Over time, many researchers have given attention to the basic requirements of construct validation we have outlined at the beginning of this chapter. There continue to be important questions, especially regarding attachment classification procedures in the preschool years; the most useful approaches to studying representational processes; and the meaning of a measure such as the AQS, which is based on unstructured home observations. As we have discussed throughout the chapter, however, these may reflect outstanding nomothetic issues as much as purely measurement-related issues. Looking to the future, we would like to consider two areas in which major change, in both practice and understanding, seems likely.

The first issue concerns the reliance on a categorical as opposed to a dimensional approach to capturing individual differences. It is well known that Ainsworth was committed to the investigation of behavioral constellations or multidimensional patterns (Ainsworth & Marvin, 1995), though she apparently was not averse to scaling based on a discriminant analysis of group differences (Ainsworth et al., 1978). Fraley and Spieker's (2003) contention that the A-B-C categories could be summarized more parsimoniously and accurately in terms of two dimensions, approach–avoidance and resistance–emotional confidence, has brought this matter to the fore once again. Fraley and Spieker argued from their findings that "it is difficult to justify the sole use of categorical models in attachment" (p. 402); this statement provoked one of the liveliest debates that the field has seen in some time (Cassidy, 2003; Cummings, 2003; Waters & Beauchaine, 2003). In rejoinders, commentators pointed out, as we have done here, that the classification approach has yielded great riches by training researchers to approach the study of relationships from the perspective of organizational and strategic differences among attachment patterns or types (Cassidy, 2003). On the other hand, there is general agreement that security scales, such as that generated for AQS scores or the emotional security scale proposed by Cummings (2003), are entirely appropriate ways of representing and simplifying individual differences in relationships.

Fraley and Spieker's article shone a much-needed spotlight on the tendency to reify attachment classifications while forgetting the underlying constructs they were meant to tap. As Waters and Beauchaine (2003) pointed out, the existence of classification categories implies the existence of testable mechanisms that underlie true categorical or taxonomic distinctions. Currently there is no evidence regarding such mechanisms. Yet the tendency to perceive and create categories to reduce a complex multidimensional reality is a pervasive human inclination. It is intriguing to consider that infants and children, like adults, may also have a bias toward simplifying experiences with a caregiver—which may lead them, in essence, to differentiate "good enough" from "not good enough" security in a more or less categorical manner.

We have suggested earlier that some experiences with parents may weigh more heavily than others in an infant or child's unconscious assessment of a relationship as basically secure ("good enough"). This proposition could lead to some testable hypotheses. For example, do infants "calculate" the ratio of accepted versus rejected bids for contact in general, or predominantly when they are distressed (McElwain & Booth-LaForce, 2006)? Do they weigh more distressing or more recent experiences more heavily than others? Certainly this "calculus," if there can be said to be one, must change over the course of development as a function of social, regulatory, and cognitive development. These are fascinating issues that we hope may be addressed in the future. In terms of measurement, however, there is no question that dimensional measures both of security and of the defensive processes that underlie patterns of attachment are more efficient to generate and statistically more flexible. Among other advantages, it is likely that the divergent estimates of relationship stability that we have highlighted throughout this chapter will converge more closely with their use, since the category system introduces a certain amount of arbitrariness regarding cutoffs for group placement. It seems often to be the fate of mature sciences that rich and complex measures become simplified as the constructs they were meant to capture become assimilated beyond their original fields. We would not be surprised, though perhaps somewhat saddened, to see the research emphasis on attachment categories fade considerably in the coming years.

The second issue concerns the assessment of attachment for children who have or are continuing to experience deprivation of attachment figures, disrupted attachments, and major or frequent separations. These are the children who were originally of great interest to Bowlby and those other researchers who contributed to our basic knowledge in this area. It is also a population of growing interest to attachment researchers (see Dozier & Rutter, Chapter 29, and B. Feeney & Monin, Chapter 39, this volume), and one that increasingly contributes to the caseloads of infant mental health and other clinical psychologists—many of whom use (or would like to use) conventional attachment measures as part of their assessments. The measurement problems in this context are twofold, requiring a new look at standard measures and the development of new, ecologically valid ones. There has long been both an implicit and an explicit understanding in attachment research that the interpretation of separation–reunion procedures is questionable when it is uncertain whether a child has developed an attachment to a particular caregiver or when the child has recently undergone a major separation. It is also a consistent finding in studies involving such children that when seen in separation–reunion contexts, the children are judged to be disorganized or unclassifiable in attachment (e.g., Jacobsen & Haight, in press; Zeanah, Smyke, Koga, & Carlson, 2005; Solomon & George, 1999c). The meaning of this disorganized attachment behavior cannot be assumed to be the same as it is for normative, home-reared children. It may reflect failure to establish attachments, separations, neurological perturbations, or interactive experiences. Furthermore, the type or manifestation of behavioral disorganization may differ as well. Careful observation may reveal behavioral variants that reflect these different factors. In short, what seems to be called for is a reexamination of the separation–reunion behavior of these children—akin to what was involved originally in detecting disorganization of attachment (Main & Solomon, 1986, 1990)—as well as the development of new, ecologically valid measures. An example of this kind of methodology is described elsewhere (Solomon & George, 1999c): We found that formerly disorganized and unclassifiable toddlers experiencing overnight visitation with their fathers in divorcing families were more likely to break down in anger toward their mothers during a cleanup task, some minutes *after* a second laboratory separation. Further investigation is yet needed to determine whether the original unclassifiability (which commonly looked like a breakdown of avoidance into a display of anger) and the later breakdown were actually functions of adverse separation–reunion experiences or of other factors.

This leads to our second point about attachment research in separation-related and other clinical contexts. The more clinicians incorporate attachment theory and research into their work, the more need they have for convenient, non-laboratory-based attachment measures. Many investigators undoubtedly hoped that the AQS could provide security data about as easily and inexpensively as conventional self-report instruments. Now that it is clear that caregivers need thorough training and observers need considerable observation time to create valid sorts, this hope has been somewhat diminished. Although clinicians may find that shortcuts such as using a one-separation procedure are adequate to their clinical needs (e.g., Hoffman et al., 2006), this procedure is less satisfactory when clinicians must contribute to legal proceedings involving the children or wish to participate in research. Researchers working in this area have already been very creative in devising alternative measures of attachment and attempting to validate them (Dozier, Stovall, Albus, & Bates, 2001; Poehlmann, 2005; Zeanah et al., 2005). We look forward to seeing more such measures—meticulously validated, of course—in the future.

NOTES

1. It must be emphasized that the construct of security is meaningful only for a relationship in which a child has already developed an attachment to a particular caregiver. In situations where this is in doubt, such as in studies involving transitions to foster care, the interpretation of any measure of security is problematic.

2. Because of space constraints, we rely for this review mainly on the published journal literature. This may have the unintended consequence of exaggerating rather than minimizing the appearance of a relation between any two variables, but it ensures that the studies have undergone peer review.

3. A similar possibility is suggested by a review of the effects of clinical interventions on attachment classification (van IJzendoorn et al., 1995). Several studies reviewed by these investigators reported improvements in maternal sensitivity to a child without a concomitant move by the child to a secure classification.

4. According to data provided by Posada, Gao, and col-

leagues (1995), the expert sort seems to describe best the 3-year-old child of mature graduate student parents in Norway. Modal security scores in this sample were the highest of any of those studied.

REFERENCES

Achermann, J., Dinneen, E., & Stevenson-Hinde, J. (1991). Clearing up at 2.5 years. *British Journal of Developmental Psychology, 9,* 365–376.

Ackerman, J. P., & Dozier, M. (2005). The influence of foster parent investment on children's representations of self and attachment figures. *Journal of Applied Developmental Psychology, 26,* 507–520.

Ainsworth, M. D. S., Blehar, M. C., Waters, E., & Wall, S. (1978). *Patterns of attachment: A psychological study of the Strange Situation.* Hillsdale, NJ: Erlbaum.

Ainsworth, M. D. S., & Marvin, R. S. (1995). On the shaping of attachment theory and research: An interview with Mary D. S. Ainsworth (Fall 1994). In E. Waters, B. E. Vaughn, G. Posada, & K. Kondo-Ikemura (Eds.), Caregiving, cultural, and cognitive perspectives on secure-base behavior and working models: New growing points of attachment theory and research. *Monographs of the Society for Research in Child Development, 60*(2–3, Serial No. 244), 3–21.

Bakermans-Kranenburg, M. J., & van IJzendoorn, M. H. (2004). No association of the dopamine D4 receptor (DRD4) and -521 C/T promoter polymorphisms with infant attachment disorganization. *Attachment and Human Development, 6,* 211–218.

Bakermans-Kranenburg, M. J., van IJzendoorn, M. H., Bokhorst, C. L., Schuengel, C. (2004). The importance of shared environment in infant–father attachment: A behavioral genetic study of the Attachment Q-Sort. *Journal of Family Psychology, 18,* 545–549.

Bar-Haim, Y., Sutton, D. B., Fox, N. A., & Marvin, R. S. (2000). Stability and change of attachment at 14, 24, and 58 months of age: Behavior, representation, and life events. *Journal of Child Psychology and Psychiatry, 41,* 381–388.

Barnett, D., Clements, M., Kaplan-Estrin, M., McCaskill, J. W., Hunt, K. H., Butler, C. M., et al. (2006). Maternal resolution of child diagnosis: Stability and relations with child attachment across the toddler to preschooler transition. *Journal of Family Psychology, 20,* 100–107.

Barnett, D., Kidwell, S. L., & Leung, K. H. (1998). Parenting and preschooler attachment among low-income urban African American families. *Child Development, 69,* 1657–1671.

Belsky, J. (1996). Parent, infant, and social-contextual antecedents of father–son attachment security. *Developmental Psychology, 32,* 905–913.

Belsky, J., Campbell, S. B., Cohn, J. F., & Moore, G. (1996). Instability of infant–parent attachment security. *Developmental Psychology, 32,* 921–924.

Belsky, J., & Rovine, M. (1990). Q-sort security and first-year nonmaternal care. *New Directions for Child Development, 49,* 7–22.

Biringen, Z., Brown, D., Donaldson, L., Green, S., Krcmarik, S., & Lovas, G. (2000). Adult Attachment Interview: Linkages with dimensions of emotional availability for mothers and their pre-kindergarteners. *Attachment and Human Development, 2,* 188–202.

Bowlby, J. (1969/1982). *Attachment and loss: Vol. 1. Attachment.* New York: Basic Books.

Bowlby, J. (1973). *Attachment and loss: Vol. 2. Separation: Anxiety and anger.* New York: Basic Books.

Bowlby, J. (1980). *Attachment and loss: Vol. 3. Loss: Sadness and depression.* New York: Basic Books.

Braungart-Rieker, J. M., Garwood, M. M., Powers, B. P., & Wang, X. (2001). Parental sensitivity, infant affect, and affect regulation: Predictors of later attachment. *Child Development, 72,* 252–270.

Bretherton, I. (2000). Emotional availability: An attachment perspective. *Attachment and Human Development, 2,* 233–241.

Bretherton, I., Grossmann, K. E., Grossmann, K., & Waters, E. (2005). In pursuit of the internal working model construct and its relevance to attachment relationships. In K. E. Grossmann, K. Grossmann, & E. Waters (Eds.), *Attachment from infancy to adulthood: The major longitudinal studies* (pp. 13–47). New York: Guilford Press.

Bretherton, I., Oppenheim, D., Buchsbaum, H., Emde, R., & the MacArthur Narrative Group. (1990). *The MacArthur Story Stem Battery.* Unpublished manuscript, University of Wisconsin–Madison.

Bretherton, I., Ridgeway, D., & Cassidy, J. (1990). Assessing internal working models of the attachment relationship: An attachment story completion task for 3-year-olds. In M. T. Greenberg, D. Cicchetti, & E. M. Cummings (Eds.), *Attachment in the preschool years* (pp. 273–308). Chicago: University of Chicago Press.

Britner, P. A., Marvin, R. S., & Pianta, R. C. (2005). Development and preliminary validation of the caregiving behavior system: Association with child attachment classification in the preschool Strange Situation. *Attachment and Human Development, 7,* 83–102.

Bureau, J.-F., Buliveau, M.-J., Moss, E., & Lépine, S. (2006). Association entre l'attachement mère–enfant et les récits d'attachement y la période scolaire [Association between mother–child attachment and attachment narratives during the school-age years]. *Revue Canadienne des Sciences du Comportement [Canadian Journal of Behavioural Sciences], 38,* 50–62.

Caldera, Y. M. (2004). Paternal involvement and infant–father attachment: A Q-set study. *Fathering, 2,* 191–210.

Campbell, D., & Fiske, D. (1959). Convergent and discriminant validation by the multitrait–multimethod matrix. *Psychological Bulletin, 56,* 81–105.

Campbell, S. B., Brownell, C. A., Hungerford, A., Spieker, S. J., Mohan, R., & Blessing, J. S. (2004). The course of maternal depressive symptoms and maternal sensitivity as predictors of attachment security at 36 months. *Development and Psychopathology, 16*(2), 231–252.

Carlson, E. A. (1998). A prospective longitudinal study of attachment disorganization/disorientation. *Child Development, 69*, 1107–1128.

Carlson, E. A., & Sroufe, L. A. (1993, Spring). Reliability in attachment classification. *Society for Research in Child Development Newsletter*, p. 12.

Carlson, V. J., & Harwood, R. L. (2003). Attachment, culture, and the caregiving system: The cultural patterning of everyday experiences among Anglo and Puerto Rican mother–infant pairs. *Infant Mental Health Journal, 24*, 53–73.

Carr, S. J., Dabbs, J. M., & Carr, T. S. (1975). Mother–infant attachment: The importance of the mother's visual field. *Child Development, 46*, 331–338.

Cassidy, J. (1988). Child–mother attachment and the self. *Child Development, 59*, 121–134.

Cassidy, J. (2003). Continuity and change in the measurement of infant attachment: Comment on Fraley and Spieker (2003). *Developmental Psychology, 39*, 409–412.

Cassidy, J., Berlin, L., & Belsky, J. (1990, April). *Attachment organization at age 3: Antecedent and concurrent correlates*. Paper presented at the biennial meetings of the International Conference on Infant Studies, Montreal.

Cassidy, J., Kirsh, S. J., Scolton, K. L., & Parke, R. D. (1996). Attachment and representations of peer relationships. *Developmental Psychology, 32*, 892–904.

Cassidy, J., & Kobak, R. R. (1988). Avoidance and its relation to other defensive processes. In J. Belsky & T. Nezworski (Eds.), *Clinical implications of attachment* (pp. 300–323). Hillsdale, NJ: Erlbaum.

Cassidy, J., & Marvin, R. S., with the MacArthur Attachment Working Group. (1992). *Attachment organization in preschool children: Coding guidelines* (4th ed.). Unpublished manuscript, University of Virginia.

Chaimongkol, N. N. & Flick, L. H. (2006). Maternal sensitivity and attachment security in Thailand: Cross-cultural validation of Western measures. *Journal of Nursing Measurement, 14*, 5–17.

Chandler, M. J. (1973). Egocentrism and antisocial behavior: The assessment and training of social perspective-taking skills. *Developmental Psychology, 9*, 326–332.

Cicchetti, D., & Barnett, D. (1991). Attachment organization in maltreated preschoolers. *Development and Psychopathology, 3*, 397–411.

Clark, S. E., & Symons, D. K. (2000). A longitudinal study of Q-sort attachment security and self-processes at age 5. *Infant and Child Development, 9*, 91–104.

Clarke, L., Ungerer, J., Chahoud, K., Johnson, S., & Stiefel, I. (2002). Attention deficit hyperactivity disorder is associated with attachment insecurity. *Clinical Child Psychology and Psychiatry, 7*, 179–198.

Cohn, D. A. (1990). Child–mother attachment of six-year-olds and social competence at school. *Child Development, 61*, 152–162.

Cox, M. J., Owen, M. T., Henderson, V. K., & Margand, N. A. (1992). Prediction of infant–father and infant–mother attachment. *Developmental Psychology, 28*, 474–483.

Crittenden, P. M. (1992a). *Preschool Assessment of Attachment*. Unpublished manuscript, Family Relations Institute, Miami, FL.

Crittenden, P. M. (1992b). The quality of attachment in the preschool years. *Development and Psychopathology, 4*, 209–241.

Crittenden, P. M. (1994). *Preschool Assessment of Attachment* (2nd ed.). Unpublished manuscript, Family Relations Institute, Miami, FL.

Crittenden, P. M., & Claussen, A. H. (1994). *Validation of two procedures for assessing quality of attachment in the preschool years*. Paper presented at the biennial meeting of the International Conference on Infant Studies, Paris.

Crittenden, P. M., & Claussen, A. H. (Eds.). (2000). *The organization of attachment relationships: Maturation, culture, and context*. New York: Cambridge University Press.

Cummings, E. M. (2003). Toward assessing attachment on an emotional security continuum: Comment on Fraley and Spieker (2003). *Developmental Psychology, 39*, 405–408.

De Wolff, M., & van IJzendoorn, M. H. (1997). Sensitivity and attachment: A meta-analysis on parental antecedents of infant attachment. *Child Development, 68*, 571–591.

Dozier, M., Stovall, K. C., Albus, K. E., & Bates, B. (2001). Attachment for infants in foster care: The role of caregiver state of mind. *Child Development, 72*, 14–67.

Easterbrooks, M. A., & Abeles, R. (2000). Windows to the self in 8-year-olds: Bridges to attachment representation and behavioral adjustment. *Attachment and Human Development, 2*, 85–106.

Easterbrooks, M. A., Biesecker, G., & Lyons-Ruth, K. (2000). Infancy predictors of emotional availability in middle childhood: The roles of attachment security and maternal depressive symptomatology. *Attachment and Human Development, 2*, 170–187.

Easterbrooks, M. A., Davidson, C. E., & Chazan, R. (1993). Psychosocial risk, attachment, and behavior problems among school-aged children. *Development and Psychopathology, 5*, 389–402.

Easterbrooks, M. A. & Goldberg, W. A. (1984). Toddler development in the family: Impact of father involvement and parenting characteristics. *Child Development, 55*, 740–752.

Erikson, E. H. (1950). *Childhood and society*. New York: Norton.

Fearon, R. M. P., van IJzendoorn, M. H., Fonagy, P., Bakermans-Kranenburg, M. J., Schuengel, C., & Bokhorst, C. L. (2006). In search of shared and non-shared environmental factors in security of attachment: A behavior-genetic study of the association between sensitivity and attachment security. *Developmental Psychology, 42*, 1026–1040.

Fish, M. (2001). Attachment in low-SES rural Appalachian infants: Contextual, infant, and maternal interaction risk and protective factors. *Infant Mental Health Journal, 22,* 641–664.

Fish, M. (2004). Attachment in infancy and preschool in low socioeconomic status rural Appalachian children: Stability and change and relations to preschool and kindergarten competence. *Development and Psychopathology, 16,* 293–312.

Fox, N. A., Susman, E. J., Feagans, L. V., & Ray, W. J. (1992). The role of individual differences in infant personality in the formation of attachment relationships. In W. J. Ray (Ed.), *Emotion, cognition, health, and development in children and adolescents* (pp. 31–52). Hillsdale, NJ: Erlbaum.

Fraley, C., & Spieker, S. J. (2003). Are infant attachment patterns continuously or categorically distributed?: A taxometric analysis of Strange Situation behavior. *Developmental Psychology, 39,* 387–404.

Fury, G. S., Carlson, E. A., & Sroufe, L. A. (1997). Children's representations of attachment in family drawings. *Child Development, 68,* 1154–1164.

George, C., Kaplan, N., & Main, M. (1984). *Adult Attachment Interview protocol.* Unpublished manuscript, University of California at Berkeley.

George, C., Kaplan, N., & Main, M. (1985). *Adult Attachment Interview protocol* (2nd ed.). Unpublished manuscript, University of California at Berkeley.

George, C., Kaplan, N., & Main, M. (1996). *Adult Attachment Interview protocol* (3rd ed.). Unpublished manuscript, University of California at Berkeley.

George, C., & Solomon, J. (1990/1996/2000). *Six-year attachment doll play classification system.* Unpublished manuscript, Mills College, Oakland, CA.

George, C., & Solomon, J. (1996a, August). *Assessing internal working models of attachment through doll play.* Paper presented at the biennial meeting of the International Society for the Study of Behavioral Development, Quebec City, QB, Canada.

George, C., & Solomon, J. (1996b). Representational models of relationships: Links between caregiving and attachment. *Infant Mental Health Journal, 17,* 18–36.

George, C., & West, M. (1999). Developmental vs. social personality models of adult attachment and mental ill health. *British Journal of Medical Psychology, 72,* 285–303.

George, C., West, M., Hilsenroth, M. J., & Segal, D. L. (2004). The Adult Attachment Projective: Measuring individual differences in attachment security using projective methodology. In M. Hersen (Series Ed.), & M. J. Hilsenroth & D. L. Segal (Vol. Eds.), *Comprehensive handbook of psychological assessment: Vol. 2. Personality assessment* (pp. 431–447). Hoboken, NJ: Wiley.

Gervai, J., Nemoda, Z., Lakatos, K., Ronai, Z., Toth, I., Ney, K., et al. (2005). Transmission disequilibrium tests confirm the link between DRD4 gene polymorphism and infant attachment. *American Journal of Medical Genetics, Part B, Neuropsychiatric Genetics, 132,* 126–130.

Gloger-Tippelt, G., Gomille, B., Koenig, L., & Vetter, J. (2002). Attachment representations in 6-year-olds: Related longitudinally to the quality of attachment in infancy and mothers' attachment representations. *Attachment and Human Development, 4,* 318–339.

Greenberg, M. T., Speltz, M. L., DeKlyen, M., & Endriga, M. C. (1991). Attachment security in preschoolers with and without externalizing behavior problems: A replication. *Development and Psychopathology, 3,* 413–430.

Hamilton, C. E. (2000). Continuity and discontinuity of attachment from infancy through adolescence. *Child Development, 71,* 690–694.

Hansburg, H. G. (1972). *Adolescent separation anxiety: Vol. 1. A method for the study of adolescent separation problems.* Springfield, IL: Thomas.

Hesse, E., & Main, M. (2006). Frightened, threatening, and dissociative parental behavior in low-risk samples: Description, discussion, and interpretations. *Development and Psychopathology, 18,* 309–343.

Hoffman, K. T., Marvin, R. S., Cooper, G., & Powell, B. (2006). Changing toddlers' and preschoolers' attachment classifications: The Circle of Security intervention. *Journal of Consulting and Clinical Psychology, 74,* 1017–1026.

Howes, C., & Hamilton, C. E. (1992). Children's relationships with child care teachers: Stability and concordance with parental attachments. *Child Development, 63,* 867–878.

Howes, P., & Markman, H. J. (1989). Marital quality and child functioning: A longitudinal investigation. *Child Development, 60,* 1044–1051.

Humber, N., & Moss, E. (2005). The relationship of preschool and early school age attachment to mother–child interaction. *American Journal of Orthopsychiatry, 75,* 128–141.

Jacobsen, T., Edelstein, W., & Hofmann, V. (1994). A longitudinal study of the relation between representations of attachment in childhood and cognitive functioning in childhood and adolescence. *Developmental Psychology, 30,* 112–124.

Jacobsen, T., & Haight, W. L. (in press). Dysfunctional responses to separation: Young children in foster care. In J. Solomon & C. George (Eds.), *Disorganized attachment and caregiving.* New York: Guilford Press.

Jacobsen, T., & Hofmann, V. (1997). Children's attachment representations: longitudinal relations to school behavior and academic competency in middle childhood and adolescence. *Developmental Psychology, 33,* 703–710.

Kaplan, N. (1987). *Individual differences in six-year-olds' thoughts about separation: Predicted from attachment to mother at one year of age.* Unpublished doctoral dissertation, University of California at Berkeley.

Kaplan, N., & Main, M. (1986). *A system for the analysis of children's family drawings in terms of attachment.* Unpublished manuscript, University of California at Berkeley.

Katsurada, E. (2007). Attachment representation of

institutionalized children in Japan. *School Psychology International, 28,* 331–345.

Kayoko, Y. (2006). Assessing attachment representations in early childhood: Validation of the attachment doll play. *Japanese Journal of Educational Psychology, 54,* 476–486.

Kirkland, J., Bimler, D., Drawneek, A., McKim, M., & Scholmerich, A. (2004). An alternative approach for the analyses and interpretation of attachment sort items. *Early Child Development and Care, 174,* 701–719.

Klagsbrun, M., & Bowlby, J. (1976). Responses to separation from parents: A clinical test for young children. *British Journal of Projective Psychology, 21,* 7–21.

Lamb, M. E. (1976). Effects of stress and cohort on mother– and father–infant interaction. *Developmental Psychology, 12,* 435–443.

Levine, R. A., & Miller, P. M. (1990). Commentary. *Human Development, 33,* 73–80.

Lounds, J. J., Borkowski, J. G., Whitman, T. L., Maxwell, S. E., & Weed, K. (2005). Adolescent parenting and attachment during infancy and early development. *Parenting: Science and Practice, 5,* 91–118.

Lyons-Ruth, K., Bronfman, E., & Parsons, E. (1999). Atypical attachment in infancy and early childhood among children at developmental risk. IV. Maternal frightened, frightening, or atypical behavior and disorganized infant attachment patterns. *Monographs of the Society for Research in Child Development, 64*(3), 67–96.

Lyons-Ruth, K., Repacholi, B., McLeod, S., & Silva, E. (1991). Disorganized attachment behavior in infancy: Short-term stability, maternal and infant correlates, and risk-related subtypes. *Development and Psychopathology, 3,* 377–396.

Lyons-Ruth, K., Yellin, C., Melnick, S., & Atwood, G. (2003). Childhood experiences of trauma and loss have different relations to maternal unresolved and hostile-helpless states of mind on the AAI. *Attachment and Human Development, 5,* 330–352.

Main, M. (1990). Cross-cultural studies of attachment organization: Recent studies, changing methodologies, and the concept of conditional strategies. *Human Development, 33,* 48–61.

Main, M. (2000). The organized categories of infant, child, and adult attachment: Flexible vs. inflexible attention under attachment-related stress. *Journal of the American Psychoanalytic Association, 48*(4), 1055–1096.

Main, M., & Cassidy, J. (1988). Categories of response to reunion with the parent at age 6: Predictable from infant attachment classifications and stable over a 1-month period. *Developmental Psychology, 24,* 415–426.

Main, M., Kaplan, N., & Cassidy, J. (1985). Security in infancy, childhood, and adulthood: A move to the level of representation. In I. Bretherton & E. Waters (Eds.), Growing points of attachment theory and research. *Monographs of the Society for Research in Child Development, 50*(1–2, Serial No. 209), 66–104.

Main, M., & Solomon, J. (1986). Discovery of a new, insecure disorganized/disoriented attachment pattern. In T. B. Brazelton & M. Yogman (Eds.), *Affective development in infancy* (pp. 95–124). Norwood, NJ: Ablex.

Main, M., & Solomon, J. (1990). Procedures for identifying infants as disorganized/disoriented during the Ainsworth Strange Situation. In M. T. Greenberg, D. Cicchetti, & E. M. Cummings (Eds.), *Attachment in the preschool years* (pp. 121–160). Chicago: University of Chicago Press.

Main, M., & Weston, D. R. (1981). The quality of the toddler's relationship to mother and to father: Related to conflict behavior and the readiness to establish new relationships. *Child Development, 52,* 932–940.

Manassis, K., Bradley, S., Goldberg, S., Hood, J., & Swinson, R. P. (1994). Attachment in mothers with anxiety disorders and their children. *Journal of the American Academy of Child and Adolescent Psychiatry, 33,* 1106–1113.

Marcovitch, S., Goldberg, S., Gold, A., Washington, J., Wasson, C., Krekewich, K., et al. (1997). Determinants of behavioral problems in Romanian children adopted in Ontario. *International Journal of Behavioral Development, 20,* 17–31.

Marvin, R. S. (1977). An ethological–cognitive model of the attenuation of mother–child attachment behavior. In T. Alloway, L. Krames, & P. Pilner (Eds.), *Advances in the study of communication and affect: Vol. 3. Attachment behavior* (pp. 25–60). New York: Plenum Press.

Marvin, R. S., & Pianta, R. C. (1996). Mothers' reactions to their child's diagnosis: Relations with security of attachment. *Journal of Clinical Child Psychology, 25,* 436–445.

McElwain, N. L., & Booth-LaForce, C. (2006). Maternal sensitivity to infant distress and nondistress as predictors of infant–mother attachment security. *Journal of Family Psychology, 20,* 247–255.

Meehl, P. E. (1973). *Psychodiagnosis: Selected papers.* Minneapolis: University of Minnesota Press.

Minde, K., Minde, R., & Vogel, W. (2006). Culturally sensitive assessment of attachment in children aged 18–40 months in a South African township. *Infant Mental Health Journal, 27,* 544–558.

Moss, E., Bureau, J.-F., Cyr, C., & Dubois-Comtois, K. (2006). Is the maternal Q-set a valid measure of preschool child attachment behavior? *International Journal of Behavioral Development, 30,* 488–497.

Moss, E., Bureau, J.-F. Cyr, C., Mongeau, C., & St.-Laurent, D. (2004). Correlates of attachment at age 3: Construct validity of the preschool attachment classification system. *Developmental Psychology, 40,* 323–334.

Moss, E., Cyr, C., Bureau, J., Tarabulsy, G. M., & Dubois-Combois, K. (2005). Stability of attachment during the preschool period. *Developmental Psychology, 41,* 773–783.

Moss, E., Cyr, C., & Dubois-Comtois, K. (2004). Attachment at early school age and developmental risk: Examining family contexts and behavior problems of controlling-caregiving, controlling-punitive, and behaviorally disorganized children. *Developmental Psychology, 40*, 519–532.

Moss, E., Gosselin, C., Parent, S., Rousseau, D., & Dumont, M. (1997). Attachment and joint problem-solving experiences during the preschool period. *Social Development, 6*, 1–17.

Moss, E., Rousseau, D., Parent, S., St.-Laurent, D., & Saintonge, J. (1998). Correlates of attachment at school age: Maternal reported stress, mother–child interaction, and behavior problems. *Child Development, 69*, 1390–13405.

Nakasawa, M., Teti, D. M., & Lamb, M. E. (1992). An ecological study of child–mother attachments among Japanese sojourners in the United States. *Developmental Psychology, 28*, 584–592.

National Institute of Child Health and Human Development (NICHD) Early Child Care Research Network. (2001). Child-care and family predictors of preschool attachment and stability from infancy. *Developmental Psychology, 31*, 847–862.

Nunnally, J. C. (1978). *Psychometric theory.* New York: McGraw-Hill.

Oppenheim, D. (1997). The attachment doll-play interview for preschoolers. *International Journal of Behavioral Development, 20*, 681–697.

Oosterman, M., & Schuengel, C. (2007). Physiological effects of separation and reunion in relation to attachment and temperament in young children. *Developmental Psychobiology, 49*, 119–128.

Poehlmann, J. (2005). Representations of attachment relationships in children of incarcerated mothers. *Child Development, 76*, 679–696.

Posada, G. (2006). Assessing attachment security at age three: Q-sort home observations and the MacArthur Strange Situation adaptation. *Social Development, 15*, 644–658.

Posada, G., Gao, Y., Wu, F., Posada, R., Tascon, M., Schoelmerich, A., et al. (1995). The secure-base phenomenon across cultures: Children's behavior, mothers' preferences, and experts' concepts. In E. Waters, B. E. Vaughn, G. Posada, & K. Kondo-Ikemura (Eds.), Caregiving, cultural, and cognitive perspectives on secure-base behavior and working models: New growing points of attachment theory and research. *Monographs of the Society for Research in Child Development, 60*(2–3, Serial No. 244), 27–48.

Posada, G., Waters, E., Crowell, J. A., & Lay, K.-L. (1995). Is it easier to use a secure mother as a secure base?: Attachment Q-Sort correlates of the adult attachment interview. In E. Waters, B. E. Vaughn, G. Posada, & K. Kondo-Ikemura (Eds.), Caregiving, cultural, and cognitive perspectives on secure-based behavior and working models: New growing points of attachment theory and research. *Monographs of the Society for Research in Child Development, 60*(2–3, Serial No. 244), 133–145.

Rauh, H., Ziegenhain, U., Muller, B., & Wijnroks, L. (2000). Stability and change in infant–mother attachment in the second year of life. In P. M. Crittenden & A. H. Claussen (Eds.), *The organization of attachment relationships: Maturation, culture, and context* (pp. 251–276). New York: Cambridge University Press.

Rheingold, H. L., & Eckerman, C. O. (1970). The infant separates himself from his mother. *Science, 168*, 78–83.

Richters, J. E., Waters, E., & Vaughn, B. E. (1988). Empirical classification of infant–mother relationships from interactive behavior and crying during reunion. *Child Development, 59*, 512–522.

Schneider-Rosen, K. (1990). The developmental reorganization of attachment relationships: Guidelines for classification beyond infancy. In M. T. Greenberg, D. Cicchetti, & E. M. Cummings (Eds.), *Attachment in the preschool years* (pp. 185–220). Chicago: University of Chicago Press.

Schneider-Rosen, K., & Rothbaum, R. (1993). Quality of parental caregiving and security of attachment. *Developmental Psychology, 29*, 358–367.

Schoppe-Sullivan, S. J., Diener, M. L., Mangelsdorf, S. C., Brown, G. L., McHale, J. L. & Frosch, C. A. (2006). Attachment and sensitivity in family context: The roles of parent and infant gender. *Infant and Child Development, 15*, 367–385.

Seifer, R., LaGasse, L. L., Lester, B., Bauer, C. R., Shankaran, S., Bada, H. S., et al. (2004). Attachment status in children prenatally exposed to cocaine and other substances. *Child Development, 75*, 850–868.

Seifer, R., & Schiller, M. (1995). The role of parenting sensitivity, infant temperament, and dyadic interaction in attachment theory and assessment. In E. Waters, B. E. Vaughn, G. Posada, & K. Kondo-Ikemura (Eds.), Caregiving, cultural, and cognitive perspectives on secure-base behavior and working models: New growing points of attachment theory and research. *Monographs of the Society for Research in Child Development, 60*, 146–174.

Shamir-Essakow, G., Ungerer, J. A., & Rapee, R. M. (2005). Attachment, behavioral inhibition, and anxiety in preschool children. *Journal of Abnormal Child Psychology, 33*, 131–143.

Shouldice, A. E., & Stevenson-Hinde, J. (1992). Coping with security distress: The Separation Anxiety Test and attachment classification at 4.5 years. *Journal of Child Psychology and Psychiatry, 33*, 331–348.

Slough, N. M., & Greenberg, M. T. (1990). Five-year olds' representations of separation from parents: Responses from the perspective of self and other. *New Directions for Child Development, 48*, 67–84.

Solomon, J., & George, C. (1996). Defining the caregiving system: Toward a theory of caregiving. *Infant Mental Health Journal, 17*, 3–17.

Solomon, J., & George, C. (1999a). The caregiving system in mothers of infants: A comparison of divorcing and married mothers. *Attachment and Human Development, 1*, 171–190.

Solomon, J., & George, C. (1999b). The place of disorganization in attachment theory: Linking classic observations with contemporary findings. In J. Solomon & C. George (Eds.), *Attachment disorganization* (pp. 3–32). New York: Guilford Press.

Solomon, J., & George, C. (1999c). The effects on attachment of overnight visitation in divorced and separated families: A longitudinal follow-up. In J. Solomon & C. George (Eds.), *Attachment disorganization* (pp. 243–264). New York: Guilford Press.

Solomon, J., & George, C. (1999d). The measurement of attachment security in infancy and childhood. In J. Cassidy & P. R. Shaver (Eds.), *Handbook of attachment: Theory, research, and clinical applications* (pp. 287–316). New York: Guilford Press.

Solomon, J., & George, C. (2000). Toward an integrated theory of maternal caregiving. In J. Osofsky & H. E. Fitzgerald (Eds.), *WAIMH handbook of infant mental health: Vol. 3. Parenting and child care* (pp. 323–368). New York: Wiley.

Solomon, J., & George, C. (2002, April). *Understanding children's attachment representations in terms of defensive process.* Paper presented at the 4th Annual Conference of the International Academy of Family Psychology, Heidelberg, Germany.

Solomon, J., & George, C. (2006). Intergenerational transmission of dysregulated maternal caregiving: Mothers describe their upbringing and childrearing. In O. Mayseless (Ed.), *Parenting representations: Theory, research, and clinical implications* (pp. 265–295). Cambridge, UK: Cambridge University Press.

Solomon, J., & George, C. (in press). Disorganization of maternal caregiving across two generations. In J. Solomon & C. George (Eds.), *Disorganized attachment and caregiving.* New York: Guilford Press.

Solomon, J., George, C., & De Jong, A. (1995). Children classified as controlling at age six: Evidence of disorganized representational strategies and aggression at home and at school. *Development and Psychopathology, 7,* 447–463.

Solomon, J., George, C., & Silverman, N. (1990). *Maternal Caretaking Q-Sort: Describing age-related changes in mother–child interaction.* Unpublished manuscript.

Speltz, M. L., Greenberg, M. T., & DeKlyen, M. (1990). Attachment in preschoolers with disruptive behavior: A comparison of clinic-referred and nonproblem children. *Development and Psychopathology, 2,* 31–46.

Sroufe, L. A. (1979). The coherence of individual development: Early care, attachment, and subsequent developmental issues. *American Psychologist, 34,* 834–841.

Sroufe, L. A., & Waters, E. (1977). Attachment as an organizational construct. *Child Development, 48,* 1184–1199.

Stevenson-Hinde, J., & Shouldice, A. (1995). Maternal interactions and self-reports related to attachment classifications at 4.5 years. *Child Development, 66,* 583–596.

Strayer, F. F., Verissimo, M., Vaughn, B. E., & Howes, C. (1995). A quantitative approach to the description

and classification of primary social relationships. In E. Waters, B. E. Vaughn, G. Posada, & K. Kondo-Ikemura (Eds.), Caregiving, cultural, and cognitive perspectives on secure-based behavior and working models: New growing points of attachment theory and research. *Monographs of the Society for Research in Child Development, 60*(2–3, Serial No. 244), 49–70.

Teti, D. M., & McGourty, S. (1996). Using mothers versus trained observers in assessing children's secure base behavior: Theoretical and methodological considerations. *Child Development, 67,* 597–605.

Teti, D. M., Sakin, J. W., Kucera, E., Corns, K. M., & Das Eiden, R. (1996). And baby makes four: Predictors of attachment security among preschool-age firstborns during the transition to siblinghood. *Child Development, 67,* 579–596.

Toth, S. L., Rogosch, F. A., Manly, J. T., & Cicchetti, D. (2006). The efficacy of toddler–parent psychotherapy to reorganize attachment in the young offspring of mothers with major depressive disorder: A randomized preventive trial. *Journal of Consulting and Clinical Psychology, 74,* 1006–1016.

Turner, P. J. (1991). Relations between attachment, gender, and behavior with peers in preschool. *Child Development, 62,* 1475–4188.

van IJzendoorn, M. H., Juffer, F., & Duyvesteyn, M. G. C. (1995). Breaking the intergenerational cycle of insecure attachment: A review of the effects of attachment-based interventions on maternal sensitivity and infant security. *Journal of Child Psychology and Psychiatry, 36,* 225–248.

van IJzendoorn, M. H., Rutgers, A. H., Bakermans-Kranenburg, M. J., van Daalen, E., Dietz, C., Buitelaar, J. K., et al. (2007). Parental sensitivity and attachment in children with autism spectrum disorder: Comparison with children with mental retardation, with language delays, and with typical development. *Child Development, 78,* 597–608.

van IJzendoorn, M. H., Schuengel, C., & Bakermans-Kranenburg, M. J. (1999). Disorganized attachment in early childhood: Meta-analysis of precursors, concomitants, and sequelae. *Development and Psychopathology, 11,* 225–249.

van IJzendoorn, M. H., Vereijken, C. M. J. L., Bakermans-Kranenburg, M. J., & Riksen-Walraven, J. M. (2004). Assessing attachment security with the Attachment Q-Sort: Meta-analytic evidence for the validity of the observer AQS. *Child Development, 75,* 1188–1213.

Vaughn, B. E., Coppola, G., Verissimo, M., Monteiro, L., Santos, A. J., Posada, G., et al. (2007). The quality of maternal secure-base scripts predicts children's secure-base behavior at home in three sociocultural groups. *International Journal of Behavioral Development, 31,* 65–76.

Vaughn, B. E., Strayer, F. F., Jacques, M., Trudel, M., & Seifer, R. (1991). Maternal descriptions of 2- and 3-year-old children: A comparison of Attachment Q-Sorts in two socio-cultural communities. *International Journal of Behavioral Development, 14,* 249–271.

Vaughn, B. E., & Waters, E. (1990). Attachment behavior at home and in the laboratory: Q-sort observations and Strange Situation classifications of one-year-olds. *Child Development, 61,* 1965–1973.

Venet, M., Bureau, J. F., Gosselin, C., & Capuano, F. (2007). Attachment representation in a sample of neglected preschool age children. *School Psychology International, 28,* 264–293.

Verschueren, K., & Marcoen, A. (1999). Representation of self and socioemotional competence in kindergartners: Differential and combined effects of attachment to mother and father. *Child Development, 70,* 183–201.

Verschueren, K., Marcoen, A., & Schoefs, V. (1996). The internal working model of the self, attachment, and competence in five-year olds. *Child Development, 67,* 2493–2511.

Völker, S., Keller, H., Lohaus, A., Cappenberg, M., & Chasiotis, A. (1999). Maternal interactive behaviour in early infancy and later attachment. *International Journal of Behavioral Development, 23,* 921–936.

Vondra, J. I., Shaw, D. S., Swearingen, L., Cohen, M., & Owens, E. B. (2001). Attachment stability and emotional and behavioral regulation from infancy to preschool age. *Development and Psychopathology, 13,* 13–33.

Wartner, U. G., Grossmann, K., Fremmer-Bombik, E., & Suess, G. (1994). Attachment patterns at age six in south Germany: Predictability from infancy and implications for preschool behavior. *Child Development, 65,* 1010–1023.

Waters, E. (1978). The reliability and stability of individual differences in infant–mother attachment. *Child Development, 49,* 483–494.

Waters, E. (1995). The Attachment Q-Set (Version 3.0). In E. Waters, B. E. Vaughn, G. Posada, & K. Kondo-Ikemura (Eds.), Caregiving, cultural, and cognitive perspectives on secure-base behavior and working models: New growing points of attachment theory and research. *Monographs of the Society for Research in Child Development, 60*(2–3, Serial No. 244), 234–246.

Waters, E., & Beauchaine, T. P. (2003). Are there re-ally patterns of attachment?: Comment on Fraley and Spiker (2003). *Developmental Psychology, 39,* 417–422.

Waters, E., & Deane, K. E. (1985). Defining and assessing individual differences in attachment relationships: Q-methodology and the organization of behavior in infancy and early childhood. In I. Bretherton & E. Waters (Eds.), Growing points of attachment theory and research. *Monographs of the Society for Research in Child Development, 50*(1–2, Serial No. 209), 41–65.

Waters, E., Merrick, S., Treboux, D., Crowell, J., & Albersheim, L. (2000). Attachment security in infancy and early adulthood: A twenty-year longitudinal study. *Child Development, 71,* 684–689.

Waters, H. S., Rodrigues, L. M., & Ridgeway, D. (1998). Cognitive underpinnings of narrative attachment assessment. *Journal of Experimental Child Psychology, 71,* 211–234.

Waters, H. S., & Waters, E. (2006). The attachment working models concept: Among other things, we build script-like representations of secure base experiences. *Attachment and Human Development, 8,* 185–198.

Webster, L., & Hackett, R. (in press). An exploratory investigation of the relationships among representation security, disorganization, and behavior in maltreated children. In J. Solomon & C. George (Eds.), *Disorganized attachment and caregiving.* New York: Guilford Press.

Zeanah, C. H., Smyke, A. T., Koga, S. F., & Carlson, E. (2005). Attachment in institutionalized and community children in Romania. *Child Development, 76,* 1015–1028.

Zimmermann, P., Becker-Stoll, F., Grossmann, K., Grossmann, K. E., Scheuerer-Englisch, H., & Wartner, U. (2000). Längsschnittliche Bindungsentwicklung von der frühen Kindheit bis zum Jugendalter [Longitudinal attachment development from infancy through adolescence]. *Psychologie in Erziehung und Unterricht, 47,* 99–117.

PART IV

ATTACHMENT IN ADOLESCENCE
AND ADULTHOOD

CHAPTER 19

The Attachment System in Adolescence

JOSEPH P. ALLEN

Adolescence is, of course, a transitional period, and this is particularly true with respect to the attachment system. The early adolescent is beginning a Herculean effort to become less dependent on primary attachment figures (i.e., parents). The late adolescent has the potential to function completely independently of parents and even to become an attachment figure to his or her own offspring. Yet adolescence is not simply a way station between these two kinds of involvement with attachment. Rather, it is a period of profound *transformation* in emotional, cognitive, and behavioral systems surrounding attachment relationships, as the adolescent evolves from being a receiver of care to becoming a self-sufficient adult and potential caregiver to peers, romantic partners, and offspring.

The psychosocial development that takes place in adolescence brings profound changes in the meaning and expression of attachment processes. As a result, one cannot begin to consider the attachment system in adolescence without immediately confronting fundamental questions about its nature. Is attachment in adolescence best conceptualized in terms of ongoing attachment relationships with parents? In terms of relationships with peers or a romantic partner? As a combination of multiple relationship experiences and behaviors? As a way of approaching new attachment relationships? As a way of *thinking* or talking about attachment experiences? Although some of these

questions also apply at earlier stages of development, adolescence brings them all to the forefront simultaneously.

This chapter begins with consideration of the normative developmental changes in attachment in adolescence. It then moves on to consider the meaning of individual differences in attachment phenomena. The chapter concludes with a discussion of the implications of what we know about continuities and discontinuities in attachment phenomena, both during adolescence and between adolescence and other phases of development. Within this overall structure, I highlight nine primary "developmental transformations," each of which reflects critical changes in the attachment system or in its conceptualization in light of the changes occurring in adolescence.

NORMATIVE DEVELOPMENT OF THE ATTACHMENT SYSTEM IN ADOLESCENCE

Developmental Transformation 1: Moving from Attachment Relationships to Generalized States of Mind Regarding Attachment

By adolescence, a milestone is reached: The attachment system can be assessed in terms of a single overarching attachment organization that has developed, displays stability, and predicts future

419

behavior and functioning both within and beyond the family (Hesse, 1999). Although adolescence is the first period during which the primary mode of assessing this overarching organization becomes available (via the Adult Attachment Interview [AAI] or its downward revision, the Attachment Interview for Childhood and Adolescence—Ammaniti, van IJzendoorn, Speranza, & Tambelli, 2000; George, Kaplan, & Main, 1984, 1985, 1996), the organization itself undoubtedly begins to develop well before adolescence. Nevertheless, there is reason to believe that "states of mind" regarding attachment—the ways that individuals conceptualize attachment experiences and relationships—develop significantly during adolescence because of teenagers' rapidly growing capacities for formal operational thinking, including logical and abstract reasoning abilities (Keating, 1990). These growing capacities allow an adolescent to begin to construct, from experiences with multiple caregivers, a more integrated and generalized stance toward attachment experiences (Hesse, 1999; Main, Kaplan, & Cassidy, 1985).

In addition, the cognitive and emotional advances of adolescence allow an adolescent to reflect upon and modify his or her states of mind regarding attachment. For example, the dramatic increases in cognitive differentiation of self and other that characterize this period (Selman, 1980) allow the teen to begin to establish a more consistent view of the self as existing apart from interactions with caregivers. The advent of formal operational thinking also allows an adolescent to contemplate abstract and counterfactual possibilities, which in turn allow him or her to compare relationships with different attachment figures, both to one another and to hypothetical ideals. Thus the adolescent gains the capacity to "de-idealize" parents—to see them in both positive and negative ways (Steinberg, 2005)—which research has linked with the security of adolescents' attachment representations (Allen et al., 2003). Adolescents not only demonstrate a capacity to think about attachment in a general way, which extends beyond any single relationship; they also have the capacity to operate metacognitively on this thinking—to begin to reconstruct (or at least tinker with) their own states of mind regarding attachment.

Developmental Transformation 2: The Continuing Role of Relationship Assessment

Having the AAI as a means of assessing attachment phenomena in adolescence does *not*, however, imply that specific qualities of individual at-

tachment relationships are no longer important or worthy of independent assessment. Although the move to the level of representation (Main et al., 1985) and consideration of states of mind regarding attachment in adolescence have been incredibly productive, they capture only certain aspects of the attachment system's operations in adolescence. As much as adolescents may at times deny the importance of relationships with attachment figures (and researchers may find these relationships difficult to assess), primary attachment relationships continue in adolescence, develop dramatically, and provide important issues worthy of study. Regardless of whether a single overarching attachment organization exists in adolescence, individual relationships can bring out related, but nevertheless potentially quite distinct, attachment "styles" during adolescence (Furman & Simon, 2004; Furman, Simon, Shaffer, & Bouchey, 2002). And although we now have increasingly well-validated measures to assess qualities of such relationships (see, e.g., Bartholomew & Shaver, 1998; Brennan, Clark, & Shaver, 1998; Crowell & Owens, 1996; Furman et al., 2002; Roisman, Collins, Sroufe, & Egeland, 2005; Treboux, Crowell, & Waters, 2004), it will be noted below just what a small proportion of research on adolescent attachment has actually focused on identifying characteristics of individual adolescent attachment relationships.

In sum, the construct of attachment in adolescence seems best viewed not as either an intrapsychic or a relationship construct, but rather as an organizational construct that is likely to be reflected both in intrapsychic development and in multiple aspects of ongoing attachment relationships (Sroufe & Waters, 1977; Thompson, 1997). The move to the level of representation that has occurred by adolescence is a fundamental transformation that has inspired an explosion of productive research in adolescence and adulthood, but the relational perspective that has so energized attachment theory earlier in the lifespan remains critical to consider.

Transformations in Parental Relationships

Developmental Transformation 3: Achieving Independence from Attachment Figures as a Developmental Goal

Kobak and Duemmler (1994) noted that one of the most important characteristics of an adolescent's attachment relationship with a parent is its potential to become increasingly goal-corrected. As the adolescent gains communication and perspective-taking skills, it becomes possible for both parent and teen to modify (or correct) their attachment-related behavior when necessary, to meet the teen's evolving attachment needs while balancing other needs as well. The increasingly goal-corrected nature of the parent–adolescent relationship provides an important context for considering one of the most important and intriguing changes of adolescence: the decreased reliance on parents as attachment figures.

Whereas the goal-corrected partnership in infancy might be described as reflecting a *coordinated* effort between parent and child, in adolescence it seems more appropriate to consider this as a *negotiated* effort. To a degree unparalleled elsewhere in childrearing (with the possible exception of early toddlerhood), the adolescent struggle for autonomy becomes an omnipresent background against which attachment processes play out. At this age, the many years of prior operation of the attachment system—and the habitual patterns of responding that have become established—present a significant threat to the adolescent's efforts to establish autonomy. Put simply, it is exquisitely difficult for a teen to strike out from his or her parents and establish independence while feeling pulled by both habit and the attachment system to retain their shoulders to cry on.

Yet, without such exploration, accomplishing the major tasks of social development in adolescence and young adulthood would be difficult if not impossible. In principle, this conflict is analogous to the competing influences of the exploratory and attachment systems on infant behavior, although the press for autonomy in adolescence may be more relentless and more directly in competition with the attachment system than is the case during infancy (Allen, Moore, & Kuperminc, 1997; Steinberg, 1990). It seems likely that a secure attachment relationship, with its goal-correcting capacities, will smooth this transition in adolescence—but it seems equally likely that there will still be significant bumps in the road that affect the teen's views of attachment and social relationships into the future (Allen, Hauser, O'Connor, & Bell, 2002).

The issue is primarily one of developing a new balance between attachment behaviors (and cognitions) regarding parents and the adolescent's exploratory needs. The adolescent's rapidly developing competence decreases his or her need for dependence on parental attachment figures, and the strong need to explore and master new environments promotes healthy growth in the exploratory system. Given that the attachment system is homeostatic, balancing safety and exploration, it makes sense that as increasing maturity increases safety, exploration will increase and overt attachment behavior will decrease. Nevertheless, most adolescents still turn to parents under conditions of extreme stress (Steinberg, 1990), and parents are still often used as attachment figures even in young adulthood (Fraley & Davis, 1997). Adolescents may be on the edge of tears far less often than infants, but when they are highly distressed, their likelihood of turning to parents for help still increases dramatically. In this respect, the attachment system operates much as it always has, albeit with a different and rapidly changing balance between attachment and exploratory behaviors.

An important secondary effect of the changing balance between attachment and exploratory behavior in adolescence is an increase in the adolescent's capacity to reevaluate the nature of his or her attachment relationship with parents. With increased independence from parents as attachment figures, there comes increased freedom from the need to monitor and assure parents' availability to meet attachment needs (Kobak & Cole, 1994). Main and colleagues (Main & Goldwyn, 1984; Main, Goldwyn, & Hesse, 2003) refer to this cognitive and emotional freedom as "epistemic space," and suggest that it allows individuals to evaluate their parents as attachment figures more objectively.

This epistemic space is likely to be as important to the emerging capacity to think autonomously about attachment relationships as are the developing cognitive capacities discussed above. For even with fully developed cognitive capacities, it is likely to be difficult to attain the critical distance needed to begin objectively evaluating the qualities of an attachment relationship on which one feels totally dependent. As independence increases, however, so too will the emotional distance needed to put developing cognitive capacities to work in reevaluating the nature of the attachment relationship with parents. Uncomfortable as this critical distance and objective evaluation may be to parents, it is likely to be fundamental to an adolescent's capacity to develop an accurate, thoughtful response to attachment experiences. This in turn may be crucial to resolving attachment difficulties in relationships with parents in ways that allow some adolescents to form more secure relationships with others in the future, and it may be necessary for allowing them to reconsider and alter their own states of mind regarding attachment (Pearson, Cohn, Cowan, & Cowan, 1994).

Transformations in Peer Relationships

Developmental Transformation 4:
Extending Attachments beyond
the Child–Caregiver Relationship

The adolescent is not simply becoming more independent of parents, however. In important respects, he or she is beginning the process of *transferring* dependencies from parental to peer relationships. Within the constellation of an infant's attachment figures, a hierarchy is believed to exist, with the most preferred attachment figure serving as the "principal" attachment figure and others as secondary figures (Bowlby, 1969/1982; Cassidy, 1999). If we begin with the premise that most adults are able to form attachment relationships with a peer, whereas almost no children can do so, then we must recognize that adolescence will be a period during which peer relationships will gradually take on more and more of the qualities of full-blown adult attachment relationships. What is not yet known is how this ontogenetically driven press to shift attachment allegiance to a peer or romantic partner unfolds in adolescence.

By midadolescence, interactions with peers have begun to take on many of the functions they will serve for the remainder of the lifespan—providing important sources of intimacy, feedback about social behavior, social influence and information, and ultimately attachment and sexual relationships and lifelong partnerships (Ainsworth, 1989; Collins & Laursen, 2000; Gavin & Furman, 1989, 1996; Hartup, 1992). The development of peer relationships in adolescence is characterized by the gradual emergence of the capacity for adult-like intimacy and supportiveness (Buhrmester, 1996; Collins, van Dulmen, Crouter, & Booth, 2006; Hartup, 1992). These well-known changes create an important challenge for our efforts to understand the operation of the attachment system during this period. The critical question is this: When do peer relationships become attachment relationships? This question can be more fruitfully, though less conventionally, phrased as follows: How do peer relationships gradually take on attachment functions?

Developmental Transformation 5: Moving from
Attachment Relationships to Attachment Processes
in Relationships

Ainsworth (1989) delineated five characteristics that distinguish attachment relationships from other enduring social relationships. These char-

acteristics help us to clarify the ways in which enduring peer relationships do and do not serve attachment functions in adolescence. These characteristics are (1) proximity seeking, (2) distress upon inexplicable separation, (3) pleasure or joy upon reunion, (4) grief at loss, and (5) secure-base behavior (comfort and freer exploration in the presence of an attachment figure). Kobak, Rosenthal, and Serwik (2005) note an additional requirement implicit in the characteristics Ainsworth described: The person must view the attachment figure as having an enduring commitment to being available if needed, regardless of changes in time or context.

Ainsworth's list of features makes clear the ways in which childhood playmates differ from attachment figures. It also makes clear the extent to which these distinctions begin to blur when adolescent peer relationships are considered. By late adolescence, long-term relationships can be formed in which peers (as romantic partners or close friends) *potentially* serve as attachment figures in all senses of the term. The change that is occurring is not just a gradual transition from one class of attachment figures (parents) to another (peers). Rather, the very nature of what it means to define a relationship as an attachment relationship must also change as both parties now take on adult or adult-like capacities. Unlike in infancy and even childhood, what spurs an adolescent to approach an attachment figure will only rarely be fundamental physical safety needs, extreme distress, or risk of imminent emotional disorganization. Rather, the spurs are now usually other, more subtle needs that may depend on complex interpretive contexts, and may be more flexibly attended to or ignored in a given situation. In addition, a relationship among equals (both of whom may be quite interested in preserving their independence) may be a context that fundamentally alters the meaning and expression of attachment behaviors that were previously directed toward a caregiver.

We now know that there is a broad array of different neural, physiological, and psychological systems underlying attachment behavior (see Coan, Chapter 11, this volume). These range from managing physiological arousal to establishing a sense of emotional security, to deactivating primitive centers of the brain that support "flight" under conditions of stress (Coan, Schaefer, & Davidson, 2006; Cummings & Davies, 1996; Hofer, 1994, 2006; Taylor et al., 2000). Given the infant's extreme vulnerability, limited capacities for self-help, and intense relationships with caregivers, these functions all come together simultaneously and powerfully under conditions of stress as a fully functioning attachment system. In adolescence, in contrast, it is not clear whether the more primitive neural circuits in the brain responsible for detecting and physically responding to threat (e.g., the amygdala and the caudate/nucleus accumbens) are fully activated by the psychosocial stressors that adolescents typically experience.

Main (1999) has posited that the attachment system evolved partly because of the value of associating with others as a source of safety, given our vulnerability as a ground-living species. Clearly, this specific function applies only rarely to modern adolescents, even if many other attachment processes still remain active. With these differences comes the likelihood that the multiple functions and features of the attachment system—which often operate powerfully and in unison during infancy—may begin to operate less synchronously in adolescence, particularly in interactions with peers. In addition, with the adolescent's increased cognitive capacity comes increased flexibility in directing attachment behavior. Adolescents increasingly gain the capacity to be "opportunistic" in seeking out a potential attachment figure, whether it be a fellow camper at a 4-week summer camp or a close-in-age sibling that a teen turns to as parents go through a divorce. Such relationships occur with enough frequency to anchor many popular books and films depicting adolescents (see, e.g., Hinton, 1967; King, 1986).

Given these changes from infancy to adolescence, trying to decide whether a given adolescent relationship is or is not an "attachment relationship" may be overly simplistic. Rather than wading into the semantic quagmire of delineating the precise conditions under which a given relationship beyond infancy becomes an "attachment relationship," it may make more sense to recognize that adolescent relationships increasingly take on critical attachment functions, even if such functions are neither as synchronous nor as intense as they were in earlier relationships with parents.

A focus on peer attachment *processes* (as opposed to the presence or absence of peer attachment relationships) allows us to formulate fruitful research questions. How does the process of "trying out" close relationships to see whether they might serve attachment functions work? Does this process differ for individuals with different attachment histories? Which facets of attachment behavior come "online" earliest in adolescent peer relationships? What happens when adolescents make precocious (or delayed) transitions to using peers to serve attachment needs? Addressing these questions can begin to build an understanding of the *development* of the attachment system during adolescence, in a way that a static dichotomizing of relationships as "attachment relationships" or not does not allow.

One of the most important endpoints of developing peer relationships in adolescence is the attainment of romantic relationships that may eventually become lifelong attachment relationships (Ainsworth, 1989; Collins, van Dulmen, et al., 2006; Furman et al., 2002). Romantic relationships do not result solely from developing interests in forming attachments with peers, of course. They also reflect the operation of a sexual/reproductive system that is every bit as biologically rooted and critical to species survival as the attachment system (Furman, Brown, & Feiring, 1999; Hazan & Shaver, 1987; Shaver, Hazan, & Bradshaw, 1988). However, the sexual and attachment systems both push toward the establishment of romantic relationships characterized by sufficient intensity, shared interests, and strong affect to begin to take over some of the functions of prior parent–child relationships. The sexual component of these relationships may also help advance the attachment component by providing consistent motivation for interaction, experience with intense, intimate affect, and a history of shared unique experience. By midadolescence, we may begin to see romantic relationships that at times meet all of the criteria Ainsworth proposed for attachment relationships—from proximity seeking to strong separation protest. And romantic partners may take turns being "stronger and wiser" for each other and thereby serving as attachment figures (Ainsworth, 1982). Whether adolescent romantic relationships do these things *enough* to be called "attachment relationships" may or may not be merely a matter of semantics, but that the development of attachment processes within these relationships is worthy of study is beyond question.

INDIVIDUAL DIFFERENCES IN ADOLESCENT ATTACHMENT STRATEGIES

Having established some notion of the transformations in attachment-related cognitions, feelings, and behavior that occur during adolescence, it is now possible to consider what we know about individual differences in the functioning of the attachment system in that age period. Somewhat ironically, given the intense relationship focus propounded by Ainsworth and Bowlby (Ainsworth, Blehar, Waters, & Wall, 1978; Bowlby,

1969/1982), by far the bulk of research on individual differences in adolescent attachment in the Ainsworth–Bowlby tradition uses the AAI to assess adolescent internal states of mind regarding attachment. Far less research has addressed individual differences in adolescents' actual attachment relationships, a point that will be considered further below. Both intrapsychic and relational approaches to adolescent attachment are considered below, however, and the preponderance of attention given to the intrapsychic approaches should not be taken as an endorsement of the primacy of those approaches, but only as a reflection of their place in the research literature to date. Unless otherwise noted, all references to security or insecurity as a property of the individual teen are based on assessments with the AAI; references to research on properties of specific relationships will note the measures used for each study considered.

Individual Differences in Family Relationships

The potential tension noted above between the adolescent's developmental push to gain autonomy and the operation of the attachment system gives rise to important individual differences in how this tension is managed. Just as the balance of exploration from a secure base has been highly informative with respect to individual differences in infant attachments, so too the balance of autonomy and attachment processes in adolescence appears as a robust marker of the quality of an adolescent's internal state of mind regarding attachment. A secure goal-corrected partnership *potentially* allows both parent and teen to recognize the teen's autonomy strivings and to support these while maintaining the relationship. For such a partnership to be successful, however, two key ingredients are required: a strong capacity to communicate across the increasingly divergent perspectives and needs of the parent and teen, and a willingness among both parties to allow the adolescent to seek autonomy while maintaining the parent–teen relationship.

Developmental Transformation 6:
Open, Full Dyadic Communication by Adolescents
with Secure Attachment States of Mind

Cassidy (2001) has suggested that a secure attachment organization beyond childhood may be reflected in part by efforts to communicate truthfully and fully in intimate relationships about important topics. Several lines of research on adolescent security bear this out.

One predictor of a secure adolescent state of mind is the presence of a parent who is highly sensitive to the adolescent's internal states. When sensitivity is assessed in terms of a mother's accuracy in predicting her teen's responses on a self-perception inventory, it is robustly linked to adolescent security in the AAI (Allen et al., 2003). In fact, the correlation of security with this marker of sensitivity was slightly higher ($r = .35$) than is typically found in studies of parental sensitivity toward infants (De Wolff & van IJzendoorn, 1997). One possible explanation is that adolescence researchers have an advantage over their infancy counterparts: In adolescence, sensitivity can be assessed directly in the form of concordance between parental report and adolescent behavior. The infancy researcher, in contrast, has the burden of trying to judge an infant's needs with sufficient accuracy to allow the presumption that any parental deviation from the researcher's judgments reflects parental insensitivity. Efforts to assess maternal sensitivity in adolescence by using the more demanding third-party approach used in infancy have been less successful (Beckwith, Cohen, & Hamilton, 1999). Infant research on sensitivity does not appear to have taken the approach of asking parents to predict their infant's behavior, although such an approach appears promising.

Although it is quite plausible that parental sensitivity leads to adolescent security, another explanation for the link between attachment and parental sensitivity during adolescence is that secure adolescents *allow* parents to be more sensitive by communicating their emotional states to the parents more accurately. Becker-Stoll, Delius, and Scheitenberger (2001) used fine-grained emotion coding during discussion tasks to observe, at a micro level, the degree to which teens are affectively communicative with their mothers. They found a reliable association between adolescents' security and the degree to which they were affectively communicative.

Further supporting this idea, we (Berger, Jodl, Allen, McElhaney, & Kuperminc, 2005) reported that adolescent insecure states of mind were linked to greater overall discrepancies between adolescents' and parents' reports of the adolescents' psychological symptoms. Notably, these discrepancies appeared not only when teen reports of symptoms were compared to parental reports, but also when teen reports of their own symptoms were compared to the reports of their closest peers regarding the teens' symptoms. This suggests that security is linked to properties of adolescents' dyadic communication both with parents and with close peers.

With respect to the dismissing attachment organization, we (Berger et al., 2005) found that communication was just generally poor and that discrepancies were not directional in nature (i.e., there was not a consistent pattern of over- or underreporting symptoms by any party). With respect to the preoccupied attachment organization, a specific form of bias in communication was found: Adolescents with preoccupied states of mind regarding attachment in the AAI consistently reported the presence of symptoms at levels that were significantly higher than those recognized by either parents or peers. These findings make sense if we view preoccupation as a manifestation of hyperactivation of the attachment system, and if we recognize that symptom reports can readily be seen as cries of distress (e.g., as attachment behaviors). From this perspective, we see that insecure-preoccupied adolescents are reporting their distress to a high degree, but not having these reports heard (or fully believed) by the people closest to them.

Clearly, both an adolescent's attachment organization and the quality of his or her relationship with parents and peers exist as parallel ongoing transactional processes, making any effort to tease out directional causal influences exceptionally difficult. What can be said, however, is that adolescents' difficulties communicating their internal states accurately to others appears as a robust marker of adolescent insecurity—whether these difficulties stem from adolescent communicative difficulties, problems in selecting receptive peer partners, parental lack of sensitivity, or some combination of all these factors.

Developmental Transformation 7:
Resolution of the Attachment–Autonomy Tension
in Adolescents with Secure Attachment States
of Mind

As noted above, the negotiation of attachment and autonomy issues may be problematic for all families at some point, but it may be especially difficult for the family of an insecure adolescent. The moodiness, changing relationships, tension, and growing emotional and behavioral independence from parents that characterize adolescent development may conspire to create chronic activation of the attachment system, thus increasing the impact of an insecure attachment organization on the adolescent's behavior. Insecure adolescents (and parents) may be overwhelmed by the affect brought on by disagreements (Kobak, Cole, Ferenz-Gillies, Fleming, & Gamble, 1993) and

may perceive disagreements as threats to otherwise shaky relationships. In addition, an insecure adolescent may have a history of less than positive experiences with attachment figures when they were called upon in times of need, which is likely to color future interactions with them.

One of the more consistent findings in the adolescent attachment literature is that teens with secure attachment states of mind tend to handle conflicts with parents by engaging in productive, problem-solving discussions that balance autonomy strivings with efforts to preserve relationships with parents (Allen & Hauser, 1996; Allen, McElhaney, Kuperminc, & Jodl, 2004; Allen et al., 2003; Allen, Porter, McFarland, McElhaney, & Marsh, 2007; Becker-Stoll & Fremmer-Bombik, 1997; Kobak et al., 1993). These discussions may be heated or intense at times, but in families with secure adolescents they are tempered by behaviors that maintain and support the parent–teen relationship. In particular, the relationship-maintaining behaviors in the midst of conflict are most consistently linked to adolescent security, and typically the behavior of the adolescents (rather than their parents) is most predictive of adolescent security. In some sense, these relationship-supporting behaviors may be viewed as "secure-base" behaviors, in which an adolescent is revisiting and refreshing the attachment bond even in the midst of exploring autonomy from parents.

Most of the research in this area has been done with mothers, although recent work suggests that similar patterns exist for fathers as well (Allen et al., 2007). Research on fathers adds one other behavior to the mix—use of harsh conflict tactics—as a marker of adolescent insecurity. As with research on mothers, the focus is less on whether an adolescent can establish autonomy in the disagreement than on the autonomy challenge as a backdrop against which relationships are either actively maintained or significantly threatened.

In terms of specific types of insecure states of mind, Becker-Stoll and Fremmer-Bombik (1997) report that dismissing adolescents show the least autonomy and relatedness in interactions with parents of all attachment groups observed. This suggests that a dismissing individual's characteristic withdrawal from engagement with attachment experiences may particularly hinder the task of renegotiating parent–adolescent relationships. Reimer, Overton, Steidl, Rosenstein, and Horowitz (1996) also noted that families of dismissing adolescents tend to be less responsive to their adolescents than do families of preoccupied adolescents.

Insecure preoccupation, in contrast, appears to be best predicted from heightened and unproductive overengagement with parents in arguments that ultimately undermine an adolescent's autonomy. We (Allen & Hauser, 1996) reported that one indicator of preoccupation with attachment in young adulthood—use of passive thought processes, reflecting mental entanglement between self and caregivers—was predicted by adolescents' overpersonalized behaviors toward fathers in arguments 10 years earlier and by adolescents' lack of simple withdrawal from or avoidance of arguments. This overengagement appears to extend well into late adolescence, as research also suggests that adolescents with insecure-preoccupied status on the AAI are likely to have more difficulty leaving home successfully for college, displaying higher levels of both conflict and contact with parents during the transition (Bernier, Larose, & Whipple, 2005). These effects were not found for adolescents who were not leaving for college, suggesting that these attachment dynamics were likely to be activated mainly in the presence of a significant stress to the attachment system.

Family interaction patterns may also predict *changes* in adolescents' states of mind over time. When autonomy-undermining, enmeshed behavior between mothers and their adolescents was observed at age 16, this predicted relative *decreases* in levels of security from age 16 to age 18 (Allen et al., 2004)—a notable finding, given evidence that insecure-preoccupied mothers may be more likely to engage in such entangled conversations (Kobak, Ferenz-Gillies, Everhart, & Seabrook, 1994). As in other attachment and family interaction studies of enmeshed and overpersonalizing behavior, the key element was the adolescents' behavior, not the mothers'. Adolescents who engage in such behavioral strategies may be struggling with autonomy issues in a highly confused way that leaves them mentally and emotionally entangled in their relationships with their mothers. Such mental entanglement during a developmental period characterized by the need to establish autonomy seems likely to produce enormous emotional stress—stress that might typically lead to seeking out an attachment figure. The catch in this case is that the stress obviously cannot be easily assuaged by mothers, given the role of the maternal relationship as the source of the stress. This unassuaged stress seems likely to make it difficult for the adolescents to step back sufficiently to engage in the thoughtful and balanced reevaluation of parental relationships that is characteristic of secure-autonomous individuals (Main, 1999).

One long-term longitudinal study has shown that infant security with mothers was more predictive of observed qualities of autonomy and relatedness in adolescent–mother interactions than it was of adolescent states of mind regarding attachment (Becker-Stoll & Fremmer-Bombik, 1997). These findings suggest that success in negotiating autonomy issues in adolescence may be a stage-specific manifestation of a long-term secure attachment relationship with parents. Notably, continuity in the qualities of an attachment *relationship* were obtained, even in the absence of continuity from an early attachment relationship to an adolescent's later internalized *state of mind* regarding attachment. This at least raises the possibility that security in adolescent–parent relationships may be distinct in important ways from security in adolescents' states of mind, and that both are worthy of study.

Individual Differences in Peer Relationships

Developmental Transformation 8: Peer Relationships as the Critical Context in Which Individual Differences in Attachment Processes Emerge

There are several reasons to expect close links between an adolescent's attachment organization and qualities of ongoing peer relationships. A secure state of mind regarding attachment, characterized by coherence in talking (and presumably thinking) about attachment-related experiences and feelings, should permit similar experiences and feelings in peer relationships to be processed more accurately and coherently as well. In contrast, the defensive exclusion of information that is characteristic of insecure organizations may lead to distorted communications and negative expectations about others, both of which have been linked to problems in social functioning at various points in the lifespan (Cassidy, Kirsh, Scolton, & Parke, 1996; Dodge, 1993; Slough & Greenberg, 1990). Similarly, discomfort with attachment-related affect and experiences may lead adolescents with dismissing attachment strategies to push away peers, particularly those who could become close friends (Larose & Bernier, 2001; Spangler & Zimmermann, 1999). This is consistent with the finding that for college students, hostility and lack of social skills as rated by close friends are linked to students' insecure attachment organizations (Kobak & Sceery, 1988). A related mechanism by which attachment organization may be linked to peer relationships is that insecure attachment organization co-occurs with (and serves to mark) problematic ongoing relationships with parents, which make it difficult to move freely beyond these relationships to establish successful new relationships with peers (Gavin & Furman, 1996).

A large, rapidly growing body of research suggests a fairly tight linkage between a secure adolescent attachment organization and competence with peers. Research indicates, for example, that secure adolescents are more comfortable with the intimate emotional interactions common in close friendships (Allen et al., 2007; Lieberman, Doyle, & Markiewicz, 1999; Sroufe, Egeland, Carlson, & Collins, 2005b; Weimer, Kerns, & Oldenberg, 2004; Zimmermann, 2004). Observational data suggest that this competence is a result of generalized comfort in handling one's own emotional reactions in challenging situations (Zimmermann, Maier, Winter, & Grossmann, 2001). Similarly, using Hazan and Shaver's (1987) three-category prototype measure of attachment style, Cooper, Shaver, and Collins (1998) found that anxious-ambivalent adolescents were prone to interpersonal hostility. And although some research suggests that security is more relevant to functioning in close relationships than in broader peer relationships (Hazan & Shaver, 1987; Lieberman et al., 1999), adolescent security has also been linked to such measures of broader social competence such as overall friendship quality, popularity, and social acceptance (Allen, Moore, Kuperminc, & Bell, 1998; Allen et al., 2007).

In some cases, peer relationship qualities (particularly the ability to seek emotional support from a peer while maintaining autonomy with respect to peer pressure) are more strongly linked with adolescent attachment states of mind than are some of the best markers of maternal and paternal relationship qualities (Allen et al., 2007). This is not necessarily surprising, given that mastering the realm of peer relationships may be the single greatest social-developmental challenge faced by most adolescents, and it does not mean that these peer relationships are causally influencing adolescent security. It does suggest, however, the extent to which peer relationships have become the central arena in which attachment processes are likely to play out during adolescence and beyond.

Individual differences in attachment organization are also linked to behavior in romantic and sexual relationships in adolescence. Furman and colleagues (2002) found that adolescents' working models of relationships with romantic partners exhibit substantial similarities to working models of relationships with parents (and with friends). Furman (2001) also noted that many of the same features of cognitive appraisal and representation that apply to thinking about relationships with parents and peers are likely to extend to romantic relationships as well. It thus seems likely that prior attachment experiences and current patterns of approach to attachment thoughts and feelings will in turn shape the nature of developing romantic relationships (Hazan & Shaver, 1994).

In late adolescence, security as assessed with the AAI has been linked to the subsequent quality of interactions with a romantic partner, as coded from videotaped observations (Roisman, Madsen, Hennighausen, Sroufe, & Collins, 2001). Assessments of the degree of self-reported insecurity in romantic relationships has been linked to greater anxiety among relationship partners, as well as to greater incidence of sexual intercourse but with less enjoyment derived from it (Tracy, Shaver, Albino, & Cooper, 2003). Moore (1997) reported that among sexually active adolescents, insecurity was associated with having more sexual partners and with less frequent use of contraception. We (Marsh, McFarland, Allen, McElhaney, & Land, 2003) found that an interaction of adolescent preoccupation and mothers' focus on their own (as opposed to their adolescents') autonomy was a predictor of adolescents' early sexual activity. Preoccupied adolescents whose mothers were focused on their own (maternal) autonomy were more likely to engage in early sexual activity, whereas preoccupied adolescents whose mothers were relatively unfocused on their own autonomy had strikingly lower rates of early sexual activity (Marsh et al., 2003). Of course, in thinking about qualities of dating relationships, partners' attachment organization will also be important to consider, as even later in adulthood only modest evidence of assortative mating with respect to attachment exists (Owens et al., 1995; Treboux et al., 2004). In this sense, predictions from the AAI-based security of one party in a relationship to overall qualities of that relationship are likely to underestimate the role of attachment, given that attachment is being assessed for only one of the two partners who together determine the qualities of the relationship (see J. Feeney, Chapter 21, this volume).

Attachment and Adolescent Mental Health

A number of recent studies suggest substantial links between adolescent attachment organization and mental health. Among the most highly disturbed adolescents—those requiring residential treatment—three studies have found links to either concurrent or future attachment insecurity, and to heightened prevalence of insecure-unresolved attachment status (Allen, Hauser, & Borman-Spurrell, 1996; Wallis & Steele, 2001). Even with less severe forms of disturbance, both the preoccupied and dismissing strategies have been implicated in problems of psychosocial functioning, although the two are associated with somewhat different patterns of problems.

Adolescents' use of preoccupied strategies has been most closely linked to internalizing problems, particularly to adolescents' self-reports of depression, anxiety disorders, and internalizing symptoms and stress during transitions (Allen et al., 1996; Bernier et al., 2005; Cole-Detke & Kobak, 1996; Kobak, Sudler, & Gamble, 1991; Larose & Bernier, 2001; Rosenstein & Horowitz, 1996). In addition, preoccupied attachment states of mind may interact with a wide array of psychosocial and environmental factors to predict critical outcomes. When preoccupied teens are confronted with intrapsychic states or environments that are confusing or enmeshing, higher levels of internalizing symptoms are found. For example, Adam, Sheldon-Keller, and West (1996) reported that suicidality in adolescence was related to a combination of preoccupied and unresolved attachment status. Similarly, preoccupied adolescents who had mothers who could not exercise their own autonomy in discussions (i.e., were passive and enmeshed) displayed higher levels of depression (Marsh et al., 2003).

Conversely, preoccupied teens are more likely to display externalizing behaviors under some circumstances. For example, when they have mothers who display extremely high levels of their own (maternal) autonomy in discussions (perhaps asserting themselves to the point of ignoring their adolescents), preoccupied teens have higher levels of drug use, engage in precocious sexual activity, and exhibit higher levels of delinquent behavior over the following year (Allen et al., 1998). Similarly, when preoccupied adolescents are exposed to poverty (perhaps another situation in which many of their needs are ignored) and/or are male, there is also an increased likelihood of delinquent behavior. Although the pattern is not yet well established, the initial research findings collectively suggest that when preoccupied adolescents are exposed to passivity or enmeshment, an internalizing, anxious/depressed pattern emerges; however, in situations where their attachment entreaties are

likely to be ignored or rebuffed, they are likely to react with externalizing behavior.

There is, of course, a third environmental possibility for preoccupied teens. They may be exposed to positive social relationships and behaviors, and in this case the outcomes look far more positive. When preoccupied and secure teens are exposed to positive friendships, they are at lower risk for delinquent behavior (McElhaney, Immele, Smith, & Allen, 2006). In addition, when exposed to effective maternal behavioral control strategies, both preoccupied and secure teens have lower levels of delinquent behavior than do dismissing teens exposed to the same maternal behavior (Allen et al., 1998).

Taken together, these results suggest that the hyperactivated state of the attachment system in preoccupied adolescents leads them to be exquisitely sensitive to their social environments. In enmeshed environments, internalizing symptoms may be a way of seeking responses from attachment figures (similar to an infant's cries of distress). When these relatively unobtrusive internalizing behaviors are likely to be completely ignored (in less responsive environments), an adolescent may "raise the volume" by turning to more dramatic externalizing behaviors as a way to engage parental attention and to express anger and resistance. Finally, a hyperactivated attachment system, although clearly problematic, is nonetheless a system that continues to function; in cases where it brings the adolescent into contact with positive social interactions, it appears to leave the teen responsive to these as well.

In contrast to preoccupied adolescents, Cole-Detke and Kobak (1996; Kobak & Cole, 1994) suggest that adolescents with dismissing strategies may take on symptoms that distract themselves and others from attachment-related cues. When examining psychiatrically hospitalized adolescents, almost all of whom were insecure, Rosenstein and Horowitz (1996) reported that dismissing strategies were associated with externalizing symptoms: Dismissing adolescents were more likely to exhibit substance abuse and conduct disorder. Similarly, my colleagues and I found that dismissing attachment strategies were predictive of increasing delinquency and externalizing behavior over both shorter and longer spans of adolescence (Allen, Marsh, et al., 2002; Allen et al., 2007).

In addition, dismissing attachment strategies have been linked to difficulty getting assistance from peers and teachers, as well as to peer-reported social withdrawal during the transition to college

(Larose & Bernier, 2001). Consistent with this finding, insecurity that manifests itself primarily as dismissal of attachment in early adolescence has been linked to relative *decreases* in social skills over time (Allen, Marsh, et al., 2002) and with less active coping strategies (Seiffge-Krenke & Beyers, 2005). Cole-Detke and Kobak (1996) also reported that eating-disordered individuals in a college population were more likely to use dismissing strategies; the attention given to their eating behaviors was hypothesized to distract them from feelings of internal emotional distress. Unlike preoccupied adolescents, dismissing adolescents do not appear to be particularly sensitive to parental behaviors: For example, a factor such as parental control of adolescent behavior, which is well established as a buffer against delinquency, did not appear to serve this role for dismissing teens (Allen et al., 1998).

Other than the few studies mentioned at the outset of this section, disorganized or unresolved states of mind have been the subject of far less research on adolescent psychopathology. This attachment status has been linked to disrupted maternal behavior with infants in adolescent–mother dyads (Madigan, Moran, & Pederson, 2006), but otherwise it remains a fertile, relatively untapped area for studying more severe forms of adolescent psychopathology.

CONTINUITY, DISCONTINUITY, AND THE CENTRAL QUESTION: WHAT IS ATTACHMENT IN ADOLESCENCE?

Thus far, this chapter has considered many of the features of adolescent attachment strategies while skirting the question raised at the outset: Just what *is* attachment in adolescence? When we are considering continuities of attachment in adolescence to attachment at other developmental stages, however, precision in defining attachment becomes critical. For example, considering the transition from the assessment of attachment *relationships* in infancy and childhood (albeit relationships that are also represented internally), to the assessment of an *internal state* in adolescence and beyond that transcends any particular relationship, makes clear that the two most common measurement approaches assess fundamentally different constructs at these two time points. Attachment as assessed with the AAI is *not* simply a more developed version of what we see in the Strange Situation. Rather, these two constructs

exist at completely different levels of analysis—the intrapsychic and the dyadic/relational—and thus by their very nature differ in fundamental and irreducible ways. The question that adolescent research brings into focus most strongly is this: How do these two different constructs relate to one another, both conceptually and empirically?

From infancy to adolescence (and from the Strange Situation to the AAI), what we find is that the continuities across measures of attachment processes are quite modest. These continuities appear most robustly when environments are generally stable and benign, and they may disappear entirely under more challenging circumstances (although assessment of intervening environmental factors can account for some apparent discontinuities) (Hamilton, 2000; Waters, Hamilton, & Weinfield, 2000; Weinfield, Sroufe, & Egeland, 2000; Weinfield, Whaley, & Egeland, 2004). Notably, observed continuities between infant attachment status and other qualities of adolescents' close relationships make clear that infant attachment status undoubtedly has implications for future relationship qualities, which in some cases are even stronger than links to future adolescent and adult attachment measures (Grossmann, Grossmann, & Kindler, 2005; Sroufe, Egeland, Carlson, & Collins, 2005b; Zimmermann, 2004; Zimmermann, Maier, Winter, & Grossmann, 2001). Within adolescence, security assessed with the AAI displays only very modest correlations with maternal security (Allen et al., 2004). These continuities and discontinuities are considered far more thoroughly in other chapters of this volume. For the purposes of this chapter, the point is that the continuities from infancy and from concurrent measures of parental attachment status to adolescent states of mind regarding attachment are relatively modest.

Evidence from within adolescence, however, suggests that the modest continuity with prior infant attachment and current maternal attachment is not due to any inherent instability in adolescent attachment organization; nor is it probably due to difficulties in assessing adolescent attachment with the AAI. Attachment as assessed with the AAI displays strong stability, with test–retest correlations between overall indices of security ranging from .51 to .61 from ages 16 to 18 in two different samples in Europe and the United States (Allen et al., 2004; Zimmermann & Becker-Stoll, 2002). Similarly, even in research using a modified AAI (the Attachment Interview of Childhood and Adolescence) with a far younger sample, similar stabilities have been found in overall security between ages 10 and 14 (kappa = .48) (Ammaniti et al., 2000).

Even the discontinuities in attachment states of mind across adolescence that have been found appear to be explained largely by environmental factors. Exposure to social and intrapsychic environments that emotionally overwhelm adolescents, while leaving them relatively unable to obtain support from attachment figures, predicts relative *increases* in insecurity over and above baseline levels across a 2-year period in adolescence (Allen et al., 2004). These environments include poverty (which stresses adolescents while draining parents), adolescent depression (a difficult-to-soothe form of distress), and emotional enmeshment (which stresses adolescents while making them want to avoid seeking comfort from a parental figure). Together, these factors account for substantial variance in the change in security during adolescence. They bring the R^2 for security at age 18 (as predicted by security and environmental factors at age 16) up to .72, which approaches the limits of the AAI's reliability. Together with the underlying stability of security, these findings suggest both the robustness of attachment during adolescence and its continuing sensitivity to qualities of the adolescent's psychosocial environment.

If the lack of strong continuity between infant Strange Situation status and adolescent attachment is not due to problems in measurement in adolescence, or to any lack of meaningfulness of the construct of adolescent attachment organization, then two explanations remain most viable. First, intervening experiences between infancy and adolescence may play a large part in altering the developmental course of the attachment system for many individuals. Recent research raises questions about whether in fact any *internal* stability in attachment actually exists from infancy to adolescence; rather, the observed continuity over this time span may primarily reflect stability in parents' attachment strategies (Belsky & Fearon, 2002; van IJzendoorn, 1996). This view is supported by evidence just reviewed showing that the attachment system remains quite open to environmental inputs well into adolescence.

Developmental Transformation 9:
The Emergence of the Caregiving System

A second explanation for the relative lack of continuity in attachment measures from infancy to adolescence is that the construct we are measuring

with the AAI is actually a *fundamentally different* (albeit related) construct from what we measure in the infant Strange Situation. Mary Main has been quite careful to describe what the AAI measures not as attachment per se, but as "states of mind with respect to attachment." And she has described the analogue to infant security not as adolescent or adult security, but as a state of mind that is "autonomous, yet valuing" of attachment (Main & Goldwyn, 1984; Main et al., 2003). Although thus far I have relied on the convenience of discussing AAI study results in terms of "security" of "adolescent attachment," this usage, while handy and defensible, may obscure several important distinctions.

If one simply examines the origin of the AAI and the validation research that led to its rapid rise to prominence, it is difficult to avoid the conclusion that the AAI is most directly tapping not the *attachment* system of the individual, but the *caregiving* system (Allen & Manning, in press). Far more than any other measure, the AAI most strongly predicts success as a caregiver in raising a secure infant—as indeed it was primarily designed and intended to do. Obviously the caregiving and attachment systems are likely to be highly interrelated, as both draw upon many of the same cognitive, behavioral, and emotional subsystems. It even appears defensible to use the terms "attachment" and "security" broadly to refer to qualities of both kinds of systems. However, equally obviously, these systems are *not* isomorphic. Although one's expectations about getting one's own attachment needs met may be linked to one's ability to meet the attachment needs of others, the two are clearly not identical (Collins, Ford, Guichard, & Allard, 2006). (See George and Solomon, Chapter 35, this volume, for an extensive discussion of the caregiving system.)

This issue comes to a head in adolescence, when individuals are making the transition from receiving care from attachment figures to gaining the capacity to be *providers* of such care to others. Notably, by far the strongest correlations of adolescent attachment assessed via the AAI with any other indicator of functioning have been with a caregiving outcome: the security of the infant offspring of adolescent mothers (Ward & Carlson, 1995). The AAI may be more strongly linked to adolescents' functioning with peers than to their relationships with parents (as initial reports suggest), because the AAI is most closely tapping a behavioral system—for meeting others' attachment needs—more relevant for relating to peers than to parents. The quality of close peer relationships may well be determined by a teen's capacity to meet a peer's emotional/attachment-like needs, whereas a teen's ability to meet the needs of a parent is of minimal importance in healthy families.

Appropriately defining the boundaries of the AAI as an indicator of adolescent attachment processes has the advantage of potentially redirecting our attention to a gaping hole that remains in research on adolescent attachment: We know remarkably little about the qualities of the actual attachment relationships adolescents form. Knowing that adolescents with autonomous states of mind regarding attachment form relationships with certain qualities is useful, but it is not the same as being able to assess security or insecurity in specific adolescent relationships (in part because secure teens may at times form insecure relationships with other teens). Our efforts to develop sophisticated approaches to assessing relationship security in adolescence (and beyond) are only just beginning (Cooper et al., 1998). Attachment relationships in adolescence clearly differ dramatically from those in infancy, as various new issues—from power and control, to gender and sexuality, to the increasing mutual capacity to provide comfort in relationships—all rise to prominence. Given these differences, it is not yet clear whether relationship assessments in adolescence will ultimately closely parallel Ainsworth's categorizations of infant attachment relationships, or whether they will need to expand upon and modify these to address the complexities of adult relationships.

From this perspective, an overly narrow focus on issues of continuity in attachment from earlier stages into adolescence, even of heterotypic continuity, may risk oversimplifying the constructs in question. It may make more sense to think of the attachment system as expanding and evolving into *multiple* new forms in adolescence—ranging from attachment functions appearing temporarily in passing relationships to complex new varieties of long-term peer relationships—than to see it as a homunculus moving from infancy into adolescence with only growth and a change in outward appearance.

To put this differently, the development of attachment theory now needs to recapitulate individual ontogeny. Adolescent development brings striking growth in capacities to maintain a diverse array of relationships meeting a diverse array of potential attachment needs, and triggering numerous systems (from primitive neural mechanisms to higher-order cognitive functions) that are typically associated with the attachment system. So too does our view of the attachment system during this period need to continue to grow and expand, to reflect this increasing complexity and sophistication.

ACKNOWLEDGMENT

This chapter was completed with the assistance of grants from the National Institute of Mental Health.

REFERENCES

Adam, K. S., Sheldon-Keller, A. E., & West, M. (1996). Attachment organization and history of suicidal behavior in clinical adolescents. *Journal of Consulting and Clinical Psychology, 64,* 264–272.

Ainsworth, M. D. S. (1982). Attachment: Retrospect and prospect. In C. Parkes & J. Stevenson-Hinde (Eds.), *The place of attachment in human behavior* (pp. 3–30). New York: Basic Books.

Ainsworth, M. D. S. (1989). Attachments beyond infancy. *American Psychologist, 44,* 709–716.

Ainsworth, M. D. S., Blehar, M. C., Waters, E., & Wall, S. (1978). *Patterns of attachment: A psychological study of the Strange Situation.* Hillsdale, NJ: Erlbaum.

Allen, J. P., & Hauser, S. T. (1996). Autonomy and relatedness in adolescent–family interactions as predictors of young adults' states of mind regarding attachment. *Development and Psychopathology, 8*(4), 793–809.

Allen, J. P., Hauser, S. T., & Borman-Spurrell, E. (1996). Attachment theory as a framework for understanding sequelae of severe adolescent psychopathology: An 11-year follow-up study. *Journal of Consulting and Clinical Psychology, 64*(2), 254–263.

Allen, J. P., Hauser, S. T., O'Connor, T. G., & Bell, K. L. (2002). Prediction of peer-rated adult hostility from autonomy struggles in adolescent–family interactions. *Development and Psychopathology, 14,* 123–137.

Allen, J. P., & Manning, N. (in press). From safety to affect regulation: Attachment from the vantage point of adolescence. *New Directions for Child and Adolescent Development.*

Allen, J. P., Marsh, P., McFarland, C., McElhaney, K. B., Land, D. J., Jodl, K. M., et al. (2002). Attachment and autonomy as predictors of the development of social skills and delinquency during midadolescence. *Journal of Consulting and Clinical Psychology, 70*(1), 56–66.

Allen, J. P., McElhaney, K. B., Kuperminc, G. P., & Jodl, K. M. (2004). Stability and change in attachment security across adolescence. *Child Development, 75,* 1792–1805.

Allen, J. P., McElhaney, K. B., Land, D. J., Kuperminc, G. P., Moore, C. M., O'Beirne-Kelley, H., et al. (2003). A secure base in adolescence: Markers of attachment security in the mother–adolescent relationship. *Child Development, 74,* 292–307.

Allen, J. P., Moore, C., & Kuperminc, G. (1997). Developmental approaches to understanding adolescent deviance. In S. S. Luthar & J. A. Burack (Eds.), *Developmental psychopathology: Perspectives on adjustment, risk, and disorder* (pp. 548–567). New York: Cambridge University Press.

Allen, J. P., Moore, C., Kuperminc, G., & Bell, K. (1998). Attachment and adolescent psychosocial functioning. *Child Development, 69*(5), 1406–1419.

Allen, J. P., Porter, M. R., McFarland, F. C., McElhaney, K. B., & Marsh, P. A. (2007). The relation of attachment security to adolescents' paternal and peer relationships, depression, and externalizing behavior. *Child Development, 78,* 1222–1239.

Ammaniti, M., van IJzendoorn, M. H., Speranza, A. M., & Tambelli, R. (2000). Internal working models of attachment during late childhood and early adolescence: An exploration of stability and change. *Attachment and Human Development, 2*(3), 328–346.

Bartholomew, K., & Shaver, P. R. (1998). Methods of assessing adult attachment: Do they converge? In J. A. Simpson & W. S. Rholes (Eds.), *Attachment theory and close relationships* (pp. 25–45). New York: Guilford Press.

Becker-Stoll, F., Delius, A., & Scheitenberger, S. (2001). Adolescents' nonverbal emotional expressions during negotiation of a disagreement with their mothers: An attachment approach. *International Journal of Behavioral Development, 25*(4), 344–353.

Becker-Stoll, F., & Fremmer-Bombik, E. (1997, April). *Adolescent–mother interaction and attachment: A longitudinal study.* Paper presented at the biennial meetings of the Society for Research in Child Development, Washington, DC.

Beckwith, L., Cohen, S. E., & Hamilton, C. E. (1999). Maternal sensitivity during infancy and subsequent life events relate to attachment representation at early adulthood. *Developmental Psychology, 35*(3), 693–700.

Belsky, J., & Fearon, R. M. P. (2002). Early attachment security, subsequent maternal sensitivity, and later child development: Does continuity in development depend upon continuity of caregiving? *Attachment and Human Development, 4*(3), 361–387.

Berger, L. E., Jodl, K. M., Allen, J. P., McElhaney, K. B., & Kuperminc, G. P. (2005). When adolescents disagree with others about their symptoms: Differences in attachment organization as an explanation of discrepancies between adolescent-, parent-, and peer-reports of behavior problems. *Development and Psychopathology, 17,* 489–507.

Bernier, A., Larose, S., & Whipple, N. (2005). Leaving home for college: A potentially stressful event for adolescents with preoccupied attachment patterns. *Attachment and Human Development, 7*(2), 171–185.

Bowlby, J. (1969/1982). *Attachment and loss: Vol. 1. Attachment.* New York: Basic Books.

Brennan, K. A., Clark, C. L., & Shaver, P. R. (1998). Self-report measurement of adult attachment: An integrative overview. In J. A. Simpson & W. S. Rholes (Eds.), *Attachment theory and close relationships* (pp. 46–76). New York: Guilford Press.

Buhrmester, D. (1996). Need fulfillment, interpersonal competence, and the developmental contexts of early adolescent friendship. In W. M. Bukowski, A. F. Newcomb, & W. Hartup (Eds.), *The company they keep: Friendship in childhood and adolescence* (pp. 158–185). Cambridge, UK: Cambridge University Press.

Cassidy, J. (1999). The nature of the child's ties. In J. Cassidy & P. R. Shaver (Eds.), *Handbook of attachment: Theory, research, and clinical applications* (pp. 3–20). New York: Guilford Press.

Cassidy, J. (2001). Truth, lies, and intimacy: An attachment perspective. *Attachment and Human Development, 3*(2), 121–155.

Cassidy, J., Kirsh, S. J., Scolton, K. L., & Parke, R. D. (1996). Attachment and representations of peer relationships. *Developmental Psychology, 32*(5), 892–904.

Coan, J. A., Schaefer, H. S., & Davidson, R. J. (2006). Lending a hand: Social regulation of the neural response to threat. *Psychological Science, 17,* 1032–1039.

Cole-Detke, H., & Kobak, R. (1996). Attachment processes in eating disorder and depression. *Journal of Consulting and Clinical Psychology, 64*(2), 282–290.

Collins, N. L., Ford, M. B., Guichard, A. M., & Allard, L. M. (2006). Working models of attachment and attribution processes in intimate relationships. *Personality and Social Psychology Bulletin, 32*(2), 201–219.

Collins, W. A., & Laursen, B. (2000). Adolescent relationships: The art of fugue. In C. Hendrick & S. S. Hendrick (Eds.), *Close relationships: A sourcebook* (pp. 59–69). Thousand Oaks, CA: Sage.

Collins, W. A., van Dulmen, M., Crouter, A. C., & Booth, A. (2006). "The course of true love(s)": Origins and pathways in the development of romantic relationships. In A. C. Crouter & A. Booth (Eds.), *Romance and sex in adolescence and emerging adulthood: Risks and opportunities* (pp. 63–86). Mahwah, NJ: Erlbaum.

Cooper, M. L., Shaver, P. R., & Collins, N. L. (1998). Attachment styles, emotion regulation, and adjustment in adolescence. *Journal of Personality and Social Psychology, 74*(5), 1380–1397.

Crowell, J. A., & Owens, G. (1996). *Current relationship interview and scoring system.* Unpublished manuscript, State University of New York at Stony Brook.

Cummings, E. M., & Davies, P. (1996). Emotional security as a regulatory process in normal development and the development of psychopathology. *Development and Psychopathology, 8*(1), 123–139.

De Wolff, M., & van IJzendoorn, M. H. (1997). Sensitivity and attachment: A meta-analysis on parental antecedents of infant attachment. *Child Development, 68*(4), 571–591.

Dodge, K. A. (1993). Social-cognitive mechanisms in the development of conduct disorder and depression. *Annual Review of Psychology, 44,* 559–584.

Fraley, R. C., & Davis, K. E. (1997). Attachment formation and transfer in young adults' close friendships and romantic relationships. *Personal Relationships, 4,* 131–144.

Furman, W. (2001). Working models of friendships. *Journal of Social and Personal Relationships, 18*(5), 583–602.

Furman, W., Brown, B. B., & Feiring, C. (Eds.). (1999). *The development of romantic relationships in adolescence.* New York: Cambridge University Press.

Furman, W., & Simon, V. A. (2004). Concordance in attachment states of mind and styles with respect to fathers and mothers. *Developmental Psychology, 40*(6), 1239–1247.

Furman, W., Simon, V. A., Shaffer, L., & Bouchey, H. A. (2002). Adolescents' working models and styles for relationships with parents, friends, and romantic partners. *Child Development, 73*(1), 241–255.

Gavin, L. A., & Furman, W. (1989). Age differences in adolescents' perceptions of their peer groups. *Developmental Psychology, 25,* 827–834.

Gavin, L. A., & Furman, W. (1996). Adolescent girls' relationships with mothers and best friends. *Child Development, 67*(2), 375–386.

George, C., Kaplan, N., & Main, M. (1984). *Adult Attachment Interview protocol.* Unpublished manuscript, University of California at Berkeley.

George, C., Kaplan, N., & Main, M. (1985). *Adult Attachment Interview protocol* (2nd ed.). Unpublished manuscript, University of California at Berkeley.

George, C., Kaplan, N., & Main, M. (1996). *Adult Attachment Interview protocol* (3rd ed.). Unpublished manuscript, University of California at Berkeley.

Grossmann, K., Grossmann, K. E., & Kindler, H. (2005). Early care and the roots of attachment and partnership representations: The Bielefeld and Regensburg longitudinal studies. In K. E. Grossmann, K. Grossmann, & E. Waters (Eds.), *Attachment from infancy to adulthood: The major longitudinal studies* (pp. 98–136). New York: Guilford Press.

Hamilton, C. E. (2000). Continuity and discontinuity of attachment from infancy through adolescence. *Child Development, 71,* 690–694.

Hartup, W. W. (1992). Friendships and their developmental significance. In H. McGurk (Ed.), *Childhood social development: Contemporary perspectives* (pp. 175–205). Hillsdale, NJ: Erlbaum.

Hazan, C., & Shaver, P. R. (1987). Romantic love conceptualized as an attachment process. *Journal of Personality and Social Psychology, 52,* 511–524.

Hazan, C., & Shaver, P. R. (1994). Attachment as an organizational framework for research on close relationships. *Psychological Inquiry, 5,* 1–22.

Hesse, E. (1999). The Adult Attachment Interview: Historical and current perspectives. In J. Cassidy & P. R. Shaver (Eds.), *Handbook of attachment: Theory, research, and clinical applications* (pp. 395–433). New York: Guilford Press.

Hinton, S. E. (1967). *The outsiders.* New York: Viking Press.

Hofer, M. A. (1994). Hidden regulators in attachment, separation, and loss. In N. Fox (Ed.), The development of emotion regulation: Biological and behavioral considerations. *Monographs of the Society for Research in Child Development, 59*(2–3), 192–207, 250–283.

Hofer, M. A. (2006). Psychobiological roots of early attachment. *Current Directions in Psychological Science, 15*(2), 84–88.

Keating, D. P. (1990). Adolescent thinking. In S. S. Feldman & G. Elliott (Eds.), *At the threshold: The developing adolescent* (pp. 54–90). Cambridge, MA: Harvard University Press.

King, S. (Writer). (1986). *Stand by me* [Motion picture]. New York: Columbia Pictures.

Kobak, R. R., & Cole, H. (1994). Attachment and meta-monitoring: Implications for adolescent autonomy and psychopathology. In D. Cicchetti & S. L. Toth (Eds.), *Rochester Symposium on Developmental Psychopathology: Vol. 5. Disorders and dysfunctions of the self* (pp. 267–297). Rochester, NY: University of Rochester Press.

Kobak, R. R., Cole, H., Ferenz-Gillies, R., Fleming, W., & Gamble, W. (1993). Attachment and emotion regulation during mother–teen problem-solving: A control theory analysis. *Child Development, 64,* 231–245.

Kobak, R. R., & Duemmler, S. (1994). Attachment and conversation: Toward a discourse analysis of adolescent and adult security. In K. Bartholomew & D. Perlman (Eds.), *Advances in personal relationships: Vol. 5. Attachment processes in adulthood* (pp. 121–149). London: Jessica Kingsley.

Kobak, R. R., Ferenz-Gillies, R., Everhart, E., & Seabrook, L. (1994). Maternal attachment strategies and emotion regulation with adolescent offspring. *Journal of Research on Adolescence, 4*(4), 553–566.

Kobak, R. R., Rosenthal, N., & Serwik, A. (2005). The attachment hierarchy in middle childhood: Conceptual and methodological issues. In K. A. Kerns & R. A. Richardson (Eds.), *Attachment in middle childhood* (pp. 71–88). New York: Guilford Press.

Kobak, R. R., & Sceery, A. (1988). Attachment in late adolescence: Working models, affect regulation and representations of self and others. *Child Development, 59,* 135–146.

Kobak, R. R., Sudler, N., & Gamble, W. (1991). Attachment and depressive symptoms during adolescence: A developmental pathways analysis. *Development and Psychopathology, 3*(4), 461–474.

Larose, S., & Bernier, A. (2001). Social support processes: Mediators of attachment state of mind and adjustment in late adolescence. *Attachment and Human Development, 3*(1), 96–120.

Lieberman, M., Doyle, A.-B., & Markiewicz, D. (1999). Developmental patterns in security of attachment to mother and father in late childhood and early adolescence: Associations with peer relations. *Child Development, 70*(1), 202–213.

Madigan, S., Moran, G., & Pederson, D. R. (2006). Unresolved states of mind, disorganized attachment relationships, and disrupted interactions of adolescent mothers and their infants. *Developmental Psychology,* 42(2), 293–304.

Main, M. (1999). Epilogue. Attachment theory: Eighteen points with suggestions for future studies. In J. Cassidy & P. R. Shaver (Eds.), *Handbook of attachment: Theory, research, and clinical applications* (pp. 845–887). New York: Guilford Press.

Main, M., & Goldwyn, R. (1984). *Adult attachment scoring and classification system.* Unpublished manuscript, University of California at Berkeley.

Main, M., Goldwyn, R., & Hesse, E. (2003). *Adult attachment scoring and classification system.* Unpublished manuscript, University of California at Berkeley.

Main, M., Kaplan, N., & Cassidy, J. (1985). Security in infancy, childhood, and adulthood: A move to the level of representation. In I. Bretherton & E. Waters (Eds.), Growing points of attachment theory and research. *Monographs of the society for research in child development,* 50(1–2, Serial No. 209), 66–104.

Marsh, P., McFarland, F. C., Allen, J. P., McElhaney, K. B., & Land, D. J. (2003). Attachment, autonomy, and multifinality in adolescent internalizing and risky behavioral symptoms. *Development and Psychopathology,* 15(2), 451–467.

McElhaney, K. B., Immele, A., Smith, F. D., & Allen, J. P. (2006). Attachment organization as a moderator of the link between peer relationships and adolescent delinquency. *Attachment and Human Development,* 8, 33–46.

Moore, C. W. (1997). *Models of attachment, relationships with parents, and sexual behavior in at-risk adolescents.* Unpublished doctoral dissertation, University of Virginia.

Owens, G., Crowell, J. A., Pan, H., Treboux, D., O'Connor, E., & Waters, E. (1995). The prototype hypothesis and the origins of attachment working models: Adult relationships with parents and romantic partners. In E. Waters, B. E. Vaughn, G. Posada, & K. Kondo-Ikemura (Eds.), Caregiving, cultural, and cognitive perspectives on secure-base behavior and working models: New growing points of attachment theory and research. *Monographs of the Society for Research in Child Development,* 60(2–3, Serial No. 244), 216–233.

Pearson, J. L., Cohn, D. A., Cowan, P. A., & Cowan, C. P. (1994). Earned- and continuous-security in adult attachment: Relation to depressive symptomatology and parenting style. *Development and Psychopathology,* 6(2), 359–373.

Reimer, M. S., Overton, W. F., Steidl, J. H., Rosenstein, D. S., & Horowitz, H. (1996). Familial responsiveness and behavioral control: Influences on adolescent psychopathology, attachment, and cognition. *Journal of Research on Adolescence,* 6(1), 87–112.

Roisman, G. I., Collins, W. A., Sroufe, L. A., & Egeland, B. (2005). Predictors of young adults' representations of and behavior in their current romantic relationship: Prospective tests of the prototype hypothesis. *Attachment and Human Development,* 7(2), 105–121.

Roisman, G. I., Madsen, S. D., Hennighausen, K. H., Sroufe, L. A., & Collins, W. A. (2001). The coherence of dyadic behavior across parent–child and romantic relationships as mediated by the internalized representation of experience. *Attachment and Human Development,* 3(2), 156–172.

Rosenstein, D. S., & Horowitz, H. A. (1996). Adolescent attachment and psychopathology. *Journal of Consulting and Clinical Psychology,* 64(2), 244–253.

Seiffge-Krenke, I., & Beyers, W. (2005). Coping trajectories from adolescence to young adulthood: Links to attachment state of mind. *Journal of Research on Adolescence,* 15(4), 561–582.

Selman, R. (1980). *The growth of interpersonal understanding: Developmental and clinical analyses.* New York: Academic Press.

Shaver, P., Hazan, C., & Bradshaw, D. (1988). Love as attachment: The integration of three behavioral systems. In R. J. Sternberg & M. Barnes (Eds.), *The psychology of love* (pp. 68–99). New Haven, CT: Yale University Press.

Slough, N. M., & Greenberg, M. T. (1990). Five-year-olds' representations of separation from parents: Responses from the perspective of self and other. *New Directions for Child Development,* 48, 67–84.

Spangler, G., & Zimmermann, P. (1999). Attachment representation and emotion regulation in adolescents: A psychobiological perspective on internal working models. *Attachment and Human Development,* 1(3), 270–290.

Sroufe, L. A., Egeland, B., Carlson, E. A., & Collins, W. A. (2005a). *The development of the person: The Minnesota Study of Risk and Adaptation from Birth to Adulthood.* New York: Guilford Press.

Sroufe, L. A., Egeland, B., Carlson, E., & Collins, W. A. (2005b). Placing early attachment experiences in developmental context: The Minnesota longitudinal study. In K. E. Grossmann, K. Grossmann, & E. Waters (Eds.), *Attachment from infancy to adulthood: The major longitudinal studies* (pp. 48–70). New York: Guilford Press.

Sroufe, L. A., & Waters, E. (1977). Attachment as an organizational construct. *Child Development,* 48, 1184–1199.

Steinberg, L. (1990). Interdependency in the family: Autonomy, conflict, and harmony in the parent–adolescent relationship. In S. S. Feldman & G. Elliott (Eds.), *At the threshold: The developing adolescent* (pp. 255–276). Cambridge, MA: Harvard University Press.

Steinberg, L. (2005). *Adolescence.* New York: McGraw-Hill.

Taylor, S. E., Klein, L. C., Lewis, B. P., Gruenewald, T. L., Gurung, R. A. R., & Updegraff, J. A. (2000). Biobehavioral responses to stress in females: Tend-and-befriend, not fight-or-flight. *Psychological Review,* 107(3), 411–429.

Thompson, R. A. (1997). Sensitivity and security: New questions to ponder. *Child Development,* 68(4), 595–597.

Tracy, J. L., Shaver, P. R., Albino, A. W., & Cooper, M. L. (2003). Attachment styles and adolescent sexuality. In P. Florsheim (Ed.), *Adolescent romantic relations and sexual behavior: Theory, research, and practical implications.* (pp. 137–159). Mahwah, NJ: Erlbaum.

Treboux, D., Crowell, J. A., & Waters, E. (2004). When "new" meets "old": Configurations of adult attachment representations and their implications for marital functioning. *Developmental Psychology, 40*(2), 295–314.

van IJzendoorn, M. H. (1996). "Attachment patterns and their outcomes": Commentary. *Human Development, 224–231.*

Wallis, P., & Steele, H. (2001). Attachment representations in adolescence: Further evidence from psychiatric residential settings. *Attachment and Human Development, 3*(3), 259–268.

Ward, M. J., & Carlson, E. A. (1995). Associations among adult attachment representations, maternal sensitivity, and infant–mother attachment in a sample of adolescent mothers. *Child Development, 66,* 69–79.

Waters, E., Hamilton, C. E., & Weinfield, N. S. (2000). The stability of attachment security from infancy to adolescence and early adulthood: General introduction. *Child Development, 71*(3), 678–683.

Weimer, B. L., Kerns, K. A., & Oldenberg, C. M. (2004). Adolescents' interactions with a best friend: Associations with attachment style. *Journal of Experimental Child Psychology, 88*(1), 102–120.

Weinfield, N. S., Sroufe, L. A., & Egeland, B. (2000). Attachment from infancy to early adulthood in a high-risk sample: Continuity, discontinuity, and their correlates. *Child Development, 71,* 695–702.

Weinfield, N. S., Whaley, G. J. L., & Egeland, B. (2004). Continuity, discontinuity, and coherence in attachment from infancy to late adolescence: Sequelae of organization and disorganization. *Attachment and Human Development, 6*(1), 73–97.

Zimmermann, P. (2004). Attachment representations and characteristics of friendship relations during adolescence. *Journal of Experimental Child Psychology, 88*(1), 83–101.

Zimmermann, P., & Becker-Stoll, F. (2002). Stability of attachment representations during adolescence: The influence of ego-identity status. *Journal of Adolescence, 25*(1), 107–124.

Zimmermann, P., Maier, M. A., Winter, M., & Grossmann, K. E. (2001). Attachment and adolescents' emotion regulation during a joint problem-solving task with a friend. *International Journal of Behavioral Development, 25*(4), 331–343.

CHAPTER 20

Pair Bonds as Attachments
Reevaluating the Evidence

DEBRA ZEIFMAN
CINDY HAZAN

When Bowlby (1979) made his oft-cited claim that attachment is an integral part of human existence "from the cradle to the grave," it was more a hypothesis than an empirically established fact. The absence of a detailed theory of attachment beyond childhood may have delayed the initiation of research into the farther reaches of the lifespan, but it did not preclude it. Since Main, Kaplan, and Cassidy (1985) first described a measure of adult states of mind with respect to attachment (see Hesse, Chapter 25, this volume), and Hazan and Shaver (1987) first applied the concept of attachment to adult romantic relationships (see J. Feeney, Chapter 21, this volume, for an overview), investigations of adult attachment have proliferated at a rate comparable to that of infant attachment studies during the years immediately following the publication of Ainsworth's findings (Ainsworth, Blehar, Waters, & Wall, 1978). Adult attachment research has proceeded largely on the faith that Bowlby and Ainsworth were right about two things: that patterns of attachment established in early life are relatively stable across development, and that pair-bond relationships are the prototypical adult instantiation of attachment (Ainsworth, 1991).

The present chapter does not address continuity in attachment patterns between infancy and adulthood (see Weinfield, Sroufe, Egeland, & Carlson, Chapter 4, this volume, for a discussion of this issue). Instead, our focus is on the second assumption—that romantic relationships qualify as attachment bonds and thus constitute the appropriate context in which to investigate adult attachment phenomena. Although these assumptions may appear to be inextricably interrelated, they represent independent issues, at least from an empirical standpoint. Consider the possible outcomes of stability studies: a finding of relative continuity in patterns of attachment from infancy to adulthood, or, alternatively, no systematic connections between infants' Strange Situation classifications and their subsequent adult attachment categorizations. Neither outcome would provide a definitive answer to the question of whether the attachment system is active in adult life or implicated in adult pair bonds. Continuity of individual differences is not the same as continuity of function; these are separate issues requiring distinct types of evidence. Thus the validity of our arguments concerning the second assumption is not dependent on the results of empirical investigations relating to the first.

The importance of the question—whether romantic bonds are attachments in the technical sense—can hardly be overestimated. The entire enterprise of adult attachment research in the field of personality and social psychology has been constructed on the premise that they are. Were it to turn out that Bowlby and Ainsworth were mistaken, either about the lifespan significance of attachment or about the preeminence of romantic partners as attachment figures in adult life, it could potentially undermine the whole body of findings. Therefore, it is crucial to the adult attachment enterprise that this foundational assumption be examined and evaluated in light of the evidence.

One reason for questioning the assumption that romantic relationships are genuine attachments concerns the presumed function of attachment bonds. In theory, the attachment behavioral system evolved in response to selection pressures in the "environment of evolutionary adaptedness" (EEA) that made it advantageous for infants to maintain proximity to protectors (Bowlby, 1958, 1969/1982). Few would argue with the adaptiveness of a system that in situations of real or perceived danger led vulnerable young to seek protection from their more mature and competent guardians, or with the necessity of such a system for human infant survival.

What is considerably less apparent is how attachment might contribute to *adult* survival (Kirkpatrick, 1998). It cannot simply be assumed that adult attachment serves the same function as infant attachment. In the adult case, attachment to a romantic partner is not necessary for survival; nor is a pair bond necessary for the survival of offspring. If, however, having an attachment to a romantic partner in adulthood enhances an individuals' chances of survival and/or the survival of two sexual partners' joint offspring, it can be said to serve a function in adulthood similar to its function in infancy. A solid foundation of evidence for the reproductive fitness advantages of adult attachment is accruing to support the already large body of findings on the functional similarity of infant and adult attachment.

Do pair-bond partners replace parents in their roles as primary attachment figures, and if so, by what processes does the transition occur? What are the unique features of attachment relationships that distinguish them from other kinds of relationships? Is there compelling evidence that the attachment system is operative in adult romantic relationships? Are adult attachment relationships the ideal mating context, or are short-term sexual pairings equally advantageous for producing and rearing offspring? How are attachment styles and sexual/mating strategies related? These are some of the questions addressed in this chapter.

In our own research, we started by investigating the process by which attachments are transferred from parents to peers. A brief summary of our findings is followed by a review of the literature as it relates to the question of whether pair bonds are attachments in the technical sense. Throughout the chapter and in the third major section especially, we address issues related to the function and evolutionary significance of the attachment system in adulthood, with particular attention devoted to how the attachment system relates to other behavioral systems. Finally, alternative evolutionary theories of mating are presented, and seeming conflicts or contradictions with an attachment perspective are addressed.

FROM PARENTAL ATTACHMENT TO PAIR BONDS

How Attachment Is Defined

Bowlby (1969/1982) took care to define the specific type of socioemotional bond to which his theory applied, and to distinguish it from other kinds of social ties. Attachment bonds have four defining features: "proximity maintenance," "separation distress," "safe haven," and "secure base." These are readily observable in the overt behavior of an infant in relation to a primary caregiver (usually the mother). She serves as a secure base from which the infant (hereafter called "he" for convenience) ventures forth and interacts with the social and physical world. He continuously monitors her proximity and availability. If he senses danger or feels anxious for any reason, he retreats to her as a source of comfort and a haven of safety. Because separations from her signal potential danger, he will object to and be distressed by them. As long as she is perceived to be sufficiently near and responsive, he will be motivated to explore his environment.

In theory, this dynamic balance between attachment and exploration is an integral part of behavior throughout the lifespan. Nevertheless, changes as a function of maturation are expected. One predictable change concerns the time and distance from the attachment figure that can be comfortably tolerated. A typical 12-month-old will exhibit greater distress (and more disrupted exploration) as the result of even brief separations from a caregiver than will a 36-month-old. By late childhood or early adolescence, longer separations are usually negotiated without undue upset, and separation distress is less apparent except in the case of unexpected and/or extended caregiver unavailability.

Perhaps the preeminent change in attachment relationships is their degree of mutuality. The asymmetrical (complementary) attachments of early life—in which infants seek and derive security from caregivers but do not provide security in return—are hypothesized to be replaced by more symmetrical (reciprocal) attachments. According to Bowlby, the pair-bond relationship—in which sexual partners *mutually* derive and provide security—is the prototype of attachment in adulthood. Thus, in the course of normative development, the sexual mating, caregiving (parenting), and attachment systems become integrated (Fraley & Shaver, 2000; Hazan & Shaver, 1994; Mikulincer & Goodman, 2006; Shaver, Hazan, & Bradshaw, 1988).

The Ontogeny of Infant Attachment

Given the opportunity, all normal human infants become attached to their primary caregivers, typically within the first 8 months of life. Attachment formation proceeds through a series of phases, beginning in the first weeks of life and ending sometime toward the end of the second year with the establishment of a "goal-corrected partnership" (Bowlby, 1969/1982). The process begins with close physical proximity, which is initially maintained by intentional actions of the caregiver and reflexive behavior on the part of the infant (e.g., crying, sucking, clinging). In time, the infant learns to associate the caregiver with comfort and distress alleviation (i.e., with viewing her as a safe haven). Typically by about 8 months of age, and concurrently with the onset of self-produced locomotion and stranger wariness, the infant begins to protest separations and to use the caregiver as a base of security for exploration. Separation distress is the accepted indicator that an attachment bond is fully formed. Note that the components, which together define attachment, do not emerge simultaneously, but rather in sequence. (See Marvin & Britner, Chapter 12, this volume, for further discussion of the ontogeny of infant attachment.)

Although multiple attachments are the norm, attachment figures are not treated equivalently. An infant shows clear discrimination among caregivers and a consistent preference for the primary caregiver (Colin, 1985, 1987; Cummings, 1980). Even if several caregivers are regularly available, an infant reliably seeks and maintains proximity to one, especially when distressed (Ainsworth, 1967, 1982). The infant also exhibits more intense protest upon being separated from the primary attachment figure as compared to others (Schaffer & Emerson, 1964), and, in unfamiliar settings, is most reassured by this figure's presence (Ricciuti, 1974; Shill, Solyom, & Biven, 1984). The primary attachment figure is thus not simply one among a coterie of possible protectors, but the individual with whom the infant has a privileged relationship. Bowlby (1958, 1969/1982) referred to this tendency to form one special attachment as "monotropy," and he considered it a crucial aspect of the survival-enhancing function of attachment.

Over the course of development, changes are to be expected in the composition and structure of individuals' attachment hierarchies. New people may be added and/or others dropped. According to Bowlby, parental figures tend to be permanent members of the attachment hierarchy, but eventually assume a position secondary in importance to the pair-bond partner. Exactly when and how this change from complementary (parental) to reciprocal (peer) attachment comes about was not specified by Bowlby. We explored these questions of timing and process in two related studies. (For more details, see Hazan & Zeifman, 1994.)

The Transfer of Attachment from Parents to Peers

Peer relationships during childhood and adolescence are usually characterized as "affiliative"—that is, functionally distinct from parental attachments and presumably regulated by a different behavioral system. Although there is obvious overlap in the behaviors that typify these two kinds of social bonds, affiliative relationships at this age primarily provide stimulation and increase arousal, in contrast to the arousal-moderating and security-enhancing provisions of attachment bonds. Yet a review of the research suggests that *some* components of attachment may be present in peer relationships fairly early in development.

By age 3, children are capable of sustaining complex social interactions with agemates (Gottman, 1983; Rubin, 1980). Not only do they possess the necessary skills for engaging their peers, but they show a growing interest in doing so. The preference for spending time with peers relative to parents increases steadily. Thus one aspect of attachment—proximity seeking—seems to be present in and typical of peer relationships by childhood, although such relationships would not qualify as attachments in the full sense of the term.

By middle childhood, youngsters are capable of developing more intimate relationships with their peers (Buhrmester & Furman, 1986, 1987; Buhrmester & Prager, 1995; Furman & Buhrmester, 1985; Hartup, 1983; Lewis, 1982) and increasingly turn to them for comfort. There is evidence that by late adolescence, peers come to be preferred over parents as sources of emotional support (Steinberg & Silverberg, 1986). The confiding and support-seeking aspects of peer relationships appear to be functionally similar to the parent-directed safe-haven behavior of infancy and early childhood.

Thus there may be normative developmental changes in the *target* of different attachment behaviors, so that during childhood and adolescence, some get redirected toward peers. On the basis of these kinds of findings, we reasoned that a key to understanding the transfer of attachment from parents to peers might lie in an analysis of attachment at the component level.

We used an interview measure of the four components of attachment (i.e., proximity seeking, safe haven, separation distress, and secure base) and administered it to over 100 children and adolescents ranging in age from 6 to 17. For each component of attachment, participants were asked several related questions about the target of the particular component of attachment, and responded by naming the single *most preferred* person in each situation. Because we were primarily interested in the distinction between parental figures and peers, responses were grouped into these two categories.

We found that nearly all children and adolescents in the sample were peer-oriented in terms of proximity seeking; that is, they preferred to spend time in the company of peers rather than parents. Regarding the safe-haven component, there was an apparent shift between the ages of 8 and 14, with peers coming to be preferred over parents as sources of comfort and emotional support. For the majority, however, parents continued to serve as bases of security and as the primary sources of separation distress. Only among the oldest adolescents (the 15- to 17-year-old group) did we find full-blown attachments to peers—relationships containing all four components. Of this minority who considered a peer to be their primary attachment figure, the overwhelming majority named a boyfriend or girlfriend (i.e., a *romantic* partner).

In a second study, we explored the time course of adult attachment formation. Research on romantic relationship formation suggests that whether and which attachment features are present may depend on how long a couple has been together. For example, romantic couples typically experience an especially strong desire for physical proximity and contact in the initial stages of a relationship (Berscheid, 1984), whereas the provision of mutual support and care becomes more important in later stages (Reedy, Birren, & Schaie, 1981; Sternberg, 1986). Similarly, reactions to separations seem to vary according to relationship length and stage (Weiss, 1988). Thus, in adult–adult as well as infant–caregiver relationships, the presence or absence of attachment components may depend on the stage of relationship development.

We administered the same interview used in our child and adolescent study to an equally diverse sample of over 100 adults ranging in age from 18 to 82, but this time we grouped subjects by *stage* of relationship development rather than by age. Three relationship status groups were identified: "not in a romantic relationship," "in a romantic relationship for less than 2 years," and "in a romantic relationship for 2 or more years." The majority of participant responses to questions about the target of attachment behaviors were covered by the following three categories: parent, adult sibling, friend, and romantic partner.

We found that these adults were clearly peer-oriented in both proximity-seeking and safe-haven behaviors. Nearly all adult respondents reported a preference for spending time with and seeking emotional support from their friends and/or partners rather than their parents. But findings for the other two components varied as a function of relationship status: Participants involved in romantic relationships of at least 2 years' duration overwhelmingly named partners in response to the items covering separation distress and secure base. Those in shorter-term romantic relationships and those without partners tended to name parents as the individuals whose absence was most distressing and whose presence served as a base of security.

In the introduction to this chapter, we have posed the question of whether romantic relationships (i.e., pair bonds) are true attachments. We reasoned that a logical starting point for addressing this question was to discover first whether romantic relationships meet the definitional criteria of attachment. In addition, it was necessary to demonstrate that romantic partners assume preeminent status in the attachment hierarchy by replacing parental figures as the predominant source of emotional security.

The results of these two studies (and a replication of the second by Fraley & Davis, 1997) are consistent with Bowlby's hypotheses. Full-blown attachments (relationships with all four defining components) were observed among adolescent as well as adult participants almost exclusively in two kinds of social relationships—with parents or romantic partners. Furthermore, and just as Bowlby predicted, pair-bond partners did assume the status of primary attachment figures (by being preferred over parents). Finally, it appears that romantic relationships require approximately 2 years to become full-blown attachments. Individuals involved in romantic relationships of at least 2 years' duration overwhelmingly looked to partners to meet their attachment needs, whereas those in shorter-term romantic relationships and those without partners tended to continue looking to parents for some of these needs. Taken together, these findings suggest that romantic relationships (after a certain length of time) qualify as bona fide attachments.

The findings may also reveal something about the basic processes by which primary attachments are transferred from parents to peers. The establishment of a goal-corrected partnership with a caregiver in early childhood facilitates social exploration. As such, the endpoint in the development of complementary attachments to parents serves as the starting point for reciprocal attachments to peers. Increased time spent in the company of peers fosters mutual confiding, comforting, and a reliance on peers as havens of safety, thereby paving the way for attachment formation. However, it is important to note that most of our adolescent and adult subjects were not attached—in the technical sense—to their friends. Peer relationships meeting the definitional criteria of attachment were almost exclusively of the romantic variety. (See Allen, Chapter 19, this volume, for additional discussion of the nature of attachment to parents and attachment to peers during adolescence.)

Sex appears to play a central role in romantic attachment. Sexual maturation may serve as a catalyst for redirecting social attention and activity toward mating, as is the case in many other species (Hinde, 1983). Furthermore, sexual exchanges create a social context that is conducive to attachment formation. (We return to this issue later.)

THE NATURE OF THE BOND IN PAIR BONDS

So far, evidence has been presented that pair-bond relationships are characterized by the same features as infant–caregiver attachments and develop according to the same process, at least in terms of the sequence in which various components come into play. These findings support the assertion that the same behavioral system is involved in pair bonds and infant–caregiver relationships. If the attachment system is operative in pair bonds, its effects should be conspicuous in other aspects of relationship functioning. In fact, the congruences are far-reaching. They include the nature of physical contact that typifies and distinguishes attachment bonds, the factors that influence the selection of attachment figures, the dynamics by which attachment affects functioning in other behavioral domains, reactions to attachment disruption and loss, and the role of attachment in biological and psychological well-being. We discuss each of these in turn.

Physical Contact

Freud was among the first to write about the striking similarities in the physical intimacy that typifies lovers and mother–infant pairs. Like caregivers and their infants, adult sexual partners (at least initially) spend much time engaged in mutual gazing, cuddling, nuzzling, sucking, and kissing in the context of prolonged face-to-face, skin-to-skin, belly-to-belly contact, and the touching of body parts otherwise considered "private." It is noteworthy that these most intimate of human interpersonal exchanges are, in virtually every culture, limited to parent–infant and pair-bond relationships (Eibl-Eibesfeldt, 1975). Although some forms of intimate contact may occur in isolation within other kinds of social relationships (e.g., kissing among friends), their collective occurrence is more restricted. When friends violate these social norms by engaging in intimate physical contact, they label themselves "friends with benefits" to denote the provision of benefits not usually associated with mere friendship (Carey, 2007).

The universal existence of prohibitions against physical intimacy outside recognized pair bonds (at least for females) has generally been attributed to the fact that copulations outside such bonds reduce confidence in paternity. Such restrictions may also reflect an implicit understanding that close physical contact with another could lead to a subsidiary emotional bond that would jeopardize the primary one. In subcultures where extrarelationship sexual contact is permitted, efforts to avoid emotional involvement are common. For example, prostitutes commonly refuse to engage in kissing, nuzzling, and other forms of intimate face-to-face contact with their clients (Nass & Fisher, 1988). Gay male couples who consensually engage in extrarelationship sexual activity usually reserve kissing and cuddling for their primary partners (Blumstein & Schwartz, 1983). And ground rules among so-called "swinging" heterosexual couples often forbid regular or frequent sexual contact with the same person (O'Neill & O'Neill, 1972). If an emotional bond is not desired in the context of a physically intimate relationship, special steps must be taken to protect against its formation. Finally, preliminary research on so-called "friends with benefits" indicates that such a relationship frequently become emotionally stressful when one party becomes more attracted than the other (Carey, 2007).

There is some evidence that the chemical basis for the effects of close physical contact may be the same for lovers and mother–infant pairs. Oxytocin, a peptide released during suckling/nursing interactions and thought to induce infant attachment and maternal caregiving, is also released at sexual climax and has been implicated in the cuddling that often follows sexual intercourse (i.e., "afterplay") (Carter, 1992, 2003). Cuddling, or contact comfort, as demonstrated by Harlow (1958), is crucial for the establishment of emotional bonds.

In sum, there are conspicuous similarities in the nature of physical contact that exemplifies pair-bond and infant–caregiver relationships and differentiates them from other classes of social relationships. Although it is the sexual system that motivates contact in the initial stages of adult romantic relationships, repeated interactions of this uniquely intimate sort foster the development of an attachment.

Selection Criteria

If pair-bond relationships involve the attachment system, one might expect some overlap between infants and adult romantic partners in the criteria on which selections are based. However, the qualities that make one a good mother or father are not necessarily the same qualities that make one appealing as a sexual partner. There is the additional complication of well-documented sex differences in mate selection criteria, which are attributed to differences in parental investment that are present and influential even before conception (Trivers, 1972; see Simpson & Belsky, Chapter 6, this volume).

Differential parental investment theory holds that sexual encounters may have vastly different consequences for males and females, resulting in different optimal mating strategies (we say more on this later) and different mate selection criteria. Males have an abundant supply of small sperm cells produced at a rate of approximately 500 million per day (Zimmerman, Maude, & Moldawar, 1965), whereas females have a far more limited supply of large egg cells, which are produced at a rate of about one per month during a much shorter period of life. Added to this are the female burdens of gestation and lactation, requiring years of investment. Because the male contribution to offspring can be so limited, the most effective reproductive strategy for males may be to take advantage of all mating opportunities with fertile partners. Females, for whom every sexual encounter is potentially quite costly, would be expected to be far choosier in accepting or encouraging copulations. Once her egg is fertilized, a female has to forgo other reproductive opportunities for a relatively long time. Traditionally it was believed that the female's most effective strategy was to limit her sexual encounters to males who possess and appear willing to share valuable resources with her and the offspring she will have to nurture. More recent research suggests that females may employ different strategies, depending on the phase of their menstrual cycle—selecting men with "good genes" in the most fertile phase, and men with "good character," or a tendency to invest in offspring, during the less fertile phase of the cycle (Gangestad, Garver-Apgar, Simpson, & Cousins, 2007). In either event, women are expected to make choices that enhance the survival and fitness of their offspring.

Numerous studies have found sex differences in mate selection criteria consistent with male–female differences in parental investment. For example, in a survey of 37 cultures, Buss (1989) found that males generally assign greater importance than females to the physical appearance of potential mates, preferring partners who look youthful and healthy—both of which may have at one time been reasonably good indices of fertility (Buss, 1989; Symons, 1979). In contrast, females typically care more than males about the social status and earning power of potential partners; this is a sensible mate selection strategy for ensuring that offspring are themselves reproductively fit and well provided for.

Sex differences are negligible, however, when it comes to evaluating potential partners for long- versus short-term relationships (Kenrick, Groth, Trost, & Sadalla, 1993). Given that humans tend to reproduce in the context of long-term relationships, it is this context that is most relevant to understanding mate selection in our species. Moreover, although sex differences in the relative importance of such traits as physical appearance and social status are reliable, *neither* trait is assigned highest priority by *either* sex. For both men and women, the most highly valued qualities in a potential mate are "kind/understanding" and "intelligent" (Buss, 1989). In choosing among potential reproductive partners, males *and* females prefer those who are responsive and competent, and these traits matter more to them than wealth or beauty.

It follows from the norm of assortative mating that men and women tend to choose partners who are similar to themselves on numerous dimensions, including socioeconomic status and physical attractiveness (Berscheid, 1984; Berscheid & Reis, 1998; Hinsz, 1989; Rubin, 1973). This may reflect the more general tendency to prefer what is familiar. In the case of mating, preexisting similarities draw potential partners into the same activities and social circles, thereby increasing familiarity. The word "familiar" comes from the Latin *familia*, which connotes "family" or "household." Others who are similar can seem like family, and may be especially appealing partners for romantic relationships.

It is noteworthy that the factors found to exert the greatest influence on the selection of pair-bond partners are similar to those used by infants in "choosing" among potential attachment figures. In the case of infants, "preference" is given to individuals who are kind, responsive, competent, and familiar—especially in the context of distress alleviation. The one who most consistently and most competently reduces the discomfort of hunger, soiled diapers, fatigue, illness, and strange environments (i.e., the *primary* caregiver) is the one to whom an infant is most likely to become attached (Bowlby, 1958, 1969/1982). Such considerations make perfect sense in the choice of attachment figures during infancy. The fact that adults are sensitive to cues of familiarity, responsiveness, and competence in potential reproductive partners, and care more about these qualities than about cues of fertility or resources, suggests that reproductive partners are evaluated as potential attachment figures. Because pair-bond relationships are relatively enduring, attachment-relevant criteria are taken into account when mates are selected.

Further evidence that mating decisions engage the attachment system comes from studies of facial attractiveness. In a series of detailed analyses involving facialmetric methods and cross-cultural samples, Cunningham, Druen, and Barbee (1997) have sought to identify the features that make potential sexual partners most appealing. Although the findings vary somewhat, sexual appeal—whether the target individual is male or female—is significantly enhanced by the co-occurrence of three types of facial features: "expressive," "neotenous," and "sexual maturational." Expressive features (e.g., size of smile area) serve as cues of warmth and sensitivity. Neotenous features (e.g., large eyes) signal vulnerability and need for nurturance. Facial features associated with sexual maturation (e.g., prominent cheekbones) function as cues of reproductive capability.

Prototypical pair bonds involve the integration of three social-behavioral systems: sexual mating, caregiving (parenting), and attachment. Cunningham and colleagues' (1997) findings lend support to this conceptualization. Clearly it is important to choose a mate who is fertile, and well over 90% of all postpubescent young people are (Symons, 1979). Expressive and neotenous features may factor into decisions about potential partners' attractiveness because they signal ability to provide care and the need for care, respectively. Attachment is relevant to mating because we humans need to select reproductive partners who will also be good companions and parents.

Reactions to Separation and Loss

Additional evidence that attachment is an integral part of pair-bond relationships comes from the literature on bereavement, as well as from studies of routine marital separation. The original inspiration for Bowlby's theory came from his observations of infants and children separated from their primary caregivers. He found it remarkable that the separations were so distressing, given that nutritional and hygienic needs were being met quite adequately by surrogates. Even more striking were the similarities across children in how they responded. Bowlby identified what appeared to be a universal pattern of reactions, which he labeled the "protest–despair–detachment" sequence. The initial reaction is characterized by agitation, hyperactivity, crying, resistance to others' offers of comfort, and extreme anxiety, often to the point of panic. Eventually, this active protest subsides, only to be replaced by a period of lethargy, inactivity, and disrupted sleeping and eating behavior. In time, a degree of emotional detachment from the lost attachment figure facilitates the resumption of normal, preseparation activities and functioning.

If the attachment system is operative in pair bonds, adult reactions to the loss of a partner should be similar, and they are. Several studies have documented essentially the same sequence in adults grieving for the loss of a spouse: initial anxiety and panic, followed by lethargy and depression, and eventually recovery through emotional detachment (Hazan & Shaver, 1992; Parkes & Weiss, 1983; Weiss, 1975) or reorganization (Fraley & Shaver, 1999, and Chapter 3, this volume). This sequence of reactions is not limited to situations of permanent loss. Even brief, routine separations are enough to trigger this pattern of response in some married individuals (Vormbrock, 1993).

It is critically important to note that the protest–despair–detachment (or reorganization) sequence is observed almost exclusively in two social-relational contexts: infant–caregiver relationships and pair bonds. The death of a relative or the decision of a friend to move away may cause sadness, but such events do not normally evoke panic. Furthermore, the reactions of caregivers to separation from or loss of their infants are qualitatively different (Bowlby, 1980). Caregivers are not attached to their offspring in the technical sense; that is, they do not rely on their young for security or protection. Caregiver behavior is regulated by a different behavioral system—the caregiving (parenting) system, the disruption of which elicits a distinct response dynamic. Even among marital partners, reactions to separation depend on which system gets activated. Partners who are left behind exhibit attachment reactions (e.g., anxiety), whereas the leavers more often experience guilt over abandoning their caregiving duties (Vormbrock, 1993).

It makes good adaptive sense to react with anxiety and protest to even the temporary "loss" of an individual who serves as a primary source of emotional and/or physical security. The fact that this reaction is the norm among adults separated from their long-term partners, and *not* the normal reaction to the loss of other kinds of social ties, is another indication that the attachment system is active in pair bonds.

Physical and Psychological Health Effects

The notion that attachment meets a very real biological need, at least early in life, was established in studies of infants reared in orphanages and other institutional settings (Robertson, 1953; Spitz, 1946). Although adults are clearly less dependent on social bonds for basic survival, there is ample evidence that they incur health benefits from having one, and suffer health decrements as a consequence of the absence or loss of such bonds. Relationship disruption (especially divorce) makes one more susceptible to a wide range of physical and psychological ills, including disease, impaired immune functioning, accidents, substance abuse, suicide, and various other forms of psychopathology (e.g., Bloom, Asher, & White, 1978; Goodwin, Hurt, Key, & Sarret, 1987; Lynch, 1977; Uchino, Cacioppo, & Kiecolt-Glaser, 1996; see B. Feeney & Monin, Chapter 39, this volume).

Among the most common stressors, attachment-related losses cause the most subjective distress. Death of a spouse is the leading stressful event on the Social Readjustment Rating Scale, followed by divorce and marital separation (Holmes & Rahe, 1967). A number of additional investigations have helped highlight the distinctiveness of attachment relationships. For instance, Weiss (1973) found that loneliness takes at least two distinct forms, depending on whether social deprivation is due to the absence of an intimate companion (which he labeled "emotional loneliness") or a lack of friends ("social loneliness"). This distinction was supported by results of a national survey that found the two types to be associated with different antecedents and symptoms (Rubenstein & Shaver, 1982). Consistent with Weiss's theory, the loss or absence of a pair-bond relationship is associated with emotional loneliness and feelings of "desperation" and anxiety. In contrast, a lack of friendships predicts social loneliness, which is experienced as "restless boredom." Additional corroboration comes from a study by Stroebe, Stroebe, Abakoumkin, and Schut (1996), who found that social support in the form of friendship did not help alleviate the distress of losing a spouse. And Vormbrock's (1993) review of the literature on war- and job-related routine marital separations led to a similar conclusion: The social provisions of pair bonds are sufficiently distinctive that other social relationships cannot compensate for their loss. Interestingly, Vormbrock did find that renewing relationships with parental *attachment* figures was helpful in moderating the anxiety caused by spousal absence.

If attachment bonds have exceptional effects on physical and psychological functioning, such effects should be absent not only in other types of relationships, but also in the kinds of relationships that typically develop into attachments but have yet to achieve that status. This appears to be the case. Early maternal deprivation is associated with long-term developmental consequences *only* if it occurs *after* an attachment bond between infant and mother has been established (Bowlby, 1958). Separations prior to 8 months of age do not increase the probability of poor developmental outcomes. Earlier in this chapter, we have reported our finding that most romantic relationships qualified as attachments only after they had endured for at least 2 years. Weiss (1988) found that widows and widowers married for less than 2 years did not show the same (protest–despair–detachment/reorganization) sequence of reactions as those grieving for the loss of longer-term bonds.

In addition to the substantial evidence that loss of an attachment figure results in health and well-being decrements, there is evidence that the presence of an attachment figure has stress-buffering effects. In a recent study, married women who held their spouses' hands while being subjected to the threat of electrical shock evidenced lower threat-related neural activation, measured by functional magnetic resonance imaging, than married women who held the hand of an unfamiliar male experimenter (Coan, Schaefer, & Davidson, 2006; see Coan, Chapter 11, this volume).

In sum, the results of a number of studies indicate that bonds between adult partners and infant–caregiver pairs are similarly and uniquely powerful in their impact on physical and psychological well-being. Other kinds of interpersonal relationships offer valuable social provisions, but emotional security does not appear to be one of them. Otherwise, disruptions would give rise to anxiety, which they do not. If separation distress is a marker of attachment, bonds between long-term adult partners clearly qualify.

THE FUNCTION OF ATTACHMENT IN ADULT LIFE

Evolutionary thinking figured prominently in Bowlby's (1969/1982) theory. The attachment system, he argued, is a species-typical characteristic that evolved to serve a protective, survival-enhancing function. Infants who identified, became attached to, and then stayed close to protectors had significantly better chances of living to reproductive age than infants who failed to develop such bonds. The survival value and evolutionary origins of adult attachment are less obvious and therefore are subject to debate in adult attachment research and theory.

Some theorists (e.g., Kirkpatrick, 1998) reject the notion that the attachment system is integral to pair bonds by reasoning that reflexive proximity seeking in the face of danger would be adaptive for infants but maladaptive for adults. Specifically, a propensity to seek protection from a mate, rather than aiding in the fight against some external threat, would be more likely to jeopardize adult survival than to enhance it. Moreover, the fact that human females are, on average, smaller and weaker than their male counterparts makes it particularly doubtful that men could gain a survival advantage by turning to their female partners for refuge in the face of danger. Therefore, attachment cannot serve the same protective function in adulthood that it does in infancy. Furthermore, given the unlikelihood that an entire system would be retained yet undergo a qualitative change in its function, pair bonds cannot involve the attachment system. There are several flaws in this line of reasoning, however.

One major shortcoming of this argument is its limited conceptualization of the protective function of attachment. Although the risk of predation in the EEA was undoubtedly reduced for infants who became attached to their caregivers, the benefits of the bond would have extended far beyond this specific type of protection. Then and now, attachments also help ensure that infants receive adequate routine care in the form of food, warmth, shelter, guidance, and monitoring—all of which enhance survival. Clearly, the protective function of attachment is not limited to brawn, even in infancy.

By relying on a narrow definition of protection, the argument also fails to take into account normative developmental changes in the behavioral manifestations of attachment. Very young and vulnerable infants do indeed rely entirely on their caregivers for protection and sustenance. But increases in maturity and competence are associated with corresponding decreases in the most primitive forms of attachment behavior, such as reflexive proximity seeking. Although older children and adolescents continue to depend on parents for many aspects of care, they do not typically run to them for physical cover at the slightest hint of danger. Their developing capacities for self-protection and self-reliance, however, do not mean that they no longer benefit from having someone who is deeply committed to and invested in their welfare looking out for them, and reliably available to help if needed. The mere fact that behavior during disparate phases of development is not identical is insufficient proof that such behavior subserves different functions (Tinbergen, 1963). Feeding behavior, for example, also changes dramatically from infancy to adulthood, but the basic function is the same.

In the preceding sections, we have reviewed a diverse set of empirical findings that together provide strong support for Bowlby's claims that the attachment system is active in adult life and integral to pair bonds. Relationships with long-term partners qualify as attachments in the technical sense by containing all four defining features. The processes by which pair-bond and infant–caregiver relationships develop appear to be quite similar. The nature of physical contact that typifies these two types of relationships also serves to distinguish them from other classes of social bonds. In addition, there is considerable overlap in the criteria used to select attachment figures in infancy and mates in adulthood. A similar sequence of reactions characterizes the responses of infants separated from primary caregivers and adults separated from long-term partners—a sequence not observed in reaction to other types of social loss. And the mental and physical health effects of infant attachments and pair-bond relationships appear to be uniquely and similarly profound and pervasive. The postulation that these multiple and diverse similarities are due to the active involvement of the same behavioral system is the most parsimonious explanation of the facts.

But what about the questions of function and evolutionary history? To seriously evaluate the possibility that attachment serves the same protective function in adulthood as in infancy requires that "protection" be defined in a manner that encompasses its full meaning and acknowledges normative developmental change. An answer to the function question, however, calls for more than simply establishing that pair-bond partners provide each other with protection. It must be established that such protection affords adaptive advantage by translating reliably into enhanced survival and reproductive success in the EEA. Hence a key to understanding the function of attachment in adulthood lies in an examination of the circumstances in which pair bonding evolved.

The Evolution of Pair Bonds

If human reproductive success required nothing more than conception, reproductive partners could part ways as soon as a viable pregnancy was achieved. In actuality, however, the vast majority of human males and females opt to remain with the same partner for a more extended period of time (Eibl-Eibesfeldt, 1989; Mellen, 1981). This trend is thought to have followed a birthing crisis in which the infant's large head, housing a more fully developed brain, could not easily pass through the birth canal of our bipedal female ancestors (Trevathan, 1987). Infants who were born prematurely, with less developed brains and smaller heads, were more likely to survive (as were their mothers). Immaturity at birth also offered the advantage of a longer period of learning during a time of heightened neural plasticity. This would have been a distinct advantage in a species with such complex social organization as our own. However, with the benefits of premature birth came new risks and challenges. The effort required to care adequately for such dependent offspring during such a protracted period of immaturity, along with the major tasks of socialization and training, made paternal investment an advantage if not a necessity. Exceptionally helpless and vulnerable offspring would have had rather poor chances of surviving to reproductive age or developing the necessary skills for their own eventual mating and parenting roles without an adequately strong force to keep fathers around and involved.

Many unique features of human sexuality appear to have evolved for the purpose of fostering and maintaining an enduring bond between reproductive partners. The most striking change in our reproductive physiology in comparison to other mammalian species is the absence of conspicuous signs of estrus in the female. Most mammals mate only during the short estrus periods of the female, but human sexual desire and activity are not so restricted. Women can be sexually receptive during any phase of their reproductive cycle, despite the fact that conception is possible only during a small fraction of it. This physiological adaptation enables a couple to maintain a continuous tie on the basis of sexual reward (Eibl-Eibesfeldt, 1975). Concealed ovulation may also serve to diminish the benefits of straying. Males of many diverse species guard their mates during periods of sexual receptivity so as to ensure paternity. When the fertile period has ended, a male can safely move on to another receptive partner. However, if ovulation is hidden, making it impossible for the male to determine just when fertilization will be possible, his optimal strategy may shift toward guarding and remaining with the same sexual partner for longer periods of time (Alcock, 1989).

The physiological changes associated with sexual climax may also stimulate bond formation between partners. As noted previously, orgasms trigger a release of oxytocin in both males and females (Carter, 1992), resulting in a state of calm and contentment. It also stimulates a desire for continued close physical contact and cuddling, again increasing the chances that a bond will develop.

When the adaptive problem of immature offspring and the corresponding need for paternal investment arose in the course of human evolution, our species—by virtue of its altricial nature—already had available a well-designed, specialized, flexible, but reliable mechanism for ensuring that two individuals would be highly motivated to stay together and vigorously resist being separated. The mechanism was attachment. In light of the generally conservative tendencies of evolution and natural selection, it is highly probable that this preexisting mechanism would have been exploited for the purpose of keeping reproductive partners together. Pair bonds are primarily reproductive relationships, but sex serves more than a reproductive function in our species. The unique features of human reproductive physiology and anatomy help to ensure that partners will engage in the kinds of intimate exchanges known to foster attachment formation.

Reproductive Advantages of Pair Bonds

In our species, reproductive success requires negotiation of at least three adaptive challenges: surviving to reproductive age, mating, and providing adequate care to offspring so that they too will survive to reproduce. We have just argued that the relative immaturity of human newborns created a situation in the EEA in which survival depended not only on their forming a strong bond to a protector, but also on a mechanism that would hold reproductive partners together for an extended period of time. The attachment system, which had evolved to ensure an enduring bond between infants and caregivers, was exploited for this additional purpose. But the advantages of pair bonding extend beyond its role in offspring survival. Benefits include enhanced survival and reproductive fitness for *mates* as well.

There is mounting evidence that offspring mating strategies may depend critically on the pair-bond status of parents, especially mothers. Adolescents from father-absent homes show precocious sexual interest, relatively early sexual maturation, more negative attitudes toward potential mates, and less interest in long-term relationships than do their counterparts reared in father-present homes (Belsky, 1999; Draper & Belsky, 1990; Draper & Harpending, 1982; Ellis, McFayden-Ketchum, Dodge, Pettit, & Bates, 1999; Surbey, 1990). Girls in father-absent homes are at increased risk for early sexual activity and teenage pregnancy (Ellis et al., 2003). In other words, if parents choose not to remain together, their children are more likely to adopt approaches to mating that emphasize quantity over quality. Parental divorce has also been found to affect offspring mating strategies and behavior (Barber, 1998). Female children of divorce tend to fear closeness and abandonment, whereas the effects for males are evidenced in a lack of achievement orientation and a greater likelihood of abandoning relationships (Henry & Holmes, 1998; Wallerstein, 1994). Thus the failure of reproductive partners to maintain long-term bonds may have a negative effect on the mating appeal and success of their offspring.

Whether opportunistic, short-term mating strategies are less advantageous than stable, long-term strategies is the source of much current debate (e.g., Belsky, 1999; Buss, 1997; Chisholm, 1996; Schmitt, 2005). According to life history theory (Stearns, 1992), organisms possess a finite amount of resources that must be allocated across various evolutionary challenges, including survival, growth, mating, and parental investment. Local circumstances determine the balance of time and energy an individual devotes to each. From this perspective, it may be most sensible for adolescents from unstable families to adopt a strategy of mating early and often. Thus both long- and short-term strategies can be viewed as reasonable and comparably adaptive responses to different ecologies, and these strategies can shift within an individual's lifetime in response to changing life circumstances.

Although it is clearly advantageous for humans to be capable of facultative mating adaptations that take account of varying ecological conditions (Daly & Wilson, 1988; Buss & Schmitt, 1993; Gangestad & Simpson, 2000), the correlates of short- and long-term mating strategies are not supportive of the view that they are different but essentially equal (see Belsky, 1999, for an alternative viewpoint). The ability to adjust behavior to nonoptimal circumstances is clearly important, but such adjustments are unlikely to produce optimal results. Consider feeding behavior, for example. Survival depends on the regular intake of food, and if humans are hungry enough, they will consume garbage to stay alive. But trash is unlikely to have the same nutritional value as a well-rounded meal; nor would it be expected to support physical development equally well. Likewise, quick and frequent copulations coupled with an avoidance of parental investment may be the best available strategy in some circumstances, but it hardly qualifies as optimal in any absolute sense. For instance, infant mortality rates are higher among children without an investing father (Hill & Hurtado, 1995). It has also been found that women suffering from infertility of unknown biological cause tend to have an avoidant attachment style (Justo, Maia, Ferreira-Diniz, Santos, & Moreira, 1997). In the currency of evolution, a superior strategy is one that enhances survival and reproductive success. It is a matter of empirical fact that pair bonds not only contribute to the survival of offspring, but also leave offspring better equipped to attract and retain mates of their own, which in turn improves their reproductive fitness.

In addition to the multiple direct and indirect benefits that accrue to the progeny of stable pair bonds, there are advantages for the mates themselves. There is at least one indication that long-term bonds between partners directly enhance their own reproductive success. It is well documented that women ovulate more regularly if they are in a stable sexual relationship (e.g., Cutler, Garcia, Huggins, & Preti, 1985; Veith, Buck, Getzlaf, Van Dalfsen, & Slade, 1983). They also tend to continue ovulating into their middle years and reach menopause significantly later if sexual activity is consistent (Kaczmarek, 2007). Earlier we have cited evidence that partners in long-term relationships enjoy more robust physical and mental health (see also Wood, Rhodes, & Whelan, 1989). Clearly, the more fit an individual is, the better able he or she is to function in all the various roles adults are required to fill—including those of mate, parent, and grandparent. A healthy member of any social group is more valued and more valuable, and more capable of protecting self as well as loved ones. A stable bond with a trusted and reliable companion also promotes the kind of exploration and productive engagement in activity on which family welfare depends (Hazan & Shaver, 1990). As for the protective aspects of this kind of companionship, adults too need someone to look out for them and keep track of them—someone to initiate a search if they fail to show up at the expected time, to take care of them when they are sick, to dress their wounds, to help defend them against external threats, to reassure them, and to keep them warm at night.

What is the function of attachment in adult life? On the basis of the evidence, we would argue that the attachment system serves essentially the same purpose in adulthood as it does in infancy. It cements an enduring emotional bond between individuals that translates today, as it did in the EEA, into differential survival and reproductive success.

A MODEL OF ADULT ATTACHMENT FORMATION

In arguing that attachment is an integral part of pair bonds, we have described some of the processes by which a sexual partner comes to supersede parents in the hierarchy of attachment figures. In this section, we offer a more detailed account of the processes. Although we have incorporated many diverse empirical findings to support our perspective, the model we propose is still largely theoretical. Firm conclusions about how two adults make the transformation from complete independence to profound psychological and physiological interdependence must await the results of future research.

Before we present the model, a few caveats are in order. In contrast to the preponderance of attachment research, which emphasizes individual differences, our model focuses on normative processes. There is good reason to expect that the processes will vary somewhat as a function of the working models that individuals bring to a relationship, but there is not space in the present chapter for a discussion of all these various possibilities. Also, in our effort to build a case that pair bonds are true attachments, we have necessarily stressed the similarities between romantic and infant–caregiver relationships over their differences. The differences are both numerous and profound, but three strike us as particularly important.

First, the reciprocal nature of prototypical adult attachments means dual roles for the partners. Each mate uses the other as an attachment figure and source of security; each also serves as an attachment figure and provider of security to the other. This implicates not only the attachment system, but the caregiving (parenting) system as well. And because pair-bond members are sexual partners, the sexual mating system is also involved. Therefore, adult attachments are qualitatively different from infant attachments by virtue of their mutuality and sexual nature.

We have referred earlier to the crucial role of physical contact in fostering attachment formation. The motivation for proximity seeking is a second major difference between infants and adults. When an infant approaches or signals the caregiver for contact, distress alleviation is often the goal. Babies are, after all, helpless to meet their own physical needs. Although adult partners also turn to each other for comfort, sexual attraction is a major impetus for contact, especially in the initial phases of relationship development.

A consideration of the evolutionary roots of pair-bond attachment highlights a third fundamental difference between lovers and parent–child pairs. Beyond the reality that infants cannot survive without protection and care, in most instances they are also biologically related to their caregivers. The issue of genetic relatedness is an important one. Although the expected fitness of mates is correlated (due to their shared genetic interests in offspring), it is generally assumed that this correlation can be reversed rather easily, as in the case of sexual infidelity, whereas the genetic interests of relatives are forever linked (Daly & Wilson, 1996). This presumes that mates are not genetically related. In fact, with the exception of first-degree relatives, a high degree of inbreeding has been the norm in our species (Thornhill, 1991). In a survey of 370 cultures, fully 26% prescribed or strongly preferred marriage between cousins (Broude, 1994). In addition, the low incidence of interracial marriage and the prevalence of look-alike partners (Hinsz, 1989) indicate that individuals tend to select mates from their own genetic pool. Although mates will not typically be first-degree relatives, they are still more likely to be "related" than two randomly selected individuals are. That said, mates do not share the genetic ties parents share with their children.

It is also worth noting that attachment is not synonymous with sexual fidelity or lifelong commitment. Results of genetic analyses provide objective evidence that even so-called "monogamous" species engage in copulations outside pair bonds (Carter et al., 1997; Mendoza & Mason, 1997). Although pair bonds are regulated by the attachment system, they are not indissoluble or even as durable as parent–offspring bonds. The current high rate of divorce, particularly in Western cultures, is but one indication that relationships between sexual partners are more fragile. Nevertheless, a close examination of the data reveals that divorce is significantly less common among couples who have at least one child (Fisher, 1992). Once partners have commingled their genes, their relationship is more likely to endure.

Bowlby identified four phases in the development of infant–caregiver attachments, and we have proposed a corresponding four-phase process model to integrate and explain the phenomenology of pair-bond development (Hazan, Gur-Yaish, & Campa, 2004). We have adopted Bowlby's labels for each of the phases and supplemented them with their hypothesized romantic relationship equivalents. (See Zeifman & Hazan, 1997, for a more detailed explication of the model.) Whether adult attachments develop in a manner that parallels attachment formation in infancy is an empirical question that awaits an answer, but we (Zeifman & Hazan, 1997) have proposed that Bowlby's four-phase model can serve as a provisional research guide. We have likened the adult counterpart of the infant preattachment phase to what Eibl-Eibesfeldt (1989) called the "proceptive program." Males and females of reproductive age are inherently interested in social interaction with potential mates and display flirtatious signals somewhat indiscriminately. It is likely that these playful, sexually charged exchanges continue when partners first become involved and are more characteristic of their interactions than attachment behaviors per se.

In contrast, the behaviors of partners in the throes of romantic infatuation show many resemblances to infant–caregiver interactions (Shaver et al., 1988), including prolonged mutual gazing, cuddling, nuzzling, and "baby talk." We have suggested that these types of exchanges may be indicative of the second phase, "attachment in the making." This is consistent with Bowlby's (1979) view that "In terms of subjective experience, the formation of a bond is described as falling in love" (p. 69). In infancy, the onset of the third phase, "clear-cut attachment," is indicated by the emergence of new attachment behaviors—and, specifically, by their organization around a single caregiver who has become the reliably preferred target of proximity maintenance and safe-haven behaviors, and elicitor of secure-base and separation distress behaviors. We have proposed that the selective orientation of these four behaviors toward a partner may signal clear-cut attachment in adulthood as well.

The childhood indicators of the fourth phase, "goal-corrected partnership," primarily reflect cognitive-developmental changes over the first 3 years of life. We have hypothesized that there nevertheless may be a comparable final phase in adult attachment formation, characterized by a decline in overt displays of attachment behavior and a redirection of attention to other aspects of life (e.g., work, hobbies, and friendships). In a goal-corrected partnership, a romantic partner has achieved the status of an attachment figure and serves as a secure base, emboldening the individual to explore his or her environment with a greater sense of security.

ATTACHMENT VERSUS OTHER EVOLUTIONARY PERSPECTIVES ON MATING

The attachment theory (AT) perspective on human mating has at times been misunderstood. For example, AT is mischaracterized as claiming that there is only one adaptive mating strategy, monogamous pair bonding (e.g., Schmitt, 2005). In this section, we address some of these misconceptions and explain areas of difference and complementarity among various evolutionary perspectives on human mating. In particular, we address two prominent theories: sexual strategies theory (SST; Buss & Schmitt, 1993), which emphasizes between-gender differences in preference for long-term versus short-term mating strategies; and strategic pluralism theory (SPT; Gangestad & Simpson, 2000), which emphasizes within-gender variability in the adoption of short- versus long-term mating strategies as a function of ecological factors.

AT posits that attachment is one of three behavioral systems operating in a pair bond, alongside the sexual/mating and caregiving systems. There is growing evidence that these three behavioral systems are distinct in their neurobiological underpinnings, as well as in their behavioral and psychological dynamics (Fisher, 2000, 2002). It is also understood that relationships can engage these systems independently, e.g., sexual behavior in the absence of attachment (Diamond, 2004, 2006). However, in the typical pair bond, all three systems become integrated. In adult attachment formation, sexual attraction motivates the kind of physical interactions that over time tend to foster mutual attachment and caregiving. If the pair bond results in the birth of a child, then caregiving is extended to offspring (Hazan & Zeifman, 1994).

AT, SST, and SPT differ in which or how many of the various behavioral systems they address. SST focuses almost exclusively on the sexual/mating system, in which there are well-documented sex differences. For example, compared to females, college-age males report greater desire for short-term matings (Buss & Schmitt, 1993). AT, in contrast, is not concerned with hypothetical mating behavior or short-term matings; attachments are, by definition, *enduring* emotional bonds. SPT, like SST, focuses on the sexual/mating system, but also indirectly on the caregiving system in the form of parental investment, and especially on tradeoffs in the effort afforded to each. The balance of effort allocated to mating versus caregiving is hypothesized to vary within gender as a function of various ecological factors. For example, in highly unstable environments, both males and females show increased interest in short-term strategies (Gangestad & Simpson, 2000). SPT acknowledges that long-term mating is the behavioral norm, but it does not address the nature of the bond that develops between long-term mates. AT is unique in that it focuses on the dynamics of a pair bond as an integration of the sexual mating, caregiving, and attachment systems.

Another common misconception regarding AT is that an enduring bond or an attachment implies sexual monogamy (Schmitt, 2005). We adopt the view common among animal researchers that "monogamy" refers to a broader constellation of social behaviors between sexual partners, such as nonsexual proximity maintenance, joint territory, prolonged association, and shared parenting (Dewsbury, 1987; Moller, 2003). Even animals that are classified as monogamous because they show a reliable preference for a specific mate engage in copulations outside pair bonds, as evidenced by studies of paternity outside such bonds (Moller, 2003). Like several other species classified as monogamous, humans form enduring bonds with sexual partners—and it is in this context that they rear their offspring, in spite of the fact that these bonds are often not sexually exclusive. Finally, across the animal kingdom, one of the most common characteristics of species classified as monogamous is having highly immature young in need of extensive parental care for a protracted maturation period, as humans do (Dewsbury, 1987; Moller, 2003). Although human mating could not be described as monogamous if monogamy were synonymous with sexual fidelity, most human mating systems qualify for less constrained definitions of monogamy (Dewsbury, 1987).

We have argued here and elsewhere that long-term pair bonds confer reproductive benefits relative to other mating strategies. This does not mean that other reproductive strategies are not also adaptive. It is important to distinguish between optimal adaptations and optimal outcomes. Ainsworth and her colleagues (1978) described three attachment styles among infants: secure, insecure-avoidant, and insecure-ambivalent. Whereas the secure attachment style is considered optimal as both an adaptation and an outcome, the two insecure attachment styles are also considered optimal adaptations to particular caregiving environments—a rejecting caregiver in the case of an avoidant infant, and an inconsistent one in the case of an ambivalent (Ainsworth et al., 1978)—but not optimal outcomes. Similarly, short-term mating strategies may be adaptive in that they optimize existing resources, particularly when resources are scarce and environments are unpredictable (Belsky, Steinberg, & Draper, 1991; Gangestad & Simpson, 2000); at the same time, they may be nonoptimal in terms of outcome, when compared to the long-term strategies typically adopted in more stable environments. From an evolutionary standpoint, the critical outcome is survival and reproductive fitness. There are numerous individual and reproductive fitness benefits associated with long-term pair bonds, which suggest that pair bonds optimize outcomes relative to short-term mating strategies.

Another source of confusion in the literature is the relation between attachment style and mating strategy. Whereas "attachment style" concerns an individual's expectations regarding the availability and responsiveness of mates, "mating strategy" concerns how mates are obtained, whether for the long or short term. Avoidant individuals have low expectations regarding the availability and responsiveness of partners (Hazan & Shaver, 1994; Mikulincer & Shaver, 2007), and are more apt than secure individuals to adopt a short-term mating strategy (Schachner & Shaver, 2004; Simpson & Gangestad, 1991). However, in spite of negative expectations, many avoidant individuals marry (a long-term strategy), as evidenced by the significant proportion of individuals in studies of attachment style and marriage who are classified as avoidant (e.g., J. Feeney, Noller, & Callan, 1994; Fuller & Fincham, 1995; Kobak & Hazan, 1991). Having a particular attachment style may predispose one toward a particular mating strategy, but it is by no means determinative.

One reason attachment style and mating strategy do not necessarily follow a single developmental trajectory (e.g., from secure attachment to monogamous, long-term mating strategy) is that each is responsive to environmental conditions at different points in development. AT locates the critical "decision point" shaping attachment style in childhood (in response to the local caregiving environment), whereas SPT locates the "decision point" for mating strategy in adulthood (in response to the local mating environment). However, neither attachment styles nor mating strategies are static entities; both accommodate ongoing events and existing resources and can change across the lifespan (Bowlby, 1980; Fuller & Fincham, 1995).

Schmitt (2005) has criticized the AT view that long-term pair bonds are adaptive, on the grounds that self-reported preferences for short-term mating strategies are associated in a college-age population with such adaptive personality traits as self-esteem, extraversion, and emotional stability. This argument assumes that for long-term bonds to be adaptive, they must also be associated with other adaptive personality traits—or, more precisely, that short-term mating strategies must not be associated with adaptive personality traits. The value of normative pair bonds, in our view, does not depend on a link between particular personality traits and preferred mating strategies. For a mating strategy to be adaptive, it need only be associated with fitness gains.

If, for the sake of argument, we accept the premise that an adaptive mating strategy is one that is associated with other adaptive personality traits, we have to consider whether the sexual behaviors of college students qualify as mating or reproductive strategies in the evolutionary sense. Insofar as mating strategies in evolutionary terms are strategies for producing and rearing offspring, sexual behavior that is intentionally uncoupled from that goal might not qualify as a mating strategy at all. In our current culture, birth control and the loosening of restrictions on premarital sex allow college-age adults to make conscious decisions about engaging in a period of sexual experimentation. This freedom from the potential consequences of sexual behavior was impossible in our EEA or in previous generations, and it may represent a behavioral "neo-phenotype"—a new pattern of behavior that was not commonly observed or that did not exist before in nature (Kuo, 1967).

Given modern means of avoiding pregnancy, preferring a short-term mate or an uncommitted sexual relationship during college or early adulthood may be distinct from adopting a similar mating strategy in the postcollege years, when decisions about long-term mates and children are often made in our culture. In fact, among men who are slightly older than college age and married, short-term mating strategies are not related to positive personality traits (Schmitt, 2005). This suggests that conclusions about mating strategies based on college-age samples may generalize poorly to marital and familial relationships—the typical contexts in which reproduction occurs.

In addition to the problem of basing conclusions about mating strategies on college-age samples, one of the weaknesses of SST is that the preponderance of SST research is based on expressed preferences or hypothetical behavior rather than actual behavior (e.g., Buss, 1989). For example, typical short-term mating measures ask respondents to indicate the number of sexual partners desired across various time frames and/or the likelihood of engaging in sexual intercourse with desirable partners after knowing them for various time intervals (Buss & Schmitt, 1993; Schmitt, Shackelford, Duntley, Tooke, & Buss, 2001). Although such preferences may tell us about the motivational systems underlying behavior, they do not tell the complete story of the behavior itself or of its effect on outcomes. For example, although humans have an evolved preference for foods high in sugar and fat content (which was highly adaptive when food was scarce), this preference in our current environment contributes to nonoptimal outcomes, such as disease and premature mortality. Similarly, a robust libido and sexual imagination may be in and of themselves associated with positive outcomes, because social, cultural, religious, and demographic constraints limit the expression of sexual behavior in most societies. The impact of restricted versus unrestricted sexual practices on various outcomes is, on the other hand, somewhat independent of the impact of restricted and unrestricted sexual desire.

When studies examine the personality profiles of those who actually engage in behavior typical of short-term strategies, rather than those who merely express a preference for doing so, the results paint a less sanguine portrait of short-term strategists. In fact, Paul, McManus, and Hayes (2000) found that individuals who reported experiencing "hookups" (i.e., casual sexual encounters with relative strangers), especially hookups involving sexual intercourse, had lower self-esteem than those who did not. The emphasis of SST on the correlates of expressed preferences rather than actual practices also downplays the negative men-

tal health consequences of short-term strategies, which are apparent from an extensive clinical literature on the harmful effects of emotional loneliness, breakups, divorce, and sexual infidelity (Hall & Fincham, 2006; Weber, 1998; Weiss, 1975). These damaging effects of relationship disruption and dissolution, coupled with growing evidence of therapeutic effects of relationship endurance, suggest that although diverse reproductive strategies exist, long-term strategies are likely to continue to be the norm.

CONCLUSIONS

The evidence reviewed in this chapter indicates that pair bonds are similar in many respects to the one type of interpersonal tie that most researchers agree does involve the attachment system—infant–caregiver bonds. Furthermore, the similarities extend far beyond the superficial to include fundamental features, functions, dynamics, and processes. From this extensive evidence, we conclude that attachment is indeed integral to pair bonds.

Critics of this viewpoint (e.g., Kirkpatrick, 1998) acknowledge the many resemblances between infant–caregiver and romantic relationships, but reject such evidence as circumstantial. Research and theory in the social sciences are built almost entirely on a foundation of circumstantial evidence. Few if any of our most interesting and cherished constructs can be directly observed or measured, and attachment is no different. Even in infancy, the evidence is circumstantial. Proximity maintenance and separation distress, as well as safe-haven and secure-base behaviors, are the data from which the existence and regulatory role of the attachment behavioral system are *inferred*. Evidence that the attachment system is operative in pair bonds is by necessity indirect, but no less solid. Alternative evolutionary theories of mating (such as SST and SPT) acknowledge that some romantic relationships involve the attachment system, but consider as well those that do not. These theories focus on the individual differences and environmental factors associated with short- versus long-term mating strategies. AT, in contrast, focuses on the nature of the bond between long-term sexual partners—the most common context for human mating and reproduction.

As for the functions of attachment in adult life, we have argued that there is significant overlap with those of attachment in infancy. The attachment system helps to ensure the development of an enduring bond that enhances survival and reproductive fitness in direct as well as indirect ways. Pair bonds are not simply mutually beneficial alliances based on the principles of reciprocal altruism. Instead, they involve such a profound psychological and physiological interdependence that the absence or loss of one partner can be literally life-threatening for the other.

Bowlby's original hypotheses concerning pair-bond attachment were based on little more than his formidable powers of observation and deep insights into human affectional behavior. In the time since their formulation, a substantial body of empirical data on relationships has been amassed—one that, on the whole, supports his initial speculations. The evidence indicates that attachment needs persist from the cradle to the grave. And, just as Bowlby surmised, in adulthood such needs are satisfied by pair bonds.

REFERENCES

Ainsworth, M. D. S. (1967). *Infancy in Uganda: Infant care and the growth of attachment.* Baltimore: Johns Hopkins University Press.

Ainsworth, M. D. S. (1982). Attachment: Retrospect and prospect. In C. M. Parkes & J. Stevenson-Hinde (Eds.), *The place of attachment in human behavior* (pp. 3–30). New York: Basic Books.

Ainsworth, M. D. S. (1991). Attachments and other affectional bonds across the life cycle. In C. M. Parkes, J. Stevenson-Hinde, & P. Marris (Eds.), *Attachment across the life cycle* (pp. 33–51). New York: Tavistock/Routledge.

Ainsworth, M. D. S., Blehar, M. C., Waters, E., & Wall, S. (1978). *Patterns of attachment: A psychological study of the Strange Situation.* Hillsdale, NJ: Erlbaum.

Alcock, J. (1989). *Animal behavior: An evolutionary approach.* Boston: Sinauer.

Barber, N. (1998). Sex differences in disposition toward kin, security of adult attachment, and sociosexuality as a function of parental divorce. *Evolution and Human Behavior, 19,* 125–132.

Belsky, J. (1999). Modern evolutionary theory and patterns of attachment. In J. Cassidy & P. R. Shaver (Eds.), *Handbook of attachment: Theory, research, and clinical applications* (pp. 141–161). New York: Guilford Press.

Belsky, J., Steinberg, L., & Draper, P. (1991). Childhood experience, interpersonal development, and reproductive strategy: An evolutionary theory of socialization. *Child Development, 62,* 647–670.

Berscheid, E. (1984). Interpersonal attraction. In G. Lindzey & E. Aronson (Eds.), *Handbook of social psychology* (3rd ed., pp. 413–484). Reading, MA: Addison-Wesley.

Berscheid, E., & Reis, H. T. (1998). Attraction and close relationships. In S. Fiske, D. Gilbert, & G. Lindzey (Eds.), *The handbook of social psychology* (4th ed., pp. 193–281). New York: McGraw-Hill.

Bloom, B. L., Asher, S. J., & White, S. W. (1978). Marital disruption as a stressor: A review and analysis. *Psychological Bulletin, 85,* 867–894.

Blumstein, P., & Schwartz, P. (1983). *American couples: Money, work and sex.* New York: Pocket Books.

Bowlby, J. (1958). The nature of the child's tie to his mother. *International Journal of Psycho-Analysis, 39,* 350–373.

Bowlby, J. (1969/1982). *Attachment and loss: Vol. 1. Attachment* (2nd ed.). New York: Basic Books.

Bowlby, J. (1979). *The making and breaking of affectional bonds.* London: Tavistock/Routledge.

Bowlby, J. (1980). *Attachment and loss: Vol. 3. Loss: Sadness and depression.* New York: Basic Books.

Broude, G. (1994). *Marriage, family, and relationships: A cross-cultural encyclopedia.* Santa Barbara, CA: ABC-Clio.

Buhrmester, D., & Furman, W. (1986). The changing functions of friends in childhood. In V. J. Derlega & B. A. Winstead (Eds.), *Friendship and social interaction* (pp. 41–62). New York: Springer-Verlag.

Buhrmester, D., & Furman, W. (1987). The development of companionship and intimacy. *Child Development, 58,* 1101–1113.

Buhrmester, D., & Prager, K. (1995). Patterns and functions of self-disclosure during childhood and adolescence. In K. J. Rotenberg (Ed.), *Disclosure processes in children and adolescents* (pp. 10–56). New York: Cambridge University Press.

Buss, D. M. (1989). Sex differences in human mate preferences: Evolutionary hypotheses tested in 37 cultures. *Behavioral and Brain Sciences, 12,* 1–49.

Buss, D. M. (1997). The emergence of evolutionary social psychology. In J. A. Simpson & D. T. Kenrick (Eds.), *Evolutionary social psychology* (pp. 387–400). Mahwah, NJ: Erlbaum.

Buss, D. M., & Schmitt, D. P. (1993). Sexual strategies theory: An evolutionary perspective on human mating. *Psychological Review, 100,* 204–232.

Carey, B. (2007, October 2). Friends with benefits, and stress too. *New York Times.* Retrieved from http://www.nytimes.com/2007/10/02/health/02sex.html

Carter, C. S. (1992). Oxytocin and sexual behavior. *Neuroscience and Biobehavioral Reviews, 16,* 131–144.

Carter, C. S. (2003). Developmental consequences of oxytocin. *Physiology and Behavior, 79,* 383–397

Carter, C. S., DeVries, A. C., Taymans, S. E., Roberts, R. L., Williams, J. R., & Getz, L. L. (1997). Peptides, steroids, and pair bonding. *Annals of the New York Academy of Sciences, 807,* 260–272.

Chisholm, J. S. (1996). The evolutionary ecology of attachment organization. *Human Nature, 7,* 1–38.

Coan, J. A., Schaefer, H. S., & Davidson, R. J. (2006). Lending a hand: Social regulation of the neural response to threat. *Psychological Science, 17,* 1032–1039.

Colin, V. (1985). *Hierarchies and patterns of infants' attachments to parents and day caregivers: An exploration.* Unpublished doctoral dissertation, University of Virginia.

Colin, V. (1987). *Infants' preferences between parents before and after moderate stress activates behavior.* Paper presented at the biennial meeting of the Society for Research in Child Development, Baltimore.

Cummings, E. M. (1980). Caregiver stability and attachment in infant day care. *Developmental Psychology, 16,* 31–37.

Cunningham, M. R., Druen, P. B., & Barbee, A. P. (1997). Angels, mentors, and friends: Trade-offs among evolutionary, social, and individual variables in physical appearance. In J. A. Simpson & D. T. Kenrick (Eds.), *Evolutionary social psychology* (pp. 109–140). Mahwah, NJ: Erlbaum.

Cutler, W. B., Garcia, C. R., Huggins, G. R., & Preti, G. (1986). Sexual behavior and steroid levels among gynecologically mature premenopausal women. *Fertility and Sterility, 45,* 496–502.

Daly, M., & Wilson, M. (1988). *Homicide.* New York: Aldine de Gruyter.

Daly, M., & Wilson, M. (1996). Evolutionary psychology and marital conflict. In D. M. Buss & N. M. Malamuth (Eds.), *Sex, power, conflict: Evolutionary and feminist perspectives* (pp. 9–28). New York: Oxford University Press.

Dewsbury, D. A. (1987). The comparative psychology of monogamy. In D.W. Leger (Ed.), *Nebraska Symposium on Motivation* (Vol. 35, pp. 6–43). Lincoln: University of Nebraska Press.

Diamond, L. M. (2004). Emerging perspectives on distinctions between romantic love and sexual desire. *Current Directions in Psychological Science, 13,* 116–119.

Diamond, L. M. (2006). How do I love thee?: Implications of attachment theory for understanding same-sex love and desire. In M. Mikulincer & G. S. Goodman (Eds.), *Dynamics of romantic love: Attachment, caregiving, and sex* (pp. 275–292). New York: Guilford Press.

Draper, P., & Belsky, J. (1990). Personality development in evolutionary perspective. *Journal of Personality, 58,* 141–161.

Draper, P., & Harpending, H. (1988). A sociobiological perspective on the development of human reproductive strategies. In K. MacDonald (Ed.), *Sociobiological perspectives on human development* (pp. 340–372). New York: Springer-Verlag.

Eibl-Eibesfeldt, I. (1975). *Ethology: The biology of behavior.* New York: Holt, Rinehart & Winston.

Eibl-Eibesfeldt, I. (1989). *Human ethology.* New York: Aldine de Gruyter.

Ellis, B. J., Bates, J. E., Dodge, K. A., Fergusson, D. M., Horwood, L. J., Pettit, G. S., et al. (2003). Does father absence place daughters at special risk for early sexual activity and teenage pregnancy? *Child Development, 74,* 801–821.

Ellis, B. J., McFadyen-Ketchum, S., Dodge, K. A., Pettit, G. S., & Bates, J. E. (1999). Quality of early family relationships and individual differences in the timing of pubertal maturation in girls: A longitudinal test of an evolutionary model. *Journal of Personality and Social Psychology, 77,* 387–401.

Feeney, J. A., Noller, P., & Callan, V. J. (1994). Attachment style, communication and satisfaction in the early years of marriage. In K. Bartholomew & D. Perlman (Eds.), *Advances in personal relationships: Vol. 5. Attachment processes in adulthood* (pp. 269–308). London: Jessica Kingsley.

Fisher, H. E. (1992). *Anatomy of love.* New York: Norton.

Fisher, H. E. (2000). Lust, attraction, attachment: Biology and evolution of the three primary emotion systems for mating, reproduction, and parenting. *Journal of Sex Education and Therapy, 25*(1), 96–104.

Fisher, H. E. (2002). Defining the brain systems of lust, romantic attraction, and attachment. *Archives of Sexual Behavior, 31,* 413–419.

Fraley, R. C., & Davis, K. E. (1997). Attachment formation and transfer in young adults' close friendships and romantic relationships. *Personal Relationships, 4,* 131–144.

Fraley, R. C., & Shaver, P. R. (1999). Loss and bereavement: Attachment theory and recent controversies concerning "grief work" and the nature of detachment. In J. Cassidy & P. R. Shaver (Eds.), *Handbook of attachment: Theory, research, and clinical implications* (pp. 735–759). New York: Guilford Press.

Fraley, R. C., & Shaver, P. R. (2000). Adult romantic attachment: Theoretical developments, emerging controversies, and unanswered questions. *Review of General Psychology, 4,* 132–154.

Fuller, T. A., & Fincham, F. D. (1995). Attachment style in married couples: Relation to current marital functioning, stability over time, and method of assessment. *Personal Relationships, 2,* 17–34.

Furman, W., & Buhmester, D. (1985). Children's perceptions of the personal relationships in their social networks. *Developmental Psychology, 21,* 1016–1024.

Gangestad, S. W., Garver-Apgar, C. E., Simpson, J. A., & Cousins, A. J. (2007). Changes in women's mate preferences across the ovulatory cycle. *Journal of Personality and Social Psychology, 92,* 151–163

Gangestad, S. W., & Simpson, J. A. (2000). The evolution of human mating: Trade-offs and strategic pluralism. *Behavioral and Brain Sciences, 23,* 573–644.

Goodwin, J. S., Hurt, W. C., Key, C. R., & Sarret, J. M. (1987). The effect of marital status on stage, treatment and survival of cancer patients. *Journal of the American Medical Association, 258,* 3125–3130.

Gottman, J. M. (1983). How children become friends. *Monographs of the Society for Research in Child Development, 48*(3, Serial No. 201).

Hall, J. H., & Fincham, F. D. (2006). Relationship dissolution following infidelity. In M. A. Fine & J. H. Harvey (Eds.), *Handbook of divorce and relationship dissolution* (pp. 153–168). Mahwah, NJ: Erlbaum.

Harlow, H. F. (1958). The nature of love. *American Psychologist, 13,* 673–685.

Hartup, W. (1983). Peer relations. In P. H. Mussen (Series Ed.) & E. M. Hetherington (Vol. Ed.), *Handbook of child psychology: Vol. 4. Socialization, personality and social development* (4th ed., pp. 301–349). New York: Wiley.

Hazan, C., Gur-Yaish, N., & Campa, M. (2004). What does it mean to be attached? In W. S. Rholes & J. A. Simpson (Eds.), *Adult attachment: Theory, research, and clinical implications* (pp. 55–85). New York: Guilford Press.

Hazan, C., & Shaver, P. R. (1987). Romantic love conceptualized as an attachment process. *Journal of Personality and Social Psychology, 52*, 511–524.

Hazan, C., & Shaver, P. R. (1990). Love and work: An attachment theoretical perspective. *Journal of Personality and Social Psychology, 59*, 270–280.

Hazan, C., & Shaver, P. R. (1992). Broken attachments. In T. L. Orbuch (Ed.), *Close relationship loss: Theoretical approaches* (pp. 90–108). Hillsdale, NJ: Erlbaum.

Hazan, C., & Shaver, P. R. (1994). Attachment as an organizational framework for research on close relationships. *Psychological Inquiry, 5*, 1–22.

Hazan, C., & Zeifman, D. (1994). Sex and the psychological tether. In K. Bartholomew & D. Perlman (Eds.), *Advances in personal relationships: Vol. 5. Attachment processes in adulthood* (pp. 151–177). London: Jessica Kingsley.

Henry, K., & Holmes, J. G. (1998). Childhood revisited: The intimate relationships of individuals from divorced and conflict-ridden families. In J. A. Simpson & W. S. Rholes (Eds.), *Attachment theory and close relationships* (pp. 280–316). New York: Guilford Press.

Hill, K., & Hurtado, M. (1995). *Demographic/life history of Ache foragers.* New York: Aldine de Gruyter.

Hinde, R. A. (1983). The human species. In R. A. Hinde (Ed.), *Primate social relationships* (pp. 334–349). Oxford, UK: Blackwell.

Hinsz, V. B. (1989). Facial resemblance in engaged and married couples. *Journal of Social and Personal Relationships, 6*, 223–229.

Holmes, T. H., & Rahe, R. H. (1967). The Social Readjustment Rating Scale. *Journal of Psychosomatic Research, 11*, 213–218.

Justo, J. M. R. M., Maia, C. B., Ferreira-Diniz, F., Santos, C. L., & Moreira, J. M. (1997, June). *Adult attachment style among women with infertility of unknown biological cause.* Paper presented at the International Network on Personal Relationships Conference, Miami University, Oxford, OH.

Kaczmarek, M. (2007). The timing of natural menopause in Poland and associated factors. *Maturitas, 57*(2), 139–153.

Kenrick, D. T., Groth, G. E., Trost, M. R., & Sadalla, E. K. (1993). Integrating evolutionary and social exchange perspectives on relationships: Effects of gender, self-appraisal, and involvement level on mate selection criteria. *Journal of Personality and Social Psychology, 64*, 951–969.

Kirkpatrick, L. A. (1998). Evolution, pair-bonding, and reproductive strategies: A reconceptualization of adult attachment. In J. A. Simpson & W. S. Rholes (Eds.), *Attachment theory and close relationships* (pp. 353–393). New York: Guilford Press.

Kobak, R. R., & Hazan, C. (1991). Attachment in marriage: Effects of security and accuracy of working models. *Journal of Personality and Social Psychology, 60*, 861–869.

Kuo, Z. Y. (1967). *The dynamics of behavior development: An epigenetic view.* New York: Random House.

Lewis, M. (1982). Social development in infancy and early childhood. In J. B. Osofsky (Ed.), *Handbook of infant development* (2nd ed., pp. 419–493). New York: Wiley.

Lynch, J. J. (1977). *The broken heart: The medical consequences of loneliness.* New York: Basic Books.

Main, M., Kaplan, N., & Cassidy, J. (1985). Security in infancy, childhood, and adulthood: A move to the level of representation. In I. Bretherton & E. Waters (Eds.), Growing points of attachment theory and research. *Monographs of the Society for Research in Child Development, 50*(1–2, Serial No. 209), 66–104.

Mellen, S. L. W. (1981). *The evolution of love.* Oxford, UK: Freeman.

Mendoza, S. P., & Mason, W. A. (1997). Attachment relationships in new world primates. *Annals of the New York Academy of Sciences, 807*, 203–209.

Mikulincer, M., & Goodman, G. S. (Eds.). (2006). *Dynamics of romantic love: Attachment, caregiving, and sex.* New York: Guilford Press.

Mikulincer, M., & Shaver, P. R. (2007). *Attachment in adulthood: Structure, dynamics, and change.* New York: Guilford Press.

Moller, A. P. (2003). The evolution of monogamy: Mating relationships, parental care and sexual selection. In U. H. Reichard & C. Boesch (Eds.), *Monogamy: Mating strategies and partnerships in birds, humans and other mammals* (pp. 29–41). Cambridge, UK: Cambridge University Press.

Nass, G. D., & Fisher, M. P. (1988). *Sexuality today.* Boston: Jones & Bartlett.

O'Neill, N., & O'Neill, G. (1972). *Open marriage: A new lifestyle for couples.* New York: M. Evans.

Parkes, C. M., & Weiss, R. S. (1983). *Recovery from bereavement.* New York: Basic Books.

Paul, E. L., McManus, B., & Hayes, A. (2000). "Hookups": Characteristics and correlates of college students' spontaneous and anonymous sexual experiences. *Journal of Sex Research, 37*, 76–88.

Reedy, M. N., Birren, J. E., & Schaie, K. W. (1981). Age and sex differences in satisfying love relationships across the adult life span. *Human Development, 24*, 52–66.

Ricciuti, H. N. (1974). Fear and the development of social attachments in the first year of life. In M. Lewis & L. Rosenblum (Eds.), *Origins of fear* (pp. 73–106). New York: Wiley.

Robertson, J. (1953). Some responses of young children to the loss of maternal care. *Nursing Times, 49*, 382–386.

Rubenstein, C., & Shaver, P. R. (1982). *In search of intimacy*. New York: Delacorte.

Rubin, Z. (1973). *Liking and loving*. New York: Holt, Rinehart & Winston.

Rubin, Z. (1980). *Children's friendships*. Cambridge, MA: Harvard University Press.

Schachner, D. A., & Shaver, P. R. (2004). Attachment dimensions and motives for sex. *Personal Relationships, 11*, 179–195.

Schaffer, H. R., & Emerson, P. E. (1964). The development of social attachments in infancy. *Monographs of the Society for Research in Child Development, 29*(3, Serial No. 94).

Schmitt, D. P. (2001). Universal sex differences in the desire for sexual variety: Tests from 52 nations, 6 continents, and 13 islands. *Journal of Personality and Social Psychology, 85*, 85–104.

Schmitt, D. P. (2005). Sociosexuality from Argentina to Zimbabwe: A 48-nation study of sex, culture, and strategies of human mating. *Behavioral and Brain Sciences, 28*, 247–311.

Schmitt, D. P., Shackelford, T. K., Duntley, J., Tooke, W., & Buss, D. M. (2001). The desire for sexual variety as a key to understanding basic human mating strategies. *Personal Relationships, 8*, 425–455.

Shaver, P. R., Hazan, C., & Bradshaw, D. (1988). Love as attachment: The integration of three behavioral systems. In R. J. Sternberg & M. L. Barnes (Eds.), *The psychology of love* (pp. 68–99). New Haven, CT: Yale University Press.

Shill, M. A., Solyom, P., & Biven, C. (1984). Parent preference in the attachment exploration balance in infancy: An experimental psychoanalytic approach. *Child Psychiatry and Human Development, 15*, 34–48.

Simpson, J. A., & Gangestad, S. W. (1991). Individual differences in sociosexuality: Evidence for convergent and discriminant validity. *Journal of Personality and Social Psychology, 60*, 870–883.

Spitz, R. A. (1946). Anaclitic depression. *Psychoanalytic Study of the Child, 2*, 313–342.

Stearns, S. (1992). *The evolution of life histories*. New York: Oxford University Press.

Steinberg, L., & Silverberg, S. B. (1986). The vicissitudes of autonomy in early adolescence. *Child Development, 57*, 841–851.

Sternberg, R. J. (1986). A triangular theory of love. *Psychological Review, 93*, 119–135.

Stroebe, W., Stroebe, M., Abakoumkin, G., & Schut, H. (1996). The role of loneliness and social support in adjustment to loss: A test of attachment versus stress theory. *Journal of Personality and Social Psychology, 70*, 1241–1249.

Surbey, M. (1990). Family composition, stress, and human menarche. In F. Bercovitch & T. Zeigler (Eds.), *The socioendocrinology of primate reproduction* (pp. 71–97). New York: Liss.

Symons, D. (1979). *The evolution of human sexuality*. New York: Oxford University Press.

Thornhill, N. W. (1991). An evolutionary analysis of rules regulating human inbreeding and marriage. *Behavioral and Brain Sciences, 14*, 247–281.

Tinbergen, N. (1963). On aims and methods of ethology. *Zeitschrift für Tierpsychologie, 20*, 410–433.

Trevathan, W. (1987). *Human birth*. New York: Aldine de Gruyter.

Trivers, R. L. (1972). Parental investment and sexual selection. In B. Campbell (Ed.), *Sexual selection and the descent of man* (pp. 1871–1971). Chicago: Aldine.

Uchino, B. N., Cacioppo, J. T., & Kiecolt-Glaser, J. K. (1996). The relationship between social support and physiological processes: A review with emphasis on underlying mechanisms and implications for health. *Psychological Bulletin, 119*, 488–531.

Veith, J. L., Buck, M., Getzlaf, S., Van Dalfsen, P., & Slade, S. (1983). Exposure to men influences the occurrence of ovulation in women. *Physiology and Behavior, 31*, 313–315.

Vormbrock, J. K. (1993). Attachment theory as applied to war-time and job-related marital separation. *Psychological Bulletin, 114*, 122–144.

Wallerstein, J. S. (1994). Children after divorce: Wounds that don't heal. In L. Fenson & J. Fenson (Eds.), *Human development, 94/95* (pp. 160–165). Guilford, CT: Dushkin.

Weber, A. L. (1998). Losing, leaving, and letting go: Coping with nonmarital breakups. In B. H. Spitzberg & W. R. Cupach (Eds.), *The dark side of close relationships* (pp. 267–306). Mahwah, NJ: Erlbaum.

Weiss, R. S. (1973). *Loneliness: The experience of emotional and social isolation*. Cambridge, MA: MIT Press.

Weiss, R. S. (1975). *Marital separation*. New York: Basic Books.

Weiss, R. S. (1988). Loss and recovery. *Journal of Social Issues, 44*, 37–52.

Wood, W., Rhodes, N., & Whelan, M. (1989). Sex differences in positive well-being: A consideration of emotional style and marital status. *Psychological Bulletin, 106*, 249–264.

Zeifman, D., & Hazan, C. (1997). A process model of adult attachment formation. In S. Duck (Eds.), *Handbook of personal relationships* (2nd ed., pp. 179–195). Chichester, UK: Wiley.

Zimmerman, S. J., Maude, M. B., & Moldawar, M. (1965). Frequent ejaculation and total sperm count, motility and forms in humans. *Fertility and Sterility, 16*, 342–345.

CHAPTER 21

Adult Romantic Attachment
Developments in the Study of Couple Relationships

JUDITH A. FEENEY

"My partner is extremely affectionate, which suits me down to the ground. I've always, always craved affection all my life, mainly through parental—*bad* parental—relationships. So, I don't know, but I put it down to that. And she's the only person I've ever gone out with that's actually given me the affection I've wanted."

It is not unusual for people, in describing their romantic and marital relationships, to emphasize the impact of early experiences with caregivers; such an emphasis is reflected in this brief quotation from a research participant. Other descriptions of romantic relationships explore in more detail the continuity between early and later social relations, including the legacy of negative experiences with caregivers. Consider the following comment, made by a participant in a study of long-term dating relationships:

"It took E. a long time to want to get close to me, because I think her mother has destroyed her trust in people and the way people express emotions. Her mother just flits in and out of moods, and she's always put E. down. So I think E. had lost the ability to get close to people. She is often really quiet and upset, and has trouble

talking about her problems. She listens, but she doesn't like to reciprocate with any discussion of her troubles. She's starting to overcome this, but only in the last couple of months, because I've raised it as a very damaging issue in our relationship. I feel separated from her because of her silence—it makes me feel like I can't make her happy. Also, E.'s never had any attention from her father. He hasn't taken an interest in what she does, and I think she feels that he hasn't had any input in her emotional development."

Comments such as these are consistent with Bowlby's (1969/1982, 1973, 1980) theory of attachment, which recognizes the enormous importance for later relationships of the bonds formed between children and their caregivers. They also support Bowlby's claim that attachment behavior plays a vital role throughout the life cycle. This chapter focuses on the proposition that romantic love and other emotions experienced in couple relationships can be conceptualized as attachment processes, which are influenced in part by earlier experiences with caregivers. The aim is to present the original theoretical and empirical work on which this proposition is based, to outline the considerable advances that have since occurred in this research area, and to explore some unresolved issues and likely future directions.

THE FIRST STUDIES OF ROMANTIC LOVE AS ATTACHMENT

Although Bowlby's attachment theory dealt primarily with the bonds that form between infants and their caregivers, theoretical work dating from the early 1980s argued for the relevance of attachment principles to adults' close relationships as well. These arguments centered on the functions of attachment bonds. Specifically, infant attachment bonds involve "proximity maintenance" and "separation protest" (seeking proximity to an attachment figure and resisting separation; see Cassidy, Chapter 1, this volume); establishment of a "secure base" (using the attachment figure as a base from which to explore the environment); and using another person as a "safe haven" (turning to an attachment figure for comfort in times of threat). According to Weiss (1982, 1986, 1991), these features of infant–caregiver bonds apply to most marital and committed nonmarital romantic relationships. That is, in such relationships a person derives comfort and security from a partner, wants to be with the partner (especially in times of stress), and protests when the partner threatens to become unavailable. Similarly, Ainsworth (1989) pointed to sexual pair bonds as the prime example of adult attachments.

Other key concepts of attachment theory suggest a link between the *quality* of infant attachment relationships and subsequent adult attachment relationships. Bowlby proposed that during the years of "immaturity" (infancy to adolescence), individuals gradually build up expectations of attachment figures, based on experiences with these individuals. Expectations about the availability and responsiveness of attachment figures are incorporated into "internal working models," which guide perceptions and behavior in later relationships (see Bretherton & Munholland, Chapter 5, this volume).

Despite claims of continuity between childhood and adult relationships, the attachment perspective on adults' romantic relationships did not become an active topic of research until Hazan and Shaver reported their seminal studies (Hazan & Shaver, 1987; Shaver & Hazan, 1988; Shaver, Hazan, & Bradshaw, 1988). In these papers, Hazan and Shaver proposed that romantic love could

be conceptualized as an attachment process. Furthermore, because variations in early social experience produce relatively lasting differences in relationship styles, the three major attachment styles described in the infant literature (see Ainsworth, Blehar, Waters, & Wall, 1978) should be manifested in romantic love. (Hazan and Shaver used the terms "secure," "avoidant," and "anxious-ambivalent" for these styles in adults; I use the same terms in this chapter.)

In support of these arguments, Hazan and Shaver presented theoretical analyses of love and attachment, integrated with new empirical data. Their theoretical analyses (Shaver & Hazan, 1988) addressed several issues, including the conceptualization of adult love as an integration of behavioral systems (attachment, caregiving, and sex), and compared the attachment perspective with previous theories of love. These issues are briefly discussed later in this chapter.

The empirical studies (Hazan & Shaver, 1987) assessed the link between attachment style and aspects of childhood and adult relationships. Hazan and Shaver developed a forced-choice, self-report measure of adult attachment consisting of three paragraphs, designed to capture the main features of the three infant attachment patterns described by Ainsworth and colleagues (1978). Participants were asked to choose the paragraph most descriptive of their feelings in close relationships. This measure was used with a large sample of respondents to a brief questionnaire printed in a local newspaper, and in a separate study with an undergraduate sample. Participants completed questions assessing general attitudes to close relationships, together with experiences specific to their "most important romance." Results showed that the frequencies of the three styles were similar to those observed among American infants from middle-class families: Just over half the adults described themselves as "secure," and of the remainder, slightly more classified themselves as "avoidant" than as "anxious-ambivalent." In line with predictions based on attachment theory, the three attachment groups differed in their reports of early family relationships, working models of attachment, and love experiences.

In reporting their results, Hazan and Shaver (1987) noted the limitations of their initial studies. Because of constraints on data collection, the measures were brief and simple. Moreover, participants described their experience of a single romantic relationship; hence, the focus was on relationship qualities that differentiated the three attachment groups. Although this focus might seem to imply a trait approach, the authors recognized that relationship qualities are influenced by "factors unique to particular partners and circumstances" (Hazan & Shaver, 1987, p. 521). This important point is addressed again later in this chapter.

EARLY STUDIES OF ROMANTIC ATTACHMENT: REPLICATIONS AND EXTENSIONS

Despite the limitations of their initial research, Hazan and Shaver succeeded in providing both a *normative* account of romantic love (i.e., an account of the typical processes of romantic attachment) and an understanding of *individual differences* in adult relationship styles. Providing a bridge between infant attachment theory and theories of romantic love, their work generated intense interest among relationship researchers, who soon set out to replicate and extend the initial findings. Two questions addressed by these early studies were the conceptual links between love and attachment, and the salience of attachment issues to individuals in romantic relationships. (Some early studies also assessed attachment-related differences in affect regulation; for a review of this topic, see Mikulincer & Shaver, Chapter 23, this volume.)

Conceptualizing Love and Attachment

The first two studies discussed here focused on the conceptualization of love and attachment. Shaver and Hazan (1988) proposed that previous theories of love (theories of "love styles"; of "anxious" love; and of separate components of love, such as passion, intimacy, and commitment) could be integrated within the attachment perspective. To test this proposition, Levy and Davis (1988) assessed the links between attachment style and measures of the love styles described by Lee (1973, 1988) and the components of love discussed by Sternberg (1986). (For a recent volume summarizing the various theories, see Sternberg & Weis, 2006.)

The love styles described by Lee are "eros" (passionate love), "ludus" (game-playing love), "storge" (friendship love), "mania" (possessive, dependent love), "pragma" (logical, "shopping-list" love), and "agape" (selfless love). Shaver and Hazan (1988) argued that this typology could be reduced to the three attachment styles. Specifi-

cally, their formulation linked secure attachment to a combination of eros and agape, avoidant attachment to ludus, and anxious-ambivalent attachment to mania (storge and pragma were not seen as forms of romantic love). Levy and Davis's results, based on ratings of each attachment and love style, largely supported this formulation. Furthermore, all three components of Sternberg's (1986) model of love (intimacy, passion, commitment) were positively related to secure attachment and negatively related to avoidant and anxious-ambivalent attachment. This finding linked secure attachment with better relationship functioning, but failed to establish a unique set of correlates for each insecure style. Other measures employed by Levy and Davis did, however, distinguish between forms of insecurity; in particular, anxious ambivalence was associated with a dominating style of response to conflict.

The second study considered here (J. A. Feeney & Noller, 1990) was designed to replicate Hazan and Shaver's (1987) work and to assess their proposed integration of theories of love. Using a large undergraduate sample, Noller and I reported attachment group differences on measures of family history and working models, which largely supported the earlier work. A new and noteworthy finding was that avoidant respondents were the most likely to report having experienced a lengthy separation from their mothers during childhood (a finding consistent with attachment theory).

Like Levy and Davis, we (J. A. Feeney & Noller, 1990) were interested in relating the attachment perspective to previous theories of love (Table 21.1 summarizes the findings of these two studies). In particular, we argued that the link between "anxious love" and anxious-ambivalent attachment warranted attention. Shaver and Hazan (1988) described theories of anxious love as unidimensional, but they did not test the structure of measures of anxious love or their relations with attachment style. Using factor analysis, we assessed the structure of a broad set of measures: self-esteem, loving, love styles, and anxious love (also called "limerence," Tennov, 1979, and "love addiction," Peele, 1975). This procedure produced 16 scales. Of particular interest was the fact that measures of anxious love were multidimensional. The limerence measure, for example, yielded four factors: "obsessive preoccupation," "self-conscious anxiety in dealing with partners," "emotional dependence," and "idealization."

TABLE 21.1. Measures of Love Associated with the Three Major Attachment Styles as of 1990

Measure	Secure	Avoidant	Anxious-ambivalent
Love styles	Eros (passionate love), agape (selfless love)	Ludus (game-playing love)	Mania (possessive love)
Components of love	High on intimacy, passion, and commitment	Low on intimacy, passion, and commitment	Low on intimacy, passion, and commitment
Higher-order factors	High on self-confidence (high on self-esteem and low on self-conscious anxiety with partners); low on avoidance of intimacy; low on neurotic love	High on avoidance of intimacy (high on ludus and low on eros, agape, and loving); low on self-confidence; low on neurotic love	High on neurotic love (high on preoccupation, dependence, and idealization); low on circumspect love (friendship, pragma); low on self-confidence; low on avoidance of intimacy

Note. Data from J. A. Feeney and Noller (1990) and Levy and Davis (1988).

Four higher-order factors emerged from the 16 scales: "neurotic love" (preoccupation, dependence, and idealization); "circumspect love" (friendship and pragma); "self-confidence" (self-esteem, lack of self-conscious anxiety); and "avoidance of intimacy" (high scores on ludus; low scores on loving, eros, and agape). All four scales strongly differentiated the attachment groups. Secure participants' experience of love was self-confident and neither neurotic nor intimacy-avoiding. Both insecure groups lacked self-confidence, but whereas avoidant participants reported avoiding intimacy, anxious-ambivalent individuals reported a somewhat desperate and impetuous approach to love. These results generally supported Shaver and Hazan's theoretical analysis. However, whereas these authors equated anxious love with anxious-ambivalent attachment, it seems that at least one aspect of anxious love (self-conscious anxiety) characterizes both insecure groups.

Salience of Attachment Issues to Perceptions of Romantic Relationships

The studies reported so far point to meaningful relations between romantic attachment style and love experiences. However, these studies relied on closed-ended, self-report measures. Because such structured measures may lead to response sets such as experimenter demand and social desirability, we (J. A. Feeney & Noller, 1991) argued that these studies had not established the *salience* of attachment issues to individuals' evaluations of their romantic relationships. That is, attachment issues may not be very important to individuals, except when they are introduced by measurement procedures.

To address this problem, we asked participants in dating relationships to provide open-ended verbal descriptions of their relationships, telling "what kind of person your partner is, and how you get along together." The descriptions were transcribed for content analysis, and participants later completed Hazan and Shaver's (1987) measure of attachment style. The salience of attachment issues was assessed by examining whether participants spontaneously referred to issues that are central to working models of attachment: openness, closeness, dependence, commitment, and affection. Each issue was mentioned by at least 25% of participants, with 89% of the sample referring to at least one of the five issues. On average, one-fifth of the content of the transcripts was devoted to discussing these issues, further supporting the salience of attachment themes.

We (J. A. Feeney & Noller, 1991) also examined the link between attachment style and open-ended reports of relationships. Attachment groups differed markedly in the content of their reports, as illustrated by the sample extracts in Table 21.2. Secure participants emphasized mutual support, but advocated "balance" in terms of the extent to which partners depended on each other. Both secure and avoidant participants described their relationships as friendship-based; unlike secure participants, however, those who were avoidant preferred clear limits to closeness, dependence, commitment, and displays of affection. Anxious-ambivalent participants, in contrast, preferred unqualified closeness, commitment and affection, and tended to idealize their partners. These results fit with findings based on structured measures of relationship experiences.

TABLE 21.2. Extracts from Open-Ended Reports of Romantic Relationships Supplied by Participants from Three Attachment Groups

Secure: "We're really good friends, and we sort of knew each other for a long time before we started going out—and we like the same sort of things. Another thing which I like a lot is that he gets on well with all my close friends. We can always talk things over. Like if we're having any fights, we usually resolve them by talking it over—he's a very reasonable person. I can just be my own person, so it's good, because it's not a possessive relationship. I think that we trust each other a lot."

Avoidant: "My partner is my best friend, and that's the way I think of him. He's as special to me as any of my other friends. His expectations in life don't include marriage, or any long-term commitment to any female, which is fine with me, because that's not what my expectations are as well. I find that he doesn't want to be overly intimate, and he doesn't expect too much commitment—which is good. ... Sometimes it's a worry that a person can be that close to you, and be in such control of your life."

Anxious-ambivalent: "So I went in there ... and he was sitting on the bench, and I took one look, and I actually melted. He was the best-looking thing I'd ever seen, and that was the first thing that struck me about him. So we went out and we had lunch in the park. ... So we just sort of sat there—and in silence—but it wasn't awkward ... like, you know, when you meet strangers and you can't think of anything to say, it's usually awkward. It wasn't like that. We just sat there, and it was incredible—like we'd known each other for a real long time, and we'd only just met for about 10 seconds, so that was—straightaway my first feelings for him started coming out."

Note. Data from J. A. Feeney and Noller (1991).

ADVANCES IN CONCEPTUALIZATION AND MEASUREMENT

Understanding recent studies of romantic attachment requires us to consider the advances in conceptualization and measurement on which they are based. In terms of measurement, Hazan and Shaver's (1987) forced-choice item had clear limitations (as they themselves noted). Reliance on a single item required assumptions about the number of attachment styles, and raised concerns about reliability of measurement. These concerns were exacerbated by the forced-choice format, which required respondents to choose from complex alternatives and seemed to imply that the styles were mutually exclusive. Given these problems, researchers soon sought more refined

measures. Before these refinements are discussed, however, two points should be noted.

First, despite the calls for more refined instruments, the three-group measure continues to be used in a considerable number of research projects. This popularity presumably reflects its ease of administration, its conceptual link with infant attachment theory, and the general appeal of simple typologies for describing individual differences. Furthermore, consistent links between the three-group measure and relationship variables support its reliability and validity. Thus the question is not whether that measure produces meaningful results, but rather how it might be improved psychometrically.

Second, it should be noted that Hazan and Shaver were not the first researchers to measure adult attachment. The Adult Attachment Interview (AAI; George, Kaplan, & Main, 1984, 1985, 1996) taps memories of childhood relationships with parents, and respondents' evaluations of the effects of these experiences on their adult personality. Interview transcripts can be used to identify three attachment patterns: "secure" (marked by the valuing of attachment experiences, and by ease and objectivity in discussing them); "dismissing" (marked by the devaluing of attachment relationships, and by difficulty in recalling specific attachment experiences); and "preoccupied" (marked by confused or incoherent accounts of attachment relationships). The validity of this measure is supported by links between parents' attachment classification, assessed by the AAI, and their children's attachment classification, assessed earlier by observers (Main & Goldwyn, 1984; Main, Goldwyn, & Hesse, 2003). AAI classifications have also been related to marital/couple relationship quality, as noted later in this chapter. Most of the measures discussed in the following sections differ from the AAI in two key respects: They focus on adult romantic or marital attachment (as opposed to current state of mind with respect to childhood attachment), and they require less in-depth training to administer and score. (For more details concerning the AAI, see Crowell, Fraley, & Shaver, Chapter 26, and Hesse, Chapter 25, this volume.)

Typologies of Attachment: Three or Four Styles?

Hazan and Shaver's (1987) original measure described three styles, based on extrapolation from studies of the major infant attachment styles. Bartholomew (1990; Bartholomew & Horowitz, 1991) subsequently proposed a four-group model of adult attachment, based on Bowlby's claim that attachment patterns reflect working models of self and others. Bartholomew argued that models of self can be dichotomized as positive or negative (the self is seen as worthy of love and attention, or as unworthy). Similarly, models of others can be positive or negative (others are seen as available and caring, or as unreliable or rejecting). Working models of self and others jointly define four attachment styles, including two avoidant styles (see Figure 21.1). "Dismissing-avoidant" individuals emphasize achievement and self-reliance, maintaining a sense of self-worth at the expense of intimacy. "Fearful-avoidant" individuals desire intimacy but distrust others, avoiding close involvements that may lead to loss or rejection.

Self-report prototypes of the four attachment styles were developed (similar in form to Hazan and Shaver's three descriptions), together with interview schedules that yield ratings on the four prototypes (Bartholomew & Horowitz, 1991). Substantial convergence has been established between Bartholomew's interview and self-report measures, and between classifications from Bartholomew's interview schedule and those based on the AAI (Bartholomew & Shaver, 1998), although this continues to be disputed (see Crowell et al., Chapter 26, this volume; that chapter also includes a discussion of couple studies based on the AAI-like Current Relationship Interview, developed by Crowell & Owens, 1996). The four-group and three-group measures also show meaningful relations with each other (Brennan, Shaver, & Tobey, 1991). Participants who choose the secure category of one measure also tend to choose the secure category of the other, and those choosing Bartholomew's preoccupied category are likely to endorse Hazan and Shaver's description of anxious ambivalence. Most fearful-avoidant individuals endorse Hazan and Shaver's description of avoidance (which emphasizes discomfort with closeness), but dismissing-avoidant individuals are drawn from both secure and avoidant groups as defined by the original measure.

The four-group model is validated by empirical support for two distinct types of avoidance. For example, the interpersonal problems of fearful-avoidant individuals involve social insecurity, need for approval, and lack of assertiveness, whereas those of dismissing-avoidant individuals involve excessive coldness (Bartholomew & Horowitz, 1991; J. A. Feeney, Noller, & Hanrahan, 1994). As a result, researchers have increasingly adopted the four-group model of adult attachment. This model is consistent with reports of a fourth infant attachment style, marked by characteristics of both avoidance and anxious ambivalence (Crittenden, 1985; Main, Kaplan, & Cassidy, 1985; Main & Solomon, 1990), in that fearful avoidant adults tend to endorse both avoidant and anxious-ambivalent prototypes (Brennan et al., 1991).

MODEL OF SELF
(Dependence)

	Positive (Low)	Negative (High)
MODEL OF OTHER (Avoidance) Positive (Low)	SECURE Comfortable with intimacy and autonomy	PREOCCUPIED Preoccupied (Main) Ambivalent (Hazan) Overly dependent
Negative (High)	DISMISSING Denial of attachment Dismissing (Main) Counterdependent	FEARFUL Fear of attachment Avoidant (Hazan) Socially avoidant

FIGURE 21.1. The four adult attachment styles defined by Bartholomew in terms of working models of self and others. From Bartholomew (1990). Copyright 1990 by Sage Publications, Inc. Reprinted by permission.

From Categorical to Dimensional Measures

Questions have been raised not only about the number of adult attachment styles, but also about the appropriate form of measurement. The first variation of Hazan and Shaver's (1987) measure involved a minor revision: The three descriptions were presented intact, but rather than having to choose among them, participants rated the relative applicability to themselves of each one (Levy & Davis, 1988). This approach recognizes that not all respondents choosing a particular attachment style (e.g., secure) will find the associated description equally applicable; some will be more "secure" than others. It also allows researchers to consider patterns of scores across attachment styles, rather than focusing only on the dominant style. Even this measure, however, assumes that the themes within each attachment description form a consistent whole.

To test this assumption, researchers began breaking each description into a number of separate statements and using factor-analytic methods to investigate the structure. Although item content varied slightly from study to study, several studies pointed to two major dimensions, tapping "comfort with closeness" and "anxiety over relationships" (J. A. Feeney, Noller, & Callan, 1994; J. A. Feeney, Noller, & Hanrahan, 1994; Simpson, Rholes, & Nelligan, 1992; Strahan, 1991). Comfort with closeness, a bipolar dimension, contrasts elements of the original secure and avoidant descriptions (e.g., "I find it easy to trust others" vs. "I am nervous when anyone gets too close"). Anxiety over relationships deals with themes central to anxious-ambivalent attachment, such as fear of rejection and the need for extreme closeness (e.g., "I often worry that my partner doesn't really love me," "I find that others are reluctant to get as close as I would like"). Similarly, a comprehensive study of all available self-report items (Brennan, Clark, & Shaver, 1998) yielded two higher-order factors: "anxiety" (about relationship issues) and "avoidance" (discomfort with closeness and interdependence). These dimensions are related to the four groups of Bartholomew's model, discussed earlier. Dismissing and fearful groups report more avoidance of intimacy than secure and preoccupied groups, suggesting that avoidance is linked to working models of others; preoccupied and fearful groups report more anxiety about rejection and unlovability than secure and dismissing groups, suggesting that relationship anxiety is linked to working models of self (J. A. Feeney, 1995).

In comparing methods of assessing adult attachment security, Griffin and Bartholomew (1994) advocated a "prototype" approach. This regards the four types as important predictors of relationship outcomes (adding to the predictive power of the two dimensions), but recognizes that the boundaries between them are "fuzzy." However, Fraley and Waller (1998) rejected this conclusion, noting that the question of whether individual differences in adult attachment should be viewed in terms of categories (latent types) or dimensions cannot be resolved by cluster analysis, by examining the distributions of attachment-related variables, or by considerations of convenience. Rather, it requires taxometric techniques, which assess patterns of covariation between measured indicators of a construct and are designed specifically to evaluate evidence of "groups" versus "dimensions." Use of such techniques suggests that differences in adult attachment are best understood in terms of dimensions (Fraley & Waller, 1998).

In summary, consensus has gradually been achieved concerning the utility and structure of dimensional self-report measures of romantic attachment. Reducing this complex construct to two dimensions, however, inevitably loses some information, as highlighted by a study employing the Attachment Style Questionnaire (ASQ; J. A. Feeney, Noller, & Hanrahan, 1994) with Italian clinical and nonclinical samples (Fossati et al., 2003). Using the minimum partial statistic to estimate the correct number of factors, this study confirmed the five factors proposed earlier (J. A. Feeney, Noller, & Hanrahan, 1994): "confidence in self and others," "need for approval," "preoccupation with relationships," "discomfort with closeness," and "relationships as secondary" (to achievement). Furthermore, discomfort with closeness was related to sample (clinical, nonclinical), but relationships as secondary was not; conversely, relationships as secondary was related to sex of respondent, but discomfort with closeness was not. Yet, when only two factors are extracted from the ASQ, items from both of these scales load on the same primary dimension (avoidance). This finding suggests that in some contexts, five scales provide more complete information than the two primary dimensions. Hence, although the two dimensions have provided a common base for researchers, especially those conducting experimental research on attachment and affect regulation (Mikulincer & Shaver, Chapter 23, this volume), the utility of measures with more complex structures should not be ignored.

STABILITY OF ADULT ATTACHMENT AND WORKING MODELS

Although studies have shown reasonable stability of attachment patterns across the early childhood years, the extent of stability remains an issue both for developmental researchers and for investigators of romantic attachment. This issue is tied to the "traits versus relationships" debate, discussed later in this section.

The stability of adult romantic attachment has been assessed over intervals ranging from 1 week to 25 years. Given the large number of studies addressing this topic, a detailed consideration of the individual findings is beyond the scope of this chapter (see Mikulincer & Shaver, 2007, for a review); however, some broad conclusions can be drawn. With forced-choice (three- or four-group) measures, approximately a quarter of participants show a change in attachment type across assessments (Baldwin & Fehr, 1995). This figure varies little with the time lag between assessments. Ratings of attachment prototypes are moderately stable, as are multiple-item scales (Collins & Read, 1990; J. A. Feeney, Noller, & Callan, 1994); when the limited reliability of multiple-item scales is considered, their stability is quite high. And interview measures (whether forced-choice or ratings) tend to be even more stable than self-reports or peer reports (Scharfe & Bartholomew, 1994).

Given that adult attachment measures are clearly not perfectly stable, researchers have considered the *meaning* of change over time. Some have argued that instability stems largely from measurement error (Scharfe & Bartholomew, 1994). Although this view fits with the finding that more refined measures are more stable, some degree of instability remains, even when the effect of unreliability is taken into account.

Other researchers argue that instability reflects "real" change, but adopt different positions on its meaning (Davila & Cobb, 2004). First, change in attachment patterns may be most likely when interpersonal circumstances change; attachment theory asserts that significant relationship experiences and life events may alter working models (see the following sections). Indeed, studies have linked instability of attachment to the formation and dissolution of couple relationships (e.g., Hammond & Fletcher, 1991; Kirkpatrick & Hazan, 1994) and to the experience of new parenthood (J. A. Feeney, Alexander, Noller, & Hohaus, 2003). A second perspective focuses on short-term instability, rather than major change.

According to this view, individuals have multiple attachment orientations, derived from their varied and complex relationship experiences; at any given time, attachment measures reflect the orientation elicited by situational factors (Baldwin, Keelan, Fehr, Enns, & Koh-Rangarajoo, 1996). A third perspective posits change in attachment style as an individual-difference variable (Davila, Burge, & Hammen, 1997). These researchers suggest that vulnerability factors make some people more susceptible to change in attachment, and that these people are similar to those who are consistently ("stably") insecure, rather than those who are secure. A longitudinal study of young women (Davila et al., 1997) supported this claim, suggesting that adverse early experiences create more tentative views of self and others.

To understand the sources of stability and change in romantic attachment, we need to consider in some detail the concept of working models. (See Bretherton & Munholland, Chapter 5, this volume, for an extensive discussion of working models.) The following sections deal with two key propositions: first, that working models shape experiences in intimate relationships, hence acting as a source of continuity (stability); and second, that working models are influenced by relational events (and hence are subject to change).

Influence of Working Models on Relationship Experiences

Theoretical and empirical work on the structure and function of working models has clarified their influence on relationship experiences. With regard to structure, Collins and Read (1994) have argued that individuals develop a hierarchy of working models. A set of generalized models lies at the top of the hierarchy, with models for particular classes of relationships (e.g., family members, peers) at an intermediate level, and models for particular relationships (e.g., father, spouse) at the lowest level. Models higher in the hierarchy apply to a wide range of others but are less predictive for any specific situation. (See Overall, Fletcher, & Friesen, 2003, for empirical confirmation of this idea.)

Collins and colleagues (Collins, Guichard, Ford, & Feeney, 2004; Collins & Read, 1994) have further suggested that working models include four components: memories of attachment-related experiences; beliefs, attitudes, and expectations of self and others in relation to attachment; attachment-related goals and needs; and strategies and plans for achieving these goals. These components vary across attachment groups, as summarized in Table 21.3 (the three-group model is used here, because much of the research is based on it). For example, secure individuals tend to remember their parents as warm and affectionate; avoidant individuals remember their mothers as cold and rejecting; and anxious-ambivalent individuals remember their fathers as unfair (e.g., J. A. Feeney & Noller, 1990; Priel & Besser, 2000; Rothbard & Shaver, 1994). These findings from retrospective reports fit with predictions from attachment theory (although not with the link in AAI research between dismissing avoidance and idealization of parents), but we cannot be sure to what extent the memories are affected by more recent experiences.

In terms of functions, working models shape our cognitive, emotional, and behavioral responses to others (Collins & Read, 1994; Collins et al., 2004; Mikulincer & Shaver, 2007, Chs. 6 and 7). Working models affect *cognitive* responses by directing us to pay attention to certain aspects of the stimuli that confront us (particularly goal-related stimuli), by creating biases in memory encoding and retrieval, and by affecting explanation process-es. For example, secure adults show faster recognition of positive-outcome words set in an interpersonal context, whereas avoidant adults show faster recognition of negative-outcome words (Baldwin, Fehr, Keedian, Siedel, & Thomson, 1993). Furthermore, explanations of relationship events by secure adults reflect their stronger perceptions of security and greater confidence in partners' availability (Collins, 1996; Gallo & Smith, 2001).

With regard to emotional response patterns, working models affect both primary and secondary appraisals of relational events (Collins et al., 2004). "Primary appraisal" refers to the immediate emotional reaction to a given situation. In "secondary appraisal," cognitive processing may maintain, amplify, or lessen the initial emotional response, depending on how the individual interprets the experience. For example, individuals who are anxious about their relationships feel more immediate distress in the face of hurtful partner behavior; furthermore, they often interpret this behavior as intentional and undeserved, which tends to amplify the distress (J. A. Feeney, 2004, 2005).

TABLE 21.3. Attachment Group Differences in Working Models

Secure	Avoidant	Anxious-ambivalent
Memories		
Parents warm and affectionate	Mothers cold and rejecting	Fathers unfair
Attachment-related beliefs, attitudes		
Few self-doubts; high in self-worth	Suspicious of human motives	Others complex and difficult to understand
Generally liked by others	Others not trustworthy or dependable	People have little control over own lives
Others generally well-intentioned and good-hearted	Doubt honesty and integrity of parents and others	
Others generally trustworthy, dependable, and altruistic	Lack confidence in social situations	
Interpersonally oriented	Not interpersonally oriented	
Attachment-related goals and needs		
Desire intimate relationships	Need to maintain distance	Desire extreme intimacy
Seek balance of closeness and autonomy in relationships	Limit intimacy to satisfy needs for autonomy	Seek lower levels of autonomy
	Place greater weight on goals such as achievement	Fear rejection
Plans and strategies		
Acknowledge distress	Manage distress by cutting off anger	Heightened displays of distress and anger
Modulate negative affect in constructive way	Minimize distress-related emotional displays; withhold intimate disclosure	Solicitous and compliant to gain acceptance

Working models affect behavioral responses through the activation of stored plans and strategies, and through the construction of new plans and strategies (Collins & Read, 1994). An example of a stored strategy that may have developed in childhood is an individual "running home to Mother" whenever conflict with the spouse arises. In the absence of an available existing strategy, new strategies may be devised for current situations. Hence working models may affect decisions about whether to discuss a conflict issue openly with one's spouse or to avoid it (J. A. Feeney, 2003).

Several factors promote the stability of working models (Bowlby, 1980). First, individuals tend to select environments that fit their beliefs about self and others (this point is revisited shortly in terms of the "traits vs. relationships" debate). Second, the information-processing biases discussed in this section lead people to perceive social events in ways that support existing models. Third, working models may be self-perpetuating; for example, someone who believes that others are untrustworthy may approach them defensively, eliciting further rejection.

Influence of Relationship Experiences on Working Models

Despite these forces promoting stability, change in working models does occur, particularly when significant events in the social environment disconfirm expectations. For example, becoming involved in a stable, satisfying relationship may lead to change for those whose working models have led to skepticism about relationship outcomes. The high percentage of secure respondents generally found in samples of stable couples supports this effect (J. A. Feeney, Noller, & Callan, 1994; Senchak & Leonard, 1992), as does the following comment made by a research participant (J. A. Feeney, 1998; this study is described more fully later):

"I had a real problem trusting anyone at the start of any relationship. A couple of things happened to me when I was young, which I had some emotional difficulties getting over. At the start of our relationship, if P. had been separated from me, I would have been constantly thinking: 'What was he doing?'; 'Was he with another girl?'; 'Was he cheating on me?'; all that would have been running through my head. Over a 3-year period of going out, you look at it in a different light; you learn to trust him."

Similarly, a secure person who is involved in a particularly negative relationship may become insecure as a result of that experience, as indicated by a comment from another participant in the same study:

"Before I started seeing T., I was in another long relationship with another fellow. ... It was good up until about 10 months, and then the last couple of months were really bad. I was always really confident about myself and secure about myself, but he made me feel in 2 months—just seemed to ruin everything I'd ever felt good about myself, and I felt bad about everything I did, and he made me feel bad. And so I've got this constant thing in the back of my head that maybe that might happen again."

Of course, the impact of such negative experiences is likely to depend on their duration and emotional significance. Working models may also change as individuals arrive at new understandings of their past experiences, particularly those that are attachment-related (Davila & Cobb, 2004).

Stability, Change, and the Conceptualization of Attachment: Traits versus Relationships

Recently Fraley and Brumbaugh (2004) have integrated theoretical and empirical work pertaining to the stability of attachment. These researchers have adopted a dynamic systems perspective, which emphasizes the dynamic mechanisms that contribute to both stability and change in attachment organization. Fraley and Brumbaugh argue that once a developmental pathway becomes established, it is less likely to change: Social environments are usually relatively stable, and intraindividual processes (e.g., assimilation of new information) operate to maintain expectations. Nevertheless, external events exert a nontrivial influence. Applying principles from developmental science and the study of biological systems, Fraley and Brumbaugh note that attachment theory cannot be "tested" by studying the stability of attachment across two points in time, because any test–retest correlation greater than zero is consistent with the theory. Hence researchers should focus less on the *degree* of stability that should be observed, and more on the *patterns* of stability. For example, the dynamic systems perspective suggests that the correlation between attachment security in infancy and at any other age gradually decays to a nonzero value, and that test–retest correlations should be higher in adulthood than in childhood. These predictions require further testing.

Fraley and Brumbaugh (2004) have also addressed an ongoing controversy about adult attachment style: Should it be conceptualized as an enduring, trait-like characteristic of the individual, or as reflecting recent experiences specific to particular relationships? Stability data (outlined earlier) support both perspectives. Stability estimates are often moderately high; indeed, some data suggest that attachment style is more stable than relationship status (Kirkpatrick & Hazan, 1994). However, the link between relationship events and change in attachment highlights the role of recent experiences in perceptions of security. Importantly, the "traits versus relationships" question does not involve mutually exclusive perspectives; rather, individual characteristics and relationship events are bound up together (Fraley & Brumbaugh, 2004). For example, by choosing particular partners, individuals may find themselves in situations that confirm their relational expectations. Supporting this claim, studies of romantic attachment have revealed a degree of "partner matching." Secure individuals tend to be paired with secure, responsive partners (e.g., J. A. Feeney, 1994; Senchak & Leonard, 1992)—a situation that should confirm positive working models. Furthermore, relationships involving an anxious female and an avoidant male seem to be quite stable, although not necessarily very happy (Kirkpatrick & Davis, 1994). Presumably the clingy, anxious female confirms the avoidant male's belief that it is unwise to let others get too close, and the avoidant male confirms the anxious female's belief that others are distant and unsupportive. Hence attachment is both trait-like and contextually fluid to an extent.

ROMANTIC ATTACHMENT SECURITY AND RELATIONSHIP QUALITY

A huge body of research attests to the link between romantic attachment security (whether assessed in terms of styles or dimensions) and the quality of couple relationships (see Mikulincer & Shaver, 2007, Ch. 10). Again, a complete presentation of individual findings is beyond the scope of this chapter; however, the following sections provide an overview of the major research questions, together with illustrative findings.

Early studies of dating relationships (Levy & Davis, 1988; Simpson, 1990) linked secure attachment with high levels of trust, commitment, satisfaction, and interdependence. By contrast (and consistent with attachment theory), avoidant and anxious-ambivalent attachment were negatively related to trust and satisfaction, and avoidant attachment was also related to low levels of interdependence and commitment.

Some studies have suggested that the implications of attachment dimensions for relationship quality are somewhat gender-specific. For example, in another study of dating relationships (Collins & Read, 1990), women's relationship anxiety was a strong correlate of their relationship evaluations, being linked with jealousy and with low levels of closeness, partner responsiveness, and satisfaction. For men, comfort with closeness was the crucial attachment dimension, being linked with most indices of relationship quality. These findings may reflect sex-role stereotypes, whereby women are socialized to value emotional closeness and men are socialized to value self-reliance. Given that relationships are rated negatively when the woman is anxious about relationships and when the man is uncomfortable with intimacy, it seems that extreme conformity to sex-role stereotypes may be detrimental to relationship quality.

Interestingly, an early longitudinal study of dating couples (Kirkpatrick & Davis, 1994) suggested that the relationships of anxious women and avoidant men are quite stable over time, despite being relatively low in quality. Why might this be? Anxious women are frequently paired with avoidant men, for whom their clingy behavior may confirm working models (as noted earlier, and as consistent with traditional gender-role stereotypes); furthermore, women tend to act as the nurturers of relationships, and anxious women may strive particularly hard in this role. Similarly, the relationships of avoidant men may be stable because they often involve secure or anxious partners; avoidant persons' tendency to shun heated negative exchanges may also defuse some tensions (J. A. Feeney, 2004). The differing implications of attachment style for current happiness and for long-term stability caution against simplistic statements about "good" or "bad" attachment styles (Kirkpatrick & Davis, 1994).

Studies of marriage have also linked attachment variables to relationship quality (both self-reported and empirically observed). For example, in Kobak and Hazan's (1991) study, spouses completed measures of working models and marital satisfaction, and engaged in interaction tasks involving confiding and problem solving. Secure working models were related to higher marital satisfaction and to ratings of less rejection and more supportiveness during problem solving. Accuracy of working models (extent of agreement with the spouse about one's own working models) was also related to marital satisfaction and to observers' ratings of marital interaction. Since Kobak and Hazan's work, many studies have confirmed the link between attachment security and marital quality (e.g., Banse, 2004; J. A. Feeney, 2002; Meyers & Landsberger, 2002). Furthermore, in an innovative approach to this topic, Roberts and Greenberg (2002) developed an interaction task that required spouses to discuss times when they had experienced positive feelings toward one another. Coding of the interactions revealed that all of the spouses in highly satisfying marriages shared feelings related to at least one of the attachment functions described earlier (proximity seeking, separation protest, secure base, and safe haven). Most referred to three or four of these functions, supporting the importance of "felt security" and of the specific themes outlined by attachment theory.

Attachment and Relationship Quality: The Role of Communication

In evaluating the implications of attachment security for relationship quality, it is important to consider the role of communication. Communication is the main avenue through which attachment relationships are maintained (Bretherton, 1990; Kobak & Duemmler, 1994), and conflict-centered communication in particular involves such attachment-related processes as affect regulation (Pietromonaco, Greenwood, & Barrett, 2004). As discussed next, many researchers have studied attachment and couple communication, using a range of methods (self-report questionnaires, behavioral observation, diary records).

Pistole (1989) investigated attachment and conflict resolution styles in a sample of students involved in love relationships, using Rahim's (1983) Organizational Conflict Inventory. Secure individuals were more likely to use an integrating (problem-solving) strategy than those who were insecure, and also compromised more than anxious-ambivalent individuals. Anxious-ambivalent participants were more likely to oblige their partners than were avoidant participants. More recently, O'Connell Corcoran and Mallinckrodt (2000) used a similar measure of conflict resolution, together with the ASQ (J. A. Feeney, Noller, & Hanrahan, 1994). Confidence in self

and others was related positively to integrating and compromising and negatively to avoiding; discomfort with closeness showed the reverse pattern of associations. These findings suggest that secure persons tend to use constructive conflict strategies, which reflect their concern both for supporting their own interests and for enhancing their relationships.

In another study of conflict-centered communication, Gaines, Work, Johnson, Youn, and Lai (1997) examined reported responses to "accommodative dilemmas"—that is, situations in which an intimate partner behaves negatively. Secure attachment was inversely related to the destructive responses of neglect (passively allowing the situation to deteriorate) and exit (actively harming the relationship). Similarly, studies by Creasey and colleagues (Creasey & Hesson-McInness, 2001; Creasey, Kershaw, & Boston, 1999) linked attachment anxiety and avoidance to questionnaire reports of negative escalation, poorer conflict management skills, and fewer positive conflict tactics. (The link between attachment and responses to severe conflict is addressed later; see "Attachment and Couple Relationships under Stress.")

Patterns of self-disclosure (another key aspect of communication) have also been linked with attachment style in studies using self-report and behavioral methods (Keelan, Dion, & Dion, 1998; Mikulincer & Nachshon, 1991). In general, secure and anxious-ambivalent individuals report more self-disclosure than avoidant individuals; security is also associated with greater ability to elicit disclosure from relationship partners. In addition, secure individuals show the most reciprocity (discussing the particular topics raised by their partners), and the most flexibility (adapting the extent of self-disclosure according to the target and the situation). Further supporting the link between security and self-disclosure, secure individuals report more open expression of feelings (both positive and negative) to their romantic partners (J. A. Feeney, 1995, 1999a).

In a more comprehensive study of communication, we (J. A. Feeney, Noller, & Callan, 1994) followed newlywed couples for 2 years, assessing attachment dimensions (comfort with closeness, relationship anxiety) and three aspects of communication: the quality of daily interactions (via diary reports), nonverbal accuracy (via the standard content paradigm), and conflict style (via questionnaires). In daily interactions, husbands' comfort with closeness was linked to their ratings of involvement, disclosure, and satisfaction, whereas wives' relationship anxiety was linked to their rat- ings of domination, conflict, and dissatisfaction. Furthermore, husbands low in relationship anxiety and wives high in comfort showed more nonver- bal accuracy. The key correlate of conflict style was relationship anxiety; highly anxious spouses rated their conflicts as coercive and distressing. Longitudinal analyses showed bidirectional rela- tions between measures of attachment and marital functioning, supporting the claim that working models and relationship experiences influence one another. Consistent with the widespread links between measures of attachment and communica- tion (J. A. Feeney, Noller, & Callan, 1994), more recent research has linked avoidance and anxiety to lower levels of "communication competence" (a composite measure of assertiveness, interpersonal sensitivity, and self-disclosure; Anders & Tucker, 2000).

Relationship Quality: Dyadic Effects

Many of the studies reported to this point have employed both members of couples, allowing researchers to assess whether perceptions of re- lationship quality are related to the attachment characteristics of the partner, as well as those of the reporter. As noted earlier, Hazan and Shaver (1987) argued that relationship quality is shaped by both partners; recognition of the dyadic nature of attachment effects has been a hallmark of re- cent research.

In early work on this topic, Collins and Read (1990) found that relationship evaluations were related to partners' attachment ratings, in ways that paralleled the effects of individuals' own at- tachment ratings: Negative evaluations were made by the partners of men who were uncomfortable with closeness and women who were anxious about relationships. Other studies of dating couples have supported these results, pointing in particular to a robust, negative effect of women's anxiety on partners' relationship evaluations (Kirkpatrick & Davis, 1994; Simpson, 1990).

Studies of married couples have also reported partner effects. Kobak and Hazan (1991) found that wives of less secure husbands were more re- jecting and less supportive than other wives, and that husbands of secure wives listened more effec- tively during problem solving. Similarly, we (J. A. Feeney, Noller, & Callan, 1994) found that com- munication patterns and marital satisfaction in newlyweds were related to both partners' attach- ment dimensions. For couples sampled across the

life cycle of marriage, spouses' marital satisfaction was again related to the comfort and anxiety lev- els of both partners, as assessed by simple correla- tions (J. A. Feeney, 1994). When the independent contribution of each attachment dimension was assessed using regression analysis, the strongest partner effect was the negative relation between wives' anxiety and husbands' satisfaction (consis- tent with studies of dating couples).

Other studies have compared "couple types," defined by combinations of attachment styles. For example, Senchak and Leonard (1992) compared three types: "secure" (in which both spouses chose the secure description of the three-group attach- ment measure), "insecure" (in which both spouses chose insecure descriptions), and "mixed" (in which one spouse chose the secure description and the other described him- or herself as insecure). They found that secure couples reported better marital adjustment (e.g., more intimacy, positive responses to conflict) than mixed and insecure couples did. Cohn, Silver, Cowan, Cowan, and Pearson (1992) linked observers' ratings of marital quality to couple types assessed with the AAI. In contrast to Senchak and Leonard's findings, mixed couples in this study were rated as similar to secure couples, and as functioning better than insecure couples. Given these conflicting findings regard- ing the adjustment of mixed couples, it remains unclear whether (or when) a secure partner can buffer the negative effects of insecurity on rela- tionship quality.

In summary, there is evidence that relation- ship quality is higher for individuals who are se- curely attached, and for those whose partners are securely attached. These findings raise a further question: Do attachment styles of individuals and their partners *interact* to predict relationship quality? That is, does the effect of an individual's attachment style depend on the style of the part- ner? This issue is implied by studies of couple types (e.g., a secure person may behave differently, de- pending on whether the person is paired with a secure or an insecure partner); however, compar- ing three couple types fails to distinguish between different forms of insecurity, and hence gives lim- ited information about interactive effects. As out- lined next, these effects have been addressed more fully by studies of hypothetical relationships, and by studies using dimensional attachment measures and regression-based analytic techniques.

Using the former approach, Pietromonaco and Carnelley (1994) conducted an experiment in which participants received a written profile of a hypothetical partner. They were asked to imagine themselves in a relationship with that partner, and to evaluate the partner and the relationship along several dimensions. Participants' attachment style was assessed with the three-category measure, and partners' attachment style was manipulated by varying the content of the profiles; thus the researchers assessed how participants responded to different kinds of partners. Relationship evaluations were related to attachment styles of both self and partner (main effects), and some dependent measures showed interactive effects. For example, secure individuals reported less positive feelings about relationships with either type of insecure partner; by contrast, insecure individuals (especially those who were avoidant) responded less favorably to an avoidant partner than to a preoccupied partner.

In one of the first studies to explore interactive attachment effects in real relationships (J. A. Feeney, 1994), couples sampled across the marital life cycle completed measures of attachment and marital satisfaction. As noted earlier, satisfaction was related to both partners' attachment dimensions (main effects). In addition, moderated regression analyses revealed interaction effects for couples married for 10 years or less. Specifically, wives' anxiety was linked with dissatisfaction for both spouses, but only if husbands were low in comfort with closeness; by contrast, husbands' anxiety was linked with dissatisfaction, regardless of wives' comfort (see Figure 21.2). It seems that in more recent marriages, anxious husbands' dependent behavior is destructive, perhaps because it violates the male sex-role stereotype. Anxious wives' dependent (and stereotype-confirming) behavior may be less harmful except when husbands struggle with intimacy, and hence provide insufficient support. (Recall, however, that several studies of dating couples have found anxiety to be more problematic in women than in men.)

Using a similar method, recent reanalyses of data from the study of newlyweds cited earlier (J. A. Feeney, Noller, & Callan, 1994) also revealed interactive attachment effects (J. A. Feeney, 2003). In particular, husbands' and wives' anxiety levels jointly predicted women's reports of several conflict behaviors, both concurrently and longitudinally. Interestingly, this effect varied in form. For example, wives reported high levels of conflict avoidance when both spouses were anxious, suggesting that their avoidance was driven by both

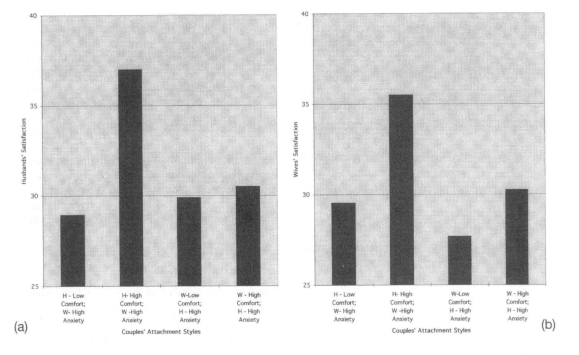

FIGURE 21.2. Relationships between couples' attachment styles on the one hand, and husband's satisfaction (a) and wives' satisfaction (b) on the other. H, Husband; W, wife.

partners' insecurities. However, anxious wives with nonanxious husbands reported *more* coercion in conflict interactions than those with anxious husbands; if anxious wives perceive nonanxious husbands as failing to understand their concerns, power struggles may result. The gender-specific nature of some dyadic attachment effects is also suggested by other studies. For example, Gallo and Smith (2001) found that husbands reported low levels of marital support when they themselves were avoidant but their partners were not. Furthermore, in a study incorporating ratings of the four attachment styles delineated by Bartholomew (1990), the positive effects of security and the negative effects of insecurity were either amplified or attenuated in specific dyadic configurations (Banse, 2004). The most consistent finding concerned husbands' dismissing attachment, which attenuated the effects of wives' preoccupied and dismissing tendencies.

Recent studies of dyadic attachment have used more sophisticated statistical techniques. For example, the "actor–partner interdependence model" (APIM; Kashy & Kenny, 2000) recognizes that in couple relationships, partners' scores on the variables of interest are likely to be correlated. The model can be used to test for "actor effects" (e.g., the effect of an individual's avoidance on his or her supportiveness), "partner effects" (e.g., the effect of an individual's avoidance on the partner's supportiveness), and interactions between these effects. In a study of disclosure patterns in dating couples (Bradford, Feeney, & Campbell, 2002), this approach yielded actor and partner effects, but no interactions between them. For example, actors' avoidance predicted their questionnaire reports of low levels of disclosure; diary records of daily interactions showed consistent negative effects (especially partner effects) of relationship anxiety. In another study using APIM analyses, Campbell, Simpson, Kashy, and Rholes (2001) assessed the effects of attachment dimensions and relationship dependence on couples' responses to a stressful situation. Their results showed interactive effects of avoidance (both actor and partner effects) and level of relationship dependence. For instance, participants who were avoidant and showed little dependence on their relationships were especially prone to displaying negative behavior (e.g., criticism), and to eliciting such behavior from their partners.

In summary, the studies outlined in this section indicate that attachment can be fully understood only at the level of the dyad. Furthermore, dyadic attachment effects are varied and complex, and are often specific to one gender. Given that the research discussed so far provides abundant evidence that attachment security promotes relationship quality, I next consider the meaning of these associations in more detail.

Mediating Variables: Exploring the Mechanisms Linking Security to Relationship Quality

The robust link between attachment security and relationship quality raises questions about the *mechanisms* involved in this association. That is, what do secure people do differently that enhances relationship quality? This question has clear implications for interventions with distressed couples; such couples may be helped not only by interventions that target working models directly, but also by approaches that focus on intervening (mediating) variables.

One of the first studies to address this issue was our study of newlyweds (J. A. Feeney, Noller, & Callan, 1994). Given that attachment security was linked with both communication and marital satisfaction, we suggested that the beneficial effects of security might stem in part from the ways in which secure individuals communicate. That is, communication patterns (e.g., conflict style, nonverbal accuracy) might mediate the link between attachment and satisfaction. Our results did not support this hypothesis; rather, in these early marriages, attachment and communication exerted independent effects on satisfaction. However, different findings emerged from the study of attachment and conflict across the marital life cycle (J. A. Feeney, 1994). In this study, the link between attachment security and marital satisfaction was mediated by mutual negotiation of conflict, although for husbands, relationship anxiety explained variance in satisfaction over and above that related to conflict patterns.

The mediating role of communication is not restricted to conflict-centered interactions. Rather, the link between attachment security and the quality of adults' close relationships also reflects the fact that secure individuals express emotions more openly (J. A. Feeney, 1999a), engage in more self-disclosure (Keelan et al., 1998), and have better overall communication competence (Anders & Tucker, 2000).

Studies exploring other potential mediators of the association between security and relationship quality have also yielded significant results. For example, evidence of full or partial media-

TABLE 21.4. Key Aspects of Relationship Quality Associated with Attachment Dimensions

Avoidance (discomfort with closeness)	Relationship anxiety
Relationship dissatisfaction	Relationship dissatisfaction
Distrust of partners	Distrust of partners
Low commitment	Jealousy
Low closeness/interdependence	High levels of conflict
Low supportiveness	Distress and hurt in the face of conflict
+Low emotional expressiveness	+Coercive and dominating conflict tactics
+Low levels of self-disclosure, including flexibility and reciprocity of disclosure	+Maladaptive (distress-maintaining) attributions for negative partner behavior
+Low tendency to forgive	+Low tendency to forgive
+Low interpersonal competence	+Low interpersonal competence

Note. + indicates there is evidence that this variable mediates the association between security and better relationship functioning.

tion has been reported for such variables as benign (relationship-maintaining) attributions for negative partner behavior (Gallo & Smith, 2001; Sumer & Cozzarelli, 2004), general tendency to forgive transgressions (Kachadourian, Fincham, & Davila, 2004), low levels of psychological distress (Meyers & Landsberger, 2002), and perceptions of the social support available from family and friends (Meyers & Landsberger, 2002).

In short, these important studies suggest that secure individuals display a more open and positive interpersonal style, as indicated by a range of affective, cognitive, and behavioral variables; these variables help to produce positive relationship outcomes. (Table 21.4 summarizes these findings.) However, it is important to note that mediation effects have often been specific to one gender, to relationship type (dating or married), and to attachment dimension (e.g., avoidance vs. anxiety). These findings again highlight the complexity of attachment-related effects in couple relationships.

Relationship Quality: Integrating Attachment, Caregiving, and Sexuality

Shaver and colleagues (1988) argued that sexuality and caregiving are independent behavioral systems that are integrated with the attachment system in prototypical romantic love. Thus romantic love involves the three components of attachment, caregiving, and sexuality, with the relative importance of these components following a predictable pattern over time (Hazan & Shaver, 1994). Because the attachment system appears very early in the course of development and shapes relational expectations, it influences the expression of care-

giving and sexuality. Hence the attachment system is pivotal to romantic bonds.

What support exists for these propositions? Empirical studies clearly support the separate importance of each of the proposed components of love. (See reviews by Shaver & Mikulincer, 2006, and the volume on romantic love edited by Mikulincer & Goodman, 2006.) We have already discussed the robust link between attachment and relationship quality. The importance of couple caregiving is supported by the finding that marital satisfaction is predicted more strongly by an index of caregiving and care receiving than by measures of personality, health, or material circumstances (Kotler, 1985). Similarly, sexual satisfaction is an acknowledged predictor of relationship quality and stability (Sprecher & McKinney, 1993). Support is also emerging for the influence of attachment on caregiving and sexuality, as discussed next.

Attachment and Caregiving

In a study of romantic couples, Carnelley, Pietromonaco, and Jaffe (1996) assessed the link between attachment and caregiving, and the implications of these variables for relationship satisfaction. Individuals' attachment security was linked with the provision of more "beneficial" (engaged and reciprocal) care to romantic partners. Moreover, individuals' own attachment security, partners' attachment security, and partners' provision of beneficial care all contributed to relationship satisfaction.

Additional support for the link between attachment and caregiving comes from Kunce and Shaver's (1994) work. These researchers developed self-report items assessing the quality of caregiving in intimate dyads. Factor analysis of the items revealed four scales: "proximity," "sensitivity," "cooperation," and "compulsive caregiving." In a student sample, these scales showed theoretically meaningful links with attachment style. For example, secure persons reported more proximity and sensitivity than dismissing persons; consistent with their need for approval, preoccupied and fearful individuals reported more compulsive (but less sensitive) caregiving. In a study using Kunce and Shaver's measure with a sample of married couples (J. A. Feeney, 1996), secure attachment was linked to beneficial caregiving to the spouse. Specifically, comfort with closeness and low relationship anxiety were related to more "responsive caregiving" (a composite scale assessing proximity, sensitivity, and cooperation) and to less compulsive caregiving. In addition, marital satisfaction was higher for secure spouses, and for those whose partners reported more responsive caregiving.

The importance of both partners' attachment characteristics is highlighted by a two-part study of spousal caregiving (J. A. Feeney & Hohaus, 2001). Each spouse first provided a semistructured account of the time when he or she had most needed to give the other spouse extra care and support. Next, spouses completed questionnaires assessing attachment dimensions, caregiving style, attachment strength (i.e., degree of reliance on the spouse for meeting attachment needs), anticipated caregiving burden, and willingness to provide ongoing spousal care in the future. Content analysis of the semistructured accounts linked attachment dimensions to perceptions of the caregiving process and its effects. For example, as caregivers, anxious wives used less problem-focused coping and more escape/avoidance, and husbands high in discomfort used less support seeking. In addition, insecurity in either partner was linked to caregivers' tendency to belittle their spouses' needs and behaviors ("tedious," "tragedy queen"). In the second part of the study, spouses' willingness to provide ongoing care was related negatively to their own and their partners' discomfort and anxiety; these effects involved relatively complex paths through caregiving style, attachment strength, and anticipated burden.

In an ongoing research program, B. C. Feeney and Collins (2004) have broadened the conceptualization of caregiving by distinguishing between two caregiving processes that are relevant to couples (see Collins, Guichard, Ford, & Feeney, 2006, for a review). "Safe-haven" caregiving involves responding to the partner's distress, and has been the focus of almost all research to date. In contrast, "secure-base" caregiving involves encouraging and supporting the partner's personal growth and exploration activities. From Bowlby's (1988) work on attachment and exploration, Feeney and Collins developed an integrated model of these processes, which recognizes the complementary roles of caregiver and care receiver. These researchers reviewed empirical evidence in support of the various paths in the model, together with evidence of attachment-related differences in caregiving and care receiving.

Attachment and Sexuality

Support is also emerging for the link between attachment style and sexual attitudes and behaviors. In an early but comprehensive study of this topic, Hazan, Zeifman, and Middleton (1994) asked adults to complete measures of attachment style and the frequency and enjoyment of various sexual behaviors. Three distinct sexual styles were identified, consistent with the three major attachment styles. Secure individuals were less likely to be involved in one-night stands or sexual activity outside of the primary relationship, and more likely to report mutual initiation and enjoyment of sex. Avoidant individuals tended to report activities reflecting low psychological intimacy (one-night stands, sex without love), as well as less enjoyment of physical contact. Anxious-ambivalent females reported involvement in exhibitionism, voyeurism, and domination/bondage, whereas anxious-ambivalent males were more sexually reticent. For both sexes, anxious-ambivalent attachment was related to enjoyment of holding and caressing, but not of more clearly sexual behaviors.

Although few studies have focused on long-term couple relationships, research continues to support the link between specific forms of insecurity and the expression of sexuality. For example, Gentzler and Kerns (2004) found that avoidant attachment was related to attitudinal and behavioral measures of "unrestricted sexuality"—that is, feeling comfortable in short-term sexual relationships that involve little commitment or emotional closeness. Similarly, researchers have reported that avoidant individuals have more accepting attitudes toward casual sex than other attachment groups (Brennan & Shaver, 1995; J. A. Feeney, Noller, & Patty, 1993). Furthermore, avoidance has been related to adolescents' rating their sexual encounters as of relatively little importance (Tracy, Shaver,

Cooper, & Albino, 2003) and to college students' reports of engaging in sex in order to impress their peers (Schachner & Shaver, 2004).

Anxious attachment also shows a unique set of sexuality correlates, particularly for women. Women's anxious attachment has been linked to measures of sexual promiscuity and recent sexual experience (Bogaert & Sadava, 2002) and to the number of sexual partners outside the primary relationship (Gangestad & Thornhill, 1997). These high rates of sexual activity may reflect anxious women's desire for intense closeness, together with fears that failure to oblige partners may drive them away (Schachner & Shaver, 2004; Tracy et al., 2003). For both sexes, anxious attachment has also been linked to perceived difficulty in negotiating sexual encounters (J. A. Feeney, Peterson, Gallois, & Terry, 2000) and to indices of unsafe sex (J. A. Feeney, Kelly, Gallois, Peterson, & Terry, 1999): Given their fear of rejection, anxious individuals may be reluctant to risk alienating partners by discussing sexual practices or by resisting pressure for unprotected sex (J. A. Feeney & Noller, 2004).

Integrating Attachment, Caregiving, and Sexuality

Little empirical work has assessed all three components of romantic bonds, despite the theoretical appeal of such integrative work. An exception is a study of the transition to parenthood (J. A. Feeney, Hohaus, Noller, & Alexander, 2001), which followed couples through pregnancy and the first 6 months of parenthood, and included a comparison sample of couples that were not planning to have children in the near future. The assessment sessions employed interview and questionnaire methods; the questionnaires assessed attachment dimensions (comfort, anxiety), caregiving (responsive and compulsive care), and sexuality (sexual desire, satisfaction with sexual communication).

Results supported the influence of attachment dimensions on caregiving and sexuality, for both transition and comparison couples. That is, security was linked to reports of better sexual functioning and more adaptive caregiving (although only the "relationship anxiety" dimension predicted compulsive care and low sexual desire). Additional analyses identified two trajectories of marital satisfaction among new parents: One group of couples showed stable levels of marital satisfaction, whereas the other struggled to deal with the restrictions on intimacy and companionship. These two groups were similar in terms of initial psychological adjustment and coping

resources, but differed in terms of husbands' attachment and caregiving patterns. The strongest finding was that husbands in couples struggling with the transition were more anxious about relationships at the beginning of the study; these husbands were also less responsive in caring for their wives. These findings support the pivotal role of the attachment system, and suggest that husbands who enter parenthood with unresolved insecurities about love and commitment put considerable pressure on both partners, perhaps by becoming overly dependent and by responding negatively to conflict.

Attachment and Couple Relationships under Stress

What can attachment theory tell us about partners' responses to stress? In addressing this question, it is important to note that most of the early research on romantic attachment linked attachment style with global evaluations of relationships. Such research implies that attachment style influences behavior across a range of settings, and indeed the findings point to pervasive differences between attachment styles. Nevertheless, there are compelling reasons for focusing on stressful situations. In infancy, the attachment system regulates the balance between proximity seeking and exploratory behavior. When attachment figures are nearby and the setting is familiar, infants tend to engage in exploratory activity. By contrast, in threatening situations, attachment behavior is likely to be evident. Three types of conditions activate infant attachment behavior: conditions in the environment, such as alarming events; conditions in the attachment relationship, such as caregivers' absence or discouraging of proximity; and conditions of the child, such as hunger and sickness (Bowlby, 1969/1982).

By analogy, three kinds of situations should activate adults' attachment behavior: stressful conditions in the social or physical environment; conditions that threaten the attachment relationship; and conditions of the individual, such as ill health. Individual differences in attachment behavior should be *most* pronounced under these conditions (Simpson & Rholes, 1994). Because conditions that threaten attachment relationships are directly relevant to couple functioning, the research discussed next focuses on these conditions: specifically, partner absence (separation and reunion behavior) and severe instances of relationship conflict.

Partner Absence

Attachment-related differences in separation and reunion dynamics have been studied in various ways. Mikulincer, Florian, Birnbaum, and Malishkevich (2002) studied responses to "separation reminders," by asking participants to imagine being separated from a relationship partner. For individuals high in relationship anxiety, this manipulation led to heightened accessibility of death-related thoughts, especially when long-term or final separations were imagined. This finding suggests that anxious individuals experience separation as quite catastrophic, and adopt a hypervigilant attitude to preventing such an outcome (Mikulincer et al., 2002).

Researchers have also studied romantic partners' responses to actual separation episodes. For instance, Cafferty, Davis, Medway, O'Hearn, and Chappell (1994) studied reunion dynamics among couples in which the husbands were deployed overseas during the 1990–1991 Gulf War. Four months after reunion, the men and their wives completed questionnaires assessing attachment style, marital satisfaction, conflict, and affect during reunion. For both deployed men and their wives, secure attachment was related to higher marital satisfaction and less postreunion conflict; preoccupied individuals showed particularly poor adjustment (low satisfaction, high conflict). Links between attachment style and affect during reunion were confined to men, perhaps because of the more stressful nature of their separation experience.

Fraley and Shaver (1998) conducted an innovative study of airport separations, finding that women who were anxious about relationships reported greater separation distress. In addition, observers' ratings indicated that when separation was imminent, highly avoidant women were less supportive and more distant, and highly anxious men were less likely to maintain contact with their partners. These associations differed from those among nonseparating couples, supporting the assertion that stressful conditions amplify the negative effects of insecurity.

Another study (J. A. Feeney, 1998) investigated three aspects of partner absence and distancing. The first aspect (physical separation) is considered here, and the others (discouraging of proximity, closeness–distance struggles) are considered in the next section. In one part of the study, participants provided open-ended reports of their experiences of being physically separated from their current dating partners. Content analyses linked secure attachment with less separation distress, with more constructive coping strategies, and with perceptions that the experience had strengthened the couple bond. For example, discomfort with closeness was strongly predictive of males' separation behavior, being related to less support seeking and more emotion-focused coping (including substance use). In contrast, relationship anxiety was associated for both genders with less diverse coping strategies, and, for women, with reports of failing to discuss relationship issues on reunion.

Severe Relationship Conflict

Like long-term or unexpected separations, severe conflict may threaten the couple bond. A laboratory study of dating couples (Simpson, Rholes, & Phillips, 1996) addressed this question by randomly assigning couples to discuss either a minor or a major relationship conflict. More anxious-ambivalent participants reported feeling more distress and hostility during the discussions; furthermore, trained raters rated more ambivalent men and women as showing more anxiety, and avoidant men as engaging in lower-quality interactions. However, these effects were stronger for couples discussing *major* problems, again highlighting the impact of relational stressors. Anxious-ambivalent participants who discussed major problems also perceived their relationships more negatively after the discussion than before; these changes were not mediated by the quality of discussion, suggesting that the negative perceptions reflect the pervasive effects of insecure working models. Interestingly, however, diary reports of everyday social interactions (Pietromonaco & Barrett, 1997) suggest that preoccupied individuals perceive high-conflict interactions as more satisfying than other individuals do, presumably because these interactions tend to involve high levels of partner attention and mutual disclosure.

In the second part of the J. A. Feeney (1998) study, couples engaged in three conflict-centered interactions. One interaction involved conflict over a specific issue (use of leisure time); the other two were designed to elicit attachment-related anxiety by having one partner rebuff the other's attempts to maintain closeness (the role of the distant, discouraging partner was adopted by the male in one interaction, and by the female in the other). Before these interactions, participants rated their expectations of their partners' behavior and motives; after each episode, they rated their own satisfaction with the interaction. In addition, trained observers rated participants' affect, nonverbal behavior, and conversation patterns. Secure attachment was related to participants' positive expectations and greater satisfaction for all interactions. In contrast, secure attachment was unrelated to observers' ratings of responses to issue-based conflict, but predicted less negative affect, less withdrawal, and more constructive conversation in response to partners' distancing. These results again integrate two key findings: Attachment style exerts pervasive effects on *global perceptions* of relationships, but it is most evident in *observable behavior* in challenging situations.

Partner distancing is also relevant to closeness–distance struggles. Closeness–distance (or autonomy–connection) is a basic relational dilemma: Intimate partners must give up some autonomy in order to forge a connection, but too much emphasis on connection may stifle partners' individual identities. Given that proximity seeking is a key function of attachment behavior, conflicts about closeness and distance are likely to activate the attachment system, and may prove intractable if partners differ markedly in their attachment orientations (Byng-Hall, 1999; Pistole, 1994). The final part of the J. A. Feeney (1998) study addressed this issue. Participants were asked to talk about their current relationships; the transcripts were coded for content relevant to the closeness–distance theme, including reports of ongoing struggles over this issue (see J. A. Feeney, 1999b). Almost all participants (92%) made some reference to the closeness–distance theme. However, ongoing struggles were reported more frequently when the male member of a couple was uncomfortable with closeness or the female member was anxious about relationships. Some couples in which both partners were insecure reported highly distressing cycles of pursuing–distancing, in which each partner's behavior exacerbated the insecurities of the other. This finding attests to the difficult emotional climate of these relationships. Similarly, Bartholomew and Allison (2006) suggested that pursuing–distancing cycles often reflect incompatible attachment needs (usually involving one anxious and one avoidant partner), whereas pursuer–pursuer struggles may arise when both partners are relatively high in relationship anxiety. With both of these patterns, failure to achieve distance regulation may result in escalating conflict and couple violence.

The relevance of attachment issues to the course of couple conflict is further evidenced by studies of hurt feelings in couple relationships. In one of these studies (J. A. Feeney, 2005), content analysis of victims' retrospective reports of hurtful events, together with ratings by expert judges, supported the proposition that hurt feelings are elicited by relational transgressions that signal a threat to positive working models. That is, the sense of personal injury that is a distinctive feature of hurt feelings reflects damage to the victim's view of the self as worthy of love and attention, and/or to core beliefs about the dependability and trustworthiness of attachment figures. There is also evidence that individual differences in attachment security predict the long-term outcomes of hurtful events (J. A. Feeney, 2004). For example, as already noted, individuals who are anxious about their relationships respond to hurtful partner behavior with high levels of distress and self-blame, which tend to maintain their fears and self-doubts. Furthermore, avoidant individuals tend to perceive their partners as lacking remorse for hurtful behavior, and this perception fuels relationship conflict.

Attachment and Relationship Quality: Further Comments

It is important to note that although attachment measures seem to tap relatively enduring individual differences, attachment style is *not* redundant with basic dimensions of personality. Relations between measures of attachment and personality tend to be modest in size (Bartholomew & Horowitz, 1991; J. A. Feeney, Noller, & Hanrahan, 1994; Noftle & Shaver, 2006; Shaver & Brennan, 1992). In addition, relationship outcomes such as satisfaction and commitment are better predicted by attachment measures than by personality measures (Noftle & Shaver, 2006; Shaver & Brennan, 1992).

Furthermore, although several studies of romantic attachment have simply correlated various self-report measures, this is by no means the only methodology that has been used. Some studies have related attachment measures to independent ratings of behavior (e.g., Mikulincer & Nachshon, 1991; Simpson et al., 1996) or to interview and diary-based reports of relationship functioning (e.g., Bradford et al., 2002; J. A. Feeney, Noller, & Callan, 1994). Others have gathered corroborative reports from friends (Bartholomew & Horowitz, 1991) or romantic partners (Kobak & Hazan, 1991), or have demonstrated the ability of attachment measures to predict relationship outcomes at later points in time (e.g., J. A. Feeney et al., 2001; Shaver & Brennan, 1992). As further evidence of the validity of self-reports of romantic attachment, these measures have been linked to indices of unconscious processes, including cognitive processing of relational information (e.g., Baldwin et al., 1993; Beinstein Miller, 2001; Mikulincer, Gillath, & Shaver, 2002; see Mikulincer & Shaver, Chapter 23, this volume) and physiological processes related to arousal and affect regulation (e.g., Diamond & Hicks, 2005; Fraley & Shaver, 1997). Finally, studies have supported specific predictions concerning the relative strength of association between attachment measures and particular behaviors—for example, responses to major versus minor conflicts (Simpson et al., 1996) and to relationship-based versus issue-based conflicts (J. A. Feeney, 1998). These studies are sufficient in number and diversity to indicate that measures of romantic attachment do not simply tap a generalized tendency to perceive or report events more or less favorably.

SUMMARY AND FUTURE DIRECTIONS

The proposition that couple relationships can be understood in terms of attachment principles has generated immense interest, and by early 2006, more than 1,000 authors had cited Hazan and Shaver's (1987) groundbreaking studies. The attachment perspective has important strengths, as Shaver and Hazan (1988) and others (e.g., Clark & Reis, 1988) have noted. Attachment theory addresses a wide range of relationship issues, including anxiety, loneliness, and grief; it enables healthy and unhealthy forms of love to be explained in terms of the same principles; and it is developmental in focus (the concept of working models can account for the continuity of early patterns of relating, and also for the possibility of change).

Attachment theory seems to be especially useful in addressing certain key issues in the study of couple relationships, such as conflict. This theory helps to explain both the sources of relationship conflict and individual differences in handling conflict. Research suggests that the relationship anxiety, or attachment anxiety, dimension of attachment style is of particular importance here. Highly anxious individuals report more relationship conflict, suggesting that much of this conflict is driven by basic insecurities over issues of love, loss, and abandonment. Those who are anxious about relationships also adopt coercive and distrusting ways of dealing with conflict, which are likely to produce the very outcomes they fear.

The studies discussed in this chapter point to considerable advances within adult attachment research. Methodological developments include the four-group model, which is grounded in Bowlby's concept of working models of self and others; and the move from categorical to continuous measures, which provide fuller and more precise description of attachment patterns.

Despite these advances, important issues remain unresolved. One issue raised in this chapter concerns the need to clarify patterns of stability and change in attachment organization, including the intraindividual and relational processes that shape these patterns. This issue may be clarified by longitudinal studies that follow individuals as their first romantic relationships develop—and, just as importantly, that track individuals who move from relationship to relationship. We are also some way from understanding the link between the experiences children have with their caregivers and the expectations they develop of romantic partners. It has been argued that whereas the matching between parent and child attachment styles is guided by identification, the matching between romantic partners may reflect self-verification processes (i.e., the tendency to prefer those who confirm expectations of the self in relation to others; see Pietromonaco & Carnelley, 1994). Although this explanation is plausible, it is not clear how or when self-verification processes become relevant to partner matching. In addition, recent data suggest the utility of exploring not only the partner characteristics that are sought by different attachment groups, but also the link between attachment style and willingness to compromise when choosing a mate (Tolmacz, 2004).

Among recent endeavors within romantic attachment research, two that stand out as particularly useful are studies of the dyadic nature of attachment effects and studies of variables that mediate the association between security and relationship functioning. As outlined in this chapter, both types of studies shed light on the complex ways in which security and insecurity are played out in couple relationships. Furthermore, these studies have vital implications for practice, and hence for enhancing relationship stability. In addition, it is important for researchers to integrate findings emerging from studies of couple relationships and from studies of the "individual mind" (see Mikulincer & Shaver, Chapter 23, this volume). Initiatives such as these will broaden the contribution made by the attachment perspective on close relationships.

REFERENCES

Ainsworth, M. D. S. (1989). Attachments beyond infancy. *American Psychologist, 44,* 709–716.

Ainsworth, M. D. S., Blehar, M. C., Waters, E., & Wall, S. (1978). *Patterns of attachment: A psychological study of the Strange Situation.* Hillsdale, NJ: Erlbaum.

Anders, S. L., & Tucker, J. S. (2000). Adult attachment style, interpersonal communication competence, and social support. *Personal Relationships, 7,* 379–389.

Baldwin, M. W., & Fehr, B. (1995). On the instability of attachment style ratings. *Personal Relationships, 2,* 247–261.

Baldwin, M. W., Fehr, B., Keedian, E., Seidel, M., & Thomson, D. W. (1993). An exploration of the relational schemata underlying attachment styles: Self-report and lexical decision approaches. *Personality and Social Psychology Bulletin, 19,* 746–754.

Baldwin, M. W., Keelan, J. P. R., Fehr, B., Enns, V., & Koh-Rangarajoo, E. (1996). Social-cognitive conceptualization of attachment working models: Availability and accessibility effects. *Journal of Personality and Social Psychology, 71,* 94–109.

Banse, R. (2004). Adult attachment and marital satisfaction: Evidence for dyadic configuration effects. *Journal of Social and Personal Relationships, 21,* 273–282.

Bartholomew, K. (1990). Avoidance of intimacy: An attachment perspective. *Journal of Social and Personal Relationships, 7,* 147–178.

Bartholomew, K., & Allison, C. J. (2006). An attachment perspective on abusive dynamics in intimate relationships. In M. Mikulincer & G. S. Goodman (Eds.), *Dynamics of romantic love: Attachment, caregiving, and sex* (pp. 102–127). New York: Guilford Press.

Bartholomew, K., & Horowitz, L. M. (1991). Attachment styles among young adults: A test of a four-category model. *Journal of Personality and Social Psychology, 61,* 226–244.

Bartholomew, K., & Shaver, P. R. (1998). Methods of assessing adult attachment: Do they converge? In J. A. Simpson & W. S. Rholes (Eds.), *Attachment theory and close relationships* (pp. 25–45). New York: Guilford Press.

Beinstein Miller, J. (2001). Attachment models and memory for conversation. *Journal of Social and Personal Relationships, 18,* 404–422.

Bogaert, A. F., & Sadava, S. (2002). Adult attachment and sexual behavior. *Personal Relationships, 9,* 191–204.

Bowlby, J. (1969/1982). *Attachment and loss: Vol. 1. Attachment.* New York: Basic Books.

Bowlby, J. (1973). *Attachment and loss: Vol. 2. Separation: Anxiety and anger.* New York: Basic Books.

Bowlby, J. (1980). *Attachment and loss: Vol. 3. Loss.* New York: Basic Books.

Bowlby, J. (1988). *A secure base.* New York: Basic Books.

Bradford, S. A., Feeney, J. A., & Campbell, L. (2002). Links between attachment orientations and dispo-

sitional and diary-based measures of disclosure in dating couples: A study of actor and partner effects. *Personal Relationships, 9,* 491–506.

Brennan, K. A., Clark, C. L., & Shaver, P. R. (1998). Self-report measurement of adult attachment: An integrative overview. In J. A. Simpson & W. S. Rholes (Eds.), *Attachment theory and close relationships* (pp. 46–76). New York: Guilford Press.

Brennan, K. A., & Shaver, P. R. (1995). Dimensions of adult attachment, affect regulation, and romantic relationship functioning. *Personality and Social Psychology Bulletin, 21,* 267–283.

Brennan, K. A., Shaver, P. R., & Tobey, A. E. (1991). Attachment styles, gender and parental problem drinking. *Journal of Social and Personal Relationships, 8,* 451–466.

Bretherton, I. (1990). Open communication and internal working models: Their role in the development of attachment relationships. In R. A. Thompson (Ed.), *Nebraska Symposium on Motivation: Vol. 36. Socioemotional development* (pp. 59–113). Lincoln: University of Nebraska Press.

Byng-Hall, J. (1999). Family couple therapy: Toward greater security. In J. Cassidy & P. R. Shaver (Eds.), *Handbook of attachment: Theory, research, and clinical applications* (pp. 625–645). New York: Guilford Press.

Cafferty, T. P., Davis, K. E., Medway, F. J., O'Hearn, R. E., & Chappell, K. D. (1994). Reunion dynamics among couples separated during Operation Desert Storm: An attachment theory analysis. In K. Bartholomew & D. Perlman (Eds.), *Advances in personal relationships: Vol. 5. Attachment processes in adulthood* (pp. 309–330). London: Jessica Kingsley.

Campbell, L., Simpson, J. A., Kashy, D. A., & Rholes, W. S. (2001). Attachment orientations, dependence, and behaviour in a stressful situation: An application of the actor–partner interdependence model. *Journal of Social and Personal Relationships, 18,* 821–843.

Carnelley, K. B., Pietromonaco, P. R., & Jaffe, K. (1996). Attachment, caregiving, and relationship functioning in couples: Effects of self and partner. *Personal Relationships, 3,* 257–277.

Clark, M. S., & Reis, H. T. (1988). Interpersonal processes in close relationships. *Annual Review of Psychology, 39,* 609–672.

Cohn, D. A., Silver, D. H., Cowan, C. P., Cowan, P. A., & Pearson, J. (1992). Working models of childhood attachment and couple relationships. *Journal of Family Issues, 13,* 432–449.

Collins, N. L. (1996). Working models of attachment: Implications for explanation, emotion, and behavior. *Journal of Personality and Social Psychology, 71,* 810–832.

Collins, N. L., Guichard, A. C., Ford, M. B., & Feeney, B. C. (2004). Working models of attachment: New developments and emerging themes. In W. S. Rholes & J. A. Simpson (Eds.), *Adult attachment: Theory, research, and clinical implications* (pp. 196–239). New York: Guilford Press.

Collins, N. J., Guichard, A. C., Ford, M. B., & Feeney, B. C. (2006). Responding to need in intimate relationships: Normative processes and individual differences. In M. Mikulincer & G. S. Goodman (Eds.), *Dynamics of romantic love: Attachment, caregiving, and sex* (pp. 149–189). New York: Guilford Press.

Collins, N. L., & Read, S. J. (1990). Adult attachment, working models, and relationship quality in dating couples. *Journal of Personality and Social Psychology, 58,* 644–663.

Collins, N. L., & Read, S. J. (1994). Cognitive representations of attachment: The structure and function of working models. In K. Bartholomew & D. Perlman (Eds.), *Advances in personal relationships: Vol. 5. Attachment processes in adulthood* (pp. 53–90). London: Jessica Kingsley.

Creasey, G., & Hesson-McInness, M. (2001). Affective responses, cognitive appraisals, and conflict tactics in late adolescent romantic relationships: Associations with attachment orientations. *Journal of Counseling Psychology, 48,* 85–96.

Creasey, G., Kershaw, K., & Boston, A. (1999). Conflict management with friends and romantic partners: The role of attachment and negative mood regulation expectancies. *Journal of Youth and Adolescence, 28,* 523–543.

Crittenden, P. (1985). Social networks, quality of childrearing, and child development. *Child Development, 56,* 1299–1313.

Crowell, J. A., & Owens, G. (1996). *Current Relationship Interview and scoring system.* Unpublished manuscript, State University of New York at Stony Brook.

Davila, J., Burge, D., & Hammen, C. (1997). Why does attachment style change? *Journal of Personality and Social Psychology, 73,* 826–836.

Davila, J., & Cobb, R. J. (2004). Predictors of change in attachment security during adulthood. In W. S. Rholes & J. A. Simpson (Eds.), *Adult attachment: Theory, research, and clinical implications* (pp. 133–156). New York: Guilford Press.

Diamond, L. M., & Hicks, A. M. (2005). Attachment style, current relationship security, and negative emotions: The mediating role of physiological regulation. *Journal of Social and Personal Relationships, 22,* 499–518.

Feeney, B. C., & Collins, N. L. (2004). Interpersonal safe haven and secure base caregiving processes in adulthood. In W. S. Rholes & J. A. Simpson (Eds.), *Adult attachment: Theory, research, and clinical implications* (pp. 300–338). New York: Guilford Press.

Feeney, J. A. (1994). Attachment style, communication patterns, and satisfaction across the life cycle of marriage. *Personal Relationships, 1,* 333–348.

Feeney, J. A. (1995). Adult attachment and emotional control. *Personal Relationships, 2,* 143–159.

Feeney, J. A. (1996). Attachment, caregiving, and marital satisfaction. *Personal Relationships, 3,* 401–416.

Feeney, J. A. (1998). Adult attachment and relationship-centered anxiety: Responses to physical and emotional distancing. In J. A. Simpson & W. S. Rholes (Eds.), *Attachment theory and close relationships* (pp. 189–218). New York: Guilford Press.

Feeney, J. A. (1999a). Adult attachment, emotional control, and marital satisfaction. *Personal Relationships, 6,* 169–185.

Feeney, J. A. (1999b). Issues of closeness and distance in dating relationships: Effects of sex and attachment style. *Journal of Social and Personal Relationships, 16,* 571–590.

Feeney, J. A. (2002). Attachment, marital interaction, and relationship satisfaction: A diary study. *Personal Relationships, 9,* 39–55.

Feeney, J. A. (2003). The systemic nature of couple relationships: An attachment perspective. In P. Erdman & T. Caffery (Eds.), *Attachment and family systems: Conceptual, empirical and therapeutic relatedness* (pp. 139–163). New York: Brunner/Mazel.

Feeney, J. A. (2004). Hurt feelings in couple relationships: Toward integrative models of the negative effects of hurtful events. *Journal of Social and Personal Relationships, 21,* 487–508.

Feeney, J. A. (2005). Hurt feelings in couple relationships: Exploring the role of attachment and perceptions of personal injury. *Personal Relationships, 12,* 253–271.

Feeney, J. A., Alexander, R., Noller, P., & Hohaus, L. (2003). Attachment insecurity, depression, and the transition to parenthood. *Personal Relationships, 10,* 475–493.

Feeney, J. A., & Hohaus, L. (2001). Attachment and spousal caregiving. *Personal Relationships, 8,* 21–39.

Feeney, J. A., Hohaus, L., Noller, P., & Alexander, R. (2001). *Becoming parents: Exploring the bonds between mothers, fathers, and their infants.* Cambridge, UK: Cambridge University Press.

Feeney, J. A., Kelly, L., Gallois, C., Peterson, C., & Terry, D. J. (1999). Attachment style, assertive communication, and safer-sex behavior. *Journal of Applied Social Psychology, 29,* 1964–1983.

Feeney, J. A., & Noller, P. (1990). Attachment style as a predictor of adult romantic relationships. *Journal of Personality and Social Psychology, 58,* 281–291.

Feeney, J. A., & Noller, P. (1991). Attachment style and verbal descriptions of romantic partners. *Journal of Social and Personal Relationships, 8,* 187–215.

Feeney, J. A., & Noller, P. (2004). Attachment and sexuality in close relationships. In J. H. Harvey, A. Wenzel, & S. Sprecher (Eds.), *Handbook of sexuality in close relationships* (pp. 183–201). Mahwah, NJ: Erlbaum.

Feeney, J. A., Noller, P., & Callan, V. J. (1994). Attachment style, communication and satisfaction in the early years of marriage. In K. Bartholomew & D. Perlman (Eds.), *Advances in personal relationships: Vol. 5. Attachment processes in adulthood* (pp. 269–308). London: Jessica Kingsley.

Feeney, J. A., Noller, P., & Hanrahan, M. (1994). Assessing adult attachment: Developments in the conceptualization of security and insecurity. In M. B. Sperling

& W. H. Berman (Eds.), *Attachment in adults: Theory, assessment, and treatment* (pp. 128–152). New York: Guilford Press.

Feeney, J. A., Noller, P., & Patty, J. (1993). Adolescents' interactions with the opposite sex: Influence of attachment style and gender. *Journal of Adolescence, 16*, 169–186.

Feeney, J. A., Peterson, C., Gallois, C., & Terry, D. J. (2000). Attachment style as a predictor of sexual attitudes and behavior in late adolescence. *Psychology and Health, 14*, 1105–1122.

Fossati, A., Feeney, J. A., Donati, D., Donini, M., Novella, L., Bagnato, M., et al. (2003). On the dimensionality of the Attachment Style Questionnaire in Italian clinical and nonclinical participants. *Journal of Social and Personal Relationships, 20*, 55–79.

Fraley, R. C., & Brumbaugh, C. C. (2004). A dynamical systems approach to conceptualizing and studying stability and change in attachment security. In W. S. Rholes & J. A. Simpson (Eds.), *Adult attachment: Theory, research, and clinical implications* (pp. 86–132). New York: Guilford Press.

Fraley, R. C., & Shaver, P. R. (1997). Adult attachment and the suppression of unwanted thoughts. *Journal of Personality and Social Psychology, 73*, 1080–1091.

Fraley, R. C., & Shaver, P. R. (1998). Airport separations: A naturalistic study of adult attachment dynamics in separating couples. *Journal of Personality and Social Psychology, 75*, 1198–1212.

Fraley, R. C., & Waller, N. G. (1998). Adult attachment patterns: A test of the typological model. In J. A. Simpson & W. S. Rholes (Eds.), *Attachment theory and close relationships* (pp. 77–114). New York: Guilford Press.

Gaines, S. O., Work, C., Johnson, H., Youn, M. S. P., & Lai, K. (2000). Impact of attachment style and self-monitoring on individuals' responses to accommodative dilemmas across relationship types. *Journal of Social and Personal Relationships, 17*, 767–789.

Gallo, L. C., & Smith, T. W. (2001). Attachment style in marriage: Adjustment and responses to interaction. *Journal of Social and Personal Relationships, 18*, 263–289.

Gangestad, S. W., & Thornhill, R. (1997). The evolutionary psychology of extrapair sex: The role of fluctuating asymmetry. *Evolution and Human Behavior, 18*, 69–88.

Gentzler, A. L., & Kerns, K. A. (2004). Associations between insecure attachment and sexual experiences. *Personal Relationships, 11*, 249–265.

George, C., Kaplan, N., & Main, M. (1984). *Adult Attachment Interview protocol.* Unpublished manuscript, University of California at Berkeley.

George, C., Kaplan, N., & Main, M. (1985). *Adult Attachment Interview protocol* (2nd ed.). Unpublished manuscript, University of California at Berkeley.

George, C., Kaplan, N., & Main, M. (1996). *Adult Attachment Interview protocol* (3rd ed.). Unpublished manuscript, University of California at Berkeley.

Griffin, D. W., & Bartholomew, K. (1994). The meta-

physics of measurement: The case of adult attachment. In K. Bartholomew & D. W. Perlman (Eds.), *Advances in personal relationships: Vol. 5. Attachment processes in adulthood* (pp. 17–52). London: Jessica Kingsley.

Hammond, J. R., & Fletcher, G. J. O. (1991). Attachment styles and relationship satisfaction in the development of close relationships. *New Zealand Journal of Psychology, 20*, 56–62.

Hazan, C., & Shaver, P. R. (1987). Romantic love conceptualized as an attachment process. *Journal of Personality and Social Psychology, 52*, 511–524.

Hazan, C., & Shaver, P. R. (1994). Attachment as an organizational framework for research on close relationships. *Psychological Inquiry, 5*, 1–22.

Hazan, C., Zeifman, D., & Middleton, K. (1994, July). *Adult romantic attachment, affection, and sex.* Paper presented at the 7th International Conference on Personal Relationships, Groningen, The Netherlands.

Kachadourian, L. K., Fincham, F., & Davila, J. (2004). The tendency to forgive in dating and married couples: The role of attachment and relationship satisfaction. *Personal Relationships, 11*, 373–393.

Kashy, D. A., & Kenny, D. A. (2000). The analysis of data from dyads and groups. In H. T. Reis & C. M. Judd (Eds.), *Handbook of research methods in social and personality psychology* (pp. 451–477). New York: Cambridge University Press.

Keelan, J. P. R., Dion, K. K., & Dion, K. L. (1998). Attachment style and relationship satisfaction: Test of a self-disclosure explanation. *Canadian Journal of Behavioural Science, 30*, 24–35.

Kirkpatrick, L. E., & Davis, K. E. (1994). Attachment style, gender, and relationship stability: A longitudinal analysis. *Journal of Personality and Social Psychology, 66*, 502–512.

Kirkpatrick, L. E., & Hazan, C. (1994). Attachment styles and close relationships: A four-year prospective study. *Personal Relationships, 1*, 123–142.

Kobak, R. R., & Duemmler, S. (1994). Attachment and conversation: Toward a discourse analysis of adolescent and adult security. In K. Bartholomew & D. Perlman (Eds.), *Advances in personal relationships: Vol. 5. Attachment processes in adulthood* (pp. 121–149). London: Jessica Kingsley.

Kobak, R. R., & Hazan, C. (1991). Attachment in marriage: Effects of security and accuracy of working models. *Journal of Personality and Social Psychology, 60*, 861–869.

Kotler, T. (1985). Security and autonomy within marriage. *Human Relations, 38*, 299–321.

Kunce, L. J., & Shaver, P. R. (1994). An attachment-theoretical approach to caregiving in romantic relationships. In K. Bartholomew & D. Perlman (Eds.), *Advances in personal relationships: Vol. 5. Attachment processes in adulthood* (pp. 205–237). London: Jessica Kingsley.

Lee, J. A. (1973). *The colors of love: An exploration of the ways of loving.* Don Mills, ON, Canada: New Press.

Lee, J. A. (1988). Love-styles. In R. J. Sternberg & M. Barnes (Eds.), *The psychology of love* (pp. 38–67). New Haven, CT: Yale University Press.

Levy, M. B., & Davis, K. E. (1988). Lovestyles and attachment styles compared: Their relations to each other and to various relationship characteristics. *Journal of Social and Personal Relationships, 5*, 439–471.

Main, M., & Goldwyn, R. (1984). *Adult attachment scoring and classification system.* Unpublished manuscript, University of California at Berkeley.

Main, M., Goldwyn, R., & Hesse, E. (2003). *Adult attachment scoring and classification system.* Unpublished manuscript, University of California at Berkeley.

Main, M., Kaplan, N., & Cassidy, J. (1985). Security in infancy, childhood, and adulthood: A move to the level of representation. In I. Bretherton & E. Waters (Eds.), Growing points of attachment theory and research. *Monographs of the Society for Research in Child Development, 50*(1–2, Serial No. 209), 66–104.

Main, M., & Solomon, J. (1990). Procedures for identifying infants as disorganized/disoriented during the Ainsworth Strange Situation. In M. T. Greenberg, D. Cicchetti, & E. M. Cummings (Eds.), *Attachment in the preschool years: Theory, research, and intervention* (pp. 121–160). Chicago: University of Chicago Press.

Meyers, S. A., & Landsberger, S. A. (2002). Direct and indirect pathways between adult attachment style and marital satisfaction. *Personal Relationships, 9*, 159–172.

Mikulincer, M., Florian, V., Birnbaum, G., & Malishkevich, S. (2002). The death-anxiety buffering function of close relationships: Exploring the effects of separation reminders on death-thought accessibility. *Personality and Social Psychology Bulletin, 28*, 287–299.

Mikulincer, M., Gillath, O., & Shaver, P. R. (2002). Activation of the attachment system in adulthood: Threat-related primes increase the accessibility of mental representations of attachment figures. *Journal of Personality and Social Psychology, 83*, 881–895.

Mikulincer, M., & Goodman, G. S. (Eds.). (2006). *Dynamics of romantic love: Attachment, caregiving, and sex.* New York: Guilford Press.

Mikulincer, M., & Nachshon, O. (1991). Attachment styles and patterns of self-disclosure. *Journal of Personality and Social Psychology, 61*, 321–331.

Mikulincer, M., & Shaver, P. R. (2007). *Attachment in adulthood: Structure, dynamics, and change.* New York: Guilford Press.

Noftle, E. E., & Shaver, P. R. (2006). Attachment dimensions and the Big Five personality traits: Associations and comparative ability to predict relationship quality. *Journal of Research in Personality, 40*, 179–208.

O'Connell Corcoran, K., & Mallinckrodt, B. (2000). Adult attachment, self-efficacy, perspective taking, and conflict resolution. *Journal of Counseling and Development, 78*, 473–483.

Overall, N. C., Fletcher, G. J. O., & Friesen, M. D. (2003). Mapping the intimate relationship mind: Comparisons between three models of attachment representations. *Personality and Social Psychology Bulletin, 29*, 1479–1493.

Peele, S. (1975). *Love and addiction.* New York: Taplinger.

Pietromonaco, P. R., & Barrett, L. F. (1997). Working models of attachment and daily social interactions. *Journal of Personality and Social Psychology, 73*, 1409–1423.

Pietromonaco, P. R., & Carnelley, K. B. (1994). Gender and working models of attachment: Consequences for perceptions of self and romantic relationships. *Personal Relationships, 1*, 63–82.

Pietromonaco, P. R., Greenwood, D., & Barrett, L. F. (2004). Conflict in adult close relationships: An attachment perspective. In W. S. Rholes & J. A. Simpson (Eds.), *Adult attachment: Theory, research, and clinical implications* (pp. 267–299). New York: Guilford Press.

Pistole, M. C. (1989). Attachment in adult romantic relationships: Style of conflict resolution and relationship satisfaction. *Journal of Social and Personal Relationships, 6*, 505–510.

Pistole, M. C. (1994). Adult attachment styles: Some thoughts on closeness–distance struggles. *Family Process, 33*, 147–159.

Priel, B., & Besser, A. (2000). Adult attachment styles, early relationships, antenatal attachment, and perceptions of infant temperament: A study of first-time mothers. *Personal Relationships, 7*, 291–310.

Rahim, M. A. (1983). A measure of styles of handling interpersonal conflict. *Academy of Management Journal, 26*, 368–376.

Roberts, L. J., & Greenberg, D. R. (2002). Observational "windows" to intimacy processes in marriage. In P. Noller & J. A. Feeney (Eds.), *Understanding marriage: Developments in the study of couple interaction* (pp. 118–149). Cambridge, UK: Cambridge University Press.

Rothbard, J. C., & Shaver, P. R. (1994). Continuity of attachment across the life span. In M. B. Sperling & W. H. Berman (Eds.), *Attachment in adults: Theory, assessment, and treatment* (pp. 31–71). New York: Guilford Press.

Schachner, D. A., & Shaver, P. R. (2004). Attachment dimensions and sexual motives. *Personal Relationships, 11*, 179–195.

Scharfe, E., & Bartholomew, K. (1994). Reliability and stability of adult attachment patterns. *Personal Relationships, 1*, 23–43.

Senchak, M., & Leonard, K. E. (1992). Attachment styles and marital adjustment among newlywed couples. *Journal of Social and Personal Relationships, 9*, 51–64.

Shaver, P. R., & Brennan, K. A. (1992). Attachment styles and the "Big Five" personality traits: Their connections with each other and with romantic relationship outcomes. *Personality and Social Psychology Bulletin, 18*, 536–545.

Shaver, P. R., & Hazan, C. (1988). A biased overview of

the study of love. *Journal of Social and Personal Relationships, 5,* 473–501.

Shaver, P. R., Hazan, C., & Bradshaw, D. (1988). Love as attachment: The integration of three behavioral systems. In R. J. Sternberg & M. Barnes (Eds.), *The psychology of love* (pp. 68–99). New Haven, CT: Yale University Press.

Shaver, P. R., & Mikulincer, M. (2006). A behavioral systems approach to romantic love relationships: Attachment, caregiving, and sex. In R. J. Sternberg & K. Weis (Eds.), *The new psychology of love* (pp. 35–64). New Haven, CT: Yale University Press.

Simpson, J. A. (1990). Influence of attachment styles on romantic relationships. *Journal of Personality and Social Psychology, 59,* 971–980.

Simpson, J. A., & Rholes, W. S. (1994). Stress and secure base relationships in adulthood. In K. Bartholomew & D. Perlman (Eds.), *Advances in personal relationships: Vol. 5. Attachment processes in adulthood* (pp. 181–204). London: Jessica Kingsley.

Simpson, J. A., Rholes, W. S., & Nelligan, J. S. (1992). Support seeking and support giving within couples in an anxiety-provoking situation: The role of attachment styles. *Journal of Personality and Social Psychology, 62,* 434–446.

Simpson, J. A., Rholes, W. S., & Phillips, D. (1996). Conflict in close relationships: An attachment perspective. *Journal of Personality and Social Psychology, 71,* 899–914.

Sprecher, S., & McKinney, K. (1993). *Sexuality.* Newbury Park, CA: Sage.

Sternberg, R. J. (1986). A triangular theory of love. *Psychological Review, 93,* 119–135.

Sternberg, R. J., & Weis, K. (Eds.). (2006). *The new psychology of love.* New Haven, CT: Yale University Press.

Strahan, B. J. (1991). Attachment theory and family functioning: Expectations and congruencies. *Australian Journal of Marriage and Family, 12,* 12–26.

Sumer, N., & Cozzarelli, C. (2004). The impact of adult attachment on partner and self-attributions and relationship quality. *Personal Relationships, 11,* 355–371.

Tennov, D. (1979). *Love and limerence: The experience of being in love.* New York: Stein & Day.

Tolmacz, R. (2004). Attachment style and willingness to compromise when choosing a mate. *Journal of Social and Personal Relationships, 21,* 267–272.

Tracy, J. L., Shaver, P. R., Cooper, M. L., & Albino, A. W. (2003). Attachment styles and adolescent sexuality. In P. Florsheim (Ed.), *Adolescent romance and sexual behavior: Theory, research, and practical implications* (pp. 137–159). Mahwah, NJ: Erlbaum.

Weiss, R. S. (1982). Attachment in adult life. In C. M. Parkes & J. Stevenson-Hinde (Eds.), *The place of attachment in human behavior* (pp. 171–184). New York: Basic Books.

Weiss, R. S. (1986). Continuities and transformations in social relationships from childhood to adulthood. In W. W. Hartup & Z. Rubin (Eds.), *Relationships and development* (pp. 95–110). Hillsdale, NJ: Erlbaum.

Weiss, R. S. (1991). The attachment bond in childhood and adulthood. In C. M. Parkes, J. Stevenson-Hinde, & P. Marris (Eds.), *Attachment across the life cycle* (pp. 66–76). London: Tavistock/Routledge.

CHAPTER 22

Same-Sex Romantic Attachment

JONATHAN J. MOHR

Without warning as a whirlwind swoops on an oak love shakes my heart.
—SAPPHO

Same-sex romantic relationships appear to have existed in most cultures throughout recorded history, regardless of prevailing attitudes toward homosexuality and bisexuality (Boswell, 1994). The scientific study of same-sex couples has evolved over the past several decades from an early emphasis on atheoretical, descriptive research to a more recent focus on the application of theories that were originally developed to explain heterosexual relationship functioning (Kurdek, 1995). The emerging empirical literature on lesbian and gay male relationships provides strong evidence that the similarities between heterosexual and same-sex relationships far outweigh the differences (Kurdek, 2005; Peplau & Spalding, 2003).

This chapter provides a basis for applying John Bowlby's attachment theory to same-sex love relationships. Although attachment researchers initially focused on the infant–caregiver bond, the past decade has witnessed a tremendous growth in the number of studies using attachment theory as a framework for investigating adult romantic relationships (see J. A. Feeney, Chapter 21, and Mikulincer & Shaver, Chapter 23, this volume; see also Mikulincer & Shaver, 2007). This research has shown not only that romantic love may be profitably conceptualized as part of an attachment-

related process, but that many aspects of relationship functioning can be reliably predicted by differences in the ways individuals internally represent their attachment relationships (i.e., differences in their working models of attachment). For example, studies have shown that positive working models of self and other are related to a wide variety of adaptive relationship behaviors, including effective conflict resolution (e.g., Campbell, Simpson, Boldry, & Kashy, 2005), support seeking and giving (Kunce & Shaver, 1994; Simpson, Rholes, & Nelligan, 1992), positive communication (J. A. Feeney, Noller, & Callan, 1994), and joint problem solving (Kobak & Hazan, 1991).

The vast majority of work on adult romantic attachment has focused on heterosexual relationships. Only a small handful of publications have acknowledged the potential relevance of attachment theory to lesbian, gay male, and bisexual (LGB) people or included empirical investigations focusing on this population. Conducting research with heterosexual couples may be less challenging (e.g., may require less effort in recruiting participants) and less controversial (i.e., more socially acceptable) than research with same-sex couples; however, the inclusion of same-sex partnerships in attachment research may lead to a broader understanding of adult attachment processes. For example, the study of same-sex attachments may help to illuminate ways in which gender and attachment interact in the dynamics of relationship functioning. Furthermore, relationship difficulties associated with the pervasive societal intolerance of same-sex partnerships (Soule, 2004) may provide an opportunity to understand the role of attachment in how couples manage chronic stress and stigma. Finally, strong arguments have been made concerning the ethical importance of including LGB individuals in mainstream psychological research (Herek, Kimmel, Amaro, & Melton, 1991).

This chapter first explores the evolutionary basis for same-sex attraction and provides an argument for the relevance of the attachment system for LGB adults. The current empirical literature on same-sex couples is then reviewed, with an emphasis on results suggestive of attachment-related processes. Finally, Bowlby's work on fear and loss is used to illustrate ways in which the study of same-sex couples may provide fertile ground for the exploration of questions about the points of intersection between contextual and intrapersonal forces.

EVOLUTION, SEXUAL ORIENTATION, AND SAME-SEX ATTACHMENT

Perhaps one of the cleverest challenges to confront evolutionary theory is homosexuality. Homosexuality seems to be a tailor-made rebuttal of the great evolutionary credo—survival of the fittest. How do we explain what is often a lifelong preference for nonreproductive sex?
—McKnight (1997, p. x)

At the core of Bowlby's theory is the idea that the human propensity for establishing affectional bonds is adaptive from an evolutionary perspective (Bowlby, 1969/1982; Simpson & Belsky, Chapter 6, this volume). The infant–caregiver bond, the romantic partnership, and the intimate friendship all ultimately serve to enhance reproductive success. It is perhaps easiest to intuitively understand the adaptive value of the infant–caregiver bond. In the environment of early humans, the chances of survival were greatest for infants who were predisposed to engage in behaviors that ensured proximity to their caregivers, so that the caregivers would be in a good position to protect them from natural threats (e.g., attack from predators, drowning). The attachment system has evolved to be activated most strongly in situations that are potentially most threatening to an infant's well-being,

such as lack of proximity to caregivers, presence of strangers, strange surroundings, and weakened infant state. Bowlby (1969/1982) offered evidence of this phenomenon in humans, nonhuman primates, and other animals (e.g., lambs and deer). From an evolutionary perspective, the survival of an infant is usually in the best interests of both the infant and his or her parents, because they all have a stake in passing along their genes. This explains the proposed survival advantage that has been accorded to parents with a readily activated caregiving system. Parents with a predisposition to maintain proximity to their infants and to respond readily to their infants' attachment behaviors are thought to have been more likely to have children who would survive into adulthood and pass along the parents' genes (see George & Solomon, Chapter 36, this volume).

To a great extent, our reproductive advantage as humans is a function of lifespan. The longer we live, the more chances we have to reproduce and raise our children into their healthy adulthood, and to provide care for our children's children. The longer we live, the more opportunities we have to offer help to our kin and thus support another venue for the survival of our genetic code. From this viewpoint, attachment relationships in adulthood may serve the same adaptive function that they do in infancy. West and Sheldon-Keller (1994) argued that the "function of attachment, the provision of safety and security, remains constant throughout the life span, although the mechanisms of achieving this function change and develop with maturation" (p. 22).

Thus, from an attachment perspective, romantic attachments provide adults with reliable relationships upon which they can depend for protection, care, and support during times of greatest need (e.g., sickness, economic hardship, violent attack). The establishment of stable romantic attachments may then increase the likelihood of surviving into old age and enjoying the reproductive advantage this affords. Furthermore, the reciprocal attachments that characterize adult romantic relationships may serve to discourage dissolution and thus provide a more secure environment for children (see Simpson & Belsky, Chapter 6, this volume).

Such propositions regarding potential functional advantages of romantic attachment have been mostly unsubstantiated because of the difficulty of testing propositions about human evolution. However, Fraley, Brumbaugh, and Marks (2005) used comparative and phylogenetic methods to identify characteristics that may have co-evolved with adult pair bonding across species. Results indicated that pair bonding coevolved with paternal investment in childrearing, whereas pair bonding did not coevolve with extended periods of childhood development. Furthermore, on the basis of evidence that paternal care developed before pair bonding, Fraley and colleagues concluded that it is more likely that pair bonding evolved from processes related to paternal care than vice versa. Although the analysis was unable to identify a specific mechanism underlying this evolutionary sequence, the authors suggested that it may be related to the greater likelihood of close and frequent contact between mates in species with high levels of paternal caregiving. This increased level of contact may have stimulated a pair-bonding process through the biobehavioral systems that had already evolved to facilitate the infant–caregiver bond. This perspective is consistent with the view that pair bonding is an adaptation of the infant–caregiver attachment system. In short, although many propositions about the function of romantic attachment remain untested, evidence from Fraley and colleagues' study clearly links pair bonding with processes associated with infant caregiving. Furthermore, the study suggests that pair bonding did not evolve to ensure protection of the young in species with an extended period of childhood development.

The existence of same-sex romantic relationships and homoerotic attraction and behavior has long posed a vexing problem for evolutionary theorists. As one writer put it, "Homosexuals were with us through antiquity and, if recent history is any guide, are a robust minority within society. So why hasn't male homosexuality died out as a less reproductive strain of humanity?" (McKnight, 1997, p. 1). Some of the earliest uses of evolutionary theory to address same-sex attractions appeared in the medical literature of the late 19th century (Gibson, 1997). At that time, a common explanation for mental disorders was degeneration theory, which proposed that weakness of the nervous system caused individuals to be especially vulnerable to the primitive impulses constituting our evolutionary legacy. Individuals unable to resist the "beast within" were thought to fall several notches on the evolutionary ladder. Homosexuality was almost always viewed as a form of degeneration in which the original "bi-sexuality of the ancestors of the race, shown in the rudimentary female organs of the male, could not fail to occasion functional, if not organic, reversions when mental or physi-

cal manifestations were interfered with by disease or congenital defect" (Kiernan, 1888, quoted in Gibson, 1997, p. 115). Although such reversions were viewed in quite negative terms (and, as demonstrated below, were often linked with masturbation), some doctors recognized the existence of genuine romantic attachments between members of the same sex:

> [Sexual perversions are] frequently produced on the neurotic soil of the male and female masturbator. The female masturbator of this type usually becomes excessively prudish, despises and hates the opposite sex, and frequently forms a furious attachment for another woman, to whom she unselfishly devotes herself. (Kiernan, 1888, quoted in Gibson, 1997, p. 116)

It is likely that this form of "furious" attachment was no more intense than those exhibited in 19th-century heterosexual love relationships. By focusing on same-sex love as a form of deviant sexuality, doctors were unable to recognize that such love was much more than a pitiable and loathsome expression of primitive sexual instincts. Although the outdated language of this example may make its absurdity evident, one does not need to look far to find similar examples from our own time. For example, same-sex couples today are sometimes accused of flaunting their sexuality when exhibiting normal attachment or courting behavior, such as holding hands in public (Herek, 1991).

Bowlby also discussed homosexuality from an evolutionary perspective, but his thinking was markedly different from that of the degeneration theorists. Whereas 19th-century doctors viewed same-sex attraction as a lapse into brutish and uncivilized instinctive behavior, Bowlby appeared to think of homosexuality as the product of an efficient but functionally ineffective behavioral apparatus. In the first volume of his trilogy, he observed that the sexual behavioral system in same-sex dyads works perfectly well, in that the predictable outcome of orgasm is routinely achieved (Bowlby, 1969/1982). The puzzle, according to Bowlby, is in why the sexual system would ever be organized in a way that runs explicitly counter to intuitive notions of reproductive fitness: "What makes it [same-sex attraction] functionally ineffective is that for some reason the system has developed in such a way that its predictable outcome is unrelated to function" (pp. 130–131). He illustrated this notion of misguided behavior by comparing homosexual sex to an antiaircraft gun that works perfectly, except that it consistently destroys friendly planes rather than enemy ones. This analogy may lack appeal for individuals in same-sex relationships, but it conveys Bowlby's idea that the sexual behavioral system of homosexuals is not serving its functional goal of reproduction.

Although Bowlby clearly saw homosexual desire as evidence of a functional mistake in the evolutionary sense, his limited discussion of the topic at no time denied that legitimate, psychologically healthy same-sex romantic attachments exist. Indeed, his writings about homosexual behavior in a variety of animals primarily reveal his curiosity about the degree to which the sexual behavioral system is environmentally labile. He did not explicitly discuss same-sex couples, but it is likely that he viewed their relationships as subject to the same psychological principles as heterosexual romantic attachment relationships. Bowlby maintained that the attachment behavioral system is active from "the cradle to the grave" (1988, p. 82), and he never gave any indication that he believed this to be true only for individuals in heterosexual couples. In her initial writings about adult attachment, Mary Ainsworth, Bowlby's collaborative partner, noted that same-sex romantic attachments are likely to function in the same manner as heterosexual attachments (Ainsworth, 1985). She stated that one of the main differences between these two kinds of romantic attachment is that only one of them (i.e., heterosexual attachment) is sanctioned by society. This observation points to the importance of context in the development of attachment bonds—a topic discussed later in this chapter.

Bowlby's (1969/1982) discussion of homosexuality was based on his understanding of evolutionary theory, which was not informed by the currently accepted notion that evolutionary success is focused on the survival of the gene (Dawkins, 1976; Kirkpatrick, 1998). As noted below, evolutionary theorists have described possible scenarios wherein homosexuality may contribute to reproductive fitness even when lesbians and gay men do not have children themselves.

Within the past several decades, a number of interesting and controversial propositions have been made regarding the evolutionary basis of homosexuality (McKnight, 1997), and these have been met with strident opposition and critique (Dickemann, 1995; McKnight, 1997; Weinrich, 1995). If homosexuality is indeed "one of the cleverest challenges to confront evolutionary theory" (McKnight, 1997, p. 1), then it is not surprising that attempts to explain it in terms of reproduc-

tive fitness have created such controversy. Bowlby himself noted that the "task of determining precisely what the function of a certain piece of instinctive behavior is may be considerable" (Bowlby, 1969/1982, p. 133). A complete discussion of recent evolutionary theories of homosexuality is beyond the scope of this chapter, but a few of the most notable theories are mentioned here.

Evolutionary theorists, faced with the problem of explaining the continued appearance of same-sex attraction throughout history, have assumed that there is a genetic component to homosexuality and bisexuality. Although many specific theories have been advanced to address this problem, a number of them come down to the proposition that "gay genes" offer a direct reproductive advantage to women and men who engage in heterosexual relations. Hutchinson (1959) was one the first theorists to offer a scientifically grounded discussion of this possibility (McKnight, 1997). He applied then-current ideas about the adaptive value of the sickle-cell mutation prevalent in some African and Asian populations to evolutionary explanations of homosexuality. The sickle-cell mutation was found to increase resistance to malaria. Although homozygous sickle-cell children (i.e., children with two sickle-cell genes) exhibited strong resistance to malaria, they would often die of severe anemia before reaching puberty. Heterozygous children (i.e., children with one sickle-cell gene and one "normal" gene) would gain a measure of protection from malaria, but would not develop the lethal anemia. These children thus had an advantage over both the children with two sickle-cell genes and those with two "normal" genes; such an advantage is called "heterozygous superior fitness."

The argument regarding homosexuality runs along similar lines, although little consensus exists regarding the ways in which a "gay gene" may contribute to evolutionary success. Theories regarding the reproductive advantages afforded by gay genetic material include the ideas that the genes are linked to (1) greater male sex drive; (2) greater female sex drive (i.e., the so-called "overloving effect"; Hamer & Copeland, 1994); and (3) traits such as charm, empathy, and intelligence that are attractive to females (McKnight, 1997). Another popular theory is that male homosexuality is somehow linked to a genetic predisposition for kin-selective altruism, although most variants of this theory do not appear to stand up to rigorous inspection (McKnight, 1997). According to one version of the kin-selective hypothesis, males with the gay gene instinctively feel at a reproductive disadvantage and decide to divert their energies into supporting the reproductive fitness of close family members (Dickemann, 1995; Salais & Fischer, 1995; Wilson, 1975). Some scientists have suggested that homosexuality is the by-product of a hypervariable mutation in the X chromosome that serves as part of a larger process of ensuring species variability (Hamer & Copeland, 1994). Observational studies of nonhuman primates have shown that sexual interactions between members of the same sex are as enduring as those between members of the opposite sexes (Pavelka, 1995). Evolutionary explanations of this phenomenon include arguments that same-sex attractions may reduce tension, promote coalition formation, reduce mating competition, and control the population.

Despite uncertainty regarding the reproductive advantages associated with the hypothesized "gay gene," many evolutionary theorists agree on the mechanisms that maintain this material in the gene pool (McKnight, 1997). A form of natural selection called "balance selection" is thought to favor a heterozygous genetic blend, in which men and women possess some homosexual genetic material, but not so much that they will favor homosexual relationships. Balance selection acts to harmonize the forces of "diversifying selection," which creates great variation in the genetic code related to sexual orientation, and "directional selection," which flushes out genes of lesser overall adaptive value (i.e., homosexual genes). The existence of a continuum of sexual preference among humans is considered to be evidence of diversifying selection, whereas the greater number of heterosexual partnerships compared to same-sex partnerships is taken as evidence of directional selection (McKnight, 1997). According to this general approach, evolution performs a balancing act in which so-called "gay genes" are actively maintained in the gene pool, while minimizing the extent to which individuals engage in exclusively same-sex sexual behavior. It is interesting to note that some theorists contend that negative attitudes toward homosexuals are an expression of directional natural selection in the social-evolutionary sphere (Gallup, 1993).

Most evolutionary theories of same-sex attraction tend to focus on the sexual behavioral system and do not explicitly address the formation of same-sex romantic attachments. What is clear from studies of love, satisfaction, and commitment, however, is that adult same-sex romantic attachments exist (Kurdek, 2005; Peplau & Spalding, 2003). Although the sexual attractions that precede or follow the formation of same-sex attachments may be the by-products of functional mistakes in the evolutionary sense (Bowlby, 1969/1982), no evidence exists to suggest that same-sex romantic attachments function in inherently different ways from their heterosexual counterparts (see next section for a review of this empirical literature). Regardless of the true evolutionary significance of same-sex attractions, it is apparent that LGB individuals have made important contributions to their families, to their communities, and to society. The attachment system offers these individuals the capacity to enjoy greater safety and security through intimate bonds, and thus to increase their chances of surviving into old age and making contributions to others' lives over time. Also, given the great variability in sexual behavior among LGB-identified individuals, as well as developments in artificial insemination and family structures, significant numbers of LGB people have children (Patterson, 1995). Thus same-sex romantic attachments may also increase individuals' ability to provide for their children, as appears to be the case for heterosexual romantic attachments (Weiss, 1982).

This discussion suggests that an evolutionary perspective on same-sex romantic couples must account for two separate but related phenomena: (1) sexual attraction toward a person of the same sex, and (2) pair bonding with a person of the same sex. Diamond (2003) has provided considerable evidence to support the idea that distinct evolutionary and biobehavioral processes underlie sexual desire and romantic love. The main evolutionary function of the sexual system seems clear: to increase inclusive fitness by orienting individuals toward potential reproductive mates. Perhaps the clearest evidence for this proposition is the rather pedestrian observation that most sexual behavior occurs between individuals of different genders (i.e., between individuals who, in principle, are capable of having offspring). Thus the sexual system has evolved to encourage gender-specific (and, in particular, heterosexual) attractions. In contrast, as noted above, the romantic attachment system is thought to have evolved so as to encourage long-lasting relationships that can serve a protective function in childrearing. Unlike reproduction, which requires partners of different genders, the provision of protection is not tied to gender. An implication of this fundamental difference between the sexual system and romantic attachment system is that the two systems have different evolutionary roots.

Diamond (2003) described a number of studies suggesting that romantic attachment has much more in common with the infant–caregiver attachment system than with the sexual system. Her review indicates that there are substantial parallels between the emotional, biological, and behavioral processes underlying infant attachment and the corresponding processes in romantic attachment. Also, it is generally believed that the capacity for adult pair bonding evolved from the infant attachment system (Fraley et al., 2005). Diamond argued that if these two manifestations of attachment do truly operate similarly, then, just as the attachment system is not gender-specific for infants, the romantic bonding system should not be gender-specific in adolescents and adults. From this perspective, the tendency to form romantic attachments should not be limited to partners of different genders, and fundamental attachment-related processes should not vary according to the gender composition of a romantic dyad.

Furthermore, because the romantic attachment system is functionally distinct from the sexual system, it should be possible for same-sex attachments to be formed in the absence of sexual desire. In fact, as Diamond noted, nonsexual attachments between people of the same sex have been documented across diverse cultures and historical periods. These passionate friendships appear to function similarly to attachment relationships that include a sexual component, featuring basic attachment behaviors such as proximity seeking in stressful situations and separation protest. Some of these nonsexual attachment relationships can even begin with the feelings of infatuation that are often associated with the early phases of traditional romantic courtships. The fact that nonsexual relationships can be "romantic," whereas sexual liaisons can occur in the absence of love, highlights the functional independence of the attachment and sexual systems.

Adding further complexity to this picture is the reality that sex and love are not altogether unrelated. Diamond (2003) offers an interesting discussion of processes through which love may lead to sex and vice versa. Interesting examples of the former are found in Diamond's (2000) longitudinal study of women, all of whom identified themselves as lesbian, bisexual, or "questioning" when the research first began. Some of the participants shared that their only experiences of same-sex attractions were in relation to emotionally intense friendships with specific women. Five years after the first interview, several of these participants had assumed a heterosexual identity. These individuals stated that their passionate friendships had ended, and consequently so had their same-sex attractions. In contrast, a few of the lesbian-identified participants shared that they had become sexually involved with a close male friend with whom they had fallen in love, despite the fact that they reported remaining mostly sexually attracted to women. Such examples underscore the importance of examining the effects of both intimate friendships and sexual attractions on the development of same-sex romantic relationships, all while keeping in mind the biological, interpersonal, and cultural influences on both sexual orientation and attachment bonds. Readers are referred to Diamond's (2003) interesting review article for more examples of the complex interplay between love and sex, as well as theory and research on this topic (see also Diamond, 2006).

Charles Darwin (quoted in Rosario, 1997, p. 9) may not have guessed how long same-sex attractions would remain a mystery when he wrote, "We do not even in the least know the final cause of sexuality: The whole subject is hidden in darkness." Although the evolutionary significance of sexual orientation is still "hidden in darkness," there appears to be no reason to assume that same-sex romantic attachments operate according to a set of different principles (e.g., set goals, functions) from those operating in heterosexual attachments. The remainder of this chapter, then, applies current knowledge regarding heterosexual romantic attachment to male and female same-sex couples.

ATTACHMENT AND SAME-SEX RELATIONSHIP QUALITY

We have been together 40 years and in these 40 years we were waiting for this.
—EIGEL AXGIL

This statement (quoted by Rule, 1989, p. A8) was made by a 67-year-old Danish citizen after marrying his longtime partner, Axel Axgil, 74, in 1989. They were the first officially registered same-sex couple in modern history. Perhaps the most remarkable feature of the modern same-sex romantic partnership is its resilience in the face of widespread societal condemnation. Recent battles over the legalization of same-sex marriage in the United States have made it eminently clear that same-sex couples are still faced with pervasive stigma, discrimination, and challenges to their legitimacy (Soule, 2004). In spite of this hostile climate, many LGB individuals manage to forge long-term intimate relationships (Kurdek, 2005) and to enjoy the sense of security afforded by growing older with a person who is invested in one's well-being over time (Mackey, Diemer, & O'Brien, 2004).

The study of romantic relationships from an attachment perspective was stimulated by the seminal work of Hazan and Shaver (1987; Shaver & Hazan, 1988), who demonstrated that the patterns of attachment found in studies of infant behavior could be profitably applied to investigations of adult love experiences. They explored individual differences in romantic attachment by translating the infant typology developed by Ainsworth, Blehar, Waters, and Wall (1978) into terms meaningful for adult relationships. Consistent with the literature on infant attachment, Hazan and Shaver defined three styles of attachment: one secure and two insecure. "Secure" romantic attachment was characterized by comfort with closeness and interdependence with one's partner, as well as by low levels of fear of being abandoned by one's partner. "Avoidant" attachment was predominantly characterized by discomfort with closeness and interdependence, whereas "anxious-ambivalent" attachment was defined by high levels of abandonment anxiety, desire to merge with one's partner, and chronic frustration with a lack of closeness. (In this chapter the terms "avoidance" and "discomfort with closeness" are used interchangeably, as are the terms "anxious ambivalence," "anxiety over relationships," and "abandonment anxiety.")

Individuals who rely on avoidant strategies are thought to minimize their attachment needs due to expectations of rebuff or rejection by romantic partners, especially in times of stress. Anxious-ambivalent strategies are conceptualized as a hyperactivation of the attachment system, in which one's expression of and vulnerability to distress are exaggerated in order to gain the attention of partners who are believed to be inconsistently available (J. A. Feeney, Chapter 21, and Mikulincer & Shaver, Chapter 23, this volume; Pietromonaco & Barrett, 2000). It is now generally believed that adult attachment patterns are best conceptualized in terms of anxiety and avoidance levels instead of the three styles originally proposed by Hazan and Shaver (Brennan, Clark, & Shaver, 1998; Mikulincer & Shaver, 2007). Four patterns corresponding to different combinations of anxiety and avoidance have been identified: "secure"

(low anxiety, low avoidance), "preoccupied" (high anxiety, low avoidance), "dismissing" (low anxiety, high avoidance), and "fearful" (high anxiety, high avoidance). A sizable body of research indicates the relevance of these attachment patterns and strategies in predicting such indices of relationship quality as satisfaction and commitment (e.g., Collins & Read, 1990; Hazan & Shaver, 1987; Kirkpatrick & Davis, 1994), as well as secure-base behavior in stressful situations (e.g., Crowell et al., 2002; Simpson et al., 1992; Simpson, Rholes, & Phillips, 1996; see Mikulincer & Shaver, 2007, for an extensive review).

As mentioned earlier, little empirical work on same-sex romantic relationships has been conducted from a perspective that is explicitly grounded in attachment theory. One of the most informative studies, however, also appears to be among the very first works on this topic. For this study, Ridge and Feeney (1998) collected data related to attachment, romantic and sexual relationships, and (to be discussed later in this chapter) self-disclosure of sexual orientation from individuals associated with LGB organizations at colleges and universities in Australia. A main goal of the study was to replicate basic attachment findings from studies of heterosexual individuals in a sample of LGB individuals. As a whole, results were consistent with findings based on heterosexual samples, adding to the considerable evidence that same-sex couples and heterosexual couples function similarly (Kurdek, 2005). Attachment security was positively associated with current romantic relationship satisfaction among participants in dating relationships. Individuals endorsing a preoccupied attachment pattern were more likely than others to report a history of intense love experiences—a finding compatible with the view that anxious strategies involve hyperactivation of the attachment system. In contrast, the opposite was true for individuals endorsing a dismissing attachment pattern, consistent with the view that avoidant strategies involve suppression of intense attachment-related feelings. Dismissing participants were most likely to endorse casual sex and to view sex solely in terms of its physical rewards, just as has been found in studies of heterosexuals (see J. A. Feeney, Chapter 21, this volume).

Other researchers have provided data on similar links between attachment patterns and romantic relationship variables in samples of LGB individuals. These studies have found associations between attachment security and ratings of relationship quality (Elizur & Mintzer, 2003; Kurdek, 2002), commitment (Kurdek, 1997, 2002), and communication patterns (Gaines & Henderson, 2002). Kurdek (1997), for example, investigated attachment variables as part of a study focusing on links between aspects of neuroticism and commitment in romantic couples. He found that positive working models of self and partner were associated with level of "attraction commitment" (the component of commitment involving factors that attract individuals to their romantic relationships). Taken together, these two facets of attachment fully explained the link found between depressive symptomatology and attraction commitment. This result duplicates results based on samples of women in heterosexual dating relationships and marriages (Carnelley, Pietromonaco, & Jaffe, 1994).

A few attachment studies have directly compared heterosexual and LGB-identified individuals. Ridge and Feeney (1998) addressed the basic question of whether the relative prevalence of attachment patterns differs in LGB individuals and heterosexuals. Using a four-category, forced-choice measure of attachment style, the researchers compared proportions of each style found in their sample of LGB college students to the corresponding proportions in their sample of heterosexual college students. No sexual orientation differences were found, regardless of whether analyses were conducted with the full sample or separately for women and men. Similarly, no differences were found sexual orientation groups were compared on dimensional ratings for each of the four attachment styles. Kurdek (1997, 2002) examined links between dimensions of attachment and relationship functioning in samples of same-sex and heterosexual couples. In neither of the studies did these associations differ for the two couple types. In short, LGB and heterosexual people have been found to be similar both in attachment style and in relational correlates of attachment style.

The development and quality of romantic relationships is believed to be a function of not only a person's own attachment pattern but also the corresponding pattern of his or her partner (J. A. Feeney, 2003). Indeed, studies of heterosexual couples have suggested that people may tend to seek relationships with partners who confirm their attachment-related schemas. For example, individuals with anxious-ambivalent styles of attachment tend to be involved with avoidantly attached partners, who give some reality-based weight to their belief that they want more closeness than their partners do (Collins & Read, 1990; Kirkpatrick & Davis, 1994). Data from a community sample of same-sex couples suggests that this may also be true for individuals in same-sex

romantic relationships (Mohr & Fassinger, 2007). In this study, individuals who were highly anxious over relationships tended to have partners who reported higher-than-average levels of anxiety and discomfort with closeness. Participants uncomfortable with closeness tended to be partnered with individuals who reported high levels of relationship anxiety. These partner-matching effects were equally strong for female and male couples, and remained significant even after relationship length was controlled for—suggesting that the similarity was not due to mutual influence over time.

For heterosexual couples, there is ample evidence that partner attachment plays a role in shaping individuals' relationship experiences and evaluations; this speaks to the value of viewing attachment-related processes as part of a dynamic and potentially complex system of mutual influence in romantic relationships (J. A. Feeney, 2003). A colleague and I (Mohr & Fassinger, 2007) recently presented evidence of similar dynamics in same-sex couples. Results were particularly robust for attachment anxiety: Both own anxiety and partner anxiety were negatively associated with indicators of relationship quality (satisfaction, commitment, intimate everyday discussion), and positively associated with indicators of relationship difficulties (perceived intensity of relationship problems, negative communication patterns). Similar results were obtained for own avoidance, but not partner avoidance. These results suggest that the partner effects of romantic attachment evident in heterosexual couples also appear in same-sex couples.

Several investigations focusing on attachment and relationship satisfaction in heterosexual couples have uncovered ways in which gender and attachment interact in predicting satisfaction. Probably the most robust result is that participants' and partners' ratings of relationship quality are best predicted by females' levels of abandonment anxiety and males' levels of avoidance and discomfort with closeness (J. A. Feeney, Chapter 21, this volume). It has been hypothesized that these effects may be due to processes related to gender-role socialization. Evidence of these gender-based effects has been found in research on gender and conflict structure in married couples. For example, one study indicated that relationship satisfaction is inversely related to the degree to which marital couples engage in a "wife demands, husband withdraws" style of conflict (Heavey, Layne, & Christensen, 1993). This dynamic is strongly suggestive of a female ambivalent and male avoidant pairing, and couples with this combination of attachment styles are precisely those that have been found to give the lowest ratings of relationship satisfaction in some studies (J. A. Feeney, 1994; Kirkpatrick & Davis, 1994). In addition to gender differences in the links between attachment and relationship functioning, differences have been found in ratings of attachment itself. For example, a study of romantic attachment across 62 cultures indicated that men reported higher levels of dismissing avoidance than women in virtually all regions sampled (Schmitt et al., 2003).

Do similar gender-related patterns emerge in same-sex couples? Even for those acquainted with the sexual orientation literature, it is difficult to make an educated guess about the answer to this question. One might guess that there would be fewer gender-related patterns in same-sex couples, given evidence that same-sex couples are less likely than their heterosexual counterparts to base their relationships on traditional gender roles (Peplau & Spalding, 2003). However, research has indicated that lesbians and gay men differ in ways that are consistent with gender socialization processes (Fassinger & Arseneau, 2007), which might suggest that attachment-related dynamics in same-sex couples may be influenced by traditional gender patterns.

Given these opposing perspectives, it is perhaps fitting that the limited empirical data on this topic offer an unclear answer to the question of gender. Contrary to gender stereotypes, studies have provided evidence of higher levels of attachment anxiety in gay and bisexual men than in lesbian and bisexual women (Mohr & Fassinger, 2007; Ridge & Feeney, 1998). Fear of abandonment may be especially high in male same-sex partners for a variety of reasons, including greater prevalence of nonmonogamy in male couples (Peplau & Spalding, 2003), expectations of lack of intimacy based on restrictive male gender roles (Brown, 1995), and exposure to the particularly negative attitudes and stereotypes associated with male homosexuality and bisexuality (Kite & Whitley, 1996). Despite the gender difference found in levels of anxiety, findings from our data indicate that links between attachment and relationship functioning tend to be quite similar for female and male same-sex couples (Mohr & Fassinger, 2007). The main gender difference that did emerge was related to interactions between own and partner attachment in predicting some relationship outcomes. For women only, the negative effects of one's own attachment insecurity depended on how insecure one's partner was. In other words, women's attachment dynamics were truly dyadic, in that the ef-

fects of one woman's attachment style depended on her partner's attachment style. It seems possible that this might be explained by gender differences in valuing relational attunement and responsiveness. Compared to men, women may be more strongly socialized to value being closely attuned to others' emotional patterns and to respond to those dynamics.

Dynamics reminiscent of traditional gender norms emerged in one study that examined attachment strength—as opposed to attachment style—in a sample of heterosexual and LGB youth (Diamond & Dubé, 2002). For each participant, a primary attachment figure was identified by asking the person to name individuals with whom he or she was most likely to exhibit four classes of attachment behavior: proximity seeking, separation distress, safe haven, and secure base. The individual who was named in relation to the most classes of attachment behavior was viewed as the participant's primary attachment figure. Strength of attachment to the attachment figure was measured as a function of the number of classes of attachment behavior in which the participant engaged with the attachment figure. When the primary attachment figure was a romantic partner (as opposed to a platonic friend), the strength of attachment was significantly higher for lesbian and bisexual women than for their gay and bisexual male counterparts. For male participants, attachment strength was somewhat higher for heterosexual youth than for sexual minority youth when the attachment figure was a romantic partner, but somewhat lower when the attachment figure was a friend. For female participants, attachment strength was somewhat higher for sexual minority youth than for heterosexual youth when the attachment figure was a romantic partner. Diamond and Dubé speculated that these differences in strength of attachment may reflect gender-role socialization practices, wherein expression of tender feelings and intimacy needs is discouraged in males and encouraged in females. Restrictive male gender-role norms may explain why attachment strength was lowest in romantic relationships with two men and highest in relationships with two women. Of course, research is needed to determine the degree to which these gender differences were in part a function of the age group studied.

One unexplored area in which attachment-related gender differences may be expected in same-sex couples is sexual exclusivity. Male same-sex couples have been found to be more likely than any other type of couple to engage in sexual activities outside the couple relationship, and no significant differences in relationship satisfaction have been found among male couples based on sexual exclusivity (Kurdek, 1995; Peplau & Spalding, 2003). This finding suggests a few interesting hypotheses about the possible moderating role of gender in links between nonmonogamy and attachment. First, it seems possible that sex outside of the relationship may be more likely to be perceived as a threat to the attachment relationship in heterosexual and female couples than in male couples. If this is true, then nonmonogamy should be more likely to activate the attachment system in heterosexual and female couples than in male couples. Second, although attachment security has been linked to sexual exclusivity in a primarily heterosexual sample (Hazan, Zeifman, & Middleton, 1994), this connection may not be as strong for men in same-sex relationships. These hypotheses are especially interesting in light of recent theory regarding the evolved functions of jealousy in heterosexual relationships. If, as has been suggested, sexual jealousy serves the evolutionary function of increasing men's paternity certainty (Buss, Larsen, Westen, & Semmelroth, 1992), then this form of jealousy may be less likely to be stimulated in relationships in which paternity certainty is not an issue (e.g., male same-sex relationships). Of course, some men in same-sex couples do view their partners' nonmonogamy as a threat to their relationships. Such reactions are probably most likely to occur in couples that have not established explicit agreements about the acceptability of sex outside the relationship.

In short, these findings suggest that basic propositions regarding attachment dynamics in romantic relationships have been supported for same-sex couples, as well as for their heterosexual counterparts. Individuals in same-sex couples who are able to establish closeness with their partners and have trust in their partners' availability tend to be more satisfied with their relationships and to report more positive communication patterns. Furthermore, individuals' reports of relationship quality appear to be related to their partners' capacity for closeness and trust. A curious mixture of results has been found regarding the interplay between gender and attachment—some consistent with traditional gender roles, and some inconsistent. Greater clarity may be gained through couple research including assessment of variables that may moderate gender effects, such as adherence to gender-role norms, adherence to traditional relationship values, and belief in negative stereotypes about same-sex couples. Differences between male and female same-sex couples with regard to sexual exclusivity may prove to be an area worthy of investigation from an attachment-theoretical perspective. Also, although it seems likely that attachment patterns play a role in the trajectory of same-sex romantic relationships (as has been found for heterosexual couples; J. A. Feeney, Chapter 21, this volume), longitudinal studies of same-sex couples are needed to establish this proposition.

There is also a need for basic research on caregiving processes in same-sex couples. Bowlby (1969/1982, 1988) viewed caregiving and attachment as complementary behavioral systems that work together to promote individuals' safety and autonomy across the lifespan. He believed that individuals' early experiences of receiving care shape not only their working models of attachment but also their internal representations of caregiving. Such links between adults' attachment and caregiving patterns have been established in parent–child relationships and, more recently, in heterosexual romantic relationships (B. C. Feeney & Collins, 2001). The few published studies on caregiving in same-sex couples have focused on identifying general aspects of caregiving in male couples affected by HIV infection, and have documented the role of emotional attunement in positive caregiving experiences (e.g., Powell-Cope, 1995; Wrubel & Folkman, 1997). Use of an attachment perspective in such studies of same-sex couples may help to ground findings in a theoretical framework and provide a basis for predictions about individual differences in caregiving behavior in same-sex couples.

FEAR, SAFETY, AND SAME-SEX RELATIONSHIPS

Throughout the assault, he talked about how he was acting for God; that what he was doing to me was God's revenge on me because I was a "queer" and getting rid of me would save children and put an end to the movement in Indiana. ... I still do not have unrestricted freedom; my significant other and I live with constant fear that it will happen again.
—SARRIS (1992, p. 202)

LGB individuals have achieved substantial political and social gains in the past several decades, but institutional intolerance for and personal antagonism toward the expression of same-sex desire remain realities throughout much of the world (Dworkin & Yi, 2003; Herek, 2003). What are the consequences of these adverse social conditions for relationship functioning in same-sex couples? Clinical writings have suggested that both external manifestations of anti-LGB prejudice (e.g., violence, discrimination, rejection) and the internalization of negative views of same-sex attraction (e.g., internalized homonegativity, discrimination expectations) can lead to diminished satisfaction and greater conflict in same-sex couples (Brown, 1995), especially when partners differ with regard to their levels of internalized homonegativity and comfort with being "out of the closet" (Brown, 1995; Patterson & Schwartz, 1994). Such propositions are beginning to receive empirical support. For example, research findings have suggested that same-sex relationship quality is inversely related to perceived discrimination and stigma sensitivity (Mohr & Fassinger, 2006; Otis, Rostosky, & Riggle, 2006), internalized homonegativity (Balsam & Szymanski, 2005; Elizur & Mintzer, 2003; Mohr & Fassinger, 2006; Otis et al., 2006), parental disapproval of individuals' sexual orientation (Murphy, 1989; Smith & Brown, 1997), and chronic nondisclosure of sexual orientation (Berger, 1990). In short, research suggests that the climate of intolerance does indeed affect same-sex couple functioning, despite the movement toward greater acceptance of homosexuality and bisexuality.

Understanding the context of LGB individuals' lives is a prerequisite to articulating the unique ways in which attachment variables may play roles in determining same-sex romantic relationship functioning. The process of developing as a lesbian, a gay male, or a bisexual person often involves confusion, anxiety, and internal conflict. Many adolescents experiencing their same-sex attractions hide this aspect of their lives and thereby suffer from a profound sense of emotional isolation (Savin-Williams, 1995). Those who do openly express their sexual orientation run the risk of ridicule, rejection, and threat. Recent data from large-scale studies in public high schools provide evidence that LGB youth experience higher levels of bullying, sexual harassment, coercive sex, dating violence, and threat or injury involving a weapon than heterosexual youth do (Goodenow, Szalacha, & Westheimer, 2006; Williams, Connolly, Pepler, & Craig, 2005). Not surprisingly, these studies also indicate that LGB youth are more likely to skip school due to feeling unsafe, as well as to report difficulties in psychosocial functioning and lower-than-average levels of social support. The climate for LGB individuals is, to a great extent, a function of formal policies regarding homosexuality.

Although a number of countries have introduced LGB-affirming policies over the past several years, a recent Amnesty International (2001) report indicated that over 70 countries have laws criminalizing homosexuality. In some counties, homosexuality or same-sex sexual behavior is punished by flogging or death. The accumulated findings of studies such as these provide a sobering view of the difficult circumstances faced by many LGB individuals.

Given these suboptimal conditions, LGB individuals must learn to identify potential sources of threat and to manage the fear, shame, and anger associated with pervasive anti-LGB stigma and hostility (de Monteflores, 1993; Troiden, 1993). The process of learning to identify sources of possible danger is an important component of the fear behavioral system. Bowlby (1973) wrote extensively about humans' predisposition to react in a self-protective fashion to certain natural or innately recognized clues to danger (e.g., darkness, sudden noise, aloneness), as well as to cultural clues to danger that are learned by observation or personal experience. According to Bowlby, fear reactions are activated both by threatening stimuli (e.g., the approach of a hostile peer) and by inaccessibility of attachment figures (including perceived threats to the accessibility of attachment figures). An individual's total fear reaction at a given time is thought to be an additive function of all the fear stimuli present in the situation. Bowlby identified three behavioral outcomes of fear reactions: immobility (i.e., freezing), increased distance from the feared situation (i.e., fleeing), and increased proximity to one's attachment figure (i.e., seeking). Individuals who are able to use their attachment figures as a secure base for exploration are believed to be less susceptible to fear stimuli than those with insecure attachments.

How might the attachment and fear systems come into play in the process of LGB identity development? If LGB identity development is conceptualized as an exploratory process, then, as a colleague and I have suggested, attachment insecurity "may increase susceptibility to fear with regard to the tasks of identity development and curtail the exploration that is often critical in forging a positive LGB identity" (Mohr & Fassinger, 2003, p. 483). Support for this hypothesis has been found in a number of studies indicating that attachment insecurity is linked to negative identity and nondisclosure of sexual orientation (Elizur & Mintzer, 2003; Jellison & McConnell, 2003; Mohr & Fassinger, 2003; Wells & Hansen, 2003). Although the data from these studies did not provide a means of exploring causal relations between the attachment and LGB identity variables, the results suggest that attachment insecurity is associated with heightened fear and anxiety about behaviors that are thought to reflect acceptance and openness regarding one's sexual orientation. Responses to this fear and anxiety may involve actively "fleeing" the challenging tasks of LGB identity development, as well as "freezing" one's identity formation process.

The developmental tasks faced by LGB individuals may present what, from an attachment perspective, might be considered double-bind situations. For example, the process of "coming out" (i.e., disclosing one's sexual orientation) to one's parents may involve risking rejection from the very figures to whom one turns in times of distress. Although disclosure to parents is probably challenging for most LGB individuals, the difficulty of the coming-out process is probably even greater to the extent that parent and child have insecure attachment patterns. Attachment insecurity could exert this effect not only through the poorer interpersonal skills associated with higher levels of anxiety and avoidance, but also through diminished capacity to negotiate intergroup contact (such as that between LGB youth and their heterosexual parents). This latter possibility is underscored by research suggesting that attachment insecurity is associated with higher levels of outgroup devaluation and threat appraisal (Mikulincer & Shaver, 2003). Few data are available on parent and child attachment dynamics in the coming-out process; however, one study of LGB adults provides evidence of links between memories of early parental caregiving style and degree of parental rejection for one's sexual orientation (Mohr & Fassinger, 2003).

Parents with anti-LGB values may reject their children, regardless of the degree to which they provided a good early caregiving environment. An interesting implication of this possibility is that the coming-out process may alter LGB individuals' working models of attachment. The change in working models need not be only negative: LGB children may actually come to view their parents as more responsive and reliable as a result of a positive coming-out experience. Such changes may then broaden into a more positive general working model of attachment. Indeed, our work has indicated that parental support for one's LGB sexual orientation is related to current romantic attachment security, identity, and outness—even when

memories of early caregiving environment are controlled for (Mohr & Fassinger, 2003). Moreover, a study of gay and bisexual men supported a model in which the association between memories of childhood gender nonconformity and current attachment security was explained by degree of anti-LGB rejection from parents and peers (Landolt, Bartholomew, & Saffrey, 2004). Although these models have yet to be tested through longitudinal research, the cross-sectional data are consistent with Bowlby's (1988) assertion that working models of attachment can change—for better or for worse—in response to significant experiences with caregivers throughout the lifespan. Regardless of the direction of causal influence between working models and experiences with caregivers, there is little question that LGB youth benefit from parental support. Indeed, Hershberger and D'Augelli (1995) provided evidence that perceived familial support can serve as a buffer against the deleterious effects of victimization, particularly in regard to more threatening acts of violence.

Just as in the parent–child relationship, same-sex romantic relationships are not immune from double-bind situations. Consider, for example, the case in which one or both partners in a same-sex couple have internalized societal anti-LGB values and attitudes (i.e., have high internalized homonegativity). Such individuals are in the position of desiring romantic attachment relationships that go against their own value systems. Those who develop romantic relationships with same-sex partners may experience a push–pull dynamic, in which they simultaneously desire same-sex intimacy while wishing for distance from partners whose sex embodies the very opposite of what they view as acceptable. As noted above, indirect evidence for this proposition has been provided by studies showing that internalized homonegativity is a risk factor for romantic relationship difficulties in same-sex couples. The potential complexity of stigma-related dynamics is underscored by evidence that stigma functions at the dyadic level in same-sex romantic relationships (Mohr & Fassinger, 2006).

Such findings, taken together with attachment research, suggest ways in which attachment and stigma-related variables may be intertwined in determining same-sex relationship functioning. For example, as noted earlier, several studies have found an association between attachment insecurity and internalized homonegativity. One interpretation of this association is that internalized homonegativity may discourage the formation of same-sex bonds in which intimate closeness and trust can be tolerated. Although this proposition has not been tested directly, one study indicated that internalized homonegativity predicted decreases in closeness and commitment over a 2-month period among college students in same-sex dating relationships (Mohr & Daly, in press). The irony of such a state of affairs is that the inability to use a partner as a secure base for exploration of an LGB identity may prevent an individual from gaining the experiences necessary to decrease levels of internalized homonegativity.

Acute stressors, such as the experience of anti-LGB violence or threats of violence, may also serve to activate the attachment behavioral system. The attachment system is believed to have evolved to ensure individuals' safety at times of greatest threat (Bowlby, 1973). Individual differences in attachment representations are expected to lead to differences in responses to threat (Simpson & Rholes, 1994). Research on responses to acute stress suggests that avoidant victims of anti-LGB violence may be expected to minimize both the impact of such an event and the need for support, whereas ambivalent victims may be expected to focus on their distress, to blame themselves, and to experience an intense need for soothing from their attachment figures (Mikulincer, Florian, & Weller, 1993; Simpson et al., 1992). Secure victims, however, may be expected to seek direct support for their distress (i.e., to use their partners as a safe haven) and to experience less symptomatology than their insecure counterparts.

These different attachment-related strategies for coping may directly affect relationship functioning, or they may affect relationship functioning indirectly through the degree to which they maintain levels of symptomatology resulting from the traumatic stressor. For example, increased use of avoidant behaviors after an incident of anti-LGB violence may affect relationship quality directly through greater avoidance of intimacy and interdependence, and indirectly by maintaining depression levels, which in turn affect couple functioning. Little research has investigated such possibilities, but we (Mohr & Fassinger, 2007) did find that the negative effects of attachment anxiety on perceived problems in the relationship were exacerbated for individuals who had experienced actual or threatened anti-LGB violence in the previous year. This result suggests that severe stigma-related stressors may leave the attachment system in a chronically activated state, which in turn may amplify negative effects of attachment insecurity on couple functioning.

Finally, the relative invisibility of committed same-sex couples may make LGB individuals more vulnerable to negative societal messages regarding prospects for long-term relationships (Brown, 1995). For example, individuals may internalize the message that same-sex partnerships are primarily defined by sex, and thus are under continual jeopardy of dissolution due to sexual temptations outside of the relationship or to sexual boredom. Individuals may also believe that same-sex relationships are less legitimate than their heterosexual counterparts because of the relative lack of public, legal, and (often) familial recognition of such relationships (Ainsworth, 1985; Brown, 1995). For LGB people with high levels of attachment anxiety, these beliefs may pose serious threats to their sense of security and lead to chronic activation of the attachment behavioral system. Avoidantly attached people, on the other hand, may respond to such beliefs by maintaining even greater distance than usual from attachment figures. Brown (1995) has speculated that individuals who have internalized these types of societal messages may be vulnerable to romantic jealousy because they typically view same-sex partnerships as inherently less stable than their heterosexual counterparts. Given evidence that insecurely attached individuals are more susceptible to romantic jealousy (Collins & Read, 1990) and to maladaptive responses to jealousy (Sharpsteen & Kirkpatrick, 1997), it is clear that the forces of societal heterosexism and attachment may be intertwined in complex ways.

Although the focus of this discussion has been on attachment, it is worth noting that similar dynamics may occur with respect to caregiving processes in same-sex couples. Research on heterosexual couples has indicated that avoidant individuals tend to demonstrate lower levels of emotional support and responsiveness compared to others, particularly when their partners are viewed as distressed and needy (B. C. Feeney & Collins, 2001). There is no reason to believe that this basic dynamic would differ in same-sex couples. However, such dynamics would be expected to emerge not only in the stressful situations that all couples face, but also in the manifestations of minority stress that are specific to same-sex couples (e.g., anti-LGB rejection, discrimination, or violence). In addition, avoidance may exert its effects on same-sex caregiving through unique mechanisms such as internalized homonegativity, given the links between avoidance and homonegativity reported above. For example, individuals with high levels of internalized homonegativity may be less motivated than others to offer sensitive and tender caregiving to their partners, because of their mixed feelings about even having same-sex partners.

This section has featured examples of attachment-related issues that are unique to same-sex couples through their association with the pervasive invisibility and hostility faced by LGB individuals. These examples may have given the impression that societal heterosexism, internalized homonegativity, and romantic attachment insecurity weave a web so pervasive and formidable that no same-sex couple can escape a miserable fate. As noted earlier, however, same-sex couples appear to be as satisfied and well adjusted as heterosexual couples (Kurdek, 2005). Brown (1995) observed that all same-sex couples must face heterosexism and internalized homonegativity, even couples that have long and happy histories: "I ... know firsthand the challenges that an oppressive reality can throw in the faces of the most happy and well-functioning couples, even when both partners are skillful communicators with a strong commitment to the functioning and health of the relationship" (p. 276). Perhaps, as Simpson and Rholes (1994) have suggested, successfully facing adversity may actually strengthen such a couple's functioning. Learning with one's same-sex partner to negotiate the challenges posed by heterosexism and internalized homonegativity may provide a basis for reworking and improving working models of attachment.

Despite such possible benefits of facing adversity, same-sex couples would probably benefit even more from systematic efforts to reduce sources of adversity through legal recognition of same-sex romantic relationships. Public legitimization of same-sex couples may strengthen relationship functioning in a number of ways (e.g., through larger support networks for couples, greater visibility of couple role models, and increased valuing of same-sex relationships). Legal recognition may also create structural barriers to relationship dissolution by increasing the seriousness with which partners take their commitment and requiring more effort of partners who wish to end a relationship. Such barriers may even lessen the effects of insecure attachment on risk of breakup. Legislation granting same-sex couples legal recognition has been passed in a number of countries, starting with Denmark, and (most recently) including Switzerland ("Timeline of same-sex marriage," 2008). At this writing, seven U.S. states provide some type of mechanism for same-sex couples to receive all or most of the state-level rights associated with heterosexual marriage. However, same-sex couples are not given any legal recognition in most parts of the world. This variability in legal status provides researchers with an opportunity to study the effects of social policy on the complex interplay between stigma and the development and maintenance of same-sex romantic bonds.

LOSS IN SAME-SEX RELATIONSHIPS

Several weeks later I was cleaning the garage and found one of his old shirts tossed in a corner. It still smelled like him—that light orange odor. I also found our old beach ball, but I could not let the air out—his breath was in it.
—McCreary (1991, p. 144)

Bowlby was deeply concerned with the psychological repercussions of losing one's attachment figure—a fact that is not surprising, given the central role he accorded to achieving a sense of security and safety through attachment bonds. The final volume of his *Attachment and Loss* trilogy, *Loss: Sadness and Depression*, is devoted to the study of loss and mourning. Bowlby (1980) attempted to explain the process of bereavement from an ethological perspective, and thus to normalize the intense affective, cognitive, and behavioral shifts that commonly accompany loss. He suggested that reactions to loss can be viewed as part of a broader category of separation from one's attachment figure. From an attachment perspective, the specific sequence of numbing, protest, despair, and reorganization found in infants following a prolonged separation is evidence of an innate behavioral system that has evolved to maximize proximity to caregivers (Bowlby, 1980); this cycle has been amply documented among infants, children, and heterosexual adults (Bowlby, 1980; Fraley & Shaver, Chapter 3, this volume).

Working models of attachment are viewed as moderators of the bereavement process. Preoccupation with attachment relationships (i.e., the ambivalent attachment pattern), for example, has been linked to chronic mourning in adults (Bowlby, 1980). A preoccupied individual who has lost a romantic partner through either death or relationship dissolution is likely to experience an extended period of yearning for the missing partner, characterized by high levels of anxiety and depression, as well as by unusual difficulty in resuming normal daily routines (Fraley & Shaver, Chapter 3, this volume). Conversely, an avoidant individual is likely to have minimal grief reactions to loss. Although Bowlby believed the suppression of grief to be associated with problems adjusting to loss, debate still continues about the degree to which this is the case (Fraley & Shaver, Chapter 3, this volume).

The attachment literature on loss and bereavement has not yet included reference to same-sex couples, but results from empirical studies of relationship dissolution can be interpreted from an attachment perspective. For example, one study of adjustment to dissolution of romantic relationships indicated that male and female same-sex couples did not differ from heterosexual couples with regard to reasons for separation or levels of separation distress (Kurdek, 1997). The finding of no difference in distress levels among types of couples suggests that the attachment system may operate similarly for same-sex and heterosexual couples in the context of relationship dissolution. Kurdek (1997) also found that predissolution levels of neuroticism (which is a correlate of attachment anxiety; Noftle & Shaver, 2006; Shaver & Brennan, 1992) predicted postdissolution levels of separation distress. This result is consistent with the notion, discussed above, that preoccupied patterns of attachment are associated with especially difficult recovery from loss and prolonged separation. In an earlier study of relationship dissolution, Kurdek (1991) found that participants who reported experiencing few postdissolution adjustment difficulties placed a low value on dyadic attachment and reported low levels of psychological distress. Given that avoidance is associated with devaluing attachment needs and underreporting symptomatology (Dozier & Lee, 1995), this result may be interpreted as suggesting that avoidant LGB individuals tend to report low levels of adjustment problems after ending a romantic relationship. Similar findings have emerged in research with individuals in heterosexual relationships. For example, Simpson (1990) found that avoidant men reported especially low levels of emotional distress 6 months after ending a romantic relationship.

The AIDS epidemic has forced many gay male couples to confront issues of death and bereavement prematurely. The literature that has emerged from this epidemic provides ample evidence of loss and grieving in the context of same-sex romantic love. Folkman, Chesney, Collette, Boccellari, and Cooke (1996) conducted one of the most intensive studies of AIDS-related bereavement to date. This study examined preloss predictors of the course of postloss depression in 110 gay men whose partners died of AIDS-related complications. Each

man was assessed bimonthly for a 10-month period, starting 3 months before the partner's death. The findings support many of Bowlby's assertions regarding loss, and they raise interesting issues that may contribute to the refinement of theory regarding bereavement. Mean scores on a measure of depression throughout the 10 months exceeded the cutoff score for risk of major depression. The levels and persistence of depression found in this study were comparable to those found in bereaved partners of heterosexual married couples, suggesting that few differences exist in the degree to which bereaved partners in same- and opposite-sex couples experience despair.

Folkman and colleagues (1996) constructed a predictive model of postloss depression that included variables representing a variety of domains: demographic, mental health, physical health, stress, resources, and coping. The only significantly predictive demographic variable was length of relationship. Interestingly, caregiver burden did not predict the course of postloss depression, but the ability to view caregiving in positive terms was predictive: Men who felt that caregiving contributed positively to their romantic relationship were likely to recover more rapidly from postloss depression than other participants. The data did not describe the patterns of caregiving observed in these men, but this result is consistent with the notion that individuals who are compulsive caregivers or ambivalent with regard to the caregiving role may be especially vulnerable to chronic mourning (Bowlby, 1980).

Level of preloss daily hassles was one of the strongest predictors of lack of recovery from postloss depression. A possible interpretation of this result is based on recent work on the role of neuroticism in exposure and reaction to daily stressors. For example, Bolger and his colleagues (Bolger & Schilling, 1991; Bolger & Zuckerman, 1995) found that high-neuroticism participants experienced more daily conflicts and hassles than their low-neuroticism counterparts did, and that they were more likely to react to these everyday stressors with anger and depression. As mentioned already, neuroticism is at least moderately associated with attachment anxiety. These findings, put together, offer a basis for a plausible attachment-related interpretation of the finding about daily hassles in the bereavement study: Men who reported high levels of preloss daily hassles may have tended to have ambivalent patterns of attachment. If this was the case, then it is not surprising that these men had a difficult bereavement process, given the association of anxious attachment with chronic mourning (Shaver & Fraley, Chapter 3, this volume). Another interpretation of the research findings, however, is that level of preloss daily hassles may reflect a more chaotic lifestyle that would make recovery from postloss depression difficult for any person, regardless of attachment style.

One important finding of the Folkman and colleagues (1996) study is that participants who reported high levels of preloss depression were more likely to have a rapid recovery from postloss depression than those who reported low levels of preloss depression. The authors interpreted this result as an example of the process referred to by Klinger (1987) as "disengagement from incentives." Interview data indicated that the caregivers were largely preoccupied with the ongoing losses associated with their partners' illness. Depressive mood in response to these losses may indicate a process wherein individuals were beginning to disengage from their partners in preparation for the impending death. Hoffman (1996) has noted that this type of depression may also reflect anticipatory grief. This process of beginning bereavement prior to the loss of a partner may be viewed as an early phase of what Bowlby (1980) referred to as the stage of "reorganization." Bowlby, in fact, initially called this stage "detachment" (Fraley & Shaver, Chapter 3, this volume). According to Bowlby, healthy recovery from loss requires an acknowledgment that the deceased is no longer available, combined with the ability to maintain a continuing secure bond with the deceased. Thus beginning to disengage from one's partner before the partner's death may facilitate the process of reorganizing one's life and working models of the partner after the loss. Evidence of continuing bonds with deceased partners is found in such important symbols as the AIDS Memorial Quilt, commemorating those who have died of AIDS-related causes in the United States (Shelby, 1994). The quilt consists of thousands of panels created by the bereaved in memory of loved ones. This memorial provides bereaved individuals an opportunity to create a relatively enduring, public symbol of their continuing bond with their partners (as well as their continuing bond with other close friends who have also died of AIDS-related causes). The quilt may also offer the bereaved a reassuring symbol of continuing social support and solidarity in the midst of a climate that is often hostile with regard to AIDS-related issues (Hoffman, 1996).

Another important finding in the Folkman and colleagues (1996) study is that levels of de-

pression in bereaved partners who were HIV+ did not decrease over the 7-month period following the loss. Similar results were found in another longitudinal study, wherein participants who were both bereaved and HIV+ reported the highest levels of distress in a large urban sample of gay men (Martin & Dean, 1991). From an attachment perspective, HIV+ caregivers may feel the need to serve as strong, reliable figures for their partners, while simultaneously experiencing attachment distress related to their own illness and to the unavailability of their partners as caregivers for them. Thus HIV+ caregivers may feel compelled to suppress their own attachment distress, which may subsequently lead to difficulties in processing the impending loss. Shelby (1994), reporting a clinical study of the impact of AIDS on male romantic relationships, found that the mourning process is often especially complex and prolonged for a surviving partner who is HIV+. He noted that such an individual may exhibit a "continued idealization of the deceased partner and an identification with his illness and death" (p. 63), which may lead to increased isolation and depressive mood. According to Shelby, the HIV+ bereaved partner may become preoccupied with the virus as a "powerful and deadly tie to the deceased partner that cannot be loosed" (p. 63). Such possibilities hint at the complex transformations that representations of self and other may undergo in response to life-threatening illness.

Although little has been written from an attachment perspective on loss in same-sex couples, the research reviewed in this section suggests that responses to loss in same-sex couples are largely consistent with Bowlby's theory. This section has featured examples from the literature on relationship dissolution and AIDS-related bereavement. Loss may also play an important role in LGB identity development. Crespi (1995), for example, writes about the role of mourning in developing a positive lesbian identity. In a society that values heterosexuality more than homosexuality, LGB individuals must face potential losses of status, respectability, physical safety, and relationships with family and friends. Loss of positive regard and support from one's parents may be especially difficult to process and could conceivably affect functioning in a romantic relationship (Murphy, 1989; Smith & Brown, 1997). Future investigations of these dynamics may be enriched by including information about the quality of parental attachment prior to disclosure of one's sexual orientation.

SUMMARY AND CONCLUSIONS

The purpose of this chapter has been to begin to articulate ways in which attachment theory may both contribute to and profit from the study of same-sex romantic relationships. Much remains to be learned about the evolutionary underpinnings of both adult attachment and homosexuality, but the steadily growing body of research on same-sex couples strongly suggests that dynamics of romantic attachment are operative for LGB individuals. The findings discussed in this chapter indicate that many parallels exist with regard to the role of attachment in same-sex and heterosexual relationship quality. Attachment-related processes may also play unique roles in same-sex couple functioning through their relations with manifestations of sexual orientation stigma. Thus the study of same-sex couples promises to illuminate points of intersection between attachment processes and stigma, stress, and societal oppression in the functioning of romantic relationships.

The lack of longitudinal work in this area, however, leaves many questions unanswered regarding these points of intersection. For example, although recent research has indicated that attachment is related to variables associated with the LGB identity formation process, it is unclear whether attachment insecurity leads to difficulties in the identity process, whether identity difficulties lead to changes in working models of attachment, or whether a third variable influences both attachment and identity. It is equally unclear what implications this may have for the formation, maintenance, and dissolution of same-sex couples. Furthermore, gender differences may contribute to the complexity of this picture. For example, research has indicated that women and men differ with regard to whether same-sex dating relationships begin via certain routes. One study found that lesbians were more likely to have met their partners in work settings, and gay men were more likely to have met their partners in bars (Bryant & Demian, 1994). Such potential differences in the contexts of romantic relationship formation for lesbians and gay men suggest the possibility that the role and salience of working models of attachment in the early stages of LGB identity formation are moderated by gender.

The examples offered in this chapter constitute a first step in identifying some possibilities for future study, but the list is hardly exhaustive. For example, longitudinal research on relationships between lesbian ex-lovers (a little-studied but much-discussed phenomenon; see Weinstock & Rothblum, 2004) may contribute to the growing literature on jealousy and attachment. Furthermore, knowledge about the interplay among the attachment, affiliative, and sexual systems may benefit from intensive study of the considerable diversity in the arrangements that LGB adults create to satisfy their emotional, romantic, and sexual needs (for an interesting discussion of such arrangements, see Rust, 1996). Another potentially interesting line of investigation may be to study the ability of LGB communities to promote secure romantic attachments through their role as a safe haven for LGB individuals and same-sex couples, particularly given evidence that individuals experience anxiety and avoidance in relation to their group attachments that are distinct from the corresponding dimensions of attachments to romantic partners (Smith, Murphy, & Coats, 1999). These examples, along with those discussed earlier, indicate that the study of same-sex couple functioning provides a rich forum for exploring the complex interplay of forces at the individual, dyadic, and societal levels—an interplay that potentially involves the attachment, fear, sex, and exploration behavioral systems. Exploration of this uncharted territory will both enhance attachment theory and provide much-needed data on same-sex romantic relationships.

ACKNOWLEDGMENTS

I would like to thank Jude Cassidy, Henry Hogue, Phillip R. Shaver, and Susan Woodhouse for their helpful comments on an earlier draft of this chapter.

REFERENCES

Ainsworth, M. D. S. (1985). Attachments across the lifespan. *Bulletin of the New York Academy of Medicine, 61*, 792–812.

Ainsworth, M. D. S., Blehar, M. C., Waters, E., & Wall, S. (1978). *Patterns of attachment: A psychological study of the Strange Situation*. Hillsdale, NJ: Erlbaum.

Amnesty International. (2001). *Crimes of hate, conspiracy of silence*. Oxford, UK: Alden Press.

Balsam, K. F., & Szymanski, D. M. (2005). Relationship quality and domestic violence in women's same-sex relationships: The role of minority stress. *Psychology of Women Quarterly, 29*, 258–269.

Berger, R. M. (1990). Passing: Impact of the quality of same-sex couple relationships. *Social Work, 35*, 328–332.

Bolger, N., & Schilling, E. A. (1991). Personality and the problems of everyday life: The role of neuroticism in exposure and reactivity to daily stressors. *Journal of Personality, 59*, 355–386.

Bolger, N., & Zuckerman, A. (1995). A framework for studying personality in the stress process. *Journal of Personality and Social Psychology, 69*, 890–902.

Boswell, J. (1994). *Same-sex unions in premodern Europe.* New York: Villard Books.

Bowlby, J. (1969/1982). *Attachment and loss: Vol. 1. Attachment.* New York: Basic Books.

Bowlby, J. (1973). *Attachment and loss: Vol. 2. Separation: Anxiety and anger.* New York: Basic Books.

Bowlby, J. (1980). *Attachment and loss: Vol. 3. Loss: Sadness and depression.* New York: Basic Books.

Bowlby, J. (1988). *A secure base: Parent–child attachment and healthy human development.* New York: Basic Books.

Brennan, K. A., Clark, C. L., & Shaver, P. R. (1998). Self-report measurement of adult attachment: An integrative overview. In J. A. Simpson & W. S. Rholes (Eds.), *Attachment theory and close relationships* (pp. 46–76). New York: Guilford Press.

Brown, L. S. (1995). Therapy with same-sex couples: An introduction. In N. S. Jacobson & A. S. Gurman (Eds.), *Clinical handbook of couple therapy* (pp. 274–294). New York: Guilford Press.

Bryant, A. S., & Demian. (1994). Relationship characteristics of American gay and lesbian couples: Findings from a national survey. In L. A. Kurdek (Ed.), *Social services for gay and lesbian couples* (pp. 101–117). New York: Haworth Press.

Buss, D. M., Larsen, R. J., Westen, D., & Semmelroth, J. (1992). Sex differences in jealousy: Evolution, physiology, and psychology. *Psychological Science, 3*, 251–255.

Campbell, L., Simpson, J. A., Boldry, J., & Kashy, D. A. (2005). Perceptions of conflict and support in romantic relationships: The role of attachment anxiety. *Journal of Personality and Social Psychology, 88*, 510–531.

Carnelley, K. B., Pietromonaco, P. R., & Jaffe, K. (1994). Depression, working models of others, and relationship functioning. *Journal of Personality and Social Psychology, 66*, 127–140.

Collins, N. L., & Read, S. J. (1990). Adult attachment, working models, and relationship quality in dating couples. *Journal of Personality and Social Psychology, 58*, 644–663.

Crespi, L. (1995). Some thoughts on the role of mourning in the development of a positive lesbian identity. In T. Domenici & R. C. Lesser (Eds.), *Disorienting sexuality: Psychoanalytic reappraisals of sexual identities* (pp. 19–32). New York: Routledge.

Crowell, J. A., Treboux, D., Gao, Y., Fyffe, C., Pan, H., & Waters, E. (2002). Assessing secure base behavior in adulthood: Development of a measure, links to adult attachment representations and relations to couples' communication and reports of relationships. *Developmental Psychology, 38*, 679–693.

Dawkins, R. (1976). *The selfish gene.* New York: Oxford University Press.

de Monteflores, C. (1993). Notes on the management of difference. In L. D. Garnets & D. C. Kimmel (Eds.), *Psychological perspectives on lesbian and gay male experiences* (pp. 218–247). New York: Columbia University Press.

Diamond, L. M. (2000). Sexual identity, attractions, and behavior among young sexual-minority women over a 2-year period. *Developmental Psychology, 36*, 241–250.

Diamond, L. M. (2003). What does sexual orientation orient?: A biobehavioral model distinguishing romantic love and sexual desire. *Psychological Review, 110*, 173–192.

Diamond, L. M. (2006). How do I love thee?: Implications of attachment theory for understanding same-sex love and desire. In M. Mikulincer & G. S. Goodman (Eds.), *Dynamics of romantic love: Attachment, caregiving, and sex* (pp. 275–292). New York: Guilford Press.

Diamond, L. M., & Dubé, E. M. (2002). Friendship and attachment among heterosexual and sexual-minority youths: Does the gender of your friend matter? *Journal of Youth and Adolescence, 31*, 155–166.

Dickemann, M. (1995). Wilson's panchreston: The inclusive fitness hypothesis of sociobiology re-examined. *Journal of Homosexuality, 28*, 147–183.

Dozier, M., & Lee, S. W. (1995). Discrepancies between self- and other-report of psychiatric symptomatology: Effects of dismissing attachment strategies. *Development and Psychopathology, 7*, 217–226.

Dworkin, S. H., & Yi, H. (2003). LGBT identity, violence, and social justice: The psychological is political. *International Journal of the Advancement of Counseling, 25*, 269–279.

Elizur, Y., & Mintzer, A. (2003). Gay males' intimate relationship quality: The roles of attachment security, gay identity, social support, and income. *Personal Relationships, 10*, 411–435.

Fassinger, R. E., & Arseneau, J. R. (2007). "I'd rather get wet than be under that umbrella": Differentiating the experiences and identities of lesbian, gay, bisexual, and transgender people. In K. J. Bieschke, R. M. Perez, & K. A. DeBord (Eds.), *Handbook of counseling and psychotherapy with lesbian, gay, bisexual, and transgender clients* (2nd ed., pp. 19–49). Washington, DC: American Psychological Association.

Feeney, B. C., & Collins, N. L. (2001). Predictors of caregiving in adult intimate relationships: An attachment theoretical perspective. *Journal of Personality and Social Psychology, 80*, 972–994.

Feeney, J. A. (1994). Attachment style, communication patterns, and satisfaction across the life cycle of marriage. *Personal Relationships, 1*, 333–348.

Feeney, J. A. (2003). The systemic nature of couple relationships: An attachment perspective. In P. Erdman & T. Caffery (Eds.), *Attachment and family systems: Conceptual, empirical, and therapeutic relatedness* (pp. 139–163). New York: Brunner-Routledge.

Feeney, J. A., Noller, P., & Callan, V. J. (1994). Attachment style, communication and satisfaction in the early years of marriage. In K. Bartholomew & D. Perlman (Eds.), *Advances in personal relationships: Vol. 5. Attachment processes in adulthood* (pp. 269–308). London: Jessica Kingsley.

Folkman, S., Chesney, M., Collette, L., Boccellari, A., & Cooke, M. (1996). Postbereavement depressive mood and its prebereavement predictors in HIV+ and HIV– gay men. *Journal of Personality and Social Psychology, 70,* 336–348.

Fraley, R. C., Brumbaugh, C. C., & Marks, M. J. (2005). The evolution and function of adult attachment: A comparative and phylogenetic analysis. *Journal of Personality and Social Psychology, 89,* 731–746.

Gaines, S. O., & Henderson, M. C. (2002). Impact of attachment style on responses to accommodative dilemmas among same-sex couples. *Personal Relationships, 9,* 89–93.

Gallup, G. G. (1993). Have attitudes toward homosexuals been shaped by natural selection? *Ethology and Sociobiology, 16,* 53–70.

Gibson, M. (1997). Clitoral corruption: Body metaphors and American doctors' constructions of female homosexuality. In V. A. Rosario (Ed.), *Science and homosexualities* (pp. 108–132). New York: Routledge.

Goodenow, C., Szalacha, L., & Westheimer, K. (2006). School support groups, other school factors, and the safety of sexual minority adolescents. *Psychology in the Schools, 43,* 573–589.

Greenberg, D. F. (1988). *The construction of homosexuality.* Chicago: University of Chicago Press.

Hamer, D. H., & Copeland, P. (1994). *The science of desire: The search for the gay gene and the biology of behavior.* New York: Simon & Schuster.

Hazan, C., & Shaver, P. (1987). Romantic love conceptualized as an attachment process. *Journal of Personality and Social Psychology, 52,* 511–524.

Hazan, C., Zeifman, D., & Middleton, K. (1994, July). *Adult romantic attachment, affection, and sex.* Paper presented at the 7th International Conference on Personal Relationships, Groningen, The Netherlands.

Heavey, C. L., Layne, C., & Christensen, A. (1993). Gender and conflict structure in marital interaction: A replication and extension. *Journal of Consulting and Clinical Psychology, 64,* 16–27.

Herek, G. M. (1991). Stigma, prejudice, and violence against lesbians and gay men. In J. C. Gonsiorek & J. D. Weinrich (Eds.), *Homosexuality: Research implications for public policy* (pp. 60–80). Newbury Park, CA: Sage.

Herek, G. M. (2003). The psychology of sexual prejudice. In L. D. Garnets & D. C. Kimmel (Eds.), *Psychological perspectives on lesbian and gay male experiences* (2nd ed., pp. 157–164). New York: Columbia University Press.

Herek, G. M., Kimmel, D. C., Amaro, H., & Melton, G. B. (1991). Avoiding heterosexist bias in psychological research. *American Psychologist, 46,* 957–963.

Hershberger, S. L., & D'Augelli, A. R. (1995). The impact of victimization on the mental health and suicidality of lesbian, gay, and bisexual youths. *Developmental Psychology, 31,* 65–74.

Hoffman, M. A. (1996). *Counseling clients with HIV disease: Assessment, intervention, and prevention.* New York: Guilford Press.

Hutchinson, G. E. (1959). A speculative consideration of certain possible forms of sexual selection in man. *American Naturalist, 93,* 81–91.

Jellison, W. A., & McConnell, A., R. (2003). The mediating effects of attitudes toward homosexuality between secure attachment and disclosure outcomes among gay men. *Journal of Homosexuality, 46,* 159–177.

Kirkpatrick, L. A. (1998). Evolution, pair-bonding, and reproductive strategies: A reconceptualization of adult attachment. In J. A. Simpson & W. S. Rholes (Eds.), *Attachment theory and close relationships* (pp. 353–393). New York: Guilford Press.

Kirkpatrick, L. A., & Davis, K. E. (1994). Attachment style, gender, and relationship stability: A longitudinal analysis. *Journal of Personality and Social Psychology, 66,* 502–512.

Kite, M. E., & Whitley, B. E. (1996). Sex differences in attitudes toward homosexual persons, behaviors, and civil rights: A meta-analysis. *Personality and Social Psychology Bulletin, 22,* 336–353.

Klinger, E. (1987). Current concerns and disengagement from incentives. In F. Halisch & J. Kuhl (Eds.), *Motivation, intention, and volition* (pp. 337–347). Berlin: Springer-Verlag.

Kobak, R. R., & Hazan, C. (1991). Attachment in marriage: Effects of security and accuracy of working models. *Journal of Personality and Social Psychology, 60,* 861–869.

Kunce, L. J., & Shaver, P. R. (1994). An attachment-theoretical approach to caregiving in romantic relationships. In K. Bartholomew & D. Perlman (Eds.), *Advances in personal relationships: Vol. 5. Attachment processes in adulthood* (pp. 205–237). London: Jessica Kingsley.

Kurdek, L. A. (1991). The dissolution of gay and lesbian couples. *Journal of Social and Personal Relationships, 8,* 265–278.

Kurdek, L. A. (1995). Lesbian and gay couples. In A. R. D'Augelli & C. J. Patterson (Eds.), *Lesbian, gay, and bisexual identities over the lifespan: Psychological perspectives* (pp. 243–261). New York: Oxford University Press.

Kurdek, L. A. (1997). Relation between neuroticism and dimensions of relationship commitment: Evidence from gay, lesbian, and heterosexual couples. *Journal of Family Psychology, 11,* 109–124.

Kurdek, L. A. (2002). On being insecure about the assessment of attachment styles. *Journal of Social and Personal Relationships, 19,* 803–826.

Kurdek, L. A. (2005). What do we know about gay and lesbian couples? *Current Directions in Psychological Science, 14,* 251–254.

Landolt, M. A., Bartholomew, K., & Saffrey, C. (2004). Gender nonconformity, childhood rejection, and adult attachment: A study of gay men. *Archives of Sexual Behavior, 33*, 117–128.

Mackey, R. A., Diemer, M. A., & O'Brien, B. A. (2004). Relational factors in understanding satisfaction in the lasting relationships of same-sex and heterosexual couples. *Journal of Homosexuality, 47*, 111–136.

Martin, J. L., & Dean, L. (1991). Effects of AIDS-related bereavement and HIV-related illness on psychological distress among gay men: A 7-year longitudinal study, 1985–1991. *Journal of Personality and Social Psychology, 61*, 94–103.

McCreary, K. (1991). Remembrance. In E. Hemphill (Ed.), *Brother to brother: New writings by black gay men* (p. 144). Boston: Alyson.

McKnight, J. (1997). *Straight science?: Homosexuality, evolution, adaptation*. London: Routledge.

Mikulincer, M., Florian, V., & Weller, A. (1993). Attachment styles, coping strategies, and posttraumatic psychological distress: The impact of the Gulf War in Israel. *Journal of Personality and Social Psychology, 64*, 817–826.

Mikulincer, M., & Shaver, P. R. (2007). *Attachment in adulthood: Structure, dynamics, and change*. New York: Guilford Press.

Mohr, J. J., & Daly, C. (in press). Sexual minority stress and changes in relationship quality in same-sex couples. *Journal of Social and Personal Relationships*.

Mohr, J. J., & Fassinger, R. E. (2003). Self-acceptance and self-disclosure of sexual orientation in lesbian, gay, and bisexual adults: An attachment perspective. *Journal of Counseling Psychology, 50*, 282–295.

Mohr, J. J., & Fassinger, R. E. (2006). Sexual orientation identity and romantic relationship quality in same-sex couples. *Personality and Social Psychology Bulletin, 32*, 1085–1099.

Mohr, J. J., & Fassinger, R. E. (2007, August). Attachment in same-sex couples: Basic processes and minority stress effects. In J. J. Mohr (Chair), *Attachment and caregiving in same-sex romantic relationships*. Symposium conducted at the meeting of the American Psychological Association, San Francisco.

Murphy, B. C. (1989). Lesbian couples and their parents: The effects of perceived parental attitudes on the couple. *Journal of Counseling and Development, 68*, 46–51.

Noftle, E. E., & Shaver, P. R. (2006). Attachment dimensions and the Big Five personality traits: Associations and comparative ability to predict relationship quality. *Journal of Research in Personality, 40*, 179–208.

Otis, M. D., Rostosky, S. S., & Riggle, E. D. B. (2006). Stress and relationship quality in same-sex couples. *Journal of Social and Personal Relationships, 23*, 81–99.

Patterson, C. (1995). Lesbian mothers, gay fathers, and their children. In A. R. D'Augelli & C. J. Patterson (Eds.), *Lesbian, gay, and bisexual identities over the lifespan: Psychological perspectives* (pp. 262–290). New York: Oxford University Press.

Patterson, D. G., & Schwartz, P. (1994). The social construction of conflict in intimate same-sex couples. In D. D. Cahn (Ed.), *Conflict in personal relationships* (pp. 3–26). Hillsdale, NJ: Erlbaum.

Pavelka, M. S. (1995). Sexual nature: What can we learn from a cross-species perspective? In P. R. Abramson & S. D. Pinkerton (Eds.), *Sexual nature, sexual culture* (pp. 17–36). Chicago: University of Chicago Press.

Peplau, L. A., & Spalding, L. R. (2003). The close relationships of lesbians, gays, and bisexuals. In L. D. Garnets & D. C. Kimmel (Eds.), *Psychological perspectives on lesbian and gay male experiences* (2nd ed., pp. 449–474). New York: Columbia University Press.

Pietromonaco, P. R., & Barrett, L. F. (2000). Attachment theory as an organizing framework: A view from different levels of analysis. *Review of General Psychology, 4*, 107–110.

Powell-Cope, G. M. (1995). The experiences of gay couples affected by HIV infection. *Qualitative Health Research, 5*, 36–62.

Ridge, S. R., & Feeney, J. A. (1998). Relationship history and relationship attitudes in gay males and lesbians: Attachment style and gender differences. *Australian and New Zealand Journal of Psychiatry, 32*, 848–859.

Rosario, V. A. (1997). Homosexual bio-histories: Genetic nostalgias and the quest for paternity. In V. A. Rosario (Ed.), *Science and homosexualities* (pp. 1–26). New York: Routledge.

Rule, S. (1989, October 2). Rights for gay couples in Denmark. *New York Times*, p. A8.

Rust, P. C. (1996). Monogamy and polyamory: Relationship issues for bisexuals. In B. A. Firestein (Ed.), *Bisexuality: The psychology and politics of an invisible minority* (pp. 127–148). Thousand Oaks, CA: Sage.

Salais, D., & Fischer, R. B. (1995). Sexual preference and altruism. *Journal of Homosexuality, 28*, 185–196.

Sarris, K. (1992). Survivor's story. In G. M. Herek & K. T. Berrill (Eds.), *Hate crimes: Confronting violence against lesbians and gay men* (pp. 201–203). Newbury Park, CA: Sage.

Savin-Williams, R. C. (1995). Lesbian, gay male, and bisexual adolescents. In A. R. D'Augelli & C. J. Patterson (Eds.), *Lesbian, gay, and bisexual identities over the lifespan: Psychological perspectives* (pp. 165–189). New York: Oxford University Press.

Schmitt, D. P., Alcalay, L., Allensworth, M., Allik, J., Ault, L., Austers, I., et al. (2003). Are men universally more dismissing than women?: Gender differences in romantic attachment across 62 cultural regions. *Personal Relationships, 10*, 307–331.

Sharpsteen, D. J., & Kirkpatrick, L. A. (1997). Romantic jealousy and adult romantic attachment. *Journal of Personality and Social Psychology, 72*, 627–640.

Shaver, P. R., & Brennan, K. A. (1992). Attachment styles and the "Big Five" personality traits: Their connections with each other and with romantic relationship outcomes. *Personality and Social Psychology Bulletin, 18*, 536–545.

Shaver, P. R., & Hazan, C. (1988). A biased overview of the study of love. *Journal of Social and Personal Relationships, 5,* 473–501.

Shelby, R. D. (1994). Mourning within a culture of mourning. In S. A. Cadwell, R. A. Burnham, Jr., & M. Forstein (Eds.), *Therapists on the front line: Psychotherapy with gay men in the age of AIDS* (pp. 53–79). Washington, DC: American Psychiatric Press.

Simpson, J. A. (1990). Influence of attachment styles on romantic relationships. *Journal of Personality and Social Psychology, 59,* 971–980.

Simpson, J. A., & Rholes, W. S. (1994). Stress and secure base relationships in adulthood. In K. Bartholomew & D. Perlman (Eds.), *Advances in personal relationships: Vol. 5. Attachment processes in adulthood* (pp. 181–204). London: Jessica Kingsley.

Simpson, J. A., Rholes, W. S., & Nelligan, J. S. (1992). Support seeking and support giving within couples in an anxiety-provoking situation: The role of attachment styles. *Journal of Personality and Social Psychology, 62,* 434–446.

Simpson, J. A., Rholes, W. S., & Phillips, D. (1996). Conflict in close relationships: An attachment perspective. *Journal of Personality and Social Psychology, 71,* 899–914.

Smith, E. R., Murphy, J., & Coats, S. (1996). Attachments to groups: Theory and measurement. *Journal of Personality and Social Psychology, 77,* 94–110.

Smith, R. B., & Brown, R. A. (1997). The impact of social support on gay male couples. *Journal of Homosexuality, 33,* 39–61.

Soule, S. A. (2004). Going to the chapel?: Same-sex marriage bans in the United States, 1973–2000. *Social Problems, 51,* 453–477.

Timeline of same-sex marriage. (2008, January 5). In *Wikipedia, The free encyclopedia*. Retrieved January 8, 2008, from *http://en.wikipedia.org/wiki/Timeline_of-same-sex_marriage*

Troiden, R. R. (1993). The formation of homosexual identities. In L. D. Garnets & D. C. Kimmel (Eds.), *Psychological perspectives on lesbian and gay male experiences* (pp. 191–217). New York: Columbia University Press.

Weinrich, J. D. (1995). Biological research on sexual orientation: A critique of the critics. *Journal of Homosexuality, 28,* 197–213.

Weinstock, J. S., & Rothblum, E. D. (Eds.). (2004). *Lesbian ex-lovers: The really long-term relationships*. New York: Haworth Press.

Weiss, R. S. (1982). Attachment in adult life. In C. M. Parkes & J. Stevenson-Hinde (Eds.), *The place of attachment in human behavior* (pp. 171–184). New York: Basic Books.

Wells, G. B., & Hansen, N. D. (2003). Lesbian shame: Its relationship to identity integration and attachment. *Journal of Homosexuality, 45,* 93–110.

West, M. L., & Sheldon-Keller, A. E. (1994). *Patterns of relating: An adult attachment perspective*. New York: Guilford Press.

Williams, T., Connolly, J., Pepler, D., & Craig, W. (2005). Peer victimization, social support, and psychosocial adjustment of sexual minority adolescents. *Journal of Youth and Adolescence, 34,* 471–482.

Wilson, E. O. (1975). *Sociobiology: The new synthesis*. Cambridge, MA: Harvard University Press.

Wrubel, J., & Folkman, S. (1997). What informal caregivers actually do: The caregiving skills of partners of men with AIDS. *AIDS Care, 9,* 691–706.

CHAPTER 23

Adult Attachment and Affect Regulation

MARIO MIKULINCER
PHILLIP R. SHAVER

The titles of the second and third volumes of Bowlby's (1973, 1980) trilogy on attachment—*Separation: Anxiety and Anger* and *Loss: Sadness and Depression*—make clear that emotions were among his central concerns. He was interested in the causes and consequences of emotions aroused by attachment to, and reunion with, attachment figures (e.g., love, tenderness, joy); separation from them (anxiety, anger); and permanent loss of them (grief, sadness, despair). Attachment theory is an attempt to explain how secure attachments develop; how they help people survive temporary bouts of pain, discomfort, doubt, and distress; and then how they help them reestablish hope, optimism, and emotional equanimity. It also explains how various forms of attachment insecurity develop and interfere with emotion regulation, social adjustment, and mental health—as explained in many other chapters in this volume.

Especially in early childhood, but also later in life ("from the cradle to the grave," in Bowlby's words; 1979, p. 129), human beings rely on attachment figures (e.g., parents, spouses/partners, mentors, therapists) for help with emotion regulation. When a security-providing mother reassuringly touches her anxious child or holds the child's hand in a novel or worrisome situation, the child's

previously heightened autonomic arousal subsides (e.g., Field, 2002; Hertenstein, 2002). When a loving husband holds his wife's hand in a painful or anxiety-provoking medical situation, neuro-images of the wife's brain reveal her return to a calmer state (Coan, Schaefer, & Davidson, 2006). (Interestingly, less loving husbands' hands do not have such beneficial effects; see Coan, Chapter 11, this volume.)

In the present chapter, we summarize our model of attachment system activation and dynamics in adulthood—a model based on what we call "adult attachment theory" and the research it has inspired (see reviews by Mikulincer & Shaver, 2003, 2007). The goal of this chapter is to use concepts and findings from attachment research, which originally focused primarily on the mother–child relationship and on children's attachment orientations (as also explained in many other chapters in this volume), to illuminate and understand the role of adult attachment relationships and mental representations of attachment experiences in adult emotion regulation. To accomplish our goal, we consult mainly the extensive research literature created by personality and social psychologists who use self-report measures of a person's hierarchy of attachment figures and attachment "style," combined with various other measures and experimental research paradigms (Shaver & Mikulincer, 2002a, 2002b), to uncover and illuminate the dynamics of the attachment behavioral system in adulthood. Research by personality and social psychologists on dyadic, relational processes related to attachment is reviewed by J. Feeney in Chapter 21 and by B. Feeney and Monin in Chapter 39 of this volume. Here we focus instead on the individual psychology of attachment-related mental processes in adulthood, which we consider to be a joint product of previous experiences in attachment relationships and current cognitive and social contexts, including contexts that are systematically manipulated in the laboratory. (There is likely to be a role for genes in these processes as well; see, e.g., Crawford et al., 2007.)

The concept of "adult attachment style" emerged from research by Hazan and Shaver (1987, 1990, 1994), who applied attachment theory to the study of adolescent and adult romantic and marital relationships. In their early studies, these authors employed a simple three-category

attachment style measure based conceptually on Ainsworth's (Ainsworth, Blehar, Waters, & Wall, 1978) descriptions of three major attachment patterns in infancy. In an influential 1991 article, Bartholomew and Horowitz argued for a four-category typology of adult attachment styles, based on two dimensions suggested by Bowlby's (1969/1982) analysis of internal working models of self and other. (Bartholomew and Horowitz divided each of these dimensions, model of self and model of others, into two regions: positive and negative.)

Bartholomew and Horowitz's theory and measures (see Bartholomew & Horowitz, 1991; Griffin & Bartholomew, 1994) inspired numerous other measures and studies, which in 1998 led Brennan, Clark, and Shaver (1998) to factor-analyze all of the self-report items written up to that time. Based on their analyses and on Bartholomew and Horowitz's (1991) findings, they created two 18-item self-report scales (the Experiences in Close Relationships [ECR] scales) to measure attachment-related anxiety and avoidance. The two dimensions are similar to the two that defined Ainsworth's infant attachment categories (see Ainsworth et al., 1978,

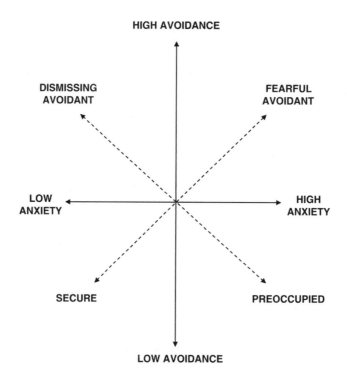

FIGURE 23.1. Diagram of the two-dimensional space defined by attachment anxiety and avoidance, showing the quadrant names suggested by Bartholomew (1990). From Mikulincer and Shaver (2007, p. 89). Copyright 2007 by The Guilford Press. Reprinted by permission.

Figure 10, p. 102). The ECR scales allow research- ers to place adolescent and adult research partici- pants into the two-dimensional attachment style space shown in Figure 23.1. Hundreds of studies (reviewed by Mikulincer & Shaver, 2007) have now used this approach to study adult attachment phenomena, including many issues related to emo- tion regulation.

We begin our review of relevant studies with a description of our model of attachment system activation and functioning in adulthood. Next, we focus on the regulatory function of attachment system activation; we review studies that have examined preconscious activation of attachment- related mental representations under threatening conditions, as well as the use of support seeking as an emotion regulation strategy. We then review studies concerned with the beneficial effects of attachment security on emotion regulation and mental health, as well as the psychological mecha- nisms that sustain these effects. We also consider the distinction between anxious/hyperactivat- ing and avoidant/deactivating strategies when no security-providing figure is available or responsive, and we summarize evidence regarding the implica- tions of these strategies for emotion regulation and mental health. At the end, we outline briefly what remains to be accomplished if we are to attain a maximally rich understanding of the influences of attachment history and attachment patterns on emotion regulation in adulthood.

A MODEL OF ATTACHMENT SYSTEM ACTIVATION AND FUNCTIONING IN ADULTHOOD

Based on a review of adult attachment studies, we (Mikulincer & Shaver, 2003) proposed the three- phase model of attachment system activation and dynamics shown in Figure 23.2. The model comprises three main components or modules. The first involves the monitoring and appraisal of threatening events, which often activate the at- tachment behavioral system (see Cassidy, Chap- ter 1, this volume). This component includes the major normative (pan-human, cross-culturally universal), evolutionarily functional features of the attachment system as conceptualized by Bowl- by (1969/1982). He proposed that this system evolved to increase an infant's chances of survival and eventual reproduction by making it likely that the infant would seek and maintain proximity to stronger and wiser attachment figures, and thereby would receive protection, emotional support, en-

couragement, guidance, and help with emotion regulation—especially when threats, stressors, or pain arose.

The second component of the model deals with the monitoring and appraisal of an attach- ment figure's availability and responsiveness. This component is responsible for individual differ- ences in the sense of attachment security ("felt se- curity"; Sroufe & Waters, 1977), which is shaped by repeated experiences with primary attachment figures, whose effective or ineffective caregiving responses cause a child to become more or less secure. By adulthood, this component of the at- tachment system is highly elaborated, based on thousands of experiences; it includes a vast store of memories related to encounters with threats and experiences with attachment figures, as well as schematic mental representations of those experiences—the "internal working models" re- ferred to by Bowlby (1969/1982) and discussed by Bretherton and Munholland (Chapter 5, this volume). Repeated security-restoring and security- enhancing experiences with attachment figures create a dispositional sense of felt security, which initiates and sustains a cascade of effects, amount- ing to a "broaden-and-build" cycle of security (Fre- drickson, 2001; Mikulincer & Shaver, 2007) that influences many aspects of mental health, personal growth, and social adjustment.

The third component of the model addresses the monitoring and appraisal of the viability and likely utility of seeking proximity to an attachment figure (either a particular figure or such figures in general) as a way of coping with worries and threats. This component is responsible for individual differ- ences in attachment style among people who are relatively insecure, and in corresponding strategies of emotion regulation, which can be characterized as "hyperactivating" or "deactivating" (Cassidy & Kobak, 1988). Hyperactivating strategies derive from previous experiences in which inattentive, self-preoccupied, or anxious attachment figures were perceived as more likely to respond favor- ably if the normative strategies of calling, crying, contacting, and clinging were up-regulated to the point of demanding a response (a behavior pattern that Bowlby, 1969/1982, called "protest"). Because such behavior, when addressed to a less than fully sensitive and responsive caregiver, is sometimes ef- fective in relieving distress and sometimes not, ac- cording to an unpredictable partial reinforcement schedule (Skinner, 1969), it is highly resistant to extinction. When consolidated over months and years, hyperactivating strategies and their effects

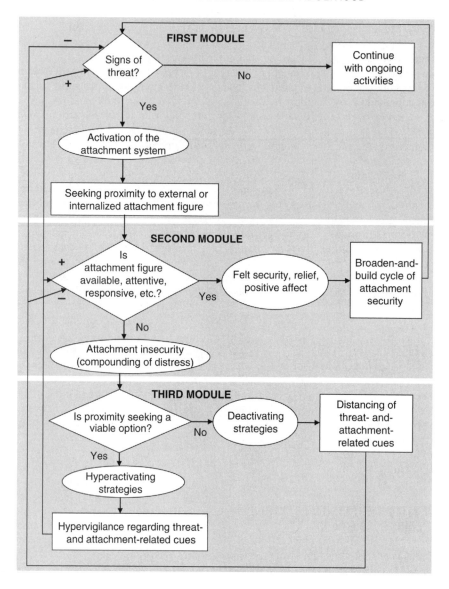

FIGURE 23.2. A model of attachment system activation and functioning in adulthood. From Mikulincer and Shaver (2007, p. 31). Copyright 2007 by The Guilford Press. Reprinted by permission.

on subjective experience and observable behavior amount to an "anxious," "anxious-ambivalent," or "anxious-resistant" pattern of attachment (Ainsworth et al., 1978; Cassidy & Berlin, 1994), which in adolescents and adults we call an "anxious" attachment style.

Deactivating strategies derive from previous experiences in which emotionally cool, distant, rejecting, or hostile caregivers reacted to normative cries for help and support by withdrawing, disapproving, or reacting with anger. This kind

of behavior, if common and persistent, makes it likely that a child will inhibit, suppress, or deactivate normal attachment behavior; this leads to an "avoidant" attachment pattern (Ainsworth et al., 1978), which Bowlby (1969/1982) called "compulsive self-reliance."

Our model includes hypothesized excitatory and inhibitory feedback loops (shown as upward arrows on the left side of Figure 23.2) that result from the recurrent use of hyperactivating or deactivating strategies. These loops affect the monitoring of threats and the appraisal of attachment figures' availability or unavailability. In particular, hyperactivating strategies lead to persisting tendencies to be especially vigilant to threats; exceptionally expressive of fears, needs, and doubts; and continually worried about attachment figure's availability and responsiveness. All of these predispose a person to excessively dependent behavior, intense and frequent proximity seeking and contact maintenance, and clinginess (Ainsworth et al., 1978; Fraley & Shaver, 1998). Deactivating strategies, in contrast, lead to dismissal or downplaying of potential threats; suppression or denial of worries, needs, and vulnerabilities; and disavowal of the need for an attachment figure's presence or support. All of these cause a person to ignore attachment figures, reject their offers of assistance, and reduce expressions of affection and engagement in intimate emotional communication (Edelstein & Shaver, 2004).

THE REGULATORY FUNCTION OF ATTACHMENT SYSTEM ACTIVATION

A core issue in attachment theory (Bowlby, 1969/1982) is the involvement of the attachment system in regulating negative emotions provoked by the appraisal of threats and dangers. Bowlby noted that reactions to such provocations include not only the classically emphasized "fight-or-flight" responses (Cannon, 1939), but also seeking proximity to a "stronger and wiser," supportive, and protective attachment figure. Main (1990) called this the "primary" attachment strategy. In adulthood (and probably childhood as well, although our concern here is adulthood), people can seek proximity to and support from an attachment figure either by requesting actual support from a real, physically present relationship partner, or by calling upon mental images, prototypes, schemas, or specific memories of interactions with real or imagined (e.g., spiritual) attachment figures. Adults can also engage in self-soothing routines learned in interactions with attachment figures (Mikulincer & Shaver, 2004). In other words, the primary attachment strategy—whether enacted in behavior or evoked internally in the form of mental representations—is often crucial for effective emotion regulation, as one might expect in the members of an intensely social species.

In constructing our model of attachment system functioning, we have postulated a two-stage process by which threat appraisals lead to activation of the primary attachment strategy. In the first stage, threat appraisals trigger preconscious activation of the system, which brings about an automatic increase in the mental accessibility of attachment-related representations in an associative memory network. In the second stage, this preconscious activation, if sufficiently robust, results in conscious thoughts about seeking proximity to attachment figures, behavioral intentions to seek proximity and support, and actual seeking of proximity and support.

According to our theory, preconscious activation of the attachment system involves heightened access to mental representations of available and responsive attachment figures; episodic memories of supportive and comforting interactions with these figures; thoughts and images related to closeness, love, comfort, relief, and support; and proximity-seeking goals. These mental processes and contents become automatically available for use in further information processing and can color a person's state of mind and influence his or her behavioral intentions and actual behaviors, even before they are consciously formulated. This theoretical model fits with many findings from social-cognitive research, which indicate that accessible cognitive elements shape a person's state of mind before they appear in the stream of consciousness (Bargh, 1990; Wegner & Smart, 1997).

Both stages of attachment system activation can be affected by a person's dispositional attachment style (Mikulincer & Shaver, 2003). For example, attachment security or insecurity can affect the nature of the attachment-related mental representations (memories, schemas, or images) that are automatically activated by threat appraisals. In the case of relatively secure adults, threat appraisals arouse thoughts and feelings related to positive interactions with attachment figures (i.e., thoughts of comfortable and reassuring proximity to such figures; memories or schematic summaries of practical and emotional support provided by them; and feelings of relief, gratitude, and emotional balance or equanimity). In the case of relatively insecure adults, however, threat appraisals can bring to mind—either consciously or unconsciously—negative, painful, dispiriting attachment-related experiences (e.g., separations, betrayals, rejections, and punishments). For such people, there are many firmly entrenched associative links in memory between thoughts of seeking proximity to attachment figures and memories or worries about separation, disapproval, or rejection. These links make it likely that attachment-system activation will arouse not only the hope of protection, closeness, and support, but also anxiety, ambivalence, and apprehension.

A person's dispositional attachment style can also affect his or her actual proximity- and support-seeking behavior (Mikulincer & Florian, 1998; Shaver & Clark, 1994). A secure person's history of interactions with available and responsive attachment figures increases his or her confidence that proximity seeking is an effective emotion regulation strategy, making it more likely that this strategy will be relied upon in times of need. Secure people maintain positive expectations about the availability and effectiveness of social support (Ognibene & Collins, 1998; Priel & Shamai, 1995), so it is easy for them to ask for help when needed.

In contrast, insecure people have learned through many painful experiences with unavailable or unresponsive attachment figures that the primary attachment strategy (proximity seeking) often fails to accomplish its emotion regulation goal, making it necessary to consider alternative secondary strategies: hyperactivation or deactivation of the attachment system. As a result, insecure individuals rely on alternative ways of regulating emotion rather than confidently seeking proximity to an attachment figure. Avoidantly attached adults are likely to deactivate their attachment systems, forgo support seeking, and rely mainly on themselves to deal with threats. Anxious adults are likely to regulate their emotions by signaling or expressing their needs and fears, exaggerating their distress, and presenting themselves as extremely vulnerable to pain and injury (Collins & Read, 1994; Shaver & Mikulincer, 2002a).

Preconscious Activation of the Attachment System in Adulthood

Preconscious activation of the attachment system has been studied in two series of experiments (Mikulincer, Birnbaum, Woddis, & Nachmias, 2000; Mikulincer, Gillath, & Shaver, 2002) in which young adults were subliminally primed with threat-related words (e.g., "death," "failure") or neutral words (e.g., "table," "hat"). The mental accessibility of cognitive and affective elements related to attachment was assessed with two well-validated cognitive techniques: a lexical decision task (deciding quickly whether particular strings of letters are words), and the Stroop color-naming task (naming, as quickly as possible, the color in which a particular word is printed on a computer

screen, which requires inhibiting the overlearned tendency to read the word and activate its associations in memory). These tasks reveal the accessibility of particular mental contents at a given moment, even if these contents are not experienced consciously; researchers can thus examine the effects of symbolic threats on the availability of attachment-related concepts without research participants' knowing what is being examined.

In Mikulincer and colleagues' (2000) studies, young adults performed a lexical decision task in which the letter strings included proximity-related words (e.g., "love," "hug"), separation-related words (e.g., "separation," "rejection"), neutral words (e.g., "office," "table"), positive non-attachment-related words (e.g., "honesty," "efficacy"), negative non-attachment-related words (e.g., "cheat," "lazy"), and nonwords (created by scrambling the letters of actual words—e.g., "btale" ["table"], "vleo" ["love"]). Before each letter string was presented, a threat-related word (e.g., "failure," "illness") or a neutral word ("hat") was flashed on the screen for 20 milliseconds, which is too short a time to allow a participant to perceive the stimulus consciously. (This procedure is called "subliminal priming.") Reaction times (RTs) served as a measure of the accessibility of thoughts related to the target words: The quicker the RT, the greater the accessibility (Meyer & Schvaneveldt, 1971).

Subliminal threat stimuli resulted in faster identification (implying greater mental availability) of proximity-related words, and the effect did not extend to neutral words or positive words with no obvious attachment-related connotations. Moreover, this heightened accessibility occurred regardless of attachment style (although individual differences in attachment style also had effects, as discussed below); this finding suggests that everyone is subject to preconscious activation of the attachment system, as would be expected if such activation is a species universal, biologically functional mental process.

Extending these studies, we (Mikulincer et al., 2002) conducted three experiments focused on the mental accessibility of the names of attachment figures. Each study participant completed the WHOTO questionnaire (Hazan & Zeifman, 1994), which identifies the people one turns to for proximity and support (e.g., "Whom do you like to spend time with?"), for a safe haven (e.g., "To whom do you turn for comfort when you're feeling down?"), and for a secure base (e.g., "Whom do you feel you can always count on?"). Each participant also named potentially close others who were not viewed as serving attachment figure functions (e.g., father, sibling, friend—if not mentioned in the WHOTO questionnaire), as well as acquaintances who were not emotionally close (e.g., coworkers, casual friends). The participants also selected names that did not apply to anyone they knew personally. Each participant then performed either a lexical decision task or a Stroop color-naming task. In the lexical decision task, they were presented with the names of their own attachment figures, names of close people who were not attachment figures, names of acquaintances, names of unknown persons, and nonwords. They were asked in each case to indicate as quickly as possible whether each string of letters was or was not a person's name. In the Stroop task, participants were exposed to the same four categories of names, each printed in one of several colors, and were asked to indicate the color in which each name was printed. Before each trial, a threat stimulus (the word "failure" or "separation") or a neutral word ("hat," "umbrella") was presented for 20 milliseconds.

Across the three experiments, participants reacted to subliminal threats with heightened accessibility of attachment figures' names. As compared with emotionally neutral words, subliminal threat words resulted in (1) faster identification of the names of attachment figures in the lexical decision task, and (2) slower color designations of attachment figures' names in the Stroop task. In both cases, short lexical decision RTs and slow color-naming RTs were interpreted as indicating heightened activation of mental representations of attachment figures' names (and probably other attachment figure qualities; Mikulincer & Shaver, 2004) in threatening contexts. Subliminal threat words had no effect on mental representations of close others or acquaintances who were not mentioned in the WHOTO questionnaire. Thus heightened accessibility of mental representations of a particular person under threatening conditions depended on the extent to which the person was viewed as a safe haven and a secure base (i.e., as an attachment figure).

Individual Differences in Preconscious Activation of the Attachment System

In addition to obtaining these overall effects, we found that more secure adults had readier access to thoughts about proximity and to the names of attachment figures, *but only in a threatening context* (Mikulincer et al., 2000, 2002). That is, se-

cure adults were not chronically or continually preoccupied with attachment-related themes or particular attachment figures. Rather, attachment-related cognitions were activated only by signals that protection might be needed. In addition, Mikulincer and colleagues (2000) found that more secure individuals' reactions to subliminal threats were limited to attachment themes with positive connotations; they displayed relatively little activation of words related to separation or rejection. We interpret these results as indicating that secure adults' favorable attachment histories resulted in a distinction in their memories between attachment system activation on the one hand, and worries about rejection on the other.

Attachment-anxious individuals' pattern of name activation was essentially the opposite of the secure individuals' pattern (Mikulincer et al., 2000, 2002). First, the more anxious people (as indicated by their scores on the ECR attachment anxiety scale) displayed heightened mental access to attachment-related themes and attachment figures' names *in both threatening and nonthreatening contexts*. Second, they displayed readier access to words related to separation and rejection. We interpret these findings as indicating hyperactivation of attachment-related thoughts, which seems to occur even in nonthreatening contexts (or perhaps alters the threshold for perceiving a situation as threatening).

Avoidant individuals produced a more complicated set of results. In general, their pattern of access to attachment-related mental contents resembled that of secure people. However, there were important differences. For avoidant people, thoughts about rejection and separation were relatively inaccessible even following subliminal exposure to the word "death," which is usually a potent activator of attachment-related fears (Kalish, 1985). Moreover, these worries suddenly became accessible to avoidant individuals in response to subliminal threats if a "cognitive load" was added to the lexical decision task. That is, when avoidant adults had to engage in an additional cognitively demanding task (rehearsing and remembering a long series of digits), they seemed to lack the resources necessary to maintain their usual defensive exclusion of attachment-related concerns. These results support the theoretical notion that avoidant people are insecure, like anxiously attached people, but are more or less continuously using defensive means to suppress or deny their insecurity.

We (Mikulincer et al., 2002) also found that when the threat word was "separation," secure individuals exhibited enhanced access to the names of their attachment figures, whereas avoidant individuals exhibited *decreased* access. There was no such difference when the subliminal threat word was "failure," which is not as closely related to attachment. It therefore seems that the attachment system is preconsciously activated under attachment-unrelated threatening conditions in both avoidant and nonavoidant people, but is preconsciously inhibited or deactivated under attachment-related threatening conditions (or at least following the threat of separation) if a person is avoidant. It seems likely that avoidant adults have learned not to appeal to attachment figures when these figures threaten to leave. This result is compatible with Ainsworth and colleagues' (1978) statement that "avoidance short circuits direct expression of anger to the attachment figure, which might be dangerous, and it also protects the baby from re-experiencing the rebuff that he has come to expect when he seeks close contact with his mother" (p. 320).

Proximity Seeking and Support Seeking as Emotion Regulation Strategies

There is extensive evidence that threats activate the seeking of proximity and support in most adults, and this evidence is found in a variety of scientific literatures. For example, studies testing Schachter's (1959) famous hypothesis that fear increases affiliation have consistently shown that anticipating noxious experiences heightens the desire to be with another person whom one perceives as similar to oneself or likely to be sympathetic (see Shaver & Klinnert, 1982, for a review). Similarly, theory and research on stress and coping indicate that a common method of coping with threats is to seek social and emotional support (see Zeidner & Endler, 1996, for a review). Recent studies of "terror management" (i.e., studies of people's management of death anxiety) have demonstrated that mortality salience (i.e., heightened death awareness) causes many people to search for proximity and support as a means of quelling death concerns and restoring emotional stability (Mikulincer, Florian, & Hirschberger, 2003).

Research has also shown that attachment style moderates the choice of proximity seeking or support seeking as an emotion regulation strategy. For example, death concerns intensify proximity-seeking efforts mainly on the part of secure rather than insecure people (Mikulincer & Florian, 2000; Taubman–Ben-Ari, Findler, & Mikulincer, 2002).

In addition, attachment security predisposes a person to seek comfort and assistance from both informal sources of support (e.g., parents, friends) and formal sources (e.g., teachers, counselors) (e.g., Larose & Bernier, 2001; Mikulincer & Florian, 1998; Seiffge-Krenke & Beyers, 2005). This tendency can also be seen in the methods used by secure people to cope with stressful events (see Mikulincer & Florian, 1998, 2001, for reviews). Across a variety of personal threats (e.g., a missile attack, combat training, chronic pain) and specifically attachment-related threats (e.g., separation from a romantic partner, interpersonal conflict, transition to parenthood), secure people report greater reliance on support seeking than do insecure people.

Secure people's support seeking has also been demonstrated in a set of three experiments examining the tendency to seek proximity to symbolic attachment figures, such as God, in times of need (Birgegard & Granqvist, 2004). Swedish undergraduates were subliminally exposed to attachment-related threats ("Mother is gone," "God has abandoned me") or subliminal control primes (e.g., "People are walking"). They then completed a measure of seeking proximity to God (e.g., "I turn to God when I am in pain," "I strive to maintain closeness to God"). In all three studies, secure individuals reacted to the subliminal separation prime (as compared to the neutral prime) with heightened seeking of proximity to God. Insecure undergraduates were less likely to seek proximity to God following a separation prime. Mikulincer, Gurwitz, and Shaver (2007) similarly found that Jewish students exposed to subliminal threats showed increased access to God-related words, and that subliminal presentation of a religious object (a Torah scroll) resulted in increased positive feelings that could be unconsciously transferred to a formerly neutral stimulus. (See Granqvist & Kirkpatrick, Chapter 38, this volume, for a review of studies on attachment and religion.)

In line with theory, other studies revealed that secure people are more likely than insecure ones to benefit from supportive interactions when coping with stress; in fact, they benefit even from mere proximity to a close relationship partner. As an example of the effects of a supportive interaction, Mikulincer and Florian (1997) found that secure people, after anticipating handling a snake, benefited from both an emotionally supportive conversation (talking about the emotions elicited by the snake) and an instrumentally supportive conversation (talking about how to deal with the snake). However, these conversations failed to improve the affective states of insecure people, and the emotionally supportive conversation was actually detrimental to avoidant individuals' affective states, whereas an instrumentally supportive conversation was detrimental to attachment-anxious individuals.

Other research has shown that symbolic proximity to a relationship partner in times of need has beneficial effects on secure individuals. For example, McGowan (2002) asked people to think about a significant other or an acquaintance while waiting to take part in a stressful task. Thinking about a significant other lowered distress among secure people, but insecure ones reported greater distress after thinking about a significant other rather than an acquaintance.

Attachment style differences have also been noted in studies of actual support seeking from dating and marital partners. In two studies, Simpson and colleagues told one member of a dating couple (women in Simpson, Rholes, & Nelligan, 1992; men in Simpson, Rholes, Orina, & Grich, 2002) that she or he would undergo a scary, painful laboratory procedure after waiting with a partner for 5 minutes. During this time, participants' behavior was unobtrusively videotaped so that raters could code the extent to which each participant sought support. A comparison of results from the two studies revealed an interesting gender difference in the link between attachment style and support seeking. For women, avoidance tended to inhibit the seeking of a partner's support mainly when anxiety was high. In such cases, avoidant women often attempted to distract themselves by reading magazines instead of seeking support. For men, however, there was no association between attachment style and support seeking. Simpson and colleagues (2002) attributed this lack of an association to social norms that inhibit men's seeking of support from women, or to men's tendency to perceive the experimental tasks as nonthreatening.

Two other observational studies provide evidence concerning avoidant and anxious people's different attitudes toward support seeking (Collins & Feeney, 2000; Fraley & Shaver, 1998). Fraley and Shaver (1998) unobtrusively coded expressions of desire for proximity and support when romantic or marital partners were about to separate from each other at a metropolitan airport, and Collins and Feeney (2000) coded support-seeking behavior while members of seriously dating couples talked about a personal problem. In both studies, avoidance was associated with less frequent seeking of proximity or support. In addition, although

attachment anxiety did not affect direct requests for partner proximity and support, it was associated with indirect methods of support seeking, such as nonverbally signaling distress (by crying, pouting, or sulking).

Overall, the evidence consistently indicates that attachment security fosters support seeking and generally does so in constructive and effective ways, whereas attachment insecurities inhibit or interfere with effective support seeking. Avoidant individuals react to threats with preconscious activation of the attachment system, but their deactivating strategies inhibit behavioral expressions of need. Anxious individuals also show strong evidence of preconscious activation of attachment-related thoughts, but for them the associated preconscious activation of worries about rejection and abandonment seems to disorganize their efforts to seek support. These worries, coupled with doubts about others' supportiveness, can interfere with direct requests for help and cause a person to rely on indirect expressions of helplessness and distress, which may not be effective. Of course, these conclusions come from integrating the findings from different studies. It would be valuable to have a single study assessing attachment style differences in both preconscious activation of support-seeking representations and actual support-seeking behavior.

Recent research has also supported another important tenet of attachment theory: that successful support seeking allows a person to become less dependent and more autonomous over time. Child development researchers had already shown that by the end of the first year of life, infants whose mothers responded regularly and promptly to their crying cried much less than infants whose mothers frequently let them cry (e.g., Ainsworth et al., 1978; Belsky, Rovine, & Taylor, 1984; Bowlby, 1988). In other words, mothers' sensitivity and responsiveness to their children's distress signals resulted in less fussy and less needy children, contrary to what many behaviorist child-rearing manuals formerly claimed (e.g., Belsky & Isabella, 1988). Moreover, attachment researchers who study adolescents have found that adolescent autonomy is most easily and effectively achieved within the context of secure attachments to parents (e.g., Allen, Chapter 19, this volume; Dykas, Ziv, Feeney, & Cassidy, 2007; Noom, Dekovic, & Meeus, 1999).

B. C. Feeney (2007) used multiple methods to test the same idea in the context of young adult romantic relationships. She hypothesized and found that a close relationship partner's acceptance of proximity seeking and dependence in times of need (i.e., being sensitively responsive to distress cues) was associated with less dependence, more autonomous functioning, and more self-sufficiency on the part of the supported individual. In two studies, she collected measures of a partner's acceptance of dependence needs and a target person's independent functioning. Measures included couple members' reports, their behavior during laboratory tasks, responses to experimentally manipulated partner assistance during an individual laboratory task, and successful goal striving over a period of 6 months. All of the results supported the hypothesis that having a dependence-accepting romantic partner allows a young adult to be more courageous and independent.

THE BROADEN-AND-BUILD CYCLE OF ATTACHMENT SECURITY

In this section, we focus on the second component of our model: the broaden-and-build cycle of attachment security produced by actual or symbolic encounters and interactions with available attachment figures in times of need. This cycle is a cascade of mental and behavioral events that enhances a person's resources for maintaining a calm and confident state of mind when dealing with life tasks, threats, and challenges, and that broadens a person's perspectives and capacities. The actual or symbolic availability of comforting, caring attachment figures, combined with their responsive provision of protection and support, generates feelings of safety and security, enhances a person's sense of self-worth and lovability, and builds confidence in the benefits of seeking support from relationship partners. Over time, repeatedly attaining felt security enhances and reinforces a person's coping capacities, creating a flexible repertoire of coping skills that increasingly functions autonomously. This security and self-confidence allow other behavioral systems (such as exploration and caregiving) to operate effectively, adding to a secure person's understanding of self and world, physical and mental health, and life skills.

Positive Mood and Mental Health

The most immediate psychological benefits of attachment figures' availability are successful regulation of distress and the restoration of emotional balance. Interactions with available and supportive attachment figures, by imparting a sense of safety, assuage distress and evoke positive emotions (relief, satisfaction, gratitude). Secure people can therefore remain relatively unperturbed under stress and experience longer periods of positive affect. Indeed, numerous studies have shown that securely attached people score higher than their insecurely attached peers on measures of joy, happiness, interest, love, and affection (see Mikulincer & Shaver, 2007, for a review). For example, in two diary studies, each lasting a week, participants completed the Rochester Interaction Record every time they engaged in a social interaction lasting 10 minutes or longer. Both sets of investigators and (Pietromonaco & Barrett, 1997; Tidwell, Reis, & Shaver, 1996) found that more secure individuals experienced more positive emotions during daily interactions.

Attachment researchers using both cross-sectional and prospective longitudinal designs have also found predicted associations between secure attachment to parents or romantic partners on the one hand, and lower levels of negative affect and less severe psychiatric symptoms on the other (see Mikulincer & Shaver, 2007, for a review). For example, Torquati and Raffaelli (2004) asked undergraduates to report their emotions six or seven times a day for 1 week and found that secure individuals (assessed with self-report scales) experienced less frequent and less intense negative emotions than insecure individuals did. Interestingly, this difference was strongest during everyday situations in which participants were not involved in social interaction. When alone, insecure undergraduates were more likely than secure ones to feel lonely, irritable, and anxious.

Several studies have also found that attachment security is associated with lower levels of distress during periods of stress and strain, whereas attachment insecurities—anxiety, avoidance, or both—are associated with heightened distress and deteriorated well-being (e.g., Birnbaum, Orr, Mikulincer, & Florian, 1997; Mikulincer & Florian, 1998; Mikulincer, Florian, & Weller, 1993). Some of these studies compared the emotional reactions of people undergoing stressful experiences with those of control samples and discovered an additional benefit of attachment security (e.g., Berant, Mikulincer, & Florian, 2001; Birnbaum et al., 1997; Mikulincer & Florian, 1998): Stressful events raise the level of negative emotion mainly among insecurely attached people, but not among people with a secure attachment style. For secure people, there is often no notable difference in emotion between neutral and stressful conditions—another indication that felt security is an effective stress buffer.

Experimental studies have shown that temporarily activating mental representations of available and responsive attachment figures (which we call "security priming") can augment a person's emotional balance and adaptability, even under fairly stressful circumstances (e.g., Mikulincer, Gillath, et al., 2001; Mikulincer, Hirschberger, Nachmias, & Gillath, 2001; Mikulincer & Shaver, 2001). In these experiments, mental representations of supportive attachment figures have been activated by well-validated social-cognitive techniques, such as subliminally presenting pictures suggestive of attachment figures' availability (e.g., a Picasso drawing of a mother lovingly cradling an infant, a couple holding hands and gazing into each other's eyes), names of people who were designated by participants as security-enhancing attachment figures, positive attachment-related words (e.g., "love," "closeness," "hug"), guided images of available and supportive attachment figures, and visualization of security-enhancing attachment figures' faces. In all of these studies, portrayals of attachment figures' availability led to more positive moods than priming with attachment-unrelated stimuli.

Mikulincer, Hirschberger, and colleagues (2001) also found that priming with representations of supportive attachment figures infused formerly neutral stimuli with positive qualities, even when the priming was done subliminally. For example, subliminal presentation of the names of people who were designated by participants as security-enhancing attachment figures, compared with the names of close others or mere acquaintances who were not designated as attachment figures, led to greater liking of previously unfamiliar Chinese ideographs. Moreover, subliminally priming mental representations of available attachment figures induced more positive evaluations of neutral stimuli, even in threatening contexts, and eliminated the detrimental effects that threats otherwise had on liking for neutral stimuli. Thus priming with mental representations of security-enhancing attachment figures has a calming, soothing effect, similar to the effects of actual interactions with available and responsive relationship partners.

Broadening Capacities and Perspectives

In his account of behavioral systems, Bowlby (1969/1982) proposed that dynamic interplay between the attachment system and other behavioral systems (such as exploration, caregiving, and sex) contributes to the development of personal knowledge and skills, opens a person's mind to new possibilities and perspectives, and helps the person adapt flexibly to a variety of situations and actualize natural talents. One reason for these beneficial effects is that security-enhancing interactions reduce anxiety, vigilance, and preoccupation with attachment, allowing a person to devote more attention and effort to growth-oriented activities. Moreover, these interactions impart a sense of safety and protection that allows a person to take calculated risks and accept important challenges. With security-enhancing relationships in mind, one can feel confident that support is available when needed, and can know that one's relationship partners will accept and love one if even some mistakes are made or some decisions prove ill-fated.

Bowlby (1973) and Ainsworth (1991) were especially interested in the relation between attachment and exploration, conceptualized as two separate behavioral systems. They proposed that an available and supportive attachment figure enhances an infant's curiosity and encourages relaxed exploration of the physical and social worlds. In adulthood, we propose, attachment security should also foster openness to new information and accommodation of one's knowledge structures when evidence indicates that accommodation is called for. In line with this hypothesis, there is evidence for associations between self-reports of attachment security and measures of curiosity (see Mikulincer & Shaver, 2007, for a review). In addition, secure adults score lower than insecure ones on self-report measures of cognitive closure, intolerance of ambiguity, and dogmatic thinking (e.g., Mikulincer, 1997). In laboratory studies, Mikulincer (1997) found that secure people were less likely than insecure ones (1) to make judgments based on early information while ignoring later data, and (2) to make stereotype-based judgments (i.e., to judge a group member based on a generalized notion about the group rather than information about the particular member).

Research has also demonstrated that experimental priming of mental representations of available and supportive attachment figures has beneficial effects on exploration and cognitive openness. For example, Green and Campbell (2000) primed representations of attachment figures' availability or unavailability (by asking people to read sentences describing secure or insecure close relationships) and found that secure primes led to stronger endorsement of exploration-related behavior and greater liking for novel pictures than insecure primes did. Moreover, Mikulincer and Arad (1999, Study 3) found that people who were asked to visualize a responsive and supportive relationship partner (as compared to those who visualized a rejecting partner) showed increased cognitive openness and were more likely to revise knowledge about a relationship partner following behavior by the partner that seemed inconsistent with prior actions.

Experimental priming of mental representations of available and responsive attachment figures also affects negative, prejudicial attitudes toward outgroups (Mikulincer & Shaver, 2001). In five experiments, we found that momentarily activating mental representations of attachment figures' availability (by subliminally presenting security-related words, such as "love" and "closeness," or by asking participants to read a story or visualize the face of a supportive relationship partner) eliminated negative responses to a variety of outgroups (as perceived by heterosexual, secular Israeli Jewish students): Israeli Arabs, ultra-Orthodox Jews, Russian immigrants, and homosexuals. That is, mental representations of available attachment figures promoted more tolerant and accepting attitudes toward people who did not belong to the study participants' own social group.

Theoretically, the security-enhancing, "broadening" effects of attachment figures' availability can also encourage people to apply their effective emotion regulation strategies to alleviate other people's distress and help them manage life hardships. As we have noted elsewhere (Shaver & Mikulincer, 2002a), securely attached people rely on constructive emotion regulation strategies, which allow them to reduce their own distress and feel confident that they can effectively deal with others' problems. As a result, attachment security improves the functioning of the caregiving system, which expresses itself in willingness to provide care to others who are suffering or otherwise in need (Gillath, Shaver, & Mikulincer, 2005). In line with this prediction, several studies have found that more securely attached people report more empathic concern for others (e.g., B. C. Feeney & Collins, 2001; Joireman, Needham, & Cummings, 2002; Lopez, 2001), stronger inclinations to take the perspective of a distressed person (e.g., Corcoran & Mallinckrodt, 2000; Joireman et al., 2002), and greater willingness to take responsibility for others' welfare (e.g., Collins & Read, 1990; Shaver et al., 1996).

In a laboratory study involving behavioral observations, Westmaas and Silver (2001) videotaped people while they interacted with a confederate of the experimenter whom they thought had recently been diagnosed with cancer. The authors found that both kinds of attachment insecurity created specific impediments to effective caregiving. As expected, avoidant participants were rated by observers as less verbally and nonverbally supportive, and as less likely to make eye contact during the interaction. Attachment anxiety was not associated with supportiveness, but more anxious participants reported greater discomfort while interacting with the confederate and were more likely to report self-critical thoughts after the interaction (as measured in free-thought listings).

Recently we examined the effects of both dispositional attachment orientations and contextually activated representations of attachment security on the way people deal with others' suffering and regulate the personal distress caused by witnessing a needy other (Mikulincer, Gillath, et al., 2001; Mikulincer, Shaver, Gillath, & Nitzberg, 2005). For example, Mikulincer, Gillath, and colleagues (2001, Study 1) performed an experiment examining the effects of security priming (having participants read a story about a loving attachment figure providing social and emotional support) on compassionate responses to a brief story about a student whose parents had been killed in an automobile accident. As expected, an enhanced sense of security led to stronger compassionate responses than the mere priming of positive affect or neutral representations. Converging findings emerged from four additional studies (Mikulincer, Gillath, et al., 2001, Studies 2–5) using different techniques for heightening security (e.g., asking participants to recall personal memories of supportive care, subliminally exposing them to proximity-related words) and measuring different dependent variables (e.g., coded descriptions of feelings elicited by others' suffering, accessibility of memories in which participants felt compassion or distress).

In a more recent series of studies, we (Mikulincer et al., 2005) examined the actual decision to help or not to help a person in distress. In the first two experiments, each participant watched a confederate while she performed a series of aversive tasks. As the study progressed, the confederate became increasingly distressed about the aversive tasks, and the actual participant was given an opportunity to take the distressed person's place, in effect sacrificing self for the welfare of another. Shortly before this scenario unfolded, participants were primed with either representations of attachment security (the name of a participant's security provider) or attachment-unrelated representations (the name of a familiar person who was not an attachment figure or the name of a mere acquaintance). This priming procedure was conducted at either a subliminal level (by very rapidly presenting the name) or supraliminal level (by asking participants to recall an interaction with a particularly supportive person). We found that either subliminal or supraliminal activation of the sense of attachment security increased participants' compassion and willingness to take the place of a distressed other.

Overall, research indicates that actual or imagined (i.e., symbolic) interactions with loving, supportive attachment figures move a person toward the ideal advocated by major religions and humanistic psychologists—a calm, confident person who is willing and able to establish intimate, caring relationships and take risks to help others and broaden personal skills and perspectives. Following Bowlby's (1988) lead, we conclude that attachment security, even in adulthood, acts as a growth-enhancing psychological agent or catalyst: It fosters prosocial motives and attitudes, and promotes personal development and improved relationships.

Mechanisms Underlying the Broaden-and-Build Cycle of Attachment Security

In theory, the broaden-and-build cycle of attachment security is maintained by mental representations of the actual or symbolic availability of sensitive and responsive attachment figures. These representations include both declarative and procedural knowledge organized around a relational prototype or script (Waters, Rodrigues, & Ridgeway, 1998), which includes something like the following if–then propositions: "If I encounter an obstacle and/or become distressed, I can approach a significant other for help; he or she is likely to be available and supportive; I will experience relief and comfort as a result of proximity to this person; I can then return to other activities." Once activated, this script serves as a guide for adaptively regulating one's own affective processes. In this section, we review four different, but related, kinds of declarative and procedural knowledge that underlie the broaden-and-build cycle of attachment security and sustain its positive effects on emotion regulation, mental health, and psychological functioning: (1) optimistic life appraisals, (2) positive

mental representations of others, (3) authentic forms of positive self-views, and (4) constructive coping strategies.

Life Appraisals

We propose that representations of attachment security include, or are associatively linked to, declarative beliefs and procedural knowledge, which play a central role in maintaining emotional stability and personal adjustment. The first set of beliefs concerns the appraisal of life problems as manageable, which helps a person maintain an optimistic and hopeful stance regarding distress management. These beliefs are a result of positive interactions with sensitive and available attachment figures, during which individuals learn that distress is manageable, external obstacles can be overcome, and the course and outcome of most threatening events are at least partially controllable. Adult attachment studies have shown that secure individuals, as identified by self-report measures, tend to appraise a wide variety of stressful events in less threatening terms than insecure people (either anxious or avoidant) do, and to hold more optimistic expectations about their ability to cope with stressful events (e.g., Berant et al., 2001; Mikulincer & Florian, 1995; Radecki-Bush, Farrell, & Bush, 1993). In addition, attachment security has been empirically associated with more positive expectations regarding the regulation of negative moods (e.g., Creasey, 2002; Creasey & Ladd, 2004); more hopeful attitudes toward life (e.g., Shorey, Snyder, Yang, & Lewin, 2003); and hardier, more stress-resistant attitudes (Mayseless, 2004; Neria et al., 2001).

Mental Representations of Others

The second kind of declarative knowledge that supports effective emotion regulation and distress alleviation consists of positive beliefs about others' intentions and traits. That is, beliefs that others will respond to one's needs can help a person manage negative emotions and managing distress. Again, these positive representations are presumably a result of interactions with available, responsive attachment figures, during which individuals learn about the sensitivity, responsiveness, and goodwill of their primary relationship partners. Regularly experiencing attachment figures' availability can assuage worries about being rejected, criticized, disapproved, or abused. Such experiences bolster a person's willingness to get close to a partner; express needs, desires, hopes, and vulnerabilities; and ask for support when needed.

This positive relational process begins with appraising an attachment figure's sensitivity and responsiveness, and then forming positive beliefs and expectations about this person's good qualities and intentions. A person who regularly has such experiences with another person gradually becomes confident that such a good and caring figure is unlikely to betray one's trust, will not react negatively or abusively to expressions of need, and will not reject bids for closeness. With such confidence, it is easy for a person to behave prosocially and become more deeply involved in a relationship. Numerous studies have shown that individuals who score low on attachment anxiety and avoidance (i.e., those who are relatively secure) possess a positive view of human nature (e.g., Collins & Read, 1990; Hazan & Shaver, 1987), use positive trait terms to describe relationship partners (e.g., J. A. Feeney & Noller, 1991; Levy, Blatt, & Shaver, 1998), perceive partners as supportive (e.g., Davis, Morris, & Kraus, 1998; Ognibene & Collins, 1998), and feel trusting toward partners (e.g., Collins & Read, 1990; Hazan & Shaver, 1987; Simpson, 1990). In addition, securely attached people have positive expectations concerning their partners' behavior (e.g., Baldwin, Fehr, Keedian, Seidel, & Thompson, 1993; Baldwin, Keelan, Fehr, Enns, & Koh-Rangarajoo, 1996) and tend to explain a partner's negative behavior in relatively positive terms (e.g., Collins, 1996).

Using priming techniques, attachment researchers have found that momentarily activating mental representations of available and supportive attachment figures has beneficial effects on expectations concerning a partner's behavior. For example, Rowe and Carnelley (2003) primed participants with representations of attachment figures' availability or unavailability (writing for 10 minutes about a relationship in which they had felt secure or insecure) and asked them to complete a questionnaire assessing general expectations about relationship partners' behavior. Priming with examples of partner availability led to more positive expectations for the current relationship than priming with insecure representations.

Authentic Self-Esteem

The third kind of declarative knowledge included in security-maintaining mental representations is authentic, well-grounded confidence in one's own worth, competence, and mastery. This solid sense of personal value is crucial for maintaining stable self-esteem and emotional balance in the face of failure, rejection, or other life difficulties. It also sustains autonomous emotion regulation by providing people with effective self-soothing procedures that can alleviate distress even in the absence of actual attachment figures.

During interactions with sensitive, available attachment figures, individuals learn to view themselves as active, strong, and competent, because they can effectively mobilize a partner's support and overcome threats that activate attachment behavior. These beliefs are tied to confidence that they can effectively overcome obstacles and manage distress. More secure individuals generally perceive themselves to be valuable, lovable, and special—thanks to having been valued, loved, and regarded as special by caring attachment figures. For example, compared to people with an anxious attachment style, secure individuals report higher self-esteem (e.g., Bartholomew & Horowitz, 1991; Mickelson, Kessler, & Shaver, 1997); view themselves as competent and efficacious (e.g., Brennan & Morris, 1997; Cooper, Shaver, & Collins, 1998); and describe themselves in positive terms and have small discrepancies between their actual self-representations and self-standards (Mikulincer, 1995).

Interactions with available, caring, and loving attachment figures in times of need constitute the primary source of an authentic, stable sense of self-worth (Kernis, 2003), which Rogers (1961) called the "real self"—that is, positive self-perceptions derived from other people's obvious and unconditional positive regard. Because securely attached people are able to feel good about themselves even under threatening conditions, there is less need for them to inflate their self-esteem defensively or reject other people's honest criticism. In fact, reliance on defensive emotion regulation strategies is an indication that a person has been forced by social experiences to cope with threats and stressors without adequate mental representations of attachment security, and has had to struggle for a sense of safety, self-worth, and lovability.

Adult attachment research provides support for these theoretical ideas. For example, Mikulincer (1995) measured the accessibility of positive and negative self-relevant traits in a Stroop task and examined the level of integration among people's different self-aspects. He found that people who scored high on attachment security could easily call to mind both positive and negative self-attributes and include all of them within a highly integrated self-structure. More avoidant participants exhibited a defensive self-organization marked by poor access to negative self-attributes and low integration among these attributes and other self-aspects.

In another series of four studies, Mikulincer (1998a) found that defensive strategies of emotion regulation (e.g., self-inflation) were most characteristic of avoidant individuals, especially under threatening conditions, and that secure individuals made relatively stable and unbiased self-appraisals even when confronted with self-relevant threats. People in these studies were exposed to various kinds of threatening or neutral situations, and self-appraisals were measured with self-report scales and other subtler cognitive techniques (e.g., RTs for trait recognition). Participants who classified themselves as secure did not differ in their self-appraisals between neutral and threatening conditions. But avoidant participants made more explicit and implicit positive self-appraisals following threatening, as compared with neutral, situations—evidence of relying on defensive strategies of emotion regulation.

Two other studies provide evidence of the effects of contextually activated representations of attachment security on self-enhancement tendencies (Arndt, Schimel, Greenberg, & Pyszczynski, 2002; Schimel, Arndt, Pyszczynski, & Greenberg, 2001). In these studies, thoughts about attachment figures' availability (e.g., thinking about an accepting and loving other) or neutral thoughts were encouraged, and participants' use of particular self-enhancement strategies was assessed. Schimel and colleagues (2001) studied defensive biases in social comparison—that is, searching for more social comparison information when it was likely to suggest that one had performed better than other people (Pyszczynski, Greenberg, & LaPrelle, 1985). Arndt and colleagues (2002) studied defensive self-handicapping—that is, emphasizing factors that impair one's performance in an effort to protect against the damage to self-esteem that might result from attributing negative outcomes to one's lack of ability (Berglas & Jones, 1978). In both studies, momentary strengthening of mental representations of attachment figures' availability weakened the tendency to make self-enhancing social comparisons or self-handicapping attributions.

Adult attachment studies also suggest ways in which securely attached people can maintain a stable sense of self-worth without pursuing defensive self-enhancement strategies. For example, we

(Mikulincer & Shaver, 2004) proposed that some components or subroutines of the self that originate in interactions with available attachment figures ("security-based self-representations") underlie the maintenance of self-worth and emotional equanimity in times of stress. Specifically, we focused on (1) representations of the self derived from how a person sees and evaluates him- or herself during interactions with an available attachment figure ("self in relation with a security-enhancing attachment figure"); and (2) representations of the self derived from identification with features and traits of a caring, supportive attachment figure ("self-caregiving representations"). We hypothesized that these representations would become accessible during encounters with threats; would have a soothing, comforting effect on the person; and would render the pursuit of defensive self-enhancement strategies unnecessary.

To test these expectations, we conducted two separate two-session studies. In the first session of each study, we asked participants to generate traits that described a security-enhancing attachment figure and themselves in relation with this figure. In the second session, we exposed participants to either a threatening or a neutral condition, noted the accessibility of various categories of traits within their self-descriptions, and then assessed their current emotional and cognitive state. As predicted, securely attached participants reacted to the threat condition with greater mental access to security-based self-representations: They rated traits that they had originally attributed to a security-enhancing attachment figure or to the "self in relation with this figure" as more descriptive of their current selves following threatening than following neutral conditions. This heightened accessibility of security-based self-representations was not observed among insecurely attached participants. More important, security-based self-representations had a soothing effect: The greater the accessibility of these self-representations, the more positive was a participant's emotional state following a threat, and the less frequent were task-related worries and other interfering thoughts. Thus it appears that secure individuals can mobilize caring qualities within themselves—qualities modeled on those of their attachment figures—as well as representations of being loved and valued. And these representations seem to provide real comfort, allowing a person to feel worthy and unperturbed without engaging in defensive forms of self-enhancement to regulate distress and maintain equanimity.

Constructive Coping Strategies

We propose further that representations of attachment security involve procedural knowledge about emotion regulation and coping effectively with stress. When regulating emotions, a secure person is able to direct most of his or her effort to changing the emotion-eliciting event (e.g., by resolving a conflict or solving a problem) or reappraising it, and is thereby able to sidestep or short-circuit many painful experiences. Specifically, when a secure person encounters internal or external stimuli or events that might provoke undesirable emotions, he or she can engage in problem solving, planning, and cognitive reappraisal; place the negative event in a broader context, making it seem less overwhelming; and mobilize support from people with additional resources or perspectives for solving the problem or reducing its painful effects. The secure person is also more likely to have developed a repertoire of self-soothing skills: calming him- or herself with implicit and explicit routines learned from security-providing attachment figures, and maintaining attention on constructive alternatives rather than becoming a victim of rumination or catastrophizing. These constructive regulatory efforts are what Epstein and Meier (1989) called "constructive ways of coping" and Gross (1999) called "antecedent-focused emotion regulation" (as distinct from suppressing an emotion after its antecedents have already had their full effects).

Research has consistently revealed an association between secure attachment and constructive, problem-focused coping. For example, self-reports of attachment security are associated with reliance on problem-focused coping strategies in studies involving a wide variety of stressors (e.g., Lussier, Sabourin, & Turgeon, 1997; Mikulincer & Florian, 1998). Moreover, people who classify themselves as securely attached tend to deal with interpersonal conflicts in their close relationships by compromising and creatively integrating their own and their partners' positions (e.g., Carnelley, Pietromonaco, & Jaffe, 1994), as well as by openly discussing the problem and resolving the conflict (e.g., Simpson, Rholes, & Phillips, 1996).

Having managed emotion-eliciting events or reappraised them in benign terms, secure people often don't have to alter or suppress other parts of the emotion process. They make what Lazarus (1991) called a "short circuit of threat," sidestepping the interfering and dysfunctional aspects of emotions while retaining their functional, adaptive qualities. They can remain open to their emotions, express and communicate feelings freely and accurately to others, and experience them fully without distortion. Secure people can also attend to their own distress without fear of losing control or becoming overwhelmed (Cassidy, 1994). For individuals whose attachment figures have been available and responsive, expression of negative emotions has usually led to distress-alleviating responses from a caregiver. The secure person learns that distress can be expressed honestly without putting the relationship at risk, and this fosters an increasingly balanced way of experiencing and expressing emotions—with a sensible goal in mind, and without undue hostility, vengeance, or anxiety about losing control or being abandoned.

In adult attachment research, there is extensive evidence that self-reports of attachment security are associated with higher scores on self-report and behavioral measures of emotional expressiveness and self-disclosure (e.g., Bradford, Feeney, & Campbell, 2002; J. A. Feeney, 1995, 1999). For example, Mikulincer and Nachshon (1991) content-analyzed participants' face-to-face verbal disclosure of personal information to another person in a laboratory situation and found that secure participants disclosed more intimate and emotion-laden information than avoidant participants did. Moreover, using a biographical memory task in which participants were asked to recall specific, early memories of positive and negative emotions, Mikulincer and Orbach (1995) found that participants who classified themselves as securely attached had ready mental access to painful memories of anger, sadness, and anxiety, and were able to reexperience some of the accompanying negative affect. However, they still had better access to positive memories of happiness and did not experience an automatic spread of associations to memories of other negative emotional experiences. This allows secure people to maintain a positive cognitive context and a well-differentiated emotion–memory architecture, which in turn allows them to process negative memories without becoming overwhelmed by negativity, as often happens in both the laboratory and real life for anxious individuals.

This functional and constructive nature of secure people's emotional experience is also evident in the way they experience and acknowledge anger. In a series of three studies, Mikulincer (1998b) found that when confronted with anger-eliciting events, secure people held optimistic expectations about a partner's subsequent behavior (e.g., "He or she will accept me") and made well-differentiated, reality-attuned appraisals of their partner's intentions. Only when there were clear contextual cues, provided by the experimenter, that a partner actually had acted with hostile intent did secure people attribute hostility to the partner and react with anger. Moreover, secure participants' accounts of anger-eliciting events were characterized by the constructive goals of repairing the relationship, engaging in adaptive problem solving, and experiencing positive affect following the temporary period of discord. Bowlby (1973) called this discord the "anger of hope," because it is intended to repair a damaged relationship. "Hope" refers to the positive expectation that a relationship partner, seeing that the securely attached person has been wronged, will be willing to discuss the matter and change accordingly.

SECONDARY ATTACHMENT STRATEGIES AND EMOTION REGULATION

"Secondary" (insecure) attachment strategies distort and damage emotion regulation, and thereby contribute to psychological and social problems. According to attachment theory (Main, 1990; Mikulincer & Shaver, 2003; Shaver & Mikulincer, 2002a, 2002b) and our model of attachment system functioning (Figure 23.2), secondary attachment strategies (hyperactivation and deactivation) include psychological defenses against the frustration and pain caused by attachment figures' unavailability. Although they are attempts at adaptation in adverse social circumstances, they end up being maladaptive when used in later relationship situations where secure strategies would be more effective. Each of the secondary strategies is aimed originally at achieving a workable relationship with an inconsistently available or consistently distant or unavailable attachment figure. In order to sustain these strategies, a person has to build otherwise distorted or constraining working models and adopt nonoptimal affect regulation strategies, which are likely to interfere with subsequent development and hamper attempts to create rewarding close relationships.

When regulating their emotions, avoidant people attempt to block or inhibit emotional states associated with threat-related thoughts (e.g., fear, sadness, shame), because these thoughts can activate unwanted attachment-related needs, memories, and behaviors. Moreover, avoidant people often view negative emotions and expressions of weakness or vulnerability as incompatible with

their desire for and maintenance of self-reliance. This causes them to inhibit natural emotional reactions to relationship threats (such as rejection, separation, and loss), and to try to keep these feelings out of consciousness. Like secure people, avoidant ones attempt to down-regulate threat-related emotions. However, whereas secure people's regulatory attempts usually promote communication, compromise, and relationship maintenance, avoidant people's efforts are aimed mainly at keeping the attachment system deactivated, regardless of the deleterious effect this can have on a relationship.

Unlike relatively secure people, those who are avoidant often cannot engage in open-minded problem solving, because this frequently requires opening one's knowledge structures (e.g., stereotypes, schemas) to new information, admitting frustration and possible defeat, dealing with uncertainty and confusion, and running freely through one's memories without attempting to block attachment system activation (Mikulincer, 1997). Avoidant people have difficulty reappraising emotion-eliciting events, because during frustrating interactions with unavailable, unresponsive, or disapproving attachment figures, they have been forced to doubt the general goodness of the world and other people's motives and intentions. They have trouble looking on the bright side of troubling events, transforming threats into challenges, and anticipating other people's support if they find themselves becoming demoralized.

Deactivating strategies cause people to avoid noticing their own emotional reactions. Avoidant individuals often deny or suppress emotion-related thoughts and memories, divert attention from emotion-related material, suppress emotion-related action tendencies, or inhibit or mask both verbal and nonverbal expressions of emotion (Kobak, Cole, Ferenz-Gillies, Fleming, & Gamble, 1993; Mikulincer & Shaver, 2003). By averting the conscious experience and expression of unpleasant emotions, avoidant individuals make it less likely that emotional experiences will be integrated into their cognitive structures and that they will use them effectively in information processing or social action. During many frustrating and painful interactions with rejecting attachment figures, they have learned that acknowledging and displaying distress lead to rejection or punishment (Cassidy, 1994).

Unlike avoidant people, who tend to view negative emotions as goal-incongruent mental states that should either be managed effectively or suppressed, anxiously attached individuals tend to perceive these emotions as congruent with attachment goals, and they therefore tend to sustain or even exaggerate them. Attachment-anxious people are guided by an unfulfilled wish to cause attachment figures to pay more attention to them and provide more reliable protection (Cassidy & Berlin, 1994; Mikulincer & Shaver, 2003). One way to attain this goal is to keep the attachment system chronically activated (i.e., in a state of hyperactivation) and intensify bids for attention until a satisfying sense of attachment security is attained. Chronically attachment-anxious individuals tend to exaggerate the presence and seriousness of threats and to remain vigilant regarding the possible unavailability of attachment figures (Kobak et al., 1993). They also tend to overemphasize their sense of helplessness and vulnerability, because signs of weakness and neediness can sometimes elicit other people's attention and care (Cassidy & Berlin, 1994). Unfortunately, this intensification of negative emotions can render problem solving irrelevant, because problem solving may thwart an anxious person's desire to perpetuate problematic situations. Moreover, problem solving works against the anxious person's self-construal as helpless and incompetent; too much competence might result in loss of attention and support from attachment figures.

How is anxious hyperactivation sustained? One method is to exaggerate the appraisal process—perceptually heightening the threatening aspects of even fairly benign events, holding onto pessimistic beliefs about one's ability to manage distress, and attributing threat-related events to uncontrollable causes and global personal inadequacies (Mikulincer & Florian, 1998). This self-defeating appraisal process is sustained by negative beliefs about both self and world (Collins & Read, 1994; Shaver & Clark, 1994). Although these beliefs are initially developed in the context of emotionally negative interactions with unavailable or unreliable attachment figures, they are sustained by cognitive biases that overgeneralize past attachment injuries and inappropriately apply memories of injuries to new situations (Mikulincer & Shaver, 2003).

Another regulatory technique that heightens the experience and expression of threat-related emotions is shifting attention toward internal indicators of distress (Cassidy & Berlin, 1994; Shaver & Mikulincer, 2002a). This maneuver involves hypervigilant attention to the physiological components of emotional states, heightened recall of

threat-related experiences, and rumination on real and potential threats (Main & Solomon, 1986; Mikulincer & Shaver, 2003). Another hyperactivating strategy is to intensify negative emotions by favoring an approach-based, counterphobic orientation toward threatening situations or making self-defeating decisions and taking ineffective courses of actions that are likely to end in failure. All of these strategies create a self-amplifying cycle of distress, which is maintained cognitively by ruminative thoughts and feelings even after a threat objectively disappears.

Interestingly, although hyperactivating and deactivating strategies lead to opposite patterns of emotional expression (intensification vs. suppression), both result in dysfunctional emotions. Avoidant people miss the adaptive aspects of emotional experiences by blocking conscious access to emotions, and anxious people miss adaptive possibilities by riveting their attention on disruptive aspects of emotional experience rather than more functional aspects. As a result, anxious individuals may perceive themselves as helpless to control the self-amplifying flow of painful thoughts and feelings, even though they are unknowingly contributing to it.

Empirical Evidence for the Regulatory Action of Secondary Attachment Strategies

There is a large body of evidence supporting the theoretical analysis above. In this section, we review this evidence while focusing on attachment style differences in coping with stress, management of attachment-related threats, experience and management of specific emotional states, and cognitive access to emotional experiences.

Coping with Stress

Several studies have supported the theoretical analysis of attachment style differences in coping with both attachment-related and attachment-unrelated stressors (e.g., Berant et al., 2001; Berant, Mikulincer, & Shaver, in press; Birnbaum et al., 1997; Mikulincer et al., 1993). Whereas anxiously attached people rely on emotion-focused coping, avoidant people are more likely to rely on distancing coping. Interestingly, three studies have revealed a significant association between avoidant attachment and emotion-focused coping. This seemingly uncharacteristic coping response for avoidant individuals may help to identify the contextual boundaries of deactivating strategies. In two studies (Lussier et al., 1997; Shapiro & Levendosky, 1999), heightened emotion-focused coping was observed in reaction to conflicts with close relationship partners. In the third study, Berant and colleagues (2001) found that avoidant mothers of newborns tended to rely on distancing coping if their infants were born healthy or with only a mild congenital heart defect (CHD), but that they seemed to use emotion-focused coping if they gave birth to children with a life-endangering CHD. It therefore seems that avoidant defenses, which are often sufficient for dealing with minor stressors, can fail when people encounter severe and persistent stressors. This conclusion is consistent with Bowlby's (1980) idea that avoidant people's segregated mental systems cannot be held outside of consciousness indefinitely, and that traumatic events can resurrect or reactivate distress that had previously been segregated and sealed off from consciousness.

Management of Attachment-Related Threats

Secondary attachment strategies are also manifested in the ways people deal with attachment-related threats. Mayseless, Danieli, and Sharabany (1996) examined the association between attachment strategies and responses to imagined separations in the projective Separation Anxiety Test; they found that whereas avoidant people refrained from dealing with the threat, anxious people reacted to separation with strong self-blame and intense distress. Similarly, when Meyer, Olivier, and Roth (2005) asked young women to imagine that their male romantic partner planned to spend time with a highly attractive woman, they found that avoidant attachment was associated with distancing responses, such as ending the relationship or avoiding contact with the partner. As expected, attachment anxiety was associated with more intense distress and more attempts to persuade the partner to change his mind.

There is also evidence that avoidant people tend to deal with attachment-related threats by suppressing separation-related thoughts. In a pair of experimental studies, Fraley and Shaver (1997) used Wegner's (1994) thought suppression paradigm and asked participants to write continuously about whatever thoughts and feelings they were experiencing while being asked to suppress thoughts about a romantic partner leaving them for someone else. In the first study, the ability to suppress these thoughts was assessed by the number of times separation-related thoughts appeared in partici-

pants' stream-of-consciousness writing following the suppression period. In the second study, this ability was assessed by the level of physiological arousal (skin conductance) during the suppression task: The lower the arousal, the greater the presumed ability to suppress the thoughts.

The findings indicated that attachment anxiety was associated with poorer ability to suppress separation-related thoughts, as indicated by more frequent thoughts of loss following the suppression task and higher skin conductance during the task. In contrast, attachment avoidance was associated with greater ability to suppress separation-related thoughts, as indicated by less frequent thoughts of loss following the suppression task and lower skin conductance during the task. A recent functional magnetic resonance imaging study (Gillath, Bunge, Shaver, Wendelken, & Mikulincer, 2005) shows that these attachment style differences are also evident in patterns of brain activation and deactivation when people are thinking about breakups/losses and when they are attempting to suppress such thoughts.

In two studies, we (Mikulincer, Dolev, & Shaver, 2004) replicated and extended Fraley and Shaver's (1997) findings while assessing, in a Stroop color-naming task, the cognitive accessibility of previously suppressed thoughts about a painful separation. Findings indicated that avoidant individuals were able to suppress thoughts related to the breakup; for them, such thoughts were relatively inaccessible, and their own positive self-traits became (presumably for defensive reasons) more accessible. However, their ability to maintain this defensive stance was disrupted when a cognitive load (remembering a seven-digit number) was added to the experimental task. Under high cognitive load, avoidant individuals exhibited ready access to thoughts of separation and negative self-traits. That is, the suppressed material resurfaced in experience and behavior when a high cognitive demand was imposed. We suspect that a similar resurfacing occurs when a high emotional demand is encountered.

Fraley, Garner, and Shaver (2000) probed the regulatory mechanisms underlying avoidant individuals' deactivation of attachment-related threats. They asked whether deactivating strategies operate in a *preemptive* manner (e.g., by deploying attention away from attachment-related threats or encoding them in only a very shallow fashion) or a *postemptive* manner (by repressing material that had been encoded). Participants listened to an interview about attachment-related threats and were asked to recall details from the interview either immediately afterward or at various delays ranging from 30 minutes to 21 days. An analysis of forgetting curves plotted over time revealed that avoidant individuals initially encoded less information about the interview than less avoidant persons did, and that the two groups forgot the information at about the same rate. Thus it seems that avoidant defenses at least sometimes act in a preemptive manner, by blocking threatening material from awareness and memory from the start.

Experiencing and Managing Anger

Several studies have examined how secondary attachment strategies affect the experience and management of anger. For example, Mikulincer (1998b) found that although avoidant individuals did not report overly intense anger in reaction to another person's negative behavior, they exhibited intense physiological arousal during discordant interactions. They also reported using distancing strategies to cope with anger-eliciting events, and displayed a tendency to attribute hostility to a partner even when there were clear contextual cues (provided by the experimenter) concerning the partner's nonhostile intent. In contrast, attachment-anxious people's recollections of anger-provoking life experiences included an uncontrollable flood of angry feelings, persistent rumination on these feelings, and sadness and despair following conflicts. Anxious people also held more negative expectations about others' responses during anger episodes, and tended to make more undifferentiated, negatively biased appraisals of a relationship partner's intentions. They attributed hostility to the partner and reacted in kind, even when there were ambiguous cues (in the experiment) concerning hostile intent.

Anxious people's problems in anger management have also been studied with physiological measures. Diamond and Hicks (2005) exposed young men to two anger-provoking experimental inductions (performance of serial subtraction accompanied by discouraging feedback from the experimenter; recollection of a recent anger-eliciting event) and measured reports of anxiety and anger during and after the inductions. The investigators also recorded participants' vagal tone, a common index of parasympathetic down-regulation of negative emotion. Diamond and Hicks found that attachment anxiety was associated with lower vagal tone—a sign that the parasympathetic nervous system responded less quickly and flexibly to the stressful tasks, and that attachment-anxious study participants recovered poorly from frustration and anger. In addition, attachment anxiety was associated with self-reports of distress and anger during and after the anger induction tasks, and vagal tone mediated the association between attachment anxiety and heightened reports of anger.

Observational studies of anger in actual social interactions also provide evidence concerning the dysfunctional nature of insecure people's anger. Simpson and colleagues (1996) examined anger reactions during conflicts in which dating partners were asked to identify an unresolved problem in their relationship and to try to resolve it via discussion. Findings revealed that attachment anxiety was associated with both displays and reports of anger and hostility during the conversation.

Rholes, Simpson, and Orina (1999) examined overt manifestations of anger among support seekers and support providers in an anxiety-provoking situation. Women were told that they would engage in an anxiety-provoking activity, and were asked to wait with their dating partners for the activity to begin. During this 5-minute stressful waiting period, the reactions of the support seekers (women) and support providers (men) were unobtrusively videotaped. Each couple was then told that the woman would not have to endure the stressful activity after all, and each couple was unobtrusively videotaped during a 5-minute "recovery" period. The videotapes documented the dysfunctional nature of insecure participants' anger during both "stress" and "recovery" periods. In the stress period, women's avoidance was associated with more intense anger toward their partners, and this was particularly common when the women were especially distressed and received relatively little support from their partners. In addition, men's avoidance was associated with more intense anger, and this was particularly common if their partners were more distressed. In the recovery period, women's attachment anxiety was associated with more intense anger toward their partners, and this was particularly true if they were more upset during the stress period or had sought more support from their partners.

These findings imply that avoidant men's lack of willingness to care for and support their distressed partners might have elicited greater anger toward them. Moreover, avoidant women's lack of confidence in their partners' support might have caused them to become more disappointed and angry while seeking support. Anxious women's lack of confidence in their partners' support seemed to elicit anger only after the threat had been lifted and support was no longer needed. Thus anxious women's strong need for support and reassurance might have counteracted or led to suppression of their angry feelings during support seeking. However, these feelings might have resurfaced once support seeking ended, which would illustrate the way hyperactivating strategies tend to perpetuate distress-related feelings. (Interestingly, this is the same kind of behavior exhibited by anxious infants after they reunite with their mothers following a laboratory separation period, as documented by Ainsworth et al., 1978.)

Cognitive Access to Emotional Experiences

Theoretically, secondary attachment strategies should influence the access a person has to emotion-relevant information, as well as the way the person encodes and organizes this information in an associative memory network (Mikulincer & Shaver, 2003). In an experimental study of emotional memories, Mikulincer and Orbach (1995) obtained support for this expectation. Participants were asked to recall early childhood experiences of anger, sadness, anxiety, or happiness, and their memory retrieval latencies were interpreted as indicators of cognitive accessibility or inaccessibility. Participants also rated the intensity of focal and nonfocal emotions in each recalled event. In the memory task, avoidant people exhibited the poorest access (longest recall latencies) to sad and anxious memories; anxious people had the quickest access to such memories, and secure people fell in between. Moreover, whereas secure individuals took more time to retrieve negative than positive emotional memories, anxious people took longer to retrieve positive than negative memories. In the emotion-rating task, avoidant individuals rated focal emotions (e.g., sadness when instructed to retrieve a sad memory) and nonfocal emotions (e.g., anger when instructed to retrieve a sad memory) as less intense than secure individuals did, whereas anxious individuals reported experiencing very intense focal *and* nonfocal emotions when asked to remember examples of anxiety, sadness, and anger.

These findings provide insight into avoidant strategies of emotion regulation. Avoidant people displayed reduced access to negative emotional memories, and the ones they recalled were fairly shallow. This unavailability of negative memories was also documented in Edelstein and colleagues'

(2005) study of long-term memories for child sexual abuse (CSA). In a sample of 102 victims of documented CSA whose cases were referred for prosecution, self-reports of avoidant attachment were negatively associated with memory accuracy for specific, well-documented, severe CSA incidents that had occurred approximately 14 years earlier. Interestingly, these memory problems were reduced among participants who reported relatively high levels of maternal support after the CSA, highlighting the buffering effect of security-enhancing interactions with supportive attachment figures. Probably such a secure base can help avoidant people to remain open to painful and even traumatic memories. We have even found that subliminal security priming can increase avoidant people's openness to memories of being hurt by relationship partners (Shaver, Mikulincer, Lavy, & Cassidy, in press).

In Mikulincer and Orbach's (1995) study, attachment anxiety was associated with ready access to negative emotional memories and impaired control of the spread of activation from one negative memory to others. These findings fit with Pietromonaco and Barrett's (1997) findings from their diary study, showing that anxious people later reported that they were globally more distressed than they had reported immediately after the distress-eliciting event. These findings also fit with Roisman, Tsai, and Chiang's (2004) findings concerning people's facial expressions during the Adult Attachment Interview (AAI; discussed by Hesse, Chapter 25, this volume). Whereas securely attached individuals' facial expressions were highly congruent with the valence of the childhood events they were describing, anxiously attached individuals exhibited marked discrepancies between the quality of the childhood experiences they described and their facial expressions (e.g., facial expressions of sadness or anger when speaking about neutral or positive childhood experiences). According to Roisman and colleagues, these discrepancies reflect anxious individuals' confusion and emotional dysregulation when being asked to talk about emotionally charged experiences.

Avoidant Attachment and Lack of Psychobiological Coherence. Avoidant people's reduced access to emotions and emotion-eliciting thoughts is also evident in studies examining the coherence between conscious self-reports of emotional experience and less conscious, more automatic expressions of these experiences. (We assume that higher concordance between these measures implies greater access to emotional experiences.) Using self-report attachment scales, Mikulincer, Florian, and Tolmacz (1990) found that avoidant individuals scored relatively low on self-reports of fear of death, but revealed heightened fear of death in the stories they wrote about Thematic Apperception Test cards. Mikulincer (1998b) also reported that avoidant people, as compared with secure ones, reacted to anger-eliciting episodes with lower levels of self-reported anger and higher levels of physiological arousal (heart rate). Three related studies examined access to emotions during the AAI, and all found that though avoidant people verbally expressed few negative feelings during the interview, they exhibited high levels of physiological arousal (heightened electrodermal activity—Dozier & Kobak, 1992; Roisman et al., 2004) and more intense facial expressions of anger, sadness, and negative surprise (Zimmermann, Wulf, & Grossmann, 1996) while speaking about their relationships with parents.

Spangler and Zimmermann (1999) examined attachment style differences (based on the AAI) in the coherence of facial muscle reactions (measured with electromyography of the smile and frown muscles) and subjective reactions (pleasantness ratings) to 24 film fragments. For each study participant, they computed the correlation between muscular and subjective reactions across the 24 scenes, with higher positive correlations reflecting higher psychobiological coherence. They found that attachment security was positively associated with psychobiological coherence, but that avoidance was associated with lower awareness of physiological state.

Sonnby-Borgstrom and Jonsson (2004) provided further evidence for avoidant individuals' lack of psychobiological coherence while processing negative emotions. In their study, participants were exposed to pictures of happy and angry faces at three different exposure times (17, 56, and 2,350 milliseconds), and their muscle reactions were assessed during exposure to each picture. When the pictures were presented subliminally and participants could not recognize the faces (at exposure times of 17 or 53 milliseconds), both avoidant and secure individuals activated muscles involved in negative emotional displays (corrugator or "frowning" muscles) when they were presented with angry faces. However, when participants were able to recognize the faces (exposure time of 2,350 milliseconds), avoidant participants showed lower levels of corrugator activity and increased zygo-

maticus muscle responses ("smiling" reactions) when exposed to angry faces. In contrast, secure people reacted to these pictures by mimicking (heightened corrugator activity). According to Sonnby-Borgstrom and Jonsson, avoidant people's heightened corrugator reaction to subliminal exposure to angry faces indicated that these pictures had automatically elicited negative emotions. Therefore, the avoidant participants' tendency to smile when they could consciously see the angry faces (at 2,350 milliseconds) suggests a defensive attempt to block cognitive access of negative emotions.

Insecure People's Problems in Attending to Emotions: The Case of Alexithymia. Studies of attachment style and "alexithymia" (difficulty in identifying and describing feelings) also reveal avoidant people's lack of conscious access to emotions. Avoidant attachment (assessed with either self-report scales or the AAI) is related to inattention to feelings (Kim, 2005; Searle & Meara, 1999) and alexithymia (Mallinckrodt & Wei, 2005; Montebarocci, Codispoti, Baldaro, & Rossi, 2004; Picardi, Toni, & Caroppo, 2005). Interestingly, these studies reveal that anxiously attached people also have difficulty identifying and describing their feelings. According to Mallinckrodt and Wei (2005), higher alexithymia scores reflect not only inhibited awareness of one's feelings, but also difficulties in differentiating global emotional arousal into more specific emotional states and communicating these specific feelings to others. It seems possible, therefore, that anxious strategies—which impair control of the spread of emotion-related activation across an associative semantic memory network, and create an undifferentiated, chaotic emotional architecture—create difficulties in differentiating and identifying specific feelings. As a result, alexithymia can reflect either blocked access to emotion (characteristic of avoidant people) or poor differentiation among emotional experiences (characteristic of anxious people).

Attachment-anxious individuals' problems in differentiating and identifying specific feelings may also result from a tendency to react with intense emotion to threatening events. Indeed, several studies have found that people who score high on attachment anxiety also score high on measures of emotional reactivity or intensity (e.g., Pietromonaco & Barrett, 1997; Searle & Meara, 1999). Similarly, J. A. Feeney (1999) reported correlations between attachment anxiety and the intensity of anger, sadness, and anxiety during daily social interactions. Interestingly, some of these studies (J. A. Feeney, 1999; Pietromonaco & Barrett, 1997) revealed that avoidant attachment was associated with lower emotional reactivity or intensity. This fits with our overall conclusion that avoidance blocks access to emotion and inhibits emotional expression, whereas anxiety intensifies affective reactions.

Problems in Mental Health and Adjustment

Attachment theorists view secondary attachment strategies as risk factors that reduce resilience in times of stress and contribute to emotional problems and poor adjustment (Bowlby, 1988; Mikulincer & Shaver, 2003). Hyperactivating strategies lead to distress intensification and a chaotic emotional architecture that impairs anxious people's ability to regulate negative emotions. As a result, the anxious person experiences an endless and uncontrollable flow of negative thoughts and emotions, which in turn can lead to cognitive disorganization and, in certain cases, culminate in psychopathology. Although avoidant, deactivating strategies contribute to defensive maintenance of a façade of security and calmness, they block access to emotions and hence can impair a person's ability to confront and cope with life's adversities. This impairment is particularly likely to be manifested during prolonged, highly demanding stressful experiences that require actively confronting a problem and mobilizing external sources of support. In addition, although deactivating strategies involve suppressing the conscious experience and display of distress, the distress can still be indirectly manifested in somatic symptoms, sleep problems, and other health problems. Moreover, negative attitudes toward close relationships and relationship partners can channel unresolved distress into feelings of hostility, loneliness, and estrangement from others.

With regard to hyperactivating strategies, a large number of studies have shown that attachment anxiety is inversely associated with well-being and positively associated with both self-reports and clinical diagnoses of global distress, depression, anxiety, eating disorders, substance abuse, conduct disorder, and severe personality disorders (for reviews, see Mikulincer & Florian, 2001; Mikulincer & Shaver, 2007). These associations have been found in different age groups (ranging from adolescents to elderly adults), community samples, psychiatric inpatients and outpatients, and individuals experiencing acute stressful events (e.g., abortion) or more chronic stressful conditions (e.g., chronic pain).

For avoidance, the findings are more complex. On the one hand, a host of studies yielded no significant associations between avoidant attachment and self-report measures of well-being and global distress (for reviews, see Mikulincer & Florian, 2001; Mikulincer & Shaver, 2007). On the other hand, several studies indicate that avoidant attachment is associated with particular patterns of emotional and behavioral problems that may result from the underlying action of deactivating strategies. Specifically, significant associations have been found between avoidance and a pattern of depression characterized by perfectionism, self-punishment, and self-criticism (e.g., Zuroff & Fitzpatrick, 1995), heightened reports of somatic complaints (e.g., Mikulincer et al., 1993), hostility toward other people (e.g., Mikulincer, 1998b), substance abuse and conduct disorder (e.g., Cooper et al., 1998; Mickelson et al., 1997), and schizoid and avoidant personality disorders (e.g., Brennan & Shaver, 1998; Crawford et al., 2006).

In addition, whereas no consistent association has been found in community samples between avoidant attachment and global distress, studies that focus on highly demanding and distressing events reveal that avoidance is related to higher levels of reported distress. For example, Berant and colleagues (2001, in press) assessed mothers' reactions to the birth of infants with a CHD and found that avoidance, as assessed at the time of the initial diagnosis of the CHD, was the most potent predictor of maternal distress a year later. It seems that deactivating strategies may contribute to mental health under fairly typical circumstances characterized by only mild encounters with stressors. Under highly demanding conditions, however, these strategies seem to collapse, and in such cases avoidant individuals may exhibit high levels of distress and emotional problems.

CONCLUSIONS

An enormous body of research—larger than we can cover here—supports an attachment-theoretical approach to understanding emotion regulation in adults. Many creative hypotheses based on the theory have been formulated and tested since 1990, using a variety of research methods—including behavioral observations, interviews, questionnaires, physiological and neuroimaging assessments, subliminal priming, implicit measures of cognitive and emotional processes, and systematic manipulations of threatening contexts and social situations. The findings are coherent, mutually reinforcing, and compatible with the model of attachment system activation and functioning presented here.

Nevertheless, there are still important issues to be resolved. Most of the social-psychological studies of adults, including our own, have involved samples of normal college students and relied on self-report measures of attachment style. As explained by Crowell, Fraley, and Shaver (Chapter 26, this volume) and by Hesse (Chapter 25), these measures often do not converge closely with the AAI, which means that more research is needed to clarify the meaning of the various measures and their associations with emotion regulation. Moreover, preliminary research by Crawford and colleagues (2007; see also Brussoni, Jang, Livesley, & MacBeth, 2000) suggests that some of the individual-difference variance in attachment anxiety (although perhaps not in avoidance) is attributable to genetic factors; if this is true, it will have implications for both theory and clinical applications. Finally, we social psychologists who study normal adults take the developmental literature on attachment for granted, but we rarely study actual links between childhood attachment and emotion regulation processes in adulthood. This means that the actual childhood roots of most of the phenomena we have studied in adults remain to be identified.

Whatever the final story turns out to be, attachment theory has already greatly advanced the study of emotion regulation in adulthood. Most of the findings summarized here are highly replicable, and many have been replicated in different countries, using stimulus materials and measures in different languages. Most of the findings are not likely to be challenged or revised in the future. Only their final, complete, and correct interpretation remains to be established.

REFERENCES

Ainsworth, M. D. S. (1991). Attachment and other affectional bonds across the life cycle. In C. M. Parkes, J. Stevenson-Hinde, & P. Marris (Eds.), *Attachment across the life cycle* (pp. 33–51). New York: Routledge.

Ainsworth, M. D. S., Blehar, M. C., Waters, E., & Wall, S. (1978). *Patterns of attachment: A psychological study of the Strange Situation*. Hillsdale, NJ: Erlbaum.

Arndt, J., Schimel, J., Greenberg, J., & Pyszczynski, T. (2002). The intrinsic self and defensiveness: Evidence that activating the intrinsic self reduces self-

handicapping and conformity. *Personality and Social Psychology Bulletin, 28*, 671–683.

Baldwin, M. W., Fehr, B., Keedian, E., Seidel, M., & Thompson, D. W. (1993). An exploration of the relational schemata underlying attachment styles: Self-report and lexical decision approaches. *Personality and Social Psychology Bulletin, 19*, 746–754.

Baldwin, M. W., Keelan, J. P. R., Fehr, B., Enns, V., & Koh-Rangarajoo, E. (1996). Social-cognitive conceptualization of attachment working models: Availability and accessibility effects. *Journal of Personality and Social Psychology, 71*, 94–109.

Bargh, J. A. (1990). Auto-motives: Preconscious determinants of social interaction. In E. T. Higgins & R. M. Sorrentino (Eds.), *Handbook of motivation and cognition: Vol. 2. Foundations of social behavior* (pp. 93–130). New York: Guilford Press.

Bartholomew, K. (1990). Avoidance of intimacy: An attachment perspective. *Journal of Social and Personal Relationships, 7*, 147–178.

Bartholomew, K., & Horowitz, L. M. (1991). Attachment styles among young adults: A test of a four-category model. *Journal of Personality and Social Psychology, 61*, 226–244.

Belsky, J., & Isabella, R. A. (1988). Maternal, infant, and social-contextual determinants of attachment security. In J. Belsky & T. Nezworski (Eds.), *Clinical implications of attachment* (pp. 41–94). Hillsdale, NJ: Erlbaum.

Belsky, J., Rovine, M., & Taylor, D. G. (1984). The Pennsylvania Infant and Family Development Project: III. The origins of individual differences in infant–mother attachment: Maternal and infant contributions. *Child Development, 55*, 718–728.

Berant, E., Mikulincer, M., & Florian, V. (2001). The association of mothers' attachment style and their psychological reactions to the diagnosis of infants' congenital heart disease. *Journal of Social and Clinical Psychology, 20*, 208–232.

Berant, E., Mikulincer, M., & Shaver, P. R. (in press). Mothers' attachment style, their mental health, and their children's emotional vulnerabilities: A seven-year study of mothers of children with congenital heart disease. *Journal of Personality*.

Berglas, S., & Jones, E. E. (1978). Drug choice as a self-handicapping strategy in response to noncontingent success. *Journal of Personality and Social Psychology, 36*, 405–417.

Birgegard, A., & Granqvist, P. (2004). The correspondence between attachment to parents and God: Three experiments using subliminal separation cues. *Personality and Social Psychology Bulletin, 30*, 1122–1135.

Birnbaum, G. E., Orr, I., Mikulincer, M., & Florian, V. (1997). When marriage breaks up: Does attachment style contribute to coping and mental health? *Journal of Social and Personal Relationships, 14*, 643–654.

Bowlby, J. (1969/1982). *Attachment and loss: Vol. 1. Attachment*. New York: Basic Books.

Bowlby, J. (1973). *Attachment and loss: Vol. 2. Separation: Anxiety and anger*. New York: Basic Books.

Bowlby, J. (1979). *The making and breaking of affectional bonds*. London: Tavistock.

Bowlby, J. (1980). *Attachment and loss: Vol. 3. Sadness and depression*. New York: Basic Books.

Bowlby, J. (1988). *A secure base: Clinical applications of attachment theory*. London: Routledge.

Bradford, S. A., Feeney, J. A., & Campbell, L. (2002). Links between attachment orientations and dispositional and diary-based measures of disclosure in dating couples: A study of actor and partner effects. *Personal Relationships, 9,* 491–506.

Brennan, K. A., Clark, C. L., & Shaver, P. R. (1998). Self-report measurement of adult romantic attachment: An integrative overview. In J. A. Simpson & W. S. Rholes (Eds.), *Attachment theory and close relationships* (pp. 46–76). New York: Guilford Press.

Brennan, K. A., & Morris, K. A. (1997). Attachment styles, self-esteem, and patterns of seeking feedback from romantic partners. *Personality and Social Psychology Bulletin, 23,* 23–31.

Brennan, K. A., & Shaver, P. R. (1998). Attachment styles and personality disorders: Their connections to each other and to parental divorce, parental death, and perceptions of parental caregiving. *Journal of Personality, 66,* 835–878.

Brussoni, M. J., Jang, K. L., Livesley, W. J., & MacBeth, T. M. (2000). Genetic and environmental influences on adult attachment styles. *Personal Relationships, 7,* 283–289.

Cannon, W. B. (1939). *The wisdom of the body* (2nd ed.). New York: Norton.

Carnelley, K. B., Pietromonaco, P. R., & Jaffe, K. (1994). Depression, working models of others, and relationship functioning. *Journal of Personality and Social Psychology, 66,* 127–140.

Cassidy, J. (1994). Emotion regulation: Influences of attachment relationships. In N. Fox (Ed.), The development of emotion regulation: Biological and behavioral considerations. *Monographs of the Society for Research in Child Development, 59*(2–3, Serial No. 240), 228–283.

Cassidy, J., & Berlin, L. J. (1994). The insecure/ambivalent pattern of attachment: Theory and research. *Child Development, 65,* 971–981.

Cassidy, J., & Kobak, R. R. (1988). Avoidance and its relationship with other defensive processes. In J. Belsky & T. Nezworski (Eds.), *Clinical implications of attachment* (pp. 300–323). Hillsdale, NJ: Erlbaum.

Coan, J. A., Schaefer, H. S., & Davidson, R. J. (2006). Lending a hand: Social regulation of the neural response to threat. *Psychological Science, 17,* 1032–1039.

Collins, N. L. (1996). Working models of attachment: Implications for explanation, emotion, and behavior. *Journal of Personality and Social Psychology, 71,* 810–832.

Collins, N. L., & Feeney, B. C. (2000). A safe haven: An attachment theory perspective on support seeking and caregiving in intimate relationships. *Journal of Personality and Social Psychology, 78,* 1053–1073.

Collins, N. L., & Read, S. J. (1990). Adult attachment, working models, and relationship quality in dating couples. *Journal of Personality and Social Psychology, 58,* 644–663.

Collins, N. L., & Read, S. J. (1994). Cognitive representations of attachment: The structure and function of working models. In K. Bartholomew & D. Perlman (Eds.), *Advances in personal relationships: Vol. 5. Attachment processes in adulthood* (pp. 53–92). London: Jessica Kingsley.

Cooper, M., Shaver, P. R., & Collins, N. L. (1998). Attachment styles, emotion regulation, and adjustment in adolescence. *Journal of Personality and Social Psychology, 74,* 1380–1397.

Corcoran, K. O., & Mallinckrodt, B. (2000). Adult attachment, self-efficacy, perspective taking, and conflict resolution. *Journal of Counseling and Development, 78,* 473–483.

Crawford, T. N., Livesley, W. J., Jang, K. L., Shaver, P. R., Cohen, P., & Ganiban, J. (2007). Insecure attachment and personality disorder: A twin study of adults. *European Journal of Personality, 21,* 191–208.

Crawford, T. N., Shaver, P. R., Cohen, P., Pilkonis, P. A., Gillath, O., & Kasen, S. (2006). Self-reported attachment, interpersonal aggression, and personality disorder in a prospective community sample of adolescents and adults. *Journal of Personality Disorders, 20,* 331–351.

Creasey, G. (2002). Psychological distress in college-aged women: Links with unresolved/preoccupied attachment status and the mediating role of negative mood regulation expectancies. *Attachment and Human Development, 4,* 261–277.

Creasey, G., & Ladd, A. (2004). Negative mood regulation expectancies and conflict behaviors in late adolescent college student romantic relationships: The moderating role of generalized attachment representations. *Journal of Research on Adolescence, 14,* 235–255.

Davis, M. H., Morris, M. M., & Kraus, L. A. (1998). Relationship-specific and global perceptions of social support: Associations with well-being and attachment. *Journal of Personality and Social Psychology, 74,* 468–481.

Diamond, L. M., & Hicks, A. M. (2005). Attachment style, current relationship security, and negative emotions: The mediating role of physiological regulation. *Journal of Social and Personal Relationships, 22,* 499–518.

Dozier, M., & Kobak, R. (1992). Psychophysiology in attachment interviews: Converging evidence for deactivating strategies. *Child Development, 63,* 1473–1480.

Dykas, M., Ziv, Y., Feeney, B., & Cassidy, J. (2007). *Parental secure base provision, adolescent secure base use, and dyadic communication: Relations with adolescent attachment security*. Manuscript submitted for publication.

Edelstein, R. S., Ghetti, S., Quas, J. A., Goodman, G. S., Alexander, K. W., Redlich, A. D., et al. (2005).

Individual differences in emotional memory: Adult attachment and long-term memory for child sexual abuse. *Personality and Social Psychology Bulletin, 31*, 1537–1548.

Edelstein, R. S., & Shaver, P. R. (2004). Avoidant attachment: Exploration of an oxymoron. In D. Mashek & A. Aron (Eds.), *Handbook of closeness and intimacy* (pp. 397–412). Mahwah, NJ: Erlbaum.

Epstein, S., & Meier, P. (1989). Constructive thinking: A broad coping variable with specific components. *Journal of Personality and Social Psychology, 57*, 332–350.

Feeney, B. C. (2007). The dependency paradox in close relationships: Accepting dependence promotes independence. *Journal of Personality and Social Psychology, 92*, 268–285.

Feeney, B. C., & Collins, N. L. (2001). Predictors of caregiving in adult intimate relationships: An attachment theoretical perspective. *Journal of Personality and Social Psychology, 80*, 972–994.

Feeney, J. A. (1995). Adult attachment and emotional control. *Personal Relationships, 2*, 143–159.

Feeney, J. A. (1999). Adult attachment, emotional control, and marital satisfaction. *Personal Relationships, 6*, 169–185.

Feeney, J. A., & Noller, P. (1991). Attachment style and verbal descriptions of romantic partners. *Journal of Social and Personal Relationships, 8*, 187–215.

Field, T. (2002). Infants' need for touch. *Human Development, 45*, 100–103.

Fraley, R. C., Garner, J. P., & Shaver, P. R. (2000). Adult attachment and the defensive regulation of attention and memory: Examining the role of preemptive and postemptive defensive processes. *Journal of Personality and Social Psychology, 79*, 816–826.

Fraley, R. C., & Shaver, P. R. (1997). Adult attachment and the suppression of unwanted thoughts. *Journal of Personality and Social Psychology, 73*, 1080–1091.

Fraley, R. C., & Shaver, P. R. (1998). Airport separations: A naturalistic study of adult attachment dynamics in separating couples. *Journal of Personality and Social Psychology, 75*, 1198–1212.

Fredrickson, B. L. (2001). The role of positive emotions in positive psychology: The broaden-and-build theory of positive emotions. *American Psychologist, 56*, 218–226.

Gillath, O., Bunge, S. A., Shaver, P. R., Wendelken, C., & Mikulincer, M. (2005). Attachment-style differences in the ability to suppress negative thoughts: Exploring the neural correlates. *NeuroImage, 28*, 835–847.

Gillath, O., Shaver, P. R., & Mikulincer, M. (2005). An attachment-theoretical approach to compassion and altruism. In P. Gilbert (Ed.), *Compassion: Conceptualizations, research, and use in psychotherapy* (pp. 121–147). London: Brunner-Routledge.

Green, J. D., & Campbell, W. (2000). Attachment and exploration in adults: Chronic and contextual accessibility. *Personality and Social Psychology Bulletin, 26*, 452–461.

Griffin, D. W., & Bartholomew, K. (1994). Models of the self and other: Fundamental dimensions underlying measures of adult attachment. *Journal of Personality and Social Psychology, 67*, 430–445.

Gross, J. J. (1999). Emotion and emotion regulation. In L. A. Pervin & O. P. John (Eds.), *Handbook of personality: Theory and research* (2nd ed., pp. 525–552). New York: Guilford Press.

Hazan, C., & Shaver, P. R. (1987). Romantic love conceptualized as an attachment process. *Journal of Personality and Social Psychology, 52*, 511–524.

Hazan, C., & Shaver, P. R. (1990). Love and work: An attachment-theoretical perspective. *Journal of Personality and Social Psychology, 59*, 270–280.

Hazan, C., & Shaver, P. R. (1994). Attachment as an organizational framework for research on close relationships. *Psychological Inquiry, 5*, 1–22.

Hazan, C., & Zeifman, D. (1994). Sex and the psychological tether. In K. Bartholomew & D. Perlman (Eds.), *Advances in personal relationships: Attachment processes in adulthood* (Vol. 5, pp. 151–177). London: Jessica Kingsley.

Hertenstein, M. J. (2002). Touch: Its communicative functions in infancy. *Human Development, 45*, 70–94.

Joireman, J. A., Needham, T. L., & Cummings, A. L. (2002). Relationships between dimensions of attachment and empathy. *North American Journal of Psychology, 4*, 63–80.

Kalish, R. A. (1985). *Death, grief, and caring relationships.* New York: Cole.

Kernis, M. H. (2003). Toward a conceptualization of optimal self-esteem. *Psychological Inquiry, 14*, 1–26.

Kim, Y. (2005). Emotional and cognitive consequences of adult attachment: The mediating effect of the self. *Personality and Individual Differences, 39*, 913–923.

Kobak, R., Cole, H. E., Ferenz-Gillies, R., Fleming, W. S., & Gamble, S. (1993). Attachment and emotion regulation during mother–teen problem solving: A control theory analysis. *Child Development, 64*, 231–245.

Larose, S., & Bernier, A. (2001). Social support processes: Mediators of attachment state of mind and adjustment in late adolescence. *Attachment and Human Development, 3*, 96–120.

Lazarus, R. S. (1991). *Emotion and adaptation.* New York: Oxford University Press.

Levy, K. N., Blatt, S. J., & Shaver, P. R. (1998). Attachment styles and parental representations. *Journal of Personality and Social Psychology, 74*, 407–419.

Lopez, F. G. (2001). Adult attachment orientations, self–other boundary regulation, and splitting tendencies in a college sample. *Journal of Counseling Psychology, 48*, 440–446.

Lussier, Y., Sabourin, S., & Turgeon, C. (1997). Coping strategies as moderators of the relationship between attachment and marital adjustment. *Journal of Social and Personal Relationships, 14*, 777–791.

Main, M. (1990). Cross-cultural studies of attachment organization: Recent studies, changing methodologies, and the concept of conditional strategies. *Human Development, 33*, 48–61.

Main, M., & Solomon, J. (1986). Discovery of an insecure-disorganized/disoriented attachment pattern. In T. B. Brazelton & M. W. Yogman (Eds.), *Affective development in infancy* (pp. 95–124). Norwood, NJ: Ablex.

Mallinckrodt, B., & Wei, M. (2005). Attachment, social competencies, social support, and psychological distress. *Journal of Counseling Psychology, 52*, 358–367.

Mayseless, O. (2004). Home leaving to military service: Attachment concerns, transfer of attachment functions from parents to peers, and adjustment. *Journal of Adolescent Research, 19*, 533–558.

Mayseless, O., Danieli, R., & Sharabany, R. (1996). Adults' attachment patterns: Coping with separations. *Journal of Youth and Adolescence, 25*, 667–690.

McGowan, S. (2002). Mental representations in stressful situations: The calming and distressing effects of significant others. *Journal of Experimental Social Psychology, 38*, 152–161.

Meyer, B., Olivier, L., & Roth, D. A. (2005). Please don't leave me!: BIS/BAS, attachment styles, and responses to a relationship threat. *Personality and Individual Differences, 38*, 151–162.

Meyer, D. E., & Schvaneveldt, R. W. (1971). Facilitation in recognizing pairs of words: Evidence of dependence between retrieval operations. *Journal of Experimental Psychology, 90*, 227–234.

Mickelson, K. D., Kessler, R. C., & Shaver, P. R. (1997). Adult attachment in a nationally representative sample. *Journal of Personality and Social Psychology, 73*, 1092–1106.

Mikulincer, M. (1995). Attachment style and the mental representation of the self. *Journal of Personality and Social Psychology, 69*, 1203–1215.

Mikulincer, M. (1997). Adult attachment style and information processing: Individual differences in curiosity and cognitive closure. *Journal of Personality and Social Psychology, 72*, 1217–1230.

Mikulincer, M. (1998a). Adult attachment style and affect regulation: Strategic variations in self-appraisals. *Journal of Personality and Social Psychology, 75*, 420–435.

Mikulincer, M. (1998b). Adult attachment style and individual differences in functional versus dysfunctional experiences of anger. *Journal of Personality and Social Psychology, 74*, 513–524.

Mikulincer, M., & Arad, D. (1999). Attachment working models and cognitive openness in close relationships: A test of chronic and temporary accessibility effects. *Journal of Personality and Social Psychology, 77*, 710–725.

Mikulincer, M., Birnbaum, G., Woddis, D., & Nachmias, O. (2000). Stress and accessibility of proximity-related thoughts: Exploring the normative and intraindividual components of attachment theory. *Journal of Personality and Social Psychology, 78*, 509–523.

Mikulincer, M., Dolev, T., & Shaver, P. R. (2004). Attachment-related strategies during thought suppression: Ironic rebounds and vulnerable self-representations. *Journal of Personality and Social Psychology, 87*, 940–956.

Mikulincer, M., & Florian, V. (1995). Appraisal of and coping with a real-life stressful situation: The contribution of attachment styles. *Personality and Social Psychology Bulletin, 21*, 406–414.

Mikulincer, M., & Florian, V. (1997). Are emotional and instrumental supportive interactions beneficial in times of stress?: The impact of attachment style. *Anxiety, Stress and Coping: An International Journal, 10*, 109–127.

Mikulincer, M., & Florian, V. (1998). The relationship between adult attachment styles and emotional and cognitive reactions to stressful events. In J. A. Simpson & W. S. Rholes (Eds.), *Attachment theory and close relationships* (pp. 143–165). New York: Guilford Press.

Mikulincer, M., & Florian, V. (2000). Exploring individual differences in reactions to mortality salience: Does attachment style regulate terror management mechanisms? *Journal of Personality and Social Psychology, 79*, 260–273.

Mikulincer, M., & Florian, V. (2001). Attachment style and affect regulation: Implications for coping with stress and mental health. In G. J. O. Fletcher & M. S. Clark (Eds.), *Blackwell handbook of social psychology: Interpersonal processes* (pp. 537–557). Oxford:, UK Blackwell.

Mikulincer, M., Florian, V., & Hirschberger, G. (2003). The existential function of close relationships: Introducing death into the science of love. *Personality and Social Psychology Review, 7*, 20–40.

Mikulincer, M., Florian, V., & Tolmacz, R. (1990). Attachment styles and fear of personal death: A case study of affect regulation. *Journal of Personality and Social Psychology, 58*, 273–280.

Mikulincer, M., Florian, V., & Weller, A. (1993). Attachment styles, coping strategies, and posttraumatic psychological distress: The impact of the Gulf War in Israel. *Journal of Personality and Social Psychology, 64*, 817–826.

Mikulincer, M., Gillath, O., Halevy, V., Avihou, N., Avidan, S., & Eshkoli, N. (2001). Attachment theory and reactions to others' needs: Evidence that activation of the sense of attachment security promotes empathic responses. *Journal of Personality and Social Psychology, 81*, 1205–1224.

Mikulincer, M., Gillath, O., & Shaver, P. R. (2002). Activation of the attachment system in adulthood: Threat-related primes increase the accessibility of mental representations of attachment figures. *Journal of Personality and Social Psychology, 83*, 881–895.

Mikulincer, M., Gurwitz, V., & Shaver, P. R. (2007, August). Attachment security and the use of God as a safe haven: New experimental findings. In L. Kirkpatrick (Chair), *Current directions in attachment, religion, and spirituality research.* Symposium conducted at the annual convention of the American Psychological Association, San Francisco.

Mikulincer, M., Hirschberger, G., Nachmias, O., & Gillath, O. (2001). The affective component of the secure base schema: Affective priming with representations of attachment security. *Journal of Personality and Social Psychology, 81*, 305–321.

Mikulincer, M., & Nachshon, O. (1991). Attachment styles and patterns of self-disclosure. *Journal of Personality and Social Psychology, 61*, 321–331.

Mikulincer, M., & Orbach, I. (1995). Attachment styles and repressive defensiveness: The accessibility and architecture of affective memories. *Journal of Personality and Social Psychology, 68*, 917–925.

Mikulincer, M., & Shaver, P. R. (2001). Attachment theory and intergroup bias: Evidence that priming the secure base schema attenuates negative reactions to out-groups. *Journal of Personality and Social Psychology, 81*, 97–115.

Mikulincer, M., & Shaver, P. R. (2003). The attachment behavioral system in adulthood: Activation, psychodynamics, and interpersonal processes. In M. P. Zanna (Ed.), *Advances in experimental social psychology* (Vol. 35, pp. 53–152). San Diego, CA: Academic Press.

Mikulincer, M., & Shaver, P. R. (2004). Security-based self-representations in adulthood: Contents and processes. In W. S. Rholes & J. A. Simpson (Eds.), *Adult attachment: Theory, research, and clinical implications* (pp. 159–195). New York: Guilford Press.

Mikulincer, M., & Shaver, P. R. (2007). *Attachment in adulthood: Structure, dynamics, and change.* New York: Guilford Press.

Mikulincer, M., Shaver, P. R., Gillath, O., & Nitzberg, R. A. (2005). Attachment, caregiving, and altruism: Boosting attachment security increases compassion and helping. *Journal of Personality and Social Psychology, 89*, 817–839.

Montebarocci, O., Codispoti, M., Baldaro, B., & Rossi, N. (2004). Adult attachment style and alexithymia. *Personality and Individual Differences, 36*, 499–507.

Neria, Y., Guttmann-Steinmetz, S., Koenen, K., Levinovsky, L., Zakin, G., & Dekel, R. (2001). Do attachment and hardiness relate to each other and to mental health in real-life stress? *Journal of Social and Personal Relationships, 18*, 844–858.

Noom, M. J., Dekovic, M., & Meeus, W. H. J. (1999). Autonomy, attachment, and psychosocial adjustment during adolescence: A double-edged sword? *Journal of Adolescence, 22*, 771–783.

Ognibene, T. C., & Collins, N. L. (1998). Adult attachment styles, perceived social support, and coping strategies. *Journal of Social and Personal Relationships, 15*, 323–345.

Picardi, A., Toni, A., & Caroppo, E. (2005). Stability of alexithymia and its relationships with the 'Big Five' factors, temperament, character, and attachment style. *Psychotherapy and Psychosomatics, 74*, 371–378.

Pietromonaco, P. R., & Barrett, L. F. (1997). Working models of attachment and daily social interactions. *Journal of Personality and Social Psychology, 73*, 1409–1423.

Priel, B., & Shamai, D. (1995). Attachment style and perceived social support: Effects on affect regulation. *Personality and Individual Differences, 19*, 235–241.

Pyszczynski, T., Greenberg, J., & LaPrelle, J. (1985). Social comparison after success and failure: Biased search for information consistent with a self-serving conclusion. *Journal of Experimental Social Psychology, 21*, 195–211.

Radecki-Bush, C., Farrell, A. D., & Bush, J. P. (1993). Predicting jealous responses: The influence of adult attachment and depression on threat appraisal. *Journal of Social and Personal Relationships, 10*, 569–588.

Rholes, W. S., Simpson, J. A., & Orina, M. (1999). Attachment and anger in an anxiety-provoking situation. *Journal of Personality and Social Psychology, 76*, 940–957.

Rogers, C. R. (1961). *On becoming a person.* Boston: Houghton Mifflin.

Roisman, G. I., Tsai, J. L., & Chiang, K. H. (2004). The emotional integration of childhood experience: Physiological, facial expressions, and self-reported emotional response during the Adult Attachment Interview. *Developmental Psychology, 40*, 776–789.

Rowe, A., & Carnelley, K. B. (2003). Attachment style differences in the processing of attachment-relevant information: Primed-style effects on recall, interpersonal expectations, and affect. *Personal Relationships, 10*, 59–75.

Schachter, S. (1959). *The psychology of affiliation.* Stanford, CA: Stanford University Press.

Schimel, J., Arndt, J., Pyszczynski, T., & Greenberg, J. (2001). Being accepted for who we are: Evidence that social validation of the intrinsic self reduces general defensiveness. *Journal of Personality and Social Psychology, 80*, 35–52.

Searle, B., & Meara, N. M. (1999). Affective dimensions of attachment styles: Exploring self-reported attachment style, gender, and emotional experience among college students. *Journal of Counseling Psychology, 46*, 147–158.

Seiffge-Krenke, I., & Beyers, W. (2005). Coping trajectories from adolescence to young adulthood: Links to attachment state of mind. *Journal of Research on Adolescence, 15*, 561–582.

Shapiro, D. L., & Levendosky, A. A. (1999). Adolescent survivors of childhood sexual abuse: The mediating role of attachment style and coping in psychological and interpersonal functioning. *Child Abuse and Neglect, 23*, 1175–1191.

Shaver, P. R., & Clark, C. L. (1994). The psychodynamics of adult romantic attachment. In J. M. Masling & R. F. Bornstein (Eds.), *Empirical perspectives on object relations theories* (pp. 105–156). Washington, DC: American Psychological Association.

Shaver, P. R., & Klinnert, M. (1982). Schachter's theories of affiliation and emotions: Implications of developmental research. *Review of Personality and Social Psychology, 3*, 37–71.

Shaver, P. R., & Mikulincer, M. (2002a). Attachment-related psychodynamics. *Attachment and Human Development, 4*, 133–161.

Shaver, P. R., & Mikulincer, M. (2002b). Dialogue on adult attachment: Diversity and integration. *Attachment and Human Development, 4,* 243–257.

Shaver, P. R., Mikulincer, M., Lavy, S., & Cassidy, J. (in press). Understanding and altering hurt feelings: An attachment-theoretical perspective on the generation and regulation of emotions. In A. L. Vangelisti (Ed.), *Feeling hurt in close relationships.* New York: Cambridge University Press.

Shaver, P. R., Papalia, D., Clark, C. L., Koski, L. R., Tidwell, M., & Nalbone, D. (1996). Androgyny and attachment security: Two related models of optimal personality. *Personality and Social Psychology Bulletin, 22,* 582–597.

Shorey, H. S., Snyder, C. R., Yang, X., & Lewin, M. R. (2003). The role of hope as a mediator in recollected parenting, adult attachment, and mental health. *Journal of Social and Clinical Psychology, 22,* 685–715.

Simpson, J. A. (1990). Influence of attachment styles on romantic relationships. *Journal of Personality and Social Psychology, 59,* 971–980.

Simpson, J. A., Rholes, W. S., & Nelligan, J. S. (1992). Support seeking and support giving within couples in an anxiety-provoking situation: The role of attachment styles. *Journal of Personality and Social Psychology, 62,* 434–446.

Simpson, J. A., Rholes, W. S., Orina, M., & Grich, J. (2002). Working models of attachment, support giving, and support seeking in a stressful situation. *Personality and Social Psychology Bulletin, 28,* 598–608.

Simpson, J. A., Rholes, W. S., & Phillips, D. (1996). Conflict in close relationships: An attachment perspective. *Journal of Personality and Social Psychology, 71,* 899–914.

Skinner, B. F. (1969). *Contingencies of reinforcement: A theoretical analysis.* New York: Appleton-Century-Crofts.

Sonnby-Borgstrom, M., & Jonsson, P. (2004). Dismissing-avoidant pattern of attachment and mimicry reactions at different levels of information processing. *Scandinavian Journal of Psychology, 45,* 103–113.

Spangler, G., & Zimmermann, P. (1999). Attachment representation and emotion regulation in adolescents: A psychobiological perspective on internal working models. *Attachment and Human Development, 1,* 270–290.

Sroufe, L. A., & Waters, E. (1977). Attachment as an organizational construct. *Child Development, 48,* 1184–1199.

Taubman–Ben-Ari, O., Findler, L., & Mikulincer, M. (2002). The effects of mortality salience on relationship strivings and beliefs: The moderating role of attachment style. *British Journal of Social Psychology, 41,* 419–441.

Tidwell, M. C., Reis, H. T., & Shaver, P. R. (1996). Attachment, attractiveness, and social interaction: A diary study. *Journal of Personality and Social Psychology, 71,* 729–745.

Torquati, J. C., & Raffaelli, M. (2004). Daily experiences of emotions and social contexts of securely and insecurely attached young adults. *Journal of Adolescent Research, 19,* 740–758.

Waters, H. S., Rodrigues, L. M., & Ridgeway, D. (1998). Cognitive underpinnings of narrative attachment assessment. *Journal of Experimental Child Psychology, 71,* 211–234.

Wegner, D. M. (1994). Ironic processes of mental control. *Psychological Review, 101,* 34–52.

Wegner, D. M., & Smart, L. (1997). Deep cognitive activation: A new approach to the unconscious. *Journal of Consulting and Clinical Psychology, 65,* 984–995.

Westmaas, J., & Silver, R. C. (2001). The role of attachment in responses to victims of life crises. *Journal of Personality and Social Psychology, 80,* 425–438.

Zeidner, M., & Endler, N. S. (Eds.). (1996). *Handbook of coping: Theory, research, and applications.* New York: Wiley.

Zimmermann, P., Wulf, K., & Grossmann, K. E. (1996). *Attachment representation: You can see it in the face.* Poster presented at the biennial meeting of the International Society for the Study of Behavioral Development, Quebec City, QB, Canada.

Zuroff, D. C., & Fitzpatrick, D. K. (1995). Depressive personality styles: Implications for adult attachment. *Personality and Individual Differences, 18,* 253–365.

CHAPTER 24

Attachment in Middle and Later Life

CAROL MAGAI

Only connect!—E. M. FORSTER (*Howard's End*, p. 148)

Bowlby's formulations about the origins and nature of human attachments (Bowlby, 1969/1982, 1973, 1980) have provided a rich corpus of theory about important aspects of close relationships and their development over time. The theory has stimulated an enormous body of research on attachment during infancy, childhood, and early adulthood (Cassidy & Shaver, 1999; Mikulincer & Shaver, 2007). However, research on relationships in later life, viewed from an attachment-theoretical perspective, has been relatively limited (Magai & Consedine, 2004). Moreover, there are no longitudinal studies of the stability of attachment styles from early adulthood to middle age and later life; nor is there any research on how attachment patterns established earlier in life may influence attitudes and behaviors later in life. Nevertheless, longitudinal research on the relation between early family circumstances (broadly construed) and later-life functioning indicates that early familial conditions predict health and illness, psychological well-being, and even mortality (Lundberg, 1993; Preston, Hill, & Drevenstedt, 1998; Shaw, Krause, Chatters, Connell, & Ingersoll-Dayton, 2004; Weisner, 2005). This research suggests that there may indeed be long-term sequelae of attachment-related bonds formed earlier in life, and that their impact may be of great consequence.

In early life, attachment bonds ensure that the infant maintains proximity to the caregiver under conditions of uncertainty or threat and develops internal working models of this figure's availability and sensitivity. As the child matures, the exploratory behavior system, which provides the scaffolding for growth and development of various skills through exploration of the environment, becomes activated; the child ventures further and further away from the caregiver, although the caregiver retains the function of a "safe haven" if the child experiences distress. The process of exploration, development, and individuation evolves over time, and a sense of autonomy is normally achieved by early adulthood. However, it is assumed that because of internal working models, the attachment figure retains his or her power to serve as a real or virtual safe haven when the individual encounters challenges in adult life. The theory also predicts that the internal working models of caregivers generalize to other people in the adult's social networks and that attachment styles are relatively enduring, although they are also responsive to new inputs (Bowlby, 1973; Davila & Cobb, 2004; Fraley & Brumbaugh, 2004). There is now a significant literature on younger adults to support these formulations. However, it is important to assess the viability of these formulations as applied to later life, given the age-graded and role-linked unique challenges that occur over the adult lifespan.

In this chapter, I take on the subject of attachments in middle adulthood and later life in the context of normative adult developmental transitions and challenges. Themes that loom large for middle-aged adults include monitoring the health of aging parents; often taking responsibility for parents' care, sometimes while still providing care to adolescent or young adult offspring (Perrig-Chiello & Hoepflinger, 2005); and eventually dealing with the loss of these primary attachment figures. Themes that loom large for later-life adults include growing social, emotional, physical, and financial dependency, dealing with bereavement of spouse and friends, facing issues of encroaching mortality, and finding personal meaning as the end of the lifespan approaches.

In the context of this review of the literature, I explore the questions of (1) whether or not attachment styles remain relatively stable in later life and (2) under what conditions they might be altered. On the basis of research on children and young adults, we can expect both stability and change in attachment patterns over time. I also examine how different attachment styles may inform salient adult developmental issues. Again on the basis of earlier research, we can perhaps expect that individual differences in attachment patterns will affect a range of experiences and behaviors—including navigating the challenges of later life, as well as providing caregiving to elderly family members.

I begin with a review of the literature regarding the distribution of attachment styles as found in studies of older adults, asking whether the distribution of attachment types observed in infancy, adolescence, and early adulthood is also found in later life, and how stable these patterns may be. Because the literature on affectional bonds in later life is so limited in terms of testing derivations from attachment theory, this review necessarily also draws on other literatures that are not grounded in attachment theory but speak to attachment issues. In this context, I review the broader literature on the nature and quality of affectional bonds in middle and later adulthood, and the ways these bonds play out in the context of the caregiving system. Finally, I focus on issues of loss and bereavement. I restrict my focus to the affectional bonds between parents and their adult children, because of space limitations and because this literature is better developed than the literature on other kinds of affectional bonds (such as those between siblings).

THE DISTRIBUTION AND STABILITY OF ATTACHMENT STYLES IN LATER LIFE

First, I consider whether the distributions of attachment patterns found in infants and young adults is replicated in samples of older adults, and whether attachment patterns are stable over time. One could argue that the distributions of attachment styles might be different, given that attachment bonds are forged not only in relational but in cultural and historical contexts as well (Weisner, 2005). In considering older adults, it is important to recognize that successive generations of adults are not only older, but are also members of successively earlier birth cohorts, which are likely to have been exposed to different historical challenges and different childrearing norms. Research involving younger samples has shown that the distribution of attachment styles varies somewhat by culture (van IJzendoorn & Kroonenberg, 1988; van IJzendoorn & Sagi-Schwartz, Chapter 37, this volume) and that these differences apparently relate to local cultural and ecological values affecting attachment socialization (Weisner, 2005). Thus the distribution of attachment patterns may be different in samples of older adults and in different generations of older adults. We also need to revisit the thesis that attachment styles are relatively stable, for it is conceivable that the unique challenges of the latter part of the lifespan create differential instability.

Distribution of Attachment Styles in Older Adults

Studies of younger adults indicate a distribution of attachment styles that resembles the one found in studies of infants and children. About 55–65% of samples studied with self-report attachment measures have been found to be secure, 22–30% avoidant (or dismissing), and 15–20% ambivalent (or preoccupied) (e.g., Davila, Burge, & Hammen, 1997; J. A. Feeney & Noller, 1990; Hazan & Shaver, 1987; Kirkpatrick & Davis, 1994). According to an early meta-analysis (van IJzendoorn & Bakermans-Kranenburg, 1996) of studies using the Adult Attachment Interview (AAI), 58% of participants were judged secure-autonomous, 24%

dismissing, and 18% preoccupied. In a more recent report of AAI results (515 adults drawn from three studies; Roisman, Fraley, & Belsky, 2007), 55.5% were found to be secure, 26.2 % dismissing, 8.5 % preoccupied, and 10.1% unresolved.

These distributions have not been replicated in the few studies of older respondents. In brief, avoidant or dismissing attachment appears to increase or to become more common in older adults, and there are low base rates of ambivalent and/or preoccupied attachment. For example, one cross-sectional study of urban adults with a mean age of 63 years (Magai, Hunziker, Mesias, & Culver, 2000) found that security of attachment as assessed by the AAI was negatively correlated with age, and that dismissing attachment was positively correlated. Another study (Diehl, Elnick, Bourbeau, & Labouvie-Vief, 1998) assessed attachment styles in a sample of young (mean age = 30 years), middle-aged (50 years), and older adults (70 years) from a relatively affluent Midwestern suburb; the results indicated that whereas 18% of the young adults were dismissing, 22% of the middle-aged adults were dismissing, and the figure for the oldest sample was 40%. In a study of attachment style and the preparedness of middle-aged adults to provide care to older adults, 56% were classified as secure, 31% as dismissive, 4% as preoccupied, and 9% as fearful (Soerensen, Webster, & Roggman, 2002). A study of patients with dementia (mean age = 76 years; Magai & Cohen, 1998), in which caregivers were asked to rate their family members' attachment style before the patients became ill, found that 56% were rated as secure, 37% as avoidant, and 6% as ambivalent. In a study of community-living older adults with a mean age of 68 years (J. D. Webster, 1997), 52% of adults were classified as dismissing, and 33% were classified as secure. In a large, randomly drawn sample of urban elders living in an economically disadvantaged community, 78% were rated as avoidant, with most of the remainder being rated as secure (Magai et al., 2001).

Although the proportion of avoidant or dismissing and secure individuals varies across samples and appears to have something to do with participants' economic background, the data clearly show that the distribution of attachment styles in older adult samples is distinctly different from the distribution in samples of younger adults. Some authors (Diehl et al., 1998) have suggested that the higher proportion of avoidant older adults may be due to a greater number of losses experienced by older persons, whereas other authors (Magai, 2001; Magai et al., 2001) have suggested that these differences may be due to cohort effects. In a test of this hypothesis, my colleagues and I (Magai, 2001; Magai et al., 2001) subdivided our own sample into a younger cohort born between 1922 and 1932, and an older cohort born between 1911 and 1921. The younger cohort had significantly lower numbers of persons with secure attachment than did the older cohort. However, there was no difference between the two age cohorts in terms of the number of close relatives or friends who had died within the past 5 years. We suggested that the differential proportions of secure attachment in the two cohorts might represent the influence of Watsonian behaviorism, which advocated the withholding of affection from children and would have reached the height of its influence between the 1920s and 1930s, thus affecting the younger cohort. In this account, the higher proportion of dismissing attachment in earlier birth cohorts might be considered evidence of cohort rather than developmental effects. Alternatively, this effect might be due to intra-individual changes in levels of dismissing, secure, ambivalent, and fearful attachment in response to age-graded developmental challenges.

In any event, the apparent existence of high rates of avoidant or dismissing attachment in older adults is grounds for some concern. Grossmann (1996) advanced the thesis that attachment relations maintained within the larger family system contribute to the survival of family members. His work, as well as that of his colleagues, suggests that particular attachment styles might confer adaptive advantage over other styles later in life. Wensauer and Grossmann (1995), for example, found that grandparents with a secure attachment orientation (in contrast to those who were avoidant) had larger social networks, named more supportive family members, and received and gave more help; avoidant individuals were significantly more self-reliant. In a related prospective, 10-year longitudinal study of older Australians, Giles, Glonek, Luscza, and Andrews (2005) found that social networks conferred an adaptive advantage over and above those provided by demographic, health, and lifestyle variables. In that study, better networks with friends (and, to a lesser extent, networks with confidants) were protective against mortality over the following decade. Somewhat surprisingly, the effects of social networks with children and relatives were not significant with respect to survival;

however, it is important to note that this study did not assess *quality of attachment* to children and other relatives—an important dimension to consider from an attachment-theoretical perspective. I return to the issue of attachment and caregiving in a later section.

Stability and Change in Attachment Styles

Although attachment styles are thought to be relatively stable, with some research even indicating that attachment styles have trait-like characteristics (e.g., Banai, Weller, & Mikulincer, 1998), Bowlby's model was quite accommodating of change (Bowlby, 1973; Davila & Cobb, 2004; Fraley & Brumbaugh, 2004), and there is an empirical literature that speaks to the issue of change. A review of the child development literature by Campos, Barrett, Lamb, Goldsmith, and Stenberg (1983) indicated that, averaged over seven studies, 32% of children showed a change in classification over time. Similar rates have been reported in young adult samples (Baldwin & Fehr, 1995), although rates as high as 46% have been reported in studies of adults undergoing particularly acute stress (Cozzarelli, Karafa, Collins, & Tagler, 2003). The literature on stability and change in later adulthood is far more limited.

Indeed, at this point there are only two studies that address this issue, both of which examined changes in attachment longitudinally over a 6-year period. One study involved a sample of 370 relatively affluent, highly educated, predominantly European American men and women between the ages of 15 and 87 years (Zhang & Labouvie-Vief, 2004). The other involved 415 less affluent, less well-educated older adults (60% African American, 40% European American) who were 72 years old at the first time of measurement and 78 years at the second (Consedine & Magai, 2006). The former study found that both secure and dismissing attachment increased over time; the latter found that both decreased over time. The discrepancy in findings is probably related to the pronounced demographic differences between the two samples, including the age ranges studied. It may also be due to the fact that the first study relied on simple paragraph measures of attachment style, whereas the latter used the 30-item Relationship Scales Questionnaire (Bartholomew & Horowitz, 1991). In the case of the exclusively later-life sample, we (Consedine & Magai, 2006) suggested that the decrease in both security and dismissiveness relates

to changes in the purposes served by attachment figures in later life and changes in patterns of social network engagement and composition. That is, the decrease in security may reflect the loss of key members of social networks due to mortality. Conversely, decreases in dismissiveness (of others in general) may reflect the developmental tendency for older adults to place increasing value on intimate, emotionally rewarding relationships when they experience their time as limited.

ATTACHMENTS BETWEEN PARENTS AND CHILDREN IN LATER LIFE

Arguably, the most powerful affectional bonds are the bidirectional ones that develop between children and their parents. In this section, I examine what the literature has to say about the nature and quality of these bonds during later life.

As Ainsworth (1989) noted, there is no reason to think that a child's attachment to his or her parent wanes once adulthood is reached, or that a parent does not continue to offer a safe haven to his or her adult offspring when needed. Although this proposition is intuitively reasonable, the attachment literature with respect to it is not well developed. Interestingly, there is much better-developed theory and research relevant to the parent–child relationship in the sociological literature. In the following paragraphs, I organize the findings about affectional bonds in later life into two categories: (1) attachment of older parents to their adult children, and (2) attachment of adult children to their aging parents. In each section, I attend first to the attachment literature and then to the sociological literature. Before I proceed, however, it will be helpful to introduce the terms I use when addressing the sociological literature.

Background: The Affective Constructs Found in the Sociological Literature

Despite the limited literature on parent–child attachment in later life viewed from an attachment perspective, there is a fair amount of sociological literature on "intergenerational solidarity" (Bengtson & Roberts, 1991; Silverstein & Bengtson, 1997). The term "solidarity" denotes the cohesion among members of families and is defined by three dimensions: "opportunity" (frequency of contact and residential propinquity between generations), "function" (flows of instrumental assistance between generations), and "affinity" (emotional closeness and perceived agreement of opinions). The literature on intergenerational solidarity, reviewed below, provides good support for the notion that adult children and their aging parents retain affectional bonds (as would be predicted from attachment theory), and also indicates that early parent–child relationships affect current solidarity.

Another, more recently evolving vein of sociological literature suggests that contemporary family relationships are diverse, fluid, and often unresolved, and that parent–child relationships can be characterized not only by intergenerational solidarity, but also by "intergenerational ambivalence" (Connidis & McMullin, 2002; Fingerman, 1996, 1998; Luescher & Pillemer, 1998). That is, an individual may experience the relationship with a parent as incorporating both affection and resentment, feelings of loyalty and distress, and other mixed emotions. Three aspects of parent–child relations in later life are especially likely to generate such ambivalence (Luescher & Pillemer, 1998): (1) tensions between dependency and autonomy motivations in both parents and children; (2) tensions resulting from conflicting norms regarding intergenerational relations, such as norms for the provision of care to disabled older persons; and (3) tensions associated with solidarity itself—for example, elder abuse has been found to evolve in the context of a nexus of mutual dependencies between parents and children in certain situations (Wolf & Pillemer, 1989).

Such research suggests that the solidarity literature does not capture the range of experiences encountered by people in close relationships. Indeed, the intergenerational ambivalence perspective suggests that we may expect an ebb and flow in the quality of affectional bonds between parents and their adult children over time, especially in later life as adults experience age-graded changes in care-seeking and caregiving roles. The parent–child bond may be robust, but it is not necessarily static. Indeed, Bowlby's (1969/1982) model of the attachment partnership in early life characterized it as evolving and "goal-corrected." This dynamic model of close relationships may also be appropriate in later life.

I turn now to a discussion of some of the findings regarding affectional bonds between parents and their adult children from both parties' perspectives, and in the context of both the attachment-theoretical literature and the more sociologically grounded literature.

The Attachment of Aging Parents to their Adult Children

Findings Based on an Attachment-Theoretical Perspective

In an interview-based assessment of attachment among elderly mothers (mean age = 72 years) (Barnas, Pollina, & Cummings, 1991), three general patterns of attachment to adult children were identified: insecure-avoidant, insecure-mixed (secure–insecure), and secure. Interestingly, an anxious or preoccupied pattern did not appear in this older cohort—a pattern that mirrors research on the distribution of attachment styles in later adulthood (largely based on self-report measures) reviewed above. What is especially interesting about this study is that while the majority of women had secure attachments with at least one child, the quality of relationships varied across children for older adults who had more than one child. Half of the mothers had insecure attachments with at least one of their children, with 31% also having very insecure attachments to at least one child. Twenty percent had insecure-avoidant attachments with all of their children, 40% were insecure-mixed with all of their children, and 40% had secure attachment relationships with all their children.

There is a similarly slim literature on the impact of early rearing experiences on adult patterns of attachment, although researchers suggest that relationship patterns forged early in life have a bearing on attachment relations in adulthood, at least as assessed by retrospective accounts. In a nationally representative sample of people between 15 and 54 years of age (Mickelson, Kessler, & Shaver, 1997), researchers found that an array of reported childhood experiences, including abuse and neglect, were associated with attachment in adulthood. Secure attachment was negatively associated with reports of physical abuse, serious neglect, and being threatened with a weapon; avoidant attachment was positively associated with serious assault, physical abuse, serious neglect, being threatened with a weapon, rape, and sexual molestation. These interpersonal traumas, with the exception of serious assault, were also positively associated with anxious attachment.

Another study (Diehl et al., 1998) examined the reported early family climate of adults ranging in age from 20 to 87 years. A positive climate in the family of origin was indexed by the extent to which participants reported family members' supporting each other and being allowed to express their feelings freely; a negative family climate was one in which the family members emphasized rules and enforced rules with punishment. Higher ratings on secure attachment were associated with a more positive evaluation of the family of origin; higher scores on fearful attachment were associated with lower scores regarding satisfaction with the family of origin, with similar trends for dismissing and preoccupied attachment styles. These self-report findings parallel those stemming from studies that explored adult reports of early life experience using the AAI (Hesse, 1999; Main, Kaplan, & Cassidy, 1985). This research indicates that childhood maltreatment of various kinds, including physical abuse, negatively influences adult attachment representations and adult attachment organization (Cicchetti, Toth, & Lynch, 1995; Lutz & Hock, 1995).

Insights from the Sociological Literature

Intergenerational Solidarity. Although there are generally affectional ties between parents and their adult children, the extent of these ties appears to be moderated by the gender of the parent and the child (Rossi & Rossi, 1990). Affectional ties between mothers and their adult daughters appear to be among the strongest and most enduring of intergenerational bonds (Rossi & Rossi, 1990, 1991). A study of 48 older mothers and their middle-aged daughters (Fingerman, 1996) replicated earlier research showing that these bonds are particularly strong, but it also showed that the relationship appeared to be slightly more important to mothers than to daughters. On a scale of 5–25, mothers rated their regard for their relationship at 21.6, and daughters rated their regard at 20.5; although mothers' scores were slightly higher, this difference was in the context of very high overall regard for the relationship.

Using another index of the relationship quality, Fingerman (1996) found that 75% of the mothers indicated that their daughters were among the three most important people in their lives; the corresponding percentage of daughters who thus nominated their mothers was 58%. Important from an attachment perspective was the finding that a mother was also more likely to name a daughter as the person she got along with best, and the person with whom she was most likely to speak when upset, than a daughter was to name a mother. Fingerman speculated that this imbalance in relationship quality from the perspectives of mothers and daughters was probably a function of the older women's narrower social networks. As networks shrink in later life, the people who remain in the network tend to become more important as sources of emotional support and gratification (Carstensen, 1995).

Affectional ties between the generations conceivably have an impact on the nature of the social and instrumental support members provide each other in times of need. A review of the literature on the factors that influence intergenerational support (Davey, Janke, & Savla, 2004) indicates that the quality of relationship history is one of several dyadic characteristics that affect a parent's tendency to supply support to his or her adult children, but it is neither a necessary nor a sufficient condition. Mothers apparently differentiate among their adult children in terms of closeness and comfort with confiding, but the literature seems to demonstrate that support exchanges between the generations, particularly instrumental exchanges, are not entirely dependent on the quality of relations between parents and children. Moreover, mothers' feelings of closeness often have little effect on their support to their adult children (Davey et al., 2004; Suitor, Pillemer, & Sechrist, 2006).

Intergenerational Ambivalence. Although the theoretical interest in intergenerational ambivalence has increased in recent years, the empirical literature is not yet well developed. In one study based on a sample of mothers 60 years of age and older (Pillemen & Suitor, 2002), about one-third of the mothers were "torn" in their ties to their oldest child and felt conflicted about the relationship. As anticipated, one source of conflict was the tension between desires for autonomy and dependency. For example, mothers were concerned about encroachments on their autonomy when adult children failed to achieve and maintain normative adult statuses and financial independence. An analysis of the Iowa Youth and Families Project (Shuey, Wilson, & Elder, 2003), which also focused on mothers' experience of ambivalence with respect to their children, found that a mother's own dependency increased her level of ambivalence.

In another study (Fingerman, 2001), older mothers were interviewed regarding both the pleasures and problems in their relationships, and one of the salient sources of tension was daughters' unsolicited advice or help. Interestingly, Fingerman also found that different mothers resolved the inherent tensions in their relationships in different ways. Three main styles were discerned: constructive, destructive, and avoidant. This distinction in styles of resolving tension finds a parallel in another study (Smith & Goodnow, 1999) of how adults responded to unasked-for support. Three styles were described: assertively ignoring or rejecting the help, active discounting, and accommodating. Although attachment styles were not measured in either study, the tripartite distinction among styles of resolving tensions and conflicts would seem to be compatible with attachment theory.

A more recent study explored intergenerational ambivalence in a sample of 75 men and women above the age of 65 (Spitze & Gallant, 2004). Participants were interviewed in focus groups, and the interviews were then transcribed verbatim and content-analyzed. One salient theme was ambivalence about the extent to which children involved themselves in their parents' affairs and health. Parents expressed annoyance at children's overprotectiveness and controllingness; at the same time, they were appreciative of the concern these behaviors expressed. Parents tended to deal with their children's overprotectiveness in one of three ways: by withholding information and confiding in others, by ignoring it, or by simply accepting it. The material also revealed a desire to be independent, coupled with a potentially conflicting desire for connection to children. In fact, the authors noted that "independence" was the most frequently used interview code, despite the fact that "independence" was not a term that was explicitly used in the questions addressed to participants. This raises a particularly important issue with respect to the measurement of attachment in older samples. Dismissing attachment is often rated on the basis of emphasis on self-reliance and autonomy. If assertion of preference for autonomy is related to a developmentally emergent theme in later adulthood linked to aging individuals' fears of becoming incapacitated and being burdensome to their children, measures that rely too heavily on evidence of older adults' preference for autonomy and independence will confound attachment with developmentally normative trends. This is an issue to which I return later.

Intergenerational ambivalence has also been examined in a study in which participants of different ages indicated the quality of their relationships with a range of individuals in their social networks (Fingerman, Hay, & Birditt, 2004). The study included two forms of a social network diagram developed by Kahn and Antonucci (1980). Participants were first asked to place social partners to whom they felt very close in the innermost

circle of three concentric circles; less close relations were to be placed in the middle, and even less close ones in the third circle. The respondents were then asked to complete a second diagram pertaining to people who bothered them, with the most problematic persons placed in the innermost circle. Participants could name any and all of their relationships in both circles. From the data, the researchers identified relationships that were solely close, solely problematic, and ambivalent. The study found that the young-old (60–69 years) and the old-old (>80 years) were more likely to describe both sets of relationships as solely close than were adolescents, young adults, and middle-aged adults. In fact, among the oldest-old, 92% rated their family relationships as close, 8% rated them as ambivalent, and none rated their relationships as solely problematic.

This apparent decline in conflicted relationships with age is consistent with socioemotional selectivity theory (Carstensen, 1992, 1995), which proposes that older adults deliberately shed their more peripheral and least emotionally gratifying social relationships in the service of regulating emotion and avoiding conflict. In terms of specific relations, the young-old—the oldest group who still had living parents—were more likely to rate the relationships with their parents as close (70%), with none rating parental relations as problematic. In the young adult sample, however, 43% rated their relationships with their parents as close, and 54% rated them as ambivalent. Sixty-three percent of the middle-aged adults rated their relationships with their parents as close, and 31% rated them as ambivalent. As in the case of the oldest-old adults, none of the parental relationships were rated as solely problematic.

Although the study was cross-sectional, the data could be taken as suggesting that people become less ambivalent about their parents as they age, perhaps reconciling differences as they confront the prospects of their own mortality. It should also be noted, however, that in some ways the data from this study would also seem to be at variance with the literature on attachment style distributions in later life; as reported above, this literature indicates that dismissiveness tends to increase with age. The difference between the two sets of data may be attributable to the fact that in Carstensen's study individuals were describing *specific* relationships, rather than a general style of relating to others, which is tapped by self-report measures of adult attachment. It may simply be that when older adults think of peripheral relationships, they downplay their significance (thereby expressing dismissive attitudes); when they think of particular family relationships, they may focus on their positive nature, especially since close relations in later life are more fundamental to their survival and well-being (and thus less likely to be probed for negative content).

Alternatively, the less ambivalent ratings of the older adults in Carstensen's study may indicate their placing a premium on avoiding negative interactions. Indeed, several studies indicate that older adults tend to shun occasions where negative affect may be aroused, and that they report higher levels of positive emotion, less interpersonal friction, lower levels of negative emotion overall, and less conflict in their close relationships than younger family members do (Akiyama, Antonucci, Takahashi, & Langfahl, 2003; Fingerman & Birditt, 2003; Lawton, Kleban, & Dean, 1993; Lawton, Kleban, Rajagopal, & Dean, 1992; Lefkowitz & Fingerman, 2003; Stimpson, Tyler, & Hoyt, 2005). Finally, another alternative explanation may be that children's behaviors toward their parents may become more positive as their parents become older, because as parents enter late life, children may become more solicitous toward them and may protect their parents by not raising issues that upset them (Fingerman & Birditt, 2003).

The Attachment of Adult Children to Their Aging Parents

The Attachment Perspective

Early in development the often exclusive mother–child attachment broadens to include the father, siblings, grandparents, and other relatives. A study involving a representative sample of Japanese and American individuals ranging in age from 8 to 93 years (Antonucci, Akiyama, & Takahashi, 2004) used the Kahn and Antonucci (1980) measure of social networks to determine how social ties were distributed at different ages. The findings were remarkably similar across the two cultures, with only slight variations. In the innermost ring (depicting closest relationships), 8- to 12-year-old children named their mothers first, followed by fathers and siblings. Adults ages 21–39 still mentioned their mothers first, but the next most frequently mentioned persons were spouses. Among 40- to 59-year-olds, spouses were the most frequently nominated as the closest relationships, with children mentioned next, and only then were mothers likely to be named. Among 60- to 79-year-olds,

the closest relationships consisted of spouses and children, with mothers no longer being nominated. Finally, among the 80- to 93-year-olds, the pattern seen in 60- to 79-year-olds continued, but with the addition of grandchildren. In Japan, grandchildren were sometimes even nominated as being very close.

To summarize the most salient shift over the generations distilled from this work, we note the prominence of the mother as the main attachment figure in early life. Although she is often displaced by a spouse later in adulthood, the mother persists as a close attachment figure through middle age. Her disappearance from the circle of closest relations later in life is likely to be due to her death.

A further literature on affectional bonds between adult children and aging parents (feelings of closeness and expressed behavior) exists in the more specific context of caregiving. This topic has become important in the context of more long-lived generations, who tend to suffer more acute and chronic illnesses, incapacitation, and growing dependency.

Insights from the Sociological Literature

Intergenerational Solidarity. There is a fairly sizable literature on solidarity with respect to adult children and their parents, and this literature supplies much evidence of mutual support and value consensus (Bengtson & Roberts, 1991; Bengtson, Rosenthal, & Burton, 1996; Davey et al., 2004). One of the most methodologically sound studies, a nationally representative survey of cross-generational relationships as reported by adult children (Silverstein & Bengtson, 1997), found that 73% of the sample described themselves as very close to their mothers (vs. somewhat close or not close at all) and 57% as being very close to their fathers. However, feelings of emotional closeness, while common, did not fully capture the range of intergenerational patterns. The same researchers (Bengtson et al., 1996) also applied a latent class analysis to six dimensions of intergenerational solidarity derived from the broader dimensions of opportunity, function, and affinity. The six dimensions were emotional closeness, similarity of opinions, geographic distance, frequency of contact, providing instrumental assistance, and receiving instrumental assistance. Five types of intergenerational relations emerged. The "tight-knit" type was indicated by relations in which adult children reported being engaged with their parents on all six indicators of solidarity. The "sociable" type was characterized by a high degree of emotional close-ness and similarity of opinion, close geographic proximity, and frequent contact, but low levels of instrumental exchange. Adult children char-acterized as "intimate but distant" were engaged with their parents in terms of emotional closeness and similarity, but not geographic proximity, fre-quency of contact, or instrumental exchange. The "obligatory" type was characterized by geographi-cal proximity and frequent contact, but was low on emotional closeness, similarity, and instrumental exchange. Finally, adult children characterized as "detached" were not engaged with their parents on any of the six indicators of solidarity.

These family solidarity characterizations offer a somewhat broader typology with which to cap-ture varieties of interpersonal relations between the generations than that offered by the bidimen-sional (Brennan, Clark, & Shaver, 1998), three-category (Hazan & Shaver, 1987), or four-category (Bartholomew & Horowitz, 1991) models found in the attachment literature. As we will see in the section on caregiving, filial relations carry with them an obligatory aspect that is probably not as salient or pronounced in other types of attachment relations; this means that the study of attachment in later life may need to revisit its "metaphysics of measurement" (Griffin & Bartholomew, 1994).

Intergenerational Ambivalence. As mentioned above, although much of the early research on in-tergenerational solidarity tends to emphasize mu-tual support and value consensus, subsequent re-search has begun to suggest a more variegated and complex picture. Earlier I have described a study of close, ambivalent, and problematic relation-ships (Fingerman et al., 2004) based on the rat-ings of older adults. That same study also gathered data on how young and middle-aged adults rated their relationships with their parents, among other family members and nonfamily individuals. In this case, there was more evidence for ambivalence. Whereas for the oldest group of adults the propor-tion of relationships with children characterized as ambivalent was quite low (only 6%), 56% of the young adults and 31% of the middle-aged adults rated their relationships with their parents as am-bivalent. The corresponding proportions of "close" relationships were 43% and 63%, respectively. Another study (Wilson, Shuey, & Elder, 2003), using data from the Iowa Youth and Families Proj-ect, focused on adult children's ambivalent feel-ings toward their parents and in-laws. The authors found that children were more ambivalent in fe-male dyads, in relations with in-laws, in relations with parents in poor health, and in cases where a daughter was serving as a caregiver to a parent.

Continuity of Relations over Time

Based on what we know about the intergenera-tional transmission of attachment styles between mothers and their young infants (e.g., Benoit & Parker, 1994; Fonagy, Steele, & Steele, 1991; van IJzendoorn, 1995), one would expect differential patterns of solidarity both to be linked to indi-viduals' relational histories and to affect current functioning. Indeed, there is much evidence to support this expectation. The bulk of literature on intergenerational solidarity and intergenerational ambivalence suggests that the history of early par-ent–child relationships, such as experiences with rejection (Stimpson et al., 2005; Whitbeck, Hoyt, & Huck, 1994), divorce, and other family prob-lems (P. S. Webster & Herzog, 1995), may affect current solidarity in various ways. These include exchanges of help and support (Parrott & Bengt-son, 1999), conflict (Clarke, Preston, Raskin, & Bengtson, 1999; Whitbeck et al., 1994), strain (Whitbeck et al., 1994), depression (Stimpson et al., 2005; Whitbeck, Hoyt, & Tyler, 2001), and reciprocity (Silverstein, Conroy, Wang, Giarrusso, & Bengtson, 2002).

GIVING AND SEEKING CARE: RELATIONS TO ATTACHMENT

Earlier I have noted that the attachment bonds be-tween parents and their children remain strong in later life, although at times there may be conflict. One occasion for conflict resides in the chang-ing nature of the relationship over developmen-tal time, due to differential engagement of two different behavioral systems—attachment (care seeking) and caregiving. We typically think of the child as the care seeker and the parent as the caregiver. But these roles often change in later life, with implications for the relations between gen-erations.

Due to demographic shifts in the popula-tion of most Western countries related to reduced mortality and longer lifespans, there is an unprec-edented lengthening of the overlap between the lifespans of children and their parents (Perrig-Chiello & Hoepflinger, 2005). Despite the exten-sion of the disability-free life expectancy within the older adult population, the last phase in the lifespan is often accompanied by physical infirmity and the resulting assumption of substantial burdens of care by middle-aged children. It has been estimated (Himes, 1994; Perrig-Chiello, & Hoepflinger, 2005) that approximately 50% of all women (who tend to be the caregivers in families) will need to deal with dependent parents during middle age, and men and women both will need to reengage psychologically with their parents in a way that activates attachment-related feelings and motivations.

Given these demographic changes, both children and parents are faced with adding new roles to their lives. In the case of a parent, he or she continues to serve as an attachment figure for the child, which represents the continuation of an old role. In addition, as the parent becomes infirm or incapacitated, the parent becomes a care seeker, representing the emergence of a new role. In the case of a middle-aged child, the parent retains his or her function as an attachment figure, which amounts to the continuation of an old role. But as the parent becomes infirm, the middle-aged adult may need to step in and provide care—generally a new role for the child. These role accretions in the parent–offspring relationship would seem to engender one of the most common sources of intergenerational ambivalence: the role reversal entailed in the transition from adult child to adult caregiver, and in the gradual, unhappy relinquishment of autonomy by the aged parent (Diehl et al., 1998; Rossi & Rossi, 1991).

Caregiver: A New Role for the Child

The quality of the child–parent bond may well affect the kind of care aged parents receive from their children, as suggested by a study that measured adult attachment styles across a broad age range (Diehl et al., 1998). The researchers found that empathy and social responsibility—traits associated with the inclination to help others—were positively associated with attachment security and negatively associated with fearful avoidance. Dismissing attachment was negatively associated with empathy, and preoccupied attachment was negatively associated with responsibility. Compatible experimental work (Mikulincer, Shaver, Gillath, & Nitzberg, 2005) has shown that increasing individuals' felt security through both implicit and explicit priming techniques fosters compassion and altruistic behavior.

Research indicates that concern for aging parents' health is highly salient in the minds of adult children, and that dealing with this concern is a pervasive aspect of relationship with parents (Cicirelli, 2000). Here I consider how adult children respond to the call for caregiving in relation to their parents; this is followed by an examination of the literature on care seeking among older adults.

Theoretical sociologists provided some of the earliest formulations about the motives and means by which adult children provide help to aging parents. From a sociological framework, helping behavior is seen as one aspect of intergenerational solidarity, and helping behavior itself is viewed as a function of a particular elderly person's dependency needs, residential propinquity to an adult child, filial obligations, and gender roles. The Longitudinal Study of Generations (Silverstein, Parrott, & Bengtson, 1995) assessed parent–child dyads participating in three waves of data collection. Structural equation modeling with lagged covariates was used to predict change in the extent of social support provided to parents. The results indicated that intergenerational affection was the factor that most motivated daughters to provide support, whereas for sons the predominant factors were filial obligation, legitimation of inheritance, and frequency of contact. Data from the same study indicated that a history of affection was also associated with equitable and reciprocal exchange of support, as well as with a greater likelihood of giving and receiving various forms of support and help (Parrott & Bengtson, 1999).

Operating from within an attachment perspective, Cicirelli (1983, 1993) proposed that caregiving by adult children is motivated by enduring affectional ties between children and their parents, and by protective motives on the part of children. That is, an adult child, who may still come to an elderly parent for instrumental or emotional support during times of stress (e.g., childrearing, job difficulties, divorce), is motivated to preserve and/or restore the threatened existence of the attachment figure as long as possible, and this may involve becoming a caregiver when the parent is ill. However, the quality of the child's attachment to the parent conceivably influences the quality of his or her caregiving.

In the literature on caregiving in dating or marital relationships (i.e., in young adult samples), secure individuals have been found to report and display more sensitive and responsive care and less controlling caregiving than avoidant and ambivalent individuals have (Carnelley, Pietromonaco, & Jaffe, 1996; Collins, Guichard, Ford, & Feeney,

2006; B. C. Feeney & Collins, 2001; J. A. Feeney, 1996). Attachment-oriented studies of caregiving in the context of adult children providing care to elderly parents are quite limited in number, but the findings are consistent in showing that secure attachment can ameliorate anticipated or experienced caregiver burden. In one of the first studies of its kind, Cicirelli (1983) proposed that affectional ties between children and their parents might be a better predictor of helping than filial obligation. He studied a sample of middle-aged adults with mothers age 60 and above. Attachment was measured by an index of feelings of closeness and perceived similarity through identification; attachment behaviors were assessed by a composite of residential proximity, frequency of visits, and frequency of telephone contacts. Path analysis revealed that caregiving behaviors were predicted by feelings of attachment, maternal dependency, and filial obligation. Current helping behaviors were a direct effect of only two variables, attachment feelings and greater dependency on the part of the parent, whereas feelings of attachment and filial obligation had indirect effects, acting through their effect on what Cicirelli described as "attachment behavior" (defined as communication over distance to maintain psychological closeness). Future help was predicted by attachment behavior, feelings of attachment, low conflict, and parental dependency; filial obligation had no direct effect on commitment to provide future help.

A more recent study assessed the degree to which middle-aged children were prepared to face the challenge of future caregiving responsibilities as a function of attachment style (Soerensen et al., 2002). This study found that security of attachment was a significant and positive predictor of feeling prepared to provide care, whereas both anxious-ambivalent and avoidant attachment predicted lower levels of feeling prepared. Three other studies have examined the actual caregiving experience and its impact on "caregiver burden" (defined as subjective experiences of stress and strain). One study assessed attachment and obligation in daughters caring for elderly mothers (Cicirelli, 1993). The data indicated that although both variables were related to the help provided by the daughters, stronger (or more secure) attachment was associated with less subjective burden, whereas stronger obligation was associated with greater burden. Another study (Crispi, Schiaffino, & Berman, 1997) found that secure (vs. insecure) attachment of middle-aged children to a parent diagnosed with dementia was associated with lower "caregiving difficulty" (a measure of subjective and objective burden) and with lower psychological distress.

Another study hinted at the possibility that the attachment style of the older parent and his or her behavior may influence the experience of caregiver burden in the child (Magai & Cohen, 1998). In this study, patients with dementia who were rated as having an anxious attachment style before they became ill displayed more anxious and depressed symptoms than patients with preillness secure or avoidant attachment styles did. Patients with the avoidant style displayed more activity disturbance than patients with the anxious style, and more paranoid symptoms than those with a secure style. Relatedly, caregivers of patients with a secure style reported lower caregiver burden than those caring for patients with avoidant or anxious attachment styles. Thus there are likely to be reciprocal and dynamic aspects of the care experience at the level of the dyad; this feature is alluded to in a recently published multicomponent conceptual model, in which both caregivers' and care recipients' characteristics and behaviors are taken into account (B. C. Feeney & Collins, 2004). Indeed, a laboratory study involving interaction with a confederate "patient with cancer" found that participants' anxious and avoidant attachment styles predicted anxiety in this particular interaction. Participants' avoidant attachment predicted low supportiveness; however, avoidant participants interacting with an avoidant confederate displayed less rejection of an avoidant than of a nonavoidant confederate (Westmaas & Silver, 2001).

Finally, there is evidence of intergenerational transmission of attachment and caregiving patterns. Longitudinal data from a Swiss study, Transitions and Life Perspectives in Middle Age (Perrig-Chiello & Hoepflinger, 2005), found that "filial autonomy" (a measure of successful coping with normative developmental tasks in adulthood) was negatively correlated with filial helpfulness and with secure relations with the adults' own children; this suggested that a strong sense of separateness between middle-aged persons and their parents was mirrored in a less secure relationship with their own children. Moreover, the strength (or security) of attachment to parents was positively associated with the strength of relationships with the middle-aged participants' own children. Another set of investigators (Wilson et al., 2003), using data from the Iowa Youth and Families Project, focused on adult children's ambivalent feelings toward their parents and in-laws, finding that there was greater ambivalence when there had been poor relations during childhood.

Help Seeking in Later Life: A New Role for the Parent

Despite older adults' clear preference for retaining their autonomy in late life, most people cannot realistically hope to avoid an increase in dependency if they live long enough. Among the potential elicitors of care seeking are (1) the various forms of chronic illness with which persons are afflicted in late life that require constant monitoring and/or care (e.g., diabetes, poor vision, and kidney disease); (2) growing limitation of activities and greater physical dependency caused by such illnesses as arthritis, circulatory disease, and stroke-related paralysis, among other conditions; and (3) anxiety and depression occurring in the context of bereavements of various kinds and the looming of the individual's own death.

Threats and illness are innate elicitors of attachment behavior in early life, and children readily turn to their parental secure base for protection and reassurance when distress arises. In later life, after decades of successful autonomy, encroaching dependency can seem a cruel denouement; as already noted, this newly emerging threat appears to elicit an internal approach–avoidance struggle between autonomy and dependence. Conceivably, this struggle is more difficult for insecurely attached individuals. Anxiously attached people are sometimes too eager to seek care and reassurance from attachment figures in general, and their potential caregivers may be put off by their sheer neediness, emotional intensity, and persistence. This may cause the caregivers to distance themselves, generating even more insecurity in their needy elderly dependents. In the case of avoidant individuals, they are likely to deny their distress and therefore unlikely to seek help. In both kinds of cases, the insecure elderly parents may perceive less social support, as has been found in studies of younger adults (Vogel & Wei, 2005). Despite the implications of such findings for later-life intergenerational relationships and their importance for the well-being of elderly adults, help-seeking behavior on the part of older adults, viewed from an attachment perspective, is virtually an unstudied phenomenon of potentially great theoretical and practical importance.

PARENTAL BEREAVEMENT

One of the most common attachment-related challenges of adulthood is coming to terms with the loss of one's parents—the ultimate separation experience. Parental death is the single most common cause of bereavement in the United States, with nearly 12 million adults, or 5% of the population, losing a parent each year (Levy, 1999). Demographic data indicate that maternal and paternal deaths are most likely to occur when children are between 45 and 64 years of age and between 35 and 54 years of age, respectively (Winsborough, Bumpass, & Aquilino, 1991). Attachment theory suggests that these losses elicit profound feelings. Oddly, although there is a good deal of literature on spousal bereavement (Stroebe, Schut, & Stroebe, 2005) and a substantial literature on bereavement experiences of parents who lose young children, there is very little empirical literature on adult children's experience of parental loss. This lack of research is especially odd, given that all of us—if we live long enough—will experience the loss of first one parent and then the other. Once both parents are deceased, feelings of being an "orphan" are common (Levy, 1999; Stroebe et al., 2005).

What limited literature exists indicates that the death of an aged parent can cause changes in an adult child's marital relationship and in the relationship with the surviving parent. Although the marital relationship can be a source of support when the spouse's parent dies, and may actually strengthen the marital relationship (Moss & Moss, 1984), it may also have a deleterious effect on that relationship. One prospective study (Umberson, 1995) found that recent maternal death was associated with a decline in social support from the adult child's marital partner and an increase in the partner's negative behaviors. In that study, recent maternal death was associated with a decline in relationship harmony and an increase in relationship strain and conflict. Another study (Lee, Dwyer, & Coward, 1993) found that father–daughter relationships deteriorated significantly after the mother's death, but that this effect was much weaker for the father–son relationship.

It appears that there are only two attachment-oriented studies of parental bereavement in later life, although in neither case were standard measures of attachment employed. One of the studies (Scharlach, 1991) tested the thesis that resolution of grief depends on the bereaved adult's attachment status relative to the parent who has died. Scharlach considered both initial and residual grief reactions in 35- to 60-year-olds. Theory would suggest that an anxious attachment orientation and a history of childhood separation would be associated with increased difficulty during the grieving process. Results of this study indicated that two of the strongest predictors of initial and residual grief were the expectedness of the parent's death and the level of the adult child's personal autonomy. The latter effect was interpreted as indexing a secure attachment, inasmuch as successful functioning as an autonomous adult is thought to be the result of a healthy separation from one's parents.

The other study (Popek & Scharlach, 1991) used interview and questionnaire data to examine the responses of adult daughters to the deaths of their elderly mothers. The authors found that a daughter's ability to resolve her grief 1–5 years after the mother's death was significantly affected by the kind of relationship she had with her mother when the mother was still alive. The personal interviews were transcribed verbatim and content-analyzed. Coders assessed the nature of each relationship (close or distant) and whether each participant's feelings regarding the mother's death were relatively resolved or unresolved. Thirty-seven percent were classified as close and resolved, 35% as close and unresolved, and 26% as distant and unresolved; one participant's relationship (0.02%) was classified as distant and resolved. Based on the authors' descriptions of other key characteristics of the groupings, the first category probably reflected a secure daughter–mother relationship, the second a preoccupied and/or fearful-avoidant relationship, and the third a dismissing relationship.

The glaring absence of research in this area, despite the ubiquity of the experience, begs for an explanation. As the literature on intergenerational ambivalence suggests, relations between children and their parents are among the strongest of intergenerational ties, although they are often fraught with tensions, unresolved issues, and mixed feeling about autonomy and dependence. The loss of a parent, therefore, will necessarily evoke intense grief, and perhaps a particularly conflicted grief that has the potential to stir up of a host of unresolved, deeply rooted mixed emotions. Perhaps it is the combination of intensity and ambivalence that helps explain the field's apparent aversion to the topic—a kind of motivated avoidance and/or forgetting on the part of researchers.

That possibility notwithstanding, and despite the physical departure of the parents from adult children's lives, there is evidence of their continued influence. In fact, one study suggests that internalized representations of parents function as "silent" attachment partners even after the parents' deaths, at least as studied within the context of dementia research (see also Shaver & Fraley, Chapter 3, this volume). The belief among many elderly patients

with dementia that one or both of their parents is still alive—called "parent fixation"—has been reported as fairly common (Miesen, 1992).

In a study of the relation between level of cognitive functioning and the expression of various forms of attachment behavior in a psychogeriatric nursing home in the Netherlands, observations of attachment behavior were made by staff members on the ward at various times of day, including during family visits (Miesen, 1992). A Standard Visiting Procedure was used, akin to Ainsworth's Strange Situation, where the person with dementia was first all alone in a room, then was with the researcher, and finally was with a family member. A critical point in this procedure occurred when the family member suddenly announced that he or she had to leave, thus creating a potentially threatening moment that should activate the attachment system. Individuals who were more cognitively intact exhibited less parent fixation (the belief that one or both parents were still alive scored as clearly present, intermittently present, or absent) and more overt forms of attachment behavior directed at a family member, such as turning toward or calling after the person. Those who were functioning at a lower level displayed more parent fixation and fewer overt attachment behaviors of any other kind.

Miesen (1992) hypothesized that the invocation of deceased parents by patients with dementia represents an attempt to regulate the fear and uncertainty that accompanies loss of cognitive function. In this view, parent fixation is an attachment behavior expressing the need for safety and security. In the early stages of dementia, he theorized, parent fixation is not observed because other, more organized forms of attachment behavior are still possible, and because of the security provided by available living attachment figures. As the illness progresses, however, the "strange situation" that is dementia becomes a more permanent condition, with the now pervasive experience of feeling unsafe being increasingly managed internally as reflected in parent fixation.

THE NEXT GENERATION OF RESEARCH

When I began writing this chapter, I was convinced that the literature on attachment and aging was so sparse, I would have trouble filling the pages allotted to me. Therefore, I cast my net wide, intending to cover all kinds of issues—including the role of religion in later life, the exploratory behavioral system, different kinds of affectional bonds (spouse, sibling, parents), mortality salience, and the like. In the end, I decided to limit my review to types of attachment patterns, their stability, and the focal theme of parent–child relationships in the latter half of life, because I found that I could not include more than this material without exceeding my page limit.

A good portion of the literature I reviewed was new to me, so writing about it was a process of discovery. I was aware of the sociological literature that speaks to attachment issues, having been introduced to it by an early mentor, Lillian Troll, who was herself mentored by some of the prominent "Chicago School" gerontologists (the trailblazers with respect to filial relations at that time). But I had lost touch with that field for more than 15 years; thus the more recent findings were new to me. I also had some background in the caregiving literature through my research on the emotional concomitants of dementia and the impact of the dementia on caregivers. But, again, new literature had emerged over the last decade or so with which I had to familiarize myself. Finally, I had never covered the issue of bereavement before, and the literature was new to me, although I had experienced the second of my own parental bereavements within the recent past and was therefore aware of some of the issues firsthand.

Even in limiting my review to patterns of attachment, stability of attachment, and the continuity of the child–parent attachment bond, I made a number of discoveries that I would like to summarize, because they signal new frontiers for attachment research. The first thing that caught my attention was a measurement issue. Specifically, this was the potential confounding of the assessment of dismissing attachment with what appeared to be a normative emergent late-life theme: that of the press to maintain independence and autonomy in the context of the encroaching depredations of later life. Researchers will need to be creative to unconfound the two—perhaps by taking advantage of a multitrait–multimethod approach involving measures of closeness and affection on the one hand, and measures of autonomy striving and comfort with dependency on the other.

Once we have a measure with discriminant validity, the next set of questions arises: What is the boundary condition between normative self-reliance and excessive self-reliance in later life? What are the social networks of secure and dismissing older adults like? Socioemotional selectivity theory (Carstensen, 1992, 1993) maintains that social networks shrink in later life and are reduced to those that are most emotionally gratifying. Is this the case for both secure and dismissing adults? Do self-reliant dismissing individuals go to extra lengths to defend their independence, causing them to retain functionality (the ability to perform the activities of daily living) longer than secure individuals, or are they ultimately more vulnerable to sudden collapse? In one study mentioned above, dismissing individuals showed no shift in attachment style in the context of increasing stress, whereas secure individuals did (Consedine & Magai, 2006); this finding suggests that avoidant individuals may be better defended. Does this make them more resilient or ultimately brittle?

The literature also suggested that there are more forms of attachment than the customary three or four categories based on studies of children and younger adults. It is an axiom of social gerontology that populations of older individuals become increasingly differentiated as they age. In other words, it is widely accepted that older adults employ a variety of strategies in adapting to the changes that accompany aging (M. M. Baltes & Carstensen, 1996; P. B. Baltes, 1987; Maddox, 1965; Thomae, 1981). As individuals age, they come to resemble one another less rather than more. Consequently, although there appear to be several normative intra- and interpersonal processes in later life, "there is not one path to [later-life] social adaptivity" (Lang, Staudinger, & Carstensen, 1998, p. 29). For the most part, older adults are not passive in dealing with the challenges they face. Instead, they actively engage in a diverse range of self-care efforts and attempt to anticipate future difficulties (Consedine, Magai, & Conway, 2004; Gignac, Cott, & Badley, 2000).

Adaptations to physical and social losses and the increased dependency that typically accompanies greater age are likely to be similarly heterogeneous, with different individuals adjusting to the aging process in diverse ways. If, as the gerontological literature suggests, people become more heterogeneous with age, we might anticipate varied kinds of dependency and interdependency in filial relationships in later life. Bowlby (1988) claimed that attachment has relevance for the entire lifespan, but he never "put flesh to bone" for this rather broad assertion, and thus we do not know whether he intended to imply cross-age applicability of all constructs and measures.

Because the literature is currently so theoretically sparse in this respect, I took an empirical approach in a recent paper prepared for a conference on attachment (Consedine, Magai, & Gillespie, 2006). In an attempt to assess variations in the structure of adult attachment across the adult lifespan, I merged archival data sets containing responses to Griffin and Bartholomew's (1994) Relationship Scales Questionnaire (age range = 18–86 years; total N = 5,130) from several studies based in New York City and conducted principal-components analyses. Both higher-order and lower-order factor structures were identified, with three and seven factors, respectively. The three-factor solution consisted of "desire for emotional closeness," "desire for independence," and "fearful avoidance." The seven-factor solution differentiated closeness and interpersonal dependency factors—"discomfort with closeness," "fear of abandonment," "desire for emotional closeness," "others as undependable," "desire for independence," "discomfort with others' dependency," and "comfort with dependency." Both factor structures were related to marital status in conceptually reasonable ways, and there were significant age differences in the factor scores. In the seven-factor solution, most factors decreased with age except for desire for independence and discomfort with others' dependency, which increased. These results raise the interesting question of whether the attachment "glove" that nicely fits the period of infancy and readily stretches to accommodate young adulthood should be further stretched to encompass later life, or whether we need to rethink our measures in the developmental contexts of middle and later life and/or the notions of attachment, autonomy, and interpersonal dependency across the lifespan.

This review also suggests that assessment of the caregiving behavioral system and its relation to the attachment behavioral system will be an important addition to the literature in future research. As some authors have suggested (B. C. Feeney & Collins, 2004), of the three behavioral systems articulated by Bowlby—the attachment, exploratory, and caregiving systems—the third has not been very well developed. Although research on younger adults (Kunce & Shaver, 1994) suggests a workable four-dimensional or four-categorical rendering of caregiving styles in the context of romantic relationships, it remains to be seen whether this system can be applied to the adult child–parent caregiving relationship. Demographic trends indicate that increasing numbers of middle-aged adults will be drawn into the task of providing care for their aging parents; in-

deed, Soerensen and colleagues (2002) suggested that caregiving for older relatives is likely to be a common developmental task of adults in middle and later life. One small but well-executed study (Thompson, Galbraith, Thomas, Swan, & Vrungos, 2002), using self-reports and direct observation of dyadic interactions, examined overprotective care among caregivers of patients recuperating from stroke. Overprotection, or a care recipient's perception that he or she is being overhelped and induced to be dependent, was found to be a function of caregiver rejection. That is, overprotection was associated with an overcontrolling caregiving style, negative affect, and resentment toward the patient. This study also included a measure of dependency and found that the patient's perception of being overprotected was associated with patient dependency, although the causal relation between the two could not be determined.

In future research, it will be important to differentiate among dependency based on a social environment that elicits and/or reinforces dependent behavior; insecurity-based dependency (similar to anxious, preoccupied attachment); and reasonable, self-accepted dependency, which may be a beneficial stance used to conserve energy and resources (Parks & Pilisuk, 1991). The field would be well served if future research on caregiving and attachment in later adulthood were directed at assessing types of caregiving, types of dependency, and their sequelae.

There is already fairly strong evidence of a relationship between social support and network structures on the one hand, and health status, mortality, and risk of entry into institutional care on the other; the effect sizes tend to be moderate to large (see Bowling & Grundy, 1998, for a review of the major longitudinal studies). Negative social interactions in later life have also been linked to depression symptoms, as found in a study of regionally representative samples from France, Germany, Japan, and the United States (Antonucci, Lansford, & Akayama, 2002). Although the existing research indicates that the quality of attachment relations varies within families, that parents apparently have "favorite" children, and that particular pairings of caregiver and care recipient may be more problematic than others (Westmaas & Silver, 2001), little is known about which child in the family becomes the caregiver and what might motivate acceptance of the role. If, as Cicirelli (1983, 1993) proposes, caregiving is motivated in part by children wanting to protect their attachment figures so as to assuage their own "fear of abandonment," we might expect more anxiously attached adult children to rise to the occasion. Providing care to a sick or disabled parent can be rewarding, but it can also be very taxing and psychologically threatening (Cicirelli, 1983, 1993). We know that innate tendencies to provide care to others in need can be overridden or suppressed by attachment insecurity (B. C. Feeney & Collins, 2001; Mikulincer et al., 2005). At such times, anxiously attached individuals are likely to be focused on their own needs rather than those of their distressed relationship partners. We also know that avoidantly attached individuals tend to be disapproving of other people's vulnerabilities, weaknesses, and needs (Collins & Read, 1994), and therefore cannot be expected to be sensitive to others' distress. This raises questions about the quality of care that will be provided by adult children with insecure styles of attachment, perhaps especially in the presence of the original cause of attachment insecurity (i.e., a parent's insecurity-arousing behavior).

Finally, my review of the literature has brought to the fore the virtual neglect of bereavement following the loss of one or both parents as a middle-life experience with potentially profound significance. Although there is little empirical literature on bereavement in this context, a keenly observed memoir by a clinical psychologist (Levy, 1999) writing about the passing of his own parents, and his subsequent exploration of relevant attachment-related thoughts and feelings with his middle-aged clients, resulted in a number of personal observations that could be a rich source of ideas for future research. Among other things, Levy (1999) suggests that when one parent dies, there may be changes in the relationship with the remaining parent; that when either parent or both parents die, there may be changes in other interpersonal relationships or changes in identity that provoke identity reorganization; and that the death of a parent refocuses an adult's sense of time.

It is likely that these issues play out in different ways for different people, and that attachment styles influence how such issues are approached, resolved, or left unresolved as people live out the remainder of their lives. Of note, a recent paper by Stroebe and colleagues (2005) offers a conceptual model—the dual-process model of coping with bereavement—that integrates coping theory and attachment theory in a very promising way. The model, which has been discussed in light of attachment research by Mikulincer and Shaver (2008), suggests that there is an array of successful and unsuccessful coping styles as well as attachment styles, some of which are loss-oriented and some of which are restoration-oriented. Furthermore, Stroebe et al. suggest that these coping orientations, when considered jointly with attachment styles, may enable researchers to understand when and for whom the process of continuing or loosening the attachment bonds with a lost loved one are likely to be adaptive or maladaptive. There is a great deal of interesting and important research to be done in this area.

ACKNOWLEDGMENTS

The writing of this chapter, and some of the research described herein, were supported by grants from the National Institute on Aging (No. KO7 AG00921, RO1 AG021017) and the National Institute of General Medical Science (No. 2SO6 GM54650).

REFERENCES

Ainsworth, M. S. (1989). Attachments beyond infancy. *American Psychologist, 44*(4), 709–716.

Akiyama, H., Antonucci, T., Takahashi, K., & Langfahl, E. S. (2003). Negative interactions in close relationships across the life span. *Journals of Gerontology: Series B: Psychological Sciences, 58B*, P70–P79.

Antonucci, T. C., Akiyama, H., & Takahashi, K. (2004). Attachment and close relationships across the life span. *Attachment and Human Development, 6*, 353–370.

Antonucci, T. C., Lansford, J. E., & Akayama, H. (2002). Differences between men and women in social relations, resource deficits, and depressive symptomatology during later life in four nations. *Journal of Social Issues, 58*, 767–783.

Baldwin, M. W., & Fehr, B. (1995). On the instability of attachment style ratings. *Personal Relationships, 2*, 247–261.

Baltes, M. M., & Carstensen, L. L. (1996). The process of successful ageing. *Ageing and Society, 16*, 397–422.

Baltes, P. B. (1987). Theoretical propositions of life-span developmental psychology: On the dynamics between growth and decline. *Developmental Psychology, 23*, 611–626.

Banai, E., Weller, A., & Mikulincer, M. (1998). Interjudge agreement in evaluation of adult attachment style: The impact of acquaintanceship. *British Journal of Social Psychology, 37*, 95–109.

Barnas, M. V., Pollina, L., & Cummings, E. M. (1991). Life-span attachment: Relations between attachment and socioemotional functioning in adult women. *Genetic, Social, and General Psychology Monographs, 117*, 175–202.

Bartholomew, K., & Horowitz, L. M. (1991). Attachment styles among young adults: A test of a four-category model. *Journal of Personality and Social Psychology, 61,* 226–244.

Bengtson, V. L., & Roberts, R. E. L. (1991). Intergenerational solidarity in aging families: An example of formal theory construction. *Journal of Marriage and the Family, 53,* 856–870.

Bengtson, V. L., Rosenthal, C. J., & Burton, L. (1996). Paradoxes of families and aging. In R. H. Binstock & L. K. George (Eds.), *Handbook of aging and the social sciences* (4th ed., pp. 253–282). San Diego, CA: Academic Press.

Benoit, D., & Parker, K. (1994). Stability and transmission of attachment across three generations. *Child Development, 65,* 1444–1456.

Bowlby, J. (1969/1982). *Attachment and loss: Vol. 1. Attachment.* New York: Basic Books.

Bowlby, J. (1973). *Attachment and loss: Vol. 2. Separation: Anxiety and anger.* New York: Basic Books.

Bowlby, J. (1980). *Attachment and loss: Vol. 3. Loss: Sadness and depression.* New York: Basic Books.

Bowlby, J. (1988). *A secure base: Parent–child attachment and healthy human development.* New York: Basic Books.

Bowling, A., & Grundy, E. (1998). The association between social networks and mortality in later life. *Reviews in Clinical Gerontology, 8,* 353–361.

Brennan, K. A., Clark, C. L., & Shaver, P. R. (1998). Self-report measurement of adult attachment. In J. A. Simpson & W. S. Rholes (Eds.), *Attachment theory and close relationships* (pp. 46–76). New York: Guilford Press.

Campos, J. J., Barrett, K. C., Lamb, M. E., Goldsmith, H. H., & Stenberg, C. (1983). Socioemotional development. In M. M. Haith (Ed.), *Handbook of child psychology: Infancy and developmental psychobiology* (Vol. 2, pp. 783–917). New York: Wiley.

Carnelley, K. B., Pietromonaco, P. R., & Jaffe, K. (1996). Attachment, caregiving, and relationship functioning in couples: Effects of self and partner. *Personal Relationships, 3,* 257–277.

Carstensen, L. L. (1992). Social and emotional patterns in adulthood: Support for socioemotional selectivity theory. *Psychology and Aging, 7,* 331–338.

Carstensen, L. L. (1992). Developmental perspectives on motivation: A theory of socioemotional selectivity. In J. E. Jacobs (Ed.), *Nebraska Symposium on Motivation: Vol. 40. Current theory and research in motivation* (pp. 209–254). Lincoln: University of Nebraska Press.

Carstensen, L. L. (1995). Evidence for a life-span theory of socioemotional selectivity. *Current Directions in Psychological Science, 4,* 151–156.

Cassidy, J., & Shaver, P. R. (Eds.). (1999). *Handbook of attachment: Theory, research, and clinical applications.* New York: Guilford Press.

Cicchetti, D., Toth, S. L., & Lynch, M. (1995). Bowlby's dream comes full circle: The application of attachment theory to risk and psychopathology. *Advances in Clinical Child Psychology, 17,* 1–75.

Cicirelli, V. G. (1983). Adult children's attachment and helping behavior to elderly parents: A path model. *Journal of Marriage and the Family, 45,* 815–825.

Cicirelli, V. G. (1993). Attachment and obligation as daughters' motives for caregiving behavior and subsequent effect on subjective burden. *Psychology and Aging, 8,* 144–155.

Cicirelli, V. G. (2000). An examination of the trajectory of the adult child's caregiving for an elderly parent. *Family Relations, 49,* 169–175.

Clarke, E. J., Preston, M., Raskin, J., & Bengtson, V. L. (1999). Types of conflicts and tensions between older parents and adult children. *The Gerontologist, 39,* 261–270.

Collins, N. L., Guichard, A. C., Ford, M. B., & Feeney, B. C. (2006). Responding to need in intimate relationships: Normative processes and individual differences. In M. Mikulincer & G. S. Goodman (Eds.), *Dynamics of romantic love: Attachment, caregiving, and sex* (pp. 149–189). New York: Guilford Press.

Collins, N. L., & Read, S. J. (1994). Cognitive representations of attachment: The structure and function of working models. In K. Bartholomew & D. Perlman (Eds.), *Advances in personal relationships: Vol. 5. Attachment processes in adulthood* (pp. 53–92). London: Jessica Kingsley.

Connidis, I. A., & McMullin, J. A. (2002). Sociological ambivalence and family ties: A critical perspective. *Journal of Marriage and the Family, 64,* 558–567.

Consedine, N. S., & Magai, C. (2006, July). *Patterns of attachment and attachment change in later life: Preliminary results from a longitudinal study of 415 older adults.* Paper presented at the Third Biennial Conference of the International Association for Relationship Research, Rethymnon, Crete, Greece.

Consedine, N. S., Magai, C., & Conway, F. (2004). Predicting ethnic variation in adaptation to later life: Styles of socioemotional functioning and constrained heterotypy. *Journal of Cross-Cultural Gerontology, 19,* 95–129.

Consedine, N. S., Magai, C., & Gillespie, M. (2006, July). *Patterns of relating in young, middle-aged, and older urban-dwelling adults: The metaphysics of attachment revisited.* Poster presented at the Third Biennial Conference of the International Association for Relationship Research, Rethymnon, Crete, Greece.

Cozzarelli, C., Karafa, J. A., Collins, N. L., & Tagler, M. J. (2003). Stability and change in adult attachment styles: Associations with personal vulnerabilities, life events, and global construals of self and others. *Journal of Social and Clinical Psychology, 22,* 315–346.

Crispi, E. L., Schiaffino, K., & Berman, W. H. (1997). The contribution of attachment to burden in adult children of institutionalized parents with dementia. *The Gerontologist, 38,* 52–60.

Davey, A., Janke, M., & Savla, J. (2004). Antecedents of intergenerational support: Families in context and families as context. *Annual Review of Gerontology and Geriatrics, 24,* 29–54.

Davila, J., Burge, D., & Hammen, C. (1997). Why does

attachment style change? *Journal of Personality and Social Psychology, 73*, 826–838.

Davila, J., & Cobb, R. J. (2004). Predictors of change in attachment security. In W. S. Rholes & J. A. Simpson (Eds.), *Adult attachment: Theory, research, and clinical implications* (pp. 133–156). New York: Guilford Press.

Diehl, M., Elnick, A. B., Bourbeau, L. S., & Labouvie-Vief, G. (1998). Adult attachment styles: Their relations to family context and personality. *Journal of Personality and Social Psychology, 74*, 1656–1669.

Feeney, B. C., & Collins, N. L. (2001). Predictors of caregiving in adult intimate relationships: An attachment theoretical perspective. *Journal of Personality and Social Psychology, 80*, 972–994.

Feeney, B. C., & Collins, N. L. (2004). Interpersonal safe haven and secure base caregiving processes in adulthood. In W. S. Rholes & J. A. Simpson (Eds.), *Adult attachment: Theory, research, and clinical implications* (pp. 300–338). New York: Guilford Press.

Feeney, J. A. (1996). Attachment, caregiving, and marital satisfaction. *Personal Relationships, 3*, 401–416.

Feeney, J. A., & Noller, P. (1990). Attachment style as a predictor of adult romantic relationships. *Journal of Personality and Social Psychology, 38*, 281–291.

Fingerman, K. L. (1996). Sources of tension in the aging mother and adult daughter relationship. *Psychology and Aging, 11*, 591–606.

Fingerman, K. L. (1998). Tight lips?: Aging mothers' and adult daughters' responses to interpersonal tensions in their relationships. *Personal Relationships, 5*, 121–138.

Fingerman, K. L. (2001). *Aging mothers and their adult daughters: A study in mixed emotions.* New York: Springer.

Fingerman, K. L., & Birditt, K. S. (2003). Do age differences in close and problematic family ties reflect the pool of available relatives? *Journals of Gerontology: Series B. Psychological Sciences, 58B*, 80–87.

Fingerman, K. L., Hay, E. L., & Birditt, K. S. (2004). The best of ties, the worst of ties: Close, problematic, and ambivalent social relationships. *Journal of Marriage and the Family, 66*, 792–808.

Fonagy, P., Steele, H., & Steele, M. (1991). Maternal representations of attachment during pregnancy predict the organization of infant–mother attachment at one year of age. *Child Development, 62*, 891–905.

Fraley, R. C., & Brumbaugh, C. C. (2004). A dynamical systems approach to conceptualizing and studying stability and change in attachment security. In W. S. Rholes & J. A. Simpson (Eds.), *Adult attachment: Theory, research, and clinical implications* (pp. 86–132). New York: Guilford Press.

Gignac, M. A. M., Cott, C., & Badley, E. M. (2000). Adaptation to chronic illness and disability and its relationship to perceptions of independence and dependence. *Journals of Gerontology: Series B. Psychological Sciences and Social Sciences, 55B*, P-62–P372.

Giles, L. C., Glonek, G. F. V., Luszcz, M. A., & Andrews, R. (2005). Effect of social networks on 10 year survival in very old Australians: The Australian longitudinal study of aging. *Journal of Epidemiology and Community Health, 59*, 574–579.

Griffin, D. W., & Bartholomew, K. (1994). The metaphysics of measurement: The case of adult attachment. In K. Bartholomew & D. Perlman (Eds.), *Advances in personal relationships: Vol. 5. Attachment processes in adulthood* (pp. 17–52). London: Jessica Kingsley.

Grossmann, K. E. (1996). Ethological perspectives on human development and aging. In C. Magai & S. McFadden (Eds.), *Handbook of emotion, adult development, and aging* (pp. 43–66). San Diego, CA: Academic Press.

Hazan, C., & Shaver, P. R. (1987). Romantic love conceptualized as an attachment process. *Journal of Personality and Social Psychology, 52*, 511–524.

Hesse, E. (1999). The Adult Attachment Interview: Historical and current perspectives. In J. Cassidy & P. R. Shaver (Eds.), *Handbook of attachment: Theory, research, and clinical applications* (pp. 395–433). New York: Guilford Press.

Himes, C. L. (1994). Parental caregiving by adult women. *Research on Aging, 16*, 191–211.

Kahn, R. L., & Antonucci, T. C. (1980). Convoys over the life course: Attachment, roles, and social support. In O. C. Brim (Ed.), *Life-span development and behavior* (pp. 254–283). New York: Academic Press.

Kirkpatrick, L. A., & Davis, K. E. (1994). Attachment style, gender, and relationship stability: A longitudinal analysis. *Journal of Personality and Social Psychology, 66*, 502–512.

Kunce, L. J., & Shaver, P. R. (1994). An attachment-theoretical approach to caregiving in romantic relationships. In K. Bartholomew & D. Perlman (Eds.), *Advances in personal relationships: Vol. 5. Attachment processes in adulthood* (pp. 205–237). London: Jessica Kingsley.

Lang, F. R., Staudinger, U. M., & Carstensen, L. L. (1998). Perspectives on socioemotional selectivity in late life: How personality and social context do (and do not) make a difference. *Journal of Gerontology: Series B. Psychological Sciences, 53B*, P21–P30.

Lawton, M. P., Kleban, M. H., & Dean, J. (1993). Affect and age: Cross-sectional comparisons of structure and prevalence. *Psychology and Aging, 8*, 165–175.

Lawton, M. P., Kleban, M. H., Rajagopal, D., & Dean, J. (1992). The dimensions of affective experience in three age groups. *Psychology and Aging, 7*, 171–184.

Lee, G., Dwyer, J., & Coward, R. (1993). Gender differences in parent care: Demographic factors and same-gender preferences. *Journal of Gerontology: Social Sciences, 48*, S9–S16.

Lefkowitz, E. S., & Fingerman, K. L. (2003). Positive and negative emotional feelings and behaviors in mother–daughter ties in late life. *Journal of Family Psychology, 17*, 607–617.

Levy, A. (1999). *The orphaned adult: Understanding and coping with grief and change after the death of our parents.* Cambridge, MA: Perseus.

Luescher, K., & Pillemer, K. (1998). Intergenerational ambivalence: A new approach to the study of parent–child relations in later life. *Journal of Marriage and the Family, 60*, 413–425.

Lundberg, O. (1993). The impact of childhood living conditions on illness and mortality in adulthood. *Social Science and Medicine, 36*, 1047–1052.

Lutz, W. J., & Hock, E. (1995). Maternal separation anxiety: Relations to adult attachment representations in mothers of infants. *Journal of Genetic Psychology, 156*, 57–72.

Maddox, G. L. (1965). Fact and artifact: Evidence bearing on disengagement theory from the Duke Geriatrics Project. *Human Development, 8*, 117–130.

Magai, C. (2001). Emotions over the lifespan. In J. E. Birren & K. W. Schaie (Eds.), *Handbook of the psychology of aging* (5th ed., pp. 310–344). San Diego, CA: Academic Press.

Magai, C., Cohen, C., Milburn, N., Thorpe, B., McPherson, R., & Peralta, D. (2001). Attachment styles in older European American and African American adults. *Journals of Gerontology: Series B. Psychological Sciences and Social Sciences, 56B*, 28–35.

Magai, C., & Cohen, C. I. (1998). Attachment style and emotion regulation in dementia patients and their relation to caregiver burden. *Journals of Gerontology: Series B. Psychological Sciences, 53B*, P147–P154.

Magai, C., & Consedine, N. S. (2004). Introduction to the special issue: Attachment and aging. *Attachment and Human Development, 6*, 349–351.

Magai, C., Hunziker, J., Mesias, W., & Culver, L. C. (2000). Adult attachment styles and emotional biases. *International Journal of Behavioral Development, 24*, 301–309.

Main, M., & Goldwyn, R. (1984). Predicting rejection of her infant from mother's representation of her own experience: Implications for the abused–abusing intergenerational cycle. *Child Abuse and Neglect, 8*, 203–217.

Main, M., Kaplan, N., & Cassidy, J. (1985). Security in infancy, childhood, and adulthood: A move to the level of representation. In I. Bretherton & E. Waters (Eds.), Growing points of attachment theory and research. *Monographs of the Society for Research in Child Development, 50*(1–2, Serial No. 209), 66–104.

Mickelson, K. D., Kessler, R. C., & Shaver, P. R. (1997). Adult attachment in a nationally representative sample. *Journal of Personality and Social Psychology, 73*, 1092–1106.

Miesen, B. (1992). Attachment theory and dementia. In B. M. L. Miesen (Ed.), *Care-giving in dementia: Research and applications* (pp. 38–56). London: Routledge/Tavistock.

Mikulincer, M., & Shaver, P. R. (2007). *Attachment in adulthood: Structure, dynamics, and change.* New York: Guilford Press.

Mikulincer, M., & Shaver, P. R. (2008). An attachment perspective on bereavement. In M. Stroebe, R. O. Hansson, H. A. W. Schut, & W. Stroebe (Eds.), *Handbook of bereavement research and practice: 21st-century perspectives.* Washington, DC: American Psychological Association.

Mikulincer, M., Shaver, P. R., Gillath, O., & Nitzberg, R. A. (2005). Attachment, caregiving, and altruism: Boosting attachment security increases compassion and helping. *Journal of Personality and Social Psychology, 89*, 817–839.

Moss, M. S., & Moss, S. Z. (1983–84). The impact of parental death on middle-aged children. *Omega: Journal of Death and Dying, 41*, 65–75.

Parks, S. H., & Pilisuk, M. (1991). Caregiver burden: Gender and the psychological costs of caregiving. *American Journal of Orthopsychiatry, 61*, 501–509.

Parrott, T. M., & Bengtson, V. L. (1999). The effects of earlier intergenerational affection, normative expectations and family conflict on contemporary exchanges of help and support. *Research on Aging, 21*, 73–105.

Perrig-Chiello, P., & Hoepflinger, F. (2005). Aging parents and their middle-aged children: Demographic and psychosocial challenges. *European Journal of Aging, 2*, 183–191.

Pillemen, K., & Suitor, J. J. (2002). Explaining mothers' ambivalence toward their adult children. *Journal of Marriage and the Family, 64*, 602–613.

Popek, P., & Scharlach, A. E. (1991). Adult daughters' relationships with their mothers and reactions to the mothers' deaths. *Journal of Women and Aging, 3*, 79–96.

Preston, S. H., Hill, M. E., & Drevenstedt, G. L. (1998). Childhood conditions that predict survival to advanced ages among African-Americans. *Social Science and Medicine, 47*, 1231–1246.

Roisman, G. I., Fraley, R. C., & Belsky, J. (2007). A taxometric study of the Adult Attachment Interview. *Developmental Psychology, 43*, 675–686.

Rossi, A. S., & Rossi, P. H. (1990). *Of human bonding: Parent–child relations across the life course.* New York: Aldine de Gruyter.

Rossi, A. S., & Rossi, P. H. (1991). Normative obligations and parent–child help exchange across the life course. In K. McCartney (Ed.), *Parent–child relationships throughout life* (pp. 201–223). Hillsdale, NJ: Erlbaum.

Scharlach, A. E. (1991). Factors associated with filial grief following the death of an elderly parent. *American Journal of Orthopsychiatry, 61*, 307–313.

Shaw, B. A., Krause, N., Chatters, L. M., Connell, C. M., & Ingersoll-Dayton, B. (2004). Emotional support from parents early in life, aging, and health. *Psychology and Aging, 19*, 4–12.

Shuey, K. M., Wilson, A. E., & Elder, G. H. Jr. (2003, August). *Ambivalence in the relationship between aging mothers and their adult children: A dyadic analysis.* Paper presented at the annual meeting of the American Sociological Association, Atlanta, GA.

Silverstein, M., & Bengtson, V. L. (1997). Intergenerational solidarity and the structure of adult child–parent relationships in American families. *American Journal of Sociology, 103*, 429–460.

Silverstein, M., Conroy, S. J., Wang, H., Giarrusso, R., & Bengtson, V. L. (2002). Reciprocity in parent–child relations over the adult live course. *Journals of Gerontology: Series B. Psychological Sciences, 57B*, S3–S13.

Silverstein, M., Parrott, T. M., & Bengtson, V. L. (1995). Factors that predispose middle-aged sons and daughters to provide social support to older parents. *Journal of Marriage and the Family, 57*, 465–475.

Smith, J., & Goodnow, J. J. (1999). Unasked-for support and unsolicited advice: Age and the quality of social experience. *Psychology and Aging, 14*, 108–121.

Soerensen, S., Webster, J. D., & Roggman, L. A. (2002). Adult attachment and preparing to provide care for older relatives. *Attachment and Human Development, 4*, 84–106.

Spitze, G., & Gallant, M. P. (2004). "The bitter with the sweet": Older adults' strategies for handling ambivalence in relations with their adult children. *Research on Aging, 26*, 387–412.

Stimpson, J. P., Tyler, K. A., & Hoyt, D. R. (2005). Effects of parental rejection and relationship quality on depression among older rural adults. *International Journal of Aging and Human Development, 61*, 195–210.

Stroebe, M., Schut, H., & Stroebe, W. (2005). Attachment in coping with bereavement: A theoretical integration. *Review of General Psychology, 9*, 48–66.

Suitor, J. J., Pillemer, K., & Sechrist, J. (2006). Within-family differences in mothers' support to adult children. *Journals of Gerontology: Series B. Psychological Sciences, 61B*, 10–17.

Thomae, H. (1981). The Bonn Longitudinal Study of Aging (BOLSA): An approach to differential gerontology. In A. E. Baert (Ed.), *Prospective longitudinal research* (pp. 165–197). Oxford, UK: Oxford University Press.

Thompson, S. C., Galbraith, M., Thomas, C., Swan, J., & Vrungos, S. (2002). Caregivers of stroke patient family members: Behavioral and attitudinal indicators of overprotective care. *Psychology and Health, 17*, S297–S312.

Umberson, D. (1995). Marriage as support or strain?: Marital quality following the death of a parent. *Journal of Marriage and the Family, 57*, 709–723.

van IJzendoorn, M. H. (1995). Adult attachment representations, parental responsiveness, and infant attachment: A meta-analysis of the predictive validity of the Adult Attachment Interview. *Psychological Bulletin, 117*, 387–403.

van IJzendoorn, M. H., & Bakermans-Kranenburg, M. (1996). Attachment representations in mothers, fathers, adolescents and clinical groups: A meta-analytic search for normative data. *Journal of Consulting and Clinical Psychology, 64*, 8–21.

van IJzendoorn, M. H., & Kroonenberg, P. M. (1988). Cross-cultural patterns of attachment: A meta-analysis of the Strange Situation. *Child Development, 59*, 147–156.

Vogel, D. L., & Wei, M. (2005). Adult attachment and help-seeking intent: The mediating roles of psychological distress and perceived social support. *Journal of Counseling Psychology, 52*, 347–357.

Webster, J. D. (1997). Attachment style and well-being in elderly adults: A preliminary investigation. *Canadian Journal on Aging, 61*, 101–111.

Webster, P. S., & Herzog, A. R. (1995). Effects of parental divorce and memories of family problems on relationships between adult children and their parents. *Journals of Gerontology: Series B. Psychological Sciences, 50B*, S24–S94.

Weisner, T. S. (2005). Attachment as a cultural and ecological problem with pluralistic solutions. *Human Development, 48*, 89–94.

Wensauer, M., & Grossmann, K. E. (1995). Quality of attachment representations, social integration, and use of network resources in old age. *Zeitschrift fuer Gerontologie und Geriatrie, 28*, 444–456.

Westmaas, J. L., & Silver, R. C. (2001). The role of attachment in responses to victims of life crises. *Journal of Personality and Social Psychology, 80*, 425–438.

Whitbeck, L. B., Hoyt, D. R., & Huck, S. M. (1994). Early family relationships, intergenerational solidarity, and support provided to parents by their adult children. *Journal of Gerontology: Social Sciences, 49*, S85–S94.

Whitbeck, L. B., Hoyt, D. R., & Tyler, K. A. (2001). Family relationship histories, intergenerational relationship quality, and depressive affect among rural elderly people. *Journal of Applied Gerontology, 20*, 214–229.

Wilson, A. E., Shuey, K. M., & Elder, G. H., Jr. (2003). Ambivalence in the relationship of adult children to aging parents and in-laws. *Journal of Marriage and the Family, 65*, 1055–1077.

Winsborough, H. H., Bumpass, L. L., & Aquilino, W. S. (1991). *The death of parents and the transition to old age* (Working Paper No. NSFH-39). Madison: University of Wisconsin, Center for Demography and Ecology.

Wolf, R. S., & Pillemer, K. (1989). *Helping elderly victims: The reality of elder abuse.* New York: Columbia University Press.

Zhang, F., & Labouvie-Vief, G. (2004). Stability and fluctuation in adult attachment style over a 6-year period. *Attachment and Human Development, 6*, 419–437.

CHAPTER 25

The Adult Attachment Interview
Protocol, Method of Analysis, and Empirical Studies

ERIK HESSE

In 1985, in an article entitled "Security in Infancy, Childhood, and Adulthood: A Move to the Level of Representation," Main, Kaplan, and Cassidy reported the results of their sixth-year follow-up study of 40 Bay Area children who had been seen with each parent in the Ainsworth Strange Situation (Ainsworth, Blehar, Waters, & Wall, 1978) at 12 (or 18) months of age. Within that presentation, special emphasis was given to verbatim texts taken from a newly developed Adult Attachment Interview (AAI; George, Kaplan, & Main, 1984, 1985, 1996). During the course of this interview, individuals are asked both to describe their attachment-related childhood experiences—especially their early relations with parents or parenting figures—and to evaluate the influence of these experiences on their development and current functioning. Main and her colleagues found that transcribed verbatim responses from these interviews could be systematically placed into one of three adult attachment classification categories (Main, 1985; Main & Goldwyn, 1984a; Main et al., 1985). The first was termed "secure-autonomous" ("valuing of attachment relationships and experiences, and yet apparently objective regarding any particular relationship experience") and was associated with infant Strange Situation security with the speaker. A second kind of interview text was associated with insecure-avoidant responses to the speaker in the Strange Situation procedure and was termed "dismissing" ("dismissing, devaluing, or cut off from attachment relationships and experiences"). The third type of interview classification category was termed "preoccupied" ("preoccupied with or by early attachments or attachment-related experiences") and was associated with insecure-resistant/ambivalent responses to the speaker. Thus a marked relation between a parent's hour-long discussion of his or her own attachment history and the offspring's Strange Situation behavior 5 years previously had been uncovered. Since that time, the AAI has been increasingly applied in both clinical and developmental research.

In this chapter, I focus not only on a description of the queries used in the AAI, but also on the associated coding scales and classification system. Although the methods of analyzing AAI transcripts have grown increasingly sophisticated over the years (e.g., Main & Goldwyn, 1984a; Main, Goldwyn, & Hesse, 2003), from the outset the scoring procedure has focused on the overall coherence of the text; it has taken into account as potential indices of insecure states of mind any major contradictions and inconsistencies in the narrative, as well as passages that are exceptionally short, long, irrelevant, or difficult to follow. Thus differences in the use of language relevant to attachment—and not retrospective inferences about the nature of the person's actual attachment history—have consistently been the basis of the analysis and the source of the AAI's predictive power.

Here I also describe the ways in which transcribed responses to the AAI are analyzed. There are five major classifications, each derived from studying the full text. These include the initial three "organized" state-of-mind classifications mentioned above ("secure," "dismissing," and "preoccupied") and two further "disorganized" classifications ("unresolved/disorganized" and "cannot classify"; see Hesse, 1996; Hesse & Main, 2000), developed later and now well delineated. (The cannot classify category has recently been expanded, see pp. 572–573.) Each of these major AAI classifications (except cannot classify) has repeatedly been associated with the security versus insecurity of the offspring's attachment to the speaker, with the speaker's responsiveness to the offspring, and with the speaker's emotional/clinical status.

Recently, among many other examples, the AAI has been used to estimate the extent to which parents in high-risk samples are willing to involve themselves in the intervention process (Heinicke et al., 2006); to determine whether, among adults, rates of insecurity are increased by disadvantages such as deafness or blindness (they are not; see van IJzendoorn & Bakermans-Kranenburg, 2008); to search for anomalous parent–infant interaction patterns related to particular AAI classifications (unresolved/disorganized parents are substantially more frightened, frightening, and dissociative than other parents; Jacobvitz, Leon, & Hazen, 2006); to ask whether the daughters of Holocaust survivors found to be insecure on the AAI in Israel are significantly more likely than daughters of control participants to be insecure (unexpectedly, and arguably due to surrounding cultural conditions, they are not; see Sagi-Schwartz, van IJzendoorn, et al., 2003); to ask whether state of mind with respect to attachment might moderate the relation between maternal postnatal depression and infant Strange Situation security (it does; McMahon, Barnett, Kowalenko, & Tennant, 2006); and to show that disorganized/disoriented attachment to the mother in a second child following stillbirth of a first is fully mediated by unresolved/disorganized status with respect to the initial loss (Hughes, Turton, Hopper, McGauley, & Fonagy, 2001).

The chapter is organized into three major sections. The first section provides a description of the AAI protocol and individual differences among the organized response patterns. I begin by introducing the ways in which the three organized classifications can be understood in terms of both attentional and—separately, albeit relatedly—linguistic (conversational or discourse) mechanisms. The former relies on the thinking of Main (e.g., 1990, 1993; see below) regarding flexibility versus inflexibility of attention under stress. The analyses of the linguistic or conversational mechanisms draw upon the work of linguistic philosopher H. P. Grice (1975, 1989). These mechanisms are well represented in the central AAI state-of-mind scales, although each of those scales (as described in a history of the Bay Area longitudinal study; Main, Hesse, & Kaplan, 2005) had been devised prior to Main's discovery of Grice's work. I conclude this section by presenting some prototypical responses to two different AAI queries that are common among "organized" speakers. As differing responses are presented, I point out how they can be understood in terms of both attentional and Gricean conversational mechanisms.

In the second section, I describe how trained coders systematically approach the analysis of an AAI transcript. This was not explicated in the first edition of this chapter (Hesse, 1999), leaving a mystery for readers who had been aware of the instrument and its connections to other phenomena, but not of the ways in which interview texts are analyzed. There are two additional approaches to analyzing the AAI, beyond the five major classifications presented in 1999. These have drawn less attention in the literature, despite the fact that they appear to be of at least equal power. First, the three organized categories of the AAI are ultimately divided into 12 subclassifications, which I describe here for the first time. This is in keeping with Ainsworth's division of her three organized infant Strange Situation classifications into eight subclassifications (Ainsworth et al., 1978), which she predicted would "in time prove even more useful than classification into the three major groups themselves" (Ainsworth et al., 1978, p. 251). As I note here, AAI and Strange Situation subclassifications have now been found to be significantly related in four different investigations (including Behrens, Hesse, & Main, 2007), but nonetheless remain underutilized. Second, from its inception, the AAI scoring system has included a set of (9-point) continuous rating scales that assess the speaker's current "state of mind with respect to attachment," whether with respect to a given parent (e.g., idealizing of the father) or with respect to discourse patterning in general (e.g., overall coherence of transcript, vague discourse usages). As researchers from several laboratories have correctly emphasized, use of these scales releases the restriction of range imposed by the presentation of findings only in terms of classifications, and hence substantially increases statistical power (Fyffe & Waters, 1997; Roisman, Fraley, & Belsky, 2007). This section brings together all three current methods of AAI text analysis.

In the third section, I review selected studies based on the AAI, beginning with Main's original investigation of a Bay Area sample (Main & Goldwyn, 1984b, 1988, 2008). I review (and then partially update) the best-replicated findings regarding the AAI, including those related to its psychometric properties, and then move on to a necessarily select group of newer studies. This selection is made with apologies to many excellent investigators whose work is not reviewed here because of space limitations. Appendix 25.1 describes training in AAI analysis.

THE AAI PROTOCOL

The AAI utilizes a prespecified format, with questions asked in a set order, accompanied by specific follow-up probes. The protocol is deliberately arranged to bring forward structural variations in the presentation of a life history, and interviewers must make certain that their own part of the conversation serves only to highlight, and not to alter, participants' natural tendencies to respond in particular ways.

The AAI normally takes about an hour to administer and currently (George et al., 1996) consists of 20 questions. The entire interview, including all comments by both the interviewer and the interviewee, is transcribed verbatim, including (timed) pauses, dysfluencies, and restarts, although cues to intonation, prosody, and nonverbal behavior are omitted. The interview opens with a call for a general description of relationships with parents during the speaker's childhood, which is followed by a request for five adjectives that would best represent the relationship with each parent. After the adjectives are provided (first for the mother), the speaker is probed for specific episodic memories that would illustrate why each descriptor was chosen. This process is then repeated for the father and, when applicable, for any other significant at-

tachment figure (e.g., stepfather or nanny). The protocol next contains questions about which parent the speaker felt closer to, and why; what the speaker did when emotionally upset, physically hurt, or ill; and how the parents responded at such times. The participant is then asked about salient separations, possible experiences of rejection, and any threats regarding discipline. Next, the speaker is queried regarding the effects of these experiences on his or her adult personality; whether any experiences constituted a significant setback to development; why the parents are believed to have behaved as they did during childhood; and whether there were any persons who did not serve as parenting figures, yet were thought of as parent-like during childhood.

An especially important feature of the AAI protocol is the section addressing experiences of loss of significant persons through death. Here the emphasis on childhood is abandoned, and important losses occurring at any point in the speaker's lifetime are addressed. Speakers are asked to describe how the death occurred, their reactions to the loss at the time, any funeral or memorial service attended, changes in feelings over time, effects on adult personality, and (where relevant) effects on their behavior with their children. In the case of persons with multiple losses, interviewers restrict their queries to those three or four that seem most significant. Descriptions of any abuse experiences (and, indeed, any overwhelmingly frightening experiences throughout a speaker's lifetime) are also sought.

Toward the close of the interview, participants are asked about the nature of the current relationship with parents (if living). In addition, they are questioned as to how they feel (or imagine they would feel if they had a child) about being separated from their child, and how experiences of being parented may have affected responses (or imagined responses) to their own child. Finally, the participant is invited to speculate regarding wishes for his or her real or imagined child 20 years from now.

Table 25.1 offers examples of some of the questions taken from the AAI protocol devised by George and colleagues (1985, 1986, 1996), but omits their follow-up probes. The current 72-page protocol is available (see Appendix 25.1), and administering the AAI requires practice with feedback from experienced interviewers.[1]

The central task the interview presents to participants is that of (1) producing and reflecting on memories related to attachment, while *simultaneously* (2) maintaining coherent, collaborative

TABLE 25.1. Brief Précis of the Adult Attachment Interview (AAI) Protocol Excerpted from George, Kaplan, and Main (1996)

1. To begin with, could you just help me to get a little bit oriented to your family—for example, who was in your immediate family, and where you lived?
2. Now I'd like you to try to describe your relationship with your parents as a young child, starting as far back as you can remember.
3–4. Could you give me five adjectives or phrases to describe your relationship with your mother/father during childhood? I'll write them down, and when we have all five I'll ask you to tell me what memories or experiences led you to choose each one.
5. To which parent did you feel closer, and why?
6. When you were upset as a child, what did you do, and what would happen? Could you give me some specific incidents when you were upset emotionally? Physically hurt? Ill?
7. Could you describe your first separation from your parents?
8. Did you ever feel rejected as a child? What did you do, and do you think your parents realized they were rejecting you?
9. Were your parents ever threatening toward you—for discipline, or jokingly?
10. How do you think your overall early experiences have affected your adult personality? Are there any aspects you consider a setback to your development?
11. Why do you think your parents behaved as they did during your childhood?
12. Were there other adults who were close to you—like parents—as a child?
13. Did you experience the loss of a parent or other close loved one as a child, or in adulthood?
14. Were there many changes in your relationship with your parents between childhood and adulthood?
15. What is your relationship with your parents like for you currently?

Note. The AAI cannot be conducted on the basis of this brief, modified précis of the protocol, which omits several questions as well as the critical follow-up probes. The full protocol, together with extensive directions for administration, can be obtained by writing to Erik Hesse or Mary Main, Department of Psychology, University of California at Berkeley, Berkeley, CA 94720. From George, Kaplan, and Main (1996). Copyright 1996 by the authors. Adapted by permission.

discourse with the interviewer (Hesse, 1996). This is not as easy as it might appear, and George and colleagues (1985, 1996) have remarked upon the potential of the protocol to "surprise the unconscious." As indicated above, the interview requires the speaker to reflect on and answer a multitude of complex questions regarding his or her life history, the great majority of which the speaker will never have been asked before. In contrast to ordinary conversations, where the interviewee has time for planning, the AAI moves at a relatively rapid pace, and usually all questions and probes have been presented within an hour's time. Ample opportunities are thereby provided for speakers to contradict themselves, to find themselves unable to answer clearly, and/or to be drawn into excessively lengthy or digressive discussions of particular topics. To maintain a consistent and collaborative narrative, a speaker must not only address the question at hand, but also be able to remember (and potentially reflect upon) what he or she has already said, in order to integrate the overall presentation as it unfurls. It is striking that although the interviewee is always informed in some detail regarding the overall topic of the interview prior to its administration, actually engaging in the process often appears to be a far more powerful experience than anticipated. This can lead to notable (and often ultimately systematic and repeated) incoherencies in linguistic aspects of the presentation, because at times the interviewee may not be able to maintain the usual degree of control over how the story unfolds.

The AAI protocol is structured to bring into relief individual differences in what are presumed to be deeply internalized strategies for regulating emotion and attention when speakers are discussing attachment-related experiences. This is achieved despite the fact that—although the interview transcripts contain the full verbatim exchange, including silences and dysfluencies—they are devoid of references to body movement, facial expression, or intonation. It is remarkable that on the basis of language use alone, AAI coders (as described below) are able to significantly predict how speakers will behave with others, including offspring, partners, friends, and even those to whom they have been newly introduced.

Finally, I should emphasize that the claim that the interview is able to elicit a particular (usually, singular—i.e., "classifiable") state of mind with respect to attachment is based on the assumption that by adulthood, what were originally independent attachments to mother and to father (e.g., Main & Weston, 1981) will have coalesced. An initial exploration of this assumption was undertaken by Furman and Simon (2004), who administered the AAI twice to 56 young adults. One interview focused on the mother only, and one on the father. As would be expected if a single state of mind does predominate in most individuals, state of mind with respect to father was found to be significantly related to state of mind with respect to mother.

Attentional and Linguistic Processes Involved in Distinguishing among the Organized AAI Categories

This section introduces two ways in which we have come to conceptualize some of the underlying mechanisms that may be responsible for the individual differences in discourse forms characteristic of secure, dismissing, and preoccupied speakers. I begin with Main's (1990) consideration of attentional flexibility versus inflexibility. I then turn to a discussion of Grice's (1975, 1989) maxims for adherence to, versus violations of, the requirements of conversational coherence and collaboration. The dovetailing of Grice's conversational maxims and the state-of-mind scales that Main and Goldwyn had devised several years prior to Main's first reading Grice has been striking. It has been highly useful heuristically, and references to Grice's maxims have appeared in all but the early versions of the AAI scoring and classification system.

The Organized Categories of the AAI Considered in Terms of Attentional Flexibility

The AAI scoring and classification system was initially grounded in the relation between the three central or organized forms of parental responses to the AAI interview queries (secure-autonomous, dismissing, or preoccupied) and the three central or organized forms of infant response to that same parent in the Strange Situation (respectively, secure, avoidant, or preoccupied), as first uncovered in Main's Bay Area study (Main & Goldwyn, 1984b, 1988, 2008; Main et al., 1985). The term "organized" is rooted in Main's (1990) contention that infants in the original three Strange Situation categories differ in flexibility versus inflexibility of attention to (1) the parent and (2) the inanimate environment—differences that are revealed in the Ainsworth separation-and-reunion procedure. The capacity for attentional flexibility was ascribed to secure babies because they readily alternate between attachment and exploratory behavior as the Strange Situation procedure unfolds, exploring in their mothers' presence and exhibiting attachment behavior (e.g., crying, calling) in the mothers' absence and again upon reunion (e.g., seeking proximity and contact). Attentional inflexibility was ascribed to insecure-avoidant infants, who focus *away from* the parent and on the toys or surroundings, and to insecure-ambivalent/resistant infants, who focus persistently *on* the parent at the expense of the toys and the surroundings.

Main later proposed that the organized AAI categories can also be viewed in terms of attentional flexibility (Main, 1993, 2000; Main et al., 2005). Thus attentional flexibility is seen in secure-autonomous parents as they fluidly shift between presenting their attachment-related experiences and responding to the request to evaluate the influences of these experiences (Hesse, 1996). In contrast, attentional inflexibility is observed (1) in dismissing responses to the AAI, in which the linguistic focus is continuously *away from* past attachment relationships and their influences; and (2) in preoccupied AAI texts, in which the focus is persistently, although confusedly, so strongly oriented *toward* attachment relationships and experiences as to prevent appropriate responses to the queries. It should be noted, however, that attentional inflexibility is relatively, albeit singularly, organized in terms of discourse strategy.

The Organized Categories of the AAI Considered in Terms of Grice's Maxims

Before methods of analyzing AAI transcripts are discussed further, a brief review of Grice's (1975, 1989) work is provided. The aim of this section is to facilitate an understanding of differing "organized" language usages within the AAI, and thus to convey what is actually being assessed when coherence versus incoherence of a given text is taken into consideration.

Although the AAI interviewer adheres to the interview questions and their probes as faithfully as possible, there are, of course, two speakers involved in the exchange. This means that the interview is a conversation as well as a response to a request for a spoken autobiography, permitting its analysis in terms of the extent to which the participant's responses approach the "Gricean" requirements for an ideally rational, coherent, and cooperative conversation. Grice (1975, 1989) proposed that these requirements are met insofar as speakers adhere to four specific "maxims" or principles. To the degree that these maxims are "violated," the conversation strays from the cooperative, rational ideal, but in fact—as Grice stressed in his later work (1989)—complete and continual adherence is not expected. For a text to be classified as secure-autonomous, coherent, cooperative discourse must simply be *relatively* well maintained, as compared to that of other conversationalists observed in this context.[2] The four maxims are as follows:

1. *Quality*: "*Be truthful, and have evidence for what you say.*" This maxim is violated when, for example, a parent is described in highly positive general terms, but the specific biographical episodes recounted subsequently contradict (or simply fail to support) the interviewee's adjectival choices. An interview of this kind can also be considered internally inconsistent, and internal inconsistency of the kind just described appears most frequently in the texts of individuals classified as dismissing.

2. *Quantity*: "*Be succinct, and yet complete.*" This maxim demands conversational turns of reasonable length—neither too short nor too long. By requiring speakers to be sufficiently "complete," Grice was saying that incomplete, excessively short answers are not acceptable. This occurs when, for example, "I don't remember" and/or "I don't know" becomes the response to several queries in sequence, cutting off further inquiry. Excessively terse responses occur most frequently in the texts of individuals classified as dismissing.

In terms of quantity, Grice also requires that so long as they are complete, responses should be reasonably succinct; consequently, the maxim of (appropriate) quantity can also be violated when a speaker takes excessively long conversational turns. Here the interviewee may hold the floor for several minutes, perhaps providing increasingly unnecessary details. Excessively lengthy responses occur most frequently in the texts of individuals classified as preoccupied.

3. *Relation*: "*Be relevant to the topic as presented.*" The maxim of relation or relevance is violated when, for example, queries regarding the childhood relationship with the speaker's mother are irrelevantly addressed with discussions of current interactions with the mother or descriptions of the speaker's relationship with his or her own children. As might be expected, violations of relevance occur most frequently in the texts of individuals classified as preoccupied.

4. *Manner*: "*Be clear and orderly.*" This maxim is violated when, for example, speech becomes grammatically entangled, psychological "jargon" is used, vague terms appear repeatedly, or the speaker does not finish sentences that have been fully started. Violations of manner appear most often in preoccupied texts.

Having concluded this discussion of Grice's conversational maxims,[3] I present two representative interview queries and provide examples of responses that would be typically associated with each of the three organized AAI classifications.

Where relevant, I discuss violations of specific maxims.

Examining Differing Responses to Selected Interview Queries as They Relate to the Organized AAI Categories

I have selected two questions that are especially useful for characterizing individual differences in response to AAI queries. The first is perhaps the best-known of all the AAI protocol questions—question 3, where the participant is addressed as follows:

"Now what I'd like you to do is to think of five adjectives, words, or phrases that would best describe your relationship with your mother during childhood—say, between the ages of 5 and 12, but even earlier if you can remember. Take a minute to think, and then I'm going to ask you why you chose them."

Notice that this question includes two parts that operate at different "mental levels": a semantic level (the descriptors, or adjectives themselves, devoid of space–time particulars); and an episodic level (what happened, and if possible, roughly when), which suggests that there will be a rationale for the adjectival choice. By implication, of course, any particular word should be readily accompanied by supportive accounts of childhood experiences.

In essence, the adjectival constellation that the speaker is asked to provide for his or her relationship with a given parent during childhood requires the person (whether consciously or unconsciously, accurately or inaccurately) to produce "on the spot" a fairly complex and incisive synopsis of the general nature of the childhood relationship. Once the first part of the question has been answered, the speaker has in effect "taken a stance" as to the kind of relationship he or she had with this particular parent. The adjectival constellation can of course vary from the extremely negative to the extremely positive, and can include mixed assessments as well. For example, with respect to the mother, if the choice of adjectives were "loving, caring, supportive, trustworthy, and warm," it will seem that the speaker is attempting to convey that he or she had a positive to highly positive experience with mother during childhood. However, it is obvious that an adjectival constellation such as "caring, interfering, warm, unpredictable, rule maker" conveys a mixed impression.

Next, the participant is systematically probed for a specific memory that would illustrate why each particular word or adjective was selected. This is the portion of the "adjectival" question in which the participant is implicitly asked to begin drawing on episodic memory. Note that even if the adjectives provided by two different speakers were identical, the narrative that emerged in the two cases could have entirely different forms.

Let us consider the "loving … " constellation above. The interviewer is now required to probe as follows:

"Okay, the first word you gave to describe your relationship with your mother during childhood was 'loving.' Can you think of a memory or incident that would illustrate for me why you chose that word?"

The range of potential responses to this request is virtually infinite, and yet it will yield information that can be approached with a view to assigning scores and ultimately a state-of-mind classification. Thus it is likely that the speaker's response bears deeply on the degree of his or her own self-awareness, and in some cases—whether or not the person is conscious of it—on the motivation to convey a particular impression to the interviewer. Consider as an example the following, and not at all uncommon, response to the interviewer's probe for any memories or incidents that could illustrate why the speaker chose "loving."

PARTICIPANT: I don't remember. … (*5-second pause*). Well, because she was caring and supportive.[4] [Notice that here the speaker is simply using similar words to describe the previous words. In essence, the speaker is repeating the word rather than answering the question.]

INTERVIEWER: Well, this can be difficult, because a lot of people haven't thought about these things for a long time, but take a minute and see if you can think of an incident or example.

PARTICIPANT: (*10-second pause*) Well … (*5-second pause*), I guess like, well, you know, she was really pretty, and she took a lot of care with her appearance. Whenever she drove me to school, I was always really proud of that when we pulled up at the playground.

INTERVIEWER: Thank you. And, I just wonder whether there might be another example?

PARTICIPANT: No, I think that pretty much takes care of it.

Here it is impossible, of course, to know whether the speaker is aware that she has not answered the question. What can be readily inferred, however, is that an attempt is being made to convey a positive impression of her childhood relationship with her mother—which, if continued throughout the interview in this fashion, will not form the basis for a believable description of the adjectives chosen. Clearly, something psychologically quite complex is taking place here, despite the brevity of the response. Although convincingly loving interactions may be recounted later in the interview, at this point we can say that if the speaker continues along these lines—that is, seeming to attempt to create a positive picture of her childhood experiences with her mother, but in fact frequently blocking discourse, yielding a paucity of substantive support for the positive adjectives chosen—it is likely that the transcript as a whole will be classified as dismissing. Thus dismissing speakers (the best-fitting classification for this speaker if only this interview extract was available) violate Grice's quality/truthfulness maxim by failing to provide evidence for what they have claimed. The responses are also overly succinct, violating quantity and perhaps involving (whether deliberate or unconscious) restrictions in attention *away from* the topic of childhood experiences with the mother.

I now turn to a second speaker who also describes the mother as "loving."

PARTICIPANT: Loving … (*5-second pause*) I don't know if this is the sort of thing you're looking for, but one thing that comes to mind is the way she stuck up for me when I got in trouble at school. Boy, if I told her about some problem at school and she thought I was in the right, or if I told her some kid or some teacher had treated me bad, she'd go out and investigate and she'd stick up for me to the teacher, or to the kid's parents, or … anybody, really. I could put it another way, too. I just knew where I stood with her, and that she'd be comforting if I was upset or crying or something.

INTERVIEWER: Thank you (*interrupted*).

PARTICIPANT: (*Interrupting and continuing*) Oh, you wanted a specific example. Um, that time I set fire to the garage, using my brother's chemistry set I absolutely positively wasn't supposed to use. Came running when the neighbors phoned the fire department about the smoke. Expected to get the life lectured out of me, but she just ran straight for me and picked me up and hugged me real hard. Guess she was so scared and so glad to see me, she just forgot the lecture. Later there were little hints at the dinner table about the incident, but I'd say, basically, what she did that time—that was very loving.

If the discussion of childhood parenting continues steadily in this vein, with well-supported (whether positive or negative) statements regarding parenting and clear responses similar to this one,[5] the trained coder will begin to suspect that the transcript is likely to be coded secure-autonomous.[6] In terms of Grice's maxims, the speaker has kept to the maxim of quality (providing evidence for "loving"), which Grice at times called the "overriding principle" for cooperative, rational discourse. There are no violations of manner or relevance (the speaker is easy to follow and stays on topic). There is a slight violation of quantity (the interviewer had considered the response complete, while the participant continued), but the speaker does wind down to a conclusion showing that he has kept the topic in mind ("but I'd say, basically, what she did that time—that was very loving"). In addition, the extra time taken is in the service of providing a *specific* example, which is what the interviewer has explicitly asked for. The passage is too brief to illustrate attentional flexibility, but no inflexibility is evident.

Finally, here is an example of a third participant, who has also chosen "loving":

PARTICIPANT: Uh, yeah, sort of very loving at times, like people were in the old days—uh, my youth, lot of changes since then. I remember home, and home was good and that. And uh, loving, that's just like my wife is with [child]—taking him out to the movies tonight, dadadada, special thing he's been wanting to see all week. Actually, it's more like a month, that turtle movie, don't like it too much myself. Saw it, though, now, when was it, um, maybe 6 months ago. Yeah, she's very loving with [child].

INTERVIEWER: Mm-hm. Okay, well, what things come to mind when you describe your childhood relationship with your mother as "very loving at times"?

PARTICIPANT: Really great things, felt really special, really grateful to her for that. My childhood, I remember just sitting on the porch, rocking, rocking back and forth watching my parents, or maybe having some lemonade—this, that, and the other. Really special sorts of things, just me and her, grateful for all she did for me. I wasn't easy, my temperament was hard on her, kind of hard. Nobody like her. Me and my cousins from [Town 1] going down soon—really big birthday, she gonna be 80, gives my age away. (*Continues*)

Although speech of this kind is not common, it provides a good example of one of the subclassifications of the preoccupied category ("passively preoccupied," subcategory E1, described later in this chapter). First, the speaker makes some strongly positive statements about the relationship with his mother during childhood, but oddly these are accompanied by the statement that his temperament was "hard on her." Second, the speaker is unable to stay with the question, which was about his childhood relationship with his mother, and he veers repeatedly to the relationship his wife has with their child. Other than drinking lemonade together, examples of how the mother was loving during childhood are not provided, largely because the speaker moves into topics irrelevant to the question (such as his mother's upcoming birthday).

Notice, then, that as in the case of the dismissing (first) speaker above, the question is not answered. However, this failure to answer appears in a very different form. These are violations of Grice's maxim of relevance (moving into topics irrelevant to the question), and implicitly the maxim of quantity as well. We also see violations of manner, with elusive additions to already completed sentences ("and that," "this, that, and the other") as well as nonsense speech ("dadadada").

Now let us briefly consider speakers who begin with a negative descriptor of the childhood relationship with mother—in this case, "troublesome." The interviewer again will have set the stage by asking whether there are any memories or incidents come to mind with respect to "troublesome."

Consider the following response taken from a first speaker who very likely will not be classified as secure.

PARTICIPANT: Troublesome. Weak, cried. Fell apart at funerals.

INTERVIEWER: I wonder if you have any specific memory of times you found her troublesome?

PARTICIPANT: Sobbed through her aunt's funeral.

Embarrassing. Couldn't wait to get away from her. Next question?

This response would most probably have come from a dismissing speaker, and it is easy to see that the speaker's attention (as seen both in the extreme brevity of the response and in the terminating suggestion, "Next question?") is inflexibly focused away from, and is dismissing of, the mother and early experiences with her. This speaker dismisses attachment relationships by casting the parent aside via derogation and refusal of further discussion.

Responses of this kind tend to come from interviewees who fall in the "derogating" subcategory of the dismissing AAI category (Ds2, described below). Notice that, like the excerpt from the transcript of the earlier dismissing speaker, who gave only brief responses and failed to support "loving" as an adjectival choice, this latest speaker also has little to say—or, in Gricean terms, violates expected quantity by being overly succinct. However, there is little violation of quality or consistency here, as there was in the previous speaker: From his own perspective, this speaker has—albeit very minimally—given an example of how the mother was troublesome.

Now consider a second speaker who also selected "troublesome" as the first adjective describing her childhood relationship with her mother:

PARTICIPANT: Troublesome. Well, she was troublesome for me when I was young, no question. She yelled a lot of the time, I remember that, and she also—she could spank really hard, and she got angry a lot. But like I said, my father left when I was 4, and she was trying to make enough of an income to support us, and trying hard to keep us on the straight and narrow at the same time that she was away such long hours. I didn't like it, what she did—like one time she slapped me in the face over something my sister had done, but she never apologized. I hated the yelling when my report card wasn't up to par. Yes, troublesome, or maybe I should have said it was a troubled relationship. But while I wish it had been different, it wasn't.

This speaker is exceptionally coherent in this passage. Her discussion is relevant and sufficiently elaborated, and her examples are consistent with her adjective, thus adhering to quality. There is no difficulty in following her reply, and hence no violations of manner. She does not violate quantity,

and since she stays on topic, there are no violations of relevance. It is hard to identify attentional flexibility in a paragraph of this length, but there is no evidence of attentional *in*flexibility.

Finally, here is a third speaker who has been asked to support "troublesome":

PARTICIPANT: That was an understatement. It was yell, yell, yell—"Why didn't you this, why didn't you that?" Well, Mom, it was because you were just at me all the time, like last week you start yelling at the only grandkid you've got when we had you over to dinner. And angry? She's angry at me, she's angry at her latest husband—that's the latest in a series—now she's angry at her neighbor about a tree that's supposed to be blocking her view, and so on and so on. She's more than troublesome; she stirs up little things, like I was saying last week at dinner, and ... (*Continues*)

This speaker has violated manner in her third sentence by suddenly addressing the mother as though she were present, and continuing to do so. If we consider what she "says" to the mother, we can see a violation of relevance as well as manner, because the interviewer has asked her to discuss her *childhood* relationship. This violation of manner is strikingly indicative of preoccupation generally, given that the speaker appears to be addressing the (absent) parent in the past rather than talking to the interviewer in the present. Finally, attentional inflexibility (relentless focus on the parent as though she were present in the room, together with untoward discussion of the present rather than the childhood relationship context) is striking.

Once again, the examples I have given are too brief to provide a coder with more than a preliminary estimate of forthcoming interview classification. They do, however, demonstrate distinctly different forms of discourse response that, if predominant across the text as a whole, would lead to placement in differing AAI categories.

Having given some initial examples of responses to the third question in the AAI, I move to question 10, which appears at the interview's midpoint. This question focuses on the speaker's view of the overall effects that experiences with the parents may have had on his or her personality, and it is accompanied by a follow-up probe regarding possible setbacks to the speaker's development. This question and probe also provide a good example of the stiff requirements the AAI places on the participant: In order to answer the question in a way that "fits properly" with the earlier description of the life history, the speaker will have to be able to recall and evaluate what he or she has said, and provide an answer consonant with that presentation. I begin with an example that might have been found in the transcript taken from a dismissing speaker, who often will have failed to convincingly describe loving experiences with either parent earlier in the interview.

INTERVIEWER: In general, how do you think your overall experiences with your parents have affected your adult personality?

PARTICIPANT: Well, like I said already, it goes hand in hand with everything I said at the beginning. You know, they were strong people, and they encouraged me to be strong and not to get upset about things and to persevere. And that's why I'm here at [prestigious university] now. I feel really good about the success I've achieved.

INTERVIEWER: Are there any aspects of your early experiences that you feel were a setback in your development?

PARTICIPANT: No, maybe some little thing like ... well, no, basically nothing that didn't just make me better, you know. I'm not saying that sometimes they didn't need to lean on me a bit to get their point across, but that's paid off in that I'm really self-motivated now.

These responses do not notably violate Grice's maxims. In terms of attentional flexibility, however, we may note that—given that all of us have limitations—to respond with essentially "no setbacks" may indicate an active and inflexible focus *away from* any problems or difficulties.

In contrast to the speaker just described, many secure-autonomous transcripts exhibit a balanced response to question 10, even if the parent was earlier described as loving. The impression given is that the speaker may have thought of the question before.

INTERVIEWER: What effects do you think your experiences with your parents have had on you?

PARTICIPANT: Well, only I guess that, like I told you, I think there was a sort of negative gender thing. I did always feel like my mom and my sister were closer than my mom and I were, because I was a boy and they could relate to each other more easily. Another thing, and I think

sometimes this gets in my way with work, is that my dad would tend to help me out maybe too much, and even when I wasn't in some kind of a jam, so that can make it harder for me to get things done by myself now. I think I depended on him a lot.

INTERVIEWER: Do you consider this a setback in your development?

PARTICIPANT: Well, for example, from my dad helping me out so much, I can be a real procrastinator, particularly if I'm anxious or under a lot of pressure. And with women, especially when they seem real close to each other, I ... stand back, I guess. Like when I watch my girlfriend with her mother, maybe.

This speaker seems to have a sufficiently ready answer to this query, so that—although both parents had earlier been described convincingly as loving—his reflection on childhood experiences and potential setbacks from childhood suggests some problems.

Other secure-autonomous speakers may, however, begin by saying they had not thought of this question before and then, perhaps following a lengthy pause, provide a coherent response. This happened with one speaker who had earlier described a difficult life, with parents who were both rejecting and neglecting:

INTERVIEWER: What effects have your experiences with your parents had on you, do you think?

PARTICIPANT: I haven't thought about that before. ... (*21-second pause*) I guess I felt unwanted and unloved. Shy. Awkward around other girls now. Guys too, of course ...

INTERVIEWER: Do you think this caused a setback in your development?

PARTICIPANT: I don't socialize that much. I guess that could come from ... (*3-second pause*) feeling unwanted when I was a child.

In neither of these examples from secure-autonomous transcripts do we see substantial violations of Grice's maxims, although admittedly the second speaker is somewhat too succinct. What is striking, however, is the ready attention to difficulties in relationships seen in both responses, together with their effects. For the first speaker, attention easily moves to negative outcomes. For the second, who finds the question new, time is taken, and then flexible attention permits access to negative outcomes.

Finally, we move to what might be an answer taken from a preoccupied transcript, this time exemplifying speakers ultimately placed in the preoccupied subclass termed "angrily preoccupied" (E2), as opposed to passively preoccupied with early attachment relationship (E1, as seen on p. 559).

INTERVIEWER: What effects do you think your experiences with your parents have had on you?

PARTICIPANT: I guess I'd have to say it affected me, you know, in almost every way, like I've been telling you about with my mother—you know, everything. It's a constant. It's something that made me completely change, shape, the way that I approach my own children. You know, like, my mother will come over and she'll say, "Why are you letting Angela run around like that and make all that noise?" and I'm like, "You raised me the way you did, and put all these constraints on me and constantly told me what to do, so I'm giving her space to be herself," you know? And with my mother, it's just like that.

INTERVIEWER: Do you think this was a setback to your development?

PARTICIPANT: Well, I'd have to say the whole thing was a setback. I mean, it's taken me years to get past it, to get to where I am now, today.

This angrily preoccupied speaker appears to use the question as an opportunity to commence on a series of complaints regarding his parents, and he becomes distracted in the process. Interestingly, this is done without adequately answering the question regarding "setbacks." Instead, the speaker appears too preoccupied with specific experiences to rise above them sufficiently to enumerate setbacks as requested (in fact, in this example the speaker implies that despite struggles he is now a success). In other words, this speaker exhibits an ongoing involvement with the parents, rather than reflection upon present setbacks stemming from childhood. This is accompanied by an unfavorable comparison wherein the speaker portrays himself as an improvement on the parent.

Notice that none of the four speakers quoted here—including those whose responses appear consistent with the dismissing or preoccupied classifications—have substantially violated Grice's maxims in response to question 10. The differences in responses observed here are, as in the examples taken from the "adjectival" question, clearly reflective of distinctively different *attentional* approaches to the interview task. The dismissing speaker seems unable even to begin to focus attention on untoward effects of parental behavior. In contrast, the fluent secure speaker readily turns attention to untoward ramifications, whereas the secure but less fluent speaker, who appears elsewhere in the transcript to have had relatively harsh experiences, has also been able slowly to "reach for and find" negative effects. However, in contrast to the preoccupied speaker, she does so in a contained manner, sticking to the query *without* repeating what had been wrong with the parent(s) other than in brief summary form. The angrily preoccupied speaker seems to use the question as an opportunity to begin a series of complaints about his parents, which results in distraction from the purposes of the question. Hence his attention seems to have become inflexibly focused upon the past with the parents again, rather than the (present) interview query itself.

In sum, the AAI protocol is designed to bring into relief what might be referred to as different "proximate working strategies" manifested in language responses to questions about early attachment-related experiences and their effects. The AAI asks the same questions of each participant—and yet, as illustrated here, very different responses appear not only regarding the same questions, but even in illustrating the same adjectives. The essence of the AAI scoring and classification system (Main et al., 2003) amounts to a systematization of the different language uses seen in response to the set questions of the protocol.

THE AAI SCORING AND CLASSIFICATION SYSTEM

The AAI scoring and classification system initially focused only on the original three "organized" classifications and subclassifications, together with an accompanying set of continuous rating scales (Main & Goldwyn, 1984a). The earliest rules for classifying and scoring AAI transcripts were based on interviews with parents (both mothers and fathers) who were visiting Main's Social Development Project laboratory at the University of California at Berkeley, together with their 6-year-old children. Five years before, when the children were between 12 and 18 months of age, each had been seen in the Strange Situation conducted separately with each parent. Scores for reunion behavior (e.g., avoidance or resistance), as well as major classifications and their associated subclassifications (Ainsworth et al., 1978), had been assigned at that time.

Out of the available sample of 103 dyads, Main and Goldwyn had selected a development sample of 36[7] for intensive study. Within this initial sample, Main and Goldwyn searched for differences and commonalities in the ways the parents of infants who had been judged secure, avoidant, or ambivalent/resistant with them in the Strange Situation 5 years earlier conversed about and described their own attachment histories and their effects.

Characteristics of each transcript were recorded and judgments were made about the speaker's probable experiences with each parent during childhood, together with the speaker's state of mind with respect to his or her attachment history. This state of mind was captured by gradually developed continuous rating scales used to assign secure-autonomous, dismissing, or preoccupied classifications, and later a set of 12 subclassifications. Both coders used their knowledge of attachment to "guess" the status of each transcript, before "deblinding" themselves to the associated Strange Situation classification and subclassification of the speaker's infant. The development sample of 36 texts was ultimately discarded, and— with no further feedback from Main—Goldwyn then continued alone through the remaining 67 texts. The results of this study are described later in this chapter (see also Main & Goldwyn, 1988, 2008). Once this first "blind" study was completed, Main and Goldwyn used all 103 available texts to expand their understanding of the relation between the adult life history narrative and infant attachment. This review led to an elaboration of the early scoring and classification system, and the new system—which included a chapter concerning the identification (Main, DeMoss, & Hesse, 1989) of speech and reasoning irregularities in the parents of infants judged as disorganized— was used by Ainsworth and Eichberg (1991) and Fonagy, Steele, and Steele (1991) in the initial parent–infant replication studies. Over the ensuing years, feedback from studies of parent–infant dyads in other samples (including, gradually, high-risk and clinical samples) has caused the system to continue to evolve, and more recently (Main et al., 2003) to include several new kinds of unclassifiability ("cannot classify").

The Organized Categories of the AAI

The organized categories of the AAI—secure-autonomous, insecure-dismissing, and insecure-preoccupied—are those in which the speaker shows a definitive, essentially singular "strategy" for getting through the interview, whether by "simply answering the questions" (as secure-autonomous speakers have been informally said to do); by blocking discourse, whether within or outside of awareness, together with refusing to reveal or discuss potentially distressing experiences (as speakers whose transcripts are assigned to the insecure-dismissing category do); or by manifesting a confused, unrelenting focus on varying incidents, feelings, and relationships aroused by the interview questions (as insecure-preoccupied speakers do). So long as a single one of these strategies seems to be at work throughout the interview, uninterrupted by a collapse of discourse or reasoning during the discussion of potentially frightening experiences, the transcript is considered organized.

As first noted in my discussion of the AAI protocol, each of the organized states of mind with respect to attachment stand—albeit at the discourse level—in attentional parallel to the secure, avoidant, and resistant forms of attachment behavior seen in the Strange Situation conducted with infants (first termed the "organized" infant attachment strategies by Main, 1990).[8] Thus parents producing inflexible, insecure-dismissing AAI texts tend to have infants who avoid them, essentially "dismissing" their comings and goings during the Strange Situation. Parents who produce inflexible, insecure-preoccupied AAI texts tend to have infants who are ambivalently (angrily or passively) preoccupied with them rather than attending to the available toys or other aspects of the surroundings. Finally, parents who produce flexible, secure-autonomous AAI transcripts ("valuing of attachment, but seemingly able to objectively evaluate any particular attachment relationship or experience") have infants whose attention in the Strange Situation is also flexible, alternating between attachment and exploratory behavior as the parents leave and then return to the room.

The AAI coder begins his or her work with the "experience scales" by assigning scores for central aspects of inferred loving versus unloving behavior of each parenting figure during the interviewee's childhood. Next, continuous scores on the scales for "overall state of mind with respect to attachment" are assigned, including a scale of primary importance (coherence), which since 1989 has increasingly referenced Grice's work. Finally, using a "feature" analysis, the coder assigns a best-fitting organized classification and associated sub-classification, even if the text will later be found primarily unresolved or even unclassifiable.

Scales Estimating a Speaker's Probable Experiences with Each Parent during Childhood

A nine-point continuous scale is provided for "loving behavior" described as occurring during childhood (not to be confused with the speaker's love for the parent or unsupported statements that the parent was loving). Evidence of four kinds of unloving behavior is also assessed (rejecting of the child's attachment; role-inverting/heightening of attachment, or, at the high end, demanding of care; neglecting; and pressuring to achieve). Every other point of each scale (i.e., 1, 3, 5, 7, and 9) is well defined, and each scale includes a lengthy introduction explaining what is meant by the con-struct. As is obvious, the higher the scores for in-ferred negative experiences, the necessarily lower are the scores for loving. Finally, the coder select-ing the score may assign a score far different from that which the speaker might have assigned—a fact most obvious when the speaker has provided extremely positive adjectives for the relationship with the mother during childhood, but when asked what the speaker did when hurt or upset during childhood has responded, "I hid. Once I had a broken arm that hurt a lot, but I didn't tell my mother; she would have been so angry." The form taken by the five scales resembles that of Ainsworth and colleagues' (1978) four "sensitiv-ity" scales (available on Everett Waters's website, www.johnbowlby.com): a long, well worked-out introduction followed by alternating point defini-tions that allow for interpolation by the coder. For each scale, behavioral examples that may be found in the transcript are offered as well.

The introduction to the "loving" scale states that no parent is expected to have been perfect—a point made in all of Ainsworth and colleagues' (1978) "maternal sensitivity" scales. A 9 can be as-signed to a parent who "fell apart" and ignored the speaker for a few weeks when a sibling was ill or in-jured, had a brief bout of substance abuse, failed to attend an important ceremony, or even slapped the speaker in the face during early adolescence. At the opposite end, a 1 can be assigned to a parent who provided well for the child materially and academi-cally, saw to it that the child's life was organized and attended to by others, and attended school meet-

ings, if the parent was also emotionally unavailable throughout the speaker's lifetime. A score of 3 is as-signed for "operational" or "instrumental" attention or assistance, such as consistently driving the child to school and helping occasionally with hobbies or homework. A list of behavioral indices of actively loving behavior, such as consistent reliable physi-cal expressions of affection, forgiving wrongdoing, or taking the child's part with peers or teachers is provided, and a score of 5 is assigned when some of these are present in mild form. Five is considered adequately loving behavior. For scores of 7, indices such as the above are definitively present.

Scales Delineating a Speaker's State of Mind with Respect to Attachment

Once a coder has scored the five scales for loving and unloving behavior, he or she moves to scoring the speaker on eight scales describing state of mind with respect to attachment. Correct scores on the state-of-mind scales cannot be assigned without careful prior assignment of scores for experience. For example, the extent to which the childhood relationship with the mother is "idealized" in the speaker's descriptions and evaluations cannot be determined until the coder has decided how "lov-ing" she probably was.

However, the eventual assignment to an overall organized state of mind with respect to at-tachment will have no further dependence on the speaker's probable experiences with the parents during childhood. This should be clear from the fact that speakers with unfavorable childhoods can be readily assigned to the secure-autonomous cat-egory, based on the coherence of their text. Simi-larly, although perhaps less frequently, a speaker with favorable experiences of childhood parenting may be incoherent during the AAI directly follow-ing a traumatic loss or a major first separation from parents at college entrance, and hence may be as-signed to an insecure organized AAI category.

In sum, the assignment of a speaker to any given organized category depends on scores on the continuous scales identifying states of mind with respect to attachment, and a feature analy-sis that follows upon it, rather than on the scales for inferred childhood experiences of parenting. The general criteria for assignment to the state-of-mind scales are displayed in Table 25.2.

Although I will soon attend to the striking associations between the original state-of-mind scales and Grice's (1975, 1989) maxims, here I briefly take a historical approach and consider our

TABLE 25.2. "State-of-Mind" Scales Used in the AAI, Related to the Three Major Categories

Scales associated with the secure-autonomous adult attachment category

Coherence of transcript. For the highest rating, the speaker exhibits a "steady and developing flow of ideas regarding attachment." The person may be reflective and slow to speak, with some pauses and hesitations, or speak quickly with a rapid flow of ideas; overall, however, the speaker seems at ease with the topic, and his or her thinking has a quality of freshness. Although verbatim transcripts never look like written narratives, there are few significant violations of Grice's maxims of quantity, quality, relation, and manner. The reader has the impression that on the whole this text provides a "singular" as opposed to a "multiple" model of the speaker's experiences and their effects (see Main, 1991).

Metacognitive monitoring (scale presently under development). For the highest rating, evidence of active monitoring of thinking and recall is evident in several places within the interview. Thus the speaker may comment on logical or factual contradictions in the account of his or her history, possible erroneous biases, and/or the fallibility of personal memory. Underlying metacognitive monitoring (Forguson & Gopnik, 1988) is active recognition of an appearance–reality distinction (the speaker acknowledges that experiences may not have been as they are being presented); representational diversity (e.g., a sibling may not share the same view of the parents); and representational change (e.g., the speaker remarks that what is said today might not have been said yesterday). This scale is included here because it does identify one of the principal aspects of speech found in secure-autonomous speakers; however, the scale needs further work at present, since criteria for high scores are overly stringent, leading to insufficient range.

Scales associated with the dismissing adult attachment category

Idealization of the speaker's primary attachment figure(s). This scale assesses the discrepancy between the overall view of the parent taken from the subject's speech at the abstract or semantic level, and the reader's inferences regarding the probable behavior of the parent. Since the reader has no knowledge of the speaker's actual history, any discrepancies come from within the transcript itself. For the highest rating, there is an extreme lack of unity between the reader's estimate of the speaker's probable experience with the primary attachment figure(s) and the speaker's positive to highly positive generalized or "semantic" description. Despite inferred experiences of, for example, extreme rejection or even abuse, the portrait of the parent is consistently positive, and gratuitous praise of the parents may be offered (e.g., references to "wonderful" or "excellent" parents).

Insistence on lack of memory for childhood. This scale assesses the speaker's insistence upon the inability to recall his or her childhood, especially as this insistence is used to block further queries or discourse. The scale focuses on the subject's direct references to lack of memory ("I don't remember"). High ratings are given to speakers whose first response to numerous interview queries is "I don't remember," especially when this reply is repeated or remains firmly unelaborated. Low scores are assigned when speakers begin a response with a reference to lack of memory, but then actively and successfully appear to recapture access to the experience they have been asked to describe.

Active, derogating dismissal of attachment-related experiences and/or relationships. This scale deals with the cool, contemptuous dismissal of attachment relationships or experiences and their import, giving the impression that attention to attachment-related experiences (e.g., a friend's loss of a parent) or relationships (those with close family members) is foolish, laughable, or not worth the time. High ratings are assigned when a speaker makes no effort to soften or disguise his or her dislike of the individual or of the topic, so that—in keeping with the apparent intent of casting the individual (or topic) aside ("My mother? A nobody. No relationship. Next question?")—the sentences used are often brief, and the topic is quickly dropped. However, only low scores are given for "gallows" humor: "Oh hell, I didn't mind another separation, I guess that one was #13." (Note: Speakers receiving high scores on this scale are assigned to a relatively rare adult attachment subcategory, Ds2, in which attachment figures are derogated rather than idealized.)

Scales associated with the preoccupied adult attachment category

Involved/involving anger expressed toward the primary attachment figure(s). Accurate ratings on this scale depend on close attention to the form of the discourse in which anger toward a particular attachment figure is implied or expressed. Direct descriptions of angry episodes involving past behavior ("I got so angry I picked up the soup bowl and threw it at her") or direct descriptions of current feelings of anger ("I'll try to discuss my current relationship with my mother, but I should let you know I'm really angry at her right now") do not receive a rating on the scale. High ratings are assigned to speech that includes, for example, run-on, grammatically entangled sentences describing situations involving the offending parent; subtle attempts to enlist interviewer agreement; unlicensed, extensive discussion of surprisingly small recent parental offenses; extensive use of psychological jargon (e.g., "My mother had a lot of material around that issue"); angrily addressing the parent as though the parent were present; and, in an angry context, slipping into unmarked quotations from the parent.

Passivity or vagueness in discourse. High scores are assigned when, throughout the transcript, the speaker seems unable to find words, seize on a meaning, or focus on a topic. The speaker may, for example, repeatedly use vague expressions or even nonsense words; add a vague ending to an already completed sentence ("I sat on his lap, and that"); wander to irrelevant topics; or slip into pronoun confusion between the self and the parent. In addition, as though absorbed into early childhood states or memories, the subject may inadvertently (not through quotation) speak as a very young child ("I runned very fast") or describe experiences as they are described to a young child ("My mother washed my little feet"). Vague discourse should not be confused with restarts, hesitations, or dysfluency.

early definitions and findings. As is clear from Table 25.2, the scale most closely identified with adult (and infant) security from our first efforts onward has been the scale for "coherence of transcript." *Webster's New International Dictionary* (1959, p. 520) states that the term "coherence" is derived from the Latin, meaning approximately "a sticking together or uniting of parts." Elaborating on this definition, Main and Goldwyn (1998) stated that "coherence" may be identified as "a connection or congruity arising from some common principle or relationship; consistency; [or] connectedness of thought, such that the parts of the discourse are clearly related, form a logical whole, or are suitable or suited and adapted to context" (p. 44).

From this point of view, coherence involves more than simply internal consistency. In other words, even if an individual speaks in a manner that is plausible and internally consistent, thereby adhering to the first aspect of the criterion, he or she may still discuss a topic at excessive length or make obscure analogies, thus failing to shape speech in a manner suitable to the discourse exchange. Thus conversational cooperation, as well as internal consistency, was an important component in Main and Goldwyn's (1984a, 1984b) original conceptualization of coherence—and, as mentioned earlier, this was true even before Main's first reading of Grice.

Recognizing Relations between the State-of-Mind Scales and Grice's Maxims

As noted earlier, in general, discourse is judged to be coherent when a speaker appears able to access and evaluate memories while *simultaneously* remaining plausible (consistent or implicitly truthful) and collaborative (Hesse, 1996). When the discussion and evaluation of attachment-related experiences is in fact reasonably consistent, clear, relevant, and succinct, this leads to relatively high AAI coherence scores and placement in the secure-autonomous category. Notably, from the inception of the AAI onward, scores for overall coherence of AAI transcripts have proven vital to analyses of the text and have been associated with infant security of attachment (see the description of the original Bay Area study, below).

As shown in Table 25.2, dismissing speakers had already been identified in the early Main and Goldwyn (1984a) scoring system as having high scores on "idealization of the parent(s)," which pointed to a violation of Grice's maxim of quality ("Be truthful, and have evidence for what you say"). Many dismissing speakers had also been described as excessively succinct, violating the quantity maxim by cutting short the conversational exchange with such statements as "I don't remember." These speech habits had been quantified as "insistence on lack of memory." Preoccupied speakers tended primarily to violate Grice's maxims of relevance, quantity, and manner, which can be termed the maxims of collaboration, and violation of each of these maxims is taken into consideration in the scales for "angrily preoccupied discourse" as well as "passive/vague discourse." For example, with respect to relevance and as seen in these scales, some preoccupied speakers wander from topic to topic or move away from the context of the query (e.g., discussing current relations with parents when asked about childhood experiences), whereas others became embroiled in excessively lengthy descriptions of past or current problems with parents. Some do both. Violations of manner also typify preoccupied speakers, as seen especially in vague speech ("sort of, sort of—and that"), excessive use of psychological jargon ("My mother had a lot of material around that issue"), and use of nonsense words ("dadadada"). Phenomena conforming to these violations and hence pointing to the preoccupied classification have been quantified in continuous scales identifying passivity or vagueness of discourse (manner) and involved/involving anger (relevance, quantity, and manner). (I have provided brief examples of speech typical of secure, dismissing, and preoccupied speakers earlier.)

Table 25.2 provides an overview of the present continuous scoring systems for states of mind (Main & Goldwyn, 1998; Main et al., 2003). I now return, however, to the remaining work of the AAI coder as he or she reviews the text.

As a close look at Table 25.2 will indicate, *an AAI coder's first estimate of category placement is based entirely on the configuration of the continuous scores for the state-of-mind scales.* The exact "expectable configuration" is given in the AAI scoring and classification manual, where, for example (ignoring the still-under-development metacognition scale), high scores on coherence and low scores on idealization, derogation, involved/involving anger, passivity, and insistence on lack of memory point to a secure-autonomous transcript, whereas low scores on coherence and high scores on (either or both) involved/involving anger or passivity of discourse point to a preoccupied speaker. An acceptable range for the configuration of scores is given for each AAI classification, and coders record their first estimate of classification from these scores. Where scores point to conflicting major classifications, the coder may begin to consider the likelihood that the text is unorganized or unclassifiable. However, importantly, it is only after recording the classification(s) emerging from the configuration of state-of-mind scores (which is termed the "bottom-up" or "score-to-classification" analysis) that the coder will turn to the "top-down" or (classificatory) feature analysis of the text, as delineated below.

The Final Step in Estimating the Best-Fitting Organized State of Mind: Application of a Feature Analysis to Classify and Subclassify AAI Texts

In the final step of interview analysis, a coder determines the applicability of all features associated with each major classification (and subclassification) to the transcript in hand. Insofar as possible, this step is carried forward independently of the continuous scores assigned to the scales for states of mind. Table 25.3 elaborates (1) scale score configurations; (2) Gricean discourse characteristics; and (3) some of the features that point to particular AAI classifications. It also presents the associated infant Strange Situation classifications.

For reasons of space, I do not elaborate on the particular features pointing to each of the three organized classifications here. Instead, examples of these features are placed in Table 25.3. In the analysis actually undertaken by coders, some of the features listed in the table are *required* for classification, whereas some are delineated as frequent correlates. In sum, features leading to a particular categorical placement, as delineated by the "top-down" analysis, should dovetail with the classification derived from the "bottom-up" configurations produced by the state-of-mind scales. If, after checking and rechecking, the classification reached by the configuration of state-of-mind scale scores (i.e., the classification suggested by the "bottom-up" analysis) continues to conflict with that arrived at by the "top-down" (feature) analysis, the coder is instructed to consider "cannot classify" as the first assignment for the transcript.

Features Delineating and Defining the 12 Subclassifications of the AAI

As the scales and features developed for the analysis of the AAI were being created, Main and Goldwyn (1984b) began to note what were at times striking differences between transcripts that had been placed in a given major classification category. Thus, for example, within the dismissing classification as a whole (which was associated with the infant avoidant classification devised by Ainsworth et al., 1978), there were four distinct subtypes of transcripts. This indicated that the AAI system differed from Ainsworth's in important ways, because her infant subclassification system contained only two subclassifications for avoidant infants (A1 and A2); these were based on the extremity of avoidance of the parent, as well as small displays of emotion (anger or distress) and even proximity seeking (soon terminated) shown by infants in the latter subcategory.

As was just noted, there are four subclassifications of dismissing adult attachment. To begin with, two types of transcripts of speakers highly dismissing of attachment—and most frequently having highly avoidant babies (A1)—were uncovered, and they differed sharply in their characteristics. In the first subtype (Ds1), speakers were highly idealizing of one or both parents, and this idealization was most frequently accompanied by moderate to strong insistence on lack of memory for childhood. In the second subtype (Ds2), rather than being idealizing of one or both parents, speakers were contemptuously derogating of one or both of them (or in some cases of attachment-related experiences, as in making fun of people who were grieving following loss). The most prevalent index of derogation was, however, attitudes expressed toward the parents that involved discarding them as without value and unworthy of consideration, or indeed of more than brief conversational consideration (e.g., "My mother was just a bitch. So, so much for her. Our next question?"). Although some insistence on lack of memory for childhood was possible for speakers in this subclassification, speakers could be placed in this relatively rare subcategory without insisting on lack of memory. It is probably not surprising that speakers in both subclassifications tended to have highly avoidant babies, because—albeit in differing ways—dismissal of attachment was equally strong.

Transcripts were assigned to the Ds3 (moderately dismissing) classification when idealization and lack of memory were marked but not necessarily extreme. At the level of features, these transcripts had another characteristic not present in Ds1 transcripts. Although expressions of hurt were usually absent, some resentment could be expressed; however, it was usually withdrawn and

TABLE 25.3. Scale Score Configurations, Feature Analyses, and Their Relations to the Organized Categories of Infant Strange Situation Behavior

Adult states of mind with respect to attachment

Secure-autonomous (F): Predictive of secure (B) Strange Situation behavior

Scale score configuration. Moderate to high scores for coherence. Low to low moderate scores on scales indicative of insecure states of mind.

Discourse characteristics. Coherent, collaborative discourse. Descriptions and evaluations of attachment-related experiences and their effects are reasonably consistent, whether the experiences appear to have been favorable or unfavorable. Discourse does not notably violate any of Grice's maxims.

Features predominating with respect to attitudes toward attachment. Avows missing, needing, and depending on others. Seems open and "free to explore" interview topic, indicating a ready flexibility of attention. States that attachment-related experiences have affected his or her development and functioning. Seems at ease with imperfections in the self. Explicit or implicit forgiveness of or compassion for parents. Can flexibly change view of person or event, even while interview is in progress, suggesting autonomy and ultimate objectivity. Sense of balance, proportion, or humor. Ruefully cites untoward flawed behavior of self, as appearing at times despite conscious intentions or efforts.

Dismissing (Ds): Predictive of avoidant (A) Strange Situation behavior

Scale score configuration. Low scores on coherence; high scores on idealization or derogation of one or both parents, often accompanied by high scores on insistence on lack of memory for childhood.

Discourse characteristics. Not coherent. Violates the maxim of quality (consistency/truthfulness), in that positive generalized representations of history are unsupported or actively contradicted by episodes recounted. Violates the maxim of quantity—either via repeated insistence on absence of memory; or via brief contemptuous derogation of, or active contemptuous refusal to discuss, a particular event or figure.

Features predominating with respect to attitudes toward attachment. Self positively described as being strong, independent, or normal. Little or no articulation of hurt, distress, or feelings of needing or depending on others. Minimizes or downplays descriptions of negative experiences; may interpret such experiences positively, in that they have made the self stronger. May emphasize fun or activities with parents, or presents and other material objects. Attention is inflexibly focused away from discussion of attachment history and/or its implications: Responses are abstract and/or seem remote from present or remembered feelings or memories, and topic of interview seems foreign. May express contempt for other person(s), or, relatedly, for events usually considered sorrowful (e.g., loss or funerals).

Preoccupied (E): Predictive of resistant/ambivalent Strange Situation behavior

Scale score configuration. Low scores for coherence; high scores for either passive or angry preoccupation with experiences of being parented (rarely, preoccupied with frightening experiences).

Discourse characteristics. Violates manner, quantity, and/or relevance, while quality/truthfulness may not be violated. In regard to quantity, sentences or conversational turns taken are often excessively long. In regard to manner, responses may be grammatically entangled or filled with vague usages ("dadadada," "and that"). In regard to relevance, the present may be brought into responses to queries regarding the past (or vice versa), or persons or events not the objects of inquiry may be brought into the discussion.

Features predominating with respect to attitudes toward attachment. Responses to interview are persistently closely and inflexibly tied to experiences with and influences of the parents, even when these are not the objects of inquiry. May attempt to involve the interviewer in agreement regarding parents' faults; may seem to weakly, confusedly praise parents, but with oscillations suggestive of ambivalence; and/or (rare) may relate frightening experiences involving them. Topic of interview is addressed, but seems inflexible and closed so that interview responses may seem memorized or unconsciously guided, as if the attachment-related history is "an old story." Unbalanced, excessive blaming of either parents or self. Indecisive—for example, evaluative oscillations ("Great mother. Well, not really, actually pretty awful. No, I mean actually, really good mother, except when she … "). May be unusually psychologically oriented, offering authoritative "insights" into motives of self or others. The lexicon of "pop" psychology may appear with excessive frequency.

Infant Strange Situation behavior

Secure (B)

Flexibility of attention: Explores or plays in parent's presence, changes attentional focus to parent on at least one separation, and seeks parent during at least one reunion. In preseparation episodes, explores room and toys with interest, with occasional returns to or checks with parent ("secure-base phenomenon"). Shows signs of missing parent during separation, often crying by the second separation. Greets parent actively, usually initiating physical contact. Usually some contact maintaining by second reunion, but then settles and returns to play.

(continued)

TABLE 25.3. *(continued)*

Avoidant (A)

Little flexibility of attention: Focuses on toys or environment, and away from parent, whether present, departing, or returning. Explores toys, objects, and room throughout the procedure. Fails to cry on separation from parent. Actively avoids and ignores parent on reunion (i.e., by moving away, turning away, or leaning out of arms when picked up). Little or no proximity or contact seeking, distress, or expression of anger. Response to parent appears unemotional. Focuses on toys or environment throughout procedure.

Resistant or ambivalent (C)

Little flexibility of attention: Focuses on parent throughout much or all of procedure; little or no focus on toys or environment. May be wary or distressed even prior to separation. Preoccupied with parent throughout procedure; may seem angry or passive. Fails to settle and take comfort in parent on reunion, and usually continues to focus on parent and cry. Signs of anger toward parent are mixed with efforts to make contact, or are markedly weak. Fails to return to exploration after reunion, as well as during separation and often preseparation as well (i.e., preoccupied by parent, does not explore).

Note. Descriptions of the adult attachment classification system are summarized from Main et al. (1985) and from Main et al. (2003). Descriptions of infant A, B, and C categories are summarized from Ainsworth et al. (1978).

accompanied by a positive reaffirmation of either parental excellence or a statement indicating that the experience just described had only made the speaker stronger. These speakers generally had A2 (only moderately avoidant) babies.

A fourth subclassification of the dismissing classification (Ds4) was very rare, but it was assigned when speakers showed extreme prospective fear of the death of the child with whom they had been observed in the Strange Situation, but were unable to trace this fear to any particular previous experience (such as loss of a previous child, or indeed any loss or illness experienced by family or friends more generally). These speakers were not necessarily either idealizing or contemptuously derogating, and insistence on absence of memory for childhood may not have been present. Nonetheless, their infants were avoidant of them in the Strange Situation in the original Bay Area study, and to my knowledge they have continued to be found avoidant in succeeding samples. It is not yet known whether their offspring will be more frequently classified as A1 or A2 in the Strange Situation.

Five subclassifications of the AAI were developed for secure-autonomous parents. Four corresponded well to the four subclassifications that Ainsworth had developed for secure infants. Prototypically secure (F3) parents—those who were the most coherent and who fit the majority of the features associated with the category—tended to have prototypically secure (B3) babies. However, so did parents who seemed somewhat conflicted or resentful (mildly angrily preoccupied) regarding their parents, yet (often somewhat humor-

ously) accepted that anger and involvement had characterized their relationship with their parents and would probably continue to do so. The parents of secure but mildly avoidant babies (B1 and B2) tended to qualify for the secure category in general, but this was accompanied by some signs of dismissal (differing for the F1 parents of B1 babies and the F2 parents of B2 babies). The parents of secure but mildly preoccupied babies (B4) tended to be slightly preoccupied with their own parents or attachment-related experiences.

Finally, three subclassifications were developed for the parents of resistant/ambivalent babies, for whom Ainsworth had developed two subclassifications. These included angrily preoccupied speakers (E2) who were expected to have angrily preoccupied babies (C1), and passively preoccupied speakers (E1), who were expected to have passively preoccupied babies (C2). In addition, a third subclassification, E3, *fearfully* preoccupied, was developed. Interestingly, it was used to discriminate just 1 of the 103 Bay Area transcripts, but it has since been found to be predominant in a study of patients with borderline personality disorder (Patrick, Hobson, Castle, Howard, & Maughan, 1994).

The Unresolved/Disorganized and Cannot Classify Categories: Local and Global Breakdowns in Discourse Strategy

The unresolved/disorganized (U/d) and cannot classify (CC) categories (see Table 25.4) were delineated only some years following the inception of the AAI, most likely because their subtlety and complexity could not be recognized until a firm grounding in the three organized categories had been established. Thus it seems likely that, as is generally true with taxonomic endeavors, an awareness of these "exceptions to the rule" were revealed in systematic ways only after much experience with the more basic entity under consideration had been acquired. The first of these two categories to be discovered was the unresolved/disorganized group.

Delineating and Refining the Unresolved/Disorganized Attachment Category

Main and Goldwyn had informally noted as early as 1984 that the parents of disorganized/disoriented infants often spoke in unusual ways about loss experiences. Unresolved or "disordered" mourning had most commonly been understood as falling into two general categories: (1) "chronic mourning," a continuing strong grief reaction that does not abate over an extended period of time (see Shaver & Fraley, Chapter 3, this volume); or (2) "failed mourning," in which expectable grief is substantially minimized or does not occur (see Bowlby, 1980). As the analysis of discussions of loss experiences within the AAI development sample proceeded, however, it became evident that the linguistic indicators of "unresolved" attachment status in adults that predicted disorganized attachment in infants did not appear as explicit manifestations of chronic or failed mourning.

Over time, it became increasingly clear that what the parents of disorganized infants had in common were various indications of what was ultimately termed "lapses in the monitoring of reasoning or discourse" during discussions of potentially traumatic experiences (Hesse & Main, 1999, 2000). More specifically, the AAI transcripts of these individuals were distinguished by the appearance of (ordinarily) brief slips in the apparent monitoring of thinking or the discourse context during the discussion of loss or (discovered later) other potentially traumatic events (see Table 25.4). Such discourse/reasoning lapses are suggestive of temporary alterations in consciousness or working memory, and are believed to represent either interference from normally dissociated memory or belief systems, or unusual absorptions involving memories triggered by the discussion of traumatic events (Hesse & Main, 1999, 2006; Hesse & van IJzendoorn, 1998, 1999).

Lapses in the monitoring of reasoning are manifested in statements suggesting that the speaker is temporarily expressing ideas that violate our usual understanding of physical causality or time–space relations. Marked examples of reasoning lapses are seen when speakers make statements indicating that a deceased person is believed simultaneously dead and not dead in the physical sense—for example, "It was almost better when she died, because then *she could get on with being dead* and I could get on with raising my family" (Main & Goldwyn, 1998, p. 118; emphasis added). This statement implies a belief, operative at least in that moment, that the deceased remains alive in the physical sense (albeit perhaps in a parallel world). Statements of this kind may indicate the existence of incompatible belief and memory systems, which, normally dissociated, have intruded into consciousness simultaneously as a result of queries regarding the nature of the experience and its effects. Lapses in the monitoring of discourse, in contrast, sometimes suggest that the topic has triggered a "state shift" indicative of considerable absorption, frequently appearing to involve entrance into peculiar, compartmentalized, or even partially dissociated states of mind (Hesse, 1996; Hesse & Main, 2006; Hesse & van IJzendoorn, 1999). Thus, for example, an abrupt alteration or shift in speech register inappropriate to the discourse context occurs when a subject moves from his or her ordinary conversational style into a eulogistic or funereal manner of speaking, or provides excessive detail. (In addition, albeit extremely rarely, individuals can also be assigned to the unresolved/disorganized category on the basis of reports of extreme and probably dissociative responses to traumatic events, which are not explained despite persistent interviewer probes.)

Both state shifts and the sudden appearance of incompatible ideas suggest momentary but qualitative changes in consciousness. Thus they appear to represent temporary/local as opposed to global breakdowns in the speaker's discourse strategy. Discourse/reasoning lapses of the kinds just described often occur in high-functioning individuals and are normally not representative of such a speaker's overall conversational style. For this reason, among others, transcripts assigned to the unresolved/disorganized (hereafter, unresolved) category are given a best-fitting alternate classification (e.g., U/Ds, or unresolved/dismissing).

Early discoveries regarding the relation between secure, dismissing, and preoccupied parental AAI status and secure, avoidant, and resistant/

TABLE 25.4. Scale Scores, Discourse Characteristics, and Features Associated with the Disorganized and Unorganized/"Cannot Classify" Categories of the AAI, and Corresponding Infant Strange Situation Categories

Adult states of mind with respect to attachment

Unresolved/disorganized (U)

Scale scores. Scores above 5 on either unresolved loss or unresolved abuse (the distinctions between these are retained) lead to category placement. At scale point 5, the coder must decide whether or not the transcript fits the unresolved/disorganized classification.

Discourse characteristics. During discussions of loss or abuse, individual shows striking lapse in the monitoring of reasoning or discourse. For example, individual may briefly indicate a belief that a dead person is still alive in the physical sense, or that this person was killed by a childhood thought. Individual may lapse into prolonged silence or eulogistic speech. The speaker will ordinarily otherwise fit Ds, E, or F categories.

Features predominating with respect to attitudes toward attachment. No particular features beyond lapse. May fit the descriptors for Ds, E, or F.

Unorganized/"cannot classify" (CC)

Scale score configuration. Scale scores may point to contradictory insecure classifications (e.g., strong idealizing and strong involved/involving anger are seen within the same transcript) as in the "original" form of CC. Alternately, all state-of-mind scores are low, none moving fully to midlevel (e.g., below midpoint for all scores indicative of insecure states of mind, as well as for coherence; see Hesse, 1996). Finally, some CC texts cannot be determined by scale scores, and rely on the use of feature analysis (Main et al., 2003).

Discourse characteristics. The early "contradictory strategies" discourse forms seen in CC texts are described below. In newer forms of CC, violations of Grice's maxims do not necessarily take the forms ordinarily seen in insecure speakers. Coherence violations are not necessarily limited to particular locations in the text, or particular persons or events. In rare and extreme cases, the transcript as a whole may be so incoherent as to be difficult to follow.

Features. In the "original" form of CC, features sufficient to fit the text to two directly contrasting classifications (e.g., dismissing and preoccupied) are observable. In one newer form of CC (Main et al., 2003), the transcript is incoherent without elevated scores for insecure states of mind. Transcripts may also now be considered unclassifiable if (a) the speaker seems to attempt to frighten the listener (e.g., with the sudden, unintroduced, detailed discussion of a murder) or (b) refuses to speak during the interview, without responding that memories are unavailable or are too painful to discuss. Finally, transcripts are considered unclassifiable if they seem to fit equally well to both a secure and insecure classification (e.g., CC/Ds/F or CC/F/E).

Infant Strange Situation behaviors

Disorganized/disoriented (D)

The infant displays disorganized and/or disoriented behaviors in the parent's presence, suggesting a temporary collapse of behavioral strategy. For example, the infant may freeze with a trance-like expression, hands in air; may rise at parent's entrance, then fall prone and huddled on the floor; or may cling while crying hard and leaning away with gaze averted. Infant will ordinarily otherwise fit A, B, or C categories. At 6 years of age, previously disorganized infants in several samples have been found to be role-inverting or "disorganized/controlling" with the parent, being either punitive or caregiving/solicitous.

Cannot classify (CC)

The infant displays aspects of more than one classification, without necessarily being primarily or even notably otherwise disorganized/disoriented. For example, the infant may fit well to the avoidant category on the first reunion, and to the resistant category on the second. Alternately, the infant's Strange Situation behavior may be so diffuse throughout the procedure that it cannot via any single reunion or separation response be found to fit to any single category.

Note. Descriptions of the U and CC categories of the adult attachment classification system are summarized from Hesse and Main (2000) and from Main et al. (2003). The description of the infant D category is summarized from Main and Solomon (1990); the description of the child D category is based on Main and Cassidy (1988); and the still new infant/child CC category has been utilized in publications by Abrams et al. (2006) and Behrens et al. (2007).

ambivalent infant attachment status have already been recounted. The next discovery regarding the AAI (Main & Hesse, 1990) was based on the simultaneous breakthrough reported by Main and Solomon (1986, 1990) that a fourth Strange Situation classification—disorganized/disoriented—could now be recognized. Infants were placed in this fourth category (see Lyons-Ruth & Jacobvitz, Chapter 28, and Solomon & George, Chapter 18, this volume) when they failed to maintain the behavioral organization characteristic of those classified as secure, avoidant, or ambivalent/resistant. Although this failure to maintain organization had previously been described as Strange Situation "unclassifiability" by Main and Weston (1981), by 1990 infants were termed disorganized/disoriented in the Strange Situation when, for example, they approached the parent with head averted, put hand to mouth in a gesture indicative of apprehension immediately upon reunion, or rose to approach the parent and then fell prone to the floor. Infants were also labeled disorganized/disoriented if they froze all movement with arms elevated, or held still for many seconds while exhibiting a trance-like expression. Disorganized attachment has now been observed in the majority of infants in maltreatment samples (Carlson, Cicchetti, Barnett, & Braunwald, 1989; Lyons-Ruth, Connell, Zoll, & Stahl, 1987). And in low-risk samples it has been associated with both externalizing and internalizing disorders (e.g., Solomon, George, & De Jong, 1995).

By 1990, it had been shown that unresolved AAI status in a parent was predictive of disorganized attachment in the infant (Main & Hesse, 1990; see Table 25.4). Specifically, we found that in a subsample of 53 mothers and infants drawn from the original Bay Area study, only 16% (3 of 19) of mothers showing no significant discourse/reasoning lapses had disorganized infants, whereas 91% (11 of 12) of adults with marked lapses (unresolved mothers) had infants who had been judged disorganized with them in the Strange Situation 5 years earlier. Thus there was now an AAI category corresponding to and predictive of each of the four Strange Situation categories in use at the time. Since this original study, 9-point scales for both indices of unresolved loss and abuse (e.g., Main et al., 2003), and similar 9-point scales for scoring infant disorganized behavior, have been developed. A recent analysis of an available subset ($n = 36$) drawn from the same Bay Area sample has shown a significant correlation between parental lapses

of monitoring in the AAI and infant disorganization (phi = .56, $p < .001$; Abrams, Rifkin, & Hesse, 2006).

Emergence of the Cannot Classify Adult Attachment Category

As mentioned earlier, a fifth interview category, "cannot classify" (CC), emerged in the early 1990s as Main and I began noticing a small percentage of transcripts that failed to meet criteria for placement in one of the three central or organized attachment categories. This was first observed in transcripts where, for example, an unsupported positive description of one or both of the parents led to a relatively high idealization score, whereas in direct contradiction to the expected global patterning, highly angrily preoccupied speech was also found. Thus the high idealization score called for placement in the dismissing category, whereas other portions of the transcript called for preoccupied category placement. Main and I (see Hesse, 1996) therefore concluded that these transcripts were unclassifiable and should be placed in a separate group. Because both this "contradictory strategies CC" and the remaining CC subtypes (see below) involve low coherence, they are necessarily defined as insecure.

Although a second CC subtype was mentioned in journal articles as early as 1996 (see, e.g., Behrens et al., 2007; Minde & Hesse, 1996), this and several other CC subtypes have only recently been added to the AAI scoring and classification manual and—given new guidelines (Main et al., 2003)—have come into use by advanced coders. Among the four new subtypes, there is one in which the coder finds coherence low (i.e., the narrative does not form a "coherent whole"), while scale scores indicative of an insecure state of mind are all too low for placement in either of the two organized insecure categories (dismissing or preoccupied). Hence this type of "low-coherence CC" text is both globally incoherent and unorganized. Put another way, the speaker appears to lack a strategy for handling the discourse task, but does not show it in a way that can be quantified by state-of-mind scores indicative of mixed or multiple states. Transcripts of this kind, like the original "contradictory strategies CC" texts, predict disorganized and unclassifiable offspring.

The additional CC subtypes have been delineated largely in highly troubled (e.g., forensic) adult samples, but have yet to be identified in parents for comparison with offspring attachment status. Space limitations prohibit elaboration here, but some kinds of discourse that can render a transcript unclassifiable are briefly referenced in Table 25.4. It should be noted as well that close reviews of particular cases involving Holocaust survivors have led Koren-Karie, Sagi-Schwartz, and Joels (2003) and Sagi-Schwartz, Koren-Karie, and Joels (2003) to consider other individual transcripts that fail to fit the organized (or even the present unresolved) categories. Stressing more specific difficulties with non-normative samples, Turton, McGauley, Marin-Avellan, and Hughes (2001) have found, for example, that *self*-derogation is sometimes seen in forensic samples.

A present difficulty with the cannot classify category is that although it is known to appear most frequently in highly troubled populations, it has not been subjected to even the most basic psychometric testing (e.g., for stability). This means that, even assuming that CC itself is stable (which, again, remains to be tested), what is currently seen as falling into a given subtype at time 1 might easily fall into another subtype at time 2. If so, there is a precedent for this in the infant literature, where (to the best of my knowledge and despite efforts in several laboratories) no subtypes of the infant D category have been identified and found stable. Thus—in parallel to infant D attachment status in the Strange Situation—CC status on the AAI may simply mean that there is no underlying, uninterrupted, and "singular" organization to the text. Nonetheless, this of course suggests an anomalous state of mind.

EMPIRICAL STUDIES INVOLVING THE AAI

This section begins with a review of findings based on the AAI that were already established by 1998. I open with a discussion of Main and Goldwyn's original (1988, 2008) parent–infant study, which differs from most succeeding studies in its emphasis on AAI state-of-mind scale scores (a direction to which the field may now be returning; see Roisman, Fraley, & Belsky, 2007) and subclassifications (as were found again matched to child subclassifications in a 2007 study by Behrens et al., conducted in Japan). I then review studies in four now-classic areas of AAI investigation, including the psychometric properties of the instrument, parent-to-offspring matches, caregiving correlates, and clinical populations. The field continues to

grow in these four "established" areas, so I mention some recent studies as well. In a separate section, I discuss what, due to space limitations, can unfortunately be only a representative sampling of the many important studies published since the first edition of this chapter (Hesse, 1999) appeared.

Early Findings and Well-Established Findings Updated

The Bay Area Study: Linking Parental AAI Responses to Infant Attachment Status

The initial Bay Area study establishing relations between parental AAIs and infant Strange Situation responses to the speaker 5 years earlier involved 32 mothers and 35 fathers and was conducted by Main and Goldwyn (1988, 2008;[9] see also Main et al., 1985; Main & Goldwyn, 1984b). In this randomly selected sample of 67 dyads (sample sizes varied slightly across analyses), 48% of parents were classified as secure, 39% as dismissing, and 13% as preoccupied. The central findings were not only the correspondence between the three then-existing organized states of mind with respect to attachment as seen in a parent's AAI and the infant's response to that parent in the Strange Situation, but also the significant match found between adult and infant subclassifications, and matches between parental state-of-mind scores and continuous dimensions of the infant's Strange Situation response. At the time the AAI texts were analyzed (1982), the infant disorganized/disoriented attachment category (Main & Solomon, 1986, 1990) had yet to be developed, and anomalous Strange Situation behavior was termed "unclassifiable" (Main & Weston, 1981). All unclassifiable infants in this study were moved to their best-fitting organized classification for purposes of analysis. A single coder who was unaware of infant Strange Situation behavior (R. Goldwyn) worked through all interviews, and interjudge agreement with two undergraduate coders was high.

- *Transcripts of interviews with the parents of children who had been secure with them in the Strange Situation 5 years before.* Infant Strange Situation security was assessed with a 3-point scale, where very secure (B3) infants scored a 3, and insecure infants a 1. With respect to scores for the then-existing state-of-mind scales (new scales were later devised), the strongest correlate of infant security of attachment for both mothers and fathers, as predicted, was the coherence observed in the AAI text overall ($r = .48$ for mothers, $r = .53$ for fathers). When Strange Situation as well as state-of-mind classifications were used, a majority of parents of both sexes were matched to their infants in terms of secure versus insecure attachment status. The effect size was $d = 1.50$ for mother–infant dyads ($d = 0.80$ marks a strong effect) and $d = 0.78$ for fathers. Interestingly, the authors reported that 3 of the 18 infants (17%) secure with their mothers had mothers for whom both parents received scores below a 3 on the loving scale. For fathers, there was no significant relation between infant security and either of his parents' loving scores on the AAI, and both parents of one father whose infant was judged secure with him in the Strange Situation had loving scores of 1.

• *Transcripts of interviews with the parents of children who had been avoidant of them in the Strange Situation 5 years before.* To explore relations between infant avoidance and parental state-of-mind characteristics, Ainsworth and colleagues' (1978) 7-point scales for infant avoidance of proximity to the parent during the two 3-minute reunion episodes of the Strange Situation 5 years previously were used. For both mothers and fathers, their infants' avoidance of them under stress was significantly correlated with their own insistence on lack of memory for childhood ($r = .41$ for mothers, $r = .47$ for fathers). For mothers, idealization of their own mothers ($r = .47$) and fathers ($r = .43$) was significantly related to their infants' avoidance of them. For fathers, relations between infant avoidance in the Strange Situation and idealization of both their mothers ($r = .53$) and their fathers ($r = .64$) were even stronger.[10] At the level of classifications, the effect sizes for the relation between parental dismissing classification and infant avoidant classification in this sample were $d = 1.22$ for mothers and $d = 0.68$ for fathers.

• *Transcripts of interviews with the parents of children who had been resistant with them in the Strange Situation 5 years before.* Scores for infant resistance to the parent on reunion in the Strange Situation were expected to be correlated with the parent's preoccupied anger toward his or her own parents. For the mother–infant sample (six infants were classified as resistant), preoccupied anger expressed in the AAI regarding both the mother's mother ($r = .56$) and father ($r = .47$) was significantly related to the infants' angry resistance 5 years earlier. Only two infants were resistant with

their fathers, and the comparable father–infant correlations were not significant.

Transcripts taken from the parents of resistant infants had most commonly been judged preoccupied. Two of the infants of the three preoccupied fathers had been resistant, as were five of the infants of the six preoccupied mothers. The effect size linking maternal preoccupied attachment status to the infant resistant/ambivalent classification was $d = 1.75$, whereas the link between paternal preoccupied attachment status and infant resistant attachment was $d = 1.08$.

The observed three-way agreement between AAI status and infant Strange Situation behavior for mother–infant dyads was 75%, whereas the agreement expected by chance was 37% (kappa = .61, $p < .001$). The three-way agreement for fathers was 69%, whereas the agreement expected by chance was 46% (kappa = .41, $p < .01$).

The match between the 12 AAI "organized" subclassifications and the 8 infant Strange Situation subclassifications was 46%, with a 17% match having been expected by chance. Here, predictions had been made in advance that, for example, both Ds1 and Ds2 interviews would be associated with A1 infant attachment status, and both F3 and F5 parents were expected to have B3 babies. This subclassification match was almost identical to that found later in Eichberg's (1989) dissertation study of middle-class mother–infant dyads (48% subclassification match, 18% expected by chance), for which Ainsworth had coded the AAI texts and her colleague Julia Green had coded the associated Strange Situations. In 2001, Pederson and Bento also found a significant subclassification to subclassification match in their study of middle-class Canadian mothers (D. R. Pederson, personal communication, 2001). Recently, in the Behrens and colleagues (2007) Sapporo sample of 39 Japanese mothers seen in the AAI and shortly thereafter in Main and Cassidy's (1988) sixth-year reunion procedure, a 49% maternal AAI subclassification to child subclassifications of reunion response was identified (24% expected by chance; kappa = .33, $p < .001$).

Psychometric Properties of the AAI

In 1996, van IJzendoorn and Bakermans-Kranenburg reported that in a combined (meta-analytic) sample of 584 nonclinical mothers, 24% were classified as dismissing, 58% as secure-autonomous, and 18% as preoccupied. With the unresolved category included, a four-way analysis of the available 487 nonclinical mothers showed the following distribution: 16% dismissing, 55% secure-autonomous, 9% preoccupied, and 19% unresolved. The combined distribution of nonclinical fathers was highly similar. A more recent meta-analysis published 12 years later by these same authors (van IJzendoorn & Bakermans-Kranenburg, 2008) yielded very similar proportions, despite the fact that the combined sample size was much larger (1,012 nonclinical mothers).

The 1996 meta-analysis examined five studies that included both wives and husbands (226 couples) and found a three-way correspondence comparable to a correlation of $r = .28$. This was accounted for by the fact that secure men and women married each other at greater than chance levels. In the four-way analysis ($n = 152$), the secure–insecure association was not found, but unresolved individuals appeared to have married each other more often than expected by chance.

AAI distributions in adolescent samples did not differ significantly from distributions in the nonclinical adult samples. However, combined samples with very low-socioeconomic-status backgrounds ($n = 995$) did differ significantly from nonclinical mother samples, with the unresolved and dismissing categories being overrepresented, and the secure-autonomous category correspondingly underrepresented. The AAI was found to be unrelated to social desirability (Bakermans-Kranenburg & van IJzendoorn, 1993; Crowell et al., 1996; Sagi et al., 1994), and showed only a modest association with social adjustment (Crowell et al., 1996). Although the AAI in general was only weakly related to content-based retrospective parenting style measures and appeared to be independent of general personality measures (van IJzendoorn, 1995), persons classified as preoccupied have been found to report more symptoms on the Minnesota Multiphasic Personality Inventory, whereas dismissing individuals report fewer (Pianta, Egeland, & Adam, 1996).

The AAI has been subjected to a series of rigorous psychometric tests of stability and discriminant validity (van IJzendoorn, 1995). Stability studies typically employ different interviewers across the time period in question, with coders unaware of one another's classifications. With interviews conducted 2 months apart ($n = 83$), Bakermans-Kranenburg and van IJzendoorn (1993) found 78% stability (kappa = .63) across the three organized attachment categories (the unresolved category was less stable), and an Israeli study of 59 college students conducted 3 months apart yielded 90% test–retest stability (kappa = .79; Sagi et al., 1994). The mean interjudge agreement for this latter study was 95%. Both studies indicated that category placement could not be attributed to the influence of a particular interviewer.

Benoit and Parker (1994) found 90% three-category stability between a prebirth interview and interviews conducted at 11 months of infant age ($n = 84$). Stability has also been tested across an 18-month period in New York (86% three-category stability, kappa = .73; Crowell et al., 1996) and across a 4-year period in Rome (95% secure–insecure correspondence, 70% three-category correspondence; Ammaniti, Speranza, & Candelori, 1996). Recently, H. Steele and M. Steele (2007) reported striking 5-year stability in a group of 51 mothers interviewed during pregnancy and again when their children were 5 years of age. The interviews were classified by independent teams of coders, and no individuals were considered "cannot classify" at either time period. Remarkably, across the remaining four major classifications (secure-autonomous, dismissing, preoccupied, and unresolved), there was 86% stability across the 5-year period.[11]

Because of the weight given to coherence scores when AAI transcripts are being assigned to secure versus insecure attachment status, it has been important to establish that in five out of six studies conducted to date, secure versus insecure adult attachment status has been unrelated to intelligence, including assessments specific to verbal fluency (van IJzendoorn, 1995). Moreover, because insistence on lack of memory for childhood is associated with the dismissing category, it has been necessary to assess general abilities involving memory. Thus, if persons assigned to the dismissing category suffer from overall difficulties with childhood memories, their insistence on lack of recall for early relationships and interactions might not pertain to state of mind specific to attachment history. This question was first examined by Bakermans-Kranenburg and van IJzendoorn (1993), who found the AAI categories to be independent of non-attachment-related memory. An Israeli study (Sagi et al., 1994) used an even broader range of memory tests. Here the accuracy of memories for childhood events was ingeniously assessed, and subjects were also examined for "immediate" memory skills in a test of (non-attachment-related) paired associates. No differences were found across the categories.

One of the most important questions pertaining to the discriminant validity of the AAI stems from its reliance on individual differences in discourse characteristics. If these characteristics were found to generalize to non-attachment-related topics, the inability of the parents of insecure infants to produce coherent and collaborative AAI narratives could not readily be attributed to an (insecure) state of mind arising specifically from a request for a review and evaluation of their attachment history. This question was addressed by Crowell, Waters, and their colleagues (1996), using an Employment Experience Interview, which followed the form of the AAI protocol but focused on technical aspects of the speaker's work history. Although transcripts of the Employment Experience Interview could be reliably classified as secure-autonomous, dismissing, or preoccupied, these classifications were orthogonal to the secure-autonomous, dismissing, and preoccupied classifications assigned to the same 53 mothers based on the AAI. Thus it appears that the attachment-related content of the AAI protocol does in fact have a direct influence on the linguistic form manifested in the interview transcript.

The Link between Adult (AAI) and Child Attachment Status

Within about a decade following the publication of Main and colleagues (1985), the relations between a parent's AAI classification and his or her infant's Strange Situation classification as first uncovered in Berkeley had been well replicated, and the association between a parent's discussion of his or her own attachment history and the infant's Strange Situation behavior was found to be robust. In the immediately succeeding years, AAI-to-Strange-Situation matches were found in both high-risk samples (e.g., Bus & van IJzendoorn, 1992, based on a Dutch sample; Ward & Carlson, 1995, based on an inner-city Hispanic and African American sample) and the low-risk samples described below. By 1995, despite its origin in close study of English speech usage, a significant AAI-to-Strange-Situation match had been found in two German samples (Grossmann, Fremmer-Bombik, Rudolph, & Grossmann, 1988). Again surprisingly, or so it has seemed to its authors, the AAI would later be found predictive of offspring attachment in language contexts differing from English more than do Dutch and German, such as Hebrew (Sagi et al., 1997), and Japanese (Behrens et al., 2007; Kazui, Endo, Tanaka, Sakagami, & Suganuma, 2000).

In 1995, van IJzendoorn used meta-analytic techniques to examine a total of 18 AAI samples,

including 854 parent–infant pairs from six different countries. This overview revealed that when the three-way analysis was used, there was a 75% two-way correspondence between parental and offspring security—a finding that held as well when the interview was conducted prior to the birth of the first child (e.g., Benoit & Parker, 1994, in Toronto; Fonagy et al., 1991, and H. Steele, Steele, & Fonagy, 1996, in London; and Ward & Carlson, 1995, in inner-city New York). The combined effect size of the secure–insecure parent-to-infant match across samples (inclusive of mother–infant and father–infant dyads) was $d = 1.06$ ($r = .47$, biserial $r = .59$). The explained variation on the basis of r was 22%, and for biserial r it was 35%. Using a statistic devised by Rosenthal (1991), van IJzendoorn calculated that it would take 1,087 studies with null results to diminish the combined one-tailed p level to insignificance.

To return to parent-to-infant matches in van IJzendoorn's (1995) meta-analysis, the combined effect size for the match between the dismissing classification and the other classifications in predicting the infant avoidant classification was $d = 1.02$ (equivalent to $r = .45$), whereas for the match between the preoccupied classification and the infant resistant/ambivalent classification the combined effect size was $d = 0.92$ ($r = .42$). Correspondence for the three-way infant and AAI classifications across the 13 samples for which it could be calculated was 70%. It is interesting as well (van IJzendoorn's [1995] Table 2, p. 393), however, that in this analysis 82% (304/369) of secure-autonomous mothers had secure offspring, and 64% of dismissing mothers had insecure-avoidant offspring; however, only 35% of preoccupied mothers had insecure-resistant/ambivalent infants.

As noted earlier, with respect to parent–child dyads, both cannot classify and unresolved/disorganized interviews are associated with the disorganized/disoriented infant Strange Situation classification (Main & Solomon, 1986, 1990). Both of these disorganized AAI categories have been found to predominate in clinical samples (van IJzendoorn & Bakermans-Kranenburg, 1996, 2008), and infants' disorganized attachment with their mothers has been associated with psychopathology assessed in the same individuals in young adulthood (Carlson, 1998), especially where intervening trauma was present (Ogawa, Sroufe, Weinfield, Carlson, & Egeland, 1997).

In his 1995 meta-analysis of nine studies including unresolved/disorganized AAI status (548 dyads), van IJzendoorn calculated $d = 0.65$

(equivalent to $r = .31$) for the relation between normally very brief lapses in speech during the AAI and similarly minimal disruptions in Strange Situation behavior. The fleeting and difficult-to-identify nature of both phenomena suggests that the association between adult unresolved status and infant disorganized status may have been attenuated in this calculation—not only by instability in the appearance of the phenomena, but also by the need for extensive training in identifying them. In keeping with this line of reasoning, van IJzendoorn found that amount of training was very strongly related to differences in effect sizes ($z = 5.59$, $p = 1.30E\text{-}08$) linking unresolved/disorganized and unclassifiable AAI texts to infant disorganization, with less training being associated with smaller effects. For example, the effect size relating unresolved AAI status in 45 mothers to infant disorganized attachment status for Ainsworth and Eichberg's (1991) study (with AAIs coded by Ainsworth following reliability training across 50 AAI transcripts, and Strange Situations coded by N. Kaplan and D. Weston following training across 75 Strange Situations) was $d = 2.32$. As a more recent example, in Behrens and colleagues' (2007) study of 43 mother–child dyads in Japan, the AAI coder (K. Behrens) had attended two training institutes and assisted Japanese participants in a third, and experts (E. Hesse and M. Main) in the sixth-year system of reunion classifications (Main & Cassidy, 1988) coded child reunion behavior; the effect size was $d = 1.50$ (equivalent to $r = .60$) for relations between mothers' unresolved or cannot classify AAI status and children's disorganized/cannot classify status.

One illustration of a study relating maternal unresolved/disorganized status to infant disorganized status may be provided (Hughes et al., 2001). This study focused on the effects of stillbirth of a first infant upon Strange Situation disorganization when mothers ($N = 53$) were seen in the Strange Situation with their next-born infant. The coder for infant attachment status for this study had attended two full Strange Situation training institutes, and the overall association between unresolved/disorganized status for the stillborn child and disorganized attachment in the following offspring was $r = .50$ ($p < .0001$). Interestingly, all the variability in disorganization associated with the stillbirth itself could be accounted for by maternal unresolved AAI status, and the association between stillbirth experience and disorganization in the next infant was not significant once unresolved maternal attachment was included in the model.

The Link between AAI Status and Caregiving

The association between infant security versus insecurity with the mother and maternal sensitivity to infant signals and communications was first discovered by Ainsworth and colleagues (Ainsworth, Bell, & Stayton, 1971; Ainsworth et al., 1978) and was based on a highly detailed scale for assessing this construct on the basis of narrative records taken from 12 hours of infant–mother observation in the home. Later studies have also assessed positive versus negative aspects of maternal responsiveness to offspring, but have often used videotaped observations lasting well under an hour and an array of at least 54 different measures. Despite these limitations, a meta-analysis recomputing the overall relation between maternal sensitivity and infant security has shown a continuing modest link (for 1,099 studies, $r = .24$; De Wolff & van IJzendoorn, 1997; see Belsky & Fearon, Chapter 13, this volume).

Since secure-autonomous parents typically have secure infants, as indicated above, they should also be especially sensitive and responsive to their infants—a point established early on by several investigators using the AAI (e.g., Haft & Slade, 1989). By 1995, van IJzendoorn's meta-analytic overview demonstrated that across studies, secure-autonomous parents were more responsive to their infants than were parents whose AAI texts had been judged dismissing or preoccupied. The combined effect size linking parental security to parental responsiveness[12] was 0.72 ($r = .34$), and it was determined that it would take more than 155 studies with null results to bring the p value to insignificance. It should be noted once again, however, that by this time assessments of parental responsiveness included many variables other than Ainsworth's (Ainsworth et al., 1978; see also www.johnbowlby.com) traditional sensitivity ratings, such as anxiety, connectedness, support with drawings, and "warmth," a parental variable that Ainsworth had twice established was unrelated to infant security[13] (Ainsworth, 1967; see also Main, 1999). Considered as a whole, these responsiveness assessments provided only a partial explanation of the relation between secure versus insecure parental attachment status and secure versus insecure infant attachment. This notably partial mediation led van IJzendoorn (1995) to point to the possibility of a "transmission gap" between adult and infant security—meaning that the kinds of behavior toward offspring that differentiated parents with secure-autonomous transcripts from others, and led to infant security, had yet to be fully identified.

Unresolved/Disorganized States of Mind and Frightening/Disruptive Behavior toward Offspring. In 1990, Main and I put forward the hypothesis that parents judged unresolved/disorganized on the AAI would exhibit frightened, frightening, and/or dissociative behavior toward their offspring. Our thinking was that if lapses in the monitoring of reasoning or discourse surrounding potentially traumatic events during the AAI occurred in conjunction with intrusions from partially dissociated frightening ideation associated with the event in question (Hesse & Main, 1999, 2006), such intrusions could also occur during interactions with an infant. The classic manifestations of primitive fear include attack, flight, and freezing—behaviors according well with the proposal that frightening (attack), frightened (flight), or directly dissociative (such as trance-like freezing) reactions might be found in unresolved/disorganized parents. A coding system identifying frightened/frightening/dissociative (FR) behavior (Main & Hesse, 1991, 1998) was therefore developed, along with a broader system identifying parental disruptive behaviors more generally (see Lyons-Ruth, Bronfman, & Parsons, 1999). Unresolved status on the AAI has now been found to predict these forms of parental behavior in several independent samples (e.g., Abrams et al., 2006; Lyons-Ruth et al., 1999; Madigan, Moran, & Pederson, 2006; see also Madigan, Bakermans-Kranenburg, et al., 2006). However, in a pioneering study of 80 dyads conducted by Schuengel, Bakermans-Kranenburg, and van IJzendoorn (1999) in the Netherlands, substantially frightening parental behavior was linked to infant disorganization only if an unresolved/disorganized mother had a secondary classification as insecure. This suggested to the authors that an underlying secure-autonomous state of mind might be protective in the context of unresolved status.

Jacobvitz and colleagues (2006) partially replicated the "protective effect" found in Schuengel and colleagues' (1999) study, as would Heinicke and colleagues (2006) in an intervention study several years later. In Jacobvitz's study, 116 prospective first-time mothers were administered the AAI during pregnancy, and they were videotaped at 8 months of infant age in their homes. Women classified as unresolved/disorganized with respect to loss and/or abuse displayed substantially higher levels of FR behavior during these interactions than did other mothers, including extended trance-like stilling and anomalous aggressive actions. However, in keeping with the Dutch study,

levels of FR behavior were lower if a mother's underlying AAI classification was secure. Unresolved/disorganized responses to loss in the AAI fully mediated the association between loss of an attachment figure other than the parent and FR behavior, and it partially mediated the relation between loss of a parent and FR behavior.

Main and Hesse (1990) had also put forward the hypothesis that parental FR behavior would mediate the relation between unresolved/disorganized lapses in speech in the AAI and infant disorganized/disoriented behavior in the Strange Situation. This would naturally be difficult to test, since, as I have already shown, there is a strong relation between the amount of training investigators have had in coding unresolved adult and disorganized infant attachment status and the effect sizes obtained in attempts to link these phenomena. Frightened, frightening, and dissociative responses, as well as more generally disruptive parental behaviors, are as fleeting as disorganized behavior in the Strange Situation—and, as noted above, the Schuengel and colleagues (1999) study had found that FR behavior mediated the relation only when the unresolved/disorganized mothers were also insecure.

Given the fleeting nature of all three phenomena (i.e., lapses in the monitoring of speech or reasoning during the AAI, frightened/frightening/dissociative behavior in parents, and infant disorganized/disoriented behavior), however, it is striking that a first meta-analysis of five samples testing the Main–Hesse hypothesis and using investigators at differing levels of training found even a partial (although still incomplete) mediation in which 42% of the variance was accounted for (Madigan, Bakermans-Kranenburg, et al., 2006). More recently, Canadian coders highly trained in the Main–Hesse system for assessing parental FR behavior found that maternal FR behavior accounted for over 50% of the variance in the association between maternal unresolved attachment status on the AAI and infant disorganized Strange Situation behavior (Evans, 2008).

Studies Comparing AAI Classifications in Clinical and Nonclinical Populations

As already explained, the central categories of the AAI were developed and refined in the mid-1980s with respect to a 1-year-old's (secure vs. insecure) response to the speaker in a stressful situation. It is therefore surprising that—without adjustment—this system was later shown to discriminate between clinical and nonclinical populations (van IJzendoorn & Bakermans-Kranenburg, 1996, 2008). However, in 1996 van IJzendoorn and Bakermans-Kranenburg showed that the effect size discriminating clinical from nonclinical populations ($d = 1.03$) was virtually identical to that discriminating the parents of secure infants from the parents of insecure infants ($d = 1.06$). Ultimately, in a four-way analysis (secure-autonomous, dismissing, preoccupied, unresolved/cannot classify), only 8% of members of clinical samples were judged secure. (I should note that "clinical samples" as used here indicates persons with specific diagnoses, not those simply in psychotherapy.)

By the mid-1990s, many studies of clinically distressed adolescents and adults had been conducted, and the predominance of the unresolved/disorganized (as well as the preoccupied) classification was striking. For example, a study of 24 closely comparable female subjects (12 with borderline personality disorder and 12 with dysthymia, none comorbid) was conducted at the Tavistock Clinic, using a coder who was unaware of either participants' diagnoses or the aims of the investigation (Patrick et al., 1994). Borderline patients were selected for having met at least seven of the eight *Diagnostic and Statistical Manual of Mental Disorders*, third edition, revised (DSM-III-R; American Psychiatric Association, 1987) criteria. All of the 12 borderline patients—but only 4 of the dysthymic patients—were classified as preoccupied (Fisher's exact test, two-tailed; $p = .001$). Moreover, 10 of the 12 borderline patients were classified into the E3 AAI subcategory, described earlier. The overall rates of experiences of trauma and loss as defined in AAI manuals did not differ between groups, but all 9 of the borderline subjects reporting loss or trauma were classified as primarily unresolved (e.g., U/E3), as compared with only 2 of the 10 dysthymic patients reporting loss or trauma (Fisher's exact test, two-tailed; $p = .0007$).

Fonagy and colleagues (1996) undertook a large study of 82 clinically distressed young adults at a national center for the inpatient treatment of severe personality disorders in London, comparing interviews to those of 85 well-matched controls. The category most strongly differentiating the groups was unresolved (76% inpatients vs. 7% controls), and—as in an earlier study of anxiety-disordered subjects conducted by Manassis, Bradley, Goldberg, Hood, and Swinson (1994; 14 of 18 or 78% unresolved)—anxiety-disordered subjects were found especially likely to be unresolved (38

of 44 or 86%). Among the subclassifications, fearful preoccupation with traumatic events (E3) was again found to be unexpectedly common in the psychiatric group (28% vs. 1%). Replicating earlier outcomes (Patrick et al., 1994), 47% of the borderline patients were classified E3.

A different and highly informative investigation was conducted by administering the AAI to 66 young adults (mean age = 26 years) who had been hospitalized 11 years earlier in adolescence, together with 76 matched (nonhospitalized) controls (Allen, Hauser, & Borman-Spurrell, 1996). Both groups came from upper-middle-class families, and individuals suffering from psychosis or organic impairment were excluded from the hospitalized sample. Any information that could provide evidence of previous hospitalization was removed from the transcripts, so that the coder (this author) successfully remained unaware of group status. The proportion of secure-autonomous transcripts among individuals hospitalized 11 years earlier (7.6%) was exceptionally low. Moreover, the interview transcripts of 25.8% of the hospitalized group were judged cannot classify, as compared with 6.6% of the comparison group. Speakers who had been hospitalized were more likely to express contempt or derogation for attachment-related experiences and attachment figures, and received higher scores for unresolved responses to abuse experiences. The state-of-mind scale for derogation was also found to be related to criminal behavior and to hard drug use. Given the success of this original study, it is perhaps not surprising that Hauser and his colleagues have recently concluded that with the development of the AAI, narrative studies have begun to come into their own in psychiatry and psychoanalysis (Hauser, Golden, & Allen, 2006).

As explained earlier, speakers are assigned to the cannot classify category whenever contradictory discourse strategies appear within the AAI. With this in mind, two early case studies are of special interest. In the first, a mother described as cannot classify (Minde & Hesse, 1996; the coder was unaware that the transcript was taken from a patient in therapy) successfully demanded to have her child removed by cesarean section 1 month early, then insisted on staying with the infant in intensive care for periods that far exceeded usual hospital practices. At later times, she was observed to alternate between periods of overinvolvement and periods of neglect. In the second, home observations of a mother judged cannot classify by Hughes and McGauley (1997) indicated marked neglect and carelessness to a degree inviting external injury, while making alternating sudden trips to the hospital occasioned by fear of germs. In keeping with the hypothesis that discourse usage in the AAI should be predictive of caregiving, then, these two case studies of unclassifiable, contradictory discourse were reflected in contradictory behavior toward the offspring.

Recently, adolescents living in the streets of Mexico City with their infants have been described by Gojman de Millán and Millán (2008). These include two coded as cannot classify, and one—whose behavior and outcome appeared far more promising—coded as unresolved/secure. Another, new kind of case study has described a patient with both narcissistic and borderline personality disorders who was classified as both unresolved and preoccupied; she is discussed in terms of both the AAI and her therapist's views (Buchheim & Kachele, 2003). Still another set of case studies has traced change over the course of psychoanalysis, considering especially the movement from unresolved/cannot classify status to organized insecurity (Ammaniti, Dazzi, & Muscetta, 2008).

In most of the above studies, individuals diagnosed with clinical disorders have been examined for their accompanying adult attachment classifications. However, Riggs and Jacobvitz (2003) examined mental health status using varying established and newly developed questionnaires in a sample of 233 expectant mothers and fathers. Preoccupied parents were the most likely of the parents in the organized attachment categories to report suicidal ideation, whereas unresolved/disorganized parents more often reported suicidal ideation, emotional distress, and substance abuse. As expected, secure-autonomous status on the AAI was linked to mental health.

Ward, Lee, and Polan (2006) investigated a *nonclinical* New York sample of 60 adult women, who were seen in the AAI and in a diagnostic setting. Using the organized (secure-autonomous, dismissing, and preoccupied) attachment categories in the analysis, the researchers found that a majority of women with insecure attachment classifications were diagnosed with some psychopathology. However, when the unresolved category was included, unresolved participants whose alternative placement was secure-autonomous—while experiencing some difficulties with daily functioning, such as marital discord or physical symptoms—were significantly less likely to be diagnosed with psychopathology than were participants with unresolved/insecure classifications.

In a recent overview of 61 clinical samples, van IJzendoorn and Bakermans-Kranenburg (2008) used a correspondence analysis to ascertain possible patterning of AAI classifications in relation to clinical diagnoses. All clinical groups with psychiatric diagnoses tended toward insecurity, as established previously with a smaller set of samples, although clinical status in general was not related to a specific organized insecure AAI category. However, when the three-way analysis was used, individuals with borderline personality disorder and those experiencing more internalizing disorders tended toward the preoccupied classification. In contrast, for more externalizing problems and disorders, such as antisocial personality disorder and conduct disorder, there was an overrepresentation of the dismissing classification. (See also Frodi, Dernevik, Sepa, Philipson, & Bragesjö, 2003, for a study that found an unusual proportion of dismissing transcripts among incarcerated males with psychopathy.) When unresolved/disorganized and unclassifiable transcripts were taken into account in a four-way analysis, an "extremely strong" association was found with borderline personality disorder, abuse, or suicide. (See also Adshead & Bluglass, 2005, for a first study of maternal factitious illness by proxy, in which 60% of mothers were found to have unresolved transcripts.)

A new direction in clinical research using the AAI may have been established in a longitudinal study of 111 middle-class Australian mothers with postnatal depression and their infants (McMahon et al., 2006). As in previous studies, chronically depressed mothers were more likely to have infants who were insecurely attached. However, the relation between maternal depression and infant insecurity was moderated by maternal response to the AAI, with secure mothers with postpartum depression being less likely to have insecure infants.

Newer Empirical Studies

In the preceding section, on earlier AAI research, I have occasionally mentioned new studies conducted along the same lines. Here, due to space limitations, I briefly discuss a selective subset of newer studies, most of which have appeared since the first edition of this chapter (Hesse, 1999) was published. I have avoided overlap with the 1999 review insofar as possible, and the reader interested in the AAI literature as a whole will need to refer to the earlier chapter. This section can be used as a roadmap to some of the territory into which the AAI has moved in recent years.

Applications of the AAI to New Populations

Adult Holocaust Survivors and Their Daughters Living in Israel. At the turn of the 21st century, a large study of female Holocaust survivors and their daughters was undertaken by Sagi-Schwartz and colleagues in Israel (Sagi-Schwartz, van IJzendoorn, et al., 2003). To avoid recruiting participants through convenience groups, population-wide demographic information from the Israeli Ministry of the Interior was used. Mothers in the Holocaust group ($N = 48$) were born between 1926 and 1937 and had lost both parents in Europe between 4 and 14 years of age. They had immigrated to Israel soon after the war, and had daughters of suitable age to be administered the AAI. A comparison group in the same age range who were born in Europe but had not experienced the Holocaust, had immigrated to Israel with their parents before the war, and had adult daughters was also studied. In the Holocaust survivors and the comparison group considered together, a majority of mothers showed the same attachment classification as their daughters (60.2%; $p = .02$). This was consonant with previous findings for adult mothers and adult daughters in Canada (Benoit & Parker, 1994).

Few Holocaust survivors were classified as secure on the AAI (22%), although this is perhaps not a surprisingly high proportion, given their early loss of parents, friends, and other family members in an atmosphere of terror and uncertainty. A very high proportion were unresolved or unclassifiable (56.3%), compared to the control group (18%). Sagi-Schwartz and colleagues have pointed out (Sagi, van IJzendoorn, Joels, & Scharf, 2002) that it is striking that disorganized lapses in reasoning or discourse surrounding trauma seemed to have endured for 50 or more years for a majority of these Holocaust survivors.

As discussed earlier in this chapter, unresolved trauma in a parent is associated with disorganized attachment in offspring, and disorganized infants in two independent samples have been found in late adolescence and early adulthood to be insecure on the AAI (Main et al., 2005). However, an unexpected and promising finding from the Sagi-Schwartz, van IJzendoorn, and colleagues study (2003) was that a substantial proportion of adult daughters of Holocaust survivors were secure, and overall did *not* differ in rates of insecurity from the comparison group. In theory, this low rate of offspring insecurity may result from the fact that, as opposed to loss experiences or other traumatic events in comparison samples, the traumatic events in question here were experienced collectively. For the Holocaust survivors, loss was not an idiosyncratic event, or hidden within an individual familial context, but originated from an outside source. For some, early family experiences were no doubt loving, and a primary representation of a bond with loving parents may have been maintained despite the loss. Finally, daughters born in Israel undoubtedly learned that what their mothers had experienced was shared with countless other residents of their country, many of whom saw Israel as a place of escape from a common enemy, as well as a newly established country sharing common hopes.

Religious/Spiritual Groups. Granqvist and colleagues at the universities of Uppsala and Göteborg in Sweden (Granqvist, Ivarsson, Broberg, & Hagekull, 2007) used the AAI with a sample of 84 adults (mean age = 29 years) drawn from religious/spiritual groups, and 46% of participants had secure-autonomous transcripts. As expected, AAI scores for mothers' loving behavior during childhood were linked to images of a loving God. However, New Age spirituality—which can include beliefs in the possibility of personal contact with the dead—was associated specifically with unresolved cannot classify and preoccupied adult attachment status. In addition (see Granqvist & Kirkpatrick, Chapter 38, this volume), strong majorities of devout Catholic laypeople and nuns have been found secure in a sample studied by Cassibba and her colleagues in Italy (Cassibba, Granqvist, Costantini, & Gatto, 2007).

Twin Studies. Two studies addressing questions of genetics, shared environment, and nonshared environment as contributors to AAI status have recently been published. In the first, 33 pairs of identical female twins (ages 13–26) and 14 of their nontwin siblings were administered the AAI (Constantino et al., 2006), with coding conducted by judges unaware of family membership. Amazingly, 22 of 33 or 67% of monozygotic twin pairs were concordant for four-category placement on the AAI (kappa = .51, $p < .0001$), and for the secure–insecure split the results were similar (26 of 33 agreements; $p < .0001$). Attachment classifications were also concordant for 13 of the 14 pairings of monozygotic twins and their nontwin siblings (who share on average 50% of their genes), and thus was as strong as for the monozygotic pairs. Because these concordance rates were similar, the results were interpreted as providing preliminary evidence that similarity in AAI classification occurs predominantly on the basis of shared environmental influences.

Torgerson, Grova, and Sommerstad (2007) conducted a pilot study of attachment patterns in same-sex adult Norwegian twins. As in the Constantino and colleagues' (2006) study, the distribution of AAI patterns for twins was essentially the same as that established for singletons, and coders were unaware of zygosity status. Although within-pair similarity was high in both zygosity groups, especially high secure–insecure correspondence was found for the 28 monozygotic twins ($p < .001$), who were also similar in scores for coherence of mind (intraclass correlation = .77). In the much smaller dizygotic group ($n = 14$), correspondence for secure–insecure status approached significance ($p < .06$), and scores for coherence of mind were significantly similar (intraclass correlation = .61, $p < .05$). It should be noted that for the three-way analysis, kappa = .79 for the monozygotic pairs, and kappa = .40 for the dizygotic pairs. However, because of the small sample size, it was not possible to carry out the most common forms of twin analysis, or to present values that could provide differentiated information about environmental versus genetic influence.

Adoptive and Foster Parent–Child Dyads. In a now-classic study, Dozier, Stovall, Albus, and Bates (2001) examined 50 foster mothers' AAI status and the Strange Situation classifications of their foster infants assessed between 12 and 24 months of age (at least 3 months following placement). The two-way correspondence between maternal secure versus insecure state of mind and infant security versus insecurity with the foster mother was 72% (kappa = .43). This result did not differ from the global norms established for biologically related dyads by van IJzendoorn (1995), and hence argued for a nongenetic process leading to secure–insecure matches for mothers and infants. There was wide variation in the time of placement (birth to 20 months of age); surprisingly, however, this was not related to the security of infant attachment, so that recently placed and early-placed infants were equally likely to be judged secure in the Strange Situation with their foster mothers as long as the foster mothers themselves were found to be secure-autonomous on the AAI.

M. Steele, Hodges, Kaniuk, Hillman, and Henderson (2003) have reported associations between AAIs obtained from adoptive mothers and emotional themes in the doll-play narratives of their previously neglected or abused 4- to 6-year-olds. Despite the children's long history of maltreatment, a strong and significant overlap was established between the mothers' AAI status and their adopted children's response to the story completion tasks. Even 3 months following placement, if a mother was secure, there was, for example, less aggression in a child's doll play. For unresolved mothers, adoptive children's doll-play themes suggested especially marked levels of emotional and relational difficulties. On a separate but important note, I add in closing this section that in an Italian study of 50 couples seeking to adopt because of infertility, a majority of couples were classified as secure on the AAI (Santona & Zavattini, 2005).

Daughters of Parents with Dementia. H. Steele, Phibbs, and Woods (2004) studied a small group ($N = 17$) of daughters caring for mothers with dementia. The AAI was administered to the daughters while the mothers waited in an adjoining room, and the most important ratings—coherence of transcript, together with coherence of mind (which additionally takes into account "irrational" even if brief intrusions into coherence, such as those seen in unresolved speech)—were examined. Upon reunion, the researchers assessed mothers' joyfulness, proximity seeking, contact maintenance, and overall responsiveness to reunion with their adult daughters now serving as caregiving figures. These indices of reunion security were each significantly correlated with the adult daughters' coherence of transcript and coherence of mind. (See Magai, Chapter 24, this volume, for discussion of attachment and the normative role reversal that occurs between aging parents and their adult children.)

Blind or Deaf Individuals. In a recent overview of clinical studies, van IJzendoorn and Bakermans-Kranenburg (2008) included as a control group individuals who (although not screened as such) were identified as suffering from physical rather than emotional or psychological impairments. Even in a four-way analysis, blind or deaf individuals were as likely to be secure as those in low-risk samples; indeed, security (over 60% secure in the four-way analysis) was, if anything, somewhat elevated. In one study, for example (McKinnon, Moran, & Pederson, 2004), normative results for AAI coherence and secure classificatory status were obtained for 50 adults whose AAIs were conducted in American Sign Language. These results were obtained not only despite hearing loss, but also in the face of long-term separations from parents, in conjunction with placement (beginning in middle childhood) in residential schools for deaf persons. Examples of loving, albeit nonverbal, behavior of parents (who were restricted from attempting substitute forms of linguistic contact) in the early years of life were convincingly described. As van IJzendoorn and Bakermans-Kranenburg conclude, the findings from blind and deaf populations provide an important corroboration for the discriminant validity of the AAI, since persons suffering from psychological difficulties have been found to be insecure on the AAI, but persons with physical impairments have not.

Intervention Studies

One of the most important uses of the AAI has been in intervention studies, two of which I described in 1999 (Fonagy et al., 1996; Korfmacher, Adam, Ogawa, & Egeland, 1997). I now briefly review four further investigations of interventions. First, Heinicke and colleagues (2006; see also Heinicke & Levine, 2008) used the AAI as a prebirth assessment for 57 high-risk mothers in an intervention project involving multiple forms of assistance, including weekly home visits for the first 2 years of life. At the end of the second year, an individual unacquainted with the dyad visited each home. This visitor (1) assessed varying aspects of maternal and child behavior (especially "child's expectation of care," measured with a scale that had proven valuable in previous work by this team), and (2) administered Waters's Observer Attachment Q-Sort. A regression analysis showed that a combined unresolved trauma/coherence scale from the prebirth AAI was the best predictor of toddler security assessed 2 years later. In addition, this combination of AAI scales predicted a mother's observed responsiveness to her 24-month-old. As in Korfmacher and colleagues' (1997) study, a mother's trauma/coherence on the prebirth AAI predicted the mother's involvement in the work of intervention from 6 months onward, and such involvement was significantly associated with positive 24-month outcomes. Put another way, the more coherent the mothers were, and the lower the scores they had received for unresolved trauma before their children's birth, the more they were able to involve themselves in the work of intervention from 6 months forward, and the more responsive they were to their children's needs at 24 months. The same (combined) variable predicted child security and expectation of care. In an in-

triguing analysis by AAI classification, Heinicke and colleagues (2006) also found that unresolved/secure mothers were the most involved in the work of intervention; that their toddlers were as secure by 24 months as were the offspring of secure mothers; and that, as would be expected, the toddlers of unresolved/dismissing and unresolved/preoccupied mothers fared worst.

Taking a different point of entry with the AAI and intervention, Levy and colleagues (2006) administered a preintervention AAI to patients with borderline personality disorder, and a second AAI following 1 year of therapy. Of the 90 participants, 30 were randomly assigned to transference-focused therapy as developed by Kernberg (1984), 30 to Linehan's (1993) dialectical behavior therapy, and 30 to supportive therapy. As predicted in advance, given the representational and relational focus of transference-focused therapy, significant change in AAI status—specifically, increases in coherence of transcript, and a more than threefold increase in number of patients coded as secure-autonomous—was established for this form of therapy. Scores for reflective functioning as seen in the AAIs (Fonagy, Steele, Steele, & Target, 1998) were also significantly increased for this group. Therapy did not reduce scores for unresolved trauma, however. Note that Moran and his colleagues in Canada (Moran, Bailey, Gleason, DeOliveira, & Pederson, 2008) also had limited success in increasing maternal sensitivity and infant Strange Situation security, due to the fact that their video feedback interventions were not successful for unresolved mothers, whose infants remained disorganized.

Recently, Bick and Dozier (2008) presented aspects of their work with 200 foster parents who were administered the AAI in conjunction with Dozier's Attachment and Biobehavioral Catch-Up Program. Just over half of these foster parents were classified as secure. One of the special features of this intervention program is that the interveners conduct the AAI at program outset, and use it both to establish rapport and to guide the continuing intervention process. Intriguing differences corresponding with AAI status occurred in responses to intervention attempts, as well as in observed behavior with the foster infants. During the intervention, as in their AAIs, foster mothers with secure-autonomous transcripts were cooperative and collaborative, and were described as exhibiting high levels of metacognitive monitoring, coherence, and openness to discussing potentially painful or sensitive topics. Foster mothers with dismissing transcripts tended to resist discussing relationship difficulties as well as the children's need for nurturance. In contrast, those classified as preoccupied on the AAI seemed relatively comfortable describing their attachment-related pasts, but this sometimes became the primary focus of the session. Foster mothers with preoccupied transcripts were described as fluctuating between seeking reassurance from the intervener and displaying annoyance, while their own concerns sometimes seemed to take precedence over those of their infants. Finally, caregivers unresolved with regard to loss or trauma seemed to have trouble developing trust in their trainers and commitment to the treatment program. In addition, they seemed to have difficulties discussing ways in which they might have been frightened as children, and within sessions had difficulty behaving in nonthreatening ways toward children in the home.

Finally, in a new examination of intervention possibilities, AAIs were administered to professional caregivers in institutions, together with institutionalized adolescents in their care (Zegers, Schuengel, van IJzendoorn, & Janssens, 2006). For the first 3 months of the clients' stay in the institution, no effects of caregiver or adolescent AAI security were found. However, after longer periods, more secure mentors were being increasingly perceived as available as a secure base, and more secure adolescents were perceived as increasing their secure-base use of their mentors.

Studies of Peer and Couple Relations

In the first edition of this chapter (Hesse, 1999), I reviewed several studies of peer and couple relations, each of which revealed that individuals with secure-autonomous AAI transcripts engaged in more positive exchanges, whereas in general those with dismissing transcripts displayed hostility, and those with preoccupied transcripts displayed anxiety. The pioneering study in this domain was that of Kobak and Sceery (1988), and similar results have now been reported by Roisman, Madsen, Hennighausen, Sroufe, and Collins (2001), Wampler, Shi, Nelson, and Kimball (2003), and Creasey and Ladd (2005).

Creasey (2002) added to more general findings concerning negative effects on couple interactions for insecurity on the AAI, reporting that individuals who were unresolved but alternatively secure engaged in positive interactions comparable to those of persons who were secure, whereas unresolved/insecure individuals were the most negative in his sample, and exhibited the most controlling behavior (as previously seen in disorganized 6-year-old children observed with their mothers;

Main & Cassidy, 1988). Crowell and colleagues (2002) developed a Secure Base Scoring System for couple interactions, which was used to assess 157 engaged couples. Members of secure couples proved able to use one another as a secure base from which to explore their relationship, and were able to turn to each other even during conflict. Bouthillier, Julien, Dubé, Bélanger, and Harmelin (2002) found that secure AAI classifications predicted proactive emotion regulation during marital conflict, whereas security on self-reported adult attachment questionnaires did not. Interestingly, in a study examining marital perceptions at 3, 12, and 24 months following the birth of a child (the AAI had been administered prenatally), a protective effect of security during stressful periods in the marriage was reported (Paley, Cox, Harter, & Margand, 2002).

Babcock, Jacobsen, Gottman, and Yerington (2000) used the AAI with nonviolent, unhappily married men as well as with violent men; the latter were especially likely to be classified as insecure. In laboratory arguments, secure husbands were, interestingly, the most defensive, whereas dismissing husbands were the most controlling and distancing, and preoccupied husbands the least distancing. In the home, wife withdrawal predicted battering for the preoccupied husbands, suggesting violent responses to abandonment fears. For dismissing husbands, wife defensiveness rather than wife withdrawal was a significant predictor of battering, suggesting use of violence to assert authority and control.

In a Minnesota study, Roisman and colleagues (2001) examined observational assessments of parent–child interactions at 13 years of age, AAIs conducted at age 19, and observed dyadic behaviors with romantic partners 1–2 years later. As expected, AAIs at age 19 predicted the quality of romantic partner interactions. In addition, however, the AAI was found to mediate the across-time correlation between parent–child behaviors at age 13 and romantic relationship behaviors in young adulthood (ages 20–21), suggesting to these authors that "salient parent–child experiences" were being internalized and on that basis carried forward into adult relationships.

In Israel, Mayseless and Sharf (2007) administered the AAI to 80 young men and interviewed them regarding their capacity for intimacy 4 years later. Questionnaires were used as well. Secure states of mind 4 years previously predicted capacities not only for romantic intimacy, but also for intimacy with friends. Furman (2001) modeled a Friendship Interview after the AAI, creating a similar scoring system, and using it with 68 high school seniors. Ratings of dyadic support from friends were related to secure working models of friendships, whereas dismissing friendship models were inversely related to dyadic support from friends. In a second study of the same group of high school seniors (Furman, Simon, Shaffer, & Bouchey, 2002), working models of friendships were related to models of romantic relationships and to relationships with parents (using the AAI); however, working models of parents and of romantic relationships were inconsistently related.

Using a sample of 11th-grade students (N = 189, 118 girls) in a large metropolitan area, Dykas, Ziv, and Cassidy (2008) examined how adolescents' AAI classifications were linked to various peer perceptions of adolescent behavior toward classmates and adolescent social status (i.e., social acceptance, social behavior). This was the first AAI study to assess multiple aspects of peer relations with a standard battery of peer report measures, in keeping with the established peer research tradition, and data were collected from 1,881 classmates. Because only 9% of these young people were classified as preoccupied, unresolved, or cannot classify, analyses focused exclusively on comparisons between adolescents whose AAI transcripts had been classified as either secure-autonomous or dismissing. Secure-autonomous adolescents were more likely than insecure-dismissing adolescents to be socially accepted by their peers, and also to be perceived as behaving prosocially. In contrast, dismissing adolescents were more likely than secure adolescents to be perceived as aggressive. Somewhat surprisingly, dismissing adolescents were also seen as more shy/withdrawn and more victimized by peers. The finding related to victimization was particularly notable, because no published study had previously examined whether adolescents' AAI classifications are linked to negative treatment by peers.

Two recent studies have used the AAI in a critical new context, examining the extent to which attachment representations are generalized to new social situations and guide behavior even during initial interactions with unfamiliar others. In one study, Roisman (2006) examined interactions between 50 same-sex stranger dyads (half women). Dyads were asked to participate in a "challenging" laboratory joint puzzle-building task. Analyses conducted after controlling for the Big Five personality dimensions revealed attachment-related differences. Secure participants demonstrated positive engagement during the task, preoccupied adults dominated the task, and dismissing adults demonstrated negative emotion. A second study examined 135 high school students who participated with unfamiliar peers in two laboratory tasks: one in which they were asked to seek support when discussing topics typically of concern to adolescents, and the other in which they were asked to provide support (Feeney, Cassidy, & Ramos-Marcuse, in press). AAI scores for coherence of mind (used in this study as the index of AAI attachment security) were predictive of behaviors exhibited during the discussions. Adolescents with higher AAI coherence scores were more likely to seek support and more receptive to the support attempts of the unfamiliar peer. With regard to support-giving behavior, adolescents with higher AAI coherence scores were less self-focused and more sensitive/responsive during the discussion. Moreover, adolescents with low AAI coherence scores strongly reciprocated expressions of negative/hostile affect from the peer during both interactions, whereas adolescents with high AAI coherence scores did not. In both of these studies, then, it was shown that even at a first meeting with another person, states of mind regarding early attachment relations with parents are evident.

Longitudinal Studies

Many kinds of longitudinal studies predictive of eventual AAI status could of course be conducted. As one example, Beckwith, Cohen, and Hamilton (1999) found that maternal insensitivity in the early months predicted dismissing AAI status at age 18. Because of limited space, however, I focus here on studies that have compared infant Strange Situation behavior with the mother to AAI status determined for the same individuals in young adulthood, and I confine even the majority of these descriptions to a secure–insecure analysis. A few of these studies were reviewed earlier (Hesse, 1999).

Four U.S. longitudinal studies have been undertaken, each indicating significant infancy-to-adulthood links. Waters, Merrick, Treboux, Crowell, and Albersheim (2000) conducted AAIs with 50 lower- to middle-class young adults seen in the Ainsworth Strange Situation at 12 months. For 72% of participants (kappa = .44, p < .001), secure versus insecure infant Strange Situation behavior was predictive of secure versus insecure AAI texts 19–21 years later. This correspondence was somewhat higher (78%; kappa = .52) when participants experiencing intervening trauma were eliminated. In the same year, Hamilton (2000) reported on the predictability of AAI responses in a sample of 30 adolescents (ages 17–19) who had been raised in unconventional settings (e.g., communal living groups). The two-way (secure vs. insecure) correspondence in this study was 77% (kappa = .49).

Using a sample of 42 participants (with some few remaining to be coded, dependent upon recovery of tapes following a mechanical defect), Main and her colleagues (Main, 2001; Main et al., 2005) compared Strange Situation classifications with mothers at 12–18 months of age to AAI status as assessed at age 19. As in Waters and colleagues' (2000) original study, a highly significant secure–insecure match was found across the 18-year period. Among the 12 participants coded as disorganized/secure during infancy, and as predicted in advance, none were secure on the AAI at age 19. Intriguingly, although most avoidant infants had become dismissing, about half of the previously disorganized infants had become dismissing as well.

In the earlier edition of this chapter, I included a first report from the Minnesota Study of Risk and Adaptation from Birth to Adulthood (57 subjects; Weinfield, Sroufe, & Egeland, 2000). The researchers had used the traditional three-way analysis of behavior in the Strange Situation (disorganized/secure infants were considered secure), and no significant relation between 12-month attachment status and AAI status at age 19 was found. Since then, more participants have been seen in the AAI (N = 125); disorganized/secure infants have been placed in the insecure infant group; and the sample has been followed to age 26. A significant 18-month Strange Situation to 26-year secure–insecure match has now been reported (p < .001), although the match from 12 months appears to remain insignificant. Interestingly, as in the Bay Area study of middle-class dyads, in this low-income sample disorganized/secure infants were only rarely found to be secure in adulthood (Sroufe et al., 2005).

Three studies conducted outside the United States have yielded insignificant relations between Strange Situation responses and AAI status in young adulthood. These include both the Regensburg and Bielefeld longitudinal studies (in which, however, disorganized/secure infants were coded as secure) as described by Grossmann, Grossmann, and Kindler (2005), and the Haifa longitudinal study (Sagi-Schwartz & Aviezer, 2005), in which the infant disorganized category seems not to have been used. Although it should be noted that only the three-way infant analysis was available to Waters and colleagues (2000) and to Hamilton

(2000) as well, it would be prudent to await a four-way analysis of infant Strange Situation responses before final conclusions are drawn regarding the German and Israeli studies.

The Concept of "Earned" Security as Inferred from the AAI

In 1999, "earned" security was just emerging as a topic within the AAI literature. The concept had originated in early AAI manuals and training institutes, which stressed that placement of texts in the secure-autonomous classification is based solely on coherence scores. Thus, it was emphasized that coherent, collaborative speakers could be judged secure-autonomous despite the coder's estimates that during childhood parents did not show loving behavior, and such transcripts were informally identified as "earned-secure." Unfortunately, no precise cutoff criteria for distinguishing earned security were provided until 1998, where a criterion of loving scores of 2.5 or below on the 9-point scale for both parents was used (recently modified to scores of 3 or below—Jacobvitz, 2008; Main, Goldwyn, & Hesse, 2008). As noted earlier, scores of 3 are assigned when a parent is seen by the coder as providing instrumental attention and assistance during childhood, *without* indices of actively loving behavior, such as reliable physical affection, forgiving misbehavior, or defending the child to others (e.g., teachers). In contrast, these indices of actively loving behavior must be present in mild form for scores of 5, which is considered sufficiently loving or "good-enough" parenting.

The current criterion for earned-secure AAI status (a coherent transcript, with both parents scoring at 3 or below for loving) was not met by any of the 19-year-old participants in the Bay Area follow-up study, and it was met extremely rarely in two other studies of participants averaging 19 years of age (Roisman, Fortuna, & Holland, 2006; Roisman, Padrón, Sroufe, & Egeland, 2002). The fact that few adolescents are judged earned-secure is probably not surprising, but suggests that given current criteria the investigation of earned security will be most feasible within samples of post-college-age adults.

Two investigations of this kind have been completed, each utilizing a cross-sectional design. Caspers, Yucuis, Troutman, and Spinks (2006) found that continuous-secure adults (identified through loving scores of 5 or above for both parents) were less likely than both insecure and earned-secure adults to abuse alcohol or other substances. However, earned-secure adults (N = 25, identified as both parents scoring at 2.5 or below for loving behavior) were more likely to have entered psychotherapy than either dismissing or continuous-secure participants. Jacobvitz (2008; see also Jacobvitz, Booher, & Hazen, 2001) also found that earned-secure adults (both parents scoring at 3 or below for loving behavior) had spent more time in therapy than either continuous-secure or insecure participants. During couple interactions, earned-secure participants were observed to more frequently reflect in the moment and appropriately modify their behavior in accordance with partner response than were continuous-secure or insecure participants—and to do so even during conflict. Thus some advantage in partner interactions appeared to accrue to coherent adults who had been inferred to have had notably difficult childhoods.

Prior to the implementation of the above guidelines, most investigators studying earned security had essentially divided their secure participants into two groups: those inferred to have had "more" versus "less" loving parents, with the latter usually being identified by one of the parents having received a score either below the sample median or below a score of 5 on the 9-point scale. In the majority of these studies mean scores for the mothers' loving behavior during childhood for participants termed earned-secure have on average been above 5, with many scores of course falling well above 5. Although ideally these might therefore best have been termed studies of participants with parents inferred to have been "more" versus "less" loving, rather than studies examining continuous- versus earned-secure participants, they have yielded interesting results.

For example, in a pioneering study conducted in 1994, Pearson, Cohn, Cowan, and Cowan found that although earned-secure participants scored higher on a depression inventory than did their continuous-secure counterparts, they were equally warm toward their 42-month-old offspring and equally providing of structure. Some years later, Phelps, Belsky, and Crnic (1998) found that self-reported "daily hassles" were not higher for earned-secure than other mothers, helping to rule out a possible "depressogenic" hypothesis that earned-secure mothers tended simply to report their experiences as being worse than did others. In addition, they found that earned-secure mothers' sensitivity to offspring held up even under high-stress conditions. Paley, Cox, Burchinal, and Payne (1999) found that earned-secure wives were no less positive and no more negative than continuous-secure wives in marital interactions. Wives responded less positively, however, to earned-secure than continuous-secure husbands.

Roisman and colleagues (2002) inspected longitudinal data from 19-year-olds in a Minnesota high-risk sample. In this study, transcripts where one parent (usually the father) fell below 5 on the loving scale were defined as earned-secure. The mean loving scores for mothers of participants identified as earned-secure was 5.46, whereas for continuous-secure participants the mean loving score for mothers was one point higher, or 6.50. In contrast, mean father-loving scores for the two groups differed substantially, being 2.56 for earned-secures and 5.73 for continuous-secures. Thus identified, earned-secure status was not significantly associated with having been insecure with mother in the Strange Situation at either 12 or 18 months, although it should be noted that the disorganized category was not utilized, so that disorganized/secure infants would have been coded as secure. In addition, earned-secure status at age 19 was not associated with significantly less positive (nor with significantly more positive) observed interactions with mother at 24 or 42 months of age, or at age 13.

It would be premature to conclude from this study, however, that AAI scores for parental loving are unrelated to childhood experiences, thereby making retrospective earned-secure assignments invalid. This is because (a) security or insecurity in infancy was identified only on the basis of Strange Situation classification with *mother*, yet (b) retrospective insecurity appears to have been determined mainly on the basis of inferred early insecurity with *father*. For the same reason, observations of father–child interactions would have been necessary to deciding whether earned-secure status did or did not correspond significantly with observed early experience.

In a recent experimental study, Roisman and colleagues (2006) attempted to induce sad or happy moods just before administering the AAI, asking participants to focus for 10 minutes on an autobiographical memory relevant to achieving a sad (or happy) state. Sad (or happy) music was played during this period, and participants were urged to achieve a mood state as intense and as real as possible. Participants were identified as earned secure if they were coherent during the AAI and if one of the two parents had received a loving score below 5, and a score above 5 for rejecting or neglecting behavior. The remaining coherent participants were regarded as continuous secure.

With the earned- versus continuous-secure categories thus defined, placement in the earned-versus continuous-secure categories was impressively related to induced mood. The mood induction procedures did not, however, affect insecure speakers, and in interpreting this finding, Roisman and colleagues (2006; see also Sroufe & Waters, 1977) suggested that perhaps only secure speakers have the ability to "tune behavior and emotion properly to contextual demands." Importantly, however, and as the investigators emphasize, coherence scores—the heart of the AAI scoring procedure—were not affected by induced mood.

It should be noted, however, that induced sad moods in this study did not in fact lead to earned-secure status as identified by loving scores of 3 or below for both parents. In the sad condition, mean father-loving scores for secure participants were at 4.45 (SD = 1.74), or on average well above 3. Also in the sad condition, the mean for mother-loving scores was 5.52 (which is, again, considered "good-enough" parenting), and readily ranged to above 7 (SD = 1.66). Thus, even in the sad condition, mother-loving scores for secure participants remained at the average for most samples, with many secure participants' mothers scoring well above it.

As yet, then, the degree to which earned-secure status reflects actual adverse experiences in childhood remains, as previously (Hesse, 1999), an open question. Currently, however, no evidence has emerged to counter the proposition that, strictly defined, earned-secure status will be found to represent a coherent AAI description of an insecure childhood. Another presently unanswered question is whether the induction of sad moods in persons with secure-autonomous status can reduce parental loving scores sufficiently to ensure that loving behavior on the part of both parents would appear inadequate.

The first of these issues will ultimately be resolved by prospective or longitudinal studies that follow participants beyond late adolescence, so that individuals insecure in adolescence will have had the opportunity to form a coherent representation of their lives despite early adverse experiences with parents. The second can be addressed by new mood induction studies, perhaps optimally by asking adult participants to focus on sad versus happy prospective events rather than elements from their autobiographies. However, many other approaches to the investigation of earned security (using current guidelines) should be undertaken as well and will likely continue to provide interesting outcomes, as has been demonstrated in the two recent cross-sectional studies of adult populations described earlier (Caspers et al., 2006: Jacobvitz,

2008). Finally, pre- to post-therapy studies that show moves from insecure to secure-autonomous attachment status (see Levy et al., 2006) appear to trace one developmental pathway to earned security within adulthood, and can also make an important contribution to our understanding of this intriguing topic.

Studies of Emotion and Emotion Regulation

The concept of "conditional behavioral strategies"—according to which individuals may be enabled through natural selection to reach the same biological ends by differing behavioral pathways, depending on circumstances—is widespread in evolutionary thinking, and Main (1990; see also Main, 1981) extended this thinking to the organized patterns of infant attachment. Specifically, Main proposed that secure infants use a primary behavioral strategy for maintaining proximity to the attachment figure(s). In contrast, she suggested that insecure infants may manipulate the level of behavioral output usually called for by the attachment system through secondary, or conditional, strategies that act to minimize or maximize that output in order to increase or maintain proximity to a caregiver who responds preferentially to indices of offspring independence or offspring dependence. Attentional/cognitive mechanisms were seen as potentially assisting offspring in minimizing or maximizing their behavioral output relative to what the system might call for at a given moment.

A few years later, Cassidy (1994) further extended this reasoning to affective responses on the part of both mother and child, and specifically to emotion regulation. This extension has been widely applied to understanding relations between attachment and emotion regulation as behaviorally expressed. Another extension of Main's (1990) reasoning is seen in the construction of Kobak's (1993) Attachment Q-Sort, which is used to score AAI interviews in terms of "hyperactivating" and "deactivating" dimensions.

The study of the AAI in relation to emotions may have begun with the work of Slade and her colleagues (Slade, Belsky, Aber, & Phelps, 1999; see also Haft & Slade, 1989), who used the AAI with 125 mothers of first-born sons, in conjunction with a Parent Development Interview (PDI) and direct observations of mothering behavior. Mothers whose transcripts were classified as secure-autonomous scored highest on the joy-pleasure/coherence dimension of the PDI, and dismissing mothers scored highest on the anger dimension.

Coping and expectations of abilities to regulate emotions were examined in two other investigations using the AAI. In a study of 88 young soldiers in Israel, Scharf, Mayseless, and Kivenson-Baron (2004) found that—according to their own reports and those of friends—secure-autonomous soldiers were able to cope better with basic training than were soldiers who were classified as insecure on the AAI. In Illinois, Creasey and Ladd (2004) reported that attachment representations moderated the association between negative mood regulation expectancies and conflict management tactics actually displayed in romantic relationships. In a small study employing the Facial Action Coding System (FACS; Ekman & Friesen, 1978) for facial expressions of emotion during videotaped AAIs (N = 14 "healthy" women), Buchheim and Benecke (2007) found that "genuine," or "Duchenne," smiles were more frequent among secure participants, who also showed positive facial affect more broadly. M. Steele, Steele, and Johansson (2002) found that mothers' secure-autonomous prebirth AAIs were linked to their 11-year-old children's acknowledgement of a pictured child's distress in peer–family situations.

DeOliveira, Moran, and Pederson (2005) followed up Cassidy's (1994) proposals regarding linkages between attachment and emotion regulation in a study of 90 adolescent mothers, linking the AAI with self-reported depressive symptomatology (Radloff, 1977) when the infants were 6 months of age, and to Gottman's metaemotion interview (Katz, Gottman, Shapiro, & Carrère, 1997) when their offspring had reached age 2. All preoccupied mothers were also unresolved, so that group differences could be assessed only for the secure-autonomous, dismissing, and unresolved AAI categories. Both dismissing and unresolved mothers had significantly higher levels of depression than autonomous mothers, and clinical depression was found in 12% of autonomous, 45% of dismissing, and 46% of unresolved mothers. Since most of the mothers were impoverished and/or single (not living in common-law relationships or marriages), perhaps the most surprising finding was the protective quality of secure-autonomous status. It is also notable that unresolved mothers reported significantly more affective/internalizing symptoms than either dismissing or autonomous mothers, whereas the dismissing and unresolved mothers reported significantly more somatic/externalizing symptoms.

In terms of mindset or awareness of their own emotions, secure mothers in this study showed the most awareness of, as well as acceptance of, fear. They also showed the greatest awareness of anger among the three groups of mothers, whereas their overall emotional regulation was better than that of unresolved mothers. With respect to fear, one dismissing mother said, "I'm not sure ... I don't really think about it. ... If I think about it, it gets worse ... so I just ignore it and it goes away" (DeOliveira et al., 2005, p. 165). In terms of responses to the *children's* emotions, secure mothers were more responsive to fear than the dismissing mothers, more responsive to anger than the unresolved mothers, and more responsive to sadness than were either dismissing or unresolved mothers. As an example of unresolved mothers' difficulties in responding to their children's anger, one mother described herself as feeling "um, uncontrollable, like I feel like I, I, I've, I have no control over her sometimes when she's angry. Um, helpless, helpless, like I mean she's angry a lot of the time" (p. 167).

Roisman, Tsai, and Chiang (2004) assessed Kobak's "hyperactivating versus deactivating" (dismissing vs. preoccupied) Q-sort dimensions, but used only coders (N = 3) who had previously been certified in Main and Goldwyn's (1998) AAI classification and scoring system. The AAI was administered to 30 European Americans and 30 Chinese Americans between 18 and 30 years of age. Physiological responses were recorded throughout the AAI, and every facial event was coded with the FACS. Interview participants were also given a self-report inventory consisting of 25 emotion terms to indicate how they felt during the interview.

In a replication and extension of Dozier and Kobak's (1992) pioneering work, elevation of skin conductance was found to be specifically associated with deactivating (dismissing) participants, whose skin conductance rose robustly from baseline as the interview progressed. Neither deactivation nor security (absence of marked hyperactivation or deactivation) was associated with the frequency of either positive or negative emotions expressed during the interview (as recorded with the FACS), but preoccupation/hyperactivation was significantly correlated with the frequency of negative expressions. Self-reported emotions ascribed to the experience of undertaking the AAI showed that only preoccupation/hyperactivation was marginally associated (negatively) with self-reported positive emotion. Security was associated with marginally less, and preoccupation with significantly more, negative emotional engagement during the interview. Despite the persistent rises in skin conductance suggestive of emotional suppression found for dismissing/deactivating speakers, dismissing orientations were not associated with self-reported negative (or positive) emotion regarding the experience.

One of the most impressive findings to emerge from this study was based on an item analysis of the Q-sort, in which positive or negative valence of childhood experiences as found in the AAIs was determined and assessed. As predicted, security was associated with matches in behaviorally (facially) expressed positive emotion and positive childhood experiences, as well as congruence between negative facial expressions and negative inferred childhood experience. In contrast, in all but one test, preoccupation was associated with discrepancies between emotion and inferred childhood experience. In summarizing the study, Roisman and colleagues (2004) suggest that "a key variable that makes secure, preoccupied, and dismissing adults different is the way that their emotional responses are tied to the valence of their memories regarding childhood experiences. Whereas secure adults appear to be 'in sync' with their recalled pasts, dismissing and preoccupied individuals do not present as emotionally integrated" (p. 788). Dismissing/deactivating participants showed subtle signs of covert emotional suppression as evidenced by electrodermal reactivity during the AAI, and preoccupied/hyperactivating adults showed reliable discrepancies. Thus only secure participants expressed and reported emotion consistent with their inferred childhood experiences (positive or negative) and their expressed as well as self-reported emotion during the AAI.

Endocrinology, Cognitive Performance, and Neuroscience

In three studies conducted at Berkeley, HPA functioning, cognitive performance, and EEG responses have been found related to AAI status. Blount-Matthews (2004) found as predicted that when the word "mother" (but not "basket" or "betray") was used as a subliminal prime, the time taken to complete a lexical decision task was significantly slowed for preoccupied, but not for dismissing or secure, participants. This AAI study provides empirical support for the notion of interference with cognitive processes via unseen attachment-related "triggers."

Rifkin-Graboi (2008) examined cortisol output in college-age men. Home assays showed little relation to overall AAI security, although passivity of discourse was significantly positively related

to elevated cortisol during the evening and night collections. In the laboratory, participants were presented with both cognitive and attachment-related challenges, the latter presenting hypothetical situations involving separation, loss, and abandonment. As expected, scores for idealization of the parents were associated with a significant rise in cortisol specific to the interpersonal (attachment) challenge.

Gribneau (2006) presented four categories of images (social positive, nature positive, blatant death/dying, and quiet cemetery images) to women who had experienced loss, half of whom (16/31) had been coded as unresolved/disorganized. As predicted, event-related potentials (ERP) demonstrated increased physiological responses to quiet cemetery images specific to unresolved women, with the anterior N2 ERP component indicating involuntary attention. A developing right-sided asymmetrical (P3 ERP) component toward all images also appeared specifically in the unresolved women.

CONCLUSIONS

With the exception of a summarized review of the pre-1999 research literature, this chapter has departed from my earlier discussion of the AAI (Hesse, 1999) in several ways. I have endeavored here to make the AAI far more accessible, both to the reader coming to the topic for the first time and to one having some familiarity with the literature who nonetheless has not been trained in the scoring and classification system (Main et al., 2003). As I reread the previous chapter prior to writing this one, I became acutely aware of how remote the AAI itself seemed to remain, despite the extensive discussion of many of its qualities and correlates. I concluded that with the increasing interest in the instrument, it has become critical for readers to gain a "living sense" of both what the AAI actually is (as provided by direct text examples) and how the process of scoring and classifying an AAI text is actually undertaken. This discussion has necessitated an extensive elaboration of both Main's (1993, 2000) views regarding attentional processes, and the work of Grice (1975, 1989).

In addition, I have said more than previously about scale scores (the continuous dimensions of the scoring system) and have presented the AAI subcategories for the first time. In future studies, I hope that both scale scores and subcategory placement will appear in print far more frequently, thereby providing a more refined understanding of processes related to attachment.

The AAI is a unique research tool with the power to tap into multiple psychological and social domains, a point that has been made amply clear by the massive expansion in research since 1999. Nevertheless, there is room for further exploration utilizing the AAI in new areas, including linguistics and, as just illustrated, cognitive psychology, biology, and neuroscience (see also Coan, Chapter 11, this volume). In 1999 I had concluded that:

> Within the AAI, the organization of language pertaining to attachment appears to be a manifestation of the "dynamics" of cognition and emotion as mediated by attention. Individual differences in attentional flexibility may therefore influence patterns of caregiving, which in turn may shape responses in the offspring that influence the organization of its own developing propensities. [T]his has no doubt permanently altered the way language will be considered within the context of clinical and developmental research. (pp. 427–428)

Happily, almost a decade later I find no need to revise or modify this statement in any way.

APPENDIX 25.1.
THE ADULT ATTACHMENT INTERVIEW: ADMINISTRATION AND TRAINING

Protocol

The most recent AAI protocol (George, Kaplan, & Main, 1996; 72 manuscript pages) is available from Erik Hesse or Mary Main at the Department of Psychology, 3210 Tolman Hall, University of California, Berkeley, CA 94720 (fax: 510-642-5293). Although it is strongly recommended that practice in the administration of the AAI take place under the guidance of an experienced coder, no special training institutes are required.

Training in the Scoring and Classification of AAI Transcripts

Training in the analysis of the AAI takes place in a 2-week institute, involving one or two certified trainers and 10–20 participants. Usually about seven institutes focused on the Main, Goldwyn, and Hesse system of interview analysis are offered per year. These are taught only by the 11 individuals who have become certified to train via (1) participation in two full conventional institutes

and (2) 2–3 weeks of participation in "training-to-train" institutes held by Mary Main and myself. These are Anders Broberg, *Anders.Broberg@psy. gu.se*; Nino Dazzi, *Nino.Dazzi@uniroma1.it*; Sonia Gojman de Millán, *sgojman@yahoo.com*; Erik Hesse, fax: 510-642-5293; Tord Ivarsson, *Tord. Ivarsson@vgregion.se*; Deborah Jacobvitz, *debj@ mail.utexas.edu*; Nancy Kaplan, *Nancy_Kaplan@ hotmail.com*; Mary Main, fax: 510-642-5293; David and Deanne Pederson, *Pederson@uwo.ca*; and June Sroufe, *jsroufe@visi.com*. Trainings are frequently offered in North America, England, Italy, Mexico, and Scandinavia.

Those wishing to become certified in the analysis of AAI transcripts not only must attend an AAI institute with one of the trainers listed above, but must also pass a reliability check in which agreement is established with Main and myself across 30 transcripts. The certification rate is high, and 50 new coders were certified in 2007. At present, trainings in the newer forms of cannot classify identification are being planned.

ACKNOWLEDGMENTS

Parts of this chapter have been adapted from Main, Hesse, and Goldwyn (2008). Copyright 2008 by The Guilford Press. Adapted by permission. I am grateful to Mary Main for her assistance and encouragement. Jennifer Arter contributed her considerable computer skills. David and Deanne Pederson made valuable suggestions regarding aspects of the presentation, as did Nino Dazzi, Avi Sagi-Schwartz, and Marinus van IJzendoorn.

NOTES

1. As noted in Appendix 25.1, copies of the full AAI protocol can be obtained from the author at the Department of Psychology, University of California, Berkeley, CA 94720. Requests may also be sent by fax to me (510-642-5293).
2. Violations of these maxims are permitted when "licensed" by the speaker (Grice, 1989; Mura, 1983). An excessively long speech turn can, for example, be licensed if the speaker begins with "Well, I'm afraid this is going to be quite a long story," whereas a very short turn can be licensed by "I'm really sorry, but I don't feel able to discuss this right now." "Dramatic license," though referenced here, is not an aspect of Mura's licensing strictures, but is used occasionally to interpret acceptable present-tense misusages within the AAI system (Main et al., 2003).
3. In the 1999 version of this chapter, I described an Italian study in which coders attempted to apply Grice's four maxims to AAI interview transcripts

(Dazzi, DeCoro, Ortu, & Speranza, 1999). Following Gricean maxims as closely as possible, but adding where necessary from the AAI manual (e.g., "passivity" indicators were added directly as violations of manner), these investigators found that, as stated in this chapter, violations of manner were most pronounced in dismissing texts, and violations of quantity, relevance, and manner were evident in preoccupied texts, whereas relatively few violations occurred in secure-autonomous texts. More recently, a group of investigators in Leiden have developed a Coherence Q-Sort, and have found that attachment-trained sorters place emphasis on different maxims than do naive sorters or linguists; this means that training in AAI institutes remains a necessary prerequisite to identifying the kinds of coherence most relevant to AAI texts (Beijersbergen, Bakermans-Kranenburg, & van IJzendoorn, 2006).

4. I have composed the quotations in this chapter, to preserve confidentiality. Nonetheless, they closely approximate actual quotations from AAI transcripts, and none would seem unusual to an experienced AAI coder.

5. This response is more elaborated than usual, but it has been seen in some interviews and is provided here for heuristic purposes.

6. This does not mean that the same speaker might not also be unresolved/disorganized (see "Empirical Studies Involving the AAI," below).

7. Within AAI manuals the development sample has been accurately described as consisting of 44 participants. However, Main and Goldwyn (1988) had referenced only the initial 36.

8. Notice that, as is the case for infant Strange Situation coding, interview transcripts are always approached first to determine the best-fitting organized category. If the first AAI category placement will ultimately be unresolved/disorganized or unorganized (cannot classify), the coder must nonetheless designate the organized category that the transcript may fit (e.g., unresolved/dismissing). The same holds for the Strange Situation, in which an infant judged primarily disorganized is also assigned to a best-fitting organized category (e.g., disorganized/avoidant).

9. The article on which this brief review is largely based was accepted for publication by a leading American Psychological Association journal in 1988, but the authors withheld the manuscript awaiting replication. The still-unpublished manuscript has been frequently cited and is available from me.

10. For both mothers and fathers, as would be expected, coherence of transcript was significantly negatively related to infant avoidance, as was angry preoccupation with either parent, except fathers' preoccupation with their mothers.

11. In a high-risk clinical sample of 37 participants followed across 13 years by Crowell and Hauser (2008), secure–insecure stability was 84%; however, all but 2 participants were insecure at both time periods, and there was considerable movement among the insecure AAI categories.

12. This effect was necessarily calculated on the basis of only 10 studies and 384 dyads.

13. It should be noted, however, that in this 1995 meta-analysis, secure-autonomous parents were usually judged to be warmer toward their offspring than were other parents.

REFERENCES

Abrams, K. Y., Rifkin, A., & Hesse, E. (2006). Examining the role of parental frightened/frightening subtypes in predicting disorganized attachment within a brief observational procedure. *Development and Psychopathology*, 18, 345–361.

Adshead, G., & Bluglass, K. (2005). Attachment representations in mothers with abnormal illness behaviour by proxy. *British Journal of Psychiatry*, 187, 328–333.

Ainsworth, M. D. S. (1967). *Infancy in Uganda: Infant care and the growth of love*. Baltimore: Johns Hopkins University Press.

Ainsworth, M. D. S., Bell, S. M., & Stayton, D. J. (1971). Individual differences in Strange Situation behaviour of one-year-olds. In H. R. Schaffer (Ed.), *The origins of human social relations* (pp. 17–57). New York: Academic Press.

Ainsworth, M. D. S., Blehar, M. C., Waters, E., & Wall, S. (1978). *Patterns of attachment: A psychological study of the Strange Situation*. Hillsdale, NJ: Erlbaum.

Ainsworth, M. D. S., & Eichberg, C. G. (1991). Effects on infant–mother attachment of mother's unresolved loss of an attachment figure or other traumatic experience. In C. M. Parkes, J. Stevenson-Hinde, & P. Marris (Eds.), *Attachment across the life cycle* (pp. 160–183). London: Routledge.

Allen, J. P., Hauser, S. T., & Borman-Spurrell, E. (1996). Attachment theory as a framework for understanding sequelae of severe adolescent psychopathology: An eleven-year follow-up study. *Journal of Consulting and Clinical Psychology*, 64, 254–263.

American Psychiatric Association. (1987). *Diagnostic and statistical manual of mental disorders* (3rd ed., rev.). Washington, DC: Author.

Ammaniti, M., Dazzi, N., & Muscetta, S. (2008). The AAI in a clinical context: Some experiences and illustrations. In H. Steele & M. Steele (Eds.), *Clinical applications of the Adult Attachment Interview* (pp. 236–269). New York: Guilford Press.

Ammaniti, M., Speranza, A. M., & Candelori, C. (1996). Stability of attachment in children and intergenerational transmission of attachment. *Psychiatria dell'Infanzia e dell'Adolescenza*, 63, 313–332.

Babcock, J. C., Jacobson, N., Gottman, J., & Yerington, T. P. (2000). Attachment, emotional regulation, and the function of marital violence: Differences between secure, preoccupied, and dismissing violent and non-violent husbands. *Journal of Family Violence*, 15, 391–409.

Bakermans-Kranenburg, M. J., & van IJzendoorn, M. H. (1993). A psychometric study of the Adult Attachment Interview: Reliability and discriminant validity. *Developmental Psychology, 29,* 870–879.

Beckwith, L., Cohen, S. E., & Hamilton, C. E. (1999). Maternal sensitivity during infancy and subsequent life events relate to attachment representation at early adulthood. *Developmental Psychology, 35,* 693–700.

Behrens, K. Y., Hesse, E., & Main, M. (2007). Mothers' attachment status as determined by the Adult Attachment Interview predicts their 6-year-olds' reunion responses: A study conducted in Japan. *Developmental Psychology, 43,* 1553–1567.

Beijersbergen, M. D., Bakermans-Kranenburg, M. J., & van IJzendoorn, M. H. (2006). The concept of coherence in attachment interviews: Comparing attachment experts, linguists, and non-experts. *Attachment and Human Development, 8,* 353–369.

Benoit, D., & Parker, K. C. H. (1994). Stability and transmission of attachment across three generations. *Child Development, 65,* 1444–1456.

Bick, J., & Dozier, M. (2008). Helping foster parents change: The role of parental state of mind. In H. Steele & M. Steele (Eds.), *Clinical applications of the Adult Attachment Interview* (pp. 452–470). New York: Guilford Press.

Blount-Matthews, K. (2004). *Attachment and forgiveness in human development: A multi-method approach.* Unpublished doctoral dissertation, University of California at Berkeley.

Bouthillier, D., Julien, D., Dubé, M., Bélanger, I., & Harmelin, M. (2002). Predictive validity of adult attachment measures in relation to emotion regulation behaviors in marital interactions. *Journal of Adult Development, 9,* 291–305.

Bowlby, J. (1980). *Attachment and loss: Vol. 3. Loss: Sadness and depression.* New York: Basic Books.

Buchheim, A., & Benecke, C. (2007). [Affective facial behavior of patients with anxiety disorders during the Adult Attachment Interview: A pilot study.] *Psychotherapie, Psychosomatik, Medizinische Psychologie, 57,* 343–347.

Buchheim, A., & Kachele, H. (2003). Adult Attachment Interview and psychoanalytic perspective: A single case study. *Psychoanalytic Inquiry, 23,* 81–101.

Bus, A. G., & van IJzendoorn, M. H. (1992). Patterns of attachment in frequently and infrequently reading mother–child dyads. *Journal of Genetic Psychology, 153,* 395–403.

Carlson, E. A. (1998). A prospective longitudinal study of attachment disorganization/disorientation. *Child Development, 69,* 1107–1128.

Carlson, V., Cicchetti, D., Barnett, D., & Braunwald, K. (1989). Disorganized/disoriented attachment relationships in maltreated infants. *Developmental Psychology, 25,* 525–531.

Caspers, K., Yucuis, R., Troutman, B., & Spinks, R. (2006). Attachment as an organizer of behavior: Implications for substance abuse problems and willingness to seek treatment. *Substance Abuse Treatment, Prevention, and Policy, 1,* 1–10.

Cassibba, R., Granqvist, P., Costantini, A., & Gatto, S.

(2007). *Attachment and God representations among devout Catholics: A matched comparison study based on the Adult Attachment Interview.* Manuscript submitted for publication.

Cassidy, J. (1994). Emotion regulation: Influences of attachment relationships. In N. Fox (Ed.), The development of emotion regulation. *Monographs of the Society for Research in Child Development, 59*(2–3, Serial No. 240), 228–283.

Constantino, J. N., Chackes, L. M., Wartner, U. G., Gross, N., Brophy, S. L., Vitale, J., et al. (2006). Mental representations of attachment in identical female twins with and without conduct problems. *Child Psychiatry and Human Development, 37,* 65–72.

Creasey, G. (2002). Association between working models of attachment and conflict management behavior in romantic couples. *Journal of Counseling Psychology, 49,* 365–375.

Creasey, G., & Ladd, A. (2005). Generalized and specific attachment representations: Unique and interactive roles in predicting conflict behaviors in close relationships. *Personality and Social Psychology Bulletin, 31,* 1026–1038.

Crowell, J. A., & Hauser, S. T. (2008). AAIs in a high-risk sample: Stability and relation to functioning from adolescence to 39 years. In H. Steele & M. Steele (Eds.), *Clinical applications of the Adult Attachment Interview* (pp. 341–370). New York: Guilford Press.

Crowell, J. A., Treboux, D., Gao, Y., Fyffe, C., Pan, H., & Waters, E. (2002). Assessing secure-base behavior in adulthood: Development of a measure, links to adult attachment relations, and relations to couples' communication and reports of relationships. *Developmental Psychology, 38,* 679–693.

Crowell, J. A., Waters, E., Treboux, D., O'Connor, E., Colon-Downs, C., Feider, O., et al. (1996). Discriminant validity of the Adult Attachment Interview. *Child Development, 67,* 2584–2599.

Dazzi, N., DeCoro, A., Ortu, F., & Speranza, A. M. (1999). L'intervista sull'attacamento in preadolescenza: Un'analisi della dimensione della coerenza. *Psicologia Clinico dello Sviluppo, 31,* 129–153.

DeOliveira, C. A., Moran, G., & Pederson, D. R. (2005). Understanding the link between maternal adult attachment classifications and thoughts and feelings about emotions. *Attachment and Human Development, 7,* 153–170.

De Wolff, M. S., & van IJzendoorn, M. H. (1997). Sensitivity and attachment: A meta-analysis on parental antecedents of infant attachment. *Child Development, 68,* 571–591.

Dozier, M., & Kobak, R. R. (1992). Psychophysiology in attachment interviews: Converging evidence for deactivating strategies. *Child Development, 63,* 1473–1480.

Dozier, M., Stovall, K. C., Albus, K. E., & Bates, B. (2001). Attachment for infants in foster care: The role of caregiver state of mind. *Child Development, 72,* 1467–1477.

Dykas, M. J., Ziv, Y., & Cassidy, J. (in press). Attachment and peer relations in adolescence. *Attachment and Human Development*.

Eichberg, C. G. (1989). Quality of infant–parent attachment: Related to mother's representation of her own relationship history and childcare attitudes. *Dissertation Abstracts International, 50*(1), 343B.

Ekman, P., & Friesen, W. V. (1978). *Unmasking the face: A guide to recognizing emotions from facial cues*. Englewood Cliffs, NJ: Prentice-Hall.

Evans, E. M. (2008). *Understanding maternal trauma: An investigation of the attachment representations, psychological symptomatology, and interactive behaviour of mothers with a trauma history*. Unpublished doctoral dissertation, University of Western Ontario, London, ON, Canada.

Feeney, B. C., Cassidy, J., & Ramos-Marcuse, F. (in press). The generalization of attachment representations to new social situations: Predicting behavior during initial interactions with strangers. *Journal of Personality and Social Psychology*.

Fonagy, P., Leigh, T., Steele, M., Steele, H., Kennedy, G., Mattoon, M., et al. (1996). The relation of attachment status, psychiatric classification, and response to psychotherapy. *Journal of Consulting and Clinical Psychology, 64*, 22–31.

Fonagy, P., Steele, H., & Steele, M. (1991). Maternal representations of attachment during pregnancy predict the organization of infant–mother attachment at one year of age. *Child Development, 62*, 891–905.

Fonagy, P., Steele, M., Steele, H., & Target, M. (1998). *Reflective-function manual: Version 5.0. For application to the Adult Attachment Interview*. Unpublished manuscript, University College, London.

Forguson, L., & Gopnik, A. (1988). The ontogeny of common sense. In J. W. Astington, P. L. Harris, & D. R. Olson (Eds.), *Developing theories of mind* (pp. 226–243). New York: Cambridge University Press.

Frodi, A., Dernevik, M., Sepa, A., Philipson, J., & Bragesjö, M. (2001). Current attachment representations of incarcerated offenders varying in degree of psychopathy. *Attachment and Human Development, 3*, 269–283.

Furman, W. (2001). Working models of friendships. *Journal of Social and Personal Relationships, 18*, 583–602.

Furman, W., & Simon, V. A. (2004). Concordance in attachment states of mind and styles with respect to fathers and mothers. *Developmental Psychology, 40*, 1239–1247.

Furman, W., Simon, V. A., Shaffer, L., & Bouchey, H. A. (2002). Adolescents' working models and styles for relationships with parents, friends, and romantic partners. *Child Development, 73*(1), 241–255.

Fyffe, C. E., & Waters, E. (1997, April). *Empirical classification of adult attachment status: Predicting group membership*. Paper presented at the biennial meeting of the Society for Research in Child Development, Washington, DC.

George, C., Kaplan, N., & Main, M. (1984). *Adult Attachment Interview protocol*. Unpublished manuscript, University of California at Berkeley.

George, C., Kaplan, N., & Main, M. (1985). *Adult Attachment Interview protocol* (2nd ed.). Unpublished manuscript, University of California at Berkeley.

George, C., Kaplan, N., & Main, M. (1996). *Adult Attachment Interview protocol* (3rd ed.). Unpublished manuscript, University of California at Berkeley.

Gojman de Millán, S., & Millán, S. (2008). The AAI and its contribution to a therapeutic intervention project for violent, traumatized, and suicidal cases. In H. Steele & M. Steele (Eds.), *Clinical applications of the Adult Attachment Interview* (pp. 297–319). New York: Guilford Press.

Granqvist, P., Ivarsson, T., Broberg, A. G., & Hagekull, B. (2007). Examining relations among attachment, religiosity, and New Age spirituality using the Adult Attachment Interview. *Developmental Psychology, 43*, 590–601.

Gribneau, N. (2006). *Event-related potentials to cemetery images distinguish electroencephalogram recordings for women unresolved for loss on the Adult Attachment Interview*. Unpublished doctoral dissertation, Department of Integrative Biology, University of California at Berkeley.

Grice, H. P. (1975). Logic and conversation. In P. Cole & J. L. Moran (Eds.), *Syntax and semantics: Vol. 3. Speech acts* (pp. 41–58). New York, Academic Press.

Grice, H. P. (1989). *Studies in the way of words*. Cambridge, MA: Harvard University Press.

Grossmann, K., Fremmer-Bombik, E., Rudolph, J., & Grossmann, K. (1988). Maternal attachment representations as related to patterns of infant–mother attachment and maternal care during the first year. In R. A. Hinde & J. Stevenson-Hinde (Eds.), *Relationships within families: Mutual influences* (pp. 241–260). Oxford, UK: Clarendon Press.

Grossmann, K., Grossmann, K. E., & Kindler, H. (2005). Early care and the roots of attachment and partnership representations: The Bielefeld and Regensburg longitudinal studies. In K. E. Grossmann, K. Grossmann, & E. Waters (Eds.), *Attachment from infancy to adulthood: The major longitudinal studies* (pp. 98–136). New York: Guilford Press.

Haft, W. L., & Slade, A. (1989). Affect attunement and maternal attachment: A pilot study. *Infant Mental Health Journal, 10*, 157–172.

Hamilton, C. E. (2000). Continuity and discontinuity of attachment from infancy through adolescence. *Child Development, 71*, 690–694.

Hauser, S. T., Golden, E., & Allen, J. P. (2006). Narrative in the study of resilience. *Psychoanalytic Study of the Child, 61*, 205–227.

Heinicke, C. M., Goorsky, M., Levine, M., Ponce, V., Ruth, G., Silverman, M., et al. (2006). Pre- and postnatal antecedents of a home visiting intervention and family developmental outcome. *Infant Mental Health Journal, 27*, 91–119.

Heinicke, C. M., & Levine, S. M. (2008). The AAI anticipates the outcome of a relation-based early intervention. In H. Steele & M. Steele (Eds.),

Clinical applications of the Adult Attachment Interview (pp. 99–125). New York: Guilford Press.

Hesse, E. (1996). Discourse, memory, and the Adult Attachment Interview: A note with emphasis on the emerging cannot classify category. *Infant Mental Health Journal, 17*, 4–11.

Hesse, E. (1999). The Adult Attachment Interview: Historical and current perspectives. In J. Cassidy & P. R. Shaver (Eds.). *Handbook of attachment: Theory, research, and clinical applications* (pp. 395–433). New York: Guilford Press.

Hesse, E., & Main, M. (1999). Second-generation effects of unresolved trauma in non-maltreating parents: Dissociated, frightened, and threatening parental behavior. *Psychoanalytic Inquiry, 19*, 481–540.

Hesse, E., & Main, M. (2000). Disorganized infant, child, and adult attachment: Collapse in behavioral and attentional strategies. *Journal of the American Psychoanalytic Association, 48*, 1097–1127.

Hesse, E., & Main, M. (2006). Frightened, threatening, and dissociative parental behavior in low-risk samples: Description, discussion, and interpretations. *Development and Psychopathology, 18*, 309–343.

Hesse, E., & van IJzendoorn, M. H. (1998). Parental loss of close family members and propensities towards absorption in offspring. *Developmental Science, 1*, 299–305.

Hesse, E., & van IJzendoorn, M. H. (1999). Propensities towards absorption are related to lapses in the monitoring of reasoning or discourse during the Adult Attachment Interview: A preliminary investigation. *Attachment and Human Development, 1*, 67–91.

Hughes, P., & MacGauley, G. (1997). Mother–infant interaction during the first year with a child who shows disorganization of attachment. *British Journal of Psychotherapy, 14*, 147–158.

Hughes, P., Turton, P., Hopper, E., McGauley, G. A., & Fonagy, P. (2001). Disorganized attachment behavior among infants born subsequent to stillbirth. *Journal of Child Psychology and Psychiatry, 42*, 791–801.

Jacobvitz, D. (2008). Afterword. In H. Steele & M. Steele (Eds.), *Clinical applications of the Adult Attachment Interview* (pp. 471–486). New York: Guilford Press.

Jacobvitz, D., Booher, C., & Hazen, N. (2001, February). *Communication within the dyad: An attachment-theoretical perspective.* Paper presented at the meeting of the Society of Social and Personality Psychologists, San Antonio, TX.

Jacobvitz, D., Leon, K., & Hazen, N. (2006). Does expectant mothers' unresolved trauma predict frightened/frightening maternal behavior?: Risk and protective factors. *Development and Psychopathology, 18*, 363–379.

Katz, L. F., Gottman, J. M., Shapiro, A. F., & Carrerre, S. (1997). *The Meta-Emotion Interview for parents of toddlers.* Unpublished manuscript, University of Washington, Seattle.

Kazui, M., Endo, T., Tanaka, A., Sakagami, H., & Suganuma, M. (2000). Intergenerational transmission of attachment: Japanese mother–child dyads. *Japanese Journal of Educational Psychology, 48*, 323–332.

Kernberg, O. F. (1984). *Severe personality disorders: Psychotherapeutic strategies.* New Haven, CT: Yale University Press.

Kobak, R. R. (1993). *The Attachment Q-Sort.* Unpublished manuscript, University of Delaware.

Kobak, R. R., & Sceery, A. (1988). Attachment in late adolescence: Working models, affect regulation, and representations of self and others. *Child Development, 59*, 135–146.

Koren-Karie, N., Sagi-Schwartz, A., & Joels, T. (2003). Absence of attachment representations (ARR) in the adult years: The emergence of a new AAI classification in catastrophically traumatized Holocaust survivors. *Attachment and Human Development, 5*, 381–397.

Korfmacher, J., Adam, E., Ogawa, J., & Egeland, B. (1997). Adult attachment: Implications for the therapeutic process in a home intervention. *Applied Developmental Science, 1*, 43–52.

Levy, K. N., Meehan, K. B., Kelly, K. M., Reynoso, J. S., Weber, M., Clarkin, J. F., et al. (2006). Change in attachment patterns and reflective function in a randomized control trial of transference-focused psychotherapy for borderline personality disorder. *Journal of Consulting and Clinical Psychology, 74*, 1027–1040.

Linehan, M. M. (1993). *Cognitive-behavioral treatment of borderline personality disorder.* New York: Guilford Press.

Lyons-Ruth, K., Bronfman, E., & Parsons, E. (1999). Maternal frightened, frightening, or atypical behavior and disorganized infant attachment patterns. In J. Vondra & D. Barnett (Eds.), Atypical patterns of infant attachment. *Monographs of the Society for Research in Child Development, 64*(3, Serial No. 258), 67–96.

Lyons-Ruth, K., Connell, D. B., Zoll, D., & Stahl, J. (1987). Infants at social risk: Relations among infant maltreatment, maternal behavior, and infant attachment behavior. *Developmental Psychology, 23*, 223–232.

Madigan, S., Bakermans-Kranenburg, M. J., van IJzendoorn, M. H., Moran, G., Pederson, D. R., & Benoit, D. (2006). Unresolved states of mind, anomalous parental behavior, and disorganized attachment: A review and meta-analysis of a transmission gap. *Attachment and Human Development, 8*, 89–111.

Madigan, S., Moran, G., & Pederson, D. R. (2006). Unresolved states of mind, disorganized attachment relationships, and disrupted interactions of adolescent mothers and their infants. *Developmental Psychology, 42*, 293–304.

Main, M. (1981). Avoidance in the service of attachment: A working paper. In K. Immelmann, G. Barlow, L. Petrinovitch, & M. Main (Eds.), *Behavioral development: The Bielefeld interdisciplinary project* (pp. 651–693). New York: Cambridge University Press.

Main, M. (Chair). (1985, April). *Attachment: A move*

to the level of representation. Symposium conducted at the meeting of the Society for Research in Child Development, Toronto.

Main, M. (1990). Cross-cultural studies of attachment organization: Recent studies, changing methodologies, and the concept of conditional strategies. *Human Development, 33,* 48–61.

Main, M. (1991). Metacognitive knowledge, metacognitive monitoring, and singular (coherent) vs. multiple (incoherent) models of attachment: Findings and directions for future research. In C. M. Parkes, J. Stevenson-Hinde, & P. Marris (Eds.), *Attachment across the life cycle* (pp. 127–159). London: Routledge.

Main, M. (1993). Discourse, prediction, and recent studies in attachment: Implications for psychoanalysis. *Journal of the American Psychoanalytic Association, 41*(Suppl.), 209–244.

Main, M. (1999). Mary D. Salter Ainsworth: Tribute and portrait. *Psychoanalytic Inquiry, 19,* 682–736.

Main, M. (2000). The organized categories of infant, child, and adult attachment: Flexible vs. inflexible attention under attachment-related stress. *Journal of the American Psychoanalytic Association, 48,* 1055–1096.

Main, M. (2001, April). *Attachment to mother and father in infancy, as related to the Adult Attachment Interview and a self-visualization task at age 19.* Poster presented at the biennial meeting of the Society for Research in Child Development, Minneapolis, MN.

Main, M. (2008, March). *The organized categories of the Adult Attachment Interview.* Paper presented at the conference on Clinical Applications of Attachment: The Adult Attachment Interview, University of California, Los Angeles.

Main, M., & Cassidy, J. (1988). Categories of response to reunion with the parent at age six: Predicted from infant attachment classifications and stable over a one-month period. *Developmental Psychology, 24,* 415–426.

Main, M., DeMoss, A., & Hesse, E. (1989). *Unresolved (disorganized/disoriented) state of mind with respect to experiences of loss.* Unpublished manuscript, University of California at Berkeley.

Main, M., & Goldwyn, R. (1984a). *Adult attachment scoring and classification system.* Unpublished manuscript, University of California at Berkeley.

Main, M., & Goldwyn, R. (1984b). Predicting rejection of her infant from mother's representation of her own experience: Implications for the abused–abusing intergenerational cycle. *International Journal of Child Abuse and Neglect, 8,* 203–217.

Main, M., & Goldwyn, R. (1988). *Interview-based attachment classifications: Related to infant–mother and infant–father attachment.* Unpublished manuscript, University of California at Berkeley.

Main, M., & Goldwyn, R. (1998). *Adult attachment scoring and classification system, Version 6.0.* Unpublished manuscript, University of California at Berkeley.

Main, M., & Goldwyn, R. (2008). [Parental states of mind and infant attachment in the Bay Area sample]. Unpublished raw data, University of California at Berkeley.

Main, M., Goldwyn, R., & Hesse, E. (2003). *Adult attachment scoring and classification system. Version 7.2.* Unpublished manuscript, University of California at Berkeley.

Main, M., Goldwyn, R., & Hesse, E. (2008). *The Adult Attachment Interview: Scoring and Classification System, Version 8.* Manuscript in preparation, University of California at Berkeley.

Main, M., & Hesse, E. (1990). Parents' unresolved traumatic experiences are related to infant disorganized attachment status: Is frightened and/or frightening parental behavior the linking mechanism? In M. T. Greenberg, D. Cicchetti, & E. M. Cummings (Eds.), *Attachment in the preschool years: Theory, research, and intervention* (pp. 161–182). Chicago: University of Chicago Press.

Main, M., & Hesse, E. (1991). *Frightening, frightened, dissociated, deferential, sexualized and disorganized parental behavior: A coding system for frightening parent–infant interactions.* Unpublished manuscript, University of California at Berkeley.

Main, M., & Hesse, E. (1998). *Frightening, frightened, dissociated, deferential, sexualized and disorganized parental behavior: A coding system for frightening parent–infant interactions.* Unpublished manuscript, University of California at Berkeley.

Main, M., Hesse, E., & Goldwyn, R. (2008). Studying differences in language usage in recounting attachment history: An introduction to the AAI. In H. Steele & M. Steele (Eds.), *Clinical applications of the Adult Attachment Interview* (pp. 31–68). New York: Guilford Press.

Main, M., Hesse, E., & Kaplan, N. (2005). Predictability of attachment behavior and representational processes at 1, 6, and 19 years of age: The Berkeley longitudinal study. In K. E. Grossmann, K. Grossmann, & E. Waters (Eds.), *Attachment from infancy to adulthood: The major longitudinal studies* (pp. 245–304). New York: Guilford Press.

Main, M., Kaplan, N., & Cassidy, J. (1985). Security in infancy, childhood, and adulthood: A move to the level of representation. In I. Bretherton & E. Waters (Eds.), Growing points of attachment theory and research. *Monographs of the Society for Research in Child Development, 50*(1–2, Serial No. 209), 66–104.

Main, M., & Solomon, J. (1986). Discovery of an insecure-disorganized/disoriented attachment pattern. In T. B. Brazelton & M. W. Yogman (Eds.), *Affective development in infancy* (pp. 95–124). Norwood, NJ: Ablex.

Main, M., & Solomon, J. (1990). Procedures for identifying infants as disorganized/disoriented during the Ainsworth Strange Situation. In M. T. Greenberg, D. Cicchetti, & E. M. Cummings (Eds.), *Attachment in the preschool years: Theory, research, and intervention* (pp. 121–160). Chicago: University of Chicago Press.

Main, M., & Weston, D. (1981). The quality of the toddler's relationship to mother and to father: Related to conflict behavior and the readiness to establish new relationships. *Child Development, 52,* 932–940.

Manassis, K., Bradley, S., Goldberg, S., Hood, J., & Swinson, R. P. (1994). Attachment in mothers with anxiety disorders and their children. *Journal of the American Academy of Child and Adolescent Psychiatry*, 33, 1106–1113.

Mayseless, O., & Scharf, M. (2007). Adolescents' attachment representations and their capacity for intimacy in close relationships. *Journal of Research on Adolescence*, 17, 23–50.

McKinnon, C. C., Moran, G., & Pederson, D. (2004). Attachment representations of deaf adults. *Journal of Deaf Studies and Deaf Education*, 9, 366–386.

McMahon, C. A., Barnett, B., Kowalenko, N. M., & Tennant, C. C. (2006). Maternal attachment state of mind moderates the impact of post-natal depression on infant attachment. *Journal of Child Psychology and Psychiatry*, 47, 660–669.

Minde, K., & Hesse, E. (1996). The role of the Adult Attachment Interview in parent–infant psychotherapy: A case presentation. *Infant Mental Health Journal*, 17, 115–126.

Moran, G., Bailey, H. N., Gleason, K., DeOliveira, C. A., & Pederson, D. R. (2008). Exploring the mind behind unresolved attachment: Lessons from and for attachment-based interventions with infants and their traumatized mothers. In H. Steele & M. Steele (Eds.), *Clinical applications of the Adult Attachment Interview* (pp. 371–398). New York: Guilford Press.

Mura, S. S. (1983). Licensing violations: Legitimate violations of Grice's conversational principle. In R. T. Craig & K. Tracy (Eds.), *Conversational coherence: Form, structure, and strategy*. Beverly Hills, CA: Sage.

Ogawa, J. R., Sroufe, L. A., Weinfeld, N. S., Carlson, E. A., & Egeland, B. (1997). Development and the fragmented self: Longitudinal study of dissociative symptomatology in a nonclinical sample. *Development and Psychopathology*, 9, 855–879.

Paley, B. J., Cox, M. J., Burchinal, M. R., & Payne, C. C. (1999). Attachment and marital functioning: Comparison of spouses with continuous-secure, earned-secure, dismissing, and preoccupied attachment stances. *Journal of Family Psychology*, 13, 580–597.

Paley, B. J., Cox, M. J., Harter, K. S., & Margand, N. A. (2002). Adult attachment stance and spouses' marital perceptions during the transition to parenthood. *Attachment and Human Development*, 4, 340–360.

Patrick, M., Hobson, R. P., Castle, D., Howard, R., & Maughan, B. (1994). Personality disorder and the mental representation of early social experience. *Development and Psychopathology*, 6, 375–388.

Pearson, J. L., Cohn, D. A., Cowan, P. A., & Cowan, C. P. (1994). Earned- and continuous-security in adult attachment: Relation to depressive symptomatology and parenting style. *Development and Psychopathology*, 6, 359–373.

Phelps, J. L., Belsky, J., & Crnic, K. (1998). Earned security, daily stress, and parenting: A comparison of five alternative models. *Development and Psychopathology*, 10, 21–38.

Pianta, R. C., Egeland, B., & Adam, E. K. (1996). Adult attachment classification and self-reported psychiatric symptomatology as assessed by the Minnesota Multiphasic Personality Inventory–2. *Journal of Consulting and Clinical Psychology*, 64, 273–281.

Radloff, L. S. (1977). The CES-D Scale: A self-report depression scale for research in the general population. *Applied Psychological Measurement*, 1, 385–401.

Rifkin-Graboi, A. (2008). Attachment status and salivary cortisol in a normal day and during simulated interpersonal stress in young men. *Stress*, 11, 210–224.

Riggs, S. A., & Jacobvitz, D. (2002). Expectant parents' presentations of early attachment relationships: Associations with mental health and family history. *Journal of Consulting and Clinical Psychology*, 70, 195–204.

Roisman, G. I. (2006). The role of adult attachment security in non-romantic, non-attachment-related first interactions between same-sex strangers. *Attachment and Human Development*, 8, 341–352.

Roisman, G. I., Fortuna, K., & Holland, A. (2006). An experimental manipulation of retrospectively defined earned and continuous attachment security. *Child Development*, 77, 59–71.

Roisman, G. I., Fraley, R. C., & Belsky, J. (2007). A taxometric study of the Adult Attachment Interview. *Developmental Psychology*, 43, 675–686.

Roisman, G. I., Holland, A., Fortuna, K., Fraley, R. C., Clausell, E., & Clarke, A. (2007). The Adult Attachment Interview and self-reports of attachment style: An empirical rapprochement. *Journal of Personality and Social Psychology*, 92, 678–697.

Roisman, G. I., Madsen, S. D., Hennighausen, K. H., Sroufe, L. A., & Collins, W. A. (2001). The coherence of dyadic behavior across parent–child and romantic relationships as mediated by the internalized representation of experience. *Attachment and Human Development*, 3, 156–172.

Roisman, G. I., Padrón, E., Sroufe, L. A., & Egeland, B. (2002). Earned-secure attachment status in retrospect and prospect. *Child Development*, 73, 1204–1219.

Roisman, G. I., Tsai, J. L., & Chiang, K. H. (2004). The emotional integration of childhood experience: Physiological, facial expressive, and self-reported emotional response during the Adult Attachment Interview. *Developmental Psychology*, 40, 776–789.

Rosenthal, R. (1991). *Meta-analytic procedures for social research* (rev. ed.). Newbury Park, CA: Sage.

Sagi, A., van IJzendoorn, M. H., Joels, T., & Scharf, M. (2002). Disorganized reasoning in Holocaust survivors: An attachment perspective. *American Journal of Orthopsychiatry*, 72, 194–203.

Sagi, A., van IJzendoorn, M. H., Scharf, M. H., Joels, T., Koren-Karie, N., Mayseless, O., et al. (1997). Ecological constraints for intergenerational transmission of attachment. *International Journal of Behavioral Development*, 20, 287–299.

Sagi, A., van IJzendoorn, M. H., Scharf, M. H., Koren-Karie, N., Joels, T., & Mayseless, O. (1994). Stability and discriminant validity of the Adult Attachment Interview: A psychometric study in young Israeli adults. *Developmental Psychology*, 30, 771–777.

Sagi-Schwartz, A., & Aviezer, O. (2005). Correlates of

attachment to multiple caregivers in kibbutz children from birth to emerging adulthood: The Haifa longitudinal study. In K. E. Grossmann, K. Grossmann, & E. Waters (Eds.), *Attachment from infancy to adulthood: The major longitudinal studies* (pp. 165–197). New York: Guilford Press.

Sagi-Schwartz, A., Koren-Karie, N., & Joels, T. (2003). Failed mourning in the Adult Attachment Interview: The case of Holocaust survivors. *Attachment and Human Development, 5*, 398–409.

Sagi-Schwartz, A., van IJzendoorn, M. H., Grossmann, K. E., Joels, T., Grossmann, K., Scharf, M., et al. (2003). Attachment and traumatic stress in female Holocaust child survivors and their daughters. *American Journal of Psychiatry, 160*, 1086–1092.

Santona, A., & Zavattini, G. C. (2005). Partnering and parenting expectations in adoptive couples. *Sexual and Relationship Therapy, 20*, 309–322.

Scharf, M., Mayseless, O., & Kivenson-Baron, I. (2004). Adolescents' attachment representations and developmental tasks in emerging adulthood. *Developmental Psychology, 40*, 430–444.

Schuengel, C., Bakermans-Kranenburg, M. J., & van IJzendoorn, M. H. (1999). Frightening maternal behavior linking unresolved loss and disorganized infant attachment. *Journal of Consulting and Clinical Psychology, 67*, 54–63.

Slade, A., Belsky, J., Aber, J. L., & Phelps, J. L. (1999). Mothers' representations of their relationships with their toddlers: Links to adult attachment and observed mothering. *Developmental Psychology, 35*, 611–619.

Solomon, J., George, C., & De Jong, A. (1995). Children classified as controlling at age six: Evidence of disorganized representational strategies and aggression at home and at school. *Development and Psychopathology, 7*, 447–463.

Sroufe, L. A., & Waters, E. (1977). Attachment as an organizational construct. *Child Development, 48*, 1184–1199.

Steele, H., Phibbs, E., & Woods, R. (2004). Coherence of mind in daughter caregivers of mothers with dementia: Links with their mothers' joy and relatedness on reunion in a Strange Situation. *Attachment and Human Development, 6*, 439–450.

Steele, H., & Steele, M. (2007, July). *Intergenerational patterns of attachment: From pregnancy in one generation to adolescence in the next.* Paper presented at the International Attachment Conference, Changing Troubled Attachment Relations: Views from Research and Clinical Work, Braga, Portugal.

Steele, H., Steele, M., & Fonagy, P. (1996). Associations among attachment classifications of mothers, fathers, and their infants. *Child Development, 67*, 541–555.

Steele, M., Hodges, J., Kaniuk, J., Hillman, S., & Henderson, K. (2003). Attachment representations and adoption: Associations between maternal states of mind and emotional narratives in previously maltreated children. *Journal of Child Psychotherapy, 29*, 187–205.

Steele, M., Steele, H., & Johansson, M. (2002). Maternal predictors of children's social cognition: An attachment perspective. *Journal of Child Psychology and Psychiatry, 43*, 861–872.

Torgerson, A. M., Grova, B. K., & Sommerstad, R. (2007). A pilot study of attachment patterns in adult twins. *Attachment and Human Development, 9*, 127–138.

Turton, P., McGauley, G., Marin-Avellan, L., & Hughes, P. (2001). The Adult Attachment Interview: Rating and classification problems posed by non-normative samples. *Attachment and Human Development, 3*, 284–303.

van IJzendoorn, M. H. (1995). Adult attachment representations, parental responsiveness, and infant attachment: A meta-analysis on the predictive validity of the Adult Attachment Interview. *Psychological Bulletin, 117*, 387–403.

van IJzendoorn, M. H., & Bakermans-Kranenburg, M. J. (1996). Attachment representations in mothers, fathers, adolescents, and clinical groups: A meta-analytic search for normative data. *Journal of Consulting and Clinical Psychology, 64*, 8–21.

van IJzendoorn, M. H., & Bakermans-Kranenburg, M. J. (2008). The distribution of adult attachment representations in clinical groups: A meta-analytic search for patterns of attachment in 105 AAI studies. In H. Steele & M. Steele (Eds.), *Clinical applications of the Adult Attachment Interview* (pp. 69–96). New York: Guilford Press.

Wampler, K. S., Shi, L., Nelson, B. S., & Kimball, T. G. (2003). The Adult Attachment Interview and observed couple interaction: Implications for an intergenerational perspective on couple therapy. *Family Process, 42*, 497–515.

Ward, M. J., & Carlson, E. A. (1995). Associations among adult attachment representations, maternal sensitivity, and infant–mother attachment in a sample of adolescent mothers. *Child Development, 66*, 69–79.

Ward, M. J., Lee, S. S., & Polan, H. J. (2006). Attachment and psychopathology in a community sample. *Attachment and Human Development, 8*, 327–340.

Waters, E., Merrick, S., Treboux, D., Crowell, J., & Albersheim, L. (2000). Attachment security in infancy and early adulthood: A twenty-year longitudinal study. *Child Development, 71*, 684–689.

Webster's new international dictionary of the English language. (1959). (2nd ed., unabridged). Springfield, MA: Merriam.

Weinfield, N. S., Sroufe, L. A., & Egeland, B. (2000). Attachment from infancy to adulthood in a high-risk sample: Continuity, discontinuity and their correlates. *Child Development, 71*, 695–7021

Zegers, M. A., Schuengel, C., van IJzendoorn, M. H., & Janssens, J. M. (2006). Attachment representations of institutionalized adolescents and their professional caregivers: Predicting the development of therapeutic relationships. *American Journal of Orthopsychiatry, 76*, 325–334.

CHAPTER 26

Measurement of Individual Differences in Adolescent and Adult Attachment

JUDITH A. CROWELL
R. CHRIS FRALEY
PHILLIP R. SHAVER

Attachment theory is a lifespan developmental theory. According to Bowlby (1969/1982), human attachments play a "vital role ... from the cradle to the grave" (p. 208). Ainsworth (1989) devoted her American Psychological Association Distinguished Scientific Contribution Award address to "attachments beyond infancy," and included discussions of adolescents' and adults' continuing relationships with parents, their relationships with especially close friends, and the role of attachment in heterosexual and homosexual "pair bonds." Although Bowlby and Ainsworth clearly acknowledged the importance of the attachment system across the lifespan, they provided relatively few guidelines concerning its specific function and expression in later life.

Early research on attachment followed Bowlby's and Ainsworth's primary focus on young children and explored the developmental roots of the attachment system, examining infants' attachment to their parents, especially their mothers. (These studies are reviewed in many other chapters in this volume.) Beginning in the mid-1980s, the groundwork was laid for examining the attachment system in older children and adults, and several new lines of research emerged. Following an interest in attachment representations, George,

Kaplan, and Main (1984, 1985, 1996) created the Adult Attachment Interview (AAI) "to assess the security of the adult's overall working model of attachment, that is, the security of the self in relation to attachment in its generality rather than in relation to any particular present or past relationship" (Main, Kaplan, & Cassidy, 1985, p. 78). As explained below, the AAI assesses adults' representations of attachment based on their discussion of childhood relationships with their parents, and of those experiences' effects on their development as adults and as parents.

At the time the AAI was being developed, Pottharst and Kessler (described in Pottharst, 1990) created an Attachment History Questionnaire (AHQ) to assess adults' memories of attachment-related experiences in childhood (e.g., separation from parents, quality of attachment relationships). In a separate research effort, Armsden and Greenberg (1987) developed the Inventory of Parent and Peer Attachment (IPPA) to assess the perceived quality of adolescents' current relationships with parents and peers. West and Sheldon-Keller (1994; West, Sheldon, & Reiffer, 1987) developed two self-report instruments, the Reciprocal Attachment Questionnaire for Adults and the Avoidant Attachment Questionnaire for

Adults, to assess individual differences in primary attachment in adulthood. Also at about this time, Hazan and Shaver (1987; Shaver, Hazan, & Bradshaw, 1988) began to consider the applicability of attachment theory in general, and of Ainsworth's infant classification scheme in particular, to the study of feelings and behavior in adolescent and adult romantic relationships.

Given the independence of these groups of investigators, and their different domains of interest and varied professional backgrounds, the lines of research they initiated developed in different ways. Each inspired variations and offshoots, so that today there are many different measures of adolescent and adult attachment—as well as a great deal of confusion about what they measure, what they are supposed to measure, and how they are related (if at all) to each other. There have been advances in the measurement literature in recent years, and guidelines can now be proposed for researchers undertaking studies of adolescent or adult attachment. Evidence continues to build (e.g., Roisman, Holland, et al., 2007) that the different kinds of measures do not converge empirically, even though they were all inspired by attachment theory and sometimes relate similarly to outcome variables (as noted in several chapters in this volume). Moreover, not all measures can be used interchangeably in research, and reviewers of attachment studies need to be clear about which measures yield which findings. Choosing an appropriate measure requires careful thought about the goals of one's study and its foundation in the literature.

This chapter begins with a brief discussion of attachment theory, especially elements that are key to understanding the attachment system in adults, and hence to assessing it. The AAI and other narrative measures derived from the developmental tradition within attachment research are discussed in the next section (and the AAI is described in more detail by Hesse, Chapter 25, this volume). After a brief section on behavioral assessments of adult attachment, the next section deals with the AHQ, the IPPA, and the Reciprocal and Avoidant Attachment Questionnaires. These instruments are considered in a single section because they all use a self-report methodology, but none is meant to capture the attachment patterns identified by Ainsworth, Blehar, Waters, and Wall (1978) in the Strange Situation. The following section deals with some of the self-report measures of romantic attachment that grew out of Hazan and Shaver's (1987) attempt to apply Ainsworth's discoveries

to the study of romantic relationships. The final section summarizes the overlaps and distinctions among measures developed in different lines of research on adolescent and adult attachment, and provides guidelines for future research.

ADULT ATTACHMENT: THEORETICAL ISSUES

The title of this chapter identifies two ideas from attachment theory that are critical to measurement. The first idea is that the attachment system is normative—that is, relevant to the development of all people, and active and important in adult life. The second idea is that there are individual differences in attachment behavior and the working models that underlie it.

Adult Attachment as Normative

Although some of Bowlby's original inspiration for attachment theory came from his work as a clinician, in developing the theory he primarily drew from research in ethology, observations of animal behavior, and cognitive psychology. He described the attachment behavioral system as an evolutionarily adaptive motivational–behavioral control system. The attachment system has the goal of promoting safety in infancy and childhood through the child's relationship with an attachment figure or caregiver (Bowlby, 1969/1982). Attachment behavior is activated in times of danger, stress, and novelty, and has the goal of gaining and maintaining proximity and contact with an attachment figure. Hence the behavioral manifestations are context-specific (evident in times of danger or anxiety), although the attachment system is considered active at all times, continuously monitoring the environment and the availability of attachment figures (Ainsworth et al., 1978; Bretherton, 1985). The child can confidently explore the environment with the active support of a caregiver, secure in the knowledge that this attachment figure is available if any need or question should arise. Ainsworth et al. (1978) termed this interaction between child and caregiver the "secure-base phenomenon," a concept central to attachment theory.

Bowlby (1969/1982) hypothesized that the attachment relationship in infancy is similar in nature to later love relationships, and he drew few distinctions among those relationships—be they child to parent, partner to partner, or aging parent to an adult child who is taking a caregiving role.

Ainsworth (1991) highlighted the function of the attachment behavioral system in adult relationships, emphasizing the secure-base phenomenon as the critical element. She stated that a secure attachment relationship is one that facilitates functioning and competence outside of the relationship: There is "a seeking to obtain an experience of security and comfort in the relationship with the partner. If and when such security and comfort are available, the individual is able to move off from the secure base provided by the partner, with the confidence to engage in other activities" (1991, p. 38).

Attachment relationships are distinguished from other adult relationships in providing feelings of security and belonging, without which there is loneliness and restlessness (Weiss, 1973, 1991). This function is distinct from aspects of relationships that provide guidance or companionship; sexual gratification; or opportunities to feel needed or to share common interests or experiences, feelings of competence, or alliance and assistance (Ainsworth, 1985; Weiss, 1974). The behavioral elements of attachment in adult life are similar to those observed in infancy, and an adult shows a desire for proximity to the attachment figure when stressed, increased comfort in the presence of the attachment figure, and anxiety when the attachment figure is inaccessible (Shaver et al., 1988; Weiss, 1991). Finally, grief is experienced following the loss of an attachment figure (Bowlby, 1980; Shaver & Fraley, Chapter 3, this volume).

A major difference between adult–adult attachment and child–parent attachment is that the attachment behavioral system in adults works reciprocally. Adult partners are not usually placed permanently in the role of "attachment figure/caregiver" or "attached individual/care receiver." Both attachment and caregiving behavior are observable in adults, and partners shift between the two roles (Ainsworth, 1991; Kunce & Shaver, 1994; Shaver et al., 1988). The potential for flexible reciprocity adds complexity to the measurement of adult attachment.

Individual Differences and Mental Representations or Working Models

The study of attachment in adults has focused largely on individual differences in the organization of attachment behavior and in expectations regarding attachment relationships, rather than on normative developmental aspects of the attachment system. The idea of individual differences emerged from the work of Ainsworth and colleagues (1978), who broadly characterized the patterns of attachment as "secure" and "insecure" (which she sometimes called "anxious"). In addition to the security–insecurity distinction, Ainsworth and colleagues drew a second distinction between "avoidance and conflict relevant to close bodily contact" (p. 298)—that is, the avoidant and resistant behaviors that distinguish two of the major insecure patterns. It is important to note that individual differences in attachment security do not represent differences in strength or quantity of attachment: "The most conspicuous dimension that has emerged so far is not strength of attachment but security vs. anxiety in the attachment relationship. This does not imply substitution of degree of security for degree of strength" (Ainsworth et al., 1978, p. 298).

Differences among attachment patterns in infancy are thought to develop primarily from different experiences in interaction with an attachment figure, rather than to be influenced by genetics, child temperament, or other child characteristics (Ainsworth et al., 1978; Finkel & Matheny, 2000; Gervai et al., 2005; Lakatos et al., 2000; see Vaughn, Bost, & van IJzendoorn, Chapter 9, this volume). The secure pattern characterizes the infant who seeks and receives protection, reassurance, and comfort when stressed. Confident exploration is optimized because of the support and availability of the caregiver. The child comes to feel secure with the attachment figure; hence the behavioral system corresponds closely with cognitions and the expression of emotion in the context of attachment-related experiences. The two major insecure patterns ("avoidant" and "ambivalent" or "resistant") develop when attachment behavior is met by rejection, inconsistency, or even threat from the attachment figure, leaving the infant "anxious" about the caregiver's responsiveness should problems arise. To reduce this anxiety, the infant's behavior evolves to fit or complement the attachment figure's behavior; in other words, it is strategic and adaptive within the context of that relationship (Main, 1981, 1990). However, the need to attend to the caregiver in this anxious, strategic way, which compromises exploratory behavior, is potentially maladaptive outside that particular relationship.

Current theory and research on adult attachment draw heavily on Bowlby's concept of "attachment representations" or "working models." Importing ideas from cognitive psychology, Bowlby (1973, 1980) hypothesized that individuals develop representations of the functioning and significance of close relationships. These representations, or models, consist of a person's beliefs and expectations about how attachment relationships operate and what he or she gains from them. As noted above, individual differences emerge in the expression of attachment behavior in the context of attachment relationships. Patterns of attachment develop in the course of behavioral interactions between an infant/child and parents (Bowlby, 1980), and reflect expectations about the child's own behavior and a parent's likely behavior in various situations. Cognitive–affective structures develop that mirror the behavioral patterns. They are called "working models" or "representations" because they are the bases for action in attachment-related situations, and because in principle they are open to revision as a function of significant attachment-related experiences. The models are relatively stable and can operate automatically without the need for conscious appraisal. They guide behavior in relationships with parents, and they influence expectations, strategies, and behavior in later relationships (Bretherton, 1985; Bretherton & Munholland, Chapter 5, this volume; Main et al., 1985).

Bowlby's incorporation of mental representations into attachment theory allows for a lifespan perspective on the attachment behavioral system, providing a way of understanding developmental change in the expression of attachment and its ongoing influence on development and behavior in relationships. An individual's model of attachment involves stable postulates about the roles of both parent and child in the relationship, because individual differences in attachment stem from a particular caregiving environment. In other words, working models are models of attachment relationships (Bretherton, 1985). Bowlby (1973) wrote:

> In the working model of the world that anyone builds, a key feature is his notion of who his attachment figures are, where they may be found, and how they may be expected to respond. Similarly, in the working model of the self that anyone builds a key feature is his notion of how acceptable or unacceptable he himself is in the eyes of his attachment figures. ... Confidence that an attachment figure is ... likely to be responsive can be seen to turn on two variables: (a) whether or not the attachment figure is judged to be the sort of person who in general responds to calls for support and protection; (b) whether or not the self is judged to be the sort of person towards whom ... the attachment figure is likely to respond in a help-

ful way. Logically these variables are independent. In practice, they are apt to be confounded. As a result, the model of the attachment figure and the model of the self are likely to develop so as to be complementary and mutually confirming. (pp. 203–204)

Bowlby (1973, 1980) also wrote about the problems that arise when a child is presented with a negative view of self and other, and/or with incompatible data about his or her experiences— that is, when the child's firsthand experience of the attachment figure is in opposition to what the parent tells the child about the meaning of the parental behavior. Because information relevant to characterizing an attachment relationship comes from multiple sources (Bowlby, 1973), a child may receive conflicting information which challenges the development of a coherent representation. Bowlby (1973) and Main (1981, 1990, 1991), among others, have described the strategies required to maintain cognitive organization in the face of stress and conflicting information. These secondary strategies (Main, 1990) (as opposed to the primary strategies of approach, contact seeking, and contact maintenance when the attachment system is activated) are defensive maneuvers that require "manipulating the level of output usually called for by the [attachment] system—[and, in addition, manipulating cognitive processes to maintain] a given attachment organization" (p. 48). Such strategies develop because there are inconsistencies, incompatibilities, and a lack of internal connectedness in the elements of the attachment representation (Bowlby, 1973; Main, 1990, 1991). Strategies may include avoidance of the attachment figure in stressful situations (Main, 1981); oscillation between the two viewpoints (i.e., "child good, parent bad," "child bad, parent good"); and acceptance of the parent's view while denying one's own experience (Bowlby, 1973).

A central idea in attachment theory is that early parent–child relationships are prototypes of later love relationships (E. Waters, Kondo-Ikemura, Posada, & Richters, 1991). Bowlby did not claim that there is a critical period in infancy that has implications across the lifespan (the most extreme interpretation of the prototype hypothesis), but rather that there is a strong tendency toward continuity in parent–child interactions, which affects the continuing development of the attachment behavioral system. That is, in addition to having effects on individual personality characteristics, child–parent relationships influence subsequent patterns of family organization and therefore play a role in the intergenerational transmission of family attachment patterns. Much of adult attachment research has been based on the assumption that there are parallel individual differences in infant and adult patterns of attachment and attachment representations (e.g., Hazan & Shaver, 1987; Main et al., 1985; Mikulincer & Shaver, 2007). However, different ideas about the origins of adult attachment patterns, and disagreement about the structure of the attachment system in adulthood, are responsible for some of the confusion in the literature on adult attachment.

Bowlby (1969/1982) also discussed change in attachment patterns, an issue relevant to adult patterns of attachment. In childhood, if an attachment pattern changes, it is assumed to have been caused by a corresponding change in the quality of parent–child interactions (Bowlby, 1969/1982). Bowlby also hypothesized that attachment patterns can change in later life through the influence of new attachment relationships and the development of formal operational thought. This combination of events allows the individual to reflect on and reinterpret the meaning of past and present experiences (Bowlby, 1973, 1980, 1988)—something that can happen in an individual's self-analysis, within a couple relationship (such as marriage), or as a consequence of psychotherapy. In a couple relationship, partners can co-construct new attachment representations, which take into account both partners' attachment representations as well as other elements of the relationship (Crowell, Treboux, & Waters, 2002; Oppenheim & Waters, 1995; Owens et al., 1995; Treboux, Crowell, & Waters, 2004). This may or may not lead to full representational change in an individual's original model of attachment.

In general, researchers have attributed the development of adult attachment patterns to three broad sources, although the relative importance and influence of the three sources are debated and are critical research issues (see, e.g., Fraley, 2002; Owens et al., 1995; E. Waters et al., 1991). The sources are (1) parent–child attachment relationships; (2) peer and romantic relationship experiences, including exposure to one's parents' marriage; and (3) a current adult attachment relationship. There is evidence that the attachment relationship between adult partners takes time to develop, and that the experience of the parents' marriage and the specific representation of the current adult relationship are integrated over time into the generalized representation that had developed earlier within the relationship with the par-

ents (Crowell, Treboux, Gao, et al., 2002; Crowell, Treboux, & Waters, 2002; Treboux et al., 2004; Zeifman & Hazan, Chapter 20, this volume).

In summary, two core propositions in attachment theory are key to understanding attachment in adulthood and to evaluating existing measures of adult attachment: The attachment system is active in adults, and there are individual differences in adult attachment behavior that have their foundations in attachment experiences and are embodied in attachment representations.

NARRATIVE ASSESSMENTS OF ADULT ATTACHMENT

The scoring systems of the measures described in this section, and in the following brief section on behavioral assessments, are based on the concept of attachment security, defined as the effectiveness of an individual's use of an attachment figure as a *secure base* from which to explore and a *safe haven* in times of distress or danger (secure). The use of narratives to assess attachment is based on the idea that "mental processes vary as distinctively as do behavioral processes" (Main et al., 1985, p. 78), and that organized behavioral and representational processes are reflected in coherent, organized language. Narrative assessments ultimately derive their validity from observations of attachment behavior in natural settings. Each of the measures discussed here was designed to assess the continuum from secure to insecure, and, secondarily, to assess differences among insecure strategies.

Adult Attachment Interview

In what Main and colleagues (1985) called "a move to the level of representation" (in contrast to the previous focus on behavior in the assessment of parent–child attachment relationships), Main and her coworkers developed a semistructured interview for adults about childhood attachment experiences and the meaning currently assigned by an individual to past attachment-related experiences (George et al., 1984, 1985, 1996). The AAI and its scoring system are based on several key ideas about attachment, including the ideas that working models operate at least partially outside of awareness; that they are based on attachment-relevant experiences; that infants begin to develop models that guide behavior in attachment relationships in the first year of life; that representations provide guidelines for behavior and affective appraisal of experience; that formal operational thought allows the individual to observe and assess a given relationship system, and hence that the model of the relationship can be altered without an actual change in experiences in the relationship; and that the models are not templates, but are processes that serve to "obtain or to limit access to information" (Main et al., 1985, p. 77). In addition, the scoring system is linked to Bowlby's and Main's ideas about secondary strategies, defensive processes, and incompatible models described earlier.

An adult is interviewed about his or her general view of the relationship with parents; ordinary experiences with parents in which the attachment system is presumed to be activated (upset, injury, illness, separation); experiences of loss; and finally the meaning that the adult attributes to these experiences in terms of the parents' behavior and the development of the interviewee's adult personality and behavior as a parent (if applicable). The resulting narrative is transcribed. The transcript is then examined for material directly expressed by the individual, and also for unintended qualities of discourse, such as incoherence and inconsistency. Scoring is based on (1) the coder's assessment of the individual's childhood experiences with parents; (2) the language used by the individual; and (3) most importantly, the individual's ability to give an integrated, believable account of experiences and their meaning. The speaker's language and discourse style are considered reflections of the "current state of mind with respect to attachment" (Main & Goldwyn, 1984; Main, Goldwyn, & Hesse, 2003; Main et al., 1985; Hesse, Chapter 25, this volume).

Main and Colleagues' Scoring System

The AAI scoring system (e.g., Main & Goldwyn, 1984; Main et al., 2003) was developed by examining 44 parental interviews for which the Strange Situation classifications of the interviewees' infants were already known, and identifying qualities of content and discourse that distinguished among them. Hence the AAI was expressly developed to capture the issues tapped by the Strange Situation, especially an individual's ability to use an attachment figure as a secure base. The system has been refined over the past 20-plus years, but it has not yet been published. Extensive training is required to administer and score the interview.

Scoring is done from a transcript, using scales that characterize the individual's childhood experiences with each parent *in the opinion of the coder*. There are two sets of scales: parental behavior scales and state-of-mind scales. Parental behavior is rated from the specific memories and descriptions given of parental behavior, and not from the general assessment of the parenting given by the individual. The parental behavior scales, rated separately for mother and father, are: loving, rejecting, neglecting, involving, and pressuring. The state-of-mind scales assess discourse style and particular forms of coherence and incoherence: idealization, insistence on lack of recall, active anger, derogation, fear of loss, metacognitive monitoring, and passivity of speech. Using these ratings and the overall coherence of the transcript, the coder also assigns scores for coherence of transcript and of mind. The concept of "coherence" is based on Grice's (1975) maxims regarding discourse. High coherence means that the narrative adheres to Grice's maxims of *quality* (it is believable, without contradictions or illogical conclusions); *quantity* (enough, but not too much, information is given to permit the coder to understand the narrative); *relevance* (the individual answers the questions asked); and *manner* (the individual uses fresh, clear language rather than jargon, canned speech, or nonsense words).

Patterns of scale scores are used to assign an adult to one of three major classifications: a secure category ("autonomous") or one of two insecure categories ("dismissing" or "preoccupied"), with the coherence scales being used to make the secure–insecure distinction. The categories parallel the three infant attachment patterns identified by Ainsworth et al. (1978), and the discourse style reflects the behavioral elements in infant attachment patterns.

Individuals classified as secure-autonomous maintain a balanced view of early relationships, value attachment relationships, and view attachment-related experiences as influential in their development. In parallel to the direct approach of the secure infant, the autonomous adult's approach to the interview is open, direct, and cooperative, regardless of how difficult the material is to discuss. The interview itself contains consistent, believable reports of behavior by parents; simply put, the adult's general descriptions of the parenting he or she received match the specific memories given of parental behavior. Because security is inferred from coherence, any kind of childhood experience may be associated with being classified as autonomous, although in many cases parental behavior is indeed summarized as loving, and there are clear and specific memories given of loving behavior by the parents.

The two major insecure classifications are associated with incoherent accounts, meaning that interviewees' assessment of experience are not matched by their descriptions of parental behavior. There is little support provided for a parent's serving as a secure base; and discourse, whether dismissing or preoccupied, mirrors the lack of exploration and inflexibility of insecure infants. The classifications reflect the strategies used to manage the anxiety of having a parent who failed in this regard. Corresponding to the behavior of avoidant infants in the Strange Situation, adults classified as dismissing are uncomfortable with the topic of the interview, deny the impact of early attachment relationships on their personality development, have difficulty recalling specific events, and often idealize experiences. The classification is associated with descriptions of rejection in the coder's opinion (pushing a child away in attachment-activating situations) in the context of an adult's giving an overarching assessment of having loving parents. Just as resistant infants are ambivalent in the Strange Situation, adults classified as preoccupied display confusion or oscillation about past experiences, and descriptions of relationships with parents are marked by active anger and/or passivity. The preoccupied classification is associated with involving, even role-reversing parenting, in which the child needed to be alert to parental needs rather than the reverse.

Individuals may be classified as "unresolved," in addition to being assigned one of the three major classifications. Unresolved adults report attachment-related traumas of loss and/or abuse, and manifest confusion and disorganization in the discussion of that topic. The unresolved classification may be given precedence over the major classification in categorizing the individual, and is considered an insecure classification. A "cannot classify" designation is assigned when the transcript does not fit any of the major classification categories, most commonly when scale scores reflect elements rarely seen together in an interview (e.g., high idealization of one parent and high active anger toward the other) (Hesse, 1996). Such interviews are often markedly incoherent, which is taken to indicate a high degree of insecurity. Fremmer-Bombik and colleagues have devised an algorithm for classification that is discussed by Hesse (Chapter 25, this volume).

Kobak's Q-Sort Scoring System

The Adult Attachment Q-Sort is an alternative method of scoring the AAI and was derived from the original scoring system (Kobak, 1993; Kobak, Cole, Ferenz-Gillies, Fleming, & Gamble, 1993). Its underlying structure parallels the Strange Situation and Main and colleagues scoring systems, but it emphasizes the relation between emotion regulation and attachment representations. The interview is scored from a transcript according to a forced distribution of descriptors, and yields scores for two conceptual dimensions: "security–anxiety" and "deactivation–hyperactivation." Security is inferred from coherence and cooperation within the interview, and often (although not necessarily) from memories of supportive attachment figures (in the coder's opinion). Deactivation corresponds to dismissing strategies, whereas hyperactivation corresponds to the excessive detail and active anger seen in the transcripts of many preoccupied subjects. These strategies lie at opposite ends of a single dimension, which is assumed to be orthogonal to the security–anxiety (insecurity) dimension. The AAI transcript is rated by two or more coders, using 100 Q-sort items and instructions that impose a forced normal distribution along a 9-point continuum (Kobak et al., 1993). The sort is correlated with an expert-based prototypic sort for each dimension. The dimensional scores can be used to classify the adult into the categories of the original system, and approximately 80% of individuals receive the same classification with the Q-sort system as with the original system (kappa = .65). There is more overlap on the deactivation–hyperactivation dimension than on the security–anxiety dimension (Kobak et al., 1993). The scoring system was created without an attempt to include the unresolved or cannot classify categories.

Fonagy and Colleagues' Reflective Functioning Scoring System

A third method of coding the AAI departs conceptually from the original classification and Q-sort systems. Fonagy, Steele, Steele, Moran, and Higgitt's (1991) system assesses "reflective functioning"—that is, an adult's quality of understanding his or her own and another's intentions, motivations, and emotions. In a study of 200 parents, the AAI self-reflection function correlated highly with AAI coherence, and was a stronger predictor of infant security. This study and many subsequent ones providing evidence for the validity and utility of measures of reflective function are reviewed by Fonagy, Gergely, and Target (Chapter 33, this volume).

Distribution of Classifications

In a meta-analysis (Bakermans-Kranenburg & van IJzendoorn, 1993), the distribution of AAI classifications in nonclinical samples of women, men, and adolescents was 58% autonomous, 24% dismissing, and 18% preoccupied. About 19% of individuals also received an unresolved classification in association with a major classification; about 11% of people classified as autonomous, 26% of the dismissing group, and 40% of the preoccupied group were also classified as unresolved. Of people classified as unresolved, 38% had a major classification of autonomous, 24% of dismissing, and 38% of preoccupied. The base rate of insecurity in clinical and at-risk samples was much higher: 8% autonomous, 26% dismissing, 25% preoccupied, and 40% unresolved. There were no gender differences in distribution of classifications (van IJzendoorn & Bakermans-Kranenburg, 1996).

Stability and Discriminant Validity

High stability of attachment classifications (78–90% for three classification groups across periods ranging from 2 weeks to 6 years) has been observed in a number of studies using the original scoring system (e.g., kappa = .73, 86%, over 21 months; Crowell, Treboux, & Waters, 2002). (See also Allen, McElhaney, Kuperminc, & Jodl, 2004; Bakermans-Kranenburg & van IJzendoorn, 1993; Benoit & Parker, 1994; Sagi et al., 1994.) The secure classification is especially stable, but the unresolved classification is often unstable. Change from insecure to secure status across the transition to marriage has been associated with positive feelings and coherent cognitions about the relationship with the partner and living away from the family of origin (Crowell, Treboux, & Waters, 2002).

Because the ability to speak coherently about attachment could conceivably be based on non-attachment-related cognitive abilities, such as intelligence or memory, the discriminant validity of the original AAI scoring system has been investigated. Security is minimally associated with intelligence in most studies and is not significantly associated with memory, social desirability, or dis-

course style on an unrelated topic (Bakermans-Kranenburg & van IJzendoorn, 1993; Crowell et al., 1996; Sagi et al., 1994).

Discriminant analysis has enabled AAI security to be represented as a continuous variable (Fyffe & Waters, 1997). The coder rating of "coherence of transcript" correlated .96 with the security function. Although this finding suggests that researchers can assess AAI security simply by reliably coding coherence of transcript, this is difficult because the other scales are used in establishing and checking the coherence rating.

Research with the AAI

The AAI had its origins in investigations of the child–parent attachment relationship, and many of the studies based on the AAI have used it for this purpose. There is a consistent link among AAI classifications, parenting behavior, and child attachment status. An increasing number of studies have used the AAI to examine attachment between adult romantic partners.

Studies of Adults as Individuals

Prospective Longitudinal Studies. To examine the idea that early attachment patterns correspond to attachment patterns in adult life, several studies have assessed the relation between infant attachment security and AAI classifications in late adolescence and young adulthood. Two studies have found a 70–75% correspondence between Strange Situation and AAI security–insecurity in late adolescents and young adults who participated as infants in studies of attachment (e.g., kappa = .44; E. Waters, Merrick, Treboux, Crowell, & Albersheim, 2000; see also Hamilton, 2000). As expected from Bowlby's ideas about change in attachment representations in childhood, lack of correspondence between infant and adult classifications was related to life stresses that significantly altered the caregiving environment, including death of a parent, life-threatening illness in subject or parent, and divorce. In a meta-analysis of all studies examining the stability of attachment, Fraley (2002) found that the continuity between security as assessed in the Strange Situation in infancy and the AAI in young adulthood ranged from $r = -.10$ to $r = .50$. Precise explanations of cross-study differences in observed continuity remain to be tested and replicated, but it seems likely that the effort to explain stability and instability will be successful.

In other words, discontinuity will turn out to be "principled" or lawful, rather than mysterious or haphazard.

The Dismissing Strategy. Adults classified as dismissing use strategies that minimize, dismiss, devalue, or deny the impact of negative attachment experiences. During the AAI, college students who used dismissing strategies showed an increase in skin conductance (Dozier & Kobak, 1992). Despite efforts to minimize negative aspects of childhood and the importance of early relationships, they showed signs of physiological distress when challenged with these topics. Indeed, adults classified as dismissing underreport distress, psychological symptoms, or problems in interpersonal relationships, compared with the reports of others who know them well (Dozier & Lee, 1995; Kobak & Sceery, 1988). The strategy of avoidance or dismissal has led to difficulties in the development of self-report assessments that discriminate the AAI dismissing group from the AAI autonomous group (Crowell, Treboux, & Waters, 1999). This may be one of several reasons, discussed later in this chapter, for the lack of high correspondence between narrative and self-report measures of attachment orientation.

Adjustment and Psychopathology. Consistent relationships have been found between security and ratings of social adjustment, social support, stress, and depression; the effect sizes have varied, depending on ecological and methodological factors (Atkinson et al., 2000; Crowell et al., 1999; Kobak & Sceery, 1988). Clinical populations have a higher proportion of insecure classifications than the general population, but few specific relations between the "organized" AAI types and psychopathology have emerged (Riggs & Jacobvitz, 2002; van IJzendoorn & Bakermans-Kranenburg, 1996; van IJzendoorn et al., 1997; Wallis & Steele, 2001; Ward et al., 2001). The unresolved group, however, is overrepresented in clinical samples, and this has led to suggestions that it is more pathological than "organized" insecure groups (van IJzendoorn & Bakermans-Kranenburg, 1996).

This complex area of investigation is not discussed further here, but as Lyons-Ruth and Jacobvitz explain in Chapter 28 of this volume, it has led to important efforts to expand the AAI coding system to address a variety of trauma-related variations in AAI discourse (Koren-Karie, Sagi-Schwartz, & Joels, 2003; Lyons-Ruth, Yellin,

Melnick, & Atwood, 2003, 2005; Sagi-Schwartz, Koren-Karie, & Joels, 2003).

"Earned Security." The subset of individuals classified as secure (because they value attachment and are coherent in their discussion of attachment relationships), despite their parents' being rated as unloving by coders, are termed "earned secure." There is some indication that such retrospectively defined earned-secure individuals may have had supportive parents, but because of current depression provide somewhat biased representations of their parents, which lead coders to rate the parents as relatively unloving (Roisman, Fortuna, & Holland, 2006; Roisman, Padrón, Sroufe, & Egeland, 2002). In contrast, *prospectively* defined earned secure individuals—that is, individuals who begin adulthood with an insecure AAI classification and over time become secure—are not found to have depressive symptoms, suggesting that the change is genuine (Pearson, Cohn, Cowan, & Cowan, 1994). (This issue has not yet been fully resolved, and different chapters in the present volume handle it differently. For further discussion, see Hesse, Chapter 25, this volume, and Roisman, Fraley, & Belsky, 2007.)

Studies of the Child–Parent Relationship

Attachment Classifications across Generations. A number of investigators have found high correspondence between parental AAI classifications and infant attachment assessed with the Strange Situation (kappa = .46 for three classifications; kappa = .44 for four classifications) and preschoolers' attachment assessed with home observations (Cassibba, van IJzendoorn, Bruno, & Coppola, 2004; Fonagy, Steele, & Steele, 1991; Posada, Waters, Crowell, & Lay, 1995; Sagi et al., 1992; Steele, Steele, & Fonagy, 1996; van IJzendoorn, 1992; see meta-analysis by van IJzendoorn, 1995). Mother–infant correspondence is greater than father–infant correspondence (Main et al., 1985; Miljkovitch, Pierrehumbert, Bretherton, & Halfon, 2004; Steele et al., 1996; van IJzendoorn, 1992).

Parents' AAI Classifications and Parental Behavior toward Children. Mothers classified as autonomous on the AAI are observed to be more responsive, perceptive, sensitive, and attuned to their infants in the first year of life (Adam, Gunnar, & Tanaka, 2004; DeOliveira, Moran, & Pederson,

2005; Goldberg, Benoit, Blokland, & Madigan, 2003; Grossmann, Fremmer-Bombik, Rudolph, & Grossmann, 1988; Haft & Slade, 1989; Macfie, McElwain, Houts, & Cox, 2005; Slade, Belsky, Aber, & Phelps, 1999; Ward & Carlson, 1995; Zeanah et al., 1993). Similarly, parental security of attachment is linked to parents' sensitivity with their preschool children, and to parents providing help and support during observed tasks and separations in both normative and clinical samples (Cohn, Cowan, Cowan, & Pearson, 1992; Crowell & Feldman, 1988, 1991; Crowell, O'Connor, Wollmers, Sprafkin, & Rao, 1991; Das Eiden, Teti, & Corns, 1995; Oyen, Landy, & Hilburn-Cobb, 2000); marital functioning appears to have moderating effects (Cohn, Cowan, et al., 1992; Das Eiden et al., 1995). Ratings of child symptoms by parents, teachers, and children themselves find that children of insecure parents have the highest ratings of problem behavior and child distress (Cowan, Cowan, Pearson, & Cohn, 1996; Crowell et al., 1991).

Adolescents classified as secure in the AAI are observed to have secure-base relationships with their mothers and to be more socially skilled than those classified as insecure (Allen et al., 2002, 2003; Kobak et al., 1993; see Allen, Chapter 19, this volume, for a review).

Studies of Romantic Relationships

Concordance of Attachment Status. A meta-analysis of AAI attachment classifications of 226 couples showed modest concordance (50–60%, equivalent to a kappa of .20, for three major classifications) between partners for attachment status, accounted for by the secure–secure pairs (van IJzendoorn & Bakermans-Kranenburg, 1996). Not surprisingly, this finding suggests that factors other than attachment security are active in partner selection and maintenance.

Little direct relation between the broad construct of marital satisfaction and AAI classification has been found, but reports of feelings of intimacy are related (Benoit, Zeanah, & Barton, 1989; Cohn, Silver, Cowan, Cowan, & Pearson, 1992; O'Connor, Pan, Waters, & Posada, 1995; Zeanah et al., 1993). In addition, feelings about the relationship are related to interactions among AAI status, representations of the adult partnership, marital behavior, and stressful events (Paley, Cox, Harter, & Margand, 2002; Treboux et al., 2004). Associations between attachment security and the use of physical aggression in couples' relationships

are consistently obtained (Crittenden, Partridge, & Claussen, 1991; O'Connor et al., 1995; Treboux et al., 2004).

There is little correspondence between the AAI and self-reports of attachment (Roisman, Holland, et al., 2007; E. Waters, Crowell, Elliott, Corcoran, & Treboux, 2002). This is discussed further in subsequent sections of this chapter.

Couples' Interactions. In the first edition of this handbook, very little research on adult relationships and the AAI had been conducted, leading some to question whether the AAI was a measure of parent–child attachment. Happily, in the intervening years, studies have found associations between the AAI and attachment/secure-base behaviors in couples' interactions, in samples of both late adolescents and adults (Cohn, Silver, et al., 1992; Creasey, 2002; Creasey & Ladd, 2004, 2005; Crowell et al., 2002; Curran, Hazen, Jacobvitz, & Feldman, 2005; Furman, Simon, Shaffer, & Bouchey, 2002; Paley, Cox, Burchinal, & Payne, 1999; Roisman, Madsen, Hennighausen, Sroufe, & Collins, 2001; Simpson, Rholes, Oriña, & Grich, 2002; Wampler, Riggs, & Kimball, 2004; Wampler, Shi, Nelson, & Kimball, 2003). These findings provide compelling support for the AAI as an assessment of a generalized representation of attachment, rather than one that is specific to a particular type of attachment relationship.

Relationship Interviews

Several interviews have been developed to assess attachment representations within romantic partnerships (e.g., Bartholomew & Horowitz, 1991; Cowan, Cowan, Alexandrov, Lyon, & Heming, 1999; Crowell & Owens, 1996; Dickstein, Seifer, Albus, & Magee, 2004; Furman & Simon, 2006). Most are rooted in the AAI tradition of examining coherence of discourse, and the findings of relations among these interviews, the AAI, self-reports of the relationship, and observed couples' behavior are similar (Alexandrov, Cowan, & Cowan, 2005; Dickstein et al., 2004; Furman & Simon, 2006; Owens et al., 1995). Of these, the Current Relationship Interview (CRI) is the most established (Crowell & Owens, 1996; Crowell, Treboux, Gao, et al., 2002; Crowell, Treboux, & Waters, 2002; Furman et al., 2002; Owens et al., 1995; Roisman, Collins, Sroufe, & Egeland, 2005; Treboux et al., 2004). The CRI investigates the representation of attachment within an adult partnership. It was developed as a way to examine the "prototype hypothesis"—the hypothesis that adult close relationships are similar in organization to parent–child attachment relationships. More specifically, it has been used to explore the process by which a new attachment relationship may be integrated into an already existing representation of attachment, or by which a new representation develops.

As a narrative assessment, the CRI is intended to examine an individual's representation of attachment and ideas regarding the partner's and his or her own attachment behavior. The interview asks the adult for descriptions of the relationship, and for instances of the use of and giving of secure-base support in the relationship. The interview is scored from a transcript, and the subject is classified into one of three groups, according to the profile of scores on a variety of rating scales. Rating scales are used to characterize (1) the participant's behavior and thinking about attachment-related issues (e.g., valuing of intimacy and independence); (2) the partner's behavior; and (3) the participant's discourse style (e.g., anger, derogation, idealization, and overall coherence). The CRI and its scoring system parallel the AAI in structure. The secure–insecure dimension is based on coherent reports of being able to use the partner as a secure base and to act as a secure base, or the coherently expressed desire to do so. Individuals who cannot coherently discuss secure-base use and support in the interview are divided between those who avoid discussion of these behaviors or dismiss their significance, and those who appear to heighten or control the attachment elements of the relationship. CRI scoring is based on state of mind regarding attachment, as well as reports of specific attachment behaviors of secure-base support and use. These factors are given primacy in the determination of attachment security, rather than the individual's reported feelings about the relationship or the behaviors of the partner.

The secure CRI interview is characterized by coherence; that is, the participant convincingly describes his or her own and the partner's secure-base behavior, or can coherently discuss negative partner behavior. The interviewee expresses the idea that an adult attachment relationship should provide support for the individuals involved and for their joint development, whether or not the relationship is actually providing these elements. The dismissing CRI classification is given when there is little evidence that the individual views attachment, support, and comfort within the relationship as important, even if the partner is convincingly described as loving. The discourse is incoherent, in that the relationship may be "normalized." A need for autonomy and separateness within the relationship may be emphasized, and there may be a focus on concrete or material aspects of the relationship (e.g., buying a house, going on vacations). The preoccupied CRI classification is given when the subject expresses strong dependence on the partner or attempts to control the partner. The individual may be dissatisfied or anxious about the partner's ability to fulfill his or her needs, and may express ambivalence or confusion about the relationship, the partner, and/or the self, regardless of the descriptions of partner behavior.

Distribution and Concordance of Classification in Couples

Empirical evidence suggests that the distribution of classifications may vary with the developmental stage of the participants and of the relationship (e.g., Alexandrov et al., 2005; Furman et al., 2002). For example, 46% of CRI transcripts were classified as secure in a sample of young engaged adults (Owens et al., 1995), whereas in a married sample with children, 71% were classified as secure with the Couple Attachment Interview (CAI; Alexandrov et al., 2005). Concordance between partners for CRI classifications was 63% premaritally (kappa = .29) and 65% after 15 months of marriage (kappa = .30); for the CAI, the concordance was 69%.

Stability and Discriminant Validity

Security on the CRI is unrelated to intelligence, education, gender, duration of relationship, or the endorsement of symptoms of depression (Owens et al., 1995). Unlike the AAI, the CRI draws upon a current relationship and is subject to life events and partner behaviors. Hence the CRI classifications are expected to be less stable than those of the AAI, especially in the early phases of relationship development (Crowell & Waters, 1997).

Research with Relationship Interviews
Reports of Relationships and Marital Satisfaction

Individuals classified as secure with relationship interviews report greater satisfaction with their relationship, greater commitment and feelings of love overall, and fewer problems in the relationship than insecure individuals do (Alexandrov et al., 2005; Owens et al., 1995; Roisman et al., 2005; Treboux et al., 2004). Investigations consistently reveal that security assessed with relationship interviews is positively related to attachment behavior in couples' interactions (Alexandrov et al., 2005; Crowell, Treboux, Gao, et al., 2002; Furman & Simon, 2006; Roisman et al., 2005).

Correspondence with the AAI

The correlation of the security scores from concurrently obtained AAIs and CRIs is $r = .51$ (Crowell, Treboux, & Waters, 2002). Evidence suggests that the configuration of AAI and relationship interview classifications within an individual is especially predictive of marital functioning, including divorce rates early in marriage (Dickstein et al., 2004; Treboux et al., 2004). For example, Treboux and colleagues (2004) reported that individuals classified as secure on both the AAI and the CRI reported more positive feelings about the relationship, low observed and reported aggression, and divorce rates consistent with the overall mean. They appeared to tolerate stressful life events without marked change in these parameters. Individuals classified as insecure on both the AAI and the CRI were the most aggressive group, by both observation and self-report. The behaviors and negative feelings about the relationship escalated in association with stressful events. Individuals classified as AAI insecure/CRI secure reported the *most positive* feelings about their relationships and had a significantly lower divorce rate in early marriage than those with other configurations did. However, when stressed, these individuals reported negative feelings about their relationships, and their conflict behavior was more aggressive. Lastly, individuals classified as AAI secure/CRI insecure reported the *most negative* feelings about their relationships and had significantly higher divorce rates than those with the other configurations did. They did not engage in aggressive conflict behaviors, however, even when stressed.

Other Narrative Assessments

The Adult Attachment Projective (AAP) is a projective narrative technique to assess adult attachment (Buchheim, George, & West, 2003; George & West, 2001). It was developed to activate a person's attachment system by presenting one neu-

tral picture (two children playing ball) and seven increasingly stressful attachment pictures (ranging from a lone child looking out a window to a child standing askance in a corner with hand and arm defensively extended, as if protecting him- or herself from a physical assault of some kind). The pictures are fairly simple line drawings, each allowing for a wide range of interpretations. Research participants tell or write brief stories about what is happening in each picture. The scoring system was developed with the AAI as a benchmark. It uses evaluations along three dimensions—discourse (specifically, merging self with a pictured character, and degree of narrative coherence); content (agentic self, and connectedness and synchrony with others); and defensive processing (deactivation, cognitive disconnection, and segregated systems)—to designate the familiar four adult classification groups: secure, dismissing, preoccupied, and unresolved.

In their 2001 article, which introduced the AAP, George and West compared 75 adults' AAI classifications with their AAP classifications, showing high interrater reliability on the AAP and good correspondence with the AAI. In a subsequent study, West and George (2002) showed that preoccupied attachment as assessed with the AAP was associated with dysthymia in a clinical sample of women. van Ecke (2006) compared the AAP classifications of a group of 69 Dutch and Belgian immigrants to California with those of 30 nonimmigrants, finding that being classified as unresolved was linked to greater perception of danger in general (in the AAP) and to a lower ability to resolve danger once it was perceived in a story stimulus picture. The immigrant group was most troubled by images of departure and isolation, whereas the nonimmigrants were most disturbed by images of illness.

The AAP has not yet been widely used in published studies, but George and colleagues (Buchheim, Erk, et al., 2006; Buchheim, George, Kächele, Erk, & Walter, 2006) have shown that it can be used successfully in a functional magnetic resonance imaging environment, with participants providing narratives about the AAP pictures while having their brains scanned. The measure seems worth examining further.

The Narrative Attachment Assessment (NAA) procedure (H. S. Waters & Rodrigues-Doolabh, 2001, 2004) was designed to access adults' possession of "secure-base scripts" regarding situations in which an attachment figure helps an individual resolve a stressful situation. These scripts are thought to be important components of internal working models (Bretherton, 1991; Bretherton & Munholland, Chapter 5, this volume; H. S. Waters & Waters, 2006). H. S. Waters, Rodrigues, and Ridgeway (1998) first tested this idea by reexamining children's responses to an attachment-related story completion task from a previous study (Bretherton, Ridgeway, & Cassidy, 1990). The children had been given a brief partial story (e.g., a child climbs a rock with a parent and hurts his knee), and they were asked to say how it would end (e.g., the child seeks and receives help from a parent). H. S. Waters and colleagues found that children who had been classified as secure at age 25 months told longer, richer, and more highly scripted stories about parents who provided a safe haven and secure base for their child when needed.

The NAA uses a similar procedure with adolescents and adults, but the story leads used with children are stripped down further and presented only in "prompt-word" outlines. (Sample outlines and resulting narratives are available in the article by H. S. Waters & Waters, 2006.) The prompt words are presented in three columns of four words each (e.g., "mother," "baby," "play," "blanket"; then "hug," "smile," "story," "pretend"; then "teddy bear," "lost," "found," "nap"). Study participants are asked to use these words to form a story. The stories are then coded for "secure-base scriptedness" on a 1–7 scale, where 1 indicates "No secure-base script content is apparent; the passage is primarily a list of events," and 7 indicates "Extensive secure-base script organization with substantial elaboration."

The scale scores have been related to AAI coherence, the Strange Situation classification of parents' infants, and the co-construction of secure-base themes during storytelling with children (see H. S. Waters & Waters, 2006, for details). The procedure has worked well in samples from several different cultures (e.g., Vaughn et al., 2006, 2007). Dykas, Woodhouse, Cassidy, and Waters (2006) found that secure-base scriptedness was related to both AAI security and self-report romantic attachment security in a study of 11th graders. Because the script construct is popular in both developmental and social/personality psychology, the NAA method may provide a domain in which both major streams of adult attachment research—one based on narrative measures and the other based on self-report measures (as described in most of the rest of this chapter)—can come together or at least be more clearly compared.

BEHAVIORAL ASSESSMENTS OF ADULT ATTACHMENT

A number of investigators have developed systems of observing attachment behaviors between adult partners, many using a standard marital interaction task as the stressor that provokes attachment behavior (Alexandrov et al., 2005; Creasey, 2002; Creasey & Ladd, 2005; Crowell, Treboux, Gao, et al., 2002; Furman & Simon, 2006; Roisman et al., 2005; Wampler et al., 2004). An external anxiety-inducing stressor has also been employed (Simpson et al., 2002). These assessments focus on support seeking and provision, rather than on positive and negative communication styles. There is evidence that the more specifically attachment behavior is assessed, as opposed to communication behaviors, the more likely it is to relate to narrative assessments of attachment (Crowell, Treboux, Gao, et al., 2002; Paley et al., 1999).

The Secure Base Scoring System (SBSS) is an example of one such behavioral assessment. Couples engage in a standard couple interaction task, which is videotaped and scored with the SBSS, an observational scoring system described in detail in Crowell, Treboux, Gao, and colleagues (2002). When a partner introduces a concern into the discussion, his or her secure-base use is scored on four subscales; scores range from "high quality" to "low quality." The subscales indicate (1) the clarity of initial signal or expression of distress, (2) maintenance of the signal as needed, (3) approach to the partner for help, and (4) the ability to be comforted. Based on these subscales and the general overview of the individual's behavior, the coder assigns a score on the Summary of Secure Base Use scale. Secure-base support is scored for the partner who is presented with the concern raised by the other. It is scored on four subscales: (1) interest in the partner, (2) recognition of distress or concern, (3) interpretation of distress, and (4) responsiveness to distress. Scores again range from "high quality" to "low quality." A Summary of Secure Base Support scale encompasses the overall support provided by the individual. Because the summary scales are often very highly correlated (women, $r = .86$; men, $r = .88$; Crowell, Treboux, Gao, et al., 2002), the average of the summary scales may be used to represent overall quality of secure-base behavior.

SELF-REPORT MEASURES OF ATTACHMENT HISTORY, ATTACHMENT TO PARENTS AND PEERS, AND DIMENSIONS OF RECIPROCAL ATTACHMENTS

The measures reviewed in this section are heterogeneous in focus and method, but all are self-report measures of adolescent and adult attachment that were not based on attempts to capture the attachment patterns identified by Ainsworth and colleagues (1978). None of the measures included in this section has generated as much published research as either the AAI and its offshoots or the Hazan and Shaver (1987) measure of romantic attachment style and its offshoots (see below), but they raise interesting questions and provide valuable leads for further research.

Attachment History Questionnaire

The AHQ was described in Pottharst (1990). It contains sections assessing demographic variables, family history, patterns of family interactions, parental discipline techniques, and friends and support systems. Most of the items are based on Bowlby's writings. Fifty-one items are answered on 7-point response scales, in addition to which there are several open-ended questions and checklists. A principal-components analysis was computed on the 51 scaled items, and four factors were obtained: "secure attachment base" (e.g., trusted parents, amount of love from mother); "parental discipline" (e.g., not allowed to see friends, parents took things away); "threats of separation" (e.g., parents threatened to leave, parents threatened to call police); and "peer affectional support" (e.g., dependability of friends, having been supported by friends). In many studies the subscales have been combined to yield a single security score with an alpha coefficient of .91. A book edited by Pottharst (1990), *Explorations in Adult Attachment*, describes several interesting studies using the measure, which showed that insecurity on one or more AHQ subscales was related to dysfunctional or pathological outcomes (e.g., being the mother in a family in which the father sexually abuses the daughter, abusing one's own children, becoming a prostitute, or having severe psychological problems following loss of a spouse).

With few exceptions (e.g., Kesner, 2000), users of the AHQ have focused on the kinds of extreme circumstances that originally captured Bowlby's interest and led to his thinking about attachment as a normative process, the disruptions or distortions of which could lead to psychopathology. It seems likely that further work with self-reports of attachment history in less troubled samples would yield interesting and useful results. (One such measure, by Parkes, 2006, is mentioned in a later section of this chapter.)

Inventory of Parent and Peer Attachment

Armsden and Greenberg (1987) developed the IPPA to assess adolescents' perceptions of their relationships with parents and close friends. The authors argued that in samples of adolescents, "the 'internal working model' of attachment figures may be tapped by assessing (1) the positive affective/cognitive experience of trust in the accessibility and responsiveness of attachment figures, and (2) the negative affective/cognitive experiences of anger and/or hopelessness resulting from unresponsive or inconsistently responsive attachment figures" (p. 431). Accordingly, the IPPA assesses three broad constructs as they apply to mothers, fathers, and peers: degree of mutual trust (e.g., "My mother respects my feelings"); quality of communication (e.g., "I like to get my mother's point of view on things I'm concerned about"); and degree of anger and alienation (e.g., "My mother expects too much from me"). The dimensions are highly correlated within each relationship type and are therefore commonly aggregated to yield a single index of security insecurity with respect to parents or peers.

Security with respect to parents and security with respect to peers correlate only about .30, indicating that adolescents relate differently to different kinds of close relationship partners, although the qualities assessed in different relationship domains may have common roots (Armsden & Greenberg, 1987). Reliability of the IPPA subscales is high. Three-week test–retest estimates and Cronbach's alphas were approximately .90. The IPPA has been used in several studies to assess security in adolescents and is related to theoretically relevant outcome variables. For example, adolescents who report secure relations with parents also report less conflict between their parents. Secure peer and parental ratings are positively associated with self-esteem and life satisfaction, use of problem-focused coping strategies, and low levels of loneliness and distress (Armsden & Greenberg, 1987). Such security is also associated with higher levels of adjustment (Bradford & Lyddon, 1993; Kenny & Perez, 1996) and identity formation (Schultheiss & Blustein, 1994). Holtzen, Kenny, and Mahalik (1995) found that among a sample of young homosexual adults, those who were secure with their parents were more likely to have disclosed their sexual orientation to their parents (see also Mohr, Chapter 22, this volume). In a sample of 10- to 16-year-old psychiatric patients, adolescents with clinical depression reported more insecure relationships with parents, but those who had recovered from depression did not (Armsden, McCauley, Greenberg, Burke, & Mitchell, 1990); this is similar to the findings for "earned security" in the AAI (Roisman et al., 2006). Lei and Wu (2007) found that parental alienation was related to adolescents' tendencies to seek attachment-like relationships via the Internet.

As mentioned, the IPPA was not designed to differentiate among the attachment patterns delineated by Ainsworth and colleagues (1978): "It is not clear what the development[al] manifestations of 'avoidant' or 'ambivalent' would be in adolescence, or if other conceptualizations of insecure attachment would be more appropriate" (Armsden & Greenberg, 1987, p. 447). Analyses by Brennan, Clark, and Shaver (1998) indicate that the IPPA subscales of trust and communication load primarily on one of the two major dimensions common to self-report measures of romantic/peer attachment, attachment anxiety. The IPPA alienation subscale loads relatively highly on both anxiety and the second dimension, avoidance (see further discussion of these dimensions later in the present chapter).

Reciprocal and Avoidant Attachment Questionnaires for Adults

West and Sheldon-Keller (West & Sheldon, 1988; West et al., 1987; West & Sheldon-Keller, 1992, 1994) have developed two multi-item instruments for measuring individual differences in adult attachment: the Reciprocal Attachment Questionnaire for Adults and the Avoidant Attachment Questionnaire for Adults. Based on Bowlby's (1980) clinical observations concerning loss and its impact on attachment behavior and functioning in children and adults, West and Sheldon-Keller's Reciprocal Attachment Questionnaire operationalizes various components of the attachment system in adults: proximity seeking (e.g., "I feel lost if I'm upset and my attachment figure is not around"); separation protest (e.g., "I feel abandoned when my attachment figure is away for a few days"); feared loss (e.g., "I'm afraid that I will lose my attachment figure's love"); availability (e.g., "I am confident that my attachment figure will try to

understand my feelings"); and use of the attachment figure (e.g., "I talk things over with my attachment figure"). It also operationalizes general patterns of attachment: angry withdrawal (e.g., "I get frustrated when my attachment figure is not around as much as I would like"); compulsive caregiving (e.g., "I put my attachment figure's needs before my own"); compulsive self-reliance (e.g., "I feel it is best not to rely on my attachment figure"); and compulsive care seeking (e.g., "I would be helpless without my attachment figure").

A unique feature of the instruments developed by West and Sheldon-Keller is that each participant is instructed to answer the questions with respect to an individual he or she considers to be a primary attachment figure. Thus the instruments do not assess attachment with respect to romantic relationships, friendship relationships, or parental relationships in general. Instead, they assess the quality of attachment to whoever is identified as an individual's most important attachment figure. (Other self-report methods have been developed to determine who a particular adult's major attachment figures are. Although we do not discuss these measures in the present chapter because of space limitations, they are worth examining. (For examples, see Doherty & Feeney, 2004; Fraley & Davis, 1997; Hazan & Zeifman, 1994; Mikulincer, Gillath, & Shaver, 2002; Trinke & Bartholomew, 1997.)

West and Sheldon-Keller created a separate questionnaire, the Avoidant Attachment Questionnaire, for adults who claim not to have a primary attachment figure. This instrument contains four subscales: "maintains distance in relationships" (e.g., "I'm afraid of getting close to others"); "high priority on self-sufficiency" (e.g., "My strength comes only from myself"); "attachment relationship is a threat to security" (e.g., "Needing someone would make me feel weak"); and "desire for close affectional bonds" (e.g., "I long for someone to share my feelings with").

The subscales of the Reciprocal Attachment Questionnaire have fairly high internal consistency and test–retest reliability over 4 months (approximately .75). Factor analyses of the items indicate that a two-factor solution provides a relatively good fit (West & Sheldon-Keller, 1994). Among the component subscales of the Reciprocal Attachment Questionnaire, availability, feared loss, and proximity seeking load highly on one factor, and use of the attachment figure and separation protest load highly on a second factor. Analyses of the general attachment patterns from the Reciprocal

Attachment Questionnaire indicate that compulsive self-reliance and angry withdrawal load highly on one factor, and that compulsive caregiving and that compulsive care seeking load highly on a second factor. A similar two-dimensional structure appears to underlie the Avoidant Attachment Questionnaire. As Brennan and colleagues (1998) showed, and as we discuss in the next section, this two-factor structure is conceptually similar to the one uncovered in analyses of most self-report measures of adult romantic attachment.

SELF-REPORT MEASURES OF ROMANTIC ATTACHMENT

The study of romantic attachment began in the late 1970s and early 1980s, in an attempt to understand the nature and etiology of adult loneliness and the various ways that people experience love. It had been noticed that many lonely adults report troubled childhood relationships with parents and either distant or overly enmeshed romantic relationships, suggesting that attachment history might play a role in the experience of adult loneliness (Rubenstein & Shaver, 1982; Shaver & Hazan, 1987; Weiss, 1973). Also, social psychologists and anthropologists had observed that there is considerable variability in the way people approach love relationships (ranging from intense preoccupation to psychological distance), and they were developing individual-difference taxonomies to capture this variability (see Sternberg & Barnes, 1988, for examples). Despite these rich descriptions, there was no compelling theoretical framework within which to organize or explain the observed individual differences (Hazan & Shaver, 1994).

In an attempt to address this issue, Hazan and Shaver (1987) published a paper in which they conceptualized romantic love (or "pair bonding," to use the term common in contemporary evolutionary psychology) as an attachment process, involving the interplay among attachment, caregiving, and sexual behavioral systems. Hazan and Shaver noted that many of the emotional and behavioral dynamics characteristic of infant–mother attachment relationships also characterize adult romantic relationships. For example, both kinds of relationships involve hugging and caressing, ventral–ventral contact, "baby talk," and cooing. More importantly, in each case an individual feels safest and most secure when the other is nearby,

accessible, and responsive. Under such circumstances, the partner may be used as a "secure base" from which to explore the environment. When an individual is feeling distressed, sick, or threatened, the partner is used as a "safe haven"—a source of safety, comfort, and protection (see Shaver et al., 1988, for further discussion of these parallels).

Hazan and Shaver (1987; Shaver & Hazan, 1988) argued that the various approaches to love and the experience of loneliness described by social psychologists reflect individual differences in the organization of the attachment system during adulthood. Specifically, they argued that the major patterns of attachment described by Ainsworth and colleagues (1978)—secure, ambivalent or resistant, and avoidant—are conceptually similar to the romantic attachment patterns observed among adults. Although Bowlby and Ainsworth had discussed the role of attachment in romantic relationships, no one had actually attempted to assess, in the adult pair-bond context, the kinds of individual differences among infants noted by Ainsworth and colleagues.

Attachment Style Questionnaires

When Hazan and Shaver (1987, 1990) began their work on romantic attachment, they adopted Ainsworth's threefold typology as a framework for organizing individual differences in the ways adults think, feel, and behave in romantic relationships. In their initial studies, Hazan and Shaver developed brief multisentence descriptions of the three proposed attachment types—avoidant, secure, and ambivalent:

"I am somewhat uncomfortable being close to others; I find it difficult to trust them completely, difficult to allow myself to depend on them. I am nervous when anyone gets too close, and often, others want me to be more intimate than I feel comfortable being" (avoidant).
"I find it relatively easy to get close to others and am comfortable depending on them and having them depend on me. I don't worry about being abandoned or about someone getting too close to me" (secure).
"I find that others are reluctant to get as close as I would like. I often worry that my partner doesn't really love me or won't want to stay with me. I want to get very close to my partner, and this sometimes scares people away" (ambivalent).

These descriptions were based on a speculative extrapolation of the three infant patterns as summarized in the final chapter of Ainsworth and colleagues' (1978) book. Research participants are asked to think back across their history of romantic relationships and say which of the three descriptions best captured the way they *generally* experience and act in romantic relationships. The descriptions refer to a person's characteristic desires, feelings, and behaviors, and to comments made by relationship partners. Because of the closed-ended nature of the measure, there is no attempt to measure discourse coherence. In other words, the manifest content of the measure is quite different from the discourse focus of the AAI and CRI, discussed earlier in this chapter.

In their initial studies, Hazan and Shaver (1987) found that people's self-reported romantic attachment patterns related to a number of theoretically relevant variables, including beliefs about love and relationships (working models of romantic relationships) and recollections of early experiences with parents. Many researchers adopted Hazan and Shaver's categorical, forced-choice measure because of its novelty, brevity, face validity, and ease of administration. Nonetheless, a few investigators quickly recognized some of its limitations (e.g., Collins & Read, 1990; Levy & Davis, 1988; Simpson, 1990). For example, the categorical measurement model assumes that variation among people within a category is unimportant or does not exist, and that individuals do not vary in the extent to which they can be characterized by each pattern. In addition, as Baldwin and Fehr (1995) pointed out, the test–retest stability of the categorical measure was only 70% (equivalent to a Pearson r of approximately .40) and did not decrease as a function of the magnitude of the test–retest interval. This suggested that the temporal instability was due to measurement error resulting from classification artifacts, not to "true" change in attachment security (Fraley & Waller, 1998; Scharfe & Bartholomew, 1994).

To address these issues, many attachment researchers began to use continuous rating scales. For example, Levy and Davis (1988) asked participants to rate how well each attachment pattern described their general approach to relationships. Test–retest reliability estimates for ratings of the three alternatives tended to be about .60 over periods ranging from 1 to 8 weeks (Baldwin & Fehr, 1995; Feeney & Noller, 1996). Subsequently, Collins and Read (1990) and Simpson (1990) de-

composed the three multisentence descriptions to form separate items that could be rated on Likert response scales. These brief multi-item scales yielded alpha and test–retest (over periods ranging from 1 week to 2 years) reliability estimates of .70 (e.g., Carpenter & Kirkpatrick, 1996; Collins & Read, 1990; Fuller & Fincham, 1995; Scharfe & Bartholomew, 1994; Simpson, Rholes, & Phillips, 1996).

A number of researchers proposed similar measures of adult romantic attachment patterns (e.g., Brennan & Shaver, 1995; Carver, 1997; J. A. Feeney, Noller, & Hanrahan, 1994; Griffin & Bartholomew, 1994a; see Brennan et al., 1998, for a comprehensive list). In the midst of these efforts, Bartholomew (1990; Bartholomew & Horowitz, 1991; Griffin & Bartholomew, 1994b) proposed a more elaborate conceptualization of what most investigators came to call "attachment orientations," "attachment patterns," or "attachment styles." The various attempts to create multi-item scales revealed that there are two major dimensions underlying self-report measures of attachment: anxiety (about abandonment or insufficient love) and avoidance (of intimacy, interdependence, and emotional openness).

These two dimensions were conceptualized by Brennan and colleagues (1998) as corresponding to the two dimensions underlying Ainsworth's infant typology (see Figure 10 of Ainsworth et al., 1978). In a discriminant analysis involving 105 infants who had been categorized and scored by coders on Ainsworth's infant behavior scales (e.g., crying, contact maintenance, exploratory behavior, resistance, avoidance), two linear combinations of coding scales were derived that discriminated well among the three infant categories (see also Fraley & Spieker, 2003). One function distinguished ambivalent (angry, tearful) from secure and avoidant infants, thereby reflecting variability in anxious or ambivalent attachment. The other distinguished avoidant from secure and anxious or ambivalent infants, thereby reflecting avoidance. Conceptually, these two dimensions can be viewed as 45-degree rotations of Kobak's security–anxiety and deactivation–hyperactivation dimensions (discussed earlier in this chapter).

Bartholomew (1990) provided an interpretation of these dimensions in terms of what Bowlby called working models of self and attachment figures. She argued that the two dimensions underlying measures of adult attachment can be conceptualized as "model of self " (positive vs. negative) and "model of others" (positive vs. negative). She also pointed out that combinations of the two dimensions can be viewed as yielding four, rather than three, attachment patterns. She chose names for the four patterns based on a mixture of Ainsworth's, Hazan and Shaver's, and Main and colleagues' (1985) typologies, calling the positive–positive group "secure," the negative–positive group "preoccupied," the positive–negative group "dismissing," and the negative–negative group "fearful."

Following Hazan and Shaver's lead, Bartholomew and Horowitz (1991) developed the Relationship Questionnaire (RQ), a short instrument containing multisentence descriptions of each of the four types:

"It is easy for me to become emotionally close to others. I am comfortable depending on them and having them depend on me. I don't worry about being alone or having others not accept me" (secure).

"I am uncomfortable getting close to others. I want emotionally close relationships, but I find it difficult to trust others completely, or to depend on them. I worry that I will be hurt if I allow myself to become too close to others" (fearful).

"I want to be completely emotionally intimate with others, but I often find that others are reluctant to get as close as I would like. I am uncomfortable being without close relationships, but I sometimes worry that others don't value me as much as I value them" (preoccupied).

"I am comfortable without close emotional relationships. It is very important to me to feel independent and self-sufficient, and I prefer not to depend on others or have others depend on me" (dismissing).

Notice that the wording of three of the four type descriptions (secure, preoccupied, and fearful) is very similar to the wording of the three Hazan and Shaver descriptions (secure, ambivalent, and avoidant). However, the compulsive self-reliance and independence depicted in Bartholomew's dismissing description are not represented in the original Hazan and Shaver taxonomy. As with Hazan and Shaver's instrument, respondents choose the RQ description that best fits them, and they rate each description according to how well it describes them. In general, reliability estimates for the RQ classifications (kappas of about .35) and ratings (r's of about .50) are comparable to those of the original Hazan and Shaver three-category instrument (Scharfe & Bartholomew, 1994).

The RQ was more fully developed by Griffin and Bartholomew (1994a) to form the Relationship Styles Questionnaire (RSQ), a 30-item inventory that contains content from both the Hazan and Shaver descriptions and the RQ descriptions. The RSQ can be scaled to create a score for each person on each of the four attachment patterns. That is, each individual can be assigned secure, fearful, preoccupied, and dismissing scores. Also, the RSQ can be used to score people on the two dimensions (model of self and model of other) that underlie these patterns. Due to its multi-item nature, the RSQ exhibits somewhat higher reliability than the RQ (r's of about .65 for the brief scales assessing each of the four attachment patterns; Fraley & Shaver, 1997).

It is worth mentioning here that Parkes (2006), in a recent book on bereavement (discussed further by Shaver & Fraley, Chapter 3, this volume), describes an interesting Retrospective Attachment Questionnaire. This instrument asks adults about their childhood relationships with parents, using only 32 yes–no questions, and about their childhood emotional experiences, using 35 additional yes–no questions. Based on responses to these questions, Parkes scored an adult sample in terms of attachment security, anxiety, avoidance, and disorganization—similar to Bartholomew's four categories (which were, of course, strongly influenced by the AAI categories). Parkes obtained many valuable insights into his sample members' reactions to bereavement. More research should be done to compare Parkes's measure, which is based on retrospective questions about childhood relationships, with ones based on Bartholomew's peer attachment measures.

Well before Parkes's (2006) measure was published, in an effort to reduce the growing number of romantic and peer attachment scales, Brennan and colleagues (1998) factor-analyzed the nonredundant items from all extant self-report attachment measures, including the RQ and RSQ. They found that two major factors (anxiety and avoidance) underlie these measures and can be represented well by two 18-item scales, each with a coefficient alpha of about .90, which are included in the Experiences in Close Relationships (ECR) inventory. The two subscales of the ECR capture the gist of the Armsden and Greenberg IPPA and the West and Sheldon-Keller Reciprocal and Avoidant Attachment Scales for Adults; this suggests that all self-report attachment scales, whether conceived originally in terms of Bowlby's specific constructs (e.g., West & Sheldon-Keller, 1994) or Ainsworth's (e.g., Hazan & Shaver, 1987), load substantially on the same two major factors. These factors can be viewed in terms of either their affective–behavioral names, "anxiety" and "avoidance," or their cognitive/representational (working-model-related) names, "model of self " and "model of other." The ECR is currently one of the most commonly used self-report measures of adult attachment, along with the ECR-R—an alternative version of the ECR developed with methods related to item response theory (Fraley, Waller, & Brennan, 2000).

Current Issues in the Measurement of Adult Romantic Attachment with Self-Reports

Despite conceptual and methodological advances in the study of romantic attachment, a number of important controversies and problems remain. The first concerns whether adult attachment patterns are best conceptualized and measured as types or dimensions (Fraley & Waller, 1998; Griffin & Bartholomew, 1994b). Taxometric work indicates that the adult attachment patterns assessed with self-report measures are best understood in terms of a latent dimensional model (Fraley & Waller, 1998). Fraley and Waller (1998) reviewed many of the problems that can arise when categorical methods are used to assess dimensional phenomena, and they recommended that researchers adopt dimensional measurement models to study adult attachment. Interestingly, this argument suggests that many published findings from research on romantic attachment might have been stronger if researchers had used dimensional rather than categorical assessment procedures (see Brennan et al., 1998, for examples). (The same kind of argument has been made with respect to the Strange Situation and the AAI; see Fraley & Spieker, 2003; Roisman, Fraley, et al., 2007.)

A second issue concerns how best to conceptualize the two dimensions that underlie adult attachment. Should measurement be focused on assessing variation in the content of working models, or variation in the functional operation of the attachment system? Within Bartholomew's framework, individual differences in adult attachment are conceptualized in terms of a person's cognitive models of self and others. Accordingly, many researchers have attempted to specify the actual beliefs that people with different attachment orientations hold (e.g., Baldwin, Fehr, Keedian, Seidel, &

Thomson, 1993; Collins, 1996; Klohnen & John, 1998). When Hazan and Shaver originally applied attachment theory to adults, however, they conceptualized individual differences in terms of the functioning of the attachment system in the domains of affect, affect regulation, and relational behavior, much of which is not very "cognitive" (Shaver et al., 1988; Shaver & Hazan, 1988; see also Mikulincer & Shaver, Chapter 23, this volume).

According to Hazan and Shaver's perspective, as elaborated by Fraley and Shaver (2000), individual differences in attachment patterns are attributable to two different components of the attachment system. One component involves anxious monitoring of the psychological proximity and availability of the attachment figure. When either the attachment figure is perceived as being available and responsive (the "secure" stance), or the attachment figure's availability is not viewed as relevant to or useful in attaining personal safety (the "avoidant" or "dismissing" stance), an individual can focus on other issues and goals (e.g., exploration). This process is closely related to individual differences on the attachment anxiety dimension. The second component of the system concerns the regulation of attachment behavior with respect to attachment-related concerns. For example, to regulate attachment-related anxiety, people can either seek contact with an attachment figure (i.e., use the figure as a safe haven) or withdraw and attempt to handle the threat alone. This decision, which is probably not usually made consciously, is responsible for individual differences on the avoidance dimension.

Viewed in these terms, further specification of the concerns, appraisals, and emotional processes that underlie adult romantic attachment experiences and behaviors need not be limited to positive and negative beliefs about self and other. Thus, although researchers from both the "internal working models" and the "behavioral systems" perspectives currently assess individual differences in terms of the same empirical dimensions (model of self/anxiety and model of other/avoidance), there are differences in the way these dimensions are conceptualized—and, accordingly, differences in the way measurement instruments are being revised and refined (see Mikulincer & Shaver, 2007 and Chapter 23, this volume, for elaborations of the attachment system model).

Finally, there is debate concerning whether attachment patterns are best assessed with self-report instruments or interviews, and whether the two kinds of methods converge on the same phenomena (Bartholomew & Shaver, 1998; Crowell & Treboux, 1995; Gjerde, Onishi, & Carlson, 2004; Roisman, Holland, et al., 2007; Shaver, Belsky, & Brennan, 2000). We return to this issue in the final section of the chapter, because it is responsible for considerable tension between the AAI and self-report traditions within the field of adult attachment research. Here, however, it is worth noting that Bartholomew (Bartholomew & Horowitz, 1991; Griffin & Bartholomew, 1994a, 1994b) and other attachment researchers (Cowan et al., 1999; Gjerde et al., 2004) have developed semistructured interview techniques for assessing adult romantic attachment. These methods are all influenced by the AAI and its scoring system, but some (most notably Bartholomew's) are scored in terms of the two dimensions discussed in the present section, anxiety (model of self) and avoidance (model of others), whereas the AAI and CRI are not. It is important to note that individual differences, when assessed with Bartholomew's interview technique, tend to correspond reasonably well with patterns assessed by self-report instruments (Bartholomew & Horowitz, 1991; Bartholomew & Shaver, 1998; Griffin & Bartholomew, 1994b).

The Nomological Network and Construct Validity

As explained earlier, the AAI coding system was initially developed empirically to maximize the prediction of an adult parent's *infant's* classification in the Strange Situation. In this sense, there was an obvious "gold standard" for the AAI's validity—the categories of the Strange Situation, which are based on naturalistic observations of infants' secure-base behavior. In contrast, the self-report instruments in the Hazan and Shaver tradition were not designed to predict any single criterion. Instead, their validity and the value of the research tradition from which they derive rest on their ability to empirically reproduce the network of covariates postulated by the theory (Cronbach & Meehl, 1955). In this section we discuss the construct validity of measures of adult romantic attachment, focusing on relationship processes, the dismissing strategy in particular, and general adjustment and psychopathology (for more detailed reviews, see Bartholomew & Perlman, 1994; J. Feeney, Chapter 21, this volume; J. A. Feeney & Noller, 1996; Mikulincer & Shaver, 2007; Reis & Patrick, 1996; Shaver & Clark, 1994; Shaver & Hazan, 1993; Shaver & Mikulincer, 2002a, 2002b;

Simpson & Rholes, 1998; Sperling & Berman, 1994). We begin with a brief rationale for the use of self-report instruments in the assessment of attachment security in adults.

The Rationale for Assessing Adult Romantic Attachment with Self-Report Methods

A number of authors have questioned the validity of assessing adult attachment with self-report instruments (Crowell & Treboux, 1995; de Haas, Bakermans-Kranenburg, & van IJzendoorn, 1994; Gjerde et al., 2004), noting the difficulty of assessing unconscious or automatic processes with measures that tap people's conscious reports. There are, however, at least three reasons why self-report instruments are appropriate for investigating individual differences in adult attachment. First, according to Bowlby, attachment plays an important role in people's emotional lives (Volumes 2 and 3 of *Attachment and Loss* [Bowlby, 1973, 1980] deal primarily with anxiety, anger, sadness, grief, and depression). Adults are able to provide valuable information about their emotional experiences and behavior. Second, most adults have sufficient experience in close relationships to recount how they behave in such relationships and the kinds of things their partners have said to them about their behavior. Third, conscious and unconscious processes typically operate in the same direction to achieve a goal (Jacoby, Toth, Lindsay, & Debner, 1992). Bowlby himself (e.g., Bowlby, 1980) talked about both conscious and unconscious forms of defense.

In some cases, however, the conscious beliefs people hold are inaccurate reflections of the organization of their attachment system. Some people defensively report that they are not anxious when actually they are; others may simply lack insight into their true motives and behavior. Nonetheless, even in these cases it is possible to use attachment theory to derive the kinds of conscious beliefs that defensive people may hold about themselves. For example, an avoidant person should believe that he or she is "independent" and "self-sufficient," does not "worry about abandonment," and does not "need close relationships." Holding such beliefs is an important part of defensively excluding attachment-related thoughts and emotions. It is a separate question whether people endorsing such statements in a questionnaire actually do or do not need close relationships to the same extent as other kinds of people, or whether they can function well without others. Although self-reports are frequently used to assess individual differences in attachment security, they are rarely used alone to investigate the dynamics of attachment and defense. In other words, placing a person in the two-dimensional attachment style space is not, by itself, the same as determining *why* the person is located in a particular region of the space. (Similarly, coding someone as having poor recall in the AAI for attachment- related events in childhood does not automatically reveal the *reasons* for poor recall.)

To probe these deeper issues, researchers typically employ behavioral observations (Fraley & Shaver, 1998), psychophysiological assessments (Carpenter & Kirkpatrick, 1996; B. C. Feeney & Kirkpatrick, 1996; Fraley & Shaver, 1997), neuroimaging (Gillath, Bunge, Shaver, Wendelken, & Mikulincer, 2005), peer reports (Banai, Weller, & Mikulincer, 1998; Bartholomew & Horowitz, 1991; Gjerde, Block, & Onishi, 1998), projective tests (Berant, Mikulincer, Shaver, & Segal, 2005; Mikulincer, Florian, & Tolmacz, 1990; Woike, Osier, & Candella, 1996), diary techniques (Pietromonaco & Barrett, 1997; Tidwell, Reis, & Shaver, 1996), and experimental cognitive research methodologies (Baldwin et al., 1993; Fraley & Shaver, 1997, 1998; Mikulincer, 1995, 1998; Mikulincer, Dolev, & Shaver, 2004; Mikulincer & Orbach, 1995). With such a diverse array of methods, the complex meanings of scores on self-report attachment measures have gradually been revealed, and the results fit coherently with attachment theory (see Mikulincer & Shaver, 2007, for a comprehensive review).

Relationship Processes

According to attachment theory, individual differences in the organization of the attachment system emerge from interactions with attachment figures (Ainsworth et al., 1978; Bowlby, 1973) and have numerous influences on relationship dynamics, potentially ranging from partner selection to mechanisms of relationship maintenance and dissolution.

Partner Selection. Cross-cultural studies suggest that the secure pattern of attachment in infancy is universally considered the most desirable pattern by mothers (see van IJzendoorn & Sagi-Schwartz, Chapter 37, this volume). For obvious reasons, there is no similar study asking infants whether they would prefer a security-inducing caregiver or attachment figure. Adults seeking

long-term relationships identify responsive caregiving qualities, such as attentiveness, warmth, and sensitivity, as most "attractive" in potential dating partners (Baldwin, Keelan, Fehr, Enns, & Koh-Rangarajoo, 1996; Chappell & Davis, 1998; Frazier, Byer, Fischer, Wright, & DeBord, 1996; Miller & Fishkin, 1997; Pietromonaco & Carnelley, 1994; Zeifman & Hazan, 1997).

Despite the attractiveness of secure qualities, however, not everyone is paired with a secure partner. Some evidence suggests that people end up in relationships with partners who confirm their existing beliefs about attachment relationships (Brennan & Shaver, 1995; Collins & Read, 1990; Frazier et al., 1996; but see Kirkpatrick & Davis, 1994). In some research that has employed social-cognitive methods for studying transference processes, Brumbaugh and Fraley (2006, 2007) found that people who held negative representations of significant others (parental or romantic) from their pasts were more likely to feel insecure with novel relationship partners. Moreover, this effect was pronounced when representations of the previous significant others were activated without the participants' awareness. This suggests that although most people would prefer a secure partner if given a choice, they tend to re-experience the same kinds of thoughts and feelings in new relationships due to the way existing representations shape new experiences.

Implications for Secure-Base and Safe-Haven Behavior. Overall, secure adults tend to be more satisfied in their relationships than insecure adults. Their relationships are characterized by greater longevity, trust, commitment, and interdependence (J. A. Feeney, Noller, & Callan, 1994; Keelan, Dion, & Dion, 1994; Kirkpatrick & Davis, 1994; Kirkpatrick & Hazan, 1994; Senchak & Leonard, 1992; Simpson, 1990), and they are more likely to use romantic partners as a secure base from which to explore the world (Fraley & Davis, 1997). A large proportion of research on adult attachment has been devoted to uncovering the behavioral and psychological mechanisms that promote security and secure-base behavior in adults. There have been two major discoveries thus far. First, and in accordance with attachment theory, secure adults are more likely than insecure adults to seek support from their partners when distressed. Furthermore, they are more likely to provide support to their distressed partners. Second, the attributions that insecure individuals make concerning their partners' behavior during and following relational conflicts exacerbate, rather than alleviate, their insecurities.

Concerning the first dynamic, Simpson, Rholes, and Nelligan (1992) found in a laboratory study that secure women who were overtly distressed were more likely than insecure women to seek emotional support from their partners. Also, secure men were more likely than insecure men to provide support to their distressed partners. In a naturalistic observational study, Fraley and Shaver (1998) found that secure women who were separating from their partners in an airport were more likely than insecure women to express their anxiety, seek comfort from their partners, and provide comfort for their partners (attending to them, holding their hands, etc.). In contrast, avoidant women were more likely to pull away or withdraw from their partners. Collins and Feeney (2000) found that secure individuals were more likely to offer care and support to their partners during a laboratory discussion of a stressful event. (For a review of related studies, see Collins, Guichard, Ford, & Feeney, 2006. For examples of extensions of these ideas well beyond romantic relationships to relationships in organizational and work contexts, see Davidovitz, Mikulincer, Shaver, Ijzak, & Popper, 2007.) Similar findings have been obtained in studies of self-reported behavioral strategies during stressful situations. For example, Pistole (1989) found that secure adults were more likely than insecure adults to use conflict resolution strategies involving compromise and integration. Gaines and colleagues (1997) found that secure individuals tended not to use defensive and destructive strategies for dealing with conflictual situations. Prospective studies corroborate these observations (e.g., Scharfe & Bartholomew, 1995).

These findings suggest that part of the reason why some individuals feel more secure in their relationships is that they openly express their worries and receive reassurance and support (B. C. Feeney, 2007). Furthermore, the data suggest that some people feel insecure in their relationships because they cannot turn to their partners for comfort and support. Existing research has not been able to tease apart the precise causal structure of these processes. It may be that having a responsive partner influences the way an individual comes to think and behave in a relationship. In addition, perhaps individuals who enter relationships with secure expectations are more likely to seek support from others and to elicit responsive behavior from them. In general, the evidence suggests that the causal relations are bidirectional (Fuller & Fincham, 1995).

In support of the first interpretation, Simpson and colleagues (1996) observed partners who were instructed to discuss and resolve a major issue in their relationship. They found that anxious adults were most likely to view their partners in a negative light after a major conflict. These adults felt more anger and hostility toward their partners than less anxious individuals, and viewed their relationship as involving less love, commitment, and mutual respect. In contrast, secure individuals viewed their partners in a more positive light after discussing a conflictual topic (see Fuller & Fincham, 1995, for related findings). Thus conflictual relationship events, despite their negative valence, may provide an opportunity for secure individuals to build their trust in each other. In contrast, such conflicts appear to magnify insecure partners' insecurities and doubts.

Research also suggests that the beliefs and expectations people hold prior to entering a relationship affect secure-base behavior and relationship development. Collins (1996) conducted an experiment in which participants were instructed to read hypothetical relationship scenarios depicting a partner behaving in ambiguous ways that could be construed in a negative light (e.g., losing track of the partner during a party). She found that anxious participants inferred hostile and rejecting intentions, whereas secure participants inferred more positive intentions. Similarly, Mikulincer (1998) found that insecure adults were more likely to attribute hypothetical trust-violating events (but not trust-validating events) to their partners' intentions. Over time, such attributional processes appear to diminish the degree of trust that both partners extend toward each other (Fuller & Fincham, 1995). For example, Keelan and colleagues (1994) found that insecure adults experienced decreases in trust and relationship satisfaction over a 4-month period.

Changes in Attachment over Time. Cross-sectional and longitudinal studies indicate that the longer partners have been together, the less anxious they become about attachment-related issues such as separation or abandonment (Fraley & Shaver, 1998; Klohnen & Bera, 1998; Mickelson, Kessler, & Shaver, 1997). In other words, scores on the anxiety dimension generally decrease over time. Cross-sectional evidence also suggests that partners become more similar to each other in security over time (Fraley & Shaver, 1998). This observation suggests that attachment security is affected by reciprocal influence processes as a relationship develops (Fuller & Fincham, 1995).

The Dismissing Strategy

According to attachment theory, people differ in the kinds of strategies they adopt to regulate the distress associated with nonoptimal caregiving. Following a separation and reunion, for example, some insecure children approach, but with ambivalence and resistance; others withdraw, apparently minimizing attachment-related feelings and behavior (Main & Weston, 1981). These different strategies have been referred to as "hyperactivating" or "maximizing" strategies and "deactivating" or "minimizing" strategies, respectively (Cassidy & Kobak, 1988; Fraley, Davis, & Shaver, 1998; Main, 1990). Researchers studying romantic attachment have attempted to illuminate some of the defense mechanisms underlying these behavioral strategies. In an experimental task in which adults were instructed to discuss losing their partners, Fraley and Shaver (1997) found that dismissing individuals were just as physiologically distressed (as assessed by skin conductance measures) as other individuals. When instructed to suppress their thoughts and feelings, however, dismissing individuals were able to do so effectively. That is, they could deactivate their physiological arousal to some degree and minimize the attention they paid to attachment-related thoughts. (Interestingly, preoccupied adults experienced an *increase* in arousal, relative to control conditions, when trying to suppress attachment-related anxiety.) Fraley and Shaver argued that such deactivation is possible because avoidant individuals (1) have less complex networks of attachment-related representations, (2) can effectively redirect their attention away from anxiety-provoking stimuli, and (3) can keep their interpersonal world structured so as to minimize attachment-related experiences.

In support of these propositions, Mikulincer and Orbach (1995) found that when asked to recall emotional childhood memories, avoidant adults recalled memories that were characterized by emotional discreteness. That is, when asked to recall a sad memory, avoidant individuals recalled memories that contained only elements of sadness and not elements of anger and anxiety, which tended to be present in the sad memories of secure and especially of preoccupied individuals. Fraley, Garner, and Shaver (2000) found that these recall processes were partly attributable to the way

information is encoded rather than the way it is retrieved per se. Indeed, using both explicit and implicit tests of memory, Fraley and Brumbaugh (2007) found that highly avoidant individuals had difficulty remembering attachment-relevant information—even when they were offered financial incentives to recall as much of the information to which they had been exposed as possible.

Research has also shown that dismissing individuals are less likely to engage in attachment behaviors with their partners (Fraley & Davis, 1997; Shaver & Fraley, Chapter 3, this volume) and are less likely to engage in behaviors thought to promote affectional bonding, such as eye-to-eye contact, kissing, and open communication about feelings (Fraley et al., 1998). In summary, individuals organize their interpersonal behavior in a way that minimizes attachment-related issues. This defensive strategy is reflected in the ways they regulate their attention, behavior, and emotions (Fraley et al., 1998).

It should be noted, however, that these defensive strategies can be undermined. Mikulincer and colleagues (2004) utilized a thought suppression paradigm similar to that used by Fraley and Shaver (1997) and found that highly avoidant people did not show even implicit indications of vulnerability after having thought about a relationship breakup; however, when they were placed under a cognitive load (having to remember a seven-digit number), concepts related to breaking up, as well as each avoidant person's own negative traits, became much more available, suggesting that avoidant defenses can be broken down. A related study (Berant, Mikulincer, & Shaver, in press) showed that avoidant women who gave birth to a child with a congenital heart defect—a persistently distressing situation that cannot be ignored—became increasingly troubled over time, as did their marriages, and their children showed detrimental effects over the first 7 years of life. Nonavoidant women in the same situation did not deteriorate over time, and their children did not show the same adverse effects. These studies suggest that some of the defensive processes used by avoidant individuals require constant cognitive effort.

General Adjustment and Psychopathology

In general, individuals who are secure with respect to attachment have high self-esteem (Bartholomew & Horowitz, 1991; Brennan & Bosson, 1998; Brennan & Morris, 1997; Collins & Read, 1990; J. A. Feeney & Noller, 1990; Shaver et al., 1996) and are considered well adjusted, nurturing, and warm by their peers (Bartholomew & Horowitz, 1991). As found in studies using the AAI (reviewed earlier in this chapter), the *kind* of self-esteem is also meaningfully related to attachment organization. For example, although autonomous and dismissing adults typically report high levels of self-esteem, Brennan and Morris (1997) found that secure adults were more likely to derive their self-esteem from internalized positive regard from others, whereas dismissing adults were more likely to derive their self-esteem from various abilities and competencies.

Not surprisingly, adults with a variety of clinical disorders are more likely to report themselves as insecure (see Mikulincer & Shaver, 2007, Ch. 13, for a review). Depressed adults are more likely to report themselves as insecure, especially preoccupied and fearful (Carnelley, Pietromonaco, & Jaffe, 1994; Hammen et al., 1995). Furthermore, individuals with eating disorders, such as bulimia nervosa and anorexia nervosa, are more likely to report themselves as insecure (Brennan & Shaver, 1995; Burge et al., 1997). College students who felt their parents had drinking problems were more likely to rate themselves as insecure (Brennan, Shaver, & Tobey, 1991) and were reportedly more likely to "drink to cope" themselves (Brennan & Shaver, 1995).

Brennan and Shaver (1998) examined the structure of self-report measures of 13 personality disorders (e.g., schizoid, paranoid, avoidant, obsessive–compulsive) and discovered that two of the three dimensions underlying these scales are the now-familiar dimensions underlying adult romantic attachment patterns. (See Crawford et al., 2006, for a related study of adult attachment orientation and personality disorders.) Woike and colleagues (1996) examined the association between self-reported attachment and the use of violent imagery in the Thematic Apperception Test (TAT). They found that anxious individuals were the most likely to use violent imagery, and they suggested that such imagery may stem from frustration with romantic partners who thwart attachment needs. Consistent with this line of reasoning, Dutton, Saunders, Starzomski, and Bartholomew (1994) found a high incidence of fearful and preoccupied men (i.e., the two groups highest on the anxiety dimension) within a sample that had been referred for treatment for wife assault. Similarly, Bookwala and Zdaniuk (1998) found that preoccupied and fearful adults were the most likely to be involved in reciprocally aggressive romantic relationships (see also Bartholomew & Allison, 2006). The anger that accompanies insecure attachment in adulthood appears to have ramifications for the way people treat their children as well. Moncher (1996) found that parents who abused their children were more likely to rate themselves as insecure than secure.

Discriminant Validity

Evidence for the construct validity of self-report measures of adult attachment comes from the nomological network (Cronbach & Meehl, 1955) of correlations between attachment measures and theoretically relevant variables. And the network corresponds with Bowlby's (e.g., 1980, 1988) belief that attachment orientation is related to many aspects of a person's life. Still, the validity of self-report attachment measures would be called into question if they overlapped too much with measures of constructs viewed as theoretically distant from attachment (Shaver & Brennan, 1992). Several constructs have been proposed as alternatives to attachment style in explaining what self-report measures of adult attachment actually measure. Some writers have expressed concern over the possibility that self-report measures of adult attachment are simply assessing relationship satisfaction (Bartholomew, 1994). Although security is correlated with relationship satisfaction, whether assessed with the AAI or with self-report attachment measures, the average magnitude of the correlation in the case of self-report attachment measures is only about .30 (e.g., Kunce & Shaver, 1994; Senchak & Leonard, 1992; Simpson, 1990). Secure people tend to be in relationships in which they are happy and satisfied, but the correlation is not high enough to suggest that self-report measures of attachment and measures of satisfaction assess the same construct. Another reason for believing that self-report measures of attachment security do not simply assess relationship satisfaction is that they show associations with other theoretically meaningful variables even when individuals are not currently involved in a romantic or couple relationship. Another factor related to close-relationship phenomena is physical attractiveness (Hatfield & Sprecher, 1986). But Tidwell and colleagues (1996) found no association between physical attractiveness (rated from photographs) and adult attachment style.

A great deal of research on adult personality has pointed to a five-factor model of personality (John, 1990; McCrae & Costa, 1990), with the factors being neuroticism, extraversion, openness to experience, agreeableness, and conscientiousness. Thus questions arise concerning how the two major attachment dimensions fit into this structure and whether they are redundant with one or more of the five factors. Noftle and Shaver (2006) examined associations between the five traits and the attachment dimensions in over 8,000 students; they found that the anxiety dimension was correlated about .42 with neuroticism, and that avoidance was correlated approximately –.22 with agreeableness. Thus the attachment dimensions, when assessed via self-reports, share variance with some of the major personality traits, but they are not simply redundant with those traits. In fact, many experimental studies of attachment processes (e.g., Mikulincer et al., 2002) find associations between the attachment dimensions and theoretically predicted outcome variables, including behavior, when, for example, neuroticism is statistically partialed out. Even in uncontrolled survey studies, the attachment variables predict relationship outcomes better than the "Big Five" trait variables (e.g., Noftle & Shaver, 2006; Shaver & Brennan, 1992). Self-report measures of adult attachment are also largely independent of verbal intelligence and social desirability response set (Fraley et al., 1998; Kunce & Shaver, 1994; Mikulincer & Orbach, 1995).

DISCUSSION

From a topic area that hardly existed before 1985, the study of adult attachment has grown over the past 20 years to become one of the most active and visible areas in developmental, social, personality, and clinical psychology. Between 1985 and 2007, nearly 1,000 journal articles dealing with "adult attachment" were published. In general, the findings obtained by adult attachment researchers have been interesting, consistent, and compatible with Bowlby's and Ainsworth's theories. Nevertheless, the issue of measurement continues to present serious challenges. One problem is the lack of convergence among different measures of adult attachment. A number of studies have included more than one measure of some aspect of adult attachment, including measures that tap different relational domains (e.g., relationships with parents, peers, or romantic partners) and embody different methods (e.g., coded interviews, self-report questionnaires). In the initial version of this chapter, published in the first edition of the *Hand-*

book of Attachment, we reported an informal meta-analysis of such studies. The results indicated that the correlation between any two measures of adult attachment were affected both by domain (i.e., whether the measures were designed to assess some aspect of romantic relationships or some aspect of relationships with parents) and by method (i.e., whether the measures were based on interviews or self-report). The correlation between different measures of security tended to be greater when there was a match between the methods used (e.g., both measures were based on self-report or both on interviews) and when there was a match in domains (e.g., both measures focused on parental representations or both on romantic representations).

One important example of this patterning is that the two most commonly used types of adult attachment measures (i.e., self-reports of the attachment dimensions and classifications based on the AAI) have only a very weak association. And this happens despite the fact that the two kinds of measures sometimes have similar correlations with other variables (e.g., Granqvist & Kirkpatrick, Chapter 38, this volume; Simpson et al., 2002). Roisman, Holland, and colleagues (2007) recently published a meta-analysis of all available studies that included both the AAI and some self-report measure of adult attachment. Aggregating data from over 900 individuals, they found a correlation of only .09, which is small by the frequently used standards proposed by Cohen (1992). Moreover, in those particular studies they found that although both measures predicted important aspects of close relationship functioning in adulthood, they did not necessarily predict the same kinds of outcomes in the same ways.

For example, in predicting interpersonal collaboration, the AAI seemed to function as a general interpersonal asset; highly autonomous or secure individuals were more likely to be collaborative in their laboratory interactions with their partners—which is not surprising when one considers that the AAI itself is measuring, in part, the ability and willingness of an interviewee to collaborate with an interviewer (see Hesse, Chapter 25, this volume). The attachment dimensions, in contrast, functioned more like what would be expected from a diathesis–stress perspective on attachment dynamics (e.g., Simpson & Rholes, 1998). Anxiety and avoidance were related to less collaborative interactions, but only among individuals who appraised the interaction as stressful or threatening to begin with (and, we suppose, were more likely to have their attachment systems activated).

Another reason for tension between researchers who use different measures of attachment is that the AAI is generally considered to be a measure of unconscious aspects of attachment-related defenses and behaviors, whereas the self-report measures are often taken to be measures only of conscious processes, since people are simply asked to answer questions based on their conscious assessments of their feelings and behaviors in close relationships. Mikulincer and Shaver, however, have conducted and reviewed numerous studies in which measures of unconscious processes (e.g., the TAT, the Rorschach, reactions to Stroop and lexical decision tasks, coded dreams, various kinds of inadvertent behavior) were systematically and predictably related to self-report measures of adult attachment (Mikulincer & Shaver, 2007, Ch. 4; Mikulincer & Shaver, Chapter 23, this volume; Shaver & Mikulincer, 2002a, 2002b, 2004). Thus the self-report measures are obviously tapping aspects of a person that are systematically associated with unconscious processes.

Although we still do not fully understand how the different measures work and why, or precisely what they measure (as inferred from their broad and largely different nomothetic networks), it is clear that they should not be viewed as substitutes for each other in particular kinds of research. We therefore encourage researchers to use assessment techniques that are most relevant to the kind of relationship or attachment-related processes they wish to study. For example, if a researcher is interested in studying romantic attachment dynamics, he or she should use either one of the multi-item self-report measures (e.g., the ECR or ECR-R) or one of the relationship interview techniques (Crowell and Owen's CRI, or Cowan and colleagues' CAI). If the focus is on coherent communication and behavioral coordination or collaboration between partners, the AAI is likely to provide stronger associations. If the focus is on relationship-related emotions and behavior under stressful circumstances, especially as experienced and reported by the person him- or herself, the self-report measures are likely to yield stronger associations. If the focus is on all of these things at once, it is possible that the two kinds of measures will both produce useful findings and insights, but they may do so without correlating with each other very highly. Investigators interested in assessing the common variance underlying adolescents' and adults' various attachment orientations will have

to assess attachment variation across multiple relationship domains (e.g., parents, close friends, romantic partners), preferably by using a variety of methods (e.g., self-reports, interviews) and latent structural modeling techniques (see Griffin & Bartholomew, 1994b).

As we have explained throughout this chapter, each measure was developed for a particular purpose. Therefore, in determining which one or more instruments to use for a particular study, a researcher should consider the theoretical assumptions underlying each instrument. The AAI classifies an adult's generalized representation of attachment based on his or her current "state of mind with respect to attachment," as inferred from narrative measures of experiences with parents during childhood—measures that require a collaborative interaction with an interviewer. Its focus on discourse is based on the assumption that the ability to describe secure-base experiences reflects either the nature of those experiences or, in the case of those who have "earned security," the ability to understand them in a coherent and believable way. It is a rich and well-validated measure. Nevertheless, the AAI is expensive and difficult to score.

The AHQ, the IPPA, and the Reciprocal Attachment Questionnaire for Adults were developed to assess attachment history, relationship behaviors, and feelings of security in relationships with parents and peers, but they were not designed to tap the attachment patterns observed in infants and children by Ainsworth and colleagues (1978). In contrast, the self-report romantic attachment measures were designed to assess patterns such as those described by Ainsworth and her colleagues, under the assumption that these patterns reflect variation in the organization of the attachment system at any age. The self-report measures assume that people can accurately describe some of their thoughts, feelings, and behaviors in romantic or other close relationships. Such measures are not ideal for investigating mechanisms and strategies per se, but they have been effectively used in conjunction with other techniques (such as psychophysiological, behavioral, and cognitive procedures) to uncover important aspects of intrapsychic processes and behavior in close relationships.

In summary, before choosing a measure to assess adult attachment, researchers should consider (1) the assumptions underlying each technique, and the conceptual connection between a technique and the concepts and propositions of attachment theory; and (2) the relationship domain to be investigated (e.g., parents, close friends, romantic partners). In light of the substantial differences among adult attachment measures, we urge caution in how researchers present their findings and in how they generalize across measures with respect to attachment theory. Furthermore, we encourage researchers to continue to investigate the many measurement issues inherent in the study of adult attachment. There is still a great deal of work to be done before we understand relations and nonrelations among the various instruments and the best ways to assess normative development and individual differences in adult attachment organization. We hope that this overview provides a useful basis for further exploration.

REFERENCES

Adam, E. K., Gunnar, M. R., & Tanaka, A. (2004). Adult attachment, parent emotion, and observed parenting behavior: Mediator and moderator models. *Child Development, 75,* 110–122.

Ainsworth, M. D. S. (1985). Attachments across the life span. *Bulletin of the New York Academy of Medicine, 61,* 792–811.

Ainsworth, M. D. S. (1989). Attachments beyond infancy. *American Psychologist, 44,* 709–716.

Ainsworth, M. D. S. (1991). Attachments and other affectional bonds across the life cycle. In C. M. Parkes, J. Stevenson-Hinde, & P. Marris (Eds.), *Attachment across the life cycle* (pp. 33–51). London: Routledge.

Ainsworth, M. D. S., Blehar, M., Waters, E., & Wall, S. (1978). *Patterns of attachment: A psychological study of the Strange Situation.* Hillsdale, NJ: Erlbaum.

Alexandrov, E. O., Cowan, P. A., & Cowan, C. P. (2005). Couple attachment and the quality of marital relationships: Method and concept in the validation for the new couple attachment interview and coding system. *Attachment and Human Development, 7,* 123–152.

Allen, J. P., Marsh, P., McFarland, C., McElhaney, K. B., Land, D. J., Jodl, K. M., et al. (2002). Attachment and autonomy as predictors of the development of social skills and delinquency during mid-adolescence. *Journal of Consulting and Clinical Psychology, 70,* 56–66.

Allen, J. P., McElhaney, K. B., Kuperminc, G. P., & Jodl, K. M. (2004). Stability and change in attachment security across adolescence. *Child Development, 75,* 1792–1805.

Allen, J. P., McElhaney, K. B., Land, D. J., Kuperminc, G. P., Moore, C. W., O'Beirne-Kelly, H., et al. (2003). A secure base in adolescence: Markers of attachment security in the mother–adolescent relationship. *Child Development, 74,* 292–307.

Armsden, G. C., & Greenberg, M. T. (1987). The Inventory of Parent and Peer Attachment: Relationships to well-being in adolescence. *Journal of Youth and Adolescence, 16,* 427–454.

Armsden, G. C., McCauley, E., Greenberg, M. T., Burke, P., & Mitchell, J. (1990). Parent and peer attachment in early adolescent depression. *Journal of Youth and Adolescence, 12,* 373–386.

Atkinson, L., Paglia, A., Coolbear, J., Niccols, A., Parker, K. C. H., & Guger, S. (2000). Attachment security: A meta-analysis of maternal mental health correlates. *Clinical Psychology Review, 20,* 1019–1040.

Bakermans-Kranenburg, M., & van IJzendoorn, M. (1993). A psychometric study of the Adult Attachment Interview: Reliability and discriminant validity. *Developmental Psychology, 29,* 870–879.

Baldwin, M. W., & Fehr, B. (1995). On the instability of attachment style ratings. *Personal Relationships, 2,* 247–261.

Baldwin, M. W., Fehr, B., Keedian, E., Seidel, M., & Thomson, D. W. (1993). An exploration of the relational schemata underlying attachment styles: Self report and lexical decision approaches. *Personality and Social Psychology Bulletin, 19,* 746–754.

Baldwin, M. W., Keelan, J. P. R., Fehr, B., Enns, V., & Koh-Rangarajoo, E. (1996). Social-cognitive conceptualization of attachment working models: Availability and accessibility effects. *Journal of Personality and Social Psychology, 71,* 94–109.

Banai, E., Weller, A., & Mikulincer, M. (1998). Interjudge agreement in evaluation of adult attachment style: The impact of acquaintanceship. *British Journal of Social Psychology, 37,* 95–109.

Bartholomew, K. (1990). Avoidance of intimacy: An attachment perspective. *Journal of Social and Personal Relationships, 7,* 147–178.

Bartholomew, K. (1994). Assessment of individual differences in adult attachment. *Psychological Inquiry, 5,* 23–27.

Bartholomew, K., & Allison, C. J. (2006). An attachment perspective on abusive dynamics in intimate relationships. In M. Mikulincer & G. S. Goodman (Eds.), *Dynamics of romantic love* (pp. 102–127). New York: Guilford Press.

Bartholomew, K., & Horowitz, L. (1991). Attachment styles among young adults: A test of a four category model. *Journal of Personality and Social Psychology, 61,* 226–244.

Bartholomew, K., & Perlman, D. (Eds.). (1994). *Advances in personal relationships: Vol. 5. Attachment processes in adulthood.* London: Jessica Kingsley.

Bartholomew, K., & Shaver, P. R. (1998). Methods of assessing adult attachment: Do they converge? In J. A. Simpson & W. S. Rholes (Eds.), *Attachment theory and close relationships* (pp. 25–45). New York: Guilford Press.

Benoit, D., & Parker, K. (1994). Stability and transmission of attachment across three generations. *Child Development, 65,* 1444–1456.

Benoit, D., Zeanah, C., & Barton, M. (1989). Maternal attachment disturbances in failure to thrive. *Infant Mental Health Journal, 10,* 185–202.

Berant, E., Mikulincer, M., & Shaver, P. R. (in press). Mothers' attachment style, their mental health, and their children's emotional vulnerabilities: A seven-year study of mothers of children with congenital heart disease. *Journal of Personality.*

Berant, E., Mikulincer, M., Shaver, P. R., & Segal, Y. (2005). Rorschach correlates of self-reported attachment dimensions: Dynamic manifestations of hyperactivating and deactivating strategies. *Journal of Personality Assessment, 84,* 70–81.

Bookwala, J., & Zdaniuk, B. (1998). Adult attachment styles and aggressive behavior within dating relationships. *Journal of Social and Personal Relationships, 15,* 175–190.

Bowlby, J. (1969/1982). *Attachment and loss: Vol. 1. Attachment.* New York: Basic Books.

Bowlby, J. (1973). *Attachment and loss: Vol. 2. Separation: Anxiety and anger.* New York: Basic Books.

Bowlby, J. (1980). *Attachment and loss: Vol. 3. Loss: Sadness and depression.* New York: Basic Books.

Bowlby, J. (1988). *A secure base.* New York: Basic Books.

Bradford, E., & Lyddon, W. J. (1993). Current parental attachment: Its relation to perceived psychological distress and relationship satisfaction in college students. *Journal of College Student Development, 34,* 256–260.

Brennan, K. A., & Bosson, J. K. (1998). Attachment-style differences in attitudes toward and reactions to feedback from romantic partners: An exploration of the relational bases of self-esteem. *Personality and Social Psychology Bulletin, 24,* 699–714.

Brennan, K. A., Clark, C. L., & Shaver, P. R. (1998). Self-report measurement of adult attachment: An integrative overview. In J. A. Simpson & W. S. Rholes (Eds.), *Attachment theory and close relationships* (pp. 46–76). New York: Guilford Press.

Brennan, K. A., & Morris, K. A. (1997). Attachment styles, self-esteem, and patterns of seeking feedback from romantic partners. *Personality and Social Psychology Bulletin, 23,* 23–31.

Brennan, K. A., & Shaver, P. R. (1995). Dimensions of adult attachment, affect regulation, and romantic relationship functioning. *Personality and Social Psychology Bulletin, 21,* 267–283.

Brennan, K. A., & Shaver, P. R. (1998). Attachment styles and personality disorders: Their connections to each other and to parental divorce, parental death, and perceptions of parental caregiving. *Journal of Personality, 66,* 835–878.

Brennan, K. A., Shaver, P. R., & Tobey, A. E. (1991). Attachment styles, gender, and parental problem drinking. *Journal of Social and Personal Relationships, 8,* 451–466.

Bretherton, I. (1985). Attachment theory: Retrospect and prospect. In I. Bretherton & E. Waters (Eds.), Growing points of attachment theory and research. *Monographs of the Society for Research in Child Development, 50*(1–2, Serial No. 209), 3–35.

Bretherton, I., Ridgeway, D., & Cassidy, J. (1990). Assessing internal working models of the attachment relationship: An attachment story-completion task

for 3-year-olds. In M. Greenberg, D. Cicchetti, & E. M. Cummings (Eds.), *Attachment during the preschool years: Theory, research, and intervention* (pp. 272–308). Chicago: University of Chicago Press.

Brumbaugh, C. C., & Fraley, R. C. (2006). Transference and attachment: How do attachment patterns get carried forward from one relationship to the next? *Personality and Social Psychology Bulletin, 32,* 552–560.

Brumbaugh, C. C., & Fraley, R. C. (2007). The transference of attachment patterns: How parental and romantic relationships influence feelings toward novel people. *Personal Relationships, 14,* 513–530.

Buchheim, A., Erk, S., George, C., Kächele, H., Ruchsow, M., Spitzer, M., et al. (2006). Measuring attachment representation in an fMRI environment: A pilot study. *Psychopathology, 39,* 144–152.

Buchheim, A., George, C., Kächele, H., Erk, S., & Walter, H. (2006). Measuring adult attachment representation in an fMRI environment: Concepts and assessment. *Psychopathology, 39,* 136–143.

Buchheim, A., George, C., & West, M. (2003). The Adult Attachment Projective (AAP): Psychometric properties and new research. *Psychotherapie, Psychosomatic Medicine, and Psychology, 53,* 419–427.

Burge, D., Hammen, C., Davila, J., Daley, S. E., Paley, B., Lindberg, N., et al. (1997). The relationship between attachment cognitions and psychological adjustment in late adolescent women. *Development and Psychopathology, 9,* 151–167.

Carnelley, K. B., Pietromonaco, P. R., & Jaffe, K. (1994). Depression, working models of others, and relationship functioning. *Journal of Personality and Social Psychology, 66,* 127–140.

Carpenter, E. M., & Kirkpatrick, L. A. (1996). Attachment style and presence of a romantic partner as moderators of psychophysiological responses to a stressful laboratory situation. *Personal Relationships, 3,* 351–367.

Carver, C. S. (1997). Adult attachment and personality: Converging evidence and a new measure. *Personality and Social Psychology Bulletin, 23,* 865–883.

Cassibba, R., van IJzendoorn, M. H., Bruno, S., & Coppola, G. (2004). Attachment of mothers and children with recurrent asthmatic bronchitis. *Journal of Asthma, 41,* 419–431.

Cassidy, J., & Kobak, R. R. (1988). Avoidance and its relation to other defensive processes. In J. Belsky & T. Nezworski (Eds.), *Clinical implications of attachment* (pp. 300–323). Hillsdale, NJ: Erlbaum.

Chappell, K. D., & Davis, K. E. (1998). Attachment, partner choice, and perceptions of romantic partners: An experimental test of the attachment-security hypothesis. *Personal Relationships, 5,* 327–342.

Cohen, J. (1992). A power primer. *Psychological Bulletin, 112,* 155–159.

Cohn, D., Cowan, P., Cowan, C., & Pearson, J. (1992). Mothers' and fathers' working models of childhood attachment relationships, parenting style, and child behavior. *Development and Psychopathology, 4,* 417–431.

Cohn, D., Silver, D., Cowan, P., Cowan, C., & Pearson, J. (1992). Working models of childhood attachment and couples relationships. *Journal of Family Issues, 13,* 432–449.

Collins, N. L. (1996). Working models of attachment: Implications for explanation, emotion, and behavior. *Journal of Personality and Social Psychology, 71,* 810–832.

Collins, N. L., & Feeney, B. C. (2000). A safe haven: Support-seeking and caregiving processes in normal relationships. *Journal of Personality and Social Psychology, 78,* 1053–1073.

Collins, N. L., Guichard, A. C., Ford, M. B., & Feeney, B. C. (2006). Responding to need in intimate relationships: Normative processes and individual differences. In M. Mikulincer & G. Goodman (Eds.), *Dynamics of love: Attachment, caregiving, and sex* (pp. 149–189). New York: Guilford Press.

Collins, N. L., & Read, S. J. (1990). Adult attachment, working models, and relationship quality in dating couples. *Journal of Personality and Social Psychology, 58,* 644–663.

Cowan, P. A., Cohn, D., Cowan, C. P., & Pearson, J. (1996). Parents' attachment histories and children's externalizing and internalizing behavior: Exploring family systems models of linkage. *Journal of Consulting and Clinical Psychology, 64,* 53–63.

Cowan, P. A., Cowan, C. P., Alexandrov, E. O., Lyon, S., & Heming, H. (1999). *Couples' Attachment Interview.* Unpublished manuscript, University of California at Berkeley.

Crawford, T. N., Shaver, P. R., Cohen, P., Pilkonis, P. A., Gillath, O., & Kasen, S. (2006). Self-reported attachment, interpersonal aggression, and personality disorder in a prospective community sample of adolescents and adults. *Journal of Personality Disorders, 20,* 331–351.

Creasey, G. (2002). Associations between working models of attachment and conflict management behavior in romantic couples. *Journal of Counseling Psychology, 49,* 365–375.

Creasey, G., & Ladd, A. (2004). Negative mood relations expectancies and conflict behaviors in late adolescent college student romantic relationships: The moderating role of generalized attachment representations. *Journal of Research on Adolescence, 14,* 235–255.

Creasey, G., & Ladd, A. (2005). Generalized and specific attachment representations: Unique and interactive roles in predicting conflict behaviors in close relationships. *Personality and Social Psychology Bulletin, 31,* 1026–1038.

Crittenden, P., Partridge, M., & Claussen, A. (1991). Family patterns of relationships in normative and dysfunctional families. *Development and Psychopathology, 3,* 491–512.

Cronbach, L. J., & Meehl, P. M. (1955). Construct validity in psychological tests. *Psychological Bulletin, 52,* 281–302.

Crowell, J., & Waters, E. (1997, April). *Couples' attach-ment representations: Stability and relation to marital behavior.* Paper presented at the biennial meeting of the Society for Research in Child Development, Washington, DC.

Crowell, J. A., & Feldman, S. S. (1988). Mothers' internal models of relationships and children's behavioral and developmental status: A study of mother–child interaction. *Child Development, 59,* 1273–1285.

Crowell, J. A., & Feldman, S. S. (1991). Mothers' working models of attachment relationships and mother and child behavior during separation and reunion. *Developmental Psychology, 27,* 597–605.

Crowell, J. A., O'Connor, E., Wollmers, G., Sprafkin, J., & Rao, U. (1991). Mothers' conceptualizations of parent–child relationships: Relation to mother–child interaction and child behavior problems. *Development and Psychopathology, 3,* 431–444.

Crowell, J. A., & Owens, G. (1996). *Current Relationship Interview and scoring system.* Unpublished manuscript, State University of New York at Stony Brook.

Crowell, J. A., & Treboux, D. (1995). A review of adult attachment measures: Implications for theory and research. *Social Development, 4,* 294–327.

Crowell, J. A., Treboux, D., & Waters, E. (1999). The Adult Attachment Interview and the Relationship Questionnaire: Relations to reports of mothers and partners. *Personal Relationships, 6,* 1–18.

Crowell, J. A., Treboux, D., & Waters, E. (2002). Stability of attachment representations: The transition to marriage. *Developmental Psychology, 38,* 467–479.

Crowell, J. A., Treboux, D., Gao, Y., Fyffe, C., Pan, H., & Waters, E. (2002). Assessing secure base behavior in adulthood: Development of a measure, links to adult attachment representations, and relations to couples' communication and reports of relationships. *Developmental Psychology, 38,* 679–693.

Crowell, J. A., Waters, E., Treboux, D., O'Connor, E., Colon-Downs, C., Feider, O., et al. (1996). Discriminant validity of the Adult Attachment Interview. *Child Development, 67,* 2584–2599.

Curran, M., Hazen, N., Jacobvitz, D., & Feldman, A. (2005). Representations of early family relationships predict marital maintenance during the transition to parenthood. *Journal of Family Psychology, 19,* 189–197.

Das Eiden, R., Teti, D., & Corns, K. (1995). Maternal working models of attachment, marital adjustment, and the parent–child relationship. *Child Development, 66,* 1504–1518.

Davidovitz, R., Mikulincer, M., Shaver, P. R., Ijzak, R., & Popper, M. (2007). Leaders as attachment figures: Their attachment orientations predict leadership-related mental representations and followers' performance and mental health. *Journal of Personality and Social Psychology, 93,* 632–650.

de Haas, M., Bakermans-Kranenburg, M., & van IJzendoorn, M. (1994). The Adult Attachment Interview and questionnaires for attachment style, temperament, and memories of parental behavior. *Journal of Genetic Psychology, 155,* 471–486.

DeOliveira, C. A., Moran, G., & Pederson, D. R. (2005). Understanding the link between maternal adult attachment classifications and thoughts and feelings about emotions. *Attachment and Human Development, 7*, 153–170.

Dickstein, S., Seifer, R., Albus, K. E., & Magee, K. D. (2004). Attachment patterns across multiple family relationships in adulthood: Associations with maternal depression. *Developmental Psychopathology, 16*, 735–751.

Doherty, N. A., & Feeney, J. A. (2004). The composition of attachment networks throughout the adult years. *Personal Relationships, 11*, 469–488.

Dozier, M., & Kobak, R. R. (1992). Psychophysiology in attachment interviews: Converging evidence for deactivating strategies. *Child Development, 63*, 1473–1480.

Dozier, M., & Lee, S. W. (1995). Discrepancies between self- and other-report of psychiatric symptomatology: Effects of dismissing attachment strategies. *Development and Psychopathology, 7*, 217–226.

Dutton, D. G., Saunders, K., Starzomski, A., & Bartholomew, K. (1994). Intimacy–anger and insecure attachment as precursors of abuse in intimate relationships. *Journal of Applied Social Psychology, 24*, 1367–1386.

Dykas, M. J., Woodhouse, S. S., Cassidy, J., & Waters, H. S. (2006). Narrative assessment of attachment representations: Links between secure base scripts and adolescent attachment. *Attachment and Human Development, 8*, 221–240.

Feeney, B. C. (2007). The dependency paradox in close relationships: Accepting dependence promotes independence. *Journal of Personality and Social Psychology, 92*, 268–285.

Feeney, B. C., & Kirkpatrick, L. A. (1996). Effects of adult attachment and presence of romantic partners on physiological responses to stress. *Journal of Personality and Social Psychology, 70*, 255–270.

Feeney, J. A., & Noller, P. (1990). Attachment style as a predictor of adult romantic relationships. *Journal of Personality and Social Psychology, 58*, 281–291.

Feeney, J. A., & Noller, P. (1996). *Adult attachment.* Thousand Oaks, CA: Sage.

Feeney, J. A., Noller, P., & Callan, V. J. (1994). Attachment style, communication, and satisfaction in the early years of marriage. In K. Bartholomew & D. Perlman (Eds.), *Advances in personal relationships: Vol. 5. Attachment processes in adulthood* (pp. 269–308). London: Jessica Kingsley.

Feeney, J. A., Noller, P., & Hanrahan, M. (1994). Assessing adult attachment: Developments in the conceptualization of security and insecurity. In M. B. Sperling & W. H. Berman (Eds.), *Attachment in adults: Clinical and developmental perspectives* (pp. 128–152). New York: Guilford Press.

Finkel, D., & Matheny, A. (2000). Genetic and environmental influences on a measure of infant attachment security. *Twin Research, 3*, 242–250.

Fonagy, P., Steele, H., & Steele, M. (1991). Maternal representations of attachment during pregnancy predict the organization of infant–mother attachment. *Child Development, 62*, 891–905.

Fonagy, P., Steele, M., Steele, H., Moran, G. S., & Higgitt, A. C. (1991). The capacity for understanding mental states: The reflective self in parent and child and its significance for security of attachment. *Infant Mental Health Journal, 12*, 201–218.

Fraley, R. C. (2002). Attachment stability from infancy to adulthood: Meta-analysis and dynamic modeling of developmental mechanisms. *Personality and Social Psychology Review, 6*, 123–151.

Fraley, R. C., & Brumbaugh, C. C. (2007). Adult attachment and preemptive defenses: Converging evidence on the role of defensive exclusion at the level of encoding. *Journal of Personality, 75*, 1033–1050.

Fraley, R. C., & Davis, K. E. (1997). Attachment formation and transfer in young adults' close friendships and romantic relationships. *Personal Relationships, 4*, 131–144.

Fraley, R. C., Davis, K. E., & Shaver, P. R. (1998). Dismissing-avoidance and the defensive organization of emotion, cognition, and behavior. In J. A. Simpson & W. S. Rholes (Eds.), *Attachment theory and close relationships* (pp. 249–279). New York: Guilford Press.

Fraley, R. C., Garner, J. P., & Shaver, P. R. (2000). Adult attachment and the defensive regulation of attention and memory: Examining the role of preemptive and postemptive defensive processes. *Journal of Personality and Social Psychology, 79*, 816–826.

Fraley, R. C., & Shaver, P. R. (1997). Adult attachment and the suppression of unwanted thoughts. *Journal of Personality and Social Psychology, 73*, 1080–1091.

Fraley, R. C., & Shaver, P. R. (1998). Airport separations: A naturalistic study of adult attachment dynamics in separating couples. *Journal of Personality and Social Psychology, 75*, 1198–1212.

Fraley, R. C., & Shaver, P. R. (2000). Adult romantic attachment: Theoretical developments, emerging controversies, and unanswered questions. *Review of General Psychology, 4*, 132–154.

Fraley, R. C., & Spieker, S. J. (2003). Are infant attachment patterns continuously or categorically distributed?: A taxometric analysis of Strange Situation behavior. *Developmental Psychology, 39*, 387–404.

Fraley, R. C., & Waller, N. G. (1998). Adult attachment patterns: A test of the typological model. In J. A. Simpson & W. S. Rholes (Eds.), *Attachment theory and close relationships* (pp. 77–114). New York: Guilford Press.

Fraley, R. C., Waller, N. G., & Brennan, K. A. (2000). An item response theory analysis of self-report measures of adult attachment. *Journal of Personality and Social Psychology, 78*, 350–365.

Frazier, P. A., Byer, A. L., Fischer, A. R., Wright, D. M., & DeBord, K. A. (1996). Adult attachment style and partner choice: Correlational and experimental findings. *Personal Relationships, 3*, 117–136.

Fuller, T. L., & Fincham, F. D. (1995). Attachment style in married couples: Relation to current marital functioning, stability over time, and method of assessment. *Personal Relationships, 2,* 17–34.

Furman, W., & Simon, V. A. (2006). Actor and partner effects of adolescents' romantic working models and styles on interactions with romantic partners. *Child Development, 77,* 588–604.

Furman, W., Simon, V. A., Shaffer, L., & Bouchey, H. A. (2002). Adolescents' representations of relationships with parents, friends and romantic partners. *Child Development, 73,* 241–255.

Fyffe, C., & Waters, E. (1997, April). *Empirical classification of adult attachment status: Predicting group membership.* Poster presented at the biennial meeting of the Society for Research in Child Development, Washington, DC.

Gaines, S. O., Reis, H. T., Summers, S., Rusbult, C. E., Cox, C. L., Wexler, M. O., et al. (1997). Impact of attachment style on reactions to accommodative dilemmas in close relationships. *Personal Relationships, 4,* 93–113.

George, C., Kaplan, N., & Main, M. (1984). *Adult Attachment Interview protocol.* Unpublished manuscript, University of California at Berkeley.

George, C., Kaplan, N., & Main, M. (1985). *Adult Attachment Interview protocol* (2nd ed.). Unpublished manuscript, University of California at Berkeley.

George, C., Kaplan, N., & Main, M. (1996). *Adult Attachment Interview protocol* (3rd ed.). Unpublished manuscript, University of California at Berkeley.

George, C., & West, M. (2001). The development and preliminary validation of a new measure of adult attachment: The Adult Attachment Projective. *Attachment and Human Development, 3,* 30–61.

Gervai, J., Nemoda, Z., Lakatos, K., Ronai, Z., Toth, I., Ney, K., et al. (2005). Transmission disequilibrium tests confirm the link between DRD4 gene polymorphism and infant attachment. *American Journal of Medical Genetics, 132B,* 126–130.

Gillath, O., Bunge, S. A., Shaver, P. R., Wendelken, C., & Mikulincer, M. (2005). Attachment-style differences and ability to suppress negative thoughts: Exploring the neural correlates. *NeuroImage, 28,* 835–847.

Gjerde, P. F., Block, J., & Onishi, M. (1998). *Personality implications of romantic attachment styles in young adults: A multi-method study.* Manuscript submitted for publication.

Gjerde, P. F., Onishi, M., & Carlson, K. (2004). Personality characteristics associated with romantic attachment: A comparison of interview and self-report methodologies. *Personality and Social Psychology Bulletin, 30,* 1402–1415.

Goldberg, S., Benoit, D., Blokland, K., & Madigan, S. (2003). Atypical maternal behavior, maternal representations, and infant disorganized attachment. *Developmental Psychopathology, 15,* 239–257.

Grice, P. (1975). Logic and conversation. In P. Cole & J. L. Moran (Eds.), *Syntax and semantics III: Speech acts* (pp. 41–58). New York: Academic Press.

Griffin, D. W., & Bartholomew, K. (1994a). The meta-physics of measurement: The case of adult attachment. In K. Bartholomew & D. Perlman (Eds.), *Advances in personal relationships: Vol. 5. Attachment processes in adulthood* (pp. 17–52). London: Jessica Kingsley.

Griffin, D. W., & Bartholomew, K. (1994b). Models of the self and other: Fundamental dimensions underlying measures of adult attachment. *Journal of Personality and Social Psychology, 67,* 430–445.

Grossmann, K., Fremmer-Bombik, E., Rudolph, J., & Grossmann, K. E. (1988). Maternal attachment representation as related to patterns of infant–mother attachment and maternal care during the first year of life. In R. A. Hinde & J. Stevenson- Hinde (Eds.), *Relationships within families: Mutual influences* (pp. 241–260). Oxford, UK: Clarendon Press.

Haft, W., & Slade, A. (1989). Affect attunement and maternal attachment: A pilot study. *Infant Mental Health Journal, 10,* 157–172.

Hamilton, C. E. (2000). Continuity and discontinuity of attachment from infancy through adolescence. *Child Development, 71,* 690–694.

Hammen, C. L., Burge, D., Daley, S. E., Davila, J., Paley, B., & Rudolph, K. D. (1995). Interpersonal attachment cognitions and prediction of symptomatic responses to interpersonal stress. *Journal of Abnormal Psychology, 104,* 436–443.

Hatfield, E., & Sprecher, S. (1986). *Mirror, mirror . . . : The importance of looks in everyday life.* Albany: State University of New York Press.

Hazan, C., & Shaver, P. R. (1987). Romantic love conceptualized as an attachment process. *Journal of Personality and Social Psychology, 52,* 511–524.

Hazan, C., & Shaver, P. R. (1990). Love and work: An attachment theoretical perspective. *Journal of Personality and Social Psychology, 59,* 270–280.

Hazan, C., & Shaver, P. R. (1994). Attachment as an organizational framework for research on close relationships. *Psychological Inquiry, 5,* 1–22.

Hazan, C., & Zeifman, D. (1994). Sex and the psychological tether. In K. Bartholomew & D. Perlman (Eds.), *Advances in personal relationships: Vol. 5. Attachment processes in adulthood* (pp. 151–177). London: Jessica Kingsley.

Hesse, E. (1996). Discourse, memory and the Adult Attachment Interview: A note with emphasis on the emerging cannot classify category. *Infant Mental Health Journal, 17,* 4–11.

Holtzen, D. W., Kenny, M. E., & Mahalik, J. R. (1995). Contributions of parental attachment to gay or lesbian disclosure to parents and dysfunctional cognitive processes. *Journal of Counseling Psychology, 42,* 350–355.

Jacoby, L. L., Toth, J. P., Lindsay, D. S., & Debner, J. A. (1992). Lectures for a layperson: Methods for revealing unconscious processes. In R. F. Bornstein & T. S. Pittman (Eds.), *Perception without awareness* (pp. 81–120). New York: Guilford Press.

John, O. P. (1990). The "Big Five" factor taxonomy: Dimensions of personality in the natural language and in questionnaires. In L. A. Pervin (Ed.), *Handbook of personality: Theory and research* (pp. 67–100). New York: Guilford Press.

Keelan, J. P. R., Dion, K. L., & Dion, K. K. (1994). Attachment style and heterosexual relationships among young adults: A short-term panel study. *Journal of Social and Personal Relationships, 11,* 201–214.

Kenny, M. E., & Perez, V. (1996). Attachment and psychological well-being among racially and ethnically diverse first-year college students. *Journal of College Student Development, 37,* 527–535.

Kesner, J. E. (2000). Teacher characteristics and the quality of child–teacher relationships. *Journal of School Psychology, 38,* 133–149.

Kirkpatrick, L. A., & Davis, K. E. (1994). Attachment style, gender, and relationship stability: A longitudinal analysis. *Journal of Personality and Social Psychology, 66,* 502–512.

Kirkpatrick, L. A., & Hazan, C. (1994). Attachment styles and close relationships: A four-year prospective study. *Personal Relationships, 1,* 123–142.

Klohnen, E. C., & Bera, S. (1998). Behavioral and experiential patterns of avoidantly and securely attached women across adulthood: A 31-year longitudinal study. *Journal of Personality and Social Psychology, 74,* 211–223.

Klohnen, E. C., & John, O. P. (1998). Working models of attachment: A theory-based prototype approach. In J. A. Simpson & W. S. Rholes (Eds.), *Attachment theory and close relationships* (pp. 115–140). New York: Guilford Press.

Kobak, R. R. (1993). *The Attachment Interview Q-Set.* Unpublished manuscript, University of Delaware.

Kobak, R. R., Cole, H., Ferenz-Gillies, R., Fleming, W., & Gamble, W. (1993). Attachment and emotional regulation during mother–teen problem solving: A control theory analysis. *Child Development, 64,* 231–245.

Kobak, R. R., & Sceery, A. (1988). Attachment in late adolescence: Working models, affect regulation, and representations of self and others. *Child Development, 59,* 135–146.

Koren-Karie, N., Sagi-Schwartz, A., & Joels, T. (2003). Absence of attachment representations in the adult years: The emergence of a new AAI classification in catastrophically traumatized Holocaust child survivors. *Attachment and Human Development, 5,* 381–397.

Kunce, L. J., & Shaver, P. R. (1994). An attachment-theoretical approach to caregiving in romantic relationships. In K. Bartholomew & D. Perlman (Eds.), *Advances in personal relationships: Vol. 5. Attachment processes in adulthood* (pp. 205–237). London: Jessica Kingsley.

Lakatos, K., Toth, I., Nemoda, Z., Ney, K., Sasvari-Szekely, M., & Gervai, J. (2000). Dopamine D4 receptor (DRD4) gene polymorphism is associated with attachment disorganization. *Molecular Psychiatry, 5,* 633–637.

Lei, L., & Wu, Y. (2007). Adolescents' paternal attach-

ment and Internet use. *Cyberpsychology and Behavior, 10,* 633–639.

Levy, M. B., & Davis, K. E. (1988). Lovestyles and attachment styles compared: Their relations to each other and to various relationship characteristics. *Journal of Social and Personal Relationships, 5,* 439–471.

Lyons-Ruth, K., Yellin, C., Melnick, S., & Atwood, G. (2003). Childhood experiences of trauma and loss have different relations to maternal unresolved and hostile-helpless states of mind on the AAI. *Attachment and Human Development, 5,* 330–352.

Lyons-Ruth, K., Yellin, C., Melnick, S., & Atwood, G. (2005). Expanding the concept of unresolved mental states: Hostile/helpless states of mind on the Adult Attachment Interview are associated with disrupted mother–infant communication and infant disorganization. *Development and Psychopathology, 17,* 1–23.

Macfie, J., McElwain, N. L., Houts, R. M., & Cox, M. J. (2005). Intergenerational transmission of role reversal between parent and child: Dyadic and family systems internal working models. *Attachment and Human Development, 7,* 51–65.

Main, M. (1981). Avoidance in the service of attachment: A working paper. In K. Immelman, G. Barlow, M. Main, & L. Petrinovitch (Eds.), *Behavioral development: The Bielefeld interdisciplinary project* (pp. 651–693). New York: Cambridge University Press.

Main, M. (1990). Cross-cultural studies of attachment organization: Recent studies, changing methodologies, and the concept of conditional strategies. *Human Development, 33,* 48–61.

Main, M. (1991). Metacognitive knowledge, metacognitive monitoring, and singular (coherent) versus multiple (incoherent) models of attachment: Findings and directions for future research. In C. M. Parkes, J. Stevenson-Hinde, & P. Marris (Eds.), *Attachment across the life cycle* (pp. 127–159). London: Routledge.

Main, M., & Goldwyn, R. (1984). *Adult attachment scoring and classification system.* Unpublished manuscript, University of California at Berkeley.

Main, M., Goldwyn, R., & Hesse, E. (2003). *Adult attachment scoring and classification system.* Unpublished manuscript, University of California at Berkeley.

Main, M., Kaplan, N., & Cassidy, J. (1985). Security of infancy, childhood, and adulthood: A move to the level of representation. In I. Bretherton & E. Waters (Eds.), Growing points of attachment theory and research. *Monographs of the Society for Research in Child Development, 50*(1–2, Serial No. 209), 66–104.

Main, M., & Weston, D. R. (1981). The quality of the toddler's relationship to mother and to father: Related to conflict behavior and the readiness to establish new relationships. *Child Development, 52,* 932–940.

McCrae, R. R., & Costa, P. T. (1990). *Personality in adulthood.* New York: Guilford Press.

Mickelson, K. D., Kessler, R. C., & Shaver, P. R. (1997). Adult attachment in a nationally representative sample. *Journal of Personality and Social Psychology*, 73, 1092–1106.

Mikulincer, M. (1995). Attachment style and the mental representation of the self. *Journal of Personality and Social Psychology*, 69, 1203–1215.

Mikulincer, M. (1998). Attachment working models and the sense of trust: An exploration of interaction goals and affect regulation. *Journal of Personality and Social Psychology*, 74, 1209–1224.

Mikulincer, M., Dolev, T., & Shaver, P. R. (2004). Attachment-related strategies during thought-suppression: Ironic rebounds and vulnerable self-representations. *Journal of Personality and Social Psychology*, 87, 940–956.

Mikulincer, M., Florian, V., & Tolmacz, R. (1990). Attachment styles and fear of personal death: A case study of affect regulation. *Journal of Personality and Social Psychology*, 58, 273–280.

Mikulincer, M., Gillath, O., & Shaver, P. R. (2002). Activation of the attachment system in adulthood: Threat-related primes increase the accessibility of mental representations of attachment figures. *Journal of Personality and Social Psychology*, 83, 881–895.

Mikulincer, M., & Orbach, I. (1995). Attachment styles and repressive defensiveness: The accessibility and architecture of affective memories. *Journal of Personality and Social Psychology*, 68, 917–925.

Mikulincer, M., & Shaver, P. R. (2007). *Attachment in adulthood: Structure, dynamics, and change*. New York: Guilford Press.

Miljkovitch, R., Pierrehumbert, B., Bretherton, I., & Halfon, O. (2004). Associations between parental and child attachment representations. *Attachment and Human Development*, 6, 305–325.

Miller, L. C., & Fishkin, S. A. (1997). On the dynamics of human bonding and reproductive success: Seeking windows on the adapted-for human–environmental interface. In J. A. Simpson & D. T. Kenrick (Eds.), *Evolutionary social psychology* (pp. 197–235). Mahwah, NJ: Erlbaum.

Moncher, F. J. (1996). The relationship of maternal adult attachment style and risk of physical child abuse. *Journal of Interpersonal Violence*, 11, 335–350.

Noftle, E. E., & Shaver, P. R. (2006). Attachment dimensions and the Big Five personality traits: Associations and comparative ability to predict relationship quality. *Journal of Research in Personality*, 40, 179–208.

O'Connor, E., Pan, H., Waters, E., & Posada, G. (1995, March). *Attachment classification, romantic jealousy, and aggression in couples*. Poster presented at the biennial meeting of the Society for Research in Child Development, Indianapolis, IN.

Oppenheim, D., & Waters, E. (1995). Narrative processes and attachment representations: Issues of development and assessment. In E. Waters, B. Vaughn, G. Posada, & K. Kondo-Ikemura (Eds.), Caregiving, cultural, and cognitive perspectives on secure-base behavior and working models: New growing points of attachment theory and research. *Monographs of the Society for Research in Child Development*, 60(2–3, Serial No. 244), 197–215.

Owens, G., Crowell, J., Pan, H., Treboux, D., O'Connor, E., & Waters, E. (1995). The prototype hypothesis and the origins of attachment working models: Adult relationships with parents and romantic partners. In E. Waters, B. Vaughn, G. Posada, & K. Kondo-Ikemura (Eds.), Caregiving, cultural, and cognitive perspectives on secure-base behavior and working models: New growing points of attachment theory and research. *Monographs of the Society for Research in Child Development*, 60(2–3, Serial No. 244), 216–233.

Oyen, A.-S., Landy, S., & Hilburn-Cobb, C. (2000). Maternal attachment and sensitivity in an at-risk sample. *Attachment and Human Development*, 2, 203–217.

Paley, B., Cox, M., Burchinal, M., & Payne, C. (1999). Attachment and marital functioning: Comparison of spouses with continuous secure, earned secure, dismissing, and preoccupied stances. *Journal of Family Psychology*, 13, 580–597.

Paley, B., Cox, M. J., Harter, K. M., & Margand, N. A. (2002). Adult attachment stance and spouses' marital perceptions during the transition to parenthood. *Attachment and Human Development*, 4, 340–360.

Parkes, C. M. (2006). *Love and loss: The roots of grief and its complications*. New York: Taylor & Francis.

Pearson, J., Cohn, D., Cowan, P., & Cowan, C. P. (1994). Earned- and continuous-security in adult attachment: Relation to depressive symptomatology and parenting style. *Development and Psychopathology*, 6, 359–373.

Pietromonaco, P. R., & Barrett, L. F. (1997). Working models of attachment and daily social interactions. *Journal of Personality and Social Psychology*, 73, 1409–1423.

Pietromonaco, P. R., & Carnelley, K. B. (1994). Gender and working models of attachment: Consequences for perceptions of self and romantic relationships. *Personal Relationships*, 1, 63–82.

Pistole, M. C. (1989). Attachment in adult romantic relationships: Style of conflict resolution and relationship satisfaction. *Journal of Social and Personal Relationships*, 6, 505–510.

Posada, G., Waters, E., Crowell, J., & Lay, K. (1995). Is it easier to use a secure mother as a secure base?: Attachment Q-Sort correlates of the Adult Attachment Interview. In E. Waters, B. Vaughn, G. Posada, & K. Kondo-Ikemura (Eds.), Caregiving, cultural, and cognitive perspectives on secure-base behavior and working models: New growing points of attachment theory and research. *Monographs of the Society for Research in Child Development*, 60(2–3, Serial No. 244), 133–145.

Pottharst, K. (Ed.). (1990). *Explorations in adult attachment*. New York: Peter Lang.

Reis, H. T., & Patrick, B. C. (1996). Attachment and intimacy: Component processes. In E. T. Higgins & A. W. Kruglanski (Eds.), *Social psychology: Handbook of basic principles* (pp. 523–563). New York: Guilford Press.

Riggs, S. A., & Jacobvitz, D. (2002). Expectant parents' representations of early attachment relationships: Association with mental health and family history. *Journal of Consulting and Clinical Psychology, 70*, 195–204.

Roisman, G. I., Collins, A. W., Sroufe, L. A., & Egeland, B. (2005). Predictors of young adults' representations of and behavior in their current romantic relationship: Prospective tests of the prototype hypothesis. *Attachment and Human Development, 7*, 105–121.

Roisman, G. I., Fortuna, K., & Holland, A. (2006). An experimental manipulation of retrospectively defined earned and continuous attachment security. *Child Development, 77*, 59–71.

Roisman, G. I., Fraley, R. C., & Belsky, J. (2007). A taxometric study of the Adult Attachment Interview. *Developmental Psychology, 43*, 675–686.

Roisman, G. I., Holland, A., Fortuna, K., Fraley, R. C., Clausell, E., & Clarke, A. (2007). The Adult Attachment Interview and self-reports of attachment style: An empirical rapprochement. *Journal of Personality and Social Psychology, 92*, 678–697.

Roisman, G. I., Madsen, S. D., Hennighausen, K. H., Sroufe, L. A., & Collins, W. A. (2001). The coherence of dyadic behavior across parent–child and romantic relationships as mediate by the internalized representation of experience. *Attachment and Human Development, 3*, 156–172.

Roisman, G. I., Padrón, E., Sroufe, L. A., & Egeland, B. (2002). Earned-secure status in retrospect and prospect. *Child Development, 73*, 1204–1219.

Rubenstein, C., & Shaver, P. R. (1982). *In search of intimacy.* New York: Delacorte.

Sagi, A., Aviezer, O., Joels, T., Korne-Karje, N., Mayseless, O., Scharf, M., et al. (1992, July). *The correspondence of mother's attachment with infant–mother attachment relationship in traditional and non-traditional kibbutzim.* Paper presented at the 25th International Congress of Psychology, Brussels.

Sagi, A., van IJzendoorn, M., Scharf, M., Korne-Karje, N., Joels, T., & Mayseless, O. (1994). Stability and discriminant validity of the Adult Attachment Interview: A psychometric study in young Israeli adults. *Developmental Psychology, 30*, 771–777.

Sagi-Schwartz, A., Koren-Karie, N., & Joels, T. (2003). Failed mourning in the Adult Attachment Interview: The case of Holocaust child survivors. *Attachment and Human Development, 5*, 398–408.

Scharfe, E., & Bartholomew, K. (1994). Reliability and stability of adult attachment patterns. *Personal Relationships, 9*, 51–64.

Scharfe, E., & Bartholomew, K. (1995). Accommodation and attachment representations in young couples. *Journal of Social and Personal Relationships, 12*, 389–401.

Schultheiss, D. E. P., & Blustein, D. L. (1994). Contributions of family relationship factors to the identity formation process. *Journal of Counseling and Development, 73*, 159–166.

Senchak, M., & Leonard, K. E. (1992). Attachment styles and marital adjustment among newlywed couples. *Journal of Social and Personal Relationships, 9*, 51–64.

Shaver, P. R., Belsky, J., & Brennan, K. A. (2000). Comparing measures of adult attachment: An examination of interview and self-report methods. *Personal Relationships, 7*, 25–43.

Shaver, P. R., & Brennan, K. A. (1992). Attachment styles and the "Big Five" personality traits: Their connections with each other and with romantic relationship outcomes. *Personality and Social Psychology Bulletin, 18*, 536–545.

Shaver, P. R., & Clark, C. L. (1994). The psychodynamics of adult romantic attachment. In J. M. Masling & R. F. Bornstein (Eds.), *Empirical perspectives on object relations theory* (pp. 105–156). Washington, DC: American Psychological Association.

Shaver, P. R., & Hazan, C. (1987). Being lonely, falling in love: Perspectives from attachment theory. *Journal of Social Behavior and Personality, 2*, 105–124.

Shaver, P. R., & Hazan, C. (1988). A biased overview of the study of love. *Journal of Social and Personal Relationships, 5*, 473–501.

Shaver, P. R., & Hazan, C. (1993). Adult romantic attachment: Theory and evidence. In D. Perlman & W. Jones (Eds.), *Advances in personal relationships* (Vol. 4, pp. 29–70). London: Jessica Kingsley.

Shaver, P. R., Hazan, C., & Bradshaw, D. (1988). Love as attachment: The integration of three behavioral systems. In R. J. Sternberg & M. L. Barnes (Eds.), *The psychology of love* (pp. 68–99). New Haven, CT: Yale University Press.

Shaver, P. R., & Mikulincer, M. (2002a). Attachment-related psychodynamics. *Attachment and Human Development, 4*, 133–161.

Shaver, P. R., & Mikulincer, M. (2002b). Dialogue on adult attachment: Diversity and integration. *Attachment and Human Development, 4*, 243–257.

Shaver, P. R., & Mikulincer, M. (2004). What do self-report attachment measures assess? In W. S. Rholes & J. A. Simpson (Eds.), *Adult attachment: Theory, research, and clinical implications* (pp. 17–54). New York: Guilford Press.

Shaver, P. R., Papalia, D., Clark, C. L., Koski, L. R., Tidwell, M., & Nalbone, D. (1996). Androgyny and attachment security: Two related models of optimal development. *Personality and Social Psychology Bulletin, 22*, 582–597.

Simpson, J. A. (1990). The influence of attachment styles on romantic relationships. *Journal of Personality and Social Psychology, 59*, 971–980.

Simpson, J. A., & Rholes, W. S. (Eds.). (1998). *Attachment theory and close relationships.* New York: Guilford Press.

Simpson, J. A., Rholes, W. S., & Nelligan, J. S. (1992). Support-seeking and support-giving within couple members in an anxiety-provoking situation: The role of attachment styles. *Journal of Personality and Social Psychology, 62*, 434–446.

Simpson, J. A., Rholes, W. S., Oriña, M. M., & Grich, J. (2002). Working models of attachment, support giving, and support seeking in a stressful situation. *Personality and Social Psychology Bulletin, 28,* 598–608.

Simpson, J. A., Rholes, W. S., & Phillips, D. (1996). Conflict in close relationships: An attachment perspective. *Journal of Personality and Social Psychology, 71,* 899–914.

Slade, A., Belsky, J., Aber, J. L., & Phelps, J. L. (1999). Mothers' representations of their relationships with toddlers: Links to adult attachment and observed mothering. *Developmental Psychology, 35,* 611–619.

Sperling, M. B., & Berman, W. H. (Eds.). (1994). *Attachment in adults: Clinical and developmental perspectives.* New York: Guilford Press.

Steele, H., Steele, M., & Fonagy, P. (1996). Associations among attachment classifications of mothers, fathers, and their infants. *Child Development, 67,* 541–555.

Sternberg, R. J., & Barnes, M. (Eds.). (1988). *The psychology of love.* New Haven, CT: Yale University Press.

Tidwell, M. C., Reis, H. T., & Shaver, P. R. (1996). Attachment, attractiveness, and social interaction: A diary study. *Journal of Personality and Social Psychology, 71,* 729–745.

Treboux, D., Crowell, J., & Waters, E. (2004). When "new" meets "old": Configurations of adult attachment representations and their implications for marital functioning. *Developmental Psychology, 40,* 295–314.

Trinke, S. J., & Bartholomew, K. (1997). Hierarchies of attachment relationships in young adulthood. *Journal of Social and Personal Relationships, 14,* 603–625.

van Ecke, Y. (2006). Unresolved attachment among immigrants: An analysis using the Adult Attachment Projective. *Journal of Genetic Psychology, 167,* 433–442.

van IJzendoorn, M. H. (1992). Intergenerational transmission of parenting: A review of studies in non-clinical populations. *Developmental Review, 12,* 76–99.

van IJzendoorn, M. H. (1995). Adult attachment representations, parental responsiveness, and infant attachment: A meta-analysis on the predictive validity of the Adult Attachment Interview. *Psychological Bulletin, 117,* 387–403.

van IJzendoorn, M. H., & Bakermans-Kranenburg, M. (1996). Attachment representations in mothers, fathers, adolescents and clinical groups: A meta-analytic search for normative data. *Journal of Clinical and Consulting Psychology, 64,* 8–21.

van IJzendoorn, M. H., Feldbrugge, J., Derks, F., de Ruiter, C., Verhagen, M., Philipse, M., et al. (1997). Attachment representations of personality disordered criminal offenders. *American Journal of Orthopsychiatry, 67,* 449–459.

Vaughn, B. E., Coppola, G., Verissimo, L. M., Santos, A. J., Posada, G., Carbonell, O. A., et al. (2007).

The quality of maternal secure-base scripts predicts children's secure-base behavior at home in three sociocultural groups. *International Journal of Behavioral Development, 31,* 65–76.

Vaughn, B. E., Waters, H. S., Coppola, G., Cassidy, J., Bost, K. K., & Verissimo, M. (2006). Script-like attachment representations and behavior in families and across cultures: Studies of parental secure base narratives. *Attachment and Human Development, 8,* 179–184.

Wallis, P., & Steele, H. (2001). Attachment representations in adolescence: Further evidence from psychiatric residential settings. *Attachment and Human Development, 3,* 259–268.

Wampler, K. S., Riggs, B., & Kimball, T. G. (2004). Observing attachment behavior in couples: The Adult Attachment Behavior Q-Set (AABQ). *Family Processes, 43,* 315–335.

Wampler, K. S., Shi, L., Nelson, B. S., & Kimball, T. G. (2003). The Adult Attachment Interview and observed couple interaction: Implications for an intergernational perspective on couple therapy. *Family Processes, 42,* 497–515.

Ward, A., Ramsay, R., Turnbull, S., Steele, M., Steele, H., & Treasure, J. (2001). Attachment in anorexia nervosa: A transgenerational perspective. *British Journal of Medicine and Psychology, 74,* 497–505.

Ward, M. J., & Carlson, E. A. (1995). Associations among adult attachment representations, maternal sensitivity, and infant–mother attachment in a sample of adolescent mothers. *Child Development, 66,* 69–79.

Waters, E., Crowell, J., Elliott, M., Corcoran, D., & Treboux, D. (2002). Bowlby's secure base theory and the social/personality psychology of attachment styles: Work(s) in progress. *Attachment and Human Development, 4,* 230–242.

Waters, E., Merrick, S., Treboux, D., Crowell, J., & Albersheim, L. (2000). Attachment security from infancy to early adulthood: A 20-year longitudinal study. *Child Development, 71,* 684–689.

Waters, E., Kondo-Ikemura, K., Posada, G., & Richters, J. (1991). Learning to love: Mechanisms and milestones. In M. Gunnar & L. A. Sroufe (Eds.), *Self processes and development* (pp. 217–255). Hillsdale, NJ: Erlbaum.

Waters, H. S., Rodrigues, L. M., & Ridgeway, D. (1998). Cognitive underpinnings of narrative attachment assessment. *Journal of Experimental Child Psychology, 71,* 211–234.

Waters, H. S., & Rodrigues-Doolabh, L. M. (2001, April). *Are attachment scripts the building blocks of attachment representations?* Paper presented at the biennial meeting of the Society for Research in Child Development, Minneapolis, MN.

Waters, H. S., & Rodrigues-Doolabh, L. M. (2004). *Manual for decoding secure base narratives.* Unpublished manuscript, State University of New York at Stony Brook.

Waters, H. S., & Waters, E. (2006). The attachment working models concept: Among other things, we build script-like representations of secure base experiences. *Attachment and Human Development, 8,* 185–197.

Weiss, R. (1973). *Loneliness: The experience of emotional and social isolation.* Cambridge, MA: MIT Press.

Weiss, R. (1974). The provisions of social relationships. In Z. Rubin (Ed.), *Doing unto others* (pp. 17–26). Englewood Cliffs, NJ: Prentice-Hall.

Weiss, R. (1991). Attachment in adult life. In C. M. Parkes, J. Stevenson-Hinde, & P. Marris (Eds.), *Attachment across the life cycle* (pp. 171–184). London: Routledge.

West, M., & George, C. (2002). Attachment and dysthymia: The contributions of preoccupied attachment and agency of self to depression in women. *Attachment and Human Development, 4,* 278–293.

West, M., & Sheldon, A. E. (1988). The classification of pathological attachment patterns in adults. *Journal of Personality Disorders, 2,* 153–160.

West, M., Sheldon, A. E. R., & Reiffer, L. (1987). An approach to the delineation of adult attachment: Scale development and reliability. *Journal of Nervous and Mental Disease, 175,* 738–741.

West, M. L., & Sheldon-Keller, A. E. (1992). The assessment of dimensions relevant to adult reciprocal attachment. *Canadian Journal of Psychiatry, 37,* 600–606.

West, M. L., & Sheldon-Keller, A. E. (1994). *Patterns of relating: An adult attachment perspective.* New York: Guilford Press.

Woike, B. A., Osier, T. J., & Candella, K. (1996). Attachment styles and violent imagery in thematic stories about relationships. *Personality and Social Psychology Bulletin, 22,* 1030–1034.

Zeanah, C., Benoit, D., Barton, M., Regan, C., Hirshberg, L., & Lipsett, L. (1993). Representations of attachment in mothers and their one-year-old infants. *Journal of the American Academy of Child and Adolescent Psychiatry, 32,* 278–286.

Zeifman, D., & Hazan, C. (1997). Attachment: The bond in pair-bonds. In J. A. Simpson & D. T. Kenrick (Eds.), *Evolutionary social psychology* (pp. 237–263). Mahwah, NJ: Erlbaum.

PART V

PSYCHOPATHOLOGY AND CLINICAL APPLICATIONS OF ATTACHMENT THEORY AND RESEARCH

CHAPTER 27

Attachment and Psychopathology in Childhood

MICHELLE DEKLYEN
MARK T. GREENBERG

The early parent–child relationship is widely believed to be central to personality development (Bowlby, 1969/1982; Bronfenbrenner, 1979; Erikson, 1963; Freud, 1965; Greenspan, 1981). Numerous empirical findings link secure attachments to caregivers in the first two years of life with sociability, compliance with parents, and effective emotion regulation (Bretherton, 1985; Richters & Waters, 1991; Weinfield, Sroufe, Egeland, & Carlson, Chapter 4, this volume). Insecure attachment to a caregiver during infancy has been related to poor peer relations, anger, and poor behavioral self-control during the preschool years and beyond (Carlson & Sroufe, 1995; Sroufe, Egeland, Carlson, & Collins, 2005).

The idea that social relationships both affect and are affected by developing psychopathology in childhood is fundamental to most modern theories of development. Object relations theorists (Mahler, Pine, & Bergman, 1975; Winnicott, 1965) and ego psychologists (Freud, 1965) hypothesized that a child's earliest and closest relationships have the greatest impact on the development of mental health and illness. Yet only after Bowlby (1969/1982, 1973) directed attention to infant and child attachment relationships did researchers begin to study the associations between the child's closest relationships and the development of vari-

ous forms of behavioral disorder. Despite Bowlby's interest in psychopathology, early attachment research focused almost entirely on normative infant development (Bretherton, 1992; Main, 1996). Although scattered projects in the 1970s and 1980s examined at-risk populations of children and adults with disorders (Belsky & Nezworski, 1988), only more recently have researchers seriously attempted to fulfill Bowlby's legacy by utilizing attachment theory in understanding and treating disorders in which relationship factors are putative causes (Cicchetti, Toth, & Lynch, 1995).

Over the last two decades, attachment theory has begun to make major contributions beyond infancy and beyond the confines of its own advocates. This is exciting, because attachment theory provides a critical developmental frame for understanding *how* caregiving relationships influence processes thought to be central to emerging psychopathology—for example, the construction of cognitive–affective expectancies, the capacity for emotional and behavioral regulation, and strategies for coping with stress. As indicated in other chapters in this volume (e.g., Dozier, Stovall, & Albus, Chapter 31; Kobak & Madsen, Chapter 2; Lyons-Ruth & Jacobvitz, Chapter 28; and Slade, Chapter 32), the regulation of emotion—particularly negative emotions, such as anxiety, anger, and sadness—plays an important role in various forms of psychopathology across the lifespan (Carlson & Sroufe, 1995; Chaplin & Cole, 2005; Fonagy et al., 1995; Izard, Youngstrom, Fine, Mostow, & Trentacosta, 2006).

This chapter reviews what is currently known about the association between attachment and psychopathology in childhood. Recent chapters in other volumes (e.g., Egeland & Carlson, 2004; Kobak, Cassidy, Lyons-Ruth, & Ziv, 2006; Ungerer & McMahon, 2005) also provide excellent discussions of this topic. Here we especially focus on disorder—that is, on psychopathological behavior serious enough to warrant clinical attention. We begin by describing principles of developmental psychopathology and risk models. We next review research involving attachment, first as a risk factor for disorder and then as perhaps the central aspect of particular disorders. In the process, two fundamental questions are addressed: How have attachment constructs contributed to our understanding of childhood disorders, and how might the study of childhood psychopathology enrich the further study of attachment? The chapter closes with suggestions for future research and a summation of what is known.

DEVELOPMENTAL PSYCHOPATHOLOGY AND MODELS OF RISK AND PROTECTION

Most of the research linking attachment with psychopathology has considered attachment as a potential risk or protective factor, examining associations between attachment measures (e.g., classification in the Strange Situation) and maladaptive behavior or disorder in a variety of populations, ranging from convenience samples to individuals with specific clinical diagnoses. The enthusiasm to utilize attachment theory has at times led to overinterpretation of findings and a fruitless search for a "Holy Grail" of psychopathology, and some researchers have employed simplistic models, looking for main effects of infant attachment on later psychopathology. As more evidence accumulates, it appears increasingly likely that attachment exerts its influence *in the context of other risk factors* within the child and in the family ecology (Cicchetti & Rogosch, 1997; Greenberg, Speltz, DeKlyen, & Jones, 2001). A short digression into key tenets of risk factor models in developmental psychopathology will provide a frame for considering the role of attachment in the etiology of psychopathology.

Basic Tenets of Risk Models in Developmental Psychopathology

Risk Factors

Research on risk factors for disorder leads to five general conclusions. First, it is unlikely that a single cause will be either a necessary or a sufficient cause for most pathology (Greenberg, Speltz, & DeKlyen, 1993); even the expression of disorders with established biochemical or genetic mechanisms will be potentiated or buffered by other biological or environmental factors. Thus it is doubtful that attachment insecurity alone will lead to disorder (Sroufe, 1983, 1990), although it may increase its likelihood. As a corollary of this principle, few childhood disorders will be eliminated by treating only causes purported to lie within the child (Rutter, 1982). Even when a powerful biological cause is implicated (e.g., autism), the parent–child relationship and, more specifically, the attachment relationship may be an appropriate focus for treatment.

A second tenet of developmental psychopathology states that *multiple pathways* exist to and from disorder (Cicchetti & Rogosch, 1997). Different combinations of risk factors may lead to the same disorder (i.e., "equifinality"), and a given risk factor may contribute to multiple disorders ("multifinality"). For example, poverty, family violence, and parental psychopathology have all been associated with a variety of childhood disorders, and attachment has been considered a risk factor for both internalizing and externalizing problems, although specific forms of insecurity may be linked to specific forms of disorder (Carlson & Sroufe, 1995). To complicate assessment further, problem behaviors often overlap with one another, resulting in comorbidities. Two corollaries of this tenet are as follows: The influence of a given risk (e.g., insecure attachment) may be moderated by other factors, such as gender and ethnicity; and a variable that confers risk for one disorder may reduce the risk for other disorders. For example, avoidant attachment may increase risk for conduct disorder, but it may decrease the risk of suicide (Adam, Sheldon-Keller, & West, 1995).

Third, risk factors occur at multiple levels, including the individual, the caregiver, and the broader ecological context (Bronfenbrenner, 1979; Kellam, 1990; Kobak et al., 2006; Weissberg & Greenberg, 1998). Some factors at each level have implications for attachment (e.g., parent employment or social support may affect sensitive caregiving), but others probably do not (e.g., peer deviance).

Fourth, the relations between risk and outcome may be nonlinear (e.g., quadratic or exponential). Although one or two risk factors may not predict poor outcomes, the rate of disorder may increase rapidly with additional risks (Greenberg et al., 2001; Rutter, 1979; Sameroff, Seifer, Barocas, Zax, & Greenspan, 1987). It is currently unclear whether certain risk factors or combinations of risks matter more than others. Several studies have included assessments of attachment in initial attempts to examine this question (Greenberg et al., 2001; Keller, Spieker, & Gilchrist, 2005; Lyons-Ruth, Alpern, & Repacholi, 1993; Shaw, Owens, Vondra, Keenan, & Winslow, 1997).

A fifth guiding principle is that certain risk factors may have differential influence in different developmental periods. For example, secure attachment may be especially important in early development, whereas cognitive ability and motivation may be more critical in middle childhood, and peer relationships and parental norms regarding behavior may be especially influential during adolescence. There is a need for basic research to elucidate the differential timing of risk factors. Although attachment theorists do not claim that there is a critical period with respect to attachment, early experience models suggest that early attachment history is of particular importance and will continue to influence later adaptation beyond what environmental continuity might explain (Fraley, 2002). These models predict, for example, that children with a secure attachment relationship in the first few years of life who later experience trauma are at less risk for disorder than those who were insecurely attached in their early years.

Protective Factors

Protective factors reduce the likelihood of poor outcomes under conditions of risk. Three kinds of protective factors have been studied, parallel to the categories of risk factors. These include characteristics of the individual (e.g., temperamental qualities and intelligence; Luthar & Zigler, 1992); the quality of the child's relationships (e.g., attachment); and ecological factors (e.g., the quality of schools, the safety of neighborhoods, and laws or regulations that protect or support children and families). Within the second domain, the importance of secure attachment to parents (Carlson & Sroufe, 1995) and of healthy relationships with peers (Parker, Rubin, Price, & DeRosier, 1995) has been demonstrated.

There is considerable controversy regarding whether specific factors should be designated as placing a child at risk or serving a protective function (Luthar, 1993; Masten, 2001; Stouthamer-Loeber et al., 1993; Zimmerman & Arunkumar, 1994). For example, socioeconomic status, attachment security, or peer group status may be conceptualized as posing risk in some studies and as protective in others, depending on which end of the spectrum is being studied, the nature of the population, and the theoretical bent of the investigator. Attachment insecurity has been conceptualized as a risk factor for disorder (Sroufe, 1983), whereas a secure attachment may be viewed as conferring protection from maladaptation under conditions of great risk (Morisset, Barnard, Greenberg, Booth, & Speiker, 1990).

Prospective longitudinal designs are critical to understanding how protective factors operate and interact with risk factors. Coie and colleagues (1993) suggest that a protective factor may work in the following ways: It may directly decrease dysfunction; it may interact with a risk factor to buffer its effect; it may disrupt the mediational chain by which risk leads to disorder; or it may prevent the initial occurrence of the risk factor. Well-planned studies can identify (1) the risk factors that predict psychopathology at various developmental stages, (2) the dynamic relation between risk and protective factors at different ages, and (3) the factors that are most likely to buffer persons with multiple risks from negative outcomes.

A Risk Factor Model Emphasizing Attachment Insecurity

On the basis of these principles of developmental psychopathology, we (Greenberg et al., 1993, 2001) have proposed a model for conceptualizing the early onset of disruptive behavior problems—a model that incorporates attachment as one critical factor. Four general risk domains for which considerable evidence has accumulated include (1) child characteristics (e.g., temperament, biological vulnerability, neurocognitive function); (2) quality of early attachment relations; (3) parental management/socialization strategies (e.g., harsh and ineffective practices, lack of warmth); and (4) family ecology (e.g., family life stress and trauma, family instrumental resources, intra- and extrafamilial social support). This risk factor model probably has generality, such that these classes of risk factors also contribute to the development of early internalizing disorders (anxiety disorders, childhood depression, and somatization). However, as Rubin, Hymel, Mills, and Rose-Krasnor (1991) and others (Manassis & Bradley, 1994; Shaw & Bell, 1993) have hypothesized, different aspects of these general risk factors may predict different disorders. For example, temperament may increase risk for certain disorders, with reactive temperament being associated with externalizing problems and inhibited and withdrawn temperaments being linked with internalizing difficulties. Furthermore, different temperamental qualities may interact differentially to moderate other risk factors. Similarly, in the domain of parental management, punitiveness and underinvolvement may create risk for externalizing problems (Patterson, DeBaryshe, & Ramsey, 1989), and overcontrol and the absence of autonomy promotion may predict internalizing difficulties (Allen, Hauser, & Borman-Spurrell, 1996; Kobak, Sudler, & Gamble, 1991). Few data, however, indicate that any one risk domain *alone* directly causes later problems. That is, in isolation, an atypical temperament, a poor home environment, an insecure attachment, or poor parent management is unlikely to result in disorder.

Figure 27.1 is a graphic model of these risk domains. The purpose of the model is not to illustrate the actual degree of overlap between risk factors (this will vary by individual and is unknown in most populations) but only to illustrate that in a particular case a child may have none of these risk factors, only one, or more than one. The circle for each of the four risk factors denotes high risk status (e.g., atypical temperament, insecure attachment, ineffective parenting, and high family risk). Thus a given child may be affected by none, one, or more of these factors. The cross-hatched area represents cases in which the probability of significant psychopathology during childhood rises significantly above the base rate. Because the model involves four major domains of risk, a two-dimensional drawing cannot adequately represent all possible interactions (e.g., behavior problems may occur in the presence of only family stressors and poor discipline—an interaction that is not visible in this figure). The model considers the assessment of risk in each domain as being both qualitative (cutoff scores for risk classification can be derived) and quantitative (levels of severity within each

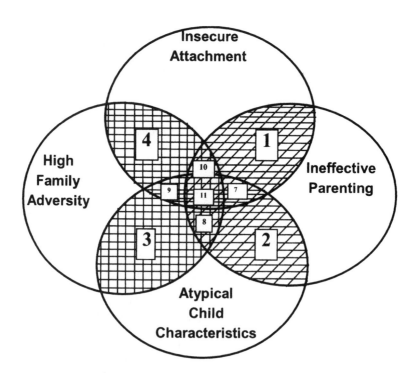

FIGURE 27.1. Factors in the etiology of childhood maladaptation. Areas 1 through 4, two-factor intersection (visible); Area 5 (high family adversity and parent management), two-factor intersection (invisible); Area 6 (insecure attachment and child characteristics), two-factor intersection (invisible); Areas 7 through 10, three-factor intersections; Area 11, four-factor intersections.

risk factor may be meaningful and would be portrayed on a fourth dimension). Although a diagram is by nature static, the relations among these four factors and maladaptation are expected to be transactional, and significant variations may occur in risk status across time—for example, in family adversity as a result of trauma.

It is likely that some domains are of more importance to certain disorders. For example, ineffective parenting may contribute more to externalizing than to internalizing disorders (Patterson et al., 1989), whereas child trauma may be especially related (via attachment processes) to dissociative disorders (Liotti, 1995; Ogawa, Sroufe, Weinfield, Carlson, & Egeland, 1997). As already noted, the type of insecurity and the nature of the atypical temperament probably help to determine what type of disorder emerges. Different combinations of risk factors (e.g., insecure attachment and family adversity vs. difficult temperament and poor parent management) may also lead to differing disorders, requiring different treatments (Speltz, 1990). For example, Campbell (1991) conducted a cluster analysis that showed how distinct sets of risk factors could be used to define three different types of families.

Figure 27.1 does not indicate proximal versus distal influences or the possible pathways by which the influence of each factor may be mediated. Indeed, these pathways will be quite different, depending on the number and types of risk factors involved and their developmental timing and sequence. Furthermore, other domains may increase in importance later in development; for instance, peer relations may become especially important at the time of school entry, and by middle childhood neighborhood ecology may become more influential.

Given the large number of possible combinations of factors identified in Figure 27.1, it may be useful to discuss a few exemplar patterns. In one possible pattern, all risk factors are present, and insecure attachment, adverse family circumstances, and child biological vulnerability interact with poor parent management. We (Greenberg et al., 2001) used this four-factor model in a comparison of clinic-referred preschoolers with diagnoses of oppositional defiant disorder (ODD) and normally behaving children. We found that this first pattern, including all four risk domains, was associated with by far the greatest risk of disorder. In logistic regression analyses, child characteristics, parental management strategies, and concurrent attachment security all provided unique information that differentiated the two groups, but the

fourth factor, family ecology, did not add unique information. Nonetheless, person-oriented analyses demonstrated that increasing the number of risk domains substantially increased the likelihood of disorder (suggesting multiplicative effects), and the clinic-referred children were 34 times more likely than the comparison children to have risk in all four domains.

Other patterns associated with elevated "relative improvement over chance" statistics included one characterized by child characteristics, poor parenting, and family adversity, and another involving poor parenting, insecure attachment, and family adversity. As we have suggested previously (Greenberg, 1999), disorder also occurred in individuals with other patterns and fewer risk factors, but none of those patterns was more common among clinic-referred than comparison boys. Very few clinic-referred children had risk in less than two domains.

It should be noted that insecure attachment may not always be of etiological significance or increase risk, as further evidenced by case studies of children with externalizing problems in which parent–child attachment appeared to be concurrently secure (Campbell, 1990; Greenberg, Speltz, DeKlyen, & Endriga, 1991). In some cases, symptoms may have been triggered by recent psychosocial stressors, uncomplicated by a history of difficult temperament, poor parent–child interaction, or parental psychopathology. In others, both biological vulnerability and family history of trauma and disorder were apparent.

In a longitudinal study of teen mothers, Keller and colleagues (2005) tested this risk model. The results of the single-domain analyses were consistent with the premise that risk in a single domain is not usually sufficient to predict disorder. In the two-domain analyses, insecurely attached children with high levels of infant negativity had a significantly greater likelihood of displaying the high-problem-behavior trajectory, whereas securely attached children with high negativity did not. The three-domain analyses provided additional specificity: The highest probability of the high-problem-behavior trajectory occurred when insecure attachment and high-risk parenting were combined with multiproblem family ecology or high infant negativity.

Process Models and the Contribution of Early Attachment to Disorder

Developmental models are most likely to be useful if they specify linkages between types of insecurity and later disorder and, further, if they indicate the processes through which early attachment is thought to influence the course of development. Theory-based process models are essential if we wish to establish that child attachment is a causal factor and not just a correlate of later behavioral maladaptation (Sroufe & Fleeson, 1986; Waters, Kondo-Ikemura, Posada, & Richters, 1991). Four interrelated mechanisms have been posited to link early attachment to later maladaptation: emotion regulation (including psychophysiological development), observed behavior, cognitive–affective structures, and motivational processes.

First, attachment may affect later disorder through its association with the emotion regulation processes that develop within the parent–child dyad. Strategies for coping with stress are believed to evolve from these early patterns, shaping the child's subsequent responses to challenging situations. As already noted, both theory and research affirm the importance of emotion regulation in the etiology and maintenance of diverse disorders (Chaplin & Cole, 2005; Izard et al., 2006). Guttmann-Steinmetz and Crowell (2006) have described the attachment behavioral system as a "relational emotional regulation system" and elaborate how the experience of a securely attached infant is likely to enhance the infant's capacity to tolerate and manage affect, whereas the strategies of avoidant and ambivalent infants (minimization and exaggeration of emotion, respectively) may interfere with effective regulation. Although some of these ideas are as yet quite speculative, several theorists have suggested ways in which dyadic interactions in early childhood may influence emotion regulation via neural organization, conditioning, and maturation (Speltz, DeKlyen, & Greenberg, 1999)—for example, by altering both the fear conditioning processes in the amygdala (LeDoux, 1995) and the development of connections between the limbic system and the prefrontal cortex (Schore, 1996). There may also be linkages among affective communication, attachment processes, and neural organization (Bretherton, 1995; Greenberg & Snell, 1997; Grossmann, 1995). Both attachment and prefrontal processing have been linked to depression (Dawson, Hessl, & Frey, 1994) and to externalizing disorders (Goleman, 1995). Associations between attachment classification and psychophysiological processes involving cortisol, heart rate, and vagal tone also suggest mechanisms common to emotion, the attachment system, and various disorders (Gunnar, 2000; Hertsgaard, Gunnar, Erickson, & Nachmias,

1995; Lyons-Ruth, Dutra, Schudar, & Bianchi, 2006; Spangler & Grossmann, 1993; Spangler & Schieche, 1998).

A second and related link between early attachment and maladaptation may occur at the level of observable behavior. We (Greenberg et al., 1993) propose that some of the behaviors labeled "disruptive" in young children may be viewed as specific attachment strategies with considerable power to regulate caregiving patterns, especially when other, potentially more adaptive strategies have been ineffective or unavailable. Thus whining, noncompliance, and other negative forms of attention seeking may in some cases serve the function of regulating parent or teacher proximity to, and monitoring of, the child under conditions of past or present nonoptimal care and/or insecurity. Although these attachment strategies have some short-term effectiveness (e.g., caregiver physical or verbal proximity may be either increased or reduced by child negativity), they probably serve as a setting condition for the development of maladaptive family processes (e.g., coercive processes; Patterson, Reid, & Dishion, 1992). In a parallel manner, Main and Hesse (1990) hypothesize that in the absence of a coherent and predictable environment, the disorganized infant begins to take control of aspects of the parent–child relationship during the preschool years. This pattern of role reversal, although helping to maintain a connection to the parent, includes some of the features that index behavioral difficulties (e.g., bossiness, domination). Similarly, the ambivalent pattern, characterized by immature behaviors that often mix anger and dependency, may illustrate how behaviors that serve the attachment system and the early need to maintain the attention of caregivers may be problematic in the larger environment (Cassidy, 1995; Cassidy & Berlin, 1994). At the family level, Marvin and Stewart (1990) discuss how patterns of child behavior may serve the attachment needs of the child and also fit maladaptive family patterns that have been identified by family theorists.

A third mechanism involves the development of social cognitions—in particular, representations of relationships. Attachment theory posits that the organization of infant attachment behavior is maintained at both behavioral and representational levels (Bowlby, 1973). Thus sensitive and responsive parenting during infancy not only results in different observable patterns of behavior directed toward caregivers, it also leads the child to develop a particular cognitive–affective schema or "working model" of both self and others. This working model includes the child's expectations regarding intimacy and care from others and is believed to selectively affect perception, cognition, and motivation (Bretherton, 1985; Sroufe & Fleeson, 1986; see also Bretherton & Munholland, Chapter 5, this volume). As the toddler's representational skills and understanding of affective states become increasingly complex, these models undergo further specification and differentiation. Main, Cassidy, and Kaplan (1985) define the internal working model "as a set of conscious and/ or unconscious rules for the organization of information relevant to attachment, and for obtaining and limiting access to that information, i.e., to information regarding attachment related experiences, feelings, ideations" (p. 66). Thus, individual differences in attachment behavior patterns are viewed as manifestations of individual differences in the child's internal working models of specific relationships.

At present there is little understanding of how resistant these working models are to revision, given changes in the quality of relationships with caregivers or traumatic experiences, or whether there are specific ages or stages during which such models may especially resist revision. With age, working models are believed to become increasingly resistant to change, as they bias perceptions of the actions and desires of others, influence the child's behavior, and set into motion a pattern of interaction that tends to reinforce and stabilize these biases (Bowlby, 1973). Another question has to do with the relative influence and organization of multiple models developed in relation to multiple caregivers (see Howes & Spieker, Chapter 14, this volume). There is controversy, reflecting a lack of empirical evidence, about whether these models operate in a hierarchical, an additive, or some other manner.

Because there are reciprocal linkages between the working models of oneself and one's attachment figures, attachment patterns are expected to lead to generalized perceptions of self-esteem and competence, as well as to expectations about caregivers' behavior. When a secure and trusting bond forms between parent and child, both parent and child develop reciprocal positive working models of the relationship, which include attributions of responsiveness, warmth, and trust and thus set the stage for cooperative interactions. Insecure attachment may play a causal role in later maladaptation through the crystallization of reciprocal working models characterized by anger, mistrust, anxiety,

and/or fear. This proposed mechanism is compatible with theory and research on the attributional biases of children with both internalizing and externalizing difficulties. For example, Dodge (1991) has hypothesized that early insecure attachments may lead to hostile working models that contain attributional biases in which hypervigilance and unresolved child anger result in reactive aggression. Support for this proposition is provided by a study of kindergarten and first-grade children (Cassidy, Kirsh, Scolton, & Parke, 1996). In response to hypothetical peer dilemmas, children with higher concurrent security scores (assessed with the Main & Cassidy [1985] procedure) exhibited more positive representations of why events happened, how the child would feel, and what would happen next, providing evidence that attachment security may be linked to representational models of the self in peer relations.

A fourth process by which attachment may contribute to maladaptation relates to its motivational function in social intercourse. Attachment may promote a generalized positive or resistant social orientation in the child, providing differential levels of readiness for socialization (Richters & Waters, 1991). Children with warm, contingent relations in early life are more likely to comply with parent controls and directives during toddlerhood and the preschool years (Maccoby & Martin, 1983; Sroufe & Fleeson, 1986). Thus attachment processes may help to explain how a prosocial orientation develops and how identification processes proceed in early and middle childhood (Waters et al., 1991). Attachment may then mediate aspects of motivation that deter children from deviance and create the positive bonding that protects children from delinquency and social and personal destructiveness, as discussed in social control theories (Hawkins, Arthur, & Catalano, 1995).

THE ROLE OF ATTACHMENT IN UNDERSTANDING CHILDHOOD PSYCHOPATHOLOGY

Attachment theory and research has informed the study of child psychopathology in two major ways. First, over the past two decades, a body of theoretical and empirical work has considered how the common forms of attachment relationships (i.e., secure, insecure-avoidant, insecure-ambivalent, and insecure-disorganized classifications) might contribute to disorder by either increasing risk or buffering the effects of other risk factors. Second, in extreme cases, atypical attachment patterns may themselves be considered disorders (Lieberman & Zeanah, 1995)—for example, when caregiving is seriously disrupted or is pathogenic due to severe maltreatment or institutionalization. Although attachment theory grew out of a concern for such extreme circumstances, surprisingly little research has carefully examined this link between attachment and psychopathology until recently. Each of these two approaches is considered below.

Theoretical Links between Early Attachment and Specific Disorders

A number of theorists have proposed models of the differing developmental pathways that might ensue from variations in the early attachment patterns described by Ainsworth, Blehar, Waters, and Wall (1978), Main and Solomon (1990), and others. According to Bowlby (1973), the avoidantly attached child learns that expressing anger in response to a caregiver's unresponsive or intrusive behavior will reduce the caregiver's proximity in stressful situations, so the child learns to redirect this anger toward the environment. The result may be hostile and aggressive behavior. In contrast, inconsistent or overprotective caregiving may engender chronic anxiety and vigilance in the ambivalently attached child, who becomes concerned that his or her needs may also not be met in other situations. Bowlby traced depression to childhood experiences of separation from and loss of attachment figures, especially if these result in hopelessness and helplessness. This might be associated with either ambivalent or avoidant patterns of attachment.

Sroufe (1983) proposed that whereas both avoidant and ambivalent infants may develop externalizing behavior problems, the meaning of their behavior and the specific manifestations may differ in predictable ways. Avoidant children may develop a hostile, antisocial pattern in response to a rejecting and emotionally unavailable caregiver. The underlying anger, which is not directed to its source, may be manifested in lying, bullying, blaming, and being insensitive to others. Ambivalent children, on the other hand, may be easily overstimulated and exhibit impulsivity, restlessness, a short attention span, and low frustration tolerance. Both kinds of children may be aggressive—but, Sroufe suggests, for different reasons.

Rubin and his colleagues (1991) suggested that avoidant children are more likely than ambivalent children to become disruptive preschoolers. In a model that included child temperament, socioecological factors, parental social setting and attitudes, as well as attachment effects, they delineated a pathway in which an unresponsive, rejecting mother responds to an avoidant infant in an authoritarian, hostile manner, sometimes resulting in aggressive child behavior. In contrast, they predicted that ambivalent infants would be more likely to develop internalizing problems.

The utility of these models may be limited if they fail to include the more recently developed disorganized/disoriented category (Main & Hesse, 1990; Main & Solomon, 1990)—a pattern that occurs at high rates in samples characterized by parent psychopathology, child abuse, or very high social risk (Carlson, Cicchetti, Barnett, & Braunwald, 1989; Crittenden, 1988; Lyons-Ruth, Connell, Zoll, & Stahl, 1987; O'Connor, Sigman, & Brill, 1987; Spieker & Booth, 1988). Given the prevalence of disorganized classifications in children at risk for psychopathology, this pattern requires further exploration in any attempt to link attachment to later psychopathology (Ogawa et al., 1997). Lyons-Ruth (1996) has reviewed the literature on the association between the disorganized classification and aggression, as well as its potential roots in intergenerational risks experienced by caregivers. With her colleagues, she has also discussed potential links between disorganization and dissociative symptoms (Lyons-Ruth et al., 2006). Unfortunately, there are as yet few data regarding the home environment in which this pattern develops. Main and Hesse (1990) postulated that the traumatized mother of the disorganized infant is unpredictably frightening to her child and that disorganization is a response to this fear and inconsistency. Egeland and Carlson (2004) noted that the child who develops a disorganized attachment has been placed in an "unresolvable paradox," in which the putative source of safety (the caregiver) is simultaneously the source of fear. In this approach–avoidance situation, the child is able neither to regulate his or her own arousal nor to enlist the caregiver's assistance in regulation; the child may therefore mentally isolate and fail to process disturbing stimuli, resulting in dissociation. Given the elevated rate of the disorganized pattern in infants with high biological risk, either perinatally (e.g., resulting from maternal alcohol abuse, smoking, multiple-drug abuse, or nutrition deficiencies), postnatally (resulting from child abuse), or both, there is a need for further investigation of potential neurological and psychological correlates of this pattern. (See Solomon & George, Chapter 18, and Lyons-Ruth & Jacobvitz, Chapter 28, this volume, for further discussion of this attachment pattern.)

Empirical Support for the Role of Infant Attachment in Disordered Behavior

In the past few decades, a growing number of studies have examined the effects of infant attachment on later development. The populations that have been studied have ranged from convenience samples (largely middle-class and low-risk) to children at high socioeconomic or medical risk, those whose caregivers have psychiatric diagnoses, and those with clinical diagnoses. As might be concluded from the preceding section on risk models, attachment is most likely to contribute to disorder in the context of other risks, so studies of disadvantaged and clinical samples have generally been most fruitful. High-risk populations with relatively high base rates of diagnoses have the advantage of facilitating longitudinal studies with early attachment measures, whereas clinical samples can test more focused hypotheses concerning specific diagnoses but usually must rely on less well-validated, contemporaneous measures of attachment.

Several studies of low-risk populations have asked whether insecure attachment in the first 2 years is related to higher rates of disruptive behavior problems. Participants in this research have generally been selected in a nonrandom manner, were primarily middle-class, included a low percentage of insecure children (30% or less), and had low base rates of psychopathology. Given their relatively small sample sizes, these studies have had little power to detect significant associations. In five illustrative studies (Bates, Bayles, Bennett, Ridge, & Brown, 1991; Bates, Maslin, & Frankel, 1985; Fagot & Kavanaugh, 1990; Goldberg, Lojkasek, Minde, & Corter, 1990; Lewis, Feiring, McGuffog, & Jaskir, 1984), no significant main effects of insecure attachment on later externalizing problems were found. There was little investigation of mediator or moderator effects except in the Lewis and colleagues (1984) study, which reported a gender–attachment interaction: 40% of insecure boys, as compared to 6% of secure boys, scored above the 90th percentile on the Child Behavior Checklist (CBCL) Total Problem score. Follow-up of this sample at age 13 revealed no main effect of infant attachment status, and no effect of interaction between attachment and exposure to stress, on teacher or maternal ratings of psychopathology (Feiring & Lewis, 1997).

These findings support the premise that main effects models will be of little interest in low-risk samples and are likely to provide little of value in understanding potential linkages between attachment and externalizing psychopathology (Fagot

& Kavanaugh, 1990). Even the large population-based National Institute of Child Health and Human Development (NICHD) Study of Early Child Care (Belsky & Fearon, 2002) found that although infant attachment predicted social competence at 3 years, its main effect on preschool behavior problems was not significant. Attachment insecurity was only predictive of problem behavior within the context of a high-risk environment.

A second and more promising strategy is to examine the effects of attachment in populations that share risk factors in other domains (e.g., difficult temperament, poor parent management strategies, socioeonomic disadvantage, and parent psychopathology) and have a high base rate of psychopathology. Several groups of investigators have studied high-risk populations (e.g., El-Sheikh & Elmore-Staton, 2004; Lyons-Ruth et al., 1987; Munson, McMahon, & Spieker, 2001; Rodning, Beckwith, & Howard, 1991; Spieker & Booth, 1988; Sroufe et al., 2005; Vondra, Shaw, Swearingen, Cohen, & Owens, 2001).

Only the Minnesota Parent–Child Project has followed a sample from infancy into early adulthood and assessed psychopathology (Sroufe et al., 2005; see also Weinfield et al., Chapter 4, this volume). In this research, the infants of primarily young, single mothers were followed from birth (long-term sample size of 174). The investigators assessed attachment at both 12 and 18 months and included only those children categorized as secure, avoidant, or ambivalent at both time periods. This use of multiple measures of attachment (unfortunately unusual in the literature) is likely to create more reliable assessment of stable patterns, avoiding inaccuracy due to error variance or to short-term fluctuations in family stressors that may affect attachment status (Vaughn, Egeland, Sroufe, & Waters, 1979). However, at different ages of follow-up, different measures (combined across time vs. only the 12-month assessment) were used as predictors. Follow-up assessments in the preschool years (Erickson, Sroufe, & Egeland, 1985; Sroufe, 1983; Troy & Sroufe, 1987), in the early elementary school years (Renken, Egeland, Marvinney, Mangelsdorf, & Sroufe, 1989; Sroufe, 1990; Sroufe, Egeland, & Kreutzer, 1990), in the preadolescent period (Urban, Carlson, Egeland, & Sroufe, 1991), and in adolescence (Carlson, 1998) have consistently shown that children in high-social-risk environments who exhibit early insecurity are significantly more likely to have poor peer relations and more symptoms of aggression, depression, and general maladjustment later than are children with early security. For externalizing outcomes, predictions from attachment and early parent–child relations were much stronger for boys than for girls (which might be expected, given the higher base rate of externalizing problems in males).

Main effects were found in this high-risk environment, and transactional processes in the preschool years were also identified that increased the risk of disruptive behavior problems for some secure infants and decreased the risk of such problems among insecure children. Compared to the secure group without behavior problems, secure infants with later behavior problems had mothers who were less supportive and encouraging at 24 and 42 months and who in the later assessment were less effective teachers, providing little support, unclear expectations, and inconsistent limits. At 30 months their homes had fewer play materials and less maternal involvement, and these mothers reported more confusion and disorganized mood states than did mothers of secure infants who did not show behavior problems later. Compared to insecurely attached infants with subsequent behavior problems, insecure infants who did not develop problems had mothers who were warmer, more supportive, and more appropriate at limit setting at 42 months. The home environments of insecure infants without later problems contained more appropriate play materials and were characterized by higher maternal involvement, and the children were more positive in their affect and more compliant and affectionate with their mothers at 42 months.

Unlike most studies of high social risk, the Minnesota project has produced several follow-up reports examining the relation of infant attachment to specific disorders and clinically significant symptoms later in childhood and in adolescence. For instance, Aguilar, Sroufe, Egeland, and Carlson (2000) identified adolescents with early-onset antisocial behavior and found that they were more likely than adolescents with later-onset antisocial behavior or nondisordered youth to have been rated avoidantly attached as infants. However, this study compared the avoidantly attached children with all others, so no clear conclusions can be drawn regarding other classifications. After controlling for such factors as maternal depression and life stress, Duggal, Carlson, Sroufe, and Egeland (2001) reported that a construct they labeled "early supportive relationship," which included infant attachment classification, independently predicted depressive symptoms in adolescence but not in childhood. Two studies using this sample have

examined the association between attachment and anxiety. Bosquet and Egeland (2006) found no direct correlation between secure attachment and childhood anxiety or clinical symptoms of anxiety at 17½ years of age, although attachment history was moderately correlated ($r = .23$) with an anxiety rating at age 16. Attachment status in infancy did predict negative representations of peer relationships in preadolescence, which in turn predicted adolescent anxiety symptoms. Warren, Huston, Egeland, and Sroufe (1997) looked for predictors of anxiety disorders in 172 individuals who received a psychiatric interview at age 17. Fifteen percent of the sample had either a current diagnosis or lifetime history of an anxiety disorder. Twenty-eight percent of ambivalent infants developed anxiety disorders, as compared with 16% of avoidant and 11% of secure infants. Even after infant temperament and maternal ratings of anxiety in infancy were accounted for, ambivalent attachment accounted for a significant but small percentage (4%) of the variance in anxiety disorder. However, secure infants did not show a lower *overall* rate of disorder (including nonanxiety disorders) than did ambivalent infants. Compared to both secure (39%), and ambivalent infants (40%), those who had been avoidant were most likely to have any disorder (70%). Overall, these findings indicate that the association between infant attachment and later anxiety disorder is moderate at best.

Ogawa and colleagues (1997) and Carlson (1998) examined the relationship of infant attachment, developmental factors, and the experience of trauma to symptoms of dissociation in adolescence (age 17) and young adulthood (age 19). Their analyses included Main's disorganized/disoriented scale and classification (Main & Solomon, 1990). Both avoidant classification and disorganization ratings and classification in infancy predicted clinical levels of dissociation in adolescence. Infancy ratings of disorganization also predicted dissociation years later, in young adulthood. These findings support the theoretical model of Liotti (1995) linking early disorganization and trauma to later dissociative disorders.

Thus, in this high-risk, low-income population, the quality of early attachment was related in a predictable manner to preschool and school-age measures of behavior problems and to adolescent measures of specific disorders. These associations were in some cases mediated by later aspects of the parent–child relationship and family circumstances. The findings clearly support a transactional, multiple-pathway model, demonstrating that information about both early security of attachment and later parent–child and family relationships may be useful in predicting later psychopathology. The fact that the Minnesota study shows more and stronger effects of infant attachment than research with low-risk samples has shown may indicate that secure attachment operates as a protective factor in high-risk environments (Morisset et al., 1990; Rutter, 1987) or that insecure attachment combined with family adversity is one potent pathway to later disruptive behavior problems (Lyons-Ruth, Zoll, Connell, & Grunebaum, 1989; but see also Greenberg et al., 2001). It should be noted that with the exception of the Ogawa and colleagues (1997) and Carlson (1998) reports, the Minnesota project did not include assessments of the infancy disorganized/disoriented classification, which may have limited its power of prediction. (The infant data were recoded for Carlson's study, after many of the other findings had already been published.)

Three other longitudinal investigations in high-risk populations have confirmed the predictive value of early attachment. Lyons-Ruth and colleagues (Lyons-Ruth et al., 1989; Lyons-Ruth, Easterbrooks, & Cibelli, 1997; Lyons-Ruth, Easterbrooks, Davidson Cibelli, & Bronfman, 1995) have followed a sample of high-risk families in which many caregivers were depressed. Follow-up assessments, including teachers' independent ratings of anxiety, hostility, and hyperactivity, revealed that preschoolers who were hostile with peers and adults were significantly more likely to have been classified as insecure (and especially disorganized) as infants; 71% of the hostile preschoolers had disorganized attachments at 18 months, while only 12% had been classified as secure. Children with disorganized classifications and mothers with psychosocial problems had a 55% rate of hostile behavior in kindergarten as compared to a 5% rate for low-income children without either risk factor. Lyons-Ruth and colleagues (1995) reported that the combination of low infant intelligence and insecure attachment was highly predictive of teacher-rated externalizing problems at age 7; however, neither factor alone was predictive. Fifty percent of the disorganized/low-intelligence group showed externalizing problems, compared to 5% of the sample with neither risk factor. In the same sample, internalizing symptoms were predicted by avoidant but not disorganized attachment, but only maternal depression predicted clinical levels of internalizing scores (Lyons-Ruth et al., 1997). In a follow-up of this Cambridge, Massachusetts, sample, Easterbrooks,

Davidson, and Chazan (1993) reported that children classified as insecure at age 7 (using the Main & Cassidy [1985] coding system) had significantly more internalizing and externalizing problems as indicated by both parent and teacher reports, and this connection was maintained even after family risk factors were accounted for.

Shaw and Vondra (1995), studying a low-income sample in Pittsburgh, found that infant attachment insecurity modestly predicted preschool behavior problems at age 3. When children were 5 years of age, insecure attachment at 12 months was uniquely associated with parent-rated behavior problems on the CBCL after other risk factors were accounted for; disorganization was predictive of externalizing problems, and ambivalent classification was predictive of internalizing problems (Shaw, Keenan, Vondra, Delliquadri, & Giovannelli, 1997). In logistic regression analyses, insecure attachment (odds ratio = 3.4) and maternal personality (odds ratio = 8.4) both contributed uniquely to predictions of clinically significant difficulties at age 5. While 60% of disorganized children had clinically elevated levels of aggression, 31% of avoidant, 28% of ambivalent, and only 17% of secure infants did. Most importantly, only when combined together were disorganized attachment and parent ratings of difficult temperament at age 2 potent predictors; children with both risk factors scored at the 99th percentile for aggression, whereas children with only disorganized attachment or only difficult temperament were within the normal range.

In both the Shaw and colleagues and the Lyons-Ruth and colleagues investigations, the insecure pattern most often related to later problems was the disorganized/disoriented attachment category, suggesting that disorganized attachment may be a general vulnerability factor for later problems in adaptation. However, Munson and colleagues (2001) followed a sample of teen mothers with a high rate of depression and found both avoidant and disorganized infancy classifications to be associated with externalizing scores at 9 years of age. Using the same sample, Keller and colleagues (2005) identified developmental trajectories that distinguished a group of children with early-starting conduct problems. In a person-oriented analysis, infant secure attachment appeared to be protective, whereas an avoidant (but not a disorganized) classification predicted a higher prevalence of conduct problems, given high personal and contextual risk. The early-starting pattern, with an escalating trajectory of behavior problems, was particularly prevalent when insecure infant attachment was combined with male gender and either high infant negativity or parenting risk, or when insecure attachment, parenting risk, and family ecological risk co-occurred. Early-starting conduct problems were significantly less likely than expected by chance under conditions of positive parenting, low family ecological risk, and secure attachment. Further evidence of the interaction between avoidant attachment and temperament was provided by Burgess, Marshall, Rubin, and Fox (2003), who found that in the context of uninhibited, fearless temperament, avoidant attachment predicted higher levels of problem behaviors.

Although they differ in the specific type of insecurity involved, each of these studies indicates that an insecure attachment may set a trajectory that, *along with other risk factors*, increases risk for either externalizing or internalizing psychopathology. To reiterate the point made earlier, they also illustrate that an insecure attachment classification is not itself a measure of psychopathology.

Focusing on medical rather than social risk, Goldberg, Gotowiec, and Simmons (1995) examined infant attachment in children without health problems, those with cystic fibrosis, and those with congenital heart defects. Two findings are of particular interest. First, both medically diagnosed groups showed lower rates of secure attachment at 12–18 months than did the healthy group; this was mostly accounted for by higher rates of disorganization in the medically diagnosed children. Second, infants who were classified as avoidant received higher internalizing *and* externalizing scores at age 4 (mother and father ratings combined) than did secure children. Neither ambivalent nor disorganized children had higher rates of problems than secure infants.

Associations between Postinfancy Attachment and Childhood Psychopathology

Classification systems developed to assess the quality of attachment in older children (e.g., Cassidy & Marvin, 1992; Crittenden, 1992; Kerns, Klepac, & Cole, 1996; Main & Cassidy, 1985, 1988; see Solomon & George, Chapter 18, this volume, for a review) have allowed the examination of contemporaneous relations between attachment and psychopathology. However, as these are concurrent measurements, they leave unresolved the question of causal direction. We first review studies from nonclinical populations and then describe findings relating concurrent attachment to functioning in samples of children with clinical diagnoses.

Nonclinical Samples

In a middle-class sample, Solomon, George, and De Jong (1995) found that 6-year-old children classified as insecure-controlling were higher in concurrent parent- and teacher-rated aggression than other children. Neither avoidant nor ambivalent children had an elevated rate of problems. Main and Cassidy (1988) and Cassidy and Marvin (1992) suggested that this controlling pattern is a developmental transformation of the infancy disorganized/disoriented pattern that occurs at elevated rates in high-risk samples.

Further evidence of the relation between the controlling classification and maladaptation was provided by a community sample of French Canadian children of mixed socioeconomic status (Moss, Cyr, & Dubois-Comtois, 2004; Moss, Rousseau, Parent, St.-Laurent, & Saintonge, 1998; Moss et al., 2006). Attachment was assessed when children were 5–7 years of age, and behavior problems were assessed concurrently and again 2 years later. At both ages, controlling children were at highest risk for both externalizing and internalizing problems, according to teacher ratings (Moss et al., 1998). Using a composite of mothers', teachers', and self-ratings when children were 7–9 years old, this research group reported that both ambivalent and controlling children were more likely to have high externalizing scores (Moss et al., 2006). Only children with controlling classifications had higher internalizing scores. Controlling children were also more likely to be above the clinical cutoff on an overall problem behavior score. Examination of subscale scores revealed that, according to mothers, ambivalent and controlling children were more aggressive, had more conduct problems, and exhibited more anxious/depressive symptoms than secure children. Predictably, compared to secure children, controlling-punitive children had more externalizing problems, whereas controlling-caregiving children had more internalizing problems (Moss et al., 2004).

Using the Crittenden (1992) preschool system for scoring attachment, Fagot and Pears (1996) examined the association between attachment security at age 3 and teacher ratings of behavioral and peer problems at age 7. Follow-up indicated that children labeled insecure-coercive at age 3 showed higher rates of behavioral problems and peer problems at age 7 than did children coded either secure or insecure-defended.

Three research reports focused on concurrent relations between attachment and peer relations. In a sample of English 4-year-olds, boys who were concurrently insecurely attached with their mothers displayed more aggression, disruption, and attention seeking in preschool than did secure boys (Turner, 1991). Insecure girls were more dependent and less assertive and controlling than secure girls but did not differ in aggression or disruptiveness. Cohn (1990) reported that 6-year-old boys with insecure attachments to their mothers were perceived by peers as more aggressive and by their teachers as having greater behavior problems. No such associations were found for girls. And using Kerns and colleagues' (1996) Security Scale to measure 10-year-old children's perception of attachment security to mothers and fathers, Booth-LaForce (2006) found that security in relation to fathers, but not mothers, was significantly associated with lower rates of peer-rated aggression.

Another study involving school-age children found contemporaneous insecure attachment with mothers to be associated with depressive symptoms (Graham & Easterbrooks, 2000). In this research, security appeared to serve a protective function: Only children with insecure attachments were at elevated risk of depression, given economic risk. Controlling children exhibited more symptoms than did children with other classifications.

Manassis, Bradley, Goldberg, Hood, and Swinson (1994) described the first study of children of mothers with diagnosed anxiety disorders—a particularly important group, given the key role of anxiety in attachment theory (Bowlby, 1973; Bretherton, 1992; Cassidy, 1995). Using the Cassidy and Marvin (1992) preschool classification system, the authors studied 20 children ages 22–51 months. Eighty percent of these children of anxious mothers were coded as insecurely attached, with a high percentage classified as controlling, disorganized, or insecure/other. Two children met criteria for childhood anxiety disorders; both were classified as avoidant. There were four secure children, distinguished from the remainder of the sample by significantly less life stress and more competent parenting, as reported by their mothers. The authors hypothesized that a measure of inhibited temperament would predict both attachment insecurity and childhood anxiety. However, they found no relation between behavioral inhibition and either attachment or anxiety disorder.

Clinical Samples

Conduct Problems. Conduct problems in early childhood have received considerable attention from attachment researchers. Reasons for this interest include their early appearance, allowing the application of existing attachment measures, and theory predicting that attachment is a significant risk factor (Greenberg et al., 1993). The theoretical grounds for expecting children classified as avoidant to be at increased risk for externalizing disorders have been reviewed above. In an alternative formulation, Solomon and colleagues (1995) hypothesized that it is the absence of a coherent strategy (i.e., disorganization) rather than insecurity per se that is linked to maladaptation. Findings in both high-risk and clinical samples indicate that children with avoidant and disorganized or controlling classifications, as well as children classified as coercive according to Crittenden's (1992) system, may be at particular risk for conduct problems.

Attachment was examined in three cohorts of clinic-referred preschool children who met criteria for ODD and comparison children matched on age, socioeconomic status, and family composition. In the first two samples (Greenberg et al., 1991; Speltz, Greenberg, & DeKlyen, 1990), approximately 80% of the clinic children were insecurely attached to their mothers (assessed concurrently with a 1989 version of the MacArthur preschool system; Cassidy & Marvin, 1992), compared to 30% of the comparison children. Although clinic children had various forms of insecurity (avoidant, ambivalent, and controlling), they exhibited a disproportionate number of controlling classifications (characterized by the child's attempt to actively control the interaction with the parent upon reunion). Many of the preschoolers who showed this pattern were punitive or rejecting toward their mothers. In a third and larger cohort of 80 clinically referred preschool boys and 80 carefully matched controls, we (Speltz et al., 1999) again found that those with ODD had higher rates of insecurity. In this sample, however, only 55% of clinic boys were coded as insecure with their mothers, and ODD diagnoses were associated with avoidant as well as controlling classifications. This study was distinctive in assessing children's attachment to fathers as well as mothers. Attachment to fathers showed a similar pattern: Clinically referred boys had higher rates of insecurity (55%) than did the comparison group (15%), and boys with insecure attachments to *both* parents were at highest risk of being in the clinic group (DeKlyen, Speltz, & Greenberg, 1998).

Several findings from these clinical samples bear discussion. First, the fact that a significant proportion of the clinic-referred boys showed secure attachments indicates that attachment is not merely assessing oppositionality and that insecure attachment is a component of only some pathways leading to ODD. This was reinforced by subsequent person-oriented analyses (described above) demonstrating that although risk of diagnosis was dramatically increased by the presence of multiple domains of risk (child characteristics, insecure attachment, poor parenting practices, and adverse family ecology), no single factor (including attachment insecurity) was either necessary or sufficient for clinic status (Greenberg et al., 2001). Campbell (1990) has similarly noted that in some families of children with high rates of aggression and hyperactivity, the mother–child relationship appears warm and trusting. Second, in the initial study (Speltz et al., 1990), the relation between attachment status and clinic status was found only among boys (there were few girls and thus little power to test the effect, but insecurity did not appear to characterize clinic girls). The second and third cohorts (Greenberg et al., 1991; Speltz et al., 1999) included only boys. Finally, the finding in the second sample of high concordance between concurrent child attachment and an independent assessment of maternal attachment using the Adult Attachment Interview (AAI) (DeKlyen, 1996) increases the likelihood that these children's attachments were also insecure in infancy and that attachment processes may therefore have influenced the development of disruptive problems.

Other research has also supported a link between parental representations of attachment and childhood externalizing problems (Crowell & Feldman, 1988; Dozier & Rutter, Chapter 29, this volume). These findings suggest that parents' attachment status may have implications for child and family treatment, and Routh, Hill, Steele, Elliot, and Dewey (1995) have reported that children of parents with autonomous (secure) adult attachment classifications showed greater clinical improvement following intervention.

Further research on the association between attachment and delinquency, criminality, and antisocial personality disorder is needed. Fonagy and colleagues (1997) presented a model that links early attachment to later attachment and to criminality. They hypothesized that internal working models of specific attachment figures become more global during the adolescent years, leading to the phenomenon often discussed as attachment or bonding to social institutions (Hawkins et al., 1995; Hirschi, 1969). That is, parent–child attachment bonds are reconfigured as bonds to so-

cial institutions (e.g., schools and businesses) and to the adults who represent them (e.g., teachers and employers). Children who lack this bonding to institutions and have deviant peer relations are at significantly greater risk for substance use and criminal careers (Brook, Whiteman, & Finch, 1993; Le Blanc, 1994). Fonagy and his colleagues posited that secure attachments facilitate awareness of the mental states of others and that this "mentalizing" inhibits malevolent acts and enhances relationship building during childhood. Thus insecure attachment is linked to criminality not only via insufficient bonding to social institutions, but also via deficient consideration of others' needs and feelings. Fonagy and colleagues further proposed that children with avoidant attachments may be especially likely to follow this pathway. Although few data exist as yet to support these propositions, they raise a number of research questions. First, what is the association between "mentalizing" or "theory of mind" and attachment relations in older children? Second, is this association specific to conduct problems, or might such associations be present in depression or other disorders as well? Third, by what developmental processes do specific working models (e.g., to mothers vs. fathers) become generalized, and when they are discrepant, what determines which model will affect the adolescent transition? Finally, what might counterexamples (i.e., children with insecure internal working models who do bond to social institutions) tell us about the process?

Anxiety Disorders. Given that anxiety may be the fundamental condition underlying insecure attachment (Bowlby, 1973), it is both surprising and curious that so little attention has been paid to anxiety disorders in childhood and their relation to attachment (Cassidy, 1995). As noted above, in the Minnesota project Warren and colleagues (1997) found that adolescents with ambivalent classifications as infants were somewhat more likely to receive anxiety diagnoses. Two recent studies have established associations between anxiety in childhood and concurrent insecure representations of attachment. Warren, Emde, and Sroufe (2000) reported that anxiety symptoms were correlated with insecure attachment working models in school-age children. Shamir-Essakow, Ungerer, and Rapee (2005) found that preschool children with disorganized or (contrary to theoretical predictions) avoidant representations of attachment had the highest levels of anxiety symptoms, after controlling for mothers' anxiety. Interestingly, although both attachment and behavioral inhibition were risk factors for anxiety, in this study they did not interact.

Although clinicians and developmental psychopathologists have theorized about the role of parent–child relations in separation anxiety disorder (SAD) (e.g., Klein, 1994; Manassis & Bradley, 1994; Thurber, 1996), little is known about the behavioral or representational attachment patterns of children with this disorder or about how these may relate to age of onset, parent–child behavior, or recent family or child trauma. Attachment theory has had little impact on either case conceptualization or treatment of SAD (but see Marvin, 1992). This is remarkable, given the attention paid to the topic by Bowlby himself, and longitudinal studies of children with SAD are clearly a next step. As the behaviors characteristic of SAD may be normal in early childhood, only when they are both excessive and developmentally inappropriate can they be considered significant. SAD is believed to be a risk factor for a variety of adult psychiatric disorders, including depression, agoraphobia, and panic disorder; thus research examining the relationship between attachment processes and SAD could illuminate the pathways to these disorders as well.

Depression. As already noted, Bowlby and others advanced theoretical arguments for the role of attachment in the pathogenesis of depression (Cicchetti & Cummings, 1990; Kobak et al., 1991); however, no investigation of attachment behavior or representational models in children with current diagnoses of dysthymia or major depression has yet appeared. Adolescent samples have exhibited the expected relations between concurrent attachment to parents (but not to peers) and depression (Essau, 2004; Nada Raja, McGee, & Staton, 1992), and children of depressive parents show higher rates of insecurity. Abela and colleagues (2005) examined self-reports of both attachment quality and reassurance seeking in a study of school-age children of depressed parents. Children with a combination of insecure attachment and high reassurance seeking were more likely to report depressive symptoms and a past history of depression than were children with only one of these risk factors. The study of children with clinically significant depression is clearly a next step in the research agenda. As with conduct problems, attachment relations may in some cases either have no relation with or be an effect of depressive disorders. Only careful case histories of

attachment patterns, as well as contemporaneous assessments, can illuminate these pathways.

Pervasive Developmental Disorder. Children with autism or other forms of pervasive developmental disorder (PDD) might be expected to exhibit unusual interpersonal relations as well as some of the bizarre behaviors associated with disorganized attachment, given the social and behavioral deficits that are diagnostic. Several studies have demonstrated that many children with PDD form secure attachments (Dissnayake & Crossley, 1996; Rogers, Ozonoff, & Maslin-Cole, 1991), although insecure and, specifically, disorganized attachments occurred more frequently than in nonclinical children, even once unusual behaviors typical of autism (e.g., stereotypies) were disregarded during coding (Capps, Sigman, & Mundy, 1994). More recently, a meta-analysis by Rutgers, Bakermans-Kranenburg, van IJzendoorn, and Van Berckelaer-Onnes (2004) indicated that although most children (53%) with PDD developed secure attachments, this rate was lower than that of normally developing children or of children with other types of developmental disorders. In a small study of toddlers with PDD, mental retardation, language delays, or typical development, van IJzendoorn and colleagues (2007) found children with PDD more likely than those without this diagnosis to be classified as disorganized. However, 72% of the children with PDD also had mental retardation, which increased the risk of both insecure attachment and disorganization. This paralleled an earlier finding that only those children with both PDD and mental retardation had elevated rates of disorganization (Willemsen-Swinkels, Bakermans-Kranenburg, Buitelaar, van IJzendoorn, & van Engeland, 2000).

Disordered Attachment: A Response to Extremes of Caregiving

For many years, clinicians have been aware of a small but often seriously impaired group of children with significant deficits of behavior, cognition, and affect believed to result from deprivation or from distorted or disrupted caregiving. These impairments are usually associated with extreme circumstances: the absence of an attachment relationship (usually due to institutional rearing), severe abuse or neglect, or traumatic disruption or loss of an attachment relationship These concerns led Bowlby and others to investigate the effects of "maternal deprivation" after World War II

(Bowlby, 1953; Goldfarb, 1955; Spitz, 1946). More recently, researchers have studied young children living in institutions (e.g., in Romania; Zeanah, Smyke, & Dumitrescu, 2002), adopted out of such institutions (O'Connor et al., 2003), or removed from their biological parents and placed with foster parents because of maltreatment or neglect (Dozier, Albus, Stovall, & Bates, 2000; Dozier & Rutter, Chapter 29, this volume).

Established diagnostic systems did not acknowledge that disorder might result from disturbed or absent attachment relations until 1980. In its first appearance in the *Diagnostic and Statistical Manual of Mental Disorders* (DSM-III; American Psychiatric Association, 1980), reactive attachment disorder (RAD) was characterized as a pervasive disturbance *across relationships*, occurring before 10 months of age, with associated "failure-to-thrive" symptoms that had little or no association with attachment (Richters & Volkmar, 1994; Zeanah, 1996). Revisions in subsequent versions of the DSM and in the *International Classification of Diseases* (ICD-10; World Health Organization, 1992) altered the age of onset (to 5 years of age or younger) and dropped the failure-to-thrive criteria. These diagnostic systems distinguish two types of the disorder: "inhibited" and "disinhibited." The inhibited subtype is marked by hypervigilance and fear, manifested in withdrawal and ambivalence. Children with the disinhibited subtype are described as indiscriminately friendly and lacking a selective attachment to a discriminated figure. DSM-IV requires, in addition, documentation of pathogenic care by the caregiver (American Psychiatric Association, 1994).

Problems in Current Nosology

Although these nosological revisions represent progress, by recognizing the pathogenesis that can result from early distortions in attachment relations, they have a number of shortcomings, reflecting the limited application of attachment theory or research in their formulation (Zeanah, 1996). First, criteria still focus on aberrant social behavior in general, rather than on the attachment relationship and its specific consequences. However, children may exhibit disordered attachment with their primary caregivers, causing considerable dysfunction, yet may react positively to other adults or peers (Lieberman & Zeanah, 1995). Second, RAD has been narrowly defined as due to severe deprivation or maltreatment, but it may also develop in a stable but unhealthy relationship not char-

acterized by severe maltreatment (Rutter, 1997). Third, as attachment disorders are by their very nature relational, they do not fit comfortably into a nosological system that characterizes disorders as person-centered. In this respect, the diagnostic classification manuals published by Zero to Three (Zero to Three Task Force, 1994, 2005) represent a significant advance. Based on the premise that the caregiver context is essential to understanding a young child's functioning, this system includes a specific axis for parent–child relationship disorders, as well as a global assessment scale for rating parent–infant relationships. Types of relationship disorders include overinvolved, underinvolved, abusive, angry/hostile, anxious/tense, and mixed. The Zero to Three system retains the traditional notion of RAD, although in the recently revised edition it has been renamed "deprivation/maltreatment disorder."

An Alternative Taxonomy of Attachment Disorders

Theory and research have led to important advances in the conceptualization of attachment disorders. It has become clear that these disorders are distinct from insecure attachment, as observed in the Strange Situation. Drawing from richly described case studies (e.g., Lieberman & Pawl, 1988, 1990; Lieberman & Zeanah, 1995), Zeanah and Boris (2000) proposed alternative criteria for attachment disorders in the early years, distinguishing among conditions of "nonattachment," "disordered attachment," and "disruption of attachments." As in the DSM-IV and ICD-10 formulations of RAD, children in the first category (nonattachment), with no discriminated attachment figure, may either fail to differentiate among adults (indiscriminate sociability) or fail to seek or respond to caregivers in a developmentally typical manner. However, in contrast to those diagnostic systems, Zeanah and Boris do not specify that these distortions must occur in most social situations (i.e., beyond the caregiving context), and they do require that the child has reached a mental age of 10 months, to aid in distinguishing attachment disorder from cognitive disorders or PDD. In the second category (disordered attachment), a selective attachment relationship exists but is disturbed, as evidenced by the child's self-endangerment, extreme inhibition, compulsive compliance, or role reversal. Finally, the third group (disruption of attachment) includes children whose attachment to a primary caregiver has been disrupted; they may display various patterns of grief reactions, ranging from protest to despair to detachment. Initial studies suggest that these criteria, grounded in both attachment theory and clinical experience, permit more reliable description of clinical cases than do the DSM-IV criteria (Boris, Fueyo, & Zeanah, 1997; Boris et al., 2004).

This advance in the development of nosology brings the study of attachment back to its clinical origins and to its concern with children who have suffered extreme deprivation in caregiving (Bowlby, 1953, 1969/1982). However, there is a need for further validation of this diagnostic system, for an examination of the developmental trajectory of children who show these extreme attachment difficulties, and for parallel work in middle childhood.

The Effects of Institutional Rearing, Late Adoption, and Maltreatment

As maternal loss and deprivation have been central to attachment theory since its inception, the dearth of studies on children who have suffered traumatic loss of attachment figures or who have been adopted after infancy is surprising. Marcovitch and colleagues (1997) used the Cassidy and Marvin (1992) system to describe the attachment security of a sample of 3- to 5-year-old Romanian children adopted into Canadian families and generally considered well adjusted. They contrasted two groups: children who spent significant time in a deprived institutional rearing setting prior to adoption and others who were adopted within the first 6 months of life. Both groups exhibited higher-than-expected rates of insecurity, but this did not relate to length of institutionalization. However, length of institutionalization and insecure attachment to adoptive parents were associated with the number of parent-reported behavior problems. Not one adoptee was classified as avoidant; the authors suggest that avoidance would be a particularly maladaptive strategy for an adoptee, and that parents who are motivated to adopt would be unlikely to have parenting patterns related to avoidance (e.g., rejection) during the relationship formation stage.

In a second study of Romanian adoptees in Canada, Chisholm, Carter, Ames, and Morison (1995) used a short form of the Attachment Q-sort (Waters & Deane, 1985) to examine attachment security. This study contrasted three groups of preschool children: those in Romanian orphanages for at least the first 8 months of life, those adopted before 4 months of age, and a home-

reared Canadian sample. Adoptive parents of the later-adopted group reported significantly more behaviors indexing insecurity and more indiscriminate sociability than either of the other groups. Parent-rated security scores were unrelated to indiscriminate friendliness. This is of interest, given the conceptualization of indiscriminate socializing with adults as a sign of nonattachment (Lieberman & Pawl, 1988). A possible limitation of this report was the use of an unvalidated parent report short form as a measure of attachment. However, the findings of this investigation are consistent with those of Singer, Brodzinsky, Ramsay, Steer, and Waters (1985), who also found that infants adopted in the first few months of life had rates of security similar to those of children reared by biological parents.

More recent studies confirm the conclusion that seriously deficient caregiving is likely to lead to insecurity and disordered attachment behavior but that standard measures of attachment do not adequately characterize children with clinically significant attachment disorders. Following another cohort of young adoptees from Romania, O'Connor and colleagues (2003) found a disproportionate rate of insecurity in a separation–reunion protocol with caring adoptive parents at age 4. These children also displayed high rates of atypical attachment behavior, not described by standard attachment classification systems, and the usual forms of insecurity did not distinguish them. Some children with disinhibited/indiscriminate sociability were nonetheless classified as securely attached, indicating that they did have preferred attachment figures.

In an effort to examine the precursors of these relationships, Zeanah and colleagues (Smyke, Dumitrescu, & Zeanah, 2002; Zeanah et al., 2002) compared young children ages 11–70 months in standard Romanian orphanages with others in a unit designed to provide more consistent care from a smaller number of caregivers, and with a third, home-reared group. Relying on information gathered from interviews with caregivers, they found more indiscriminate behavior among the children in the standard orphanage group, followed by those in the special unit. Withdrawal was also observed, but a mixed pattern of inhibited and disinhibited behavior was most typical. Also of interest, only the children in institutional care exhibited *severe* aggression, although caregivers also reported that many of these children displayed no aggression at all. Home-reared children had a relatively high rate of "moderate" aggression, helping to explain why indiscriminate behavior was not statistically related to aggressive behavior.

Two recent studies applied these concepts and measures of attachment disorder to maltreated youngsters—the attachment-disordered population clinicians are most likely to encounter. Using the interview developed for their earlier investigations of Romanian orphans (Smyke et al., 2002; Zeanah et al., 2002), Zeanah and colleagues (2004) demonstrated that RAD could be reliably diagnosed, with a prevalence of 38–40% in a sample of 94 American toddlers in foster care. A significant number displayed both withdrawn and indiscriminate social behavior, and some children who otherwise met criteria for indiscriminate/disinhibited RAD nonetheless appeared to have a selective attachment to a caregiver, according to interviews with the clinicians who were treating them. (No direct observations of the children with their caregivers were conducted.) There was considerable concordance in diagnosis across siblings.

Boris and colleagues (2004) compared three groups of young children (ages 18–48 months): one with a history of maltreatment, a second from a homeless shelter, and the last from Head Start programs. Using Zeanah and Boris's (2000) alternative criteria, the researchers found maltreated children to be the most likely to qualify for a diagnosis of RAD. Children with an attachment disorder were also less likely to be concurrently classified as securely attached (to foster mothers, in the maltreated sample) via the Cassidy and Marvin (1992) system and had lower Q-sort security scores. However, the difference in disorganized attachment between children with and without attachment disorders was not significant.

Summary

Relatively few researchers have used standard laboratory assessments of attachment in studies of attachment disorders, but these measures appear to be of relatively limited value in diagnosis (Boris et al., 2004; Chisholm et al., 1995; Marcovitch et al., 1997). Although many children with attachment disorders may exhibit insecure attachment behaviors in such situations, others do not (O'Connor et al., 2003), and overall very few children with insecure attachments have an attachment disorder. The DSM and ICD diagnostic systems for attachment disorder also appear to be insufficient. However, many children who have experienced extremely deficient caregiving clearly do exhibit disordered behavior that relates to their caregiving

history. The alternative criteria proposed by Zeanah and Boris (2000) represent a major step forward in describing these children. However, they also require further investigation and validation; in some respects (e.g., the description of indiscriminately sociable children as necessarily lacking an attachment figure), they also appear inaccurate. Much more research is needed, particularly with respect to children in the child protective system, to clarify the forms that attachment disorders are likely to take and to inform the design of more effective interventions. Such investigations are also likely to contribute to a deeper understanding of basic processes critical to social and emotional development and to the etiology of various psychopathologies.

DEVELOPMENTAL PSYCHOPATHOLOGY AND A RESEARCH AGENDA: ASSESSING ATTACHMENT

Developmental psychopathology has provided a rich and more nuanced perspective within which to consider attachment processes and their associations with disorder. It informed the general tenets enumerated earlier, which allow a more sophisticated approach to attachment research and theory building. This perspective has suggested new approaches and raised new questions that promise to extend our understanding of attachment. As attachment researchers have begun to work in closer collaboration with researchers and theorists from different traditions (e.g., temperament, neuropsychology, and family processes), their work has been increasingly integrated into the larger framework of developmental psychopathology, and the role of attachment in psychopathology has become more clearly delineated.

The Measurement Roadblock

Attachment theory derives, in part, from a long tradition of utilizing clinical case studies as a means of developing hypotheses about pathways to disorder. One of its unique aspects is that it bridges basic theory and research in developmental, evolutionary, and cognitive psychology (Bowlby, 1969/1982, 1973, 1980). Unfortunately, in its transition from the child clinic to the normative study of childhood, attachment has often been so reified that research has been limited to a few validated paradigms in which aspects of attachment have been carefully assessed, but the larger picture has been insufficiently attended to. This was surely not the intention of Ainsworth or others (Ainsworth & Marvin, 1995), and it has led to limitations in the study of both normal and clinical populations and in the potential contribution of attachment theory to our understanding of psychopathology.

Since Ainsworth first developed the Strange Situation, measurement has been a central concern of attachment researchers. We have three suggestions that relate to this concern and illustrate the productive relationship between a developmental-psychopathology framework and attachment theory and research. First, the development of alternative measures of attachment processes may open new opportunities and permit new understandings of the role of attachment in the development of psychopathology. In developing such measures, it may be useful to focus on the processes that presumably form the links between early caregiving (e.g., sensitivity and responsivity) and later measures of attachment—that is, to extend the exciting progress that has been made in understanding what happens *while* the infant is developing a secure or insecure attachment relationship with a caregiver. As noted earlier, among the mechanisms that have been examined in this regard are emotion regulation and coping strategies, cognitive–affective schema (e.g., internal working models), and (perhaps underlying both of these) the development of brain structures and neurophysiological processes. Second, a return to the clinic might facilitate the development of useful measures; note, for example, the progress that has been made in describing disrupted attachment and attachment disorders. Finally, attention to the systems in which attachment relationships are embedded (e.g., the family) will ultimately be essential.

Alternative Measures

As detailed by others (Ainsworth, 1989; Cicchetti et al., 1995; Crowell, Fraley, & Shaver, Chapter 26, this volume; Greenberg, Cicchetti, & Cummings, 1990; Main & Cassidy, 1988; Solomon & George, Chapter 18, this volume), dramatic advances have been made in the measurement of attachment in early childhood, later adolescence, and adulthood. The use of separation–reunion situations as well as Q-sort assessments with preschool children has led to significant findings, and the AAI (George, Kaplan, & Main, 1984, 1985, 1996) in late adolescence and adulthood has quickly been appropriated by clinical researchers and is providing important information regarding the contribution

of representations of close relationships to adult psychopathology (see Dozier et al., Chapter 30, this volume).

Considerably less progress has been made in the development of measures for school-age children. Three types of measures have been developed. The first are behavioral measures of reunion behavior (Main & Cassidy, 1985, 1988). To date, however, they have not been utilized after age 7 (Easterbrooks et al., 1993). The second type are representational measures of attachment, which have primarily been used with 3- to 6-year-olds (Bretherton, Ridgeway, & Cassidy, 1990; Cassidy, 1988; Main et al., 1985; Oppenheim, Nir, Warren, & Emde, 1995; Oppenheim & Waters, 1995; Slough & Greenberg, 1990). Some studies have shown these to be concurrently related to measures of reunion behavior in community samples (Cassidy, 1988; Shouldice & Stevenson-Hinde, 1992; Slough & Greenberg, 1997). Representational measures have rarely been applied to the study of children with disorders. However, in a preschool sample, we (Greenberg, DeKlyen, Speltz, & Endriga, 1997) found that attachment narratives underestimated insecurity (as assessed in a separation–reunion paradigm) in a clinic-referred group and somewhat overestimated insecurity in a normal comparison group.

For children above age 6, various self-report measures have been utilized, but without other validated measures of attachment to relate them to, their validity is uncertain (Cook, Greenberg, & Kusche, 1995; Kerns et al., 1996; Lynch & Cicchetti, 1991). A number of difficulties impede the development of assessment tools for this age range. The first is the assumption that observational paradigms will not reveal individual differences in this period of life. Observational measures may ultimately prove useful in middle childhood, but they will require fine-grained analyses and age-appropriate stressors. Second, at this age children may be less able or willing to reveal their representations of relationships in an interview format. Although measures that are sensitive in normative school-age populations are sorely needed, they may be particularly valuable in the investigation of children with disorders in which attachment is believed to play a role. Furthermore, measures of attachment that can provide assessment benchmarks in the many clinical situations involving decisions regarding removal of children from their homes, the effects of foster care, and adaptation to late adoption are essential (Pilowsky & Kates, 1995).

Reliability and validity are major concerns to be addressed regarding all of these measures. There is minimal evidence that measures at different ages are in fact assessing the same construct (e.g., infancy to preschool), and that which exists derives from relatively stable, low-risk populations. The field would benefit greatly from measurement development and validation. This should focus on elucidating the relationships between measures at different ages, using a variety of methodologies (e.g., behavioral observations and interviews), and using multiple measures concurrently, to assure more reliable assessment of the attachment construct.

Careful attention to how caregiver–child interactions and biological processes at each stage of life relate to established measures of attachment and to the development of psychopathology may help to advance research and theory to the next level. In the 1980s, the move to the level of representation (Bretherton, 1985) invigorated the field and permitted tremendous progress in revealing how attachment might relate to psychopathology. Similarly, the examination of physiological correlates of attachment-related measures may suggest new avenues of research and fresh insights into how early caregiving experiences affect functioning.

Evolving Standardized Measurement Models from the Clinical Setting

Studying clinical samples in which insecure attachment is more common and patterns of insecurity are especially marked may be a useful strategy for identifying such patterns in middle childhood. Such a strategy would also deal with a further concern: Because both child and adult measures of attachment have been developed with normative samples, they may not capture important aspects of attachment relationships in clinical populations (Adam et al., 1995; Crittenden, 1995; Goldberg, 1997; Levine & Tuber, 1993). Given these potential benefits, it is remarkable that there has been so little study in middle childhood of disorders that are believed to relate to attachment.

Family Systems, Attachment, and Psychopathology

As the study of attachment in childhood has evolved, interest has increased in studying systems larger than the dyad. This is especially important in clinical settings, given the central role of family systems in the treatment of childhood disorders. There have been several illuminating formulations of the relation between attachment theory and family systems theory (Byng-Hall, 1995, 1999; Byng-Hall & Stevenson-Hinde, 1991; Jacobvitz, Morgan, Kretchmar, & Morgan, 1991; Marvin & Stewart, 1990; Johnson, Chapter 34, this volume). Empirical research has demonstrated that a father's behavior affects infant–mother attachment (perhaps indirectly; Das Eiden & Leonard, 1996) and that father–child attachment influences child adjustment (Cowan, Cohn, Cowan, & Pearson, 1996; DeKlyen et al., 1998). Grandparents also help to shape their grandchildren's attachment styles (Benoit & Parker, 1994; Spieker & Bensley, 1994). The role of attachment processes in psychopathology is complicated, and family system considerations will be essential to elucidating these processes (Radke-Yarrow, Cummings, Kuczynski, & Chapman, 1995). The development of diagnostic models of attachment at the level of the family system, and of measures with which to assess the impact of these processes, is a considerable challenge. However, the role of emergent properties at this level of analysis may be crucial in explaining how unexpected patterns of attachment between children and their individual parents are linked to the development of psychopathology.

CONCLUSIONS

Attachment insecurity appears to be an important but nonspecific factor that increases risk for several forms of childhood psychopathology. There are insufficient longitudinal data from infancy to establish with certainty that specific pathways exist between early attachment types and differing forms of psychopathology. The research examining specific linkages between avoidant attachment and later externalizing problems and between ambivalent attachment and internalizing disorders is suggestive but inconclusive. The strongest links are found in the Minnesota Parent–Child Project, in which infant avoidance predicted teacher-rated aggressiveness in middle childhood and ambivalence predicted passive withdrawal; however, these associations were significant only for boys (Renken et al., 1989). Ambivalent attachment in infancy was also modestly linked to anxiety disorders at age 17 (Warren et al., 1997). At other ages (later preschool years and early adolescence), clear differentiation was not detected. Findings by other researchers (e.g., Goldberg, 1997; Moss et al.,

1996) do not consistently support these differential pathways. Similarly, disorganized attachment appears to be a potent risk factor for disorder, but its specific association with, for example, externalizing problems has also not been uniformly found. This is an area that requires further research.

It is clear that insecure attachment is not itself a form of psychopathology but may set a trajectory that, along with other risk factors, can increase the risk for either externalizing or internalizing psychopathology (Rutter, 1985). Further study of the role of attachment as both a mediator and moderator in developmental psychopathology is warranted.

Attachment theory has been mistakenly understood by some to indicate that early attachment relations are necessarily stable and inexorably lead to either healthy or pathological outcomes. As our review indicates, attachment processes have shown both predictive and concurrent associations with maladaptation in childhood and early adolescence. With few exceptions, however, insecure attachment is unlikely to be either a necessary or a sufficient cause of later disorder, and in some cases it may be an effect of the disorder itself (Cicchetti et al., 1995). It appears evident that with the intersection of two, three, or four risk factors in a child's ecology, there is an increasing probability of later problems. Numerous studies reviewed above have demonstrated this empirically. Although epidemiological samples are critical to further illuminating how multiple risks interact with each other and contribute to psychopathology, longitudinal case studies and studies of samples selected with strong theoretical rationales can make important contributions as well.

The role that child gender plays in potentiating risk is as yet unclear. Current findings indicate that the effect of attachment is often moderated by gender: Insecure attachment is more often linked to the development of identifiable (usually externalizing) problems in early and middle childhood in boys. These findings fit well with the generally greater vulnerability of boys to high-risk environments (Duncan, Brooks-Gunn, & Klebanov, 1994; Zaslow & Hayes, 1986). It is not clear whether this greater vulnerability is due to the higher base rate of such problems in boys in middle childhood or to some particular interactional mechanism, and further research with both boys and girls and in the adolescent period will be necessary to clarify this issue.

The study of attachment and its relation to developmental pathways of normality and psychopathology has made significant advances in the past decade. Research with both normal and clinical populations has improved our knowledge base. Advances have been made in attachment theory regarding processes of transmission and in developmental psychopathology regarding risk models; both offer the prospect of a better understanding of how attachment might affect divergent pathways for different forms of maladaptation. Greater attention to the development and validation of attachment indices in early and middle childhood is necessary to fully investigate the transactional relations linking attachment, risk, and psychopathology. A renewed emphasis on attachment-informed studies of children who have experienced extremes of caregiving is also critical in order to address urgent clinical and public health demands; it also promises to enrich our understanding of attachment processes. Longitudinal studies of representative normative populations, high-risk populations, and samples in which there are specific forms of maladaptation are needed to provide a fuller picture of the role of attachment in risk for psychopathology in childhood.

REFERENCES

Abela, J. R. Z., Hankin, B. L., Haigh, E. A. P., Adams, P., Vinokuroff, T., & Treyhern, L. (2005). Interpersonal vulnerability to depression in high-risk children: The role of insecure attachment and reassurance seeking. *Journal of Clinical Child and Adolescent Psychology, 34,* 182–192.

Adam, K. S., Sheldon-Keller, A. E., & West, M. (1995). Attachment organization and vulnerability to loss, separation, and abuse in disturbed adolescents. In S. Goldberg, R. Muir, & J. Kerr (Eds.), *Attachment theory: Social, developmental, and clinical perspectives* (pp. 309–341). Hillsdale, NJ: Analytic Press.

Aguilar, B., Sroufe, L. A., Egeland, B., & Carlson, E. (2000). Distinguishing the early-onset/persistent and adolescence-onset antisocial behavior types: From birth to 16 years. *Development and Psychopathology, 12,* 109–132.

Ainsworth, M. D. S. (1989). Attachments beyond infancy. *American Psychologist, 44,* 709–716.

Ainsworth, M. D. S., Blehar, M. C., Waters, E., & Wall, S. (1978). *Patterns of attachment: A psychological study of the Strange Situation.* Hillsdale, NJ: Erlbaum.

Ainsworth, M. D. S., & Marvin, R. S. (1995). On the shaping of attachment theory and research: An interview with Mary D. S. Ainsworth (Fall 1994). In E. Waters, B. E. Vaughn, G. Posada, & K. Kondo-Ikemura (Eds.), Caregiving, cultural, and cognitive perspectives on secure-base behavior and working models: New growing points of attachment theory and research. *Monographs of the Society for Research in Child Development, 60*(2–3, Serial No. 244), 3–21.

Allen, J. P., Hauser, S. T., & Borman-Spurrell, E. (1996). Attachment theory as a framework for understanding sequelae of severe adolescent psychopathology: An 11-year follow-up study. *Journal of Consulting and Clinical Psychology, 64,* 254–263.

American Psychiatric Association. (1980). *Diagnostic and statistical manual of mental disorders* (3rd ed.). Washington, DC: Author.

American Psychiatric Association. (1994). *Diagnostic and statistical manual of mental disorders* (4th ed.). Washington, DC: Author.

Bates, J. E., Bayles, K., Bennett, D. S., Ridge, B., & Brown, M. M. (1991). Origins of externalizing behavior problems at eight years of age. In D. J. Pepler & K. H. Rubin (Eds.), *The development and treatment of childhood aggression* (pp. 93–120). Hillsdale, NJ: Erlbaum.

Bates, J. E., Maslin, C. A., & Frankel, K. A. (1985). Attachment security, mother–child interaction, and temperament as predictors of behavior problem ratings at age three years. In I. Bretherton & E. Waters (Eds.), Growing points of attachment theory and research. *Monographs of the Society for Research in Child Development, 50*(1–2, Serial No. 209), 167–193.

Belsky, J., & Fearon, R. M. P. (2002). Infant–mother attachment security, contextual risk, and early development: A moderational analysis. *Development and Psychopathology, 14,* 293–310.

Belsky, J., & Nezworski, T. (Eds.). (1988). *Clinical implications of attachment.* Hillsdale, NJ: Erlbaum.

Benoit, D., & Parker, K. C. H. (1994). Stability and transmission of attachment across three generations. *Child Development, 65,* 1444–1456.

Booth-LaForce, C., Oh, W., Kim, A. H., Rubin, K. H., Rose-Krasnor, L., & Burgess, K. (2006). Attachment, self-worth, and peer-group functioning in middle childhood. *Attachment and Human Development, 8,* 309–325.

Boris, N. W., Fueyo, M., & Zeanah, C. H. (1997). The clinical assessment of attachment in children less than five. *Journal of the American Academy of Child and Adolescent Psychiatry, 36,* 291–293.

Boris, N. W., Hinshaw-Fuselier, M. S. W., Smyke, A. T., Scheeringa, M. S., Heller, S. S., & Zeanah, C. H. (2004). Comparing criteria for attachment disorders: Establishing reliability and validity in high-risk samples. *Journal of the American Academy of Child and Adolescent Psychiatry, 43,* 568–577.

Bosquet, M., & Egeland, B. (2006). The development and maintenance of anxiety symptoms from infancy through adolescence in a longitudinal sample. *Development and Psychopathology, 18,* 517–550.

Bowlby, J. (1953). *Child care and the growth of love.* Harmondsworth, UK: Penguin.

Bowlby, J. (1969/1982). *Attachment and loss: Vol. 1. Attachment.* New York: Basic Books.

Bowlby, J. (1973). *Attachment and loss: Vol. 2. Separation: Anxiety and anger.* New York: Basic Books.

Bowlby, J. (1980). *Attachment and loss: Vol. 3. Loss: Sadness and depression.* New York: Basic Books.

Bretherton, I. (1985). Attachment theory: Retrospect and prospect. In I. Bretherton & E. Waters (Eds.), Growing points of attachment theory and research. *Monographs of the Society for Research in Child Development, 50*(1–2, Serial No. 209), 3–35.

Bretherton, I. (1992). The origins of attachment theory: John Bowlby and Mary Ainsworth. *Developmental Psychology, 28,* 759–775.

Bretherton, I. (1995). Attachment theory and developmental psychopathology. In D. Cicchetti & S. Toth (Eds.), *Rochester Symposium on Developmental Psychopathology: Vol. 6. Emotion, cognition, and representation* (pp. 231–260). Rochester, NY: University of Rochester Press.

Bretherton, I., Ridgeway, D., & Cassidy, J. (1990). Assessing internal working models of the attachment relationship. In M. T. Greenberg, D. Cicchetti, & M. Cummings (Eds.), *Attachment in the preschool years: Theory, research, and intervention* (pp. 273–308). Chicago: University of Chicago Press.

Bronfenbrenner, U. (1979). *The ecology of human development.* Cambridge, MA: Harvard University Press.

Brook, J. S., Whiteman, M., & Finch, S. (1993). Role of mutual attachment in drug use: A longitudinal study. *Journal of the American Academy of Child and Adolescent Psychiatry, 32,* 982–989.

Burgess, K. B., Marshall, P. J., Rubin, K. H., & Fox, N. A. (2003). Infant attachment and temperament as predictors of subsequent externalizing problems and cardiac physiology. *Journal of Child Psychology and Psychiatry, 44,* 819–831.

Byng-Hall, J. (1995). *Rewriting family scripts.* New York: Guilford Press.

Byng-Hall, J. (1999). Family and couple therapy: Toward greater security. In J. Cassidy & P. R. Shaver (Eds.), *Handbook of attachment: Theory, research, and clinical applications* (pp. 625–645). New York: Guilford Press.

Byng-Hall, J., & Stevenson-Hinde, J. (1991). Attachment relationships within a family system. *Infant Mental Health Journal, 12,* 187–200.

Campbell, S. B. (1990). *Behavior problems in preschool children: Clinical and developmental issues.* New York: Guilford Press.

Campbell, S. B. (1991). Longitudinal studies of active and aggressive preschoolers: Individual differences in early behavior and outcome. In D. Cicchetti & S. L. Toth (Eds.), *Rochester Symposium on Developmental Psychopathology: Vol. 2. Internalizing and externalizing expressions of dysfunction* (pp. 57–90). Hillsdale, NJ: Erlbaum.

Capps, L., Sigman, M., & Mundy, P. (1994). Attachment security in children with autism. *Development and Psychopathology, 6,* 249–261.

Carlson, E. A. (1998). A prospective longitudinal study of attachment disorganization/disorientation. *Child Development, 59,* 121–134.

Carlson, E. A., & Sroufe, L. A. (1995). Contributions of attachment theory to developmental psychopathology. In D. Cicchetti & D. J. Cohen (Eds.), *Developmental psychology* (Vol. 1, pp. 581–617). New York: Wiley.

Carlson, V., Cicchetti, D., Barnett, D., & Braunwald, K. (1989). Disorganized/disoriented attachment relationships in maltreated infants. *Developmental Psychology, 25*, 525–531.

Cassidy, J. (1988). Child–mother attachment and the self in six-year-olds. *Child Development, 59*, 121–134.

Cassidy, J. (1995). Attachment and generalized anxiety disorder. In D. Cicchetti & S. Toth (Eds.), *Rochester Symposium on Developmental Psychopathology: Vol. 6. Emotion, cognition, and representation* (pp. 343–370). Rochester, NY: University of Rochester Press.

Cassidy, J., & Berlin, L. J. (1994). The insecure/ambivalent pattern of attachment: Theory and research. *Child Development, 65*, 971–981.

Cassidy, J., Kirsh, S. J., Scolton, K., & Parke, R. D. (1996). Attachment and representation of peer relationships. *Developmental Psychology, 32*, 892–904.

Cassidy, J., & Marvin, R. S., with the MacArthur Working Group. (1992). *Attachment organization in preschool children: Coding guidelines* (4th ed.). Unpublished manuscript, University of Virginia.

Chaplin, T. M., & Cole, P. M. (2005). The role of emotion regulation in the development of psychopathology. In B. L. Hankin & J. R. Z. Abela (Eds.), *Development of psychopathology: A vulnerability–stress perspective* (pp. 49–74). Thousand Oaks, CA: Sage.

Chisholm, K. M., Carter, M. C., Ames, E. W., & Morison, S. J. (1995). Attachment security and indiscriminately friendly behavior in children adopted from Romanian orphanages. *Development and Psychopathology, 7*, 283–294.

Cicchetti, D., & Cummings, E. M. (1990). Towards a transactional model of relations between attachment and depression. In M. T. Greenberg, D. Cicchetti, & M. Cummings (Eds.), *Attachment in the preschool years: Theory, research, and intervention* (pp. 339–374). Chicago: University of Chicago Press.

Cicchetti, D., & Rogosch, F. A. (1997). Equifinality and multifinality in developmental psychopathology. *Development and Psychopathology, 8*, 597–600.

Cicchetti, D., Toth, S. L., & Lynch, M. (1995). Bowlby's dream comes full circle: The application of attachment theory to risk and psychopathology. In T. H. Ollendick & R. J. Prinz (Eds.), *Advances in clinical child psychology* (Vol. 17, pp. 1–75). New York: Plenum Press.

Cohn, D. A. (1990). Child–mother attachment of six-year-olds and social competence at school. *Child Development, 61*, 152–162.

Coie, J. D., Watt, N. F., West, S. G., Hawkins, J. D., Asarnow, J. R., Markman, H. J., et al. (1993). The science of prevention: A conceptual framework and some directions for a national research program. *American Psychologist, 48*, 1013–1022.

Cook, E. T., Greenberg, M. T., & Kusche, C. A. (1995, March). *People in my life: Attachment relationships in middle childhood.* Paper presented at the biennial meeting of the Society for Research in Child Development, Indianapolis, IN.

Cowan, P. A., Cohn, D. A., Cowan, C. P., & Pearson, J. L. (1996). Parents' attachment histories and children's externalizing and internalizing behaviors: Exploring family systems models of linkages. *Journal of Consulting and Clinical Psychology, 64*, 53–63.

Crittenden, P. M. (1988). Relationships at risk. In J. Belsky & T. Nezworski (Eds.), *Clinical implications of attachment* (pp. 136–176). Hillsdale, NJ: Erlbaum.

Crittenden, P. M. (1992). Quality of attachment in the preschool years. *Development and Psychopathology, 4*, 209–241.

Crittenden, P. M. (1995). Attachment and psychopathology. In S. Goldberg, R. Muir, & J. Kerr (Eds.), *Attachment theory: Social, developmental, and clinical perspectives* (pp. 367–406). Hillsdale, NJ: Analytic Press.

Crowell, J. A., & Feldman, S. S. (1988). Mothers' internal models of relationships and children's behavioral and developmental status: A study of mother–child interaction. *Child Development, 59*, 1273–1285.

Das Eiden, R., & Leonard, K. E. (1996). Paternal alcohol use and the mother–infant relationship. *Development and Psychopathology, 8*, 307–324.

Dawson, G., Hessl, D., & Frey, K. (1994). Social influences of early developing biological and behavioral systems related to risk for affective disorder. *Development and Psychopathology, 6*, 759–779.

DeKlyen, M. (1996). Disruptive behavior disorders and intergenerational attachment patterns: A comparison of normal and clinic-referred preschoolers and their mothers. *Journal of Consulting and Clinical Psychology, 64*, 357–365.

DeKlyen, M., Speltz, M. L., & Greenberg, M. T. (1998). Fathers and early starting conduct problems: Positive and negative parenting, father–son attachment, and the marital context. *Clinical Child and Family Psychology Review, 1*, 3–21.

Dissanayake, C., & Crossley, S. A. (1996). Proximity and sociable behaviours in autism: Evidence for attachment. *Journal of Child Psychology and Psychiatry, 37*, 149–156.

Dodge, K. A. (1991). The structure and function of reactive and proactive aggression. In D. J. Pepler & K. H. Rubin (Eds.), *The development and treatment of childhood aggression* (pp. 201–218). Hillsdale, NJ: Erlbaum.

Dozier, M., Albus, K. E., Stovall, K. C., & Bates, B. (2000). Attachment for infants in foster care: The role of caregiver state of mind. *Child Development, 72*, 1467–1477.

Duggal, S., Carlson, E. A., Sroufe, L. A., & Egeland, B. (2001). Depressive symptomatology in childhood and adolescence. *Development and Psychopathology, 13*, 143–164.

Duncan, G. J., Brooks-Gunn, J., & Klebanov, P. K. (1994). Economic deprivation and early childhood development. *Child Development, 65*, 296–318.

Easterbrooks, M. A., Davidson, C. E., & Chazan, R. (1993). Psychosocial risk, attachment, and behavior problems among school-aged children. *Development and Psychopathology, 5,* 389–402.

Egeland, B., & Carlson, B. (2004). Attachment and psychopathology. In L. Atkinson & S. Goldberg (Eds.), *Attachment issues in psychopathology and intervention* (pp. 27–48). Mahwah, NJ: Erlbaum.

El-Sheikh, M., & Elmore-Staton, L. (2004). The link between marital conflict and child adjustment: Parent–child conflict and perceived attachments as mediators, potentiators, and mitigators of risk. *Development and Psychopathology, 16,* 631–648.

Erickson, M. F., Sroufe, L. A., & Egeland, B. (1985). The relationship between quality of attachment and behavior problems in preschool in a high-risk sample. In I. Bretherton & E. Waters (Eds.), Growing points of attachment theory and research. *Monographs of the Society for Research in Child Development, 50*(1–2, Serial No. 209), 147–156.

Erikson, E. H. (1963). *Childhood and society* (2nd ed.). New York: Norton.

Essau, C. A. (2004). The association between family factors and depressive disorders in adolescents. *Journal of Youth and Adolescence, 33,* 365–372.

Fagot, B. I., & Kavanaugh, K. (1990). The prediction of antisocial behavior from avoidant attachment classifications. *Child Development, 61,* 864–873.

Fagot, B. I., & Pears, K. C. (1996). Changes in attachment during the third year: Consequences and predictions. *Development and Psychopathology, 8,* 325–344.

Feiring, C., & Lewis, M. (1997). Finality in the eye of the beholder: Multiple sources, time points, multiple paths. *Development and Psychopathology, 8,* 721–733.

Fonagy, P., Steele, M., Steele, H., Leigh, T., Kennedy, R., Mattoon, G., et al. (1995). Attachment, the reflective self, and borderline states. In S. Goldberg, R. Muir, & J. Kerr (Eds.), *Attachment theory: Social, developmental, and clinical perspectives* (pp. 233–278). Hillsdale, NJ: Analytic Press.

Fonagy, P., Target, M., Steele, M., Steele, H., Leigh, T., Levinson, A., et al. (1997). Crime and attachment: Morality, disruptive behavior, borderline personality, crime, and their relationships to security of attachment. In L. Atkinson & K. Zucker (Eds.), *Attachment and psychopathology* (pp. 223–274). New York: Guilford Press.

Fraley, R. C. (2002). Attachment stability from infancy to adulthood: Meta-analysis and dynamic modeling of developmental mechanisms. *Personality and Social Psychology Review, 6,* 123–151.

Freud, A. (1965). *The writings of Anna Freud: Vol. 6. Normality and pathology in childhood: Assessments of development.* New York: International Universities Press.

George, C., Kaplan, N., & Main, M. (1984). *Adult Attachment Interview protocol.* Unpublished manuscript, University of California at Berkeley.

George, C., Kaplan, N., & Main, M. (1985). *Adult Attachment Interview protocol* (2nd ed.). Unpublished manuscript, University of California at Berkeley.

George, C., Kaplan, N., & Main, M. (1996). *Adult Attachment Interview protocol* (3rd ed.). Unpublished manuscript, University of California at Berkeley.

Goldberg, S. (1997). Attachment and childhood behavior problems in normal, at-risk, and clinical samples. In L. Atkinson & K. Zucker (Eds.), *Attachment and psychopathology* (pp. 171–195). New York: Guilford Press.

Goldberg, S., Gotowiec, A., & Simmons, R. J. (1995). Infant–mother attachment and behavior problems in healthy and chronically ill preschoolers. *Development and Psychopathology, 7,* 267–282.

Goldberg, S., Lojkasek, M., Minde, K., & Corter, C. (1990). Predictions of behavior problems in children born prematurely. *Development and Psychopathology, 1,* 15–30.

Goldfarb, W. (1955). Emotional and intellectual consequences of psychological deprivation in infancy: A reevaluation. In P. Hoch & D. Zubin (Eds.), *Psychopathology in childhood* (pp. 105–119). New York: Grune & Stratton.

Goleman, D. (1995). *Emotional intelligence.* New York: Bantam.

Graham, C. A., & Easterbrooks, M. A. (2000). School-aged children's vulnerability to depressive symptomatology: The role of attachment security, maternal depressive symptomatology, and economic risk. *Development and Psychopathology, 12,* 201–213.

Greenberg, M. T. (1999). Attachment and psychopathology in childhood. In J. Cassidy & P. R. Shaver (Eds.), *Handbook of attachment: Theory, research, and clinical applications* (pp. 469–497). New York: Guilford Press.

Greenberg, M. T., Cicchetti, D., & Cummings, E. M. (Eds.). (1990). *Attachment in the preschool years: Theory, research, and intervention.* Chicago: University of Chicago Press.

Greenberg, M. T., DeKlyen, M., Speltz, M. L., & Endriga, M. C. (1997). The role of attachment processes in externalizing psychopathology in young children. In L. R. Atkinson & K. J. Zucker (Eds.), *Attachment and psychopathology* (pp. 196–222). New York: Guilford Press.

Greenberg, M. T., & Snell, J. (1997). The neurological basis of emotional development. In P. Salovey (Ed.), *Emotional development and emotional literacy* (pp. 93–119). New York: Basic Books.

Greenberg, M. T., Speltz, M. L., & DeKlyen, M. (1993). The role of attachment in the early development of disruptive behavior problems. *Development and Psychopathology, 5,* 191–213.

Greenberg, M. T., Speltz, M. L., DeKlyen, M., & Endriga, M. C. (1991). Attachment security in preschoolers with and without externalizing problems: A replication. *Developmental and Psychopathology, 3,* 413–430.

Greenberg, M. T., Speltz, M. L., DeKlyen, M., & Jones, K. (2001). Correlates of clinic referral for early conduct problems: Variable- and person-oriented approaches. *Development and Psychopathology, 13,* 255–276.

Greenspan, S. I. (1981). *Psychopathology and adaptation in infancy and early childhood: Principles of clinical diagnosis and preventive intervention.* New York: International Universities Press.

Grossmann, K. E. (1995). The evolution and history of attachment research and theory. In S. Goldberg, R. Muir, & J. Kerr (Eds.), *Attachment theory: Social, developmental, and clinical perspectives* (pp. 85–121). Hillsdale, NJ: Analytic Press.

Gunnar, M. R. (2000). Early adversity and the development of stress reactivity and regulation. In C. A. Nelson (Ed.), *Minnesota Symposium on Child Psychology: Vol. 31. The effects of early adversity on neurobehavioral development* (pp. 163–200). Mahwah, NJ: Erlbaum.

Guttmann-Steinmetz, S., & Crowell, J. A. (2006). Attachment and externalizing disorders: A developmental psychopathology perspective. *Journal of the American Academy of Child and Adolescent Psychiatry, 45,* 440–450.

Hawkins, J. D., Arthur, M. W., & Catalano, R. F. (1995). Preventing substance abuse. In M. Tonry & D. Farrington (Eds.), *Crime and justice: A review of research. Vol. 19. Building a safer society: Strategic approaches to crime prevention* (pp. 343–427). Chicago: University of Chicago Press.

Hertsgaard, L., Gunnar, M., Erickson, M. F., & Nachmias, M. (1995). Adrenocortical responses to the Strange Situation in infants with disorganized/disoriented attachment relationships. *Child Development, 66,* 1100–1106.

Hirschi, T. (1969). *Causes of delinquency.* Berkeley: University of California Press.

Izard, C. E., Youngstrom, E. A., Fine, S. E., Mostow, A. J., & Trentacosta, C. J. (2006). Emotions and developmental psychopathology. In D. Cicchetti & D. J. Cohen (Eds.), *Developmental psychopathology: Vol. 1. Theory and method* (2nd ed., pp. 244–292). Hoboken, NJ: Wiley.

Jacobvitz, D. B., Morgan, E., Kretchmar, M. D., & Morgan, Y. (1991). The transmission of mother–child boundary disturbances across three generations. *Development and Psychopathology, 3,* 513–527.

Kellam, S. G. (1990). Developmental epidemiological framework for family research on depression and aggression. In G. R. Patterson (Ed.), *Depression and aggression in family interaction* (pp. 11–48). Hillsdale, NJ: Erlbaum.

Keller, T. E., Spieker, S. J., & Gilchrist, L. (2005). Patterns of risk and trajectories of preschool problem behaviors: A person-oriented analysis of attachment in context. *Development and Psychopathology, 17,* 349–384.

Kerns, K. A., Klepac, L., & Cole, A. K. (1996). Peer relationships and preadolescents' perceptions of security in the child–mother relationship. *Developmental Psychology, 32,* 457–466.

Klein, R. G. (1994). Anxiety disorders. In M. Rutter, E. Taylor, & L. Hersov (Eds.), *Child and adolescent psychiatry* (pp. 351–374). London: Blackwell.

Kobak, R., Cassidy, J., Lyons-Ruth, K., & Ziv, Y. (2006). Attachment, stress, and psychopathology: A developmental pathways model. In D. Cicchetti & D. J. Cohen (Eds.), *Developmental psychopathology: Vol. 1. Theory and method* (2nd ed., pp. 333–369). Hoboken, NJ: Wiley.

Kobak, R. R., Sudler, N., & Gamble, W. (1991). Attachment and depressive symptoms during adolescence: A developmental pathways analysis. *Development and Psychopathology, 3,* 461–474.

Le Blanc, M. (1994). Family, school, delinquency and criminality: The predictive power of an elaborated social control theory for males. *Criminal Behavior and Mental Health, 4,* 101–117.

LeDoux, J. E. (1995). Emotion: Clues from the brain. *Annual Review of Psychology, 46,* 209–235.

Levine, L. V., & Tuber, S. B. (1993). Measures of mental representation: Clinical and theoretical considerations. *Bulletin of the Menninger Clinic, 57,* 69–87.

Lewis, M., Feiring, C., McGuffog, C., & Jaskir, J. (1984). Predicting psychopathology in six-year-olds from early social relations. *Child Development, 55,* 123–136.

Lieberman, A. F., & Pawl, J. H. (1988). Clinical applications of attachment theory. In J. Belsky & T. Nezworski (Eds.), *Clinical implications of attachment* (pp. 327–347). Hillsdale, NJ: Erlbaum.

Lieberman, A. F., & Pawl, J. H. (1990). Disorders of attachment and secure base behavior in the second year of life: Conceptual issues and clinical intervention. In M. T. Greenberg, D. Cicchetti, & M. Cummings (Eds.), *Attachment in the preschool years: Theory, research, and intervention* (pp. 375–398). Chicago: University of Chicago Press.

Lieberman, A. F., & Zeanah, C. H. (1995). Disorders of attachment in infancy. *Child and Adolescent Psychiatric Clinics of North America, 4,* 571–687.

Liotti, G. (1995). Disorganized/disoriented attachment in the psychotherapy of dissociative disorders. In S. Goldberg, R. Muir, & J. Kerr (Eds.), *Attachment theory: Social, developmental, and clinical perspectives* (pp. 343–366). Hillsdale, NJ: Analytic Press.

Luthar, S. S. (1993). Annotation: Methodological and conceptual issues in research on childhood resilience. *Journal of Child Psychology and Psychiatry, 34,* 441–453.

Luthar, S. S., & Zigler, E. (1992). Intelligence and social competence among high-risk adolescents. *Development and Psychopathology, 4,* 287–299.

Lynch, M., & Cicchetti, D. (1991). Patterns of relatedness in maltreated and nonmaltreated children: Connections among multiple representational models. *Development and Psychopathology, 3,* 207–226.

Lyons-Ruth, K. (1996). Attachment relationships among children with aggressive behavior problems: The role of disorganized early attachment patterns. *Journal of Consulting and Clinical Psychology, 64,* 64–73.

Lyons-Ruth, K., Alpern, L., & Repacholi, B. (1993). Disorganized infant attachment classification and maternal psychological problems as predictors of hostile-aggressive behavior in the preschool classroom. *Child Development, 64*, 572–585.

Lyons-Ruth, K., Connell, D., Zoll, D., & Stahl, J. (1987). Infants at social risk: Relationships among infant maltreatment, maternal behavior, and infant attachment behavior. *Developmental Psychology, 23*, 223–232.

Lyons-Ruth, K., Dutra, L., Schuder, M. R., & Bianchi, I. (2006). From infant attachment disorganization to adult dissociation: Relational adaptations or traumatic experiences? *Psychiatric Clinics of North America, 29*, 63–86.

Lyons-Ruth, K., Easterbrooks, M. A., & Cibelli, C. D. (1997). Infant attachment strategies, infant mental lag, and maternal depressive symptoms: Predictors of internalizing and externalizing problems at age 7. *Developmental Psychology, 33*, 681–692.

Lyons-Ruth, K., Easterbrooks, M. A., Davidson Cibelli, C. E., & Bronfman, E. (1995, April). *Predicting school-age externalizing symptoms from infancy: Contributions of disorganized attachment strategies and mild mental lag.* Paper presented at the biennial meeting of the Society for Research in Child Development, Indianapolis, IN.

Lyons-Ruth, K., Zoll, D., Connell, D., & Grunebaum, H. U. (1989). Family deviance and family disruption in childhood: Associations with maternal behavior and infant maltreatment during the first years of life. *Development and Psychopathology, 1*, 219–236.

Maccoby, E. E., & Martin, J. A. (1983). Socialization in the context of the family: Parent–child interaction. In P. H. Mussen (Series Ed.) & E. M. Hetherington (Vol. Ed.), *Handbook of child psychology: Vol. 4. Socialization, personality, and social development* (4th ed., pp. 469–546). New York: Wiley.

Mahler, M. S., Pine, F., & Bergman, A. (1975). *The psychological birth of the human infant.* New York: Basic Books.

Main, M. (1996). Introduction to the special section on attachment and psychopathology: 2. Overview of the field of attachment. *Journal of Consulting and Clinical Psychology, 64*, 237–243.

Main, M., & Cassidy, J. (1985). *Assessments of child–parent attachment at six years of age.* Unpublished manuscript, University of California at Berkeley.

Main, M., & Cassidy, J. (1988). Categories of response to reunion with the parent at age six: Predictable from infant attachment classifications and stable over a one-month period. *Developmental Psychology, 24*, 415–426.

Main, M., Cassidy, J., & Kaplan, N. (1985). Security in infancy, childhood and adulthood: A move to the level of representation. In I. Bretherton & E. Waters (Eds.), Growing points of attachment theory and research. *Monographs of the Society for Research in Child Development, 50*(1–2, Serial No. 209), 66–104.

Main, M., & Hesse, E. (1990). Parents' unresolved traumatic experiences are related to infant disorganized attachment status: Is frightened and/or frightening parental behavior the linking mechanism? In M. T. Greenberg, D. Cicchetti, & M. Cummings (Eds.), *At-*

tachment in the preschool years: Theory, research, and intervention (pp. 161–184). Chicago: University of Chicago Press.

Main, M., & Solomon, J. (1990). Procedures for identifying infants as disorganized/disoriented during the Ainsworth Strange Situation. In M. T. Greenberg, D. Cicchetti, & M. Cummings (Eds.), *Attachment in the preschool years: Theory, research, and intervention* (pp. 121–160). Chicago: University of Chicago Press.

Manassis, K., & Bradley, S. (1994). The development of childhood anxiety disorders: toward an integrated model. *Journal of Applied Developmental Psychology, 15*, 345–366.

Manassis, K., Bradley, S., Goldberg, S., Hood, J., & Swinson, R. P. (1994). Attachment in mothers with anxiety disorder and their children. *Journal of the American Academy of Child and Adolescent Psychiatry, 33*, 1106–1113.

Marcovitch, S., Goldberg, S., Gold, A., Washington, J., Wasson, C., Krekewich, K., et al. (1997). Determinants of behavioral problems in Romanian children adopted in Ontario. *International Journal of Behavioral Development, 20*, 17–31.

Marvin, R. S. (1992). Attachment and family systems-based intervention in developmental psychopathology. *Development and Psychopathology, 4*, 697–711.

Marvin, R. S., & Stewart, R. B. (1990). A family systems framework for the study of attachment. In M. T. Greenberg, D. Cicchetti, & M. Cummings (Eds.), *Attachment in the preschool years: Theory, research, and intervention* (pp. 51–86). Chicago: University of Chicago Press.

Masten, A. S. (2001). Ordinary magic: Resilience processes in development. *American Psychologist, 56*, 227–238.

Morisset, C. T., Barnard, K. E., Greenberg, M. T., Booth, C. L., & Spieker, S. J. (1990). Environmental influences on early language development: The context of social risk. *Development and Psychopathology, 2*, 127–149.

Moss, E., Cyr, C., & Dubois-Comtois, K. (2004). Attachment at early school age and developmental risk: Examining family contexts and behavior problems of controlling-caregiving, controlling-punitive, and behaviorally disorganized children. *Developmental Psychology, 40*, 519–532.

Moss, E., Rousseau, D., Parent, S., St.-Laurent, D., & Saintonge, J. (1998). Correlates of attachment at school-age: Maternal reported stress, mother–child interaction, and behavior problems. *Child Development, 69*, 1390–1405.

Moss, E., Smolla, N., Cyr, C., Dubois-Comtois, K., Mazzarello, T., & Berthiaume, C. (2006). Attachment and behavior problems in middle childhood as reported by adult and child informants. *Development and Psychopathology, 18*, 425–444.

Munson, J. A., McMahon, R. J., & Spieker, S. J. (2001). Structure and variability in the developmental trajectory of children's externalizing problems: Impact of infant attachment, maternal depressive symptomatology, and child sex. *Development and Psychopathology, 13,* 277–296.

Nada Raja, S., McGee, R., & Staton, W. R. (1992). Perceived attachment to parents and peers and psychological well-being in adolescence. *Journal of Youth and Adolescence, 21,* 471–485.

O'Connor, M. J., Sigman, M., & Brill, N. (1987). Disorganization of attachment in relation to maternal alcohol consumption. *Journal of Consulting and Clinical Psychology, 55,* 831–836.

O'Connor, T. G., Marvin, R. S., Rutter, M., Olrick, J. T., Britner, P. A., & the English and Romanian Adoptees Team. (2003). Child–parent attachment following early institutional deprivation. *Development and Psychopathology, 15,* 19–38.

Ogawa, J. R., Sroufe, L. A., Weinfield, N. S., Carlson, E. A., & Egeland, B. (1997). Development and the fragmented self: Longitudinal study of dissociative symptomatology in a nonclinical sample. *Development and Psychopathology, 9,* 855–879.

Oppenheim, D., Nir, A., Warren, S., & Emde, R. N. (1997). Emotion regulation in mother–child narrative co-construction: Association with children's narratives and adaptation. *Developmental Psychology, 33,* 284–294.

Oppenheim, D., & Waters, H. S. (1995). Narrative processes and attachment representations: Issues of development and assessment. In E. Waters, B. E. Vaughn, G. Posada, & K. Kondo-Ikemura (Eds.), Caregiving, cultural, and cognitive perspectives on secure-base behavior and working models: New growing points of attachment theory and research. *Monographs of the Society for Research in Child Development, 60*(2–3, Serial No. 244), 197–215.

Parker, J. G., Rubin, K. H., Price, J. M., & DeRosier, M. E. (1995). Peer relations, child development, and adjustment: A developmental psychopathology perspective. In D. Cicchetti & D. J. Cohen (Eds.), *Developmental psychopathology* (Vol. 2, pp. 96–161). New York: Wiley.

Patterson, G. R., DeBaryshe, B. D., & Ramsey, E. (1989). A developmental perspective on antisocial behavior. *American Psychologist, 44,* 329–335.

Patterson, G. R., Reid, J. B., & Dishion, T. J. (1992). *Antisocial boys.* Eugene, OR: Castalia.

Pilowsky, D. J., & Kates, W. G. (1995). Foster children in acute crisis: Assessing critical aspects of attachment. *Journal of the American Academy of Child and Adolescent Psychiatry, 35,* 1095–1097.

Radke-Yarrow, M., Cummings, E. M., Kuczynski, L., & Chapman, M. (1985). Patterns of attachment in two-and three-year-olds in normal families and families with parental depression. *Child Development, 56,* 884–893.

Renken, B., Egeland, B., Marvinney, D., Mangelsdorf, S., & Sroufe, L. A. (1989). Early childhood antecedents of aggression and passive-withdrawal in early elementary school. *Journal of Personality, 57,* 257–281.

Richters, J. E., & Waters, E. (1991). Attachment and socialization: The positive side of social influence. In M. Lewis & S. Feinman (Eds.), *Social influences and socialization in infancy* (pp. 185–213). New York: Plenum Press.

Richters, M. M., & Volkmar, F. R. (1994). Reactive attachment disorder of infancy or early childhood. *Journal of the American Academy of Child and Adolescent Psychiatry, 33,* 328–332.

Rodning, C., Beckwith, L., & Howard, J. (1991). Quality of attachment and home environments in children prenatally exposed to PCP and cocaine. *Development and Psychopathology, 3,* 351–366.

Rogers, S. J., Ozonoff, S., & Maslin-Cole, C. (1991). A comparative study of attachment behavior in young children with autism or other psychiatric disorders. *Journal of the American Academy of Child and Adolescent Psychiatry, 30,* 483–488.

Routh, C. P., Hill, J. H., Steele, H., Elliot, C. E., & Dewey, M. E. (1995). Maternal attachment status, psychosocial stressors and problem behavior: Follow-up after parent training courses for conduct disorder. *Journal of Child Psychology and Psychiatry, 36,* 1179–1198.

Rubin, K. H., Hymel, S., Mills, S. L., & Rose-Krasnor, L. (1991). Conceptualizing different developmental pathways to and from social isolation in childhood. In D. Cicchetti & S. L. Toth (Eds.), *Rochester Symposium on Developmental Psychopathology: Vol. 2. Internalizing and externalizing expressions of dysfunction* (pp. 91–122). Hillsdale, NJ: Erlbaum.

Rutgers, A. H., Bakermans-Kranenburg, M. J., van IJzendoorn, M. H., & Van Berckelaer-Onnes, I. A. (2004). Autism and attachment: A meta-analytic review. *Journal of Child Psychology and Psychiatry, 45,* 1123–1134.

Rutter, M. (1979). Protective factors in children's responses to stress and disadvantage. In M. W. Kent & J. Rolf (Eds.), *Primary prevention of psychopathology: Vol. 3. Social competence in children* (pp. 49–74). Hanover, NH: University Press of New England.

Rutter, M. (1982). Prevention of children's psychosocial disorders: Myth and substance. *Pediatrics, 70,* 883–894.

Rutter, M. (1985). Resilience in the face of adversity: Protective factors and resistance to psychiatric disorder. *British Journal of Psychiatry, 147,* 598–611.

Rutter, M. (1987). Psychosocial resilience and protective mechanisms. *American Journal of Orthopsychiatry, 57,* 316–331.

Rutter, M. (1997). Clinical implications of attachment concepts: Retrospect and prospect. In L. Atkinson & K. Zucker (Eds.), *Attachment and psychopathology* (pp. 17–46). New York: Guilford Press.

Sameroff, A. J., Seifer, R., Barocas, R., Zax, M., & Greenspan, S. (1987). Intelligence quotient scores of 4-year-old children: Social-environmental risk factors. *Pediatrics, 79,* 343–350.

Schore, A. N. (1996). The experience-dependent maturation of a regulatory system in the orbital prefrontal cortex and the origin of developmental psychopathology. *Development and Psychopathology, 8,* 59–87.

Shamir-Essakow, G., Ungerer, J. A., & Rapee, R. M.

(2005). Attachment, behavioral inhibition, and anxiety in preschool children. *Journal of Abnormal Child Psychology, 33*, 131–143.

Shaw, D. S., & Bell, R. Q. (1993). Developmental theories of parental contributions to antisocial behavior. *Journal of Abnormal Child Psychology, 21*, 493–518.

Shaw, D. S., Keenan, K., Vondra, J. I., Delliquadri, E., & Giovannelli, J. (1997). Antecedents of preschool children's internalizing problems: A longitudinal study of low-income families. *Journal of the American Academy of Child and Adolescent Psychiatry, 36*, 1760–1767.

Shaw, D. S., Owens, E. B., Vondra, J. I., Keenan, K., & Winslow, E. B. (1996). Early risk factors and pathways in the development of early disruptive behavior problems. *Development and Psychopathology, 8*, 679–699.

Shaw, D. S., & Vondra, J. I. (1995). Infant attachment security and maternal predictors of early behavior problems: A longitudinal study of low-income families. *Journal of Abnormal Child Psychology, 23*, 335–357.

Shouldice, A. E., & Stevenson-Hinde, J. (1992). Coping with security distress: The Separation Anxiety Test and attachment classifications at 4.5 years. *Journal of Child Psychology and Psychiatry and Allied Disciplines, 33*, 331–348.

Singer, L. M., Brodzinsky, D. M., Ramsay, D., Steer, M., & Waters, E. (1985). Mother–infant attachment in adoptive families. *Child Development, 56*, 1543–1551.

Slough, N. M., & Greenberg, M. T. (1990). Five-year-olds' representations of separation from parents: Responses from the perspective of self and other. *New Directions for Child Development, 48*, 67–84.

Slough, N. M., & Greenberg, M. T. (1997, April). *Assessment of attachment in five-year-olds: Validation of a revised version of the Separation Anxiety Test*. Paper presented at the biennial meeting of the Society for Research in Child Development, Washington, DC.

Smyke, A. T., Dumitrescu, A., & Zeanah, C. H. (2002). Attachment disturbances in young children. I: The continuum of caretaking casualty. *Journal of the American Academy of Child and Adolescent Psychiatry, 41*, 972–982.

Solomon, J., George, C., & De Jong, A. (l995). Children classified as controlling at age 6: Evidence of disorganized representational strategies and aggression at home and at school. *Development and Psychopathology, 7*, 447–463.

Spangler, G., & Grossmann, K. E. (1993). Biobehavioral organization in securely and insecurely attached infants. *Child Development, 64*, 1439–1450.

Spangler, G., & Schieche, M. (1998). Emotional and adrenocortical responses of infants to the Strange Situation: The differential function of emotional expression. *International Journal of Behavioral Development, 22*, 681–706.

Speltz, M. L. (1990). The treatment of preschool conduct problems: An integration of behavioral and attachment concepts. In M. T. Greenberg, D. Cicchet-

ti, & M. Cummings (Eds.), *Attachment in the preschool years: Theory, research, and intervention* (pp. 399–426). Chicago: University of Chicago Press.

Speltz, M. L., DeKlyen, M., & Greenberg, M. T. (1999). Attachment in boys with early onset conduct problems. *Development and Psychopathology, 11*, 269–286.

Speltz, M. L., Greenberg, M. T., & DeKlyen, M. (1990). Attachment in preschoolers with disruptive behavior: A comparison of clinic-referred and nonproblem children. *Development and Psychopathology, 2*, 31–46.

Spieker, S. J., & Bensley, L. (1994). Roles of living arrangement and grandmother social support in adolescent mothering and infant attachment. *Developmental Psychology, 30*, 102–111.

Spieker, S. J., & Booth, C. L. (1988). Maternal antecedents of attachment quality. In J. Belsky & T. Nezworski (Eds.), *Clinical implications of attachment* (pp. 95–135). Hillsdale, NJ: Erlbaum.

Spitz, R. (1946). Anaclitic depression: An inquiry into the genesis of psychiatric conditions in early childhood—II. *Psychoanalytic Study of the Child, 2*, 313–342.

Sroufe, L. A. (1983). Infant caregiver attachment and patterns of adaptation in preschool: The roots of maladaptation and competence. In M. Perlmutter (Ed.), *Minnesota Symposium on Child Psychology: Vol. 16. Development and policy concerning children with special needs* (pp. 41–81). Hillsdale, NJ: Erlbaum.

Sroufe, L. A. (1990). Pathways to adaptation and maladaptation: Psychopathology as developmental deviation. In D. Cicchetti (Ed.), *Rochester Symposium on Developmental Psychopathology: Vol. 1. The emergence of a discipline* (pp. 13–40). Hillsdale, NJ: Erlbaum

Sroufe, L. A., Egeland, B., Carlson, E., & Collins, A. (2005). *The development of the person: The Minnesota Study of Risk and Adaptation from Birth to Adulthood*. New York: Guilford Press.

Sroufe, L. A., Egeland, B., & Kreutzer, T. (1990). The fate of early experience following developmental change: Longitudinal approaches to individual adaptation in childhood. *Child Development, 61*, 1363–1373.

Sroufe, L. A., & Fleeson, J. (1986). Attachment and the construction of relationships. In W. W. Hartup & Z. Rubin (Eds.), *The nature of relationships* (pp. 51–71). Hillsdale, NJ: Erlbaum.

Stouthamer-Loeber, M., Loeber, R., Farrington, D. P., Zhang, Q., Van Kammen, W., & Maguin, E. (1993). The double edge of protective and risk factors for delinquency: Interrelations and developmental patterns. *Development and Psychopathology, 5*, 683–701.

Thurber, C. A. (1996). Separation anxiety disorder and the collapse of anxiety disorders of childhood and adolescence. *Anxiety Disorders Practice Journal, 2*, 115–135.

Troy, M., & Sroufe, L. A. (1987). Victimization among preschoolers: The role of attachment relationship history. *Journal of the American Academy of Child and Adolescent Psychiatry, 26*, 166–172.

Turner, P. (1991). Relations between attachment, gender, and behavior with peers in the preschool. *Child Development, 62,* 1475–1488.

Ungerer, J., & McMahon, C. (2005). Attachment and psychopathology: A lifespan perspective. In J. L. Hudson & R. M. Rapee (Eds.), *Psychopathology and the family* (pp. 33–52). Oxford, UK: Elsevier.

Urban, J., Carlson, E., Egeland, B., & Sroufe, L. A. (1991). Patterns of individual adaptation across childhood. *Development and Psychopathology, 3,* 445–460.

van IJzendoorn, M. H., Rutgers, A. H., Bakermans-Kranenburg, M. J., Swinkels, S. H. N., van Daalen, E., Dietz, C., et al. (2007). Parental sensitivity and attachment in children with autism spectrum disorder: Comparison with children with mental retardation, with language delays, and with typical development. *Child Development, 78,* 597–608.

Vaughn, B., Egeland, B., Sroufe, L. A., & Waters, E. (1979). Individual differences in infant–mother attachment at 12 and 18 months: Stability and change in families under stress. *Child Development, 50,* 971–975.

Vondra, J. I., Shaw, D. S., Swearingen, L., Cohen, M., & Owens, E. B. (2001). Attachment stability and emotional and behavioral regulation from infancy to preschool age. *Development and Psychopathology, 13,* 13–33.

Warren, S. L., Emde, R., & Sroufe, L. A. (2000). Predicting anxiety from children's play narratives. *Journal of the American Academy of Child and Adolescent Psychiatry, 39,* 100–107.

Warren, S. L., Huston, L., Egeland, B., & Sroufe, L. A. (1997). Child and adolescent anxiety disorders and early attachment. *Journal of the American Academy of Child and Adolescent Psychiatry, 36,* 637–644.

Waters, E., & Deane, K. E. (1985). Defining and assessing individual differences in attachment relationships: Q-sort methodology and the organization of behavior in infancy and early childhood. In I. Bretherton & E. Waters (Eds.), Growing points of attachment theory and research. *Monographs of the Society for Research in Child Development, 50*(1–2, Serial No. 209), 41–65.

Waters, E., Kondo-Ikemura, K., Posada, G., & Richters, J. E. (1991). Learning to love: Mechanisms and milestones. In M. Gunnar & L. A. Sroufe (Eds.), *Minnesota Symposium on Child Psychology: Vol. 23. Self processes and development* (pp. 217–255). Hillsdale, NJ: Erlbaum.

Weissberg, R., & Greenberg, M. T. (1998). School and community competence-enhancement and prevention programs. In W. Damon (Series Ed.) & I. Sigel & A. Renninger (Vol. Eds.), *Handbook of child psychology: Vol. 4. Child psychology in practice* (5th ed., pp. 877–954). Hoboken, NJ: Wiley.

Willemsen-Swinkels, S. H. N., Bakermans-Kranenburg, M. J., Buitelaar, J. K., van IJzendoorn, M. H., & van Engeland, H. (2000). Insecure and disorganized attachment in children with a pervasive developmental disorder: Relationship with social interaction and heart rate. *Journal of Child Psychology and Psychiatry, 41,* 759–767.

Winnicott, D. W. (1965). *The maturational processes and the facilitating environment.* New York: International Universities Press.

World Health Organization. (1992). *The ICD-10 classification of mental and behavioural disorders: Clinical descriptions and diagnostic guidelines.* Geneva: Author.

Zaslow, M. S., & Hayes, C. D. (1986). Sex differences in children's reposes to psychosocial stress: Toward a cross-context analysis. In M. Lamb, A. Brown, & B. Rogoff (Eds.), *Advances in developmental psychology* (Vol. 4, pp. 298–337). Hillsdale, NJ: Erlbaum.

Zeanah, C. H. (1996). Beyond insecurity: A reconceptualization of attachment disorders in infancy. *Journal of Consulting and Clinical Psychology, 64,* 42–52.

Zeanah, C. H., & Boris, N. W. (2000). Disturbances and disorders of attachment in early childhood. In C. H. Zeanah (Ed.), *Handbook of infant mental health* (2nd ed., pp. 353–368). New York: Guilford Press.

Zeanah, C. H., Scheeringa, M., Boris, N. W., Heller, S. S., Smyke, A. T., & Trapani, J. (2004). Reactive attachment disorder in maltreated toddlers. *Child Abuse and Neglect, 28,* 877–888.

Zeanah, C. H., Smyke, A. T., & Dumitrescu, A. (2002). Attachment disturbances in young children: II. Indiscriminate behavior and institutional care. *Journal of the American Academy of Child and Adolescent Psychiatry, 41,* 983–989.

Zero to Three Task Force on Diagnostic Classification in Infancy. (1994). *Diagnostic classification of mental health and developmental disorders of infancy and early childhood (DC:0–3).* Arlington, VA: Zero to Three.

Zero to Three Task Force on Diagnostic Classification in Infancy. (2005). *Diagnostic classification of mental health and developmental disorders of infancy and early childhood—Revised (DC:0–3R).* Arlington, VA: Zero to Three.

Zimmerman, M. A., & Arunkumar, R. (1994). Resiliency research: Implications for schools and social policy. *Social Policy Report, 8,* 1–20.

CHAPTER 28

Attachment Disorganization
Genetic Factors, Parenting Contexts, and Developmental Transformation from Infancy to Adulthood

KARLEN LYONS-RUTH
DEBORAH JACOBVITZ

The conceptual cornerstone of our understanding of disorganized attachment in infancy was laid when Main and Solomon (1990) chose the term "disorganized/disoriented" to describe an array of previously unrecognized fearful, odd, disorganized, or overtly conflicted behaviors exhibited by infants during Ainsworth's Strange Situation procedure (Ainsworth, Blehar, Waters, & Wall, 1978). Infants are considered "disorganized/disoriented" when, for example, they appear apprehensive, cry and fall huddled to the floor, or put their hands to their mouths with hunched shoulders in response to their parents' return following a brief separation. Still others appear disoriented, freezing all movements while exhibiting a trance-like expression. Main and colleagues' descriptions of disorganized/disoriented behavioral patterns in infancy (e.g., Main & Solomon, 1990; Main & Weston, 1981) led to an explosion of empirical and theoretical publications on the developmental origins, correlates, and outcomes of disorganized attachment (see van IJzendoorn, Schuengel, & Bakermans-Kranenberg, 1999).

Since the first edition of this handbook was published, several new frontiers have emerged in the study of attachment disorganization. First, genetic contributions, and gene–environment interactions in particular, are being actively explored. Second, the forms of parent–infant communication thought to be related to infant disorganization are the subjects of active debate, with a substantial body of new literature accrued. The importance of assessing these early communication patterns has been underscored both by the emerging work on gene–environment interaction and by longitudinal studies of predictors of maladaptive outcomes in young adulthood. Third, the interface between disorganized attachment displayed in relation to the caregiver and indiscriminate attachment behavior displayed toward relative strangers is yielding unexpected findings. Fourth, new work has examined outcomes of early attachment disorganization in adolescence and young adulthood, as well as the ways disorganization may present behaviorally in adolescence.

We begin with a review of the literature on attachment disorganization in infancy; we cover its definition, prevalence, and associated infant characteristics, including potential genetic underpinnings. The second section, on family correlates of disorganized attachment, summarizes studies of family risk factors; parental states of mind regarding attachment, assessed with the Adult Attachment Interview (AAI; George, Kaplan, & Main,

1984, 1985, 1996; Main & Goldwyn, 1984; Main, Goldwyn, & Hesse, 2003; Main, Kaplan, & Cassidy, 1985); and frightened, frightening, or disrupted parental behavior toward an infant. This section also considers recent work assessing interactions between genetic factors and the early caregiving environment. In the third section, we review data on the longitudinal reorganization of disorganized infant behavior into controlling forms of attachment behavior, along with evidence linking both disorganized and controlling forms of attachment behavior with internalizing or externalizing behavior problems and dissociative behaviors evident by school age. The subsequent section describes recent longitudinal work identifying sequelae of infant disorganization in adolescence and young adulthood, as well as work assessing adolescent disorganization directly. We conclude with issues raised by the new literature and questions that need attention over the next decade.

DISORGANIZED ATTACHMENT BEHAVIOR IN INFANCY: DEFINITION, PREVALENCE, AND ASSOCIATED INFANT CHARACTERISTICS

Definition of Disorganized/Disoriented Behavior

Understanding the central role of fear in attachment theory is critical to the theoretical framework of attachment disorganization (Hesse & Main, 2006; Main & Hesse, 1990). Bowlby's (1969/1982) initial formulation of attachment theory emphasized the organization of an infant's observable behaviors around the set goal of maintaining physical proximity to the parent. Signs of danger or potential danger, such as unfamiliarity, hunger, fatigue, illness, or injury, result in higher levels of activation of this attachment behavioral system. When the system is strongly aroused, physical contact with a caregiver (e.g., touching, clinging, cuddling) may be necessary to terminate the infant's attachment behavior. When the environment is benign and the mother's whereabouts are well known, the child typically ceases to exhibit attachment behavior and instead explores the environment (Bowlby, 1969/1982).

Ainsworth and colleagues (1978) discovered three patterns of behavior displayed by infants when they are distressed by a separation from their caregivers in the Strange Situation. Some infants, termed "avoidant," show minimal displays of affect; for example, they direct attention toward objects and away from their caregivers; they turn away or look away rather than seek contact and

comfort (Ainsworth et al., 1978). Other infants, termed "resistant" or "ambivalent," mingle proximity and contact seeking with angry behavior and continued distress on reunion. Finally, "secure" infants seek proximity and contact with little or no avoidance or angry resistance toward their caregivers. The contact and comfort they receive are effective in calming them, allowing them to return to play. (For comprehensive reviews, see Thompson, Chapter 16; van IJzendoorn & Sagi-Schwartz, Chapter 37; and Weinfield, Sroufe, Egeland, & Carlson, Chapter 4, this volume).

However, for many years, researchers noted that some infants did not fit these three organized attachment patterns (Crittenden, 1985; Lyons-Ruth, Connell, Zoll, & Stahl, 1987; Main & Weston, 1981; Radke-Yarrow, Cummings, Kuczynski, & Chapman, 1985). Based on ethologists descriptions of "conflict behaviors" arising from the simultaneous activation of incompatible systems, Main (1973, 1979) developed a scale for assessing "disorganized/disordered" behavior. Infants who were unclassifiable in the Strange Situation showed the most pronounced disorganized behavior when exposed to an initially silent, unmoving masked clown (Main & Weston, 1981). A description of the disorganized/disoriented attachment category was undertaken following the realization that many infants, particularly from high-risk environments, were difficult or impossible to place into the three organized categories (Main, 1973; Main & Solomon, 1986, 1990; Main & Weston, 1981). To gain a better understanding of why some infants were unclassifiable, Main and Solomon (1990) reexamined over 200 anomalous Strange Situation videotapes. They concluded that most of the children lacked any organized strategy for dealing with the stress of separation. For example, unclassifiable infants were observed approaching the parent with head averted; rocking on hands and knees following an abortive approach; or screaming by the door for the parent, then moving silently away on reunion. What unclassifiable infants appeared to have in common was contradictory intentions (approaching a parent with head averted), or behaviors that involved apprehension either directly (fearful facial expressions, oblique approaches) or indirectly (disoriented behaviors, including dazed and trance-like expressions; freezing of all movement at the parent's entrance). Main and Solomon viewed these contradictory or out-of-context behaviors as indicating that an infant was unable to organize a consistent secure, avoidant, or ambivalent strategy toward the care-

...en experiencing a need for comfort. This view was subsequently elaborated to describe "fear without solution" as the heart of the disorganized infant's dilemma in seeking comfort.

Main and Solomon (1990) proposed that infants be categorized as disorganized/disoriented when, in the presence of the caregiver in the Strange Situation, they display behaviors falling under one or more of the following headings:

1. Sequential display of contradictory behavior patterns, such as very strong attachment behavior suddenly followed by avoidance, freezing, or dazed behavior.
2. Simultaneous display of contradictory behaviors, such as strong avoidance with strong contact seeking, distress, or anger.
3. Undirected, misdirected, incomplete, and interrupted movements and expressions—for example, extensive expressions of distress accompanied by movement away from, rather than toward, the mother.
4. Stereotypies, asymmetrical movements, mistimed movements, and anomalous postures, such as stumbling for no apparent reason and only when the parent is present.
5. Freezing, stilling, and slowed "underwater" movements and expressions.
6. Direct indices of apprehension regarding the parent, such as hunched shoulders or fearful facial expressions.
7. Direct indices of disorganization and disorientation, such as disoriented wandering, confused or dazed expressions, or multiple rapid changes in affect.

The directions for assigning a disorganized classification include instructions to assign a secondary "best-fitting" organized attachment classification—either secure, avoidant, or resistant. In the disorganized-secure subgroup, the infant seeks contact with the caregiver without marked avoidance or ambivalence and is soothed by her presence, but shows other unusual signs of hesitation, confusion, apprehension, dysphoria, or conflict in relation to her. Disorganized-avoidant and disorganized-ambivalent infants often display unexpected combinations of distress, contact seeking, avoidance, resistance, or other apprehensive or conflict behaviors. Good interrater reliability on classification of infant behavioral patterns as disorganized/disoriented is well documented (van IJzendoorn et al., 1999).

Prevalence and Stability of Disorganized Attachment Patterns

van IJzendoorn and colleagues (1999) conducted a meta-analysis indicating that the percentage of infants classified as disorganized was 14% in middle-class, nonclinical groups ($N = 1,882$) and 24% in low-socioeconomic-status samples ($N = 493$). In 20 studies across 25 samples ($N = 1,219$), van IJzendoorn and colleagues found that disorganized attachment was accompanied by a secondary classification of ambivalent in 46% of the cases, avoidant in 34% of the cases, and secure in 14% of the cases. However, these subtypes may be differentially distributed in low- and high-social-risk environments. In middle-income samples, more disorganized infants have been reported to be classified as disorganized-secure (62%, $N = 268$, Main & Solomon, 1990; and 52%, $N = 1,131$, K. McCartney, personal communication, 2005; data from National Institute of Child Health and Human Development [NICHD] Early Child Care Research Network, 2001). Modest but significant overall stability of disorganized attachment over a 1- to 60-month period ($r = .36$, $N = 515$) was also found (van IJzendoorn et al., 1999). Less stable and less supportive family contexts have been associated with instability in attachment classification across all categories (Egeland & Farber, 1984; Lamb, Thompson, Gardner, & Charnov, 1985). Vondra and colleagues (Vondra, Hommerding, & Shaw, 1999; Vondra, Shaw, Swearingen, Cohen, & Owens, 2001) found that disruptive family events were specifically related to change to a disorganized classification from 12 to 18 months of age.

Temperament and Disorganized Attachment Behavior

Given the behavioral inconsistency that characterizes many disorganized attachment behaviors, an important question is whether temperamental differences underlie a disorganized classification. However, studies have shown that infants are unlikely to be classified as disorganized with more than one caregiver (Main & Solomon, 1990; Fonagy et al., 1996; van IJzendoorn et al., 1999). For example, Main and Solomon (1990) reported that 31 of 34 infants classified as disorganized with one parent were not so classified with the other parent. Based on a meta-analysis of 12 samples ($N = 1,877$), van IJzendoorn and colleagues (1999) reported a nonsignificant association between disorganized attachment in infancy and constitutional and temperamental variables ($r = .003$). In the eight studies ($N = 1,639$) that examined the association between the construct of "difficult temperament" in particular and disorganized attachment classifications, the effect size ($r = .02$) was small and not significant.

One still unexplored possibility is that neonatal temperamental effects interact with caregiving risk, so that temperamental differences are more evident in low-risk samples (Spangler, Fremmer-Bombik, & Grossmann, 1996; Spangler & Schieche, 1998; see Vaughn, Bost, & van IJzendoorn, Chapter 9, this volume), but are overridden by caregiving effects in higher-risk samples (Carlson, 1998). However, the findings accrued to date indicate that attachment disorganization emerges within a particular relationship; they do not support the notion of attachment disorganization as an individual trait or inborn characteristic of the infant.

Genetic Effects and Infant Disorganized Attachment Behavior

An important new area of study concerns possible genetic influences on disorganized attachment behavior. Bokhorst and colleagues (2003), using behavioral genetic methods in a study of 138 twin pairs at 1 year of age, found that only nonshared environmental factors accounted for the variance in twin concordances of disorganized versus organized attachment, whereas both shared and nonshared environmental factors accounted for the variance in secure versus insecure attachment. This led these authors to surmise that nonshared factors, such as trauma or differential parental treatment (and/or error variance due to the difficulty of coding disorganization), may be important in the etiology of disorganized attachment. In a second study of 110 twin pairs at age 3½ years (O'Connor & Croft, 2001), only shared and nonshared environmental effects on attachment classification were significant. Due to the small sample size, however, O'Connor and Croft (2001) declined to test genetic influences on disorganized/ controlling attachment separately (see also Finkel & Matheny, 2000).

Behavioral genetic methods examine genetic effects by statistically comparing monozygotic and dizygotic twin correlations. However, a good deal of power is needed to detect significant differences

between correlations, making large sample sizes necessary. With only one modestly sized twin study reporting on disorganized forms of attachment, no firm conclusions on heritability estimates for infant disorganization can yet be drawn.

With the recent advent of molecular genetic techniques, it is easier to detect small effects of particular genes with modest sample sizes. The dopamine D4 receptor (DRD4) gene has been considered a candidate gene for infant attachment behavior, because it is preferentially expressed in the brain regions of the mesocorticolimbic dopamine pathway mediating reward related to social interaction, including mother–infant attachment (Insel, 2003; Muller, Brunelli, Moore, Myers, & Shair, 2005). A review by Swanson, Flodman, and Kennedy (2000) confirmed the likely role of the 7-repeat allele of this gene in making the postsynaptic dopamine receptor subsensitive, and further suggested that dopamine underactivity compromises attentional and reward systems.

In the first studies to use molecular genetic techniques in research on attachment, Lakatos and colleagues (2000, 2002) found associations between the DRD4 7-repeat genotype and disorganized attachment in a low-risk sample. Analysis of a second polymorphism affecting dopamine system efficiency (the –521 C/T promoter polymorphism) revealed that the association between the 7-repeat allele and disorganized attachment was observed only in the presence of the –521T allele. In the presence of both risk alleles, incidence of disorganized attachment was 40%, compared to 11% for the rest of the sample (Lakatos et al., 2002). The same research team found that an independent method, the family-based transmission disequilibrium test, also indicated significant nontransmission of the 7-repeat allele from parent to child among securely attached infants, as well as a trend for preferential transmission of the 7-repeat allele to disorganized infants (Gervai et al., 2005). Their interpretation of their findings overall was that the short form of the DRD4 allele (2,4-repeat) facilitated secure attachment in a low-risk sample. However, two subsequent studies failed to replicate the main effect of the DRD4 7-repeat allele on disorganization (Bakermans-Kranenburg & van IJzendoorn, 2004; Spangler & Zimmermann, 2007).

It is important to note that gene–environment interaction was not assessed in these studies. If caregiver behavior affects the expression of genes related to fearful arousal, as has been demonstrated in other species (e.g., Francis, Champagne, Liu, & Meaney, 1999), overlap between infant genotype and atypical caregiver behavior in a small sample of disorganized infants will greatly influence the obtained association between genotype and disorganization. Therefore, it is now critical to account for quality of caregiving in the model. These recent studies are reviewed as part of the section on family influences.

Stress Hormone Levels and Disorganized Attachment Behaviors

In animal models, cortisol secretion is correlated with an animal's inability to mobilize an effective strategy to cope with a stressor (e.g., Levine, Wiener, & Coe, 1993). To date, three studies have examined the association between infants' attachment behavior and their stress levels as indexed by salivary cortisol levels. In two of the three studies, infants with insecure or disorganized attachment classifications displayed significantly higher cortisol levels in response to brief separations than did secure infants (Hertsgaard, Gunnar, Erickson, & Nachmias, 1995; Spangler & Grossmann, 1993). These findings are consistent with Main and Solomon's (1990) view that disorganized infant behavior reflects the lack of an effective strategy for coping with stress.

Disorganized Attachment and Indiscriminate Attachment Behavior

An important new area of study concerns how disorganized attachment may intersect with indiscriminate attachment behavior—another form of atypical attachment behavior most often seen among severely deprived infants reared in orphanages with multiple caregivers (O'Connor, Rutter, & The English and Romanian Adoptees Study Team, 2000; see Dozier & Rutter, Chapter 29, this volume). Indiscriminate attachment behavior is seen when young children seek close contact with people other than a few preferred caregivers, and it is typically assessed by caregiver report rather than direct observation. A few studies have begun to examine how such indiscriminate attachment behavior is related to the disorganized attachment behaviors described above.

A study of attachment among 12- to 31-month-old institutionalized children in Romania revealed a high incidence of disorganization (78%) and a low incidence of organized-insecure classifications (Zeanah, Smyke, Koga, Carlson, &

The Bucharest Early Intervention Project Core Group, 2005). Based on a rating of "nonattachment," 65% of the children showed a clear but passive preference for the familiar caregiver over the stranger, but only 3% showed a recognizable pattern of attachment behavior consistent with one of the four traditional attachment patterns. The authors concluded that among institutionally reared infants, both secure and disorganized behavior may have different presentations and meanings from those seen in a noninstitutional group. Surprisingly, caregiver reports of indiscriminate attachment behavior toward relative strangers were unrelated either to disorganized attachment behavior or to the rating of nonattachment to the caregiver. Therefore, a child's indiscriminately intimate behavior toward others may be somewhat independent of the degree and patterning of focused attachment behavior toward the preferred caregiver.

Whereas most studies have used caregiver reports of indiscriminate attachment behavior (Boris et al., 2004; Zeanah et al., 2005), two studies have looked at the relation between disorganized attachment behavior and directly observed engagement with the stranger during the Strange Situation procedure. In a study by Lyons-Ruth and colleagues (Lyons-Ruth, Bureau, Riley, & Atlas-Corbett, in press; Riley, Atlas-Corbett, Bureau, & Lyons-Ruth, 2007), both disorganized and avoidant attachment were associated with degree of engagement with the stranger. However, after both avoidant and disorganized attachment behavior were controlled for, engagement with the stranger in the Strange Situation was independently and significantly associated with higher levels of clinically judged caregiving risk (with higher levels of maternal disrupted communication also assessed in the Strange Situation; the rating of disrupted communication is described later in this chapter); and with later child hyperactivity rated by teachers at age 5 (see also DeKlyen & Greenberg, Chapter 27, this volume, regarding hyperactivity and indiscriminate behavior). O'Connor and colleagues (2003), studying 4- to 6-year-old Romanian orphans who had been adopted into British households, used preschool Strange Situation assessments conducted in a home setting and found a relation between controlling/disorganized attachment in the Strange Situation and caregiver-reported indiscriminate behavior. It was noted, however, that the preschool coding system was modified to include directly observed overly intimate engagement with the stranger in the

Strange Situation as a form of disorganization (insecure/other behavior), rather than maintaining the focus of the Strange Situation coding system on anomalous behavior toward the caregiver.

Other studies of severely maltreated infants also raise the question of whether traditional attachment behaviors have the same correlates and meaning in low- and high-risk samples. In a study of 38 infants placed in foster care between 5 and 28 months of age, Stovall-McClough and Dozier (2004) found a high rate of secure attachment behavior in the Strange Situation among maltreated infants in foster care within 4 months of placement. However, Dozier and colleagues (2006) also reported atypical diurnal cycles of cortisol release among infants in foster care. The literature as a whole suggests that among infants with multiple caregivers, apparently secure behavioral patterns are displayed in concert with other atypical indicators, such as lack of strong attachment behavior, socially indiscriminate behavior toward strangers, or atypical physiological responses. More work is needed to determine whether such anomalous indicators are better understood as distinct from disorganized forms of attachment behavior, or whether they will be seen to be part of the spectrum of pathways leading to intergenerational transmission of disorganized attachment (see Dozier & Rutter, Chapter 29, this volume, for further discussion).

FAMILY CORRELATES OF DISORGANIZED ATTACHMENT BEHAVIOR

Disorganized Attachment Behavior and Family Risk Factors

The incidence of disorganized attachment in infancy has ranged from 13% to 82%, depending on the presence and type of family risk factors. In both middle- and low-income samples, parental maltreatment has been associated with infant disorganization (Carlson, Cicchetti, Barnett, & Braunwald, 1989; Cicchetti, Rogosch, & Toth, 2006; George & Main, 1979; Lyons-Ruth, Connell, Grunebaum, & Botein, 1990). For example, in the Carlson and colleagues (1989) study, 82% of maltreated infants were classified as disorganized, compared to 18% of those in a low-income control group; in the Cicchetti and colleagues (2006) study, 90% of maltreated infants were disorganized, compared to 43% of low-income controls.

Several studies have examined the relation between maternal depression and attachment disorganization, because maternal depression has been associated with both hostile and inconsistent caregiving (Lyons-Ruth, Lyubchik, Wolfe, & Bronfman, 2002). The results of such studies have been mixed. A meta-analysis of 16 studies (N = 1,053) examining the association between maternal depressive symptoms and infant disorganization found only a marginally significant relationship (r = .06, p = .06; van IJzendoorn et al., 1999). In the large NICHD Study of Early Child Care (N = 1,131), infant attachment disorganization was not significantly related to mothers' psychological adjustment, as assessed by the Center for Epidemiologic Studies Depression Scale and the Neuroticism, Extraversion, and Openness Personality Inventory (NICHD Early Child Care Research Network, 1997). However, a second meta-analysis found a significant effect of maternal depression when only serious depressive disorders requiring treatment were considered (Martins & Gaffan, 2000; see also Toth, Rogosch, Manly, & Cicchetti, 2006). It appears that more chronic and severe maternal depression resulting in significant clinical impairment is necessary before associations with infant disorganization become apparent.

A few studies have examined associations between maternal substance abuse and attachment disorganization. Infants of middle-income mothers who had consumed moderate to heavy amounts of alcohol prior to pregnancy (vs. abstinent mothers or light drinkers) were more often classified as disorganized (O'Connor, Sigman, & Brill, 1987). Replication of this finding is still needed. Drug-addicted mothers maintained on methadone were also more likely to have infants classified as disorganized than were nonaddicted low-income controls (Finger, 2006; Melnick, Finger, Hans, Patrick, & Lyons-Ruth, 2008).

In one of the few studies examining anxiety-disordered mothers and their children (ages 18–59 months), Manassis, Bradley, Goldberg, Hood, and Swinson (1994) found that 78% of such mothers were classified on the AAI as "unresolved with respect to loss or trauma," and that 65% of their children (n = 20) were classified as disorganized. Moreover, 65% of offspring were also classified as behaviorally inhibited (Manassis, Bradley, Goldberg, Hood, & Swinson, 1995). However, no statistical relation between behavioral inhibition and insecure attachment emerged, with three of the four secure children classified as inhibited. Since there was no control group, these figures were compared to established norms. Finally, Hobson, Patrick, Crandell, García-Pérez, and Lee (2005) found that infants of mothers with borderline personality disorder (BPD; $n = 10$) were more likely to be classified as disorganized than were infants of nondisordered controls ($n = 23$). In addition, mothers in the BPD group more often displayed intrusive behavior in a play setting.

Other family risk factors may also play a role in attachment disorganization. For example, Hughes, Turton, Hopper, McGauley, and Fonagy (2001) compared women during pregnancy whose most recent prior pregnancy ended in stillbirth after 18 weeks' gestation with a matched control group of pregnant women. Across the entire sample, there was a significant association between mothers' unresolved status on the AAI (see below) and attachment disorganization in their infants (effect size $r = .50$). However, among the women who experienced a stillbirth, infant disorganization was also independently predicted by a mother having seen the stillborn child and by her having elective termination of the pregnancy.

Disorganized Attachment and Parental States of Mind on the AAI

Unresolved Parental States of Mind on the AAI

Exploring parents' attachment-related mental representations associated with particular infant attachment classifications has deepened our understanding of the intergenerational transmission of attachment patterns. According to attachment theory, as patterns of interaction are repeated in close relationships over time, children build expectations about future interactions with parents and others that guide their interpretations and behaviors in new situations. As these largely unconscious expectations become elaborated and organized, they are termed "internal working models" (Bowlby, 1973; Bretherton & Munholland, Chapter 5, this volume).

Main and colleagues (1985) found that when parents' representations of their childhood attachment relationships are explored in an open-ended interview, four broad classifications of adults' states of mind regarding attachment can be reliably assigned (see Hesse, Chapter 25, this volume, for a review). These four classifications, labeled "autonomous," "dismissing," "preoccupied," and "unresolved/disorganized," predict the four infant attachment classifications, labeled "secure," "avoidant," "resistant," and "disorganized."

The unresolved/disorganized (U) classification is assigned to adults who show signs of disori-

entation and disorganization during discussions of potentially traumatic events (i.e., deaths of relatives, physical abuse, or sexual abuse). As detailed by Main and colleagues (2003), one such sign is a lapse in the monitoring of discourse, whereby the speaker no longer appears conscious of the interview situation and has "lost awareness of the discourse context." Examples include falling silent in midsentence and then completing the sentence 20 seconds or more later as if no time had passed, or failing to finish the sentence entirely.

Another sign of unresolved loss or trauma is a lapse in the monitoring of reasoning. Lapses in the monitoring of reasoning are usually brief and should not be confused with "irrational" thinking in the transcript as a whole. These lapses can take several forms, including indications of a belief that a lost person is simultaneously dead and alive (in a physical rather than a religious sense). For example, one speaker said, "It's probably better that he is dead, because he can get on with being dead and I can get on with raising a family" (Main et al., 2003, p. 118). Such lapses may also include disbelief that the person is dead (e.g., discussing a parent in the present tense even though the parent died 20 years earlier). Similar to disorganized infants, parents judged unresolved are also given a best-fitting alternate classification, identifying the pattern most closely corresponding to the overall organization of the interview (e.g., unresolved-secure).

Unresolved lapses in the monitoring of reasoning and discourse are notable, because they involve a sudden shift or alteration in the quality of discourse. Hesse (1996) suggested that these lapses involve "frightening and/or overwhelming experiences that may momentarily be controlling or altering discourse" (p. 8). Hesse and Main (2006) proposed that parents who are unresolved with respect to loss or trauma on the AAI are still overwhelmed either by the trauma itself, which is inherently frightening, or by "incompletely remembered loss experiences." Unresolved states of mind have been associated empirically with altered states of consciousness, such as trance-like states. Among 140 low-risk subjects, those classified as unresolved on the AAI showed significantly elevated scores on Tellegen's Absorption Scale, which includes such items as "I sometimes 'step outside' my usual self and experience an entirely different state of mind" (Hesse & van IJzendoorn, 1999; see also Granqvist & Kirkpatrick, Chapter 38, this volume). In a study of two low-risk samples ($N = 138$, $N = 308$), adults whose mothers had experienced familial loss within 2 years of their births also showed a significant propensity toward absorption, as assessed on the Absorption Scale (Hesse & van IJzendoorn, 1998).

Early loss of a parent through death has been associated with infant disorganization (Lyons-Ruth, Yellin, et al., 2005; Main et al., 1985). However, a mother's early loss of an attachment figure does not inevitably lead to infant disorganization. Rather, Ainsworth and Eichberg (1991) found that the lack of resolution of loss, as revealed in parents' lapses in the monitoring of reasoning and discourse, was a more powerful predictor of attachment disorganization than loss per se. A meta-analysis of nine studies ($N = 548$) revealed an effect size of $d = 0.65$ ($r = .31$) for the relation between child disorganization and parental unresolved status (van IJzendoorn, 1995). Unresolved states of mind have been associated with infant disorganization in studies conducted throughout North America, Western Europe, the Middle East, Africa, and Mexico, and this association occurs even when an adult's attachment status is assessed prior to the child's birth.

In one of the few studies to examine the transmission of the unresolved state of mind from mother to adult daughter, the intergenerational transmission of unresolved attachment status was examined among 48 Holocaust survivors and a matched comparison group of 50 women who had not experienced the Holocaust. Although Holocaust survivors were significantly more likely to be classified as unresolved, unresolved status was not transmitted to the next generation (Sagi-Schwartz et al., 2003). The authors noted that it may be important that the traumatic events were not created by attachment figures, but emerged from an outside destructive force (the Nazis). The basic trust the survivors had developed with their parents prior to the Holocaust may have empowered them to cope with the war, adapt to normal life after the war, and become attachment figures themselves.

Cannot Classify and Hostile-Helpless States of Mind

The meta-analysis cited above of 548 mother–infant dyads revealed that 53% of disorganized infants had mothers with unresolved responses to loss and trauma (van IJzendoorn, 1995). Although this is a robust effect, it also means that 47% of disorganized infants did not have unresolved mothers. This lack of correspondence between mother and infant attachment may have stemmed in part from measurement error, since stronger links were un-

covered when Strange Situation coders had more training, or in part from the fact that some mothers did not discuss experiences of loss or trauma in enough detail for lapses in discourse to occur. In addition, assigning an unresolved classification on the AAI depends on a participant's report of a specific loss or abuse experience. If no loss or abuse is identified by the participant, then adult state of mind cannot be coded unresolved. Therefore, discourse about loss or abuse per se may constitute too narrow a window for capturing all anomalous attachment states of mind seen among adults with more difficult childhood experiences.

In one approach to this dilemma, Hesse (1996) developed interview-wide criteria for designating an AAI as "cannot classify" (CC). This may occur if both a dismissing and a preoccupied attachment strategy are evident in different parts of the interview (e.g., in discussing mother vs. father or present vs. past), or if the participant exhibits low coherence across the interview. Subtypes of CC have been linked to specific psychiatric diagnoses (Ivarsson, 2008), but have not been examined in relation to infant disorganization (see Hesse, Chapter 25, this volume, for an extended discussion).

In another interview-wide approach to coding disorganized states of mind, "hostile-helpless" (HH) states of mind on the AAI have been described, based on transcript-wide criteria for contradiction and global devaluation of attachment relationships themselves in discourse (Lyons-Ruth, Yellin, Melnick, & Atwood, 2005). Theoretically, the coding system operationalizes the clinically described defense mechanism of splitting, in which contradictory affective evaluations of the same figure are stored in segregated memory systems, unintegrated with one another but available to consciousness in alternation. This defense mechanism is seen as distinct from the mechanism of repression, in which negative or disturbing evaluations are more consistently maintained out of awareness.

The central feature of an HH state of mind is the extent to which the individual has positively identified with the psychological stance of a childhood caregiver whom he or she also globally devalues elsewhere in the interview. In addition to evidence of identification with a globally devalued figure, HH interviews may combine "hot" but unelaborated devaluation, a concise narrative, apparently frank discussion of both positive and negative aspects of childhood attachment relationships, and an entertaining quality—a combination that provides a poor fit with other existing classifications and may erroneously lead to placement in the "earned-secure" subgroup (see Lyons-Ruth, Yellin, et al., 2005, for details). Both "hostile" and "helpless" subtypes may be seen. In the hostile subtype, one or more attachment figures are represented in globally devalued terms as hostile or malevolent, but there is also evidence of a competing positive representation of or continued identification with the same attachment figure. For example, one speaker said, "We were friends, ... we were enemies. We're just alike but we fought all the time." Individuals in this subgroup may describe themselves as very close to, in daily contact with, or "just like" one or more attachment figures, so that the attachment relationship itself is not consistently devalued. However, contradictory mental contents are seen in the juxtaposition of positive and globally devaluing evaluations of the same caregiver over the course of the interview. Theoretically, such a hostile adult state of mind is viewed as a potential outgrowth of a controlling/ punitive stance in childhood (see the discussion of controlling stances below).

In the helpless subtype, the participant globally devalues but also positively identifies with a helpless or parentally abdicating caregiver—for example, "We're best friends. ... She's a basket case" (see George & Solomon, Chapter 35, this volume). Individuals with a helpless state of mind may describe having adopted a vigilant and protective caregiving role toward the parent in childhood. Anger is inhibited or expressed in assertions that are not integrated with the more predominant caregiving attitude. Theoretically, a helpless state of mind in adulthood is viewed as a potential outgrowth of a caregiving attachment stance in childhood.

A "mixed" HH subtype is also commonly seen. Hostile and helpless subtypes are viewed theoretically as alternate expressions of a single underlying unbalanced HH model of dyadic relationships (Lyons-Ruth, Bronfman, & Atwood, 1999).

The infant and adult correlates of parental HH states of mind have been examined in three high-risk samples, all of them also coded independently with the Main and colleagues (2003) coding system. In the first study of HH states of mind among 45 mothers with high rates of childhood trauma, a mother's HH state of mind on the AAI was significantly related to the extent of disorganized attachment behavior displayed by her infant,

and HH classification explained a significant portion of variance in infant disorganization not accounted for by unresolved, fearfully preoccupied, and CC status (Lyons-Ruth, Yellin, et al., 2005). In addition, unresolved and HH states of mind were similarly good predictors of disorganized-secure infant behavior, but HH states of mind were stronger predictors of disorganized-avoidant or disorganized-ambivalent infant classifications (Lyons-Ruth, Yellin, et al., 2005). Severity of maternal trauma in childhood was related strongly to HH states of mind, but the experience of trauma itself did not directly predict infant disorganization in the absence of such states of mind (Lyons-Ruth, Yellin, Melnick, & Atwood, 2003).

In a second study, 62 mothers receiving treatment for methadone dependence were compared to 87 women in a nonaddicted matched control group (Finger, 2006; Melnick et al., 2008). An HH state of mind on the AAI was significantly associated with infant disorganization, even when unresolved status on the AAI was controlled for.

It was further proposed that HH states of mind would be especially prevalent among patients with BPD (Lyons-Ruth, Melnick, Patrick, & Hobson, 2007). Previous work with a sample of 12 adult outpatients with BPD and 11 with dysthymia had revealed that unresolved states of mind were more frequent in the BPD group (Patrick, Hobson, Castle, Howard, & Maughan, 1994). In the current work, significantly more women in the BPD group (100%) also displayed an HH state of mind, compared to 55% of the dysthymic group. In addition, patients with BPD made significantly more globally devaluing statements concerning attachment figures, and significantly more patients with BPD (75%, compared to 27% in the dysthymic group) conveyed that in childhood they had engaged in punitive or caregiving forms of controlling behavior toward parents. These results indicate that in addition to the previously described unresolved lapses while discussing loss or trauma, patients with BPD exhibit a pervasive lack of integration in affective evaluations of attachment figures.

In summary, rather than elaborating on current criteria for unresolved or CC categories, the HH codes appear to delineate new ways in which contradictory and pervasively unintegrated affective evaluations of attachment relationships may be displayed on the AAI and contribute to infant disorganization. This work suggests that not only experiences of unintegrated loss or trauma, but also pervasively unbalanced relationship patterns, may contribute to the intergenerational transmission of disorganization.

Caregiver–Infant Interaction, Parental States of Mind, and Infant Disorganization

Why are unresolved or HH states of mind in parents related to their infants' display of disorganized attachment behavior? In one theory of the etiology of infant disorganization, Main and Hesse (1990; Hesse & Main, 2006) have hypothesized that when the still-traumatized parent responds to memories or ideas related to loss or trauma, the parent may engage in inexplicably frightened or frightening behavior with the infant. Main and Hesse (1990) further theorized that some attachment figures engage in directly frightening behavior, ranging from creeping up from behind the infant and sliding both hands around the infant's neck and throat to incidents of physical or sexual abuse. Other attachment figures, however, appear frightened of their own infants. Main and Hesse (1990; Hesse & Main, 2006) describe frightened parental behaviors as including entrance into dissociative or trance-like states (e.g., freezing of all movement with a "dead" stare, unblinking); seeking safety and comfort from the infant (e.g., showing deferential behavior); and viewing the infant as the source of alarm (e.g., backing away, as one parent did, while stammering in an unusual and frightened voice, "D-don't follow me, d-don't"). Main and Hesse (1990; Hesse & Main, 2006) proposed that frightened parental behavior occurs spontaneously and is triggered internally, stemming from the parent's thoughts or from events or objects in the environment associated with their own traumatic and/or frightening experiences. According to these authors, the apparent inexplicability of such frightened parental behavior will inevitably be alarming to an infant.

A frightened or frightening attachment figure is thought to provoke conflict for the infant, because the attachment figure is "at once the source of and the solution to its alarm" (Main & Hesse, 1990, p. 163). Unable to maintain a single coherent strategy of approaching or fleeing, the infant shows disorganized and/or disoriented attachment behavior. Although Hesse and Main (2006) have specified that disorganized attachment behavior may stem from experiences other than frightened or frightening caregiving, the central conflict thought to distinguish disorganized infants from other insecurely attached infants is that they cannot find a solution

to the paradox of fearing the figure whom they must approach for comfort in times of stress.

Studies have not yet been conducted to examine whether an infant experiences a focused fear of a caregiver, such as might be indicated by disorganized infants displaying fearful expressions toward their parents more often than other infants do, or by cortisol elevations when the infant is exposed to such parental behavior. Studies are needed that differentiate a specific fear of the caregiver, which should activate attachment behavior whether or not separations have occurred, from parental failure to provide comfort for fear aroused by other sources, including separation.

Lyons-Ruth and her colleagues (Lyons-Ruth, Bronfman, & Atwood, 1999; Lyons-Ruth, Bronfman, & Parsons, 1999) have suggested that for the disorganized infant fear arises from a variety of sources, not simply from parental behavior, but the parent of a disorganized infant engages in disrupted and contradictory forms of affective communication around the infant's need for comfort (e.g., failing to comfort a distressed infant while asking tenderly, "What's the matter?"). In this view, disrupted parental responses to infant attachment behavior are extreme enough, and contradictory enough, that avoidant or ambivalent strategies cannot be organized in relation to the caregiver; that is, such strategies do not work well enough to maintain a modicum of proximity and protection. These disrupted and contradictory parental responses, in turn, generate complementary patterns of disorganized helpless and contradictory responses from the infant around the need for closeness and comfort.

Frightened or Frightening Parental Behavior, Unresolved States of Mind, and Infant Disorganization

Main and Hesse (1992, 2006) have developed six scales to identify subtypes of "frightened or frightening" (FR) parental behavior:

1. *Threatening.* Postures, facial expressions, and movements that appear aggressive—for example, sudden movements into the area immediately surrounding the infant's face and eyes.
2. *Frightened.* Behaviors indicating that a mother is inexplicably frightened—for example, a retreat sequence, as in pulling or backing away from the infant.
3. *Dissociative.* Indications of possible entrance into an altered state of consciousness, such as

stilling or freezing in trance-like postures or haunted voice tones.

4. *Timid or deferential*. Behavior in which the parent appears submissive to the infant, such as very timid or deferential handling of the infant.

5. *Spousal or romantic*. For example, excessive intimate or sexualized caressing of the baby.

6. *Disorganized*. Parental behavior fitting Main and Solomon's (1990) description of infant disorganized/disoriented behaviors.

Jacobvitz, Leon, and Hazen (2006), Schuengel, Bakermans-Kranenburg, and van IJzendoorn (1999), and Abrams, Rifkin, and Hesse (2006) examined FR behavior in studies that also included the AAI. Jacobvitz, Hazen, and Riggs (1997) and Jacobvitz and colleagues (2006) administered the AAI to 116 pregnant women and later observed them at home for 30–40 minutes interacting with their firstborn 8-month-olds. Mothers classified as unresolved with respect to loss and/or abuse displayed significantly higher levels of FR behavior with their infants at 8 months. However, mothers classified as unresolved did not differ significantly from other mothers on any other negative parenting interaction patterns observed in the mothers' homes, including maternal insensitivity, interference, or rejection (Jacobvitz et al., 2006). This difference between unresolved mothers and other mothers in FR behavior occurred regardless of whether the unresolved mothers were given a secondary secure or insecure AAI classification (Jacobvitz et al., 2006).

In a sample of 85 mother–child dyads, Schuengel and colleagues (1999) found a relation between maternal unresolved loss on the AAI when an infant was 12 months old and maternal display of FR behaviors toward the infant at 10 or 11 months. However, this finding occurred only among the subgroup of mothers classified as unresolved-insecure on the AAI (analogous to the disorganized-insecure infant subgroup). Schuengel and colleagues found that mothers classified as unresolved-insecure displayed significantly more frightened or frightening behavior than mothers classified as unresolved-secure.

Bowlby (1980) suggested that the earlier the loss and the closer the relationship with the person lost, the more difficult the resolution process might be. However, Ainsworth and Eichberg (1991) did not find a significant association between unresolved states of mind and either a mother's age

when the loss occurred or her relationship to the deceased (attachment figure vs. someone else). Replicating Ainsworth and Eichberg's study with a larger sample ($N = 116$), Jacobvitz and colleagues (2006) also found that a mother's age when the loss occurred was unrelated to her resolution of the loss, but they did find that mothers who were unresolved were more likely to have lost a parent than to have lost a less important figure. Moreover, both a mother's age when the loss occurred and the mother's relationship to the deceased discriminated between unresolved mothers who engaged in FR behavior toward their infants and those who did not. Ninety-one percent of unresolved mothers who either lost an attachment figure or were younger than 17 when the unresolved loss occurred engaged in FR behavior toward their infants. In contrast, only 20% of the unresolved mothers who were older than 16 when the loss occurred and did not lose an attachment figure displayed FR behavior. Therefore, kinship and timing of the loss may be important in predicting whether a mother's unresolved state of mind impinges on her caregiving behavior.

Abrams and colleagues (2006) were the first to explore associations between unresolved loss or trauma and particular subtypes of FR parental behavior. They studied a sample of 32 middle-class mother–infant and father–infant dyads. The six unresolved parents had significantly higher scores on the dissociative FR subscale than did the other parents. Interestingly, unresolved loss or trauma in the parents was not associated with any of the other FR subscales. Since mothers and fathers were combined and only six parents were classified as unresolved, this finding requires replication in a larger study.

Frightened or Frightening Parental Behavior and Disorganized Attachment Behavior

Studies in several countries provide evidence for Main and Hesse's (1990) hypothesis that maternal FR behavior is related to the *infant's* attachment disorganization, as well as to the parent's unresolved state of mind (Abrams et al., 2006; Jacobvitz, 2007; Lyons-Ruth, Bronfman, & Parsons, 1999; Schuengel et al., 1999; Tomlinson, Cooper, & Murray, 2005; True, Pasani, & Oumar, 2001). In the study by Schuengel and colleagues (1999), maternal FR behavior marginally predicted infant disorganized attachment. However, the subscale for maternal dissociative behavior more strongly predicted infant disorganized behavior, as did a broader set of maternal "disorganized" behaviors (Schuengel, van IJzendoorn, Bakermans-Kranenburg, & Blom, 1997). In light of this finding, it is notable that both Lyons-Ruth and Block (1996) and Schuengel and colleagues (1999) failed to find a relation between maternal scores on the Dissociative Experiences Scale and infant disorganization. Schuengel and colleagues (1997, 1999) did not examine maternal FR behavior separately for the two subgroups of disorganized infants, as they had for the two subgroups of unresolved mothers. It was also notable that the closeness of kin of the mother's experienced loss did not predict infant disorganization. Similarly, Jacobvitz (2007) reported a relation between mothers' FR behavior with their 8-month-old infants and infant disorganized attachment at 12 or 15 months.

The Abrams and colleagues (2006) study is the only study to date that has examined FR behavior in both father–infant (n = 25) and mother–infant (n = 50) dyads. Both maternal and paternal FR behavior was significantly related to attachment disorganization. Parents of disorganized infants received significantly higher scores on the threatening and dissociative FR scales. For mothers only, those who had disorganized infants scored higher on the disorganized FR scale. When all six FR subscales were considered simultaneously, only dissociative FR parental behavior uniquely predicted infant disorganization.

In the only high-risk study to date, Lyons-Ruth, Bronfman, and Parsons (1999) also found that FR behavior was significantly related to infant disorganization. When the two subgroups of disorganized infants were examined separately, however, only the mothers of disorganized-insecure infants differed significantly from mothers of infants with organized patterns of attachment, differing in particular on FR behavior. None of the FR scores differentiated infants with a disorganized-secure pattern of behavior. This finding paralleled Schuengel and colleagues' (1999) identification of elevated FR behavior only among mothers in the unresolved-insecure subgroup.

A study of 20 village-living mother–infant dyads in the Dogon ethnic group in Mali, Africa, provides preliminary support cross-culturally for a relationship between FR maternal behavior and attachment disorganization (True et al., 2001). Although none of the mothers scored above the midpoint on the overall FR scale, infants whose mothers scored above 1 on the scale were more often classified as disorganized in the Strange Situation.

In a recent meta-analysis of studies using the FR system, the combined effect size for the relation between unresolved attachment and FR behavior was r = .28 (N = 242). The combined effect size for the relation between FR and disorganized infant attachment was r = .32 (N = 325) (Madigan, Bakermans-Kranenburg, et al., 2006).

Disrupted Parental Affective Communication, Parental States of Mind, and Infant Disorganized Attachment

Lyons-Ruth, Bronfman, and Parsons (1999) expanded on Main and Hesse's construct of "fright without solution" to develop a coding system for disrupted forms of affective communication between parent and infant—the Atypical Maternal Behavior Instrument for Assessment and Classification (AMBIANCE). This coding system includes aspects of caregiving behavior not included in the FR system that are also theoretically related to unmodulated infant fear and attachment disorganization. Lyons-Ruth and colleagues reasoned that maternal unavailability to comfort the infant should lead to unmodulated infant fear and contradictory approach–avoidance behavior, whether or not the mother herself is the source of fear. Caregiver nonresponse to infant fearful arousal can take a variety of forms, including negative intrusive or self-referential responses at moments of infant need, dissociative or withdrawing behavior, or contradictory cues as to the caregiver's availability. Accordingly, five broad dimensions of disrupted parental affective communication with the infant are assessed:

1. *Negative-intrusive behavior*. For example, mocking or teasing the infant.
2. *Role confusion*. For example, reassurance elicited from the infant at time of reunion.
3. *Withdrawal*. For example, silent interaction with the infant.
4. *Affective communicative errors*. Contradictory cues or nonresponse to clear infant cues, such as verbal invitation for the infant to approach followed by physical distancing.
5. *Disorientation* (from Main & Hesse, 1992, 2006). For example, unusual changes in pitch and intonation of voice when interacting with the infant.

Lyons-Ruth, Bronfman, and Parsons (1999) used the AMBIANCE system to code disrupted affective communication in the Strange Situation at

18 months among 65 mother–infant dyads. Level of disrupted communication significantly predicted infant attachment disorganization. In addition, with all FR behaviors excluded from the computations, the frequency of disrupted communications still significantly predicted infant disorganization. This suggests that FR behavior is occurring within a broader matrix of disturbed communication between mother and child. Only 17% of maternal behaviors coded on the AMBIANCE in this study were FR behaviors.

As with the FR codes, when the two infant disorganized subgroups were examined, only mothers of infants in the disorganized-insecure subgroup showed significantly higher rates of disrupted communication, including negative-intrusive behavior, affective communication errors, and role confusion. However, mothers of disorganized-secure infants were found to be significantly more withdrawing from the infant than were mothers of disorganized-insecure infants, without showing higher levels of frightening, intrusive, dissociated, or role-reversed behavior (Lyons-Ruth, Bronfman, & Parsons, 1999).

The association between maternal disrupted affective communication and attachment disorganization has been replicated by researchers in several countries (Gervai et al., 2007; Goldberg, Benoit, Blokland, & Madigan, 2003; Grienenberger, Kelly, & Slade, 2005; Madigan, Moran, & Pederson, 2006). Studying adolescent mothers and their 12-month-olds, Madigan, Moran, and colleagues (2006) assessed disrupted communication in two post-Strange Situation play sessions, the first without toys and the second with a standard set of toys. Mothers of infants classified as disorganized scored higher on disrupted communication than did mothers of organized infants in the play-without-toys condition. Following these mother–child dyads over the next year, Forbes, Evans, Moran, and Pederson (2007) assigned attachment classifications to toddlers. Disrupted communication at 24 months was associated with concurrent assessments of attachment disorganization. Moreover, change in disrupted communication predicted change in disorganization from 12 to 24 months. When maternal AAI classifications were considered among these dyads, Madigan, Moran, Schuengel, Pederson, and Otten (2007) further found a robust relation between disorganization and maternal disrupted communication rated in play sessions among 45 adolescent mothers who were not classified as unresolved on the AAI.

Therefore, the AMBIANCE may be helpful in identifying dyads at risk who do not exhibit lapses of monitoring when discussing loss or trauma on the AAI. The authors also demonstrated that disorganized attachment mediated a significant relation between disrupted maternal communication and behavior problems assessed at 24 months.

In a middle-income sample of 45 mother–infant dyads, Grienenberger, Kelly, and Slade (2005) found that mothers who were assigned low AMBIANCE scores on disrupted maternal communication were more likely to have securely attached infants. However, high scores on disrupted communication did not differentiate infants classified as disorganized ($n = 10$) from those classified as resistant ($n = 4$). Interestingly, disrupted maternal behavior partially mediated the relation between a mother's reflective functioning—that is, her capacity to consider her child's subjective intentions, and infant attachment disorganization (see Fonagy, Gergely, & Target, Chapter 33, and Slade, Chapter 32, this volume, for more discussion of reflective functioning).

In another low-risk sample ($N = 197$), Goldberg and colleagues (2003) found that mothers who showed high levels of disrupted communication with their infants during the Strange Situation more often had infants who were classified as disorganized (62%) than secure (32%). It is important to note, however, that a sizable number (32%) of secure infants in this large sample had mothers who displayed high levels of disrupted behavior. Furthermore, disrupted affective communication did not mediate the relation between unresolved attachment and attachment disorganization. Finally, Gervai and colleagues (2007), in a low-risk Hungarian sample of 96 infants, also reported a significant relation between levels of disrupted communication and infant disorganization. A meta-analysis of the published studies using the AMBIANCE (Madigan, Bakermans-Kranenburg, et al., 2006) has confirmed a significant relation between maternal disrupted communication and unresolved classification on the AAI ($r = .20$, $N = 311$), and between maternal disrupted communication and infant disorganization ($r = .35$, $N = 384$). In addition, stability of the AMBIANCE over periods ranging from 18 to 60 months was high ($r = .56$, $N = 203$).

Taylor and colleagues (2000) have advanced the hypothesis that gender differences occur in responses to threat. Whereas "fight–flight" responses are stronger among males in response to threat, "tend–befriend" responses are stronger among females. David and Lyons-Ruth (2005) assessed this hypothesis in relation to frightening or withdrawing maternal behavior in a high-risk sample. Maternal behavior did not differ by infant gender (Lyons-Ruth, Bronfman, & Parsons, 1999). Consistent with the hypothesis, however, infant gender interacted significantly with maternal behavior: When maternal frightening or withdrawing behavior was high, female infants were more likely than male infants to continue to approach mothers at reunion and were less likely to show disorganized conflict behavior. Males, in contrast, showed more disorganized conflict behavior and avoidance to high levels of frightening or withdrawing behavior. Since gender differences have not been observed in low-risk samples, gender differences in response to threat may emerge only in the context of more frightening or abandoning maternal behavior. Because of girls' tendencies to continue to approach a frightening or withdrawing caregiver, boys' disorganized attachment responses were more reliable indicators of the quality of the parent–infant interaction than were girls' attachment responses.

Finally, in an innovative extension of work using the AMBIANCE, Crawford and Benoit (in press) developed criteria for coding the five dimensions of maternal disrupted affective communication at a representational rather than a behavioral level on the Working Model of the Child Interview (Zeanah, Benoit, & Barton, 1986). Among 35 dyads, mothers' level of disrupted communication at the representational level in the third trimester of pregnancy significantly forecast their infants' disorganization at 12 months, as well as mothers' levels of observed disrupted communication with their infants at 12 months, and their own unresolved classification on the AAI at 12 months. Due to the small sample size, however, this work needs replication in other samples.

In summary, across all the literature (12 studies, 851 families), infants whose parents displayed anomalous behavior (i.e., FR or AMBIANCE) were 3.7 times more likely to display disorganized attachment behavior than other infants ($r = .34$; Madigan, Bakermans-Kranenburg, et al., 2006). In addition, it appears that the patterning of parental behavior within the disorganized spectrum may take quite different forms. Future work is needed to explore whether different correlates and developmental pathways characterize infants whose parents are more dissociative, more withdrawn, or more pervasively frightening.

It is important to note that ratings of maternal insensitivity (made with Ainsworth's sensitivity–insensitivity scale) have not been associated with attachment disorganization in infancy. In a meta-analysis of 12 studies, van IJzendoorn and colleagues (1999) reported no significant association between disorganized attachment in infants and ratings of parental insensitivity. The sensitivity–insensitivity scale, which is a global rating of maternal caregiving, does not appear to be specific enough about the affective communications involved in fear-related behavior to predict infant disorganization.

Unfortunately, few studies have examined relations between disorganized attachment strategies at 1 year and characteristics of infant and maternal affective communication in the first 6 months of life. In one exception, Tomlinson and colleagues (2005) assessed maternal depression and caregiving behavior of 147 mothers with their infants at 2 and 18 months in a periurban settlement in Cape Town, South Africa. Maternal depression at 2 months and all three maternal behavior codes—sensitivity, maternal remote/disengaged behaviors, and maternal intrusive coerciveness—assessed at 2 and 18 months predicted infant disorganization. However, examining predictor variables together in the same model revealed that only remote/disengaged and intrusive maternal behavior at 2 months uniquely predicted attachment disorganization at 18 months. Jaffe, Beebe, Feldstein, Crown, and Jasnow (2001) found that "hypervigilant" tight vocal rhythm tracking by both mother and baby at 4 months of age, combined with the baby's postural and visual avoidance, was a predictor of attachment disorganization at 12 months. They postulated that hypervigilance was an indicator of maternal stress or anxiety. Jaffe and colleagues also found that babies who became disorganized at 12 months showed more vocal and facial distress at 4 months. In addition, Kelly, Ueng-Hale, Grienenberger, and Slade (2003) found that maternal disrupted communication rated in a face-to-face play assessment with the infant at 4 months of age predicted disorganized attachment behavior at 1 year.

It will now be critical to explore further whether disrupted or FR behavior begins early in the first year. In addition, it will be important to assess whether these early parent–infant interactive processes affect the infant's stress physiology, and whether there are particular early physiological adaptations that precede and predict the emergence of behavioral disorganization in relation to the caregiver by the end of the first year.

Interaction between Genes and Quality of Parental Care in Disorganized Attachment Behavior

Several potential models of gene–environment interaction have received support in recent studies of disorganized attachment, including a diathesis–stress model and a differential susceptibility-to-care model. A diathesis–stress model would posit that genetic vulnerability to stress makes some infants more vulnerable to insensitive care than others. In a low-risk sample (N = 96), Spangler and Zimmermann (2007) investigated the interaction between maternal responsiveness and the serotonin transporter polymorphism (5HTTLPR) in relation to infant disorganization. The serotonin transporter polymorphism is related to the regulation of fear and anxiety (e.g., Caspi et al., 2002; Hariri, 2006). They found that infants who carried the short form of the polymorphism were significantly more likely to display disorganization at 12 months, but that this genetic effect was evident only among infants whose mothers were low in responsiveness. No genetic effect was evident among infants of highly responsive mothers. Maternal genotype was not evaluated as a potential correlate of both maternal responsiveness and infant genotype.

van IJzendoorn and Bakermans-Kranenburg (2006) explored a diathesis–stress model in relation to the DRD4 polymorphism. Dopamine is a neurotransmitter related to reward processing and to attention-deficit/hyperactivity disorder, and the long variant of the DRD4 polymorphism (the DRD4 7-repeat allele) has been related to less efficient dopamine function (for a review, see Swanson et al., 2000). In a middle-income sample of 63 mothers who had experienced a significant loss, the authors did not find a relation between the DRD4 polymorphism and infant disorganization; nor did the interaction between maternal FR behavior and the DRD4 polymorphism predict infant disorganized attachment. There was also no main effect of maternal FR behavior on infant disorganization, as found in previous research (Madigan, Bakermans-Kranenburg, et al., 2006), mitigating the likelihood of finding genetic moderation (should it exist).

Using the same sample, van IJzendoorn and Bakermans-Kranenburg (2006) also examined relations among maternal unresolved attachment, infant DRD4 polymorphism, and infant disorganized attachment. There was no overall effect of

maternal unresolved loss on infant disorganization in this sample; maternal unresolved attachment was associated with infant disorganization only when the infant carried the long allele of the DRD4 gene. The patterning of this interaction term was also consistent with a diathesis–stress hypothesis. Maternal genotype was not assessed as a potential correlate of both maternal unresolved status and infant disorganization.

In a sample of 138 mother–infant dyads, 42 of whom were socioeconomically at risk, Gervai and colleagues (2007) examined whether the interaction between disrupted mother–infant affective communication (assessed with the AMBIANCE) and the DRD4 7-repeat allele predicted infant disorganized attachment. Consistent with the literature, there was a significant main effect of maternal disrupted communication on infant disorganization, but no main effect of infant DRD4 genotype. However, infant genotype significantly interacted with maternal disrupted communication. The pattern of the interaction supported a differential susceptibility-to-care model rather than a diathesis–stress model. The more common and efficient short allele conferred the expected sensitivity to maternal affective communication, with a strong relation (r = .56) between quality of maternal communication and infant disorganization. Among infants with the less efficient long allele, however, the relation between maternal communication and infant disorganization was not significant, suggesting less sensitivity to the reward value of maternal cues in this group. Maternal DRD4 genotype was also assessed and found to be unrelated both to maternal disrupted communication and to infant disorganization.

To date, no studies of disorganized attachment have found a pattern of interaction effects consistent with an environmental override model. In this model, genetic effects are expressed in low-risk environments but overridden by environmental factors in high-risk settings (e.g., Turkheimer, Haley, Waldron, D'Onofrio, & Gottesman, 2003).

Should the gene–environment interaction effects described above prove reliable with replications, a more complex model of genetic effects will be needed than the model of main effects reviewed in an earlier section of this chapter. In particular, infant genetic factors may interact differently with maternal state of mind and with quality of maternal affective communication, producing some of their nonshared variance in relation to infant disorganization (the "transmission gap"; van IJzendoorn, 1995). Given the wide spectrum of maternal and infant behavior encompassed within the disorganized spectrum, the presence of specific risk groups with different genetic and environmental contributors would not be surprising.

DISORGANIZED/CONTROLLING BEHAVIOR IN PRESCHOOL AND MIDDLE CHILDHOOD

In a study of 33 families, Main and Cassidy (1988) developed an assessment of parent–child attachment at age 6. Children's behavioral and verbal responses to a reunion with a parent after an hourlong separation were classified into four categories that corresponded to the four infant attachment classifications: "secure-confident," "insecure-avoidant," "insecure-ambivalent," and "insecure-controlling." Children were classified as insecure-controlling if they "seem to actively attempt to control or direct the parent's attention and behavior and assume a role which is usually considered more appropriate for a parent with reference to a child" (Main & Cassidy, 1988, p. 418; see Solomon & George, Chapter 18, this volume). Two prospective longitudinal studies in low-risk samples documented a shift from disorganized behavior with the mother during infancy to disorganized/controlling behavior of either a punitive or a caregiving type at age 6 (Main & Cassidy, 1988; Wartner, Grossmann, Fremmer-Bombik, & Suess, 1994). Combining data from the two studies, van IJzendoorn and colleagues (1999) reported a strong association ($r = .55$) between attachment disorganization in infancy and later controlling attachment behavior in low-risk settings. Studies exploring correlates of controlling/disorganized attachment behavior after infancy are summarized in Table 28.1 and are reviewed in subsequent sections.

Age, Gender, and Disorganized/Controlling Behavior

Gender differences have not generally been obtained in the prevalence of disorganized/controlling attachment behavior (for an exception at age 3, see NICHD Early Child Care Research Network, 2001); nor have gender differences been reported in the types of controlling attachment behaviors displayed (caregiving vs. punitive), although small N's limit the power of the latter analyses. In relation to age, Moss, Cyr, and Dubois-Comtois (2004) found that at age 3, two-thirds of the preschoolers classified as disorganized/controlling in their

middle-income sample displayed disorganized behavior rather than controlling behavior. However, at age 6, two-thirds of the disorganized/controlling group displayed controlling behavior. As Moss and her colleagues noted, one possible explanation for this developmental shift is that older preschoolers' increased role-taking capacities facilitate the development of controlling behavior among formerly disorganized infants.

Disorganized/Controlling Attachment Patterns and Cognitive Correlates

Bowlby's (1969/1982) formulation of the complementary relations between attachment and exploration predicts that continued activation of the attachment system will inhibit exploration of the environment. Several studies have demonstrated associations between disorganized/controlling attachment patterns and the quality of children's cognitive functioning. In a 10-year study assessing 85 Icelandic children at ages 7, 9, 12, 15, and 17, Jacobsen, Edelstein, and Hofmann (1994) examined the association between attachment security on a representational measure at age 7 and later cognitive functioning. On the subset of formal operational measures that assessed syllogistic reasoning, disorganized/controlling children differed significantly from other secure and insecure children from ages 9 to 17, and these differences remained when self-confidence, IQ, and attention problems were included in the analyses. Disorganized/controlling children were particularly likely to give contradictory responses on these tasks, compared to children in other attachment groups, and disorganized/controlling adolescents as a group never reached the formal operational level. These results need replication, however, because of the small number of disorganized/controlling participants ($n = 6$).

These difficulties with cognitive functioning suggest that disorganized children may be at risk for academic problems. Moss and colleagues (Moss, Rousseau, Parent, St.-Laurent, & Saintonge, 1998; Moss & St.-Laurent, 2001; Moss, St.-Laurent, & Parent, 1999) found that despite the similarity in IQ between 5- to 7-year-old children classified as disorganized/controlling and those in other attachment groups, controlling children showed the poorest school performance at 5–7 years and at 7–9 years. Moreover, controlling children had low academic self-esteem and metacognitive deficits at ages 5–7 and demonstrated poorer math performance and difficulty becoming cognitively en-

TABLE 28.1. Longitudinal Outcomes of Disorganization in Infancy and Correlates of Controlling/Disorganized Behavior in Preschool and Elementary School: Studies since 1998

Reference	Children's ages	Assessment methods/instruments	Outcomes and correlates of disorganization
Carlson (1998)	18, 24, and 42 months; 4½–5 years; grades 1, 2, 3, 6; 17½ years	Strange Situation; birth complications; Neonatal Behavioral Assessment Scale; Carey Infant Temperament Questionnaire; observations of mother–child interactions; preschool behavior problem index; teachers' completion of Child Behavior Checklist (CBCL) and emotional health rank; Kiddie Schedule of Affective Disorders and Schizophrenia (K-SADS)	Less confident with mother (24 months); avoidance of mother (42 months); dissociation and internalizing behavior (grades 1, 2, 3, 6); lower emotional health rank (grades 1, 2, 3, 6); overall behavior problems, internalizing problems, and dissociative symptoms (17½ years); and higher ratings of psychopathology in general and dissociation specifically on the K-SADS (17½ years)
Hazen, Jacobvitz, Allen, Higgins, & Jin (in press)	12 and 15 months; 7 years	Strange Situation; CBCL	Internalizing behavior problems; externalizing problems, social problems, and thought problems for boys, but not girls, classified as disorganized during infancy
Jacobvitz & Hazen (1999)	18, 20, 24, 30, 36, 42, and 54 months	Strange Situation; observations of mother–child and father–child interactions, of family dinners, of interactions with two different peers, and of peer interactions in preschool classrooms	Emergence of controlling behavior between 24 and 30 months; timing linked to severity of disorganization in infancy; fearful/disorganized behavior, emotional disconnection, and aggression toward peers
Main, Hesse, & Kaplan (2005)	1 year; 6 years; 19 years	Strange Situation; Main & Cassidy 6-year reunion; Adult Attachment Interview (AAI) at age 19	Secure vs. insecure attachment at 1 year predicted attachment security at age 19; controlling behavior at 6 years predicted attachment disorganization at age 19
Madigan, Goldberg, Moran, & Pederson (2004)	2 years; 7 years	Strange Situation; family drawings	Family drawings scored high on family chaos, bizarreness, disorganization, carelessness, uneasiness, and dysfunction; naive observers reacted with less positive and more negative emotions to the drawings
Moss, Bureau, Cyr, Mongeau, & St.-Laurent (2004)	3–5 years; 5–7 years	Main and Cassidy 6-year reunion; observations of mother–child interactions; questionnaires completed by parents and teachers, including the Preschool Socio-Affective Profile, CBCL, Parenting Stress Index, Life Experiences Survey, Beck Depression Inventory, and Dyadic Adjustment Scale	Unbalanced mother–child interactions predicted controlling patterns; controlling/caregiving behavior predicted internalizing problems; controlling/punitive behavior predicted externalizing patterns; controlling patterns and maternal depression were unrelated
Moss, Rousseau, Parent, St.-Laurent, & Saintonge (1998)	5–7 years; 9–11 years	Main and Cassidy 6-year reunion; observations of mother–child interactions; questionnaires completed by parents and teachers, including the Social Behavior Questionnaire, CBCL, Parenting Stress Index, and Beck Depression Inventory	Controlling/other children were at the highest risk for externalizing and internalizing problems across the age periods

(continued)

TABLE 28.1. *(continued)*

Reference	Children's ages	Assessment methods/instruments	Outcomes and correlates of disorganization
Moss et al. (2006)	5–7 years; 9–11 years	Main and Cassidy 6-year reunion measure; during middle childhood, Social Behavior Questionnaire (teacher report), CBCL (teacher report), and Dominic Questionnaire (child report) of internalizing and externalizing behaviors	Insecure-ambivalent and insecure-controlling children scored higher on composite (teacher, mother, and child) measure of externalizing problems; only controlling children scored higher on composite measure (teacher and mother report) of internalizing problems and child report of internalizing problems.
Moss & St.-Laurent (2001)	5–7 years; 9–11 years	Main and Cassidy 6-year reunion measure; observation of a joint planning task; Goal Orientation Questionnaire; school grades in language and math; child IQ	School underachievement; poor cognitive engagement
Paulo-Pott, Pott, & Beckmann (2007)	4, 8, 12, and 30 months	Observational ratings of temperament at 4, 8, and 12 months; Strange Situation; Mannheim Parent Interview	Ratings of child negative emotionality over the first year combined with attachment disorganization was marginally related to behavior problems at 30 months
Weinfeld, Whaley, & Egeland (2004)	3, 6, 24, and 42 months; 6, 13, and 19 years	Strange Situation; infant temperament; maternal personality; parenting attitudes; maternal depression; life stress; Home Observation for Measurement of the Environment; parent–child observations at 24 and 42 months and 13 years; AAI at age 19	Disorganized infants were more often insecure and unresolved at age 19, even after early maltreatment was controlled for

gaged in a problem-solving task at ages 7 to 9. In a recent follow-up of these children, Bureau, Moss, and St.-Laurent (2006) reported that the punitive subgroup of controlling children were evaluated by teachers as having poorer academic performance than secure children in middle childhood, even after the children's sex, IQ, and family socioeconomic status were controlled for. The association between disorganized/controlling attachment and mathematics performance disappeared after the researchers controlled for children's self-confidence regarding schoolwork.

Disorganized/Controlling Attachment Behavior and Parental Internal Models

Several researchers have reported an association between controlling/disorganized behavior in childhood and maternal unresolved loss or trauma as assessed on the AAI (George & Solomon, 1996; Greenberg, Speltz, DeKlyen, & Endriga, 1991). A recent study of 43 mothers and 6-year-olds in Sap-

poro, Japan, demonstrated a 77% match between mothers' unresolved or CC status on the AAI and their children's disorganized/controlling classification on the 6-year reunion measure (Behrens, Hesse, & Main, 2007).

George and Solomon (1996) also developed a semistructured Caregiving Interview, probing mothers' relationships to their 6-year-olds. They found that a helpless parental stance on this interview was related to children's controlling attachment behavior. In some cases this helpless stance involved failing to provide reassurance and protection to a child, while in other cases the helpless stance included fear either of the child or of their own loss of control in relation to the child. Others described feeling that the child was in control of the relationship, because of either the child's precocious capabilities or his or her unmanageability. Moreover, 62% of parents with unresolved loss or trauma described their relationships with their children in helpless terms. Helpless stances on this interview have not yet been related to disorganized attachment behavior in infancy, however (see also George & Solomon, Chapter 35, this volume).

Disorganized/Controlling Attachment Patterns and Children's Internal Representations of Attachment Figures

As described earlier, infants are thought to display disorganized attachment behavior because they are unable to obtain adequate comfort for fearful arousal from their caregivers, either because the caregivers themselves are alarming or because they cannot adequately soothe their infants. Several studies examining children's depictions of themselves and caregivers show that significantly more children classified as disorganized in infancy display fright without solution at age 6 on story tasks. Kaplan (see Main et al., 1985) administered her Separation Anxiety Test (SAT; Kaplan, 1987) to children in the Berkeley sample to assess the children's responses to drawings of parent–child separations. The responses of children classified as disorganized in infancy were more likely to be coded as fearful and disorganized, as indicated by remaining silent, elaborating fearful or passive themes, or engaging in catastrophic fantasies.

In another middle-income sample, 69 kindergartners were asked to respond to a set of doll-play stories about attachment-related themes (Solomon, George, & De Jong, 1995). Compared to other children, those classified as controlling depicted themselves as helpless and their caregivers as frightening more often. Such helplessness at kindergarten age is theoretically compatible with the collapse of attachment strategies seen among disorganized children as infants.

Finally, Madigan, Goldberg, Moran, and Pederson (2004) examined the family drawings of 7-year-old high-risk children previously classified as disorganized in infancy. Compared to the drawings produced by the rest of the sample, the drawings of these children were rated higher on scales measuring disorganization, carelessness, family chaos, bizarreness, uneasiness, and dysfunction. Moreover, these drawings evoked less positive and more negative reactions from naive observers (untrained college students) than did the drawings made by children in the other attachment groups.

Disorganized/Controlling Attachment Patterns and the Development of Peer Relationships

Most studies of the relation between attachment disorganization and peer interaction have relied on behavior problem checklists completed by mothers and/or teachers, as shown in Table 28.1. Only a few studies have obtained ratings of friendship quality from the peers themselves or from trained observers (Cohn, 1990; Jacobvitz & Hazen, 1999; Wartner et al., 1994). In one cross-sectional study of 40 children, trained observers rated 6-year-olds classified as disorganized/controlling as less competent in the quality of their play and ability to resolve conflict than secure children. However, ratings of these children's friendship quality did not differ from those of avoidant children (Wartner et al., 1994). In another cross-sectional study, in which ratings of peer liking, sociometric status, and peer nominations were obtained from the children themselves, disorganized/controlling children did not differ from the other attachment groups (Cohn, 1990). However, contrary to other studies, nine children who were considered disorganized-unclassifiable were eliminated from the study, creating a small and possibly unrepresentative group of children in the disorganized/controlling category.

Few studies have examined the development of peer relationships among children classified as disorganized in infancy. As part of a larger longitudinal study, Jacobvitz and Hazen (1999) followed 66 infants with attachment classifications at 18 months. Mother–child, father–child, and peer interactions were videotaped when the children were 20, 26, 32, 44, and 56 months old, in play, cleanup (parent–child), and problem-solving (parent–child) situations. In addition, at all five ages, children were videotaped in their day care classrooms and in dyadic play and cleanup with two different peers identified by their teachers as "friends." Preschoolers classified as secure, avoidant, or resistant in infancy behaved in similar ways with the two different peers. However, based on case study data, children classified as disorganized at 18 months were observed to act quite differently with one peer as compared to another at both the 44- and 56-month assessments. For example, one child spent much of his time with one peer trying to annoy him, whereas the same child did not interact at all with the other peer and progressively withdrew. Jacobvitz and Hazen proposed that disorganized children may be more likely than other children to carry unintegrated models of the same caregiver into their interactions with peers, so that they draw on different models with different peers. Children who took longer to establish a more consistently controlling pattern with their caregivers also took longer to sustain peer interactions, even aggressive or passive interchanges.

Disorganized/Controlling Attachment Patterns and the Development of Behavior Problems

Kochanska (2001) observed the emotional development of disorganized infants at 22 and 33 months. Consistent with earlier findings linking infant attachment disorganization with later aggression, a substantial increase in anger was found from 22 to 33 months, and by 33 months (but not earlier), disorganized infants showed higher levels of anger than infants classified as avoidant, resistant, or secure.

Consistent with more recent work (e.g., Hazen, Jacobvitz, Allen, Higgins, & Jin, in press), van IJzendoorn and colleagues (1999), in a meta-analysis of 12 studies ($N = 734$) of both normative and high-risk samples, found that children classified as disorganized (with the infant, preschool, or school-age assessment procedures) were more likely than other children to have aggressive and externalizing behavior problems during preschool and early school age, with a combined effect size of $r = .29$. Researchers have also noted increased risk for internalizing problems for this group during childhood and adolescence (Carlson, 1998; Moss, Bureau, Cyr, Mongeau, & St.-Laurent, 2004; Moss, Cyr, & Dubois-Comtois, 2004). In the NICHD Study of Early Child Care, following more than 1,000 children from birth through preschool, kindergarten, and first grade, children who had been classified as avoidant or disorganized at 15 months were rated by their teachers as showing more internalizing behaviors than other children (NICHD Early Child Care Research Network, 2006). Dissociative symptomatology has also been investigated as a longitudinal outcome of early disorganization. Carlson (1998) found that disorganization in infancy was related to teacher reports of dissociation, internalizing behavior, and poorer overall emotional health in grades 1, 2, and 3.

Recent work has examined differential correlates of the three disorganized/controlling subtypes at preschool age (punitive, caregiving, and behaviorally disorganized). After child sex, IQ, and socioeconomic status were controlled for, the punitive subtype of attachment was a significant predictor of children's externalizing behavior at ages 4, 5, and 8 (Moss et al., 2006). Analyses of behavior problem profiles revealed significantly higher rates of internalizing behavior problems for the caregiving subgroup than for secure children. For the behaviorally disorganized subgroup, by age 8 a significant difference on the externalizing scale was found in comparison with the secure group. These results converge with previous findings indicating concurrent maladaptive behavior among children with a behaviorally disorganized profile in the preschool years (Cicchetti & Barnett, 1991; Teti, 1999). Moss, Bureau, St.-Laurent, and Tarabulsy (in press) also found that parents of caregiving children were more likely to have experienced a loss, whereas parents of behaviorally disorganized children engaged in more marital conflicts.

Longitudinal antecedents of the three disorganized subgroups also appear to be different. Bureau, Easterbrooks, Killam, Miranda, and Lyons-Ruth (2007), in a high-risk sample of 43 children, found that children with higher behaviorally disorganized scores at age 8 were significantly more likely to come from families who were clinically referred in infancy for concerns about quality of infant care. In addition, behaviorally disorganized children produced more disorganized representations of attachment relationships on the SAT (Kaplan, 1987) at age 8. Higher punitive scores at age 8 were associated with higher levels of maternal disrupted affective communication in infancy, with disorganized classifications on the SAT, and with greater child unresponsiveness in a free-play session with mother at age 8. Higher caregiving scores at age 8 were associated with greater maternal withdrawal in infancy on the AMBIANCE, and with more child overresponsive behavior to mother in free play.

Additional work is needed to track the developmental pathways associated with controlling/disorganized forms of attachment behavior beyond the early school years. Almost nothing is known about the forms these behaviors take across the transitions from middle childhood to adolescence and from adolescence to adulthood. It is also of particular interest to explore whether controlling strategies may allow more advantageous behavioral and hypothalamic–pituitary–adrenocortical axis functioning than occurs among children who continue to exhibit behaviorally disorganized attachment responses.

ATTACHMENT DISORGANIZATION IN ADOLESCENCE AND YOUNG ADULTHOOD

Adolescent and Young Adult Outcomes Associated with Earlier Disorganization

Dissociation is one internalizing symptom that has been related to early disorganized attachment strategies both theoretically and empirically. Liotti (1992) has pointed out the phenotypic similarity between the unintegrated quality of disorganized behaviors in infancy and the unintegrated nature of dissociated mental states in adulthood, and has proposed that disorganization in infancy will increase a child's vulnerability to later altered states or dissociative disorders (e.g., trance states, multiple personality disorder/dissociative identity disorder, and experiences of depersonalization and derealization).

Empirical support for Liotti's hypothesis comes from a prospective longitudinal study following a low-income sample of 129 children from birth to age 17½ (Carlson, 1998). Infants classified as disorganized at 12 and 18 months of age (vs. the other infants) more often displayed dissociative behavior in high school, as reported by teachers on the Teacher Report Form of the CBCL and by the adolescents themselves on the Kiddie Schedule of Affective Disorders and Schizophrenia at age 17½.

Ogawa, Sroufe, Weinfield, Carlson, and Egeland (1997) further explored this hypothesis by studying the same sample from infancy to age 19. From a wide array of potential predictors from infancy to middle childhood, including measures of sexual and physical abuse, the best predictors of symptoms on the Dissociative Experiences Scale (Bernstein & Putnam, 1986) at age 19 were disorganized attachment at 12–18 months and mothers' psychological unavailability from 0 to 24 months. Experience of sexual or physical abuse did not continue to predict dissociative symptoms after the quality of early caregiving was accounted for. Only in elementary school did the occurrence of physical abuse add to the explained variance in dissociative symptoms.

The most surprising aspect of both these findings is that the prediction from infancy to adolescence was direct; it was not mediated by a number of other well-chosen variables, such as the incidence of abuse or childhood behavior problems, which would be expected to "carry forward" or mediate relations between infant disorganization and later adaptation. Instead, the early caregiving relationship appears to create a broader vulnerability to dissociative symptoms than is captured by later assessments of childhood risk factors and symptoms.

Ogawa and colleagues (1997) also compared scores on the Dissociative Experiences Scale of young adults classified as disorganized during infancy who had not faced trauma (n = 10); young adults classified as disorganized during infancy who were faced with later trauma (n = 35); and other young adults not previously classified as disorganized (n = 83). This group was not further divided by trauma history. A significant elevation in dissociation scores was found only among those who were both disorganized and had experienced trauma. It is also notable that 78% of those classified as disorganized during infancy had experienced later trauma. This high rate suggests that caregiving environments associated with infant disorganization also place an infant at risk for further exposure to trauma or loss. However, the preceding multivariate analyses had already established that the effect of trauma on dissociation was better accounted for by the earlier history of maternal emotional unavailability.

In a second study of dissociative symptoms among 56 young adults followed prospectively from infancy (Dutra, Bureau, Holmes, Lyubchik, & Lyons-Ruth, 2008; Dutra & Lyons-Ruth, 2005), the three measures of quality of care accounted for half of the variance (50%) in dissociation after gender and demographic risk were controlled for. Within the quality-of-early-care cluster, level of disrupted communication in the lab, mothers' lack of positive affective involvement at home, and mothers' flatness of affect at home significantly predicted dissociative symptoms in young adulthood. Infant disorganization in itself was not significantly related to later dissociation. Only extent of verbal abuse in childhood and adolescence, but not physical or sexual abuse or witnessed violence, added to the prediction of dissociation once quality of early care was considered. As in the Ogawa and colleagues (1997) study, then, quality of parent–infant interaction before 24 months of age was a stronger predictor of dissociative symptoms than later maltreatment experiences.

Other papers from the Minnesota Study of Risk and Adaptation from Birth to Adulthood examining predictors of depression, anxiety disorders, substance abuse, and antisocial behavior in late adolescence did not report on the relation with disorganized attachment in infancy (Aguilar, Sroufe, Egeland, & Carlson, 2000; Bosquet & Egeland, 2006; Duggal, Carlson, Sroufe, & Egeland, 2001; Siebenbruner, Englund, Egeland, & Hudson, 2006). However, contributions of the compromised quality of early care were found in all of these studies, as compared to a specific contribution of infant disorganized attachment behavior. Bureau, Easterbrooks, and Lyons-Ruth (in press) also examined prospective predictors from infancy to depressive symptoms in late adolescence. Mothers' depressive symptoms in infancy, but not in childhood or young adulthood, predicted young adult depression, but infant attachment did not add to the model. Sroufe, Egeland, Carlson, and Collins (2005) concluded from the pattern of Minnesota results that the overall context of early care is quite important for later development.

Continuity of Disorganized Attachment into Adolescence and Young Adulthood

Whereas attachment assessments in infancy and childhood have focused primarily on direct observation of parent–child interaction, attachment assessments in adolescence and adulthood have relied on the AAI (see Allen, Chapter 19; Crowell, Fraley, & Shaver, Chapter 26; and Hesse, Chapter 25, this volume). However, early studies of adolescent attachment used low-risk samples and did not code for unresolved attachment status (e.g., Kobak & Sceery, 1988). In addition, most studies of adolescent attachment began in adolescence, so the relation between measures of attachment in infancy or childhood and adolescent attachment on the AAI could not be evaluated.

In one adolescent-to-adult longitudinal study, Allen, Hauser, and Borman-Spurrell (1996) followed a cohort of psychiatrically hospitalized adolescents and their controls longitudinally from age 14. Maternal behaviors promoting adolescent autonomy and relatedness at age 14 predicted coherence of transcript on the AAI 11 years later. However, attachment classifications in adulthood, including unresolved status, were not predicted by autonomy and relatedness in adolescence.

The very few attachment-oriented longitudinal studies extending from infancy to adolescence have used the AAI to index attachment in late adolescence. Most of these longitudinal samples have involved low-risk cohorts with a low incidence of disorganized attachment (Grossmann et al., 2002; Hamilton, 2000; Waters, Merrick, Treboux, Crowell, & Albersheim, 2000). However, two longitudinal studies have examined continuity and discontinuity in attachment disorganization from infancy to age 19 (Main, Hesse, & Kaplan, 2005; Sampson, 2004; Weinfeld, Whaley, & Egeland, 2004) and age 26 (Sroufe et al., 2005). In their low-income sample, Weinfeld and colleagues (2004) found that infants classified as disorganized (n = 42) were more likely to be classified as insecure (either dismissing or preoccupied) and less likely to be classified as autonomous on the AAI at age 19 than participants who were classified as organized in their attachment during infancy (n = 83). Eighty-six percent of the infants classified as disorganized were later considered insecure on the AAI. The lack of specificity from infant disorganization to unresolved status at age 19 occurred partly because of the atypical distribution of attachment classifications on the AAI, with 55% classified as dismissing and only 15% as unresolved, despite the high-risk nature of the sample.

By age 26, infants classified as disorganized were more likely to be classified as unresolved on the AAI in the high-risk Minnesota study (Sroufe et al., 2005). In addition, among low-risk families, Main and colleagues (2005) reported a significant tendency for infants classified as disorganized to be placed in the unresolved category at age 19. Weinfeld and colleagues (2004) reported that when they used the highest score on the nine-point infant disorganization scale and included only participants who experienced loss or abuse, infant disorganization was significantly associated with unresolved abuse at age 19, but not with unresolved loss. Continuity between disorganized/controlling behavior at age 6 and insecure attachment at age 19 has also been reported (Main et al., 2005). Ninety percent of the children who were classified as disorganized/controlling based on the 6-year reunion measure were insecure on the AAI at age 19.

Changes in attachment security over time have also shown significant correlates (Waters, Weinfeld, & Hamilton, 2000). Correlates of change in attachment security have included composite measures of attachment-related life events, as well as separate assessments of maltreatment, caregiver depression, parental life stress, and quality of family interaction (Egeland & Sroufe, 1981; Schneider-Rosen, Braunwald, Carlson, & Cicchetti, 1985; Weinfeld, Sroufe, & Egeland, 2000).

Assessment of Attachment in Adolescence

The above-noted limitations in using the AAI with high-risk adolescents and young adults may also stem from the AAI coding issues noted earlier—namely, that if adolescents with a history of attachment disorganization in infancy and controlling patterns in preschool do not report loss or abuse on the AAI, they cannot be judged unresolved/disorganized in young adulthood. In addition, they would not be expected to transmit disorganized attachment patterns to their own infants. This has been termed a "transmission block" in the developmental model pertaining to disorganization of attachment (Hennighausen & Lyons-Ruth, 2005).

Therefore, an important conceptual and methodological problem arises: How should we assess disorganized attachment in adolescence and young adulthood? One approach to this dilemma is to move away from sole reliance on narrative assessments and develop a direct observational measure of the attachment strategies used by adolescents when interacting with their parents. The advantage of observational measures is that they are conceptually and methodologically much closer to *in vivo* assessment of how adolescents regulate attachment-oriented affects in the parent–adolescent dialogue itself. Availability of such an observational measure would also allow a more direct assessment of how disorganized and controlling behavioral patterns continue over time or change during adolescence.

A goal-corrected partnership or secure base in adolescence has been conceptualized as a sense of freedom to explore thoughts and feelings with parents in a collaborative way (Allen et al., 1996; Kobak & Sceery, 1988). Similar to earlier observational assessments of attachment that focus on children's behavior when their attachment system is activated, secure-base behavior during adolescence may become most salient during times of negotiation, conflict, and stress.

Four high-risk longitudinal studies have examined aspects of parent-adolescent interaction theoretically related to disorganization. In the Minnesota longitudinal study, adolescent–parent interaction across a series of tasks was observed at age 13 and coded on a number of attachment-related scales. Parents and adolescents (175 mothers and 44 fathers/father substitutes) were asked to plan an antismoking campaign or an antishoplifting campaign designed to appeal to teenagers; each teenager was directed to help a parent put together objects while the parent was blindfolded, and the pair was asked to discuss a hypothetical question and to complete a Q-set of the ideal person. In the 44 families with two parents present, the three family members were asked to arrive at a joint solution for a hypothetical problem involving the teen and to plan a vacation together. These videotaped tasks were rated on a number of scales for engagement, affect, conflict, conflict resolution, role/boundary maintenance, and balance in the relationship. Parent–child boundary dissolution at age 13 predicted change in behavior problems between grade 6 and age 16 (Hiester, 1993; Nelson, 1994). Parental hostility at age 13 also discriminated heavy drinkers at age 16 (Englund, Hudson, & Egeland, 2003; Sroufe et al., 2005).

In the second study, a coding system was developed for assessing adolescent–parent goal-corrected partnership, to be applied to a 10-minute revealed-differences procedure in which the parent and adolescent discuss an area of disagreement (the Goal-Corrected Partnership in Adolescence Coding System [GPACS]; Lyons-Ruth, Hennighausen, & Holmes, 2005). Criteria for attachment classifications in adolescence, including several variants of disorganized/controlling behavior, were specified based on 12 rating scales indexing parent and adolescent collaborative communication, warmth, role confusion, disorientation, odd out-of-context behavior, and hostility. In an initial validity study, the coding system was applied in a stratified random sample of 40 psychiatrically hospitalized and nonhospitalized adolescents and their families, selected from the larger study of Allen and colleagues (1996). At age 14, adolescents and their parents had completed an audiotaped conflict resolution task in which they discussed their differing opinions regarding solutions to moral dilemmas. At age 25, previously coded AAIs were available from the study database. Transcripts of the audiotapes were classified by evaluators using the GPACS classifications who were unaware of all other data from the study. A significant four-way correspondence (73%; kappa = .57) was obtained. Correspondence was to be obtained between each category individually, from the four GPACS categories assessed at age 14 (facilitating, deflecting, entangled, and disorganized/controlling) to the corresponding four AAI categories assessed at age 25 (secure, dismissing, preoccupied, and unresolved/CC) (Hennighausen, Bureau, David, & Lyons-Ruth, in press).

In a third study of 104 low-income young adults, parents and young adults were videotaped in a 5-minute unstructured reunion and a 10-minute discussion of an area of disagreement in their relationship. Controlling/caregiving forms of adolescent–parent attachment relationships coded on the GPACS were significantly related to extent of borderline features, and to suicidality/self-injury in particular, displayed in young adulthood on the Structured Clinical Interview for DSM-IV, Axis II. Controlling/caregiving attachment patterns were not related either to depressive diagnoses or to antisocial features, demonstrating discriminant validity for this caregiving pattern. The variance in borderline features related to controlling/caregiving attachment was independent of variance related to later abuse. Thus directly observed adolescent–parent interactions revealed a paradoxical relation between hypervigilant management of the relationship within the dyad, but impulsive and self-damaging behavior displayed outside the dyad (Lyons-Ruth, Bureau, Henninghausen, & Holmoes, in press).

A final study by Kobak and his colleagues (Kobak, Lyons-Ruth, Zajac, & Rosenthal, 2007; Kobak & Zajac, 2006) assessing 166 low-income adolescents longitudinally from 13 to 15 years of age also found that adolescent–parent interaction on the GPACS, assessed in a parent–teen conflict discussion task at age 13, predicted increases in problem behavior by age 15. In that study, the 12 GPACS continuous scales were factored into four factors indexing adolescent–parent collaborative communication, caregiving/role reversal, hostility, and odd/disoriented behavior. In particular, caregiving/role reversal ratings at age 13 predicted increases in impulsive self-damaging behavior by age 15, including substance abuse and risky sexual behavior, particularly among boys.

SUMMARY AND IMPLICATIONS

Main and Solomon's (1990) identification of a disorganized attachment pattern in infancy has opened up new ground for understanding the interface between development and psychopathology. Disorganized attachment behavior is one of the few predictors of later psychopathology that have been identified as early as infancy among biologically normal individauals. Although parental psychopathology, low socioeconomic status, and other indices of low-resource family environments also predict elevated rates of psychopathology, these are distal processes that need more proximal mediating mechanisms to explain psychopathology in a child.

One of the most important recent developments reviewed in this chapter is the further validation of coding systems for assessing parental behavior related to infant disorganization. FR or disrupted maternal behavior has received meta-analytic support from more than 12 studies as a correlate of both infant disorganization and maternal lack of resolution of loss or trauma. The availability of these validated instruments opens an array of theoretical issues for further exploration. One important set of questions concerns whether there are specific kinds of disruption in early communication (such as frightening vs. dissociative vs. withdrawn patterns) that foster specific kinds of child developmental difficulties in cognitive investment, affect regulation, interpersonal func-

tioning, and self- or other-damaging behavior. Conversely, are some forms of disrupted or FR behavior more characteristic of parents with particular clinical characteristics, such as BPD or depression? Arriving at more specific characterizations of such potential subgroups of parents and children in the disorganized spectrum will be important to the development of more specific interventions for particular forms of caregiving risk.

Another important question raised in recent work is whether the quality of parental behavior associated with infant disorganization is a more stable factor, and hence is more predictive of later outcomes, than infant disorganization itself (e.g., Ogawa et al., 1997; NICHD Early Child Care Research Network, 2006; Sroufe et al., 2005). Conversely, is an additive model that includes both infant behavior and parental behavior a better fit to the data than the use of parental behavior alone (e.g., Ogawa et al., 1997)? Further multivariate modeling is needed to evaluate which models best apply to which domains of development.

A third important question to be addressed with these new measures of parental behavior is the question of gene–environment interaction in the genesis and maintenance of disorganized attachment relationships. Since the first edition of this handbook was published, animal models have definitively demonstrated the impact of quality of early care on gene expression (e.g., Francis et al., 1999). Such findings call for the careful assessment of early care to be given priority in human studies of gene–environment interaction. Recent research reviewed here is beginning to explore such interaction effects, although the literature is still too meager to yield a body of replicated findings.

As can also be seen from this review, the relation between attachment disorganization and later outcomes is complex. In work to date, disorganized attachment processes are early predictors of both internalizing and externalizing forms of psychopathology from infancy into school age. As such, attachment disorganization is likely to index a broad relational contribution to maladaptation and psychopathology that cuts across conventional diagnostic categories and interacts with individual biological vulnerability to contribute to a range of psychiatric disorders.

However, as pointed out in this chapter, our understanding of attachment processes and longitudinal trajectories is particularly weak in middle childhood and adolescence. In an effort to address these gaps, recent work has produced new observational coding systems for disorganized and controlling forms of parent–child interaction in middle childhood and adolescence, and has begun to relate these forms of interaction to the emergence of impulsive, self-damaging forms of problem behavior, including risky sexual behavior, substance abuse, and suicidality.

One notable omission in the reviewed literature is a more explicit developmental framework for understanding shifts and reorganizations in the expression of disorganized attachments. With the extension of research on disorganization into later childhood and adolescence, developmental factors need to be more strongly integrated into the theoretical framework for understanding attachment processes. As developmental challenges are engaged during particular periods, we would expect that opportunities for reorganization would be more likely to arise (Sroufe et al., 2005). This clearly seems to be the case in the shift from disorganized to predominantly controlling presentations from infancy to childhood. To some extent, such developmental transformations have been anticipated and taken account of in the construction of the attachment measures themselves. Thus any finding of "continuity" from one age to another should be understood not as continuity in a phenotypic presentation across ages, but as continuity at a broader organizational level in the lack of integration and coherence underlying a child's representations and interactions. Nevertheless, more attention should be paid to how new developmental capacities interact with such unintegrated mental states to transform the child's approach to regulating fearful arousal at both relational and representational levels.

Although predictors of disorder are of great social importance, we should not lose sight of the likelihood that disorganized and controlling attachment behavior constitutes an advantageous adaptation to particular family and social circumstances. Consistent with evolutionary arguments advanced by Belsky (2005) and Hrdy (2005), these adaptations may contribute to the survival of the kinship group as a whole, while still generating considerable biological and social costs for the individual. Decreasing maternal commitment to a particular child may be adaptive for a single mother with few social and emotional resources to invest. In turn, the child's taking over direction of the parent–child relationship through controlling attachment strategies may contribute to the care of the parent and the larger family group. Enhanced parental functioning, in turn, may benefit the child. In addition, controlling attachment

strategies ensure that parental attention and interaction will occur, even if fear modulation or actual protection remains seriously compromised. Thus, in very-low-resource environments, child disorganized/controlling strategies may be adaptive both for the individual and the family unit as a whole from an evolutionary perspective, even though they are costly to the child in terms of physiological regulation of stressful arousal and integration of mental states.

We would like to call the reader's attention to related work reviewed by Berlin, Zeanah, and Lieberman (Chapter 31, this volume), in which recent randomized controlled intervention trials provide strong experimental evidence that disorganized attachment processes are amenable to change. Among both depressed middle-income mothers and low-income maltreating mothers, thoughtful and sustained interventions (>40 sessions) were associated with significant reductions in infant disorganized attachment relative to randomized untreated controls (Cicchetti et al., 2006; Toth et al., 2006). Contrary to expectations, however, intervention models expected to produce change in maternal representationals were not more effective than those aimed at improving parent–child interactions (Cicchetti et al., 2006); this finding suggests that a relatively broad array of intensive intervention formats may be effective. Despite the success of these models, however, the mechanisms contributing to the changes—such as changes in caregiver representations or interaction patterns—have not yet been identified. Therefore, the next generation of intervention work should carefully evaluate the mechanisms mediating such changes in disorganized attachment. In particular, the new methods of assessing FR or disrupted parent–infant interaction were not available at the time these studies were designed. However, changes in these aspects of parent–child interaction would constitute one candidate for a mediating mechanism with strong theoretical and empirical grounding.

Finally, given exciting new advances in neuroscience, we need to understand the dynamic interplay between neurobiological and behavioral attachment processes. With the advent of neurobiological assessment, adequate measurement of attachment outcomes may need to include physiological measures, as well as behavioral and representational assessments. Differing biological vulnerabilities interacting with differing experiences of loss, abuse, and/or chronically hostile or neglecting relationships may lead to quite different biobehavioral developmental trajectories and adult outcomes. In summary, with the current confluence of neurobiological, genetic, and relational assessments, there is now the potential to delineate many of the interactions between biological and relational processes that contribute to the emergence of child and adult psychopathology. Disorganized attachment processes are likely to play a prominent role in those developmental trajectories.

REFERENCES

Abrams, K., Rifkin, A., & Hesse, E. (2006). Examining the role of parental frightened/frightening subtypes in predicting disorganized attachment within a brief observational procedure. *Development and Psychopathology, 18,* 344–362.

Aguilar, B., Sroufe, L. A., Egeland, B., & Carlson, E. (2000). Distinguishing the early-onset/persistent and adolescent-onset antisocial behavior types: From birth to 16 years. *Development and Psychopathology, 12,* 109–132.

Ainsworth, M. D. S., Blehar, M., Waters, E., & Wall, S. (1978). *Patterns of attachment: A psychological study of the Strange Situation.* Hillsdale, NJ: Erlbaum.

Ainsworth, M. D. S., & Eichberg, C. G. (1991). Effects on infant–mother attachment of mother's unresolved loss of an attachment figure or other traumatic experience. In C. M. Parkes, J. Stevenson-Hinde, & P. Marris (Eds.), *Attachment across the life cycle* (pp. 160–183). London: Routledge.

Allen, J. P., Hauser, S. T., & Borman-Spurrell, E. (1996). Attachment theory as a framework for understanding sequelae of severe adolescent psychopathology: An 11-year follow-up study. *Journal of Consulting and Clinical Psychology, 64,* 254–263.

Bakermans-Kranenburg, M. J., & van IJzendoorn, M. H. (2004). No association of dopamine D4 receptor (DRD4) and–521 C/T promoter polymorphisms with infant attachment disorganization. *Attachment and Human Development, 6,* 211–218.

Behrens, K. Y., Hesse, E., & Main, M. (2007). Mothers' attachment status as determined by the Adult Attachment Interview predicts their 6-year-olds' reunion responses: A study conducted in Japan. *Developmental Psychology, 43,* 1553–1567

Belsky, J. (2005). The development and evolutionary psychology of intergenerational transmission of attachment. In S. Carter, L. Ahnert, K. E. Grossmann, S. Hrdy, M. Lamb, S. Porges, et al. (Eds.), *Attachment and bonding: A new synthesis* (pp. 269–301). Cambridge, MA: MIT Press.

Bernstein, E. M., & Putnam, F. W. (1986). Development, reliability, and validity of a dissociation scale. *Journal of Nervous and Mental Disease, 174,* 1769–1782.

Bokhorst, C. L., Bakermans-Kranenburg, M. J., Fearon, R. M. P., van IJzendoorn, M. H., Fonagy, P., & Schuengel, C. (2003). The importance of shared environment in mother–infant attachment security: A behavioral genetic study. *Child Development, 74,* 1769–1782.

Boris, N. W., Hinshaw-Fuselier, S. S., Smyke, A. T., Sheeringa, M. S., Heller, S. S., & Zeanah, C. H. (2004). Comparing criteria for attachment disorders: Establishing reliability and validity in high-risk samples. *Journal of the American Academy of Child and Adolescent Psychiatry, 45,* 568–577.

Bosquet, M., & Egeland, B. (2006). The development and maintenance of anxiety symptoms from infancy through adolescence in a longitudinal sample. *Development and Psychopathology, 18,* 517–550.

Bowlby, J. (1969/1982). *Attachment and loss: Vol. 1. Attachment.* New York: Basic Books.

Bowlby, J. (1973). *Attachment and loss: Vol. 2. Separation: Anxiety and anger.* New York: Basic Books.

Bowlby, J. (1980). *Attachment and loss: Vol. 3. Loss: Sadness and depression.* New York: Basic Books.

Bureau, J.-F., Easterbrooks, M. A., Killam, S., Miranda, C., & Lyons-Ruth, K. (2007, March). *Behavioral manifestations of attachment disorganization and role-reversal in middle childhood: Validity of a new coding system.* Paper presented at the biennial meeting of the Society for Research in Child Development, Boston.

Bureau, J.-F., Easterbrooks, M. A., & Lyons-Ruth, K. (in press). Maternal depressive symptoms in infancy: Unique contribution to children's depressive symptoms in childhood and adolescence? *Development and Psychopathology.*

Bureau, J.-F., Moss, E., & St.-Laurent, D. (2006, June). The roles of attachment and individual and familial processes in the prediction of academic and cognitive functioning. In F. Lamb-Parker (Chair), *Attachment, adult–child relationships, and affect regulation: Contributions to children's later cognitive, social, and behavioral competence.* Symposium conducted at the Head Start Eighth National Research Conference, Washington, DC.

Carlson, E. A. (1998). A prospective longitudinal study of attachment disorganization/disorientation. *Child Development, 69,* 1107–1128.

Carlson, V., Cicchetti, D., Barnett, D., & Braunwald, K. (1989). Disorganized/disoriented attachment relationships in maltreated infants. *Developmental Psychology, 25,* 525–531.

Caspi, A., McClay, J., Moffitt, T. E., Mill, J., Martin, J., Craig, I. W., et al. (2002). Role of genotype in the cycle of violence in maltreated children. *Science, 297,* 851–854.

Cicchetti, D., & Barnett, D. (1991). Attachment organization in maltreated preschoolers. *Development and Psychopathology, 3,* 397–411.

Cicchetti, D., Rogosch, F. A., & Toth, S. L. (2006). Fostering secure attachment in infants in maltreating families through preventative interventions. *Development and Psychopathology, 18,* 623–649.

Cohn, D. A. (1990). Child–mother attachment of six-year-olds and social competence at school. *Child Development, 61,* 152–162.

Crawford, A., & Benoit, D. (2007, March). Caregivers' disrupted representations of their unborn child predict later infant–caregiver disorganized attachment and disrupted interactions. *Infant Mental Health Journal.*

Crittenden, P. M. (1985). Maltreated infants: Vulnerability and resilience. *Journal of Child Psychology and Psychiatry, 26,* 85–96.

David, D., & Lyons-Ruth, K. (2005). Differential attachment responses of male and female infants to frightening maternal behavior: Tend or befriend versus fight or flight? *Infant Mental Health Journal, 26,* 1–18.

Dozier, M., Manni, M., Gordon, M. K., Peloso, E., Gunnar, M. R., Stovall-McClough, K. C., et al. (2006). Foster children's diurnal production of cortisol: An exploratory study. *Child Maltreatment, 2,* 189–197.

Duggal, S., Carlson, E. A., Sroufe, L. A., & Egeland, B. (2001). Depressive symptomatology in childhood and adolescence. *Development and Psychopathology, 13,* 143–164.

Dutra, L., Bureau, J. F., Holmes, B., Lyubchik, A., & Lyons-Ruth, K. (2007). *Prospectively assessed infancy and childhood predictors of dissociative symptoms in young adulthood.* Manuscript under review.

Dutra, L., & Lyons-Ruth, K. (2005, April). Maltreatment, maternal and child psychopathology, and quality of early care as predictors of adolescent dissociation. In J. Borrelli (Chair), *Interrelations of attachment and trauma symptoms: A developmental perspective.* Symposium conducted at the biennial meeting of the Society for Research in Child Development, Atlanta, GA.

Egeland, B., & Farber, E. A. (1984). Infant–mother attachment: Factors related to its development and changes over time. *Child Development, 55,* 753–771.

Egeland, B., & Sroufe, L. A. (1981). Developmental sequelae of maltreatment in infancy. In R. Rizley & D. Cicchetti (Eds.), *Developmental perspectives in child maltreatment* (pp. 77–92). San Francisco: Jossey-Bass.

Englund, M., Hudson, K., & Egeland, B. (2003, April). *Common pathways to heavy alcohol use and abstinence in adolescence.* Paper presented at the biennial meeting of the Society for Research in Child Development, Tampa, FL.

Finger, B. (2006). *Exploring the intergenerational transmission of attachment disorganization.* Unpublished doctoral dissertation, University of Chicago.

Finkel, D., & Matheny, A. P., Jr. (2000). Genetic and environmental influences on a measure of infant attachment security. *Twin Research, 3,* 242–250.

Fonagy, P., Leigh, T., Steele, M., Steele, H., Kennedy, G., Mattoon, M., et al. (1996). The relation of attachment status, psychiatric classification, and response to psychotherapy. *Journal of Consulting and Clinical Psychology, 64,* 22–31.

Forbes, L. M., Evans, E. M., Moran, G., & Pederson, D. R. (2007). Change in atypical maternal behavior predicts change in attachment disorganization from 12 to 24 months in a high-risk sample. *Child Development, 78,* 955–971.

Francis, D. D., Champagne, F. A., Liu, D., & Meaney, M. J. (1999). Maternal care, gene expression, and the development of individual differences in stress reactivity. *Annals of the New York Academy of Sciences, 896,* 66–84.

George, C., Kaplan, N., & Main, M. (1984). *Adult Attachment Interview protocol.* Unpublished manuscript, University of California at Berkeley.

George, C., Kaplan, N., & Main, M. (1985). *Adult Attachment Interview protocol* (2nd ed.). Unpublished manuscript, University of California at Berkeley.

George, C., Kaplan, N., & Main, M. (1996). *Adult Attachment Interview protocol* (3rd ed.). Unpublished manuscript, University of California at Berkeley.

George, C., & Main, M. (1979). Social interaction of young abused children: Approach, avoidance, and aggression. *Child Development, 50,* 306–318.

George, C., & Solomon, J. (1996). Representational models of relationships: Links between caregiving and attachment. *Infant Mental Health Journal, 17,* 198–216.

Gervai, J., Nemoda, Z., Lakatos, K., Ronai, Z., Toth, I., Ney, K., et al. (2005). Transmission disequilibrium tests confirm the link between DRD4 gene polymorphism and infant attachment. *American Journal of Medical Genetics: Part B. Neuropsychiatric Genetics, 132B,* 126–130.

Gervai, J., Novak, A., Lakatos, K., Toth, I., Danis, I., Ronai, Z., et al. (2007). Infant genotype may moderate sensitivity to maternal affective communications: Attachment disorganization, quality of care, and the DRD4 polymorphism. *Social Neuroscience, 2,* 1–13.

Goldberg, S., Benoit, D., Blokland, K., & Madigan, S. (2003). Atypical maternal behavior, maternal representations, and infant disorganized attachment. *Development and Psychopathology, 15,* 239–257.

Greenberg, M. T., Speltz, M. L., DeKlyen, M., & Endriga, M. C. (1991). Attachment security in preschoolers with and without externalizing behavior problems: A replication. *Development and Psychopathology, 3,* 413–430.

Grienenberger, J. F., Kelly, K., & Slade, A. (2005). Maternal reflective functioning, mother–infant affective communication, and infant attachment: Exploring the link between mental states and observed caregiving behavior in the intergenerational transmission of attachment. *Attachment and Human Development, 7,* 299–311.

Grossmann, K., Grossmann, K. E., Fremmer-Bombik, E., Kindler, H., Scheuerer-Englisch, H., & Zimmermann, P. (2002). The uniqueness of the child–father attachment relationship: Fathers' sensitive and challenging play as a pivotal variable in a 16-year longitudinal study. *Social Development, 11,* 307–331.

Hamilton, C. (2000). Continuity and discontinuity of attachment from infancy through adolescence. *Child Development, 71,* 690–694.

Hariri, A. R. (2006). Genetically driven variation in serotonin function: Impact on amygdala reactivity and individual differences in fearful and anxious personality. In T. Canli (Ed.), *Biology of personality and individual differences* (pp. 295–313). New York: Guilford Press.

Hazen, N., Jacobvitz, D., Allen, S., Higgins, K., & Jin, M. K. (in press). Pathways from disorganized attachment to later social-emotional problems: The role of gender and parent–child interaction patterns. In J. Solomon & C. George (Eds.), *Attachment disorganization* (2nd ed.). New York: Guilford Press.

Hennighausen, K., Bureau, J.-F., David, D., & Lyons-Ruth, K. (in press). Attachment disorganization in adolescence. In J. Solomon & C. George (Eds.), *Attachment disorganization* (2nd ed.). New York: Guilford Press.

Hennighausen, K., & Lyons-Ruth, K. (2005). Disorganization of behavioral and attentional strategies toward primary attachment figures: From biologic to dialogic processes. In S. Carter, L. Ahnert, K. E. Grossmann, S. Hrdy, M. Lamb, S. Porges, et al. (Eds.), *Attachment and bonding: A new synthesis* (pp. 269–301). Cambridge, MA: MIT Press.

Hertsgaard, L., Gunnar, M., Erickson, M. F., & Nachmias, M. (1995). Adrenocortical response to the Strange Situation in infants with disorganized/disoriented attachment relationships. *Child Development*, *66*, 1100–1106.

Hesse, E. (1996). Discourse, memory, and the Adult Attachment Interview: A note with emphasis on the emerging cannot classify category. *Infant Mental Health Journal*, *17*, 4–11.

Hesse, E., & Main, M. (2006). Frightened, threatening, and dissociative parental behavior in low-risk samples: Description, discussion, and interpretations. *Development and Psychopathology*, *18*, 309–343.

Hesse, E., & van IJzendoorn, M. (1998). Parental loss of close family members and propensities toward absorption in offspring. *Developmental Science*, *1*, 299–305.

Hesse, E., & van IJzendoorn, M. (1999). Propensities towards absorption are related to lapses in the monitoring of reasoning or discourse during the Adult Attachment Interview: A preliminary investigation. *Attachment and Human Development*, *1*, 67–91.

Hiester, M. (1993). *Generational boundary dissolution between mothers and children in early childhood and early adolescence: A longitudinal study.* Unpublished doctoral dissertation, University of Minnesota.

Hobson, R. P., Patrick, M., Crandell, L., García-Pérez, R., & Lee, A. (2005). Personal relatedness and attachment in infants of mothers with borderline personality disorder. *Development and Psychopathology*, *17*, 329–347.

Hrdy, S. (2005). Evolutionary context of human development: The cooperative breeding model. In S. Carter, L. Ahnert, K. E. Grossmann, S. Hrdy, M. Lamb, S. Porges, et al. (Eds.), *Attachment and bonding: A new synthesis* (pp. 269–301). Cambridge, MA: MIT Press.

Hughes, P., Turton, P., Hopper, E., McGauley, G. A., &

Fonagy, P. (2001). Disorganized attachment behavior among infants born subsequent to stillbirth. *Journal of Child Psychology and Psychiatry*, *42*, 791–801.

Insel, T. R. (2003). Is social attachment an addictive disorder? *Physiology and Behavior*, *79*, 351–357.

Ivarsson, T. (2008). Obsessive–compulsive disorder in adolescence: An AAI perspective. In H. Steele & M. Steele (Eds.), *Clinical applications of the Adult Attachment Interview* (pp. 213–235). New York: Guilford Press.

Jacobsen, T., Edelstein, W., & Hofmann, V. (1994). A longitudinal study of the relation between representations of attachment in childhood and cognitive functioning in childhood and adolescence. *Developmental Psychology*, *30*, 112–124.

Jacobvitz, D. (2007, April). *Parental correlates of attachment disorganization in infancy.* Paper presented at a preconference at the biennial meeting of the Society for Research in Child Development, Boston.

Jacobvitz, D., & Hazen, N. (1999). Developmental pathways from infant disorganization to childhood peer relationships. In J. Solomon & C. George (Eds.), *Attachment disorganization* (pp. 127–159). New York: Guilford Press.

Jacobvitz, D., Hazen, N., & Riggs, S. (1997, April). *Disorganized mental processes in mothers, frightening/frightened caregiving, and disoriented/disorganized behavior in infancy.* Paper presented at the biennial meeting of the Society for Research in Child Development, Washington, DC.

Jacobvitz, D., Leon, K., & Hazen, N. (2006). Does expectant mothers' unresolved trauma predict frightening/frightened maternal behavior?: Risk and protective factors. *Development and Psychopathology*, *18*, 363–379.

Jaffe, J., Beebe, B., Feldstein, S., Crown, C. L., & Jasnow, M. D. (2001). Rhythms of dialogue in infancy: Coordinated timing in development. *Monographs of the Society for Research in Child Development*, *66*(2, Serial No. 265).

Kaplan, N. (1987). *Individual differences in 6-year-olds' thoughts about separation: Predicted from attachment to mother at age 1.* Unpublished doctoral dissertation, University of California at Berkeley.

Kelly, K., Ueng-McHale, J., Grienenberger, J., & Slade, A. (2003, April). *Atypical maternal behavior and their relation to infant attachment disorganization.* Poster presented at the biennial meeting of the Society for Research in Child Development, Tampa, FL.

Kobak, R. R., Lyons-Ruth, K., Zajac, K., & Rosenthal, N. (2007). *Adolescent–caregiver attachment: Adaptation and risk in an economically disadvantaged sample.* Manuscript submitted for publication.

Kobak, R. R., & Sceery, A. (1988). Attachment in late adolescence: Working models, affect regulation and representations of self and others. *Child Development*, *59*, 135–146.

Kobak, R. R., & Zajac, K. (2006, March). *Attachment and psychopathology among economically disadvantaged teens: The contribution of interviews and teen–parent in-*

teractions. Paper presented at the annual meeting of the Society for Research in Adolescence, San Francisco.

Kochanska, G. (2001). Emotional development in children with different attachment histories: The first three years. *Child Development, 72,* 474–490.

Lakatos, K., Nemoda, Z., Toth, I., Ronai, Z., Ney, K., Sasvari-Szekely, M., et al. (2002). Further evidence for the role of the dopamine D4 receptor gene (DRD4) in attachment disorganization: Interaction of the III exon 48 bp repeat and the–521 C/T promoter polymorphisms. *Molecular Psychiatry, 7,* 27–31.

Lakatos, K., Toth, I., Nemoda, Z., Ney, K., Sasvari-Szekely, M., & Gervai, J. (2000). Dopamine D4 receptor (DRD4) gene polymorphism is associated with attachment disorganization. *Molecular Psychiatry, 5,* 633–637.

Lamb, M. E., Thompson, R. A., Gardner, W., & Charnov, E. L. (1985). *Infant–mother attachment.* Hillsdale, NJ: Erlbaum.

Levine, S., Wiener, S. G., & Coe, C. L. (1993). Temporal and social factors influencing behavioral and hormonal responses to separation in mother and infant squirrel monkeys. *Psychoneuroendocrinology, 18,* 297–306.

Liotti, G. (1992). Disorganized/disoriented attachment in the etiology of the dissociative disorders. *Dissociation, 5,* 196–204.

Lyons-Ruth, K., & Block, D. (1996). The disturbed caregiving system: Relations among childhood trauma, maternal caregiving, and infant affect and attachment. *Infant Mental Health Journal, 17,* 257–275.

Lyons-Ruth, K., Bronfman, E., & Atwood, G. (1999). A relational diathesis model of hostile-helpless states of mind: Expressions in mother–infant interaction. In J. Solomon & C. George (Eds.), *Attachment disorganization* (pp. 33–69). New York: Guilford Press.

Lyons-Ruth, K., Bronfman, E., & Parsons, E. (1999). Maternal frightened, frightening, or atypical behavior and disorganized infant attachment patterns. In J. I. Vondra & D. Barnett (Eds.), Atypical patterns of infant attachment: Theory, research, and current directions. *Monographs of the Society for Research in Child Development, 64*(3, Serial No. 258), 67–96.

Lyons-Ruth, K., Bureau, J., Hennighausen, K., & Holmes, B. (2008). *Disorganized/controlling attachment behavior among young adults: Relations to borderline features and suicidality/self-injury.* Manuscript submitted for publication.

Lyons-Ruth, K., Bureau, J.-F., Riley, C., & Atlas-Corbett, A. (in press). Socially indiscriminate attachment behavior in the Strange Situation: Convergent and discriminant validity in relation to caregiving risk, later behavior problems, and attachment insecurity. *Development and Psychopathology.*

Lyons-Ruth, K., Connell, D. B., Grunebaum, H. U., & Botein, S. (1990). Infants at social risk: Maternal depression and family support services as mediators of infant development and security of attachment. *Child Development, 61,* 85–98.

Lyons-Ruth, K., Connell, D., Zoll, D., & Stahl, J. (1987). Infants at social risk: Relations among infant maltreatment, maternal behavior, and infant attachment behavior. *Developmental Psychology, 23,* 223–232.

Lyons-Ruth, K., Hennighausen, K., & Holmes, B. (2005). *Goal-Corrected Partnership in Adolescence Coding System (GPACS): Coding manual, Version 2.* Unpublished manuscript, Harvard Medical School.

Lyons-Ruth, K., Lyubchik, A., Wolfe, R., & Bronfman, E. (2002). Parental depression and child attachment: Hostile and helpless profiles of parent and child behavior among families at risk. In S. Goodman & I. Gotlib (Eds.), *Children of depressed parents: Alternative pathways to risk for psychopathology* (pp. 89–121). Washington, DC: American Psychological Association.

Lyons-Ruth, K., Melnick, S., Patrick, M., & Hobson, R. P. (2007). A controlled study of hostile-helpless states of mind among borderline and dysthymic women. *Attachment and Human Development, 9,* 1–16.

Lyons-Ruth, K., Yellin, C., Melnick, S., & Atwood, G. (2003). Childhood experiences of trauma and loss have different relations to maternal unresolved and hostile-helpless states of mind on AAI. *Attachment and Human Development, 5,* 330–352.

Lyons-Ruth, K., Yellin, C., Melnick, S., & Atwood, G. (2005). Expanding the concept of unresolved mental states: Hostile/helpless states of mind on the Adult Attachment Interview are associated with atypical maternal behavior and infant disorganization. *Development and Psychopathology, 17,* 1–23.

Madigan, S., Bakermans-Kranenburg, M. J., van IJzendoorn, M. H., Moran, G., Pederson, D. R., & Benoit, D. (2006). Unresolved states of mind, anomalous parental behavior, and disorganized attachment: A review and meta-analysis of a transmission gap. *Attachment and Human Development, 8,* 89–111.

Madigan, S., Goldberg, S., Moran, G., & Pederson, D. (2004). Naïve observers' perceptions of family drawings by 7-year-olds with disorganized attachment histories. *Attachment and Human Development, 6,* 223–239.

Madigan, S., Moran, G., & Pederson, D. R. (2006). Unresolved states of mind, disorganized attachment relationships, and disrupted interactions of adolescent mothers and their infants, *Developmental Psychology, 42,* 293–304.

Madigan, S., Moran, G., Schuengel, C., Pederson, D., & Otten, R. (2007). Unresolved maternal attachment representations, disrupted maternal behavior and disorganized attachment in infancy: Links to toddler behavior problems. *Journal of Child Psychology and Psychiatry, 48,* 1042–1050.

Main, M. (1973). *Exploration, play, and cognitive functioning as related to child–mother attachment.* Unpublished doctoral dissertation, Johns Hopkins University.

Main, M. (1979). *Scale for disordered/disoriented infant behavior in response to the Main and Weston clown sessions.* Unpublished manuscript, University of California at Berkeley.

Main, M., & Cassidy, J. (1988). Categories of response to reunion with the parent at age 6: Predicted from infant attachment classifications and stable over a 1-month period. *Developmental Psychology, 24,* 415–426.

Main, M., & Goldwyn, R. (1984). *Adult attachment scoring and classification system.* Unpublished manuscript, University of California at Berkeley.

Main, M., Goldwyn, R., & Hesse, E. (2003). *Adult attachment scoring and classification system.* Unpublished manuscript, University of California at Berkeley.

Main, M., & Hesse, E. (1990). Parents' unresolved traumatic experiences are related to infant disorganized attachment status: Is frightened and/or frightening parental behavior the linking mechanism? In M. T. Greenberg, D. Cicchetti, & E. M. Cummings (Eds.), *Attachment in the preschool years: Theory, research and intervention* (pp. 161–182). Chicago: University of Chicago Press.

Main, M., & Hesse, E. (1992). *Frightened, threatening, dissociative, timid-deferential, sexualized, and disorganized parental behavior: A coding system for frightened/frightening (FR) parent–infant interactions.* Unpublished manuscript, University of California at Berkeley.

Main, M., & Hesse, E. (2006). *Frightened, threatening, dissociative, timid-deferential, sexualized, and disorganized parental behavior: A coding system for frightened/frightening (FR) parent–infant interactions.* Unpublished manuscript, University of California at Berkeley.

Main, M., Hesse, E., & Kaplan, N. (2005). Predictability of attachment behavior and representational processes at 1, 6, and 18 years of age: The Berkeley longitudinal study. In K. E. Grossmann, K. Grossmann, & E. Waters (Eds.), *Attachment from infancy to adulthood* (pp. 245–304). New York: Guilford Press.

Main, M., Kaplan, N., & Cassidy, J. (1985). Security in infancy, childhood, and adulthood: A move to the level of representation. In I. Bretherton & E. Waters (Eds.), Growing points of attachment theory and research. *Monographs of the Society for Research in Child Development, 50*(1–2, Serial No. 209), 66–104.

Main, M., & Solomon, J. (1986). Discovery of a new, insecure-disorganized/disoriented attachment pattern. In T. B. Brazelton & M. W. Yogman (Eds.), *Affective development in infancy* (pp. 95–124). Norwood, NJ: Ablex.

Main, M., & Solomon, J. (1990). Procedures for identifying infants as disorganized/disoriented during the Ainsworth Strange Situation. In M. T. Greenberg, D. Cicchetti, & E. M. Cummings (Eds.), *Attachment in the preschool years: Theory, research, and intervention* (pp. 121–160). Chicago: University of Chicago Press.

Main, M., & Weston, D. R. (1981). The quality of the toddler's relationship to mother and to father: Related to conflict behavior and the readiness to establish new relationships. *Child Development, 52,* 932–940.

Manassis, K., Bradley, S., Goldberg, S., Hood, J., & Swinson, R. (1994). Attachment in mothers with anxiety disorders and their children. *Journal of the American Academy of Child and Adolescent Psychiatry, 33,* 1106–1113.

Manassis, K., Bradley, S., Goldberg, S., Hood, J., & Swinson, R. (1995). Behavioral inhibition, attachment, and anxiety in children of mothers with anxiety disorders. *Canadian Journal of Psychiatry, 40,* 87–92.

Martins, C., & Gaffan, E. A. (2000). Effects of early maternal depression on patterns of infant–mother attachment: A meta-analytic investigation. *Journal of Child Psychology and Psychiatry, 41,* 737–746.

Melnick, S., Finger, B., Hans, S., Patrick, M., & Lyons-Ruth, K. (2008). Hostile–helpless states of mind in the AAI: A proposed additional AAI category with implications for identifying disorganized infant attachment in high-risk samples. In H. Steele & M. Steele (Eds.), *Clinical applications of the Adult Attachment Interview* (pp. 399–424). New York: Guilford Press.

Moss, E., Bureau, J.-F., Cyr, C., Mongeau, C., & St.-Laurent, D. (2004). Correlates of attachment at age 3: Construct validity of the preschool attachment classification system. *Developmental Psychology, 40,* 323–334.

Moss, E., Bureau, J.-F., St.-Laurent, D., & Tarabulsy, G. M. (in press). Understanding disorganized attachment at preschool and school age: Examining divergent pathways of disorganized and controlling children. In J. Solomon & C. George (Eds.), *Attachment disorganization* (2nd ed.). New York: Guilford Press.

Moss, E., Cyr, C., & Dubois-Comtois, K. (2004). Attachment at early school age and developmental risk: Examining family contexts and behavior problems of controlling-caregiving, controlling-punitive, and behaviorally disorganized children. *Developmental Psychology, 40,* 519–532.

Moss, E., Rousseau, D., Parent, S., St.-Laurent, D., & Saintonge, J. (1998). Correlates of attachment at school age: Maternal reported stress, mother–child interaction, and behavior problems. *Child Development, 69,* 1390–1405.

Moss, E., Smolla, N., Cyr, C., Dubois-Comtois, K., Mazzarello, T., & Berthiaume, C. (2006). Attachment and behavior problems in middle childhood as reported by adult and child informants. *Development and Psychopathology, 18,* 425–444.

Moss, E., & St.-Laurent, D. (2001). Attachment at school age and academic performance. *Developmental Psychology, 37,* 863–874.

Moss, E., St.-Laurent, D., & Parent, S. (1999). Disorganized attachment and developmental risk at school age. In J. Solomon & C. George (Eds.), *Attachment disorganization* (pp. 160–187). New York: Guilford Press.

Muller, J. M., Brunelli, S. A., Moore, H., Myers, M. M., & Shair, H. N. (2005). Maternally modulated infant separation responses are regulated by D2-family dopamine receptors. *Behavioral Neuroscience, 119,* 1384–1388.

National Institute of Child Health and Human Development (NICHD) Early Child Care Research Network. (1997). The effects of infant child care on infant–mother attachment security: Results of the NICHD Study of Early Child Care. *Child Development, 68,* 860–879.

National Institute of Child Health and Human Development (NICHD) Early Child Care Research Network. (2001). Child-care and family predictors of preschool attachment and stability from infancy. *Developmental Psychology, 37,* 847–862.

National Institute of Child Health and Human Development (NICHD) Early Child Care Research Network. (2006). Infant–mother attachment classification: Risk and protection in relation to changing maternal caregiving quality. *Developmental Psychology, 42,* 38–58.

Nelson, N. (1994). *Predicting adolescent behavior problems in late adolescence from parent–child interactions in early adolescence.* Unpublished doctoral dissertation, University of Minnesota.

O'Connor, M. J., Sigman, M., & Brill, N. (1987). Disorganization of attachment in relation to maternal alcohol consumption. *Journal of Consulting and Clinical Psychology, 55,* 831–836.

O'Connor, T. G., & Croft, C. M. (2001). A twin study of attachment in preschool children. *Child Development, 72,* 1501–1511.

O'Connor, T. G., Marvin, R. S., Rutter, M., Olrick, J. T., Britner, P. A., & The English and Romanian Adoptees Study Team. (2003). Child–parent attachment following early institutional deprivation. *Development and Psychopathology, 15,* 19–38.

O'Connor, T. G., Rutter, M., & The English and Romanian Adoptees Study Team. (2000). Attachment disorder behavior following early severe deprivation: Extension and longitudinal follow-up. *Journal of the American Academy of Child and Adolescent Psychiatry, 39,* 702–712.

Ogawa, J. R., Sroufe, L. A., Weinfield, N. S., Carlson, E. A., & Egeland, B. (1997). Development and the fragmented self: Longitudinal study of dissociative symptomatology in a nonclinical sample. *Development and Psychopathology, 9,* 855–879.

Patrick, M., Hobson, R. P., Castle, P., Howard, R., & Maughan, B. (1994). Personality disorder and mental representation of early social experience. *Development and Psychopathology, 6,* 375–388.

Paulo-Pott, U., Pott, A., & Beckmann, D. (2007). Negative emotionality, attachment quality, and behavior problems in early childhood. *Infant Mental Health Journal, 28,* 39–53.

Radke-Yarrow, M., Cummings, E. M., Kuczynski, L., & Chapman, M. (1985). Patterns of attachment in two- and three-year-olds in normal families and families with parental depression. *Child Development, 56,* 884–893.

Riley, C., Atlas-Corbett, A., Bureau, J.-F., & Lyons-Ruth, K. (2007, March). *Caregiving risk, behavior problems, and socially indiscriminate attachment behaviors assessed in the Strange Situation.* Poster presented

at the biennial meeting of the Society for Research in Child Development, Boston.

Sagi-Schwartz, A., van IJzendoorn, M., Grossmann, K. E., Joels, T., Grossmann, K., Scharf, M., et al. (2003). Attachment and traumatic stress in female Holocaust child survivors and their daughters. *American Journal of Psychiatry, 160,* 1086–1092.

Sampson, M. (2004). *Continuity and change in patterns of attachment between infancy, adolescence, and early adulthood in a high risk sample.* Unpublished doctoral dissertation, University of Minnesota.

Schneider-Rosen, K., Braunwald, K., Carlson, V., & Cicchetti, D. (1985). Current perspectives in attachment theory: Illustration from the study of maltreated infants. In I. Bretherton & E. Waters (Eds.), *Growing points of attachment theory and research. Monographs of the Society for Research in Child Development, 50*(1–2, Serial no. 209), 194–210.

Schuengel, C., Bakermans-Kranenburg, M. J., & van IJzendoorn, M. H. (1999). Frightening maternal behavior linking unresolved loss and disorganized infant attachment. *Journal of Consulting and Clinical Psychology, 67,* 54–63.

Schuengel, C., van IJzendoorn, M., Bakermans-Kranenburg, M., & Blom, M. (1997, April). Frightening, frightened and/or dissociated behavior, unresolved loss, and infant disorganization. In D. Jacobvitz (Chair), *Caregiving correlates and longitudinal outcomes of disorganized attachments in infants.* Symposium conducted at the biennial meeting of the Society for Research in Child Development, Washington, DC.

Siebenbruner, J., Englund, M. M., Egeland, B., & Hudson, K. (2006). Developmental antecedents of late adolescence substance use patterns. *Development and Psychopathology, 18,* 551–571.

Solomon, J., George, C., & De Jong, A. (1995). Children classified as controlling at age six: Evidence of disorganized representational strategies and aggression at home and at school. *Development and Psychopathology, 7,* 447–463.

Spangler, G., Fremmer-Bombik, E., & Grossmann, K. (1996). Social and individual determinants of infant attachment security and disorganization. *Development and Psychopathology, 17,* 127–139.

Spangler, G., & Grossmann, K. E. (1993). Biobehavioral organization in securely and insecurely attached infants. *Child Development, 64,* 1439–1450.

Spangler, G., & Schieche, M. (1998). Emotional and adrenocortical responses of infants to the Strange Situation: The differential function of emotional expression. *International Journal of Behavioral Development, 22,* 681–706.

Spangler, G., & Zimmerman, P. (2007, March). *Genetic contribution to attachment disorganization and temperament.* Paper presented at the biennial meeting of the Society for Research in Child Development, Boston.

Sroufe, L. A., Egeland, B., Carlson, E., & Collins, W. A. (2005). *The development of the person: The Minnesota Study of Risk and Adaptation from Birth to Adulthood.* New York: Guilford Press.

Stovall-McClough, K. C., & Dozier, M. (2004). Forming attachments in foster care: Infant attachment behaviors during the first 2 months of placement. *Development and Psychopathology, 16,* 253–271.

Swanson, J. M., Flodman, P., & Kennedy, J. (2000). Dopamine genes and ADHD. *Neuroscience and Biobehavioral Reviews, 24,* 21–25.

Taylor, S. E., Klein, L. C., Lewis, B. P., Gruenewald, T. L., Gurung, A. R., & Updegraff, J. A. (2000). Behavioral responses to stress in females: Tend-and-befriend, not fight-or-flight. *Psychological Review, 107,* 411–429.

Teti, D. M. (1999). Conceptualizations of disorganization in the preschool years: An integration. In J. Solomon & C. George (Eds.), *Attachment disorganization* (pp. 213–242). New York: Guilford Press.

Tomlinson, M., Cooper, P., & Murray, L. (2005). The mother–infant relationship and infant attachment in a South African peri-urban settlement. *Child Development, 76,* 1044–1054.

Toth, S. L., Rogosch, F. A., Manly, J. T., & Cicchetti, D. (2006). The efficacy of toddler–parent psychotherapy to reorganize attachment in the young offspring of mothers with major depressive disorder: A randomized preventive trial. *Journal of Consulting and Clinical Psychology, 74,* 1006–1016.

True, M., Pasani, L., & Oumar, F. (2001). Infant–mother interactions among the Dogon of Mali. *Child Development, 72,* 1451–1466.

Turkheimer, E., Haley, A., Waldron, M., D'Onofrio, B., & Gottesman, I. I. (2003). Socioeconomic status modifies heritability of IQ in young children. *Psychological Science, 14,* 623–628.

van IJzendoorn, M. H. (1995). Adult attachment representations, parental responsiveness, and infant attachment: A meta-analysis on the predictive validity of the Adult Attachment Interview. *Psychological Bulletin, 117,* 387–403.

van IJzendoorn, M. H., & Bakermans-Kranenburg, M. (2006). DRD4 7-repeat polymorphism moderates the association between maternal unresolved loss or trauma and infant disorganization. *Attachment and Human Development, 8,* 291–307.

van IJzendoorn, M. H., Schuengel, C., & Bakermans-Kranenburg, M. J. (1999). Disorganized attachment in early childhood: A meta-analysis of precursors,

concomitants, and sequelae. *Development and Psychopathology, 11,* 225–249.

Vondra, J., Hommerding, K. D., & Shaw, D. S. (1999). Stability and change in infant attachment in a low-income sample. In J. Vondra & D. Barnett (Eds.), Atypical attachment in infancy and early childhood among children at development risk. *Monographs of the Society for Research in Child Development, 64*(3, Serial No. 258), 119–144.

Vondra, J., Shaw, D. S., Swearingen, L., Cohen, M., & Owens, E. B. (2001). Attachment stability and emotional and behavioral regulation from infancy to preschool age. *Development and Psycopathology, 13,* 13–33.

Wartner, U. G., Grossmann, K., Fremmer-Bombik, E., & Suess, G. (1994). Attachment patterns at age six in south Germany: Predictability from infancy and implications for preschool behavior. *Child Development, 65,* 1014–1027.

Waters, E., Merrick, S., Treboux, D., Crowell, J., & Albersheim, L. (2000). Attachment security in infancy and early adulthood: A twenty-year longitudinal study. *Child Development, 71,* 684–689.

Waters, E., Weinfield, N. S., & Hamilton, C. (2000). The stability of attachment security from infancy to adolescence and early adulthood: General discussion. *Child Development, 71,* 703–706.

Weinfield, N. S., Sroufe, L. A., & Egeland, B. (2000). Attachment from infancy to adulthood in a high-risk sample: Continuity, discontinuity, and their correlates. *Child Development, 71,* 695–702.

Weinfeld, N. S., Whaley, G. J. L., & Egeland, B. (2004). Continuity, discontinuity, and coherence in attachment from infancy to late adolescence: Sequelae of organization and disorganization. *Attachment and Human Development, 6,* 73–97.

Zeanah, C., Benoit, D., & Barton, M. L. (1986). *Working model of the child interview.* Unpublished manuscript, Brown University Program in Medicine, Providence, RI.

Zeanah, C. H., Smyke, A. T., Koga, S. F., Carlson, E., & The Bucharest Early Intervention Project Core Group. (2005). Attachment in institutionalized and community children in Romania. *Child Development, 76,* 1015–1028.

CHAPTER 29

Challenges to the Development of Attachment Relationships Faced by Young Children in Foster and Adoptive Care

MARY DOZIER
MICHAEL RUTTER

Children are born biologically prepared to develop attachment relationships to primary caregivers. Parents are likewise biologically prepared to provide care for their young children (Numan & Insel, 2003). Foster care and adoption represent deviations from the more typical situation in which a child is raised continuously by birth parents. In some species foster care and adoption do not occur, and in many other species such care is rare (Maestripieri, 2005). The human caregiving system appears relatively flexible in this regard; nonetheless, there are challenges involved for both surrogate parents and children. Depending on the nature of the preplacement conditions, the postplacement conditions, and a child's vulnerabilities and strengths, different effects are seen across behavioral and biological systems.

In this chapter, we discuss young children in foster care, as well as those adopted both nationally and internationally. Although children in these groups experience different challenges, they are all raised by someone other than birth parents for at least part of their lives. Some of the challenges include institutional care, changes in caregivers, early experiences of maltreatment, and prenatal or genetic factors that confer vulnerability. We include a discussion of animal models of separation

and neglect, because they richly inform our understanding of the effects of infants' early experience.

TYPES OF SURROGATE CARE

Foster Care

Over 500,000 children are in formal foster care in the United States (U.S. Department of Health and Human Services [DHHS], 2006). In 2004, the last year for which national statistics are available, the count was 518,000. This number is substantially higher than the 280,000 reported to be in care in 1985, but there has nonetheless been a linear decrease each year since 2000 (U.S. DHHS, 2006). Many children living in informal foster care arrangements (e.g., with relatives or neighbors) are not counted in this number. In the United States, about 14% of children entering foster care are less than a year old, and 26% are between 1 and 5 years of age. Thus the associated disruptions in care and the forming of attachment relationships to new caregivers occur for many at a developmental point when forming and maintaining attachment relationships are key biologically programmed tasks. Children enter foster care with a range of previous caregiving experiences, both prior to entering the foster care system and within the foster care system. With the exception of those placed into foster care at birth, most have been neglected by their birth parents, and some have experienced abuse, either by itself or in combination with neglect.

Although foster care is intended to be a temporary solution, children of all ages tend to stay in care for relatively long periods in the United States. Only 5% stay in foster care less than a month, with an additional 34% staying for less than a year. Twenty-one percent stay in foster care between 1 and 2 years, and 40% longer than 2 years. When children leave foster care, approximately 55% are reunited with birth parents, and 18% are placed with adoptive parents (U.S. DHHS, 2006). For those reunifying, about one-third return to foster care within 3 years.

Adoption

The population of adopted children overlaps with the population of children who have been in foster care. The number of children adopted from the foster care system in the United States was between 50,000 and 53,000 in each of the years from 2000 to 2004, with no significant change during this period. About 22,000 children were adopted internationally during each of the years 2004 and 2005 (U.S. Department of State, 2005). The number of children adopted internationally increased dramatically and consistently each year after 1990, when about 7,000 children were adopted. Most recent adoptions were from China, Russia, Guatemala, and Korea. Policies within various nations have partially driven these numbers. For example, China's policy limiting families in urban areas to only one child, combined with the preference for male infants, has made many female infants available for adoption in recent years. In the early 1990s, many children were adopted from Romania, following the fall of the Ceaucescu regime (U.S. Department of State, 2005). Many of the children adopted internationally have been in institutional care for at least some period of time prior to adoption.

EXPERIENCES PRIOR TO PLACEMENT IN FOSTER OR ADOPTIVE CARE

Human young have a long period of immaturity and therefore remain dependent on caregivers for a number of years. Nonetheless, the period when the formation of initial selective attachments has the most biological significance is probably the first several years of life. During the second half of the first year of life, children typically develop attachment relationships to specific caregivers. From an evolutionary perspective, one of the functions of attachment behaviors is to keep children close to caregivers under potentially dangerous circumstances. Even before children develop selective attachment relationships, caregivers play critical roles in helping their infants begin to regulate physiological and behavioral states. For example, neonates are typically dependent upon their mothers for temperature regulation, and young infants are dependent upon parents for physiological regulation. Thus experiences of separation, maltreatment, and privation, even early in the first year of life, may have long-term developmental consequences.

Children experience a range of conditions prior to placement in foster care and adoptive care. At one end of a continuum are children who have lacked a caregiver altogether and experienced minimal stimulation. Although privation at this level is most often associated with institutional care, it is also sometimes seen among children reared with birth parents or foster parents. At the other end of the continuum are children who have been cared for by loving, committed caregivers who for some reason (e.g., death, imprisonment) were not able to continue parenting. Many children who enter surrogate care fall between these two extremes; they have not been starkly deprived, nor have they received consistently nurturing care. In the following sections, we consider experiences of institutional care, neglect, abuse, and separation from caregivers.

Institutional Care

Historically, many children who did not have parents to care for them lived in group care or institutional care settings (Bowlby, 1951). Attention to the effects of these conditions in the 1940s and 1950s ended the wide-scale use of institutional care in the United States and the United Kingdom. Nonetheless, such institutional care continues to exist in some places within the United States, where it is often referred to as "group care" or "congregate care." About 19% of all children who are removed from their parents' care are placed in facilities that house more than 11 children (U.S. DHHS, 2006). Older children are especially likely to be placed in institutional care, although infants and young children are placed in such facilities as well. Reasons given for these placements include the shortage of foster parents, the desire to keep siblings together, and the high quality of the facilities. Even high-quality institutional care, however, has problematic effects (Kaufman et al., 2004).

Compared to the United States and the United Kingdom, institutional care is seen more often in a number of other countries. The World Health Organization (WHO) defines "institutional care" as care that occurs in any facility providing care to at least 11 children. Nearly 44,000 children under the age of 3 are in institutional care in the 46 European nations for which WHO data are available (Browne, Hamilton-Giachritsis, Johnson, & Ostergren, 2006). Countries with the highest number of young children in institutional care include Russia, Romania, Ukraine, Spain, and France (Browne et al., 2006).

In 1945, Spitz described the conditions of orphanages in the United States. In an attempt to reduce infection and in response to low staff-to-child ratios, institutional environments had become increasingly sterile. Babies were handled as little as possible, kept in cribs from which they could not interact with each other or with staff members, and fed and changed in perfunctory fashion. Bowlby (1951) conducted a study of institutions in Europe for the WHO, describing similar conditions. Orphanages in Romania and St. Petersburg, Russia, were described in similar ways over 50 years later (Groark, Muhamedrahimov, Palmov, Nikiforova, & McCall, 2005; Rutter, Kreppner, & O'Connor, 2001). For example, bottles were propped up so that babies could be fed without being held, and children were left lying in their cribs for extended periods.

Effects of Institutional Care on Development

Starkly depriving conditions are associated with the most pervasive effects on child functioning. At the very basic level, death rates are high. Furthermore, these children are often delayed in physical growth. They show deficits in motor development, with many of them crawling and walking well behind schedule (Johnson et al., 1996). Extensive delays in cognitive functioning and language development are also seen (Carlson & Earls, 1997; Johnson et al., 1996). In addition to developmental delays, institutionalized children show highly anomalous behaviors, including stereotypies such as rocking and self-stimulating behaviors. Social behaviors are odd and often include one of two

extremes: Some children are withdrawn and depressed in appearance, whereas others are indiscriminate in their attachment behaviors (Chisholm, 1998; Chisholm, Carter, Ames, & Morison, 1995; O'Connor, Rutter, & the English and Romanian Adoptees Study Team, 2000; Tizard & Rees, 1975).

Nonhuman primates raised under isolated conditions show similar deficits in functioning (Suomi, Chapter 8, this volume). For example, rhesus infants reared without appropriate mother surrogates show highly anomalous behaviors that persist when the infants are placed back in their home cages. These monkeys show stereotypies, inappropriate social behaviors, and (when mating does occur) inadequate parenting. Reintegrating these isolates with other animals is difficult, because their inappropriate behavior patterns often make them targets for abuse (Suomi & Harlow, 1972).

Differences among Institutions

There are differences among institutions and even within institutions in the care provided (Groark et al., 2005; Gunnar, Bruce, & Grotevant, 2000). Key differences among institutions include different staff-to-child ratios and philosophies regarding staff interactions with children (Groark et al., 2005). There may be exceptions, and staff-to-child ratios and philosophies can be manipulated (Groark et al., 2005). Indeed, Groark and colleagues found that conditions in institutions can be substantially improved, resulting in changes in child behavioral outcomes. Reducing staff-to-child ratios, combined with altering expectations of child care workers, can result in profoundly altered interaction patterns.

Despite such results, even high-quality institutional care appears to have deleterious effects on young children's development (Kaufman et al., 2004). As a rule, children often miss the opportunity to develop selective attachment relationships to caregivers in institutions, and institutional care discourages caregivers from committing themselves to children. A number of forces operate to make caring for children in institutions perfunctory. Developing faster ways to feed and change children becomes important under such conditions. Institutional care seems to have specific adverse effects on children that other depriving conditions do not. In particular, the disinhibited attachment seen among institutionalized children is rarely seen among children who have experienced other forms of deprivation, as will be discussed later.

Neglect

Neglect accounts for 63% of all substantiated cases of child maltreatment. "Neglect" is a care-giver's failure to provide for his or her child's basic safety or welfare. Examples include leaving young children home alone, failing to provide adequate food or shelter, and failing to protect children from dangerous conditions (e.g., exposure to violence). Although this may seem similar to the description of institutional care, neglecting parents usually have relationships with their children, and their children typically form selective attachments to them or to other caregivers in the home. From an evolutionary perspective, it makes sense that the attachment system is adaptable to a range of care-giving conditions. We expect that the formation of a selective attachment protects neglected children from the long-term effects seen among some institutionalized children.

On the other hand, although neglect is less toxic than conditions of privation, it has perva-sive, long-term effects (for a review, see Smith & Fong, 2004). Children who experience early ne-glect are at increased risk for a host of problem-atic outcomes. During school-age years, children who have experienced early neglect exhibit more internalizing and externalizing behavior problems and have greater difficulties in relationships with peers than other children do (Egeland, Sroufe, & Erickson, 1983). As adolescents and adults, these children continue to be at significantly increased risk for a range of problems, including depression, anxiety, eating disorders, substance abuse, post-traumatic stress disorder, suicide, and criminal ac-tivities (e.g., Spertus, Yehuda, Wong, Halligan, & Seremetis, 2003). There is some evidence that the consequences are most serious for children who experience neglect early in life (e.g., Keiley, Howe, Dodge, Bates, & Pettit, 2001; U.S. DHHS, 2006).

Abuse

When abuse is documented, children are often removed from the home, at least for a period of time. As with children who experience neglect, abused children typically form selective attach-ment relationships with caregivers. In fact, Roth and Sullivan (2005) argued that abuse heightens the connectedness children feel with their care-givers. They found, studying rodent pups, that the pairing of pain with the mother's presence is as-sociated with enhanced positive feelings for the mother (see also Polan & Hofer, Chapter 7, this

volume). Rajecki, Lamb, and Obmascher (1978) reported similar findings with a broader range of animal species.

Nonetheless, children who experience abuse are involved in a "paradoxical situation," in the words of Hesse and Main (2006, p. 336). When children experience abuse at the hands of a care-giver, they are frightened of the person from whom they would normally seek support. Under more typical parenting conditions, young children are frightened by a variety of things, including the dark, being left alone, and a dog barking, but they can typically turn to a caregiver to protect and soothe them. For example, when children receive inoculations, they are likely to be both hurt and frightened; caregivers, however, can buffer the ef-fects of the stress (Gunnar, Brodersen, Krueger, & Rigatuso, 1996). When caregivers are the source of the fear, they fail to protect their children effec-tively from danger. Children's "paradoxical situa-tion" is seen in their behavior when reunited with abusive caregivers in the Strange Situation (Hesse & Main, 2006). Typical responses include freezing upon reunion or moving away from, rather than toward, the parent. The fear that children expe-rience interferes with their approach to parents. Thus such children behave in odd, inexplicable behaviors that are classified as disorganized or dis-oriented (see also Lyons-Ruth & Jacobvitz, Chap-ter 28, and George & Solomon, Chapter 35, this volume).

Repeated exposure to frightening conditions may result in children developing a sensitized neu-robiology, whereby minor threats elicit strong be-havioral and physiological reactions. Other effects of maltreatment include children's difficulty in developing a trusting relationship with a caregiver (Milan & Pinderhughes, 2000), differential pro-cessing of angry faces (Cicchetti & Curtis, 2005; Pollak & Tolley-Schell, 2003), lack of empathy for distressed peers (George & Main, 1979), nega-tive attributional biases (Dodge, Pettit, Bates, & Valente, 1995; Gibb, 2001), and later dissociative and externalizing symptoms (Lyons-Ruth, Alpern, & Repacholi, 1993).

Separations from Caregivers

Except when children are placed in foster or adop-tive care at birth, placement involves separation from caregivers. Infants have a number of biologi-cal systems that maximize the likelihood of ob-taining care from their biological mothers in par-ticular. For example, at birth an infant prefers the mother's smell to other smells, and this facilitates turning toward the nipple for breast feeding (Roth & Sullivan, 2005). Under benign conditions, the infant comes to anticipate certain rhythms of activity and responsiveness from the mother or caregiver (Beebe, Lachman, & Jaffe, 1997; Gianino & Tronick, 1988). Even prior to the development of a selective attachment, separations are likely to be experienced as dysregulating (see Polan & Hofer, Chapter 7, this volume).

Animal studies demonstrate how powerfully nonhuman primate and rodent young respond to separations from their mothers. Levine, Weiner, and Coe (1993) showed that infant squirrel monkeys never habituated to separations from their mothers. Even when infants had been separated many times, they continued to show neuroendocrine distress responses to the separations. A number of researchers (e.g., Levine et al., 1993; Sanchez, Ladd, & Plotsky, 2001) have found that these early separations have short-term and long-term effects on neuroendocrine regulation. For example, when rodent pups were separated from their mothers for periods of time longer than they would be separated in the wild, they developed a hyperreactive neuroendocrine system. Presumably, rodent pups' stress systems are not designed to deal with these long separations, because there would be little chance of survival if their mothers did not return to the nest. Although these separations have been described as unnaturally long and thus of limited usefulness in generalizing to the human condition, these longer separations may in fact be analogous to a human child's experience when placed in foster or adoptive care.

Experiences of maltreatment and separation are often confounded for young children placed into foster and adoptive care, making it difficult to isolate effects. Animal studies may help point to which experiences are critical and which are not, although developing adequate models of abuse and separation remains complex, as does the generalization across species.

FACTORS AFFECTING HOW CHILDREN COPE WITH ADVERSITY

Child Vulnerabilities

A number of prenatal and genetic factors affect how children cope with adversity. Some of these factors, such as prenatal exposure to alcohol and premature birth, may be overrepresented in the population of children that enter foster and adop-

tive care (e.g., Barth & Needell, 1996). There are also high rates of prior maternal substance abuse among children placed into foster care and domestic adoptive care in the United States. The rates of prenatal substance exposure are often highest among children placed at birth, because detection of maternal use of illegal substances is often a cause for placement into foster care. This is important, because there is often an inverse association between prenatal and postnatal risk factors for children placed in domestic foster and adoptive care. For example, children who are placed in foster or adoptive care at birth are likely to have higher levels of prenatal substance exposure, but lower levels of postnatal risk (e.g., abuse, neglect, separations), than children placed at later ages.

The incidence of maternal smoking and drinking, as well as maternal use of illegal substances (e.g., cocaine and amphetamines), is high for children placed into foster and adoptive care in the United States (Barth, 1991). Prenatal exposure to substances has been linked with a wide range of problems for children, including attentional problems (Savage, Brodsky, Malmud, Giannetta, & Hurt, 2005), substance abuse (Glantz & Chambers, 2006), and conduct disorder (Wakschlag & Hans, 2002).

The preponderance of evidence suggests that the effects of risk are generally additive, with each additional factor increasing the odds of problematic outcomes (Appleyard, Egeland, van Dulmen, & Sroufe, 2005; Sameroff, Bartko, Baldwin, Baldwin, & Seifer, 1998). Some investigators, in fact, have found that the effects of risk factors are multiplicative, with three or four risk factors showing a much stronger effect than fewer risk factors (e.g., Appleyard et al., 2005). There is growing evidence for gene–environment interactions. Genetic variants often have little or no main effect on maladaptive psychological outcomes, but nonetheless are associated with an increased vulnerability to such risks as child abuse (Rutter, Moffitt, & Caspi, 2006). For example, Caspi et al. (2002, 2003) reported evidence for a gene–environment interaction involving the monoamine oxidase A (MAOA) gene that affects antisocial behavior and another gene (the short-allele variant of the serotonin transporter gene) that affects rates of depression (see also Kaufman et al., 2006). Suomi (2003) similarly found that the short-allele version of the serotonin transporter gene in rhesus monkeys was associated with maladaptive outcomes in peer-reared, but not mother-reared, monkeys. Bakermans-Kranenburg and van IJzendoorn (2006) found a significant interaction between the 7-repeat variant of the dopamine D4 receptor (DRD4) gene and maternal insensitivity in relation to externalizing behavior. Most recently, the same genetic variant has been found to moderate the effects of an intervention to promote sensitive parenting and positive discipline (Bakermans-Kranenburg, van IJzendoorn, Mesman, Alink, & Juffer, in press).

Quality of Surrogate Caregiving Experiences

Among children in intact families and children who have been placed in foster or adoptive care, the later caregiving environment has proven to be important in affecting many outcomes (Ackerman, Kogos, Youngstrom, Schoff, & Izard, 1999; Duyme, Dumaret, & Tomkiewicz, 1999; Sinclair & Wilson, 2003). Children who are moved to privileged adoptive families after institutional care typically show a rapid catch-up in physical growth, followed by rapid cognitive development. Nonetheless, there are some domains of development that do not necessarily improve when children are placed into stable foster or adoptive homes (van IJzendoorn & Juffer, 2006). These issues are considered in more depth in a later section.

Sroufe and colleagues (Sroufe, Egeland, Carlson, & Collins, 2005; Weinfield, Sroufe, & Egeland, 2000) have suggested that when conditions in children's lives change, developmental outcomes follow rules of "lawful discontinuity." For the most part, the changes that have been studied have included parental death, divorce, and other similar life stressors. Although these changes are significant, they often pale in comparison with the changes in the lives of children who enter surrogate care. Such children typically change caregivers, sibling groups, neighborhoods, socioeconomic statuses, and sometimes even nations, cultures, and languages spoken. We expect that for infants and young children, the caregivers' characteristics are most critical to children's adjustment.

Hinde and McGinnis (1977) found that rhesus infants adjusted much more quickly following separations if their mothers' behavior returned to normal rather than if mothers exhibited distressed or aberrant behavior. This is similar to findings regarding a child's ability to adjust to such stressors as death and divorce. When the remaining caregiver is able to function as an effective support to the child, the child's adjustment is much better than if the caregiver cannot serve this role (Harris, Brown, & Bifulco, 1986).

Adoptive, Foster, and Kinship Caregivers

In general, adoptive parents, traditional foster caregivers, and kinship caregivers represent somewhat different populations. Parents adopting across national boundaries are screened most extensively, and kinship caregivers are screened least extensively. Parents seeking to adopt internationally are typically screened to ensure that they do not present risks to any adopted child through their pattern of rearing. At the time of adoption, adopting parents have rates of psychopathology that are low by general population standards (Rutter, 2006). Accordingly, it might be expected that this population would mirror the general population with regard to attachment state of mind, or indeed might show high rates of autonomous states of mind. But many adoptive parents have experienced the stress of infertility and of failed attempts at assisted conception. These issues may be largely unresolved at the point of adoption, perhaps leading to parenting behaviors more akin to those shown by parents with an unresolved state of mind. So far as we are aware, studies reporting the differential effects of adoptive parents' states of mind with respect to attachment (see Hesse, Chapter 25, this volume) have not been published. In addition, nothing systematic is known about how adoptive parents' attachment representations influence the handling of adoptive children's concerns over their origins.

Screening Caregivers

Screening of foster parents is somewhat variable. Most child welfare agencies attempt to place children in foster homes within the same city or county system from which children were removed. Therefore, in areas where removal of children is high per capita (such as in high-poverty areas), the available pool of foster parents is often much smaller than the number needed. A smaller foster parent pool typically results in less screening. When one is considering why individuals would choose to become foster parents, a number of hypotheses might be made regarding parents' own attachment issues. For example, given the challenging task of parenting potentially difficult children for undetermined lengths of time, one could hypothesize that parents with autonomous states of mind might be overrepresented (e.g., because the task is difficult and requires strength); that parents with dismissing states of mind might be overrepresented (e.g., because some distance would be required to accept that the relationship will end); or that parents with unresolved states of mind might be overrepresented (e.g., because of the motivation to overcome their own unresolved issues). For the most part, however, such differences have not emerged between foster parents' states of mind and those of other adults (e.g., Dozier, Stovall, Albus, & Bates, 2001). Dozier and colleagues' (2001) sample was small, leaving the possibility that differences might emerge with a larger sample.

Qualifications for becoming kin caregivers depend upon whether the caregiver is licensed as a foster parent or the arrangement is informal. Combined with the fact that kin caregivers are often the parents of the child's parents (who were unable to care for the child), it is not surprising that these kin caregivers have fewer resources and experience more stressors than traditional foster parents do (Brooks & Barth, 1998; Cuddleback, 2004). The distribution of kin caregivers' attachment state of mind of kin has not been reported in the literature. We anticipate that these caregivers might be expected to show a distribution of states of mind somewhat intermediate between that of high-risk birth parents and that of foster parents.

CHALLENGES FOR CHILDREN FORMING ATTACHMENTS TO NEW CAREGIVERS

To this point, we have considered the conditions associated with foster and adoptive care likely to affect children's adjustment. We now consider the challenges children face in developing attachments to new caregivers. The literature on attachment in relation to foster care and adoption falls into three general categories: foster placement, adoptive placement at birth or soon after, and adoptive care following institutional care. We consider each of these in turn.

Attachments of Children in Foster Care

The Process of Forming New Attachment Relationships

When developing in typical mother–child dyads, children form selective attachments as a result of maturation and an extended history of interactions. In contrast, children who are placed into foster or adoptive care are often at a developmental stage in which selective attachment relationships would already have been formed with caregivers. Therefore, the process by which new selective attachments are formed is likely to move along a different trajectory, or to take a form different from the usual one.

To study this process, Stovall and Dozier (2000) developed a diary method for tracking children's attachment behaviors. They examined the formation of attachment relationships from as close to the first day of a child's placement in a new home as possible. Foster parents were asked to report on children's behaviors during incidents likely to elicit attachment behaviors. In particular, they recorded how children responded to being frightened, hurt, and separated from them. Foster parents also recorded their own reactions to their children's behaviors and children's subsequent responses. These behaviors were recorded on a checklist developed to be as complete as possible. Parents also provided a short narrative of each incident, to ensure that they were completing the checklist thoughtfully and to assist coders with interpreting events.

Children who were classified as secure in the Strange Situation had lower avoidance scores in the diary than other children, and children who were classified as avoidant in the Strange Situation had higher avoidance scores than other children (Stovall-McClough & Dozier, 2004). Security scores in the diary were also related, although less strongly than avoidance, to Strange Situation classifications. Resistance scores in the diary were not linked with Strange Situation classifications.

Stovall and Dozier used the attachment diary to study children's developing attachment relationships in a new foster home (Stovall & Dozier, 2000; Stovall-McClough & Dozier, 2004). For children placed into care before about 1 year of age, placements became stable quickly. Within 1–2 weeks, most infants and toddlers developed a consistent pattern of responding to their caregivers (Stovall & Dozier, 2000). For children placed later than approximately 1 year of age, the process appeared to take longer than for younger children. Even after 2 months, these children often did not show stable patterns of attachment behavior. Furthermore, in this early period of attachment formation, diary data suggested that the children "led the dance" (Stern, 2002). That is, children's avoidant and resistant behaviors elicited rejecting behaviors from caregivers, even for caregivers with an autonomous state of mind.

These findings regarding the formation of attachments to new caregivers are probably neither as encouraging as they seem for the younger infants, nor as discouraging as they seem for the older infants. First, the finding that children younger than about a year of age show secure behaviors quickly with an autonomous foster parent is promising in terms of children's ability to organize their behavior in relation to a new caregiver. A period of 1–2 weeks (i.e., the length of time it appears to take young infants to develop expectations concerning a new caregiver's availability) is probably a long time in the life of a young infant. Although infants adapt to the new caregivers by organizing attachment behaviors in relation to caregiver availability, disruptions may still have had dysregulating effects, as discussed below in the section on the neuroendocrine system. Second, the findings suggest that children who are more than about a year of age at the time of placement have some difficulty trusting new caregivers and behaving in ways that elicit nurturing behaviors. Stovall and Dozier (2000) were concerned, based on these early findings, that the children's behaviors would be self-perpetuating—that children who behaved in avoidant or resistant ways would fail to elicit nurturance from caregivers, and thus would not experience an environment that could positively challenge and change their expectations. As we discuss below in the section on consolidated attachment relationships, however, these children are eventually able to develop attachment relationships that reflect their caregivers' state of mind rather than the children's anticipation of a non-nurturing world.

Consolidated Attachment Relationships among Foster Children

Dozier and colleagues (2001) studied the consolidated attachment relationships of children placed into foster care for at least 2 months. Infant attachment quality in this study was assessed in the Strange Situation, and foster mother state of mind with respect to attachment was assessed with the Adult Attachment Interview (George, Kaplan, & Main, 1984, 1985, 1996; see Hesse, Chapter 25, this volume). Based on the diary findings, Dozier et al. had anticipated that maternal state of mind would predict child attachment, but only for children who were placed into foster care early (i.e., before 12 months of age). Contrary to those expectations, foster mothers' state of mind predicted children's attachment, but age at placement was unrelated to attachment (either as a main effect or in interaction with foster mothers' state of mind). The two-way match between parental state of mind and child attachment was nearly as strong as seen among intact dyads in van IJzendoorn's (1995) meta-analysis that included intact mother–child dyads. Foster mothers' state of mind was concordant with infant attachment 72% of the time (kappa = .43) in the Dozier and colleagues

study, as compared with 76% (kappa = .49) in the meta-analysis.

When children are placed with autonomous foster parents, it seems that experiences of maltreatment and separation do not affect their ability to form organized attachment relationships. These results are surprising in one sense, but are also consistent with the evidence that attachment formation is a relationship-specific construct for young children. For example, the quality of attachment relationships that children form with mothers, fathers, and preschool teachers have been found to be relatively independent (e.g., Goossens & van IJzendoorn, 1990; Howes & Hamilton, 1992; see Howes & Spieker, Chapter 14, this volume, for a review). We expect that there is an age limit after which it may be difficult for children to develop trusting relationships with new caregivers, but we do not yet have data to support that expectation. In the small Dozier and colleagues (2001) sample, children placed into care up to the age of 20 months appeared able to organize attachment in relation to their new caregivers' availability when caregivers had autonomous states of mind.

Whereas the attachment outcomes for children placed with autonomous foster parents were quite positive, children placed with nonautonomous caregivers were disproportionately likely to develop disorganized attachment relationships. This disproportionate distribution resulted from foster children developing disorganized attachment relationships when parented by foster parents with either dismissive or unresolved states of mind. Among biologically intact dyads, disorganized infant attachment is predicted only by parental unresolved state of mind and not by a dismissive state of mind. Dozier and colleagues (2001) interpreted these results as suggesting that children who have experienced early adversity are especially in need of nurturing care. Without such care, they do not appear to be able to organize their attachment relationships.

Meaning of Attachment Security for Children in Foster Care

It is important to remember that we do not know whether foster children's new attachment relationships have the same predictive power that attachment relationships with parents in intact dyads have. To this point, Dozier and colleagues (Dozier, 2005) have not been able to predict later outcomes from secure attachments with surrogate caregivers. That is, even though child attachment quality can be predicted from foster parents' states of mind, child attachment does not then predict later child cooperation during problem-solving tasks or representations of self and others, for example (Dozier, 2005). Thus the findings that children can organize attachment behaviors in relation to the availability of new caregivers do not mean that these attachment relationships confer the usual benefits of stable, intact attachment relationships. This finding may have important implications for the further development of attachment theory.

Attachment among Adopted Children

Children Adopted Early in Infancy

Among children adopted at birth, Singer, Brodzinsky, Steir, and Waters (1985) found no significant difference in the distribution of attachment classifications compared with children from intact biological dyads. A meta-analysis of unpublished data suggests that attachment security (as measured in the Strange Situation) is somewhat less frequent in adopted children than in nonclinical nonadopted samples (47% vs. 67%) (van IJzendoorn & Juffer, 2006).

Children Adopted Following Extended Institutional Care

The only published research to investigate attachment in institutional settings and postadoption attachment was undertaken by Vorria and colleagues (2003, 2006). Their sample was made up of children initially cared for in the Greek Metera Babies Centre and then adopted from that institution at a mean age of 20 months (range = 11 months to 3 years, 5 months). The comparison group comprised children attending a day care center in the same city (Athens). The children were followed up at a mean age of 50 months, some 28 months after adoption. The findings revealed a high rate of disorganized attachment (64% vs. 28%) while the children were in residential care, as found in other studies (van IJzendoorn, Schuengel, & Bakermans-Kranenburg, 1999; Zeanah, Smyke, Koga, Carlson, & the Bucharest Early Intervention Project Core Group, 2005). At follow-up, some 2 years after adoption, attachment security as measured with the Waters and Deane (1985) Attachment Q-Sort procedure (based on observer ratings) showed a lower level of security in the former Metera children than in the comparison group (a difference of over half a standard deviation), and less coherence and greater avoidance on the Bretherton (1985) Attachment Story Completion Task (ASCT). Thus, even after 2 years, there were continuing

differences in attachment security associated with early institutional rearing. Strikingly and surprisingly, however, there was no effect of preadoption attachment security on the ACST, and a negative effect on Q-sort-rated security. Disorganized attachment before adoption, as compared with security before adoption, was more likely to be associated with security after adoption.

This finding needs to be replicated, and the Zeanah and colleagues (2005) study should provide that opportunity (albeit with *fostering* of formerly institutionalized children, rather than adoption). Also, the Vorria and colleagues (2006) study is limited by the fact that using the Q-sort procedure at follow-up meant that there was no measure of postadoption disorganized attachment. If confirmed by others, the finding raises challenging questions about the concept of disorganized attachment. Does it have the same meaning for children in institutions as it does for maltreated children in family settings? Could the disorganization, usually regarded as dysfunctional, be adaptive in the context of institutional rearing? Alternatively, did the presence of a secure attachment relationship in the institution make it more difficult for a child to develop such a relationship with a new caregiver after adoption?

ATYPICAL ATTACHMENTS

Sroufe and colleagues (2005) have emphasized that among intact dyads, strength of attachment is irrelevant. Except under very atypical circumstances, all infants in intact parent–child dyads are expected to become attached to their primary caregivers. Even when children have maltreating parents, they appear to develop specific attachment relationships with those parents (e.g., Crittenden, 1985; Egeland & Sroufe, 1981). It is quality of attachment that differentiates most children, rather than whether they have developed attachment relationships of a certain relative strength or intensity. Among children who have been placed into foster or adoptive care, however, it appears critical to consider the *extent* to which children develop attachment relationships to new caregivers. The Strange Situation, the standard way of assessing attachment quality, does not assess whether the child is attached to the caregiver.

Failure to Develop Specific Attachments

When children do not have an opportunity to develop early primary attachment relationships, they may fail to develop specific attachments to subsequent caregivers or may show odd behaviors with regard to those caregivers. Zeanah and colleagues (2005) have developed a coding system for assessing the extent to which a child shows attachment behaviors toward a particular figure in the Strange Situation. Ratings are made on the basis of the child's display of such behaviors, ranging from behaviors typically shown by children from intact parent–child dyads (at the high end of the scale) to no display of attachment behaviors (at the low end of the scale). This system is important in considering differences among children who spent the early months of their lives in institutional care. In particular, Zeanah and colleagues found that early-institutionalized children displayed less discriminating attachment behaviors than never-institutionalized children. In fact, 100% of the never-institutionalized children showed clear attachment behavior patterns (coded as secure, avoidant, resistant, or disorganized), whereas only 3.2% of the institutionalized children showed clear attachment behaviors.

Indiscriminate Friendliness and Disinhibited Attachment

Related to this failure to develop discriminating attachment relationships are disinhibited attachment and indiscriminate friendliness or indiscriminate sociability. Indiscriminate sociability was first described by Tizard and Hodges (1978); children who display it approach strangers as if they are attachment figures. Rutter and colleagues (2007) provided a multisource assessment of disinhibited attachment at age 11 years, after at least 7½ years in adoptive families. Among Romanian adoptees entering the United Kingdom between 6 and 42 months of age, after having experienced institutional rearing, 26% showed marked disinhibition as assessed by parental report, as compared with 9% of those who had not experienced institutional rearing or who had entered the United Kingdom below 6 months of age, and 4% in domestic adoptees who had not experienced institutional care and who had been adopted under the age of 6 months. Investigator ratings showed that the features most strongly associated with disinhibited attachment were socially inappropriate physical contact, a lack of social reserve, an unusual relationship with the examiner, verbal and social violation of conventional boundaries, and a high rate of spontaneous comments. At age 6 years, disinhibited attachment had been associated with a high proportion of disorganized, insecure/other, and unclassifiable

classifications, with 41% rated as secure. It was also noteworthy that the majority of the children with disinhibited attachment exhibited problems in several other domains of behavior.

Indiscriminate sociability and disinhibited attachment are seen relatively frequently among children who were previously institutionalized for longer than 6 months of the first 2 years of life (e.g., Chisholm, 1998; Zeanah & Smyke, 2005). Most of the existing evidence suggests that children who were in foster care do not show high rates of indiscriminate sociability.

The Meaning of Disinhibited Attachment

Four features of these findings stand out. First, disinhibited attachment constitutes a clinically significant problem that is remarkably persistent many years after adoption for children who were once in institutional care, and almost exclusively so for this population. In the Bucharest early intervention project, Zeanah and Smyke (2005) reported that although inhibited attachment disorders were not disproportionately represented in frequency 18 months after the children were placed in foster families, disinhibited attachment disorders did not remit.

Second, it would be inappropriate to view this pattern as one of attachment insecurity. Rather, it seems to represent an attachment *disorder* that involves a relative failure to develop normal attachment relationships.

Third, although the pattern was strongly associated with institutional deprivation, a substantial proportion of institutionally deprived children did *not* show this pattern. So far, the reasons for the individual differences in response remain obscure. Stevens, Sonuga-Barke, Asherson, Kreppner, and Rutter (2006) have suggested that genetic influences in susceptibility to environmental hazards may be implicated. The possibility of gene–environment interactions (see Rutter, 2006) will need further study and may prove to be an important source of individual differences.

Fourth, it seems that the pattern rarely develops if the institutional deprivation does not persist beyond 6 months of age, but it is common with any persistence beyond 6 months (and apparently does not become more common with increasing periods of institutional deprivation—at least up to the age of 42 months). This implies that some form of biological programming is involved in disinhibited attachment. The findings call for study of the biological processes that may be involved, but they also raise questions about possible sensitive periods in the development of selective attachment relationships.

EFFECTS OF EARLY ADVERSITY ON THE NEUROENDOCRINE SYSTEM

The neuroendocrine system, particularly the hypothalamic–pituitary–adrenocortical (HPA) axis, appears especially susceptible to the effects of relationship disturbance. Glucocorticoids (cortisol in primates, corticosterone in rodents) are end products of the HPA system. Cortisol has received a great deal of attention because it is a product that we can easily measure; it is sequestered in saliva and can therefore be assessed noninvasively, which is critical in studying human youngsters.

The HPA system has two primary functions. One is the more familiar function of responding to stress, and the second is the equally important maintenance of a diurnal rhythm. We describe these two functions below and discuss findings regarding their disturbance.

Stress Reactivity

When an animal experiences a stressor, the limbic system signals to the hypothalamus, which releases corticotropin-releasing hormone (CRH). This signals the pituitary to release adrenocorticotropic hormone (ACTH), which signals the adrenal cortex to produce glucocorticoids (cortisol in humans). This is a negative feedback system, such that the release of glucocorticoids signals to the pituitary to stop releasing ACTH, thus essentially shutting itself off. The system is designed for short, transient stressors, preparing an animal for a fight-or-flight response. Long periods of high levels of glucocorticoids result in damage to the hippocampus and perhaps to the prefrontal cortex—two brain regions with a high density of glucocorticoid receptors (Sapolsky, Romero, & Munck, 2000). Furthermore, high levels of glucocorticoids may result in the long-term down-regulation of the HPA system, such that low levels of glucocorticoids are produced (Gunnar, Fisher, & the Early Experience, Stress, and Prevention Network, 2006).

Among rodents, there is a stress-hyporesponsive period, during which the pup shows minimal response to most stressors. In particular, in the face of threat, the rat pup shows a muted response in terms of producing ACTH and glucocorticoids. This hyporesponsive reaction is likely to be adaptive, in that the rodent pup does not need to mount a stress response. Rather, the pup is helpless to predators and therefore requires the attention of the dam (mother) to survive. Chances of survival are increased if the pup is passive. Evidence is mounting that human infants and toddlers show a hyporeactive period that resembles rodents' hyporesponsive period (e.g., Dozier, Peloso, et al., 2006; Gunnar et al., 2006). Like rodent pups, human infants are helpless in the face of danger without protection from caregivers.

In a number of experimental studies with normally developing young children, Gunnar and colleagues (2006) have found that stressors are not associated with rises in cortisol. Indeed, such activities as going into the lab, going to preschool, and even getting into a car seat are associated with decreases rather than increases in cortisol levels. By the age at which a child could be expected to fend for him- or herself more effectively, the HPA system becomes more stress-reactive, but is hyporesponsive when the child is of an age where he or she can do little to participate in self-protection. Given this hyporesponsive period, it is probably not surprising that differences in stress responsiveness have not been reported for infants and young children in foster or adoptive care relative to other infants.

Maintaining Diurnal Pattern

The second function of the HPA system is to maintain a diurnal pattern. Other systems, such as temperature, also serve in this capacity by ensuring that the animal is awake when others of the species are awake. For diurnal creatures such as humans, there is a high morning level of cortisol that helps an animal wake up, followed by decreasing levels throughout the day, reaching a nadir at night. This diurnal pattern is seen by the time children are 6 weeks old (Gunnar, Brodersen, Nachmias, Buss, & Rigatuso, 1996). For nocturnal creatures such as rodents, this pattern is similar, but with high evening levels (of corticosterone) and low morning levels. In considering human cortisol levels, it is therefore important to remember that the high morning and low evening levels do not reflect differential stress, but rather the diurnal properties of the system.

Dozier, Manni, and colleagues (2006) and Fisher (2005) have found that the maintenance of an abnormal diurnal pattern differentiates young foster children from other young children. In both labs, young children were found to disproportionately show atypical diurnal patterns. Some children showed low levels of cortisol across the day, and others children showed high levels of cortisol. Gunnar, Morison, Chisholm, and Schuder (2001) reported high levels of cortisol production among children who had previously been institutionalized.

Significance of Findings

Thus a young child appears to be in a stress-hyporeactive period, and the stress-reactive property of the HPA system appears largely protected. It seems that the maintenance of the diurnal rhythm is what is disrupted by early adversity. This disruption has not yet been linked with differences in the attachment system. Essentially, regardless of whether foster children can organize their behavior in relation to the availability of new caregivers, they may nonetheless be dysregulated at the neuroendocrine level.

Although we are only beginning to understand the effects of early adversity on neuroendocrine regulation, the preliminary findings are concerning. There is some evidence that low morning cortisol levels are associated with conduct disorder (e.g., McBurnett, Lahey, Rathouz, & Loeber, 2000; Pajer, Gardner, Rubin, Perel, & Neal, 2001), as well as with posttraumatic stress disorder (Davies, Sturge-Apple, Cicchetti, & Cummings, 2007; Yehuda et al., 2000; Yehuda, Halligan, & Bierer, 2002), both contemporaneously and predictively. Thus it is possible that adverse early experiences affect brain development in ways that confer vulnerability for later disorder.

HPA Functioning and Brain Development

Links between HPA functioning and brain development are being studied, with a number of connections seeming plausible. Both the hippocampus and the prefrontal cortex seem especially important regions for study (e.g., De Bellis, 2001). The long-term problems with emotion regulation on the one hand, and with attention and impulse control on the other, make these two regions of particular interest. Animal studies suggest that early adversity can affect hippocampal and prefrontal cortex development, with some suggestion that this is mediated by high levels of glucocorticoids. As mentioned above, it is possible that the low levels seen most often among older foster children result from a system that has been down-regulated in response to high levels of circulating glucocorticoids. At this point, it is important to recognize

that our field still has much to learn about how these systems function in human children. Animal studies are critical, but their results should be applied to humans with caution. Because humans are born more altricial than most other primates, they may have a more extended hyporesponsive period, thus making a monkey model nonoptimal. Rodents may provide a better model for this aspect of the system, however much they differ with respect to the complexity of the caregiving system.

CAREGIVER COMMITMENT

In biologically intact families, commitment is often assumed on the part of the children and parents. It is relatively rare to hear of parents who threaten their children with placement outside the family (e.g., in a juvenile delinquency center, with the gypsies, or on the street), or for underage children to think seriously about leaving home. For foster parents and foster children, however, these issues are often salient. Foster parents have the option of giving the children back to the agency for care. Although adoption is intended as a permanent solution, nearly 8% of adoptions are disrupted annually, mostly because parents request the children's removal. Whereas young children form attachment relationships with their new caregivers, some children retain a sense of connection to other parents or to members of another family. These issues are considered in the sections below.

Under typical conditions, we would rarely expect to see a lack of commitment on a parent's part. Humans produce relatively few young and invest an enormous amount of resources in each. There are rare conditions when commitment appears low on the part of biological parents. When children are placed into foster care or with adoptive parents, however, parents' commitment can be variable.

Among some species, infants are adopted, but only under fairly limited conditions. For example, typically only lactating females and biologically related females appear to adopt orphaned or abandoned rhesus macaque infants (M. Gerald, personal communication, February 14, 2004). In general, humans are less under the control of hormonal influences than other species, perhaps partly because of a more highly developed prefrontal cortex. Nonetheless, it is important to remember that fostering and adopting occur without the usual biological preparedness that accompanies parenting under more typical conditions.

At one end of the continuum, some foster parents appear to think of their foster children as their own, investing emotionally in their children in ways not unlike parents with their birth children. At the other end of the continuum, some foster parents appear to think of themselves as temporary caregivers who should not invest emotionally in their children (Dozier & Lindhiem, 2006).

We have assessed commitment through an interview called the This Is My Baby Interview (Bates & Dozier, 1997) with foster parents. In the interview, a foster mother is asked to describe her child, and to indicate how much she would miss the child if he or she were removed from her care, among other things. Differences in commitment are associated with how many children parents have fostered in the past, with the number of children fostered in the past being inversely related to commitment to current children (Dozier & Lindhiem, 2006). For example, some foster parents have fostered more than 100 children in the past, whereas others are fostering their first children. Foster parents who have fostered more children are less likely than first-time foster parents to commit to the children currently in their care. Also, commitment differs for children of different ages, with caregivers showing higher levels of commitment to children placed at younger ages.

Dozier and Lindhiem (2006) have suggested that having a committed caregiver is even more important to the child's sense of security than is the caregiver's responsiveness to the child's bids for reassurance. The two constructs of commitment and responsiveness to distress are largely orthogonal. For example, it is possible for a foster mother to be dismissing (and not responsive to child cues), but yet highly committed to a child. From an evolutionary perspective, it is critical that the child have a caregiver who will be there to protect him or her under threatening conditions. Although it is optimal if the caregiver is also soothing and responsive, it may be less essential than the caregiver's commitment to the child. We do not know precisely how differences in commitment are communicated to children. Commitment is associated with whether the relationship endures or is disrupted, but there are probably subtle as well as more obvious ways of communicating commitment or its absence. Placements are more likely to be disrupted when caregivers are less highly committed than when caregivers are more committed (Dozier & Lindhiem, 2006).

OPEN ADOPTION AND CONTACT WITH THE BIOLOGICAL FAMILY

When foster children have visitation with birth parents, and/or move back and forth between birth parent homes and foster homes, issues of "Whose child am I?" sometimes arise. For example, birth mothers may want children to think of themselves as their children's mothers, but children often refer to their foster mothers as their mothers. The younger the child, the harder it is for the child to hold onto any notion of another parent at all (Piaget, 2000). As children become older, they may be raised by one set of parents while knowing about the existence of another set of parents. A similar set of circumstances faces children who are adopted.

These issues are more salient in this era of open adoption, when there is the possibility for both biological parents and adopted children to search for each other. The research undertaken up to now regarding open adoption, although very useful in its own right, has not used attachment measures or assessed attachment issues. The move to open adoption was driven initially by the view that this would be beneficial for a child (Hale & Fortin, 2008). Nonetheless, open adoption has implications for all three groups of participants in the adoption triangle (Triseliotis, Feast, & Kyle, 2005)—the biological family, the adoptive family, and the adopted individual. What is the effect on the biological parents' attachment representations of giving up a child for adoption? What is the parallel effect on the adoptive parents having to share parenthood with another set of parents? What is the effect on the adopted child if the circumstances of international adoption mean that continuing contact with the biological family is not possible in practice? What is the effect on attachment representations when, after an initially closed adoption, contact with the biological family is made after years of no contact? Attachment theory provides no clear guide to what is likely to happen or what should happen. What it does do, however, is help us to recognize that contact or the impossibility of contact is likely to impinge on people's internal working models of themselves and of their relationships with other people.

The literature on search and reunion has been well summarized by Triseliotis and colleagues (2005). Howe and Feast (2001) focused primarily on the adopted individual—comparing 394 who had searched for their biological parents with 78 who had not, and who had been sought out and approached on behalf of a birth relative. Of those searchers who found a birth relative, few (7%) were rejected outright, and few (9%) had the contact terminated within a year after only one or two contacts, which was also experienced as a rejection. Nevertheless, most (71%) evaluated the reunion as emotionally satisfying, and nearly half claimed that it had improved their self-esteem. Few (11%) of the searchers and a quarter of the nonsearchers felt that the reunion experience had been upsetting. Howe and Feast (2001) concluded that adopted individuals who did *not* search were on the whole well integrated into their adoptive families. Those placed transracially were less likely (56% vs. 71% in same-race placements) to report that they felt they "belonged" in their adoptive family.

Triseliotis and colleagues (2005) examined the outcome of contact with respect to all three members of the adoption triangle. Data were derived from a large-scale postal questionnaire, and a matched-sample design was employed, focusing only on adopted children included in the first study. A high participation rate (82%) was achieved.

Approximately one-half of the birth mothers were under the age of 20 at the time of the adopted children's birth, and a minority (11%) were 16 or under. Most became pregnant during the 1950s and early 1960s, when social attitudes toward pregnancies outside marriage tended to be very censorious. Most of the girls' parents were initially shocked and upset, but eventually approximately one-third were supportive (despite usually keeping the pregnancies secret). Most women reported that they felt they had no choice about giving up their babies. Emotional support was usually lacking at the time of parting with their children, and most of the biological mothers came to feel lonely and abandoned. Nevertheless, many (70%) of the mothers said that as they looked back, they felt that adoption had been the right decision. Most did not think the experience had affected their capacity to make new relationships (but 14% said that it had). Similarly, some three-fifths did not think parting with their adopted children had affected the quality of their relationships with their other children, but two-fifths thought it had. These findings suggest that a more detailed study of social relationships, including a use of attachment concepts, would be worthwhile.

Regarding the contact with the adopted children many years later, mothers who were sought out were more likely than seekers to report that the contact felt comfortable. In two-thirds of cases,

contact was stopped at the initiative of the adopted persons, especially in the case of seeker mothers. For most birth mothers, contact and reunion were happy and satisfying experiences, with about half feeling that their ability to relate to others had been improved by the reunion; however, some (1 in 10) were dissatisfied, and about the same proportion felt angrier since contact than before.

Most adopted people rated their relationships with their adoptive parents as close, but some (nearly 20%) described them as not close. Those who felt that their relationships were close were least likely to feel rejected by their biological parents. In cases in which there was a feeling of rejection, however, this tended to peak in adolescence. Some adopted persons reported a sense of loss. The experience of reunion with their biological mothers was reported by a third as having enhanced their relationships with their adoptive families, but some (1 in 6) said that it had led to deterioration in these relationships. Eight years after the reunion, about three-quarters were still in contact with the biological relatives. Some (1 in 3) came to look upon their birth mothers as parents, but just over half viewed them as friends or friends/relatives. For the remaining subset (18%), the relationships were distant or their birth mothers felt like strangers. Many (80%) were pleased to have made contact, and where contact had been established, feelings of rejection or loss tended to diminish. Nevertheless, some (10–20%) of adopted people felt that adoption had adversely affected their marriage and social relationships.

Most (nearly 90%) adopting parents had disclosed the adoption when their children were 4 years of age or younger, and most felt that this had been the right time. Most adoptive parents talked (sometimes or often) with their children about the children's birth families, but a minority (1 in 5) felt that their children were reluctant to do this. Almost all adopting parents felt close to their adopted children and felt very happy about their relationship. Over three-quarters of adopters described their children's motivation to search as strong, and most were supportive of it. However, a few (1 in 6) felt frightened and worried. A prominent concern was that their children might be hurt by the contact, but some felt worried that reunion would mean that they would "lose" their children.

Most (70%) adopters reported that their relationships with their children were unchanged by the search and reunion, and for almost everyone else it had been enhanced. Nevertheless, some (1 in 8) said that, especially in the early stages of the search, their relationships were under strain. Overall, most (nearly 70%) reported that the contact experience had been positive, and very few (3%) reported it as clearly negative.

Viewed as a whole, the search and reunion were positive experiences. For an appreciable minority, the experience of parting with their children may have had an adverse effect on their social relationships. Similarly, for a minority of adopted individuals, there were concerns over some aspects of social relationships. A more detailed study of these variations would benefit from an attachment perspective, but it would be a mistake to ignore the broader social context, and the attachment features would need to be examined alongside other perspectives.

INTERVENTIONS TO ENHANCE ATTACHMENT AMONG FOSTER AND ADOPTED CHILDREN

Harlow found that isolate-reared monkeys engaged in odd, aggressive, and self-destructive behaviors when placed back into their home cages following extended isolation. It turned out that younger monkeys best served as "therapist monkeys" for these isolate-reared monkeys; these younger monkeys allowed close contact while tolerating aberrant behavior without reprisal (Suomi & Harlow, 1972; Suomi, Harlow, & McKinney, 1972). The principle here might be that contact was needed, but in a context that would not result in injury. For children in institutional care, foster care and adoption represent interventions that often meet these two criteria. A reasonably stimulating but tolerant environment appears to result in excellent physical catch-up, as well as reasonable cognitive catch-up for children who had been institutionalized (Gunnar et al., 2000).

Even when provided with the company of "therapist monkeys," Harlow's isolate-reared monkeys continued to show odd behavior. Most did not mate as adults, and most that did mate showed very inappropriate parenting behaviors. Similarly, children adopted from orphanages continue to show anomalous behaviors, especially with regard to social behaviors and inhibitory control. Without nurturing parents, foster children may develop cognitively but have difficulty organizing attachment behaviors (Gunnar et al., 2000) The aspects of functioning that appear problematic, at least for some children, are regulation of neuroendocrine functioning, inhibitory control, and behavioral control (including risk for substance

abuse and related problems), as well as disorganized attachment, nondiscriminating attachment relationships, and odd social behaviors (Gunnar et al., 2000). There has been relatively little research investigating how best to alter these behavioral trajectories. We suggest that interventions need to target the behaviors identified as specifically problematic. In some instances there will be overlap in intervention strategies for foster children, domestically adopted children, and internationally adopted children, and in other instances there will not be. The last two decades have seen an explosion of attachment-based interventions for young children (e.g., Hoffman, Marvin, Cooper, & Powell, 2006). A smaller number of interventions target the needs of children in foster or adoptive care (Dozier, Lindhiem, & Ackerman, 2005; Fisher & Chamberlain, 2000; Juffer, Hoksbergen, Riksen-Walraven, & Kohnstamm, 1997).

Evidence-Based Interventions for Adopted Children

Juffer and colleagues (1997) assessed the effectiveness of an intervention for internationally adopted children who were placed before 6 months of age. Adoptive parents were randomly assigned to one of two groups. Half of the parents received a book describing appropriately sensitive behavior, and half received, in addition to the book, video feedback designed to enhance sensitivity. Children in the video feedback condition showed lower rates of disorganized attachment than children in the control condition did. This study is impressive in its use of a randomized clinical trial and a brief intervention. Still, the findings target early-placed adopted children, who are at low risk for development of disorganized attachment.

Evidence-Based Interventions for Foster Children

Two attachment-based interventions that have been developed for foster children are Dozier and colleagues' (2005) Attachment and Biobehavioral Catch-Up intervention and Zeanah and colleagues' (2005) New Orleans intervention for maltreated children in foster care. These two programs (mainly focused on fostered children, but relevant for adopted children from similar backgrounds) share with other attachment-based interventions the aim of guiding parents to help their children regulate emotions, respond effectively to the children's distress, and understand the children's signals.

The efficacy of the Attachment and Biobehavioral Catch-Up intervention has been assessed in a small, randomized clinical trial. In the trial, young foster children were randomly assigned to Attachment and Biobehavioral Catch-Up or to a control intervention of the same duration and frequency (10 in-home sessions). Children whose foster parents received the experimental intervention showed less avoidance than other children did, as well as more typical daily patterns of cortisol production (Dozier, Peloso, et al., 2006).

A behavioral intervention that was designed for older children (i.e., preschoolers) has also shown effects on attachment outcomes as well. Fisher, Burraston, and Pears (2005) assessed the efficacy of a behavioral home-based intervention, Multidimensional Treatment Foster Care (Fisher & Chamberlain, 2000), for caregivers of preschoolers in foster care. The children targeted often had significant behavioral problems that interfered with caregivers' attempts to form relationships. Foster parents using this procedure are taught to provide an environment with reliable contingencies for children. Although a behavioral intervention may not seem relevant to attachment, one of the striking findings of the Fisher and colleagues work is that children showed secure behaviors more, and remained in stable placements longer, than children who did not receive the intervention. We suggest that helping foster parents and children gain control over children's behavioral problems allows the dyads to develop relationships that would not otherwise be possible. The behavioral problems interfere with parents' ability to respond in nurturing ways and to commit to the children's long-term development, and this interference in turn undermines the children's ability to trust in the caregivers' availability.

HARMFUL INTERVENTIONS FOR FOSTER AND ADOPTED CHILDREN

In parallel with these positive developments in evidence-based interventions that target specific needs of foster and adopted children, there have been various coercive interventions claiming to be attachment-based, but actually using concepts that are antithetical to attachment theory. These approaches, known as "attachment therapy" or "holding therapy," lack empirical support and indeed have led to adverse effects, as suggested by Lillienfield (2007), Pignotti and Mercer (2007), and O'Connor and Zeanah (2003). Lillienfield

includes holding therapy as one of the "potentially harmful therapies (PHTs)" (p. 53) in his 2007 *Psychological Science* review. Holding therapy is included as a level 1 PHT, classified as "probably produc[ing] harm in some individuals" (Lillienfield, 2007, p. 59). Several deaths have been associated with the use of this treatment (Pignotti & Mercer, 2007), and no randomized clinical trials have been conducted that support its efficacy (Lillienfield, 2007). Despite claims to the contrary, holding therapy does not provide a useful basis for further developments in the design of treatments for attachment disorders in adopted or nonadopted children. This treatment is unfortunately often referred to as "attachment therapy." It seems critical to differentiate it from treatments derived from attachment theory.

CONCLUSIONS

From an evolutionary perspective, it is advantageous that the human attachment system can adapt to a range of caregiving conditions. Children can form attachment relationships to new caregivers when a previous relationship has been disrupted or after the experience of adversity. When new caregivers are nurturing, children can organize their attachment behavior in relation to the new caregivers' availability. Nonetheless, when children experience conditions that are beyond those the attachment system is designed to deal with, it seems that rigid means of coping (e.g., disinhibited attachment), or a neurobiology that predisposes to later disorder, become more likely. Interventions need to target the specific issues with which children struggle most.

REFERENCES

Ackerman, B. P., Kogos, J., Youngstrom, E., Stroff, K., & Izard, C. (1999). Family instability and the problem behaviors of children from economically disadvantaged families. *Developmental Psychology, 35,* 258–268.

Appleyard, K., Egeland, B., van Dulmen, M. H. M., & Sroufe, L. A. (2005). When more is not better: The role of cumulative risk in child behavior outcomes. *Journal of Child Psychology and Psychiatry, 46,* 235–245.

Bakermans-Kranenburg, M. J., & van IJzendoorn, M. H. (2006). Gene–environment interaction of the dopamine D4 receptor (DRD4) and observed maternal insensitivity predicting externalizing behavior in preschoolers. *Developmental Psychobiology, 48,* 406–409.

Bakermans-Kranenburg, M. J., van IJzendoorn, M. H., Mesman, J., Alink, L. R., & Juffer, F. (in press). Effects of an attachment-based intervention on daily cortisol moderated by DRD4: A randomized control trial on 1–3-year-olds screened for externalized behavior. *Development and Psychopathology.*

Barth, R. P. (1991). Adoption of drug-exposed children. *Children and Youth Services Review, 13*, 323–342.

Barth, R. P., & Needell, B. (1996). Outcomes for drug-exposed children four years post-adoption. *Children and Youth Services Review, 18*, 37–56.

Bates, B., & Dozier, M. (1997). *This Is My Baby Interview.* Unpublished manuscript, University of Delaware.

Beebe, B., Lachmann, F., & Jaffe, J. (1997). Mother–infant interaction structures and presymbolic self- and object representations. *Psychoanalytic Dialogues, 7*, 133–182.

Bowlby, J. (1951). *Maternal care and mental health.* Geneva: World Health Organization.

Bretherton, I. (1985). Attachment theory: Retrospect and prospect. In I. Bretherton & E. Waters (Eds.), Growing points of attachment theory and research. *Monographs of the Society for Research in Child Development, 50*(1–2, Serial No. 209), 3–35.

Brooks, D., & Barth, R. P. (1998). Characteristics and outcomes of drug-exposed and non-drug exposed children in kinship and non-relative foster care. *Children and Youth Services Review, 20*, 475–501.

Browne, K., Hamilton-Giachritsis, C., Johnson, R., & Ostergren, M. (2006). Overuse of institutional care for children in Europe. *British Medical Journal, 332*, 485–487.

Carlson, M., & Earls, F. (1997). Psychological and neuroendocrinological sequelae of early social deprivation in institutionalized children in Romania. *Annals of the New York Academy of Sciences, 807*, 419–428.

Caspi, A., McClay, J., Moffitt, T. E., Mill, J., Martin, J., Craig, et al. (2002). Role of genotype in the cycle of violence in maltreated children. *Science, 297*, 851–854.

Caspi, A., Sugden, K., Moffitt, T. E., Taylor, A., Craig, I. W., Harrington, H., et al. (2003). Influence of life stress on depression: Moderation by a polymorphism in the 5-HTT gene. *Science, 301*, 386–389.

Chisholm, K. (1998). A three year follow-up of attachment and indiscriminate friendliness in children adopted from Romanian orphanages. *Child Development, 69*, 1092–1106.

Chisholm, K., Carter, M. C., Ames, E. W., & Morison, S. J. (1995). Attachment security and indiscriminately friendly behavior in children adopted from Romanian orphanages. *Development and Psychopathology, 7*, 283–294.

Cicchetti, D., & Curtis, W. J. (2005). An event-related potential study of the processing of affective facial expressions in young children who experienced maltreatment during the first year of life. *Development and Psychopathology, 17*, 641–677.

Crittenden, P. M. (1985). Maltreated infants: Vulner-

ability and resilience. *Journal of Child Psychology and Psychiatry, 26*, 85–96.

Cuddleback, G. S. (2004). Kinship family foster care: A methodological and substantive synthesis of research. *Children and Youth Services Review, 26*, 623–639.

Davies, P. T., Sturge-Apple, M. L., Cicchetti, D., & Cummings, E. M. (2007). The role of child adrenocortical functioning in pathways between interparental conflict and child maltreatment. *Developmental Psychology, 43*, 918–930.

De Bellis, M. D. (2001). Developmental traumatology: The psychobiological development of maltreated children and its implications for research, treatment, and policy. *Development and Psychopathology, 13*, 539–564.

Dodge, K. A., Pettit, G. S., Bates, J. E., & Valente, E. (1995). Social information-processing patterns partially mediate the effect of early physical abuse on later conduct problems. *Journal of Abnormal Psychology, 104*, 632–643.

Dozier, M. (2005). [Attachment security and later outcomes.] Unpublished raw data, University of Delaware.

Dozier, M., & Lindhiem, O. (2006). This is my child: Differences among foster parents in commitment to their young children. *Child Maltreatment, 11*, 338–345.

Dozier, M., Lindhiem, O., & Ackerman, J. P. (2005). Attachment and Biobehavioral Catch-up: An intervention targeting empirically identified needs of foster infants. In L. J. Berlin, Y. Ziv, L. Amaya-Jackson, & M. T. Greenberg (Eds.), *Enhancing early attachments: Theory, research, intervention, and policy* (pp. 178–194). New York: Guilford Press.

Dozier, M., Manni, M., Gordon, M. K., Peloso, E., Gunnar, M. R., Stovall-McClough, K. C., et al. (2006). Foster children's diurnal production of cortisol: An exploratory study. *Child Maltreatment, 11*, 189–197.

Dozier, M., Peloso, E., Lindhiem, O., Gordon, M. K., Manni, M., Sepulveda, S., et al. (2006). Preliminary evidence from a randomized clinical trial: Intervention effects on foster children's behavioral and biological regulation. *Journal of Social Issues, 62*, 767–785.

Dozier, M., Stovall, C., Albus, K., & Bates, B. (2001). Attachment for infants in foster care: The role of caregiver state of mind. *Child Development, 72*, 1467–1477.

Duyme, M., Dumaret, A.-C., & Tomkiewicz, S. (1999). How can we boost IQs of "dull children"?: A late adoption study. *Proceedings of the National Academy of Sciences USA, 96*, 8790–8794.

Egeland, B., & Sroufe, L. A. (1981). Attachment and early maltreatment. *Child Development, 52*, 44–52.

Egeland, B., Sroufe, L. A., & Erickson, M. (1983). The developmental consequence of different patterns of maltreatment. *Child Maltreatment, 7*, 459–469.

Fisher, P. A. (2005, April). *Translational research on underlying mechanisms of risk among foster children: Implications for prevention science.* Paper presented at the biennial meeting of the Society for Research on Child Development, Washington, DC.

Fisher, P. A., Burraston, B., & Pears, K. (2005). The Early Intervention Foster Care Program: Permanent placement outcomes from a randomized trial. *Child Maltreatment, 10,* 61–71.

Fisher, P. A., & Chamberlain, P. (2000). Multidimensional Treatment Foster Care: A program for intensive parent training, family support, and skill building. *Journal of Emotional and Behavioral Disorders, 8,* 155–164.

George, C., Kaplan, N., & Main, M. (1984). *Adult Attachment Interview protocol.* Unpublished manuscript, University of California at Berkeley.

George, C., Kaplan, N., & Main, M. (1985). *Adult Attachment Interview protocol* (2nd ed.). Unpublished manuscript, University of California at Berkeley.

George, C., Kaplan, N., & Main, M. (1996). *Adult Attachment Interview protocol* (3rd ed.). Unpublished manuscript, University of California at Berkeley.

George, C., & Main, M. (1979). Social interactions of young abused children: Approach, avoidance, and aggression. *Child Development, 50,* 306–318.

Gianino, A., & Tronick, E. Z. (1988). The mutual regulation model: The infant's self and interactive regulation coping and defensive capacities. In T. Field, P. McCabe, & N. Schneiderman (Eds.), *Stress and coping* (pp. 47–68). Hillsdale, NJ: Erlbaum.

Gibb, B. E. (2001). Childhood maltreatment and negative cognitive styles. *Clinical Psychology Review, 22,* 223–246.

Glantz, M. D., & Chambers, J. C. (2006). Prenatal drug exposure effects on subsequent vulnerability to drug abuse. *Development and Psychopathology, 18,* 893–922.

Goossens, F., & van IJzendoorn, M. H. (1990). Quality of infants' attachments to professional caregivers: Relation to infant–parent attachment and daycare characteristics. *Child Development, 61,* 832–837.

Groark, C. J., Muhamedrahimov, R. J., Palmov, O. I., Nikiforova, N. V., & McCall, R. B. (2005). Improvements in early care in Russian orphanages and their relationship to observed behaviors. *Infant Mental Health Journal, 26,* 96–109.

Gunnar, M. R., Brodersen, L., Krueger, K., & Rigatuso, J. (1996). Dampening of adrenocortical responses during infancy: Normative changes and individual differences. *Child Development, 67,* 877–888.

Gunnar, M. R., Brodersen, L., Nachmias, M., Buss, K., & Rigatuso, J. (1996). Stress reactivity and attachment security. *Developmental Psychology, 29,* 191–204.

Gunnar, M. R., Bruce, J., & Grotevant, H. D. (2000). International adoption of institutionally reared children: Research and policy. *Development and Psychopathology, 12,* 677–693.

Gunnar, M. R., Fisher, P. A., & the Early Experience, Stress, and Prevention Network. (2006). Bringing basic research on early experience and stress neurobiology to bear on preventative interventions for neglected and maltreated children. *Development and Psychopathology, 18,* 651–677.

Gunnar, M. R., Morison, S. J., Chisholm, K., & Schuder, M. (2001). Salivary cortisol levels in children adopted from Romanian orphanages. *Development and Psychopathology, 13,* 611–628.

Hale, B., & Fortin, J. (2008). Legal issues in the care and treatment of children with mental health problems. In M. Rutter, D. Bishop, D. Pine, S. Scott, J. Stevenson, E. Taylor, et al. (Eds.), *Rutter's child and adolescent psychiatry* (5th ed.). Oxford, UK: Blackwell.

Harris, T., Brown, G. W., & Bifulco, A. (1986). Loss of parent in childhood and adult psychiatric disorder: The role of lack of adequate parental care. *Psychological Medicine, 16,* 641–659.

Hesse, E., & Main, M. (2006). Frightening, threatening, and dissociative behavior in low-risk parents: Description, discussion, and interpretations. *Development and Psychopathology, 18,* 309–343.

Hinde, R. A., & McGinnis, L. (1977). Some factors influencing the effects of temporary mother–infant separation: Some experiments with rhesus monkeys. *Psychological Medicine, 7,* 197–212.

Hoffman, K. T., Marvin, R. S., Cooper, G., & Powell, B. (2006). Changing toddlers' and preschoolers' attachment classifications: The Circle of Security intervention. *Journal of Consulting and Clinical Psychology, 74,* 1017–1026.

Howe, D., & Feast, J. (2001). The long-term outcome of reunions between adult adopted people and their birth mothers. *British Journal of Social Work, 31,* 351–368.

Howes, C., & Hamilton, C. E. (1992). Children's relationships with child care teachers: Stability and concordance with parental attachments. *Child Development, 63,* 867–878.

Johnson, D., Albers, L., Iverson, S., Mathers, M., Dole, K., Georgieff, M., et al. (1996). Health status of U.S. adopted Eastern European (EE) orphans. *Pediatric Research, 39,* 134A.

Juffer, F., Hoksbergen, R. A. C., Riksen-Walraven, J. M., & Kohnstamm, G. A. (1997). Early intervention in adoptive families: Supporting maternal sensitive responsiveness, infant–mother attachment, and infant competence. *Journal of Child Psychology and Psychiatry, 38,* 1039–1050.

Kaufman, J., Yang, B., Douglas-Palumberi, H., Grasso, D., Lipschitz, D., Houshyar, S., et al. (2006). Brain-derived neurotrophic factor-5-HHTLPR gene interactions and environmental modifiers of depression in children. *Biological Psychiatry, 59,* 673–680.

Kaufman, J., Yang, B., Douglas-Palumberi, H., Houshyar, S., Lipschitz, D., Krystal, J. H., et al. (2004). Social supports and serotonin transporter gene moderate depression in maltreated children. *Proceedings of the National Academy of Sciences USA, 101,* 17316–17321.

Keiley, M. K., Howe, T. R., Dodge, K. A., Bates, J. E., & Pettit, G. S. (2001). The timing of child physical maltreatment: A cross-domain growth analysis of impact on adolescent externalizing and internalizing problems. *Development and Psychopathology, 13,* 891–912.

Levine, S., Weiner, S. G., & Coe, C. L. (1993). Temporal and social factors influencing behavioral and hormonal responses to separation in mother and infant squirrel monkeys. *Psychoneuroendocrinology, 4,* 297–306.

Lillienfield, S. O. (2007). Psychological treatments that cause harm. *Psychological Science, 2,* 53–70.

Lyons-Ruth, K., Alpern, L., & Repacholi, B. (1993). Disorganized infant attachment classification and maternal psychosocial problems as predictors of hostile-aggressive behavior in the preschool classroom. *Child Development, 64,* 572–585.

Maestripieri, D. (2005). Early experience affects the intergenerational transmission of infant abuse in rhesus monkeys. *Proceedings of the National Academy of Sciences USA, 102,* 9726–9719.

McBurnett, K., Lahey, B. B., Rathouz, P. J., & Loeber, R. (2000). Low salivary cortisol and persistent aggression in boys referred for disruptive behavior. *Archives of General Psychiatry, 57,* 38–43.

Milan, S. E., & Pinderhughes, E. E. (2000). Factors influencing maltreated children's early adjustment in foster care. *Development and Psychopathology, 12,* 63–81.

Numan, M. J., & Insel, T. R. (2003). *The neurobiology of parental behavior* (3rd ed.). New York: Springer.

O'Connor, T. G., Marvin, R. S., Rutter, M., Olrick, J. T., & Britner, P. A. (2003). Child–parent attachment following institutional deprivation. *Development and Psychopathology, 15,* 19–38.

O'Connor, T. G., Rutter, M., & the English and Romanian Adoptees Study Team. (2000). Attachment disorder behaviour following early severe deprivation: Extension and longitudinal follow-up. *Journal of the American Academy of Child and Adolescent Psychiatry, 39,* 703–712.

O'Connor, T. G., & Zeanah, C. (2003). Attachment disorders: Assessment strategies and treatment approaches. *Attachment and Human Development, 5,* 223–244.

Pajer, K., Gardner, W., Rubin, R. T., Perel, J., & Neal, S. (2001). Decreased cortisol levels in adolescent girls with conduct disorder. *Archives of General Psychiatry, 58,* 297–302.

Piaget, J. (2000). Childhood cognitive development: The essential readings. In K. Lee (Ed.), *Essential readings in cognitive development* (pp. 33–47). Oxford, UK: Blackwell.

Pignotti, M., & Mercer, J. (2007). Holding therapy and dyadic developmental psychotherapy are not supported and acceptable social work interventions: A systematic research synthesis revisited. *Research on Social Work Practice, 17,* 513–519.

Pollak, S. D., & Tolley-Schell, S. A. (2003). Selective attention to facial emotion in physically abused children. *Journal of Abnormal Psychology, 112,* 323–338.

Rajecki, D. W., Lamb, M. E., & Obmascher, P. (1978). Toward a general theory of infantile attachment: A comparative review of aspects of the social bond. *Behavioral and Brain Sciences, 3,* 417–464.

Roth, T. L., & Sullivan, R. M. (2005). Memory of early maltreatment: Neonatal behavioral and neuronal correlates of maternal maltreatment within the context of classical conditioning. *Biological Psychiatry, 57,* 823–831.

Rutter, M. (2006). *Genes and behavior: Nature–nurture interplay explained.* Oxford, UK: Blackwell.

Rutter, M., Colvert, E., Kreppner, J., Beckett, C., Castle, J., Groothues, C., et al. (2007). Early adolescent outcomes for institutionally-deprived and non-deprived adoptees: I. Disinhibited attachment. *Journal of Child Psychology and Psychiatry, 48,* 17–30.

Rutter, M., Kreppner, J. M., & O'Connor, T. G. (2001). Specificity and heterogeneity in children's responses to profound institutional privation. *British Journal of Psychiatry, 179,* 97–103.

Rutter, M., Moffitt, T. E., & Caspi, A. (2006). Gene–environment interplay and psychopathology: Multiple varieties by real effects. *Journal of Child Psychology and Psychiatry, 47,* 226–261.

Sameroff, A. J., Bartko, W. T., Baldwin, A., Baldwin, C., & Seifer, R. (1998). Family and social influences on the development of child competence. In M. Lewis & C. Feiring (Eds.), *Families, risk, and competence* (pp. 161–185). Mahwah, NJ: Erlbaum.

Sanchez, M. M., Ladd, C. O., & Plotsky, P. M. (2001). Early adverse experience as a developmental risk factor for later psychopathology: Evidence from rodent and primate models. *Development and Psychopathology, 13,* 419–449.

Sapolsky, R. M., Romero, L. M., & Munck, A. U. (2000). How do glucocorticoids influence stress responses?: Integrating permissive, suppressive, stimulatory, and preparative actions. *Endocrine Reviews, 21,* 55–89.

Savage, J., Brodsky, N. L., Malmud, E., Giannetta, J. M., & Hurt, H. (2005). Attentional functioning and impulse control in cocaine-exposed and control children at age ten years. *Journal of Developmental and Behavioral Pediatrics, 26,* 42–47.

Sinclair, I., & Wilson, K. (2003). Matches and mismatches: The contribution of carers and children to the success of foster placements. *British Journal of Social Work, 33,* 871–884.

Singer, L., Brodzinsky, D., Steir, M., & Waters, E. (1985). Mother–infant attachment in adoptive families. *Child Development, 56,* 1543–1551.

Smith, M. G., & Fong, R. (2004). *The children of neglect: When no one cares.* New York: Brunner-Routledge.

Spertus, I. L., Yehuda, R., Wong, C. M., Halligan, S., & Seremetis, S. V. (2003). Childhood emotional abuse and neglect as predictors of psychological and physical symptoms in women presenting to a primary care practice. *Child Abuse and Neglect, 27,* 1247–1258.

Spitz, R. (1945). Hospitalism: An inquiry into the genesis of psychiatric conditions in early childhood. *Psychoanalytic Study of the Child, 1,* 53–74.

Sroufe, L. A., Egeland, B., Carlson, E. A., & Collins, W. A. (2005). *The development of the person: The Minnesota Study of Risk and Adaptation from Birth to Adulthood.* New York: Guilford Press.

Stern, D. N. (2002). *The first relationship: Infant and mother.* Cambridge, MA: Harvard University Press.

Stevens, S., Sonuga-Barke, E., Asherson, P., Kreppner, J., & Rutter, M. (2006). A consideration of the potential role of genetic factors in individual differences in response to early institutional deprivation: The case of inattention/overactivity in the English and Romanian Adoptees Study. *ACAMH Occasional Papers: Genetics, 25,* 63–76.

Stovall, K. C., & Dozier, M. (2000). The development of attachment in new relationships: Single subject analyses for 10 foster infants. *Development and Psychopathology, 12,* 133–156.

Stovall-McClough, K. C., & Dozier, M. (2004). Forming attachments in foster care: Infant attachment behaviors during the first 2 months of placement. *Development and Psychopathology, 16,* 253–271.

Suomi, S. J. (2003). Gene–environment interactions and the neurobiology of social conflict. *Annals of the New York Academy of Sciences, 1008,* 132–139.

Suomi, S. J., & Harlow, H. F. (1972). Social rehabilitation of isolate-reared monkeys. *Developmental Psychology, 6,* 487–496.

Suomi, S., Harlow, H. F., & McKinney, W. T. (1972). Monkey psychiatrists. *American Journal of Psychiatry, 128,* 927–932.

Tizard, B., & Hodges, J. (1978). The effect of early institutional rearing on the development of eight year old children. *Journal of Child Psychology and Psychiatry, 19,* 99–118.

Tizard, B., & Rees, J. (1975). The effect of early institutional rearing on the behavioral problems and affectional relationships of four-year-old children. *Journal of Child Psychology and Psychiatry, 27,* 61–73.

Triseliotis, J., Feast, J., & Kyle, F. (2005). *The adoption triangle revisited: A study of adoption, search and reunion experiences.* London: British Association for Adoption and Fostering.

U.S. Department of Health and Human Services (DHHS), Administration on Children, Youth and Families. (2006). *Child welfare outcomes 2004: Annual report.* Washington, DC: U.S. Government Printing Office.

U.S. Department of State. (2005). *International adoption.* Retrieved from *travel.state.gov/family/adoption/notices/notices_473.html*

van IJzendoorn, M. H. (1995). Adult attachment representations, parental responsiveness and infant attachment: A meta-analysis on the predictive validity of the Adult Attachment Interview. *Psychological Bulletin, 117,* 387–403.

van IJzendoorn, M. H., & Juffer, F. (2006). The Emanual Miller Memorial lecture 2006: Adoption as intervention. Meta-analytic evidence for massive catch-up and plasticity in physical, socio-emotional and cognitive development. *Journal of Child Psychology and Psychiatry, 47,* 1228–1245.

van IJzendoorn, M. H., Schuengel, C., & Bakermans-Kranenburg, M. J. (1999). Disorganized attachment in early childhood: Meta-analysis of precursors, concomitants, and sequelae. *Development and Psychopathology, 11,* 225–249.

Vorria, P., Papaligoura, Z., Dunn, J., van IJzendoorn, M. H., Steele, H., Kontopoulou, A., et al. (2003). Early experiences and attachment relationships of Greek infants raised in residential group care. *Journal of Child Psychology and Psychiatry, 44,* 1–13.

Vorria, P., Papaligoura, Z., Sarafidou, J., Kopakaki, M., Dunn, J., van IJzendoorn, M. H., et al. (2006). The development of adopted children after institutional care: A follow-up study. *Journal of Child Psychology and Psychiatry, 47,* 1246–1253.

Wakschlag, L. S., & Hans, S. L. (2002). Maternal smoking during pregnancy and conduct problems in high-risk youth: A developmental framework. *Development and Psychopathology, 12,* 351–369.

Waters, E., & Deane, K. E. (1985). Defining and assessing individual differences in attachment relationships: Q-methodology and the organization of behavior in infancy and early childhood. In I. Bretherton & E. Waters (Eds.), Growing points of attachment theory and research. *Monographs of the Society for Research in Child Development, 50*(1–2, Serial No. 209), 41–65.

Weinfield, N. S., Sroufe, L. A., & Egeland, B. (2000). Attachment from infancy to early adulthood in a high-risk sample: Continuity, discontinuity, and their correlates. *Child Development, 71,* 695–702.

Yehuda, R., Bierer, L. M., Schmiedler, J., Aferiat, D. H., Breslau, I., & Dolan, S. (2000). Low cortisol and risk for PTSD in adult offspring of Holocaust survivors. *American Journal of Psychiatry, 157,* 1252–1259.

Yehuda, R., Halligan, S. L., & Bierer, L. M. (2002). Cortisol levels in adult offspring of Holocaust survivors: Relation to PTSD symptom severity in the parent and child. *Psychoneuroendocrinology, 27,* 171–180.

Zeanah, C. H., & Smyke, A. T. (2005). Building attachment relationships following maltreatment and severe deprivation. In L. J. Berlin, Y. Ziv, L. Amaya-Jackson, & M. T. Greenberg (Eds.), *Enhancing early attachments: Theory, research, intervention, and policy* (pp. 195–216). New York: Guilford Press.

Zeanah, C. H., Smyke, A. T., Koga, S. F., Carlson, E., & the Bucharest Early Intervention Project Core Group. (2005). Attachment in institutionalized and community children in Romania. *Child Development, 76,* 1015–1028.

CHAPTER 30

Attachment and Psychopathology in Adulthood

MARY DOZIER
K. CHASE STOVALL-McCLOUGH
KATHLEEN E. ALBUS

Bowlby (1969/1982, 1973, 1980) proposed a model of development with clearly articulated implications for psychopathology. According to this model, an infant's formation of an attachment to a caregiver is a key developmental task that influences not only the child's representations of self and other, but also strategies for processing attachment-related thoughts and feelings. Attachment-related events, such as loss and abuse, lead to modifications in these internal representations and affect a child's strategies for processing thoughts and feelings. Bowlby (1973, 1980) suggested that when children develop negative representations of themselves or others, or when they adopt strategies for processing attachment-related thoughts and feelings that compromise realistic appraisals, they become more vulnerable to psychopathology. In this chapter, we consider how the quality of an infant's attachment to his or her caregiver, subsequent attachment-related experiences, and concurrently assessed states of mind with respect to attachment (Main & Goldwyn, 1984; Main, Goldwyn, & Hesse, 2003) may be related to risk for psychopathology or to psychological resilience in adulthood.

ATTACHMENT TO CAREGIVERS

Infants develop expectations about their primary caregivers' availability through interactions with those caregivers. According to Bowlby (1969/1982), these expectations then serve as the basis for an infant's working models of self and others. When infants' experiences lead to expectations that caregivers will be responsive to their needs, they develop secure strategies for seeking out their caregivers when distressed or in need, with the expectation that their needs will be met. When infants instead have experiences that lead them to expect caregivers to be rejecting or undependable, they do not expect that caregivers will be available when needed, and they develop alternative, insecure strategies for coping with their distress.

Insecure strategies vary primarily along the dimension of attempts to minimize or maximize the expression of attachment needs. When children use minimizing strategies, they defensively turn attention away from their distress and from issues of caregiver availability. They therefore have limited access to their own feelings and develop an unrealistic portrayal of parents' availability. When children use maximizing strategies, they defensively turn their attention to their own distress and to issues of caregiver availability. Because they are so "enmeshed" (Main & Goldwyn, 1984; Main et al., 2003) in issues of caregiver availability, they are unable to appraise accurately whether threats exist and whether caregivers are available. Either of these strategies may leave children at increased risk for psychopathology. Minimizing strategies may predispose a child to externalizing disorders because attention is turned away from the self, without the resolution of negative representations. Maximizing strategies may predispose a child to internalizing disorders because attention is riveted on caregiver availability, and negative representations remain painfully alive.

Sroufe and colleagues (e.g., Sroufe, 1997, 2005; Sroufe, Egeland, Carlson, & Collins, 2005b) have emphasized the importance of the organizational function of the attachment system in integrating affective, motivational, and behavioral components of experience. As representational capacities change, so too do the processes of thinking about attachment figures and experiences. Various factors make continuity in development likely, including continuity in quality of care and the limitations of previous levels of adaptation (Crowell & Waters, 2005; Sroufe, 1996; Sroufe, Egeland, Carlson, & Collins, 2005a, 2005b). Nonetheless, changes in environmental quality can result in changes in developmental trajectories. According to Sroufe and colleagues (2005a, 2005b), discontinuity, as well as continuity, is lawful. Bowlby (1973) considered issues such as loss of caregivers, traumatic experiences, and the continuing level of caregiver availability as critical to continuity and discontinuity. For example, experiences of loss or abuse may leave a child vulnerable and without emotionally available attachment figures. The child may then revise earlier models of trusting caregivers. The family context, however, appears central to the likelihood and the nature of traumatic events such as abuse, and may be integral to the child's ability to cope with loss. For example, ongoing abuse may be unlikely to occur if the child has a competent and emotionally available caregiver (Alexander, 1992).

OVERVIEW OF THE CHAPTER

If we were to limit our discussion in this chapter to evidence linking attachment behavioral strategies in infancy with adult psychopathology, this would be a relatively brief chapter. The evidence specifically linking infants' attachment behavioral strategies to psychopathology in adulthood is limited to a few longitudinal studies (e.g., Carlson, 1998; Dutra & Lyons-Ruth, 2005; Grossmann, Grossmann, & Waters, 2005; Sroufe et al., 2005a, 2005b). In this chapter, therefore, we cast our net more broadly, looking at associations between attachment-relevant events in childhood (e.g., trauma and separation from parents) and later psychopathology. In addition, we examine the association between concurrently assessed attachment states of mind and psychopathology.

We limit our consideration of attachment states of mind to Main and colleagues' (Main & Goldwyn, 1984; Main et al., 2003) formulation and operationalization. Although the constructs of "attachment style" (Hazan & Shaver, 1987, 1994) and "attachment states of mind" share a conceptual framework, there are key differences that lead to different operationalizations (see Crowell, Fraley, & Shaver, Chapter 26, this volume). Main and colleagues' system assesses state of mind with respect to attachment as a function of discourse coherence and defensive strategy. By contrast, attachment style assesses the individual's self-reported style of forming adolescent and adult attachments. As expected, given the different operationalizations, these variables are not strongly related to each other (Bartholomew & Shaver, 1998; Crowell et al., Chapter 26, this volume; Shaver, Belsky, & Brennan, 2000). Because we are interested in differences in processing attachment-related thoughts and feelings, we deal only with findings linking attachment states of mind with psychopathology in this chapter. The links between self-report attachment measures and psychopathology have been thoroughly reviewed by Mikulincer and Shaver (2007, Ch. 13), and the links between those measures and studies of emotion regulation are discussed by Mikulincer and Shaver in Chapter 23 of this volume.

We progress through the major psychopathological disorders, considering first the Axis I disorders, or clinical syndromes. We start with mood disorders, followed by anxiety disorders. Both of these groups of disorders are heterogeneous with regard to heritability and symptomatology; therefore, it would be surprising if clear findings emerged with regard to attachment-related issues without further specification of parameters. We move from there to a discussion of dissociative disorders. Although dissociative phenomena have been discussed throughout the 20th century, the recognition of dissociative disorders as a bona fide diagnostic category is relatively recent. Nonetheless, the evidence linking attachment in infancy and attachment-related traumas to later dissociative symptoms, and the evidence linking concurrent states of mind with dissociative symptoms, converge to form a compelling picture. We consider eating disorders next; these disorders are often comorbid with personality disorders and mood disorders. We end the discussion of Axis I disorders with schizophrenia, a disorder that is highly heritable.

From there, we move to a consideration of two of the most prevalent Axis II, or personality, disorders: borderline personality disorder and antisocial personality disorder. We include these two disorders because they are prevalent and largely distinct from Axis I disorders. (As we discuss later, rates of borderline personality disorder and depression comorbidity are high, but the disorders themselves are distinguishable.) Genetic involvement in personality disorders is variable, with relatively high heritability for antisocial personality disorder and low heritability for borderline personality disorder. The concept of borderline personality disorder emerged from the perspective of problematic early relationships with caregivers.

For each disorder or group of disorders considered, we begin with a general description of the disorder(s) and with evidence regarding genetic involvement. We then discuss attachment theory's contributions to an understanding of the disorder(s). From there we move to a consideration of the empirical evidence linking attachment phenomena to the disorder(s).

MOOD DISORDERS

Unipolar and bipolar mood disorders are very different with respect to symptomatology, genetic involvement, course, level of associated dysfunction, and the probable role of attachment in the etiology and course of the disorders. The basic distinction between unipolar and bipolar mood disorders is that unipolar disorders are characterized only by a depressed mood, whereas bipolar disorders are also characterized by elevated (manic or hypomanic) mood.

When unipolar mood disorder is severe and disabling, and represents a change from a previous level of functioning, major depressive disorder is

diagnosed. When unipolar mood disorder is milder but more chronic (of at least 2 years' duration), dysthymic disorder is diagnosed. The heritability of unipolar disorders may be linearly related to severity, with severe unipolar disorders more heritable than less severe ones, and moderately severe disorders intermediate in heritability (Moldin, Reich, & Rice, 1991; Nigg & Goldsmith, 1994; Sullivan, Neale, & Kendler, 2000). In a large Danish sample, the concordance among monozygotic twins was 43%, as contrasted with 20% for dizygotic twins (Bertelsen, Harvald, & Hauge, 1977).

The primary category of bipolar disorders (bipolar I) is characterized by the presence of manic episodes and possibly (but not necessarily) depressive episodes. Although bipolar disorders can be quite debilitating when untreated, treatment with lithium allows many people with bipolar disorders to function well, with relatively little dysfunction. Bipolar disorders are highly heritable, with the concordance among monozygotic twins estimated to be as high as 70–86%, as contrasted with 25% concordance or lower for dizygotic twins (e.g., McGuffin & Katz, 1986). Although there are several theories with regard to the involvement of specific genes in bipolar disorders, the findings are as yet inconclusive (Nurnberger & Gershon, 1992). Because very little work on the involvement of family factors in bipolar disorders has been reported in the literature, most of our comments concern unipolar disorders.

The heterogeneity among the unipolar mood disorders is important to consider in relation to attachment. First, major depression and dysthymia differ with regard to heritability; it is therefore reasonable to expect that they may differ with regard to the importance of attachment-related issues as well. Second, even within diagnostic categories, severity seems an important dimension to consider (Brown & Harris, 1993). Third, within diagnostic categories, the differential reliance on internalizing versus externalizing coping strategies is important, and central to states of mind with respect to attachment. Some people with unipolar disorders show predominantly internalizing symptoms, with self-blame and self-deprecation primary. Others show a preponderance of externalizing symptoms, with interpersonal hostility primary. Preoccupied states of mind, which involve a preoccupation with one's own thoughts and feelings, are consistent with internalizing symptoms. On the other hand, dismissing states of mind, which involve a turning away from one's own distress, are consistent with externalizing symptoms. Findings of different treatment responsiveness between people with depression who use internalizing versus externalizing coping strategies suggest the importance of the distinction we are making (Barber & Muenz, 1996; Beutler et al., 1991). Unfortunately, distinctions between internalizing and externalizing symptoms are not frequently made within a diagnosis of depression, and this dimension has not been considered in research relating states of mind to depression.

Attachment and Mood Disorder: Theoretical Links

Bowlby (1980) suggested that three major circumstances are most likely to be associated with the later development of depression. First, when a child's parent dies, and the child experiences little control over ensuing events, he or she is likely to develop a sense of hopelessness and despair in reaction to traumatic events. Second, when a child is unable (despite many attempts) to form stable and secure relationships with caregivers, he or she develops a model of the self as a failure. Any subsequent loss or disappointment is then likely to be perceived as reflecting that the child is a failure. Third, when a parent gives a child the message that he or she is incompetent or unlovable, the child develops complementary models of the self as unlovable and of others as unloving (Bretherton, 1985). Thus the child and later the adult will expect hostility and rejection from others when in need. Cummings and Cicchetti (1990) have suggested that these experiences of having a psychologically unavailable parent are similar to the experience of actually losing a caregiver, in that the child experiences frequent or even chronic losses of the parent.

Bowlby's formulation is compatible with Seligman's learned helplessness theory of depression (Seligman, Abramson, Semmel, & von Baeyer, 1979), as Bowlby (1980) himself noted. Seligman proposed that hopelessness (and hence depression) develops when noxious events occur that are experienced as uncontrollable. Each of the sets of circumstances specified by Bowlby involves a sense of uncontrollability on the part of the child. In the second and third sets of circumstances, the child feels a sense of uncontrollability as the result of the parent's disappointing responses to the child. In circumstances involving parental death, the child feels lack of control over the loss of the caregiver and over subsequent caregiving experiences.

Children's Attachment-Related Experiences and Later Depression

The circumstances Bowlby proposed as central to the development of depression have received strong empirical support. Insecure attachment (both resistant and avoidant) predicts depression in adolescence (Duggal, Carlson, Sroufe, & Egeland, 2001), though to our knowledge those findings have not been extended to adulthood. Moreover, several studies provide converging evidence that the death of a parent in early childhood puts an individual at risk for later depression (e.g., Harris, Brown, & Bifulco, 1990; Kivela, Luukinin, Koski, Viramo, & Pahkala, 1998; Takeuchi et al., 2003). Harris and colleagues (1990) found that when a girl's mother died before the child was 11 years old, she was at increased risk for later depression. Indeed, of those women whose mothers died before they were 11 years old, 42% were later diagnosed with depression, contrasted with 14% of those whose mothers died after they were 11. Furthermore, loss by death was associated with more severe forms of depression, which were accompanied by vegetative signs such as psychomotor retardation. Loss by separation was associated with less severe, but angrier, forms of depression. Bowlby (1980) suggested that the death of a child's mother may well lead to a sense of total despair, whereas separation from the mother may lead to a belief that events are reversible (i.e., that there is still hope).

Just as important as the loss itself are the child's subsequent experiences with caregivers (Harris, Brown, & Bifulco, 1986; Kendler, Sheth, Gardner, & Prescott, 2002; Oakley-Browne, Joyce, Wells, Bushnell, & Hornblow, 1995). Harris and colleagues (1986) found that inadequate care following the loss doubled the risk of depression in adulthood, particularly in cases of separation rather than death. Inadequate care often consisted of neglect, indifference, and low levels of parental control. Consistent with the Harris and colleagues findings, Kendler and colleagues (2002) found that risk for depression returned to baseline levels sooner for children who experienced parental death rather than separation, presumably because problems in family functioning were less severe in such cases.

Depressed individuals' retrospective recall of parental support and rejection provides some support for Bowlby's hypothesized relation between parental emotional availability and depression. In several studies (e.g., Fonagy et al., 1996; Raskin, Boothe, Reatig, Schulterbrandt, & Odel, 1971), depressed individuals described their parents as having been less supportive and more rejecting than did people without diagnosed psychiatric disorders. In Fonagy and colleagues' (1996) study, ratings of "probable experience" of parenting were made by coders on the basis of interview data. Parents of depressed individuals were rated as unloving and as moderately rejecting; this did not differentiate the depressed people from others with psychiatric diagnosis, but it did differentiate them from people without psychiatric diagnoses.

Attachment States of Mind and Unipolar Depression

Main and colleagues (Main & Goldwyn, 1984; Main et al., 2003) have proposed that different attachment states of mind are associated with different patterns of processing attachment-related thoughts, feelings, and memories. The classification system they developed involves discourse analysis of transcribed responses to the Adult Attachment Interview (AAI; George, Kaplan, & Main, 1984, 1985, 1996). Responses are coded primarily for "state of mind" with respect to attachment experiences, and secondarily for "probable experiences" with parents. (See Hesse, Chapter 25, and Crowell et al., Chapter 26, this volume.) "Autonomous" transcripts are characterized by coherence; the speaker's representation of attachment experiences is straightforward, clear, and consistent with evidence presented.

Nonautonomous transcripts fall into several categories, including "dismissing," "preoccupied," "unresolved," and "cannot classify." Dismissing transcripts are characterized most especially by lack of recall, idealization of one or both parents, or (less frequently) derogation of attachment experiences. Preoccupied transcripts are characterized by current angry involvement with attachment figures, or by passive speech, such as rambling discourse (Main & Goldwyn, 1984; Main et al., 2003). The category "unresolved with respect to loss or trauma" is used for transcripts in which the speaker experiences lapses in reasoning or lapses in monitoring discourse regarding a loss or trauma. When an unresolved classification is given, a secondary classification (of autonomous, preoccupied, or dismissing) is also made.

Recently, the "cannot classify" category has received increasing attention (see Hesse, Chapter 25, this volume; Hesse & Main, 2006). This catego-

ry represents a mixture, or shifting, of information-processing strategies that are inconsistent with one another. For example, the individual may describe one parent in a highly dismissing way and relate incidents of distress concerning the other parent in an enmeshed way. The cannot classify category has been associated with high rates of psychopathology (e.g., Allen, Hauser, & Borman-Spurrell, 1996; Holtzworth-Munroe, Stuart, & Hutchinson, 1996; Riggs et al., 2007), but sample sizes are rarely large enough to examine associations between this category and specific forms of psychopathology. In some studies, the cannot classify and unresolved groups are combined into a single group to maximize statistical power. The reliable coding of transcripts as cannot classify requires training additional to that required for the other four categories. Therefore, many investigators have not used the category, or have used it in a way that may not be standard across studies. Nonetheless, recent evidence suggests the importance of this category as a predictor of psychopathology.

These state-of-mind categories are sometimes considered as autonomous or nonautonomous (with nonautonomous including dismissing, preoccupied, unresolved, and cannot classify transcripts), referred to as a two-category scheme. Unresolved and cannot classify transcripts are typically grouped with nonautonomous transcripts, although there are exceptions to this practice. A three-group classification typically forces unresolved (and sometimes cannot classify) transcripts into autonomous, dismissing, or preoccupied categories. A four-group classification scheme includes autonomous, dismissing, preoccupied, and unresolved (sometimes combined with cannot classify). In almost no instances are five categories (i.e., autonomous, dismissing, preoccupied, unresolved, cannot classify) included in analyses, because statistical power is inadequate.

The findings regarding the association between states of mind and depressive disorders have been somewhat inconsistent, with some studies reporting depression associated with preoccupied states of mind (Cole-Detke & Kobak, 1996; Fonagy et al., 1996; Rosenstein & Horowitz, 1996), but others reporting depression associated more closely with dismissing states of mind (Patrick, Hobson, Castle, Howard, & Maughan, 1994). Many others have found that people with insecure states of mind are depressed more than others, but have inadequate power to examine differences between dismissing and preoccupied states of mind (e.g., McMahon, Barnett, Kowalenko, & Tennant,

2006). Consistent with the point made by Sroufe and colleagues (2005a), we suggest that there may be systematic differences on the internalizing–externalizing dimension in the groups labeled as "depressed" in these studies, and that these may account for the discrepancies in findings.

First, Rosenstein and Horowitz (1996) examined the states of mind of adolescents who had been admitted to a psychiatric hospital. Adolescents were classified as having "affective disorders" if they met diagnostic criteria for major depressive disorder, dysthymia, or schizoaffective disorder, and if they did not meet criteria for conduct disorder. Adolescents were classified as having conduct disorder if they met criteria for conduct disorder or oppositional defiant disorder, but not criteria for depression. Adolescents were classified in a third group (comorbid affective disorder and conduct disorder) if they met criteria for both disorders. Thus the "pure affective disorder" group excluded people who showed externalizing symptoms of conduct disorder, but did not exclude those who were comorbid for a more internalizing disorder. Those in the pure affective disorder group were classified as having preoccupied states of mind significantly more often than those in the comorbid or the conduct disorder group. More specifically, 69% of the pure affective disorder group was classified as preoccupied, whereas 25% of the comorbid group and 14% of the conduct disorder group were classified as preoccupied. (See Table 30.1.)

Cole-Detke and Kobak (1996) examined the states of mind of women who reported depressive symptoms, eating disorder symptoms, both types of symptoms, or neither. The distribution of women who reported only depressed symptoms was relatively even across the three categories of attachment. Although depressed women were classified as preoccupied more often than were women with eating disorders, the majority fell into categories other than preoccupied. Again, the criteria for the depressed group excluded at least some with comorbid externalizing, but not internalizing, symptoms.

On the other hand, Patrick and colleagues (1994) limited their depressed group to women inpatients without any borderline personality disorder symptomatology, thus excluding some with internalizing symptomatology. Patrick and colleagues assessed the states of mind of 24 female inpatients who had diagnoses of either dysthymia or borderline personality disorder. Women were included in the dysthymic group only if they met none of the criteria for borderline personality dis-

order. The distribution of states of mind was significantly different for the two groups. All of the women in the borderline group were classified as preoccupied, as contrasted with 50% of those in the dysthymic group.

Several points are worth making with regard to these findings. First, the distribution of state-of-mind classifications among people with depressive symptoms in two of the studies (Cole-Detke & Kobak, 1996; Patrick et al., 1994) was quite similar, but the findings have been cited in the literature as if they suggest opposite conclusions. Second, the exclusion criteria in each of these three studies created depressed groups that were systematically different from one another. For example, Rosenstein and Horowitz (1996) excluded people from their pure affective disorder group who were comorbid for antisocial disorders. This comorbid group was classified primarily as dismissing. Although the remaining group was indeed more diagnostically "pure," the exclusion process systematically excluded people likely to have dismissing classifications, and not those likely to have preoccupied classifications. The exclusion criteria used by Patrick and colleagues (1994) were likely to have had the opposite effect, because those who met any criteria for borderline personality disorder were excluded. On a related issue, it is likely in each of these studies that the apparently diagnostically "pure" depressive group included a number of people who had other relevant diagnoses. For example, in the Rosenstein and Horowitz study, 75% of the pure affective disorder group had Axis II (personality disorder) diagnoses, and most of those with personality disorders were classified as having preoccupied states of mind with regard to attachment. We suggest, therefore, that these several studies yield very important data relating states of mind to eating disorders, conduct disorder, and borderline personality disorder. Conclusions regarding states of mind and depression, however, are more complicated.

Given that the experience of loss is hypothesized to be a significant vulnerability factor for depression, it follows that people with unipolar mood disorders may be unresolved with respect to loss. In the several studies that have examined unresolved status among depressed people, the results have been inconsistent. In Fonagy and colleagues' (1996) large sample of inpatients, 72% of people with depression were classified as unresolved, versus 18% in Rosenstein and Horowitz's (1996) adolescent inpatient sample and 16% of Patrick and colleagues' (1994) outpatient sample.

TABLE 30.1. Diagnostic Groups and AAI Classifications

	Three-way classifications			Four-way classifications			
	F	E	Ds	F	E	Ds	U
Axis I							
Mood disorders							
Unipolar							
Cole-Detke & Kobak (1996) (dep. symp.)	4	6	4				
Rosenstein & Horowitz (1996) (mixed)	0	22	10	0	19	8	6
Tyrrell & Dozier (1997) (MDD)	5	1	0	3	1	0	2
Patrick et al., 1994 (dysthymia)	2	4	6				
Bipolar							
Tyrrell & Dozier (1997)	0	0	7	0	0	3	4
Mixed							
Fonagy et al. (1996)	18	41	13	9	6	5	52
Adam et al. (1996) (suicidality)	16	29	16	16	29	16	43
Schizoaffective							
Tyrrell & Dozier (1997)	1	1	6	1	0	5	2
Anxiety disorders							
Fonagy et al. (1996)	7	29	8	2	1	3	38
Eating disorders							
Cole-Detke & Kobak (1996)	3	1	8				
Fonagy et al. (1996)	1	9	4	0	0	1	13
Manassis et al. (1994)	7	5	2	0	3	1	14
Stovall-McClough & Cloitre (2006) (PTSD)	12	15	3	5	3	3	19
Zeijlmans van Emmichoven et al. (2003)	8	8	12	8	6	11	3
Substance abuse							
Fonagy et al. (1996)	6	23	8	4	3	2	28
Ward et al. (2001)	1	4	15	0	1	11	8
Schizophrenia							
Tyrrell & Dozier (1997)	3	0	24	1	0	16	12
Comorbid groups							
Eating disorders and depression							
Cole-Detke & Kobak (1996)	4	10	5				
Conduct disorder and depression							
Rosenstein & Horowitz (1996)	0	3	9	0	1	6	5
Axis II							
Borderline personality disorder							
Fonagy et al. (1996)	3	27	6	2	1	1	32
Patrick et al. (1994)	0	12	0				
Barone (2003)				3	9	8	20
Diamond et al. (2003)	1	4	5	1	1	2	6 (1 CC)
Rosenstein & Horowitz (1996)	1	9	4				
Stalker & Davies (1995)	0	5	3			7	
Stovall-McClough & Cloitre (2003)	4	8	1	1	2	0	10

(continued)

TABLE 30.1. *(continued)*

	Three-way classifications			Four-way classifications			
	F	E	Ds	F	E	Ds	U
Axis II *(continued)*							
Antisocial personality disorder							
Rosenstein & Horowitz (1996) (CD)	0	1	6	0	1	6	0
Fonagy et al. (1996)	8	9	5	3	1	1	17
Levinson & Fonagy (2004) (violent prisoners)							
Holtzworth-Munroe et al. (1997) (DV)				4	6	4	5 (11 C)
Babcock et al. (2000) (DV)	6	10	7	6	7	6	2 (2 CC)

Note. F, autonomous; E, preoccupied; Ds, dismissing; U, unresolved; dep. symp., dep. symp., depressive symptoms; mixed, mixed unipolar mood disorder diagnoses; MDD, major depressive disorder; CC, cannot classify; CD, conduct disorder; DV, domestic violence.

Fonagy and colleagues (1996) found that different subtypes of depression were differentially related to states of mind. Compared with other mood disorders, major depression in the Fonagy and colleagues study was more often associated with autonomous states of mind. In Tyrrell, Dozier, Teague, and Fallot's (1999) study of people with serious psychopathological disorders, five of six individuals with major depression were classified as autonomous when the three-category system was used, and three were classified as autonomous when the four-category system was used. Fonagy and colleagues suggested that these findings could be attributable to the episodic nature of major depression. Major depression may not interfere with the maintenance of coherent states of mind as pervasively as chronic dysthymia does. Another possibility is that major depression is more heritable than dysthymia, so that it takes less unfavorable caregiving for the disorder to emerge.

The primary criterion for autonomous states of mind is coherence. It is possible to have coherent states of mind even if life experiences are described as difficult and caregivers are described as generally unavailable. People who seem to have developed autonomous states of mind despite describing difficult life circumstances are termed "earned-secure" (Main & Goldwyn, 1984; Main et al., 2003), as contrasted with those who describe having had loving parents throughout their lives, who are termed "continuous-secure." Pearson, Cohn, Cowan, and Cowan (1994) studied differences in reported depression, measured with the Center for Epidemiologic Studies Depression Scale (Radloff, 1977), among women with these two types of autonomous classifications. Women in the earned-secure group reported significantly

more depressive symptomatology than women in the continuous-secure group. These results have generally been assumed to reflect the overcoming of difficult experiences among these earned-secure women. Roisman, Padron, Sroufe, and Egeland (2002), however, found that earned-secure adults had actually experienced very supportive relationships with caregivers as children. The earned security (i.e., the combination of coherent discourse with the recall of difficult experiences) seemed a function of current depressive symptoms rather than unsupportive early caregivers.

Dickstein, Seifer, Albus, and Magee (2004) assessed the association between adult attachment states of mind, indices of family functioning including maternal depression, and marital attachment as measured with the Marital Attachment Interview (MAI; Dickstein, 1993). Although depression was unrelated to attachment states of mind as measured with the AAI, discordant attachment classifications (specifically, a secure classification on the AAI coupled with an insecure classification on the MAI) were associated with increased severity of maternal depressive symptoms. Dickstein and colleagues suggested two possible explanations for this finding. First, consistent state of mind across relationship domains may be associated with increased predictability, and predictability may be conducive to healthier emotional functioning. Second, individuals who are depressed may be more likely to form relationships that are incongruent with previous internal working models, yielding greater likelihood of the secure AAI/insecure MAI pattern observed in this study.

Findings relating state of mind and bipolar disorders are limited. Fonagy and colleagues

(1996) found that people with bipolar disorders were significantly more likely to be classified as dismissing than were those with other mood disorders. Tyrrell and colleagues (1999) found that all seven people with bipolar disorders were classified as dismissing when Main and colleagues' (Main & Goldwyn, 1984; Main et al., 2003) three-category system was used, and that four of those seven were classified as unresolved when the four-category system was used.

These various findings point to the importance of diagnostic issues when one is considering linkages between attachment states of mind and mood disorders. The first critical distinction is between unipolar and bipolar mood disorders. These disorders are quite different in a number of ways. Preliminary findings suggest that these disorders can also be distinguished by the states of mind with which they are associated. Second, several distinctions among the unipolar mood disorders appear important. Compared with dysthymia, major depression is less frequently associated with autonomous states of mind. Within the categories of major depressive disorder and dysthymia, we suggest that differences in the extent to which disorders are self-blaming (internalizing) versus other-blaming (externalizing) are important in terms of states of mind. A related issue is comorbidity. Although a diagnosis of unipolar mood disorder may not provide evidence of the extent to which symptoms are internalizing or externalizing, other comorbid diagnoses (such as borderline personality disorder, eating disorders, and particular anxiety disorders) may provide such evidence. Several studies have highlighted how important it is to consider comorbid diagnoses in analyses.

ANXIETY DISORDERS

As are mood disorders, anxiety disorders are quite heterogeneous. Most are characterized by a combination of fear and avoidance, with the balance differing for different disorders. We suggest that when fear predominates, the disorder involves primarily internalizing symptoms, whereas when avoidance predominates, the disorder involves primarily externalizing symptoms. As discussed previously, strategies that maximize the expression of attachment needs are expected to be associated with more internalizing disorders, and strategies that minimize the expression of attachment needs are expected to be associated with more externalizing disorders. The disorder in which fear most

clearly predominates is generalized anxiety disorder. Individuals who have this disorder experience chronic anxiety regarding at least several life circumstances. Panic disorder is often characterized primarily by fear. Yet, given that agoraphobia accompanies panic disorder more often than not in clinical samples (American Psychiatric Association, 2000), avoidance is often associated with panic disorder. Phobic disorders (including specific phobia, social phobia, and agoraphobia) are characterized by fear when the individual does not successfully avoid the feared stimulus, but avoidance often predominates. Similarly, in obsessive–compulsive disorder, fear is experienced to the extent that self-prescribed compulsive behaviors are not engaged in. Posttraumatic stress disorder (PTSD) is characterized by vacillation between (1) emotional numbing and efforts to avoid reminders of the trauma, and (2) fear and anxiety associated with reexperiencing the trauma. Underlying this emotional instability is a generalized hypervigilance. Fear and anxiety predominate in this disorder.

Comorbidity of anxiety disorders with other diagnoses is common; in particular, anxiety disorders and depressive disorders often co-occur (Hettema, Neale, & Kendler, 2001; Kendler, Heath, Martin, & Eaves, 1987). The estimates of heritability of anxiety disorders vary from study to study. Different anxiety disorders may be more heritable than others (Cassidy, 1995; Torgersen, 1988), although a meta-analysis conducted by Hettema and colleagues (2001) found similar heritability across most mood disorders.

Attachment and Anxiety Disorders: Theoretical Links

Bowlby (1973) proposed that all forms of anxiety disorders (with the exception of specific animal phobias) are best accounted for by anxiety regarding the availability of the attachment figure. Several types of family environments were specified as most likely by Bowlby, all of which involve parental control through overprotection or rejection. Included among these are family environments in which a child worries about a parent's survival in the child's absence (because of parental fighting or suicide attempts); environments in which the child worries about being rejected or abandoned (because of threats from parents); environments in which the child feels the need to remain home as a companion to a parent; and environments in which a parent has difficulty letting the child go because of overwhelming feelings that harm will come to the child.

Infant Attachment and Later Anxiety Disorders

The Minnesota Study of Risk and Adaptation from Birth to Adulthood (Bosquet & Egeland, 2006; Warren, Huston, Egeland, & Sroufe, 1997) examined the association between attachment in infancy and later anxiety disorders. Anxiety disorders were diagnosed when children were 17½. Infants with resistant attachments were significantly more likely than infants with secure or avoidant attachments to be diagnosed with anxiety disorders as adolescents. Warren and colleagues (1997) also assessed whether this relation between resistant attachment and anxiety disorders was attributable to temperamental differences, as indicated by neonatal nurse ratings of reactivity (Terreira, 1960) as well as the Neonatal Behavioral Assessment Scale (Brazelton, 1973). Even when differences in temperament were controlled for, resistant attachments emerged as significant predictors of later anxiety disorders.

Children's Attachment-Related Experiences and Later Anxiety Disorder

Consistent with Bowlby's position, problematic family environments have been linked with anxiety disorders. Brown and Harris (1993) found that patients with panic disorder had more frequently experienced early loss of a caregiver or extremely inadequate caregiving than people with no psychiatric diagnosis had. Faravelli, Webb, Ambonetti, Fonnesu, and Sessarego (1985) found that people with agoraphobia had experienced early separation from their mothers or parental divorce significantly more often than a control group with no psychiatric disorder. de Ruiter and van IJzendoorn (1992) conducted a meta-analysis of studies examining the association between early childhood separation anxiety and later agoraphobia. They found that adults with agoraphobia reported more childhood separation anxiety than controls, but were not more likely to suffer from separation anxiety disorder as children. Adults with agoraphobia were also more likely to rate their parents as low on affection and high on overprotection than controls. de Ruiter and van IJzendoorn argued that this provided indirect support of Bowlby's hypothesized association between ambivalent (resistant) infant attachment and later agoraphobia.

Cassidy (1995) found that people with generalized anxiety disorder reported more rejection by their parents and role reversal than people who did not report symptoms of generalized anxiety. Similarly, Chambless, Gillis, Tran, and Steketee (1996) found that most people with anxiety disorders described their parents as unloving and controlling. Specific anxiety disorder diagnosis (obsessive–compulsive disorder vs. panic disorder with agoraphobia) was not differentially associated with parental care (Chambless et al., 1995). The underlying personality cluster, as assessed with the Structured Clinical Interview for DSM-III-R (Spitzer, Williams, & Gibbon, 1987), was related to reported care, however. People who engaged in more avoidant behavior reported that their mothers had been neglectful, whereas those who engaged in dependent or passive–aggressive behavior reported that their mothers had been overprotective.

Bandelow and colleagues (2002) compared histories of patients with panic disorder ($n = 115$) and normal controls ($n = 124$). Based on retrospective report, the patients with panic disorder had experienced significantly more traumatic early life events, including parental death and separation, than adults without panic disorder had. Such individuals also reported more parental restriction and less love than controls. In a study of adults with social anxiety disorder (social phobia), Bandelow and colleagues (2004) obtained similar results and concluded that, beyond a family history of mental illness, separation experiences in childhood were among the most important contributing factors to adult social anxiety.

Attachment States of Mind and Anxiety Disorders

Of adolescents with clinically elevated scores on the anxiety scale of the Millon Multiaxial Personality Inventory (Millon, 1983), 65% had preoccupied states of mind (Rosenstein & Horowitz, 1996). Similarly, Fonagy and colleagues (1996) found that most adults with anxiety disorders were classified as preoccupied in the three-category system, although that did not differentiate them from other clinical groups (Lichtenstein & Cassidy, 1991). What did differentiate them was that they were disproportionately unresolved with respect to loss or trauma, relative to other clinical groups. Cassidy (1995) found that, contrasted with people without symptoms of generalized anxiety disorder, those with generalized anxiety disorder reported greater anger and vulnerability on the Inventory of Adult Attachment (Lichtenstein & Cassidy, 1991). Feelings of anger and vulnerability are consistent with preoccupied states of mind. Manassis, Bradley, Goldberg, Hood, and Swinson (1994) found that all of the 18 women with anxiety disorders included in their study were classified as nonautonomous, with 78% rated as unresolved. The women were diagnosed with a variety of anxiety disorders (panic, obsessive–compulsive disorder, and generalized anxiety disorder). Because of the small sample size, it was not possible to analyze relations between specific anxiety disorders and attachment state of mind.

Zeijlmans van Emmichoven, van IJzendoorn, de Ruiter, and Brosschot (2003) examined attachment state of mind among 28 adults with anxiety disorders and 56 adult outpatients without such disorders. In the sample of outpatients, 39% were classified as dismissing, 29% as autonomous, 21% as preoccupied, and 11% as unresolved. Most (86%) of the adults with anxiety disorders were diagnosed with panic disorder and agoraphobia, supporting our contention that anxiety disorders that involve mainly avoidance may be best characterized by dismissing states of mind.

PTSD falls under anxiety disorders in the *Diagnostic and Statistical Manual of Mental Disorders*, fourth edition, text revision (DSM-IV-TR; American Psychiatric Association, 2000). We include discussion of the one study linking adult attachment classifications with PTSD in this section. However, we note that PTSD may have more in common with dissociative disorders (considered in the next section) than with anxiety disorders in terms of etiology. Stovall-McClough and Cloitre (2006) examined attachment in a sample of 60 women with histories of childhood abuse, 30 of whom were diagnosed with child-abuse-related PTSD and the other 30 of whom had no trauma-related diagnosis. Sixty-three percent of those with PTSD were classified as unresolved regarding trauma, compared to 27% of those without PTSD; this represented a 7.5-fold increase in risk for PTSD. Unresolved status, rather than preoccupied status, predicted a PTSD diagnosis. Finally, unresolved trauma on the AAI was associated specifically with PTSD avoidance symptoms, and not with reexperiencing or hypervigilant symptoms. See Kobak, Cassidy, and Ziv (2004) for further discussion of attachment and PTSD.

DISSOCIATIVE DISORDERS

Dissociative disorders, as the name suggests, are characterized by a dissociation of parts of the self that are usually integrated. Minor dissociative states are commonplace—for example, becoming so absorbed in a conversation while driving as to be unaware of the passing landscape. The dissociative disorders specified in the DSM-IV-TR (American Psychiatric Association, 2000) involve dissociation of one's identity (dissociative identity disorder and dissociative fugue), memory (dissociative amnesia), and consciousness (depersonalization disorder). Transient experiences of depersonalization are seen in about 40% of hospitalized patients (American Psychiatric Association, 2000) and appear to be experienced at some point by many nonpatients as well. The more serious dissociative disorders have been diagnosed relatively rarely until recently, when there has been a sharp rise in such diagnoses (Johnson, Cohen, Kasen, & Brook, 2006). Waller and Ross (1997) found no evidence for genetic influences in dissociative disorders.

Attachment and Dissociation: Theoretical Links

Dissociation involves turning away, presumably not volitionally, from some aspect of the environment. Dissociation clearly has an adaptive function, in that it allows a person not to become overwhelmed by trauma. Evolution has predisposed infants and children to experience dissociative states readily when threatened. The cost of experiencing dissociative states frequently as a child, however, is a sensitized and compromised neurobiology (De Bellis, 2001). This is especially true because children pass through critical periods for the organization of brain systems. Once sensitization has occurred, less is required to evoke dissociative states (De Bellis, 2001). Thus a child who repeatedly enters dissociative states will more readily enter such states under conditions of mild stress.

When a traumatic event (e.g., a natural disaster, loss, or abuse at the hands of an adult) is experienced, but the caregiver can provide sensitive care and a sense of protection, the child is not in a position of experiencing "fright without solution" (Main & Hesse, 1990). In these cases, a child can continue to rely on a caregiver for protection. If, however, the caregiver cannot protect the child under conditions that the child experiences as threatening, or if the parent is actually the source of the threat, the child may experience the threat as overwhelming and enter a dissociative state (Main & Morgan, 1996).

One predictor of dissociative symptoms is disorganized/disoriented attachment in infancy (Carlson, 1998). Evidence of dissociation can be seen among some infants in the Strange Situation (see Lyons-Ruth & Jacobvitz, Chapter 28, this volume; Main & Morgan, 1996). For most children, the Strange Situation is distressing, but an organized attachment system orchestrates behaviors with the caregiver. Some infants experience a breakdown of attachment strategies. Abused infants, as well as infants of caregivers who are unresolved with respect to trauma or loss, are likely to show this breakdown in strategies (Carlson, Cicchetti, Barnett, & Braunwald, 1989; Main & Morgan, 1996). Main and Hesse (1990) proposed that frightened or frightening parental behavior leaves these children "frightened without solution." According to Main and Hesse (1990) and Liotti (2004), early experiences with a frightened or frightening caregiver cause a child to develop multiple, incompatible models of the self and the other. In interactions with the caregiver, the child experiences rapid shifts in which the caregiver is at first frightened, then no longer frightened, then caring for the child. With each shift, a different model of self (perpetrator of fright, rescuer, loved child) and of the caregiver (victim, rescued victim, competent caregiver) is operative. These multiple models of the self and other cannot be integrated by young children and are retained as multiple models (Liotti, 2004; Main & Hesse, 1990). These children have an unsolvable dilemma when distressed: They are neither able to go to their caregivers for nurturance, nor able to turn away and distract themselves. Because they experience this continued threat without resolution, they are at risk for entering a minor dissociative state during the Strange Situation and under other threatening conditions. Liotti pointed out that these behaviors are most phenotypically similar to dissociative states in adulthood, thus suggesting a possible connection between early trance-like states and later dissociative disorders. Given evidence that the experience of dissociative states in childhood leads to a sensitized neurobiology that predisposes individuals to experiencing later dissociative states, disorganized attachment in infancy and childhood experiences of abuse without caregiver protection may predispose individuals to dissociative states in adulthood (Carlson, 1998).

Infant Attachment and Dissociation in Adulthood

Carlson (1998) and Ogawa, Sroufe, Weinfield, Carlson, and Egeland (1997) examined the association between disorganized attachment in infancy and dissociative symptoms during childhood and adolescence in the Minnesota longitudinal study. Infants in this study had originally been classified with Ainsworth's three-category system (Ains-

worth, Blehar, Waters, & Wall, 1978), because the fourth category of disorganized/disoriented attachment had not yet been conceptualized or operationalized (Main & Solomon, 1986). Carlson recoded these infants for disorganized/disoriented behavior, finding that 35% of the infants could be classified as disorganized/disoriented at 12 months, and 43% could be classified as disorganized at 18 months. To create a teacher assessment of dissociative symptoms, Carlson selected items from the Teacher Report Form of the Child Behavior Checklist (Achenbach & Edelbrock, 1986) that were consistent with a diagnosis of a dissociative disorder. Infant disorganization was associated with higher teacher ratings of dissociative symptoms both in elementary school and in high school and in adulthood (Carlson, 1998). Furthermore, disorganized/disoriented behavior in the Strange Situation predicted the self-report of more dissociative symptomatology at age 19 (Carlson, 1998) and into adulthood (Sroufe et al., 2005a). Thus two sets of raters converged in pointing to symptoms of dissociation for adolescents who were assessed as disorganized/disoriented in infancy, and the relations persisted over time. Ogawa et al. found that, combined with indices of maternal emotional availability, disorganized attachment accounted for 34% of the variance in later dissociative symptoms. One might wonder whether some gross neurological deficit contributed to the ratings of dissociation in both infancy and adolescence. No associations emerged between disorganized/disoriented attachment and any of the variables assessing endogenous vulnerability, such as prenatal difficulties, difficulties during childbirth, or maternal drug and alcohol use (Carlson, 1998; Ogawa et al., 1997).

Dutra and Lyons-Ruth (2005) obtained similar findings in their longitudinal study. Fifty-six late adolescents who had participated in the Strange Situation as infants were administered the Dissociative Experiences Scale. Measures of parent–infant affective communication, quality of care, parental psychopathology, and maltreatment history were also administered at several time periods. The strongest predictors of adolescent dissociative symptoms were disorganization of attachment during infancy, disrupted affective communication with the mother, and maternal neglect.

Children's Attachment-Related Experiences and Later Dissociative Disorders

As noted earlier, Main and Hesse (1990) proposed that disorganized or disoriented behavior in the

Strange Situation results from the caregiver behaving in a frightened or frightening manner toward the child. This caregiver, who is often unresolved with respect to attachment, is unable to protect the child adequately from later threats, or may even perpetrate threats. Thus it seems that a child who is disorganized in infancy may be at increased risk for later abuse because of the caregiver's qualities. Children who have formed disorganized attachments to caregivers in infancy, and are later repeatedly abused, may be particularly susceptible to later dissociative disorders (Liotti, 2004). Two findings provide preliminary support for this hypothesis. First, E. A. Carlson (personal communication, August 1996) found that the three adolescents in the Minnesota sample who had dissociative disorders (rather than only dissociative symptoms) each had disorganized/disoriented attachments to caregivers as infants. Second, the incidence of abuse among people with dissociative disorders is extremely high, with figures as high as 97% reported in some studies (e.g., Putnam, 1991).

Main and Hesse (1990) proposed an intergenerational model of the transmission of dissociative symptoms. They suggested that unresolved loss and trauma are the underlying causes of parent behaving in frightening or frightened ways with their children. Indirect support for this idea is suggested by the finding that unresolved loss on the AAI is associated with levels of absorption as measured by Tellegen's Absorption Scale (Hesse & van IJzendoorn, 1998). Losses require some time to resolve, according to Main and colleagues (Main & Goldwyn, 1984; Main et al., 2003). Very recent losses are not considered in the scoring of unresolved status in the Main and colleagues system, because lack of resolution in such cases is normative. Even recent losses can have disorganizing effects on parental behavior, however. Therefore, it follows that a parent's experiencing the death of someone close may make disorganized attachment and even later dissociative states in a child more likely. Indeed, Liotti (2004) found that 62% of adults diagnosed with dissociative disorders had mothers who had lost a close relative within 2 years of their children's birth. In a follow-up study, Pasquini, Liotti, Mazzotti, Fassone, and Picardi (2002) compared a sample of patients with dissociative disorders to clinical controls. Patients whose mothers had suffered a loss or other traumatic life event within 2 years of the patients' births had an increased risk of 2.6 for a dissociative disorder diagnosis.

Attachment States of Mind and Dissociative Disorders

Attachment states of mind are classified as unresolved with respect to loss or trauma when some notable lapse of reasoning or monitoring of discourse is evident in the AAI. Thus, like the classification of disorganized/disoriented attachment in the Strange Situation, the classification of unresolved status is based on behavior that is similar to dissociative phenomena. For example, when a person becomes lost in recounting episodes of abuse or loss and appears frightened in the retelling, he or she may be experiencing a dissociation-like state. When a person gives details at one point in the discourse regarding loss or trauma that contradict other details, he or she may be once again experiencing a dissociation-like state. Thus it seems likely that unresolved status may be associated with dissociative disorders and symptoms.

Several studies have examined unresolved attachment status and the presence of dissociative symptoms in patient samples. West, Adam, Spreng, and Rose (2001) found that adolescent inpatients with higher dissociation scores were classified as unresolved or cannot classify in the AAI more often than adolescent inpatients with lower dissociation scores were. Riggs and colleagues (2007) found that psychiatric inpatients with unresolved trauma showed more dissociative symptomatology than inpatients without unresolved trauma. Stovall-McClough and Cloitre (2006) found that continuous scores for unresolved status were marginally associated with self-report of dissociative symptoms ($r = .27$, $p = .05$).

Although to our knowledge there are no published studies documenting the distribution of attachment classifications among adults with dissociative disorders per se (rather than dissociative symptoms more generally), Steele (2003) reported that the AAI was routinely administered to patients at the Clinic for Dissociative Studies in London. When it was administered to people diagnosed with dissociative identity disorder, the transcripts were characterized by multiple organizational strategies. More specifically, separate identifiable personalities appear to be linked with their own personal histories and strategies for managing the affect and content elicited by AAI questions.

EATING DISORDERS

Eating disorders include anorexia nervosa and bulimia nervosa. Anorexia nervosa is characterized by maintaining a body weight that is dangerously low, accompanied by distorted body image and fears of becoming fat. Bulimia nervosa is characterized by binge eating accompanied by behaviors intended to compensate for the bingeing, such as purging and taking laxatives. Typically these disorders emerge in adolescence, particularly at stressful times such as college entry. The vast majority (90%) of those diagnosed with eating disorders are women (American Psychiatric Association, 2000). Many women with eating disorders are also depressed, with rates of reported comorbidity as high as 75% (Mitchell & Pyle, 1985).

Attachment and Eating Disorders: Theoretical Links

Bowlby (1973) suggested that a child feels inadequate and out of control if given the message that he or she will have difficulty functioning independently or is unlovable. As discussed previously, children who receive such messages may feel their own anxiety exquisitely—developing generalized anxiety disorder or agoraphobia, for example. If these children have developed an avoidant strategy of turning their attention away from their own distress, however, they may be at increased risk for developing externalizing symptoms. Cole-Detke and Kobak (1996) suggested that young women who develop eating disorders may be attempting to control their world through eating behavior by directing attention away from their own feelings of distress.

Children's Attachment-Related Experiences and Later Eating Disorders

Much of the evidence linking early attachment-related experiences to eating disorders relies on retrospective accounts of parenting availability. The findings that emerge are complicated but relatively consistent. First, women with anorexia nervosa typically describe both their parents negatively (e.g., Palmer, Oppenheimer, & Marshall, 1988; Ratti, Humphrey, & Lyons, 1996; Rowa, Kerig, & Geller, 2001; Vidovic, Juresa, Begovac, Mahnik, & Tocilkj, 2005; Wade, Treloar, & Martin, 2001; Wallin & Hansson, 1999; Woodside et al., 2002). Second, fathers are often described as emotionally unavailable and rejecting (Cole-Detke & Kobak, 1996; Rhodes & Kroger, 1992). Third, mothers are described as domineering, overprotective, and perfectionistic (Minuchin, Rosman, & Baker, 1980; Woodside et al., 2002). Finally, parents appear to

act in ways that thwart efforts at independence (Ratti et al., 1996). Kenny and Hart (1992) found that women with eating disorders described their parents as generally unsupportive of their independence.

An observational study conducted by Humphrey (1989) provided converging evidence for this pattern of family interaction. In interactional analyses, parents were found to communicate double messages, suggesting support for daughters while simultaneously undermining their confidence. The effects of such interactions can be seen in the daughters' feelings of inadequacy. For example, Armstrong and Roth (1989) found that women with eating disorders responded to imagined minor separations from loved ones in extreme ways.

Thus a picture generally emerges of an over-controlling, perfectionistic mother who communicates lack of support for her daughter's autonomy striving; an emotionally rejecting father; and a daughter who feels rejected, controlled, and inadequate. Although sexual abuse has been suggested as a causal factor for eating disorders, the preponderance of evidence suggests that such abuse is not strongly related to the development of either anorexia nervosa or bulimia nervosa (e.g., Carter, Bewell, Blackmore, & Woodside, 2006; Pope, Mangweth, Negrao, Hudson, & Cordas, 1994; Welch & Fairburn, 1994).

Attachment States of Mind and Eating Disorders

Several studies have examined the association between AAI states of mind and eating disorders, with somewhat contradictory results. As reviewed previously, Cole-Detke and Kobak used the self-reports of a sample of college women for the assessment of eating disorders. The methodology yielded information about preoccupied, dismissing, and autonomous states of mind, but not about the unresolved or cannot classify categories. The breakdown of states of mind differed significantly for women reporting eating disorders, depression, a combination of the two, or neither. Women who reported eating disorders only were most frequently classified as dismissing. Women who reported a combination of eating disorders and depression were most frequently classified as preoccupied (similar to women who reported only depression). Similarly, Ward and colleagues (2001) found that the overwhelming majority (95%) of patients were classified as nonautonomous (or insecure) on the AAI, and that 79% were classified as dismissing.

In contrast, Fonagy and colleagues (1996) found that 64% of people with eating disorders were classified as preoccupied. When the four-category system was used, 13 of the 14 individuals with eating disorders were classified as unresolved with respect to loss or trauma. Those with eating disorders did not differ significantly from those with other psychiatric disorders in the breakdown of state-of-mind classifications. In the Cole-Detke and Kobak (1996) study, over half (61%) of the women reporting eating disorders also reported depression, and were thus not included in the "pure" eating disorder group. If a similar proportion of people in Fonagy et al.'s study were comorbid for depression, the majority of the remaining "pure" eating disorder group might have been classified as dismissing, thus matching Cole-Detke and Kobak's results.

Consistent with the patterns of family interaction described above, Cole-Detke and Kobak (1996) and Ward and colleagues (2001) have argued that women with eating disorders are attempting to control their worlds through their eating behavior, and that the type of control exerted is externally oriented. This type of control is chosen because women with eating disorders do not have the ability to examine their own psychological states, and cope instead by diverting their distress to focus on their own bodies. Cole-Detke and Kobak have therefore proposed that eating disorders allow the diversion of attention away from attachment-related concerns, and toward the more external and more "attainable" goal of body change.

SCHIZOPHRENIA

The various types of schizophrenia are the disorders associated with the greatest dysfunction of any of the Axis I disorders. They are characterized most especially by psychosis (i.e., loss of touch with reality), as manifested often in delusions or hallucinations. The schizophrenias appear to have high heritability (e.g., Thompson, Watson, Steinhauer, Goldstein, & Pogue-Geile, 2005). For example, the concordance for monozygotic twins is usually estimated at about 50%, as opposed to 15% for dizygotic twins (Gottesman, 1991). Even in adoption studies, when the influence of the environmental effects associated with biological parents is minimized, the influence of biological parents appears more predictive of the development of schizophrenia than the influence of adop-

tive parents (Gottesman, 1991). The mechanism for the transmission has not been clearly specified as a single-gene or single-chromosome locus. Many researchers are now exploring what seems the more likely explanation that multiple genes are involved, and that the involvement of specific genes will be variable across the schizophrenias (Baron, 2001; Gottesman, 1991).

Children's Attachment-Related Experiences and Later Schizophrenia

The family environment variable that has been most widely suggested as causal in the etiology of schizophrenia is "expressed emotion" (Goldstein, 1985). High levels of expressed emotion are characterized by familial overinvolvement and/or criticality. Communication deviance and expressed emotion assessed in the families of adolescents with mild to moderate clinical disturbances predicted schizophrenia and schizophrenia spectrum disorders (schizoid, schizotypal, and paranoid personality disorders) 15 years later (Goldstein, 1985). Even though these results suggest that parental behavior is important in the onset of schizophrenia, it is equally plausible that the parents' behaviors reflected sensitivity to different premorbid behaviors of their children who later developed schizophrenia. For example, Walker, Grimes, Davis, and Smith (1993) found that in home videotapes taken years before the onset of schizophrenia, the children who later developed schizophrenia could be reliably differentiated from their siblings who did not develop schizophrenia.

The evidence regarding familial influences on the recurrence of schizophrenia is more compelling, and findings have been replicated in a number of studies (e.g., Brown, Birley, & Wing, 1972; Butzlaff & Hooley, 1998; Leff & Vaughn, 1985). Indeed, people in high-expressed-emotion families relapse at about four times the rate of those in low-expressed-emotion families. Even in studies where expressed emotion is manipulated through family intervention, high expressed emotion is strongly related to relapse (Goldstein, 1985).

Attachment States of Mind and Schizophrenia

In our lab, we have examined states of mind among individuals with schizophrenia (Dozier, Cue, & Barnett, 1994; Tyrrell et al., 1999). Tyrrell and colleagues (1999) found that 89% of individuals with schizophrenia were classified as dismissing when unresolved status was not considered, but

44% were classified as unresolved when that category was included. The cannot classify category was not used in these studies.

We argue, however, that these results tell us little about factors predisposing individuals to schizophrenia. First, we suggest that findings of higher rates of unresolved status among people with schizophrenia should be interpreted with caution. Indeed, schizophrenia, characterized most especially by thought disorder, involves "lapses in monitoring of reasoning and discourse" (Main & Goldwyn, 1984; Main et al., 2003)—the characteristics that define unresolved status. Thus people with thought disorder may appear unresolved with respect to loss or abuse *because* of their thought disorder. Second, we suggest that the failure to find many autonomous transcripts among people with schizophrenia is to be expected, because the incoherence associated with thought disorder is inconsistent with a coherent transcript. Although we urge caution in thinking of states of mind as preceding psychopathology when measured concurrently, we suggest that differences in states of mind are important in how relationships are approached and how treatment is used (see Slade, Chapter 32, this volume).

BORDERLINE PERSONALITY DISORDER

People with borderline personality disorder have a notably unstable sense of self (American Psychiatric Association, 2000). Similarly, representations of others are undeveloped and unstable; that is, others are idealized at times and devalued at other times. A central issue is the fear of abandonment by an idealized other. Because the unstable sense of self is dependent on validation from the idealized other, the threat of abandonment is experienced as potentially devastating. This instability of internal representations is often associated with emotional volatility. In particular, strong feelings of anger and dysphoria can be readily precipitated by subtle suggestions of rejection. Thus a number of factors contribute to create conditions in which interpersonal relationships are likely to be intense and tumultuous. Such factors also point to probable attachment-relevant influences on the etiology of borderline personality disorder (Agrawal, Gunderson, Holmes, & Lyons-Ruth, 2004).

Although borderline personality disorder afflicts only about 1% of the general population, the prevalence among people receiving treatment is much greater—about 15% among outpatients

and 50% among outpatients diagnosed with personality disorders (Widiger, 1993). Thus people with borderline personality disorder are relatively more likely than others to seek treatment; this is not surprising, given that "crying out for help" is characteristic of the disorder.

There has been less research on genetic involvement in borderline personality disorder than in most other disorders. Nigg and Goldsmith (1994) concluded, on the basis of a number of family studies, that the incidence of borderline personality disorder among first-degree relatives of someone with a borderline diagnosis is about 11%. Studies investigating concordance among twins have not found evidence for genetic transmission (Torgersen, 1984). The diagnostic label "borderline" was originally intended to refer to the border between neurosis and psychosis, and this suggests a possible link between borderline and psychotic disorders (i.e., schizophrenia). There is, however, little evidence for a genetic link between BPD and schizophrenia (Nigg & Goldsmith, 1994). Borderline and mood disorders are often comorbid, though, with rates of comorbidity as high as 50% in clinic samples (Alnaes & Torgersen, 1988).

Attachment and Borderline Personality Disorder: Theoretical Links

Main and Hesse (1990) have suggested that the experience of trauma in the absence of a supportive caregiver predisposes individuals to develop either borderline or dissociative pathology. As described previously, Main and Hesse have proposed that a child cannot integrate the various qualities of a caregiver into single models of self and other when the caregiver behaves in a frightened or frightening way; thus unintegrated models are maintained. This formulation is consistent with Gunderson, Kerr, and Englund's (1980) characterization of borderline pathology, in which attentional and behavioral processes are described as unintegrated.

Borderline pathology is generally associated with exaggeration of symptomatology and negative affect, as well as a "preoccupation" with concerns about current and previous relationship difficulties. The readiness to report distress is consistent with maximizing the expression of attachment needs, seen in infants with resistant attachment and in adults who are preoccupied with respect to attachment. Internalized models of caregivers as incompetent or inconsistently available, and of the self as inconsistently valued, seem as central to a diagnosis of borderline personality disorder as to a classification of preoccupied attachment (Agrawal et al., 2004).

Fonagy and colleagues (e.g., Fonagy, 2000; Fonagy & Bateman, 2005; Fonagy, Target, Gergely, Allen, & Bateman, 2003) have proposed that security of attachment fosters the development of the capacity to understand one's own and others' mental states. The emotional environment associated with security of attachment provides a child with opportunities to come to know his or her own intentional states, and to know him- or herself through caregivers' accurate reflection or mirroring of intentions. The ability to link interpersonal behavior and affect with underlying mental states is critical to the development of emotion regulation, impulse control, self-awareness, empathy, and agency (Fonagy & Target, 1997). Insecure and disorganized early relationships create interpersonal environments that force the child to inhibit reflection. According to Fonagy, the affective lability, interpersonal instability, absence of empathy, identity diffusion, and tendency toward concrete thinking that characterize borderline personality disorder can be understood as resulting from a severe impairment in the capacity to mentalize.

Children's Attachment-Related Experiences and Later Borderline Personality Disorder

The evidence for problematic family conditions in the development of borderline personality disorder is compelling. Indeed, the family histories of people with this disorder are difficult to distinguish from those of persons with dissociative disorders. Most especially, as in dissociative disorders, early abuse is often seen in the histories of people diagnosed with borderline personality disorder. For example, Herman, Perry, and van der Kolk (1989) found that 81% of people with borderline personality disorder reported physical or sexual abuse, or were witnesses to such abuse when they were children. For 57% of these children, the trauma occurred before age 7. Similarly, Ogata and colleagues (1990) found that 71% of women with borderline personality disorder were sexually abused, contrasted with only 22% of women with mood disorders. The only notable exception to these very high rates is Brown and Anderson's (1991) finding that 29% of inpatients with borderline personality disorder reported that they had been abused as children. Sanders and Giolas (1991) found evidence of higher rates of documented abuse histories in the hospital records of patients

with this disorder than in the histories of other patients. Thus these results do not appear to reflect a reporting bias only.

People with borderline personality disorder report high rates of prolonged separations from caregivers during their childhoods (Zanarini, Gunderson, Marino, Schwartz, & Frankenburg, 1989), especially from their mothers (Soloff & Millward, 1983). They also report emotional neglect when their caregivers were physically present (Patrick et al., 1994; Zanarini et al., 1989). Liotti and Pasquini (2000) found a 2.5-fold increase in the risk for borderline personality disorder for individuals whose mothers had suffered a loss within 2 years of their birth, and a 5.3-fold increase for those with early maltreatment.

To our knowledge, only one longitudinal study to date has examined the association between infant attachment quality and later borderline symptoms. Lyons-Ruth, Yellin, Melnick, and Atwood (2005) reported on the development of borderline personality disorder features in a group of 56 high-risk infants in early adulthood. Early attachment status, including attachment disorganization, did not predict later borderline personality disorder symptoms as measured by a psychiatric interview. Rather, early maltreatment and disrupted parent–infant communication were associated with a greater likelihood of developing borderline symptoms.

Attachment States of Mind and Borderline Personality Disorder

A number of studies have reported on the association between attachment state of mind, as measured by the AAI, and the incidence of diagnosed borderline personality disorder in clinical samples (Barone, 2003; Diamond, Stovall-McClough, Clarkin, & Levy, 2003; Fonagy et al., 1996; Patrick et al., 1994; Rosenstein & Horowitz, 1996; Stalker & Davies, 1995; Stovall-McClough & Cloitre, 2003). Using the three-way classification system, Fonagy and colleagues (1996) found that 75% of people with borderline personality disorder had preoccupied states of mind, and that half of those with preoccupied states of mind fell into a rarely used subgroup, "fearfully preoccupied with respect to trauma" (E3). In Patrick and colleagues' (1994) study, all women with borderline personality disorder were classified as preoccupied, and 10 of the 12 were classified as E3. Preoccupied attachment often co-occurs with unresolved status. Not surprisingly, when the four-way classification system was used, 89% and 75% of people with borderline personality disorder were classified as unresolved in the Fonagy and colleagues and Patrick and colleagues studies, respectively. In a study of inpatient adolescents, Rosenstein and Horowitz (1996) found that the majority of those diagnosed with borderline personality disorder (64%) were also classified as preoccupied on the AAI. This study did not include the unresolved category. Barone (2003) examined attachment status in a sample of 80 subjects, 40 of whom were patients diagnosed with borderline personality disorder and 40 of whom were nonclinical controls. Using the four-way attachment classification system, he identified only 7% of those with borderline personality disorder as autonomous, whereas 23% were preoccupied, 20% were dismissing, and 50% were unresolved. This distribution was significantly different from that found in the control group, where 62% were identified as autonomous, 10% as preoccupied, and only 7% as unresolved.

ANTISOCIAL PERSONALITY DISORDER

Antisocial personality disorder, as described in the DSM-IV-TR (American Psychiatric Association, 2000), is characterized by a consistent disregard for the rights and feelings of others and for the basic laws of society. Characteristics of antisocial personality disorder include deceitfulness, impulsivity, irresponsibility, irritability, and lack of remorse. The links between childhood and adolescent conduct disorder and later adult antisocial personality disorder have been noted in numerous studies (e.g., McCord, 1979; Robins, 1966). Indeed, one of the criteria for antisocial personality disorder is the presence of earlier conduct disorder.

Attachment and Antisocial Personality Disorder: Theoretical Links

Bowlby (1973) proposed that when children experience separations from parents, and when parents threaten abandonment, children feel intense anger. Ordinary but stressful separations are often met with anger, which is functional in communicating to the parents the children's feelings about the separation. When prolonged separations are combined with frightening threats, however, Bowlby suggested that children are likely to feel a dysfunctional level of anger toward parents, often

involving intense hatred. Initially the anger may be directed toward the parents. Because that may prove dangerous in maintaining the relationship with the parents, however, the anger is often repressed and directed toward other targets (Bowlby, 1973).

Children's Attachment-Related Experiences and Later Antisocial Personality Disorder

Prolonged separations from primary caregivers (as the result of divorce or separation rather than death); fathers' antisocial or deviant behavior; and mothers' unaffectionate, neglectful care are associated with antisocial personality disorder (McCord, 1979; Robins, 1966). Robins (1966) found that parental desertion, divorce, or separation was associated with the diagnosis of antisocial personality disorder. Zanarini and colleagues (1989) found that 89% of people with antisocial personality disorder had experienced prolonged separations from a caregiver at some point in childhood. Given that loss by death was not associated with later antisocial personality disorder, however, it does not seem to be simply the absence of a caregiver that is important (Robins, 1966). McCord (1979) found that antisocial personality disorder was a likely outcome only when mothers were also unaffectionate and did not provide adequate supervision, and when fathers were deviant. Many people with antisocial personality disorder report that they experienced physical abuse, or at least harsh discipline, during childhood (e.g., Zanarini et al., 1989).

Attachment States of Mind and Antisocial Personality Disorder

Most of the empirical evidence suggests that antisocial personality disorder (or conduct disorder in adolescents) is associated with unresolved and dismissing states of mind (Allen et al., 1996; Levinson & Fonagy, 2004; Rosenstein & Horowitz, 1996). Allen and colleagues (1996) assessed states of mind among adolescents who were psychiatric inpatients and a control group of high school students. Criminality and use of "hard drugs" were then assessed approximately 10 years later. The most impressive finding was that ratings from the adolescents' attachment interviews predicted criminality 10 years later, even after previous psychiatric hospitalization was accounted for. In particular, derogation of attachment and lack of resolution of trauma predicted criminal behavior. "Derogation of attachment" is a rarely occurring feature of dismissing attachment, in which the person derogates attachment figures or attachment experiences. Among the sample of psychiatric inpatients in the Allen and colleagues study, 15% of the interviews were categorized as cannot classify because they met criteria for multiple, incompatible categories. This group of people reported the most criminal behavior, followed by people classified as dismissing and unresolved. Post hoc analyses revealed that the cannot classify (termed "unclassifiable" at that time) group showed higher levels of criminal behavior than the secure and preoccupied groups, and that the dismissing group showed significantly higher levels than the secure group.

Rosenstein and Horowitz (1996) found that among adolescents with conduct disorder only, six of seven were classified as dismissing, and none was classified as unresolved. Among adolescents comorbid for conduct disorder and mood disorder, half were classified as dismissing, and nearly half were classified as unresolved with respect to loss or trauma. Fonagy and colleagues (1996) obtained very different results for a combined group made up of people with antisocial and paranoid personality disorders, however. When the three-category system was used, more were classified as preoccupied and autonomous than as dismissing. When the four-category system was used, most were classified as unresolved.

Findings have been relatively consistent when researchers have considered violence rather than antisocial personality disorder. In a study examining the association between attachment status and propensity toward domestic violence, Holtzworth-Munroe and colleagues (1997) administered the AAI to maritally distressed violent men (n = 30) and nonviolent men (n = 30). Men with histories of domestic violence were more likely than nonviolent men to be classified as nonautonomous (or insecure), and 37% were rated as cannot classify. Babcock, Jacobson, Gottman, and Yerington (2000) conducted a study with a group of martially distressed men with a history of domestic violence (n = 23) and those without such a history (n = 13). Similar to Holtzworth-Munroe and colleagues' findings, domestically violent men were more likely to be rated as nonautonomous (or insecure). Moreover, the dismissing category was associated with higher scores on an antisocial scale than were other categories. Only 9% of the domestically violent men could not be classified on the AAI—a lower rate than that reported by Holtzworth-Munroe and colleagues, but higher than that seen in the general population.

SUMMARY AND CONCLUSIONS

Attachment in Infancy

At this point, the only clear connections between infant attachment and adult psychopathology are between disorganized attachment and dissociative symptoms in adolescence and early adulthood (Carlson, 1998; Sroufe et al., 2005a) and between resistant attachment and anxiety disorders in adolescence (Warren et al., 1997). These associations are compelling for a number of reasons. First, the "phenotypic similarity" of the phenomena is striking when one considers the link between disorganized attachment and dissociative symptoms (Liotti, 2004; Main & Morgan, 1996) and between resistant attachment and anxiety (Cassidy, 1995). Second, the caregiving experiences predictive of disorganized and resistant attachment are similar to the caregiving experiences predictive of dissociative symptoms and anxiety symptoms, respectively. More specifically, the occurrence of attachment-related trauma, especially abuse, is known to be associated with both disorganized attachment (Carlson et al., 1989) and dissociative disorders (e.g., Putnam, 1991). This connection between abuse and later dissociation may be accounted for partially by the development of a sensitized neurobiology when a child experiences frightening events from which escape is not possible. Similarly, unavailable or inconsistently available caregiving appears predictive of both resistant attachment and symptoms of anxiety (Cassidy, 1995). Carlson (1998) has suggested that a child who frequently becomes hyperaroused (rather than disorganized) when threatened with an unavailable caregiver develops a sensitized neurobiology that predisposes him or her to later anxiety.

Finally, the categories of adult attachment that parallel infant disorganized and resistant attachment are characterized by behaviors consistent with the predicted symptomatology (Sroufe et al., 2005a). Adults who are unresolved with respect to loss or trauma are characterized by a "lapse in reasoning or in the monitoring of discourse" when discussing loss or trauma (Main & Goldwyn, 1984; Main et al., 2003). Similarly, the discourse of adults who are preoccupied with respect to attachment is affected by anxiety that may be either more diffuse (e.g., similar to the anxiety associated with generalized anxiety disorder; Cassidy, 1995) or more focused (e.g., similar to the anxiety associated with a phobic disorder). Thus the categories of adult attachment that parallel infant disorganized and resistant attachment are themselves characterized by some level of dissociation and anxiety, respectively.

Attachment-Related Circumstances

Loss

Loss predicts multiple disorders, including depression, anxiety, and antisocial personality disorder. To some degree, the type of loss experienced appears to affect the development of psychopathology differentially. Depression is associated generally with early loss of the mother. Major depression in particular, or depression involving vegetative signs, has been related to permanent loss of a caregiver, whereas depression characterized by anger and other externalizing symptoms has been related to separation (Brown & Harris, 1993). Anxiety appears to be associated more closely with threats of loss and instability than with permanent loss (Monroe & Simons, 1991). Antisocial personality disorder is associated with loss through desertion, separation, and divorce (McCord, 1979).

For mood and anxiety disorders, the circumstances prior to and subsequent to the loss appear to be as important in determining risk or resilience as the loss itself. With regard to vulnerability to depression and anxiety, experiences with the mother prior to the loss and with other caregivers subsequent to the loss affect the child's resilience or vulnerability (Brown & Harris, 1993; Crowell & Waters, 2005). A nurturing relationship with the mother, and nurturing continuous relationships with the father or other caregivers, seem to protect the child from the effects of the loss. An emotionally unavailable mother and/or neglectful care subsequent to the loss can leave the child desperately vulnerable, and thus at risk for later depression and anxiety (Harris et al., 1986). Bowlby (1980) suggested that children who have had rejecting caregivers may then experience a subsequent loss as overwhelming.

Caregiving experiences prior and subsequent to loss appear central to the development of antisocial personality disorder as well. Paternal deviance and inadequate maternal caregiving are correlates of divorce and desertion. The results of several studies (McCord, 1979; Robins, 1966) suggest that these caregiving conditions themselves, rather than loss, are what predict antisocial personality disorder.

Abuse

Reports of abuse are consistently high among people with borderline personality disorder, dissociative disorders, and antisocial personality disorder. When children have caregivers who do them harm, they experience unresolvable conflicts, because the very people who should be providing protection from threat are themselves threatening. Thus Liotti (2004) has proposed that multiple models of caregivers develop for several reasons. First, the actual behavior of a caregiver often vacillates quickly from hurtful to loving, in ways that cannot be accommodated by a single model of the caregiver (Liotti, 2004; Main & Morgan, 1996). When parents' behavior remains menacing, children often "fix parents up" (Harris, 1995, p. 57) so that they can derive some security from them, however illusory that security might be. The act of "fixing them up" involves a distortion too great to be accommodated within a single model of such a parent.

Alexander (1992) argued that abuse is often symptomatic of the caregiving system within the family. The nature and duration of the abuse are not random, therefore, but systematically related to the family's functioning (Alexander, 1992). Furthermore, the system of caregiving may be as important to later adjustment as the abuse itself, if not more so. For instance, dismissing parents may minimize the evidence or effects of abuse, according to Alexander, thus allowing the abuse to continue over time. Preoccupied parents may get their own needs met by role reversal with their children, so that they fail to take a competent position in protecting children. Parents with unresolved states of mind who abuse their children may be acting out their models of their own caregivers internalized as children (Sroufe, 1988), whereas their unresolved partners may be too disoriented to protect children (Alexander, 1992). Thus extended abuse often occurs in a context of disordered caregiving. When abuse occurs in a caregiving context in which caregivers are competent and emotionally available, however, the caregivers are likely to intervene quickly, providing support and protection so that children can successfully resolve the effects of the trauma.

Quality of Caregiving

Reports of inadequate caregiving of one kind or another are associated with all forms of psychopathology. Considering combinations of rejection and/or neglect with overprotection or inadequate control allows some specificity in the prediction of specific disorders. Mood and anxiety disorders tend to be associated most frequently with parental rejection combined with loss. Antisocial personality disorder is most frequently associated with parental rejection, harsh discipline, and inadequate control. Eating disorders are associated with maternal rejection and overprotection combined with paternal neglect, and borderline personality disorder is associated most consistently with parental neglect.

Attachment States of Mind

There are relatively few findings regarding the distribution of attachment states of mind among people with psychiatric disorders. The findings that do exist are consistent in some respects, as described below, but are inconsistent in others. We suggest that there may be several important reasons for the discrepancies. First, the classification system has been evolving in recent years. An especially important recent development is the refinement of the category of cannot classify, particularly because of its apparent strong association with psychopathology. Few raters have yet completed reliability testing on this coding category. As additional laboratories meet reliability criteria and begin to use this system of coding, some discrepancies in findings may be resolved.

A second possible reason for discrepancies in findings is that diagnostic groups are defined differently in different studies. We suggest the creation of diagnostic groupings that are as specific as possible, with researchers systematically assessing the effects of other comorbid diagnoses and symptomatology. Furthermore, we urge attention to heterogeneity within disorders. In particular, we expect that differences related to the internalization–externalization dimension that cuts across some disorders may be quite important to consider in relation to states of mind (see also Sroufe et al., 2005a).

Nonetheless, several consistent findings have emerged. One such finding is that psychiatric disorders are nearly always associated with nonautonomous (or insecure) states of mind. Furthermore, unresolved status is the most overrepresented state of mind among people with psychiatric disorders. What these findings mean in terms of the causal connection between attachment state of mind and psychiatric disorders is unclear. Only the Allen and colleagues (1996) study provided evidence

that ratings of derogation and ratings of lack of resolution of abuse can predict problematic behaviors (in particular, criminal behavior and hard-drug use) in a high-risk sample. Some of the longitudinal studies now being conducted with high-risk samples will address the association between states of mind and the emergence of different psychiatric disorders more comprehensively.

We suggest that the classification of unresolved status may be more meaningful for some psychiatric disorders than for others. For disorders where disorganization is not a key feature, we expect that unresolved classifications are more likely to indicate lack of resolution of loss or trauma. In contrast, individuals with schizophrenia and bipolar mood disorders are at times highly disorganized in speech. Therefore, disorganization when discussing loss or trauma is consistent with this general presentation, rather than suggesting anything more specific about their states of mind.

Dismissing states of mind reflect attempts to minimize attachment needs, whereas preoccupied states of mind reflect the maximizing of attachment needs (Cassidy, 1994; Main, 1990). Therefore, dismissing states of mind should be associated with disorders that involve turning attention away from one's own feelings (such as antisocial personality disorder, eating disorder, substance abuse and dependence, hostile forms of depression, and externalizing forms of anxiety disorders). Preoccupied states of mind should be associated with disorders that involve absorption in one's own feelings (such as internalizing forms of depression and anxiety, as well as borderline personality disorder). The evidence available thus far generally supports this hypothesis, with some exceptions. As discussed previously, the findings of Rosenstein and Horowitz (1996), Cole-Detke and Kobak (1996), and Patrick and colleagues (1994) can be interpreted as consistent in suggesting that some externalizing disorders (i.e., eating disorders and conduct disorder) are associated with dismissing states of mind, and that an internalizing disorder (i.e., borderline personality disorder) is associated with preoccupied states of mind. We suggest that both depression and anxiety are more heterogeneous disorders, subsuming those who are more self-focused (i.e., internalizing) and those who are less self-focused (i.e., externalizing).

The Metaphor of the Branching Railway Lines

Bowlby (1973) described "branching railway lines" as a metaphor for the development of psychopathology and psychological health. Infants with emotionally available caregivers begin their development by moving out from the "metropolis" in different directions from those with emotionally unavailable caregivers. Future experiences with caregivers, and experiences of loss and abuse, have differential effects on these children because they are on different branching pathways (Sroufe, 1997). No circumstances, including the quality of early caregiving or the experiences of loss or abuse, fully constrain development. Nonetheless, certain pathways become more or less likely, because there develops within a child an organized system for coping with his or her experiences (Sroufe et al., 2005a). The research we have examined in this chapter provides tentative support for this model. Over time, we expect fuller tests of this model of "psychopathology as an outcome of development" (Sroufe, 1997, p. 251).

ACKNOWLEDGMENT

Support for this work was provided by National Institute of Mental Health Grant Nos. R01 52135 and K02 74374 to Mary Dozier.

NOTE

1. Relations between self-report romantic attachment and various forms of psychopathology are discussed in Brennan and Shaver (1995, 1998); Cooper, Shaver, and Collins (1998); Mickelson, Kessler, and Shaver (1997); Mikulincer and Shaver (2007); Shaver and Clark (1994); and Shaver, Belsky, and Brennan (2000).

REFERENCES

Achenbach, T., & Edelbrock, C. (1986). *Manual for the Teacher's Report Form and Teacher Version of the Child Behavior Profile*. Burlington: University of Vermont, Department of Psychiatry.

Adam, K. S., Sheldon-Keller, A. E., & West, M. (1996). Attachment organization and history of suicidal behavior in clinical adolescents. *Journal of Consulting and Clinical Psychology, 64*, 264–272.

Agrawal, H. R., Gunderson, J., Holmes, B. M., & Lyons-Ruth, K. (2004). Attachment studies with borderline patients: A review. *Harvard Review of Psychiatry, 12*, 94–104.

Ainsworth, M. D. S., Blehar, M., Waters, E., & Wall, S. (1978). *Patterns of attachment: A psychological study of the Strange Situation*. Hillsdale, NJ: Erlbaum.

Alexander, P. C. (1992). Application of attachment theory to the study of sexual abuse. *Journal of Consulting and Clinical Psychology, 60*, 185–195.

Allen, J. P., Hauser, S. T., & Borman-Spurrell, E. (1996). Attachment theory as a framework for understanding sequelae of severe adolescent psychopathology: An 11-year follow-up study. *Journal of Consulting and Clinical Psychology, 64*, 254–263.

Alnaes, R., & Torgersen, S. (1988). The relationship between DSM-III symptom disorders (Axis I) and personality disorders (Axis II) in an outpatient population. *Acta Psychiatrica Scandinavica, 78*, 485–492.

American Psychiatric Association. (2000). *Diagnostic and statistical manual of mental disorders* (4th ed., text rev.). Washington, DC: Author.

Armstrong, J. G., & Roth, D. M. (1989). Attachment and separation difficulties in eating disorders: A preliminary investigation. *International Journal of Eating Disorders, 8*, 141–155.

Babcock, J. C., Jacobson, N. S., Gottman, J. M., & Yerington, T. P. (2000). Attachment, emotional regulation, and the function of marital violence: Differences between secure, preoccupied, and dismissing violent and nonviolent husbands. *Journal of Family Violence, 15*, 391–409.

Bandelow, B., Spath, C., Tichauer, G. A., Broocks, A., Hajak, G., & Ruther, E. (2002). Early traumatic life events, parental attitudes, family history, and birth risk factors in patients with panic disorder. *Comprehensive Psychiatry, 43*, 269–278.

Bandelow, B., Torrente, A. C., Wedekind, D., Broocks, A., Hajak, G., & Ruther, E. (2004). Early traumatic life events, parental rearing styles family history of mental disorders, and birth risk factors in patients with social anxiety disorder. *European Archives of Psychiatry and Clinical Neuroscience, 254*, 397–405.

Barber, J. P., & Muenz, L. R. (1996). The role of avoidance and obsessiveness in matching patients to cognitive and interpersonal psychotherapy: Empirical findings from the Treatment for Depression Collaborative Research Program. *Journal of Consulting and Clinical Psychology, 64*, 951–958.

Baron, M. (2001). Genetics of schizophrenia and the new millennium: Progress and pitfalls. *American Journal of Human Genetics, 68*, 299–312.

Barone, L. (2003). Developmental protective and risk in borderline personality disorder: A study using the Adult Attachment Interview. *Attachment and Human Development, 5*, 64–77.

Bartholomew, K., & Shaver, P. R. (1998). Measures of attachment: Do they converge? In J. A Simpson & W. S. Rholes (Eds.), *Attachment theory and close relationships* (pp. 25–45). New York: Guilford Press.

Bertelsen, A., Harvald, B., & Hauge, M. (1977). A Danish twin study of manic depressive disorders. *British Journal of Psychiatry, 130*, 330–351.

Beutler, L. E., Engle, D., Mohr, D., Daldrup, R. J., Bergan, J., Meredith, K., et al. (1991). Predictors of differential response to cognitive, experiential, and self-directed psychotherapeutic procedures. *Journal of Consulting and Clinical Psychology, 59*, 333–340.

Bosquet, M., & Egeland, B. (2006). The development and maintenance of anxiety symptoms from infancy through adolescence in a longitudinal sample. *Development and Psychopathology, 18*, 517–550.

Bowlby, J. (1969/1982). *Attachment and loss: Vol. 1. Attachment.* New York: Basic Books.

Bowlby, J. (1973). *Attachment and loss: Vol. 2. Separation: Anxiety and anger.* New York: Basic Books.

Bowlby, J. (1980). *Attachment and loss: Vol. 3. Loss: Sadness and depression.* New York: Basic Books.

Brazelton, T. B. (1973). *Neonatal Behavioral Assessment Scale.* Philadelphia: Lippincott.

Brennan, K. A., & Shaver, P. R. (1995). Dimensions of adult attachment, affect regulation, and romantic functioning. *Personality and Social Psychology Bulletin, 21*, 267–283.

Brennan, K. A., & Shaver, P. R. (1998). Attachment styles and personality disorders: Their connections to each other and to parental divorce, parental death, and perceptions of parental caregiving. *Journal of Personality, 66*, 835–878.

Bretherton, I. (1985). Attachment theory. Retrospect and prospect. In I. Bretherton & E. Waters (Eds.), Growing points of attachment theory and research. *Monographs of the Society for Research in Child Development, 50*(1–2, Serial No. 209), 3–35.

Brown, G. R., & Anderson, B. (1991). Psychiatric morbidity in adult inpatients with childhood histories of sexual and physical abuse. *American Journal of Psychiatry, 148*, 55–61.

Brown, G. W., Birley, J. L. T., & Wing, J. K. (1972). Influence of family life on the course of schizophrenic disorders: A replication. *British Journal of Psychiatry, 121*, 241–258.

Brown, G. W., & Harris, T. O. (1993). Aetiology of anxiety and depressive disorders in an inner city population: 1. Early adversity. *Psychological Medicine, 23*, 143–154.

Butzlaff, R. L., & Hooley, J. M. (1998). Expressed emotion and psychiatric relapse: A meta-analysis. *Archives of General Psychiatry, 55*, 547–552.

Carlson, E. A. (1998). A prospective longitudinal study of disorganized/disoriented attachment. *Child Development, 69*, 1107–1128.

Carlson, V., Cicchetti, D., Barnett, D., & Braunwald, K. (1989). Disorganized/disoriented attachment relationships in maltreated infants. *Developmental Psychology, 25*, 525–531.

Carter, J. C., Bewell, C., Blackmore, E., & Woodside, D. B. (2006). The impact of childhood sexual abuse in anorexia nervosa. *Child Abuse and Neglect, 30*, 257–269.

Cassidy, J. (1994). Emotion regulation: Influences of attachment relations. In N. A. Fox (Ed.), The development of emotion regulation: Biological and behavioral considerations. *Monographs of the Society for Research in Child Development, 59*(2–3, Serial No. 240), 228–249.

Cassidy, J. (1995). Attachment and generalized anxiety disorder. In D. Cicchetti & S. Toth (Eds.), *Rochester Symposium on Developmental Psychopathology: Vol. 6. Emotion, cognition, and representation* (pp. 343–370). Rochester, NY: University of Rochester Press.

Chambless, D. L., Gillis, M. M., Tran, G. Q., & Steketee, G. S. (1996). Parental bonding reports of clients with obsessive compulsive disorder and agoraphobia. *Clinical Psychology and Psychotherapy, 3*, 77–85.

Cole-Detke, H., & Kobak, R. (1996). Attachment processes in eating disorder and depression. *Journal of Consulting and Clinical Psychology, 64*, 282–290.

Cooper, M. L., Shaver, P. R., & Collins, N. L. (1998). Attachment styles, emotion regulation, and adjustment in adolescence. *Journal of Personality and Social Psychology, 74*, 1380–1397.

Crowell, J., & Waters, E. (2005). Attachment representations, secure-base behavior, and the evolution of adult relationships: The Stony Brook Adult Relationship Project. In K. E. Grossmann, K. Grossmann, & E. Waters (Eds.), *Attachment from infancy to adulthood: The major longitudinal studies* (pp. 223–244). New York: Guilford Press.

Cummings, E. M., & Cicchetti, D. (1990). Toward a transactional model of relations between attachment and depression. In M. T. Greenberg, D. Cicchetti, & E. M. Cummings (Eds.), *Attachment in the preschool years* (pp. 339–372). Chicago: University of Chicago Press.

De Bellis, M. D. (2001). Developmental traumatology: The psychobiological development of maltreated children and its implications for research, treatment, and policy. *Development and Psychopathology, 13*, 539–564.

de Ruiter, C., & van IJzendoorn, M. H. (1992). Agoraphobia and anxious-ambivalent attachment: An integrative review. *Journal of Anxiety Disorders, 6*, 365–381.

Diamond, D., Stovall-McClough, K. C., Clarkin, J. F., & Levy, K. N. (2003). Patient–therapist attachment in the treatment of borderline personality disorder. *Bulletin of the Menninger Clinic, 67*, 227–259.

Dickstein, S. (1993). *Marital Attachment Interview.* Unpublished manuscript.

Dickstein, S., Seifer, R., Albus, K. E., & Magee, K. D. (2004). Attachment patterns across multiple family relationships in adulthood: Associations with maternal depression. *Development and Psychopathology, 16*, 735–751.

Dozier, M., Cue, K., & Barnett, L. (1994). Clinicians as caregivers: Role of attachment organization in treatment. *Journal of Consulting and Clinical Psychology, 62*, 793–800.

Duggal, S., Carlson, E. A., Sroufe, L. A., & Egeland, B. (2001). Depressive symptomatology in childhood and adolescence. *Development and Psychopathology, 13*, 143–164.

Dutra, L., & Lyons-Ruth, K. (2005). *Maltreatment, maternal and child psychopathology, and quality of early care as predictors of adolescent dissociation.* Paper presented at the biennial meeting of the Society for Research in Child Development, Atlanta, GA.

Faravelli, C., Webb, T., Ambonetti, A., Fonnesu, F., & Sessarego, A. (1985). Prevalence of traumatic early life events in 31 agoraphobic patients with panic attacks. *American Journal of Psychiatry, 142,* 1493–1494.

Fonagy, P. (2000). Attachment and borderline personality disorder. *Journal of the American Psychoanalytic Association, 48,* 1129–1146.

Fonagy, P., & Bateman, A. W. (2005). Attachment theory and mentalization-oriented model of borderline personality disorder. In J. Oldham, A. Skodol, & D. S. Bender (Eds.), *The American Psychiatric Publishing textbook of personality disorders* (pp. 187–207). Washington, DC: American Psychiatric Publishing.

Fonagy, P., Leigh, T., Steele, M., Steele, H., Kennedy, R., Mattoon, G., et al. (1996). The relation of attachment status, psychiatric classification, and response to psychotherapy. *Journal of Consulting and Clinical Psychology, 64,* 22–31.

Fonagy, P., & Target, M. (1997). Attachment and reflective function: Their role in self-organization. *Development and Psychopathology, 9,* 679–700.

Fonagy, P., Target, M., Gergely, G., Allen, J. G., & Bateman, A. (2003). The developmental roots of borderline personality disorder in early attachment relationships: A theory and some evidence. *Psychoanalytic Inquiry, 23,* 412–459.

George, C., Kaplan, N., & Main, M. (1984). *Adult Attachment Interview protocol.* Unpublished manuscript, University of California at Berkeley.

George, C., Kaplan, N., & Main, M. (1985). *Adult Attachment Interview* (2nd ed.). Unpublished manuscript, University of California at Berkeley.

George, C., Kaplan, N., & Main, M. (1996). *Adult Attachment Interview protocol* (3rd ed.). Unpublished manuscript, University of California at Berkeley.

Goldstein, M. J. (1985). Family factors that antedate the onset of schizophrenia and related disorders: The results of a fifteen year prospective study. *Acta Psychiatrica Scandinavica, 71,* 7–18.

Gottesman, I. I. (1991). *Schizophrenia genesis.* New York: Freeman.

Grossmann, K. E., Grossmann, K., & Waters, E. (Eds.). (2005). *Attachment from infancy to adulthood: The major longitudinal studies.* New York: Guilford Press.

Gunderson, J. G., Kerr, J., & Englund, D. W. (1980). The families of borderlines: A comparative study. *Archives of General Psychiatry, 37,* 27–33.

Harris, M. (1995). *The loss that is forever.* New York: Dutton.

Harris, T. O., Brown, G. W., & Bifulco, A. (1986). Loss of parent in childhood and adult psychiatric disorder: The Walthamstow Study. 1. The role of lack of adequate parental care. *Psychological Medicine, 16,* 641–659.

Harris, T. O, Brown, G. W., & Bifulco, A. T. (1990). Depression and situational helplessness/mastery in a sample selected to study childhood parental loss. *Journal of Affective Disorders, 20,* 27–41.

Hazan, C., & Shaver, P. R. (1987). Romantic love conceptualized as an attachment process. *Journal of Personality and Social Psychology, 52,* 511–524.

Hazan, C., & Shaver, P. R. (1994). Attachment as an organizational framework for research on close relationships. *Psychological Inquiry, 5,* 1–22.

Herman, J. L., Perry, J. C., & van der Kolk, B. A. (1989). Childhood trauma in borderline personality disorder. *American Journal of Psychiatry, 146,* 490–495.

Hesse, E., & Main, M. (2006). Frightened, threatening, and dissociative parental behavior: Theory and associations with parental Adult Attachment Interview status and infant disorganization. *Development and Psychopathology, 18,* 309–343.

Hesse, E., & van IJzendoorn, M. H. (1998). Parental loss of close family members and propensities towards absorption in offspring. *Developmental Science, 1,* 299–305.

Hettema, J. M., Neale, M. C., & Kendler, K. S. (2001). A review and meta-analysis of the genetic epidemiology of anxiety disorders. *American Journal of Psychiatry, 158,* 1568–1578.

Holtzworth-Munroe, A., Stuart, G. L., & Hutchinson, G. (1997). Violent versus nonviolent husbands: Differences in attachment patterns, dependency, and jealousy. *Journal of Family Psychology, 11,* 314–331.

Humphrey, L. L. (1989). Observed family interactions among subtypes of eating disorders using Structural Analysis of Social Behavior. *Journal of Consulting and Clinical Psychology, 57,* 206–214.

Johnson, J. G., Cohen, P., Kasen, S., & Brook, J. S. (2006). Dissociative disorders among adults in the community, impaired functioning, and Axis I and II comorbidity. *Journal of Psychiatric Research, 40,* 131–140.

Kendler, K. S., Heath, A. C., Martin, N. G., & Eaves, L. J. (1987). Symptoms of anxiety and symptoms of depression. *Archives of General Psychiatry, 44,* 451–457.

Kendler, K. S., Sheth, K., Gardner, C. O., & Prescott, C. A. (2002). Childhood parental loss and risk for first-onset of major depression and alcohol dependence: The time-decay of risk and sex differences. *Psychological Medicine, 323,* 1187–1194.

Kenny, M. E., & Hart, K. (1992). Relationship between parental attachment and eating disorders in an inpatient and a college sample. *Journal of Counseling Psychology, 39,* 521–526.

Kivela, S., Luukinin, H., Koski, K., Viramo, P., & Pahkala, K. (1998). Early loss of mother or father predicts depression in old age. *International Journal of Geriatric Psychiatry, 13,* 527–530.

Kobak, R., Cassidy, J., & Ziv, Y. (2004). Attachment related trauma and post-traumatic stress disorder: Implications for adult adaptation. In W. S. Rholes & J. A. Simpson (Eds.), *Adult attachment: Theory, research, and clinical implications* (pp. 388–407). New York: Guilford Press.

Leff, J., & Vaughn, C. (1985). *Expressed emotion in families.* New York: Guilford Press.

Levinson, A., & Fonagy, P. (2004). Offending and attachment: The relationship between interpersonal awareness and offending in a prison population with psychiatric disorder. *Canadian Journal of Psychoanalysis, 12,* 225–251.

Lichtenstein, J., & Cassidy, J. (1991). *The Inventory of Adult Attachment: Validation of a new measure.* Paper presented at the biennial meeting of the Society for Research in Child Development, Seattle, WA.

Liotti, G. (2004). Trauma, dissociation, and disorganized attachment: Three strands of a single braid. *Psychotherapy: Theory, Research, Practice, Training, 41,* 472–486.

Liotti, G., & Pasquini, P. (2000). Predictive factors for borderline personality disorder: Patients' early traumatic experiences and losses suffered by the attachment figure. *Acta Psychiatrica Scandinavica, 102,* 282–289.

Lyons-Ruth, K., Yellin, C., Melnick, S., & Atwood, G. (2005). Expanding the concept of unresolved mental states: Hostile/helpless states of mind on the Adult Attachment Interview are associated with disrupted mother–infant communication and infant disorganization. *Development and Psychopathology, 17,* 1–23.

Main, M. (1990). Cross-cultural studies of attachment organization: Recent studies, changing methodologies, and the concept of conditional strategies. *Human Development, 33,* 48–61.

Main, M., & Goldwyn, R. (1984). *Adult attachment scoring and classification system.* Unpublished manuscript, University of California at Berkeley.

Main, M., Goldwyn, R., & Hesse, E. (2003). *Adult attachment scoring and classification system.* Unpublished manuscript, University of California at Berkeley.

Main, M., & Hesse, E. (1990). Parents' unresolved traumatic experiences are related to infant disorganized attachment status: Is frightened and/or frightening parental behavior the linking mechanism? In M. T. Greenberg, D. Cicchetti, & E. M. Cummings (Eds.), *Attachment in the preschool years* (pp. 161–182). Chicago: University of Chicago Press.

Main, M., & Morgan, H. (1996). Disorganization and disorientation in infant Strange Situation behavior. In L. K. Michelson & W. J. Ray (Eds.), *Handbook of dissociation: Theoretical, empirical, and clinical perspectives* (pp. 107–138). New York: Plenum Press.

Main, M., & Solomon, J. (1986). Discovery of a new, insecure-disorganized/disoriented attachment pattern. In T. B. Brazelton & M. Yogman (Eds.), *Affective development in infancy* (pp. 95–124). Norwood, NJ: Ablex.

Manassis, K., Bradley, S., Goldberg, S., Hood, J., & Swinson, R. P. (1994). Attachment in mothers with anxiety disorders and their children. *Journal of the American Academy of Child and Adolescent Psychiatry, 33,* 1106–1113.

McCord, J. (1979). Some child-rearing antecedents of criminal behavior in adult men. *Journal of Personality and Social Psychology, 37,* 1477–1486.

McGuffin, P., & Katz, R. (1986). Nature, nurture, and affective disorder. In J. F. W. Deakin (Ed.), *The biology of depression* (pp. 26–52). London: Royal College of Psychiatrists/Gaskell Press.

McMahon, C. A., Barnett, B., Kowalenko, N. M., & Tennant, C. C. (2006). Maternal attachment state of mind moderates the impact of postnatal depression on infant attachment. *Journal of Child Psychology and Psychiatry, 47,* 660–669.

Mickelson, K. D., Kessler, R. C., & Shaver, P. R. (1997). Adult attachment in a nationally representative sample. *Journal of Personality and Social Psychology, 73,* 1092–1106.

Mikulincer, M., & Shaver, P. R. (2007). *Attachment in adulthood: Structure, dynamics, and change.* New York: Guilford Press.

Millon, T. (1983). *The Millon Clinical Multiaxial Inventory manual* (3rd ed.). Minneapolis, MN: National Computer Systems.

Minuchin, S., Rosman, B. L., & Baker, L. (1980). *Psychosomatic families: Anorexia nervosa in context.* Cambridge, MA: Harvard University Press.

Mitchell, J. E., & Pyle, R. L. (1985). Characteristics of bulimia. In J. E. Mitchell (Ed.), *Anorexia nervosa and bulimia: Diagnosis and treatment* (pp. 29–47). Minneapolis: University of Minnesota Press.

Moldin, S. O., Reich, T., & Rice, J. P. (1991). Current perspectives on the genetics of unipolar depression. *Behavior Genetics, 21,* 211–242.

Monroe, S. M., & Simons, A. D. (1991). Diathesis–stress theories in the context of life stress research: Implications for the depressive disorders. *Psychological Bulletin, 110,* 406–425.

Nigg, J. T., & Goldsmith, H. H. (1994). Genetics of personality disorders: Perspectives from personality and psychopathology research. *Psychological Bulletin, 115,* 346–380.

Nurnberger, J. I., & Gershon, E. S. (1992). Genetics. In E. S. Paykel (Ed.), *Handbook of affective disorders* (2nd ed., pp. 131–148). New York: Guilford Press.

Oakley-Browne, M. A., Joyce, P. R., Wells, J. E., Bushnell, J. A., & Hornblow, A. R. (1995). Adverse parenting and other childhood experiences as risk factors for depression in women aged 18–44 years. *Journal of Affective Disorders, 34,* 13–23.

Ogata, S. N., Silk, K. R., Goodrich, S., Lohr, N. E., Westen, D., & Hill, E. M. (1990). Childhood sexual and physical abuse in adult patients with borderline personality disorder. *American Journal of Psychiatry, 147,* 1008–1013.

Ogawa, J., Sroufe, L. A., Weinfield, N. S., Carlson, E. A., & Egeland, B. (1997). Development and the fragmented self: A longitudinal study of dissociative symptomatology in a non-clinical sample. *Development and Psychopathology, 9,* 855–879.

Palmer, R. L., Oppenheimer, R., & Marshall, P. D. (1988). Eating disordered patients remember their parents: A study using the Parental Bonding Instrument. *International Journal of Eating Disorders, 7,* 101–106.

Pasquini, P., Liotti, G., Mazzotti, E., Fassone, G., & Picardi, A. (2002). Risk factors in the early family life of patients suffering from dissociative disorders. *Acta Psychiatrica Scandinavica, 105,* 110–116.

Patrick, M., Hobson, R. P., Castle, D., Howard, R., & Maughan, B. (1994). Personality disorder and the mental representation of early social experience. *Development and Psychopathology, 6,* 375–388.

Pearson, J. A., Cohn, D. A., Cowan, P. A., & Cowan, C. P. (1994). Earned- and continuous-security in adult attachment: Relation to depressive symptomatology and parenting style. *Development and Psychopathology, 6,* 359–373.

Pope, H. G., Mangweth, B., Negrao, A. B., Hudson, J. I., & Cordas, T. A. (1994). Childhood sexual abuse and bulimia nervosa: A comparison of American, Austrian, and Brazilian women. *American Journal of Psychiatry, 151,* 732–737.

Putnam, F. W. (1991). Recent research on multiple personality disorder. *Psychiatric Clinics of North America, 14,* 489–502.

Radloff, L. S. (1977). The CES-D scale: A self-report depression scale for research in the general population. *Applied Psychological Measurement, 1,* 385–401.

Raskin, A., Boothe, H. H., Reatig, N. A., Schulterbrandt, J. G., & Odel, D. (1971). Factor analyses of normal and depressed patients' memories of parental behavior. *Psychological Reports, 29,* 871–879.

Ratti, L. A., Humphrey, L. L., & Lyons, J. S. (1996). Structural analysis of families with a polydrug-dependent, bulimic, or normal adolescent daughter. *Journal of Consulting and Clinical Psychology, 64,* 1255–1262.

Rhodes, B., & Kroger, J. (1992). Parental bonding and separation–individuation difficulties among late adolescent eating disordered women. *Child Psychiatry and Human Development, 22,* 249–263.

Riggs, S. A., Paulson, A., Tunnell, E., Sahl, G., Atkison, H., & Ross, C. A. (2007). Attachment, personality, and psychopathology among adult inpatients: Self-reported romantic attachment style versus Adult Attachment Interview states of mind. *Development and Psychopathology, 19,* 263–291.

Robins, L. (1966). *Deviant children grown up.* Baltimore: Williams & Wilkins.

Roisman, G. I., Padron, E., Sroufe, L. A., & Egeland, B. (2002). Earned-secure attachment status in retrospect and prospect. *Child Development, 73,* 1204–1219.

Rosenstein, D. S., & Horowitz, H. A. (1996). Adolescent attachment and psychopathology. *Journal of Consulting and Clinical Psychology, 64,* 244–253.

Rowa, K., Kerig, P. K., & Geller, J. (2001). The family and anorexia nervosa: Examining parent–child boundary problems. *European Eating Disorders Review, 9,* 97–114.

Sanders, B., & Giolas, M. H. (1991). Dissociation and childhood trauma in psychologically disturbed adolescents. *American Journal of Psychiatry, 148,* 50–54.

Seligman, M. E. P., Abramson, L. Y., Semmel, A., & von Baeyer, C. (1979). Depressive attributional style. *Journal of Abnormal Psychology, 88,* 242–247.

Shaver, P. R., Belsky, J., & Brennan, K. A. (2000). The Adult Attachment Interview and self-reports of romantic attachment: Associations across domains and methods. *Personal Relationships, 7,* 25–43.

Shaver, P. R., & Clark, C. L. (1994). The psychodynamics of adult romantic attachment. In J. M. Masling & R. F. Bornstein (Eds.), *Empirical perspectives on object relations theories* (pp. 105–156). Washington, DC: American Psychological Association.

Soloff, H. P., & Millward, J. W. (1983). Developmental histories of borderline patients. *Comprehensive Psychiatry, 24,* 574–588.

Spitzer, R. L., Williams, J. B., & Gibbon, M. (1987). *Instruction manual for the Structured Clinical Interview for DSM-III-R (SCID).* New York: Biometrics Research Department, New York State Psychiatric Institute.

Sroufe, L. A. (1988). The role of infant–caregiver attachment in development. In J. Belsky & T. Nezworski (Eds.), *Clinical implications of attachment* (pp. 18–38). Hillsdale, NJ: Erlbaum.

Sroufe, L. A. (1996). *Emotional development.* New York: Cambridge University Press.

Sroufe, L. A. (1997). Psychopathology as development. *Development and Psychopathology, 9,* 251–268.

Sroufe, L. A. (2005). Attachment and development: A prospective, longitudinal study from birth to adulthood. *Attachment and Human Development, 7,* 349–367.

Sroufe, L. A., Egeland, B., Carlson, E., & Collins, W. A. (2005a). *The development of the person: The Minnesota Study of Risk and Adaptation from Birth to Adulthood.* New York: Guilford Press.

Sroufe, L. A., Egeland, B., Carlson, E., & Collins, W. A. (2005b). Placing early attachment experiences in developmental context: The Minnesota longitudinal study. In K. Grossmann, K. Grossmann, & E. Waters (Eds.), *Attachment from infancy to adulthood: The major longitudinal studies* (pp. 48–70). New York: Guilford Press.

Stalker, C. A., & Davies, F. (1995). Attachment organization and adaptation in sexually-abused women. *Canadian Journal of Psychiatry, 40,* 234–240.

Steele, H. (2003). Unrelenting catastrophic trauma within the family: When every secure base is abusive. *Attachment and Human Development, 5,* 353–366.

Stovall-McClough, K. C., & Cloitre, M. (2003). Reorganization of unresolved childhood traumatic memories following exposure therapy. *Annals of the New York Academy of Sciences, 1008,* 297–299.

Stovall-McClough, K. C., & Cloitre, M. (2006). Unresolved attachment, PTSD, and dissociation in women with childhood abuse histories. *Journal of Consulting and Clinical Psychology, 74,* 219–228.

Sullivan, P. F., Neale, M. C., & Kendler, K. S. (2000). Genetic epidemiology of major depression: Review and meta-analysis. *American Journal of Psychiatry, 157,* 1552–1562.

Takeuchi, H., Hiroe, T., Kanai, T., Morinobu, S., Kitamura, T., Takahashi, K., et al. (2003). Childhood parental separation experiences and depressive symptomatology in acute major depression. *Psychiatry and Clinical Neurosciences, 57*(2), 215–219.

Terreira, A. (1960). The pregnant woman's attitude and its reflection on the newborn. *American Journal of Orthopsychiatry, 30*, 553–561.

Thompson, J. L., Watson, J. R., Steinhauer, S. R., Goldstein, G., & Pogue-Geile, M. F. (2005). Indicators of genetic liability to schizophrenia: A sibling study of neuropsychological performance. *Schizophrenia Bulletin, 31*, 85–96.

Torgersen, S. (1984). Genetic and nosological aspects of schizotypal and borderline personality disorders. *Archives of General Psychiatry, 41*(6), 546–554.

Torgersen, S. (1988). Genetics. In C. Last & M. Hersen (Eds.), *Handbook of anxiety disorders* (pp. 159–170). New York: Pergamon Press.

Tyrrell, C., & Dozier, M. (1997). *The role of attachment in therapeutic process and outcome for adults with serious psychiatric disorders.* Paper presented at the biennial meeting of the Society for Research in Child Development, Washington, DC.

Tyrrell, C., Dozier, M., Teague, G. B., & Fallot, R. D. (1999). Effective treatment relationships for persons with serious psychiatric disorders: The importance of attachment states of mind. *Journal of Consulting and Clinical Psychology, 67*, 725–733.

Vidovic, V., Juresa, V., Begovac, I., Mahnik, M., & Tocilkj, G. (2005). Perceived family cohesion, adaptability and communication in eating disorders. *European Eating Disorders Review, 13*, 19–28.

Wade, T. D., Treloar, S. A., & Martin, N. G. (2001). A comparison of family functioning, temperament, and childhood conditions in monozygotic twin pairs discordant for lifetime bulimia nervosa. *American Journal of Psychiatry, 158*, 1155–1157.

Walker, E. F., Grimes, K. E., Davis, D. M., & Smith, A. J. (1993). Childhood precursors of schizophrenia: Facial expressions of emotion. *American Journal of Psychiatry, 150*, 1654–1660.

Waller, N. G., & Ross, C. (1997). The prevalence and biometric structure of pathological dissociation in the general population: Taxonomic and behavior genetic findings. *Journal of Abnormal Psychology, 106*, 499–510.

Wallin, U., & Hansson, K. (1999). Anorexia nervosa in teenagers: Patterns of family function. *Nordic Journal of Psychiatry, 53*, 29–35.

Ward, A., Ramsay, R., Turnbull, S., Steele, M., Steele, H., & Treasure, J. (2001). Attachment in anorexia nervosa: A transgenerational perspective. *British Journal of Medical Psychology, 74*, 497–505.

Warren, S. L., Huston, L., Egeland, B., & Sroufe, L. A. (1997). Child and adolescent anxiety disorders and early attachment. *Journal of the American Academy of Child and Adolescent Psychiatry, 36*, 637–644.

Welch, S. L., & Fairburn, C. G. (1994). Sexual abuse and bulimia nervosa: Three integrated case control comparisons. *American Journal of Psychiatry, 15*, 402–407.

West, M., Adam, K., Spreng, S., & Rose, S. (2001). Attachment disorganization and dissociative symptoms in clinically treated adolescents. *Canadian Journal of Psychiatry, 46*, 627–631.

Widiger, T. A. (1993). The DSM-III-R categorical personality diagnoses: A critique and an alternative. *Psychological Inquiry, 4*, 75–90.

Woodside, D. B., Bulik, C. M., Halmi, K. A., Fichter, M. M., Kaplan, A., Berrettini, W. H., et al. (2002). Personality, perfectionism, and attitudes toward eating in parents of individuals with eating disorders. *International Journal of Eating Disorders, 31*, 290–299.

Zanarini, M. C., Gunderson, J. G., Marino, M. F., Schwartz, E. O., & Frankenberg, F. R. (1989). Childhood experiences of borderline patients. *Comprehensive Psychiatry, 30*, 18–25.

Zeijlmans van Emmichoven, I. A., van IJzendoorn, M. H., de Ruiter, C., & Brosschot, J. F. (2003). Selective processing of threatening information: Effects of attachment representation and anxiety disorder on attention and memory. *Development and Psychopathology, 15*, 219–237.

CHAPTER 31

Prevention and Intervention Programs
for Supporting Early Attachment Security

LISA J. BERLIN
CHARLES H. ZEANAH
ALICIA F. LIEBERMAN

Supporting early child–parent relationships is an increasingly prominent goal of mental health practitioners, community-based service providers, and policymakers (Sameroff, McDonough, & Rosenblum, 2004; Shonkoff & Phillips, 2000; Zeanah, 2000). This goal in turn reflects two burgeoning bodies of research: (1) research illustrating the influence of children's earliest experiences—and especially their earliest relationships—on their later development (Shonkoff & Phillips, 2000; Sroufe, Egeland, Carlson, & Collins, 2005); and (2) research indicating that attachment disturbances are at the root of many child and adult disorders (DeKlyen & Greenberg, Chapter 27, this volume; Greenberg, 1999; Sroufe et al., 2005).

Theory, research, and interventions focusing on early child–parent attachments offer powerful tools for pursuing the goal of enhancing early child–parent relationships. Attachment theory and research have generated important findings concerning early child development and spurred the creation of programs to support early child–parent relationships (Berlin, Ziv, Amaya-Jackson, & Greenberg, 2005; Oppenheim & Goldsmith,

2007). Although best known as the originator of attachment theory, Bowlby (1969/1982) was also a practicing psychiatrist and psychoanalyst. Attachment theory and many of the programs it has spawned bear the unmistakable imprint of the object relations approach to psychoanalysis that was the prevailing clinical *Zeitgeist* of Bowlby's era.

In the past 20 years, prevention and intervention programs grounded in attachment theory and research and explicitly focusing on supporting attachment security have proliferated. In this chapter, we review these programs and their contributions to theory, research, practice, and policy. We begin with a discussion of the implications of attachment theory and research for prevention and intervention programs. We then discuss a number of promising prevention and intervention programs for supporting early attachment security, including public health and criminal justice programs that have incorporated attachment assessments and attachment-focused treatments. We conclude with several suggestions for developing the next generation of prevention and intervention programs in this area.

745

IMPLICATIONS OF ATTACHMENT THEORY AND RESEARCH FOR PREVENTION AND INTERVENTION

The Attachment "Transmission Model"

Attachment theory and research on the origins of individual differences in child–parent attachment have direct implications for prevention and intervention. van IJzendoorn's (1995) "transmission model" and his identification of a "transmission gap" concisely summarize this theory and research. According to the transmission model, a parent's internal working models of attachment drive parenting behaviors, which in turn influence the quality of the child's attachment to that parent. The parent's internal working models shape parenting behaviors by guiding the parent's interpretations of and responses to the child's needs (Main, 1990). In particular, the parent's sensitive responsiveness to the child's needs is what directly fosters emotional security in the child. Conversely, less supportive parenting is characterized by insensitivity to the child's needs and by partial or inconsistent responsiveness.

Through two meta-analyses, van IJzendoorn (1995; De Wolff & van IJzendoorn, 1997) provided strong support for direct links between (1) parents' internal working models and their sensitive parenting behaviors, (2) parents' internal working models and their children's attachment to them, and (3) sensitive parenting behaviors and child attachment. Sensitive parenting behaviors, however, accounted for a relatively small proportion of the association between parental internal working models and child attachment (van IJzendoorn, 1995). Thus sensitive parenting, at least as typically measured, does not appear to be the principal mediator of the effects of parental working models on child attachment. This "transmission gap" has since been replicated in several other investigations (for reviews, see Atkinson et al., 2000, 2005; Madigan, Bakermans-Kranenburg, et al., 2006).

Studies in several new areas of attachment research are helping to elucidate the processes underlying the development of individual differences in attachment. To the extent that they help close the transmission gap, they also yield implications for prevention and intervention. The first area of research expands conceptualizations of adults' internal working models to include "reflective functioning" and "insightfulness." These two concepts refer to the ways in which parents think about their children's behaviors and emotions. Reflective functioning focuses on "the parent's capacity to reflect on her own and her child's internal mental experience" (Slade, 2005, p. 269). Insightfulness is described as "the capacity to see things from the child's point of view" (Oppenheim & Koren-Karie, 2002, p. 599), which involves an appreciation of the "emotional needs underlying the child's behavior" (Oppenheim, Goldsmith, & Koren-Karie, 2004, p. 354). There is initial evidence that reflective functioning examined in a parent interview relates to adult state of mind with respect to attachment, parenting behaviors, and child attachment (Slade, Grienenberger, Bernbach, Levy, & Locker, 2005). Similarly, maternal insightfulness has been found to relate to mothers' sensitive parenting behaviors and to their infants' attachment to them (Koren-Karie, Oppenheim, Dolev, Sher, & Etzion-Carasso, 2002).

A second relatively new area of inquiry concerns specific types of insensitive parenting behaviors, rather than the absence of parental sensitivity per se. For example, Lyons-Ruth and her colleagues assess several kinds of disrupted affective communications in mothers' interactions with their infants during the Strange Situation procedure (Lyons-Ruth, Bronfman, & Parsons, 1999). These maternal behaviors, which include withdrawal, negative intrusiveness, role confusion, disorientation, and conflicting cues, are viewed as stemming from mothers' insecure internal working models and difficulties in managing their own stress in the face of their infants' arousal during the Strange Situation. Several studies have supported this view by illustrating relations between mothers' disrupted communications and their internal working models ("states of mind with respect to attachment," identified with the Adult Attachment Interview [AAI]) and/or infant attachment quality (e.g., Goldberg, Benoit, Blokland, & Madigan, 2003; Grienenberger, Kelly, & Slade, 2005; Lyons-Ruth, Yellin, Melnick, & Atwood, 2005). There is also some evidence that mothers' insensitive parenting behaviors can mediate associations between maternal state of mind and infant attachment quality, especially in high-risk samples (Bailey, Moran, Pederson, & Bento, 2007; Lyons-Ruth et al., 2005; Madigan, Moran, & Pederson, 2006).

A third new area of attachment research examines gene–environment interactions, drawing on theorizing by Belsky (2005) and Rutter (2006) about the possibility that all children are not equally susceptible to rearing influences (e.g., to their parents' internal working models and/or parenting behaviors). For example, a recent study found that mothers' unresolved loss or trauma predicted infant attachment disorganization only in the presence of a specific genetic polymorphism (the dopamine D4 receptor [DRD4] 7-repeat allele; van IJzendoorn & Bakermans-Kranenburg, 2006). This striking finding, though awaiting replication, suggests that genetic variation may be one source of differential susceptibility to rearing influence. By extension, one reason for the transmission gap may be that the transmission model is more relevant to some children than others. Furthermore, the implications of the transmission model for attachment programs may be more relevant to some children than to others.

In sum, the transmission model highlights parents' internal working models and parenting behaviors as the principal drivers of child–parent attachment quality. The mechanisms through which parents' working models affect child–parent attachment are not well understood, however. Recent research that may help to close the transmission gap highlights parents' reflective capacity, or insightfulness, and their insensitivity/dysregulation. In addition, recent gene–environment research suggests that because of genetically based differential susceptibility to rearing influence, the transmission model and its implications for prevention and intervention may not be equally relevant to all children. These theoretical and empirical advances are reflected in the attachment programs we review and in our suggestions for developing future attachment programs.

Three Therapeutic Tasks

In 1988, Bowlby published a collection of lectures instructing clinical practitioners in conceptualizing and treating child and family disorders according to attachment theory and research. Considering his instructions along with research on the transmission model leads us to suggest that prevention and intervention programs for supporting early attachment security focus on three therapeutic tasks (see also Berlin, 2005). The first two tasks concern intervention targets: (1) the parent's internal working models and (2) parenting behaviors. The parent's rather than the child's working models and behaviors are the proposed foci of intervention, because the latter are so responsive to the former. That is, if changes in the parent's behavior and subjective experience of the child can be sustained, then changes in the child's behavior and working models should follow. The third task concerns the intervention process. We argue that the parent's relationship with the intervener serves as the engine of therapeutic change.

With respect to the first task, targeting the parent's internal working models means helping the parent (usually the mother) gain insight into her working models of self and others, especially in intimate and emotionally charged contexts. The intervener can help the parent examine how these working models affect her interactions with her child, as well as the extent to which they are accurate and helpful in achieving parenting goals. Bowlby (1988) argued that this insight often comes through discussion of the parent's early family relationships, current close relationships, and the influences of early relationships on current ones. In particular, the intervener can help the parent understand the extent to which strategies developed in early relationships may undermine current ones.

Slade and her colleagues have further argued that helping parents gain insight depends on the parents' capacity for reflection, and that reflective functioning itself can be an intervention target (Slade, Sadler, & Mayes, 2005). In Slade and Sadler's Minding the Baby program (to be described later in this chapter), home visitors continually describe and link the child's behaviors and mental states—such as noting, "[Your baby] keeps looking around, I'll bet he's wanting to know where you are" (Slade et al., 2005, p. 160). In so doing, home visitors not only model a reflective stance, but also frame infant behaviors in terms of normal attachment needs for attention and support from the parent. This framing can in turn challenge a parent's insecure working models. For example, a father who thinks that an infant who cries when he leaves the room is "bad" or manipulative may consider the alternative that his baby simply missed him. A mother who is irritated by a toddler who wants to eat off her plate and try on her best shoes may consider that instead of being greedy and selfish, her daughter adores her and wants to be just like her mother.

With respect to the second therapeutic task, although many parenting programs exist, targeting parenting behaviors according to attachment theory and research means helping the parent to interpret accurately her child's needs for both comfort and exploration, and to respond contingently. The intervener can teach the parent about the many ways in which children express their needs, and the extent to which specific parenting behaviors satisfy as well as thwart these needs. As demonstrated by the Circle of Security program (Cooper, Hoffman, Powell, & Marvin, 2005; Hoffman, Marvin, Cooper, & Powell, 2006), it can be especially useful to teach parents basic attachment theory. This program (described later in this chapter) presents a parent's two principal parenting tasks as (1) providing closeness in response to the child's attachment needs and (2) facilitating autonomy in response to the child's need to explore. Most important is the balancing of comforting and facilitating exploration in response to the child's needs. In addition, as discussed earlier, the work of Lyons-Ruth and her colleagues highlights the importance of parents' own emotion regulation. The Circle of Security program focuses on building parents' emotion regulation skills, especially in response to children's distress. As both parental and child regulation improve, a child learns not only that difficult feelings *can* be resolved, but also that his or her parent is there to help.

With respect to the third therapeutic task, according to Bowlby and others, success in addressing parental internal working models and parenting behaviors depends on the quality of the relationship between the intervener and the parent. Especially important is the extent to which the intervener serves as a "secure base" from which the parent can mentally explore herself and her relationship with her child (Bowlby, 1988). Bowlby (1980, 1988) purported that new attachments are one of the factors most likely to alter internal working models. Thus a secure attachment to an intervener should facilitate a parent's insights into her own history and her attempts at new parenting behaviors. As noted by Lieberman and her colleagues, the intervener can also serve as a model of supportive behavior (Lieberman, 1991; Lieberman, Silverman, & Pawl, 2000). In the intervener's care, "parents learn, often for the first time, ways of relating that are characterized by mutuality and caring" (Lieberman & Zeanah, 1999, p. 558).

In sum, we propose that prevention and intervention programs for early attachment security establish supportive relationships between interveners and parents that help the parents examine (1) their internal working models and (2) their actual parenting behaviors. Depending on the approach of a particular prevention or intervention program, the distinction between targeting internal working models and targeting parenting behaviors may quickly blur. In addition, success in one task can quickly inform another. For example, the sense of accomplishment that a parent may gain from observing how changes in her own parenting behavior lead to changes in her child's behavior toward her may provide a powerful lever for reworking insecure working models about the child and the self (Lieberman, Ippen, & Van Horn, 2006). We also recognize that one "size" does not fit all, and that different approaches and services will be differentially helpful to different families. As the field of attachment programs grows, the question of "What works for whom?" remains key.

PROMISING PREVENTION AND INTERVENTION PROGRAMS

Since the late 1980s, prevention and intervention programs designed to support early attachment security have proliferated. Despite, or perhaps because of, this proliferation, a unified sense of the field has been difficult to achieve. In 2000, Egeland and his colleagues reviewed 15 attachment programs and suggested that such programs must address internal working models and parenting behaviors through "lengthy, intensive, and carefully timed" services (Egeland, Weinfield, Bosquet, & Cheng, 2000, p. 70). In short, they argued that "more is better" (Egeland et al., 2000, p. 79), especially for multiple-risk families. This conclusion contrasts sharply with the title of a 2003 meta-analysis of attachment programs, "Less Is More" (Bakermans-Kranenburg, van IJzendoorn, & Juffer, 2003). Bakermans-Kranenburg and her colleagues conducted a meta-analysis of 29 studies including 1,503 participants. The authors concluded that "less broad interventions that only focus on sensitive maternal behavior appear rather successful in improving insensitive parenting as well as infant attachment insecurity" (Bakermans-Kranenburg et al., 2003, p. 208). A 2005 meta-analysis focusing on the prevention of disorganized attachment led these authors to a similar conclusion—namely, that interventions focusing on maternal sensitivity are more effective than interventions that also provide support and target parents' working models (Bakermans-Kranenburg, van IJzendoorn, & Juffer, 2005).

In part to reconcile these disparate views, Berlin (2005) reviewed a subset of the programs examined by Egeland and his colleagues (2000) and Bakermans-Kranenburg and her colleagues (2003). All of the programs reviewed were published and evaluated through randomized trials. Berlin concluded that when focusing on attachment security as an outcome, the field has been moderately successful. When defining success as improving either attachment quality or maternal sensitivity, however, the field has been highly successful. This contrast highlights the need for clearly defined goals and criteria for success for attachment programs—an issue that we discuss later in this chapter. With respect to whether "more" or "less" intense services are better, both Berlin (2005) and Greenberg (2005) argue that both can be true, because "less is more" for some families, whereas "more is better" for others.

Since 2005, the development and evaluation of attachment programs has progressed rapidly. Empirical support has emerged for five intensive attachment programs. Three of these programs are both long-lasting (at least 1 year long) and comprehensive in scope, targeting parents' internal working models and parenting behaviors through supportive relationships between parents and interveners: Child–Parent Psychotherapy (CPP), the UCLA Family Development Project, and Minding the Baby (MTB). Two of the programs are briefer (10 or 20 weeks long), although also intensive: the Circle of Security (COS) and Attachment and Biobehavioral Catch-Up (ABC). Empirical support has also emerged for a cadre of very brief (three- or four-session) and narrowly focused programs, all developed at Leiden University in the Netherlands. We review all of these programs and their evaluation findings. Unless otherwise noted, evidence of program effects on infant–parent attachment refer to findings based on Strange Situation classifications. We also describe several initiatives devoted to supporting early attachment security within the context of public health or criminal justice programs.

Child–Parent Psychotherapy

CPP is a dyadic intervention based on "infant–parent psychotherapy," Fraiberg's (1980) psychoanalytic approach to treating disturbances in infant–parent relationships during the first 3 years of life. The premise of Fraiberg's model is that such disturbances are the manifestation in the present of unresolved conflicts between one or both parents and important figures from their own childhoods. Fraiberg described these families as haunted by "old 'ghosts' that have invaded the nursery" (p. 61). In infant–parent psychotherapy, the "patient" is the infant–parent relationship. The principal goals are to (1) help the parent come to grips with the pain, fear, anger, and helplessness evoked by difficult childhood experiences; and (2) help the parent connect these experiences to feelings of ambivalence, anger, rejection, and fear toward her own infant. The therapist's empathic understanding is considered the essential ingredient in giving

the parent the courage to explore herself and to test new parenting behaviors.

Lieberman and her colleagues expanded the infant–parent psychotherapy model into CPP, a manualized intervention that has been delivered primarily to impoverished and traumatized families with children younger than 5 years of age (Lieberman & Van Horn, 2005). CPP retains the emphasis on the links between the parents' early childhood experiences and their current feelings, perceptions, and behaviors toward their infants. It adds a focus on the parents' current stressful life circumstances and on the parents' culturally derived values. CPP interveners are master's-level and pre- and postdoctoral therapists. The sessions involve both the parent and the child, and take place either in the home or in an office playroom. Sessions are unstructured, with the themes largely determined by the parent and by the unfolding interactions between the parent and child.

Five randomized trials have supported the efficacy of CPP. In the first, Lieberman and her colleagues randomly assigned 59 insecurely attached 1-year-olds from low-income, newly immigrated families to 1 year of weekly, 90-minute home-based CPP or to a control group (Lieberman, Weston, & Pawl, 1991). At age 2, although there were no significant differences in intervener-rated attachment security according to the Attachment Q-Sort (AQS), there were significant differences between the CPP and control groups in observed maternal empathy; dyadic goal-corrected partnership; and children's avoidance, resistance, and anger toward their mothers, with all differences favoring the intervention group. Moreover, in the CPP group, a rating of the "level of therapeutic process," based on case reviews conducted by the intervener and her supervisor, predicted attachment security; maternal empathy, initiation, and involvement; dyadic goal-corrected partnership; and children's (lower) avoidance.

CPP has also been successful in fostering attachment security in infants and preschoolers from maltreating families (Cicchetti, Rogosch, & Toth, 2006; Toth, Maughan, Manly, Spagnola, & Cicchetti, 2002). One study included 137 infants either known to be maltreated or living in maltreating families with their biological mothers. Those who received CPP between 12 and 24 months were significantly more likely to be securely attached at 26 months than control infants. The CPP infants were as likely to be secure as those who had received a home-based, didactic, psychoeducational parenting intervention (Cicchetti et al., 2006).

There were not significant changes in maternal sensitivity in either intervention group.

Another study applied a similar design to 87 maltreated preschoolers (Toth et al., 2002). Those who received CPP during their fourth year showed a significantly greater decline in negative self-representations than either the control children or those who had received the didactic parenting intervention. Thus, interestingly, CPP was as efficacious in fostering attachment security as the didactic intervention during infancy, whereas CPP seemed to offer an advantage over the didactic intervention during the preschool years. By the preschool years, the authors speculate, children's working models may be harder to change and may thus require more intensive treatment to do so.

Weekly CPP for an average of approximately 1 year has also been successful in fostering attachment security in toddlers of depressed mothers (Cicchetti, Toth, & Rogosch, 1999; Toth, Rogosch, Manly, & Cicchetti, 2006). Among the same children, CPP also promoted cognitive development, according to IQ tests at age 3 (Cicchetti, Rogosch, & Toth, 2000). None of these studies found effects of CPP on maternal depression. Similarly, there was no evidence of maternal depression during CPP participation moderating any intervention effects.

Among 75 preschool-age children exposed to marital violence, those who received weekly CPP for 1 year, compared to case management plus community treatment as usual, showed a reduction in mother-reported behavior problems and traumatic stress symptoms (Lieberman, Van Horn, & Ippen, 2005). The children were also significantly less likely to meet criteria for a diagnosis of posttraumatic stress disorder (PTSD), and their mothers reported significantly fewer symptoms of PTSD-related avoidance (Lieberman et al., 2005).

A follow-up study reexamining 50 of these dyads 6 months after the intervention ended showed that significant reductions in the CPP group were maintained for children's behavior problems—a finding confirmed by rigorous intent-to-treat analyses with all participants. In addition, analyses of the 50 follow-up participants only revealed significant fewer self-reported psychiatric symptoms among mothers in the CPP group (Lieberman et al., 2006). This finding is notable because CPP does not focus on maternal mental health per se, and because 73% of the mothers in the control group reported that they *had* received individual psychotherapy. This finding thus suggests that the therapeutic focus on the mother–child relationship contributed to better maternal mental health—perhaps, the authors speculate, through the CPP therapists' specific attention to helping the mothers and their children create a joint narrative of their shared trauma, and/or through the mothers' increased satisfaction with their children's (improved) functioning.

UCLA Family Development Project

Heinicke and his colleagues have designed and evaluated the UCLA Family Development Project, a randomized trial with 64 high-risk pregnant women and their firstborn infants (Heinicke et al., 1999, 2000, 2006; Heinicke, Fineman, Ponce, & Guthrie, 2001). The intervention consisted of weekly home visits by master's-level interveners from the second trimester of pregnancy through the infant's first year, followed by biweekly home visits during the second year. There were also weekly mother–infant groups from 3 to 15 months. The control condition consisted of developmental evaluations with feedback and referrals. The therapeutic foci of the program were a mother's relationships—with the intervener, her family of origin, her partner, and her child. The relationship between the intervener and mother was viewed as the driving mechanism of the intervention.

Findings to date have been wide-ranging and supportive of program efficacy. Program infants were significantly more likely to be securely attached than control infants. At 24 months, program toddlers were significantly more compliant than control toddlers. At both 12 and 24 months, program mothers were observed to be more responsive and encouraging of autonomy, less intrusive, and less punitive. Unlike the effects of CPP, there were no significant effects of the UCLA program on children's cognitive development. Similar to CPP, however, the UCLA program provides tentative support for the role of the intervener–mother relationship in driving this program's positive outcomes. Interveners' ratings of each mother's "ability to work with the intervener" were related significantly to maternal responsiveness and child attachment security (Heinicke et al., 2001). Potential bias in interveners' ratings of their own work suggests that this finding should be interpreted with caution, however. Interestingly, program effects persisted for the 24-month outcomes, even above and beyond the positive effects of mothers' own prenatal adult attachment classifications (Heinicke et al., 2006). The small sample sizes in the UCLA studies make replication of these findings especially important.

Minding the Baby

MTB is a home visiting program serving first-time, very-high-risk mothers, 80% of whom reported a history of abuse at enrollment (Slade et al., 2005, 2007). The intervention consists of weekly home visits provided by one of two interveners (a pediatric nurse-practitioner or a clinical social worker) on an alternating basis. Both interveners aim to serve as a secure base for the parent. Weekly home visits begin during pregnancy and continue through the infant's first year. Biweekly visits are conducted throughout the infant's second year. The manualized intervention addresses mothers' internal working models and parenting behaviors, with a specific and novel emphasis on building mothers' reflective functioning. Preliminary (unpublished) analyses of 60 families randomly assigned to receive MTB services as opposed to routine prenatal and primary care have focused on program participants only (Slade et al., 2007). These analyses indicate significant increases in mothers' reflective functioning between pregnancy and 18 months, and a 76% rate of attachment security at 12 months—a rate typically observed in low-risk samples.

Attachment and Biobehavioral Catch-Up

Developed by Dozier and her colleagues, ABC is a brief home visiting program for foster parents and their foster infants and toddlers (Dozier, Lindheim, & Ackerman, 2005). Master's-level social workers provide 10 weekly 1-hour home visits organized according to three themes. The first of these themes is that infants in foster care often appear rejecting of care; the second is that caregivers' own histories may interfere with their providing nurturing care; and the third is that infants in foster care need special help with self-regulation. These themes are woven into four didactic modules, emphasizing the importance of (1) caregiver/parental nurturance, (2) following the child's lead, (3) "overriding" one's own history and/or non-nurturing instincts, and (4) nonthreatening caregiving. Videotaped interactions between the foster parent and foster child are used throughout. The ABC program also promotes foster parents' com-

fort with their foster children's negative emotions. In addition, there are two home visits that draw heavily on the concept of "shark music," borrowed from the COS program (see below). Interveners use this concept to raise caregivers' awareness of defensive responses to their children that may be based more on caregivers' own histories than on their children's behavior per se. Initially designed for foster infants as a particularly vulnerable group, the ABC program is being adapted and tested by Dozier and her colleagues for use with high-risk birth parents and their infants.

Although the ABC program is brief and does not explicitly target foster parents' internal working models, the program can be viewed as addressing two of the three therapeutic tasks described earlier, by targeting parenting behaviors and foster parents' histories. Moreover, although the relationship between the intervener and the mother is not an explicit component of the ABC program, Dozier emphasizes the interpersonal context in which the intervention occurs; she argues that "it is critical to consider the interaction of what the foster mother and the treatment provider bring to the intervention context" (Dozier & Sepulveda, 2004, p. 372). Furthermore, interveners attend carefully to foster mothers' states of mind with respect to attachment, and tailor their approach accordingly (Dozier & Sepulveda, 2004). Thus the ABC program packs considerable intensity into its 10 sessions.

Findings from two randomized studies offer initial evidence of program efficacy. One preliminary study focused on attachment security in 86 children who had been placed in foster care between birth and 18 months of age (Dozier, Peloso, Zirkel, & Lindheim, 2007). Preliminary (unpublished) analyses indicated that, compared to the control foster infants, ABC infants were significantly more likely to be securely attached to their foster mothers. Moreover, 60% of the infants in the ABC group were securely attached—a rate typically observed in much lower-risk populations. A second study focused on cortisol production (a key index of stress regulation, which often reaches atypical levels in traumatized children) in 60 foster children between the ages of 3 months and 3 years (Dozier et al., 2006). Compared to controls, the ABC children exhibited more normal patterns of morning and evening cortisol production; moreover, this pattern was not significantly different from that observed in a comparison group of 104 children who had never been in foster care.

Circle of Security

Of all of the attachment programs we have examined, the COS is the one most directly derived from attachment theory and research. The COS is a 20-week, group-based program for parents or primary caregivers of infants, toddlers, or preschoolers; it has also been used as a dyadic intervention (Cooper et al., 2005). Highly trained and experienced master's-level therapists deliver the intervention in 75-minute weekly sessions to six to eight parents at a time. The COS begins with two attachment assessments: the Strange Situation and the Circle of Security Interview (COSI), which taps parents' working models of attachment. Strange Situation classifications and parents' responses to the COSI are used to guide individualized treatment. COS treatment focuses on five parental "relationship capacities": (1) understanding of children's relationship needs, (2) observational and inferential skills, (3) reflective functioning, (4) emotion regulation, and (5) empathy (Cooper et al., 2005). The centerpiece of the COS program is the COS graphic, a remarkably simple yet comprehensive pictorial depiction of attachment theory's key constructs about parenting. The COS also focuses on children's needs, cues, and miscues, emphasizing that children sometimes "miscue" their parents about their true needs. In addition, group leaders provide extensive, carefully guided review of videotaped child–parent interactions for each parent in the group. As noted earlier, the COS program uses the concept of "shark music" to help parents think about why specific child behaviors that are not blatantly negative might evoke parental feelings of danger/threat and elicit negative parental responses (i.e., activate a parent's "shark music").

Initial findings from a pre–post study of 65 toddlers and preschoolers offer initial evidence of the program's efficacy (Hoffman et al., 2006). The children were recruited from Head Start and Early Head Start programs and identified by program staff as (1) regular participants in the program and (2) neither low- nor high-functioning compared to other families in the program. It is important to note that this recruitment strategy may have resulted in a particularly motivated group of parents. All of the participants were from low-income families, and most of the parents reported that they had experienced childhood maltreatment or trauma. Comparisons of pre- and postintervention Strange Situation classifications revealed significant decreases in both disorganized classifications

in particular and insecure classifications in general. Whereas 80% of the children were classified as insecure at baseline, 46% of the children were classified as insecure after the intervention (54% were classified as secure). This study's small sample size and pre–post design makes replication of these findings—particularly in the context of a randomized trial—especially important. Meanwhile, as will be discussed later (see "Public Health and Criminal Justice Programs"), the COS has also shown initial promise as a supplemental treatment in a jail diversion program for pregnant women.

The Leiden Programs

van den Boom's "Skill-Based Treatment"

van den Boom (1994, 1995) developed the first of a Dutch cadre of very brief attachment programs. She herself (a professor of developmental and educational psychology) delivered three home visits to low-income mothers and their 6- to 9-month-old temperamentally irritable infants. Lasting about 2 hours apiece, the home visits focused on mothers' sensitive responsiveness to their infants' cues. Findings from a randomized trial of 100 infant–mother pairs were wide-ranging and impressive (van den Boom, 1994, 1995). For example, when infants were 9 months old, program mothers were significantly more responsive, stimulating, and visually attentive. When infants were 12 and 18 months old, program children were significantly more likely to be securely attached than control children. When the infants were 18, 24, and 42 months old, program mothers continued to demonstrate significantly more sensitivity and responsiveness than control mothers. At 42 months, program children received comparable scores on an observer-rated AQS to those of control children, but were significantly more likely than control children to interact harmoniously with an unfamiliar peer. Finally, 12-month attachment mediated the program's effect on some maternal behaviors and on children's peer interactions (van den Boom, 1995).

Video-Feedback Intervention to Promote Positive Parenting

Juffer, Bakermans-Kranenburg, van IJzendoorn, and their colleagues have developed and evaluated several versions of Video-Feedback Intervention to Promote Positive Parenting (VIPP; Juffer, Bakermans-Kranenburg, & van IJzendoorn, 2007). VIPP is delivered in four home visits to parents of infants less than 1 year old by pre-master's-level through doctoral-level interveners. VIPP home visits last approximately 90 minutes and focus on promoting maternal sensitivity through interveners' presentation of written materials and review of in-home, videotaped infant–parent interactions. An expanded version, VIPP-R, provides 3-hour home visits that add a component focusing on parents' internal working models through discussion of the parents' childhood attachment experiences.

Findings are supportive of program efficacy, if somewhat mixed. A recent study focused on 81 first-time mothers tentatively classified as having insecure states of mind with respect to attachment, according to review of these mothers' pre-intervention AAI audiotapes (Klein Velderman, Bakermans-Kranenburg, Juffer, & van IJzendoorn, 2006). Mothers were randomly assigned to VIPP, VIPP-R, or a control group. VIPP and VIPP-R mothers received home visits between their infants' 7th and 10th months. When their infants were 11 and 13 months old, mothers who received either VIPP or VIPP-R were rated as significantly more sensitive than control mothers. There were no significant differences, however, in infant–mother attachment at 13 months. In no case were there differential effects of VIPP and VIPP-R. Interestingly, paralleling van den Boom's studies of irritable infants, mothers of "highly reactive" infants derived most benefit from the interventions, showing significantly greater increases in sensitivity from pre- to postintervention.

In a follow-up study conducted when these children were of preschool age, only children who had received VIPP during infancy (and not VIPP-R) were less likely to meet clinical criteria for externalizing behavior problems (Klein Velderman, Bakermans-Kranenburg, Juffer, van IJzendoorn, et al., 2006). These effects were not mediated by earlier maternal sensitivity. In addition, there were no program effects on maternal sensitivity or observer-rated AQS scores at this time; nor was there any evidence of moderation of program effects by infant reactivity.

Another randomized trial examined 130 adoptive parents with and without birth children. Among the adoptive parents without birth children, only those who had participated in VIPP-R (and not VIPP) evinced greater maternal sensitivity and a higher proportion of securely attached infants compared to the control group (Juffer, Hoksbergen, Riksen-Walraven, & Kohnstamm, 1997). Among the adoptive parents with birth children,

there were positive effects of VIPP-R on maternal sensitivity but not infant attachment (Juffer, Rosenboom, Hoksbergen, Riksen-Walraven, & Kohnstamm, 1997), and positive long-term effects on behavior problems at age 7 (Stams, Juffer, van IJzendoorn, & Hoksbergen, 2001). In recent analyses of both groups of adoptive parents combined, only those who had received VIPP-R (and not VIPP) were significantly less likely to have infants classified as insecure-disorganized than those in the control group (Juffer, Bakermans-Kranenburg, & van IJzendoorn, 2005).

VIPP-SD, a version of VIPP emphasizing sensitive disciplinary practices for children showing early signs of externalizing problems, has been developed recently (Mesman et al., 2007). In a randomized trial of 237 families included on the basis of their 1- to 3-year-old children's high scores for externalizing behaviors, program mothers exhibited significantly more sensitive disciplinary attitudes and behaviors 1 year after completing treatment than control mothers did (van Zeijl et al., 2006). More recently, VIPP-SD has been shown to have stronger effects on child cortisol production and externalizing behavior for children with a specific genetic polymorphism (the DRD4 7-repeat allele; Bakermans-Kranenburg, van IJzendoorn, Mesman, Alink, & Juffer, in press; Bakermans-Kranenburg, van IJzendoorn, Pijlman, Mesman, & Juffer, in press).

Thus the various versions of VIPP show promise. VIPP-R increases intensity by adding a component focusing on parents' internal working models. In Klein Velderman's studies, however, VIPP-R did not show significantly greater efficacy than VIPP (Klein Velderman, Bakermans-Kranenburg, Juffer, & van IJzendoorn, 2006; Klein Velderman, Bakermans-Kranenburg, Juffer, van IJzendoorn, et al., 2006). In the follow-up study, in fact, it was only the less intensive version (VIPP) that fostered longer-term effects (Klein Velderman, Bakermans-Kranenburg, Juffer, van IJzendoorn, et al., 2006). For these families, the less intensive approach appears to have been more helpful, at least in terms of children's externalizing disorders. In contrast, among adoptive families, only the more intensive version (VIPP-R) predicted attachment organization/disorganization.

Summary

The field of attachment intervention has matured significantly in the recent past. Several programs have now rigorously demonstrated success in supporting early attachment security and in positively affecting other important outcomes, including children's neuroendocrine regulation (according to cortisol levels), IQ scores, and behavior problems. Both more and less intensive programs have demonstrated promise. With the exception of Dozier's ABC program for foster parents, the more intensive programs have typically served high-risk, multiproblem families. And whereas some of these programs targeted participants such as low-income parents with irritable infants or (tentatively classified) parents with insecure internal working models, the less intensive Leiden programs typically served lower-risk families. In addition, the positive effects of the Leiden programs were concentrated among families with irritable or highly reactive infants and/or those with specific genetic polymorphisms such as the DRD4 7-repeat allele. Supporting Belsky's (2005) and Rutter's (2006) hypotheses, these findings suggest that some infants are more susceptible to intervention, and that such susceptibility is temperamentally and/or genetically based. These population differences and moderated effects may explain how both more and less intensive programs have produced measurable effects. Further examination of "what works for whom" should prove valuable. For example, researchers could examine the extent to which a less intensive program such as VIPP is adequate for high-risk families, or the extent to which infant irritability moderates more intensive programs' effects.

Other issues that call for further investigation are programs' essential "ingredients" and the mechanisms underlying program success. Interestingly, two VIPP studies have examined but found no evidence for maternal sensitivity as a mediator of program effects (Bakermans-Kranenburg, van IJzendoorn, Mesman, et al., in press; Klein Velderman, Bakermans-Kranenburg, Juffer, van IJzendoorn, et al., 2006). Bakermans-Kranenburg and her colleagues have speculated that the key ingredient in the VIPP programs is the use of video feedback (i.e., showing parents videotaped interactions of themselves and their children) (Bakermans-Kranenburg, van IJzendoorn, Mesman, et al., in press). Describing the child as becoming a "co-intervener," they state, "Video feedback intervention stimulates the parent to have an eye for the feedback from the child. ... When the parent begins to see the grateful smile on the [child's] face ... as a reaction to sensitive parenting, the child takes the intervener's place. ... The process of feedback may continue after the inter-

vener leaves the home" (Bakermans-Kranenburg, van IJzendoorn, Mesman, et al., in press). Notably, all of the short-term attachment programs reviewed in this chapter (VIPP, ABC, and COS) include video feedback procedures.

van IJzendoorn and Bakermans-Kranenburg have also suggested several other reasons why less intensive attachment programs may succeed, including (1) the setting of precisely defined, short-term goals; (2) a good fit between program requirements and the capabilities of typical interveners; and (3) relative ease of adherence to treatment (van IJzendoorn, Bakermans-Kranenburg, & Juffer, 2005). These factors deserve careful investigation. Last, as described earlier, both CPP and the UCLA program have yielded some (albeit tentative) evidence that the quality of the intervener–parent relationship contributes to positive program outcomes (Heinicke et al., 2006; Lieberman et al., 1991). If, how, for whom, and under what circumstances the intervener–parent relationship has positive effects in attachment programs are also important areas for further research—not only for the sake of future program development, but also because of the centrality in attachment theory of the notion of relationships as engines of change.

SUPPORTING EARLY ATTACHMENT SECURITY IN THE CONTEXT OF PUBLIC HEALTH AND CRIMINAL JUSTICE PROGRAMS

In response to the increasing emphasis in both practice and policy on supporting early child development, a number of public programs have sought to integrate attachment-focused assessments and intervention protocols into their services. Here we describe four such efforts: the Tulane Infant Team, the Florida Infant Mental Health Pilot Program, Early Head Start with Parent–Child Communication Coaching, and Tamar's Children.

Tulane Infant Team

In Jefferson Parish, Louisiana, through contracts with the state and private foundations, every child younger than 5 years old who has been maltreated and placed into foster care is referred to a program developed by Zeanah and his colleagues called the Tulane Infant Team (Larrieu & Zeanah, 1998, 2003; Smyke, Wajda-Johnston, & Zeanah, 2004; Zeanah et al., 2001). The program treats 40–80 children per year. To date, more than 250 families have participated. The program is staffed by a multidisciplinary team of faculty members and trainees. It works collaboratively with the legal, child welfare, educational, health, and mental health systems to provide assessment and treatment for these high-risk young children and their foster and biological parents.

Assessments and treatment are heavily informed by attachment theory and research. There are two principal assessments. The first is the "Crowell procedure," a semistructured videotaped observation of a 12- to 60-month-old child interacting with the parent/caregiver, based on the work of Crowell and Feldman (1988). The procedure includes nine episodes designed to elicit key child and parent/caregiver behaviors related to attachment and exploration (e.g., parent/caregiver emotional availability, child security, child curiosity). A similar procedure (the "Baby Crowell") is followed for infants between 6 and 12 months old. For infants younger than 6 months, an infant–parent face-to-face interaction assessment is administered. The Crowell procedure is not used to classify attachment security. Attachment behaviors are carefully noted, however, as are indices of attachment disorganization. These and other behaviors are used to guide treatment.

The second principal assessment is the Working Model of the Child Interview (WMCI; Zeanah & Benoit, 1995), administered to biological parents and foster parents. Derived from the AAI, the WMCI focuses on a parent or caregiver's internal working model of the child and of him- or herself as a parent. The WMCI has been validated in several published studies that have shown it to be stable, to be associated with both parent and child interactive behaviors, and to be meaningfully associated with both risk conditions and clinical status (Benoit, Zeanah, Parker, Nicholson, & Coolbear, 1997; Rosenblum, McDonough, Muzik, Miller, & Sameroff, 2002; Schechter et al., 2005; Zeanah, Benoit, Hirshberg, Barton, & Regan, 1994). Like the AAI, the WMCI includes a formal coding system focusing on qualitative features of the parent's discourse (Zeanah, Larrieu, Heller, & Valliere, 2000). The Tulane Infant Team uses both the formal codes and parents' or caregivers' uncoded responses to guide treatment.

The Infant Team provides simultaneous treatment to the child and foster parent, who must co-construct a new attachment relationship, and to the child and birth parents, with whom the child has disrupted and usually disturbed relationships. Treatment plans are individualized and consist of a variety of interventions, including CPP, COS, and Interaction Guidance, a dyadic psychotherapy developed by McDonough (2004).

Following their placement in foster care, about half of the children treated by the Tulane Infant Team are returned to their parents or relatives, and about half are freed for adoption following voluntary or involuntary termination of parental rights (Zeanah et al., 2001). Although randomized assignment to the intervention is not possible, Zeanah and his colleagues have conducted a study of a 4-year cohort, comparing outcomes for maltreated children in the 4 years following the intervention to the 4 years that immediately preceded the intervention. They found that prior to the intervention, the rate of the same child being maltreated (substantiated for maltreatment) was 13.1%, whereas after the intervention it was 4.2%—a 68% reduction in recidivism. In addition, they found that prior to the intervention, 14.1% of mothers maltreated a subsequent child, but after the intervention, the recidivism rate for a subsequent child was 5.2%—a 75% reduction in maltreatment recidivism for a child born subsequently to the same mother (Zeanah et al., 2001). These findings illustrate the value of using attachment theory, assessments, and treatments as the essential building blocks of services for maltreated young children and their caregivers.

Florida Infant Mental Health Pilot Program

A similar effort exists under the auspices of the Florida Infant Mental Health Pilot Program, a three-site project funded by the Florida state legislature (Osofsky et al., 2007). Participants were 57 mothers with infants or young children (up to age 52 months) who had been investigated or substantiated for child maltreatment. The principal treatment for the mothers and children was CPP. Pre- and posttreatment assessments included the Crowell procedure. During and immediately after 25 treatment sessions, there were no further maltreatment reports on participants. In addition, there were also some positive changes in (four of nine) maternal behaviors and (two of seven) child behaviors coded from the Crowell procedure. This study's small sample size and pre–post design makes replication of these findings—particularly in the context of a randomized trial—especially important.

With partial funding from several Florida state agencies, this project is continuing in one site, now known as the Miami Court Team Model Program. Under the auspices of the national advocacy organization Zero to Three, similar court teams are being established in five other states. And federal legislation (the Safe Babies Act) has recently been introduced to fund a National Court Teams Resource Center, which would create more court teams in other locations.

Early Head Start with Parent–Child Communication Coaching

Another example of a public program integrating attachment-focused assessments and intervention protocol into its services comes from Spieker and her colleagues, who augmented an Early Head Start program with a brief home-based attachment protocol (Spieker, Nelson, DeKlyen, & Staerkel, 2005). Parent–Child Communication Coaching consisted of 33 "steps" in 10 topic areas targeting parents' internal working models, parenting behaviors, and the relationships between parents and their home visitors. Each step included an activity, an informational handout, and "homework." Some activities included the use of videotaped parent–child interactions with feedback. A randomized trial found no significant differences in observed parenting behavior or 19-month Strange Situation classifications between those families who had received Early Head Start with Parent–Child Communication Coaching and control families who had received community services as usual. Spieker and her colleagues attribute this null finding in part to considerable program staff turnover and general difficulties with engaging multiple-risk mothers in sustained participation in the program. Despite this null finding, the work of Spieker and her colleagues represents a very important first step toward understanding the extent to which a theoretically grounded and evidence-based attachment protocol can add value to a widely disseminated, publicly funded program such as Early Head Start.

Tamar's Children

A final notable example of a public program augmenting its services with an attachment protocol comes from Tamar's Children, a pilot program of the Maryland Department of Health and Mental Hygiene and the city of Baltimore. Tamar's Children is a jail diversion program for pregnant women with a history of substance abuse who have become involved in the criminal justice system. A prenatal–early infancy version of the COS, cre-

ated for this program, the COS: *Marycliffe Institute Perinatal/First Year Protocol*, provided by doctoral-level therapists, has been added to the program's other services (e.g., substance abuse treatment, trauma treatment, job training). Preliminary (unpublished) analysis of the first 19 infants to complete 12-month outcome assessments illustrated a 68% rate of secure infant–mother attachment—a rate typically found in low-risk samples (Cassidy et al., 2007).

Summary

These four examples reflect the growing interest and promise in integrating attachment-focused assessments and interventions into public health and criminal justice programs. Such initiatives are extremely important for practice, policy, and research. In terms of practice and policy, Greenberg (2005) notes that transforming new evidence-based interventions into widespread practice requires integrating the interventions into existing systems. The initiatives we have described begin this integration. These initiatives also bring attachment theory- and research-based treatments to publicly funded programs whose goals often mirror those of attachment programs, yet whose services often are not theory- or research-based. For example, in fiscal year 2006, there were over 650 Early Head Start programs serving almost 62,000 children throughout the United States (Administration for Children and Families, 2007). Early Head Start was designed in part by a federal advisory committee recommending that the program focus on supporting infant–parent relationships (U.S. Department of Health and Human Services, 1994). Yet most Early Head Start programs' "attachment" services are not explicitly theory-based, research-based, or implemented or documented in such a way as to allow for rigorous evaluation.

In addition, two separate U.S. federal laws—the Individuals with Disabilities Education Improvement Act and the Child Abuse Prevention and Treatment Act—have recently been amended to mandate that children under 3 with substantiated child abuse or neglect, and children under 5 with substantiated trauma due to exposure to family violence, be referred for public early intervention services. This landmark legislation not only recognizes the urgent mental health needs that child maltreatment and exposure to family violence trigger, but also requires new collaborations among mental health, early education, and child welfare systems to provide early intervention services to young victims of attachment-related traumas. Attachment-focused assessments and treatments can and should facilitate these efforts.

With respect to research, public programs with attachment-focused assessments and intervention protocols offer unprecedented opportunities not only to examine the added value of attachment treatments, but also to examine a wide range of outcomes, both individually and in combination. For example, the Tamar's Children pilot program has demonstrated preliminary success in terms of infant attachment outcomes. This program will also be able to examine its successes in terms of maternal substance abuse and criminal recidivism. Then the extent to which attachment outcomes relate to and possibly mediate other maternal outcomes will also be important to examine.

CONCLUSIONS AND SUGGESTIONS FOR RESEARCH AND PROGRAM DEVELOPMENT

Prevention and intervention programs for supporting early attachment security have made tremendous strides in the past 20 years and especially quite recently. Our suggestions for next steps center on three sets of research questions, which, if answered, could significantly advance the next generation of programs for supporting early attachment security. First, what works for whom? Second, what drives program success? Third, what *is* program success?

With respect to what works for whom, understanding how to tailor intervention components to participating families is important both for initially engaging families and for sustaining their participation in services. It is also important for the allocation of often scarce resources, so that the most intensive services will go to those most likely to benefit from them. Clearly, different services fit some families better than others, depending on characteristics of the program (e.g., more or less intensive), characteristics of the family (e.g., irritable or nonirritable infant), and interactions among these characteristics. One fruitful method for addressing what works for whom may center on rigorously assessing parents' preintervention internal working models and the extent to which they moderate program outcomes. As noted earlier, several attachment programs (e.g., ABC, COS, the Tulane Infant Team) target participants or tailor services on the basis of parents' formally and informally assessed working models. There is also increasing evidence that adult attachment classi-

fications can moderate program engagement (e.g., Spieker et al., 2005) and program outcomes (e.g., Heinicke et al., 2006). Given the central role of parents' internal working models in their children's development, further studies along these lines could be very useful for future program development, especially for broad-based public programs that may have limited resources for directly targeting attachment processes.

With respect to what drives program success, as discussed earlier, practitioners and scholars have speculated on such factors as the use of video feedback, parents' engagement in program services, and the quality of the relationships between parents and interveners. All of these factors merit further study. It would also be interesting to assess program participants' views on what factors make a program more or less helpful to them.

Last, with respect to defining program success, criteria have included (1) preventing or changing the development of insecure attachments; (2) altering parents' internal working models; (3) altering parenting behaviors; (4) altering important childhood outcomes shown to be forecast by attachment security (e.g., social skills, behavior problems); or (5) some combination of the preceding. These criteria need to be more clearly articulated and studied, ideally through longitudinal investigations that include pre- and postintervention assessments of attachment and nonattachment outcomes. Lieberman and Zeanah (1999) noted that "no single investigation to date has simultaneously assessed maternal representations, maternal sensitivity, and infant representations (i.e., [Strange Situation] classifications) before and after intervention" (p. 571). This is still the case. In addition, the extent to which attachment programs have long-term effects on children's development, with or without changes in early child–parent attachments, is another question for future research. Such research will in turn help illuminate the role of early attachments in human development and how best to support them.

ACKNOWLEDGMENTS

Portions of this chapter are based on Berlin (2005). Copyright 2005 by The Guilford Press. Other portions are based on Lieberman and Zeanah (1999). Copyright 1999 by The Guilford Press. Adapted by permission. We thank Naomi Jean-Baptiste for help with manuscript preparation. Lisa Berlin's work was supported by National Institute of Mental Health Grant No. K01MH 70378.

REFERENCES

Administration for Children and Families. (2007, April). *Head Start Program fact sheet: Fiscal year 2007.* Retrieved from *www.acf.dhhs.gov/programs/hsb/research/2007.htm*

Atkinson, L., Goldberg, S., Raval, V., Pederson, D. R., Benoit, D., Moran, G., et al. (2005). On the relation between maternal state of mind and sensitivity in the prediction of infant attachment security. *Developmental Psychology, 41,* 42–53.

Atkinson, L., Niccols, A., Paglia, A., Coolbear, J., Parker, K. C. H., Poulton, L., et al. (2000). A meta-analysis of time between maternal sensitivity and attachment assessments: Implications for internal working models of infancy/toddlerhood. *Journal of Social and Personal Relationships, 17,* 791–810.

Bailey, H. N., Moran, G., Pederson, D. R., & Bento, S. (2007). Understanding the transmission of attachment using variable- and relationship-centered approaches. *Development and Psychopathology, 19,* 313–343.

Bakermans-Kranenburg, M. J., van IJzendoorn, M. H., & Juffer, F. (2003). Less is more: Meta-analyses of sensitivity and attachment interventions in early childhood. *Psychological Bulletin, 129,* 195–215.

Bakermans-Kranenburg, M. J., van IJzendoorn, M. H., & Juffer, F. (2005). Disorganized infant attachment and preventive interventions: A review and meta-analysis. *Infant Mental Health Journal, 26,* 191–216.

Bakermans-Kranenburg, M. J., van IJzendoorn, M. H., Mesman, J., Alink, L. R., & Juffer, F. (in press). Effects of an attachment-based intervention on daily cortisol moderated by DRD4: A randomized control trial on 1-3-year-olds screened for externalizing behavior. *Development and Psychopathology.*

Bakermans-Kranenburg, M. J., van IJzendoorn, M. H., Pijlman, F. T. A., Mesman, J., & Juffer, F. (in press). Experimental evidence for differential susceptibility: Dopamine D4 receptor polymorphism (DRD4 VNTR) moderates intervention effects on toddlers' externalizing behavior in a randomized control trial. *Developmental Psychology.*

Belsky, J. (2005). The developmental and evolutionary psychology of intergenerational transmission of attachment. In C. S. Carter, L. Ahnert, K. E. Grossmann, S. B. Hrdy, M. E. Lamb, S. W. Porges, et al. (Eds.), *Attachment and bonding: A new synthesis* (pp. 169–198). Cambridge, MA: MIT Press.

Benoit, D., Zeanah, C. H., Parker, K. C. H., Nicholson, E., & Coolbear, J. (1997). Working Model of the Child Interview: Related to clinical status of infants. *Infant Mental Health Journal, 18,* 107–121.

Berlin, L. (2005). Interventions to enhance early attachments: The state of the field today. In L. J. Berlin, Y. Ziv, L. Amaya-Jackson, & M. T. Greenberg (Eds.), *Enhancing early attachments: Theory, research, intervention, and policy* (pp. 3–33). New York: Guilford Press.

Berlin, L. J., Ziv, Y., Amaya-Jackson, L., & Greenberg,

M. T. (Eds.). (2005). *Enhancing early attachments: Theory, research, intervention, and policy.* New York: Guilford Press.

Bowlby, J. (1969/1982). *Attachment and loss: Vol. 1. Attachment.* New York: Basic Books.

Bowlby, J. (1980). *Attachment and loss: Vol. 3. Loss: Sadness and depression.* New York: Basic Books.

Bowlby, J. (1988). *A secure base.* New York: Basic Books.

Cassidy, J., Ziv, Y., Cooper, G., Hoffman, K., Powell, B., & Karfgin, A. (2007). Enhancing attachment security in the infants of women in a jail-diversion program. In J. A. Poehlmann (Chair), *Incarcerated mothers, their children, and families: Attachment and parenting.* Symposium conducted at the biennial meeting of the Society for Research in Child Development, Boston.

Cicchetti, D., Rogosch, F. A., & Toth, S. L. (2000). The efficacy of toddler–parent psychotherapy for fostering cognitive development in offspring of depressed mothers. *Journal of Abnormal Child Psychology, 28,* 135–148.

Cicchetti, D., Rogosch, F. A., & Toth, S. L. (2006). Fostering secure attachment in infants in maltreating families through preventive interventions. *Development and Psychopathology, 18,* 623–649.

Cicchetti, D., Toth, S. L., & Rogosch, F. A. (1999). The efficacy of toddler–parent psychotherapy to increase attachment security in offspring of depressed mothers. *Attachment and Human Development, 1,* 34–66.

Cooper, G., Hoffman, K., Powell, B., & Marvin, R. (2005). The Circle of Security intervention: Differential diagnosis and differential treatment. In L. J. Berlin, Y. Ziv, L. M. Amaya-Jackson, & M. T. Greenberg (Eds.), *Enhancing early attachments: Theory, research, intervention, and policy* (pp. 127–151). New York: Guilford Press.

Crowell, J. A., & Feldman, S. S. (1988). Mothers' internal models of relationships and children's behavioral and developmental status: A study of mother–child interaction. *Child Development, 59,* 1273–1285.

De Wolff, M. S., & van IJzendoorn, M. H. (1997). Sensitivity and attachment: A meta-analysis on parental antecedents of infant attachment. *Child Development, 68,* 571–591.

Dozier, M., Lindhiem, O., & Ackerman, J. P. (2005). Attachment and Biobehavioral Catch-up. In L. J. Berlin, Y. Ziv, L. Amaya-Jackson, & M. T. Greenberg (Eds.), *Enhancing early attachments: Theory, research, intervention, and policy* (pp. 178–194). New York: Guilford Press.

Dozier, M., Peloso, E., Lindhiem, O., Gordon, M. K., Manni, M., Sepulveda, S., et al. (2006). Developing evidence-based interventions for foster children: An example of a randomized clinical trial with infants and toddlers. *Journal of Social Issues, 62,* 767–785.

Dozier, M., Peloso, E., Zirkel, S., & Lindheim, O. J. (2007). Intervention effects on foster infants' attachments to new caregivers. In L. J. Berlin (Chair), *Interventions to support early attachments: New findings.*

Symposium conducted at the biennial meeting of the Society for Research in Child Development, Boston.

Dozier, M., & Sepulveda, S. (2004). Foster mother state of mind and treatment use: Different challenges for different people. *Infant Mental Health Journal, 25,* 368–378.

Egeland, B., Weinfield, N. S., Bosquet, M., & Cheng, V. K. (2000). Remember, repeating, and working through: Lessons from attachment-based interventions. In J. Osofsky & H. E. Fitzgerald (Eds.), *WAIMH handbook of infant mental health* (Vol. 4, pp. 35–89). New York: Wiley.

Fraiberg, S. (1980). *Clinical studies in infant mental health: The first year of life.* New York: Basic Books.

Goldberg, S., Benoit, D., Blokland, K., & Madigan, S. (2003). Atypical maternal behavior, maternal representations, and infant disorganized attachment. *Development and Psychopathology, 15,* 239–257.

Greenberg, M. T. (1999). Attachment and psychopathology in childhood. In J. Cassidy & P. R. Shaver (Eds.), *Handbook of attachment: Theory, research, and clinical applications* (pp. 469–496). New York: Guilford Press.

Greenberg, M. T. (2005). Enhancing early attachments: Synthesis and recommendations for research, practice, and policy. In L. J. Berlin, Y. Ziv, L. Amaya-Jackson, & M. T. Greenberg (Eds.), *Enhancing early attachments: Theory, research, intervention, and policy* (pp. 327–343). New York: Guilford Press.

Grienenberger, J., Kelly, K., & Slade, A. (2005). Maternal reflective functioning, mother–infant affective communication, and infant attachment: Exploring the link between mental states and observed caregiving behavior in the intergenerational transmission of attachment. *Attachment and Human Development, 7,* 299–311.

Heinicke, C. M., Fineman, N. R., Ponce, V., & Guthrie, D. (2001). Relation-based intervention with at-risk mothers: Outcome in the second year of life. *Infant Mental Health Journal, 22,* 431–462.

Heinicke, C. M., Fineman, N. R., Ruth, G., Recchia, S. L., Guthrie, D., & Rodning, C. (1999). Relationship-based intervention with at-risk mothers: Outcome in the first year of life. *Infant Mental Health Journal, 20,* 349–374.

Heinicke, C. M., Goorsky, M., Levine, M., Ponce, V., Ruth, G., Silverman, M., et al. (2006). Pre- and postnatal antecedents of a home-visiting intervention and family developmental outcome. *Infant Mental Health Journal, 27,* 91–119.

Heinicke, C. M., Goorsky, M., Moscov, S., Dudley, K., Gordon, J., Schneider, C., et al. (2000). Relationship-based intervention with at-risk mothers: Factors affecting variations in outcome. *Infant Mental Health Journal, 21,* 133–155.

Hoffman, K. T., Marvin, R. S., Cooper, G., & Powell, B. (2006). Changing toddlers' and preschoolers' attachment classifications: The Circle of Security intervention. *Journal of Consulting and Clinical Psychology, 74,* 1017–1026.

Juffer, F., Bakermans-Kranenburg, M. J., & van IJzendoorn, M. H. (2005). The importance of parenting in the development of disorganized attachment: Evidence from a preventive intervention study in adoptive families. *Journal of Child Psychology and Psychiatry, 46,* 263–274.

Juffer, F., Bakermans-Kranenburg, M. J., & van IJzendoorn, M. H. (Eds.). (2007). *Promoting positive parenting: An attachment-based intervention.* Mahwah, NJ: Erlbaum.

Juffer, F., Hoksbergen, R. A. C., Riksen-Walraven, J. M., & Kohnstamm, G. A. (1997). Early intervention in adoptive families: Supporting maternal sensitive responsiveness, infant–mother attachment, and infant competence. *Journal of Child Psychology and Psychiatry, 38,* 1039–1050.

Juffer, F., Rosenboom, L. G., Hoksbergen, R. A. C., Riksen-Walraven, J. M. A., & Kohnstamm, G. A. (1997). Attachment and intervention in adoptive families with and without biological children. In W. Koops, J. B. Hoeksma, & D. C. van den Boom (Eds.), *Development of interaction and attachment: Traditional and non-traditional approaches* (pp. 93–108). Amsterdam: North-Holland.

Klein Velderman, M., Bakermans-Kranenburg, M. J., Juffer, F., & van IJzendoorn, M. H. (2006). Effects of attachment-based interventions on maternal sensitivity and infant attachment: Differential susceptibility of highly reactive infants. *Journal of Family Psychology, 20,* 266–274.

Klein Velderman, M., Bakermans-Kranenburg, M. J., Juffer, F., van IJzendoorn, M. H., Mangelsdorf, S. C., & Zevalkink, J. (2006). Preventing preschool externalizing behavior problems through video-feedback intervention in infancy. *Infant Mental Health Journal, 27,* 466–493.

Koren-Karie, N., Oppenheim, D., Dolev, S., Sher, E., & Etzion-Carasso, A. (2002). Mothers' insightfulness regarding their infants' internal experience: Relations with maternal sensitivity and infant attachment. *Developmental Psychology, 38,* 534–542.

Larrieu, J. A., & Zeanah, C. H. (1998). Intensive intervention for maltreated infants and toddlers in foster care. *Child and Adolescent Psychiatric Clinics of North America, 7,* 357–371.

Larrieu, J. A., & Zeanah, C. H. (2003). Treating parent–infant relationships in the context of maltreatment: An integrated systems approach. In A. J. Sameroff, S. C. McDonough, & K. L. Rosenblum (Eds.), *Treating parent–infant relationship problems: Strategies for intervention* (pp. 243–264). New York: Guilford Press.

Lieberman, A. F. (1991). Attachment theory and infant–parent psychotherapy: Some conceptual, clinical and research issues. In D. Cicchetti & S. Toth (Eds.), *Rochester Symposium on Developmental Psychopathology: Vol. 3. Models and integrations* (pp. 261–288). Hillsdale, NJ: Erlbaum.

Lieberman, A. F., Ippen, C. G., & Van Horn, P. (2006). Child–Parent Psychotherapy: 6-month follow-up of a randomized controlled trial. *Journal of the Ameri-*

can *Academy of Child and Adolescent Psychiatry, 45,* 913–917.

Lieberman, A. F., Silverman, R., & Pawl, J. H. (2000). Infant–parent psychotherapy: Core concepts and current approaches. In C. H. Zeanah (Ed.), *Handbook of infant mental health* (2nd ed., pp. 472–484). New York: Guilford Press.

Lieberman, A. F., & Van Horn, P. (2005). *Don't hit my mommy: A manual for Child–Parent Psychotherapy with young witnesses of family violence.* Washington, DC: Zero to Three Press.

Lieberman, A. F., Van Horn, P., & Ippen, C. G. (2005). Toward evidence-based treatment: Child–Parent Psychotherapy with preschoolers exposed to marital violence. *Journal of the American Academy of Child and Adolescent Psychiatry, 44,* 1241–1248.

Lieberman, A. F., Weston, D. R., & Pawl, J. H. (1991). Preventive intervention and outcome with anxiously attached dyads. *Child Development, 62,* 199–209.

Lieberman, A. F., & Zeanah, C. H. (1999). Contributions of attachment theory to infant–parent psychotherapy and other interventions with infants and young children. In J. Cassidy & P. R. Shaver (Eds.), *Handbook of attachment: Theory, research, and clinical applications* (pp. 555–574). New York: Guilford Press.

Lyons-Ruth, K., Bronfman, E., & Parsons, E. (1999). Maternal frightened, frightening, or atypical behavior and disorganized infant attachment patterns. *Monographs of the Society for Research in Child Development, 64*(3, Serial No. 258), 67–96.

Lyons-Ruth, K., Yellin, C., Melnick, S., & Atwood, G. (2005). Expanding the concept of unresolved mental states: Hostile-helpless states of mind on the Adult Attachment Interview are associated with disrupted mother–infant communication and infant disorganization. *Development and Psychopathology, 17,* 1–23.

Madigan, S., Bakermans-Kranenburg, M. J., van IJzendoorn, M. H., Moran, G., Pederson, D. R., & Benoit, D. (2006). Unresolved states of mind, anomalous parental behavior, and disorganized attachment: A review and meta-analysis of a transmission gap. *Attachment and Human Development, 8,* 89–111.

Madigan, S., Moran, G., & Pederson, D. R. (2006). Unresolved states of mind, disorganized attachment relationships, and disrupted mother–infant interactions of adolescent mothers and their infants. *Developmental Psychology, 42,* 293–304.

Main, M. (1990). Cross-cultural studies of attachment organization: Recent studies, changing methodologies, and the concept of conditional strategies. *Human Development, 33,* 48–61.

McDonough, S. C. (2004). Interaction guidance: Promoting and nurturing the caregiving relationship. In A. J. Sameroff, S. C. McDonough, & K. L. Rosenblum (Eds.), *Treating parent–infant relationship problems: Strategies for intervention* (pp. 79–96). New York: Guilford Press.

Mesman, J., Stolk, M. N., van Zeijl, J., Alink, L. R. A., Juffer, R., Bakermans-Kranenburg, M. J., et al. (2007). Extending the video-feedback intervention to sensitive discipline: The early prevention of antisocial behavior. In F. Juffer, M. J. Bakermans-Kranenburg, & M. H. van IJzendoorn (Eds.), *Promoting positive parenting: An attachment-based intervention* (pp. 171–192). Mahwah, NJ: Erlbaum.

Oppenheim, D., & Goldsmith, D. F. (2007). *Attachment theory in clinical work with children: Bridging in the gap between research and practice.* New York: Guilford Press.

Oppenheim, D., Goldsmith, D. F., & Koren-Karie, N. (2004). Maternal insightfulness and preschoolers' emotions and behavior problems: Reciprocal influences in a therapeutic preschool program. *Infant Mental Health Journal, 25,* 352–367.

Oppenheim, D., & Koren-Karie, N. (2002). Mothers' insightfulness regarding their children's internal worlds: The capacity underlying secure child–mother relationships. *Infant Mental Health Journal, 23,* 593–605.

Osofsky, J. D., Kronenberg, M., Hammer, J. H., Lederman, C., Katz, L., Adams, S., et al. (2007). The development and evaluation of the intervention model for the Florida Infant Mental Health Pilot Program. *Infant Mental Health Journal, 28,* 259–280.

Rosenblum, K. L., McDonough, S., Muzik, M., Miller, A., & Sameroff, A. (2002). Maternal representations of the infant: Associations with infant response to the still face. *Child Development, 73,* 999–1015.

Rutter, M. (2006). *Genes and behavior: Nature–nurture interplay explained.* Oxford, UK: Blackwell.

Sameroff, A. J., McDonough, S., & Rosenblum, K. (Eds.). (2004). *Treating parent–infant relationship problems: Strategies for intervention.* New York: Guilford Press.

Schechter, D. S., Coots, T., Zeanah, C. H., Davies, M., Coates, S. W., Trabka, K. A., et al. (2005). Maternal mental representations of the child in an inner-city clinical sample: Violence-related posttraumatic stress and reflective functioning. *Attachment and Human Development, 7,* 313–331.

Shonkoff, J., & Phillips, D. (Eds.). (2000). *From neurons to neighborhoods: The science of early childhood development.* Washington, DC: National Academy Press.

Slade, A. (2005). Parental reflective functioning: An introduction. *Attachment and Human Development, 7,* 269–281.

Slade, A., Grienenberger, J., Bernbach, E., Levy, D., & Locker, A. (2005). Maternal reflective functioning, attachment, and the transmission gap: A preliminary study. *Attachment and Human Development, 7,* 283–298.

Slade, A., Sadler, L., deDios-Kenn, C., Fitzpatrick, S., Webb, D., & Mayes, L. (2007). Minding the Baby: The promotion of attachment security and reflective functioning in a nursing/mental health home visiting program. In L. J. Berlin (Chair), *Interventions to support early attachments: New findings.* Symposium conducted at the biennial meeting of the Society for Research in Child Development, Boston.

Slade, A., Sadler, L. S., & Mayes, L. C. (2005). Minding

the Baby: Enhancing parental reflective functioning in a nursing/mental health home visiting program. In L. J. Berlin, Y. Ziv, L. Amaya-Jackson, & M. T. Greenberg (Eds.), *Enhancing early attachments: Theory, research, intervention, and policy* (pp. 152–177). New York: Guilford Press.

Smyke, A. T., Wajda-Johnston, V., & Zeanah, C. H. (2004). Working with traumatized infants and toddlers in the child welfare system. In J. D. Osofsky (Ed.), *Young children and trauma: Intervention and treatment* (pp. 260–284). New York: Guilford Press.

Spieker, S., Nelson, D., DeKlyen, M., & Staerkel, F. (2005). Enhancing early attachments in the context of Early Head Start: Can programs emphasizing family support improve rates of secure infant–mother attachments in low-income families? In L. J. Berlin, Y. Ziv, L. Amaya-Jackson, & M. T. Greenberg (Eds.), *Enhancing early attachments: Theory, research, intervention, and policy* (pp. 250–275). New York: Guilford Press.

Sroufe, L. A., Egeland, B., Carlson, E. A., & Collins, W. A. (2005). *The development of the person: The Minnesota Study of Risk and Adaptation from Birth to Adulthood.* New York: Guilford Press.

Stams, G. J., Juffer, F., van IJzendoorn, M. H., & Hoksbergen, R. A. C. (2001). Attachment-based intervention in adoptive families in infancy and children's development at age seven: Two follow-up studies. *British Journal of Developmental Psychology, 19*, 159–180.

Toth, S. L., Maughan, A., Manly, J. T., Spagnola, M., & Cicchetti, D. (2002). The relative efficacy of two interventions in altering maltreated preschool children's representational models: Implications for attachment theory. *Development and Psychopathology, 14*, 877–908.

Toth, S. L., Rogosch, F. A., Manly, J. T., & Cicchetti, D. (2006). The efficacy of toddler–parent psychotherapy to reorganize attachment in the young offspring of mothers with major depressive disorder: A randomized preventive trial. *Journal of Consulting and Clinical Psychology, 74*, 1006–1016.

U.S. Department of Health and Human Services. (1994). *Statement of the Advisory Committee on Services for Families with Infants and Toddlers* (DHHS Publication No. 1994-615-032/03062). Washington, DC: U.S. Government Printing Office.

van den Boom, D. C. (1994). The influence of temperament and mothering on attachment and exploration: An experimental manipulation of sensitive respon-

siveness among lower-class mothers with irritable infants. *Child Development, 65*, 1457–1477.

van den Boom, D. C. (1995). Do first-year intervention effects endure?: Follow-up during toddlerhood of a sample of Dutch irritable infants. *Child Development, 66*, 1798–1816.

van IJzendoorn, M. H. (1995). Adult attachment representations, parental responsiveness, and infant attachment: A meta-analysis on the predictive validity of the Adult Attachment Interview. *Psychological Bulletin, 117*, 387–403.

van IJzendoorn, M. H., & Bakermans-Kranenburg, M. J. (2006). DRD4 7-repeat polymorphism moderates the association between maternal unresolved loss or trauma and infant disorganization. *Attachment and Human Development, 8*, 291–307.

van IJzendoorn, M. H., Bakermans-Kranenburg, M. J., & Juffer, F. (2005). Why less is more: From the dodo bird verdict to evidence-based interventions on sensitivity and early attachments. In L. J. Berlin, Y. Ziv, L. Amaya-Jackson, & M. T. Greenberg (Eds.), *Enhancing early attachments: Theory, research, intervention, and policy* (pp. 297–312). New York: Guilford Press.

van Zeijl, J., Mesman, J., van IJzendoorn, M. H., Bakermans-Kranenburg, M. J., Juffer, F., Stolk, M. N., et al. (2006). Attachment-based intervention for enhancing sensitive discipline in mothers of 1- to 3-year-old children at risk for externalizing behavior problems: A randomized controlled trial. *Journal of Consulting and Clinical Psychology, 74*, 994–1005.

Zeanah, C. H. (Ed.). (2000). *Handbook of infant mental health* (2nd ed.). New York: Guilford Press.

Zeanah, C. H., & Benoit, D. (1995). Clinical applications of a parent perception interview. *Child Psychiatric Clinics of North America, 4*, 539–554.

Zeanah, C. H., Benoit, D., Hirshberg, L., Barton, M. L., & Regan, C. (1994). Mothers' representations of their infants are concordant with infant attachment classifications. *Developmental Issues in Psychiatry and Psychology, 1*, 9–18.

Zeanah, C. H., Larrieu, J. A., Heller, S. S., & Valliere, J. (2000). Infant–parent relationship assessment. In C. H. Zeanah (Ed.), *Handbook of infant mental health* (2nd ed., pp. 222–235). New York: Guilford Press.

Zeanah, C. H., Larrieu, J. A., Heller, S. S., Valliere, J., Hinshaw-Fuselier, S., Aoki, Y., et al. (2001). Evaluation of a preventive intervention for maltreated infants and toddlers in foster care. *Journal of the American Academy of Child and Adolescent Psychiatry, 40*, 214–221.

CHAPTER 32

The Implications of Attachment Theory and Research for Adult Psychotherapy
Research and Clinical Perspectives

ARIETTA SLADE

Attachment theory began with John Bowlby's (1944, 1969/1982, 1973, 1979, 1980, 1988) elegant and parsimonious ideas about the nature and function of human attachments. These ideas began to shape the course of developmental psychology as early as the 1960s, largely through the work of his colleague and friend Mary Ainsworth (Ainsworth, Blehar, Waters, & Wall, 1978; see also Karen, 1998, and Slade, 1999a, 2000, for reviews). However, despite the fact that Bowlby was a psychoanalyst and psychotherapist, his work was largely ignored by clinicians and clinical researchers for decades. Late in his life, Bowlby expressed his dismay at this state of affairs:

> It is a little unexpected that, whereas attachment theory was formulated by a clinician for use in the diagnosis and treatment of emotionally disturbed patients and families, its usage hitherto has been mainly to promote research in developmental psychology. Whilst I welcome the findings of this research as enormously extending our understanding of personality development and psychopathology, and thus as of the greatest clinical relevance, it has not the less been disappointing that clinicians have been so slow to test the theory's uses. (1988, pp. ix–x)

The failure of clinicians to embrace Bowlby's work had largely (although not entirely) to do with his rift with the psychoanalytic community—a rift that was the result of his challenging some of the basic tenets of psychoanalysis, in particular drive theory, and the privileging of the impact of fantasy (rather than reality) on psychological functioning and psychopathology. The unfortunate consequences of this breach have been well documented (Karen, 1998; Slade, 1999a).

However, thanks largely to the pioneering work of Ainsworth's student Mary Main, as well as that of psychoanalyst Peter Fonagy and his colleagues, the tide began to turn toward the end of the 1980s. Their work emerged at a time when psychoanalysis had begun to abandon its exclusive focus on the drives and to embrace an increasingly relational and intersubjective perspective. Psychoanalysis was finally ready for attachment theory: Nearly 50 years after the publication of Bowlby's (1944) paper on the experience of parental loss in 44 juvenile thieves, his wish for dialogue became a reality, and attachment theory could return to its ancestral home, psychoanalysis.

As a consequence of these shifts, interest in the clinical implications of attachment theory and research has grown exponentially over the last two decades. When I wrote about adult psychotherapy[1] and attachment theory for the first edition of the *Handbook of Attachment* (Slade, 1999a), the literature was—relative to today—in its infancy. Over the course of the last decade, however, interest in the interface among adult attachment, mentalization (Fonagy, Gergely, Jurist, & Target, 2002), and dynamic psychotherapy has grown dramatically. Today the influence of attachment theory and research can be seen across a number of domains of clinical research, theory, and practice. In addition to the publication of numerous books (e.g., Atkinson & Goldberg, 2004; Fonagy, 2001; Oppenheim & Goldsmith, 2007; Sable, 2000; Wallin, 2007) and articles on the topic, several leading clinical and research journals have devoted entire special issues to bridging the gap between attachment theory and clinical work. These include the *Journal of the American Psychoanalytic Association* (2000); *Infant Mental Health Journal* (2004); *Psychoanalytic Inquiry* (1999 and 2003); *Journal of Infant, Child, and Adult Psychotherapy* (2002); and, most recently, *Journal of Clinical and Consulting Psychology* (2006). And since its inception in 2000, the journal *Attachment and Human Development* has made this interface one of its abiding concerns. Thus, whereas my task in the late 1990s was complex, it was relatively contained. Today, almost a decade later, this is no longer the case.

There are essentially two bodies of literature exploring the clinical implications of attachment theory and research for adult psychotherapy. The first is a research literature examining the various links between attachment classification or style and the process and outcome of psychotherapy. The second is a clinical literature, in which individual practitioners describe the various ways that the constructs and methods of attachment theory and research have influenced their clinical work. In this chapter, I try to do justice to elements of both literatures.

My perspective here is that attachment theory and research have the potential to *enrich* (rather than dictate) a therapist's understanding of particular patients. Attachment theory does not dictate a particular form of treatment; rather, understanding the nature and dynamics of attachment and of mentalization informs rather than defines intervention and clinical thinking. Attachment theory offers a broad and far-reaching view of human functioning that has the potential to change the way clinicians think about and respond to their patients, and the way they understand the dynamics of the therapeutic relationship (Slade, 1999a, 1999b, 2000, 2004a, 2004b, 2007). This perspective provides yet another template with which a therapist can understand and make meaning of the

patient's experience, without needing to jettison other, equally important and valid kinds of clinical understanding. Thus attachment constructs can be useful in making sense of some, but by no means all, psychotherapy patients. For some, the qualities of relatedness, modes of defense and affect regulation, and/or failures in mentalization that are associated with insecure attachment will shape the treatment and its course in numerous ways. For other patients, these are background issues that—although they may inform the treatment—will not dominate the clinical work.

I begin with a brief introduction to the theoretical work that has been essential to latter-day attachment theory and research.

BOWLBY, AINSWORTH, AND MAIN: A BRIEF REVIEW

Over the course of his career, Bowlby (e.g., 1969/1982, 1979, 1988) established the basic assumptions of attachment theory: (1) that children are predisposed to become attached to their caregivers; and (2) that because these primary attachment relationships are vital to the child's survival, they must be maintained *at whatever cost to the child*. Throughout his writings, Bowlby suggested that when such crucial adaptations result in disrupted or distorted primary attachment relationships, the child's basic capacities for both relatedness and autonomy will be affected, sometimes resulting in psychopathology (see DeKlyen & Greenberg, Chapter 27, this volume, for the complex conditions under which psychopathology emerges). These early formulations made a powerful impression on Ainsworth, who was inspired to study the natural development of mother–infant attachment in the first year of life (Ainsworth et al., 1978). One of her most significant contributions was the development of a simple laboratory separation procedure—the Strange Situation—that allowed her to delineate the core elements of both insecure and secure attachment organization in children. Out of this seminal work emerged a description of individual differences in attachment organization that were the sequelae of maternal care in the first year: the "secure" pattern and its two insecure counterparts, the "avoidant" and "resistant" patterns.

Main, a student of Ainsworth's, made two key contributions that expanded upon Bowlby and Ainsworth's work significantly. The first was the delineation of a fourth category of infant attachment, the disorganized/disoriented pattern

(Main & Solomon, 1990). The second—the development of the Adult Attachment Interview (AAI: George, Kaplan, & Main, 1984, 1985, 1996)—revolutionized attachment research. The AAI (described in detail by Hesse, Chapter 25, this volume) is a 16-question interview that asks parents to describe their early experiences with their parents. It is remarkably successful in evoking "states of mind with respect to attachment," and is in many respects a verbal analogue of the Strange Situation. Main and her colleagues' analysis of the AAI revealed patterns of narrative organization that were analogous to infantile patterns of behavior in the Strange Situation (Main, Kaplan, & Cassidy, 1985). These narrative patterns, which Main saw as reflections of internal working models of attachment, were manifest not in adults' descriptions of the *events* of their lives, but in the way such events were remembered and organized in the telling of their attachment stories.

The analysis of narrative patterns led Main and her colleagues (Hesse, Chapter 25, this volume; Main & Goldwyn, 1984; Main, Goldwyn, & Hesse, 2003; Main et al., 1985) to describe three adult attachment classifications, each of which had its analogue in Ainsworth's original classification system, supplemented by the later-discovered (Main & Solomon, 1990) disorganized attachment pattern: "secure-autonomous" (analogous to the secure infant classification), "dismissing" (avoidant infant classification), "preoccupied" (resistant infant classification), and "unresolved" (disorganized/disoriented infant classification). Hesse (1996) described the "cannot classify" category several years later.

In their original research, Main and her colleagues were able to document high levels of concordance between the attachment status of mothers and their infants. Given that mothers were interviewed 5 years after their children were assessed in infancy, these findings were particularly striking. Multiple studies have since confirmed the essential aspects of Main's research (see reviews by van IJzendoorn, 1995; van IJzendoorn & Bakermans-Kranenburg, 1996).

FONAGY AND MENTALIZATION THEORY

The revolution in attachment theory and research that Main set in motion with her "move to the level of representation" laid the foundation for the work of Fonagy and his colleagues (notably Mary Target, Anthony Bateman, Miriam Steele, and Howard Steele), and initiated another revolution in attachment research—one that was to have a particular impact in clinical research and practice. Rather than focus on classification, as Ainsworth, Main, and (to some extent) Bowlby had, Fonagy instead described the development and function of a unitary but complex capacity—"reflective functioning" or "mentalization"[2]—and its presence, absence, or distortion in psychopathology. (For fuller discussions of mentalization theory and research, see Fonagy, Gergely, & Target, Chapter 33, this volume; Fonagy et al., 1995, 2002.)

Mentalization and Reflective Functioning

The construct of mentalization emerged from Fonagy and colleagues' initial attempts to operationalize and expand upon Main's (1991) notions of "metacognitive monitoring." What, they wondered, was the core capacity that was present in secure individuals but absent or distorted in insecure individuals? As experienced clinicians, they recognized a set of psychological capacities that were crucial to what Main had described as a secure state of mind in relation to attachment. "Reflective functioning" or "mentalization" refers to the capacity to envision mental states in oneself and another, and to understand one's own and another's behavior in terms of underlying mental states and intentions. Inherent in high-level mentalizing is the capacity to regulate and envision negative and disruptive mental states, as well as to appreciate the interpersonal, intrapersonal, causal, and dynamic aspects of mental states.

According to Fonagy and his colleagues (2002), mentalization is a basic human capacity intrinsic to affect regulation and productive social relationships. It allows one to understand that one's own or another's behaviors are linked in meaningful, predictable ways to underlying, often unobservable, changing and dynamic feelings and intentions. The more a person is able to envision mental states in self and others (and thus to distinguish between what is internal to the self and what is particular to the other) the more likely the person is to engage in productive, intimate, and sustaining relationships; to feel connected to others at a subjective level; and also to feel autonomous and of a separate mind. Indeed, failure to engage with the minds of others, or with one's own mental experience, is one of the markers of a range of insecure attachment-related states of mind.

In their research, Fonagy and his colleagues (1995) demonstrated that adults who are highly reflective during the AAI (i.e., able to mentalize about themselves and their parents when asked about early childhood relationships) are more likely to be classified as secure in relation to attachment. Their infants are also more likely to be secure. In fact, mothers' reflective functioning was more predictive of infant security than were their adult attachment classifications. (See also Slade, 2005; Slade, Grienenberger, Bernbach, Levy, & Locker, 2005.) In later research with clinical populations, Fonagy and his colleagues (1996) were able to link failures of mentalization with psychopathology—particularly with more severe forms of personality disorder, notably borderline personality disorder (Fonagy et al., 2002). They were also able to show that the development of mentalizing is protective in instances of trauma, such that individuals whose mentalizing capacities are intact are unlikely to develop borderline personality disorder, even in instances where there has been severe and early relational trauma (Fonagy et al., 1995).[3]

Unlike the AAI scoring system (Main & Goldwyn, 1984; Main et al., 2003), which relies on the categorical scoring of interview material, reflective functioning is coded along a continuous scale from –1 ("bizarre") to 9 ("full reflective functioning") (Fonagy, Target, Steele, & Steele, 1998). Even though this coding system is based on a single continuum, running from high to low reflective functioning, it allows for the differentiation of dismissing and preoccupied forms of disrupted or deficient mentalization.

As I describe in the following three sections, Main's work on adult attachment and Fonagy's work on mentalization have both had a significant effect on clinical research and practice.[4] I begin by examining the impact of adult attachment theory and methods on psychotherapy research, and then turn to a description of the ways these theories and methods have been adopted and understood by clinical practitioners. In the final major section, I briefly review some of the ways that Fonagy's work has influenced clinical theory and led specifically to the development of "mentalization-based therapy."

ADULT ATTACHMENT AND PSYCHOTHERAPY RESEARCH

The past decade has seen an enormous increase in research on the links between attachment and psychotherapy. Although this literature raises more questions than it answers, and provides few clear guidelines for practitioners (see Mallinckrodt, Porter, & Kivlighan, 2005), its breadth alone speaks to the degree to which Main's work on adult attachment has captured the imagination of psychotherapy researchers. (For an excellent and comprehensive review of this literature, see Daniel, 2006.)

In the sections that follow, I review the research in several broad areas: (1) relations between patient attachment and psychotherapy process variables (alliance, transference, attachment to therapist, therapist response); (2) relations between therapist variables (attachment organization, attachment to patient) and therapy process and outcome; (3) attachment as a measure of change in psychotherapy; and (4) relations between patient attachment and therapy outcome. Before beginning, however, I would like to contextualize this review in several respects.

The literature in this area is still quite recent and continues to develop. Although a number of studies have been conducted to assess various relations between patient attachment classification and therapy process and outcome, there has been little consistency in types of patients, treatments, or therapists studied. Moreover, numerous different measures have been used to measure adult attachment, many of which measure slightly different underlying constructs. A relatively small number of researchers have used the AAI and the classification system developed by Main and colleagues (Main & Goldwyn, 1984; Main et al., 2003). Yet another small group of studies have used the AAI, but have classified patients by using Kobak's attachment Q-set rather than Main's scoring system (Kobak, Cole, Ferenz-Gillies, & Fleming, 1993). Kobak's method yields scores along two axes: the "deactivation–hyperactivation" axis and the "secure–anxious" axis. Data can be analyzed continuously or categorically. The third and most widely used approach is the self-report, which obviously has great advantages over the AAI in terms of time and cost efficiency. Over the past 20 years, a number of self-report instruments have been developed to measure adult attachment (see Daniel, 2006, and Crowell, Fraley, & Shaver, Chapter 26, this volume). These measures include the Adult Attachment Scales, developed by Collins and Read (1990); the Relationship Styles Questionnaire, developed by Bartholomew and colleagues (Bartholomew & Horowitz, 1991; Griffin & Bartholomew, 1994); and the Experiences in Close Relationships inventory (Brennan, Clark,

& Shaver, 1998). They are scored in a variety of different ways: Some yield three prototypes, some four; and of these, the prototypes are not necessarily the same. For the most part, these prototypes do not map directly onto AAI categories. Thus the various measures available to assess adult attachment are only partially correlated (Shaver, Belsky, & Brennan, 2000), and likely to assess overlapping but not identical constructs.

At present, most researchers describe adult attachment along two orthogonal dimensions—avoidance and anxiety—and as falling into one of four prototypes derived from scores along these two dimensions (Mikulincer & Shaver, Chapter 23, this volume). Space limitations preclude the review of the particular methods used in the studies cited below. For the sake of clarity, however, I use the terms "avoidant," "deactivating," and "dismissing" to refer to the state of mind typically associated with the dismissing category described by Main and colleagues (1985), and the terms "anxious," "hyperactivating," and "preoccupied" to refer to what they have described as preoccupied states of mind. With rare exception, the AAI-based studies reviewed here address only differences between organized secure and insecure states of mind, and not those between organized and disorganized (unresolved or cannot classify) insecure states of mind.

Does Patient Attachment Organization Affect the Process of Psychotherapy?

One of the first questions researchers asked in the years following Main's introduction of the AAI was whether a patient's attachment classification would predict the patient's willingness to engage in treatment, his or her capacity to form a working alliance, and (finally) the capacity to develop an attachment to the therapist. The short answer—in line with theoretical assumptions—is yes. Bowlby believed that the willingness to seek and accept care would be associated with attachment security. This notion has received support from a number of empirical studies. In two different studies, Dozier and her colleagues (Dozier, 1990; Dozier, Lomax, Tyrrell, & Lee, 2001) found that secure patients were comfortable seeking therapy and were able to commit themselves to the process. This was in contrast to dismissing patients, who denied their need for help, and preoccupied patients, whose neediness and dependency made it difficult for them to use the therapist productively. Dozier and her colleagues' findings with regard to the impact of secure and dismissing states of mind were confirmed in a num-

ber of later studies (Dolan, Arnkoff, & Glass, 1993; Lopez, Melendez, Sauer, Berger, & Wyssmann, 1998; Riggs, Jacobvitz, & Hazen, 2002; Tasca et al., 2006). None of these studies were able to identify the effects of preoccupied or hyperactivating states of mind on process variables, however.

Secure attachment has also been found to facilitate a positive alliance in several studies (Kivlighan, Patton, & Foote, 1998; Mallinckrodt, Coble, & Gantt, 1995; Satterfield & Lyddon, 1995). Only one (Mallinckrodt, Coble, & Gantt, 1995) described differences *within* insecure groups. In this study, the alliance ratings of anxiously attached (i.e., more preoccupied) patients were lower than those of secure or avoidant patients.

Given the fact that the vast majority of psychotherapy patients are insecure (see Dozier, Stovall-McClough, & Albus, Chapter 30, this volume, for a review), the establishment of a link between secure attachment and positive alliance is not particularly informative, because it sheds little light on why or how insecure patients fail to create such alliances, and how type of insecurity might affect the nature of treatment ruptures.[5] Only a few studies—which examined fluctuations in the therapeutic alliance *over time*—have offered a more nuanced assessment of the relation between type of insecurity and the evolving treatment alliance. Kanninen, Salo, and Punamaki (2000) found that whereas secure patients reported few shifts in therapeutic alliance over the course of treatment, there was a steep drop in therapeutic alliance ratings for preoocupied patients in the middle of therapy, with a steep rise at the end of therapy. Dismissing patients, by contrast, showed a drop in alliance ratings at the end of therapy. In related work, Eames and Roth (2000) have examined the link between attachment organization and patterns of treatment rupture. In their research, preoccupied patients reported more frequent ruptures, whereas dismissing patients reported lower rates of rupture. These patterns are consistent with theoretical predictions and suggest that the ebb and flow of the therapeutic alliance takes on different shapes, depending on a patient's attachment organization.

A small number of studies have suggested—again in line with theoretical expectations—that attachment organization predicts differences in the development of the transference. Specifically, it predicts the patient's tendency to project his or her own interpersonal expectations and childhood fantasies onto the therapist. Bradley, Heim, and Westen (2005) describe a typology of transference dimensions ("angry/entitled," "anxious/

preoccupied," "secure/engaged," "avoidant/counterdependent," and "sexualized") that map onto Main's attachment classifications in predictable ways. Woodhouse, Schlosser, Crook, Ligiero, and Gelso (2003) reported that anxiously attached patients were more inclined toward splitting in the transference, as they experienced swings between idealizing the therapist on the one hand and being angry, frustrated, and disappointed in him or her on the other. These transference manifestations also influenced the therapist in significant ways.

Several research groups have considered questions of alliance and transference from the vantage point of the patient's *attachment* to the therapist. Mallinckrodt, Gantt, and Coble (1995) developed a self-report measure (the Client to Therapist Attachment Scale) that distinguishes among "secure," "avoidant-fearful," and "preoccupied-merger" attachment to the therapist. Parish and Eagle (2003) developed a self-report measure to assess the patient's experience of the therapist in terms of nine central components of attachment, among them proximity seeking, secure base, availability, and stronger/wiser. It yields a series of continua, rather than a typology. Finally, Diamond and her colleagues developed an interview (the Patient–Therapist AAI [PT-AAI]; see Diamond, Stovall-McClough, Clarkin, & Levy, 2003) that is based directly on the AAI, but that assesses the relationship to the therapist rather than the parents and yields an attachment classification in a typology analogous to Main's.

Using the term "attachment" to describe a patient's relationship to the therapist raises a number of complex issues about what kind of relationship can reasonably be called an attachment relationship (see Eagle & Wolitzky, in press; Farber, Lippert, & Nevas, 1995). In general, however, it seems that in most successful treatments the therapist becomes very significant to the patient, that the relationship has many elements of an attachment relationship, and that the therapist fulfills many of the functions of an attachment figure. Indeed, as Eagle and Wolitzky (in press) point out, the development of both positive and negative transference manifestations indicates that the therapist is becoming an attachment figure—"i.e., that he or she is activating internal working models (associative networks) originally formed in relation to [a patient's] initial attachment figures." Optimally, the patient develops a "secure" attachment to the therapist, meaning, on the one hand, that he or she uses the security inherent in the current relationship with the therapist to rework previously established insecure working models. On the other

hand, a secure attachment makes it possible for the patient to tolerate and make sense of feelings of disappointment, anger, or even fear (of being abandoned, misunderstood, etc.) in relation to the therapist. Ultimately, these are incorporated into a positive and integrated representation of the therapist and of the self-as-patient. The research in this area supports these various assumptions—namely, that patients with insecure attachment histories are more likely to form insecure attachments with their therapists and to have difficulty seeing a therapist as a secure base, or as a reliable, caring attachment figure, regardless of the therapist's behavior (Diamond et al., 2003; Eagle & Wolitzky, in press; Hamilton, 1987; Sable, 2000; Slade, 2004b). At the same time, to the degree that patients are able to experience a therapist as an available safe haven and secure base, they are likely to engage more fully and successfully in treatment (Parish & Eagle, 2003).

Unsurprisingly, research suggests that not only do patients' attachment organizations affect their capacity to engage in treatment and trust their therapists; it also affects the therapists and their responses to their patients. This is reflected in the results of two separate studies indicating that attachment classification predicts whether therapists respond in more "cognitive" or "affective" ways. In both studies, therapists were more likely to respond with interpretations to dismissing patients, and with reflection of feelings to preoccupied patients (Hardy et al., 1999; Rubino, Barker, Roth, & Fearon, 2000).

Both of these studies indicate that therapists are predisposed to respond "in style" to patients, offering more cognitive comments to dismissing or avoidant individuals and more exploration of feelings to preoccupied patients. Although these reports make intuitive sense—we would expect therapists to mirror their patients' affective styles in responding to them—there remain a number of questions as to (1) whether it is more therapeutic to respond "in style" and (2) what factors other than patient characteristics determine a therapist's responses. These are discussed more fully in the next section.

Does Therapist Attachment Organization Affect the Process of Psychotherapy?

Most training in psychotherapy emphasizes that being a successful therapist depends on managing one's own emotional reactions to patients; this means both that one remains aware of one's own feelings and reactions in relation to a patient, and that one is able to make *use* of these feelings in the treatment without being disrupted by them or provocatively expressing them to the patient. Presumably, attachment insecurity in the therapist would interfere with all of these processes. And indeed it does. Attachment theory would predict that the predilection to care is as vulnerable to distortion in the insecure therapist as it is in the insecure patient.[6] And, regardless of the degree to which a therapist is secure in relation to attachment, different patients will engage the therapist's attachment representations in different ways. Thus, in the intersubjective field that is at the heart of good psychotherapy, attachment representations are very likely to be evoked in the therapist, and may well have to do with the emergence of problematic countertransference reactions.[7]

These assumptions have been confirmed by a number of research studies. Dozier, Cue, and Barnett (1994) led the way in this work, reporting that secure therapists were more able than insecure therapists to hear and respond to the dependency needs of their dismissing patients, and were thus less vulnerable to countertransference reactions toward them. Secure therapists were also more able to manage the overt demands and explicit dependency needs of patients who were preoccupied in relation to attachment. Insecure therapists were also likely to see their preoccupied/hyperactivating patients as more needy and dependent than were secure therapists, and were thus more likely to become entangled with such patients, responding to their overt reactions rather than their underlying needs. Later work by Dunkle and Friedlander (1996), Black, Hardy, Turpin, and Parry (2005), and Rubino and colleagues (2000) confirmed many of these findings. Only two studies (Ligiero & Gelso, 2002; Sauer, Lopez, & Gormley, 2003) suggested that therapist attachment anxiety might actually improve the alliance. Whereas these results could be interpreted to mean that anxious therapists establish better working alliances, it is more likely that therapists who are less secure in their own attachment organization try too hard to make patients like them and feel connected to them at the beginning of treatment. Although this may have a superficially positive impact at the start of treatment, these effects are unlikely to last over its full course.

A therapist's attachment organization also plays a role in determining whether he or she responds "in style" or "out of style" with a patient. As described above, researchers report that therapists are typically inclined to respond in the styles of their patients—namely, to respond with more cognitive interventions (interpretations and suggestions) with dismissing/deactivating patients, and with more affective interventions (reflection of feelings, empathy) to more preoccupied/hyperactivating patients. These linear trends do not obtain when the therapist's attachment organization is considered as part of the equation, however. In their original study, Dozier and colleagues (1994) reported that secure case managers were less likely than insecure case managers to become enmeshed with hyperactivating patients or to shut down in concert with their deactivating patients. In fact, secure therapists were inclined to adopt styles that were noncomplementary to those of their patients. In another study of the interaction between patient and therapist, Tyrrell, Dozier, Teague, and Fallot (1999) reported similar findings. Even though therapists in this sample were without exception secure, those who were less dismissing/deactivating were able to form stronger alliances with patients who were more dismissing/deactivating. And there was a trend for more dismissing practitioners to form weaker alliances with patients who were more dismissing/deactivating. These same researchers also reported that more dismissing patients did better with more preoccupied/hyperactivating clinicians, and vice versa.

What this research suggests is that a more secure therapist can respond "out of style" with a patient as necessary and appropriate. In many instances, such gentle challenges to the patient's attachment organization have the effect of softening rather than provoking characteristic defensive styles, thereby enhancing flexibility and change (see also Bernier & Dozier, 2002; Daniel, 2006). Indeed, moving between these two strategies—sometimes mirroring the patient's experience (responding "in style"), and at other times challenging his or her state of mind (responding "out of style")—seems an important component of any successful therapy. The research to date suggests that such flexibility is much more typical of therapists who are themselves secure in relation to attachment. It is important to note, however, that experience plays a role in the degree to which therapists take a flexible stance in relation to their patients, regardless of their particular therapeutic orientation (Daly & Mallinckrodt, 2008). Thus security and experience are two therapist variables that are likely to play a crucial role in treatment outcome.

In their work using the PT-AAI, Diamond and her colleagues (2003) assessed not only a patient's internal working model of a therapist, but also a therapist's internal working model of a patient. In a small pilot study, they found that all therapists were secure in their representations of their patients, whereas the majority of patients were insecure in their therapist representations. The fact that therapists develop internal working models of their patients does not, however, suggest that patients become attachment objects for their therapists (Eagle & Wolitzky, in press). Indeed, it could well be argued that the development of an *attachment* to a patient—which might, for instance, preclude mentalizing about the patient (see Fonagy, 2006)—would inhibit certain kinds of therapeutic work. But therapists certainly do have strong feelings for their patients; whether these are best described as attachments remains open to discussion.

Does Patient Attachment Organization Predict Psychotherapy Outcomes?

Another way to address the link between attachment organization and psychotherapy outcome is to examine whether psychotherapy results in a change in attachment status. The results of the small number of studies in this area are mixed and complex. In their study of 82 inpatients, Fonagy and his colleagues (1995) reported that whereas all patients were insecure at the start of treatment, 40% were securely attached upon discharge. Travis, Bliwise, Binder, and Horne Meyer (2001) likewise noted increases in the number of patients who were secure and a decrease in those who were fearful. However, the bulk of the patients whose attachment style changed moved from one form of insecurity to another. Also, the patients who changed to a secure attachment style were those who had the lowest levels of symptomatology before treatment. Mirroring these findings, Diamond and her colleagues (1999) also reported complex shifts in attachment organization over the course of a year of treatment in a small sample of hospitalized patients with borderline personality disorder. Within a group of 10 patients, some moved from insecure to secure, some did not change, and some moved from insecure to "cannot classify."

Clearer evidence for the utility of the AAI as an outcome measure recently emerged in a large-sample randomized clinical trial conducted by Levy and his colleagues (2006). This group compared the effectiveness of transference-focused psychotherapy with that of dialectical behavior therapy and modified psychodynamic supportive psychotherapy in treating individuals with borderline personality disorder. They reported that after 1 year, transference-focused psychotherapy

(but not dialectical behavior therapy or supportive psychotherapy) led to a significant increase in the number of individuals classified as secure in relation to attachment; narrative coherence and reflective functioning also improved significantly.

Nevertheless, it is worth asking whether it is a reasonable idea to use attachment classification as a way of assessing treatment outcome. Attachment classifications are probably overt manifestations of deep structures that will take some time to change, even in the most successful of treatments. Also, as is evident from two of the studies described above (Diamond et al., 1999; Travis et al., 2001), there are shifts from one type of defensive organization to another over the course of treatment. In addition, changes in attachment patterns are not necessarily accompanied by changes in real-life behavior or relationships (Eagle & Wolitzky, in press). Thus a change in attachment security may or may not accompany symptom remission, structural change, or behavioral change.

Researchers have also examined whether patient attachment classification is linked to treatment outcome, or (importantly) should dictate treatment type. In the first large-scale outcome study of the relation between attachment classification and psychotherapy outcome, Fonagy and his colleagues (1996) found that dismissing or avoidant patients did better in psychotherapy than did those who were preoccupied or unresolved. In a recent study, McBride, Atkinson, Quilty, and Bagby (2006) found that that depressed patients who were high on avoidant attachment did better than their anxiously attached (i.e., more preoccupied) peers.[8]

It is interesting that both of these studies (Fonagy et al., 2006; McBride, 2006) indicate that dismissing/avoidant patients are likely to do better in psychotherapy than their preoccupied/anxious peers. Preoccupied or anxiously attached individuals are presumably *more* in touch with their feelings, and dismissing patients obviously pose challenges to the basic assumptions of therapy (namely, that one will talk about one's problems and be open to forming a therapeutic relationship). Nevertheless, the latter group appears for the most part to do better in psychotherapy. Fonagy and his colleagues (1996) speculate that whereas therapy gradually *exposes* dismissing patients to their emotional experience, preoccupied patients have already "well-formed and self-serving opinions" (Daniel, 2006, p. 979) about their feelings and life experiences that are resistant to change.

This general finding may also be attributable to the fact that preoccupied/anxious and unresolved patients are often more disturbed than those who are dismissing, making them particularly challenging to treat. Evidence for this assumption can be found in the fact that individuals with borderline personality disorder are most likely to be preoccupied or unresolved with respect to attachment (see Agrawal, Gunderson, Holmes, & Lyons-Ruth, 2004, and Westen, Nakash, Thomas, & Bradley, 2006, for reviews). Indeed, the fact that these individuals are notoriously difficult to work with in therapy has led to the development of a number of treatment modalities aimed specifically at working with them (Bateman & Fonagy, 2004; Kernberg, Diamond, Yeomans, Clarkin, & Levy, in press; Linehan, 1993), each of which in one way or another addresses the sequelae of insecure attachment.

The next question raised by the Fonagy and colleagues and McBride and colleagues studies is whether attachment organization should dictate treatment type. Fonagy and his colleagues (1996) suggested that dismissing patients did better with psychoanalytically oriented psychotherapy. By contrast, McBride and her colleagues (2006) reported that avoidant depressed patients did better with cognitive-behavioral therapy than with more traditional interpersonal dynamic therapy. In related work, Borman-Spurrell (1996) found that whereas preoccupied patients with binge-eating disorder did better with cognitive-behavioral than with psychodynamic treatment, dismissing patients benefited from both.

On the one hand, it is difficult to compare these reports because of the differences in measures used and in types of treatments and patients studied. Still, they interestingly raise again the question of whether a treatment type that is *noncomplementary* to the patient's attachment style may be most therapeutic. For instance, as Daniel (2006) suggests, a more deactivating treatment (such as cognitive-behavioral therapy) may be more effective for patients who are preoccupied/anxious, whereas hyperactivating treatments (such as psychodynamically oriented psychotherapy) may be more useful for dismissing/avoidant patients. On the other hand, experienced therapists are likely to adjust their stance in subtle ways and from moment to moment, depending on the needs of their patients (Daly & Mallinckrodt, 2008). Thus they may be likely—regardless of their orientation—to respond in more deactivating or hyperactivating ways as a patient's own orientation to his or her inner life shifts within the course of a therapy session or over the course of an entire treatment.

The studies reviewed in this section exem-plify a point I made earlier—namely, that it is very difficult, if not impossible, to quantify the multiple factors that contribute to treatment success insofar as patient attachment is concerned. At the same time, several general provisos can be derived from the studies discussed here. First, different insecure strategies are likely to influence the treatment in a variety of ways. It seems that preoccupied individuals experience more fluctuations in forming therapeutic relationships, as opposed to their dismissing peers, who only warm to treatment and to the therapist slowly. Preoccupied patients are also more likely to experience intense and sometimes primitive affects within the context of the treatment relationship. Second, these differences probably have a powerful impact on therapists—an impact that is moderated by a therapist's own attachment proclivities. The global tendency to respond "in style" with the patient is more modulated and nuanced in a secure (and even better, experienced) therapist, who can also respond "out of style" as needed. Finally, while treatment certainly has an impact on the way a patient manages needs for and fears of intimacy and autonomy, these shifts are probably best measured in noncategorical ways.

Although many practicing clinicians are intrigued by attachment research, they remain unsure of how to apply it in their day-to-day work with patients. Obviously, simply classifying one's patients is of limited value, especially since some of the research suggests that patients actually shift in the ways they are insecure over the course of treatment. In any event, as noted by Waters, Hamilton, and Weinfield (2000), adult attachment patterns are particularly unstable in clinical populations. Thus knowledge of a patient's attachment organization is useful if and only if such knowledge is tied to technique in a meaningful way. As I describe below, a small number of clinicians have attempted to tackle this issue in recent years. Within the context of this review, I also consider some of the ways that the more radical and potentially transforming aspects of attachment theory and research have yet to be incorporated into latter-day clinical thinking.

ADULT ATTACHMENT THEORY AND RESEARCH: IMPLICATIONS FOR PSYCHOTHERAPY PRACTICE

From the moment Main and her colleagues (1985) published their seminal paper on the intergenerational transmission of attachment, which established the link between early experience and current "state of mind with respect to attachment," the exile of attachment theory and research from psychoanalytic psychology ended. With the "move to the level of representation," Main and colleagues described the development of the internal world in ways that were entirely consistent with object relations and other contemporary psychoanalytic theories (i.e., relational and intersubjective perspectives). In addition, Main's methods, which were quite "clinical" (unlike those, for instance, developed to assess infant attachment), emphasized defense, representation, and affect regulation in ways that were entirely familiar to dynamically oriented clinicians. It was easy for such clinicians to find themselves, their patients, and their theoretical beliefs in Main's work.

This was partly due to the fact that by documenting links between early experience and the development of internal, representational structures, Main affirmed assumptions that had been at the core of psychoanalytic developmental theory for nearly a century but had never been empirically validated. In this, she accomplished something that psychoanalytic researchers had tried to do for decades: develop qualitative and clinical methods providing evidence that (1) the quality of early experience, and particularly early relationships, influences adult ways of thinking, knowing, and feeling; and (2) the effect of such influences is routinely transmitted from one generation to the next at the level of *structure*, rather than *content*. And she did so simply, eloquently, and brilliantly. The term "attachment" became a code word for early experience—a code word that now had empirical validation and support. A field that had long shunned Bowlby, and even the term "attachment," was suddenly eager to identify itself with his ideas.

Nevertheless, as much as psychoanalytically oriented clinicians have in recent years incorporated the *terms* of attachment theory into their thinking, relatively few (notably Diana Diamond, Morris Eagle, Jeremy Holmes, Pat Sable, David Wallin, and—as I describe toward the end of this chapter—Peter Fonagy) have really integrated the *core* elements of an attachment perspective into their clinical thinking. Thus a good deal of the work on the clinical implications of attachment has, in my view, focused on those elements of attachment theory that that can be assimilated into extant thinking, rather than grappling with its other, potentially more controversial, aspects. Aside from the work by those listed above, attachment has become synonymous with early relationship difficulties, and implicitly with difficulties in

the pre-Oedipal period; otherwise, it has not added much to clinical dialogue.

Adult attachment research rests in large part on the core distinctions among secure, dismissing, preoccupied, and unresolved states of mind in relation to attachment. Whether measured categorically or continuously, these dimensions and *their dynamic properties* are at the heart of nearly all attachment research, and it is in the "deep" structure of these coding approaches that the true contributions of attachment theory and research to clinical work become most apparent. Embedded in the approaches of both Main and Ainsworth (and their various methodological "cousins") is a way of thinking about how anxiety about basic needs for closeness and nurture are managed as a function of the early relationship climate.

In latter-day attachment research, two crucial dimensions are seen to underlie all adult and infant attachment classification systems. The first is the dismissing/deactivating versus preoccupied/hyperactivating dimension, which refers to an individual's defensive style, or particular way of regulating affective experience. The dismissing end of the continuum refers to the tendency to favor defenses that downplay or minimize affect, whereas the preoccupied end refers to the tendency to favor defenses in which affects are maximized and intensified, usually in an attempt to establish closeness. From an attachment perspective, these modes of defense are particularly prominent when negative affects are aroused within an attachment-related context. The second dimension, the organized versus disorganized dimension, refers to the level and degree of psychological structure the individual has available for containing and regulating emotional experience. It is, in essence, an assessment of *level* of functioning; those who fall at the low end of the organization axis are likely to be more disturbed and lower-functioning.

Implicit in this dimensional approach to attachment classification is the notion that an individual can favor dismissing or preoccupied modes of defense in a more secure or organized way, or in a more insecure or disorganized way. Many of the psychotherapy patients for whom thinking in terms of attachment will be particularly important are those whose defensive strategies are most rigid and self-defeating, and whose organizational capacities are inflexible and vulnerable.

In my opinion, these core dimensions are what have been least understood by clinicians (again, notable exceptions are the work of Holmes, Sable, and Wallin). This is partly due to the fact that few have any real familiarity with the methods and measures of attachment research. In addition, most clinicians are unsure of how to apply research methods and findings in their clinical work, and are uncomfortable with structured assessments, with coding systems, and certainly with classification. Indeed, thinking about patients in terms of their attachment organization has rarely captured the imagination of clinicians. In fact, many see the parameters inherent in classification (as well as many other research assessments) as *limiting* rather than expanding clinical understanding (Doctors, 2007; Slade, 2004b). Unfortunately, this concern about reductionism has obscured what I see as the potential therapeutic value of using the underlying *principles* of attachment organization in clinical work. It must also be said, of course, that this disjunction reflects the fact that the methods and sensibilities of researchers and clinicians are often quite distinct, making a full dialogue at best challenging and often ephemeral.

Interestingly, the distinctions that underlie attachment classification are actually very familiar to psychodynamically oriented clinicians, who regularly distinguish patients in terms of obsessional or deactivating defenses on the one hand and hysterical or hyperactivating defenses on the other, and between higher-level or more reliable and consistent defense and character structure on the one hand, and more primitive, fluid, and chaotic defenses and personality structure on the other (Daly & Mallinckrodt, 2008; Westen et al., 2006). Clinicians also develop hypotheses about the origins of these defenses and levels of psychic structure all the time (see Daly & Mallinckrodt, 2008). Indeed, these kinds of distinctions are at the heart of what Shapiro long ago referred to as "neurotic styles" (Shapiro, 1965/1999; see also Mikulincer & Shaver, Chapter 23, this volume; Mikulincer, Shaver, & Cassidy, in press).[9]

This raises the following question: If in fact clinicians are already aware of and responsive to these dimensions, what is the particular contribution of attachment theory and research to an individual practitioner's clinical work? As I hope will become clear in the following sections, there are many answers to that question.

A Theory of Early Development and Defense

Inherent in the notion of attachment classification is the notion that human beings develop regular and stable ways of defending against the feelings that arise from disruptions in care. The resulting "patterns" or "internal working models of attach-

ment" (Bowlby, 1969/1982) are necessary adaptations to the caregiving environment that allow the infant or child to maintain contact with and proximity to the caregiver, ensuring that basic needs for basic comfort and nurture are met, and that survival is guaranteed. They also protect the self from further disruptions and disappointments. Importantly, such patterns are *dynamic* rather than *static* entities. They are activated in (some) attachment-related situations, and function to maintain a particular state of mind in the self or the other. Thus, for instance, deactivation or detachment functions to control others and their proximity (and thus their potential to reject or hurt), to promote one's sense of self-reliance and independence, and to regulate unbearable emotions.

Such patterns are also dynamic in the sense that they sometimes elicit *opposing* tendencies in others, and may actually give way to *opposing* tendencies in the self. Imagine, for instance, a withdrawn husband and his needy, hyperactivating wife. Related to this is the notion that even the most dismissing individuals crave intense emotionality (hence they sometimes seek romantic partners who are their polar opposites), and that they themselves will shift strategies and in fact become quite hyperactivating when under pressure, or when trying to undo the effects of their withdrawal and isolation. The obverse is obviously true for preoccupied individuals.

Main locates these patterns in early interactions with the caregiver—interactions that have been internalized, and that form the basis for internal working models of attachment. It is crucial to understand that these models are inherently dyadic; the caregiver's response is encoded as part of the experience of seeking closeness and nurture. In other words, the activation of the attachment system is experienced both at an internal level and in a relational frame. Doctors (2007) has referred to these as "organizing principles." Here are two examples: "When I feel very hungry and mad, Mom puts me down and looks away, and I am scared," and "When I crawl around and get interested in things away from Mom, she gets sad and doesn't pay enough attention to me. If I start to cry, she gets very excited and picks me right up. That makes me feel safe." These represent the unconscious expectations that are generated in the face of particular affects or affect dysregulation.

The dynamics inherent in attachment organization (which Fonagy et al., 1995, refer to as "cognitive–affective schema[s]") and the organizing principles that arise from an adult's early relationships (and possibly later relationships and/or traumas) will be central issues in psychotherapy with patients struggling with the sequelae of insecure or disorganized attachment. Presumably, these patterns and their dynamics are what the therapist hopes will change.[10] Thus recognizing how and when these dynamics are activated in a patient's real-life relationships, and how they are activated in the therapeutic relationship, is an essential part of any good treatment (for clinical examples, see Holmes, 1998, 2000, 2001, 2004; Slade, 1999b, 2004b, 2007).

Tracking Attachment Processes in Language

One of the most important aspects of Main's work was her development of techniques to track the manifestations of insecure attachment in narratives. She noted that the various forms of insecure attachment are directly discernible in the dysfluencies and incoherence in narrative process, markers of which include changes in voice, contradictions, lapses, irrelevancies, and breakdowns in meaning during discussions of familial relationships. These are overt manifestations, in her view, of the "organizing principles" of an individual's early relationship experiences.

Main's methods of analysis are geared to identifying crucial elements of a particular attachment style or classification—the deactivating–hyperactivating dimension and the organized–disorganized dimension—with specific linguistic markers being linked to specific sorts of defensive operations. For instance, contradiction, shifts in voice, and idealization are linked to dismissing or deactivating strategies, and incoherence, breakdowns in meaning, and oscillation are linked to preoccupied or hyperactivating strategies.

In many ways, Main's work on narrative analysis provided empirical validation for crucial psychoanalytic assumptions: that flexible ego organization is key to adaptation, and that unintegrated thoughts and feelings affect the sense of self and other in important ways. In addition, the privileging of cognitive and linguistic rather than behavioral patterns, and the emphasis on the *organization* rather than the *content* of narratives, were entirely consistent with dynamic, clinical ways of listening to text, and with attention to meaning and defensive processes in the telling of a story. In these ways, by providing a number of linguistic and other markers to track defensive and integrative processes, Main operationalized some of the most subtle aspects of defense analysis and clinical listening.

And yet Main linked particular types of narratives to particular organizing principles about relationships in ways that were quite revolutionary. Essentially, her work suggests that listening for particular linguistic patterns, *as these reflect dismissing, preoccupied, or disorganized defensive organizations*, offers a direct view of how the adult regulates strong emotion experienced in the context of intimate (attachment) relationships. This obviously has direct relevance to the clinical enterprise. Thus, for instance, attending to language at this level invariably helps the therapist to imagine how the patient lives in the world and in relation to others, what he or she can tolerate feeling, and what he or she needs to make others feel in order to feel personally safe. What can be known, what can be felt, what can be spoken, and what cannot be contained? It further allows the therapist to understand the *function* of particular patterns of thought and feeling, as they protect the patient from intolerable experiences, and as they are designed to elicit ways of thinking and behaving in others (in both real and transferential aspects of such relationships).

Along these same lines, listening for attachment processes also offers the therapist a view to how early attachment relationships have been internalized and represented, and how nodal experiences of seeking comfort and care have been encoded in the structure and function of language. Thus attending both to *what* can and cannot be told, and to *how* it is told, helps the therapist to imagine patients' early experience in crucial ways. It helps the therapist to imagine the dynamic patterns that evolved in early childhood, to understand early empathic breaks with caregivers, and to identify islands of dissociated, unintegrated affective experience. It makes it possible to think much more closely about how early interactive experiences may be affecting responses to emotional upheaval and conflict, and may be affecting the way a patient thinks or does not think about emotion. Obviously, finding ways to imagine and describe a patient's ways of being in his or her primary relationships is crucial to helping the patient make meaning of early, often forgotten or unformulated experience.

The Impact on the Therapist of Listening for Attachment

There are several ways to think about how listening for and thinking in terms of attachment may affect the therapist and the therapeutic process. At one level, it will help him or her use language and metaphors that will be meaningful, evocative, and experience-near for the patient. Hearing patterns that reflect something essential about psychological organization, and about an individual's sense of how his or her emotions affect crucial others in his or her life, may provide a particularly direct entrée into the patient's experience. The more the therapist speaks in ways that reflect the patient's experience—that resonate with his or her way of being in the world—the deeper and more effective the work will be. And the more likely it is that the therapist will be experienced as a truly secure base for the patient's experience.

Equally important, it will help the therapist become more aware of the ways in which attachment-related strategies and dynamics are being activated in the patient's life, and/or within the context of the treatment hour. This raises the issue of how to respond to such dynamics when they occur. What is most likely to shift the patient's way of responding in a more "secure," balanced, and organized direction? For example, should the therapist respond "in style" or "out of style" when attachment-related defenses are activated? Although this issue is necessarily simplified in research, it is actually more complex when examined in a clinical context. Both Holmes and I have suggested, on the one hand, that there is value in gently challenging an individual's predominant defensive style. This means (to put it very simplistically) using more feeling-based or empathic responses for dismissing patients, and more intellectual or structuring responses for preoccupied patients. This is based on the assumption that dismissing or deactivating patients are likely to require more "attuning" (Holmes, 2000) responses than their preoccupied counterparts, for whom attunement is actually counterproductive and regressive. For dismissing patients, the goal of treatment will be to tolerate and express emotional experience that has been denied access to consciousness. Preoccupied or hyperactivating patients, by contrast, require more "containing" (Holmes, 2000) responses from the therapist, and have a greater need for organization and structure. The goal of treatment will be to contain and regulate that which remains overwhelming and possibly traumatizing (Holmes, 2001, 2004; Slade, 2004b, 2007).

Holmes (1998) has suggested that another, related way of describing these differences is as pathologies of narrative capacities. He sees the therapist's relation to narrative disruption as central to the work of therapy, which he suggests involves both "story making and story breaking"—helping the patient to tell a coherent story and allowing this story to be told in a different, perhaps more healing light. "Implicit in my argument so far is the view that psychological health (closely linked to secure attachment) depends on a dialectic between story making and story breaking, between the capacity to form narrative, and to disperse it in light of new experience" (Holmes, 1998, p. 59). Holmes defines "three prototypical pathologies of narrative capacity: clinging to rigid stories (the dismissing pattern); being overwhelmed by unstoried experience (the preoccupied pattern); or being unable to find a narrative strong enough to contain traumatic pain (the unresolved pattern)." By definition, insecure representational models preclude either story making (knitting together the events of one's life in a coherent way) or story breaking (examining the events of one's life anew in the light of new insight).

At the same time, it must be said that there is equal value in mirroring the patient's defensive organization when developing and strengthening the therapeutic alliance. One can hardly press a dismissing patient to express emotion until trust has been *well* established; likewise, one can hardly address a preoccupied patient's anxieties rationally and pragmatically until an alliance has been formed. And in both sorts of patients, this alliance is hard-won. Ruptures and fluctuating alliances are *de rigeur* in work with patients who are insecure in relation to attachment. Although it may be that ruptures are more tangible in working with preoccupied patients (Eames & Roth, 2000), the kinds of ruptures that take place with dismissing patients are more subtle, but just as disruptive. They are not, in some sense, ruptures at all; rather, it is only after a long period of time that the relationship is acknowledged to the point that a rupture can even be registered. In any event, working both with and in opposition to a patient's attachment style seems essential to the establishment and maintenance of an alliance, as well as to the promotion of therapeutic change.

Experienced therapists, and particularly those who are more secure in their own attachment organization, make these sorts of adjustments all the time, modulating their responses so as to most effectively engage an individual patient at a given moment in time (Daly & Mallinckrodt, 2008). And regardless of a patient's attachment organization, therapeutic success involves finding a way to help the patient become less rigid and inflexible, and more open to change. Thus, for instance, a therapist would hope that a more dismissing patient would be able to tolerate affects more readily, and that a preoccupied patient would be able to regulate intense affects and tolerate separateness more effectively. In this light, it is interesting to recall that in both the Diamond and colleagues (1999) and Travis and colleagues (2001) studies cited earlier, outcome assessments indicated that some patients had not become secure over the course of treatment, but rather had shifted to a different *insecure* attachment organization. What I would suggest is that these patients were evaluated in the middle of forming more flexible internal working models of attachment; that is, perhaps these patients were assessed at a time in therapy when their old ways of regulating affects and relationships had been destabilized. Only a later assessment would have revealed whether these patients were in fact "on the way" to developing more stable and secure modes of organization.

Therapists do not necessarily make these adaptations—from story making and story breaking, from mirroring to challenging—at a conscious level. Nor do they necessarily make them easily. As Hamilton (1987) noted, it is easy to get lost in a patient's characteristic way of responding, lost in the patterns. This is particularly true for beginning therapists. As a student therapist remarked to me recently, "It is very difficult to think and feel with patients at the same time" (L. Trub, personal communication, October 3, 2007). It is for this reason that it is important to describe these processes as clearly as possible—both because such clarity can help even seasoned therapists become more sensitive listeners and observers (Pine, 1985), and because such observations are of vital utility in training. Equally important, understanding these dynamics will be helpful in making sense of countertransference and other negative therapeutic reactions, even in a secure therapist. Each patient has the potential to evoke the therapist's own internal working models of attachment in a unique way: A dismissing patient's rejection of the therapist may make an insecure therapist feel hurt and thus withholding, whereas a preoccupied patient's neediness and dependency may make *that same therapist* respond in overly gratifying ways. Presumably, security affords a therapist the capacity to manage these experiences in such a way as to limit their impact on the treatment, but this does not mean that the therapist is impervious to their effects.

The construct of "coherence" offers another useful way to think about therapeutic outcome.

From Main's perspective, narrative coherence is one of the most robust markers of a secure attachment organization. Coherence is a construct that implies both a high level of organization and a flexible defensive style. This perspective is mirrored in many latter-day analytic approaches, which suggest that one outcome of a successful psychotherapy is the eventual discovery or creation of a "coherent" narrative—one that is "co-constructed" by patient and therapist. The development of a coherent narrative in this context refers to the idea that aspects of self-experience that have been defended against, distorted, or otherwise kept out of awareness can be integrated into a singular, organized sense of self. Defensive styles are softened, and structures for regulation of self and affect are more organized. This perspective seems totally in keeping with the notion of security and coherence arising out of a safe and collaborative attachment relationship. In fact, Bowlby's (1988) notion of a secure base seems especially well suited to describing the ways that the therapist provides a foundation from which the patient can explore the breadth and depth of his or her experience, without fear of loss or reprisal.

Attachment Theory and the Privileging of Fear

Finally, I turn to what is perhaps the most radical and least appreciated element of attachment theory—the privileging of fear in the development of psychopathology. Essential to attachment theory is the notion that psychopathology and maladaptation arise largely as a function of fear in the face of actual or perceived threats to a child's survival: fear of danger, fear of loss, fear of abandonment. Often these threats come from a primary caregiver; at other times they are external to this relationship. Such disruptions may be mild and transient, or they may be severe and chronic. In either case, because a child is biologically programmed to seek care from those to whom he or she is attached, the child's recourse in the face of fear is to do whatever is necessary to maintain a relationship with an attachment figure, even if the caregiver is the source of fear. In the latter case, the child must adapt to the implicit demands of this relationship in order to survive. Insecure attachment organizations are manifestations of this adaptive capacity; that is, the distortions in behavior, thinking, and feeling that typify each insecure category are manifestations of a primary attachment figure's unique demands.

In a variety of ways, Bowlby's view of what constitutes core and formative infantile experiences was vastly different from those of his more classical psychoanalytic contemporaries. Bowlby's privileging of fear rather than aggression challenges the notion of the infant (or patient) as having to relinquish the pleasure principle largely against his or her will, and replaces it with the notion of the infant as clinging to what is known and relatively safe (or to beliefs that, while maladaptive, preserve some sense of safety), while fearing the dangers and losses inherent in change. In the traditional model, anxiety is the result of threatened aggression from within; in the attachment model, aggression is a response to anxiety about both internal and external threats to one's essential safety and integrity. From this perspective, the "deep structure" for understanding others revolves around fear rather than anger.

The fact that Freud privileged aggression in his motivational system has much to do with the fact that he viewed most psychopathology through an Oedipal lens. This way of conceiving of psychopathology may be helpful in understanding the conflicts of more Oedipally organized neurotic patients for whom attachment difficulties are not central. For patients who are more pre-Oedipally organized, however—who struggle with dyadic regulation, who have difficulty with issues of intimacy and autonomy, or who have been disorganized by interpersonal trauma and/or loss[11]—Bowlby's privileging of fear makes far more sense.

Although many contemporary psychoanalysts view individuals who have suffered early disruptions in this way, the ramifications of this shift in emphasis have, from my perspective, been largely unelaborated in psychoanalytic theory. The emphasis on attachment and survival, which is of course *the* foundation upon which all attachment theory and classification rests, *implicitly* defines psychotherapy and psychoanalysis as attempting to help the patient relinquish maladaptive ways of being that were at one time essential to survival. From an attachment perspective, an individual's problematic ways of regulating emotion and relationships, as well as his or her resistance to change, are viewed as driven by the fear of losing what the person desperately needs to survive, literally and psychologically. From this perspective, the defenses not only function to protect the ego from unbearable affects, but also to protect the *other* from unbearable affects (e.g., rage at a caregiver for absence or abandonment), and to protect the self from thus *losing* the other (even if only internally). And aggression is seen as *reactive* to fear, rather than fear being the result of inherent aggression.

From this perspective, patients for whom attachment is a primary issue may best be understood as organized around fear rather than aggression. This reframing will have a major impact on the way we think about these patients, what we say to them, and how we manage the therapeutic encounter. It changes our therapeutic stance in subtle but profound ways. In particular, placing fear at the core of our understanding with these types of patients positions a therapist in sympathy with rather than opposition to a patient's defenses and resistance; these defenses were arrived at quite honestly, and they make enormous sense given the context of the patient's history. This sympathetic or compassionate (which does not mean gratifying) stance assumes that because the patient's adaptations to relationships and to his or her emotional life emerged in meaningful and purposeful ways, relinquishing them will undoubtedly be painful, difficult, and anxiety-provoking. In this sense, the therapist is more a collaborator than one digging for the unacknowledged "truth." This difference in stance will very much shape the therapeutic relationship and the patient's feeling of being held and understood.

In line with this argument, Bowlby's (1988) notion of the therapist as secure base is also actually quite radical (see Eagle, 2003; Eagle & Wolitzky, in press). To extrapolate the attachment–exploration balance to the clinical situation, a patient will not be free to explore his or her inner world until the patient is relatively free of anxiety. Relative freedom from anxiety emerges as a function of the development of a mutative and transforming relationship with a more benign and trustworthy attachment figure *who does not threaten the patient's safety or psychic integrity*. Although this perspective is in many ways concordant with contemporary analytic views of the therapist–patient relationship, there remain many vestiges of the notion that the patient's unconscious aggression must be confronted rather than held (see Breger, 2000) by the analyst. This perspective cannot help invading the work at a number of levels, and for insecure adults, this can only reify defenses and other adaptive mechanisms. This is not to say that there is no place within psychotherapy or psychoanalysis to confront aggression, infantile sexuality, and other forms of enactment and acting out. Rather, for patients who are insecure in relation to attachment, because aggression is a symptom and sequela of fear, the fear must be seen as the root rather than secondary issue. Then and only then can the patient explore his or her inner world and take ownership of aggression and other elements of emotional experience. It is my sense that even in the 21st century, elements of Freud's developmental theory continue to affect psychotherapists in powerful ways. The failure to fully rethink what is essential in early development continues to resonate throughout psychoanalytic theory, with what I believe is a distorting effect on technique. The next generation of psychoanalysts must grapple with the multiple ramifications of the emphasis on adaptation and fear that is unique to attachment theory.

MENTALIZATION-BASED THERAPIES

In this final major section, I briefly review work by Fonagy and his colleagues on clinical applications of mentalization theory (for a fuller description, see Fonagy et al., Chapter 33, this volume). Perhaps because Fonagy is a psychoanalyst writing from *within* psychoanalytic psychology, and because his contributions revolve around a construct that is explicitly noncategorical and more rooted in a psychoanalytic understanding of emotional functioning (as opposed to the more cognitive perspective of Main's construct of coherence, for instance), he has produced work on mentalization that has been far more widely accepted by psychodynamically oriented clinicians than Main's work. The construct of mentalization captures an essential difference between normal/neurotic individuals and those who are more disturbed, less emotionally accessible, and far more difficult to treat. It also beautifully captures what actually shifts and ultimately *changes* in good clinical work. As is self-evident to any experienced psychotherapist, "Any reasonable and effective psychotherapy is likely to enhance mentalizing capacity" (Allen, 2006, p. 19). Also, because of its relative methodological simplicity and clinical relevance, Fonagy's reflective functioning scale has been successfully used as an outcome measure in psychotherapy research (Diamond et al., 1999; Kernberg et al., 2008).

Over the past 10 years, Fonagy and his colleagues have focused on developing ways of enhancing mentalization in clinical populations. His efforts have led to the development of "mentalization-based therapy," which—although initially developed for use with borderline and other severe personality disorders—has been increasingly and widely adapted and disseminated for use in other treatment settings (see Allen & Fonagy, 2006; Fearon et al., 2006; Sadler, Slade, & Mayes, 2006; Slade, 2008; Slade, Sadler, & Mayes, 2005).

Mentalization-based therapy is an empirically validated treatment approach resting on the assumption that the maintenance of a mentalizing attitude is most compromised at times of intense affective arousal or stress. Failures of mentalization, reflected in nonmentalizing narratives, lead to coercive and controlling interactions with others (Allen, 2006; Bateman & Fonagy, 2004; Fearon et al., 2006; Fonagy, 2006). Thus therapy is designed to (1) develop the capacity to distinguish between mentalizing and nonmentalizing narratives, and support skillful mentalization; (2) develop the capacity to pause and reflect in the course of describing a nonmentalizing interaction or experience; (3) elicit and facilitate curiosity about the mental states of others; and (4) clarify and label acknowledged and unacknowledged feeling states. Importantly, the therapist and the therapeutic relationship are crucial to all versions of mentalization-based therapy. Just as secure attachment promotes mentalization in the early mother–child relationship, so will a "secure attachment climate promote mentalizing in psychotherapy" (Allen, 2006, p. 19). In initial clinical trials, this therapeutic approach has been effective in enhancing mentalization, as well as bringing about symptom remission in severely ill psychiatric patients (Bateman & Fonagy, 2004).

Although it might seem from this necessarily brief discussion that mentalization-based therapy is distinct from other psychotherapeutic efforts to modulate attachment-related defenses and dynamics, these approaches are in fact quite compatible and complementary. Helping patients to mentalize is an essential part of any good therapy, and indeed likely has much to do with the creation of a coherent treatment narrative, and other positive treatment outcomes. What I have argued here is that the *particular* understanding that comes from an attachment perspective, from attention to the dynamics of attachment-related defenses both in and out of the treatment context, will be especially helpful to the therapist in enhancing mentalization, and in guiding efforts to relax rigid and maladaptive ways of knowing, feeling, and being in the patient.

CLOSING NOTES

As a whole, the research, theory, and clinical work reviewed here suggests strongly that the dynamics of an individual's attachment organization, *as well as* his or her capacities for mentalization, will play a crucial role in the openness to and capacity to be helped by treatment. Given the complexities of the issues involved, however, there is still a good deal of work to be done to translate what has essentially been a research literature into the clinical domain. What I think would be most helpful at this juncture is to find a way to expose clinicians to the measures and methods of attachment research, so that they can more fully appreciate its core elements (see Slade, 2004a). The aim of such an effort would not be to teach clinicians to administer research measures per se, but to use methods to inform clinical listening and formulation.

The understanding of defense, affect regulation, motivation, and the dynamics of relationships that is provided by latter-day attachment theory does not replace other ways of understanding developmental and relational processes, but it can add to therapists' ways of listening to and understanding clinical material, and can be helpful with some (though not necessarily all) patients. Attachment and attachment processes constitute only one (admittedly very important) aspect of human functioning, and although attachment processes define an aspect of human experience, they do not *define* an individual in all his or her complexity. Nevertheless, an understanding of the processes so richly described by Bowlby, Ainsworth, Main, and Fonagy, along with a broad array of attachment theorists and researchers, can shed much light on the clinical enterprise and can serve as a valuable adjunct to good clinical work.

ACKNOWLEDGMENTS

I would like to acknowledge the many colleagues, students, and patients who have helped me understand the subtleties and complexities of the issues I have written about here. In particular, I would like to thank Jeremy Holmes and Morris Eagle, as well as Jude Cassidy and Phillip R. Shaver, who—as truly exceptional editors—have given me both a secure base from which to explore and the help I needed along the way to do this fully and thoughtfully.

NOTES

1. "Psychotherapy" is a term used to describe a wide range of therapeutic approaches that vary in duration, intensity, and goals, and that can be administered to families, couples, groups, and individual children or adults. A discussion of the complexity of and overlap among different forms of psychotherapy is beyond the scope of this chapter. Here I limit myself to a consideration of what is variously called "psychoanalytically oriented psychotherapy," "insight-oriented psychotherapy," and "dynamic psychotherapy." All of these terms refer to the idea that there exists a dynamic relation between early childhood experience and current adaptation; the aim of treatment in this form of psychotherapy is to illuminate the emotional and structural links between past and present experience. Bowlby himself was a psychoanalytic psychotherapist; thus an emphasis on the representation of early childhood experience is intrinsic to both attachment theory and psychoanalytic psychotherapy.

2. Although these two terms are used interchangeably in this chapter, it is important to note that Fonagy reserves the term "mentalization" to describe the process of envisioning mental states. The term "reflective functioning" refers to the operationalization of the mentalizing capacity.

3. It should be noted, however, that this finding does not make clear whether mentalizing capacities develop prior or subsequent to the trauma, or how one develops mentalizing capacities in the face of trauma.

4. Obviously research on attachment and psychotherapy is related to research on attachment and psychopathology. This is reviewed by DeKlyen & Greenberg, Chapter 27, this volume, and by Dozier, Stovall-McClough, & Albus, Chapter 30, this volume.

5. Interestingly, the failure to link *type* of insecurity with particular disruptions in the therapeutic relationship is consistent with the relative failure of both infant and adult attachment research to reliably distinguish the antecedents or sequelae of avoidant/dismissing and resistant/preoccupied attachment. This probably has to do with the substantial overlap between the resistant/preoccupied, disorganized/unresolved, and cannot classify categories—overlap that makes it difficult to delineate fine-grained distinctions between these insecure categories. Also, perhaps the assumption (see Main, 2000) that the preoccupied pattern is a form of "organized" insecurity needs to be reexamined.

6. As Main (1995) has suggested, this raises important issues for the training and supervision of therapists. Obviously, the expectation within virtually all psychodynamic schools of thought that personal psychoanalysis or psychotherapy is a crucial part of any therapist's training is meant to address some of these concerns. See also Daly and Mallinckrodt (2008) for a discussion of the value of clinical experience in remaining flexible in the therapeutic situation.

7. Importantly, the issue of how therapist attachment organization is specifically linked to the countertransference—while mentioned in a small number of studies—has yet to be investigated in its own right.

8. It is difficult to interpret the results of two other outcome studies (Horowitz, Rosenberg, & Bartholomew, 1993; Meyer, Pilkonis, Proietti, Heape, & Egan, 2001) as the result of differences in measures used to derive patient attachment organization.

9. It is important to note that this way of thinking is quite distinct from the effort to link attachment organization to diagnostic category, which has been largely unsuccessful (see Dozier et al., Chapter 30, this volume), because diagnosis does not necessarily imply one or another type of defense or level of character organization.

10. Westen et al. (2006) have noted in this regard that attachment organization is in this sense the "target" of change, rather than an indicator of outcome per se.

11. Sadly, this would include many of Freud's own patients (Breger, 2000).

REFERENCES

Agrawal, H. R., Gunderson, J., Holmes, B., & Lyons-Ruth, K. (2004). Attachment studies with borderline patients. *Harvard Review of Psychiatry, 12*(2), 94–104.

Ainsworth, M. D. S., Blehar, M. C., Waters, E., & Wall, S. (1978). *Patterns of attachment: A psychological study of the Strange Situation*. Hillsdale, NJ: Erlbaum.

Allen, J. G. (2006). Mentalizing in practice. In J. G. Allen & P. Fonagy (Eds.), *Handbook of mentalization-based treatment* (pp. 3–30). Chichester, UK: Wiley.

Allen, J. G., & Fonagy, P. (Eds.). (2006). *Handbook of mentalization-based treatment*. Chichester, UK: Wiley.

Atkinson, L., & Goldberg, S. (Eds.). (2004). *Attachment issues in psychopathology and intervention*. Mahwah, NJ: Erlbaum.

Bartholomew, K., & Horowitz, L. M. (1991). Attachment styles among young adults: A test of a four-category model. *Journal of Personality and Social Psychology, 61*, 226–244.

Bateman, A., & Fonagy, P. (2004). *Psychotherapy for borderline personality disorder: Mentalization-based treatment*. Oxford, UK: Oxford University Press.

Bernier, A., & Dozier, M. (2000). The client–counselor match and the corrective emotional experience: Evidence from interpersonal and attachment research. *Psychotherapy: Theory, Research, Practice, Training, 39*, 32–43.

Black, S., Hardy, G., Turpin, G., & Parry, G. (2005). Self-reported attachment styles and therapeutic orientation of therapists and their relationship with reported general alliance quality and problems in therapy. *Psychology and Psychotherapy, 78*, 363–377.

Borman-Spurrell, E. (1996). *Patterns of adult attachment and psychotherapy outcomes for patients with binge eating disorder*. Unpublished doctoral dissertation, Yale University.

Bowlby, J. (1944). Forty-four juvenile thieves: Their characters and home life. *International Journal of Psycho-Analysis, 25*, 19–52, 107–127.

Bowlby, J. (1969/1982). *Attachment and loss: Vol. 1. Attachment*. New York: Basic Books.

Bowlby, J. (1973). *Attachment and loss: Vol. 2. Separation: Anxiety and anger*. New York: Basic Books.

Bowlby, J. (1979). *The making and breaking of affectional bonds*. London: Tavistock/Routledge.

Bowlby, J. (1980). *Attachment and loss: Vol. 3. Loss: Sadness and depression*. New York: Basic Books.

Bowlby, J. (1988). *A secure base: Parent–child attachment and healthy human development*. New York: Basic Books.

Bradley, R., Heim, A. K., & Westen, D. (2005). Transference patterns in the psychotherapy of personality disorders: Empirical investigation. *British Journal of Psychiatry, 186*, 342–349.

Breger, L. (2000). *Freud: Darkness in the midst of vision*. New York: Wiley.

Brennan, K. A., Clark, C. L., & Shaver, P. (1998). Self-report measures of adult romantic attachment. In J. A. Simpson & W. S. Rhodes (Eds.), *Attachment theory and close relationships* (pp. 46–76). New York: Guilford Press.

Collins, N. L., & Read, S. J. (1990). Adult attachment, working models, and relationship quality in dating couples. *Journal of Personality and Social Psychology, 58*, 644–663.

Daly, K., & Mallinckrodt, B. (2008). *A grounded-theory model of experts' approach to psychotherapy for clients with attachment avoidance or attachment anxiety*. Manuscript submitted for publication.

Daniel, S. I. F. (2006). Adult attachment patterns and individual psychotherapy: A review. *Clinical Psychology Review, 26*, 968–984.

Diamond, D., Clarkin, J., Levine, H., Levy, K., Foelsch, P., & Yeomans, F. (1999). Borderline conditions and attachment: A preliminary report. *Psychoanalytic Inquiry, 19*, 831–884.

Diamond, D., Stovall-McClough, C., Clarkin, J., & Levy, K. N. (2003). Patient–therapist attachment in the treatment of borderline personality disorder. *Bulletin of the Menninger Clinic, 67*, 227–259.

Doctors, S. (2007). On utilizing attachment theory and research in self psychological/intersubjective clinical work. In P. Buirski & A. Kottler (Eds.), *New developments in self psychology practice* (pp. 23–48). Lanham, MD: Aronson.

Dolan, R. T., Arnkoff, D. B., & Glass, C. R. (1993). Client attachment style and the psychotherapist's interpersonal stance. *Psychotherapy, 30*, 408–412.

Dozier, M. (1990). Attachment organization and treatment use for adults with serious psychopathological disorders. *Development and Psychopathology, 2*, 47–60.

Dozier, M., Cue, K., & Barnett, L. (1994). Clinicians as caregivers: Role of attachment organization in treatment. *Journal of Consulting and Clinical Psychology, 62*, 793–800.

Dozier, M., Lomax, L., Tyrrell, C., & Lee, S. (2001). The challenge of treatment for clients with dismissing states of mind. *Attachment and Human Development, 3*, 62–76.

Dunkle, J. H., & Friedlander, M. L. (1996). Contribution of therapist experience and personal characteristics to the working alliance. *Journal of Counseling Psychology, 43*, 456–460.

Eagle, M. (2003). Clinical implications of attachment theory. *Psychoanalytic Inquiry, 23,* 27–53.

Eagle, M., & Wolitzky, D. (in press). The perspectives of attachment theory and psychoanalysis: Adult psychotherapy. In J. H. Obegi & E. Berant (Eds.), *Clinical applications of adult attachment research.* New York: Guilford Press.

Eames, V., & Roth, A. (2000). Patient attachment orientation and the early working alliance: A study of patient and therapist reports of alliance quality and ruptures. *Psychotherapy Research, 10,* 421–434.

Farber, B. A., Lippert, R. A., & Nevas, D. B. (1995). The therapist as attachment figure. *Psychotherapy, 32,* 204–212.

Fearon, R. M. P., Target, M., Sargent, J., Williams, L., McGregor, J., Bleiberg, E., et al. (2006). Short-term mentalization and relational therapy (SMART): An integrative family therapy for children and adolescents. In J. Allen & P. Fonagy (Eds.), *Handbook of mentalization-based treatment* (pp. 201–222). Chichester, UK: Wiley.

Fonagy, P. (2001). *Attachment theory and psychoanalysis.* New York: Other Press.

Fonagy, P. (2006). The mentalization-focused approach to social development. In J. Allen & P. Fonagy (Eds.), *Handbook of mentalization-based treatment* (pp. 53–100). Chichester, UK: Wiley.

Fonagy, P., Gergely, G., Jurist, E., & Target, M. (2002). *Affect regulation, mentalization, and the development of the self.* New York: Other Press.

Fonagy, P., Leigh, T., Steele, M., Steele, H., Kennedy, R., Mattoon, G., et al. (1996). The relation of attachment status, psychiatric classification and response to psychotherapy. *Journal of Consulting and Clinical Psychology, 64,* 22–31.

Fonagy, P., Steele, M., Steele, H., Leigh, T., Kennedy, R., Mattoon, G., et al. 1995). Attachment, the reflective self, and borderline states: The predictive specificity of the Adult Attachment Interview and pathological emotional development. In S. Goldberg, R. Muir, & J. Kerr (Eds.), *Attachment theory: Social, developmental, and clinical perspectives* (pp. 233–279). Hillsdale, NJ: Analytic Press.

Fonagy, P., Target, M., Steele, H., & Steele, M. (1998). *Reflective functioning manual, versions 5.0, for application to Adult Attachment Interviews.* London: University College London.

George, C., Kaplan, N., & Main, M. (1984). *Adult Attachment Interview protocol.* Unpublished manuscript, University of California at Berkeley.

George, C., Kaplan, N., & Main, M. (1985). *Adult Attachment Interview protocol* (2nd ed.). Unpublished manuscript, University of California at Berkeley.

George, C., Kaplan, N., & Main, M. (1996). *Adult Attachment Interview protocol* (3rd ed.). Unpublished manuscript, University of California at Berkeley.

Griffin, D., & Bartholomew, K. (1994). Models of the self and other: Fundamental dimensions underlying measures of adult attachment. *Journal of Personality and Social Psychology, 67,* 430–445.

Hamilton, V. (1987). Some problems in the clinical application of attachment theory. *Psychoanalytic Psychotherapy, 3,* 7–83.

Hardy, G. E., Aldridge, J., Davidson, C., Rowe, C., Reilly, S., & Shapiro, D. A. (1999). Therapist responsiveness to client attachment styles and issues observed in client-identified significant events in psychodynamic–interpersonal psychotherapy. *Psychotherapy Research, 9,* 36–53.

Hesse, E. (1996). Discourse, memory, and the Adult Attachment Interview: A note with emphasis on the emerging cannot classify category. *Infant Mental Health Journal, 17,* 4–11.

Holmes, J. (1998). Defensive and creative uses of narrative in psychotherapy: An attachment perspective. In G. Roberts & J. Holmes (Eds.), *Narrative in psychotherapy and psychiatry* (pp. 49–68). Oxford, UK: Oxford University Press.

Holmes, J. (2000). Attachment theory and psychoanalysis: A rapprochement. *British Journal of Psychotherapy, 17,* 157–172.

Holmes, J. (2001). *The search for the secure base: Attachment theory and psychotherapy.* London: Taylor & Francis.

Holmes, J. (2004). Disorganized attachment and borderline personality disorder: A clinical perspective. *Attachment and Human Development, 6,* 181–190.

Horowitz, L. M., Rosenberg, S. E., & Bartholomew, K. (1993). Interpersonal problems, attachment styles, and outcome in brief dynamic psychotherapy. *Journal of Consulting and Clinical Psychology, 61,* 549–560.

Kanninen, K., Salo, J., & Punamaki, R. L.(2000). Attachment patterns and working alliance in trauma therapy for victims of political violence. *Psychotherapy Research, 10,* 435–449.

Karen, R. (1998). *Becoming attached: First relationships and how they shape our capacity to love.* New York: Oxford University Press.

Kernberg, O., Diamond, D., Yeomans, F. E., Clarkin, J. R., & Levy, K. N. (2008). Mentalization and attachment in borderline patients in transference focused psychotherapy. In E. Jurist, A. Slade, & S. Bergner (Eds.), *Mind to mind: Infant research, neuroscience, and psychoanalysis* (pp. 167–201). New York: Other Press.

Kivlighan, D. M., Jr., Patton, M. J., & Foote, D. (1998). Moderating effects of client attachment on the counselor experience–working alliance relationship. *Journal of Counseling Psychology, 45,* 274–278.

Kobak, R. R., Cole, H. E., Ferenz-Gillies, R., & Fleming, W. S. (1993). Attachment and emotion regulation during mother–teen problem solving: A control theory analysis. *Child Development, 64,* 231–245.

Levy, K. N., Meehan, K., Kelly, K. M., Reynoso, J., Weber, M., Clarkin, J., et al. (2006). Changes in attachment patterns and reflective function in a randomized control trial of transference-focused psychotherapy for borderline personality disorder. *Journal of Consulting and Clinical Psychology, 74,* 1027–1040.

Ligiero, D. P., & Gelso, C. J. (2002). Countertransference, attachment, and the working alliance: The therapist's contribution. *Psychotherapy: Theory, Research, Practice, Training, 39,* 3–11.

Linehan, M. M. (1993). *Cognitive-behavioral treatment of borderline personality disorder.* New York: Guilford Press.

Lopez, F. G., Melendez, M. C., Sauer, E. M., Berger, E., & Wyssmann, J. (1998). Internal working models, self-reported problems, and help-seeking attitudes among college students. *Journal of Counseling Psychology, 45,* 79–83.

Main, M. (1991). Metacognitive knowledge, metacognitive monitoring, and singular (coherent) vs. multiple (incoherent) model of attachment: Findings and directions for future research. In C. Parkes, J. Stevenson-Hinde, & P. Marris (Eds.), *Attachment across the life cycle* (pp. 127–160). London: Routledge.

Main, M. (1995). Recent studies in attachment: Overview, with selected implications for clinical work. In S. Goldberg, R. Muir, & J. Kerr (Eds.), *Attachment theory: Social, developmental, and clinical perspectives* (pp. 407–475). Hillsdale, NJ: Analytic Press.

Main, M. (2000). The organized categories of infant, child, and adult attachment: Flexible vs. inflexible attention under attachment-related stress. *Journal of the American Psychoanalytic Association, 48,* 1055–1096.

Main, M., & Goldwyn, R. (1984). *Adult attachment scoring and classification system.* Unpublished manuscript, University of California at Berkeley.

Main, M., Goldwyn, R., & Hesse, E. (2003). *Adult attachment scoring and classification system.* Unpublished manuscript, University of California at Berkeley.

Main, M., Kaplan, N., & Cassidy, J. (1985). Security in infancy, childhood, and adulthood: A move to the level of representation. In I. Bretherton & E. Waters (Eds.), Growing points of attachment theory and research. *Monographs of the Society for Research in Child Development, 50*(1–2, Serial No. 209), 66–104.

Main, M., & Solomon, J. (1990). Procedures for identifying infants disorganized/disoriented during the Ainsworth Strange Situation. In M. T. Greenberg, D. Cicchetti, & E. M. Cummings (Eds.), *Attachment in the preschool years: Theory, research, and intervention* (pp. 95–124). Chicago: University of Chicago Press.

Mallinckrodt, B., Coble, H. M., & Gantt, D. L. (1995). Working alliance, attachment memories, and competencies of women in brief therapy. *Journal of Counseling Psychology, 42,* 79–84.

Mallinckrodt, B., Gantt, D. L., & Coble, H. M. (1995). Attachment patterns in the psychotherapy relationship: Development of the Client Attachment to Therapist Scale. *Journal of Counseling Psychology, 42,* 307–317.

Mallinckrodt, B., Porter, M. J., & Kivlighan, D. M., Jr. (2005). Client attachment to therapist, depth of in-session exploration, and object relations in brief psychotherapy. *Psychotherapy: Theory, Research, Practice, Training, 42,* 85–100.

McBride, C., Atkinson, L., Quilty, L. C., & Bagby, R. M. (2006). Attachment as moderator of treatment outcome in major depression: A randomized control trial of interpersonal psychotherapy vs. cognitive behaviour therapy. *Journal of Consulting and Clinical Psychology, 74,* 1041–1054.

Meyer, B., Pilkonis, P. A., Proietti, J. M., Heape, C. L., & Egan, M. (2001). Attachment styles and personality disorders as predictors of symptom course. *Journal of Personality Disorders, 15,* 371–389.

Mikulincer, M., Shaver, P. R., & Cassidy, J. (in press). Attachment-related defensive processes. In J. H. Obegi & E. Berant (Eds.), *Clinical applications of adult attachment research.* New York: Guilford Press.

Oppenheim, D., & Goldsmith, D. (Eds.). (2007). *Attachment theory in clinical work with children: Bridging the gap between research and practice.* New York: Guilford Press.

Parish, M., & Eagle, M. N. (2003). Attachment to the therapist. *Psychoanalytic Psychology, 20,* 271–286.

Pine, F. (1985). *Developmental theory and clinical process.* New Haven, CT: Yale University Press.

Riggs, S. A., Jacobvitz, D., & Hazen, N. (2002). Adult attachment and history of psychotherapy in a normative sample. *Psychotherapy: Theory, Research, Practice, Training, 39,* 344–353.

Rubino, G., Barker, C., Roth, T., & Fearon, R. M. P. (2000). Therapist empathy and depth of interpretation in response to potential alliance ruptures: The role of therapist and patient attachment styles. *Psychotherapy Research, 10,* 408–420.

Sable, P. (2000). *Attachment and adult psychotherapy.* Northvale, NJ: Aronson.

Sadler, L. S., Slade, A., & Mayes, L. C. (2006). Minding the Baby: A mentalization-based parenting program. In J. G. Allen & P. Fonagy (Eds.), *Handbook of mentalization-based treatment* (pp. 271–288). Chichester, UK: Wiley.

Satterfield, W. A., & Lyddon, W. J. (1995). Client attachment and perceptions of the working alliance with counselor trainees. *Journal of Counseling Psychology, 42,* 187–189.

Sauer, E. M., Lopez, F. G., & Gormley, B. (2003). Respective contributions of therapist and client adult attachment orientations to the development of the early working alliance: A preliminary growth modeling study. *Psychotherapy Research, 13,* 371–382.

Shapiro, D. (1999). *Neurotic styles.* New York: Perseus. (Original work published 1965)

Shaver, P. R., Belsky, J., & Brennan, K. A. (2000). The Adult Attachment Interview and self-reports of romantic attachment: Associations across domains and methods. *Personal Relationships, 7,* 25–43.

Slade, A. (1999a). Attachment theory and research: Implications for the theory and practice of individual psychotherapy with adults. In J. Cassidy & P. R. Shaver (Eds.), *Handbook of attachment: Theory, research, and clinical applications* (pp. 575–594). New York: Guilford Press.

Slade, A. (1999b). Representation, symbolization, and affect regulation in the concomitant treatment of a mother and child: Attachment theory and child psychotherapy. *Psychoanalytic Inquiry, 19,* 797–830.

Slade, A. (2000). The development and organization of attachment: Implications for psychoanalysis. *Journal of the American Psychoanalytic Association, 48,* 1147–1174.

Slade, A. (2004a). The move from categories to phenomena: Attachment processes and clinical evaluation. *Infant Mental Health Journal, 25,* 1–15.

Slade, A. (2004b). Two therapies: Attachment organization and the clinical process. In L. Atkinson & S. Goldberg (Eds.), *Attachment issues in psychopathology and intervention* (pp. 181–206). Mahwah, NJ: Erlbaum.

Slade, A. (2005). Parental reflective functioning: An introduction. *Attachment and Human Development, 7,* 269–281.

Slade, A. (2007). Disorganized mother, disorganized child: The mentalization of affective dysregulation and therapeutic change. In D. Oppenheim & D. Goldsmith (Eds.), *Attachment theory in clinical work with children: Bridging the gap between research and practice* (pp. 226–250). New York: Guilford Press.

Slade, A. (2008). Working with parents in child psychotherapy: Engaging reflective capacities. In E. Jurist, A. Slade, & S. Bergner (Eds.), *Mind to mind: Infant research, neuroscience, and psychoanalysis* (pp. 307–334). New York: Other Press.

Slade, A., Grienenberger, J., Bernbach, E., Levy, D., & Locker, A. (2005). Maternal reflective functioning and attachment: Considering the transmission gap. *Attachment and Human Development, 7,* 283–292.

Slade, A., Sadler, L., & Mayes, L. C. (2005). Minding the Baby: Enhancing parental reflective functioning in a nursing/mental health home visiting program. In L. Berlin, Y. Ziv, L. Amaya-Jackson, & M. T. Greenberg (Eds.), *Enhancing early attachments: Theory, research, intervention, and policy* (pp. 152–177). New York: Guilford Press.

Tasca, G. A., Ritchie, K., Conrad, G., Balfour, L., Gayton, J., Lybanon, V., et al. (2006). Attachment scales predict outcome in a randomized controlled trial of two group therapies for binge eating disorder: An aptitude by treatment interaction. *Psychotherapy Research, 16,* 106–121.

Travis, L. A., Bliwise, N. G., Binder, J. L., & Horne Meyer, H. L. (2001). Changes in clients' attachment styles over the course of time-limited dynamic psychotherapy. *Psychotherapy: Theory, Research, Practice, and Training, 38,* 149–159.

Tyrrell, C. L., Dozier, M., Teague, G. B., & Fallot, R. D. (1999). Effective treatment relationships for persons with serious psychiatric disorders: The importance of attachment states of mind. *Journal of Consulting and Clinical Psychology, 67,* 725–733.

van IJzendoorn, M. H. (1995). Adult attachment representations, parental responsiveness, and infant attachment: A meta-analysis on the predictive validity of the Adult Attachment Interview. *Psychological Bulletin, 117,* 387–403.

van IJzendoorn, M. H., & Bakermans-Kranenburg, M. J. (1996). Attachment representations in mothers, fathers, adolescents, and clinical groups: A meta-analytic search for normative data. *Journal of Consulting and Clinical Psychology, 64,* 8–21.

Wallin, D. (2007). *Attachment and psychotherapy.* New York: Guilford Press.

Waters, E., Hamilton, C. E., & Weinfield, N. S. (2000). The stability of attachment from infancy to adolescence and early adulthood: General introduction. *Child Development, 71,* 678–683.

Westen, D., Nakash, O., Thomas, C., & Bradley, R. (2006). Clinical assessment of attachment patterns and personality disorder in adolescents and adults. *Journal of Consulting and Clinical Psychology, 74,* 1065–1085.

Woodhouse, S. S., Schlosser, L. Z., Crook, R. E., Ligiero, D. P., & Gelso, C. J. (2003). Client attachment to therapist: Relations to transference and client recollections of parental caregiving. *Journal of Counseling Psychology, 50,* 395–408.

CHAPTER 33

Psychoanalytic Constructs
and Attachment Theory and Research

PETER FONAGY
GEORGE GERGELY
MARY TARGET

Over the last 15–20 years, attachment theory has become a topic "of the highest importance for psychoanalysis and psychoanalysts" (Sandler, 2003, p. 13). Hundreds of papers, special issues of journals, and a slew of monographs integrating psychodynamic clinical work with attachment theory and research have appeared. In the first edition of this handbook (Fonagy, 1999b) and in a separate monograph (Fonagy, 2001a), Fonagy identified points of contact and divergence between attachment theory and psychoanalytic theories as a whole. This chapter presents a more selective consideration of the issue. First, we analyze the overarching relation between attachment theory and psychoanalysis, exploring common general assumptions and changes in psychoanalytic thinking that may account for the increasing acceptance of attachment theory. We then closely examine two areas of active integrative work: relational psychoanalysis, where the move is from a well-established set of psychoanalytic ideas toward attachment theory and research; and mentalization-based theory and treatment, where research originally undertaken from an attachment theory and laboratory-based perspective aims to make contact with clinical concerns and ideas.

ANALYZING THE RELATIONSHIP BETWEEN PSYCHOANALYSIS AND ATTACHMENT THEORY

The recent rapprochement between psychoanalysis and attachment theory results from (1) the common ground between the two theoretical frameworks, as elaborated systematically by attachment theorists and researchers; (2) a shift in what psychoanalysts implicitly consider core to their discipline (Canestri, Fonagy, Bohleber, & Dennis, 2006); and (3) the emergence of both a psychoanalytically rooted exploration of the attachment system (relational psychoanalysis) and an attachment-rooted psychoanalytic clinical approach (mentalization-based theory and treatment).

Common Foundations

Although unlikely to be embraced by all psychoanalytic theorists, the following precepts may constitute a common terrain for attachment theory and psychoanalytic approaches (Holmes & Bateman, 2002; Person, Gabbard, & Cooper, 2005):

1. *A shared notion of psychological causation.* All psychodynamic approaches, including attach-

ment theory, assume that mental disorders can be meaningfully understood as specific organizations of an individual's conscious or unconscious beliefs, thoughts, and feelings. Whereas Bowlby argued that interpersonal experiences, particularly in the family context, could account for many disorders, he was equally clear that in his psychological model, social influences are understood to act on cognitive structures (Bowlby, 1988a). Thus, whereas both psychoanalytic and attachment theories acknowledge a wide range of influences on personality development, both assume that we need (also) to understand and address these influences at the level of the individual's beliefs, wishes, and feelings.

2. *The central role of the first object in psychic functioning.* Even those who are hostile to attachment theory acknowledge a shared concern in Bowlby's insistence on the formative nature of the mother–infant relationship (e.g., Zepf, 2006). Both theoretical frameworks claim that the first years of life play a fundamental role in personality development, and they agree that maternal sensitivity is a key causal factor in determining psychic development. Both also claim that the infant–caregiver relationship is based on an independent need for a relationship that creates the biological context within which mental functions can develop (Fonagy, 2001a, pp. 158–164).

3. *Limitations of consciousness and the influence of nonconscious mental states.* Psychodynamic clinicians and attachment theorists both generally assume that to understand conscious experiences, we need to refer to other mental states of which the individual is unaware. In both theoretical frameworks, nonconscious narrative-like experiences, analogous to conscious fantasies, are assumed implicitly and explicitly to influence behavior and the capacity both to regulate affect and to handle interpersonal environments. This should not be taken to diminish the emphasis placed on consciousness by either attachment theory or psychoanalysis. For both Bowlby and Freud, it is the effect that *awareness* of unconscious expectations can have on behavior that places work with what is nonconscious at the heart of the dynamic approach.

4. *The assumption of internal representations of interpersonal relationships.* Attachment theorists and psychodynamic clinicians are by no means alone in considering interpersonal relationships (and family relationships in particular) to be key to the organization of personality. Both theoretical frameworks, however, differ from other social-psychological approaches in which current interpersonal relationships are emphasized, because they assume that intense relationship experiences are internalized and aggregated over time, thereby forming schematic mental structures that shape both later interpersonal expectations and self-representations. Within both attachment theory and many psychoanalytic models, self–other relationship representations are also considered as the organizers of emotion, and particular feelings are thought to characterize particular patterns of interpersonal relating.

5. *The ubiquity of psychological conflict.* It is axiomatic for both theoretical frameworks that wishes, affects, and ideas will at times come into conflict. Both theories see incompatibilities of motive, thought, and feeling as key causes of distress and the lack of a sense of safety (Main & Morgan, 1996). Clinical experience shows that such conflicts are frequently associated with adverse environmental conditions (Hennighausen & Lyons-Ruth, 2005). For example, neglect or abuse is likely to aggravate a child's arguably natural but mild predisposition to relate with mixed feelings to the caregiver, who is perceived as vital to the child's continuing existence. Attachment and psychodynamic models often diverge in their clinical foci: The former aims to address conflicts between an individual's needs and expectations regarding the attachment figure; the latter focuses on the conflict between the need for and the internal rejection of the attachment figure and the contempt that subsequently arises (Eagle, 2006). In both theoretical contexts, however, conflicts are thought not only to cause distress, but also potentially to undermine the normal development of key psychological capacities (Fonagy & Target, 2003; Freud, 1965).

6. *The assumption of psychic defenses.* Both attachment theory and psychoanalysis are organized around the idea of mental operations that distort conscious mental states to reduce their capacity to generate anxiety, distress, or displeasure. Self-serving distortions of mental states are generally accepted and are frequently demonstrated experimentally in an attachment context (Blagov & Singer, 2004; Lyons-Ruth, 2003). Internal working models are often defensive; for example, traumatic experiences may give rise to omnipotent internal working models to address a feeling of helplessness. Deactivating (dismissing or avoidant) attachment strategies include defensively suppressing ideas related to painful attachment experiences, repressing painful memories, minimizing stress and dis-

tress, and segregating mental systems to exclude distressing material from the stream of consciousness (Bowlby, 1980; Cassidy & Kobak, 1988; Mikulincer, Shaver, & Cassidy, in press).

7. *The assumption of complex meanings.* In terms of the specific meanings that clinicians assign to particular pieces of behavior, there are major differences between many psychodynamic approaches and attachment theory. However, both frames of reference assume that behavior may be understood in terms of mental states that are not explicit within the awareness of the person concerned.

8. *The emphasis on the therapeutic relationship.* There is a consensus that aspects of relationships with supportive, respectful, and empathic people will benefit patients. Within different clinical models, the significance of establishing an attachment relationship with a clinician may be understood differently. Ferenczi (1922/1980) and Winnicott (1965) both emphasized the mutative aspects of the new personal and emotional experiences provided by therapy. Bowlby's (1988b) suggestion that therapists function as a secure base implies that psychodynamic therapists are, in part, conducting attachment therapy. There is accumulating evidence for this claim (Diamond, Stovall-McClough, Clarkin, & Levy, 2003; Parish & Eagle, 2003). Converging theorization and research data suggest that engagement with an understanding and sympathetic adult triggers a basic set of human capacities for relatedness and generates an alliance that appears therapeutic—apparently almost regardless of content—and that the quality of the alliance is one of the better predictors of outcome (Orlinsky, Ronnestad, & Willutski, 2004).

9. *A developmental perspective.* Psychodynamic psychotherapies are formulated in developmental terms, although specific assumptions concerning normal and abnormal child and adolescent development vary (Fonagy, Target, & Gergely, 2006). This developmental orientation generates a shared clinical orientation with attachment theory, because therapists are invariably interested in the developmental aspects of their patients' presenting problems, and work at least in part to optimize developmental processes, sometimes in the somewhat naive hope of rekindling an aborted developmental process (e.g., Gedo, 1979).

Reviews of longitudinal studies of attachment confirm that the quality of early experiences with caregivers is reflected in adaptation to salient life tasks at least through young adulthood (Grossmann, Grossmann, & Waters, 2005; see Wein-

field, Sroufe, Egeland, & Carlson, Chapter 4, this volume), although a number of influential scholars continue to express doubts about this (e.g., Bruer, 2002). In any case, neither psychoanalytic nor attachment theories are developmentally deterministic models. Attachment research reveals the ongoing impact of early experiences even when later experiences are controlled for. It also gives ample indication of complex developmental paths with cumulative effects, as well as of the increasingly active role of the individual in determining his or her environment, including the interpersonal world.

In asserting the connections between childhood and adulthood, psychoanalytic approaches often go considerably beyond attachment research, which warns us about the danger of making unequivocal links between past and present. For example, Adult Attachment Interview (AAI) accounts of childhood highlight that even when there is a "fit" between attachment classification in infancy and adult attachment, the historical construction is less than perfect. Adults with so-called "earned-secure" attachment status (i.e., those who, according to their attachment narratives, appear to have struggled out of insecure relationships to achieve adult attachment security) are most likely to have been secure in infancy as well, and the historical account of "earning security" is more of an indication of their *current* states of mind than of their actual childhood experiences (Grossmann et al., 2005).

Changes in Psychoanalytic Ideas

Changes in psychoanalytic thinking may have contributed to the recent rapprochement of psychoanalysis and attachment theory. Psychoanalysis has become more pluralistic and accepting of differences (e.g., Wallerstein, 2005), but there are other factors:

1. The increasing hegemony of object relations models has created a psychoanalytic culture in which attachment theory's emphasis on an autonomous need for a relationship is increasingly embraced by all (with a few notable exceptions; e.g., Widlocher & Fairfield, 2004). This shift has been one of those implicit theoretical changes in psychoanalysis to which Sandler (1983) alerted us, and it has only recently become a subject of systematic study (Canestri, 2006).

2. Closely linked with the dominance of object relations theory is the increasing interest

in infant development as a legitimate way of explaining differences in adult behavior. Although this interest is controversial (see Geyskens, 2003), the opportunity that attachment theory affords to systematize infant–caretaker behavior and to make it emotionally meaningful undoubtedly assists in integrating such concepts as affect regulation, sensitivity, and bonding into clinical psychoanalytic vocabulary. The work of Beebe (e.g., Jaffe, Beebe, Feldstein, Crown, & Jasnow, 2001), Emde (e.g., Emde & Spicer, 2000), and others has been reviewed frequently and systematically (Gergely, 2000; Tyson & Tyson, 1990)—and there has been a gradual modification of the image of the "psychoanalytic infant" from a hypothetical creature based on speculative reconstruction from adult narratives, to a picture that is constrained and moderated by actual systematic observations of children.

3. Main (e.g., Main, 2000) identified narrative coherence, which was a similar research-led force for integration, as an indicator of attachment security, thereby bringing attachment researchers and psychoanalysts closer together. Clinically, psychoanalysts have increasingly utilized their knowledge of the nature and form of patients' internalized representations, and appear to be able to make reliable judgments about these (Westen, Nakash, Thomas, & Bradley, 2006). Attachment research findings have given more confidence to psychoanalytic clinicians that they were not simply creating useful fictions with their patients, and that attachment narratives had predictive value when studied systematically (Cortina, 1999).

4. Driven initially by the embarrassment of the apparently endemic neglect of childhood maltreatment (Masson, 1984), psychoanalysts subsequently embraced the trauma concept with enthusiasm (e.g., Person & Klar, 1994). The hegemony of object relations theory also contributed to increasing recognition of the formative nature of the child's external, social environment. Perhaps clinicians also increasingly encountered clients who had endured serious deprivation (e.g., Downey, 2000). Engaging with the psychological consequences of childrearing patterns characteristic of families with serious social disadvantages has forced psychoanalysts to rethink the concept of trauma (e.g., Bohleber, 2007), bringing their conceptualization closer to attachment formulations.

5. There is increasing recognition of the need for measurement in relation to the outcomes of psychoanalytic therapy (PDM Task Force, 2006). Psychoanalysts now generally accept that system-

atic research must be carried out on all mental health interventions, including psychoanalysis, and that the combination of clinical and quantitative research on psychoanalytic ideas is the only way to ensure that Freud's insights are developed (Mayes, Fonagy, & Target, 2007).

A number of issues related to attachment research may have played a part in the shift in psychoanalysis toward attachment theory:

1. Attachment theory has helped psychoanalysis respond to charges of being a pseudoscience (Grünbaum, 1993), by providing evidence for the view that human development and the construction of meaning are indeed law-governed if not deterministic processes (Cortina, 1999, p. 562).

2. The strong psychometric contributions of attachment researchers have quickly been recognized and further developed by psychoanalytic researchers. In particular, the links between the adult attachment construct and object relations patterns of self–other representation have been carefully studied (Priel & Besser, 2001). In general, self-report measures of attachment tend to predict consciously regulated behavior, whereas narrative-based and other implicit assessment measures often turn out to be better predictors of behavior over time (Westen, 1998).

3. Adult attachment measurement tools are also increasingly applied in clinical settings (Buchheim & Kachele, 2003; Steele et al., 2007). For example, the AAI was creatively used in the context of psychoanalytic parent–infant psychotherapy (Baradon et al., 2005) as an indicator of mental functioning in relation to unresolved attachment issues that could be unconsciously repeated in parents' interactions with their infants (Steele & Baradon, 2004). The integration of attachment measures into routine clinical work seems both clinically desirable and empirically justified. A landmark study from Westen's laboratory demonstrated that a nationally representative sample of doctoral-level clinicians could reliably assess attachment patterns on the basis of ongoing psychotherapy hours (Westen et al., 2006).

4. The past decade has seen a significant rise in attachment-theory-oriented randomized controlled trials (RCTs) and preventive interventions that psychoanalytically oriented reviewers (Fonagy, Target, Cottrell, Phillips, & Kurtz, 2002) have claimed as evidence for the general effectiveness of the psychodynamic approach. In a large-scale

RCT, toddler–parent psychotherapy reduced the rate of insecure attachment in the 3-year-old children of chronically depressed mothers (Toth, Rogosch, Manly, & Cicchetti, 2006). A similar RCT of mother–child therapy with excellent outcomes was reported earlier by Lieberman, Van Horn, and Ippen (2005). A further, well-controlled RCT found that parent–infant psychotherapy for maltreating families was effective, relative to a standard community control, in increasing secure attachment and reducing disorganized attachment in the infants (Cicchetti, Rogosch, & Toth, 2006). Open-label trials of psychodynamically rooted interventions have found attachment-focused interventions for high-risk groups to be effective in reducing insecure-disorganized attachment (Hoffman, Marvin, Cooper, & Powell, 2006). It should be noted that not all psychodynamically informed attachment-security-focused RCTs yielded significant effects (Brisch, Bechinger, Betzler, & Heinemann, 2003). In general, psychodynamic treatments are more likely to be effective in populations that carry high psychosocial risk (e.g., victims of maltreatment, severe neglect, or abuse).

5. Attachment may enable us to predict which individuals are better suited to psychoanalytically oriented treatments. There is some evidence from RCTs that patients with binge-eating disorder and high attachment anxiety benefit more from psychodynamic group therapy, whereas those patients with lower attachment anxiety benefit more from group cognitive therapy (Tasca et al., 2006). In a study of depression contrasting interpersonal therapy (IPT) with cognitive-behavioral therapy (CBT), patients with higher scores on avoidant attachment also exhibited significantly greater reduction in depression severity with CBT than with IPT (McBride, Atkinson, Quilty, & Bagby, 2006). In a unique study that experimentally manipulated the frequency of transference interpretations in psychodynamic psychotherapy, patients with poor pretreatment social networks (arguably greater attachment problems) did well when randomized to the high-transference-interpretation group (Hoglend, Johansson, Marble, Bogwald, & Amlo, 2007). In an observational study of IPT, fearfully avoidant women also responded more slowly to treatment (Cyranowski et al., 2002). The attachment research framework has enabled the extension of the researchable domain of psychoanalytic work, through exploration of personality structure, RCTs of psychoanalytically informed treatments, and identifying the personality types best suited to this kind of work.

6. A number of research-driven theoretical developments have brought attachment theory and psychoanalytic ideas closer together. One of these—the mentalization-based approach that emerged from attachment research—is discussed in detail later in this chapter, but there have been many other important advances. Among the most notable is the work of Blatt, who has integrated a psychoanalytic and a cognitive-developmental perspective to create an epigenetic view of the development of self- and other-representation (Blatt, 1995). Blatt suggested that personality development involves two fundamental, parallel developmental lines: (a) an anaclitic or relatedness line, which involves the development of the capacity to establish increasingly mature and mutually satisfying interpersonal relationships; and (b) an introjective or self-definitional line, which involves the development of a consolidated, realistic, essentially positive, differentiated self-identity (Blatt & Blass, 1990). Normal development throughout the life cycle involves a complex, reciprocal transaction between these two developmental sequences, but they get out of kilter in most forms of psychopathology (Blatt, 2004; Blatt & Blass, 1990). This dichotomy overlaps with the two common forms of attachment insecurity: avoidant and anxious.

RELATIONAL AND RELATIONSHIP-FOCUSED PSYCHOANALYSIS

Arguably the most radical change in psychoanalytic thinking has been the emergence of an interpersonal relationship-focused perspective—perhaps best exemplified by the so-called "relational school," partly rooted in the work of Sullivan (Benjamin, 1998; Bromberg, 1998; Mitchell & Aron, 1999; Sullivan, 1953). Mitchell (1988) introduced a framework including a range of theoretical developments that collectively may be termed "relational psychoanalytic theories." This framework formed a "relational matrix" of self–object relational configurations, which include as ingredients the self, the other, and the relatedness they co-construct. These elements can be configured and reconfigured to create multiple new theories. The theory is more of an orientation than a coherent body of ideas, and many great theoreticians and clinicians who emphasize relational issues do not necessarily identify themselves as "relational psychoanalysts." Each of the major theorists with this orientation has offered a slightly different integration of the relational matrix (e.g., Mitchell's theory of relational conflict, Ogden's intersubjectivity theory, and Hoffman's social-constructivist theory), meaning that there is no single, unifying relational psychoanalytic theory. Relational theories are metatheories, in which human relations are considered to play a superordinate role in the creation of human character.

Relational psychoanalysis often appears to combine the concerns of modern psychoanalysis with the traditional concerns of attachment theory. Psychodynamic therapists who wish to embrace the relational approach often move toward an attachment model, albeit unwittingly (Cortina, 2001). Buechler (1997), herself a relational psychoanalyst, has elaborated 12 points of contact between relational psychoanalytic theory and attachment theory. For example, both regard emotional problems as the result of interference with an innate potential for interrelatedness; both view patterns of relating as crucial for diagnosis and treatment; and both consider the meaning of behavior in terms of its interpersonal functions. Looking at the growth points of relational and attachment theories, we see a marked convergence between the two, and little by way of fundamental incompatibility. Both see the dynamic transactions between people (rather than what transpires within the individual mind) as the primary context for theory building and analytic technique. Furthermore, relational psychoanalysis and modern attachment theory both argue for the following: (1) attachment and intersubjectivity as motivational systems; (2) subtle aspects of interpersonal interaction in the creation of identity and thus also in therapeutic change; (3) a systemic perspective in which the subject and object have interchanging roles (i.e., the baby affects the parent just as the parent influences the baby); (4) an emphasis on the dyadic nature of affect representations; (5) the dynamics of recognition and otherness that grow out of a transactional understanding of relationships; and (6) the central role of reality in development.

The Developmental Perspective

Relational psychoanalysis emerged as psychoanalysis moved toward the developmental framework established within attachment theory and other dynamic psychological approaches rooted in observing early development. Mitchell's early papers (e.g., Mitchell, 1984) explicitly argued *against* the "developmental tilt" of psychoanalytic writings—not because of an antipathy toward the developmental approach, but through impatience with the tendency to exclude the current relational perspective from the "high table" of psychoanalytic theorizing. Typically, it was relegated to the early years of development, only to be overshadowed by traditional concerns regarding drive-related and Oedipal issues that could readily preclude the self, other, and interaction relational perspectives. Relational analysts have also traditionally been concerned that a focus on early development might lead to a (defensive) avoidance of the participation of the real adults in the therapeutic relationship. However, Mitchell's work, and that of other relational analysts such as Benjamin (1998), increasingly focused on developmental theory. The developmental approach of relational theory, unlike most other psychoanalytic formulations, does not rely on a conception of the child's mind as organized by endogenous infantile givens that are preserved directly into adulthood (particularly in cases where development goes awry); rather, developmental and relational models are brought together by the "transactional systems perspective" (Sameroff & Chandler, 1975).

From the transactional systems perspective, factors such as temperament transform the impact of other factors, such as parental sensitivity; these factors interact over time, creating new patterns. In other words, development involves factors whose effects are measured only through their interaction with other factors, which is exactly the kind of interpersonal dynamic that relational psychoanalytic theorists wanted to capture in their writings. This transactional perspective was generally adopted by developmental psychopathologists influenced by attachment research (e.g., Belsky, 2005). Transactional interaction patterns emerged clearly in the study of temperament and attachment in primates, where the genetic predisposition of both caregivers and infants could be experimentally manipulated (Suomi, 2000, and Chapter 8, this volume; Vaughn, Bost, & van IJzendoorn, Chapter 9, this volume).

Intersubjectivity and the Self

The relational model starts from the assumption that subjectivity is interpersonal—that is, the intersubjective replaces the intrapsychic (Mitchell, 1988). This renders the human mind a contradiction in terms, since subjectivity is invariably rooted in an intersubjective matrix of relational bonds within which personal meanings are embedded (Mitchell, 2000), rather than in biological drives.

Unlike most other psychoanalytic theories, the relational model lacks a specific explanation of how relationality and intersubjectivity may develop. For this reason, attachment theory and conclusions drawn from the observation of attachment relationships may be helpful.

Bowlby was a quintessential relational theorist, thanks to his unwavering focus on child–caregiver interaction as the primary driver of social development. Among others, Bowlby clearly influenced Trevarthen (e.g., Trevarthen & Aitken, 2001), who argues that infants are innately predisposed to social relationships and that primary intersubjectivity characterizes the mental experience of infants during infant–caregiver interactions (Trevarthen, 1993; Trevarthen, Aitken, Vandekerckhove, Delafield-Butt, & Nagy, 2006). In addition to a predisposition to relate, attachment theory posits and describes other adaptations—including defensive processes—that develop in the context of specifically elaborated relational processes, which themselves occur at the interface between infant distress and the caregiver's response. That is, attachment theory, like relational theory, is a two-person theory of conflict and defense, which sees defensive mechanisms as arising from the conflict between the infant's needs and the caregiver's responses (Lyons-Ruth, 1999, 2003).

The Relational Baby

Following from Bowlby's work, in the 1980s the relational approach was augmented and modified by the intersubjectivist vision of philosophically oriented psychoanalysts such as Stolorow (1997) and infant researchers such as Emde (e.g., Emde, Kubicek, & Oppenheim, 1997). Relational theory posits that the infant is oriented toward the outside world from birth, and that the baby's mind is already organized and becomes increasingly complex and integrated as it meets a fully supportive caregiving environment and interacts in dyadic structures such as the infant–parent relationship.

These structures can be manifested internally, externally, or in the intersubjective spaces between them. For example, Tronick's (1989, 2007) mutual regulation model of infant–adult interaction, and Beebe's (Beebe, Lachmann, & Jaffe, 1997) interactive regulation model, focus on the subtle, nonverbal, microregulatory, and socioemotional processes that unfold in mother–infant interactions. They allow us to operationalize such concepts as the "holding environment" (Winnicott, 1965) and "background of safety'" (Sandler,

1960), and take us toward a genuinely relational model of change in psychoanalytic treatment. Furthermore, studies of the contingency between the mother's and infant's vocalizations can help us to predict secure attachment relationships (Jaffe et al., 2001).

Both attachment theory and relational psychoanalysis posit self-with-other schemas as the organizing structures of the mental world. The infant's development is molded by its dependence on the caregiver and by the latter's special sensitivity. Similarly, the therapeutic process is thought to be shaped by the therapist's sensitivity in a clinical context. We are thought to become aware of ourselves as seen by others, and we come to develop a sense of ourselves in the process of becoming aware of the other's awareness of us. The subjective self cannot develop self-understanding without the experience of having been reflected on by another and "understood."

The Subjectivity of the Mother

Attachment theory placed maternal behavior and the subjective experiences of mothering at center stage (George & Solomon, 1999 and Chapter 35, this volume), with some theorists analyzing the impact of the mother's conscious and unconscious beliefs and fantasies on parenting (Lieberman, 1999). Main's work on the AAI (Hesse & Main, 2006; Main, 2000), together with Slade's (2005) mapping of the parent's conception of the child's mind with the Parent Development Interview (PDI), also opened up new ground.

Psychoanalysts, however, were slow to focus on maternal experience, even in the tradition of British object relations theory. It was the feminist influence within relational theory that finally generated interest in the independent role of maternal subjectivity. Within this frame, there has been considerable interest in the intergenerational transmission of the mothering role (Chodorow, 1994), the developmental process underpinning this role, and the fundamental dynamics of submission and dominance entailed in how mothers help their babies to establish their subjectivity (Benjamin, 1998).

The Intersubjective and Therapy

Relational analysts have adapted infant research to apply the principle of ongoing dyadic regulation to the therapeutic situation (Stern et al., 1998). The therapist and the patient supposedly create a dyadic state of consciousness through mutual affect regulation; each patient–therapist dyad is different, but will influence future exchanges for both parties—both with each other and with other people. Therapy happens when existing states of consciousness are reintegrated and reconfigured for the patient.

The hypothesis of procedural representations of implicit relational knowing raises the theory of internal object relations to a more general "systems" conception. The implicit relational knowing of two partners or of a patient and an analyst will be altered by moments of "meeting"—by the enactment of a new potential that will come to be represented as a future possibility. The best-documented forms of procedural implicit relational knowing are displayed during the first 2 years of life, when interactions are registered in representations of interpersonal events in a nonsymbolic form. The unique configuration of adaptive strategies that emerges from the attachment relationship comes to constitute the initial organization of the child's domain of implicit relational knowing (internal working models, proto-narrative envelopes, themes of organization, relational scripts).

The Pragmatics of Therapy

If traditional psychoanalytic approaches emphasize fantasy (poetics) as a core explanatory construct, then relational psychoanalysis, after Sullivan, supplements this by paying greater attention to pragmatics (descriptions of experience). Sullivan's break from traditional psychoanalysis mirrors Bowlby's conflict with the British psychoanalytic community: Bowlby shared an emphasis on dyadic relationships with interpersonalists, but he also shared with Sullivan (1964) an interest in observable behavior. Neither Bowlby nor Sullivan could specifically be labeled "behaviorist," but they shared a systematic and consistent interest in what happens between people. For Sullivan, this entailed a detailed inquiry into who said what to whom, whereas Bowlby's focus was on what happened in the past to explain the current state of affairs. In general, both attachment theorists and interpersonalists are reluctant to privilege fantasy over actuality. Interpersonal and intrapsychic factors are seen as equally important.

Current relational thinking often uses psychopathological accounts of trauma to highlight the relational aspects of actual experience (e.g., Davies, 1996). "What really happened" is combined with attention to the subjective experience of the

patient, not in order to separate veridical events from distortions associated with unconscious fantasy, but rather to elaborate the overwhelming nature of the experience itself—especially because the context of trauma is assumed to preclude awareness of its meanings (Pizer, 2003). It is the inherent paradox of attachment trauma (i.e., an apparently unintended trauma perpetrated by a figure on whom one depends) that a stance of "not knowing what one knows" (Bowlby, 1988b, p. 99) may be adopted to keep the crucial relationship intact. Relational psychoanalytic (Stern, 1997) and attachment-inspired (Hesse & Main, 2006) clinical descriptions provide similar formulations of dissociation linked with traumatic experience.

The Presymbolic

Mitchell (2000) has identified a number of basic modes through which relationality can generate psychiatric disorder. Nonreflective, presymbolic behavior (or what people actually do with each other) involves reciprocal influence and mutual regulation, which are key to the organization of relational fields. This topic area includes work on the representation of interpersonal interactions in procedural memory (Crittenden, 1997), whether relegated to this by repression of trauma (Davies & Frawley, 1994) or constraints imposed by cognitive development (Stern, 1994).

Many of these ideas resonate with attachment theory. Defensive attachment strategies also involve nonconscious, implicit representations that develop in earliest childhood, before the explicit memory system begins to function properly (Stern et al., 1998). As Lyons-Ruth (2003, p. 888) has pointed out, these implicit two-person representations contain within them the "deep structure of the early parent–infant affective dialogue, including deletions and distortions ... that will eventually become intrapsychic defenses." The relational approach also meshes well with Lyons-Ruth's work on maternal behaviors associated with disorganized infant attachment (e.g., Lyons-Ruth & Spielman, 2004).

Bowlby's original concept of internal working models was elaborated and expanded within the relational framework. Its essence was incorporated into Stern's (1985) concept of generalized representations of interactions, Lyons-Ruth's (1998) concept of implicit interpersonal knowledge, and Lichtenberg's (1989) concept of model scenes. For both attachment and relational psychoanalytic theories, there is a linear progression of developmental stages, although the development of procedural systems is likely to be task-organized under the sway of increasingly complex control or meaning systems. These concepts both emphasize nondeclarative psychological patterns that operate on a nonreflective level of personality organization. We cannot reflect on the specific dyadic interactions that have shaped our patterns of relating. Rather, it is the "way of being with" another that is made explicit, reflected upon, and modified within the therapeutic context (Fonagy, 1999a).

Affective Permeability

"Affective permeability" refers to a shared experience of intense affect across permeable boundaries where direct resonances emerge in interpersonal dyads (Bromberg, 1998). The attachment-based work of Lyons-Ruth has once again fleshed out this idea: In developing a new coding system for the AAI, she and her colleagues have described an atypical state of mind that can predict infant disorganization in the absence of loss or trauma (Lyons-Ruth, Yellin, Melnick, & Atwood, 2005). Lyons-Ruth and colleagues (2005) thave argued that some individuals' unintegrated and fearful affect is rooted solely in their relationship with their caregivers, and is generated, for example, by implacably hostile parental affect. They have proposed a relational diathesis model of the intergenerational transmission of disorganized attachment, where unintegrated states of mind in the caregiver are thought to be primary mediators of fear-inducing experiences, deviant caregiving, or a combination of both. This is in line with a relational approach to conflict, which is no longer seen as within the individual, but as produced by contradictory signals and values in the environment (Sullivan, 1964).

A General Relational Model of Therapeutic Change in Psychodynamic Psychotherapy

The emphasis on the mutual influence of infant and caregiver informs an emerging relational model of therapy as a two-person process, with little room for a detached analyst with pretensions of "objectivity." The assumption that people are predisposed toward co-constructed systems that provide a context for psychic change led to the view that the quality of engagement between therapist and patient is part of the core of therapeutic action—in keeping with attachment theory. The relational therapist, like the therapist offering developmental help, does not seek simply to impart

understanding; his or her style is more active and participatory and aims to explore the nature of and reasons for maladaptive patterns of behavior. The emphasis is on the mutativeness of the combination of relatedness and interpretative insights—with one depending on the other for therapeutic effectiveness. An interpretation is thought of as "performative," in the sense that it always partially reflects or enacts the relationship itself. Similarly, the relationship itself is considered to be a form of interpretation, which may be explored and understood once it has been experienced. What changes the mind, then, is not just the insights gained, but learning from the interactional experience of being with another person. The interplay between relatedness, reflection on that relatedness, co-constructed interpretation of its symbolic meanings, and a similar exploration of "there and then" and extratherapeutic life is considered mutative in treatment. Neither the analyst nor the patient can be considered as forging meaning; rather, meaning is co-constructed.

Overall, developmental research implies that patient and therapist affect each other in myriad mutually influencing ways, including both a rapid flux of moment-to-moment changes and slower-changing parameters. Projective identification is seen as occurring in a bidirectional interpersonal field between analyst and patient—a model clearly adapted from Kleinian approaches to infant–caregiver interaction (Seligman, 1999). If we take this perspective seriously, we have to concede that all analytic interventions change the situations into which they are introduced, and that their content and style always reflect the analyst's countertransference or response to the treatment situation (e.g., Hoffman, 1998). Relational psychoanalysis advocates making explicit the interactional influence of analyst upon patient. As Levenson (1983, p. ix) put it, the key therapeutic question is not "What does this mean?", but rather, "What is going on around here?" The therapist will "act" on the patient; this is not a therapeutic disaster, but rather a potentially progressive and certainly inevitable part of the process. This too, of course, mirrors the infant–parent interaction, where disruption and repair create the potential for the expansion of dyadic consciousness (Tronick, 2007).

The most intriguing relational model of therapy was advanced a decade ago by the Process of Change Study Group (Nahum et al., 2002; Stern et al., 1998). Its members proposed that change in therapy is the consequence of the impact of the shared implicit relationship between patient and therapist on the patient's implicit relational knowledge. Repetitive behavior by the patient— for example, expectation of nonresponse, indifference, and rejection—is engaged and potentially disconfirmed as part of a process of ongoing mutual regulation (Beebe & Lachmann, 1994). The emphasis on relational knowledge is based on attachment theory's assumption that the capacity for self-regulation in infancy is acquired through the internalization of mutual but asymmetrical mother–infant interactions (Sroufe, 1996; Tronick, 2007). The goals of the interaction are both physiological (coordinating sleeping and feeding) and intersubjective (mutual recognition and sharing). By analogy, changes in implicit relational knowledge in the course of therapy are through "moments of meeting"—moments when the shared implicit knowledge of both parties is altered.

Present moments become represented as schemas of "ways of being with" another. "Now moments" occur when the traditional frame of the therapy is (or should be) broken (e.g., when the patient makes the analyst laugh or when major life events call for the therapist to react). At such moments of meeting the protagonists of the therapy are able to encounter each other "unhidden by their usual therapeutic roles" (Stern et al., 1998, p. 913). The idea of heightened affective moments in the course of therapy is not new (Fenichel, 1941; Pine, 1981; Strachey, 1934), but defining the idea in terms of discontinuity of implicit relational knowing is. The relational space opens, and the change in the intersubjective environment causes a dyadic expansion of consciousness, which in turn permits a change in the patient's relational knowing (Tronick, 2001). Importantly, this shared relational knowing is considered as distinct from traditional constructions based on transference and countertransference. Disruptions are not solely a consequence of the patient's resistance; nor are they solely a result of the analyst's countertransference. The analyst's spontaneous, personal, nontechnical response may be the most important component in bringing about the desired shift, since repairs are jointly constructed (Harrison, 2003).

The technical implications of this new model are far from clear (Fonagy, 1998). Ryle has advanced a model of psychotherapy based on the realization that unconscious relationship procedures can be described, and that the resulting descriptions can be of considerable value in psychotherapy (Ryle, 2003; Ryle & Fawkes, 2007). Cogni-tive analytic therapy identifies and represents a relatively small number of underlying relationship patterns, including issues of care, dependency, control, submission, love, and anger, as "reciprocal role procedures." Reciprocal role procedures are addressed explicitly by the therapy, including through formal correspondence between therapist and patient. Relational ideas also underpin IPT (Klerman, Weissman, Rounsaville, & Chevron, 1984), which has a strong evidence base in the adult literature on depression, albeit a somewhat more meager one for its adolescent adaptation (see Mufson, Dorta, Olfson, Weissman, & Hoagwood, 2004; Mufson, Dorta, Wickramaratne, et al., 2004; Mufson, Gallagher, Dorta, & Young, 2004; Mufson & Moreau, 1999; Warner, Weissman, Mufson, & Wickramaratne, 1999; Young, Mufson, & Davies, 2006). IPT may have moved too far from its origins to be considered a genuine psychodynamic approach (even in the broad sense of that term); yet the clearly psychoanalytic adaptations of the interpersonal psychodynamic tradition retain the focus on the relationship-seeking aspect of human character, and remain the key pragmatic concern of both the child and the therapeutic relationship in this context.

Having looked at the common ground between relational psychoanalysis and attachment theory, let us now develop our argument further by introducing a new concept that has itself sprung from considerations of attachment theory: "mentalization."

ATTACHMENT THEORY AND THE DEVELOPMENT OF MENTALIZATION

Mentalization-based theory and treatment represent a recent psychoanalytic extension of attachment theory and research. This extension specifically concerns itself with the parent's understanding and reflection on the infant's internal world; it claims a vital synergistic relationship between attachment processes and the growth of the child's capacity to understand interpersonal behavior in terms of mental states (Fonagy, Gergely, Jurist, & Target, 2002). This capacity is referred to as "mentalization." It is operationalized for research (usually based on AAI narratives) as "reflective function."

Our model was first outlined in the context of a large empirical study, in which security of infant attachment with each parent proved to be strongly predicted not only by that parent's security of attachment during the pregnancy (Fonagy, Steele, & Steele, 1991), but even more by the parents' capacity to understand their own childhood relationships with their own parents in terms of states of mind (Fonagy, Steele, Moran, Steele, & Higgitt, 1991). On the basis of empirical observations and theoretical elaboration, we proposed that the capacity to mentalize is a key determinant of self-organization and affect regulation, and that it emerges in the context of early attachment relationships. We have tried to describe how a child's understanding of itself as a mental agent grows out of interpersonal experience, particularly in the child–caregiver relationship (Fonagy, Gergely, et al., 2002).

Mentalization involves both a self-reflective and an interpersonal component, is both implicit and explicit, and concerns both feelings and cognitions (Lieberman, 2007). In combination, these skills enable a child to distinguish inner from outer reality; to construct representations of his or her own mental states from perceptible cues (arousal, behavior, context); and to infer and attribute others' mental states from subtle behavioral and contextual cues. In our view, the mind is not transparent to itself. All too often we have presumed an innate capacity for primary introspective access to our internal mental states, providing us with "first-person authority" over the contents of our private subjective mental lives; this presumption means that the role of attachment relationships in the emergence of subjectivity has been ignored (see Carpendale & Lewis, 2006). We contend that the full development of mentalization depends on interaction with more mature and sensitive minds. In this section, we consider some of the evidence linking mentalization to the quality of attachment relationships, and we outline our psychoanalytic model inspired by attachment theory and research.

Attachment Experience and Mentalization

Linking the attachment and mentalization constructs has been made easier by recent research in biological psychology, including behavior genetics and functional neuroimaging.

Genetics of Mentalization

Can attachment influence social cognition? Not if, as with most cognitive capacities, genetics leaves little room for attachment (Carpendale & Lewis, 2006). There is, however, evidence that environ-

mental factors have a substantial effect on attachment. In a longitudinal sample of 1,116 twin pairs (age 60 months) who completed a comprehensive battery of theory-of-mind (ToM) tasks, behavioral genetic models of the data showed that environmental factors explained the largest part (85%) of the variance in ToM performance (Hughes et al., 2005). Bivariate genetic analysis revealed that, to the extent that genetic factors can be said to influence ToM, these were the same as those that determine verbal ability and account for a relatively small proportion of the variance in this ability (15%). Forty-four percent of the variance in ToM was nonshared and specific to ToM.

If mentalization is not predominantly genetically determined, then factors influencing it should be largely environmentally determined. Attachment classification shows little heritability in twin studies (Fearon et al., 2006), and shared environmental influence accounts for the biggest proportion of the variance (53%). Attachment is associated with the quality of the infant–caregiver relationship, which is consistent with an environmental focus. Roisman and Fraley (2006) reported from the nationally representative Early Childhood Longitudinal Study data set that observed variation in the quality of the infant–caregiver relationship also could not be accounted for by genetic variation (heritability = .01), and that both shared and unique environmental contributions were substantial (shared = .40 and nonshared = .59). There appears to be a selective advantage to leaving early attachment and social cognition maximally open to environmental influence and social heredity. Behavior genetic studies are helpful not only in indicating the social determinants, but also in specifying that in looking for social influence on both infant attachment and mentalization, we are searching for a combination of family-level (shared) and relationship-level or dyad-specific (nonshared) factors.

Functional Neuroimaging of Attachment and Mentalization

Recent neuroimaging studies have confirmed the association between the attachment system and mentalization. The vasopressin and oxytocin systems play a vital role in establishing social bonds and regulating emotional behavior (Fries, Ziegler, Kurian, Jacoris, & Pollak, 2005). Investigations of pair bonding as well as mother–infant attachment in rodent models have linked them to the oxytocin and vasopressin mediated activation of the mesocorticolimbic dopaminergic reward circuit (e.g., Lim, Murphy, & Young, 2004). Because this circuit plays a key role in mediating the process of addiction (Panksepp, 1998), attachment has even been interpreted as an addiction (Insel, 2003). Functional magnetic resonance imaging studies also indicate specific activation of these reward-sensitive pathways in the brain when people see their own partners or offspring (but not the partners or children of other people) (Nitschke et al., 2004).

Bartels and Zeki (2000, 2004) have shown that when the areas of the brain that mediate maternal and/or romantic attachments are stimulated, brain activity in regions mediating different aspects of cognitive control are simultaneously suppressed. They suggest that attachment suppresses two neural systems. The first includes the medial prefrontal, inferior parietal, and medial temporal cortices (mainly in the right hemisphere), as well as the posterior cingulate cortex, which specializes in attention and long-term memory (Cabeza & Nyberg, 2000), and which has variable involvement in both positive (Maddock, 1999) and negative (Mayberg et al., 1999) emotions. Some propose that these regions may specifically be responsible for integrating emotion and cognition (Maddock, 1999), whereas lesion studies suggest that they play a role in judgments involving negative emotions (Adolphs, Damasio, Tranel, Cooper, & Damasio, 2000). The second system deactivated by the activation of the attachment system includes the temporal poles, parietotemporal junction, amygdala, and mesial prefrontal cortex. This system constitutes the primary neural network that allows us to identify and to interpret mental states (both thoughts and feelings) in other people (Gallagher & Frith, 2003), as well as in ourselves (Lieberman, 2007).

The way in which activation of the attachment system interferes with the two systems identified by Bartels and Zeki (2000, 2004) sheds light on the nature of individual differences in attachment representations, on the relationship of attachment and mentalization, and consequently on our understanding of dysfunctions associated with problems in mentalizing. Broadly speaking, we may envision three types of associations between aspects of social cognition and attachment. These are created by attachment relationships based on intense romantic and maternal love, attachment relationships based on threat/fear, and secure and predictable attachment relationships. More specifically, (1) associations mediated by dopaminergic

structures of the reward system in the presence of oxytocin and vasopressin (i.e., love-related activation of the attachment system) can inhibit the neural systems that underpin the generation of negative affect; (2) threat-related activation of the attachment system may also evoke intense arousal and overwhelming negative affect, activating posterior cortical and subcortical areas and switching off frontal cortical activity, including mentalization (Mayes, 2000); and (3) a secure and predictable attachment relationship may be most effective in *preempting* threat, which possibly reduces the need for frequent activation of the attachment system, thus enhancing mentalization (Coan, Schaefer, & Davidson, 2006; see also Coan, Chapter 11, this volume).

It is perhaps worth noting that Bowlby, (1969/1982, 1973) assumed fear—in particular the loss of the attachment figure, to be the primary reason for activation of the attachment system. An unpredictable, insecure caregiver–infant relationship is likely to result in frequent activation of the attachment system, accompanied by deactivation of neural structures underpinning aspects of social cognition. Evidence also suggests that the level of attachment anxiety is positively correlated with activation in emotion-related areas of the brain (e.g., the anterior temporal pole, which is activated when an individual is sad) and inversely correlated with activation in a region associated with emotion regulation (orbitofrontal cortex) (Gillath, Bunge, Shaver, Wendelken, & Mikulincer, 2005). These findings suggest that anxiously attached people may underrecruit the brain regions normally used to down-regulate negative emotions. Because insecure, unpredictable parent–child relationships are most likely to activate the attachment system, we may predict on the basis of recent neuroimaging data alone that a stable parent–child relationship should facilitate the development of mentalization, since it is likely to be associated with limited inhibitory interference with the brain mechanisms subserving mentalization.

Prediction of Mentalizing by Secure Attachment

Many studies support the suggestion that secure children are better than insecure ones at mentalization (measured as passing ToM tasks earlier in development) (e.g., de Rosnay & Harris, 2002). Children with secure attachment relationships assessed by the Separation Anxiety Test do better than children with disorganized attachment on a test of emotion understanding (Fonagy, Redfern,

& Charman, 1997). The first of these findings reported from the London Parent–Child Project (Fonagy, Steele, Steele, & Holder, 1997) found that 82% of children who were secure with their mothers in the Strange Situation passed Harris's Belief–Desire–Reasoning Task at 5½ years, compared to 50% of those who were avoidant and 33% of the small number who were ambivalent/resistant. Findings along these lines are not always consistent (see, e.g., Meins et al., 2002), but it generally seems that secure attachment and mentalization are subject to similar social influences. In the next section, we briefly explore some of these influences.

Understanding Why Secure Attachment Predicts Mentalizing

Mentalizing and Parenting

Two decades of research have confirmed parenting as the key determinant of attachment security. Can aspects of parenting account for the overlap between mentalization and attachment security? In particular, does parental mentalization of the child have an influence? Researchers designate the mother's capacity to take a psychological perspective on her child by different terms, including maternal "mind-mindedness," "insightfulness," and reflective function. These overlapping attributes appear to be associated with both secure attachment and mentalization (Sharp, Fonagy, & Goodyer, 2006).

Meins (e.g., Meins, Fernyhough, Fradley, & Tuckey, 2001), Oppenheim (e.g., Oppenheim & Koren-Karie, 2002), and Slade (e.g., Slade, Grienenberger, Bernbach, Levy, & Locker, 2005) have sought to link parental mentalization with the development of affect regulation and secure attachment by analyzing interactional narratives between parents and children. Although Meins and colleagues (2001) assessed parents' quality of narrative about their children in real time (while the parents were playing with their children), and Oppenheim's group did this in a more "offline" manner (while parents narrated a videotaped interaction), both groups concluded that maternal mentalizing was a more powerful predictor of attachment security than, say, global sensitivity. Meins and colleagues found that mind-related comments by mothers at 6 months predicted attachment security at 12 months (Meins et al., 2001), mentalizing capacity at 45 and 48 months (Meins et al., 2002), and stream-of-consciousness

performance at 55 months (Meins et al., 2003). Oppenheim and Koren-Karie (2002) found that a secure mother–child relationship was predicted by high levels of mentalization about the child's behavior.

Slade and colleagues (2005; see also Slade, Chapter 32, this volume) also observed a strong association between infant attachment and the quality of the parent's mentalizing about the child. Rather than using an episode of observed interaction, Slade et al. used an autobiographical memory-based interview about the child, the PDI. High scorers on the PDI's mentalizing scale are aware of the characteristics of their infants' mental functioning, and they grasp the complex interplay between their own mental states and their children's putative inner experience. They are likely to have secure relationships with infants whom they describe in a mentalizing way. Low-scoring mothers on the mentalizing scale in Slade's studies were more likely to show atypical maternal behavior on the Atypical Maternal Behavior Instrument for Assessment and Classification system (Bronfman, Parsons, & Lyons-Ruth, 1999), which relates not only to infants' attachment disorganization, but also to unresolved (disorganized) attachment status in the mothers' AAI (Grienenberger, Kelly, & Slade, 2005).

Taken together, these results suggest that a mentalizing style of parenting may well facilitate the development of mentalization. Mindful parenting probably enhances both attachment security and mentalization in a child. Consistent with this conclusion is a range of findings covering aspects of parenting that have been shown to predict performance on ToM tasks. Precocious understanding of false beliefs is predicted by more reflective parenting practices (Ruffman, Perner, & Parkin, 1999), including the quality of parental control (Ruffman et al., 1999); parental discourse about emotions (Meins et al., 2002); the depth of parental discussion involving affect (Dunn, Brown, & Beardsall, 1991); parents' beliefs about parenting (Vinden, 2001); and non-power-assertive disciplinary strategies (Pears & Moses, 2003) that focus on mental states (e.g., a victim's feelings, or the nonintentional nature of transgressions) (Charman, Ruffman, & Clements, 2002). All of these measures reflect concern with a child's subjective state.

We should, however, be cautious about these correlations. They are as readily explained by child-to-parent as by parent-to-child effects. For example, less power-assertive parenting may be associated with mentalization not because it facilitates it, but because less mentalizing children are more likely to elicit controlling parenting behavior. Moreover, the same aspects of family functioning that facilitate secure attachment may also facilitate the emergence of mentalizing. For example, tolerance for negative emotions is a marker of secure attachment (Sroufe, 1996) and precocious mentalizing (Hughes & Dunn, 2002).

The process of acquiring mentalization is so ordinary and normal that it may be more correct to consider secure attachment as removing obstacles rather than actively and directly facilitating its development. The key to understanding the interaction of attachment with the development of mentalization may be to look at instances where normally available catalysts for mentalization are absent.

Family Discourse

Exposure to normative conversational and social opportunities appears to be a precondition for mentalization. For example, deaf Nicaraguan adults who grew up without hearing references to beliefs appear incapable of passing false-belief tests (Pyers, 2003, cited in Siegal & Patterson, in press). It is fair to say that under normal circumstances, conversations with frequent and accurate elaboration of psychological themes may be the "royal road" to understanding minds (Harris, 2005). Main's (2000) groundbreaking work has linked attachment to this kind of communication with words. Coherent family discourse characteristic of secure attachment (Hill, Fonagy, Safier, & Sargent, 2003) helps to generate explanatory schemas by means of which the behavior of others can be understood and predicted.

Playfulness

Classical work links quality of play with attachment (Steele, Fonagy, Yabsley, Woolgar, & Croft, 1995; see Grossmann, Grossmann, Kindler, & Zimmermann, Chapter 36, this volume). Play may also be important in acquiring mentalizing. The impact of lack of playfulness is most obvious in extreme cases. In blind children, active pretend play is quite limited (Tröster & Bambring, 1994), and they also understand pretend play poorly (Lewis, Norgate, Collis, & Reynolds, 2000). They are delayed on false-belief tests (Green, Pring, & Swettenham, 2004), and pass only when they reach a verbal mental age of 11 as opposed to the more

normal 5 (McAlpine & Moore, 1985). Hobson (2002) has explored the social and developmental implications of blindness in this context. Blind infants miss out on access to parental nonverbal information about internal states, such as facial expression, and can experience problems of identity, which are perhaps associated with mentalization problems. For example, they may refer to themselves as "you" while speaking (Dunlea, 1989).

Maltreatment

Maltreatment disorganizes the attachment system (see Cicchetti & Valentino, 2006, for a comprehensive review). There is also evidence to suggest that it may disrupt mentalization. Young maltreated children manifest certain characteristics that could suggest problems with mentalization: (1) Like blind children, they engage in less symbolic and dyadic play (Alessandri, 1991); (2) they sometimes fail to show empathy when witnessing distress in other children (Klimes-Dougan & Kistner, 1990); (3) they have poor affect regulation (Maughan & Cicchetti, 2002); (4) they make fewer references to their internal states (Shipman & Zeman, 1999); and (5) they struggle to understand emotional expressions, particularly facial ones (During & McMahon, 1991), even when verbal IQ is controlled for (Camras et al., 1990). Maltreated children tend to misattribute anger (Camras, Sachs-Alter, & Ribordy, 1996) and show elevated event-related potentials to angry faces (Cicchetti & Curtis, 2005). The evidence for significant developmental delay in the emotional understanding of maltreated young children is consistent (Pears & Fisher, 2005), if slightly reduced, when IQ and socioeconomic status are controlled for (Smith & Walden, 1999).[1] Understanding sad and angry emotions at age 6 predicts social competence and social isolation at age 8 (Rogosch, Cicchetti, & Aber, 1995).

In addition to problems of emotional understanding, there have been reports of delayed ToM understanding in maltreated children (Cicchetti, Rogosch, Maughan, Toth, & Bruce, 2003; Pears & Fisher, 2005). The capacity to parse complex and emotionally charged representations of the parent and of the self may even deteriorate with development (Toth, Cicchetti, Macfie, Maughan, & Vanmeenen, 2000).

Considered in relation to attachment, mentalization deficits associated with childhood maltreatment may be a form of decoupling, inhibition, or even a phobic reaction to mentalizing. First, adversity may undermine cognitive development in general (Cicchetti, Rogosch, & Toth, 2000; Crandell & Hobson, 1999). Mentalization problems may also reflect arousal problems associated with exposure to chronic stress (see Cicchetti & Walker, 2001). Finally, a child may avoid mentalization to avoid perceiving an abuser's frankly hostile and malevolent thoughts and feelings about him or her (e.g., Fonagy, 1991).

Maltreatment can contribute to an acquired partial "mind-blindness" by compromising open reflective communication between parent and child. Maltreatment may undermine the benefit derived from learning about the links between internal states and actions in attachment relationships (e.g., a child may be told that he or she "deserves," "wants," or even "enjoys" the abuse). This is more likely to be destructive if the maltreatment is perpetrated by a family member. Even when this is not the case, parents' ignorance of maltreatment taking place outside the home may invalidate the child's communications with the parents about his or her feelings. The child finds that reflective discourse does not correspond to these feelings— a consistent misunderstanding that could reduce the child's ability to understand/mentalize verbal explanations of other people's actions. In such circumstances, the child is likely to struggle to detect mental states behind actions and will tend to see these actions as inevitable rather than intended. This formulation implies that treatments should aim to engage maltreated children in causally coherent psychological discourse.

Summary

It would be absurd to suggest (from either a scientific or a common-sense perspective) that secure attachment is the only relationship influence on the development of mentalization. Many important influences may work in the opposite direction. For example, being able to mentalize may enable children maliciously to tease each other, thereby increasing vulnerability to relational aggression (e.g., Cutting & Dunn, 2002), or, worse, to bully each other (Sutton, Smith, & Swettenham, 1999a, 1999b). Negative experiences (e.g., emotionally charged conflict) may facilitate the rapid development of mentalizing *as readily as* the positive emotions linked to secure attachment (Newton, Reddy, & Bull, 2000). The reality is that numerous aspects of relational influence are likely to be involved in the emergence of mentalizing, some of which correlate with secure attachment. Each of these correlates of secure attachment in-

terface with one or more of a series of components of mentalizing, so relationship influences on the development of mentalization should be thought of as limited and specific rather than broad and unqualified (Hughes & Leekham, 2004).

The Social-Cognitive Influence of Attachment Security from the Viewpoint of the "Pedagogical Stance"

The attachment figure's pedagogical role has thus far been neglected as an aspect of human attachment relationships. This facet of the relationship may hold essential clues to the association of attachment and social cognition. The evolutionary underpinnings of human culture require that the infant turn to the caregiver for information about the internal and external nature of the world (Csibra & Gergely, 2006). Correspondingly, the caregiver is biologically prepared to act as a teacher. We all grow up within a cognitive system that was collaboratively designed and that has evolved to ensure the efficient transmission of relevant cultural information from knowledgeable people to ignorant ones, but specifically to receptive human babies (Gergely & Csibra, 2006). Gergely and Csibra (2006) have suggested the term "pedagogical stance" for the ability to teach and to learn from teaching, which is a fundamental attitude in social interaction within the caregiver–infant relationship. We have recently elaborated this model to incorporate the potential moderating influence of quality of attachment on the pedagogical aspect of infant and caregiver interaction (Fonagy, Gergely, & Target, 2007). Below, we briefly review the theory of natural pedagogy before presenting some ideas about its potential interface with psychoanalytic ideas related to the emergence of social cognition.

The Theory of Natural Pedagogy

Adults produce two kinds of pedagogical communicative cues to which infants are specifically receptive: cues of "referential knowledge manifestation" (a teacher transmitting knowledge—e.g., the name of an object) and "ostensive" cues that alert the infant to the speaker's intention to communicate. Ostensive cues trigger a specific receptive attitude (the pedagogical stance) in the infant. They tell the infant that new and relevant knowledge is about to be communicated about the object, and also that the communication is specifically addressed to him or her. They may include establishing eye contact, knowingly raising one's eyebrows, momentarily widening one's eyes, tilting one's head slightly forward toward the infant, calling the infant by name, and using "motherese." Turn taking and contingent reactivity also function as essential addressing and alerting cues (Csibra & Gergely, 2006). Thus early turn taking, joint attention, proto-declarative pointing, social referencing (Egyed, Király, & Gergely, 2004), and imitative learning (Gergely & Csibra, 2006) are all examples of pedagogical communication whose primary function is to facilitate fast and efficient transfer of knowledge about the world, rather than (or perhaps as well as) enabling intersubjective sharing of internal psychological states (see Tronick, 2007).

The Natural Pedagogy of Subjective States

Children need to learn not only about physical objects in the external world, but also about their own and others' subjective states. Affect-mirroring interactions between infant and caregiver are critical to the development of this capacity for introspection. The human infant is equipped at birth with the capacity to exchange affective signals with the caregiver (Jaffe et al., 2001). To achieve normal self-experience, the infant requires his or her emotional signals to be accurately or contingently mirrored by an attachment figure (Gergely & Watson, 1996). Such mirroring is far more than acceptance and validation of the experience by a significant adult; it must support the child's sense of agency as someone who can make something happen (Ryan, 2005). The experience of control that ensues from inducing the attachment figure to mirror the infant's automatic affect expressions generates a sense of agency and pleasure in the infant, which can counteract emotional distress (Watson, 1984).

In mirroring the infant, the caregiver must achieve more than contingency (in time, space, and emotional tone). The mirroring must be "marked"; in other words, the way the infant's affect display is mirrored must involve a slightly distorted or transformed (e.g., exaggerated or schematized) rendering of the emotion expression if the infant is to understand the caregiver's display as referring to the infant's emotional experience rather than being an expression of the caregiver's actual affective state (Gergely, 2004). The unmarked form of the caregiver's emotion display would indicate to the child that the emotional display is not part of a communicative act of teaching, but an expression of the caregiver's own current dispositional state. The ostensive cues activate a search for the intended referent ("What is she trying to teach me?"). Since the caregiver is clearly oriented toward the infant while responding to the infant's internal states, the infant's attention will be directed toward his or her own face and body (Gergely, 2007b). This social biofeedback system of pedagogical interactions enables infants to internalize their caregivers' representations of the reflection of their experience, and thus to generate a representational system for internal states (Gergely & Watson, 1996).

The quality of the parent–infant relationship in particular and attachment security in general predict both theoretically (Fonagy, 2001b) and empirically (Fearon & Belsky, 2004) the capacity for self-control. If ostensive cues indeed reflect the quality of parent–child relations, then variation in the quality of these cues provides us with a possible mechanism for explaining the covariation of mentalization and attachment. We now turn to the issue of these individual differences.

Consequences of Referential Knowledge and Ostensive Cues for Affect Regulation and Mentalization

Parents may fail in the pedagogical process in two ways: They may not mirror the child's internal states congruently, or they may not "mark" their mirroring. In the absence of appropriate ostensive cues, an expression of affect congruent with the baby's state may overwhelm the infant. Disruptions in communication—such as frightening behavior, grossly noncontingent emotional responding, or role reversals involving seeking comfort from the infant—are clear failures of the pedagogical stance, and these are precisely the behaviors that may suggest a significant parental failure in mentalizing the child (Grienenberger et al., 2005). Such behaviors will fail to direct the infant's attention toward his or her internal experience. From this perspective, disorganization of attachment can be understood as the consequence of a baby being presented frequently with a contingent (relevant), but either grossly incongruent (inaccurate) or unmarked (realistic), negative emotional display.

The quality of parenting in this framework can be specified as the quality of teaching about *internal* states. We believe that a caregiver's capacity to focus on an infant in a way that enables the infant to focus on his or her current experience is the crucial and operationalizable aspect of the elusive construct of parental sensitivity. Quality of ostensive and referential cuing will predict both attachment security and many of the developmental advantages that appear to flow from it. This model of infant–parent interaction is an elaboration of the general principle that the child's capacity to create a coherent image of mind depends on an experience of being perceived as having a mind by the contingently responsive attachment figure. More generally, social understanding of the subjective self can then be seen as an emergent property of the child's experience of "marked" mirroring interactions with the caregiver, which form the foundation for the eventual discovery that others have differing beliefs about the world from one's own.

Neglect

The speculations above clearly imply that the foundations of subjective selfhood will be less robustly established in individuals who have experienced early neglect. Such individuals will find it harder to learn about how subjective experiences inevitably vary between people. In some longitudinal investigations, low parental affection or nurturing in early childhood appears more strongly associated with elevated risk for borderline, antisocial, paranoid, and schizotypal personality disorders diagnosed in early adulthood than even physical or sexual abuse in adolescence (Johnson, Cohen, Kasen, Ehrensaft, & Crawford, 2006). A number of studies have pointed to the importance of neglect, low parental involvement, and emotional maltreatment rather than the presence of abuse as the critical predictor of severe personality disorder (e.g., Johnson et al., 2001). Studies of family context of childhood trauma in borderline personality disorder tend to see the unstable, non-nurturing family environment as the key social mediator of abuse (Bradley, Jenei, & Westen, 2005), whereas underinvolvement is the best predictor of suicide (Johnson et al., 2002) and personality dysfunction (Zweig-Frank & Paris, 1991). The primary task of pedagogy is to draw attention to and represent the infant's experience, thus facilitating the appropriate development of self-organization and social cognition (as suggested in Lyons-Ruth et al., 2005).

The Adaptive Value of Insecure Attachment and Low Mentalization

We have argued that insecure and unpredictable attachment relationships between parent and infant may create an adverse social environment that limits the infant's opportunity to acquire "mind reading." But why should evolution allow for such variation if mentalizing is such a valuable adaptive capacity? In social environments where resources are limited, nonmentalizing may be adaptive. A parent's lack of mirroring behavior may serve as a signal for limited resources, warning a child that he or she will need to use physical force (even interpersonal violence) to survive. Violence is incompatible with mentalization (Fonagy, 2003a, 2003b). If violence rather than collaboration is required to survive, and violence is only possible when we avoid contemplating the mental state of the victim, then a child's lack of mentalizing capacity may increase his or her chances of survival. By contrast, in resource-rich environments, adult carer-teachers are in a better position to facilitate children's access to subjectivity. If parent–child interaction lacks marking, contingency, and other ostensive cues, mentalization will be less firmly established and more readily abandoned under emotional stress. A child may then manifest early aggression and conduct problems (Lyons-Ruth, 1996). From the point of view of appropriate intervention, it is probably more helpful to view this kind of aggression as an understandable adaptation than to demonize it as an incomprehensible genetic aberration, even if these behaviors are primed in some individuals by a very sizable genetic component acting transactionally (e.g., Silberg, Rutter, Tracy, Maes, & Eaves, 2007).

Natural Pedagogy and a Theory of the Differentiation of the Self

Pedagogy theory predicts that young children will initially view everything they are taught as generally available cultural knowledge—that is, as shared by everyone (Csibra & Gergely, 2006b). Thus, when they are taught a word for a new referent, they do not need to check who else knows it. Young children assume that knowledge of subjective states is also common and that there is nothing unique about their own thoughts or feelings. A sense of the uniqueness of one's own perspective develops only gradually.

The gradual nature of this development was underscored by developmental discussion of the phenomenon that has been termed the "curse-of-knowledge bias" (Birch & Bloom, 2004). This refers to the common enough observation that if one knows something about the world, one expects that everyone else should know it too (e.g., Birch & Bloom, 2003). Young children commonly report that other children will know facts that they themselves have just learned. The curse-of-knowledge bias explains the apparent egocentrism of young children who cannot appreciate another person's perspective: It is not the overvaluing of private knowledge, as Piaget's concept of egocentrism implies, but rather the undifferentiated experience of shared knowledge that hinders them from taking the perspective of the other. Of course, this makes sense from a social-constructionist perspective. We are correct to assume universal knowledge during development, since our representations of our own subjectivity were indeed someone else's beliefs about us before their social mirroring enabled us to make them our own. This phenomenon will gradually be less and less true as we mature; yet, even as adults, we may occasionally catch ourselves assuming that others think the same way as we do.

Young children do not yet know that they can choose whether or not to share their thoughts and feelings with adults. Toddlers may be prone to tantrums because they fully expect other people to know what they are thinking and feeling, and to see situations in the same way as they do. Disagreement cannot yet be understood as the result of different points of view, so if other people thwart toddlers, the others must be either malign or wilfully obtuse. Thus conflict is not just hurtful but intolerable and maddening, since it denies this probably highly valued shared reality. We have suggested that a toddler equates the internal world with the external (Target & Fonagy, 1996). What exists in the mind must exist "out there," and what exists out there must also exist in the mind. This "psychic equivalence," as a mode of experiencing the internal world, can cause intense distress, since the projection of fantasy can be terrifying. The acquisition of a sense of pretend in relation to mental states is therefore essential. Repeated experience of affect-regulative mirroring helps the child to learn that feelings do not inevitably spill out into the world. They are decoupled from physical reality. At first this decoupling is complete (what we have called the "pretend" mode): Although it is focused on the internal, no connection with physical reality is possible. Only gradually, by engaging in playful interaction with a concerned adult who seriously entertains the child's pretend world, will the "pretend" and psychically equivalent modes integrate to form genuine subjectivity.

In understanding the emergence of mentalization, we do not need to account for how children come to understand that other people

have minds. They assume, once they acquire introspectively accessible representations, that this is always the case. Recent ToM research, using a specially adapted version of the displacement task, suggests that awareness of other minds is present from as early as 15 months (e.g., Onishi & Baillargeon, 2005). The new theoretical perspective of pedagogy theory focuses developmental attention on children's understanding that others have *separate minds* with different contents. The question is what social conditions might help infants to learn when to suspend their default assumption of universal knowledge.

Psychotherapists are invariably (and at times painfully) confronted with the recognition that their patients think in different ways. Yet they also quickly encounter the "childish" expectation of certain patients that they should be "totally" understood. More generally, an element of the significance of therapeutic alliance in psychotherapy (Orlinsky et al., 2004) is surely related to the creation of an illusion of shared consciousness with another person. It should be noted that the intersubjectivity construct implied here has a somewhat different and more specific meaning than in other usages. It refers to the recreation of a regressive illusory state of universally shared knowledge. Therapeutic alliance is often thought to be essential to therapeutic progress (although the evidence for this claim is modest) (Safran & Muran, 2000). In the light of our theory, therapeutic alliance can be seen as at least sometimes indicating a *failure* of mentalization and the reemergence of a psychic equivalent mode of thinking where others' thoughts and feelings were assumed to be the same as one's own. We would argue that the *rupture* of this illusion may have greater therapeutic potential than its mere presence. The devastation of feeling that one has not been accurately perceived (Safran & Muran, 1996) has therapeutic potential precisely because it forces therapist and patient to step beyond the illusion of shared consciousness. It creates an opportunity for each to have a mind of his or her own—at least in the patient's experience.

Pedagogy theory clarifies the role of early attachment relationships in the emergence of individual subjectivity and perspective taking. We have seen that the establishment of subjectivity is linked to attachment via the overlap between consistent ostensive and accurate referential cuing, and what attachment theorists have designated as sensitive parenting (Fearon et al., 2006). By building second-order representations on the one hand, and providing mental reasoning schemes to make sense of action on the other, the relationship with the mind-minded reflective caregiver transforms the child's implicit and automatic mentalizing competence into an explicit, potentially verbally expressible, and systematized ToM. Aspects of secure attachment (e.g., attunement sensitivity) appear to have a pedagogical function, teaching children what they cannot learn about the world by simple observation. Subjectivity of course belongs to this class of phenomena. Secure attachment and the mind-minded reflective mirroring environment extend awareness to include internal states, thereby making self-prediction and emotional self-control possible. Pedagogical referential communication applied to the domain of the emotional and dispositional/intentional states of the self creates the context wherein a caregiver can teach a child about the subjective self. The benign effects of secure attachment arise at least in part out of superior competence at ostensive cuing.

There is a second aspect of this process, however, in which the attachment relationship may play a crucial part: competition with other people, which is potentially a primary driver of the evolution of mentalization (Alexander, 1989). The pedagogical function needs to be protected from deliberate misinformation by competitors who do not have genetic material in common with the infant, and are therefore not invested in their survival. Sensitivity to false beliefs suggests that a 3- to 4-year-old child has become aware not only that knowledge is not invariably shared, but also that it is not necessarily communicated with benign intent. In Mascaro and Sperber's (2006) study, preschool children responded differentially to information supplied by a "good guy" versus a "bad guy." Passing the false-belief test—that is, having a ToM—was associated with sensitivity to information coming from positively versus negatively connoted sources.

We monitor the mental states of others in part to establish the possible motives behind any giving of information. The quality of relationship between parent and child plays an important role in establishing our capacity to do this. Children who have experienced disorganized attachment will be disadvantaged because of confusion about the possibility of trust. Secure children, by contrast, have already developed a robust sense of shared subjectivity and may also be most open to learning about the uniqueness and separateness of their self-experience. Attachment may well be a helpful behavioral marker of shared genetic makeup (Belsky & Jaffee, 2006), and consequently

a kind of "hallmark of authenticity of knowledge." The indications of generic cognitive benefits associated with secure attachment are in line with the assumption of more reliable processing of pedagogical information in caregiving environments that engender attachment security (Cicchetti et al., 2000).

Summary

In summary, we suggest that the advantage of secure attachment for the precocious development of mentalization and the stronger establishment of an agentive sense of self is the consequence of an infant's general predisposition to learn from adults. As learning is triggered by ostensive cues that share characteristics with secure parenting, the teaching of secure infants may be smoother than that of insecure ones. By contrast, disorganized attachment interferes with ostensive cues and may be expected to disrupt learning. It is expected that the influence of secure attachment will be particularly crucial in teaching infants about their own subjectivity. Finally, the characteristics of communication associated with sensitive caregiving also reassure infants about the trustworthiness of the information to be communicated. From an evolutionary standpoint, we may consider such ostensive cues (at least in infancy) to trigger a "basic epistemic trust" in a caregiver as a benevolent, cooperative, and reliable source of cultural information (Gergely, 2007a). This enables an infant to learn quickly what is communicated, without the need to test for social trustworthiness (Gergely & Csibra, 2005). Adults mainly teach infants they look after, about whom they have genetic reasons to care. Infants are also selective, identifying attachment figures to teach them what in the world is safe and trustworthy—and, furthermore, how they can think about their thoughts and feelings, and how knowledge of such internal states can eventually form a bridge to understanding and prediction in the wider social world.

CONCLUSION

In this chapter, we have reviewed the relationship of attachment theory and psychoanalysis in two stages. First, we have analyzed the relationship between these two domains, noting with some satisfaction that since the first edition of this handbook was published, accumulating work suggests a definite increase in common ground. Attachment research and theory have acquired sophistication in relation to unconscious determinants of behavior, and psychoanalysis has recognized the importance of attachment theory for many reasons, among them its contribution to ensuring the empirical legitimacy of psychoanalysis. Although the vast majority of psychoanalytic assumptions are disputed by those who adopt nondynamic approaches, few dispute the importance of attachment, or the close and appropriate tie between the psychodynamic frame of reference and the data that emerge from attachment research.

Second, rather than providing a comprehensive review of the role of attachment theory in a variety of analytic orientations, we have focused on two models, each of which illustrates how attachment theory and psychoanalysis may consolidate their rapprochement. First, we have considered relational psychoanalysis, arguably the most popular current psychodynamic approach. Close analysis of the key constructs of relational theory shows that many ideas from both attachment theory and research are implied by its constructs and observations. In particular, the process of change proposed by relational theorists is connected closely to new developments in parent–infant research inspired by attachment theory.

An alternative framework for integration is provided by a theory that moves from attachment research toward a clinical application, via developmental constructs that build on both traditional psychoanalytic ideas and developmental science. Mentalization-based treatment is rooted in attachment theory and is consistent with many findings from attachment research; its clinical technique leans heavily on psychoanalytic practice, including a relatively free therapeutic discourse about current events, particularly in an interpersonal attachment context. The focus of the approach, however, is provided by attachment-theory-inspired developmental research into the enhanced understanding of mental states in the self and in others.

We have advanced a model of the development of social cognition that pays adequate regard to the role of attachment relationships as the primary teaching context within which the understanding of minds in self and others occurs. This may help to explain why individuals in a situation of psychological distress tend to seek an understanding person with whom they recreate the pedagogical configuration of one mind teaching another mind about aspects of subjectivity. We have tried to show how the dual components of attachment and interpersonal understanding are the key ingredients for recovering the equilibrium—a kind of recalibration of understanding of mental phenomena. Psychoanalysis, in its concern with the intensive study of human subjectivity, and attachment theory, which has made the dyadic human relationship its particular focus, are thus inseparably linked in providing a model for psychological therapy.

Attachment theory cannot and does not aspire to specify the full richness of the subjective contents that preoccupy the ordinary mind, let alone the mind in distress. This is the ambition of psychoanalysis (see Slade, Chapter 32, this volume). Attachment theory, however, does offer the best theoretical and research framework for understanding and elaborating the interpersonal process within which the human mind is best able to explore the subtleties of subjectivity. Attachment theory provides an understanding of the frame, as well as some key facets of the contents; psychoanalysis guides, systematizes, and inspires the mind's understanding of the mind. It is the achievement of such understandings, regardless of specific contents, that brings about change. In seeking to describe the relationship between attachment theory and psychoanalysis, we could say that the former offers a narrative framework, while the latter provides the thickness of description required to create a complete story. Attempting to reduce one to the other will inevitably generate partial accounts and paradoxes. Neither is complete without the other.

NOTE

1. The appropriateness of IQ control is not entirely clear, given that IQ itself will also reflect social and emotional deprivation (e.g., Crandell & Hobson, 1999).

REFERENCES

Adolphs, R., Damasio, H., Tranel, D., Cooper, G., & Damasio, A. R. (2000). A role for somatosensory cortices in the visual recognition of emotion as revealed by three-dimensional lesion mapping. *Journal of Neuroscience, 20,* 2683–2690.

Alessandri, S. M. (1991). Play and social behaviors in maltreated preschoolers. *Development and Psychopathology, 3,* 191–206.

Alexander, R. D. (1989). Evolution of the human psyche. In P. Mellars & C. Stringer (Eds.), *The human revolution: Behavioral and biological perspectives on the origins of modern humans* (pp. 455–513). Princeton, NJ: Princeton University Press.

Baradon, T., Woodhead, J., Joyce, A., James, J., Gibbs, I., & Broughton, C. (2005). *The practice of psychoanalytic parent infant psychotherapy*. London: Taylor & Francis.

Bartels, A., & Zeki, S. (2000). The neural basis of romantic love. *NeuroReport, 11*, 3829–3834.

Bartels, A., & Zeki, S. (2004). The neural correlates of maternal and romantic love. *NeuroImage, 21*, 1155–1166.

Beebe, B., & Lachmann, F. M. (1994). Representation and internalization in Infancy: Three principles of salience. *Psychoanalytic Psychology, 11*, 127–166.

Beebe, B., Lachmann, F. M., & Jaffe, J. (1997). Mother–infant interaction structures and presymbolic self and object representations. *Psychoanalytic Dialogues, 7*, 113–182.

Belsky, J. (2005). The development and evolutionary psychology of intergenerational transmission of attachment. In C. S. Carter, L. Ahnert, K. E. Grossmann, S. B. Hrdy, M. E. Lamb, S. W. Porges, et al. (Eds.), *Attachment and bonding: A new synthesis* (pp. 169–198). Cambridge, MA: MIT Press.

Belsky, J., & Jaffee, S. R. (2006). The multiple determinants of parenting. In D. Cicchetti & D. J. Cohen (Eds.), *Developmental psychopathology: Vol. 3. Risk, disorder, and adaptation* (2nd ed., pp. 38–85). Hoboken, NJ: Wiley.

Benjamin, J. (1998). *The shadow of the other: Intersubjectivity and gender in psychoanalysis*. New York: Routledge.

Birch, S. A., & Bloom, P. (2003). Children are cursed: An asymmetric bias in mental state attributions. *Psychological Science, 14*, 283–286.

Birch, S. A., & Bloom, P. (2004). Understanding children's and adults' limitations in mental state reasoning. *Trends in Cognitive Sciences, 8*, 255–260.

Blagov, P. S., & Singer, J. A. (2004). Four dimensions of self-defining memories (specificity, meaning, content, and affect) and their relationships to self-restraint, distress, and repressive defensiveness. *Journal of Personality, 72*, 481–511.

Blatt, S. J. (1995). Representational structures in psychopathology. In D. Cicchetti & S. L. Toth (Eds.), *Rochester Symposium on Developmental Psychopathology: Vol. 6. Emotion, cognition, and representation* (pp. 1–33). Rochester, NY: University of Rochester Press.

Blatt, S. J. (2004). *Experiences of depression: Theoretical, clinical, and research perspectives*. Washington, DC: American Psychological Association.

Blatt, S. J., & Blass, R. B. (1990). Attachment and separateness: A dialectical model of the products and processes of development throughout the life cycle. *Psychoanalytic Study of the Child, 45*, 107–127.

Bohleber, W. (2007). Remembrance, trauma and collective memory: The battle for memory in psychoanalysis. *International Journal of Psycho-Analysis, 88*(Pt. 2), 329–352.

Bowlby, J. (1969/1982). *Attachment and loss: Vol. 1. Attachment*. London: Hogarth Press and the Institute of Psycho-Analysis.

Bowlby, J. (1973). *Attachment and loss: Vol. 2. Separation: Anxiety and anger*. London: Hogarth Press and the Institute of Psycho-Analysis.

Bowlby, J. (1980). *Attachment and loss: Vol. 3. Loss: Sadness and depression*. London: Hogarth Press and the Institute of Psycho-Analysis.

Bowlby, J. (1988a). Developmental psychiatry comes of age. *American Journal of Psychiatry, 145*, 1–10.

Bowlby, J. (1988b). *A secure base: Clinical applications of attachment theory*. London: Routledge.

Bradley, R., Jenei, J., & Westen, D. (2005). Etiology of borderline personality disorder: Disentangling the contributions of intercorrelated antecedents. *Journal of Nervous and Mental Disease, 193*, 24–31.

Brisch, K. H., Bechinger, D., Betzler, S., & Heinemann, H. (2003). Early preventive attachment-oriented psychotherapeutic intervention program with parents of a very low birthweight premature infant: Results of attachment and neurological development. *Attachment and Human Development, 5*, 120–135.

Bromberg, P. M. (1998). *Standing in the spaces*. Hillsdale, NJ: Analytic Press.

Bronfman, E., Parsons, E., & Lyons-Ruth, K. (1999). *Atypical Maternal Behavior Instrument for Assessment and Classification (AMBIANCE): Manual for coding disrupted affective communication, Version 2*. Unpublished manuscript, Harvard Medical School.

Bruer, J. T. (2002). *The myth of the first three years: A new understanding of early brain development and lifelong learning*. New York: Free Press.

Buchheim, A., & Kachele, H. (2003). Adult Attachment Interview and psychoanalytic perspective: A single case study. *Psychoanalytic Inquiry, 23*, 81–101.

Buechler, S. (1997). Attachment theory as a secure base for psychoanalytic exploration. *Contemporary Psychoanalysis, 33*, 157–161.

Cabeza, R., & Nyberg, L. (2000). Neural bases of learning and memory: Functional neuroimaging evidence. *Current Opinion in Neurology, 13*, 415–421.

Camras, L. A., Ribordy, S., Hill, J., Martino, S., Sachs, V., Spaccarelli, S., et al. (1990). Maternal facial behavior and the recognition and production of emotional expression by maltreated and nonmaltreated children. *Developmental Psychology, 26*, 304–312.

Camras, L. A., Sachs-Alter, E., & Ribordy, S. C. (1996). Emotion understanding in maltreated children: Recognition of facial expressions and integration with other emotion cues. In M. D. Lewis & M. Sullivan (Eds.), *Emotional development in atypical children* (pp. 203–225). Mahwah, NJ: Erlbaum.

Canestri, J. (Ed.). (2006). *Psychoanalysis: From practice to theory*. London: Whurr.

Canestri, J., Fonagy, P., Bohleber, W., & Dennis, P. (2006). The map of private (implicit, preconscious) theories in clinical practice. In J. Canestri (Ed.), *Psychoanalysis: From practice to theory* (pp. 29–43). London: Whurr.

Carpendale, J. I. M., & Lewis, C. (2006). *How children develop social understanding*. Oxford, UK: Blackwell.

Cassidy, J., & Kobak, R. R. (1988). Avoidance and its relation to other defensive processes. In J. Belsky & T. Nezworski (Eds.), *Clinical implications of attachment* (pp. 300–323). Hillsdale, NJ: Erlbaum.

Charman, T., Ruffman, T., & Clements, W. (2002). Is there a gender difference in false belief development? *Social Development, 11*, 1–10.

Chodorow, N. (1994). *Femininities, masculinities, sexualities: Freud and beyond*. London: Free Association Books.

Cicchetti, D., & Curtis, W. J. (2005). An event-related potential study of the processing of affective facial expressions in young children who experienced maltreatment during the first year of life. *Developmental Psychopathology, 17*, 641–677.

Cicchetti, D., Rogosch, F. A., Maughan, A., Toth, S. L., & Bruce, J. (2003). False belief understanding in maltreated children. *Developmental Psychopathology, 15*, 1067–1091.

Cicchetti, D., Rogosch, F. A., & Toth, S. L. (2000). The efficacy of toddler–parent psychotherapy for fostering cognitive development in offspring of depressed mothers. *Journal of Abnormal Child Psychology, 28*, 135–148.

Cicchetti, D., Rogosch, F. A., & Toth, S. L. (2006). Fostering secure attachment in infants in maltreating families through preventive interventions. *Developmental Psychopathology, 18*, 623–649.

Cicchetti, D., & Valentino, K. (2006). An ecological–transactional perspective on child maltreatment: Failure of the average expectable environment and its influence on child development. In D. Cicchetti & D. J. Cohen (Eds.), *Developmental psychopathology: Vol. 3. Risk, disorder, and adaptation* (2nd ed., pp. 129–201). Hoboken, NJ: Wiley.

Cicchetti, D., & Walker, E. F. (2001). Editorial: Stress and development: Biological and psychological consequences. *Development and Psychopathology, 13*, 413–418.

Coan, J. A., Schaefer, H. S., & Davidson, R. J. (2006). Lending a hand: Social regulation of the neural response to threat. *Psychological Science, 17*, 1032–1039.

Cortina, M. (1999). Causality, adaptation, and meaning: A perspective from attachment theory and research. *Psychoanalytic Dialogues, 9*, 557–596.

Cortina, M. (2001). Sullivan's contributions to understanding personality development in light of attachment theory and contemporary models of the mind. *Contemporary Psychoanalysis, 37*, 193–238.

Crandell, L. E., & Hobson, R. P. (1999). Individual differences in young children's IQ: A social-developmental perspective. *Journal of Child Psychology and Psychiatry, 40*, 455–464.

Crittenden, P. M. (1997). Toward an integrative theory of trauma: A dynamic-maturation approach. In D. Cicchetti & S. L. Toth (Eds.), *Rochester Symposium on Developmental Psychopathology: Vol. 8. Developmental perspectives on trauma* (pp. 33–84). Rochester, NY: University of Rochester Press.

Csibra, G., & Gergely, G. (2006). Social learning and social cognition: The case for pedagogy. In M. H. Johnson & Y. M. Munakata (Eds.), *Attention and performance: Vol. 21. Processes of change in brain and cognitive development* (pp. 249–274). Oxford, UK: Oxford University Press.

Cutting, A. L., & Dunn, J. (2002). The cost of understanding other people: Social cognition predicts young children's sensitivity to criticism. *Journal of Child Psychology and Psychiatry, 43*, 849–860.

Cyranowski, J. M., Bookwala, J., Feske, U., Houck, P., Pilkonis, P., Kostelnik, B., et al. (2002). Adult attachment profiles, interpersonal difficulties, and response to interpersonal psychotherapy in women with recurrent major depression. *Journal of Social and Clinical Psychology, 21*, 191–217.

Davies, J. M. (1996). Linking the "pre-analytic" with the postclassical: Integration, dissociation, and the multiplicity of unconscious processes. *Contemporary Psychoanalysis, 32*, 553–576.

Davies, J. M., & Frawley, M. G. (1994). *Treating the adult survivor of childhood sexual abuse: A psychoanalytic perspective*. New York: Basic Books.

de Rosnay, M., & Harris, P. L. (2002). Individual differences in children's understanding of emotion: The roles of attachment and language. *Attachment and Human Development, 4*, 39–54.

Diamond, D., Stovall-McClough, C., Clarkin, J. F., & Levy, K. N. (2003). Patient–therapist attachment in the treatment of borderline personality disorder. *Bulletin of the Menninger Clinic, 67*, 227–259.

Downey, W. T. (2000). Little Orphan Anastasia. *Psychoanalytic Study of the Child, 55*, 145–179.

Dunlea, A. (1989). *Vision and the emergence of meaning*. Cambridge, UK: Cambridge University Press.

Dunn, J., Brown, J., & Beardsall, L. (1991). Family talk abut feeling states and children's later understanding of others' emotions. *Developmental Psychology, 27*, 448–455.

During, S., & McMahon, R. (1991). Recognition of emotional facial expressions by abusive mothers and their children. *Journal of Clinical and Consulting Psychology, 20*, 132–139.

Eagle, M. N. (2006). Attachment, psychotherapy, and assessment: A commentary. *Journal of Consulting and Clinical Psychology, 74*, 1086–1097.

Egyed, K., Király, I., & Gergely, G. (2004, May). *Object-centered versus agent-centered interpretations of referential attitude expressions in 14-month-olds*. Poster presented at the 14th Biennial International Conference on Infant Studies, Chicago.

Emde, R. N., Kubicek, L., & Oppenheim, D. (1997). Imaginative reality observed during early language development. *International Journal of Psycho-Analysis, 78*, 115–133.

Emde, R. N., & Spicer, P. (2000). Experience in the midst of variation: New horizons for development and psychopathology. *Development and Psychopathology, 12,* 313–332.

Fearon, R. M. P., & Belsky, J. (2004). Attachment and attention: Protection in relation to gender and cumulative social-contextual adversity. *Child Development, 75,* 1677–1693.

Fearon, R. M. P., van IJzendoorn, M. H., Fonagy, P., Bakermans-Kranenburg, M. J., Schuengel, C., & Bokhorst, C. L. (2006). In search of shared and nonshared environmental factors in security of attachment: A behavior-genetic study of the association between sensitivity and attachment security. *Developmental Psychology, 42,* 1026–1040.

Fenichel, O. (1941). *Problems of psychoanalytic technique.* New York: Psychoanalytic Quarterly.

Ferenczi, S. (1980). The further development of an active therapy in psychoanalysis. In S. Ferenczi, *Further contributions to the theory and technique of psychoanalysis* (pp. 198–216). London: Karnac Books. (Original work published 1922)

Fonagy, P. (1991). Thinking about thinking: Some clinical and theoretical considerations in the treatment of a borderline patient. *International Journal of Psycho-Analysis, 72,* 1–18.

Fonagy, P. (1998). Moments of change in psychoanalytic theory: Discussion of a new theory of psychic change. *Infant Mental Health Journal, 19,* 163–171.

Fonagy, P. (1999a). Memory and therapeutic action [Guest editorial]. *International Journal of Psycho-Analysis, 80,* 215–223.

Fonagy, P. (1999b). Psychoanalytic theory from the viewpoing of attachment theory and research. In J. Cassidy & P. R. Shaver (Eds.), *Handbook of attachment: Theory, research, and clinical applications* (pp. 595–624). New York: Guilford Press.

Fonagy, P. (2001a). *Attachment theory and psychoanalysis.* New York: Other Press.

Fonagy, P. (2001b). The human genome and the representational world: The role of early mother–infant interaction in creating an interpersonal interpretive mechanism. *Bulletin of the Menninger Clinic, 65,* 427–448.

Fonagy, P. (2003a). The developmental roots of violence in the failure of mentalization. In F. Pfäfflin & G. Adshead (Eds.), *A matter of security: The application of attachment theory to forensic psychiatry and psychotherapy* (pp. 13–56). London: Jessica Kingsley.

Fonagy, P. (2003b). Towards a developmental understanding of violence. *British Journal of Psychiatry, 183,* 190–192.

Fonagy, P., Gergely, G., Jurist, E., & Target, M. (2002). *Affect regulation, mentalization, and the development of the self.* New York: Other Press.

Fonagy, P., Gergely, G., & Target, M. (2007). The parent–infant dyad and the construction of the subjective self. *Journal of Child Psychology and Psychiatry, 48,* 288–328.

Fonagy, P., Redfern, S., & Charman, T. (1997). The relationship between belief–desire reasoning and a projective measure of attachment security (SAT). *British Journal of Developmental Psychology, 15,* 51–61.

Fonagy, P., Steele, H., Moran, G., Steele, M., & Higgitt, A. (1991). The capacity for understanding mental states: The reflective self in parent and child and its significance for security of attachment. *Infant Mental Health Journal, 13,* 200–217.

Fonagy, P., Steele, H., & Steele, M. (1991). Maternal representations of attachment during pregnancy predict the organization of infant–mother attachment at one year of age. *Child Development, 62,* 891–905.

Fonagy, P., Steele, H., Steele, M., & Holder, J. (1997). Attachment and theory of mind: Overlapping constructs? *Association for Child Psychology and Psychiatry Occasional Papers, 14,* 31–40.

Fonagy, P., & Target, M. (2003). *Psychoanalytic theories: Perspectives from developmental psychopathology.* London: Whurr.

Fonagy, P., Target, M., Cottrell, D., Phillips, J., & Kurtz, Z. (2002). *What works for whom?: A Critical review of treatments for children and adolescents.* New York: Guilford Press.

Fonagy, P., Target, M., & Gergely, G. (2006). Psychoanalytic perspectives on developmental psychopathology. In D. Cicchetti & D. J. Cohen (Eds.), *Developmental psychopathology: Vol. 1. Theory and methods* (2nd ed., pp. 701–749). Hoboken, NJ: Wiley.

Freud, A. (1965). *Normality and pathology in childhood: Assessments of development.* New York: International Universities Press.

Fries, A. B., Ziegler, T. E., Kurian, J. R., Jacoris, S., & Pollak, S. D. (2005). Early experience in humans is associated with changes in neuropeptides critical for regulating social behavior. *Proceedings of the National Academy of Sciences USA, 102,* 17237–17240.

Gallagher, H. L., & Frith, C. D. (2003). Functional imaging of "theory of mind." *Trends in Cognitive Sciences, 7,* 77–83.

Gedo, J. E. (1979). *Beyond interpretation.* New York: International Universities Press.

George, C., & Solomon, J. (1999). A comparison of attachment theory and psychoanalytic approaches to mothering. *Psychoanalytic Inquiry, 19,* 618–646.

Gergely, G. (2000). Reapproaching Mahler: New perspectives on normal autism, normal symbiosis, splitting, and libidinal object constancy from cognitive developmental theory. *Journal of the American Psychoanalytic Association, 48,* 1197–1228.

Gergely, G. (2004). The role of contingency detection in early affect-regulative interactions and in the development of different types of infant attachment. *Social Behavior, 13,* 468–478.

Gergely, G. (2007a). Learning "about" versus learning "from" other minds: Human pedagogy and its implications. In P. Carruthers, S. Laurence, & S. Stich (Eds.), *The innate mind: Foundations and the future* (pp. 170–199). Oxford, UK: Oxford University Press.

Gergely, G. (2007b). The social construction of the subjective self: The role of affect-mirroring, markedness, and ostensive communication in self development. In L. Mayes, P. Fonagy, & M. Target (Eds.), *Developmental science and psychoanalysis* (pp. 45–82). London: Karnac Books.

Gergely, G., & Csibra, G. (2005). The social construction of the cultural mind: Imitative learning as a mechanism of human pedagogy. *Interaction Studies, 6,* 463–481.

Gergely, G., & Csibra, G. (2006). Sylvia's recipe: Human culture, imitation, and pedagogy. In N. J. Enfield & S. C. Levinson (Eds.), *Roots of human sociality: Culture, cognition, and human interaction* (pp. 229–255). London: Berg Press.

Gergely, G., & Watson, J. (1996). The social biofeedback model of parental affect-mirroring. *International Journal of Psycho-Analysis, 77,* 1181–1212.

Geyskens, T. (2003). Imre Hermann's Freudian theory of attachment. *International Journal of Psycho-Analysis, 84,* 1517–1529.

Gillath, O., Bunge, S. A., Shaver, P. R., Wendelken, C., & Mikulincer, M. (2005). Attachment-style differences in the ability to suppress negative thoughts: exploring the neural correlates. *NeuroImage, 28,* 835–847.

Green, S., Pring, L., & Swettenham, J. (2004). An investigation of first-order false belief understanding of children with congenital profound visual impairment. *British Journal of Developmental Psychology, 22,* 1–17.

Grienenberger, J. F., Kelly, K., & Slade, A. (2005). Maternal reflective functioning, mother–infant affective communication, and infant attachment: Exploring the link between mental states and observed caregiving behavior in the intergenerational transmission of attachment. *Attachment and Human Development, 7,* 299–311.

Grossmann, K. E., Grossmann, K., & Waters, E. (Eds.). (2005). *Attachment from infancy to adulthood: The major longitudinal studies.* New York: Guilford Press.

Grünbaum, A. (1993). *The validation of the clinical theory of psychoanalysis.* Madison, CT: International Universities Press.

Harris, P. (2005). Conversation, pretence, and theory of mind. In J. Astington & J. Baird (Eds.), *Why language matters for theory of mind* (pp. 70–83). New York: Oxford University Press.

Harrison, A. M. (2003). Change in psychoanalysis: Getting from A to B. *Journal of the American Psychoanalytic Association, 51,* 221–256.

Hennighausen, K., & Lyons-Ruth, K. (2005). Disorganization of behavioral and attentional strategies toward primary attachment figures: From biologic to dialogic processes. In C. S. Carter, L. Ahnert, K. E. Grossmann, S. B. Hrdy, M. E. Lamb, S. W. Porges, et al. (Eds.), *Attachment and bonding: A new synthesis* (pp. 269–300). Cambridge, MA: MIT Press.

Hesse, E., & Main, M. (2006). Frightened, threatening, and dissociative parental behavior in low-risk samples: Description, discussion, and interpretations. *Developmental Psychopathology, 18,* 309–343.

Hill, J., Fonagy, P., Safier, E., & Sargent, J. (2003). The ecology of attachment in the family. *Family Process, 42,* 205–221.

Hobson, P. (2002). *The cradle of thought: Explorations of the origins of thinking.* Oxford, UK: Macmillan.

Hoffman, I. Z. (1998). *Ritual and spontaneity in the psychoanalytic process.* Hillsdale, NJ: Analytic Press.

Hoffman, K. T., Marvin, R. S., Cooper, G., & Powell, B. (2006). Changing toddlers' and preschoolers' attachment classifications: The Circle of Security intervention. *Journal of Consulting and Clinical Psychology, 74*(6), 1017–1026.

Hoglend, P., Johansson, P., Marble, A., Bogwald, K.-P., & Amlo, S. (2007). Moderators of the effect of transference interpretation in brief dynamic psychotherapy. *Psychotherapy Research, 17,* 162–174.

Holmes, J., & Bateman, A. (2002). *Integration in psychotherapy: Models and methods.* Oxford, UK: Oxford University Press.

Hughes, C., & Dunn, J. (2002). "When I say a naughty word." Children's accounts of anger and sadness in self, mother and friend: Longitudinal findings from ages four to seven. *British Journal of Developmental Psychology, 20,* 515–535.

Hughes, C., Jaffee, S. R., Happe, F., Taylor, A., Caspi, A., & Moffitt, T. E. (2005). Origins of individual differences in theory of mind: From nature to nurture? *Child Development, 76,* 356–370.

Hughes, C., & Leekham, S. (2004). What are the links between theory of mind and social relations?: Review, reflections, and new directions for studies of typical and atypical development. *Social Behavior, 13,* 590–619.

Insel, T. R. (2003). Is social attachment an addictive disorder? *Physiology and Behavior, 79,* 351–357.

Jaffe, J., Beebe, B., Feldstein, S., Crown, C. L., & Jasnow, M. D. (2001). Rhythms of dialogue in infancy. *Monographs of the Society for Research in Child Development, 66*(2, Serial No. 131).

Johnson, J. G., Cohen, P., Gould, M. S., Kasen, S., Brown, J., & Brook, J. S. (2002). Childhood adversities, interpersonal difficulties, and risk for suicide attempts during late adolescence and early adulthood. *Archives of General Psychiatry, 59,* 741–749.

Johnson, J. G., Cohen, P., Kasen, S., Ehrensaft, M. K., & Crawford, T. N. (2006). Associations of parental personality disorders and Axis I disorders with child-rearing behavior. *Psychiatry, 69,* 336–350.

Johnson, J. G., Cohen, P., Smailes, E., Skodol, A., Brown, J., & Oldham, J. (2001). Childhood verbal abuse and risk for personality disorders during adolescence and early adulthood. *Comprehensive Psychiatry, 42,* 16–23.

Klerman, G. L., Weissman, M. M., Rounsaville, B. J., & Chevron, E. S. (1984). *Interpersonal psychotherapy of depression.* New York: Basic Books.

Klimes-Dougan, B., & Kistner, J. (1990). Physically abused preschoolers' responses to peers' distress. *Developmental Psychology, 25,* 516–524.

Levenson, E. (1983). *The ambiguity of change.* New York: Basic Books.

Lewis, V., Norgate, S., Collis, G., & Reynolds, R. (2000). The consequences of visual impairment for children's symbolic and functional play. *British Journal of Developmental Psychology, 18,* 449–464.

Lichtenberg, J. (1989). *Psychoanalysis and motivation.* Hillsdale, NJ: Analytic Press.

Lieberman, A. F. (1999). Negative maternal attributions: Effects on toddlers' sense of self. *Psychoanalytic Inquiry, 19,* 737–756.

Lieberman, A. F., Van Horn, P., & Ippen, C. G. (2005). Toward evidence-based treatment: Child–parent psychotherapy with preschoolers exposed to marital violence. *Journal of the American Academy of Child and Adolescent Psychiatry, 44,* 1241–1248.

Lieberman, M. D. (2007). Social cognitive neuroscience: A review of core processes. *Annual Review of Psychology, 58,* 259–289.

Lim, M. M., Murphy, A. Z., & Young, L. J. (2004). Ventral striatopallidal oxytocin and vasopressin V1a receptors in the monogamous prairie vole (*Microtus ochrogaster*). *Journal of Comparative Neurology, 468,* 555–570.

Lyons-Ruth, K. (1996). Attachment relationships among children with aggressive behavior problems: The role of disorganized early attachment patterns. *Journal of Consulting and Clinical Psychology, 64,* 32–40.

Lyons-Ruth, K. (1998). Implicit relational knowing: Its role in development and psychoanalytic treatment. *Infant Mental Health Journal, 7,* 127–131.

Lyons-Ruth, K. (1999). The two-person unconscious: Intersubjective dialogue, enactive relational representation, and the emergence of new forms of relational organization. *Psychoanalytic Inquiry, 19,* 576–617.

Lyons-Ruth, K. (2003). Dissociation and the parent–infant dialogue: A longitudinal perspective from attachment research. *Journal of the American Psychoanalytic Association, 51,* 883–911.

Lyons-Ruth, K., & Spielman, E. (2004). Disorganized infant attachment strategies and helpless-fearful profiles of parenting: Integrating attachment research with clinical intervention. *Infant Mental Health Journal, 25,* 318–335.

Lyons-Ruth, K., Yellin, C., Melnick, S., & Atwood, G. (2005). Expanding the concept of unresolved mental states: Hostile/helpless states of mind on the Adult Attachment Interview are associated with disrupted mother–infant communication and infant disorganization. *Developmental Psychopathology, 17,* 1–23.

Maddock, R. J. (1999). The retrosplenial cortex and emotion: New insights from functional neuroimaging of the human brain. *Trends in Neurosciences, 22,* 310–316.

Main, M. (2000). The organized categories of infant, child and adult attachment: Flexible vs. inflexible attention under attachment-related stress. *Journal of the American Psychoanalytic Association, 48,* 1055–1096.

Main, M., & Morgan, H. (1996). Disorganization and disorientation in infant strange situation behavior: Phenotypic resemblance to dissociative states. In L.

K. Michelson & W. J. Ray (Eds.), *Handbook of dissociation: Theoretical, empirical, and clinical perspectives* (pp. 107–138). New York: Plenum Press.

Mascaro, O., & Sperber, D. (2006, October). *Mindreading, comprehension, and epistemic vigilance: An evolutionary and developmental perspective.* Paper presented at the AHRC Workshop on "Culture and the Mind," Sheffield, UK.

Masson, J. (1984). *The assault on truth: Freud's suppression of the seduction theory.* New York: Farrar, Straus & Giroux.

Maughan, A., & Cicchetti, D. (2002). Impact of child maltreatment and interadult violence on children's emotion regulation abilities and socioemotional adjustment. *Child Development, 73,* 1525–1542.

Mayberg, H. S., Liotti, M., Brannan, S. K., McGinnis, S., Mahurin, R. K., Jerabek, P. A., et al. (1999). Reciprocal limbic–cortical function and negative mood: Converging PET findings in depression and normal sadness. *American Journal of Psychiatry, 156,* 675–682.

Mayes, L. C. (2000). A developmental perspective on the regulation of arousal states. *Seminars in Perinatology, 24,* 267–279.

Mayes, L. C., Fonagy, P., & Target, M. (Eds.). (2007). *Developmental science and psychoanalysis.* London: Karnac Books.

McAlpine, L. M., & Moore, C. L. (1985). The development of social understanding in children with visual impairments. *Journal of Visual Impairment and Blindness, 89,* 349–358.

McBride, C., Atkinson, L., Quilty, L. C., & Bagby, R. M. (2006). Attachment as moderator of treatment outcome in major depression: A randomized control trial of interpersonal psychotherapy versus cognitive behavior therapy. *Journal of Consulting and Clinical Psychology, 74,* 1041–1054.

Meins, E., Fernyhough, C., Wainwright, R., Clark-Carter, D., Das Gupta, M., Fradley, E., et al. (2003). Pathways to understanding mind: Construct validity and predictive validity of maternal mind-mindedness. *Child Development, 74,* 1194–1211.

Meins, E., Fernyhough, C., Wainwright, R., Das Gupta, M., Fradley, E., & Tuckey, M. (2002). Maternal mind-mindedness and attachment security as predictors of theory of mind understanding. *Child Development, 73,* 1715–1726.

Meins, E., Fernyhough, C., Fradley, E., & Tuckey, M. (2001). Rethinking maternal sensitivity: Mothers' comments on infants mental processes predict security of attachment at 12 months. *Journal of Child Psychology and Psychiatry, 42,* 637–648.

Mikulincer, M., Shaver, P. R., & Cassidy, J. (in press). Attachment-related defensive processes. In J. H. Obegi & E. Berant (Eds.), *Clinical applications of adult attachment research.* New York: Guilford Press.

Mitchell, S. A. (1984). Object relations theories and the developmental tilt. *Contemporary Psychoanalysis, 20,* 473–499.

Mitchell, S. A. (1988). *Relational concepts in psychoanaly-*

sis: An integration. Cambridge, MA: Harvard University Press.

Mitchell, S. A. (2000). *Relationality: From attachment to intersubjectivity.* Hillsdale, NJ: Analytic Press.

Mitchell, S. A., & Aron, L. (Eds.). (1999). *Relational psychoanalysis: The emergence of a tradition.* Hillsdale, NJ: Analytic Press.

Mufson, L., Dorta, K. P., Olfson, M., Weissman, M. M., & Hoagwood, K. (2004). Effectiveness research: Transporting interpersonal psychotherapy for depressed adolescents (IPT-A) from the lab to school-based health clinics. *Clinical Child and Family Psychology Review, 7,* 251–261.

Mufson, L., Dorta, K. P., Wickramaratne, P., Nomura, Y., Olfson, M., & Weissman, M. M. (2004). A randomized effectiveness trial of interpersonal psychotherapy for depressed adolescents. *Archives of General Psychiatry, 61,* 577–584.

Mufson, L., Gallagher, T., Dorta, K. P., & Young, J. F. (2004). A group adaptation of interpersonal psychotherapy for depressed adolescents. *American Journal of Psychotherapy, 58,* 220–237.

Mufson, L., & Moreau, D. (1999). Interpersonal psychotherapy for depressed adolescents (IPT-A). In S. W. Russ & T. H. Ollendick (Eds.), *Handbook of psychotherapies with children and families* (pp. 239–253). New York: Kluwer.

Nahum, J. P., Bruschweiler-Stern, N., Harrison, A. M., Lyons-Ruth, K., Morgan, A. C., Sander, L. W., et al. (2002). Explicating the implicit: The local level and the microprocess of change in the analytic situation. *International Journal of Psycho-Analysis, 83*(Pt. 5), 1051–1062.

Newton, P., Reddy, V., & Bull, R. (2000). Children's everyday deception and performance on false-belief tasks. *British Journal of Developmental Psychology, 18,* 297–317.

Nitschke, J. B., Nelson, E. E., Rusch, B. D., Fox, A. S., Oakes, T. R., & Davidson, R. J. (2004). Orbitofrontal cortex tracks positive mood in mothers viewing pictures of their newborn infants. *NeuroImage, 21,* 583–592.

Onishi, K. H., & Baillargeon, R. (2005). Do 15-month-old infants understand false beliefs? *Science, 308,* 255–258.

Oppenheim, D., & Koren-Karie, N. (2002). Mothers' insightfulness regarding their children's internal worlds: The capacity underlying secure child–mother relationships. *Infant Mental Health Journal, 23,* 593–605.

Orlinsky, D. E., Ronnestad, M. H., & Willutski, U. (2004). Fifty years of psychotherapy process–outcome research: Continuity and change. In M. Lambert (Ed.), *Bergin and Garfield's handbook of psychotherapy and behavior change* (5th ed., pp. 307–390). New York: Wiley.

Panksepp, J. (1998). *Affective neuroscience: The foundations of human and animal emotions.* Oxford, UK: Oxford University Press.

Parish, M., & Eagle, M. N. (2003). Attachment to the therapist. *Psychoanalytic Psychology, 20,* 271–286.

PDM Task Force. (2006). *Psychodynamic diagnostic manual.* Silver Spring, MD: Alliance of Psychoanalytic Organizations.

Pears, K. C., & Fisher, P. A. (2005). Emotion understanding and theory of mind among maltreated children in foster care. *Development and Psychopathology, 17,* 47–65.

Pears, K. C., & Moses, L. J. (2003). Demographics, parenting, and theory of mind in preschool children. *Social Development, 12,* 1–20.

Person, E. S., Gabbard, G. O., & Cooper, A. M. (Eds.). (2005). *The American Psychiatric Publishing textbook of psychoanalysis.* Washington, DC: American Psychiatric Publishing.

Person, E. S., & Klar, H. (1994). Establishing trauma: The difficulty distinguishing between memories and fantasies. *Journal of the American Psychoanalytic Association, 42,* 1055–1081.

Pine, F. (1981). In the beginning: Contributions to a psychoanalytic developmental psychology. *International Review of Psycho-Analysis, 8,* 15–33.

Pizer, B. (2003). When the crunch is a (k)not: A crimp in relational dialogue. *Psychoanalytic Dialogues, 13,* 171–192.

Priel, B., & Besser, A. (2001). Bridging the gap between attachment and object relations theories: A study of the transition to motherhood. *British Journal of Medical Psychology, 74*(Pt. 1), 85–100.

Rogosch, F. A., Cicchetti, D., & Aber, J. L. (1995). The role of child maltreatment in early deviations in cognitive and affective processing abilities and later peer relationship problems. *Development and Psychopathology, 7,* 591–609.

Roisman, G. I., & Fraley, R. C. (2006). The limits of genetic influence: A behavior-genetic analysis of infant–caregiver relationship quality and temperament. *Child Development, 77,* 1656–1667.

Ruffman, T., Perner, J., & Parkin, L. (1999). How parenting style affects false belief understanding. *Social Development, 8,* 395–411.

Ryan, R. M. (2005). The developmental line of autonomy in the etiology, dynamics, and treatment of borderline personality disorders. *Developmental Psychopathology, 17,* 987–1006.

Ryle, A. (2003). Something more than the 'something more than interpretation' is needed: A comment on the paper by the Process of Change Study Group. *International Journal of Psycho-Analysis, 84*(Pt. 1), 109–118.

Ryle, A., & Fawkes, L. (2007). Multiplicity of selves and others: Cognitive analytic therapy. *Journal of Clinical Psychology, 63,* 165–174.

Safran, J. D., & Muran, J. C. (1996). The resolution of ruptures in the therapeutic alliance. *Journal of Consulting and Clinical Psychology, 64,* 447–458.

Safran, J. D., & Muran, J. C. (2000). The therapeutic alliance: Introduction. *Journal of Clinical Psychology, 56,* 159–161.

Sameroff, A. J., & Chandler, M. J. (1975). Reproductive risk and the continuum of caretaking causality.

In F. D. Horowitz (Ed.), *Review of child development research* (pp. 187–244). Chicago: University of Chicago Press.

Sandler, J. (1960). The background of safety. *International Journal of Psycho-Analysis, 41*, 191–198.

Sandler, J. (1983). Reflections on some relations between psychoanalytic concepts and psychoanalytic practice. *International Journal of Psycho-Analysis, 64*, 35–45.

Sandler, J. (2003). On attachment to internal objects. *Psychoanalytic Inquiry, 23*, 12–26.

Seligman, S. (1999). Integrating Kleinian theory and intersubjective infant research. *Psychoanalytic Dialogues, 9*, 129–159.

Sharp, C., Fonagy, P., & Goodyer, I. (2006). Imagining your child's mind: Psychosocial adjustment and mothers' ability to predict their children's attributional response styles. *British Journal of Developmental Psychology, 24*, 197–214.

Shipman, K. L., & Zeman, J. (1999). Emotional understanding: A comparison of physically maltreating and nonmaltreating mother–child dyads. *Journal of Clinical Child Psychology, 28*, 407–417.

Siegal, M., & Patterson, C. C. (in press). Language and theory of mind in atypically developing children: Evidence from studies of deafness, blindness, and autism. In C. Sharp, P. Fonagy, & I. Goodyer (Eds.), *Social cognition and developmental psychology*. Oxford, UK: Oxford University Press.

Silberg, J. L., Rutter, M., Tracy, K., Maes, H. H., & Eaves, L. (2007). Etiological heterogeneity in the development of antisocial behavior: The Virginia Twin Study of Adolescent Behavioral Development and the Young Adult Follow-Up. *Psychological Medicine, 37*(8), 1193–1202.

Slade, A. (2005). Parental reflective functioning: An introduction. *Attachment and Human Development, 7*, 269–281.

Slade, A., Grienenberger, J., Bernbach, E., Levy, D., & Locker, A. (2005). Maternal reflective functioning, attachment, and the transmission gap: A preliminary study. *Attachment and Human Development, 7*, 283–298.

Smith, M., & Walden, T. (1999). Understanding feelings and coping with emotional situations: A comparison of maltreated and nonmaltreated preschoolers. *Social Development, 8*, 93–116.

Sroufe, L. A. (1996). *Emotional development: The organization of emotional life in the early years*. New York: Cambridge University Press.

Steele, M., & Baradon, T. (2004). The clinical use of the Adult Attachment Interview in parent–infant psychotherapy. *Infant Mental Health Journal, 25*, 284–299.

Steele, M., Fonagy, P., Yabsley, S., Woolgar, M., & Croft, C. (1995, May). *Maternal representations of attachment during pregnancy predict quality of children's doll play at 5 years of age*. Paper presented at the biennial meeting of the Society for Research in Child Development, Indianapolis, IN.

Steele, M., Henderson, K., Hodges, J., Kaniuk, J., Hillman, S., & Steele, H. (2007). In the best interest of the late placed child: A report from the attachment representations and adoption outcome study. In L. C. Mayes, P. Fonagy, & M. Target (Eds.), *Developmental science and psychoanalysis* (pp. 159–182). London: Karnac Books.

Stern, D., Sander, L., Nahum, J., Harrison, A., Lyons-Ruth, K., Morgan, A., et al. (1998). Non-interpretive mechanisms in psychoanalytic therapy: The 'something more' than interpretation. *International Journal of Psycho-Analysis, 79*, 903–921.

Stern, D. B. (1997). *Unformulated experience: From dissociation to imagination in psychoanalysis*. Hillsdale, NJ: Analytic Press.

Stern, D. N. (1985). *The interpersonal world of the infant: A view from psychoanalysis and developmental psychology*. New York: Basic Books.

Stern, D. N. (1994). One way to build a clinically relevant baby. *Infant Mental Health Journal, 15*, 36–54.

Stolorow, R. D. (1997). Review of "A dynamic systems approach to the development of cognition and action." *International Journal of Psycho-Analysis, 78*, 620–623.

Strachey, J. (1934). The nature of the therapeutic action of psychoanalysis. *International Journal of Psycho-Analysis, 50*, 275–292.

Sullivan, H. S. (1953). *The interpersonal theory of psychiatry*. New York: Norton.

Sullivan, H. S. (1964). *The fusion of psychiatry and social science*. New York: Norton.

Suomi, S. J. (2000). A biobehavioral perspective on developmental psychopathology: Excessive aggression and serotonergic dysfunction in monkeys. In A. J. Sameroff, M. Lewis, & S. Miller (Eds.), *Handbook of developmental psychopathology* (pp. 237–256). New York: Plenum Press.

Sutton, J., Smith, P. K., & Swettenham, J. (1999a). Bullying and "theory of mind": A critique of the "social skills deficit" view of anti-social behaviour. *Social Development, 8*, 117–127.

Sutton, J., Smith, P. K., & Swettenham, J. (1999b). Social cognition and bullying: Social inadequacy or skilled manipulation? *British Journal of Developmental Psychology, 17*, 435–450.

Target, M., & Fonagy, P. (1996). Playing with reality: II. The development of psychic reality from a theoretical perspective. *International Journal of Psycho-Analysis, 77*, 459–479.

Tasca, G. A., Ritchie, K., Conrad, G., Balfour, L., Gayton, J., Lybanon, V., et al. (2006). Attachment scales predict outcome in a randomized controlled trial of two group therapies for binge eating disorder: An aptitude by treatment interaction. *Psychotherapy Research, 16*, 106–121.

Toth, S. L., Cicchetti, D., Macfie, J., Maughan, A., & Vanmeenen, K. (2000). Narrative representations of caregivers and self in maltreated pre-schoolers. *Attachment and Human Development, 2*, 271–305.

Toth, S. L., Rogosch, F. A., Manly, J. T., & Cicchetti, D.

(2006). The efficacy of toddler–parent psychotherapy to reorganize attachment in the young offspring of mothers with major depressive disorder: A randomized preventive trial. *Journal of Consulting and Clinical Psychology, 74*, 1006–1016.

Trevarthen, C. A. (1993). The self born in intersubjectivity: An infant communicating. In U. Neisser (Ed.), *The perceived self* (pp. 121–173). New York: Cambridge University Press.

Trevarthen, C. A., & Aitken, K. J. (2001). Infant intersubjectivity: Research, theory, and clinical applications. *Journal of Child Psychology and Psychiatry, 42*, 3–48.

Trevarthen, C. A., Aitken, K. J., Vandekerckhove, M., Delafield-Butt, J., & Nagy, E. (2006). Collaborative regulations of vitality in early childhood: Stress in intimate relationships and postnatal psychopathology. In D. Cicchetti & D. J. Cohen (Eds.), *Developmental psychopathology: Vol. 2. Developmental neuroscience* (2nd ed., pp. 65–126). Hoboken, NJ: Wiley.

Tronick, E. Z. (1989). Emotions and emotional communication in infants. *American Psychologist, 44*, 112–119.

Tronick, E. Z. (2001). Emotional connection and dyadic consciousness in infant–mother and patient–therapist interactions: Commentary on paper by Frank M. Lachman. *Psychoanalytic Dialogues, 11*, 187–195.

Tronick, E. Z. (2007). *The neurobehavioral and social-emotional development of infants and children*. New York: Norton.

Tröster, H., & Bambring, M. (1994). Play behavior and play materials in blind and sighted infants and preschoolers. *Journal of Visual Impairment and Blindness, 88*, 421–433.

Tyson, P., & Tyson, R. L. (1990). *Psychoanalytic theories of development: An integration*. New Haven, CT: Yale University Press.

Vinden, P. G. (2001). Parenting attitudes and children's understanding of mind: A comparison of Korean American and Anglo-American families. *Cognitive Development, 16*, 793–809.

Wallerstein, R. S. (2005). Will psychoanalytic pluralism be an enduring state of our discipline? *International Journal of Psycho-Analysis, 86*(Pt. 3), 623–626.

Warner, V., Weissman, M. M., Mufson, L., & Wickramaratne, P. J. (1999). Grandparents, parents, and grandchildren at high risk for depression: A three generation study. *Journal of the American Academy of Child and Adolescent Psychiatry, 38*, 289–296.

Watson, J. S. (1984). Bases of causal inference in infancy: Time, space, and sensory relations. In L. P. Lipsitt & C. Rovee-Collier (Eds.), *Advances in infancy research* (pp. 152–165). Norwood, NJ: Ablex.

Westen, D. (1998). Affect regulation and psychopathology: Applications to depression and borderline personality disorder. In W. F. Flack & J. Laird (Eds.), *Emotions in psychopathology: Theory and research* (pp. 394–406). New York: Oxford University Press.

Westen, D., Nakash, O., Thomas, C., & Bradley, R. (2006). Clinical assessment of attachment patterns and personality disorder in adolescents and adults. *Journal of Consulting and Clinical Psychology, 74*, 1065–1085.

Widlocher, D., & Fairfield, S. (Eds.). (2004). *Infantile sexuality and attachment* (2nd ed.). London: Karnac Books.

Winnicott, D. W. (1962). The aims of psychoanalytic treatment. In *The maturational processes and the facilitating environment* (pp. 166–170). London: Hogarth Press.

Winnicott, D. W. (1965). *The maturational process and the facilitating environment*. London: Hogarth Press.

Young, J. F., Mufson, L., & Davies, M. (2006). Impact of comorbid anxiety in an effectiveness study of interpersonal psychotherapy for depressed adolescents. *Journal of the American Academy of Child and Adolescent Psychiatry, 45*, 904–912.

Zepf, S. (2006). Attachment theory and psychoanalysis: Some remarks from an epistemological and from a Freudian viewpoint. *International Journal of Psycho-Analysis, 87*, 1529–1548.

Zweig-Frank, H., & Paris, J. (1991). Parents' emotional neglect and overprotection according to the recollections of patients with borderline personality disorder. *American Journal of Psychiatry, 148*, 648–651.

CHAPTER 34

Couple and Family Therapy
An Attachment Perspective

SUSAN M. JOHNSON

At the turn of this century, the editor of the journal *Family Process*, Carol Anderson, began her plenary speech at the 2000 annual meeting of the American Association for Marital and Family Therapy by noting that family therapists have "set out on a vast and troubled ocean in a very small theoretical boat." In the couple and family therapy (C&FT) field, systems theory (von Bertalanffy, 1968) has been used as the primary guide to understanding and promoting change in close relationships. Therapists have viewed problems in terms of rigid, constricted response patterns that evolve into self-maintaining negative feedback loops, such as critical complaint followed by defensive withdrawal. The systems theory of change has contributed a great deal to the C&FT field, and has also contributed to the development of Bowlby's initial theorizing about attachment (Bowlby, 1969/1982). However, the strength of systems theory, which is to capture the nature of patterned interactions in a group such as a family, can also be viewed as a limitation. In practice, systemic therapies have sometimes been viewed as impersonal and mechanistic (Merkel & Searight, 1992), focusing as they do on the structure of the relational "dance" rather than the dancers' lived experience, on triangles rather than dyads, and on interaction positions rather than inner motives and emotions.

To make headway in what Anderson has called the "troubled ocean" of conflictual couple and family relationships, the field needs a broad, clinically relevant theory that elucidates the specific nature of close relationships and the motivations of the individuals who continually create and recreate these relationships—a theory that incorporates the systemic perspective, but also adds to it. Attachment theory is the ideal candidate. It offers a broad and well-researched perspective on parent–child and couple relationships that guides a therapist to the heart of the matter, elucidating the task of restructuring key interactions, cognitions, and emotional responses. Attachment theory views the need for secure emotional connections with irreplaceable loved ones, and the regulation of emotions such as fear of loss and disconnection, as the implicit organizing elements in the dramas that play out in C&FT. Bowlby (1973, p. 180) spoke of the relation between an individual and his or her environment (most essentially loved ones) as the "outer ring" of a system, proposing that this outer ring is complementary to the "inner ring" that maintains an emotional "homeostasis" within each person's body and mind. Attachment is systemic in the traditional sense, and it also adds this "inner ring" to our understanding of relationships.

Despite its many strengths, until recently attachment theory has not played a large role in C&FT. The reasons for this neglect are many. Attachment theory blossomed as a theory of personality development and affect regulation (e.g., Ainsworth, Blehar, Waters, & Wall, 1978; Grossmann, Grossmann, & Waters, 2005; Main, Kaplan, & Cassidy, 1985; Mikulincer & Shaver, Chapter 23, this volume) rather than a theory of clinical intervention, and for many years mother–child interactions were attachment theorists' main focus. Also, as Mackey (1996) suggested, issues of nurturance and connection tended to be neglected in C&FT in favor of a focus on power, control, and autonomy. In addition, in our culture and in the C&FT field, the need for others has generally been pathologized, and the focus has been on self-definition and the creation of boundaries between self and others. So, although Bowlby (1944) wrote what is arguably the first professional treatise on family therapy, called "Forty-Four Juvenile Thieves: Their Characters and Home Life," the impact of attachment theory on C&FT remained limited.

This is now beginning to change as the key concepts of child and adult attachment become integrated into existing models, such as behavioral couple therapy (Davila, 2003) and multidimensional family therapy (Liddle, 1999). More significantly, over the last decade prototypical attachment-centered C&FT interventions have been developed and tested. These include attachment-based family therapy (ABFT; Diamond, Siqueland, & Diamond, 2003), as well as emotionally focused therapy (EFT) for couples and emotionally focused family therapy (EFFT) (Johnson, 2004).

The great promise of attachment theory is that it offers answers to some of the most fundamental questions of human emotional life, most of which arise in the context of close relationships (Karen, 1998). For instance, how do we learn what to expect from others? How does a couple relationship specifically affect the emotional lives of children (Davis & Cummings, 1994)? How do we become caught in futile strategies that rob us of the love we desire from our partners and family members? Why does distancing fail to cool down conflictual interactions with attachment figures? Why do certain events define the nature of relationships more than others? How does the self get constructed in interactions with significant others, and how can we best repair bonds with those we love?

Attachment theory and research are also crucial parts of a new relationship science (Ber-

scheid, 1999) that has begun to address the "core mysteries of human relationships." In this new science, many different kinds of research, relationship concepts, and clinical findings are coming together to form a coherent whole. For example, data on the nature of satisfaction and distress in couple partnerships (Huston, Caughlin, Houts, Smith, & George, 2001), research on the nature of love as outlined by attachment theory and research (Johnson, 2003), new understandings of emotion and the "panic" triggered by disconnection (Panksepp, 1998), and research on the process of relationship repair in therapy sessions viewed in terms of EFT (Johnson, Hunsley, Greenberg, & Schindler, 1999)—all of these now point in the same direction. This research suggests that emotional responsiveness between adult partners predicts stability and satisfaction in relationships, and that positive cycles of interactions in which each partner responds to the other's attachment vulnerabilities are key to relationship repair and the regulation of the primal panic that arises in negative interactions. There is also increasing emphasis on relatively short, efficient, and verifiably effective interventions in the field of psychotherapy. Attachment theory meets the urgent need for a perspective that allows a therapist to hone in on and bring into focus the organizing elements in the drama of close relationships and the ongoing definition of self in these relationships.

In this chapter, I outline the unique contributions of attachment theory to C&FT and explain how these contributions represent significant departures from the field's traditions. I then present prominent clinical models of C&FT based on attachment theory, along with relevant outcome research. Potential limitations of attachment theory as it relates to C&FT are then outlined, together with future promising directions for attachment-oriented interventions in both the couple therapy and family therapy domains.

ATTACHMENT: A NEW PERSPECTIVE ON COUPLE AND FAMILY SYSTEMS

What Attachment Theory Offers to C&FT

First, on a general level, attachment theory offers couple and family therapists a broad, integrated theory of close relationships and normal growth within such relationships, including a clear outline of basic human needs and emotional processes from the cradle to the grave. For a therapist, this is invaluable. The theory is specific enough to guide the formulation of individual couples' or families' problems, and then to shape interventions enacted in therapy sessions. Attachment anxiety and avoidance can be viewed as natural responses to the lack of a felt sense of secure connection with a partner, rather than, for example, a lack of skill or insight. The process of change will also include helping partners to recognize and "own" their attachment needs and guide partners to ask for these needs to be met, in a clear, congruent way that fosters partner responsiveness.

Attachment theory also provides a compass in the intrapsychic and interpersonal maelstrom of couple and family distress. Clients enter therapy with many different issues, at different levels of complexity. A central question is this: What should be the focus, the target, of intervention? From an attachment viewpoint, the core problem in a troubled relationship is the struggle to create a relationship that serves as a reliable safe haven and secure base—that is, to create a certain kind of connection or learn to cope better with its absence. Attachment theory offers a therapist a way to get to the heart of the matter: It facilitates not just the modification of particular symptoms (such as transforming loud arguments into less hostile negotiations), but also the creation of new, potent, positive interaction cycles of emotional responsiveness that can redefine the relationship as a whole.

By providing a picture of relationship health, attachment theory offers an answer to the longstanding clinical question: What constitutes necessary and sufficient change? Relapse after apparently successful treatment has long been an issue in couple therapy. Attachment theory is arguably the only systematic relational theory that offers a large body of research detailing the key interactions in healthy relationships (between adults and between adults and children) and documents the specific results of these interactions. For example, research on couples pinpoints a soothing emotional presence as a key factor determining relationship satisfaction (Gottman, Coan, Carrère, & Swanson, 1998), and much of the research summarized in the present volume establishes links between early attachment security in relationships with parents and later social and emotional functioning (e.g., Weinfield, Sroufe, Egeland, & Carlson, Chapter 4, this volume).

Furthermore, practitioners have often found theory and outcome research to be relatively useless for providing specific guidance in creating change during a C&FT session. Attachment theory and research inform a therapist about the nature of the pivotal processes and watershed events that define close relationships, and they offer guidance about how to restructure these events in therapy. In all the attachment-oriented models of C&FT described in this chapter, key change events and specific interventions are detailed.

Finally, primary relationships have great healing power. Attachments to key other people provide our "primary protection against feelings of helplessness and meaninglessness" (McFarlane & van der Kolk, 1996). Attachment theory empowers a therapist to link self and system, and to create interactions that not only change a relationship but address individual problems within that relationship. Attachment-oriented interventions have been used successfully to address a variety of clinical issues, including depression in adults and adolescents (Dessaulles, Johnson, & Denton, 2003; Diamond, 2005), traumatic stress in adults (MacIntosh & Johnson, in press), and negative, defiant behaviors in adolescents (Moretti & Holland, 2003).

The remainder of this section provides a closer examination of how the main tenets of attachment theory are relevant for couple and family therapists, and an explanation of why they constitute a change in this field. First, attachment theory depathologizes dependency. Second, it emphasizes the power of emotion in attuning individuals to their own attachment needs and in organizing interactions in attachment relationships, suggesting that emotion is both a target and an agent of change. Third, attachment theory has clear implications for the therapeutic alliance and the role of the therapist in C&FT. Fourth, the theory offers a therapist a map, so that individual differences in relationship style can be respected and addressed. This map is able to accommodate individual and relationship variables in a sophisticated and relevant manner that guides the change process in C&FT. Fifth, the concept of "working models" (Bretherton & Munholland, Chapter 5, this volume) adds a cognitive component to the focus on emotional response and interaction patterns, and it helps to explain how behaviors are passed on and perpetuated in families. Finally, the integrative model offered by attachment theory is inclusive and shapes C&FT interventions in a manner that is highly relevant to the lived realities clients bring into therapy. Focusing on attachment issues fosters engagement in therapy, which in turn predicts change in attachment responses (Johnson & Talitman, 1996). These points are discussed briefly below and then illustrated in the models of therapy described later in this chapter.

Depathologizing Dependency

The dominant discourse in the field of C&FT has long been one that promotes autonomy and is critical of dependency (Fishbane, 2005). In contrast, the central tenet of attachment theory is that seeking and maintaining contact with significant others is an innate, primary motivating force in human beings at all phases of the lifespan. Dependency is an innate part of being human, rather than a childhood trait that we outgrow; it is not necessarily a sign of enmeshed relationships and/ or of lack of differentiation from others. Rejection and emotional isolation are inherently painful, and can sometimes be traumatizing. A sense of connection with loved ones can be maintained more readily on a representational (working-model) level as we mature (Main et al., 1985), but contact is still a primary need. This need is universal across cultures (van IJzendoorn & Sagi-Schwartz, Chapter 37, this volume), although it may be expressed somewhat differently in different contexts. Whereas this view of dependency has been increasingly accepted for children and their parents, recognition that adult romantic relationships are also based on this kind of need, rather than being essentially friendships or rational exchanges of resources, has been slower. The first articles framing romantic love as an attachment process were published in the 1980s (e.g., Hazan & Shaver, 1987; Johnson, 1986), and they have generated a great deal of research since then. The attachment perspective, with its focus on effective dependency as positive and growth-promoting, departs significantly from many models of C&FT. The attachment perspective focuses the therapy on issues of connection and disconnection, and allows for the active validation of needs and fears concerning attachment. It offers the therapist a language for the "emotional starvation" (Levy, 1937) that characterizes an insecure relationship.

For couple and family therapists, whose training so often focuses on the need to help family members differentiate from each other to prevent "enmeshment," this perspective suggests that members grow and differentiate *with* each other rather than *from* each other. A felt sense of secure connection is seen as the best route to confident autonomy—a state that is often a key goal in family therapy, especially with adolescents. The *secure base* provided by a loving attachment figure encourages a cognitive openness to new information (Mikulincer, 1997). It promotes the confidence necessary to risk, learn, and continually update models of self and others, so that adjustment to new contexts is facilitated. It also strengthens the ability to stand back and reflect on oneself, including one's behavior and mental states (Fonagy, Gergely, & Target, Chapter 33, this volume; Fonagy & Target, 1997; Slade, Chapter 32, this volume). An increase in emotional accessibility and responsiveness is therefore a key goal in attachment-oriented C&FT, rather than focusing only on setting boundaries and developing assertiveness skills.

The Pivotal Role of Emotion

Emotion is central to attachment, and attachment theory provides a guide for understanding and normalizing many of the extreme emotions that accompany distressed relationships. As Bowlby (1979) suggested, "The psychology and psychopathology of emotion [are] ... in large part the psychology and psychopathology of affectional bonds" (p. 130).

Separation distress, indicated by powerful emotions of anger, panic at rejection, and abandonment and sadness, results from the perception that an attachment figure is inaccessible or does not care. Attachment relationships are where our strongest emotions arise and where they seem to have the most impact. They are the music of our most intimate relationships. When an individual is threatened—either by traumatic events or by a sense of disconnection in an attachment relationship—powerful affect arises, attachment needs for comfort and connection become particularly compelling, and attachment behaviors are activated.

A positive sense of connection with a loved one is a primary emotion regulation device (Mikulincer & Shaver, Chapter 23, this volume). The attachment view of family members as "hidden regulators" of each other's physiological and emotional worlds is supported by recent studies; for example, Coan, Schaefer, and Davidson (2006) demonstrated that in happy couples, holding hands in a stressful situation calms "jittery neurons" in the brain and lessens the perception of pain.

Attachment theory focuses the therapist on emotional experience and elucidates the logic and meaning of emotional responses. The valuing and active recognition of emotion has not, until very recently, been a primary focus in C&FT. Emotion was either considered to be part of the problem, or to be epiphenomenal and irrelevant to changes in family systems or individual behavior. In contrast, the models mentioned in this chapter entail a "bold swinging" (Hughes, 2007) toward and into the subjective experience of couple and family members, to explore and reprocess key emotions, use emotion as a key change mechanism, and focus on barriers to emotional responsiveness.

The Nature of the Therapeutic Alliance

The tenet of attachment theory that outlines the need for a safe haven and a secure base suggests that the creation of safe emotional engagement with a therapist is a key part of the clinical change process (Bowlby, 1988). Although C&FT has long espoused therapeutic alliances of a collaborative nature, the explicit validation and careful creation of a secure base in the therapies presented in this chapter, as well as the level of emotional engagement fostered between therapist and client, reflects the attachment perspective. An attachment-oriented therapist also acts as a surrogate attachment figure by actively helping clients regulate emotion, particularly the attachment-related anxiety or panic (Panksepp, 1998) that triggers negative emotional flooding or requires strongly avoidant suppression in insecure relationships.

Emotion is also more differentiated in the attachment perspective and so can be addressed and regulated in a more specific fashion by an emotionally present and attuned therapist. Bowlby (1973) viewed anger in close relationships as often being an attempt to make contact with an inaccessible attachment figure, and he distinguished between the more positive anger of hope, which leads to a clear assertion of needs, and the anger of despair, which becomes desperate and coercive. In secure relationships, protest concerning inaccessibility is recognized and accepted (Bowlby, 1969/1982; Holmes, 1996). Therapists who understand the process of separation distress can tune in to clients' emotional perspective, look beyond disruptive responses such as hostile criticism or stonewalling, and place them in the context of legitimate attachment needs and fears. In the context of a secure base, a therapist can translate what might appear to be intractable characterological deficits or lack of social skills into context-specific responses to loss of connection—responses that can be validated and restructured.

Bowlby (1988) noted that human beings are "strongly inclined towards self-healing" (p. 152). The therapist's job is to provide the context—namely, a secure base—that allows this natural healing process to occur. This is a very different theoretical frame from the one that casts the therapist as a magician or creator of miraculous reversals of negativity, which has been popular in the C&FT field.

Understanding and Addressing Individual Differences

Attachment theory also offers the couple and family therapist a way to understand and address individual differences in affect regulation and engagement with partners. There has been an increasing emphasis in this field on respecting individual differences and moving away from a one-size-fits-all set of interventions. There are only so many ways of coping with disconnection—that is, with a negative response to the question "Can I depend on you when I need you?" Attachment strategies in both parent–child and adult relationships can be described in terms of two main dimensions, anxiety and avoidance (Ainsworth et al., 1978; Brennan, Clark, & Shaver, 1998; see also Crowell, Fraley, & Shaver, Chapter 26, this volume).

When the connection with an irreplaceable other is threatened but not yet severed, the attachment system may become hyperactivated (Cassidy & Berlin, 1994). Attachment behaviors become heightened and intense as anxious clinging, pursuit, and even aggressive attempts to obtain a response from the loved one escalate (Bartholomew & Allison, 2006). The second strategy for dealing with the lack of safe emotional engagement, especially when hope for responsiveness has been lost, is to deactivate the attachment system (Cassidy & Kobak, 1988) and suppress attachment needs. This is done by focusing on other issues, such as work, and avoiding distressing attempts to engage emotionally with attachment figures (Mikulincer & Shaver, Chapter 23, this volume). These two strategies, anxious clinging and detached avoidance, can develop into habitual styles of engagement with intimate others.

A third insecure pattern has been identified—a combination of yearning for closeness and then fearfully avoiding reliance on a relationship partner because of potential emotional pain. This pattern is referred to as "disorganized" in the child literature (Lyons-Ruth & Jacobvitz, Chapter 28, this volume) and "fearfully avoidant" in the adult social-psychological literature (Bartholomew & Horowitz, 1991; Crowell et al., Chapter 26, this volume). This failure to establish a coherent, organized strategy is associated with chaotic or traumatic attachment experiences with frightening, abusive, or ineffectual relationship partners (Main & Hesse, 1990).

All of these insecure patterns, which begin as accommodations to the behaviors of key attachment figures, can be rigidly and inappropriately applied in subsequent relationships, thereby generating ongoing negative cycles of interaction and lack of connection with loved ones. These adaptations become "self-maintaining patterns of social interaction and emotion regulation" (Shaver & Clark, 1994, p. 119). They echo the display rules for emotion—namely, exaggerating, substituting one feeling for another (as when we focus on anger rather than fear), and minimizing (Ekman & Friesen, 1975). Knowing about these strategies, or breakdown of strategies, helps us as couple and family therapists understand the positions individuals take in the midst of couple and family distress. They allow us to understand not only the "unique meaning of disruptive behavior" in child–parent relationships (Byng-Hall, 1991) and adult partnerships (Johnson, 2004), but also the compelling nature of habitual strategies and styles.

For example, when a partner anxiously demands contact and then withdraws when it is offered, a therapist sees a pattern of fearful avoidance and understands the dilemma of the client who longs for closeness but also turns it down, unable to regulate the fear and pain associated with it. The ambiguous meanings behind closeness can then be unpacked, and emotions and responses can be validated and clarified and shared with the other partner. This kind of process empowers the couple therapist to work with people who have been damaged and traumatized in close relationships (Johnson, 2002).

Couple and family therapists, in particular, tend to see attachment processes and attachment styles from a transactional perspective—that is, as being continually constructed and reconstructed in interactions with loved ones. If internal models and modes of regulating emotion remain stable, it is because they seem to a person to be confirmed in ongoing interactions; they are not just fixed models that get projected onto new relationships (Shaver & Hazan, 1993). Attachment research has shown that these habitual forms of engagement can be modified by new or changed relationships (e.g., Davila, Burge, & Hammen, 1997; Davila, Karney, & Bradbury, 1999), suggesting that new interaction patterns created in therapy can have a significant impact on individuals and their re-

lationships. Attachment theory is especially helpful in being concerned with "a reality-regulating and reality-creating, not just a reality-reflecting system" (Bretherton & Munholland, 1999, p. 98). In distressed relationships, attachment processes and attachment-related styles of perceiving social interactions and responding to them often operate outside awareness (Bowlby, 1980) and are so habitual that they cannot easily be modified by the skill-building and cognitive reframing interventions so often used in C&FT. In the attachment-oriented models presented later in this chapter, the focus is expanded to include new attachment-related emotional experiences; a clearer addressing of attachment needs; and the potential alteration of working models of self, partner, and relationship.

Working Models: The Self in the System

Secure attachment is theoretically characterized by a working model of self as worthy of love and care and as competent. Research has strongly supported this aspect of the theory by showing that measured attachment security is associated with greater self-efficacy and a more coherent, articulated, and positive view of self (e.g., Mikulincer, 1995). Secure individuals, who have experienced their attachment figures as responsive and supportive when needed, also tend to have working models of others as dependable and trustworthy. These models of self and others are based on thousands of social interactions. They are carried forward into new interactions and new relationships not as one-dimensional cognitive schemas, but as emotionally charged procedural scripts for how to create relatedness under particular conditions. A person may have multiple and conflicting models, but most often one is dominant in a given context.

Working models are formed, elaborated, maintained, and—most importantly for the couple and family therapist—*changed* through emotional communication. Attachment theory offers a specific explanatory framework that allows the therapist to infer and understand models of self and other, which can then be highlighted, reconceived in relation to changed interaction patterns, and gradually transformed. The therapist can point out the pitfalls of specific perceptions that arise from negative working models, showing how they prohibit openness toward loved ones, block relationship change, and ultimately keep a person stuck with self-damaging perceptions and behaviors. At the end of therapy, for example, a 13-year-old boy might be able to say to his new stepfather, "When I was little, with my first dad, I decided I was a bad kid. That was why he was so mad at me. Now I assume you think I'm bad, and when you get upset with me, I just tell you I don't care. I'll never please you anyway. I just give up." His stepfather can now tell him, "I don't want you to feel like you're a bad kid. You are my kid now—my special son. I don't want you to give up with me. And I want to learn to be a kinder dad."

A Relevant Focus for Intervention

Bowlby began his career as a health care professional by studying the effects of maternal deprivation and separation on children. Attachment theory describes and explains the trauma of deprivation, loss, rejection, and abandonment by those we need most. Couple and family therapists know about the stress of deprivation and separation. They can see, for example, what Bowlby described in his 1944 article, "Forty-Four Juvenile Thieves"—that "behind the mask of indifference [of avoidant children] is bottomless misery and behind apparent callousness, despair." Bowlby saw his young charges as frozen in the attitude "I will never be hurt again" and paralyzed by their isolation and rage. Attachment theory encourages a therapist to reach, with empathic questions, reflections, and conjectures, behind couple and family members' masks and unpack separation distress, anger about rejections and hurts, and the attachment longings that color emotional reactions. Attachment theory has supreme relevance to the lived experience and dilemmas of couple and family members in distressed relationships.

ATTACHMENT-ORIENTED MODELS OF INTERVENTION IN FAMILY THERAPY

Although there are some emerging attachment-based family interventions with adolescents (Mackey, 2003; Moretti & Holland, 2003) and younger children (Hughes, 2007), there are only two family therapy models that have preliminary empirical validation of their effectiveness and that systematically use an attachment framework to assess and address problems in families. These are ABFT (Diamond, 2005) and EFFT (Johnson & Lee, 2000; Johnson, Maddeaux, & Blouin, 1998). These approaches assume that adolescents who enter therapy need to reconnect with parents in

order to move toward more confident autonomy, and that a new level of emotional communication is necessary for this to occur. They address a wide range of symptoms, both internalizing (such as depression) and externalizing (such as conduct disorder). Both assume that attachment issues such as rejection, neglect, and abandonment are often obscured by conflicts related to behavioral problems (e.g., neglecting chores or homework), and that therapy must foster empathic, attuned conversations about relationship ruptures and attachment injuries.

Attachment-Based Family Therapy

For adolescents, secure attachment nurtures healthy development, whereas insecure attachment is associated with depression and other forms of problems in adaptation (Herring & Kaslow, 2002; Rosenstein & Horowitz, 1996). Practitioners of ABFT—an approach whose clinical procedures draw from many systems approaches, including EFT (Diamond et al., 2003)—have specialized in working with depressed adolescents, who benefit from more direct communication with parents. Secure attachment is characterized by this kind of communication, which fosters perspective taking and effective, collaborative problem solving (Allen, Chapter 19, this volume; Kobak & Duemmler, 1994).

Diamond and colleagues (2003) note that depressed adolescents usually talk in the first therapy session about feeling hopeless, alone, and angry at their parents. The parents speak of frustration about their own perceived failure to help their children. The parents' lack of availability at critical moments has often become a source of injury and alienation for the adolescents. ABFT is an attempt to help parents and adolescents address these "relational ruptures," address core attachment concerns (including increasing the adolescents' sense of entitlement to care), and develop a coherent understanding of attachment events. All of this increases the adolescents' sense of felt security and helps them to revise negative working models of self and other. A major challenge in this approach, and in all attachment-based family interventions, is to build the parents' capacity for providing a sense of security in their children. Diamond and colleagues point out that an adolescent's ability to express vulnerability and attachment needs often rekindles the desire for a parent's care, and the parent can then be helped by the therapist to connect with the child. This approach targets parental criticism—a factor often labeled "expressed emotion" and linked to depression (Asarnow, Goldstein, Tompson, & Guthrie, 1993), as well as to ineffective parenting and to the adolescent's withdrawal/hopelessness, sense of disconnection from parents, inability to regulate emotions, and negative self-concept. The first session involves the family unit; the second is with the adolescent alone; and the third is with the parent(s) alone. The remaining sessions involve combinations of one or both parents and the adolescent, the adolescent alone, or a parent alone.

Treatment focuses on several tasks. The first task is reframing the problem in terms of negative interaction cycles, such as parental reaching out, adolescent rejection of help, parental expression of frustration or criticism, and adolescent withdrawal while feeling rejected. The therapist helps the adolescent describe his or her unhappiness and attempts to create a more compassionate emotional climate in the family. The therapist also attempts to build an alliance with the adolescent, including validating any sense of abandonment, acknowledging the burden of being "parentified" (i.e., having to take care of a parent), and empathizing with the frustration and pain of being triangulated in conflicts between the parents. The therapist helps the adolescent communicate his or her concerns, and then, in a meeting with the parents alone, prepares them to listen to and respond to the adolescent's concerns; this can then move the attachment relationships in the family toward greater security. The therapist sets up a conversation addressing core relationship failures, encouraging parents to respond to the adolescent's grievances with empathy so that a new kind of encounter can occur. Finally, the therapist promotes competency by encouraging parents to challenge and support the adolescent, and urging the adolescent to take more responsibility for his or her behavior. This may allow important goals, such as returning to school, to be attained. Parents can become more "authoritative" (to use Baumrind's [1991] well-known concept, which she contrasted with being either too authoritarian or too permissive), and adolescents can become more mature, autonomous, and responsible.

Emotionally Focused Family Therapy

The goals of EFFT are to modify the distressing cycles of interaction that amplify conflict and undermine the potentially secure connection between parents and children, and to shape positive cycles of accessibility and responsiveness that offer the developing adolescent a safe haven and secure base (Johnson, 2004: Johnson & Lee, 2000). As in EFT for couples, therapy takes place in three stages: deescalation of negative cycles, restructuring of attachment interactions, and consolidation. Therapy usually involves approximately 10–12 sessions. The first two of these include the entire family. Once the network of alliances has been mapped out, the family members' views of the problem have been grasped, and the adolescent's problematic behavior has been placed in the context of family attachment patterns, sessions may be conducted with the adolescent alone or with any combination of family members. The emotionally focused therapist focuses on two tasks: the elucidation and reprocessing of key attachment-related emotions and emotional responses (the "music" of the relational "dance"), and the gradual revision of key patterns of interaction to create a more secure attachment. The therapist focuses on emotion as the organizing element in interactions and acts as less of a coach than the therapist does in ABFT, relying instead on the power of new emotional signals to evoke new behaviors and revise expectations, perceptions, and models of relationships in both parents and children. The recognition, validation, and expression of attachment needs is a key part of EFFT, as is addressing the adolescent's frustration and despair over disconnection.

EFFT follows the same steps as the more developed EFT for couples, which is discussed later in this chapter. Perhaps the best way to illustrate this treatment process is to offer a brief overview of key moves in the change process in a particular case. James was 16 years old and had been expelled from school for haranguing teachers. Moira, James's mother, was clinically depressed, had chronic pain from a back problem, and was preoccupied with her four younger children. James was excluded from the family group because of his aggressive and bullying behavior, which had started in childhood and had become especially severe with respect to Tim, his father. Tim admitted that he had been overly critical and even "abusive" with his son; however, he reported that this had stopped when he gave up drinking about 4 years ago. James was dismissive in his discussion of relationships, stating that he did not need anyone and that everyone was "against" him anyway.

After two initial sessions, it became clear that two main negative interaction patterns were fueling the conflict and maintaining distance in this family. The first was that James bullied his younger brother because he perceived him to be his mother's favorite. When this brother was out of the home, James was able to connect with his mother and occasionally confide in her about his "problems." When he bullied his brother, his mother confronted him and then withdrew. James then "gave up" trying to reach his mother and teased his brother at every opportunity. In his relationship with his father, James felt "accused" and either refused to talk or openly defied him. His father then became angry, set up rules, and withdrew in frustration.

The third session was an individual session with James. He described many responses consonant with depression, including deciding that he was "useless," that no one cared about him, and that he had no future. He spoke longingly of the times he could "chat a little" with his mother, but he expressed only cold hostility toward his father. He felt most comfortable at home when he played with his younger sisters. The therapist mapped out the patterns of connection and disconnection that James helped to create but was also victimized by, and framed these patterns as problems for the family. James, expecting to be labeled as a "bad kid," was surprised and intrigued by this reframing. Using many empathic reflections, the therapist then helped James "unpack" his responses to his family—looking with him at his frustration and anger, his more primary responses of sadness and "not belonging," and the action tendencies fueled by these emotions (either to attack and "fight" to "show them," or to "shut them out" and "not care"). The therapist validated James's strategies as being the only way he had found to deal with his sense of isolation in his family. James's aggression was framed in terms of his sense of hopelessness and despair.

In the fourth session, James and his mother were able to identify the negative interaction pattern they repeatedly generated together. James would feel abandoned by his mother and direct his anger toward his brother or her. She would then withdraw and focus more on protecting the brother. In therapy, they talked about more superficial reactive feelings that arose in this cycle (frustration and numbing out), but then moved into formulating and sharing deeper feelings of sadness and fear. The therapist helped them clarify the responses each made that contributed to their negative cycle, and also to identify and understand the emotions underlying these responses. The therapist then set up enactments that challenged this cycle and promoted more appropriate emotional

contact. Moira shared that she was now physically afraid of James, especially when he shouted, and this caused her to be wary around him. His complaint concerning her distance was therefore seen to be legitimate. James was surprised at this, and, following his mother's lead, he began to share his fear that he could not "compete" with his "perfect" younger brother. He expressed deep sadness, especially about a time several years ago when his mother seemed to turn away from him. His mother moved into reassuring and comforting James, and he responded by telling her how much he needed her support and how afraid he became when she "went away" from him.

In the fifth session, with James, his mother, and his younger brother present, James was able to consolidate his new relationship with his mother and own his aggression toward his brother. He could also hear his brother's hurt and fear concerning the bullying. The therapist helped James admit his jealousy and respond with understanding to his brother's expressions of fear. The therapist then framed James as an older protective figure who was important to his brother; he could be a safe haven and secure base, and could respond favorably when his brother expressed a need for respect and caring. The sixth and seventh sessions focused on the relationship between Moira and Tim, and on how their marital issues sometimes undermined their ability to work as a team when dealing with James's behavior. The eighth session focused on Tim and his considerable grief and shame at how he had parented his son, especially when James was younger and Tim had been drinking heavily. A main objective of the therapy in this session and the next one was to restructure James's relationship with his father. Research informs us that a father's current frame of mind concerning attachment is a powerful predictor of his child's externalizing behaviors (Cowan, Cohn, Cowan, & Pearson, 1996). Modifying Tim's attachment responses to his son thus seemed to be an obvious route to changing James's aggressive behavior.

Again the therapist focused first on containing and reframing the negative cycle of Tim becoming critical while James shut him out or occasionally exploded aggressively, and Tim then also withdrew. This cycle was described as taking over their relationship and hurting them both. Both were able to grasp the "game" as a whole, rather than focusing on the "ball"—the other's responses. James found it difficult to open up to his father, beginning by telling him that he was indifferent to him and his opinions. Tim was able to take the lead and respond nondefensively, telling his son that he had many feelings about the mistakes he had made as a parent and that he could understand James's being guarded around him. This enabled James to access deeper emotions and begin to tell his father about how he did not want to hurt any more, so he had decided to give up on his father's approval or love. James and his father were then able to move into a process of accessing hurts and past injuries, and then through a sequence in which Tim showed his son his grief and shame and asked for his forgiveness (both for his aggression and for his absence as a supportive parent).

James at first tried to stop his father's disclosures, as if protecting himself from his own and Tim's feelings. However, after a while he became engaged and was able to share a particular painful moment of disconnection, when he decided he could never please his father and there was therefore "probably something wrong with me." Tim was able to respond with empathy and sorrow. He then began to share that listening to James's pain affected him deeply, and to describe how his own problems had blocked his ability to be the father he wanted to be. He again apologized, and James was gradually able to hear and accept Tim's apologies. James expressed his own long-denied longings and needs for Tim's comfort and care. He was also able to formulate in a new way how his sense of isolation and rejection in his family was beginning to "poison" him with anger and despair. Tim responded to his son with caring and empathy, describing the parent he wanted to be and asking James for a chance to be that parent. They were then able to reflect on this new way of connecting, and to plan new ways to keep this connection in their everyday life.

In a final session, the changes described above were integrated into the family as a whole. A coherent story of how the family had become "stuck" was created, and each person described the changes that had occurred and what they meant to their sense of family. They then described how their new sense of connection was translating into everyday cooperation and problem solving. In a follow-up session a few months later, James confided that he was learning that he could trust other people more and that he didn't need to be the "tough guy" at school or in his family.

There are some similarities between both EEFT and ABFT and the work of John Gottman on emotional communication between parents and children. However, Gottman's model is more focused on teaching parents how to coach their children directly about emotions and emotion regulation (e.g., Gottman, Katz, & Hooven, 1997). Both EEFT and ABFT promote a particular way of being emotionally present with and attuning to family members. Trevarthen and Aitken's (2001) concept of "primary intersubjectivity" within an attachment framework, which explains how children's view of themselves emerges from their experience of what their parents tune in to and respond to in them, would also appear to be relevant here. In both EFFT and ABFT, there is more recognition of emotion than has been customary in the majority of family therapies; even so, ABFT appears to be somewhat more cognitive than EFT and to use heightened emotion less when creating new kinds of interactions between parent and child. All attachment-oriented models and interventions referred to in this chapter seem to focus on helping parents and children repair attachment rifts and injuries, and elucidate interaction patterns and responses in a way that makes "the attachment needs that underlie problem behaviors visible" (Moretti & Holland, 2003, p. 245).

EMPIRICAL SUPPORT FOR ATTACHMENT-BASED FAMILY INTERVENTIONS

A randomized trial of ABFT (12 sessions) was conducted with 32 adolescents, half of whom were assigned to a wait list (Diamond, 2005). Of those treated, 62% scored in the nonclinical range on the Beck Depression Inventory after treatment, compared to only 19% of controls. Of those who responded to treatment, only 13% met criteria for depression at a 6-month follow-up. Treatment also significantly influenced levels of anxiety and also family conflict. Interventions as implemented were checked by coders for fit with the ABFT model and were reliably different from cognitive-behavioral therapy. When parents were shown videotapes of sessions and asked to discuss changes that had occurred, the key factor seemed to be that the parents had come to understand how ruptures in their relationships with their adolescents contributed to the depression, and that their adolescents desired and needed their love. In a "reattachment" stage of therapy, the change process was studied by using ratings of statements made in sessions. The process as mapped seems similar to that outlined in recent work on forgiveness in the second stage of EFT (Johnson, 2004; Makinen & Johnson, 2006). In ABFT, an adolescent first discloses anger about relationship failures. A parent is supported to remain nondefensive, apologize, and explain his or her own inability to make better choices. The parent and adolescent then share more vulnerable feelings and needs, and come to a better appreciation of each other's struggles.

There are preliminary data on the effectiveness of EFFT in a study of 13 young women diagnosed with bulimia nervosa at an outpatient hospital clinic (Johnson et al., 1998). Most also met criteria for clinical depression, and several had attempted suicide. All subjects except one rated themselves as having either an anxious or a fearfully avoidant attachment to their parents on an attachment questionnaire (Bartholomew & Horowitz's [1991] Relationship Questionnaire). A cognitive-behavioral educational group (n = 4) was compared with an EFFT group (n = 9). Both treatments (10 sessions) were supervised by experts in these interventions, and implementation checks were conducted. Both were found to result in decreased severity of bulimic symptoms, lower scores on the Beck Depression Inventory, and reduced general psychiatric symptomatology. Remission rates for bingeing and vomiting were better than those reported by Garner, Olmsted, and Polivy (1983) for individual therapy. The size of this study was curtailed by institutional changes, and differential effects are difficult to find with such a small number of subjects. Nevertheless, the results were encouraging. In clinical practice, EFFT is used with both internalizing and externalizing disorders, mostly with adolescents and their families.

ATTACHMENT-ORIENTED COUPLE THERAPY

The couple therapy field appears to be moving slowly toward greater recognition of adult attachment needs and the desirability of promoting emotional connection and nurturance in couples. However, although a few commentators (e.g., Davila, 2003) have suggested ways in which the attachment perspective could be used to enhance behavioral couple therapy—for example, by measuring attachment patterns and predicting and explicating negative behavior and its consequences—the attachment perspective does not seem to have influenced interventions in couple therapy, except as used in EFT (Johnson, 2004, 2008).

Attachment theory suggests that many relationship problems are essentially due to the insecurity of the bond between partners and to the struggle to define the relationship as a potential safe haven and a secure base (Bowlby, 1969/1982,

1988). The key issue in distressed relationships is seen as the negative cycles that maintain disconnection and limited responsiveness to emotional signals and attachment cues. As a distressed woman remarked to her husband, "It's not the fights that really matter. I could handle disagreements if I felt like you were there for me. But I can never find you when I need you. I feel alone in this relationship."

There is now a sizable body of research on the relevance of attachment theory to adult relationships (reviewed, e.g., by Mikulincer & Shaver, 2007). Secure attachment, whether measured by questionnaires or interviews (see Crowell et al., Chapter 26, this volume, for a review of measures), has been found to predict such positive aspects of relationship functioning as greater interdependence, commitment, trust, and satisfaction in couples (e.g., J. Feeney, Chapter 21, this volume; Kirkpatrick & Davis, 1994); higher levels of support seeking and providing (e.g., Simpson, Rholes, & Nelligan, 1992); greater intimacy and less withdrawal and verbal aggression (Senchak & Leonard, 1992); more sensitive and appropriate caregiving behavior (B. C. Feeney, 2004, 2007; Kunce & Shaver, 1994); less jealousy (Hazan & Shaver, 1987); and more satisfying sexual interactions (e.g., Brassard, Shaver, & Lussier, 2007). Individuals with insecurely attached partners also report lower satisfaction, and couples in which both partners are securely attached report better adjustment than couples in which either or both partners are insecurely attached (Lussier, Sabourin, & Turgeon, 1997). This research parallels other findings indicating the pivotal importance of soothing and supportive responses in high-functioning relationships and the absolute requirement for safe emotional engagement (e.g., Gottman, 1994; Pasch & Bradbury, 1998).

EFT uses systemic and experiential interventions to promote change in couple relationships, but places these in the context of an attachment-theoretical understanding of adult love relationships. As a couple therapy based on attachment theory, EFT is characterized by the following:

1. A focus on and validation of attachment needs and fears, and the promotion of safe emotional engagement, comfort, and support.
2. A privileging of emotional responses and communication, and direct addressing of attachment vulnerabilities and fears so as to foster emotional attunement and responsiveness.
3. The creation of a respectful collaborative alli-

ance, so that the therapy setting itself is a safe haven and a secure base.

4. An explicit shaping of responsiveness and accessibility (withdrawn partners are to be reengaged, and blaming partners will be guided to ask for attachment needs to be met in a positive manner, so that bonding events can occur and serve as an antidote to negative cycles and insecurity).
5. A focus on self-definitions that can be redefined through emotional communication with partners (attachment figures).
6. An explicit shaping of pivotal attachment responses that redefine a relationship (as each person asks that attachment needs be met, and the other partner responds to ensure that positive bonding interactions occur).
7. Addressing and healing specific attachment injuries (Johnson, Makinen, & Millikin, 2001), including betrayals and abandonment at key moments of need (e.g., at the time of a miscarriage).

This approach has received extensive empirical validation, both in terms of outcomes and in terms of defined change processes. It has been found to be more effective than skill-building cognitive-behavioral approaches (Johnson & Greenberg, 1985), and at present it obtains what are arguably the best results of any couple intervention in the literature. A meta-analysis of the most rigorous studies of EFT found that 70–73% of couples recovered from relationship distress after 10–12 sessions (with therapists who were receiving clinical supervision), and that 86% rated their relationship as significantly improved (Johnson et al., 1999). The effectiveness of EFT does not appear to be as heavily influenced by initial distress levels as other approaches are. Specifically, initial distress was found to account for only 4% of the variance in satisfaction at follow-up, compared to an estimated 46% in the behavioral approaches tested (Whisman & Jacobson, 1990).

Attachment theory and Bowlby's (1988) book about its application in psychotherapy lead us to believe that a positive alliance with the therapist is a crucial factor in the change process. The quality of the alliance has been found to predict 20% of the variance in outcome in EFT, but it is the task relevance aspect of this alliance that seems to be the most powerful predictor of outcome, rather than the bond with the therapist or a sense of shared goals (Johnson & Talitman, 1996). This suggests that couples find the focus on

attachment relevant and compelling. In particular, in clinical practice, partners repeatedly inform us that attachment as a framework and a language captures and orders their experience and the nature of their relationship in a powerful and unique way. The validation of attachment fears and needs seems to be especially powerful.

The attachment framework offers us (as both clinicians and scientists) a way of understanding how we create lasting changes and avoid relapse, even in a brief therapy. EFT does not seem to have the same problem with relapse as other approaches do. There is evidence that results are stable, even in very stressed, high-risk relationships where relapse might be expected (Clothier, Manion, Gordon-Walker, & Johnson, 2002), and there is a trend toward continuing improvement after therapy ends (Johnson et al., 1999). If interventions reach to the heart of the matter, they are more likely to create lasting change. Also, after an intervention such as EFT, ongoing crises and stressors that would undermine a relationship in which attachment issues had not been focused on and effectively addressed become opportunities for partners to turn to each other and make bids for attachment responsiveness—bids that, if accepted, can continue to add to the security of the couple's bond.

The steps in EFT are well documented in the couple therapy literature (Johnson, 2004; Johnson et al., 2005). The process of change moves from outlining negative interaction patterns and their attachment consequences to deepening the awareness of the core attachment-related emotions underlying these interaction patterns. A silent, withdrawn partner (typically a man) is able to attune to and express his helplessness and hopelessness when he sees the anger in the other partner, and he can link this anger to his tendency to remain silent. He also begins to understand that his silence creates panic in his partner, which then fuels her critical complaining. In Stage One of EFT, both partners begin to express newly accessed and formulated emotions, and to frame the negative cycle and disconnection as a mutual enemy. Once this cycle is deescalated, partners are guided in Stage Two of EFT to engage authentically with their emotions and to express the fear, sadness, or shame that keeps them blaming or distancing. Wired-in longings for connection and comfort can then emerge and be used to create more explicit and coherent bids for responsiveness from each other. This process is crystallized into key change events in Stage Two, where the focus is on restructuring attachment responses and building positive cycles of connection. Here, more withdrawn, avoidant partners can assert their needs for validation and safety, and more anxiously attached, blaming partners can ask that their needs for comfort and connection be met. Stage Two of therapy ends with a new kind of safe emotional engagement for both partners. These changes are then consolidated in Stage Three: A new narrative or story about of how the relationship was threatened and repaired is created, new attachment behaviors are highlighted; and it becomes easier to solve pragmatic problems from a position of safety.

In the key change events of Stage Two, change occurs on many levels. As a blaming partner (typically a woman) finds herself asking that her attachment needs be met, she moves to a new level of affect regulation where vulnerable emotions can be encountered, ordered, and expressed congruently, so that her attachment needs are made clear. She also moves away from her attributions of weakness and accepts her "softer side" as legitimate, integrating attachment fears and needs into her sense of self. As her partner responds favorably, her image of others as untrustworthy is challenged. As new, more secure interactions occur, a new pattern of attuned responsiveness is created that expands the couple's behavioral repertoire and model of relatedness.

In a typical session, attachment is not used just as an overall perspective on a couple's problems; it also elicits specific interventions. Empathic reflection of emotional responses and interaction processes, validation, and empathic questioning are used to create a sense of safety and focus the process on attachment needs. Here is an example: "Peter, you said you try not to react so as to stop the fights. You also said, 'I put up a wall, and that is kind of sad.' The word 'sad' really struck me. It *is* sad. It's a loss to you when you wall out someone you love. Yes? I wonder what it feels like behind that wall? The wall that Mary then rails against and 'hurls' herself toward with more and more fury. Do you ever talk to *her* about that sadness?" The therapist then distills inner emotions and outer moves with the client, and clarifies attachment-oriented messages to the other while promoting new, more attachment-friendly interactions: "So you say that Mary sees this 'cool' guy, but inside you feel small and sad and lonely. You just don't know what to do when she tells you she isn't happy. You're scared of making a mistake, so you freeze up. You freeze not because she is unimportant, as she believes, but because she has such an impact on you. Can

you tell her, please, 'When I feel small and scared, I do shut you out, and I see now how that upsets and frustrates you. I am so unsure of how to please you, I shut down before I can even think'?" The therapist then turns to the other partner and helps him or her respond to this new kind of interaction. Attachment theory has great breadth, but it is also specific enough to focus on the agreed-upon priority for most clinicians (Beutler, Williams, & Wakefield, 1993)—that is, to specify the therapist and client behaviors that create important moments of change.

The latest development in EFT (Johnson et al., 2001)—the focus on the forgiveness of attachment injuries that create blocks to the creation of new levels of trust—speaks to the fact that a powerful theoretical map elucidates the nature of impasses in the therapeutic process and suggests how to deal with these impasses. Attachment theorists have pointed out that incidents in which one partner responds or fails to respond at times of urgent need seem to influence the quality of an attachment relationship disproportionately (Simpson & Rholes, 1994). Such incidents either shatter or confirm one partner's assumptions about attachment relationships and the dependability of the other partner. Negative attachment-related events, particularly abandonments and betrayals, cause seemingly irreparable damage to close relationships. Many partners enter therapy not only in general distress, but also with the goal of bringing closure to such events and thereby restoring lost intimacy and trust. During therapy, these events, even if they are long past, often reemerge in an alive and intensely emotional manner (much as a traumatic flashback does) and overwhelm the injured partner, creating an impasse and hindering the process of change. These incidents usually occur in the context of life transitions, loss, physical danger, or uncertainty (e.g., after a medical diagnosis or miscarriage), when attachment needs are most salient and compelling; as such, they can be considered relationship traumas. Attachment theory offers an explanation of why certain painful events, such as specific abandonments, become pivotal in a relationship, as well as offering an understanding of what the key features of such events will be, how they will affect a particular couple's relationship, and how such events can be optimally resolved. Such events are taken into account throughout therapy, but are focused on and worked through in Stage Two of EFT.

The steps in the forgiveness process are as follows: The injury is placed in the context of attachment needs, and the evolution of the incident is examined in terms of attachment strategies and assumptions. The injured party is then encouraged to clarify his or her pain associated with the event and to frame it in attachment terms. The other partner is then guided to respond with empathy and regret in a congruent and engaged manner. The injured party is supported to face his or her fears of becoming vulnerable again, and is able to ask that the attachment needs aroused by the incident be addressed. The other partner can now respond empathically, creating a positive reenactment of the original injuring event. This process is then integrated into the couple's story of the injury and their new ability to repair it. In a recent study (Makinen & Johnson, 2006), all distressed couples with a single attachment injury recovered from relationship distress, reduced the pain caused by the injury, and reached positive levels of forgiveness. These results were maintained over a 3-year period. Couples with more than one attachment injury and very low initial levels of trust did experience reduced pain, but had less positive results in the domains of forgiveness and relationship satisfaction. Dealing with these more seriously damaged kinds of relationships presumably requires more sessions than the limited number offered in this study.

POSSIBLE LIMITS OF THE ATTACHMENT PERSPECTIVE FOR C&FT

There are certain ways in which attachment theory is not an obvious fit with the field of C&FT interventions as it has developed to date. For one thing, as Byng-Hall (1999) pointed out, the focus in attachment theory has been on the dyad rather than the family group. Even family interventions such as ABFT or EFFT often involve sessions with dyads or a dyadic focus when other family members are present. In both approaches, however, this dyadic process is meant to be gradually integrated into family interactions as a whole. Some theorists have suggested conceptualizations that address this issue. Marvin and Stewart (1990) speak of a family "shared working model." Byng-Hall discusses the network of attachment relationships in a family and describes how this network might be influenced by articulating a family script—for example, stating that care is always given priority when it is needed and that members will collaborate to ensure this.

A consistent, shared family script would seem to be a natural part of a secure family, whereas a less secure family would be less likely to have a shared script focused on connection and care. Although we can theorize about this, research suggests that attachment strategies and models are relationship-specific, so in our pursuit of family change, perhaps a mainly dyadic focus makes sense. Still, in practice, family therapists have to deal with the issue of integrating dyadic changes into the family group (Sroufe & Fleeson, 1988). This issue needs future attention from both researchers and clinicians.

Some forms of family therapy (e.g., functional family therapy; Sexton & Alexander, 2005) do not address attachment per se, but focus on teaching and practicing the behavioral skills involved in parenting or in negotiating about rules and ways of establishing rules. Other approaches place more emphasis on cultural issues and the stresses associated with such events as immigration, which might seem to be ignored in attachment-oriented treatments. The assumption in attachment-oriented C&FT is that attachment processes, organized by powerful emotions and working models, provide the core scaffolding on which other elements in relationships depend. Deficits in attachment security will affect communication, negotiation, problem solving, and strategies for coping with stress. Although there is some education involved—about the nature of love, innate needs for support, and the methods of sensitive, responsive parenting—the basic assumption in attachment-oriented models is that once the bond between intimates is made more secure, other elements of the relationship will also improve. We know that secure attachment is associated with such factors as assertiveness, empathy, and caregiving (Johnson & Whiffen, 1999). In the first study of EFT (Johnson & Greenberg, 1985), couples whose members were able to share attachment needs also, in a final session, demonstrated problem-solving skills at the same level as those displayed by couples that had received the behavioral intervention offering specific training in this area.

When the attachment approach was first presented at C&FT conferences, therapists often commented that this approach was overly focused on individual characteristics, attachment styles, and unconscious processes rather than on interaction contexts and patterns. Methods of measurement have indeed focused on individuals and their general attachment orientation. For example, the Adult Attachment Interview (George, Kaplan, & Main, 1984, 1985, 1996) focuses on characteristics of narrative discourse about past attachment experiences, mostly with parents; and self-report questionnaires such as the Experiences in Close

Relationships scales (Brennan et al., 1998) ask about experiences and behaviors in "romantic" or "close" relationships (see Crowell et al., Chapter 26, this volume). Although other more relationship-specific and transactional measures now exist, such as the Current Relationship Interview and the Secure Base Scoring System (see Crowell et al., Chapter 26, this volume), much theory and research still focus on internal processes, working models, and features of an individual's personality rather than on behavioral transactions in current attachment relationships—the couple and family therapist's main concern.

Attachment theory and research do not offer a specific blueprint for intervention (Eagle & Wolitzky, in press), although useful ideas have been proposed (e.g., Berlin, Zeanah, & Lieberman, Chapter 31, and Slade, Chapter 32, this volume). Nor does attachment theory offer a specific theory of therapeutic change. It does not tell the couple therapist, for example, exactly how to help clients move from distress and distance to a supportive, secure connection. Bowlby (1988) did write about the nature of the alliance between therapist and client and about the importance of emotion in the change process: "First and foremost, he [the therapist] accepts and respects his patient warts and all as a fellow human being in trouble," and "it is the emotional communication between patient and therapist that plays the crucial part" in therapy (pp. 152, 156). But there is no manual that operationalizes "respect" and explains how to use "emotional communication" and revise working models. It is striking, however, that the forms of C&FT described briefly in this chapter share important features. All are collaborative; stress empathic responses on the part of the therapist; focus on attachment issues and events; respect emotion; integrate emotional responses with shifts in cognitive meanings; and encourage loved ones to interact in new ways that encourage emotional attunement, flexible responsiveness, and repair of conflict and disconnection.

ATTACHMENT AND C&FT: WHERE DO WE GO FROM HERE?

The attachment perspective is changing the field of C&FT. It is giving rise to systematic, empirically validated interventions; as part of the new science of relationships, it is also offering the field an explanatory framework for relationship problems, a detailed researched model of health, and a map for intervention. There are still many other developments on the horizon, and of course there are still many questions to answer.

One potential development is that attachment theory and research can contribute to our understanding of and ability to address pivotal transitions in close relationships. The transition to parenthood—a time when many relationships begin to unravel, and many women begin a journey into depression—is being examined through the lens of attachment. As Cowan and Cowan (2000, p. 161) note, "as men and women cross the great divide from couplehood to parenthood, they tend to get divided from each other." The emotional support offered by the new father, and his level of awareness of his partner and their relationship, seem to be key factors in determining how this transition is managed (Shapiro, Gottman, & Carrère, 2000) and appear to affect the number of women who become more anxiously attached at this time (Simpson, Rholes, Campbell, Tran, & Wilson, 2003). As attachment theory predicts, such transitions bring attachment needs to the fore. If we understand these transitions in attachment terms, rather than simply in terms of factors such as role change or general stress, we can more effectively help struggling couples and reduce the likelihood of clinical problems such as postpartum depression (Whiffen, 2003).

Attachment theory is also being used as a framework for understanding reactions to traumatic stress and general depression (Johnson, 2002). As this work continues, it should contribute to the refinement of C&FT interventions in relationships where distress is complicated by such symptomatology. Most distressed families and couples have other problems. Attachment theory gives us a way of seeing the coherence in the web of symptoms and interpersonal difficulties that our clients present; it therefore helps us identify the most effective targets for change. Rather than addressing problems piecemeal with a focus on one person's depression, another's disengagement, and a third's anger or conduct disorder, attachment theory allows us to see how all parts of the system are linked to the fundamental problem of emotional unavailability—of attachment insecurity (Whiffen, 2003b).

There are also many fascinating questions to be answered. For example, are there ways that C&FT can not only reduce conflict and negativity and increase responsiveness, but can also influence and change attachment styles and guide family members into the state of "earned security" (Pearson, Cohn, Cowan, & Cowan, 1994)? Can we create refinements to help partners generalize from new interactions in a specific relationship to more positive working models of self and other, and more general flexible and positive prototypes for relationships? If this is possible, it will raise the issue of the time needed to shift habitual perceptions and expectations; we will need to learn how best to facilitate the integration of new experience into new cognitive models and interactions.

Another question concerns what exactly constitutes change in attachment relationships. One focus in the field has been on working models, viewed as cognitive representations of interactions. It might be beneficial to focus more on the pivotal role of modes of affect regulation (see Mikulincer & Shaver, Chapter 23, this volume). Insight, however relevant, and relationship narratives, however coherent, do not seem to change affect-laden interaction patterns in families and couples. A change in the level of emotional engagement, and the creation of new attachment interactions where needs are expressed and responded to, appear to be necessary. The ability to regulate emotions, to move flexibly from reactive anger to sadness or fear, and to grasp and communicate these emotions in a way that moves the loved one to respond appears to be at the heart of change in attachment-oriented C&FT.

The attachment perspective is changing the face of C&FT. Two of the great leaders of the field, Salvador Minuchin and his colleague Mike Nichols, ended their 1993 book with a comment that would have been out of place and unacceptable only a few years earlier. They suggested (Minuchin & Nichols, 1993, p. 287) that family and couple therapists need the "courage to renounce the illusion of the autonomous self and to accept the limitations of belonging." Even here, there was still the word "limitation." To understand the essence of attachment and belonging is surely more liberating and empowering than constraining. This is also, however, a large and perhaps endless task. In relationships with those we love, as the poet e. e. cummings observed, "There is always a more beautiful answer that asks a more beautiful question."

REFERENCES

Ainsworth, M. D. S., Blehar, M. C., Waters, E., & Wall, S. (1978). Patterns of attachment: A psychological study of the Strange Situation. Hillsdale, NJ: Erlbaum.

Asarnow, J. R., Goldstein, M. J., Tompson, M., & Guthrie, D. (1993). One-year outcomes of depressive disorders in child psychiatric inpatients: Evaluation of the prognostic power of a brief measure of expressed emotion. Journal of Child Psychology and Psychiatry, 34, 129–137.

Bartholomew, K., & Allison, C. J. (2006). An attachment perspective on abusive dynamics in intimate relationships. In M. Mikulincer & G. S. Goodman (Eds.), Dynamics of romantic love (pp. 102–127). New York: Guilford Press.

Bartholomew, K., & Horowitz, L. (1991). Attachment styles among young adults. Journal of Personality and Social Psychology, 61, 226–244.

Baumrind, D. (1991). The influence of parenting style on adolescent competency and substance abuse. Journal of Adolescence, 11, 56–95.

Berscheid, E. (1999). The greening of relationship science. American Psychologist, 54, 260–266.

Beutler, L., Williams, R., & Wakefield, P. (1993). Obstacles to disseminating applied psychological science. Applied and Preventative Psychology, 2, 53–58.

Bowlby, J. (1944). Forty-four juvenile thieves: Their characters and home life. International Journal of Psycho-Analysis, 25, 19–52, 107–127.

Bowlby, J. (1969/1982). Attachment and loss: Vol. 1. Attachment. New York: Basic Books.

Bowlby, J. (1973). Attachment and loss: Vol. 2. Separation: Anxiety and anger. New York: Basic Books.

Bowlby, J. (1979). The making and breaking of affectional bonds. London: Tavistock.

Bowlby, J. (1980) Attachment and loss: Vol. 3. Loss: Sadness and depression. New York: Basic Books.

Bowlby, J. (1988). A secure base: Clinical applications of attachment theory. London: Routledge.

Brassard, A., Shaver, P. R., & Lussier, Y. (2007). Attachment, sexual experience, and sexual pressure in romantic relationships: A dyadic approach. Personal Relationships, 14, 475–494.

Brennan, K. A., Clark, C. L., & Shaver, P. R. (1998). Self-report measurement of adult romantic attachment: An integrative overview. In J. A. Simpson & W. S. Rholes (Eds.), Attachment theory and close relationships (pp. 46–76). New York: Guilford Press.

Bretherton, I., & Munholland, K. A. (1999). Internal working models in attachment relationships: A construct revisited. In J. Cassidy & P. R. Shaver (Eds.), Handbook of attachment: Theory, research, and clinical applications (pp. 89–111). New York: Guilford Press.

Byng-Hall, J. (1991). The application of attachment theory to understanding and treatment in family therapy. In C. M. Parkes, J. Stevenson-Hinde, & P. Harris (Eds.), Attachment across the life cycle (pp. 199–215). New York: Routledge.

Byng-Hall, J. (1999). Family and couple therapy: Toward greater security. In J. Cassidy & P. R. Shaver (Eds.), Handbook of attachment: Theory, research, and clinical applications (pp. 625–645). New York: Guilford Press.

Cassidy, J., & Berlin, L. J. (1994). The insecure/ambivalent pattern of attachment: Theory and research. Child Development, 65, 971–981.

Cassidy, J., & Kobak, R. (1988). Avoidance and its relation to other defensive processes. In J. Belsky & T. Nezworski (Eds.), Clinical implications of attachment (pp. 300–323). Hillsdale, NJ: Erlbaum.

Clothier, P., Manion, I., Gordon-Walker, J., & Johnson,

S. M. (2002). Emotionally focused interventions for couples with chronically ill children: A two year follow-up. *Journal of Marital and Family Therapy*, 28, 391–399.

Coan, J., Schaefer, H., & Davidson, R. (2006). Lending a hand. *Psychological Science*, 17, 1–8.

Cowan, C. P., & Cowan, P. A. (2000). *When partners become parents*. Mahwah, NJ: Erlbaum.

Cowan, P. A., Cohn, D. A., Cowan, C. P., & Pearson, J. L. (1996). Parents' attachment histories and children's externalizing and internalizing behaviors: Exploring family systems models of linkage. *Journal of Consulting and Clinical Psychology*, 64, 53–63.

Davila, J. (2003). Attachment processes in couple therapy: Informing behavioral models. In S. Johnson & V. Whiffen (Eds.), *Attachment processes in couple and family therapy* (pp. 124–143). New York: Guilford Press.

Davila, J., Burge, D., & Hammen, C. (1997). Why does attachment style change? *Journal of Personality and Social Psychology*, 73, 826–838.

Davila, J., Karney, B. R., & Bradbury, T. N. (1999). Attachment change processes in the early years of marriage. *Journal of Personality and Social Psychology*, 76, 783–802.

Davis, P. T., & Cummings, M. E. (1994). Marital conflict and child adjustment: An emotional security hypothesis. *Psychological Bulletin*, 116, 387–411.

Dessaulles, A., Johnson, S. M., & Denton, W. H. (2003). Emotion-focused therapy for couples in the treatment of depression: A pilot study. *American Journal of Family Therapy*, 31, 345–353.

Diamond, G. (2005). Attachment–based family therapy for depressed and anxious adolescents. In J. Lebow (Ed.), *Handbook of clinical family therapy* (pp. 17–41). Hoboken, NJ: Wiley.

Diamond, G., Siqueland, L., & Diamond, G. M. (2003). Attachment-based family therapy for depressed adolescents: Programmatic treatment development. *Clinical Child and Family Psychology Review*, 6, 107–128.

Eagle, M., & Wolitzky, D. L. (in press). Adult psychotherapy from the perspectives of attachment theory and psychoanalysis. In J. Obegi & E. Berant (Eds.), *Clinical applications of adult attachment theory and research*. New York: Guilford Press.

Ekman, P., & Friesen, W. (1975). *Unmasking the face*. Englewood Cliffs, NJ: Prentice-Hall.

Feeney, B. C. (2004). A secure base: Responsive support of goal strivings and exploration in adult intimate relationships. *Journal of Personality and Social Psychology*, 87, 631–648.

Feeney, B. C. (2007). The dependency paradox in close relationships: Accepting dependence promotes independence. *Journal of Personality and Social Psychology*, 92, 268–285.

Fishbane, M. (2005). Differentiation and dialogue in intergenerational relationships. In J. Lebow (Ed.), *Handbook of clinical family therapy* (pp. 543–568). Hoboken, NJ: Wiley.

Fonagy, P., & Target, M. (1997). Attachment and reflective function: Their role in self-organization. *Development and Psychopathology*, 9, 679–700.

Garner, D. M., Olmsted, M. P., & Polivy, J. (1983). Development and validation of a multidimensional Eating Disorder Inventory for anorexia nervosa and bulimia. *International Journal of Eating Disorders*, 2, 15–34.

George, C., Kaplan, N., & Main, M. (1984). *Adult Attachment Interview protocol*. Unpublished manuscript, University of California at Berkeley.

George, C., Kaplan, N., & Main, M. (1985). *Adult Attachment Interview protocol* (2nd ed.). Unpublished manuscript, University of California at Berkeley.

George, C., Kaplan, N., & Main, M. (1996). *Adult Attachment Interview protocol* (3rd ed.). Unpublished manuscript, University of California at Berkeley.

Gottman, J. M. (1994). *What predicts divorce?* Hillsdale, NJ: Erlbaum.

Gottman, J. M., Coan, J., Carrère, S., & Swanson, C. (1998). Predicting marital happiness and stability from newlywed interactions. *Journal of Marriage and the Family*, 60, 5–22.

Gottman, J. M., Katz, L. F., & Hooven, C. (1997). *Meta-emotion: How families communicate emotionally*. Hillsdale, NJ: Erlbaum.

Grossmann, K. E., Grossmann, K., & Waters, E. (Eds.). (2005). *Attachment from infancy to adulthood: The major longitudinal studies*. New York: Guilford Press.

Hazan, C., & Shaver, P. R. (1987). Romantic love conceptualized as an attachment process. *Journal of Personality and Social Psychology*, 52, 511–524.

Herring, M., & Kaslow, N. J. (2002). Depression and attachment in families: A child-focused perspective. *Family Process*, 41, 494–506.

Holmes, J. (1996). *Attachment, intimacy, autonomy: Using attachment theory in adult psychotherapy*. Northvale, NJ: Aronson.

Hughes, D. A. (2007). *Attachment-focused family therapy*. New York: Norton.

Huston, T. L., Caughlin, J. P., Houts, R. M., Smith, S. E., & George, L. J. (2001). The connubial crucible: Newlywed years as predictors of marital delight, distress, and divorce. *Journal of Personality and Social Psychology*, 80, 237–252.

Johnson, S. M. (1986). Bonds or bargains: Relationship paradigms and their significance for marital therapy. *Journal of Marital and Family Therapy*, 12, 259–267.

Johnson, S. M. (2002). *Emotionally focused couple therapy with trauma survivors: Strengthening attachment bonds*. New York: Guilford Press.

Johnson, S. M. (2003). Attachment theory: A guide for couple therapy. In S. Johnson & V. Whiffen (Eds.), *Attachment processes in couple and family therapy* (pp. 103–123). New York: Guilford Press.

Johnson, S. M. (2004). *The practice of emotionally focused couple therapy: Creating connection* (2nd ed.). New York: Brunner-Routledge.

Johnson, S. M. (2008). *Hold me tight: Seven conversations for a lifetime of love*. New York: Little, Brown.

Johnson, S. M., Bradley, B., Furrow, J., Lee, A., Palmer,

G., Tilley, D., et al. (2005). *Becoming an emotionally focused couple therapist: The workbook.* New York: Brunner-Routledge.

Johnson, S. M., & Greenberg, L. S. (1985). Differential effects of experiential and problem-solving interventions in resolving marital conflict. *Journal of Consulting and Clinical Psychology, 53,* 175–184.

Johnson, S. M., Hunsley, J., Greenberg, L., & Schlindler, D. (1999). Emotionally focused couples therapy: Status and challenges. *Clinical Psychology: Science and Practice, 6,* 67–79.

Johnson, S. M., & Lee, A. (2000). Emotionally focused family therapy: Restructuring attachment. In C. E. Bailey (Ed.), *Children in therapy: Using the family as a resource* (pp. 112–136). New York: Norton.

Johnson, S. M., Maddeaux, C., & Blouin, J. (1998). Emotionally focused family therapy for bulimia: Changing attachment patterns. *Psychotherapy, 35,* 238–247.

Johnson, S. M., Makinen, J., & Millikin, J. (2001). Attachment injuries in couple relationships: A new perspective on impasses in couples therapy. *Journal of Marital and Family Therapy, 27,* 145–155.

Johnson, S. M., & Talitman, E. (1996). Predictors of success in emotionally focused marital therapy. *Journal of Marital and Family Therapy, 23,* 135–152.

Johnson, S. M., & Whiffen, V. (1999). Made to measure: Attachment styles in couples therapy. *Clinical Psychology: Science and Practice, 6,* 366–381.

Karen, R. (1998). *Becoming attached.* Oxford, UK: Oxford University Press.

Kirkpatrick, L. A., & Davis, K. E. (1994). Attachment style, gender, and relationship stability: A longitudinal analysis. *Journal of Personality and Social Psychology, 66,* 502–512.

Kobak, R., & Duemmler, S. (1994). Attachment and conversation: Toward a discourse analysis of adolescent security. In K. Bartholomew & D. Perlman (Eds.), *Advances in personal relationships: Vol. 5. Attachment processes in adulthood* (pp. 121–149). London: Jessica Kingsley.

Kunce, L. J., & Shaver, P. R. (1994). An attachment theoretical approach to care-giving in romantic relationships. In K. Bartholomew & D. Perlman (Eds.), *Advances in personal relationships: Vol. 5. Attachment processes in adulthood* (pp. 205–237). London: Jessica Kingsley.

Levy, D. (1937). Primary affect hunger. *American Journal of Psychiatry, 94,* 643–652.

Liddle, H. A. (1999). Theory development in a family-based therapy for adolescent drug abuse. *Journal of Clinical Child Psychology, 28,* 521–532.

Lussier, Y., Sabourin, S., & Turgeon, C. (1997). Coping strategies as moderators of the relationship between attachment and marital adjustment. *Journal of Social and Personal Relationships, 14,* 777–791.

MacIntosh, H., & Johnson, S. M. (in press). Emotionally focused couple therapy with couples dealing with childhood trauma. *Journal of Marital and Family Therapy.*

Mackey, S. K. (1996). Nurturance: A neglected dimension in family therapy with adolescents. *Journal of Marriage and Family Therapy, 22,* 489–508.

Mackey, S. K. (2003). Adolescence and attachment: From theory to treatment implications. In P. Erdman & T. Caffery (Eds.), *Attachment and family systems: Conceptual, empirical, and therapeutic relatedness* (pp. 79–113). New York: Brunner-Routledge.

Main, M., & Hesse, E. (1990). Parents' unresolved traumatic experiences are related to infant disorganized attachment status: Is frightened and/or frightening parental behavior the linking mechanism? In M. T. Greenberg, D. Cicchetti, & E. M. Cummings (Eds.), *Attachment in the preschool years: Theory, research, and intervention* (pp. 161–182). Chicago: University of Chicago Press.

Main, M., Kaplan, N., & Cassidy, J. (1985). Security in infancy, childhood, and adulthood: A move to the level of representation. In I. Bretherton & E. Waters (Eds.), Growing points of attachment theory and research. *Monographs of the Society for Research in Child Development, 50*(1–2, Serial No. 209), 66–104.

Makinen, J. A., & Johnson, S. M. (2006). Resolving attachment injuries in couples using emotionally focused therapy: Steps toward forgiveness and reconciliation. *Journal of Consulting and Clinical Psychology, 74,* 1055–1064.

Marvin, R. S., & Stewart, R. B. (1990). A family systems framework for the study of attachment. In M. T. Greenberg, D. Cicchetti, & E. M. Cummings (Eds.), *Attachment in the preschool years: Theory, research, and intervention* (pp. 51–86). Chicago: University of Chicago Press.

McFarlane, A. C., & van der Kolk, B. A. (1996). Trauma and its challenge to society. In B. A. van der Kolk, A. C. McFarlane, & L. Weisaeth (Eds.), *Traumatic stress: The effects of overwhelming experience on mind, body, and society* (pp. 24–46). New York: Guilford Press.

Merkel, W., & Searight, H. (1992). Why families are not like swamps, solar systems, or thermostats: Some limits of systems theory as applied to family therapy. *Contemporary Family Therapy, 14,* 33–50.

Mikulincer, M. (1995). Attachment style and the mental representation of self. *Journal of Personality and Social Psychology, 69,* 1203–1215.

Mikulincer, M. (1997). Adult attachment style and information processing. *Journal of Personality and Social Psychology, 72,* 1217–1230.

Mikulincer, M., & Shaver, P. R. (2007). *Attachment in adulthood: Structure, dynamics, and change.* New York: Guilford Press.

Minuchin, S., & Nichols, M. P. (1993). *Family healing: Tales of hope and renewal from family therapy.* New York: Free Press.

Moretti, M. M., & Holland, R. (2003). The journey of adolescence: Transitions in self in the context of attachment relationships. In S. M. Johnson & V. Whiffen (Eds.), *Attachment processes in couple and family therapy* (pp. 234–257). New York: Guilford Press.

Panksepp, J. (1998). *Affective neuroscience: The founda-*

tions of human and animal emotions. New York: Oxford University Press.

Pasch, L. A., & Bradbury, T. N. (1998). Social support, conflict, and the development of marital dysfunction. *Journal of Consulting and Clinical Psychology, 66,* 219–230.

Pearson, J. L., Cohn, D. A., Cowan, P. A., & Cowan, C. P. (1994). Earned and continuous security in adult attachment: Relation to depressive symptomatology and parenting style. *Development and Psychopathology, 6,* 359–613.

Rosenstein, D. S., & Horowitz, H. A. (1996). Adolescent attachment and psychopathology. *Journal of Consulting and Clinical Psychology, 64,* 244–253.

Senchak, M., & Leonard, K. E. (1992). Attachment styles and marital adjustment among newlywed couples. *Journal of Social and Personal Relationships, 9,* 51–64.

Sexton, T., & Alexander, J. (2005). Functional family therapy for externalizing disorders in adolescents. In J. L. Lebow (Ed.), *Handbook of clinical family therapy* (pp. 164–191). Hoboken, NJ: Wiley.

Shapiro, A. F., Gottman, J. M., & Carrère, S. (2000). The baby and the marriage: Identifying factors that buffer against decline in marital satisfaction after the first baby arrives. *Journal of Family Psychology, 14,* 59–70.

Shaver, P. R., & Clark, C. L. (1994). The psychodynamics of adult romantic attachment. In J. M. Masling & R. F. Bornstein (Eds.), *Empirical perspectives on object relations theories* (pp. 105–156). Washington, DC: American Psychological Association.

Shaver, P. R., & Hazan, C. (1993). Adult romantic attachment: Theory and evidence. In D. Perlman & W. Jones (Eds.), *Advances in personal relationships* (Vol. 4, pp. 29–70). London: Jessica Kingsley.

Simpson, J. A., & Rholes, W. S. (1994). Stress and secure base relationships in adulthood. In K. Bartholomew & D. Perlman (Eds.), *Advances in personal relationships: Vol. 5. Attachment processes in adulthood* (pp. 181–204). London: Jessica Kingsley.

Simpson, J. A., Rholes, W. S., Campbell, L., Tran, S., & Wilson, C. L. (2003). Adult attachment, the transition to parenthood, and depressive symptoms. *Journal of Personality and Social Psychology, 84,* 1172–1187.

Simpson, J. A., Rholes, W. S., & Nelligan, J. S. (1992). Support seeking and support giving within couples in an anxiety-provoking situation: The role of attachment styles. *Journal of Personality and Social Psychology, 62,* 434–446.

Sroufe, L. A., & Fleeson, J. (1988). The coherence of family relationships. In R. A. Hinde & J. Stevenson-Hinde (Eds.), *Relationships within families: Mutual influences* (pp. 27–47). Oxford, UK: Oxford University Press.

Trevarthen, C., & Aitken, K. J. (2001). Infant intersubjectivity: Research, theory, and clinical applications. *Journal of Child Psychology and Psychiatry, 42,* 3–48.

Whiffen, V. (2003). Adult attachment and child bearing depression. In S. M. Johnson & V. Whiffen (Eds.), *Attachment processes in couple and family therapy* (pp. 321–341). New York: Guilford Press.

Whiffen, V. (2003b). What attachment theory can offer marital and family therapists. In S. M. Johnson & V. Whiffen (Eds.), *Attachment processes in couple and family therapy* (pp. 389–398). New York: Guilford Press.

Whisman, M. A., & Jacobson, N. S. (1990). Power, marital satisfaction, and response to marital therapy. *Journal of Family Psychology, 4,* 202–212.

von Bertalanffy, L. (1968). *General system theory: Foundations, development, applications.* New York: George Braziller.

PART VI

SYSTEMS, CULTURE, AND CONTEXT

CHAPTER 35

The Caregiving System
A Behavioral Systems Approach to Parenting

CAROL GEORGE
JUDITH SOLOMON

An 8-month-old infant clambers on … a fallen tree while its mother sits about 7 feet below. The infant slips and hangs by two hands. [His mother] looks up, stands on two legs, and barely reaches the foot of her infant. She pulls it to her chest but it wriggles free, repeats the climb only to slip at the same place again, to be rescued once more by its mother.
—SCHALLER (1963, p. 263, describing gorillas)

Gremlin's concern for Gimble went way beyond merely responding to his appeals for help: like a good mother she would anticipate trouble. … Once, as she was carrying him along a trail, she saw a small snake ahead. Carefully she pushed Gimble off her back and kept him behind her as she shook branches at the snake until it glided away.
—GOODALL (1990, p. 169, describing chimpanzees)

One day Effie was observed contentedly feeding about twenty feet behind the group, while Poppy, some six feet behind her mother, was solo playing and swinging in a Seneco tree. … [S]uddenly Effie twirled around and stared at Poppy. … Poppy had fallen and was hanging by her neck in a narrow fork of the tree. The infant could only feebly kick her legs and flail her arms as the stranglehold began cutting off her oxygen. Instantly Effie ran to her baby. With considerable effort she tugged at Poppy, trying to release her from a potentially fatal position. Effie was wearing a horrified expression of fear similar to that of a human parent whose child is in mortal danger. … At last Effie succeeded in releasing her infant from the tree's stranglehold. Immediately upon regaining her breath, Poppy began to whimper, then attached herself to Effie's nipple for four minutes before her mother carried her off, in a protective ventral position, toward the group, which were unaware of the drama that had unfolded behind them.
—FOSSEY (1983, p. 88, describing gorillas)

Bowlby's attachment theory inspired a dramatic shift in the way we understand the development of the early infant–caregiver relationship and other relationships across the lifespan. By reframing attachment in terms of the ethological concept of behavioral systems, attachment theory added a new perspective to developmental inquiries about relationships. The attachment system is one of many behavioral systems that have evolved to promote survival and reproductive success (Hinde, 1982). The goal of attachment behavior is to seek protec- tion by maintaining proximity to an attachment figure in response to real or perceived stress or danger (Bowlby, 1969/1982). The goal of that behavior remains the same across the lifespan, although the actual behavior varies according to context and age. The empirical evidence supporting the role of attachment in the child's development is impressive. Almost four decades of research have shown that attachment contributes importantly to an individual's ability to accomplish age-appropriate socioemotional and cognitive tasks in childhood

833

and adulthood. Marked aberrations in attachment organization are associated with developmental and mental health risks in children and adults (see DeKlyen & Greenberg, Chapter 27, this volume; Lyons-Ruth & Jacobvitz, Chapter 28, this volume; Solomon & George, 1999a, in press-a).

According to attachment theory, the most important factor guiding the formation of the attachment relationship is the child's experience with caregivers. All infants who receive some form of regular care select attachment figures, suggesting that simple propinquity and social interactions with a caregiver are sufficient for an attachment to develop (Bowlby, 1969/1982). The quality of care determines the organization of the relationship through its effect on a child's confidence in the availability of a caregiver (i.e., security; see Ainsworth, Blehar, Waters, & Wall, 1978; De Wolff & van IJzendoorn, 1997). But what are the origins of the attachment figure's sensitivity? What causes parents to provide care for their infants—care that sometimes requires costly personal sacrifices on the part of parents?

Bowlby proposed that an attachment figure's behavior is organized by a caregiving behavioral system reciprocal to the care recipient's attachment behavior (Bowlby, 1969/1982, 1988). Historically, it was unusual to view caregiving as the result of an organized behavioral system. There is a large literature on parenting that covers a wide range of topics (e.g., Bornstein, 2003; Hoghughi & Lond, 2004). What this literature lacks, however, is a theory that integrates the internal organization of a parent's caregiving behavior with a child's outcomes.

We were part of a small group of attachment researchers in the late 1980s through the mid-1990s who were interested in describing the caregiving system. During that era, attachment research moved "to the level of representation" (Main, Kaplan, & Cassidy, 1985); that is, it moved from observations of infant behavior with a caregiver to an examination of how relationships are mentally represented, remembered, and described (see Hesse, Chapter 25, this volume). The purpose of the present chapter is to provide a comprehensive framework for understanding caregiving as a behavioral system in its own right—that is, as an organized set of behaviors guided by a representation of the current parent–child relationship (George & Solomon, 1989, 1996; Solomon & George, 1996, 2000).

A unique contribution of this chapter is to emphasize the importance for the parent of making a shift away from *seeking protection and proximate care from attachment figures* (the function and goal of attachment for the child) to *providing protection, comfort, and care for a child* (the function and proximate goal for the parent). This shift is fundamental to understanding the meaning of and motivation underlying critical aspects of parental behavior, cultural differences in providing care, the development of the child's quality of attachment, and the mechanisms of intergenerational transmission.

The first section of this chapter outlines the components of a behavioral systems approach to caregiving. We next describe the caregiving system in relation to interactions and competition among behavioral systems. This discussion leads us to define the construct of "flexible care." We next discuss what little is known about the ontogeny of a mother's caregiving system, including potential influences in childhood, adolescence, and the transition to parenthood (pregnancy and childbirth). The final major section discusses representational models of caregiving. The predominant focus of caregiving researchers to date has been on describing the representational mechanisms that underlie maternal sensitivity. We complete our caregiving model by contrasting these approaches with our own, which defines caregiving representation in terms of flexibility and of organizing and disorganizing forms of defensive exclusion.

DEFINING THE CAREGIVING BEHAVIORAL SYSTEM

A Behavioral Systems Model of Caregiving

This section describes the behavioral system concept, guided by Hinde's (1982) method of defining elements. A behavioral system is a biologically based motivational control system that governs the rules and behaviors associated with a specific proximate goal (see Marvin & Britner, Chapter 12, this volume). Important to this approach is the distinction among levels of causality (e.g., ultimate, proximate, ontogenic). Behavioral systems (1) comprise behaviors coordinated to achieve specific goals and adaptive functions; (2) are activated and terminated by endogenous and environmental cues; (3) are "goal-corrected" (i.e., regulated by goals that extend over long periods of time and are served by nonrandom behavior that flexibly adjusts to a wide range of environments and an individual's level of development); (4) are "activated" and "terminated" at the biological level by a feedback system that monitors internal cues (central nervous system activity, hormones) as well as environmental cues; (5) are related to and interact with other behavioral systems; (6) are developmentally integrated behavioral sequences that become functional (i.e., mature) over time as the product of organism–environment interaction; and (7) are organized and integrated by specific cognitive control systems (in the case of humans, mental representations).

We begin our discussion of caregiving by examining the first four principles. The remaining principles are discussed in later sections.

The behavioral systems approach to caregiving begins with Bowlby's (1969/1982, 1973) belief that the caregiving system is reciprocal to, and evolved in parallel with, the attachment system. The ways in which the infant's behavioral systems (e.g., attachment, exploration, affiliation) interact with each other were outlined thoroughly in Bowlby's and Ainsworth's original work and have become standard features of attachment theory and research (see Cassidy, Chapter 1, this volume). The ways in which the infant's behavioral systems interact with those of the caregiver, and the ways in which the caregiver's behavioral systems interact with each other, are as yet largely unexplored.

The first step in defining the caregiving system is to delineate its adaptive function and behavioral goal. We adopt Bowlby's position that the adaptive function of the caregiving system, as with attachment, is protecting the young and thereby ultimately increasing one's own reproductive fitness (Solomon & George, 1996; see Simpson & Belsky, Chapter 6, this volume). Following ethological theory and paralleling Bowlby's (1969/1982) discussion of attachment, we assume that the behavioral goal of the caregiving system is to provide protection for the child.

Central to Bowlby's theory was his identification of factors involved in the activation, termination, and regulation of the child's attachment system. The attachment system is activated by internal or external cues that the child perceives as frightening, dangerous, or stressful. It follows that the caregiving system is activated by internal or external cues associated with situations that the *parent* perceives as frightening, dangerous, or stressful for the child. These situations include (but are not limited to) separation, child endangerment, and the child's signals of discomfort and distress.

Once activated, the parent's caregiving system can call upon a repertoire of behaviors that serve the system's protective function. These be-

haviors may include retrieval, maintaining proximity, carrying, following, signaling the child to follow, calling, looking, and in humans, smiling, all of which work to establish proximity, care, and comfort.[1] The child's attachment system is terminated by proximity, or physical or psychological contact with the attachment figure, when the caregiver responds to the child's attachment needs in a satisfactory manner. Again following Bowlby's template for attachment, we propose that the parent's caregiving system is terminated by physical or psychological proximity and signs that the child is comforted, contented, or satisfied. Just as Bowlby proposed that attachment is associated with and regulated by strong feelings, including joy and anger in response to whether or not the caregiver is within proximity, caregiving is also associated with and regulated by strong emotions. Mothers express intense feelings of pleasure and satisfaction when they are able to protect and comfort their children; they experience heightened anger, sadness, anxiety, or despair when they are separated from the children, or when their ability to protect and comfort the children is threatened or blocked.

Behavioral systems are goal-corrected—a feature that potentially allows for maximum behavioral flexibility—and guided by a biological feedback system. Bowlby (1973) proposed that flexibly integrated attachment behavior is the foundation of physiological homeostasis (see Polan & Hofer, Chapter 7, this volume). Individual differences in the way the goal is achieved, operationally defined as individual differences in security, should therefore be evidenced in neural and hormonal activity. There is now excellent research on mothering in humans and other mammals that demonstrates the role of hormones and neural activation patterns in the regulation of attachment and caregiving (e.g., Bartels & Zeki, 2004; Hrdy, 1999; Lorberbaum et al., 1999; Novakov & Fleming, 2005).

Once the caregiving system is activated, the caregiver must "decide" whether and how to behave. The caregiver's behavior depends on his or her conscious and unconscious evaluation of competing sources of information. One source of information is the caregiver's evaluation of the child's signals. Another is the caregiver's appraisal of danger or threat. The parent must always be vigilant, scanning regularly for cues from these sources. He or she must then organize the various perceptions and select a response. This requires a capacity to flexibly integrate these sources of information in order to achieve the goals of the caregiving system.

We turn now to the parent's perspective on caregiving. The parent has access to more information than the child, including a wealth of information drawn from his or her evaluation of the context and personal past experience both as a child and as a parent. There are many situations in which the parent's caregiving system is activated, but the child's attachment system is not. These situations may lead to occasions of parent–child conflict. For example, the desire of parents of adolescents to protect and care for their teenagers often conflicts with the teens' view that their parents are controlling or intrusive.

The Caregiving System: Interaction and Competition among Behavioral Systems

According to ethological theory, behavior is the product of the *interaction* among behavioral systems (Hinde, 1982; Marvin & Britner, Chapter 12, this volume). Another important step in defining the caregiving system, therefore, is to examine the interaction between the parent's caregiving system and other behavioral systems that may compete with providing care for any particular child (Bowlby, 1969/1982; Solomon & George, 1996; Stevenson-Hinde, 1994). Just as flexible integration of sources of information is important, flexibility and the ability to balance competing behavioral systems are essential to accomplishing caregiving goals. This is true at the ultimate (functional) as well as at the proximate (psychological and physiological) level of analysis. From a functionalist view, a parent and child have overlapping interests and inherent and inevitable conflicts (Cassidy, 2000; Simpson & Belsky, Chapter 6, this volume; Solomon & George, 1996; Trivers, 1974). In addition to being a caregiver to one child, a parent may be a caregiver for other children (competing caregiving), a friend (affiliative system), a sexual partner (sexual system), a worker (exploratory system), or a person who seeks care from his or her own attachment figures (attachment system). A parent must strike a balance among these competing demands, as constrained by developmental, ecological, cultural, and individual factors that have been detailed elsewhere (Cassidy, 2000; Hrdy, 1999; Simpson & Belsky, Chapter 6, this volume; Solomon & George, 1996, 2000).

Flexible care appears to be characteristic of all humans, despite vast differences in caregiving behavior (e.g., Posada, Gao, Wu, & Posada, 1995). Care is elevated through toddlerhood and followed by less direct supervision as the child matures.

Flexibility is thought to contribute to selective advantage under difficult environmental conditions (Kermoian & Liederman, 1986). A parent may need to develop alternative or compromise strategies that are manipulations of a primary behavioral system strategy (Hinde & Stevenson-Hinde, 1991). Main (1990) proposed that an infant's behavior associated with security is the primary attachment strategy; patterns of behavior associated with avoidant and ambivalent attachment are conditional secondary behavioral strategies that sacrifice feelings of security but permit a child to maintain proximity to the mother for protection. Following this thinking, we propose that mothers of avoidant and ambivalent children develop complementary alternative, conditional caregiving strategies, including heightened or minimized care (i.e., strategies that keep children close or at a distance), which may be culturally promoted in relation to overarching cultural socialization goals (George & Solomon, 1999; Solomon & George, 1996).

If we are correct in assuming that the goal of caregiving is protection of the young, then a very broad range of caregiving strategies may be considered "good enough," to the extent that the mother's behavior *under conditions of risk or threat to the child* is organized around protection. Mothers of infants classified as avoidant and resistant, as well as those of infants classified as secure, may be considered "good enough" under normal rearing conditions (i.e., in the absence of multiple or severe threats). In contrast to these relationships, we discuss later in this chapter how mothers of infants classified as disorganized may properly be labeled "disabled" caregivers, because they intermittently or persistently "abdicate" their protective role. This view is supported indirectly by well-established evidence that disorganized attachment, in contrast to the organized secure, avoidant, and ambivalent patterns, is associated with children's developmental risk (e.g., Lyons-Ruth & Jacobvitz, Chapter 28, this volume; Solomon & George, in press-a).

A Note about Caregiving in Mothers versus Fathers

It is likely that there are differences in interaction and competition among behavioral systems, depending on a parent's gender. Attachment research has focused primarily on mothers, although there is evidence that fathers can also be sensitive and involved caregivers (Bakermans-Kranenburg, van IJzendoorn, Bokhorst, & Schuengel, 2004; Belsky, Jaffee, Sligo, Woodward, & Silva, 2005;

Grossmann, Grossmann, Kindler, & Zimmermann, Chapter 36, this volume). A few recent attachment studies describe fathers' views of their parenting activities (e.g., Bretherton, Lambert, & Golby, 2005). No attention has been devoted, however, to defining the caregiving system in relation to a father's other behavioral systems.

ONTOGENY OF MATERNAL CAREGIVING

The behavioral systems framework includes discussion of how caregiving behavior becomes an integrated, organized behavioral system. The most prominent explanations within attachment research assert that maternal caregiving is the transmission of the mother's attachment to the next generation (George, Kaplan, & Main, 1984, 1985, 1996; Main & Goldwyn, 1984, 2003; see Hesse, Chapter 25, for an overview). A view that this pathway is linear has become widely accepted in the field. We call this the assimilation model of caregiving (Solomon & George, 1996). Assimilation is the process by which new experiences and information are integrated into existing schemes; attachment theorists suggest that under normal circumstances, a mother integrates her experiences with the child into her mental representation of attachment.

At first glance, the assimilation model is appealing and appears to be supported empirically by findings that report statistically significant concordance patterns between a mother's Adult Attachment Interview (AAI) classification and a child's attachment classification (e.g., Benoit, Parker, & Zeanah, 1997; van IJzendoorn, 1995). More careful examination of this data shows that concordance is found predominantly for mothers who are judged secure or autonomous with regard to attachment on the AAI (see discussion by Solomon & George, 1996, in press-b). Concordance is lowest for mothers of disorganized children. The assimilation model predicts that mothers of disorganized children should be unresolved with respect to their own attachment-related loss or trauma; yet this is frequently not the case. Another striking mismatch that challenges the assimilation model has been demonstrated in attachment trauma research. Mothers who have "earned security" (see Hesse, Chapter 25, this volume) with respect to childhood trauma have been described as disorganized parents. As we discuss in detail in the section on disorganized caregiving at the end of this chapter, caring for their own children dysregulates

these mothers' caregiving system and reactivates personal traumatic fears and memories (Fisher, 2000).

Development of Maternal Behavior

Many contributions to the understanding of caregiving from outside the field of attachment bear on the development of the caregiving system and caregiving behavior. Central to our argument is that this development is the product of a complex transaction among biological and experiential factors. The biological foundation of mothering is regulated by neurological mechanisms associated with effective protection and care (Bell, 2001; Gobbini & Haxby, 2006; Kinsley et al., 1999; Leibenluft, Gobbini, Harrison, & Haxby, 2004; Lorberbaum et al., 1999; Nitschke, Heller, Etienne, & Miller, 2004; Swain, Lorberbaum, Kose, & Strathearn, 2007).

Comparative researchers describe the similarities among mammals in maternal behavior as due to common brain regions and mechanisms (e.g., Carter et al., 2005; Kinsley & Lambert, 2006; Poindron, Terrazas, de la Luz Navarro Montes de Oca, Serafán, & Hernández, 2007). Kerverne (1995) emphasized the similarity across species of hormonal priming associated with pregnancy and birth, especially the role of oxytocin (see also Carter et al., 2005).

Pryce (1995) has developed the only comprehensive model of mothering that describes the developmental pathways that may lead to individual differences in mothering. Pryce stresses the importance of interacting influences, including the caregiving environment (e.g., social support, stress), characteristics of the infant, and "maternal motivation" (defined as the mother's motivation to provide care, based on the reward value of the baby). Following attachment theory, and similar to the position advanced by Pryce, we propose that the caregiving system has important roots in childhood as well as more contemporary adult influences (see also Simpson & Belsky, Chapter 6, this volume).

In the remainder of this section, we outline ontogenetic factors beyond the mother's own childhood experience that are likely to be important to the development of the caregiving system. Some of these influences have been considered briefly by other researchers interested in maternal behavior (e.g., Fraiberg, 1980; Sroufe & Fleeson, 1986), but not in terms of their relation to the caregiving system. We consider the following discussion to be a work in progress and do not intend it to be a definitive statement on caregiving. Our primary goal is to stimulate future thinking about the development of the caregiving system.

Factors Important to the Development of the Caregiving System

Childhood Influences

All behavioral systems begin with immature forms of behavior that gradually become integrated and "mature." Behavioral systems contribute to an individual's fitness, but they do not develop at the same rate or at the same time during the life course. Behavioral systems essential for survival of the young (e.g., attachment, feeding) mature quickly. Behavioral systems important to later stages of development (e.g., caregiving, sex) mature more slowly. Immature, isolated, and incomplete forms of behavior associated with a behavioral system can be observed before the system has reached maturity (Bowlby, 1969/1982; Marvin & Britner, Chapter 12, this volume). Behavior resulting from immature systems differs qualitatively from behavior resulting from mature systems. The stimuli activating immature behavioral systems are more varied than those that activate mature behavioral systems. Upon maturity, stimulus discrimination and organization improve, which results in a system that is potentially flexibly integrated and goal-corrected (Bowlby, 1969/1982)

The first expressions of the caregiving system appear as isolated, immature, nonfunctional forms of care and affection. These elements are observable at early ages in human and nonhuman primates. For example, "play-mothering" is common among juveniles, especially females (Pryce, 1995). The presence of babies, including dolls and baby animals, elicits interest and caregiving behavior in human children. There are important differences, however, between play-mothering and mature caregiving. The behavioral sequences in play-mothering are fragmented and incomplete, and a child's attention is easily distracted away from the baby (Pryce, 1995). As a result, the child is not likely to follow through in providing complete or satisfactory care, and the baby may be placed in jeopardy.

Behavioral biologists emphasize that maternal behavior in juveniles is likely to be cued not only by the presence of an infant, but also by the child's own experiences of maternal care (Pryce, 1995). Play-mothering does not occur, for example, in rhesus macaques that are isolated from their own mothers during the first year of life. Furthermore, these monkeys fail to show normal preferences for their own infants over infants of other females when they become mothers themselves (Pryce, 1995). Attachment theory proposes that children develop a sense of caregiving through their experiences with their mothers (Bowlby, 1969/1982; Bretherton & Munholland, Chapter 5, this volume).

Although there is no research on caregiving behavior during middle childhood (roughly ages 5–11), we expect that the caregiving system matures gradually under childrearing conditions in which a child is not placed in the position to assume *principal* responsibility for the care and protection of siblings or the child's own parents. In many cultures, children take on major responsibility for sibling care, tutored by their mothers or guided by older siblings. The degree to which this experience contributes to the early maturity of a child's caregiving system (i.e., causing it to become fully organized and integrated) is an empirical question.

Adolescence

It is likely that the caregiving system begins a transformation toward maturity during adolescence (Solomon & George, 1996). This view fits with the developmental perspective that adolescence is the period during which many of a child's characteristics (e.g., physical, mental) mature into adult forms. Fullard and Reiling (1976) found that children between the ages of 7 and 12 preferred to look at pictures of adults when given a choice between adults and infants. They report a shift to adult-like preferences for pictures of infants in girls ages 12–14 and boys ages 14–16. These shifts in preferences coincide with the average ages at which girls and boys become capable of reproduction. It suggests that the adolescent transformation of the caregiving system may be partly based on the biological changes associated with puberty. In girls, the changes in the hypothalamus, pituitary, and ovaries associated with menarche result in dramatic changes in primary and secondary sexual characteristics, including ovulation, placental development, and the production of adrenocorticotropic hormones. Given the influence of hormones on mammalian and primate mothering, we speculate that these changes may be a catalyst toward maturity of the caregiving system during adolescence; this speculation is supported by observations of earlier maturity of caregiving in girls than boys (Kerverne, 1995).

This transition is also influenced by experience. Stressful childhood experiences, for example, may provoke the early onset of menarche and an early interest in infants (Dario, 2005; Ellis & Garber, 2000; Kim & Smith, 2000; Moffitt, Caspi, Belsky, & Silva, 1992; Wierson, Long, & Forehand, 1993). The influence of mores and taboos in cultures that discourage adolescent sexual behavior and pregnancy may override a girl's biological predisposition to become a mother. In our experience, however, despite cultural pressures against adolescents having babies, many older adolescent girls (e.g., ages 17–19) demonstrate remarkable interest and thoughtfulness regarding mothering that extends beyond the intellectual knowledge of reproduction. Girls at this age are often consumed by questions about whether or not they will be good mothers, how it is that a mother comes to love a baby, and what it would be like to be responsible for an infant.

Transition to Parenthood

The caregiving system probably undergoes its greatest development during the transition to parenthood (pregnancy, birth, and the months following birth). Developmentalists conceptualize a transition as a "crisis" or "bio-social-behavioral shift" that results from the transaction among unique biological, psychological, and social factors (Emde, Gaensbauer, & Harmon, 1976; Lee, 1995). We view the development of the caregiving system as a similar kind of qualitative shift. At the biological level, this period in a woman's life is accompanied by intense hormonal and neurological changes (Pryce, 1995), especially influences on neural networks considered to be the "maternal circuit" (i.e., hypothalamus and orbitofrontal cortex; Kinsley et al., 1999). Ovarian steroids (e.g., oxytocin, progesterone, oestradiol), adrenal hormones, and endorphins produced during this period are thought to activate "motherly impulses" (Gintzler, 1980, as cited by Kinsley et al., 1999) and to influence sensory acuity, emotional calm, and closeness (Fleming & Li, 2002). Finally, many psychologists have noted an enormous upsurge in thoughts, doubts, and worries about the self as a parent, the spouse, and the past during this period. Some theorists propose that this upwelling of anxiety is essential for the mother's reorganization of self (Ammaniti, 1994; Benedict, 1959; Bibring, Dwyer, Huntington, & Valenstein, 1961; Brazel-

ton, 1981; Cohen & Slade, 2000; Coleman, Nelson, & Sundre, 1999; Cowan, 1991; Deutscher, 1971; Ilicali & Fisek, 2004; Lee, 1995; Liefer, 1980).

The caregiving system is influenced by the experience of childbirth itself, including the hormonal milieu and stimuli emanating from the young, and shifts in hormone production that reduce mothers' fear and facilitate acceptance of their offspring (e.g., Fleming & Li, 2002; Hrdy, 1999; Klaus, Kennell, & Klaus, 1995). Factors surrounding a baby's birth are thought to be critical to human mothering, although the strong interpretation of these effects has now been tempered (Klaus et al., 1995). Providing human mothers with bonding experiences (i.e., the opportunity for extended closeness and physical contact with the infant immediately following birth) enhances touching, kissing, talking to their babies, and nursing, especially for mothers at risk (e.g., those experiencing economic risk, high stress, unplanned or unwanted pregnancies) (e.g., Tallandini & Scalembra, 2006). Mothers' bonding experiences, however, have not been found to be related to their children's attachment security later in infancy (Rode, Chang, Fisch, & Sroufe, 1981).

The degree to which childbirth and other influences associated with the transition to parenthood influence the caregiving system is an issue that needs further investigation. The experiences that a mother brings to her baby's birth, her representation of herself as a caregiver, her interpretation of the birth experience, and her experience of the birth itself (e.g., birthing technique—Manning-Orenstein, 1997; miscarriage—Hughes, Turton, McGauley, & Fonagy, 2006; Slade et al., 1995; premature birth—Borghini et al., 2006; foster care—Stovall-McClough & Dozier, 2004) may be synergistic factors that together influence (positively or negatively) the caregiving system.

The Baby

Other factors that may influence the development of the caregiving system are associated with the baby him- or herself (e.g., Bell, 1968; Sameroff, 1993). The baby has enormous power to evoke caregiving behavior. Physical features of "babyness," including a combination of the prominent features of an infant (e.g., rounded, oversized head; large eyes) and distinctive emotional expressiveness, evoke caregiving in adults (Fullard & Reiling, 1976; Lorenz, 1943; Suomi, 1995). Infant cues (e.g., odor, cries) and proximity (including touching the baby) influence both the patterning of behavior and the mother's motivation to respond in rats and humans (Carter et al., 2005; Corter & Fleming, 2002; Fleming & Li, 2002). A mother's perception of her baby as physically unattractive or abnormal can elicit rejection, neglect, abandonment, or infanticide (Clutton-Brock, 1991; Langlois, Ritter, Cassey, & Sawin, 1995; Miller, 1987; Scheper-Hughes, 1987; Volk, Lukjanczuk, & Quinsey, 2005). Intervention techniques developed to increase parents' propensity to paying attention to infant cues, such as "kangaroo care" (i.e., ventral physical contact with the infant through a soft baby carrier), increase sensitivity, mood, and touching for mothers and fathers (Feldman, 2004; Feldman, Weller, Sirota, & Eidelman, 2003; Magill-Evans, Harrison, Rempel, & Slater, 2006), and attachment security with mothers at 1 year (Anisfeld, Casper, Nozyce, & Cunningham, 1990).

The mother's perception of her infant and of their relationship appear to be more important factors than any single quality of the baby, including temperament (Belsky & Rovine, 1987; Bokhorst et al., 2003; Egeland & Farber, 1984; Pianta, Marvin, Britner, & Borowitz, 1996; Vaughn, Bost, & van IJzendoorn, Chapter 9, this volume). Furthermore, her perceptions are likely to be integrated into a transactional feedback loop that is heavily influenced by other factors associated with the mother herself, including her memories and feelings about her own childhood attachment experiences.

Social-Contextual Factors Related to Providing Care

Social-contextual variables—including the extent of a mother's satisfaction with her social support network, her marriage/couple relationship, or economic factors—can support or compete with the mother's ability to focus on providing care for her child (Cowan, Bradburn, & Cowan, 2005; Cox, Paley, Payne, & Burchinal, 1999; Huth-Bocks, Levendosky, Bogat, & von Eye, 2004; Lundy, 2002; Meyers, 1999; Moss, Cyr, Bureau, Tarabulsy, & Dubois-Comtois, 2005; Solomon & George, 1999c). According to Bowlby (1969/1982), it is likely that the mother's partnership with the baby's father or another coparent especially influences her ability to provide care (see also Gable, Belsky, & Crnic, 1992; Lundy, 2002). From a behavioral systems perspective, the mother's partner can enhance or compete directly with the mother's ability or desire to be caregiver. Marital satisfaction, in and of itself, has not been found

to be a strong predictor of child attachment with the mother (Belsky, Rosenberger, & Crnic, 1995). Other aspects of a marriage or relationship may, however, influence child attachment and maternal caregiving, especially each parent's ability to work together in a coparenting relationship and to buffer the child from insensitivity in the other parent (Cowan et al., 2005; Edwards, Eiden, & Leonard, 2006; Solomon & George, 1999c).

REPRESENTATIONAL MODELS OF CAREGIVING

The final specification of the caregiving behavioral system requires describing the internal guidance system that regulates the parent's thinking and behavior regarding providing care and protection. In humans, this internal system is conceived of as an internal working model or mental representation, following Bowlby (1969/1982). The reader is referred to Bretherton and Munholland (Chapter 5, this volume) for a comprehensive discussion of mental representation in attachment theory. Here we provide an overview of the key points related to our thinking about caregiving representations.

Bowlby (1969/1982) proposed that the attachment behavioral system is regulated by internal working models that evaluate, emotionally appraise, and organize the infant's real-life experience. He believed that these models are updated and reworked to achieve internal consistency and available for use in novel situations or as the basis of future plans. We have emphasized that if caregiving is a behavioral system in its own right, then it should be guided by a representational model, separate from other models (e.g., the parent's model of attachment) (George & Solomon, 1989; Solomon & George, 1996). That is, the parent's caregiving representation is specific to the child. Caregiving representations capture the parent's immediate "retranscription" (West & Sheldon-Keller, 1994) or reconstruction of the past and current experiences with the child, in intersection with memories of the parent's attachment past, in terms of the current appraisal or thinking about the parent–child relationship (Solomon & George, 1996, 2006). The importance of relationship-specific models in current relationships has been more recently echoed in models of adult romantic attachment (see, e.g., Crowell et al., 2002; J. Feeney, Chapter 21, this volume).

Representation is conceived by Bowlby (1973) as contributing to biological system homeostasis. Representational flexibility, then, should be the hallmark of a truly goal corrected relationship—one of the defining behavioral systems constructs described at the beginning of this chapter. Representational flexibility would be expected to contribute to integration and balance, and thus to maintain caregiving homeostasis. Optimally, these processes enable sensitivity, and they fortify the parent's commitment to the child with feelings of competence and joy. Representational flexibility should facilitate the parent's ability and desire to detect and differentiate among the signals and events associated with competing behavioral systems and goals. Such differentiation should be evidenced by thinking and behavior that demonstrate understanding of the fundamental boundaries between and intersections among systems, including protection and care of the child (caregiving system), seeking protection and care from others (attachment system), peer friendships (affiliative system), sexual activity (sexual system), and exploration (exploratory system) (George & Solomon, 1999; Solomon & George, 1996). Flexibility and balance are undermined when defensive processes distort and exclude information and feelings to the extent that the parent is not able to detect and integrate the signals associated with caregiving, attachment, and other behavioral system. This results in exclusion, confusion, or breakdown.

This integrative quality is captured by concepts related to the flexibly integrated states of mind. "State of mind" refers to how an individual integrates thoughts and feelings about relationships, as well as to the processes that support or exclude relationship-related information from the individual's thinking. State of mind was first defined in attachment theory through use of the AAI (George, Kaplan, & Main, 1984, 1985, 1996; Main & Goldwyn, 1984, 2003; Main, Goldwyn, & Hesse, 2003). Main has proposed that AAI attachment security represents maximal representational integration, reflected best by the interview's "coherence" ratings (the strongest predictor of security on the AAI—see Hesse, Chapter 25, this volume, and Main, Hesse, & Kaplan, 2005). The relation between integrative flexibility and security is integral to two other state-of-mind constructs. The "internalized secure base" is defined as the individual's capacity to draw upon internalized attachment figures to explore and integrate thoughts and feelings about attachment distress and possible solutions (i.e., as a safe internal haven for secure-base explorations of attachment) (George & West, 2001, in press). Reflective functioning, a

form of psychoanalytic intersubjectivity, is defined as the individual's ability to conceive of and integrate the mind of the self and parent (e.g., Fonagy, Steele, & Steele, 1991; see Fonagy, Gergely, & Target, Chapter 33, and Slade, Chapter 32, this volume).

Table 35.1 provides a chronological summary of the different representational approaches to caregiving in the field of attachment. These approaches share an emphasis on describing a parent's *current* relationship-specific state of mind regarding a child, and all use structured clinical interviews to elicit narrative descriptions of affect, experience, and appraisals of the child or the child–parent relationship. The reader will see that there is no single approach, and that interviews and analysis dimensions overlap considerably across methods. Some approaches address the phenomenon that van IJzendoorn and colleagues have termed "the transmission gap" (De Wolff & van IJzendoorn, 1997; van IJzendoorn, 1995)—the fact that a mother's state of mind regarding her childhood attachment experiences is not as powerful a predictor of maternal sensitivity and child security as was expected. Caregiving researchers tested hypotheses that parents' representations of their children would be a strong contributor to explaining the "gap," and found that integrated "mentalizing" features of caregiving representations were important mediators between mothers' representations of their past and sensitive interactions with their children in the present. The mentalizing dimensions defined by this body of research fit what we have described in this chapter as representational flexibility, including coherence (derived from the AAI), mind-mindedness (Bernier & Dozier, 2003, following Meins, 1999), insightfulness (Oppenheim, Koren-Karie, & Sagi, 2001; Oppenheim & Koren-Karie, 2002), and reflective functioning (Slade, Grienenberger, Bernbach, Levy, & Locker, 2005, following Fonagy et al., 1991). Other approaches have examined representational dimensions of parenting related to a child's attachment and developmental correlates, including parents' resolution of their child's disability diagnosis (Marvin & Pianta, 1996; Pianta et al., 1996), quality of care in foster mothers (Ackerman & Dozier, 2005; Bates & Dozier, 2002; Bernier & Dozier, 2003), intrusive infant interaction (Grienenberger, Kelly, & Slade, 2005), and psychosocial adjustment in adolescence (Mayseless & Scharf, 2006).

Classification groups are the primary conceptual and methodological foundation in child and adult *developmental* attachment research. (See

TABLE 35.1. Approaches to Measuring Caregiving Representations

Reference	Interview summary	What is measured?	Age group and population	Research findings
Aber, Slade, Berger, Bresgi, & Kaplan (1985)	Parent Development Interview (PDI), 1½–2 hours. Patterned after the AAI. Includes questions about mother's affective states, words to describe the relationship, how mother appraises separations from child.	Mother's representation of affective experience: *coherence*, joy/pleasure, anger, guilt/separation distress.	Prenatal, infants, toddlers. Married and divorced mothers.	(Aber et al., 1999; Slade et al., 1999) Joy/pleasure was correlated with positive maternal behavior and attachment security. Anger was correlated with maternal dismissing status and daily hassles.
Bretherton, Biringen, Ridgeway, Maslin, & Sherman (1989)	Parent Attachment Interview, 1 hour. Obtains mother's descriptions and emotional appraisals of specific caregiving events.	Parenting sensitivity/insight (content analysis).	Toddlers.	(Bretherton, 2005) Sensitivity/insight was significantly correlated with concurrent attachment security at 18 mos. and with attachment representation 1½ years later.
George & Solomon (1988)	Caregiving Interview, 1 hour. (Modified PDI; see Aber et al., 1989.)	Defensive processes: flexible integration, deactivation, cognitive disconnection, helplessness/segregated systems.	Infants to age 12.	(George & Solomon, 1989, 1996; Fisher, 2000; Solomon & George, 1999b, 2006, in press-a) Significant concurrent concordance with security and protection ratings at 12 mos. and age 5: 91% concordance with secure–insecure status at 12 mos.; 81% concordance with four-group reunion classification at age 5. Helplessness/segregated systems ratings predicted child attachment disorganization at age 6. Helplessness/segregated systems ratings predicted poor parenting outcomes for mothers with sexual abuse histories.
Cox, Owen, Henderson, & Margand (1992)	Excerpts from a longer postnatal parent interview.	Modified from Ainsworth scales, including sensitivity, acceptance–rejection, parenting investment.	Infants.	(Cox, Paley, Payne, & Burchinal, 1999) Mothers: Attitudes toward babies did not contribute significant information to overall security rating beyond observation of other–baby interaction. Fathers: Significant independent contributions of attitudes toward babies to overall security rating beyond behavioral observations.
Zeanah, Benoit, Hirschberg, & Barton (1993)	Working Model of the Child Interview (WMCI), 1 hour. Assesses emotional reactions to pregnancy; perceptions of infant's personality and development.	Three-group classification scheme: balanced, disengaged, distorted.	Prenatal, infants.	(Benoit et al., 1997; Zeanah et al., 1994) 69% concordance between prenatal interview and Strange Situation classification at 1 year; 74% concurrent concordance between three mother caregiving groups and three-group infant classification.
Pianta, O'Connor, & Marvin (1993)	Child–Parent Attachment Project Parent Development Interview (CPAP-PDI), 45 minutes. (Modified PDI; see Aber et al., 1989.)	Parent's representation of affective experience, compliance, caretaking, achievement, perspective taking.	Toddlerhood–middle childhood; typical and atypical development.	(Button, Pianta, & Marvin, 2001; Messina Sayre, Pianta, Marvin, & Saft, 2001; Steinberg & Pianta, 2006) Validity for typical and disabled children. Overall PDI score was correlated with maternal sensitivity at 36 mos. and 54 mos.

(continued)

TABLE 35.1. *(continued)*

Reference	Interview summary	What is measured?	Age group and population	Research findings
Pianta, Marvin, Britner, & Horowitz (1996)	Reaction to Diagnosis Interview, 15 minutes. Covers parents' memories, beliefs, and feelings about learning about their child's diagnosis.	Resolved or unresolved.	Atypical development.	(Marvin et al., 1996; Pianta et al., 1996) Unresolved diagnosis representation was unrelated to AAI classification.
Sharf & Mayseless (1997, 2000)	The Parenting Representations Interview— Adolescents, 1–1½ hours. (Modified PDI; see Aber et al., 1989.)	Three-group classification scheme: adequate/ balanced, flooded, restricted.	Adolescence	(Mayseless & Scharf, 2006) 52% concordance with three AAI groups (autonomous, dismissing, preoccupied).
Bates & Dozier (1998)	This is My Baby Interview, 10 minutes. Includes questions on baby's personality and feelings about the baby.	Acceptance, commitment, belief in influence on baby. Also, mind-mindedness: ability to think about and treat the child as having an autonomous mind (Meins, 1999)	Foster infants and toddlers.	(Ackerman & Dozier, 2005; Bates & Dozier 2002; Bernier & Dozier, 2003) Secure (AAI) mothers were more accepting of and had greater belief of influence on early-placed babies than late-placed babies; not found for insecure (AAI) mothers. No relation for commitment. Mother investment at age 6: Acceptance + commitment investment → emotional security. Negative correlations between maternal (AAI) security, child (Strange Situation) security, and mind-mindedness.
Oppenheim, Koren-Karie, & Sagi (2001)	Insightfulness Assessment (IA). Examines mother's views of child's thoughts after viewing video segments from a 1½-hour laboratory visit at age 4–5.	Insightfulness: mother's insight into child's motives and complexity, and openness to new information about the child. Four-group classification scheme: balanced, one-sided, disengaged, mixed.	Preschoolers (4–5 years).	(Koren-Karie, Oppenheim, Dolev, & Etzion-Carasso, 2002; Oppenheim et al., 2001; Oppenheim & Koren-Karie, 2002) 56% secure–insecure concordance rate between parent representation at 4–5 years and infant at 12 mos. Strange Situation (no avoidant children in sample) and parent empathy. No association between infant attachment classification and disengaged parent representation.
Slade, Grienenberger, Bernbach, Levy, & Locker (2005)	Parent Development Interview (PDI). (See Aber et al., 1989.)	Parental reflective functioning (RF): mother's capacity to understand and coordinate mother's own and child's mental states.	Infants.	(Grienenberger et al., 2005; Slade et al., 2005) RF was measured when infants were 10 months old. Organized (AAI) mothers' RF > unresolved (AAI) mothers' RF. Secure (AAI) mothers had highest RF ratings. No differences in RF ratings between dismissing and preoccupied mothers. Infant attachment was measured at 14 mos. Mothers of secure infants had RF ratings > mothers of insecure infants, but RF ratings did not differentiate between mothers of secure and avoidant infants. Negative correlation between RF and AMBIANCE communication and disruption scales.

Crowell, Fraley, & Shaver, Chapter 26, this volume, for a discussion of developmental and social–personality approaches to adult attachment, and the merits of classification groups vs. rating scales as tools for analysis.) Four caregiving approaches have produced a caregiving classification system (see Table 35.1). Three systems report moderate concordances (52–74%) between caregiving representations and child attachment classifications (B, A, C classification groups—Mayseless & Scharf, 2006; Zeanah, Benoit, Hirschberg, & Barton, 1993; B, C, D classification groups—Oppenheim et al., 2001).

All of these approaches (parent representation dimensions, mentalizing, and classification systems) have provided new and important insights into parenting. Theory and research in attachment draws heavily from the four-group infant classification system. As we have noted earlier, models of parenting have either emphasized caregiving dimensions associated with security, or developed three- or four-group classification systems that are only weakly associated with identifying the insecure attachment groups. We have developed a different approach to classification based on Bowlby's (1980) view of defensive exclusion, which we describe more fully in the discussion below and which has demonstrated a high secure–insecure (91%) and four-group classification (81%) concordance rate (George & Solomon, 1996).

With Table 35.1 in mind, we now complete our behavioral systems model of caregiving by describing how caregiving is related to the child's secure, avoidant, ambivalent, or disorganized attachment. Studies describing parent and child dimensions not specifically related to attachment are beyond the scope of this discussion. We begin by discussing the representations of caregiving for the mothers of secure children.

The Relation of Caregiving to Secure Attachment

We have tied the child's attachment security to behavioral and representational caregiving flexibility and balance, which contribute to a goal-corrected partnership. Caregiving representation studies converge in describing mothers of secure children as flexible, balanced, and integrated (Ackerman & Dozier, 2005; Bernier & Dozier, 2003; George & Solomon, 1996; Grienenberger et al., 2005; Oppenheim & Koren-Karie, 2002; Oppenheim et al., 2001; Slade, Belsky, Aber, & Phelps, 1999; Slade et al., 2005; Solomon & George, 1999c, 1999d; Steinberg & Pianta, 2006). Mothers' narratives

describe other features of a goal-corrected parent–child relationship as well, including commitment, trust, cooperation, knowledge of self and child as individuals, the ability and desire to communicate clearly about caregiving and attachment goals (especially when these goals are in conflict), and the joy associated with being a parent (Bernier & Dozier, 2003; George & Solomon, 1996, 1999; Grienenberger et al., 2005; Slade et al., 1999, 2005; Steinberg & Pianta, 2006). Many of these representational characteristics coincide with recent behavioral descriptions of maternal caregiving behavior with preschoolers in the Strange Situation (Britner, Marvin, & Pianta, 2005).

Research demonstrates as well that the caregiving representations of mothers of insecure children are not flexible, balanced, or integrated. Mothers of insecure children receive lower ratings for insight and sensitivity, maternal reflective function, and mind-mindedness than mothers of secure children (Bernier & Dozier, 2003; Bretherton, Biringen, Ridgeway, Maslin, & Sherman, 1989; Slade et al., 2005). There is little systematic research or theory building regarding individual differences in caregiving representation related to insecure attachment. This shortage is likely due in part to the primary research focus on representational dimensions, especially in relation to the quest for the roots of maternal sensitivity. Slade (2004) has argued that dimensional processes are more informative about an individual's representation of interpersonal experience than categories. We have always found that understanding processes in the context of classification groups provides a more structured framework of understanding caregiving in relation to attachment than dimensions alone, and a "compass," so to speak, that orients us to the fundamental differences among caregiving–attachment relationships (e.g., Solomon & George, 2006). We now describe mothers of insecure children, predominantly drawing on our own work, and integrating other research findings when available. This discussion requires a brief discussion of our approach. Our goal, as with the chapter as a whole, is to stimulate theory building in relation to the caregiving system.

The Relation of Caregiving to Avoidant and Ambivalent Attachment: Defensive Processes

Our approach is built on Bowlby's model of defense. Bowlby (1973) defined defense as "contributing to the maintenance of what can ... be termed a steady 'representational' state" (p. 149).

He described three forms of defensive exclusion—deactivation, cognitive disconnection, and the segregated system (Bowlby, 1980). We have defined how patterns of Bowlby's defenses are manifested in mothers' descriptions of parenting during the Caregiving Interview, and how these patterns are related to individual differences in child attachment (George & Solomon, 1988/1993/2005/2007, 1996). This approach has also been validated in our doll-play assessment procedure for young school-age children (Solomon, George, & De Jong, 1995) and in a projective assessment for adults (the Adult Attachment Projective; George & West, 2001, in press).

We have conceived of deactivation and cognitive disconnection as "organizing" defenses (George & Solomon, 1996; Solomon et al., 1995). We have shown that these forms of defensive exclusion serve to protect an individual from breakdown and keep internal working models of caregiving and attachment organized—that is, to protect the individual from representational and behavioral disorganization. Bowlby (1980) defined deactivation as a defensive process that removes distress from conscious awareness. This form of defensive exclusion characterizes the interviews of mothers of avoidant children. We understand deactivation as the exclusion mechanism that permits circumventing activation (arousal) of the caregiving system, resulting in evaluations of self and child that diminish the importance of caregiving and attachment experiences, and in descriptions of caregiving practices we have called "distanced protection" (Solomon & George, 1996). Mothers in this group express disdain for clingy children and do not enjoy caregiving closeness; they describe caregiving strategies that emphasize overseeing their children from afar or assigning care to someone else. Psychological distance is maintained through emphasizing negative portrayals of self and child (e.g., that the mother is not doing a good job, or that the child is manipulative and requires authoritarian discipline). Similar emphases on lack of intimacy and on discipline have been noted in behavioral observations of mothers of avoidant preschoolers in the Strange Situation (Britner et al., 2005).

Cognitive disconnection is the dominant defensive process that we have found to characterize the mothers of ambivalent/resistant children (George & Solomon, 1996). Bowlby (1980) defined cognitive disconnection as a form of splitting (literally disconnecting) attachment information and affect from their sources. Whereas deactiva-

tion is likely to block or redefine caregiving experiences in order to keep distress and need out of conscious thinking, it is helpful in understanding Bowlby's conceptualization of disconnection to view this process as "chopping up" events and affects. This form of exclusion leads to a different quality of limited awareness and narrative descriptions from that characterizing deactivation. Complete events and their associated affects are neither fully remembered nor fully excluded; disconnection prevents these mothers from seeing "the bigger picture." We view disconnection as the underlying mechanism that heightens activation of the caregiving system, leading to caregiving practices we have described as "close protection" (Solomon & George, 1996). Keeping children close presumably affords mothers maximum opportunity to detect caregiving and attachment signals. We have found that most mothers of ambivalent/resistant children endorse the advantages of closeness, emphasizing descriptions of the positive aspects of the relationship (e.g., enjoying a child's sweet nature, happy togetherness) and attempts to stop thinking about distressing aspects of caregiving (George & Solomon, 1996). The disadvantage of this level of physical and psychological closeness, however, is that mothers are not able to turn fully away from their children's unhappiness or from their own caregiving failures. They are ultimately unable to integrate or deactivate, and they describe how they are worried, guilty, and anxious about their misunderstandings and confusing ineffectiveness. This mixed or confused quality of thinking is consistent with features of caregiving classification typologies that have been relatively successful in identifying the mothers of ambivalent infants (Oppenheim et al., 2001; Zeanah et al., 1993); it has also been described in observations of maternal behavior in the Strange Situation (Britner et al., 2005).

Now that we have described the mental representations of caregiving that we propose to be associated with children with organized attachments, we return to examining our proposition that these forms of caregiving representational processes are associated with "good enough" protection and care. The reader will recall that when viewed from a behavioral systems framework, maternal behavior is the product not only of activation and termination of the mother's caregiving system, but also of the mother's integration of her own and the child's competing behavioral systems. We have found that the flexibly integrated mother clearly understands the boundaries and intersections of behavioral systems. The mother attempts and is successful in balancing competing behavioral systems' goals without threatening caregiving and attachment, investing in or putting other goals aside as context and the child's development permits (George & Solomon, 1988/1993/2005/2007).

What we have found in the interviews of mothers of avoidant and ambivalent children is the degree to which defensive exclusion permits representational approximations of behavioral system integration, despite being out of balance. Mothers of avoidant children are clear in their minds about the boundaries among competing behavior systems, attending to caregiving goals as necessary or through distanced protection and elevating the attention and energy invested in the exploratory system (e.g., personal achievement, contributing role in a child's education) and affiliative system (e.g., being with friends). Mothers of ambivalent/resistant children elevate caregiving at the expense of exploration and affiliation. Thus, although their system integration is out of balance, mothers of organized insecure children describe providing some degree of care and protection for their children, as compared with the mothers we consider in the next section.

The Disabled Caregiving System: Abdication of Care, Helplessness, and Disorganized Attachment

There are several overlapping views of attachment disorganization in children. These views agree that a child's fear, of the mother herself or of the context created in her care, is central to the child's disorganized attachment (George & Solomon, 1999; Lyons-Ruth & Jacobvitz, Chapter 28, this volume). In contrast to mothers of children with organized attachments, we have proposed that the caregiving representations of mothers of disorganized and controlling children are characterized by "abdicated caregiving," "failures of protection," and "helplessness" (George & Solomon, 1996; Solomon & George, 1996). Following Bowlby (1980), we conceive of abdicated caregiving in terms of the breakdown of regulated normative defenses (i.e., deactivation, cognitive disconnection) that he termed "segregated systems." Linked to attachment trauma (Bowlby, 1980) and caregiving trauma or threats (Solomon & George, 2000), the defensive processes that are developed to maintain a "steady representational state" can be achieved only if painful and threatening memories and their associated affects are blocked from consciousness. Bowlby likened segregated systems to repression,

and he proposed that the contents of segregated memories are maintained as a separate representational model. He conceived of segregated systems as the psychological foundation of "pathological mourning," because this mental state blocks memories (failure to mourn) or floods the individual with memories of traumatic events (chronic mourning). In either manifestation, segregated systems create a situation in which the individual cannot face or integrate traumatic attachment events in a way that makes them available to consciousness and subject to monitoring by executive processing control mechanisms. Bowlby proposed that segregated systems are the most extreme and brittle forms of defensive exclusion—acting behind the scenes, so to speak, and suddenly subject to defensive breakdown when the attachment system is activated. Segregated systems, therefore, are more likely to interfere with a steady representational state than to help maintain it.

Bowlby's description of segregated systems is consistent with contemporary thinking in attachment theory (e.g., Hesse & Main, 2006; Liotti, in press). Attachment studies using functional magnetic resonance imaging have demonstrated, in adults with unresolved states of mind regarding attachment (analogous to disorganized child attachment) in community and psychiatric samples, a failure of the prefrontal cortex to modulate limbic system activity when attachment was activated (Buchheim et al., 2006, in press; Buchheim & George, in press). These patterns were interpreted as indicative of the effects of attachment distress on the mental states of "disorganized" individuals, such that autobiographical memories, especially trauma, flooded and overwhelmed their executive control processes.

We conceive of disorganization and dysregulation of caregiving as the failure to use adaptive, normative forms of defense (and the executive control mechanisms associated with normative defenses) to regulate segregated caregiving experience (George & Solomon, 1988/1993/2005/2007; Solomon et al., 1995). Disorganization of caregiving marks the potential for *failure* to protect (functional goal) and to provide care and comfort (proximate goal) (Solomon & George, 1996). We return to this idea shortly when we discuss "abdication of caregiving."

We believe that segregated systems are evident in two forms of processing that we have identified in mothers' caregiving interviews: "dysregulation" and "constriction." Dysregulated caregiving is conceived of as "unleashed" segregated systems—a mental state characterized by flooding and by mothers becoming overwhelmed by their worst fears about themselves and their children. When dysregulated, mothers describe their helplessness to care for or protect themselves or their child from threats and danger. Their interviews include strong themes of vulnerability, inadequacy, loss of control, and inability to provide assurance or comfort when children are frightened. In some instances, these inadequacies are "not their fault," but rather the result of individuals or contexts that prevented them from providing care and protection for their children (e.g., court-imposed visitation with a father whom a mother does not trust; Solomon & George, 1999b). Mothers' descriptions of their children emphasize many of the qualities they describe of themselves. Their children are viewed as being as out of control (e.g., acting like "maniacs," defiant, hysterical, threatening)—descriptions conveying the message that these children are "devils" who rendered mothers helpless to combat or organize their children's behavior. As a result, at the behavioral systems level, these mothers are markedly out of balance, desperately struggling to remain in control.

Constricted caregiving is conceived of as a brittle defensive guard or heightening of segregating exclusion processes that prevents dysregulated representational and behavioral states from emerging (Solomon et al., 1995). Constriction appears to prevent a mother from thinking about how she and the child together contribute to their caregiving–attachment relationship. Constricted mothers describe constricted caregiving practices. They describe how they remove themselves from caregiving situations (e.g., taking a bath in a locked bathroom), often leaving their children in distress, in order to prevent breaking down and losing self-control. They describe situations in which their children take over caregiving responsibilities, evaluating the children as possessing precocious and amazing (sometimes supernatural) abilities to manage and control people and situations in which the mothers would be incompetent (i.e., adultification, role reversal; see also Ackerman & Dozier, 2005). They also describe the converse: psychologically merging with the child or taking on the child's distress as their own (e.g., "We have a special understanding of each other," "The child and I are one"). We view constriction as a mechanism that blocks integration of self and child. Such mothers can think of their children only in relation to themselves—the children are invisible.

It appears from the interviews that invisibility permits mothers to block from their awareness potential evaluations of their children that might dysregulate caregiving and unleash feelings of helpless and being of out of control. It is evident from the interviews that this form of defensive exclusion releases mothers from the difficulties of caregiving. Constriction is associated with descriptions of children as "angels" who never create any problems or conflicts. Like the behavioral systems of dysregulated mothers, those of constricted mothers are also markedly out of balance; the caregiving system, like the children, is essentially invisible.

In contrast to the interviews with mothers of avoidant and ambivalent children, the interviews with mothers of disorganized children have failed to reveal any predominant organizing defensive processing strategies. Rather, these mothers describe their own extreme behavioral reactions or feelings of impotence or constriction, and their inability to select, evaluate, or modify their own behavior or that of their children. They view themselves as helpless—an appraisal that is often associated with strong, uncontrollable emotions and affective dysregulation.[2]

Two studies support our approach to disorganized caregiving. First, Britner and colleagues (2005) adapted our concept of "abdication of care" for the Strange Situation. Mothers of disorganized/controlling preschoolers were described as not taking the "executive role" and as incompetent, passive, frightened, and inappropriately accepting of their children's punitive or caregiving behavior. Drawing from our prior discussion, we would characterize the mothers in this preschool sample as helpless.

Second, we (George & Solomon, in press) examined disorganized caregiving in a sample of mothers of children ages 3–11. Disorganization was measured with a Helplessness Questionnaire that we derived from and validated with the Caregiving Interview. The questionnaire measures three dimensions of disorganized caregiving: mother helpless (e.g., "When I am with my child, I feel out of control"), mother and child frightened (e.g., "My child does scary and dangerous things"), and child as caregiving (e.g., "My child is good at tending to or caring for others," "My child is always trying to make others laugh"). The first two dimensions appear to indicate dysregulated caregiving; the third dimension taps constricted caregiving. Disorganized caregiving (each of the three dimensions) was significantly associated with mothers' self-reported distress, including parenting stress and depressive symptomatology. There were important differences, however, between the correlates of the dysregulated and constricted dimensions. Dysregulated caregiving was significantly related to mothers' reports of their children as troublesome and as causing their distress (e.g., failing to meet mothers' expectations, moody, hyperactive/distractible; Child Behavior Checklist externalizing behavior). These associations were not found for constricted caregiving. Caregiving constriction was associated with precocious adultification and perceived goodness in the children, but was not linked to mothers' distress.

We now return to the concept of abdicated care. We have defined "abdication" as a breakdown in the caregiving system, and the result is a disorganized and dysfunctional form of care (Solomon & George, 1996, in press-b). Dysfunction as associated with attachment disorganization has been defined in the field only in terms of developmental or mental health risk. Dysfunction from a functionalist view (i.e., an evolutionary perspective) would take into consideration caregiving that undermines a mother's adaptive fitness. It may sometimes be in a mother's interest to abdicate care, and even to abandon or kill her infant (Clutton-Brock, 1991; Hrdy, 1999; Miller, 1987; Scheper-Hughes, 1987); however, these forms of physical abdication are relatively rare after the immediate neonatal period, and in our own culture they are considered pathological. Of particular interest to psychologists is a subset of mothers who do not dispose of their infants physically, but nevertheless behave in ways that are antithetical to protection, including frightening, maltreating, neglecting, or leaving the children unprotected from threats by others or the environment. Taken together, these are all examples of abdication of care. For these mothers, in whom the caregiving system is disabled, their attachment and caregiving systems are dysequilibrated and unintegrated. This means that the caregiving and attachment behavioral systems are not working reciprocally and are failing to mutually inform each other. We propose that it is under conditions of failed protection—that is, abdication of the caregiving system—that a mother fails to provide "good enough" care for a child.

This may occur especially when mothers are overwhelmed by their own distress (and their attachment system is activated). Flooded, distressed mothers are blocked from detecting the attachment needs of their children (a function of the caregiving system). As a result, these mothers

experience caregiving and their relationship with their children in terms of profound helplessness and fear. Our recent study of mothers of disorganized children showed that even if a mother's adult attachment classification was not unresolved, memories of being frightened and unprotected as a child were associated with disorganized and helpless representations of the self as a mother (Solomon & George, in press-b).

In sum, evidence from these studies suggests that these mothers are afraid, although they need not be constantly preoccupied with or consciously aware of their fear. We have proposed, however, that for a full understanding of attachment disorganization, mother–child interaction must also be examined from the perspective of the caregiving system. Based on this perspective, two important questions arise: What is the mother afraid of? And what is it about the mother's caregiving behavior that frightens the child?

We suggest that the mother is afraid of her own profound helplessness—a helplessness that may be the product of overlapping fears. She may be afraid for the safety and protection of herself and/or her child. She may also fear losing control of her emotions and her behavior, and/or of circumstances or people (self, child, or others) that threaten her fragile resources. Determining the immediate causes of the mother's fear—that is, the situational cues eliciting the mother's fear in the moment—is more difficult; these causes may be rooted in either the mother's childhood or her current experiences. Unresolved childhood loss and trauma have been linked with attachment disorganization (Hesse & Main, 2006). However, as described earlier in this chapter, this link is not fully supported by research, and there are many gaps in this model. Further research is needed to examine how lack of resolution is linked explicitly to a mother's fears and helplessness.

In addition to childhood trauma, we propose that the mother's caregiving system may be immobilized by "assaults to the caregiving system" (Solomon & George, 2000). These may include, but are not limited to, parental divorce (Solomon & George, 1999b), child disability (Pianta et al., 1996), prematurity (Borghini et al., 2006), perinatal loss of a child (Bakermans-Kranenburg, Schuegel, & van IJzendoorn, 1999; Cote-Arsenault & Dombeck, 2001; Heller & Zeanah, 1999; Hughes, Turton, Hopper, McGauley, & Fonagy, 2004; O'Leary, 2005; Turton, Hughes, Fonagy, & Fainman, 2004), or brutal urban violence, war, and terrorism (Almqvist & Broberg, 2003; Schechter et al., 2005; Stovall-McClough & Cloitre, 2006). Fear is known to increase stress and arousal, and thus hypervigilance (Perry, Pollard, Blakley, Baker, & Vigilante, 1995).

We propose that isolating the particular causes of attachment disorganization requires observing a mother and child under stressful circumstances—specifically, in situations that threaten the mother's ability to manage (regulate) either her child's negative affect and behavior or her own. Our data suggest that mothers of disorganized children can sometimes provide organized protective care (Solomon & George, in press-b), and that under some circumstances they evaluate themselves as effective. Observations of mother–child interaction under low-stress conditions have failed to differentiate between organized and disorganized groups (Lyons-Ruth & Jacobvitz, Chapter 28, this volume). Links between stress and helplessness have also been found in studies directly measuring parents' perceived stress as related to their children (George & Solomon, in press-b). According to our model, a mother's fear can be understood only in the context of the stressful events or cues that dysregulate her and leave her feeling vulnerable, unprotected, and helpless.

In order to understand what in a mother's behavior frightens a child, we must examine the chain of events that prevail during mother–child interactions in disorganized dyads. Our thinking is that because she is hypervigilant and lacking robust, organized defenses—and perhaps is also constricted and shut off from the child—the mother is susceptible to being overwhelmed by helplessness and fear (e.g., affective flooding). The panic or helplessness disables caregiving, because the mother becomes closed or shut off from the child's attachment cues. Thus the mother does not detect the child's need and is not able to care for or respond to these needs. We propose that *what frightens the child is the mother's simultaneous abdication of care and impermeability to the child's cues or bids for care*. The mother is unavailable to her child during the moments that her child needs her the most. It is under conditions of failed protection—that is, abdication of the caregiving system—that the mother fails to provide "good enough" care for the child.

CONCLUSIONS AND IMPLICATIONS

We believe that consideration of the caregiving system offers important insights into the parent–child relationship that are missed in a focus on attachment system alone. This chapter has been dedicated to describing some of those insights. Attachment researchers, and more broadly developmental psychologists and psychoanalysts, have historically approached the mother as a "variable." Maternal behavior has been carved into an infinite list of qualities and behaviors. Attachment theorists have described mothers, for example, as sensitive, rejecting, accepting, intrusive, or frightened. In this chapter, we have argued that in order to understand caregiving, theorists need to move from the level of considering the mother as a "variable" to seeking to understand her as an individual in her own right. Mothers as individuals represent a complex interplay of developmental factors and challenges—including, as we emphasize in this chapter, an integration of competing behavioral systems.

What is added to our understanding of maternal caregiving and attachment by looking at the mother and her behavior through the lens of the caregiving behavioral system? We propose that this lens has important implications for understanding the development of caregiving behavior throughout the lifespan, and we have made specific suggestions for future research as related to the parent–child relationship throughout this chapter. We still know little about the caregiving system in fathers, and in parents of children beyond early childhood, including adolescents. Other questions concern caregiving in relationships other than the primary parent–child relationship. In what ways is caregiving by a parent's partner or relatives (e.g., a grandmother), or by caregiving professionals (e.g., day care providers, preschool teachers), similar to and different from the caregiving system for parents?

Some attachment theorists have described caregiving in the context of other relationships, including adult attachments (e.g., Crowell et al., 2002; J. Feeney, Chapter 21, this volume; Mikulincer & Shaver, Chapter 23, this volume) and the relationships between middle-aged adults and their elderly parents (e.g., Magai, Chapter 24, this volume; Steele, Phibbs, & Woods, 2004). With regard to adult attachments, the reciprocal balance is defined in terms of peer relationships. These relationships among equals are qualitatively different from the hierarchical caregiver–child relationship, in which relationship members are not equal. The caregivers in parent–child attachment are thought to be "stronger and wiser" (Bowlby, 1969/1982; West & Sheldon-Keller, 1994). In relationships among equals, adult partners are likely to change roles—sometimes acting in the role of the stronger and wiser support provider, and sometimes in the role of the one who is troubled and needs support. With regard to adult children and their elderly parents, we might be especially interested in the question of whether or how the children may change roles to become caregivers for the parents (see Magai, Chapter 24, this volume). Is this role reversal or parentification, as it would be conceived for children, or a more normative chain of events that may be precipitated by the parent's loss of all other attachment figures (e.g., spouse)?

The overlaps in discrete behaviors (caring for the other, paying attention to signals of distress) and motivation among the different kinds of relationships generate questions about the etiology of caregiving behaviors. A discussion of the many different relationships in which caregiving is a component is beyond the scope of this chapter. We hope that the principles we have described will prove helpful in understanding the overlaps and differences among caregiving behaviors in these other relationships, including their relation to the biological function and goal of caregiving.

We end with a major clinical implication of our approach to the caregiving system. The caregiving system provides clinicians with a powerful tool—a tool that frames a mother's behavior and perceptions of her child in terms of *protection*. The mother's desire and ability to provide protection are the central organizing features of the child's attachment. Behavioral interventions usually focus on changing the mother's "bad" behavior. Furthermore, as we have discussed earlier, attachment theory (and therefore attachment-related interventions) has assumed that maternal sensitivity is the strongest determinant of attachment security. Captivated by this concept, the field has focused on getting mothers to be more sensitive to their children in a variety of interactive settings (e.g., play, problem solving, or feeding), and has strayed away from the kind of sensitivity that is fundamental to attachment—sensitivity to a child's need for protection.

Even mothers with very traumatic and disturbed attachment histories are strongly motivated to protect their children (Fraiberg, 1980). In our experience, mothers with serious intellectual, behavioral, or adjustment problems, who may not be able to benefit immediately from insight-oriented therapy or some forms of didactic parent education, have been able to understand what it means to provide or fail to provide protection for their children. Attachment theory suggests that there may be other ways to influence mother–child attachment. We propose that one powerful influence that has been overlooked is intervention organized around the framework of the caregiving system—that is, a mother's evaluation of herself as effective in providing protection for her child.

NOTES

1. A good question is raised here as to whether other maternal caregiving behaviors, also central to the baby's survival, may be considered "parts" of this system (e.g., nursing, cleaning, behavioral thermo-regulation, "affectionate" behavior, grooming/licking/washing). Whether or not these behaviors are included, it is clear that a much wider variety of maternal behaviors can and must be brought to bear (organized) to serve the goal of protection, especially when the infant is immature and immobile.

2. We note that one might expect the interviews of these mothers to resemble the AAI discourse patterns of lack of resolution, since the unresolved adult attachment category is viewed as analogous to child disorganization (e.g., George, West, & Pettem, 1999; Hesse & Main, 2006), and mothers' lack of resolution is associated with attachment disorganization in their children (Main & Hesse, 1990; Lyons-Ruth & Jacobvitz, Chapter 28, this volume). The hallmark of lack of resolution in the AAI is an individual's inability to monitor discourse or reasoning. We have not observed these monitoring-related features of thought in the caregiving interviews of mothers of disorganized/controlling children, despite the fact that many of these mothers are classified as unresolved with respect to loss on the AAI (George & Solomon, 1996). We see this as further support for our view that a mother's thinking about her caregiving and her attachment experiences are regulated by separate representational models, which are distinct components of the attachment and caregiving behavioral systems.

REFERENCES

Aber, J. L., Belsky, J., Slade, A., & Crnic, K. (1999). Stability and change in mothers' representations of their relationship with their toddlers. *Developmental Psychology, 35*, 1038–1047.

Aber, J. L., Slade, A., Berger, B., Bresgi, I., & Kaplan, M. (1985). *The Parent Development Interview.* Unpublished manuscript.

Ackerman, J. P., & Dozier, M. (2005). The influence of foster parent investment on children's representations of self and attachment figures. *Journal of Applied Developmental Psychology, 26*, 507–520.

Ainsworth, M. D. S., Blehar, M., Waters, E., & Wall, S. (1978). *Patterns of attachment: A psychological study of the Strange Situation*. Hillsdale, NJ: Erlbaum.

Almqvist, K., & Broberg, A. G. (2003). Young children traumatized by organized violence together with their mothers: The critical effects of damaged internal representations. *Attachment and Human Development, 5*, 367–380.

Ammaniti, M. (1994). Maternal representations during pregnancy and early infant–mother interaction. In M. Ammaniti & D. S. Stern (Eds.), *Psychoanalysis and development: Representations and narratives* (pp. 79–96). New York: New York University Press.

Anisfeld, E., Casper, V., Nozyce, M., & Cunningham, N. (1990). Does infant carrying promote attachment? An experimental study of the effects of increased physical contact on the development of attachment. *Child Development, 61*, 1617–1627.

Bakermans-Kranenburg, M. J., Schuegel, C., & van IJzendoorn, M. H. (1999). Unresolved loss due to miscarriage: An addition to the Adult Attachment Interview. *Attachment and Human Development, 1*, 157–170.

Bakermans-Kranenburg, M. J., van IJzendoorn, M. H., Bokhorst, C. L., & Schuengel, C. (2004). The importance of shared environment in infant–father attachment: A behavioral genetic study of the attachment Q-Sort. *Journal of Family Psychology, 18*, 545–549.

Bartels, A., & Zeki, S. (2004). The neural correlates of maternal and romantic love. *NeuroImage, 21*, 1155–1166.

Bates, B. C., & Dozier, M. (1998). *"This is My Baby" coding manual*. Unpublished manuscript, University of Delaware, Newark.

Bates, B. C., & Dozier, M. (2002). The importance of maternal state of mind regarding attachment and infant age at placement to foster mothers' representations of their foster infants. *Infant Mental Health Journal, 23*, 417–431.

Bell, D. C. (2001). Evolution of parental caregiving. *Personality and Social Psychology Review, 5*, 216–229.

Bell, R. (1968). A reinterpretation of the direction of effects in studies of socialization. *Psychological Review, 75*, 81–95.

Belsky, J., Jaffee, S. R., Sligo, J., Woodward, L., & Silva, P. A. (2005). Intergenerational transmission of warm-sensitive-stimulating parenting: A prospective study of mothers and fathers of 3-year-olds. *Child Development, 76*, 384–396.

Belsky, J., Rosenberger, K., & Crnic, K. (1995). *The origins of attachment security: 'Classical' and contextual determinants*. Hillsdale, NJ: Analytic Press.

Belsky, J., & Rovine, M. (1987). Temperament and attachment security in the Strange Situation: An empirical rapprochement. *Child Development, 58*, 787–796.

Benedict, T. (1959). Parenthood as a developmental phase: A contribution to the libido theory. *Journal of the American Psychoanalytic Association, 7*, 389–417.

Benoit, D., Parker, K. C. H., & Zeanah, C. H. (1997). Mothers' internal representations of their infants assessed prenatally: Stability over time and association with infants' attachment classifications at 12 months. *Journal of Child Psychology and Psychiatry, 38*, 307–313.

Bernier, A., & Dozier, M. (2003). Bridging the attachment transmission gap: The role of maternal mind-mindedness. *International Journal of Behavioral Development, 27*, 355–365.

Bibring, G., Dwyer, T., Huntington, D., & Valenstein, A. (1961). A study of the psychological processes in pregnancy and of the earliest mother–child relationship. *Psychoanalytic Study of the Child, 16*, 9–24.

Bokhorst, C. L., Bakermans-Kranenburg, M. J., Fearon, R. M. P., van IJzendoorn, M. H., Fonagy, P., & Schuengel, C. (2003). The importance of shared environment in mother–infant attachment security: A behavioral genetic study. *Child Development, 74*, 1769–1782.

Borghini, A., Pierrehumbert, B., Milkjkovitch, R., Muller-Nix, C., Forcada-Guex, M., & Ansermet, F. (2006). Mother's attachment representations of their premature infant at 6 and 18 months after birth. *Infant Mental Health Journal, 27*, 494–508.

Bornstein, M. H. (Ed.). (2003). *Handbook of parenting: Children and parenting* (2nd ed.). Mahwah, NJ: Erlbaum.

Bowlby, J. (1969/1982). *Attachment and loss: Vol. 1. Attachment*. New York: Basic Books.

Bowlby, J. (1973). *Attachment and loss: Vol. 2. Separation: Anxiety and anger*. New York: Basic Books.

Bowlby, J. (1980). *Attachment and loss: Vol. 3. Loss: Sadness and depression*. New York: Basic Books.

Bowlby, J. (1988). *A secure base*. New York: Basic Books.

Brazelton, T. B. (1981). *On becoming a family*. New York: Delacorte Press/Lawrence.

Bretherton, I. (2005). In pursuit of the internal working model construct and its relevance to attachment relationships. In K. E. Grossmann, K. Grossmann, & E. Waters (Eds.), *Attachment from infancy to adulthood: The major longitudinal studies* (pp. 13–47) New York: Guilford Press.

Bretherton, I., Biringen, Z., Ridgeway, D., Maslin, D., & Sherman, M. (1989). Attachment: The parental perspective. *Infant Mental Health Journal, 10*, 203–221.

Bretherton, I., Lambert, J. D., & Golby, B. (2005). Involved fathers of preschool children as seen by themselves and their wives: Accounts of attachment, socialization, and companionship. *Attachment and Human Development, 7*, 229–251.

Britner, P. A., Marvin, R. S., & Pianta, R. C. (2005). Development and preliminary validation of the caregiving behavior system: Association with child attachment classification in the preschool Strange Situation. *Attachment and Human Development, 7*, 83–102.

Buchheim, A., Erk, S., George, C., Kächele, H., Kircher, T., Martius, P., et al. (in press). Neural correlates of attachment dysregulation in borderline personality disorder using functional magnetic resonance imaging. *Psychiatry Research: Neuroimaging.*

Buchheim, A., Erk, S., George, C., Kächele, H., Ruchsow, M., Spitzer, M., et al. (2006). Measuring attachment representation in an fMRI environment: A pilot study. *Psychopathology, 39,* 144–152.

Buchheim, A., & George, C. (in press). The representational, neurobiological, and emotional foundation of attachment disorganization in borderline personality disorder and anxiety disorder. In J. Solomon & C. George (Eds.), *Disorganized attachment and caregiving.* New York: Guilford Press.

Button, S., Pianta, R. C., & Marvin, R. S. (2001). Mothers' representations of relationships with their children: Relations with parenting behavior, mother characteristics, and child disability status. *Social Development, 10,* 455–472.

Carter, C. S., Ahnert, L., Grossmann, K. E., Hrdy, S. B., Lamb, M. E., Porges, S. W., et al. (Eds.). (2005). *Attachment and bonding: A new synthesis.* Cambridge, MA: MIT Press.

Cassidy, J. (2000). The complexity of the caregiving system: A perspective from attachment theory. *Psychological Inquiry, 11,* 86–92.

Clutton-Brock, T. H. (1991). *The evolution of parent care.* Princeton, NJ: Princeton University Press.

Cohen, L. J., & Slade, A. (2000). The psychology and psychopathology of pregnancy: Reorganization and transformation. In C. H. Zeanah (Ed.), *Handbook of infant mental health* (2nd ed., pp. 20–36). New York: Guilford Press.

Coleman, P., Nelson, E. S., & Sundre, D. L. (1999). The relationship between prenatal expectations and postnatal attitudes among first-time mothers. *Journal of Reproductive and Infant Psychology, 17,* 27–39.

Corter, C. M., & Fleming, A. S. (2002). *Psychobiology of maternal behavior in human beings.* Mahwah, NJ: Erlbaum.

Cote-Arsenault, D., & Dombeck, M.-T. B. (2001). Maternal assignment of fetal personhood to a previous pregnancy loss: Relationship to anxiety in the current pregnancy. *Health Care for Women International, 22,* 649–665.

Cowan, P. A. (1991). Individual and family life transitions: A proposal for a new definition. In P. Cowan & M. Hetherington (Eds.), *Family transitions* (Vol. 2, pp. 3–30). Hillsdale, NJ: Erlbaum.

Cowan, P. A., Bradburn, I., & Cowan, C. P. (2005). *Parents' working models of attachment: The Intergenerational context of parenting and children's adaptation to school.* Mahwah, NJ: Erlbaum.

Cox, M., Owen, M. T., Henderson, V. K., & Margand, N. A. (1992). Prediction of infant–father and infant–mother attachment. *Developmental Psychology, 28,* 474–483.

Cox, M. J., Paley, B., Payne, C. C., & Burchinal, M. (1999). The transition to parenthood: Marital conflict and withdrawal and parent–infant interactions. In M.

J. Cox & J. Brooks-Gunn (Eds.), *Conflict and cohesion in families: Causes and consequences* (pp. 87–104). Mahwah, NJ: Erlbaum.

Crowell, J., Treboux, D., Pan, H., Gao, Y., Fyffe, C., & Waters, E. (2002). Assessing secure base behavior in adulthood: Development of a measure, links to adult attachment representations, and relations to couples' communication and reports of relationships. *Developmental Psychology, 38,* 679–693.

Dario, M. (2005). Effects of early experience on female behavioural and reproductive development in rhesus macaques. *Proceedings of the Royal Society of London: Series B. Biological Sciences, 272,* 1243–1248.

De Wolff, M. S., & van IJzendoorn, M. H. (1997). Sensitivity and attachment: A meta-analysis on parental antecedents of infant attachment. *Child Development, 68,* 571–591.

Deutscher, M. (1971). First pregnancy and family formation. In D. Milmen & G. Goldman (Eds.), *Psychoanalytic contributions to community psychology* (pp. 233–255). Springfield, IL: Thomas.

Edwards, E. P., Eiden, R. D., & Leonard, K. E. (2006). Behavior problems in 18- to 36-month-old children of alcoholic fathers: Secure mother–infant attachment as a protective factor. *Development and Psychopathology, 18,* 395–407.

Egeland, B., & Farber, E. A. (1984). Infant–mother attachment: Factors related to its development and changes over time. *Child Development, 55,* 753–771.

Ellis, B. J., & Garber, J. (2000). Psychosocial antecedents of girls' pubertal timing: Maternal depression, stepfather presence, and marital and family stress. *Child Development, 71,* 485–501.

Emde, R. N., Gaensbauer, T. J., & Harmon, R. J. (1976). Emotional expression in infancy: A behavioral study. *Psychological Issues: Monograph Series, 10*(1, No. 37).

Feldman, R. (2004). Mother–infant skin-to-skin contact (kangaroo care). *Infants and Young Children: An Interdisciplinary Journal of Special Care Practices, 17,* 145–161.

Feldman, R., Weller, A., Sirota, L., & Eidelman, A. I. (2003). Testing a family intervention hypothesis: The contribution of mother–infant skin-to-skin contact (kangaroo care) to family interaction, proximity, and touch. *Journal of Family Psychology, 17,* 94–107.

Fisher, N. K. (2000). *Mental representations of attachment and caregiving in women sexually abused during childhood: Links to the intergenerational transmission of trauma?* Unpublished doctoral dissertation, City University of New York.

Fleming, A. S., & Li, M. (2002). *Psychobiology of maternal behavior and its early determinants in nonhuman mammals.* Mahwah, NJ: Erlbaum.

Fonagy, P., Steele, H., & Steele, M. (1991). Maternal representations of attachment during pregnancy predict the organization of attachment at one year of age. *Child Development, 62,* 891–905.

Fossey, D. (1983). *Gorillas in the mist.* Boston: Houghton Mifflin.

Fraiberg, S. (1980). *Clinical studies in infant mental health: The first year of life*. New York: Basic Books.

Fullard, W., & Reiling, A. M. (1976). An investigation of Lorenz's "babyness." *Child Development, 47*, 1191–1193.

Gable, S., Belsky, J., & Crnic, K. (1992). Marriage, parenting, and child development: Progress and prospects. *Journal of Family Psychology, 5*, 276–294.

George, C., Kaplan, N., & Main, M. (1984/1985/1996). *Adult Attachment Interview protocol*. Unpublished manuscript, University of California at Berkeley.

George, C., & Solomon, J. (1988/1993/2005/2007). *The Caregiving Interview: Caregiving representation rating manual*. Unpublished manuscript, Mills College, Oakland, CA.

George, C., & Solomon, J. (1989). Internal working models of caregiving and security of attachment at age six. *Infant Mental Health Journal, 10*, 222–237.

George, C., & Solomon, J. (1996). Representational models of relationships: Links between caregiving and attachment. *Infant Mental Health Journal, 17*, 198–216.

George, C., & Solomon, J. (1999). Attachment and caregiving: The caregiving behavioral system. In J. Cassidy & P. R. Shaver (Eds.), *Handbook of attachment: Theory, research, and clinical applications* (pp. 649–670). New York: Guilford Press.

George, C., & Solomon, J. (in press). The disorganized caregiving system: Mothers' helpless state of mind. In J. Solomon & C. George (Eds.), *Disorganized attachment and caregiving*. New York: Guilford Press.

George, C., & West, M. (2001). The development and preliminary validation of a new measure of adult attachment: The Adult Attachment Projective. *Attachment and Human Development, 3*, 30–61.

George, C., & West, M. (in press). *The Adult Attachment Projective Picture System*. New York: Guilford Press.

George, C., West, M., & Pettem, O. (1999). The Adult Attachment Projective: Disorganization of adult attachment at the level of representation. In J. Solomon & C. George (Eds.), *Attachment disorganization* (pp. 462–507). New York: Guilford Press.

Gobbini, M. I., & Haxby, J. V. (2006). Neural response to the visual familiarity of faces. *Brain Research Bulletin, 71*, 76–82.

Goodall, J. (1990). *Through a window: My thirty years with the chimpanzees of Gombe*. Boston: Houghton Mifflin.

Grienenberger, J., Kelly, K., & Slade, A. (2005). Maternal reflective functioning, mother–infant affective communication, and infant attachment: Exploring the link between mental states and observed caregiving behavior in the intergenerational transmission of attachment. *Attachment and Human Development, 7*, 299–311.

Heller, S. S., & Zeanah, C. H. (1999). Attachment disturbances in infants born subsequent to perinatal loss: A pilot study. *Infant Mental Health Journal, 20*, 188–199.

Hesse, E., & Main, M. (2006). Frightened, threatening, and dissociative parental behavior in low-risk samples: Description, discussion, and interpretations. *Development and Psychopathology, 18*, 309–343.

Hinde, R. A. (1982). *Ethology*. New York: Oxford University Press.

Hinde, R. A., & Stevenson-Hinde, J. (1991). Perspectives on attachment. In C. M. Parkes, J. Stevenson-Hinde, & P. Marris (Ed.), *Attachment across the life cycle* (pp. 52–65). New York: Routledge.

Hoghughi, M., & Lond, N. (Eds.). (2004). *Handbook of parenting: Theory, research and practice*. London: Sage.

Hrdy, S. B. (1999). *Mother nature: History of mothers, infants, and natural selection*. New York: Random House.

Hughes, P., Turton, P., Hopper, E., McGauley, G. A., & Fonagy, P. (2004). Factors associated with the unresolved classification of the Adult Attachment Interview in women who have suffered stillbirth. *Development and Psychopathology, 16*, 215–230.

Hughes, P., Turton, P., McGauley, G. A., & Fonagy, P. (2006). Factors that predict infant disorganization in mothers classified as U in pregnancy. *Attachment and Human Development, 8*, 113–122.

Huth-Bocks, A. C., Levendosky, A., Bogat, G. A., & von Eye, A. (2004). The impact of maternal characteristics and contextual variables on infant–mother attachment. *Child Development, 75*, 480–496.

Ilicali, E. T., & Fisek, G. O. (2004). Maternal representations during pregnancy and early motherhood. *Infant Mental Health Journal, 25*, 16–27.

Kermoian, R., & Liederman, P. H. (1986). Infant attachment to mother and child caretaker in an east African community. *International Journal of Behavioral Development, 9*, 455–469.

Kerverne, E. B. (1995). Neurochemical changes accompanying the reproductive process: Their significance for maternal care in primates and in other mammals. In C. R. Pryce, R. D. Martin, & D. Skuse (Eds.), *Motherhood in human and nonhuman primates* (pp. 69–77). Basel: Karger.

Kim, K., & Smith, P. D. (2000). Retrospective survey of marital relations and child reproductive development. *International Journal of Behavioral Development, 22*, 729–751.

Kinsley, C. H., Gifford, G. W., Madonia, L., Tureski, K., Griffin, G. R., Lowry, C., et al. (1999). Motherhood improves learning and memory. *Nature, 402*, 137–138.

Kinsley, C. H., & Lambert, K. G. (2006). The maternal brain. *Scientific American, 294*, 72–79.

Klaus, M. H., Kennell, J. H., & Klaus, P. H. (1995). *Bonding*. Reading, MA: Addison-Wesley.

Koren-Karie, N., Oppenheim, D., Dolev, S., & Etzion-Carasso, A. (2002). Mothers' insightfulness regarding their infants' internal experience: Relations with maternal sensitivity and infant attachment. *Developmental Psychology, 38*, 534–542.

Langlois, J. H., Ritter, J. M., Cassey, R. J., & Sawin, D. B. (1995). Infant attractiveness predicts maternal behaviors and attitudes. *Developmental Psychology, 31,* 464–472.

Lee, R. E. (1995). Women look at their experience of pregnancy. *Infant Mental Health Journal, 16,* 192–205.

Leibenluft, E., Gobbini, M. I., Harrison, T., & Haxby, J. V. (2004). Mothers' neural activation in response to pictures of their children and other children. *Biological Psychiatry, 56,* 225–232.

Liefer, M. (1980). *Psychological effects of motherhood.* New York: Praeger.

Liotti, G. (in press). Attachment disorganization and the clinical dialog: Theme and variations. In J. Solomon & C. George (Eds.), *Disorganized attachment and caregiving.* New York: Guilford Press.

Lorberbaum, J. P., Newman, J. D., Dubno, J. R., Horwitz, A. R., Nahas, Z., Teneback, C. C., et al. (1999). Feasibility of using fMRI to study mothers responding to infant cries. *Depression and Anxiety, 10,* 99–104.

Lorenz, K. (1943). Die angeboren formen moglichend Erfahrun. *Zeitschrift für Tierpsychologie, 5,* 233–409.

Lundy, B. L. (2002). Paternal socio-psychological factors and infant attachment: The mediating role of synchrony in father–infant interactions. *Infant Behavior and Development, 25,* 221–236.

Magill-Evans, J., Harrison, M. J., Rempel, G., & Slater, L. (2006). Interventions with fathers of young children: Systematic literature review. *Journal of Advanced Nursing, 55,* 248–264.

Main, M. (1990). Cross-cultural studies of attachment organization: Recent studies, changing methodologies and the concept of conditional strategies. *Human Development, 33,* 48–61.

Main, M., & Goldwyn, R. (1984/2003). *Adult attachment scoring and classification system.* Unpublished manuscript, University of California at Berkeley.

Main, M., & Hesse, E. (1990). Parents' unresolved traumatic experiences are related to infant disorganized attachment status: Is frightened and/or frightening parental behavior the linking mechanism? In M. T. Greenberg, D. Cicchetti, & E. M. Cummings (Eds.), *Attachment in the preschool years* (pp. 161–182). Chicago: University of Chicago Press.

Main, M., Hesse, E., & Kaplan, N. (2005). Predictability of attachment behavior and representational processes at 1, 6, and 19 years: The Berkeley longitudinal study. In K. E. Grossmann, K. Grossmann, & E. Waters (Eds.), *Attachment from infancy to adulthood: The major longitudinal studies* (pp. 245–304). New York: Guilford Press.

Main, M., Kaplan, M., & Cassidy, J. (1985). Security in infancy, childhood, and adulthood: A move to the level of representation. In I. Bretherton & E. Waters (Eds.), Growing points in attachment theory and research. *Monographs of the Society for Research in Child Development, 50*(1–2, Serial No. 209), 66–104.

Manning-Orenstein, G. (1997). *A birth intervention: Comparing the influence of doula assistance at birth versus Lamaze birth preparation on first-time mothers' working models of caregiving.* Unpublished doctoral dissertation, Saybrook Institute, San Francisco.

Marvin, R. S., & Pianta, R. C. (1996). Mothers' reaction to their child's diagnosis: Relations with security of attachment. *Journal of Clinical Child Psychology, 25,* 436–445.

Mayseless, O., & Scharf, M. (2006). Maternal representations and psychosocial functioning. In O. Mayseless (Ed.), *Parenting representations: Theory, research, and clinical implications* (pp. 208–238). New York: Cambridge University Press.

Meins, E. (1999). Sensitivity, security, and internal working models: Bridging the transmission gap. *Attachment and Human Development, 1,* 325–342.

Messina Sayre, J., Pianta, R. C., Marvin, R. S., & Saft, E. W. (2001). Mothers' representations of relationships with their children: Relations with mother characteristics and feeding sensitivity. *Journal of Pediatric Psychology, 26,* 375–384.

Meyers, S. A. (1999). Mothering in context: Ecological determinants of parent behavior. *Merrill–Palmer Quarterly, 45,* 332–357.

Miller, B. D. (1987). Female infanticide and child neglect in rural North India. In N. Scheper-Hughes (Ed.), *Child survival: Anthropological perspectives on the treatment and maltreatment of children* (pp. 164–181). Boston: Reidel.

Moffitt, T. E., Caspi, A., Belsky, J., & Silva, P. A. (1992). Childhood experience and the onset of menarche. *Child Development, 63,* 47–58.

Moss, E., Cyr, C., Bureau, J., Tarabulsy, G. M., & Dubois-Comtois, K. (2005). Stability of attachment during the preschool period. *Developmental Psychology, 41,* 773–783.

Nitschke, J. B., Heller, W., Etienne, M. A., & Miller, G. A. (2004). Prefrontal cortex activity differentiates processes affecting memory in depression. *Biological Psychology, 67,* 125–143.

Novakov, M., & Fleming, A. S. (2005). The effects of early rearing environment on the hormonal induction of maternal behavior in virgin rats. *Hormones and Behavior, 48,* 528–536.

O'Leary, J. (2005). The trauma of ultrasound during a pregnancy following perinatal loss. *Journal of Loss and Trauma, 10,* 183–204.

Oppenheim, D., & Koren-Karie, N. (2002). Mothers' insightfulness regarding their children's internal worlds: The capacity underlying secure child–mother relationships. *Infant Mental Health Journal, 23,* 593–605.

Oppenheim, D., Koren-Karie, N., & Sagi, A. (2001). Mothers' empathic understanding of their preschoolers' internal experience: Relations with early attachment. *International Journal of Behavioral Development, 25,* 16–26.

Perry, B. D., Pollard, R. A., Blakley, T. L., Baker, W. L., & Vigilante, D. (1995). Childhood trauma, the neurobiology of adaptation, and "use dependent" development of the brain: How "states" become "traits." *Infant Mental Health Journal, 16,* 271–289.

Pianta, R. C., Marvin, R. S., Britner, P., & Borowitz, K. (1996). Parents' reactions to their child's diagnosis: Relations with security of attachment. *Infant Mental Health Journal, 17,* 239–256.

Pianta, R. C., O'Connor, T. G., & Marvin, R. S. (1993). *Measuring representations of parenting: An interview-based system.* Unpublished manuscript, University of Virginia.

Poindron, P., Terrazas, A., de la Luz Navarro Montes de Oca, M., Serafán, N., & Hernández, H. (2007). Sensory and physiological determinants of maternal behavior in the goat (*Capra hircus*). *Hormones and Behavior, 52,* 99–105.

Posada, G., Gao, Y., Wu, F., & Posada, R. (1995). The secure-base phenomenon across cultures: Children's behavior, mother's preferences, and experts' concepts. In E. Waters, B. E. Vaughn, G. Posada, & K. Kondo-Ikemura (Eds.), Caregiving, cultural, and cognitive perspectives on secure-base behavior and working models: New growing points of attachment theory and research. *Monographs of the Society for Research in Child Development, 60*(2, Serial No. 244), 27–48.

Pryce, C. R. (1995). Determinants of motherhood in human and nonhuman primates: A biosocial model. In C. R. Pryce, R. D. Martin, & D. Skuse (Eds.), *Motherhood in human and nonhuman primates* (pp. 1–15). Basel, Switzerland: Karger.

Rode, S. E., Chang, P., Fisch, R. O., & Sroufe, L. A. (1981). Attachment patterns in infants separated at birth. *Developmental Psychology, 17,* 188–191.

Sameroff, A. J. (1993). Models of development and developmental risk. In C. H. Zeanah (Ed.), *Handbook of infant mental health* (pp. 3–14). New York: Guilford Press.

Schaller, G. B. (1963). *The mountain gorilla: Ecology and behavior.* Chicago University of Chicago Press.

Schechter, D. S., Coots, T., Zeanah, C. H., Davies, M., Coates, S. W., Trabka, K. A., et al. (2005). Maternal mental representations of the child in an inner-city clinical sample: Violence-related posttraumatic stress and reflective functioning. *Attachment and Human Development, 7,* 313–331.

Scheper-Hughes, N. (1987). Culture, scarcity and maternal thinking: Mother love and child death in Northeast Brazil. In N. Scheper-Hughes (Ed.), *Child survival: Anthropological perspectives on treatment and maltreatment of children* (pp. 291–317). Boston: Reidel.

Sharf, M., & Mayseless, O. (1997/2000). *Parenting Representations Interview—Adolescence (PRI-A).* Unpublished manuscript, University of Haifa, Haifa, Israel.

Slade, A. (2004). The move from categories to process: Attachment phenomena and clinical evaluation. *Infant Mental Health Journal, 25,* 269–283.

Slade, A., Belsky, J., Aber, J. L., & Phelps, J. L. (1999). Mothers' representations of their relationships with their toddlers: Links to adult attachment and observed mothering. *Developmental Psychology, 35,* 611–619.

Slade, A., Dermer, M., Gerber, J., Gibson, L., Graf, F., Siegal, N., et al. (1995, March). *Prenatal representa-*

tion, dyadic interaction, and the quality of attachment. Paper presented at the biennial meeting of the Society for Research in Child Development, Indianapolis, IN.

Slade, A., Grienenberger, J., Bernbach, E., Levy, D., & Locker, A. (2005). Maternal reflective functioning, attachment, and the transmission gap: A preliminary study. *Attachment and Human Development, 7,* 283–298.

Solomon, J., & George, C. (1996). Defining the caregiving system: Toward a theory of caregiving. *Infant Mental Health Journal, 17,* 183–197.

Solomon, J., & George, C. (Eds.). (1999a). *Attachment disorganization.* New York: Guilford Press.

Solomon, J., & George, C. (1999b). The caregiving system in mothers of infants: A comparison of divorcing and married mothers. *Attachment and Human Development, 1,* 171–190.

Solomon, J., & George, C. (1999c). The development of attachment in separated and divorced families: Effects of overnight visitation, parent and couple variables. *Attachment and Human Development, 1,* 2–33.

Solomon, J., & George, C. (1999d). The effects on attachment of overnight visitation in divorced and separated families: A longitudinal follow-up. In J. Solomon & C. George (Eds.), *Attachment disorganization* (pp. 243–264). New York: Guilford Press.

Solomon, J., & George, C. (2000). Toward an integrated theory of caregiving. In J. Osofsky & H. Fitzgerald (Eds.), *WAIMH handbook of infant mental health* (pp. 323–368). New York: Wiley.

Solomon, J., & George, C. (2006). Intergenerational transmission of dysregulated maternal caregiving: Mothers describe their upbringing and childrearing. In O. Mayseless (Ed.), *Parenting representations: Theory, research, and clinical implications* (pp. 265–295). New York: Cambridge University Press.

Solomon, J., & George, C. (Eds.). (in press-a). *Disorganized attachment and caregiving.* New York: Guilford Press.

Solomon, J., & George, C. (in press-b). Dysregulation of maternal caregiving across two generations. In J. Solomon & C. George (Eds.), *Disorganized attachment and caregiving.* New York: Guilford Press.

Solomon, J., George, C., & De Jong, A. (1995). Children classified as controlling at age six: Evidence of disorganized representational strategies and aggression at home and at school. *Development and Psychopathology, 7,* 447–463.

Sroufe, L. A., & Fleeson, J. (1986). Attachment and the construction of relationships. In W. Hartup & Z. Rubin (Eds.), *The nature and development of relationships* (pp. 51–71). Hillsdale, NJ: Erlbaum.

Steele, H., Phibbs, E., & Woods, R. (2004). Coherence of mind in daughter caregivers of mothers with dementia: Links with their mothers' joy and relatedness on reunion in the Strange Situation. *Attachment and Human Development, 6,* 439–450.

Steinberg, D. R., & Pianta, R. C. (2006). Maternal representations of relationships: Assessing multiple parenting dimensions. In O. Mayseless (Ed.), *Parenting representations: Theory, research, and clinical implications* (pp. 41–78). New York: Cambridge University Press.

Stevenson-Hinde, J. (1994). An ethological perspective. *Psychological Inquiry, 5,* 62–65.

Stovall-McClough, K. C., & Cloitre, M. (2006). Traumatic reactions to terrorism: The individual and collective experience. In L. A. Schein, H. I. Spitz, G. M. Burlingame, P. R. Muskin, & S. Vargo (Eds.), *Psychological effects of catastrophic disasters: Group approaches to treatment* (pp. 113–153). New York: Haworth Press.

Stovall-McClough, K. C., & Dozier, M. (2004). Forming attachments in foster care: Infant attachment behaviors during the first 2 months of placement. *Development and Psychopathology, 16,* 253–271.

Suomi, S. J. (1995). Attachment theory and nonhuman primates. In S. Goldberg, R. Muir, & J. Kerr (Eds.), *Attachment theory: Social, developmental, and clinical perspectives* (pp. 185–201). Hillsdale, NJ: Analytic Press.

Swain, J. E., Lorberbaum, J. P., Kose, S., & Strathearn, L. (2007). Brain basis of early parent–infant interactions: Psychology, physiology, and *in vivo* functional neuroimaging studies. *Journal of Child Psychology and Psychiatry, 48,* 262–287.

Tallandini, M. A., & Scalembra, C. (2006). Kangaroo mother care and mother–premature infant dyadic interaction. *Infant Mental Health Journal, 27,* 251–275.

Trivers, R. L. (1974). Parent–offspring conflict. *American Zoologist, 11,* 249–264.

Turton, P., Hughes, P., Fonagy, P., & Fainman, D. (2004). An investigation into the possible overlap between PTSD and unresolved responses following stillbirth: An absence of linkage with only unresolved status predicting infant disorganization. *Attachment and Human Development, 6,* 241–253.

van IJzendoorn, M. H. (1995). Adult attachment representations, parental responsiveness, and infant attachment: A meta-analysis. *Psychological Bulletin, 117,* 387–403.

Volk, A. A., Lukjanczuk, J. M., & Quinsey, V. L. (2005). Influence of infant and child facial cues of low body weight on adults' ratings of adoption preference, cuteness, and health. *Infant Mental Health Journal, 26,* 459–469.

West, M., & Sheldon-Keller, A. E. (1994). *Patterns of relating: An adult attachment perspective.* New York: Guilford Press.

Wierson, M., Long, P. J., & Forehand, R. L. (1993). Toward a new understanding of early menarche: The role of environmental stress in pubertal timing. *Adolescence, 28,* 913–924.

Zeanah, C. H., Benoit, D., Hirschberg, L., & Barton, M. L. (1993). *Working Model of the child Interview: Rating scales and classification.* Unpublished manuscript, Louisiana State University School of Medicine.

Zeanah, C. H., Benoit, D., Hirschberg, L., & Barton, M. L. (1994). Mothers' representations of their infants are concordant with infant attachment classification. *Developmental Issues in Psychiatry and Psychology, 1,* 1–14.

CHAPTER 36

A Wider View of Attachment and Exploration

The Influence of Mothers and Fathers on the Development of Psychological Security from Infancy to Young Adulthood

KARIN GROSSMANN
KLAUS E. GROSSMANN
HEINZ KINDLER
PETER ZIMMERMANN

Attachment research has come of age. In the 1970s, only a few years after Bowlby's (1969/1982) first comprehensive formulation of attachment theory and Ainsworth's translation of attachment theory into observational, empirical research (e.g., Ainsworth, Blehar, Waters, & Wall, 1978), many studies of infant attachment (usually to mothers) were initiated. Now four of them have succeeded in following infants all the way into young adulthood: the Minnesota Study of Risk and Adaptation from Birth to Adulthood (Sroufe, Egeland, Carlson, & Collins, 2005a, 2005b); the Berkeley longitudinal study (Main, Hesse, & Kaplan, 2005); the Stony Brook Adult Relationship Project (Crowell & Waters, 2005); and our own research in northern and southern Germany (K. Grossmann, Grossmann, & Kindler, 2005). The researchers involved in these projects, as well as many other attachment researchers, came from diverse backgrounds (K. E. Grossmann, Grossmann, & Waters, 2005). Research at Klaus E. Grossmann's lab, which is particularly relevant to the present chapter, was primarily rooted in ethology, which had also played a major role in Ainsworth's and Bowlby's thinking (Ainsworth & Bowlby, 1991; Hinde, 2005).

Here we advocate a broad perspective on attachment and exploration, as influenced by children's experiences with both mothers and fathers. For each issue we discuss, we present studies exploring the influence of fathers alongside those exploring the influence of mothers. It was Bowlby's (1969/1982) premise that exploration, competent play, and mastery of the environment are facilitated when a child feels secure in relationships with caregivers. In this chapter, the concept of "security of exploration" as a companion to secure attachment is introduced. We define "secure exploration" in the early years as confident, attentive, eager, and resourceful exploration of materials or tasks, especially when a child is facing disappointment. Such exploration is accompanied by persistence and tolerance of frustration in the service of goal-corrected action. This type of security allows a person to ask for help if his or her competency is insufficient for a particular task.

A study with 3-year-olds may serve as an example. Each child in a group of 3-year-olds was observed in a competitive game with an experimenter that involved stacking rings on a pole. The procedure caused the child to win the first round, lose the second round, and win again on the third round (Luetkenhaus, Grossmann, & Grossmann, 1985). The children's responses to becoming aware that they would lose were related to the quality of tachment to their mothers in infancy (assessed 2 years earlier). Secure children carefully increased their speed of stacking the rings and maintained eye contact with the experimenter. They openly showed him their disappointment when he asked after the round who had won the game. Insecure children also tried to increase their speed, but became confused and less well organized in their motor coordination, resulting in a slower building speed. When the experimenter asked who won, they hid their faces from him and attended to other issues.

Concentration and engagement in unfamiliar tasks, even when individuals are facing obstacles, are hallmarks of secure exploration at any age—in toddlerhood, childhood, or adolescence. We posit that secure attachment and secure exploration function together in the service of "psychological security." Here we review research showing that trust in reliably available and supportive attachment figures—fathers as well as mothers—fosters an optimal balance and smooth transition between attachment and exploration at all ages, even under stressful circumstances.

As to assessing the quality of child–father attachment, we propose on the basis of many studies that the security of such attachment may be more evident in smooth cooperation between child and father than in an infant's reaction to separation from and reunion with the father as assessed in the Strange Situation. Our review of many studies suggests that the father's functioning as a sensitive, trusted, and dependable companion when the child is faced with challenges seems to be the central marker of a secure relationship. Even though many early studies examining the implications of infant–father relationship quality for the child's later development used the Strange Situation only, the particularly close link between the quality of the child–father relationship and children's quality of exploration became more clearly evident in studies that assessed fathers' sensitivity during play situations. The unique role of fathers' sensitive support during joint play in children's security of exploration seems to be supported by many studies, independent of the method used to assess child–father relationship quality.

We begin this chapter by discussing the concept of secure exploration in greater detail. In the next section, we review studies showing that both a secure child–mother attachment and a father's sensitive and challenging support of a child's exploration influence the child's (and, later, the adolescent's) secure exploration of cognitive challenges. An interesting corollary is also discussed: An increasing number of studies provide evidence that a secure child–mother attachment and a supportive father–child relationship are associated with less gender-stereotypic behavior in both girls and boys.

In the subsequent section, we review research exploring the relation between secure child–parent relationships and a child's resourceful transition and adaptation to new social as well as intellectually challenging situations in which the parents are not present. These situations include transitions into and adaptation to preschool, kindergarten, later school grades, and college. Secure exploration based on secure attachment to the mother and/or the father seems to be a fruitful basis for successful adaptation to age-appropriate institutionalized group situations. Insecurity, evidenced by problem behaviors, may interfere with the attainment of academic competence in such situations.

Some additional evidence reveals a link between quality of the father–child relationship and a child's quality of relationships with close friends and siblings. These findings have been missing from discussions of the impact of fathers on older children's close relationships. We close the chapter with a short summary of the findings from our two German longitudinal studies (see K. Grossmann et al., 2005, for a detailed account), and with a description of the current status of our wider view of attachment.

THE CONCEPT OF SECURITY OF EXPLORATION

A young child's confidence in an adult caregiver's solicitude promotes exploration and competence—a notion central to attachment theory (Bowlby, 1969/1982). During development, the child must balance exploratory motivation with appropriate fear of novelty and danger, while becoming familiar with new environments and developing new skills. Human infancy, childhood, and adolescence last much longer than the comparable periods in the lives of other primate species. Many biological and cultural anthropologists have speculated about the function of such an extended period of learning before adult sexual maturity. Some ethologists have inferred from the prominent childlike appearance of even some adult characteristics that prolonged openness and immaturity may help to maintain curiosity, which in other playful species is restricted to much briefer juvenile periods. Much of human exploratory behavior is playful, and "play [is] only possible in a tension-free field" (Lorenz, 1977, p. 147). Attachment theory provides insight into what is necessary to allow a child to feel safe and tension-free: a protective, responsive, supportive, reliably available, stronger, and wiser attachment figure. With this kind of nurturance, a child is likely to explore the world confidently, to initiate warm and sociable interactions with others, and to find solace in the knowledge that a caregiver is available (Ainsworth et al., 1978).

Ainsworth (1990, p. 463) emphasized early that "attachment theory as originated by Bowlby is an open-ended theory; open to extension, revision, and refinement through research." With this in mind, we proposed the concept of security of exploration (K. E. Grossmann, Grossmann, & Zimmermann, 1999). Main (1983) and her colleagues, as well as Belsky's research group (e.g., Belsky, Garduque, & Hrncir, 1984), were the first to notice a close association between quality of infant attachment to mother and/or father and quality of exploration, as indicated by concentration, enthusiastic play, and better cognitive functioning within the ranges of a given mental capacity.

Security of exploration seems to rest on (1) a child's ability to organize emotions and behaviors open-mindedly, nondefensively, and with concentration when responding to "curious" events, and to do so with care; and (2) the child's confidence in an attachment figure's availability and helpfulness, should help be needed. Both factors are based on (3) attachment figure's observable sensitivity and support during distressing situations, when the child's attachment system or need to explore is aroused. In our opinion, security of exploration is not the same as mastery motivation, because the motive to master tasks may be a strategy to divert attention from attachment issues (Frodi, Bridges, & Grolnick, 1985). Mastery motivation is believed to represent a less relational and more intrinsic infant characteristic. Empirically, quality of attachment has proven not to be related to mastery motivation (Seifer, Schiller, Hayden, & Geerher, 1993; Zeanah et al., 1999).

Parents' willingness and ability to support their child's exploration sensitively and appropriately provide the child with realistic self-confidence in his or her competence in new situations. A psychologically secure child is eager to engage the world, knowing that a secure base is available. Supporting secure exploration has much in common with what Ryan and his colleagues call "supporting autonomy in relatedness"

(Grolnick, Deci, & Ryan, 1997; Ryan & Lynch, 1989). Neither concept implies that children will be wholly self-reliant, independent, or detached. Grolnick and colleagues (1997) argued that autonomy is facilitated by attachment and trust in the supportiveness of parents, not by detachment. Regarding adolescence, they suggested that among the primary reasons adolescents detach from, and refuse to rely on, parents is that parents have been overly controlling and/or underinvolved. According to this analysis, adolescents whose parents provide a good caregiving environment do not need to relinquish their attachment in order to become more autonomous and self-regulated.

It is noteworthy that in the coding system for the Adult Attachment Interview (AAI; see Hesse, Chapter 25, this volume), the concept of "freedom to explore" and its companion "freedom to evaluate experiences" are included. Expanding on this idea, Bretherton and Munholland (Chapter 5, this volume) suggest that secure attachment leaves a person relatively free from attachment-related preoccupations (e.g., the struggle in late childhood to find a balance between personal autonomy and continuing connectedness with parents) (see also Ryan, Kuhl, & Deci, 1997). Adolescents with an autonomous state of mind regarding attachment thus have more emotional and cognitive resources available to invest in stage-salient tasks, such as adjusting to and succeeding in the social and cognitive challenges presented by committed friendships and by institutions of formal learning. Throughout this chapter, we highlight the idea that freedom to explore the external and internal worlds is an important marker of security across the lifespan.

QUALITY OF ATTACHMENT TO FATHER AND SECURE EXPLORATION

Most fathers are attachment figures for their infants, even though in most families around the world fathers are not primary caregivers and do not spend as much time with their infants as mothers do. In all known cultures, fathers prefer playing with their infants (see Horn, 2000, and Lamb & Lewis, 2004, for reviews). In this section, we provide arguments that the Strange Situation may not be the most appropriate method for assessing quality of child–father attachment. We propose instead that the extent of fathers' warm, supportive, and sensitive challenges during joint play may best reflect their attachment quality. Ainsworth (1967, p. 352) may have had similar thoughts when she noted in describing her Uganda study: "One can assume that there was some special quality in the father's interaction with his child—whether of tenderness or intense delight—which evoked in turn a strength of attachment disproportionate to the frequency of his interaction with the baby."

Most infant–father Strange Situation studies have focused on fathers' sensitivity in interactions with their infants as a predictor of a secure pattern. For more than 80% of infant–father pairs studied to date, results have failed to confirm findings obtained with mother–infant pairs (see van IJzendoorn & De Wolff, 1997, for a meta-analysis, and Braungart-Rieker, Garwood, Powers, & Wang, 2001, for additional results). Antecedents and correlates of infant–father attachment security are different from correlates of infant–mother security (see Horn's [2000] review). Evidence to date suggests that the quality of the infant–father attachment relationship is more closely associated with a father's attitudes toward fathering and the family than with his observable sensitivity during caregiving interactions with his child during the child's first year of life.

Likewise, in our north German longitudinal study of 47 families, fathers' sensitivity, effectiveness in soothing their babies, and quality of interactions assessed three times during the first year were all unrelated to the quality of infant–father patterns of attachment at 18 months (K. Grossmann & Grossmann, 1991). In addition, very few studies using the Strange Situation have found robust links between patterns of infant–father attachment and indices of children's later socioemotional development (Parke et al., 2004). Although patterns of infant–father interaction can be assessed with the same instruments as patterns of infant–mother attachment, the classifications do not have the same meaning as those for mother–infant pairs. Thus the Strange Situation does not seem to be equally valid for fathers, as previously noted by Youngblade and Belsky (1992).

The weak association between paternal sensitivity during the first year and infant–father attachment security in the Strange Situation has been repeatedly documented (see reviews by K. Grossmann, Grossmann, Fremmer-Bombik, Kindler, Scheuerer-Englisch, & Zimmermann, 2002; Lamb & Lewis, 2004; Parke, 1996). However, if a father's positive involvement and sensitive, supportive, and challenging play interactions with his child are used as indices of a secure infant–father attachment relationship, then other factors are associated with this quality. Involvement in care-

giving activities is predicted by factors other than caregiving sensitivity (National Institute of Child Health and Human Development [NICHD] Early Child Care Research Network, 2000), such as a father working fewer hours, his degree of involvement with his child, the father's younger age, his child's gender, the father's personality, his less traditional childrearing beliefs, the quality of his relationship with the mother, his degree of stress, and his sense of being supported both at home and at work (see also Horn, 2000, for a review).

Supportive evidence has been gathered in studies in Germany, Israel, and the United States. K. E. Grossmann and Volkmer (1984) asked husbands of wives in their last trimester of pregnancy whether they wanted to be present at the birth or not. The hospital's policy was to force fathers into the delivery room. Only fathers who wanted to participate were found to be more involved in infant care 9 months later, regardless of whether they were present for their children's birth.

Fathers' involvement in caregiving and their sensitivity during play with their toddlers were both associated with a father's recollection of his own attachment experiences as a child in another German study (K. Grossmann, Grossmann, Fremmer-Bombik, Kindler, Scheuerer-Englisch, & Zimmermann, 2002). Fathers who valued attachments as a result of their own experiences were more often present at the birth of their infants, participated more in infant care, and more often had infants who developed a secure attachment relationship to them. All three variables, in turn, were closely linked to a father's sensitive challenging behavior during play with his 24-month-old. In addition, fathers' sensitivity during play was found to be highly stable across 4 years. If a father had been sensitive during play with his toddler, he was also very likely to be a better play partner and more sensitive guide during a teaching task when the child reached age 6. Thus, as a measure of quality of the child–father relationship in this study, play sensitivity was found to be pivotal. Patterns of infant–father attachment in the Strange Situation were found to have only very limited predictive power.

U.S. and Israeli studies yield similar conclusions. Fathers' who valued secure, supportive attachment experiences were more sensitive to their preschoolers during play (Cohn, Cowan, Cowan, & Pearson, 1992). Fathers who recalled their own fathers as nurturant (Sagi, 1982) and as involved in childrearing (Cabrera, Tamis-LeMonda, Bradley, Hofferth, & Lamb, 2000) were more involved with their own children, took more paternal responsibility, and showed greater warmth. They also monitored their children's behavior and activities more closely, seeming to care more about the children's health and safety.

Our interest in the unique role of fathers is based on our longitudinal findings over more than 22 years (K. Grossmann et al., 2005; Kindler & Grossmann, 2004). Our findings suggest that the quality and predictive power of child–father and child–mother attachment relationships derive from different sets of early social experiences, and consequently should be assessed differently. A secure attachment relationship to the mother provides comfort and relaxation, including at the physiological level, when the child is distressed (Spangler & Grossmann, 1993). In contrast, the father provides security in the context of monitored, controlled excitement, through sensitive and challenging support when the child's exploratory system is aroused (K. Grossmann, Grossmann, Fremmer-Bombik, Kindler, Scheuerer-Englisch, & Zimmermann, 2002). We have developed an instrument called the Sensitive and Challenging Interactive Play (SCIP) scale, and have used it to assess joint play interactions between a mother or father and a 24-month-old infant. The SCIP scale assesses emotional supportiveness, encouragement, meshing, attentiveness, positive affect, praise, and nonintrusiveness as markers of play sensitivity, as well as age-appropriate challenges and responsive instructions. These interactive qualities can be interpreted as organizing an infant's positive and negative emotions during exploration and play. They also help to maintain the child's concentration on the task during curiosity–wariness conflicts.

We found that individual differences in fathers' ratings on the SCIP scale were significantly related to (1) a composite index of fathers' quality of caregiving during their infants' first year, and (2) fathers' state of mind with respect to attachment (assessed with the AAI). These differences were stable across 4 years. Longitudinally, fathers' play sensitivity and infant–mother attachment quality predicted 10-year-olds' state of mind with respect to attachment. Moreover, fathers' higher SCIP scores significantly predicted fewer behavioral problems when the children were in kindergarten, and predicted higher ratings on personality characteristics associated with secure exploration when the children were 16 years old (see details later in this chapter). Fathers' SCIP scores were also associated with children's AAI classifications at age 16 and 22 years. Even the internal represen-tation of partnership at age 22 had its firm roots in fathers' much earlier play sensitivity (K. Grossmann et al., 2005; see also Parke et al., 2004).

Interestingly, Harry Harlow's experiments (using Peggy Harlow's "nuclear family apparatus"; Harlow, Harlow, & Suomi, 1971; Harlow & Mears, 1979; see also Blum, 2002) revealed a similar potential in rhesus monkey fathers. In these experiments, a rhesus monkey mother, father, and children were forced to live together in "home-like" cages (unlike the usual rhesus social system, in which mothers spend most of the time with children, and fathers are relatively independent). The rhesus children could move in and out of the "house," but their parents could not. To the researchers' surprise, "even an arrogant alpha macaque could find untapped potential. They took part in protection and rearing" (Blum, 2002, p. 202). For example, the nuclear fathers did not allow mothers, their mates, or their neighbors to abuse or abandon their infants. The fathers guarded the group against "predators"—primarily the human experimenters. Many monkey fathers engaged in reciprocal play with their infants at a level far surpassing that of the mothers (Harlow et al., 1971, p. 541). "Harry would remark that of all the animals in his laboratory, these [infants] were the most confident, the most socially adept, the most outgoing—and, surprisingly, the smartest. ... Their minds seemed sharper and more flexible, as if learning to handle a multitude of social relationships had built their brains to handle other challenges well, too" (Blum, 2002, p. 203).[1]

A recent press release by *ScienceDaily* (February 7, 2008) reports on the surprising influence of baboon fathers on their daughters' fitness, according to research done at Duke University and Princeton University. Paternity information became available as genetic research on baboon feces was included. The yellow baboon males at the Amboseli site could recognize their own offspring and exhibited paternal care by protection and supporting their own sons and daughters in disputes with other juveniles. The researchers found that fathers' protection gave their daughters an advantage in reproductive fitness. For sons, reproductive success was supported by fathers' protection only if the father was high ranking in the group (Duke University, 2008).

In summary, we propose that a father's play sensitivity, rather than quality of attachment as assessed in the Strange Situation, is the best and most valid measure of the quality of a child–father relationship.

SECURE PARENT–CHILD RELATIONSHIPS AND LATER SECURITY OF EXPLORATION

Our wider view of attachment and exploration, as well as our broader perspective on the influence of mothers and fathers, guides our interpretation of studies showing close associations between security of attachment and security of exploration. As a child grows older, "security of exploration" refers mainly to situations in which a parent is not present. We focus here on developmental outcomes that are likely to be related to the child's security with the mother and/or the father, even if the mother and father exert their influences on the functioning of their child's attachment system in different ways (K. Grossmann, Grossmann, Fremmer-Bombik, Kindler, Scheuerer-Englisch, & Zimmermann, 2002; Lamb & Lewis, 2004).

Security of Exploration in the Early Years

We begin this section with evidence concerning the association between secure child–mother attachment and secure exploration, and then document this association for child–father relationships.

Links to Child–Mother Attachment

In the Minnesota longitudinal study, toddlers who were insecurely attached to their mothers also displayed insecure exploration. They were less effective in their efforts to master challenging tasks, were less enthusiastic and less curious, and showed less endurance (Arend, Gove, & Sroufe, 1979; Matas, Arend, & Sroufe, 1978). In a follow-up study at age 3½, the children were challenged with more difficult tool-using tasks in the absence of the parent. Those who had been stably secure with their mothers were more likely to be placed later into the most competent group, whose members also exhibited higher self-esteem, more positive affect, and greater flexibility and agency. These are all markers of secure exploration at this developmental level (Arend, 1984; summarized in Sroufe et al., 2005a, pp. 125–126). As toddlers, the securely attached group had been more competent in successfully enlisting their mothers' support to achieve a solution, and their mothers' support was more appropriately attuned to the children's needs and exploratory goals. The follow-up study demonstrated the enduring effect of such maternal support for a child's later security of exploration as a part of his or her personality. The child's cumula-

tive history of care was the best predictor of his or her curiosity at 4½ years of age.

Van Bakel and Riksen-Walraven (2004) found, in a sample of Dutch 15-month-olds, that high levels of infant task orientation and pleasure were related to the Attachment Q-Sort security score (Waters, 1995). In part, this was due to low levels of infant anger; anger proneness was particularly characteristic of disorganized infants. Likewise, Vondra, Shaw, Swearingen, Cohen, and Owens (2001) reported, for a high-risk sample, that stable security across 12, 18, and 24 months was associated with better behavioral and emotional regulation in challenging tasks.

Ego resiliency can be interpreted as an aspect of secure exploration. Ego resiliency during the preschool-age period was strongly associated with a secure infant attachment history (Sroufe et al., 2005a). A similar finding emerged from a study of low-risk preschoolers by Easterbrooks and Goldberg (1990). Recently, Fish (2004) again explored the relation between attachment and preschool and kindergarten competence. She challenged a group of low-socioeconomic-status, rural Appalachian 4-year-olds with puzzles, one of which was too difficult for them. Initiative, persistence, attention, positive affect, enthusiasm, and animation were predicted by infant attachment security. (See also Belsky & Fearon, 2002.)

Spontaneous exploring or "reading" of books by preschool children was observed more frequently in securely attached 5-year-old Dutch preschoolers than in insecurely attached preschoolers (Bus, Belsky, van IJzendoorn, & Crnic, 1988). Toddlers in a German sample who had been securely attached to their mothers in infancy showed more adequate task-oriented problem-solving strategies than did toddlers with avoidant or disorganized attachment (Schieche & Spangler, 2005). In addition, task orientation and intensity of exploration were significantly associated with lower cortisol levels after the task, whereas off-task behavior was positively correlated with higher cortisol levels, indicating physiological distress.

An insecure-resistant pattern of attachment to mothers (or other female caregivers) seems to pose a special risk for insecure exploration. Less attention, exploration, and make-believe during solitary play at 36 months were observed in a U.S. study of young children with an insecure-resistant attachment history (McElwain, Cox, Burchinal, & Macfie, 2003). Five-year-old Israeli children who had displayed an insecure-resistant pattern of attachment to their regular kibbutzim caregivers in infancy were less ego-controlled, less achievement-oriented, and less independent than children with a secure attachment to their caregivers during infancy (Oppenheim, Sagi, & Lamb, 1988).

In a study of German 5-year-olds, the quality and length of a child's concentrated play were predicted by secure attachment to their mothers during infancy and, less strongly, by secure attachment to their fathers as assessed in the Strange Situation (Suess, Grossmann, & Sroufe, 1992). Specifically, children with a secure attachment to both parents in infancy produced more than twice the amount of concentrated play produced by children classified as insecure-avoidant with both parents. In this study, security of attachment to mother was more influential than security of attachment to father; however, as we have already mentioned, the Strange Situation may not be the most appropriate assessment for child–father relationship quality. In addition, the effect on concentrated play was significant only for girls. We will return to the interaction between attachment and gender in a later section.

Child–father attachment security became more important when the preschoolers were asked to participate in a picture story task with an unfamiliar experimenter. The stories were designed as a projective assessment of hostile attributional bias (Dodge, Pettit, McClaskey, & Brown, 1986). In this study, 88% of the children who were securely attached to their fathers in infancy, but only 62% of the children with an avoidant attachment to their fathers, were willing to participate (Suess, 1987). In this study, even a secure pattern of attachment to fathers as assessed in the Strange Situation was related to more secure exploration. Sensitivity of fathers' play quality was not assessed in this study.

Even in a village on a remote South Sea Island, secure infant–mother attachment was significantly related to secure exploration in a study of toddlers between the ages of 12 and 36 months (K. E. Grossmann, Grossmann, & Keppler, 2005). Secure exploration was indicated by active interest in strange and unfamiliar objects placed on the floor during the Strange Situation procedure. This finding was confirmed by our field observations in the toddlers' home village. Securely attached toddlers explored and engaged in concentrated play with both familiar and unfamiliar objects significantly more often than insecurely attached toddlers did.

The connection between security of mother–child attachment and secure exploration may be related to particular aspects of maternal care. A Canadian study (Whipple, Bernier, Mageau, & Ouellet-Gagnon, 2007) provided evidence that maternal autonomy support in the context of infant exploration contributed independently of maternal sensitivity to the prediction of infant attachment security. Meins, Fernyhough, Russell, and Clark-Carter (1998) observed the tutoring strategies of mothers of preschoolers and tested the children's mentalizing ability longitudinally. Mothers in the secure group used more sensitive tutoring strategies, and, consistent with predictions, their children were better able to incorporate an experimenter's play suggestions and had superior mentalizing abilities at age 5. The Minnesota group (Sroufe et al., 2005a) discovered significant links between child–mother attachment security and a number of personality dimensions that are characteristic of secure exploration: appropriate self-esteem, agency, self-confidence, ego resiliency, and social competence.

What about Fathers?

Research on the unique contribution of fathers to children's development is growing in complexity (see Cabrera et al., 2000, for a review). A generation ago, positive, engaged fathering was largely attributable to a harmonious family context (Lamb, 1986). But recently, studies of fathers from less optimal family contexts have also been conducted, and more sophisticated statistical methods have been applied. The results show convincingly that fathers contribute uniquely to child development (Parke et al., 2004).

A father's sensitivity can be best defined by his accessibility to his infant or toddler, his positive engagement and supportive involvement, and his warmth and closeness to the child (for extended reviews, see Lamb, 2002; Lamb & Lewis, 2004). A number of early father–infant interaction studies established the link between fathers' sensitivity during playful interactions with their toddlers and the quality of their toddlers' solitary play (Belsky et al., 1984; Easterbrooks & Goldberg, 1984). More recent research reconfirms the link. Cox, Paley, and Towe (2003) observed toddlers' enthusiastic and confident exploration of a challenging task in interactions with both mother and father. Enthusiastic exploration was defined as "Child acts with vigor, confidence, and eagerness in exploring the materials and the task." Both a father's affect and his sensitive, supportive involvement predicted his toddler's enthusiastic, confident exploration, independently of maternal variables. In a study by Verschueren and Marcoen (1999), Belgian preschoolers displayed less secure exploration if they had represented their attachment to their fathers as insecure in narratives responding to attachment-related stories.

In one study examining laboratory free-play behavior, both mothers' and fathers' support of exploration and interpretation of infant communications varied according to patterns of infant–parent attachment (K. E. Grossmann, Scheuerer-Englisch, & Loher, 1991). Mothers' and fathers' interactive behavior with their 1-year-olds was rated for sensitivity and cooperation 1 month prior to their assessment of attachment security in the Strange Situation. Parents in dyads later classified as secure interfered less with their infants' exploratory activity while engrossed in play. But when their infants signaled discontent, these parents assisted them in finding new exploratory enjoyment (e.g., by offering a new toy). Parents in secure attachment relationships helped their infants sustain interest in exploration by stepping in before the infants' exploration–attachment balance tipped away from exploration and toward attachment behavior. Parents in avoidant dyads also noticed negative emotional expressions in their infants, but reacted very differently. They would join the infants during concentrated exploration or play, offer a toy, or redirect the infants' attention. As a result of such untimely interference, the infants became frustrated and distressed. However, when the infants' negative mood became evident and their exploration ceased, these parents would more often than not withdraw and wait for the infants to overcome their distress alone (K. E. Grossmann, Scheuerer-Englisch, & Loher, 1991).

In a study of low-income, ethnically diverse families, fathers' behaviors were rated during play with their 24-month-old children. Several behaviors were aggregated to form a scale labeled Responsive–Didactic, which was unrelated to paternal education. Toddlers of high-scoring fathers expressed more positive affect during joint play, were more involved with toys, and scored higher on symbolic and creative play. Moreover, fathers with high scores on this scale were nearly five times as likely as low-scoring fathers to have children within the normal range on the Mental Developmental Index of the Bayley Scales of Infant Development (Shannon, Tamis-LeMonda, London, & Cabrera, 2002).

Parke and colleagues (2004) reviewed a number of studies linking fathers' more or less sensitive play with their children's affect management

skills. They concluded that "being able to read a play partner's emotional signals and to send clear emotional cues is critical for successfully sustaining ongoing play activities. These skills allow partners to modulate their playful behavior so that neither becomes overly aroused or too understimulated. ... Father–child play may be a particularly important context because its range of excitement and arousal is higher than in the more modulated mother–child play" (p. 315). Fathers' sensitivity during play, as well as fathers' responsiveness and appropriate teaching behavior, supports toddlers' secure exploration and ability to profit from sensitive, didactic, and challenging interactions.

In sum, young children who are secure in their attachment relationship with their mothers and/or fathers have longer attention spans and are more affectively positive during free play. They exhibit greater curiosity and more autonomous exploration. They also show less frustration in problem-solving situations and are more enthusiastic. In contrast, children who are insecure about the availability and support of their attachment figures are more readily frustrated, more negativistic, less eager to explore, and less likely to play with high concentration.

Secure Exploration of Cognitive Challenges in Childhood and Adolescence

In this section, we consider the importance of child–parent interactions and attachment in predicting academic competence. Children's competence in mastering classroom academic tasks reflects the extent to which basic task-related skills such as attention, conceptual development, communication skills, and reasoning emerge from, and remain embedded within, a matrix of interactions with caregivers and other adults (Pianta, Hamre, & Stuhlman, 2003). Enjoying the challenge, being motivated to learn, tolerating frustration and sometimes boredom, and developing appropriate social skills all correspond to our concept of secure exploration in school-age children.

Several studies suggest that mothers' sensitivity and support of their children can enhance early school achievement through enhancing the learning-related skills that children bring to the classroom. In a NICHD (in press) study, for example, the association between stimulating and sensitive care in the family and in the child care environment on the one hand, and individual differences in attention and memory (but not planning in first grade) on the other hand, was supported. At least two more studies provided evidence that child–mother attachment quality is associated with academic performance during later developmental periods (Moss & St.-Laurent, 2001; Teo, Carlson, Mathieu, Egeland, & Sroufe, 1996). In the Minnesota study of children born into poverty, performing well at school (particularly in mathematics and reading) was related both to caregiver sensitivity and cooperation when the children were 6 months old, and to stable infant–mother attachment security. Furthermore, quality of the home environment when the children entered school consistently predicted achievement scores (Teo et al., 1996; see also Sroufe et al., 2005a).

Moss and St.-Laurent (2001) assessed patterns of attachment to mothers in 6-year-olds, along with other affective qualities of child–mother interaction, and related them to mastery motivation and academic performance at age 8. Securely attached children had higher scores than their insecure peers on cognitive engagement, communication, and mastery motivation. Children showing the insecure-disorganized pattern evidenced by high controlling behavior were at greatest risk for school underachievement, with the poorest performance on all measures except mastery motivation. The results of this study are concordant with our concept of secure exploration, which includes cognitive engagement and communication skills, but not mastery motivation.

A special test for secure exploration, or appropriate behavioral and emotional organization during a complex problem-solving task, was given to adolescents whose attachment states of mind had been assessed with the AAI (Zimmermann, Maier, Winter, & Grossmann, 2001). The task was a computer simulation of ecological conditions in a fictitious Third World country (the "Moro" country game devised by Doerner & Wearing, 1995). Due to many discordant subgoals and a large number of interconnected variables, the task was complex and not transparent to the study participants. Inherent in the program were catastrophes that either were responses to "inappropriate" decisions made by a participant or "just happened" independently of his or her actions.

Participants were asked to rate their emotional states on scales four times during the session—before the task, during Phase I, during Phase II, and after the simulation. An interesting interaction was noted: If insecure adolescents rated themselves high on negative emotions (e.g., anger, disappointment, and annoyance) during Phase II, their behavior became more erratic and less thoughtful, leading to more catastrophes. The

opposite pattern was observed in secure adolescents: If they rated themselves high on negative emotions, they slowed down, thought more about the consequences of their actions, and became more careful, resulting in fewer catastrophes. Thus, especially in conditions of high levels of stress or anxiety, a secure attachment representation of adolescents was closely related to secure, circumspect exploration.

Relatively few research groups have included the quality of child–father relationships in studies of the determinants of academic performance or achievement. The first such study was conducted by Radin (1982), who found a positive correlation between the degree of father involvement and verbal intelligence scores for both boys and girls. However, the quality of paternal involvement was not specified. The NICHD Study of Early Child Care and Youth Development (2004) included ratings of fathers' sensitive support of autonomy during interactions with their children at age 54 months. Controlling for mothers' sensitive support for autonomy, and for boys' and girls' reading and mathematics achievement at 54 months, this study found that fathers' sensitive support for autonomy had a significant and unique effect on children's achievement, over and above the mothers' sensitive support for autonomy, but only for boys. This effect was mediated by higher self-reliance in boys at first grade and greater increases in self-reliance from first to third grade (NICHD, in press).

During middle childhood, paternal involvement in children's school performance, in both single-father and two-parent families, was found to be associated with children's greater academic achievement and enjoyment of school (Nord, Brimhall, & West, 1997). Seginer (1985) examined the contributions made to Israeli adolescents' scholastic achievement by perceived quality of relationships with and closeness to fathers and mothers. She used two relationship measures: perceived similarity to each parent and emotional closeness to each parent. Results showed that perceived similarity to fathers related to females' academic performance, whereas emotional closeness to fathers was negatively related to males' academic performance. Perceived relationship to mothers was not found to be related to academic performance in this study. Based on their review of research addressing fathers' differential impact on adolescent boys' and girls' attainment of developmental tasks, Shulman and Seiffge-Krenke (1997) inferred that males have a greater need for some sort of push toward independence from their fathers than do girls, but that girls also benefit from paternal and maternal support and participation. For both sexes, paternal acceptance was often combined with paternal support of adolescents' striving toward autonomy.

The children of our north German longitudinal study were visited at home when they were 16 years old (Zimmermann & Grossmann, 1997; Zimmermann, 2000). The adolescents responded to the AAI and to various other assessments, such as the Coping Questionnaire (Seiffge-Krenke, 1989). Longitudinal analyses revealed an impact of child–father relationship quality, as assessed by many different indices at several ages. The indices were a secure pattern of infant–father attachment at 18 months, a father's sensitivity during play with his toddler, and a father's secure attachment state of mind when the child was 8 years old. The composite of these indices was related to a more active and less avoiding coping style in adolescence, to higher ego resiliency, and to less anxiousness and helplessness (K. Grossmann, Grossmann, Fremmer-Bombik, Kindler, Scheuerer-Englisch, Winter, et al., 2002; Zimmermann & Grossmann, 1997). The coping styles of the 16-year-olds were not related to any of the earlier mother–child assessments, however.

Zimmermann (1994) also asked the mother, the father, and a friend of each adolescent to describe the adolescent on the California Adult Q-Set (Block, 1978), which the home visitor did as well after the visit. A set of items indicating "security of exploration" was preselected and related to qualities of early child–parent relationships. The preselected items were "Is uncomfortable with uncertainties and complexities," "Seeks reassurance from others (lacks self-confidence)," "Is productive, gets things done (regardless of speed)," "Gives up and withdraws when possible in the face of frustration and adversity," "Thinks and associates to ideas in unusual ways; has unconventional thought processes (either pathological or creative)," and "Has [a] brittle ego-defense system." The composite score of the positive poles on this dimension of an adolescent's personality was significantly related across 14 years to a father's ratings on the SCIP scale (described earlier) with his 24-month-old (K. Grossmann, Grossmann, Fremmer-Bombik, Kindler, Scheuerer-Englisch, Winter, et al., 2002). Again, the data support the importance of fathers to children's healthy self-reliance and confidence in challenging situations.

A strong indication of competent mastering of academic and vocational challenges should be an individual's level of functioning at a later stage in life. Snarey (1993) studied the educational and occupational development of children whose fathers' behavior was evaluated during their childhood and adolescence. Engaged, involved, and challenging fathers had children whose adult educational or occupational achievement was higher than that of their fathers. Furstenberg's (1976; Furstenberg & Harris, 1993) longitudinal study on the development of young unwed mothers, their children, and the fathers of those children supported Snarey's finding, even in a group at risk for developmental deficits. This 17-year follow-up of children whose teenage mothers were recruited into the study during pregnancy revealed a strong impact of father involvement: A stable and close relationship with a male figure (biological father or stepfather) in the home produced high rates of successful adjustment in early adulthood. The indices of adjustment were educational and employment attainment, as well as avoidance of teen birth, no imprisonment, and no depression. By contrast, the youth living with their biological fathers who were not as close were actually doing worse than the average for this sample (Furstenberg & Harris, 1993).

In the Minnesota longitudinal study of high-risk children, the children also experienced many permutations of fathers' residency, involvement, and number of male figures in their lives (Pierce, 2000, 2003; Sroufe & Pierce, 1999). Despite the large variations of male presence in the home, analyses showed that support from a father figure during early childhood predicted more adaptive adolescent behavior, beyond support from mothers and beyond early family disruption. Girls from stepfather homes and boys from single-mother homes during their early years showed the highest level of behavioral problems, as rated by their teachers.

In sum, the evidence supports a strong link between secure child–parent relationships—as indexed by the child's trust in the availability, support, and acceptance of the mother as well as the father—and a more pronounced eagerness to meet the challenges of autonomous exploration and a greater ability to use cognitive skills efficiently. In the next section, we extend this review to the domain of gender-role behavior.

Secure Attachment to Mothers, Supportive Fathering, and Gender-Role Behavior

When attachment researchers have included observations of children without their parents present, they have found that children's attachment security to their mothers or the mothers' caregiving quality, assessed either in infancy or concurrently, is positively related to peer competence (see Berlin, Cassidy, & Appleyard, Chapter 15, this volume, and Thompson, 2006 and Chapter 16, this volume, for reviews). Complementing these findings, Parke and colleagues (2004) have provided ample evidence for the unique contribution of fathers to children's peer competence, evaluation of their acceptance by their peers, and their social adaptation.

However, in the studies reviewed by Thompson (2006) and Parke and colleagues (2004), gender-specific differential effects of attachment or relationship quality on boys and girls were rarely reported. This lack may be justified, because attachment theory is not gender-specific. For Simpson (1999), this came as no surprise, given the roots of attachment theory in evolutionary biology. Situations posing threats to survival should have been similar for infants of both sexes. In fact, as Simpson comments, "One of the most striking features of research on attachment is the paucity of systematic sex differences ... , particularly in children" (p. 122).

The question of whether the security or insecurity of child–mother attachment or the quality of the child–father relationship affects girls differently from boys has also been explored very little (Greenberg, 1999). Some studies have found links between infant–mother attachment or maternal sensitivity and some specific outcome variables only for one gender (Cohn, 1990; Suess et al., 1992). In the NICHD study, fathers' sensitive support for autonomy of their preschool children had a significant and unique effect on boys' but not on girls' third-grade achievement (NICHD, in press). Evidence suggests that insecure child–parent relationships may be a risk factor for behavior problems—usually externalizing problems—in boys. It may also imply that secure attachment in boys protects them from acting out masculine and dominant behaviors with more vigor than is socially appropriate. However, findings for only one gender may also imply that the variety of child behaviors assessed has been too restricted for links to attachment quality to be found for the other gender. Internalizing behaviors of girls are much less often reported than externalizing behaviors as problematic by teachers.

Thought-provoking interaction effects between gender and attachment have been found in a few studies of preschool children that assessed a wide range of child behaviors. The finding that securely attached preschool boys and girls showed less gender-stereotypic behaviors than children with insecure patterns of attachment to their mothers has been reported in a British study (Turner, 1991, 1993). More aggressive, disruptive, assertive, controlling, and attention-seeking behaviors, and significantly fewer positive behaviors, were observed in insecurely attached boys than in secure boys. The teachers responded accordingly with fewer positive interactions. Insecurely attached boys received less guidance, instruction, or help, but elicited the most discipline and were least compliant with teachers' discipline. On the other hand, insecurely attached girls were overly "good girls." They showed more positive expressions, reminding the observer of appeasement behaviors, and were unassertive, compliant, and quietly observant bystanders. Teacher behaviors reflected these behaviors: Insecure girls received more help, guidance, and instruction from the teachers. In contrast, securely mother-attached girls were more self-assertive and showed leadership qualities, whereas secure boys were more cooperative and compliant than their insecure peers. Thus secure girls and boys did not differ significantly in any of the assessed behaviors or in the responses they elicited from their teachers, but insecure girls and boys differed widely. Differences in gender-stereotypic behaviors were mostly due to the behaviors of insecurely attached children.

In their study of 4½-year-old preschoolers from postdivorce families, Bretherton and her colleagues (e.g., Page & Bretherton, 2001) asked the children to complete attachment-related stories. As expected, boys generated significantly more aggressive stories than girls. But girls' and boys' story codes correlated in opposite directions with quality of maternal guidance as rated from mothers' Parental Attachment Interview (PAI results), maternal ratings of fathers' coparenting, and teacher ratings of social competence. For boys, all correlations between aggression and attachment were in the expected direction. Especially noteworthy was the fact that boys' father–child attachment themes correlated positively with maternal PAI effectiveness and firmness, father coparenting support, and teacher ratings of social competence at the preschool. In contrast, girls' father–child attachment themes were associated with ineffective maternal PAI guidance, low maternal ratings for father coparenting, and lower teacher ratings for social competence. Examining the story patterns for clarification of these unexpected findings, the authors noted that girls with high scores for father–child attachment themes also tended to enact a relatively high number of parental discord themes in long, rambling stories. They were preoccupied with divorce issues. In contrast, boys whose stories contained many father–child attachment themes tended to create coherent, to-the-point story resolutions. And boys who portrayed few father–child attachment themes tended to enact much aggression, especially unmotivated aggression by both parent and child protagonists.

Both gender differences and interactions with gender in relation to story completions were also reported by Steele and coworkers (M. Steele et al., 2003). They administered the MacArthur Story Stem Battery to 6-year-old children, and their theme scores were consolidated into three scales: nonphysical maternal discipline or limit setting; affection and other positive maternal representations; and physical aggression/punishment. The children's mothers had been interviewed with the AAI during pregnancy. In addition, mothers and children had been seen in the Strange Situation at 12 months. Analysis of variance (secure–insecure AAI by gender) showed a significant gender main effect: Boys enacted more antisocial themes, and girls more prosocial themes. In addition, there was a significant interaction between gender and prenatal AAI for prosocial themes: As expected, boys whose mothers had insecure AAIs received the lowest prosocial scores for their stories, whereas girls whose mothers had insecure AAIs received the highest prosocial scores. Boys *and* girls of mothers with secure AAIs, in contrast, had intermediate prosocial theme scores. The patterns of findings were similar when secure versus insecure patterns of attachment in 12-month Strange Situations were used in the analysis.

Together, these studies provide evidence that a secure child–mother attachment exerts an important influence on preschool children's behaviors, rendering them more flexible and less gender-stereotypic. Within the concept of secure exploration, we posit that secure attachment, implying healthy self-confidence and self-esteem, allows boys and girls to explore and enact a full range of behavioral options across gender boundaries. Of course, many other experiences also influence gender-typical behavior—such as role behaviors prescribed by a child's societal and home culture, and the extent of sex-typed interaction between the child's parents (Money & Ehrhard, 1972).

What about the influence on males of involved, caring, supportive, and dependable fathers? Do these boys and men explore more behavior patterns thought to be typical of women? In a study of a large sample of sixth graders, the children were asked to evaluate the supportive qualities of their mothers and fathers (East, 1991). Peer sociometric nominations were used to group the children into "withdrawn," "aggressive," and "sociable" groups. Children's ratings of their father–child relationships (not their mother–child relationships) revealed a significant peer group × gender interaction. Sociable girls and boys rated their father–child relationships very similarly in warmth and closeness. However, withdrawn girls and aggressive boys perceived less support in their father–child relationships than other children did.

Some studies also explored the relation between sensitive and appropriate father engagement and adolescents' professional and social development. Fathers' influence on gender-role behavior may become especially apparent in early adulthood, when young women may opt for professional careers and young men are challenged with the role of fatherhood. One study found, for example, that high paternal involvement in preschool years predicted adolescent approval of nontraditional employment patterns, and high paternal involvement in middle childhood predicted adolescent approval of nontraditional childrearing patterns (Williams, Radin, & Allegro, 1992). Other studies specified the outcome separately for women and men. Highly achieving college women who enjoyed intimate relationships and were accomplished in interpersonal skills had supportive fathers who described their daughters as intelligent, energetic, and talented, and encouraged them to use their abilities (Lozoff, 1974). Aloof and perfectionist fathers had daughters who were academically successful but incompetent in interpersonal relations, and daughters of uninvolved fathers were not achievement-oriented.

"Achieved upward mobility" (i.e., the extent to which an individual's educational or occupational achievement is higher than that of his or her father) was one of the outcome measures in Snarey's (1993) longitudinal study. Snarey analyzed the development of males and females whose fathers' behavior had been evaluated during the study participants' childhood and adolescence. The domains examined were "physical-athletic," "social-emotional," and "intellectual-academic." Age and domain-specific support were found to differ in their effects on daughters' and sons' upward mobility (see also Shulman & Seiffge-Krenke, 1997). Fathers who supported their daughters' physical-athletic development made a positive contribution to their daughters' educational upward mobility—a link not found for sons. A higher achievement motivation in women who report highly and appropriately involved fathers may be part of a broader non-gender-stereotypic orientation that emerges from valuing their fathers' behavior. Sagi (1982) obtained related findings in his study of paternal involvement in childrearing in Israel. Girls who reported at least an intermediate level of father involvement scored higher on masculinity than daughters of low-involvement fathers. Although this relation also held for boys, a ceiling effect was evident. Sagi stressed, however, that involved fathers do not eliminate the feminine tendencies of their daughters, but provide them with a masculine perspective as well.

Complementary influences of fathers on their sons' adult behavior have also been reported. Men's experiences with their fathers and their current evaluation of their early care experiences were shown to influence clearly the meaning and practices of their own fatherhood. Men who perceived their fathers as more involved in rearing them were themselves more involved in rearing their own children. This relationship was found for Israeli fathers (Sagi, 1982), U.S. fathers (Cohn et al., 1992; see also Cabrera et al., 2000, for an extended review), German fathers (K. Grossmann, Grossmann, Fremmer-Bombik, Kindler, Scheuerer-Englisch, & Zimmermann, 2002), and British fathers (H. Steele & Steele, 2005). Evidence suggests that a man's positive memories of being cared for, especially by his own father, and his positive and negative feelings as a child, contribute to his being more understanding and responsive to his own child's needs and feelings. This in turn makes him a better, more sensitive play partner for his child. Although caring for and being responsive to children are mostly thought of as female activities, well-cared-for fathers seem to develop a more gender-equitable attitude, thus expanding their behavioral repertoire to include sensitivity toward their own children.

A caring, supportive relationship with at least one reliable adult was found to foster resiliency in the well-known Kauai longitudinal study (Werner & Smith, 2001). In their 30s, the resilient men and women in the study had developed similar values, such as being highly achievement-oriented and valuing the support of a mate. However, the women in this group made more transitions into multiple life trajectories than the men. Eighty-six percent of the women were married at that point, had children, *and* worked full time, whereas only half of the men were married and had children. For the women and men who became parents, their expectations for their children differed according

to gender, although both expected high achievement. A higher proportion of mothers stressed early independence in their children, whereas a higher proportion of fathers tolerated dependence in their offspring instead of emphasizing independence.

In sum, although attachment theory does not provide gender-specific hypotheses, a growing body of work supports the idea that secure attachment to their mothers and/or a reliably supportive relationship with their fathers will allow girls and boys to explore a wider domain of behaviors than is typical for their traditional gender roles. Several studies of people ranging from preschool age to adulthood show that securely mother-attached girls and boys do not differ significantly in gender-typical behaviors or attachment story contents, whereas girls and boys with insecure attachment to their mothers conform more to stereotypic gender roles. Studies of child–father relationship quality and its influence on gender-typical behavior reveal that daughters who experience involved, caring, supportive, and encouraging fathers explore behavior patterns that were traditionally thought to be typical of men: They are more achievement-oriented and more likely to exceed their fathers' occupational status. Sons who remember caring fathers during their childhood are themselves more involved, sensitive fathers. Thus it seems that psychologically secure children can afford to be less gender-typed in their behavior, which is another sign of secure exploration.

SECURE PARENT–CHILD RELATIONSHIPS AND CHILDREN'S ADAPTATION TO GROUP SITUATIONS IN FORMAL LEARNING

In familiar, everyday situations, learned behavior is usually sufficiently adaptive. In new, unfamiliar, and challenging situations, however, the quality of a child's emotional and behavioral organization is challenged. Age-appropriate challenges for the developing child include transitions to preschool, school, and college. The child must keep attention focused on coping with the new social and mental challenges, instead of turning attention away as a result of rising emotional tension. Difficulties may include engaging in disruptive behaviors, avoiding communication, failing to enlist help, or becoming an uninvolved bystander. Such behaviors may hinder academic success in institutional group settings. There is evidence that children who have developed security of exploration through sensitive parental support are better prepared for such challenges.

Security of Exploration, Resourceful Transition, and Adaptation to Preschool and Early Schooling

Observations of children in transition to institutions of learning provide critical tests of the proposition that relationship experiences provide the foundation for a resourceful organization of relational behaviors and mental capacities that will facilitate constructive adjustment. Sroufe and colleagues (2005a) were impressed by the predictive power of attachment history when they examined children participating in a university preschool. Those who had secure histories were rated by their teachers as dramatically more resilient than those with histories of either resistant or avoidant attachment. Children "in the avoidant group showed a rather uniform lack of flexibility in adjusting their behavior and expressiveness to fit circumstances" (p. 139). In an Israeli study, both a stable history of secure child–mother attachment and the number of secure attachments within a network of early extended attachment relations (mother, father, caregiver) were associated with children's adjustment to kindergarten (Sagi-Schwartz & Aviezer, 2005). Ego resiliency, field independence, empathy, dominance, and goal-directed behaviors were all examined, and all can be interpreted as elements of secure exploration. Similar results were obtained in a Dutch study (van IJzendoorn, Sagi, & Lambermon, 1992).

Some years ago, Pianta and Harbers (1996) reviewed studies that predicted adjustment to the requirements of formal and informal learning in school from measures of child–mother interaction in problem-solving situations. They concluded, in support of the wider view of attachment, that higher-quality mother–child interactions accompanied secure, confidant exploration of the world of learning. Cox and Paley (2003) more recently advocated that studies of children's competence during formal learning should consider the broader perspective by including both mothers and fathers, if not whole families. In a German study, the security of infants' attachment to mothers and then to fathers, in that order, was reflected in children's duration of concentration, conflict management skills, and ego resiliency as rated by their preschool teachers (Suess et al., 1992). This is one of the few studies linking infant–father attachment quality as observed in the Strange Situation to competent preschool behavior.

Security of attachment to mothers as a protective factor against the development of behavioral problems in preschool and primary grades has been amply demonstrated (see Thompson, Chapter 16, this volume). The role of fathers in this process has been studied much less (Parke et al., 2004; Phares, 1996). Low paternal play sensitivity during toddlerhood was found to be a reliable predictor of teacher-rated behavioral problems in preschoolers and early school-age children (K. Grossmann, Grossmann, Fremmer-Bombik, Kindler, Scheuerer-Englisch, Winter, et al., 2002; NICHD Early Child Care Research Network, 2004). In addition, a Belgian longitudinal study explored qualities of child–mother and child–father attachment representations (assessed by attachment story completion tasks) as predictors of later behavioral adaptation in school. The relative predictive power of the representations of attachment with each parent differed according to the domain of child functioning. Preschool children's positive self-image was better predicted by child–mother attachment representations, whereas anxious/withdrawn behavioral problems were better predicted by child–father attachment representations (Verschueren & Marcoen, 1999). At age 9, the quality of children's representations of attachment to fathers proved even more influential in the children's peer nominations as "shy/withdrawn," same-sex peer acceptance, and peer sociometric ratings (Verschueren & Marcoen, 2003, 2005).

For a competent transition to formal schooling, the quality of a child's relationships with both parents seems to be important. The quality of preschool father–child interaction uniquely predicts a child's social adjustment in the classroom, even when mother–child interaction is also used as a predictor (NICHD Early Child Care Research Network, 2004). The NICHD study explored mothers' and fathers' parenting behaviors and beliefs as predictors of their children's social adjustment during the transition to school. Children's social skills with peers and teachers, and their behavioral regulation during preschool and the first two school grades, were related to parental sensitivity during problem-solving situations. The most competent and least problematic children, from the teachers' viewpoint, were those whose fathers were sensitive and supportive of their children's autonomy, those whose mothers' parenting beliefs supported self-directed child behavior, and those whose parents maintained an emotionally intimate relationship. Together with other studies, this one supports the notion that child–father interactions are not simply redundant with child–mother interactions, but offer children unique and enriching experiences (Cowan & Cowan, 2005).

Relationship Qualities with Both Parents and Adaptive Functioning in School and College

There is growing research interest in the association between attachment (however it may be assessed) and different indices of scholastic achievement throughout the school years, including college (Bernier, Larose, Boivin, & Soucy, 2004; Moss & St.-Laurent, 2001; Teo et al., 1996).[2] By first grade, children have assumed the full role of students, with a new set of supervisors (their teachers and principals), a new set of peers, and a new set of role obligations (Entwisle & Alexander, 1999). The way in which children fulfill the student role in these early school years is an important predictor of their future academic and behavioral adjustment. For this reason, early experiences at home and current mental models of the supportiveness of close relationships are increasingly seen as contributors during this important period, which involves the consolidation of the important cognitive, literacy, and social skills that form the foundation for current and later academic functioning.

In early adolescence, adjustment to school in Israel is linked with representations of relationships, as well as with IQ and self-perceived scholastic competence (Sagi-Schwartz & Aviezer, 2005). Beyond these concurrently assessed variables and life event control variables (parental reports of marital relationships, extent of exposure to collective sleeping in early childhood), infant–mother attachment contributed significantly to the explained variance in verbal skills and curiosity, as well as in emotional maturity (Aviezer, Sagi, Resnick, & Gini, 2002). In a British study, the quality of the child–father relationship as perceived by preschool and young school-age children contributed uniquely to friendship and adjustment, as did the quality of child–mother and child–sibling relationships (Sturgess, Dunn, & Davies, 2001).

A longitudinal study of school children from 7 to 15 years of age in Reykjavik, Iceland, investigated the link between children's attachment representations on the one hand and their school behavior and academic competence on the other (Jacobsen & Hofmann, 1997). Security of attachment representation was significantly associated

with attention and participation at ages 9 and 15; security about self at ages 9, 12, and 15; and grade point average (GPA) at ages 7, 9, 12, and 15. The relationship of attachment representations to GPA at age 15 was partially mediated by prior attention and participation in school, but not completely. An Israeli study by Granot and Mayseless (2001) provided additional support: They assessed children's representations of attachment concurrently, and found that secure children were perceived by their teachers to be better adjusted than insecure children in the scholastic, emotional, social, and behavioral domains. These children were also rated by their peers as being higher in social status.

Besides children's representations of attachment, observed support from both parents affected early achievement in school (NICHD, in press). Mothers' sensitive support for autonomy uniquely predicted both boys' and girls' reading and mathematics achievement in third grade, after achievement in these areas at age 54 months was controlled for. The effect was mediated by the level of self-reliance the children showed in first- and third-grade classrooms. This result confirmed earlier findings indicating that mothers' sensitivity and support of their children enhanced their early school achievement, through the mediation of the children's learning-related skills (Pianta & Harbers, 1996). In addition, the study showed that fathers' preschool sensitive support for autonomy, over and above the mothers' sensitive support for autonomy, had a significant and unique effect on children's third-grade achievement, but only for boys. The authors suggested that the sensitive support of fathers during transition to school may have been particularly important for boys, who were initially lower in self-reliance.

Transition to college is a further challenge that requires adaptation to a new world of learning and may be facilitated by secure exploration. A Canadian longitudinal study of adjustment to college explored the process, linking attachment state of mind (assessed via the AAI) to academic achievement, students' learning disposition, and academic performance during the college transition (Bernier et al., 2004; Larose & Bernier, 2001; Larose, Bernier, & Tarabulsy, 2005; Larose & Boivin, 1998). Learning disposition was assessed by a questionnaire tapping students' beliefs, emotional reactions, and behaviors in learning situations. Learning dispositions of autonomous students (i.e., students with a secure attachment state of mind) were less negatively affected by the college transition than were those of nonauto-nomous students. Autonomous students showed better learning dispositions throughout the transition, and they were less likely than dismissing and preoccupied students to experience a decrease in these dispositions between the end of high school and their first year of college. The mediating factors were anxiousness, quality of attention, willingness to seek help, examination preparation, and giving priority to studies. In an exploratory analysis, the authors found that these self-reported components of learning varied as a function of type of insecurity. Preoccupied students experienced more fear of failure in the middle of the first semester of college than at the end of high school, felt less comfortable seeking help from teachers, and gave less priority to their studies. In addition, preoccupied students who left home for college reported having a more negative relationship with their parents and experienced more family-related stress (Bernier, Larose, & Whipple, 2005). Feeling a lack of support from their attachment figures while being separated from them seemed to undermine the security of their exploration of the social and academic challenges in the new college situation. In contrast, dismissing students experienced a decrease in their examination preparation and in their quality of attention during the same period of time. As to academic performance, students with a dismissing attachment state of mind obtained the lowest average grades in college. This association was mediated by changes in quality of attention during the transition.

In discussing the conceptual implications of their results, Larose and colleagues draw on the concept of secure exploration as developed by us (K. E. Grossmann et al., 1999), by Moss and St. Laurent (2001), and by Thompson, Easterbrooks, and Padilla-Walker (2003): "Security of attachment in late adolescence appears to favor *security of exploration* by providing the student with the emotional, cognitive, and behavioral resources that have been shown to favor college success" (Larose et al., 2005, p. 287; emphasis added).

ADDITIONAL CONSIDERATIONS AND CONCLUSIONS

This last section addresses three issues: (1) the underemphasized effects of fathers on children's relationships with close friends and siblings; (2) the influence of parent–child relationships during infancy, childhood, and adolescence on young adults' attachment and partnership representations

in our north German longitudinal study; and (3) the present status of the wider view of attachment, including security of exploration and the unique contributions of mothers and fathers to general psychological security.

Fathers' Influence on Children's Relationships with Special Friends and Siblings

A far-reaching impact of early, and probably ongoing, infant–father relationships on relationships with siblings and friends was demonstrated in the London Parent–Child Project (H. Steele & Steele, 2005). In the 11-year follow-up phase of the research, children were interviewed about their relationships with siblings and best friends. The 11-year-olds who gave the most convincing or "truthful" accounts of their positive and negative views of themselves and others were likely to have mothers whose attachment state of mind during pregnancy (assessed via the AAI) was judged to be secure-autonomous. In addition, but for boys only, they were likely to have fathers whose attachment state of mind before the birth of the child were judged secure-autonomous. Notably, the study found long-term connections between the expectant fathers' AAIs and their daughters' and sons' interviews only in the domain of relations with siblings and friends (H. Steele, Steele, & Fonagy, 1996). The most coherent and resourceful accounts of how social disagreements were negotiated and resolved came from 11-year-olds whose fathers had provided secure-autonomous AAIs more than 11 years before. The authors supposed, however, that this longitudinal link was probably based on positive, ongoing father–child relationships.

In our north German longitudinal study, adolescents' friendship concepts were significantly related to the quality of their early interactive play with their fathers (K. Grossmann, 2001; K. Grossmann & Grossmann, 2004). The 16-year-olds were interviewed about their friendships. The maturity of their conception of friendship was rated in terms of such issues as integration into peer groups in and outside of school, trust in at least one friend, conflict management, social anxiety, and hostile attributional bias (Zimmermann & Grossmann, 1995). Early paternal play sensitivity (assessed with the SCIP scale, described earlier) was significantly associated with adolescents' attachment state of mind, which in turn was strongly related to adolescents' friendship concepts. Still, a specific analysis revealed a significant relation between fathers' play sensitivity when the now-adolescents were 2 years old and the adolescents' conception of friendship, even after we accounted statistically for the adolescents' attachment state of mind.

Earlier, Volling and Belsky's study (1992) provided evidence for the proposition that the quality of the child–father relationship during play is more important than patterns of infant–father attachment in the Strange Situation. They found no main effect of infant–father attachment on quality of sibling interaction 5 years later. Instead, the predictive utility of the father–child relationship became more apparent by the time a child was 3 years of age, and when the quality of father–child interaction was observed during teaching and free-play episodes. This longitudinal study also investigated sibling interactions across 5 years. Conflict and aggression between a 6-year-old and his or her younger sibling were related to an insecure pattern of attachment to the mother in infancy and to less supportive mothering during the preschool period. In addition, the father's more pronounced affection toward the younger sibling also contributed to more sibling conflict, whereas the father's observed facilitative and supportive behavior toward the firstborn was reflected in more prosocial sibling interactions.

The Impact of Parent–Child Interactions from Infancy through Adolescence on Attachment and Partnership Representations in Young Adulthood

The young adults in our studies (22 years old in the north German study, 20 years old in the south German study) responded to the AAI (see Hesse, Chapter 25, this volume) and to the Current Relationship Interview (Crowell & Owens, 1996) regarding their best and most stable partnership or intimate relationship (K. E. Grossmann, Grossmann, Winter, & Zimmermann, 2002). In both of our studies of low-risk samples, we failed to find a one-to-one correspondence between infant patterns of organized attachment in the Strange Situation and later attachment or partnership representations. But there were connections through more diverse pathways. For longitudinal analyses in the north German study, we combined attachment assessments with assessments of appropriate parental stimulation (for each parent separately). A composite index of mother–child as well as father–child relationship quality was formed for infancy (0–3 years), childhood (5–10 years), and adolescence (16 years).

The children's attachment and exploratory experiences with their mothers and fathers throughout their years of immaturity were found to be the major influences on the young adults' attachment states of mind and their partnership representations (K. Grossmann et al., 2005; Stoecker, Strasser, & Winter, 2003). Using a variance decomposition analysis (Amato, 1996), we determined that mothers' and fathers' sensitive support during infancy, childhood, and adolescence contributed uniquely and jointly to offspring's attachment and partnership representations as young adults. The findings suggest that psychological security in early adulthood depends on a long history of secure emotional organization *and* freedom to explore and evaluate past and present attachment relationships with parents and/or partners. (See also Simpson, Collins, Tran, & Haydon, 2007.)

Present Status of the Wider View of Attachment

The wider view of attachment is based on (1) the interdependence of the attachment and exploration behavioral systems (Bowlby, 1969/1982); (2) Bowlby's (1969/1982) premise that exploration, competent play, and mastery of the environment are facilitated when a child feels secure in the relationship with the mother, and a little later with the father; and (3) empirical support for these ideas in studies in multiple cultures (K. E. Grossmann & Grossmann, 2005). We propose that security eventually depends on both attachment security and safe familiarity with the real world. Finding a large number of studies that provide support for this broader view, we advocate the concept of "psychological security," which includes both security of attachment and security of exploration, as emerging from sensitive support from both mother and father.

We define "secure exploration" as confident, attentive, eager, and resourceful exploration of materials or tasks, especially in the face of disappointment. Secure exploration implies a social orientation, particularly when help is needed. Here we have reviewed studies of the precursors of secure exploration. The empirical link between secure attachment and secure exploration provides the basis for a concept of psychological security. Maternal sensitivity and cooperation during play, as well as quality of child–mother attachment, are linked with secure exploration, even in a traditional society such as the Trobrianders of Papua New Guinea (K. E. Grossmann, Grossmann, & Keppler, 2005; Liegel, 2001). There is a unique contribution of the quality of fathers' role as a play partner, which adds to the effects of security of attachment to mothers. Fathers' play sensitivity, rather than security of infant–father attachment as assessed in the Strange Situation, is an important predictor of a child's long-term psychological security. In addition, studies of children, adolescents, and young adults provide ample evidence that secure child–mother attachment and supportive fathering allow boys and girls the liberty to challenge the boundaries of narrow gender stereotypes.

Psychological security seems to facilitate secure exploration in challenging new situations by providing a child with the needed emotional, cognitive, and behavioral resources. This in turn results in resourceful transitions and adaptation to preschool, school, and eventually college. Longitudinal data also point to the importance of the quality of the child–father relationship for a child's or adolescent's ability to form close relationships; again, this is in addition to the mother's influence, especially when it comes to a son's readiness to be an involved, supportive father.

The quality of representations of attachment and partnership at age 22 is similarly rooted in attachment experiences with mother *and* father, their respect for the child, and their support of the child's striving for competence. These roots can be traced back to the child's first 3 years of life. Early experiences influence later experiences and mental representation measures, in line with attachment theory (Bowlby, 1979).

In terms of the proposed wider view of attachment and exploration, mothers *and* fathers both contribute to the lengthy, complex developmental process of achieving psychological security or insecurity. Security of child–mother attachment involves tender, loving care; comfort and consolation; and external help with emotion regulation, particularly during times of threat or stress. This security, however, does not suffice to create psychological security in children, who must explore to gain knowledge and skills for successful psychological and cultural adjustment. Security in attachment relationships needs to be supplemented by the equally necessary security of exploration, based on sensitive support for exploration from both mother and father. With secure exploration, a person can remain open more often and for longer periods to new challenges, experiences, communications, and reflections, resulting in healthy psychological adjustment. A psychologically secure person, in contrast to an insecure person, is able to respond appropriately to a wider variety of challenging situations and emotional states, while keeping the goal of cooperative partnership in mind.

ACKNOWLEDGMENTS

Throughout the more exploratory parts of our longitudinal research, we received generous financial support from the Koehler Foundation. David George provided much help on an early draft of this chapter, and we are grateful for the helpful comments from Jude Cassidy and Phillip R. Shaver.

NOTES

1. We are grateful to Sir Richard Bowlby for suggesting that we take a fresh look at the section on rhesus monkey fathers in Blum's (2002) book *Love at Goon Park*.
2. We acknowledge that social skills in relating to teachers and peers constitute the most important resources for successful adjustment to institutions of learning, but a review of the association between quality of parental care, support, and encouragement on the one hand and social skills on the other is beyond the scope of this chapter.

REFERENCES

Ainsworth, M. D. S. (1967). *Infancy in Uganda: Infant care and the growth of love*. Baltimore: Johns Hopkins University Press.
Ainsworth, M. D. S. (1990). Some considerations regarding theory and assessment relevant to attachment beyond infancy. In M. T. Greenberg, D. Cicchetti, & E. M. Cummings (Eds.), *Attachment in the preschool years: Theory, research, and intervention* (pp. 463–488). Chicago: University of Chicago Press.
Ainsworth, M. D. S., Blehar, M. C., Waters, E., & Wall, S. (1978). *Patterns of attachment: A psychological study of the Strange Situation*. Hillsdale, NJ: Erlbaum.
Ainsworth, M. D. S., & Bowlby, J. (1991). An ethological approach to personality development. *American Psychologist, 46,* 333–341
Amato, P. R. (1996). More than money?: Men's contributions to their children's lives. In A. Booth & A. C. Crouter (Eds.), *Men in families: When do they get involved? What difference does it make?* (pp. 241–278). Mahwah, NJ: Erlbaum.
Arend, R. (1984). *Preschoolers' competence in a barrier situation: Patterns of adaptation and their precursors in infancy*. Unpublished doctoral dissertation, University of Minnesota.
Arend, R., Gove, F. L., & Sroufe, L. A. (1979). Continuity of individual adaptation from infancy to kindergarten: A predictive study of ego-resiliency and curiosity of preschoolers. *Child Development, 50,* 950–959.
Aviezer, O., Sagi, A., Resnick, G., & Gini, M. (2002). School competence in young adolescence: Links to early attachment relationships beyond concurrent self-perceived competence and representations of re-

lationships. *International Journal of Behavioral Development*, *26*, 397–409.

Belsky, J., & Fearon, R. M. P. (2002). Infant–mother attachment security, contextual risk, and early development: A moderational analysis. *Development and Psychopathology*, *14*, 293–310.

Belsky, J., Garduque, L., & Hrncir, E. (1984). Assessing performance, competence, and executive capacity in infant play: Relations to home environment and security of attachment. *Developmental Psychology*, *20*, 406–417.

Bernier, A., Larose, S., Boivin, M., & Soucy, N. (2004). Attachment state of mind: Implications for adjustment and academic counseling in college. *Journal of Adolescent Research*, *19*, 783–806.

Bernier, A., Larose, S., & Whipple, N. (2005). Leaving home for college: A potentially stressful event for adolescents with preoccupied attachment patterns. *Attachment and Human Development*, *7*, 171–185.

Block, J. (1978). *The Q-sort method in personality assessment and psychiatric research* (2nd ed.). Palo Alto, CA: Consulting Psychologists Press.

Blum, D. (2002). *Love at Goon Park: Harry Harlow and the science of affection*. Cambridge, MA: Perseus.

Bowlby, J. (1969/1982). *Attachment and loss: Vol. 1. Attachment*. New York: Basic Books.

Bowlby, J. (1979). *The making and breaking of affectional bonds*. London: Tavistock/Routledge.

Braungart-Rieker, J., Garwood, M. M., Powers, B. P., & Wang, X. (2001). Parental sensitivity, infant affect, and affect regulation: Predictors of later attachment. *Child Development*, *72*, 252–270.

Bus, A. G., Belsky, J., van IJzendoorn, M. H., & Crnic, K. (1997). Attachment and bookreading patterns: A study of mothers, fathers, and their toddlers. *Early Childhood Quarterly*, *12*, 81–98.

Cabrera, N. J., Tamis-LeMonda, C. S., Bradley, R. H., Hofferth, S., & Lamb, M. E. (2000). Fatherhood in the twenty-first century. *Child Development*, *71*, 127–136.

Cohn, D. A. (1990). Child–mother attachment of six-year-olds and social competence in school. *Child Development*, *61*, 152–162.

Cohn, D. A., Cowan, P. A., Cowan, C. P., & Pearson, J. (1992). Mothers' and fathers' working models of childhood attachment relationships, parenting styles, and child behavior. *Development and Psychopathology*, *4*, 417–431.

Cowan, P. A., & Cowan, C. P. (2005). Five-domain models: Putting it all together. In P. A. Cowan, C. P. Cowan, J. C. Ablow, V. K. Johnson, & J. R. Measelle (Eds.), *The family context of parenting in children's adaptation to elementary school* (pp. 315–334). Mahwah, NJ: Erlbaum.

Cox, M., & Paley, B. (2003). Understanding families as systems. *Current Directions in Psychological Science*, *12*, 193–196.

Cox, M., Paley, B., & Towe, N. (2003). *Fathers' and mothers' supportive involvement and their toddlers' enthusiastic exploration: A family perspective*. Paper presented at the biennial meeting of the Society for Research in Child Development, Tampa, FL.

Crowell, J., & Owens, G. (1996). *Current relationship interview and scoring system*. Unpublished manuscript, State University of New York at Stony Brook.

Crowell, J., & Waters, E. (2005). Attachment representations, secure base behavior, and the evolution of adult relationships: The Stony Brook Adult Relationship Project. In K. E. Grossmann, K. Grossmann, & E. Waters (Eds.), *Attachment from infancy to adulthood: The major longitudinal studies* (pp. 223–244). New York: Guilford Press.

Dodge, K. A., Pettit, G. S., McClaskey, C. L., & Brown, M. M. (1986). Social competence in children. *Monographs of the Society for Research in Child Development*, *51*(2, Serial No. 213), 1–80.

Doerner, D., & Wearing, A. J. (1995). Complex problem solving: Towards a (computer simulated) theory. In P. A. French & J. Funke (Eds.), *Complex problem solving: The European perspective* (pp. 65–99). Hillsdale, NJ: Erlbaum.

Duke University. (2008, February 7). Baboon dads have surprising influence on daughters' fitness. *ScienceDaily*. Retrieved February 8, 2008, from *www.sciencedaily.com/releases/2008/02/080204172226.htm*

East, P. L. (1991). The parent–child relationships of withdrawn, aggressive, and sociable children: Child and parent perspectives. *Merrill–Palmer Quarterly*, *37*, 423–443.

Easterbrooks, M. A., & Goldberg, W. A. (1984). Toddler development in the family: Impact of father involvement and parenting characteristics. *Child Development*, *55*, 740–752.

Easterbrooks, M. A., & Goldberg, W. A. (1990). Security of toddler–parent attachment. In M. T. Greenberg, D. Cicchetti, & M. E. Cummings (Eds.), *Attachment in the preschool years* (pp. 221–244). Chicago: University of Chicago Press.

Entwisle, D. R., & Alexander, K. L. (1999). Early schooling and social stratification. In R. C. Pianta & M. J. Cox (Eds.), *The transition to kindergarten* (pp. 13–38). Baltimore: Brookes.

Fish, M. (2004). Attachment in infancy and preschool in low socioeconomic status rural Appalachian children: Stability and change in relations to preschool and kindergarten competence. *Development and Psychopathology*, *16*, 293–312.

Frodi, A., Bridges, L., & Grolnick, W. (1985). Correlates of mastery related behavior: A short term longitudinal study. *Child Development*, *56*, 1291–1298.

Furstenberg, F. F. (1976). *Unplanned parenthood*. New York: Free Press.

Furstenberg, F. F., & Harris, F. M. (1993). When and why fathers matter: Impacts of father involvement on the children of adolescent mothers. In R. I. Lerman & T. J. Ooms (Eds.), *Young unwed fathers* (pp. 150–176). Philadelphia: Temple University Press.

Granot, D., & Mayseless, O. (2001). Attachment security and adjustment to school in middle childhood. *International Journal of Behavioral Development*, *25*, 530–541.

Greenberg, M. T. (1999). Attachment and psychopathology in childhood. In J. Cassidy & P. R. Shaver (Eds.), Handbook of attachment: Theory, research, and clinical applications (pp. 469–496). New York: Guilford Press.

Grolnick, W. S., Deci, E. L., & Ryan, R. M. (1997). Internalization within the family: The self-determination theory perspective. In J. E. Grusec & L. Kuczynski (Eds.), Parenting and children's internalization of values (pp. 135–161). New York: Wiley.

Grossmann, K. (2001). Child–father attachment relationship: Quality of joint play as the pivotal variable in a 22-year longitudinal study of attachment development. Paper presented at the University of Jyväskylä, Jyväskylä, Finland.

Grossmann, K., & Grossmann, K. E. (1991). Newborn behavior, early parenting quality, and later toddler–parent relationships in a group of German infants. In J. K. Nugent, B. M. Lester, & T. B. Brazelton (Eds.), The cultural context of infancy (Vol. 2, pp. 3–38). Norwood, NJ: Ablex.

Grossmann, K., & Grossmann, K. E. (2004). Bindungen: Das Gefüge psychischer Sicherheit [Attachment: The composition of psychological security]. Stuttgart: Klett-Cotta.

Grossmann, K., Grossmann, K. E., Fremmer-Bombik, E., Kindler, H., Scheuerer-Englisch, H., Winter, M., et al. (2002). Väter und ihre Kinder: Die "andere" Bindung und ihre längsschnittliche Bedeutung für die Bindungsentwicklung, das Selbstvertrauen und die soziale Entwicklung des Kindes [Fathers and their children: A different attachment and its longitudinal significance for the child's attachment development, self-reliance, and social development]. In K. Steinhardt, W. Datler, & J. Gstach (Eds.), Die Bedeutung des Vaters in der frühen Kindheit [The significance of the father in early childhood] (pp. 43–72). Gießen, Germany: Psychosozial Verlag.

Grossmann, K., Grossmann, K. E., Fremmer-Bombik, E., Kindler, H., Scheuerer-Englisch, H., & Zimmermann, P. (2002). The uniqueness of the child–father attachment relationship: Fathers' sensitive and challenging play as the pivotal variable in a 16-year longitudinal study. Social Development, 11, 307–331.

Grossmann, K., Grossmann, K. E., & Kindler, H. (2005). Early care and the roots of attachment and partnership representation in the Bielefeld and Regensburg longitudinal studies. In K. E. Grossmann, K. Grossmann, & E. Waters (Eds.), Attachment from infancy to adulthood: The major longitudinal studies (pp. 98–136). New York: Guilford Press.

Grossmann, K. E., & Grossmann, K. (2005). Universality of human social attachment as an adaptive process. In C. S. Carter, L. Ahnert, K. E. Grossmann, S. B. Hrdy, M. E. Lamb, S. W. Porges, et al. (Eds.), Attachment and bonding: A new synthesis (pp. 199–229). Cambridge; MA: MIT Press.

Grossmann, K. E., Grossmann, K., & Keppler, A. (2005). Universal and culturally specific aspects of human behavior: The case of attachment. In W. Friedlmeier, P.

Chakkarath, & B. Schwarz (Eds.), Culture and human development: The importance of cross-cultural research to the social sciences (pp. 75–97). Hove, UK: Psychology Press.

Grossmann, K. E., Grossmann, K., & Waters, E. (Eds.). (2005). Attachment from infancy to adulthood: The major longitudinal studies. New York: Guilford Press.

Grossmann, K. E., Grossmann, K., Winter, M., & Zimmermann, P. (2002). Attachment relationships and appraisal of partnership: From early experience of sensitive support to later relationship representation. In L. Pulkkinen & A. Caspi (Eds.), Paths to successful development (pp. 73–105). Cambridge, UK: Cambridge University Press.

Grossmann, K. E., Grossmann, K., & Zimmermann, P. (1999). A wider view of attachment and exploration: Stability and change during the years of immaturity. In J. Cassidy & P. R. Shaver (Eds.), Handbook of attachment: Theory, research, and clinical applications (pp. 760–786). New York: Guilford Press.

Grossmann, K. E., Scheuerer-Englisch, H., & Loher, I. (1991). Die Entwicklung emotionaler Organisation und ihre Beziehung zum intelligenten Handeln [The development of emotional organization and its relationship to intelligent behavior]. In F. J. Mönks & G. Lehwald (Eds.), Neugier, Erkundung und Begabung bei Kleinkindern [Curiosity, exploration, and talent in young children] (pp. 66–76). München: Ernst Reinhardt Verlag.

Grossmann, K. E., & Volkmer, J. J. (1984). Fathers' presence during birth of their infants and paternal involvement. International Journal of Behavioral Development, 7, 157–165.

Harlow, H. F., Harlow, M. K., & Suomi, S. J. (1971). From thought to therapy: Lessons learned from a primate laboratory. American Scientist, 59, 538–549.

Harlow, H. F., & Mears, C. (1979). The human model: Primate perspectives. New York: Wiley.

Hinde, R. A. (2005). Ethology and attachment theory. In K. E. Grossmann, K. Grossmann, & E. Waters (Eds.), Attachment from infancy to adulthood: The major longitudinal studies (pp. 1–12). New York: Guilford Press.

Horn, W. F. (2000). Fathering infants. In J. D. Osofsky & H. E. Fitzgerald (Eds.), WAIMH handbook of infant mental health: Vol. 3. Parenting and child care (pp. 270–297). New York: Wiley.

Jacobsen, T., & Hofmann, V. (1997). Children's attachment representations: Longitudinal relations to school behavior and academic competency in middle childhood and adolescence. Developmental Psychology, 33, 703–710.

Kindler, H., & Grossmann, K. (2004). Vater–Kind-Bindung und die Rolle der Väter in den ersten Lebensjahren ihrer Kinder [Father–child attachment and the role of the father in their children's first years of life]. In L. Ahnert (Ed.), Frühe Bindung: Entstehung und Entwicklung [Early attachments: Their origins and development] (pp. 240–255). München, Germany: E. Reinhardt Verlag.

Lamb, M. E. (Ed.). (1986). The father's role: Applied perspectives. New York: Wiley.

Lamb M. E. (2002). Infant–father attachments and their impact on child development. In C. S. Tamis-LeMonda & N. Cabrera (Eds.), *Handbook of father involvement: Multidisciplinary perspectives* (pp. 93–117). Mahwah, NJ: Erlbaum.

Lamb, M. E., & Lewis, C. (2004). The development and significance of father–child relationships in two-parent families. In M. E. Lamb (Ed.), *The role of the father in child development* (4th ed., pp. 272–306). Hoboken, NJ: Wiley.

Larose, S., & Bernier, A. (2001). Social support processes: Mediators of attachment state of mind and adjustment in late adolescence. *Attachment and Human Development, 3,* 96–120.

Larose, S., Bernier, A., & Tarabulsy, G. M. (2005). Attachment state of mind, learning dispositions, and academic performance during the college transition. *Developmental Psychology, 41,* 281–289.

Larose, S., & Boivin, M. (1998). Attachment to parents, social support, expectations, and socioemotional adjustment during the high school–college transition. *Journal of Research on Adolescence, 8,* 1–27.

Liegel, M. (2001). *Beobachtungen zum Explorations und Bindungsverhalten Ein bis Dreijähriger Trobriand Kinder* [*Observations of exploratory and attachment behaviors of one- to three-year-old Trobriand children*]. Unpublished thesis, Universität Regensburg, Regensburg, Germany.

Lorenz, K. (1977). *Behind the mirror: A search for a natural history of human knowledge.* New York: Harcourt Brace Jovanovich.

Lozoff, M. M. (1974). Fathers and autonomy in women. In R. B. Kundsin (Ed.), *Women and success* (pp. 103–109). New York: Morrow.

Luetkenhaus, P., Grossmann, K. E., & Grossmann, K. (1985). Infant–mother attachment at twelve months and style of interaction with a stranger at the age of three years. *Child Development, 56,* 1538–1542.

Main, M. (1983). Exploration, play, and cognitive functioning related to infant–mother attachment. *Infant Behavior and Development, 6,* 167–174.

Main, M., Hesse, E., & Kaplan, N. (2005). Predictability of attachment behavior and representational processes at 1, 6, and 19 years of age: The Berkeley longitudinal study. In K. E. Grossmann, K. Grossmann, & E. Waters (Eds.), *Attachment from infancy to adulthood: The major longitudinal studies* (pp. 245–304). New York: Guilford Press.

Matas, L., Arend, R., & Sroufe, L. A. (1978). Continuity of adaptation in the second year: The relationship between quality of attachment and later competence. *Child Development, 49,* 547–556.

McElwain, N. L., Cox, M. J., Burchinal, M. R., & Macfie, J. (2003). Differentiating among insecure mother–infant attachment classifications: A focus on child–friend interaction and exploration during solitary play at 36 months. *Attachment and Human Development, 5,* 136–164.

Meins, E., Fernyhough, C., Russell, J., & Clark-Carter, D. (1998). Security of attachment as a predictor of symbolic and mentalising abilities: A longitudinal study. *Social Development, 7,* 1–24.

Money, J., & Ehrhard, A. (1972). *Man and woman, boy and girl: Differentiation and dimorphism of gender identity from conception to maturity.* Baltimore: Johns Hopkins University Press.

Moss, E., & St.-Laurent, D. (2001). Attachment at school age and academic performance. *Developmental Psychology, 37,* 863–874.

National Institute of Child Health and Human Development (NICHD) Early Child Care Research Network. (2000). The relation of child care to cognitive and language development. *Child Development, 71,* 960–980.

National Institute of Child Health and Human Development (NICHD) Early Child Care Research Network. (2004). Father's and mother's parenting behavior and beliefs as predictors of child social adjustment in the transition to school. *Journal of Family Psychology, 18,* 628–638.

National Institute of Child Health and Human Development (NICHD) Early Child Care Research Network. (in press). Mothers' and fathers' support for child autonomy and early school achievement. *Developmental Psychology.*

Nord, C., Brimhall, C. A., & West, J. (1997). *Fathers' involvement in their children's schools.* Washington, DC: Office of Educational Research and Improvement, U.S. Department of Education.

Oppenheim, D., Sagi, A., & Lamb, M. E. (1988). Infant–adult attachments on the kibbutz and their relation to socioemotional development four years later. *Developmental Psychology, 24,* 427–433.

Page, T., & Bretherton, I. (2001). Mother– and father–child attachment themes as represented in the story completions of preschoolers in postdivorce families: Linkages with teacher ratings of social competence. *Attachment and Human Development, 3,* 1–29.

Parke, R. D. (1996). *Fatherhood.* Cambridge, MA: Harvard University Press.

Parke, R. D., Dennis, J., Flyr, M. L., Morris, K. L., Killian, C., McDowell, D. J., et al. (2004). Fathering and children's peer relationships. In M. E. Lamb (Ed.), *The role of the father in child development* (4th ed., pp. 307–340). Hoboken, NJ: Wiley.

Phares, V. (1996). *Fathers and developmental psychopathology.* New York: Wiley.

Pianta, R. C., Hamre, B., & Stuhlman, M. (2003). Relationships between teachers and children. In I. B. Weiner (Series Ed.) & W. Reynolds & G. Miller (Vol. Eds.), *Handbook of psychology: Vol. 7. Educational psychology* (pp. 199–234). New York: Wiley.

Pianta, R. C., & Harbers, K. L. (1996). Observing mother and child behavior in a problem-solving situation at school entry: Relations with academic achievement. *Journal of School Psychology, 34,* 307–322.

Pierce, S. L. (2000). *The role of fathers and men in the development of child and adolescent externalizing behavior.* Unpublished doctoral dissertation, University of Minnesota.

Pierce, S. L. (2003). *Emotional support from fathers: Predicting adolescent behavior.* Paper presented at the biennial meeting of the Society for Research in Child Development, Tampa, FL.

Radin, N. (1982). Primary caregiving and role-sharing fathers of preschoolers. In M. E. Lamb (Ed.), *Nontraditional families: Parenting and child development* (pp. 173–204). Hillsdale, NJ: Erlbaum.

Ryan, R. M., Kuhl, J., & Deci, E. L. (1997). Nature and autonomy: An organizational view of social and neurobiological aspects of self-regulation in behavior and development. *Development and Psychopathology, 9,* 701–728.

Ryan, R. M., & Lynch, J. H. (1989). Emotional autonomy versus detachment: Revisiting the vicissitudes of adolescence and young adulthood. *Child Development, 60,* 340–356.

Sagi, A. (1982). Antecedents and consequences of various degrees of paternal involvement in child rearing: The Israeli Project. In M. E. Lamb (Ed.), *Nontraditional families: Parenting and child development* (pp. 205–232). Hillsdale, NJ: Erlbaum.

Sagi-Schwartz, A., & Aviezer, O. (2005). Correlates of attachment to multiple caregivers in Kibbutz children from birth to emerging adulthood: The Haifa longitudinal study. In K. E. Grossmann, K. Grossmann, & E. Waters (Eds.), *Attachment from infancy to adulthood: The major longitudinal studies* (pp. 165–197). New York: Guilford Press.

Schieche, M., & Spangler, G. (2005). Individual differences in biobehavioral organization during problem-solving in toddlers: The influence of maternal behavior, infant–mother attachment, and behavioral inhibition on the attachment-exploration balance. *Developmental Psychobiology, 46,* 293–306.

Seginer, R. (1985). Family learning environment: The subjective view of adolescent males and females. *Journal of Youth and Adolescence, 14,* 121–131.

Seifer, R., Schiller, M., Hayden, L. C., & Geerher, C. (1993). *Mastery motivation, temperament, attachment and maternal interaction.* Paper presented at the biennial meeting of the Society for Research in Child Development, New Orleans, LA.

Seiffge-Krenke, I. (1989). Bewältigung alltäglicher Problemsituationen: Ein Coping-Fragebogen für Jugendliche. *Zeitschrift für Differentielle und Diagnostische Psychologie, 10,* 201–220.

Shannon, J. K., Tamis-LeMonda, C. S., London, K., & Cabrera, N. (2002). Beyond rough and tumble: Low-income fathers' interactions and children's cognitive development at 24 months. *Parenting Science and Practice, 2,* 77–104.

Shulman, S., & Seiffge-Krenke, I. (1997). *Fathers and adolescents.* New York: Routledge.

Simpson, J. A. (1999). Attachment theory in modern evolutionary perspective. In J. Cassidy & P. R. Shaver (Eds.), *Handbook of attachment: Theory, research, and clinical applications* (pp. 115–140). New York: Guilford Press.

Simpson, J. A., Collins, W. A., Tran, S., & Haydon, K. C. (2007). Attachment and the experience and expression of emotions in romantic relationships: A developmental perspective. *Journal of Personality and Social Psychology, 92,* 355–367.

Snarey, J. (1993). *How fathers care for the next generation: A four-decade study.* Cambridge, MA: Harvard University Press.

Spangler, G., & Grossmann, K. E. (1993). Biobehavioral organization in securely and insecurely attached infants. *Child Development, 64,* 1439–1450.

Sroufe, L. A., Egeland, B., Carlson, E., & Collins, W. A. (2005a). *The development of the person: The Minnesota Study of Risk and Adaptation from Birth to Adulthood.* New York: Guilford Press.

Sroufe, L. A., Egeland, B., Carlson, E. A., & Collins, W. A. (2005b). Placing early attachment experiences in developmental context: The Minnesota longitudinal study. In K. E. Grossmann, K. Grossmann, & E. Waters (Eds.), *Attachment from infancy to adulthood: The major longitudinal studies* (pp. 48–70). New York: Guilford Press.

Sroufe, L. A., & Pierce, S. (1999). Man in the family: Associations with juvenile conduct. In G. Cunningham (Ed.), *Just in time research: Children, youth, and families* (pp. 19–22). Minneapolis: University of Minnesota Extension Service.

Steele, H., & Steele, M. (2005). Understanding and resolving emotional conflict: The London Parent–Child Project. In K. E. Grossmann, K. Grossmann, & E. Waters (Eds.), *Attachment from infancy to adulthood: The major longitudinal studies* (pp. 137–164). New York: Guilford Press.

Steele, H., Steele, M., & Fonagy, P. (1996). Associations among attachment classifications of mothers, fathers, and their infants. *Child Development, 67,* 541–555.

Steele, M., Steele, H., Woolgar, M., Yabsley, S., Johnson, D., Fonagy, P., et al. (2003). An attachment perspective on children's emotion narratives: Links across generations. In R. N. Emde, D. P. Wolf, & D. Oppenheim (Eds.), *Revealing the inner worlds of young children: The MacArthur Story Stem Battery and parent–child narratives* (pp. 163–181). New York: Oxford University Press.

Stoecker, K., Strasser, K., & Winter, M. (2003). Bindung und Partnerschaftsrepräsentation. In I. Grau & H. W. Bierhoff (Eds.), *Sozialpsychologie der Partnerschaft* [*Social psychology of partnership*] (pp. 138–163). New York: Springer.

Sturgess, W., Dunn, J., & Davies, L. (2001). Young children's perceptions of their relationships with family members: Links with family setting, friendships, and adjustment. *International Journal of Behavioral Development, 25,* 521–529.

Suess, G. (1987). *Auswirkungen frühkindlicher Bindungserfahrungen auf die Kompetenz im Kindergarten* [*Consequences of early attachment experiences for children's competence in preschool*]. Unpublished doctoral dissertation, Universität Regensburg, Regensburg, Germany.

Suess, G., Grossmann, K. E., & Sroufe, L. A. (1992).

Effects of infant attachment to mother and father on quality of adaptation in preschool: From dyadic to individual organization of self. *International Journal of Behavioral Development, 15*, 43–65.

Teo, A., Carlson, E., Mathieu, P., Egeland, B., & Sroufe, L. A. (1996). A prospective longitudinal study of psychosocial predictors of achievement. *Journal of School Psychology, 34*, 285–306.

Thompson, R. A. (2006). The development of the person: Social understanding, relationships, self, conscience. In W. Damon & R. M. Lerner (Series Eds.) & N. Eisenberg (Vol. Ed.), *Handbook of child psychology: Vol. 3. Social, emotional, and personality development* (6th ed., pp. 25–98). Hoboken, NJ: Wiley.

Thompson, R. A., Easterbrooks, M. A., & Padilla-Walker, L. (2003). Social and emotional development in infancy. In I. B. Weiner (Series Ed.) & R. Lerner, M. A. Easterbrooks, & J. Mistry (Vol. Eds.), *Handbook of psychology: Vol. 6.* (pp. 91–112). New York: Wiley.

Turner, P. J. (1991). Relations between attachment, gender, and behavior with peers in preschool. *Child Development, 62*, 1457–1488.

Turner, P. J. (1993). Attachment to mother and behavior with adults in preschool. *British Journal of Developmental Psychology, 11*, 75–89.

Van Bakel, H. J. A., & Riksen-Walraven, J. M. (2004). AQS security scores: What do they represent? A study in construct validation. *Infant Mental Health Journal, 25*, 175–193.

van IJzendoorn, M. H., & De Wolff, M. S. (1997). In search of the absent father: Meta-analysis of infant–father attachment: A rejoinder to our discussants. *Child Development, 68*, 604–609.

van IJzendoorn, M. H., Sagi, A., & Lambermon, M. W. E. (1992). The multiple caretaker paradox: Data from Holland and Israel. *New Directions in Child Development, 57*, 5–24.

Verschueren, K., & Marcoen, A. (1999). Representation of self and socioemotional competence in kindergarteners: Differential and combined effects of attachment to mother and to father. *Child Development, 70*, 183–201.

Verschueren, K., & Marcoen, A. (2003). *Kindergartners' representations of attachment to father and to mother: Differential effects on later socioemotional functioning*. Paper presented at the biennial meeting of the Society for Research in Child Development, Tampa, FL.

Verschueren, K., & Marcoen, A. (2005). Perceived security of attachment to mother and father: Developmental differences and relations to self-worth and peer relationships at school. In K. Kerns & R. Richardson (Eds.), *Attachment in middle childhood* (pp. 212–230). New York: Guilford Press.

Volling, B. L., & Belsky, J. (1992). Infant, father, and marital antecedents of infant–father attachment security in dual-earner and single-earner families.

International Journal of Behavioral Development, 15, 83–100.

Vondra, J. I., Shaw, D. S., Swearingen, L., Cohen, M., & Owens, E. B. (2001). Attachment stability and emotional and behavioral regulation from infancy to preschool age. *Development and Psychopathology, 13*, 13–33.

Waters, E. (1995). The Attachment Q-Set. In E. Waters, B. E. Vaughn, G. Posada, & K. Kondo-Ikemura (Eds.), Caregiving, cultural, and cognitive perspectives on secure-base behavior and working models. *Monographs of the Society for Research in Child Development, 60*(2–3, Serial No. 244, 247–254.

Werner, E. E., & Smith, R. S. (2001). *Journeys from childhood to midlife: Risk, resilience, and recovery.* Ithaca, NY: Cornell University Press.

Whipple, N., Bernier, A., Mageau, G. A., & Ouellet-Gagnon, D. (2007, April). *Broadening the study of infant security of attachment: Maternal autonomy–support in the context of infant exploration.* Poster presented at the biennial meeting of the Society for Research in Child Development, Boston.

Williams, E., Radin, N., & Allegro, T. (1992). Sex role attitudes of adolescents reared primarily by their fathers: An 11-year follow-up. *Merrill–Palmer Quarterly, 38*, 457–476.

Youngblade, L. M., & Belsky, J. (1992). Parent–child antecedents of 5-year-olds' close friendships: A longitudinal analysis. *Developmental Psychology, 28*, 700–713.

Zeanah, C., Danis, B., Hirshberg, L., Benoit, D., Miller, D., & Scott Heller, S. (1999). Disorganized attachment associated with partner violence: A research note. *Infant Mental Health Journal, 20*, 77–86.

Zimmermann, P. (1994). *Bindung im Jugendalter: Entwicklung und Umgang mit aktuellen Anforderungen [Attachment in adolescence: Development while coping with actual challenges].* Unpublished doctoral dissertation, Universität Regensburg, Regensburg, Germany.

Zimmermann, P. (2000). Attachment in adolescence: Development, assessment, and adaptation. In S. Larose & G. M. Tarabulsy (Eds.), *Attachment and development* (pp. 181–204). Quebec: University of Quebec Press.

Zimmermann, P., & Grossmann, K. E. (1995, April). *Attachment and adaptation in adolescence.* Poster presented at the biennial meeting of the Society for Research in Child Development, Indianapolis, IN.

Zimmermann, P., & Grossmann, K. E. (1997). Attachment and adaptation in adolescence. In W. Koops, J. B. Hoeksma, & D. C. van den Boom (Eds.), *Development of interaction and attachment: Traditional and non-traditional approaches* (pp. 271–280). Amsterdam: North-Holland.

Zimmermann, P., Maier, M., Winter, M., & Grossmann K. E. (2001). Attachment and adolescents' emotion regulation during a joint problem-solving task with a friend. *International Journal of Behavioral Development, 25*, 331–343.

CHAPTER 37

Cross-Cultural Patterns of Attachment
Universal and Contextual Dimensions

MARINUS H. VAN IJZENDOORN
ABRAHAM SAGI-SCHWARTZ

It was in Uganda, a former British protectorate in East Africa, that Mary Ainsworth (1967) began to create the famous tripartite classification system of "avoidant" (A), "secure" (B), and "resistant" or "ambivalent" (C) infant–mother attachment relationships. In her short-term longitudinal field study, carried out in 1954–1955, she found three patterns of attachment behavior in a small sample of 28 infants. The "securely attached group," consisting of 16 children, cried infrequently and seemed especially content when they were with their mothers. Secure children also used their mothers as a secure base from which to explore the environment. The "insecurely attached group," consisting of 7 babies, cried frequently, not only when left alone by their mothers but also in the mothers' presence; they cried to be picked up and then cried when they were put down. These babies wanted continuous physical contact with their mothers, but at the same time seemed ambivalent about their mothers' presence. A "nonattached" group consisting of 5 infants responded similarly to their mothers and to other adults. For example, they were not upset about being left alone by their mothers and did not respond to the mothers' return in any specific way. In fact, from Ainsworth's detailed case studies of these 5 "nonattached" infants, it can be

inferred that in the Strange Situation procedure (Ainsworth, Blehar, Waters, & Wall, 1978) they would have been classified as avoidant.

Ainsworth's Uganda study raised some important cross-cultural issues, the first being the universality of the infant–mother attachment relationship and the tripartite classification system. The second issue was the universality of the nomological network surrounding the concept of attachment. Ainsworth (1967) clearly initiated her famous Baltimore study (Ainsworth & Wittig, 1969) to test the replicability of her Uganda results in another, Western culture. In so doing, she was particularly interested in documenting the crucial role of maternal sensitivity as an antecedent of attachment. The third issue raised by the Uganda research was the culture-specific or contextual dimension of attachment development. It is surprising to see that even in the Uganda study, the presence of multiple caretakers did not interfere with the development of a secure attachment (Weisner & Gallimore, 1977). After Bowlby's (1951; see also Robertson & Robertson, 1971) report on the disastrous effects of fragmented institutional care, the Uganda study showed for the first time that the decisive factors for attachment security were not the number of caretakers per se, but the continu-

880

ity and quality of the mother–infant interaction. Ainsworth (1967) considered her study as the beginning of a cross-cultural search for antecedents and sequelae of attachment security. The question now is this: What results have four decades of cross-cultural attachment research yielded?

Cross-cultural attachment research has been using the "etic" approach more often than the "emic" approach (Jackson, 1993; van IJzendoorn, 1990). Pike (1967) derived the terms "emic" and "etic" from the two different approaches to the study of sound in language: "phonemics" and "phonetics." Phonetics concerns the sound characteristics of language that are supposed to be universal, whereas phonemics concerns the meaningful, and therefore culture-specific, sound properties of a language. In cross-cultural research, the "etic" approach leads to an emphasis on theories and assessments that have been developed in a specific culture (often a Western, industrialized society). These theories and assessments are then applied in other cultures to test whether the phenomena under scrutiny are really cross-culturally valid rather than culture-specific. The "emic" approach focuses on social and behavioral configurations and developmental trajectories that are specific to the culture, and it tries to understand this culture from within its own frame of reference (see also Berry, 1969).

Most cross-cultural attachment research can be characterized as "etic," because in many cases Bowlby's conceptualization of attachment and Ainsworth's operationalization of attachment have been applied to various non-Western cultures. One of the reasons for this "etic" emphasis may be the ethological foundation of attachment theory. Because attachment processes have also been observed in nonhuman primates and in other species, Bowlby (1969/1982) suggested that the formation of an attachment relationship between infants and their protective caregivers is the outcome of evolution; "inclusive fitness" (Trivers, 1974) was deemed to be facilitated by an innate bias to become attached to a conspecific (see Simpson & Belsky, Chapter 6, this volume). Therefore, a core element of attachment theory is the idea of the universality of this bias in infants to become attached, regardless of their specific cultural niche.

From this universality thesis, however, it does not follow that the development of attachment is insensitive to culture-specific influences and idiosyncrasies. On the contrary, the evolutionary perspective leaves room for globally adaptive behavioral propensities that are realized in a specific way,

depending on the cultural niche in which children have to survive (Hinde & Stevenson-Hinde, 1990, 1991). If a cultural niche requires the suppression of negative emotions, infants may develop an avoidant attachment pattern to meet this cultural demand. In such a culture, the avoidant attachment pattern may well be normative in the sense that it promotes inclusive fitness and general adaptation, and it may be observed in the majority of cases. That is, the universality thesis predicts only that attachment bonds will be established in any known culture, regardless of childrearing arrangements and family constellations. It does not imply that one of the three principal attachment patterns is universally normative; evolution may not have equipped human beings with rigid behavioral strategies that would have made it difficult to adapt to changing (natural and social) environments (see Simpson & Belsky, Chapter 6, this volume). Nevertheless, one may wonder whether the secure attachment pattern is the primary strategy for adapting to a social environment that is basically supportive of the infant, and whether the insecure strategies should be considered as secondary, in that they constitute deviating but adaptive patterns provoked by less supportive contexts (Main, 1990).

In this chapter, we describe and evaluate the cross-cultural attachment studies that have followed Ainsworth's Uganda example. We limit our discussion to cultures other than the Anglo-Saxon and European cultures. The outcomes of attachment studies in the major English-speaking countries and Europe are of course presupposed in the "etic" application of attachment theory and assessments to non-Western cultures, but we refer to other chapters in this volume for reviews (see Belsky & Fearon, Chapter 13; Thompson, Chapter 16; and Weinfield, Sroufe, Egeland, & Carlson, Chapter 4). In particular, we presuppose the following findings:

1. In Western countries all infants—when given any opportunity at all—become attached to one or more specific (parental or nonparental) caregivers, except perhaps in the most extreme cases of neurophysiological impairments, such as extreme mental retardation. For the purpose of cross-cultural research, this finding may be translated into the "universality hypothesis."

2. In Western societies the majority of infants are securely attached, although a considerable number of infants (up to 40%) have been found to be insecurely attached (van IJzendoorn

& Kroonenberg, 1988; van IJzendoorn, Sagi, & Lambermon, 1992), and the number of secure infants may vary considerably across samples within a culture (e.g., Grossmann, Grossmann, Huber, & Wartner, 1981). In stressful circumstances, secure infants appear to settle more easily than insecure infants, as shown by several psychophysiological studies (Hertsgaard, Gunnar, Erickson, & Nachmias, 1995; Spangler & Grossmann, 1993; Verweij-Tijsterman, 1996). Secure attachment therefore seems to be normative in both the numerical and the physiological senses; this may be called the "normativity hypothesis."

3. Attachment security is dependent on childrearing antecedents, particularly sensitive and prompt responses to the infants' attachment signals, although other factors may be relevant as well (De Wolff & van IJzendoorn, 1997; van IJzendoorn & De Wolff, 1997). The causal relation between sensitive childrearing and attachment security has been documented in several experimental intervention studies (for meta-analytic evidence, see Bakermans-Kranenburg, van IJzendoorn, & Juffer, 2003; see also Belsky & Fearon, Chapter 13, this volume). This is the "sensitivity hypothesis."

4. Attachment security leads to differences in children's competence to regulate their negative emotions (absence of aggression, ego control; Cassidy, 1986, 1994), to establish satisfactory relationships with peers and teachers (Bretherton, 1991), and to develop cognitive abilities (emergent literacy, metacognition; for reviews, see Meins, 1997; van IJzendoorn, Dijkstra, & Bus, 1995). (See Thompson, Chapter 16, this volume, for further discussion.) This is the "competence hypothesis."

The universality, normativity, sensitivity, and competence hypotheses constitute the core hypotheses of attachment theory (Ainsworth et al., 1978; Belsky & Cassidy, 1995; Bowlby, 1969/1982; Bretherton, 1985, 1991; Main, 1990; van IJzendoorn, 1990). "Etic" studies on attachment in various cultures may be heuristically fruitful in documenting (1) the universality of attachment in infancy, (2) the culture-specific dimensions and normativity of the three attachment patterns, and (3) the generalizability of the nomological network of attachment-related constructs across cultures (see Main, 1990, and van IJzendoorn, 1990, for preliminary analyses). From this point on, we discuss attachment studies in several non-European, non-Anglo-Saxon societies: various African cultures, the People's Republic of China,

Israel, Japan, and Indonesia. The time has come to describe, evaluate, and integrate the growing points and directions in the cross-cultural study of attachment.

INFANT–MOTHER ATTACHMENT IN A NETWORK OF CAREGIVERS: THE AFRICAN CASE

In her Uganda study, Ainsworth (1967, 1977) described the development of attachment in a multiple-caregiver context. Even in a childrearing environment in which mothers share their caregiving responsibilities with several other adults and older children, infants nevertheless become attached to their mothers and use them as a secure base to explore the world. The Uganda study, however, was rather small and exploratory, and certainly not representative of the various African cultures (Jackson, 1993).

In this section we discuss some other studies of attachment in Africa, conducted in the years following Ainsworth's (1967) research. We place special emphasis on child development in a network of (child and adult) caregivers, in order to test the idea that a multiple-caregiver environment is in no way incompatible with a unique attachment relationship between child and parent. Attachment in a network of multiple caregivers is of crucial importance, because cross-cultural evidence shows that in most societies nonparental caretaking is either the norm or a frequent form (Weisner & Gallimore, 1977). Only a few studies on attachment in Africa have been published as yet, and of course they cannot be considered representative of the vast African continent. Nevertheless, they may provide cumulative evidence for some of the core hypotheses of attachment theory.

Uganda Revisited

Family life in Africa has changed drastically in recent years, due to the HIV/AIDS pandemic. In particular, mothers of young children often become victims of this infection, for which no medical treatment is yet available in Africa on a large scale; many infants are born with HIV. Peterson, Drotar, Olness, Guay, and Kiziri-Mayengo (2001) investigated a Ugandan sample of 35 HIV-positive mothers with or without AIDS, and 25 HIV-negative mothers, all with infants in their first year of life. The researchers used the Attachment Q-Sort (AQS; Vaughn & Waters, 1990; see Solomon & George, Chapter 18, this volume) to rate the attachment security of the infants during a 4-hour home visit. The AQS consists of 90 specific behavioral descriptions of 12- to 48-month-old children in the natural home setting, with special emphasis on secure-base behavior (Vaughn & Waters, 1990). Peterson and colleagues conducted the AQS observations at home, with a potentially higher ecological validity (van IJzendoorn, Vereijken, Bakermans-Kranenburg, & Riksen-Walraven, 2004), and they also measured maternal display of positive affect to an infant. They found that 32% of the variance of AQS attachment security in the Ugandan sample was predicted by maternal affect. Almost half a century after the original Uganda study, the new Ugandan findings support Ainsworth's (1967) central thesis that maternal sensitivity is strongly associated with infant attachment security.

The Gusii Study

Childrearing among the Gusii of Kenya is different from childrearing in Western, industrialized countries in at least two ways. First, mothers share their childrearing tasks and responsibilities with other caregivers to a larger extent than in many other non-Western cultures; in particular, child caregivers such as older siblings take care of the infants during a large part of the day. Second, the division of tasks between mothers and other caregivers is rather strict, in that mothers provide most of the physical care and are responsible for their children's health, whereas the activities of child caregivers are limited to social and playful interactions (Kermoian & Leiderman, 1986). The strict division of caregiving tasks between mothers and other caregivers provided Kermoian and Leiderman with the opportunity to test whether different attachment relationships would develop between an infant and his or her mother and between that infant and another caregiver, as well as whether the influence of a specific attachment relationship would be restricted to a specific area of competence.

Kermoian and Leiderman (1986) included 26 families in their study, with infants between the ages of 8 and 27 months (mean age = 14½ months). Outside each mother's hut, a modified Strange Situation procedure was implemented, with two separation–reunion episodes for mother, caregiver, and stranger each. The lack of a strange laboratory environment was meant to be compensated for by the extra separations. Gusii infants are used to being greeted with a handshake by their mothers and caretakers. During the reunions, the Gusii infants anticipated the handshake in the same way as North American or European infants anticipate a hug. The secure Gusii infants would reach out to an adult with one arm, to receive the handshake enthusiastically, whereas the insecure infants would avoid the adult or reach and then pull away after the adult approached. The insecure children's exploratory behavior was also different: They explored the environment visually instead of manipulatively.

Although the Gusii infants used culture-specific attachment behaviors to express their emotions about the separations and reunions, the distribution of patterns of attachment was comparable with Western findings. Sixteen of the infants (61%) were classified as securely attached to their mothers at the first assessment, and 14 infants (54%) were classified as securely attached to their nonmaternal caregivers. Kermoian and Leiderman (1986) did not differentiate between the two insecure categories. The percentage of secure infants is almost identical to the percentage found in a Dutch study on infants' attachment to mothers, fathers, and professional caregivers (Goossens & van IJzendoorn, 1990). The authors concluded that the development of differential or person-specific attachment behaviors for "polymatric" infants is similar to that observed in "monomatric" Western societies, that is, infants do become uniquely attached to a protective adult caregiver, regardless of the presence of one or more mother figures (Reed & Leiderman, 1981).

Because the mothers developed their attachment relationship with their infants in the context of physical care, it was expected that attachment security with mothers would be related to the infants' health status. The child caregivers developed their bond with the infants in the context of stimulating social, verbal, and playful interactions, and attachment security with the caregivers was therefore expected to be associated with the infants' cognitive-developmental status. Indeed, the infants who were securely attached to their nonmaternal caregivers had higher scores on the Bayley Scales of Infant Development than the insecurely attached infants. For the infant–mother relationship, there was no association between security and cognitive development. Furthermore, the nutritional or health status of the infants was related to the security of the infant–mother attachment and not to the security of the infant–caregiver attachment. Infants who were securely attached to their mothers had a recent history of higher nutritional status than insecurely attached infants. In this respect, the infant–caregiver bond appeared to be irrelevant. Thus attachment security appeared to have a different impact on the infants' development, depending on the context in which the bond emerged. (In the section below on the Israeli kibbutzim, we report a similar finding.) Kermoian and Leiderman (1986) suggested that the pervasive influence of the infant–mother attachment relationship in Western cultures may be caused by the absence of role differentiation and task division in most Western families.

The Gusii study also provided some evidence in favor of the sensitivity hypothesis. Kermoian and Leiderman (1986) hypothesized that mothers would be more sensitive to the signals of their infants if they were older, because Gusii women gain status with age, and thus older mothers might be more likely to be emotionally balanced themselves. Furthermore, in a larger household the mothers would be able to share their burden of tasks with more people, and therefore would be able to devote more time and energy to their infants. Lastly, the birth of a new baby was expected to decrease a mother's sensitivity to her older infant (Trivers, 1974). As predicted, maternal age and household density were associated with infants' secure attachment to their mothers. Similar correlations were absent in the case of the caregivers. The birth of a new baby increased the risk for insecure attachment. These results support the cross-cultural validity of the sensitivity hypothesis.

The Hausa Study

The Hausa, who populate a large market town in Nigeria, represent a polymatric culture in which the distribution of child care tasks is somewhat less strict than in the Gusii. Because Hausa men (as Muslims) are allowed to marry as many as four wives, and because these wives do not have to work in the fields, polymatric care is provided mainly by adults instead of children.

An average of four caregivers share with the mothers the tasks of social, verbal, and playful interactions. Mothers also contribute to a substantial part of these activities. The biological mothers, however, take almost complete responsibility for physical care activities, such as feeding and bathing (Marvin, VanDevender, Iwanaga, LeVine, & LeVine, 1977). Agriculture is the main economy in this flat-savannah, orchard–bush part of the country. The Hausa live in small, round, walled compounds with separate huts for each of the

wives. In the middle of each compound is an open common cooking and working area, where open fires and freely accessible tools and other utensils constitute a continuous risk for infants.

Marvin and colleagues (1977) included 18 infants in their descriptive study, which focused on the occurrence of attachment and exploratory behaviors in the natural setting. When not asleep, these Hausa infants were almost always in close physical contact with or in close proximity to one or more adult caregivers. The infants were not allowed to explore the wider environment alone, because of the dangers involved. The high social density of the Hausa compound led to prompt adult or older sibling responses to any infant attachment signals, such as crying. The Hausa caregivers therefore appeared to be indulgent and sensitive, and at the same time restrictive toward their infants, who were not allowed to move around freely. The restriction of locomotion also led to a different use of adult caregivers as a secure base: Hausa infants explored their immediate environment in visual and manipulative ways, but only in close proximity to an attachment figure, and they ceased to explore as soon as the caregiver had left. The Hausa infants studied by Marvin and colleagues thus differed from Western infants not only in their preference for manipulative exploration, but also in their use of passive or signaling attachment behaviors, instead of more active proximity-seeking or following behaviors. Nevertheless, the Hausa infants clearly appeared to use adult caregivers as safe bases from which to explore, and they differentiated between attachment figures and strangers.

Furthermore, all infants displayed attachment behavior to more than one caregiver, and on the average they appeared to be attached to three or four different figures, including their fathers. Although they were raised in a network of attachment relationships, most Hausa infants were primarily attached to one attachment figure, to whom they addressed their attachment behaviors most frequently. This principal attachment figure was in most cases the person who held the baby most and who otherwise interacted with him or her most frequently (Marvin et al., 1977). The most important attachment figure was not necessarily the biological mother. Unfortunately, Marvin and colleagues (1977) did not use the Ainsworth tripartite system to classify the infant–caregiver relationships. It is therefore unclear how attachment security was affected by the prompt and sensitive responses to the infants' signals. However, the Hausa study clearly documents the existence of multiple attachments in a multiple-caregiver context, as well as the infants' preference for one of the attachment figures. The Hausa study provides further support for the universality hypothesis, and shows how attachment serves to protect infants from the dangers of their environment. The culture-specific attachment and exploratory behaviors appear to leave room for the universal occurrence of the secure-base phenomenon.

The Dogon Study

In a more recent cross-cultural study of 26 mothers and their 1-year-old infants, True (1994), in cooperation with Pisani and Oumar (True, Pisani, & Oumar, 2001), tested the hypothesis that secure and insecure dyads among the Dogon of Mali (West Africa) would be characterized by different communication patterns in attachment-related circumstances. Traditionally, the Dogon economy is based on subsistence farming of a single crop, millet, which makes the members of the Dogon society vulnerable to malnutrition. The sample included in True's study was derived from a more acculturated and economically diverse town population. With a few exceptions, these infants were living in compounds with their extended families. The fathers usually had children with several wives. During the first year of their lives, the infants were nursed by their biological mothers. Maternal care was supplemented with care from siblings and other family members (True, 1994). In particular with a firstborn male infant, the primary caregiver during the day was the paternal grandmother; however, the mother was available when the child was hungry, and the mother slept at night with the infant. For other infants, the mothers were mainly responsible during the day and night, but they readily shared the child care with female relatives or older children. Infant mortality was high during the first years of life: 25% of the children did not survive the first 5 years. This threatening ecology may have been one of the reasons why these Dogon mothers breast-fed their infants on demand and very frequently, and kept them in close proximity almost all the time. Physical interaction was favored above verbal or visual interaction, and infant distress signals were met with immediate responses. The process of weaning during the end of the second year was gradual, with fathers and older siblings becoming more important (True, 1994).

The Dogon dyads were filmed in the traditional Strange Situation procedure, and they were also observed twice in the stressful setting of a standardized well-baby examination, the Weigh-In. For the first time in cross-cultural research in Africa, not only were the Strange Situation data classified into the classic tripartite A-B-C system, but the additional coding system for disorganized/disoriented attachment behaviors (Main & Solomon, 1990; see Lyons-Ruth & Jacobvitz, Chapter 28, and George & Solomon, Chapter 35, this volume) was also applied. The Weigh-In setting was used to assess the communication patterns of the infant–mother dyads during a stressful but naturalistic situation. The mutual orientation ("directness") and cooperation between mothers and infants were rated, and scales assessing violations of communication (e.g., infant avoidance of the mother or maternal withdrawal from the infant) were applied. The most extreme score of a dyad on the communication violation scales was used post hoc to calculate a summary rating (True, 1994).

The Dogon study showed a high percentage of disorganized infants (24%), compared to the percentages in normal Western samples (15–20%). The percentage of secure infant–mother dyads was also high (69%), whereas the avoidant classification appeared to be absent, and few resistant infant–mother dyads were found (8%). True (1994) also "forced" the infants into the best-fitting attachment classification of the tripartite coding system, regardless of the disorganized behaviors (see Lyons-Ruth & Jacobvitz, Chapter 28, this volume). The forced attachment classification distribution was as follows: 88% secure, 12% resistant, and 0% avoidant. The study supports the universality hypothesis in showing how the Strange Situation procedure remains classifiable with the A-B-C-D coding system, even in an African culture. Furthermore, True also demonstrated that the majority of her participants were classified as securely attached, which provides some further cross-cultural evidence for the normativity hypothesis.

To explain the lack of avoidant attachments, True (1994) hypothesized that the Strange Situation procedure in the Dogon society may have been experienced as highly stressful instead of mildly stressful. The stress of two separations from the mother and two encounters with a stranger may have forced the avoidant infants to seek proximity, and may also have increased the number of disorganized infants. The association between attachment security and communication violations, however, only partly supports this argument. True found a negative correlation ($r = -.40$) between attachment and communication: That is, secure infant–mother dyads were less likely to violate the rules of open communication than were the insecure infant–mother dyads. This outcome is in line with findings in Western societies, and therefore supports the validity of the Strange Situation in the Dogon society. This post hoc outcome was, however, limited to part of the sample—that is, to those participants who did not show strong avoidance in the Weigh-In and therefore were unable to violate communication rules (True, 1994).

The Environment of Evolutionary Adaptedness: The !Kung and Efé Studies

Bowlby (1969/1982) developed his evolutionary theory of attachment on the basis of speculations about child development and child rearing in the original environment in which the human species spent about 99% of its historical time as hunters and gatherers. In this "environment of evolutionary adaptedness," an infant would be protected against predators and other dangers by staying in close proximity to a protective adult. Only a few societies are left that might resemble this original way of living, and still fewer have been studied from the viewpoint of attachment. Konner's (1977) study of the !Kung San or Bushmen of northwestern Botswana, and Morelli and Tronick's (1991) study on the Efé or Pygmies of the Ituri forest in northeastern Zambia, are outstanding examples of attachment research on hunter–gatherer societies. Hunters and gatherers are characterized by their living in small seminomadic groups with a fluid group structure, absence of strict social rules, and flexible subsistence strategies (Konner, 1977).

The general rules of childrearing in the !Kung society are indulgence, stimulation, and nonrestriction (Konner, 1977). The !Kung infants studied by Konner were fed whenever they cried and whenever they reached for the breast. This feeding on demand led to brief but frequent feeds, amounting to several times an hour during the day. At night the infants slept in close proximity to their mothers, and they were also fed on demand—even without the mothers' awakening. The extent of physical contact was large compared to that in Western infant–mother dyads. An infant was carried around in a sling, which left the infant with constant access to the mother's breast and to decorative objects hanging around her neck. The infant was able to look around freely and to experience extensive physical and cognitive stimulation. Konner found that this stimulating environment led to advanced neuromotor development in the !Kung infants.

The 2- and 3-year-old children studied by Konner were involved in multiage peer groups, in which they spent more time than with their mothers, and in which they readily established new bonds. Konner (1977) suggested that the great social density of this childrearing environment enabled the mothers to be extremely indulgent and sensitive to the infants' signals, and that at the same time this social network facilitated the gradual transition into the peer group, in which the older peers took responsibility for the care and protection of the younger toddlers. The !Kung study thus provides support for the universality as well as the sensitivity hypothesis. In this hunter–gatherer society, the infant–mother bond seems to fulfill a unique function of protection and stimulation, even in the context of a wider social network of caregivers. Furthermore, a basic tenet of attachment theory is confirmed—namely, that sensitive responses to infants' signals foster independence instead of dependence later on in life.

The Efé employ a system of multiple caregivers throughout the first few years of life (Morelli & Tronick, 1991). Beginning at birth, the newborn is allowed to suckle other adult females besides the mother, and childrearing remains the responsibility of a larger network of adult caregivers (Tronick, Morelli, & Winn, 1987). Even the physical care is shared with other caregivers, in contrast with the Hausa and the Gusii, where the mothers are mainly responsible for feeding, bathing, and other physical care activities. Multiple caregiving is not necessarily related to the unavailability of the mother: Other caregivers may nurse an infant even in the presence of the mother. Morelli and Tronick (1991) reported that the percentage of time the infants they studied spent with other individuals increased from 39% at 3 weeks to 60% at 18 weeks. The number of caregivers in the first 18 weeks amounted to 14.2 on average. This extremely dense social network led to prompt responses to any sign of infant distress.

During the second half of the first year, the infants in this study began to show preference for the care of their own mothers, and they were more likely to be carried by their mothers on trips out of the camp and to protest against their leaving. Morelli and Tronick (1991) proposed that Efé cultural beliefs about infants' growing competence to discriminate between mothers and other caregivers may have been a reason for this shift. They also pointed to the 1-year-olds' interference with adults' work activities, which prevented nonmaternal caregivers from taking on caregiving responsibility during work. Another intriguing reason for the emergence of a special infant–mother bond, despite the multiple-caregiver context, may have been the care provided during the night. At night, only the mothers cared for their infants, and sleep was regularly interrupted by episodes of playful interaction exclusively between infants and their mothers (Morelli & Tronick, 1991). From the perspective of attachment theory, the night may be an especially stressful time during which infants in general need a protective caregiver most (see the description of the Israeli communal kibbutzim, below).

The Khayelitsha Study

In South Africa, Tomlinson, Cooper, and Murray (2005) studied attachment in a black sample of 98 mother–infant dyads, and assessed them at 2, 6, and 18 months postpartum. Families were living in Khayelitsha, an impoverished black settlement close to Cape Town, with a high proportion of migrants from rural areas. Only 4% of mothers were born in Cape Town; 58% of the families had no regular income. Only 5% lived in brick houses, and 49% of the houses were without modern plumbing. Fifty-one percent of the pregnancies were unplanned. The researchers undertook the challenging job of conducting the Strange Situation; the Home Observation for Measurement of the Environment (developed by Caldwell & Bradley, 1984) was used to assess the quality of the childrearing environment); and a structured play procedure was used to assess sensitive responsiveness. Despite the poor living circumstances, the majority of infants were securely attached to their mothers (62%), although a rather large number of infants did develop a disorganized attachment (26%); only 4% were avoidantly attached, and the remaining 8% were resistantly attached. The forced attachment classification distribution (see the description of the Dogon study, above) was as follows: 17% avoidant, 72% secure, and 11% resistant attachments (Tomlinson et al., 2005). Furthermore, a remarkably high incidence of postpartum depression was found in the mothers (35% when infants were 2 months old), compared to similar samples in Western countries (with about 10% of mothers experiencing postpartum depression). The presence of postpartum depression was strongly associated with attachment insecurity and disorganization, and sensitivity at 2 months as well

as at 18 months predicted attachment security significantly and independently of depression, again providing support for one of the basic hypotheses of attachment theory.

ATTACHMENT IN THE ONLY CHILD: THE CHINESE CASE

Research on socioemotional development in general, and on attachment in particular, is almost nonexistent in the People's Republic of China (Wang, 1993; Wu, 1985; Zhu & Lin, 1991). The dearth of studies on socioemotional development in China is distressing, in view of Kagitcibasi's (1996) suggestion that the Chinese culture favors interdependence instead of independence, and that in Chinese childrearing the model of emotional interdependence is dominant (cf. Chen, Rubin, & Li, 1995; Li-Repac, 1982)—emphases comparable to those in Japanese cultural and parental beliefs (see below). This observation concurs with Ho's (1986) conclusion that Chinese parents tend to emphasize emotional harmony and control in social relationships, whereas Western parents are inclined to stress individuality and spontaneity.

Because China represents one-fifth of the world's population (with more than 1,300,000,000 inhabitants in 2007), and is unique in its birth restriction policy of one child per family (Kuotai & Jing-Hwa, 1985), we have decided to discuss the relevant attachment studies, despite the fact that so few have been carried out to date. It should be kept in mind that the vast population of China is not homogeneous, although the majority of the Chinese are said to belong to the ethnic group of the Han. For political reasons, the common ethnicity of the Chinese has often been stressed at the cost of ethnic differentiation. China is composed of at least 56 nationalities (Wang, 1993). The first studies on psychological characteristics of different nationalities have shown remarkable similarities (Wang, 1993), but socioemotional research on intranational differences has yet to be conducted.

The Beijing Q-Sort Study

In their cross-cultural study on attachment in China, Gao and Wu (Posada et al., 1995) addressed the following questions: Does the secure-base phenomenon exist in Beijing? Do mothers and experts evaluate secure attachment in ways similar to those of Western mothers and experts? And do mothers and experts agree with each other about the "ideal" typical secure child? The authors used a Chinese version of the AQS (Vaughn & Waters, 1990) to stimulate mothers and experts to provide descriptions of real and ideal children from the perspective of attachment theory. The sample consisted of 41 mothers living in the city of Beijing; all but one mother had only one child (age range = 13–44 months). Each Chinese mother was asked to sort the 90 behavioral descriptions of her own child and of the "ideal" child in two separate runs. Mothers were asked to sort the descriptions into nine piles, ranging from "not descriptive of the [ideal] child at all" to "very descriptive of the [ideal] child." Only some of the 90 behavioral descriptions pertain to the secure-base phenomenon, and are thus related to attachment instead of dependence or sociability.

If Chinese mothers or experts had not selected the security descriptions as relevant to a real or ideal Chinese child, there would have been some doubt about the universality of the secure-base phenomenon in general, and its applicability in Chinese culture in particular. The patterning of the attachment behaviors in the range of the more or less pertinent descriptors showed, however, that Chinese parents as well as experts found the concept of attachment applicable in their cultural context. Furthermore, the Chinese mothers' descriptions of their own children were not more highly correlated with one another than with descriptions from various Western (Germany, Norway, United States) and non-Western (Colombia, Japan) societies (Posada et al., 1995). The implication is that Chinese mothers do not systematically deviate from mothers living in a variety of other societies in terms of their descriptions of the relevance of the secure-base phenomenon to their own children. The same appeared to be true for the Chinese mothers' descriptions of the ideal child. This outcome concurs with the results of an anthropological study of Chinese families living in Papua New Guinea; this study focused on attachment behaviors and the parental responses, and did find interactive patterns predicted by attachment theory (Wu, 1985).

The experts' opinion about the "optimally secure" child was also highly associated with the mothers' view of the "ideal" child. That is, Chinese mothers perceived the ideal child as a securely attached child, just as the Chinese experts did, and the experts' descriptions of the optimally secure Chinese child were strongly associated with similar descriptions by experts from various Western and non-Western societies. These results clearly support the universality hypothesis of attachment theory. It is important to note that among these Chinese experts and parents, the idea of emotional interdependence did not seem to regulate their views of the ideal child, at least in certain domains.

This finding appears to replicate the unexpected outcome of the Lin and Fu (1990) study of childrearing attitudes in Chinese, Chinese American, and European American parents of kindergarten-age and elementary-school-age children. In this study, the Chinese and Chinese American parents rated the importance of encouragement of independence higher than their European American counterparts did. Lin and Fu suggested that valuing interdependence and filial piety within the family is not necessarily incompatible with individual independence in the wider social context, such as school or work. In fact, being successful in school and at work may be a filial obligation to be reached only through personal autonomy. Furthermore, children's age may be an important factor. Whereas Chinese parents are considered to be indulgent and overprotective of younger children, this parenting attitude changes drastically when the children are deemed to be responsible for their own actions. From that point in time (which may be located anywhere between 2 and 6 years), impulse control and harsh discipline begin to dominate (Ho, 1986).

The First Chinese Strange Situation Study

A pioneering study of attachment in China using the Strange Situation procedure was conducted by Hu and Meng (1996) of the Psychology Department of Peking University in Beijing. The authors' aim was to describe patterns of attachment in Chinese infants, as well as the association between attachment and temperament. They also focused on associations between the mothers' involvement in the care of their infants and the quality of the infant–mother attachment relationship. The sample consisted of 31 mother–infant dyads (16 of the infants were boys) from intact families with a "middle-class" background. Each infant was an only child, and all but one family lived with the grandparents. Filial piety has remained functional in the Chinese context of housing shortages, especially for the younger generations. In fact, this is the reason why parents and children tend to live with the grandparents instead of the grandparents with their offspring (C.-F. Yang, 1988; K.-S. Yang, 1988).

The distribution of attachment classifications in this Chinese sample was remarkably similar to the global distribution (van IJzendoorn & Kroonenberg, 1988). The percentage of secure infant–mother dyads was 68%; the avoidant classification was assigned in 16% of the cases; and the resistant classification was used in 16% of the cases. In view of the strict birth control policy and the traditional preference for a male child, it is important to note that the distributions of attachment classifications for male and female infants were virtually the same (Hu & Meng, 1996). Paradoxically, the policy of one child per family may enhance the importance of the only child to such a degree that it overrides the traditional sex-specific preferences (the "little emperor" phenomenon described by Stafford, 1995; see also Kuotai & Jing-Hwa, 1985).

Hu and Meng (1996) expressed some doubts about the validity of the avoidant category. They noted that the avoidant infants did not show stranger anxiety, and they commented on the indifference the avoidant infants expressed toward their mothers at reunion. The Chinese mothers' stress on early independence in their infants, as well as their reliance on nonparental caregivers, may have been responsible for this "indifferent attachment." In some cases, grandparents may have served as the primary attachment figures. An alternative interpretation, however, may refer to the subtle avoidant behaviors that are difficult for even well-trained coders to observe in infants. Without more details about this study, it is difficult to evaluate the authors' claim of the invalidity of the avoidant classification. In this respect, the outcome of this study does not seem to fit easily with Kagan, Kearsly, and Zelazo's (1978) finding that Chinese (American) infants tended to be more apprehensive toward strangers and unfamiliar situations than European American infants—in other words, that Chinese infants were more inhibited (Hsu, 1985).

In this Chinese sample, attachment appeared to be associated with mothers' involvement in the care of their infants. Mothers of avoidant and secure infants worked outside the home every day, whereas mothers of resistant babies stayed at home. Furthermore, mothers of avoidant infants were less involved in child care than mothers of secure infants, and the grandparents played an even larger role as substitute caregivers in the former cases. This outcome may be considered an indirect confirmation of the sensitivity hypothesis of attachment theory, as secure Chinese infants seemed to receive the most continuous and involved care by their mothers.

ATTACHMENT IN THE KIBBUTZ: THE ISRAELI CASE

Following a visit to Israeli kibbutzim in the early 1950s, Bowlby (1951) noted the rich opportunities for research provided by kibbutz upbringing and predicted that this childrearing context, though clearly different from institutional care, might produce higher rates of attachment insecurity.

Until about 20 years ago, collective sleeping arrangements for children away from their parents constituted probably the most distinctive characteristic of Israeli kibbutz practices in collective childrearing. Whereas most institutionalized childrearing in Western cultures involves clinical and multiproblem populations, the collective sleeping arrangements in the kibbutzim were designed for healthy, middle-class, well-functioning, intact families. Many cultures practice multiple caregiving; the patterns are in many ways similar to the practice in kibbutzim (Rabin & Beit-Hallahmi, 1982). However, a worldwide sample of 183 societies showed that none of them maintained a system of having infants sleep away from their parents (Barry & Paxton, 1971). Communal sleeping can be conceived as a unique natural experiment in extremely extended nonparental care with normal children (Beit-Hallahmi & Rabin, 1977). Thus studying attachment in the Israeli kibbutz, especially where collective sleeping arrangements for infants were practiced, has provided a unique opportunity to examine the four major working hypotheses discussed at the beginning of this chapter (Aviezer, van IJzendoorn, Sagi, & Schuengel, 1994).

Collective Sleeping Arrangements

The children's house on a kibbutz still serves as the place in which children spend most of their time, eat their meals, and are bathed, in much the same way as they might do at home—hence the term "children's house." Because in the past many kibbutzim adhered to communal sleeping arrangements for children during the night, the children's house was physically designed to fulfill all such functions. Therefore, it consisted of a number of bedrooms (each of which was shared by three or four children), a dining area, showers, and a large space for play activities and learning. Children had private corners in their bedrooms where they kept their personal things, and which were decorated according to each child's preference. When collective sleeping was still in effect, family time was in the afternoon and evening, when both parents tried to be available. Children were returned to the children's house for the night by their parents, who put them to bed; a caregiver or a parent then remained with them until the night watchwomen took over. Communal sleeping started a few months after birth (Aviezer et al., 1994).

Attachment and Collective Sleeping Practices

Sagi and colleagues (1985) were the first to use the Strange Situation and its classification system to study the attachments of communally sleeping kibbutz infants to their parents and caregivers. Sagi, Koren-Karie, Gini, Ziv, and Joels (2002) also examined infant–mother attachment in 758 Israeli infants representing various types of early child care in the city. They found that only 59% of kibbutz infants were securely attached to their mothers, as compared with 72% of Israeli city infants, and with the 65–70% found in most studies worldwide. Among children with insecure attachments in both Israeli samples, ambivalent relationships were overrepresented (see below). Communal sleeping in children's houses—the unique characteristic of a collective upbringing—was postulated by Sagi and his colleagues to be a possible antecedent for the development of insecure attachments, and a second study was designed to investigate this hypothesis.

In a quasi-experimental study, 23 mother–infant dyads from kibbutzim with communal sleeping arrangements, and 25 dyads from kibbutzim where family-based sleeping had been instituted, were observed in the Strange Situation (Sagi, van IJzendoorn, Aviezer, Donnell, & Mayseless, 1994). The distribution of attachment patterns for communally sleeping infants was confirmed: Only 48% of the infants were securely attached to their mothers. It should be noted, however, that even in the communal sleeping context, all children appeared to be attached to their mothers; this finding supports the universality hypothesis. The attachment distribution for infants in the family-based sleeping arrangements was completely different. Eighty percent of these infants were securely attached to their mothers—a rate similar to that found among urban Israeli infants (Sagi et al., 1985, 2002), as well as to that found in other international samples (van IJzendoorn & Kroonenberg, 1988). As for the normativity hypothesis, across studies the

majority of the infants living in the collective sleeping arrangement were still securely attached to their mothers. The disorganized classification was, however, not included in this study.

In order to rule out alternative explanations for the effect of communal sleeping arrangements, assessments were also made of the ecology of the children's house during the day, maternal separation anxiety, infants' temperaments, and mother–infant play interactions. The two groups (i.e., family-based and communal sleepers) were found to be comparable on all of these variables. Thus it was concluded that collective sleeping, experienced by infants as a time during which mothers were largely unavailable and inaccessible, was responsible for the greater insecurity found in this group. Inconsistent responsiveness was inherent in the reality of these infants, given that sensitive responding by a mother or caregiver during the day contrasted sharply with the presence of an unfamiliar person at night. Inconsistent responsiveness has been described as an important antecedent of ambivalent attachment (Ainsworth et al., 1978; Cassidy & Berlin, 1994). This confirms the sensitivity hypothesis, as did the city study, where maternal sensitivity was found to predict security of attachment (Sagi et al., 2002)

It should be noted that in several Israeli studies (Sagi et al., 1985, 1994, 1997, 2002), the ambivalent classification appeared to be overrepresented and the avoidant classification to be underrepresented, compared to the global distribution (van IJzendoorn & Kroonenberg, 1988). In fact, this finding has been replicated consistently across different Israeli childrearing arrangements and different kinds of caregivers. We offer two speculations concerning the Israeli bias toward ambivalent attachments. First, the ambivalent attachment strategy may be elicited in the context of continual threats to national and personal security more readily than the avoidant strategy may be. Parental preoccupation with these daily stresses may lead to exaggerated overprotectiveness and impaired sensitivity to children's attachment signals. Second, there is growing evidence that emotional reactivity may be more closely associated with ambivalent attachment than with avoidant attachment (Belsky & Rovine, 1987; Vaughn et al., 1992). The overrepresentation of ambivalent attachment and the near-absence of avoidant attachment may therefore also be attributed to a possible predominance of a high degree of emotional reactivity in Israeli society. To our knowledge, sound empirical evidence on temperament in Israel is still absent. As long as studies of temperament in this cultural context have not yet provided a test of this bold conjecture, our interpretation remains speculative. The finding of a substantial number of adults with an avoidant stance (classified as dismissing on the Adult Attachment Interview ([AAI]; George, Kaplan, & Main, 1984, 1985, 1996; see Hesse, Chapter 25, this volume) complicates the matter even further (Sagi et al., 1995, 1997).

Networks of Attachment Relationships

The kibbutz context has also made a unique contribution to the evaluation of the competence hypothesis. Oppenheim, Sagi, and Lamb (1990) assessed a broad spectrum of socioemotional skills in most of the subjects in the Sagi and colleagues (1985) sample when they were 5 years old, in an attempt to understand the sequelae of early relationships. They found that secure attachment to a nonparental caregiver (the *metapelet*) during infancy was the strongest predictor of a child's being empathic, dominant, independent, achievement-oriented, and behaviorally purposive in kindergarten. On the other hand, no significant associations were found between these socioemotional developments and the quality of children's attachment to their parents. These results suggest that the influence of attachment relationships may be viewed as domain-specific (for similar results, see the Gusii study described earlier in this chapter). Because the infants' relations with caregivers had been formed in the context of the infant house, they were the best predictor of children's socioemotional behavior in similar contexts.

One can expect attachment relationships in a multiple-caregiver environment, however, to interact in such a way that the predictive power of individual relationships is weaker than that of their combination (Howes, Rodning, Galluzzo, & Myers, 1988; Tavecchio & van IJzendoorn, 1987). Thus we proposed a model of testing multiple-caregiver environments based on the kibbutz experience (Sagi & van IJzendoorn, 1996; van IJzendoorn et al., 1992), in which the interrelations between multiple attachments were examined. More specifically, we examined in the group of kibbutz children the predictive power of the "extended" network of infants' attachments to the three types of caregivers (i.e., attachments to mothers, fathers, and *metaplot*), in comparison to the family network (attachments to mothers and fathers) and the infants' attachment to their mothers only.

We found that an extended network was the best predictor of later advanced functioning.

This outcome may be interpreted as support for the "integration" model, which assumes that in a network consisting of two or more attachment relationships, secure attachments may compensate for insecure attachments in a linear way (van IJzendoorn et al., 1992). Beyond kindergarten, however, networks of infant attachment relations did not contribute as much to the explanation of later behavior (Sagi-Schwartz & Aviezer, 2005). Instead, the data were more supportive of the hierarchy model (van IJzendoorn et al., 1992), suggesting that early relations with mother as the primary caregiver contributed most to later adaptive functioning at all ages (except in kindergarten), even in the kibbutz environment, where additional caregivers were introduced to be extensively involved in childcare. The relations with father and metapelet also contributed, but to a lesser degree. In the city study, infant–mother attachment was consistently found to predict various developmental outcomes at ages 4 and 7 (Gini, Oppenheim, & Sagi-Schwartz, 2007; Oppenheim, Koren-Karie, & Sagi-Schwartz, 2007; Ziv, Oppenheim, & Sagi-Schwartz, 2004).

Ecological Constraints on Intergenerational Transmission of Attachment

The kibbutz is the most unusual cultural setting in which the intergenerational transmission of attachment has been studied. "Intergenerational transmission of attachment" refers to the process through which parents' mental representations of their past attachment experiences influence their parenting behavior and the quality of their children's attachment to them (Bowlby, 1969/1982; Fonagy, Steele, & Steele, 1991; Main, Kaplan, & Cassidy, 1985; see Hesse, Chapter 25, this volume). In several studies of Western cultures, a strong association (concordance rate of about 75%) was found between the security of the parents' mental representation of attachment and the security of the child–parent attachment (for a review, see van IJzendoorn, 1995).

In an Israeli study, we (Sagi et al., 1997) presented the AAI to 20 mothers from kibbutzim maintaining collective sleeping arrangements, and to 25 mothers from home-sleeping kibbutzim (same design and participants as in Sagi et al., 1994). Parent–child concordance in attachment classifications was low for the communally sleeping group (40%), whereas it was rather high for the home-sleeping group (76%). Thus our data appear to be compatible with a model of intergenerational transmission of attachment in which the ecological context plays a facilitative or inhibiting role. Transmission of attachment across generations appears to depend on the specific child-rearing arrangements, and contextual factors such as communal sleeping may override the influence of parents' attachment representation and their sensitive responsiveness. This finding indicates the limits of a context-free, universal model of transmission.

AMAE, DEPENDENCE AND ATTACHMENT: THE JAPANESE CASE

One of the most severe critiques of attachment theory has come in the form of an accusation of "cultural blindness" among attachment researchers to alternative conceptions of relatedness (Rothbaum, Weisz, Pott, Miyake, & Morelli, 2000). This accusation of a Western bias in attachment theory was based specifically on the Japanese case.

The Japanese case can indeed be considered a real challenge to attachment theory's universality, normativity, and sensitivity hypotheses. From research on attachment in Japan, three issues have come to the fore. First, researchers studying attachment in Japan have claimed that ambivalent attachment relationships are overrepresented and that avoidant attachments are underrepresented (Miyake, Chen, & Campos, 1985; Takahashi, 1986). Second, the stressful Strange Situation, including two separations from the attachment figure, is criticized for being an invalid assessment of attachment in Japanese infants, who are used to continuous close proximity to their mothers. Third, the concept of attachment may not be relevant to the Japanese culture, in which the idea of *amae* (Doi, 1973, 1992) seems to play a more prominent and more adequate role in describing family relationships and their societal implications (Emde, 1992). Doi (1989) emphasizes that *amae* covers the same area as attachment, but that the bond with the parent inevitably implies dependence as well—an implication that, according to Doi, is denied in attachment theory (see Ainsworth, 1969). He argues that "*amae* definitely has an advantage over attachment precisely because it implies a psychological dependence" (Doi, 1989, p. 350). Therefore, an important preliminary question is how attachment, *amae*, and dependence are interpreted and evaluated in Japan.

Amae *and Attachment*

In Rothbaum and colleagues' (2000) challenge to the cross-cultural validity of attachment theory, the authors overlooked some crucial evidence (van IJzendoorn & Sagi, 2001). One piece of evidence is the Q-sort study by Vereijken (1996), in which eight native Japanese behavioral scientists were asked to describe the concepts of *amae*, attachment, and dependence with the help of the AQS procedure (Vaughn & Waters, 1990). The AQS cards contain descriptions of 90 different behaviors and can be regarded as a standard vocabulary pertinent to children's behavior in a wide variety of settings. The experts were asked to describe a child whom they considered prototypical for *amae* by sorting the 90 cards. Relevant behavioral descriptions of *amae* were "fussiness after playing in presence of mother," "demanding and impatient with the mother," and "enjoys having mother hug or cuddle him [or her]." The experts were strongly in agreement on the description of *amae*. They were also asked to provide ideal typical profiles of a dependent child and of a securely attached child. The descriptions of *amae* and dependence appeared to be very similar, whereas the descriptions of attachment security and *amae* were not associated at all (Vereijken, 1996, p. 85). Furthermore, when the descriptions of the ideal child according to Japanese mothers were compared with the experts' definitions of *amae*, attachment, and dependence, only attachment security appeared to be desirable, whereas *amae* and dependence were not associated with the ideal Japanese child in the eyes of mothers.

In another Japanese study of 42 mothers and 18 experts, the similarity of Japanese mothers' description of the ideal child with the experts' profile of the most secure child was striking ($r = .86$; Posada et al., 1995). Thus, in regard to a culture-specific evaluation of the importance of *amae*, we may conclude that even from a Japanese perspective, attachment security seems to be more desirable to mothers than the behavioral characteristics included in *amae*. It should be noted, however, that the domain of 90 behavioral descriptions may have restricted the range of potential definitions and evaluations of the concepts for which the AQS was not originally constructed (i.e., *amae* and dependence). In an observational study of Japanese sojourners in the United States, however, Mizuta, Zahn-Waxler, Cole, and Hiruma (1996; see also Nakagawa, Teti, & Lamb, 1992) confirmed Vereijken's (1996) conclusion that *amae* and attachment appear to be orthogonal dimensions that can be reliably distinguished (see also Behrens, 2004). This empirical evidence is in contrast with Johnson's (1993) speculation that the concept of attachment may be similar to the intrapsychical dimension of *amae*—that is, a desire to be held, fed, bathed, made safe, and emotionally comforted.

Two studies using the Strange Situation procedure to assess attachment security in Japan have been reported in the international literature. Durrett, Otaki, and Richards (1984) studied a middle-class sample of 39 intact families with their 12-month-old firstborns in Tokyo. Miyake, Takahashi, Nakagawa, and others studied a total of 60 middle-class intact families with their 12-month-old infants in Sapporo, a large city in the northern part of Japan (Miyake et al., 1985; Nakagawa, Lamb, & Miyake, 1992; Takahashi, 1986). An earlier report of a Strange Situation study by Takahashi (1982) did not focus on attachment classifications but on attachment behaviors, particularly toward the stranger. In both studies, the mothers were the primary caregivers of the infants, and in both cases the large majority of the mothers were full-time homemakers. The results of these two studies are rather discrepant.

The Tokyo study showed a pattern of avoidant, secure, and resistant infant–mother attachments consistent with the global distribution (13% A, 61% B, and 18% C, with 8% unclassifiable cases). The Sapporo study did not include avoidantly attached children, and it showed a distribution of either 68% securely attached and 32% resistantly attached infants (Takahashi, 1986), or 75% securely attached and 21% resistantly attached infants, with 4% unclassifiable cases and 4 damaged videotapes (Nakagawa, Lamb, & Miyake, 1992). The two studies also differed markedly in their conclusions about the validity of the Strange Situation procedure for use in the Japanese context. It is of course needless to say that Japan cannot be represented adequately by only two attachment studies of modest size.

The Tokyo Study

The Tokyo study investigated the relation between the security of infant–mother attachment and the mothers' perception of the positive support they received from their husbands. In accordance with previous studies of social support and attachment, Durrett and colleagues (1984) hypothesized that mothers who felt supported by their husbands would be more sensitive to their infants' needs and attachment signals, and therefore would be better able to foster the secure attachment of their infants.

The mothers of securely attached infants indeed indicated that they felt more supported by their husbands than did the mothers of avoidantly attached infants, but they did not differ in this regard from the mothers of resistantly attached infants. The differences in support were especially large with respect to a husband's pride in his wife's accomplishments, enjoyment in her activities, and sensitivity to her needs (Durrett et al., 1984). The authors concluded "that in Japan as well as in America the adequacy of mothering seems to be influenced by the support perceived by the mother and the family context" (Durrett et al., 1984, p. 174). The sensitivity hypothesis is only partially and indirectly supported, because the assessment of perceived social support was not equivalent to observed maternal sensitivity. Furthermore, on the basis of perceived support, the resistant category could not be discriminated from the secure category. The Tokyo study confirms the universality and normativity hypotheses more definitively, because it did not report difficulties in applying the attachment coding system to this population, and because the normative "modal" category was secure.

The First Sapporo Study

The first Sapporo study to be described in this chapter provides a more complicated picture, in particular because the various reports do not converge in terms of the basic data or in terms of the number of cases involved. If we leave out the interim reports on part of the sample (Miyake et al., 1985, included only approximately 20 subjects in most of their analyses), we should concentrate on the longitudinal data provided by Nakagawa, Lamb, and Miyake (1992), who focused on maternal sensitivity. But first we should examine the suggestion that the Strange Situation procedure may be too stressful for Japanese infants, and therefore invalid.

In order to examine whether the stress level induced by the complete Strange Situation procedure might be a cause of the overrepresentation of resistantly attached infants, Takahashi (1986) decided to classify the infant–mother attachments also on the basis of the first five Strange Situation episodes, which include only one separation from the mother and no episode in which the child is alone in the strange room. With this modified procedure, she found that 83% of the infants could be classified as securely attached to their mothers, and only 17% as resistantly attached. Again, she did not find infants who qualified for the avoidant category. More importantly, however, Takahashi also reported that in the absence of clear instructions about the curtailing of episodes in case of excessive crying behavior, the maximum duration of a crying episode was set at 2 minutes. This is considerably longer than in most attachment studies elsewhere, as Takahashi (1986, p. 266) conceded, because normally crying leads to a curtailed episode after only 20–30 seconds. The absence of avoidance in the Sapporo study may therefore be explained by the "more than mild" stress level induced in the Japanese version of the Strange Situation procedure. We are reminded of Ainsworth and colleagues' (1978) report on a short-term test–retest study of the original procedure, in which at the second assessment most avoidant infants appeared to behave in a "secure" way, and many secure infants showed resistant behavior.

Because the status of the Sapporo attachment classifications is unclear (Grossmann & Grossmann, 1989), it is difficult to evaluate the Nakagawa, Lamb, and Miyake (1992) report on the antecedents of attachment security in this sample. In part of the sample (25–29 families), researchers rated videotaped home interactions at 4 and 8 months after birth; they also conducted 8-month laboratory assessments on scales for maternal accessibility, acceptance, cooperation, and sensitivity. The authors found no association between attachment security and antecedent maternal interactive behavior at home or in the laboratory. They suggested that the ratings of maternal behavior may have been less valid, because the Japanese mothers looked very self-conscious during the observations, although they were asked to behave naturally. Mizuta and colleagues (1996) have also remarked that the Japanese mothers in their study were inclined to show strong deference, compliance, and reserve toward the experimenter as an authority figure.

In sum, the Sapporo Strange Situation study does not seem to undermine either the universality or the normativity hypothesis; in fact, the absence of avoidant infants may have been an artifact of the rigid procedure and/or the unique characteristics of this sample, which were not shared by the Tokyo sample (van IJzendoorn & Kroonenberg, 1988). The sensitivity hypothesis is of course not supported by the results of this study, although

plausible alternative interpretations of the absence of an association between maternal sensitivity and attachment security have been proposed. It may be added that in a meta-analysis of more than 65 studies, the association between sensitivity and attachment was found to be $r = .24$ (De Wolff & van IJzendoorn, 1997). A sample of fewer than 30 cases does not provide sufficient power to detect this medium effect size.

Takahashi (1990) followed the Sapporo sample for 21/2 years after the attachment assessment, and she focused on the children's compliance to their mothers' requests, their curiosity, their social competence, and their cognitive development. The assessments during the second year of life showed that the secure infants complied more with their mothers' directions and demands; they also showed more curiosity about a new object and were more competent in relating to unfamiliar peers than the resistantly attached infants. During the third year of life, however, the resistantly attached children no longer differed from the securely attached children in terms of social competence and cognitive development.

Takahashi (1990) concluded that the Strange Situation procedure does not predict competence after infancy, and thus appears to lack cross-cultural validity. However, studies in Western countries on the long-term sequelae of attachment security after infancy have not always yielded strong differences between the secure and insecure groups, either; in most comparisons, the resistant group was too small to be studied separately from the avoidant group (see Thompson, Chapter 16, this volume). Furthermore, during the first 5 years of life, changes in attachment security should be considered to be the outcome of the interaction between the developing child and the changing environment (Bowlby, 1969/1982). The follow-up studies presented by Takahashi (1990) did not include assessments of the potentially changing childrearing context (van IJzendoorn, 1996).

The AQS Study

The cross-cultural debate on attachment in Japan has focused on the validity of the Strange Situation procedure, and in fact has been based on the outcomes of only one study using this procedure, the Sapporo study. As we have shown earlier, the Tokyo study does not confirm the results of the Sapporo study. Fortunately, the Strange Situation procedure is no longer the only measure to be used in cross-cultural research. The AQS (Vaughn &

Waters, 1990) is a viable alternative, particularly in cases where separations between parents and children may be uncommon (van IJzendoorn et al., 2004). Vereijken (1996) constructed a Japanese version of the AQS, and he studied the association between sensitivity and attachment security in a Tokyo sample of 48 intact families with 14-month-old infants. More sensitive mothers had more secure children, and the association between sensitivity and attachment was impressively strong (all correlations—based on reports from independent coders—were .59 or higher). In a follow-up study 10 months later, the association between sensitivity and attachment was replicated (Vereijken, 1996). The Vereijken study indeed supports the validity of attachment theory—in particular, the universality and the sensitivity hypotheses—and, again, this study did not get the attention it deserved in the Rothbaum and colleagues (2000) critique.

The Osaka and Sapporo Studies on Adult Attachment

Another set of findings that Rothbaum and colleagues (2000) did not take into account in their critique emerged from a pioneering study by Kazui, Endo, Tanaka, Sakagami, and Suganuma (2000). Their study of the intergenerational transmission of attachment between 50 Japanese mothers and their preschool-age children was the first Japanese replication of the well-established association between mothers' attachment security and their children's security (Hesse, Chapter 25, this volume). They showed that the children of secure mothers as assessed with the AAI had the highest security scores on the AQS, whereas the children of unresolved mothers had the lowest AQS scores. The children of the dismissing and preoccupied mothers scored in between. The majority of the mothers were classified as secure (66%). If we assume that secure mothers generally have more sensitive interactions with their children than insecure mothers do, this outcome may be interpreted as another confirmation of attachment theory's sensitivity hypothesis.

Following the first Sapporo study reporting a predominance of ambivalent attachment among insecure Sapporo infants, the generalizability of attachment theory to Japanese infants was further tested in a replication and extension study by Behrens, Main, and Hesse (2007). In this second study of Sapporo mother–child dyads (N = 43), attachment distributions were presented for both the children, based on Main and Cassidy's 6th-year reunion assessment procedure (see Solomon & George, Chapter 18, this volume), and the mothers, based on the AAI (see Hesse, Chapter 25, this volume). In contrast to the previous Sapporo study, children's three-way or forced "organized" attachment classification distribution did not differ from the global distribution: 28 secure (B) infants (70%), 9 avoidant (A) infants (23%), and 3 ambivalent (C) infants (7%), with 3 children remaining unclassified. However, a high proportion of controlling (D) children was found: 19 of 41 cases (46%) were classified as D or as Unclassifiable. The adult attachment classification distributions for Japanese mothers deviated only slightly from the global norm, with the majority of Japanese mothers being classified as secure-autonomous (77%). Furthermore, mothers' AAI classification predicted child reunion classification, with proportions very similar to matches reported worldwide. This is support for the sensitivity hypothesis, because secure mothers have been shown to be more sensitive than insecure mothers. Notably, even mothers' unresolved attachment status strongly predicted child D status ($r = .65$).

It is remarkable that an assessment of discourse coherence during the AAI, developed in the English language, shows similar predictive validity in Japanese and in two independent investigations. Competent indigenous researchers have thus demonstrated that it is possible to cross both cultural and language barriers to test and confirm hypotheses based on attachment theory—and, contrary to Rothbaum and colleagues' (2000) assertions, to do this even in Japan. In fact, Rothbaum and colleagues' attack on the universality hypothesis of attachment theory clearly missed its target, considering the overwhelming empirical support in favor of the universality hypothesis, including in all but one Japanese study of attachment. Rothbaum and colleagues did not take into account crucial evidence from recent attachment studies on Japanese families conducted by or in close cooperation with Japanese investigators. The only empirical study in partial support of Rothbaum and colleagues' attack is the first Sapporo study discussed above, which we have shown to be seriously flawed because of ill-informed use of the Strange Situation procedure. The Japanese studies fit well with the global picture of cross-cultural attachment research in various parts of the world, and as a whole they disconfirm Rothbaum and colleagues' critique of attachment theory's universality claim.

On a theoretical level, Rothbaum and colleagues (2000) claimed that "[m]any ... features of ambivalent behavior characterize the normal *amae* relationship in Japan" (p. 1100). In other words, children's behaviors called ambivalent in attachment studies in the Western world would probably be viewed as *amae* behaviors in Japan, which in that culture would be considered appropriate. In a ground-breaking and comprehensive treatise on the concept of *amae*, Behrens (2004), a psychologist of Japanese origin, has presented a totally different, context-based, multifaceted view of the construct of amae. She has analyzed the use of the term and related terminology in natural Japanese discourse, and concluded that attachment and *amae* can be readily distinguished and often serve different purposes. Behrens (2004; Behrens et al., 2007) states that for many native Japanese speakers, *amae* has a negative connotation involving social enforcement of obligations. Theoretically, she argues that *amae* lacks the biological roots of the attachment concept and is not associated with the regulation of stress, but can occur any time there is a desire or a motive on the part of the *amae* provider (Behrens, 2004; Behrens et al., 2007). *Amae* is tied to a specific social role and is culturally unique. Because of the fundamental linguistic and biological differences between the two constructs, attachment research in Japan should not be considered a challenge to the concept of *amae*, and *amae* should not be considered a refutation of the concept of attachment. Considering attachment and *amae* as competing concepts—as Rothbaum and colleagues did—is making a logical category error.

ATTACHMENT IN MUSLIM FAMILIES IN INDONESIA

Indonesia is the fourth most populous country in the world, with a population of approximately 200 million persons, most of them Muslim. Indeed, it has the largest Islamic population of any country in the world. Zevalkink (1997) conducted the first attachment study on Islamic families of Sundanese-Indonesian origin in West Java. Sundanese-Indonesian children generally experience relatively extensive periods of close physical proximity to their mothers, being carried in a carrying cloth or *slendang* during the first year; they are breast-fed on demand until 2 or 3 years of age, and sleep in the same beds as their mothers during the first 4 years of life. When an infant is fussy or cries, the mother promptly responds with soothing or feeding. Sundanese-Indonesian women, however, marry at a very young age, and their divorce rate is high. A stable income and a permanent job are rare, which adds to the instability of family life. Poverty and health problems lead to rather high infant mortality (56 per 1,000 births in 1993) (Zevalkink, Riksen-Walraven, & Van Lieshout, 1999).

Zevalkink and colleagues (1999) reported Strange Situation assessments of 46 children, ages 12–30 months. They also conducted extensive home observations on maternal sensitivity and observed maternal support in structured play sessions. The distribution of attachment classifications was as follows: 3 avoidantly attached, 24 securely attached, 9 resistantly attached, and 10 disorganized. The forced classification distribution was this: 7% avoidant, 57% secure, 33% resistant, and 4% other (Zevalkink et al., 1999). The majority of the children were securely attached, but the number of avoidant children was relatively low. The distribution of the 25 children between 12 and 18 months of age was similar. More maternal support in structured play sessions was associated with attachment security; disorganized children received low maternal support. Thus in these Muslim families, a majority of children appeared to be securely attached, and secure attachment was associated with maternal support in the predicted way.

UNIVERSAL AND CONTEXTUAL DIMENSIONS OF ATTACHMENT

In this section, we review the findings of cross-cultural attachment research in two ways. First, we discuss the use of the *concept* of attachment security across cultures. Second, we summarize the cross-cultural support for the core *hypotheses* of attachment theory. Of course, the most powerful test of the universality of attachment theory is the cross-cultural confirmation of its nomological network.

The Concept of Attachment

To start with cross-cultural use of the concept of attachment, we focus on the conceptual normativity of attachment security. The AQS (Vaughn & Waters, 1990) provides the opportunity to test whether experts and parents conceptualize attachment security in a similar manner, within as well as across societies. Posada and colleagues (1995) performed exactly this test, in a cross-cultural comparison of expert and mother samples from China, Colombia, Germany, Israel, Japan, and the United States. They correlated the descriptions of the "optimally secure" child as sorted by the experts from the different societies and the descriptions of the "ideal" child in the eyes of the mothers in each culture. Without exception, the correlations were substantial, indicating that across cultures the experts' conceptualization of attachment was very similar to the mothers' ideas about the ideal child (Posada et al., 1995). Similarly, the experts' opinions about the most secure child and the mothers' views of the most ideal child converged strongly across cultures. It seems, therefore, that across cultures experts as well as mothers interpret attachment security in a similar manner; they also appear to evaluate it in the same way, although the reasons for their preference of secure instead of insecure attachments may be different (Harwood, Miller, & Irizarry, 1995).

The conceptual similarity of attachment security across diverging cultures does not mean that exactly the same infant attachment behaviors are considered to be indicative of secure or insecure attachment. In some cultures, distal attachment behaviors may be stressed somewhat more than proximal behaviors, or vice versa. The secure-base phenomenon, however, is located at the level of behavior patterns or behavioral organization, at which separate behaviors play only a minor role (Waters, 1978). Gusii infants, for example, are accustomed to being greeted with a handshake instead of a hug by their mothers, as noted earlier. After separations the Gusii infants expect the handshake, whereas Western infants look forward to "more intimate" physical contact. The patterning of attachment behaviors demonstrating the secure base remains the same, regardless of the specific behaviors. The secure Gusii infants studied by Kermoian and Leiderman (1986) would reach out to the adult with one arm, to receive the handshake enthusiastically, whereas the insecure infants would avoid the adult or would reach and then pull away as the adult approached. This is a powerful demonstration of the culture-specific behavioral markers of a universal and normative phenomenon.

A Cross-Cultural Test of the Nomological Network

The evidence for the cross-cultural validity of attachment theory is impressive. In Table 37.1, we present the findings of the cross-cultural studies as they pertain to the four core hypotheses of attach-

ment theory: the universality, normativity, sensitivity, and competence hypotheses. The overview is limited to the studies discussed above.

The universality hypothesis appears to be supported most strongly. In every cross-cultural study, similar patterns of attachment behavior have been observed. Some children may have been difficult to rate—for example, because of the stresses of the assessment procedure—but reports of children who did not show attachment behavior in stressful circumstances are absent. Furthermore, the numbers of children who were difficult to rate do not differ across cultures. In the studies discussed here, these children were exceptions rather than the rule, and the application of the coding system for disorganized attachment behavior (Main & Solomon, 1990) might have rendered their interactions interpretable.

The cross-cultural studies included here support Bowlby's (1969/1982) idea that attachment is indeed a universal phenomenon, and an evolutionary explanation seems to be warranted. Although in many cultures children grow up with a network of attachment figures, the parent or caregiver who takes responsibility for the care of a child during part of the day or the night becomes the favorite target of infant attachment behaviors. Not only the attachment phenomenon itself, but also the different types of attachment, appear to be present in various Western and non-Western cultures. Avoidant, secure, and resistant attachments have been observed in the African, Chinese, Indonesian, and Japanese studies; even in the extremely diverging childrearing context of the Israeli communal kibbutzim, the differentiation between secure and insecure attachment could be made.

The cross-cultural evidence for the normativity hypothesis is rather strong as well. In all cross-cultural studies included here, the majority of infants were classified as securely attached. In Table 37.2, the attachment classification distributions of the studies discussed above are presented. When these are combined with AQS findings about the cross-cultural preference among experts as well as mothers for securely attached children, we may be confident that secure attachment is not just a North American invention or a Western ideal, but a rather widespread and preferred phenomenon. As we have described in the introductory section, the category of secure attachments emerged from Ainsworth's Uganda study, not from her Baltimore study (as is often suggested). Scrutinizing Ainsworth's (1967) report on the Uganda sample, we became acutely aware of its importance in estab-

TABLE 37.1. Evidence from Africa, China, Israel, Japan, and Indonesia for the Cross-Cultural Validity of Attachment Theory

Society	Hypothesis			
	Universality	Normativity	Sensitivity	Competence
Africa				
Uganda (Ainsworth, 1967)	+	+	+	0
Gusii (Kermoian & Leiderman, 1986)	+	+	+	0
Dogon (True, 1994; True et al., 2001)	+	+	0	+
Hausa (Marvin et al., 1977)	+	0	0	0
!Kung San (Konner, 1977)	+	0	(+)	0
Efé (Morelli & Tronick, 1991)	+	0	(+)	0
Uganda (Peterson et al., 2001)	+	0	+	0
Khayelitsha (Tomlinson et al., 2005)	+	+	+	0
China				
Beijing (Posada et al., 1995)	+	+	0	0
Beijing (Hu & Meng, 1996)	+	+	+	0
Israel				
Communal kibbutzim (Sagi et al., 1985, 1995)	+	+	+	+
Family-based kibbutzim (Sagi et al., 1995)	+	+	+	0
City (Sagi et al., 2002)	+	+	+	+
Japan				
Tokyo (Durrett et al., 1984)	+	+	±	0
Sapporo (Takahashi, 1986)	+	+	−	±
Tokyo (Vereijken, 1996)	+	+	+	0
Osaka (Kazui et al., 2000)	+	+	+	0
Sapporo (Behrens et al., 2007)	+	+	+	0
Indonesia				
West Java (Zevalkink et al., 1999)	+	+	+	0

Note. +, positive evidence; 0, no evidence available; ±, mixed positive and negative evidence; −, negative evidence; (+), indirect positive evidence.

lishing the Strange Situation procedure and its coding system. In fact, the Baltimore study should be considered much more of a replication than a pioneering exploration into uncharted territory, as others have noted (e.g., Lamb, Thompson, Gardner, Charnov, & Estes, 1984).

The sensitivity and competence hypotheses receive less support. A meta-analysis of more than 65 studies showed that the association between attachment and sensitivity is important but modest: The combined effect size in a selected set of pertinent studies was equivalent to $r = .24$ (De Wolff & van IJzendoorn, 1997). Cross-cultural studies on attachment are by necessity small, and the lack of

statistical power may have been one of the most important causes for the disconfirming results in the first Sapporo study (Takahashi, 1990). Nevertheless, in 12 studies unequivocal support for the sensitivity hypothesis was found, and in 2 other studies support may be indirectly derived from the reports (Konner, 1977; Morelli & Tronick, 1991). The most striking disconfirming data have been found in the first Sapporo study, but at the same time supporting evidence has been presented in the second Sapporo study and in the Tokyo study. That is, whether findings support or disconfirm the sensitivity hypothesis does not depend on culture, but seems to be associated with specific

TABLE 37.2. Distributions of Infant–Mother Attachment Classifications in Africa, China, Israel, Japan, and Indonesia Compared with Western Europe and the United States

Society	N	Avoidant (A)	Secure (B)	Resistant (C)	Other
Africa					
Uganda (Ainsworth, 1967)	28	18%	57%	25%	—
Gusii (Kermoian & Leiderman, 1986)	26	—[a]	61%	—[a]	—
Dogon (True, 1994; True et al., 2001)	26	0%	69%	8%	23%
Khayelitsha (Tomlinson et al., 2005)	98	17%	72%	11%	—
China					
Beijing (Hu & Meng, 1996)	31	16%	68%	16%	—
Israel					
Communal kibbutzim (Sagi et al., 1985, 1995)	104	7%	56%	37%	—
Family-based kibbutzim (Sagi et al., 1995)	25	0%	80%	20%	—
City (Sagi et al., 2002)	758	3%	72%	21%	3%
Japan					
Tokyo (Durrett et al., 1984)	39	13%	61%	18%	8%
Sapporo (Takahashi, 1986)	60	0%	68%	32%	—
Sapporo (Behrens et al., 2007)	40	23%	70%	7%	—
Indonesia					
West Java (Zevalkink et al., 1999)	46	7%	57%	33%	4%
Western Europe					
9 samples combined (van IJzendoorn & Kroonenberg, 1988)	510	28%	66%	6%	—
United States					
21 samples combined (van IJzendoorn et al., 1992)	1,584	21%	67%	12%	—

[a]No differentiation between avoidant and resistant attachments available.

studies or samples. The first Sapporo results cannot be used to invalidate the Strange Situation or attachment theory's claim of universality, because of the presence of more positive support in other Japanese research (in the same as well as in other cities; Vereijken, 1996), unless there are good reasons to suspect that intracultural differences play an important role. In the discussions of the Sapporo findings, this line of reasoning has never been stressed (Miyake et al., 1985; Takahashi, 1990). Although the sensitivity hypothesis does not appear to be refuted in cross-cultural research, more studies on the antecedents of attachment security are needed to settle the issue more definitively (see also Bakermans-Kranenburg, van IJzendoorn, & Kroonenberg, 2004).

The competence hypothesis has been tested only sporadically in cross-cultural research; this concurs with the relative lack of Western studies on the association between attachment and (later) competence (Meins, 1997; van IJzendoorn, Dijkstra, & Bus, 1995). In the Gusii study (Kermoian & Leiderman, 1986), the nutritional status of the secure infants was better than that of the insecure infants. This outcome has been replicated by Valenzuela (1990) in her Chilean study of undernourished infants. Although the relation between attachment and health status is truly remarkable, it is still not clear whether attachment security serves only as the cause and nutritional status only as the effect. A more intricate causal pattern cannot be completely excluded on the basis of the correlational evidence that Kermoian and Leiderman (1986) and Valenzuela have provided. The Dogon study (True, 1994; True et al., 2001) does not allow for differentiation between cause and effect, either. We should therefore conclude that the cross-cultural support for the competence hypothesis is still insufficient. The concept of attachment networks may be fruitfully applied in further cross-cultural studies of the competence hypothesis.

CONCLUSIONS

Our analysis and integration of cross-cultural attachment research suggest a balance between universal trends and contextual determinants. Attachment theory without contextual components is as difficult to conceive of as attachment theory without a universalistic perspective. If across cultures all infants used the same fixed strategies to deal with attachment challenges, it would leave no room for adaptation to dynamic changes of the environment (Hinde & Stevenson-Hinde, 1990) and to the constraints imposed by different developmental niches (DeVries, 1984; Harkness & Super, 1992, 1996; LeVine & Miller, 1990; see Simpson & Belsky, Chapter 6, this volume). Without variation, selection of optimal behavioral strategies would become obsolete (Darwin, 1859/1985; see van IJzendoorn, Bakermans-Kranenburg, & Sagi-Schwartz, 2006, for an evolutionary attachment model integrating universal and contextual dimensions of attachment). The three basic attachment patterns—avoidant, secure, and ambivalent—can be found in every culture in which attachment studies have been conducted thus far. Even in the Israeli research, some avoidant infant–parent relationships have been found, albeit at a much lower than usual rate.

What seems to be universal are the general cultural pressure toward selection of the secure attachment pattern in the majority of children, and the preference for the secure child in parents across cultures. Even in the extremely deviating context of the communal sleeping arrangement, the majority of children develop secure attachments to their parents. The most dramatic demonstration of the adaptive value of attachment security is its role as a protective factor against malnutrition (True, 1994; True et al., 2001). Dixon, LeVine, and Brazelton (1982) even identified malnutrition as a symptom of a "disorder of attachment." Furthermore, in many cultural contexts, the secure attachment strategy seems to emerge from the most

sensitive parenting. Although the cross-cultural evidence pertaining to the competence hypothesis is still scarce, secure attachment seems to increase the likelihood of better social competence in the future. Thus the universal validity of attachment theory appears to be confirmed in cross-cultural research. Cross-cultural studies on attachment have made us sensitive to the importance of wider social networks in which children grow and develop (Harkness & Super, 1996; Nsamenang, 1992; Thompson, 1993). We need a radical change from a dyadic perspective to an attachment network approach (Tavecchio & van IJzendoorn, 1987). In Western as well as non-Western cultures, most children communicate with several attachment figures (Lamb, 1977; Main & Weston, 1981), including siblings (Weisner & Gallimore, 1977). Examining the competence hypothesis only on the basis of infant–mother attachment may decrease predictive power substantially.

If Kermoian and Leiderman (1986) had included only mothers in their study, they would not have been able to predict cognitive competence on the basis of their attachment assessments. In the Israeli case, infant–mother attachment did not predict aspects of competence as assessed in a kindergarten context, whereas the extended attachment network was found to predict social competence at age 5 more strongly than any single attachment relationship (Sagi & van IJzendoorn, 1996; van IJzendoorn et al., 1992). Because child–mother attachment became a stronger predictor of functioning beyond kindergarten (Sagi-Schwartz & Aviezer, 2005), more conceptual and empirical work is needed to determine how experiences with different attachment figures become organized to form a coherent internal working model.

Cross-cultural studies on attachment require major investments on the part of the researchers. It is remarkable that so many studies in various parts of the world have been performed. The cross-cultural studies are rather small-scale, in-depth observational studies, often combined with a longitudinal component. The validity of the cross-cultural data can be regarded as high, because in general the researchers have been carefully adapting their assessments to the particular culture. In this respect, cross-cultural attachment research is not only "etic"; it also contains elements of the "emic" approach, and the two approaches appear compatible (Pike, 1967). For example, the use of the naturally occurring Weigh-In procedure for the purpose of assessing communication patterns between parents and infants (True, 1994; True et al., 2001) is ecologically valid as well as replicable. Nevertheless, the current cross-cultural database is almost absurdly small, compared to the domain that should be covered. In cultural anthropology, the number of different cultures (past and present) has been estimated at more than 1,200. Systematic anthropological data are available on at least 186 different cultural areas in the Standard Cross-Cultural Sample (Murdock & White, 1969). In this chapter, we have covered only a few cultural areas in China, Japan, Israel, Indonesia, and Africa. Data on attachment in India and most Islamic countries are still lacking. Furthermore, large parts of China, Indonesia, and Africa are uncharted territories with respect to the development of attachment. For example, we have been able to present data from only two Chinese studies. Although these studies represent admirable contributions to the attachment literature, they cannot be considered to be representative of a population of more than 1 billion people from at least 56 nationalities.

Of course, cross-cultural attachment research is not meant to produce representative demographic data. Its most important contribution is the test of some core propositions of attachment theory. The central issue is whether attachment theory is just a middle-class Western invention with no relevance at all to other cultures, or whether its universalistic perspective can be confirmed in non-Western childrearing circumstances. The cross-cultural studies have not (yet) refuted the bold conjectures of attachment theory about the universality and normativity of attachment, and about its antecedents and sequelae. In fact, taken as a whole, the studies are remarkably consistent with the theory. Attachment theory may therefore claim cross-cultural validity.

ACKNOWLEDGMENT

Support for the preparation of this chapter was provided by a fellowship from the Netherlands Institute for Advanced Study in the Humanities and Social Sciences (NIAS) and the Spinoza Prize of the Netherlands' Foundation for Scientific Research (NW)) to Marinus H. van IJzendoorn.

REFERENCES

Ainsworth, M. D. S. (1967). *Infancy in Uganda: Infant care and the growth of love.* Baltimore: Johns Hopkins University Press.

Ainsworth, M. D. S. (1969). Object relations, dependency, and attachment: A theoretical review of the infant–mother relationship. *Child Development, 40,* 969–1025.

Ainsworth, M. D. S. (1977). Infant development and mother–infant interaction among Ganda and American families. In P. H. Leiderman, S. R. Tulkin, & A. H. Rosenfeld (Eds.), *Culture and infancy* (pp. 119–150). New York: Academic Press.

Ainsworth, M. D. S., Blehar, M. C., Waters, E., & Wall, S. (1978). *Patterns of attachment.* Hillsdale, NJ: Erlbaum.

Ainsworth, M. D. S., & Wittig, B. A. (1969). Attachment and exploratory behavior of one year olds in a strange situation. In B. M. Foss (Ed.), *Determinants of infant behavior* (Vol. 4, pp. 113–136). London: Methuen.

Aviezer, O., van IJzendoorn, M. H., Sagi, A., & Schuengel, C. (1994). "Children of the dream" revisited: 70 years of collective early child care in Israeli kibbutzim. *Psychological Bulletin, 116,* 99–116.

Bakermans-Kranenburg, M. J., van IJzendoorn, M. H., & Juffer, F. (2003). Less is more: Meta-analyses of sensitivity and attachment interventions in early childhood. *Psychological Bulletin, 129,* 195–215.

Bakermans-Kranenburg, M. J., van IJzendoorn, M. H., & Kroonenberg, P. M. (2004). Differences in attachment security betwen African-American and white children: Ethnicity or socio-economic status? *Infant Behavior and Development, 27,* 417–433.

Barry, H. I., & Paxton, L. M. (1971). Infancy and early childhood: Cross-cultural codes 2. *Ethnology, 10,* 466–508.

Behrens, K. (2004). A multifaceted view of the concept of *amae:* Reconsidering the indigenous Japanese concept of relatedness. *Human Development, 47,* 1–27.

Behrens, K., Main, M., & Hesse, E. (2007). Mothers' attachment status as determined by the Adult Attachment Interview predicts their 6-year-olds' responses to separation and reunion: A study conducted in Japan. *Developmental Psychology, 43,* 1553–1567.

Beit-Hallahmi, B., & Rabin, A. (1977). The kibbutz as a social experiment and as a child-rearing laboratory. *American Psychologist, 12,* 57–69.

Belsky, J., & Cassidy, J. (1995). Attachment: Theory and evidence. In M. Rutter, D. Hay, & S. Baron-Cohen (Eds.), *Developmental principles and clinical issues in psychology and psychiatry* (pp. 373–402). Oxford, UK: Blackwell.

Belsky, J., & Rovine, M. (1987). Temperament and attachment security in the Strange Situation: An empirical rapprochement. *Child Development, 58,* 787–795.

Berry, J. W. (1969). On cross-cultural comparability. *International Journal of Psychology, 4,* 119–128.

Bowlby, J. (1951). *Maternal care and mental health.* Geneva: World Health Organization.

Bowlby, J. (1969/1982). *Attachment and loss: Vol. 1. Attachment.* New York: Basic Books.

Bretherton, I. (1985). Attachment theory: Retrospect and prospect. In I. Bretherton & E. Waters (Eds.),

Growing points of attachment theory and research. *Monographs of the Society for Research in Child Development, 50*(1–2, Serial No. 209), 3–35.

Bretherton, I. (1991). The roots and growing points of attachment theory. In C. M. Parkes, J. Stevenson-Hinde, & P. Marris (Eds.), *Attachment across the life cycle* (pp. 9–32). London: Tavistock/Routledge.

Caldwell, B., & Bradley, R. (1984). *Home Observation for Measurement of the Environment.* Little Rock: University of Arkansas at Little Rock.

Cassidy, J. (1986). The ability to negotiate the environment: An aspect of infant competence as related to quality of attachment. *Child Development, 57,* 331–337.

Cassidy, J. (1994). Emotion regulation: Influences of attachment relationships. In N. A. Fox (Ed.), The development of emotion regulation: Biological and behavioral considerations. *Monographs of the Society for Research in Child Development, 59*(2–3, Serial No. 240), 228–249.

Cassidy, J., & Berlin, L. J. (1994). The insecure/ambivalent pattern of attachment: Theory and research. *Child Development, 65,* 971–991.

Chen, X. Y., Rubin, K. H., & Li, B. S. (1995). Social and school adjustment of shy and aggressive children in China. *Development and Psychopathology, 7,* 337–349.

Darwin, C. (1985). *On the origin of species by means of natural selection, or the preservation of favoured races in the struggle for life.* Harmondsworth, UK: Penguin. (Original work published 1859)

DeVries, M. W. (1984). Temperament and infant mortality among the Masai of East Africa. *American Journal of Psychiatry, 141,* 1189–1194.

De Wolff, M. S., & van IJzendoorn, M. H. (1997). Sensitivity and attachment: A meta-analysis on parental antecedents of infant attachment. *Child Development, 68,* 571–591.

Dixon, S. D., LeVine, R. A., & Brazelton, T. B. (1982). Malnutrition: A closer look at the problem in an East African village. *Developmental Medicine and Child Neurology, 24,* 670–685.

Doi, T. (1973). *The anatomy of dependence.* New York: Kodansha.

Doi, T. (1989). The concept of *amae* and its psychoanalytic implications. *International Review of Psychoanalysis, 16,* 349–354.

Doi, T. (1992). On the concept of *amae. Infant Mental Health Journal, 13,* 7–11.

Durrett, M. E., Otaki, M., & Richards, P. (1984). Attachment and the mother's perception of support from the father. *International Journal of Behavioral Development, 7,* 167–176.

Emde, R. N. (1992). *Amae*, intimacy, and the early moral self. *Infant Mental Health Journal, 13,* 34–42.

Fonagy, P., Steele, H., & Steele, M. (1991). Maternal representations of attachment during pregnancy predict the organization of infant–mother attachment at one year of age. *Child Development, 62,* 891–905.

George, C., Kaplan, N., & Main, M. (1984). *Adult At-

tachment Interview protocol.* Unpublished manuscript, University of California at Berkeley.

George, C., Kaplan, N., & Main, M. (1985). *Adult Attachment Interview protocol* (2nd ed.). Unpublished manuscript, University of California at Berkeley.

George, C., Kaplan, N., & Main, M. (1996). *Adult Attachment Interview protocol* (3rd ed.). Unpublished manuscript, University of California at Berkeley.

Gini, M., Oppenheim, D., & Sagi-Schwartz, A. (2007). Negotiation styles in mother–child narrative co-construction in middle childhood: Associations with early attachment. *International Journal of Behavioral Development, 31,* 149–160.

Goossens, F. A., & van IJzendoorn, M. H. (1990). Quality of infants' attachments to professional caregivers: Relation to infant–parent attachment and day-care characteristics. *Child Development, 61,* 832–837.

Grossmann, K. E., & Grossmann, K. (1989). Preliminary observations on Japanese infants' behavior in Ainsworth's Strange Situation. *Annual Report of the Research and Clinical Center for Child Development,* no. 13, 1–12.

Grossmann, K. E., Grossmann, K., Huber, F., & Wartner, U. (1981). German children's behavior towards their mothers at 12 months and their fathers at 18 months in Ainsworth's Strange Situation. *International Journal of Behavioral Development, 4,* 157–181.

Harkness, S., & Super, C. M. (1992). Shared child care in East Africa: Sociocultural origins and developmental consequences. In M. E. Lamb, K. J. Sternberg, C. P. Hwang, & A. G. Broberg (Eds.), *Child care in context: Cross-cultural perspectives* (pp. 441–459). Hillsdale, NJ: Erlbaum.

Harkness, S., & Super, C. M. (Eds.). (1996). *Parents' cultural belief systems: Their origins, expressions, and consequences.* New York: Guilford Press.

Harwood, R. L., Miller, J. G., & Irizarry, N. L. (1995). *Culture and attachment: Perceptions of the child in context.* New York: Guilford Press.

Hertsgaard, L., Gunnar, M., Erickson, M. F., & Nachmias, M. (1995). Adrenocortical responses to the Strange Situation in infants with disorganized/disoriented attachment relationships. *Child Development, 66,* 1100–1106.

Hinde, R. A., & Stevenson-Hinde, J. (1990). Attachment: Biological, cultural, and individual desiderata. *Human Development, 33,* 62–72.

Hinde, R. A., & Stevenson-Hinde, J. (1991). Perspectives on attachment. In C. M. Parkes, J. Stevenson-Hinde, & P. Marris (Eds.), *Attachment across the life cycle* (pp. 52–65). London: Tavistock/Routledge.

Ho, D. Y. F. (1986). Chinese patterns of socialization: A critical review. In M. H. Bond (Ed.), *The psychology of the Chinese people* (pp. 1–37). Hong Kong: Oxford University Press.

Howes, C., Rodning, C., Galluzzo, D. C., & Myers, L. (1988). Attachment and child care: Relationships with mother and caregiver. *Early Childhood Research Quarterly, 3,* 403–416.

Hsu, C. C. (1985). Characteristics of temperament in

Chinese infants and young children. In W. S. Tseng & D. Y. H. Wu (Eds.), *Chinese culture and mental health* (pp. 135–152). Orlando, FL: Academic Press.

Hu, P., & Meng, Z. (1996). *An examination of infant–mother attachment in China.* Poster presented at the meeting of the International Society for the Study of Behavioral Development, Quebec City, QB, Canada.

Jackson, J. F. (1993). Multiple caregiving among African Americans and infant attachment: The need for an emic approach. *Human Development, 36,* 87–102.

Johnson, F. A. (1993). *Dependency and Japanese socialization: Psychoanalytic and anthropological investigations into amae.* New York: New York University Press.

Kagan, J., Kearsley, R. B., & Zelazo, P. R. (1978). *Infancy: Its place in human development.* Cambridge, MA: Harvard University Press.

Kagitcibasi, C. (1996). *Family and human development across cultures: A view from the other side.* Hillsdale, NJ: Erlbaum.

Kazui, M., Endo, T., Tanaka, A., Sakagami, H., & Suganuma, M. (2000). Intergenerational transmission of attachment Japanese mother–child dyads. *Japanese Journal of Educational Psychology, 48,* 323–332.

Kermoian, R., & Leiderman, P. H. (1986). Infant attachment to mother and child caretaker in an East African community. *International Journal of Behavioral Development, 9,* 455–469.

Konner, M. (1977). Infancy among the Kalahari Desert San. In P. H. Leiderman, S. R. Tulkin, & A. Rosenfeld (Eds.), *Culture and infancy: Variations in the human experience* (pp. 287–328). New York: Academic Press.

Kuotai, T., & Jing-Hwa, C. (1985). The one-child-per-family policy: A psychological perspective. In W. S. Tseng & D. Y. H. Wu (Eds.), *Chinese culture and mental health* (pp. 153–166). Orlando, FL: Academic Press.

Lamb, M. E. (1977). The development of mother–infant and father–infant attachments in the second year of life. *Developmental Psychology, 13,* 637–648.

Lamb, M. E., Thompson, R. A., Gardner, W. P., Charnov, E. L., & Estes, D. (1984). Security of infantile attachment as assessed in the "Strange Situation": Its study and biological interpretation. *Behavioral and Brain Sciences, 7,* 127–171.

LeVine, R. A., & Miller, P. M. (1990). Commentary. *Human Development, 33,* 73–80.

Lin, C. Y. C., & Fu, V. R. (1990). A comparison of child-rearing practices among Chinese, immigrant Chinese, and Caucasian-American parents. *Child Development, 61,* 429–433.

Li-Repac, D. C. (1982). *The impact of acculturation on the child-rearing attitudes and practices of Chinese-American families: Consequences for the attachment process.* Unpublished doctoral dissertation, University of California at Berkeley.

Main, M. (1990). Cross-cultural studies of attachment organization: Recent studies, changing methodologies, and the concept of conditional strategies. *Human Development, 33,* 48–61.

Main, M., Kaplan, N., & Cassidy, J. (1985). Security in infancy, childhood, and adulthood: A move to the level of representation. In I. Bretherton & E. Waters (Eds.), Growing points of attachment theory and research. *Monographs of the Society for Research in Child Development, 50* (1–2, Serial No. 209), 66–104.

Main, M., & Solomon, J. (1990). Procedures for identifying infants as disorganized/disoriented during the Ainsworth Strange Situation. In M. T. Greenberg, D. Cicchetti, & E. M. Cummings (Eds.), *Attachment in the preschool years: Theory, research, and intervention* (pp. 121–160). Chicago: University of Chicago Press.

Main, M., & Weston, D. R. (1981). The quality of the toddler's relationship to mother and to father: Related to conflict behavior and the readiness to establish new relationships. *Child Development, 52,* 932–940.

Marvin, R. S., VanDevender, T. L., Iwanaga, M. I., LeVine, S., & LeVine, R. A. (1977). Infant–caregiver attachment among the Hausa of Nigeria. In H. McGurk (Ed.), *Ecological factors in human development* (pp. 247–259). Amsterdam: North-Holland.

Meins, E. (1997). *Security of attachment and the social development of cognition.* Hove, UK: Psychology Press.

Miyake, K., Chen, S. J., & Campos, J. J. (1985). Infant temperament, mother's mode of interaction, and attachment in Japan: An interim report. In I. Bretherton & E. Waters (Eds.), Growing points of attachment theory and research. *Monographs of the Society for Research in Child Development, 50*(1–2, Serial No. 209), 276–297.

Mizuta, I., Zahn-Waxler, C., Cole, P. M., & Hiruma, N. (1996). A cross cultural study of preschoolers' attachment: Security and sensitivity in Japanese and U.S. dyads. *International Journal of Behavioral Development, 19,* 141–159.

Morelli, G. A., & Tronick, E. Z. (1991). Efé multiple caretaking and attachment. In J. L. Gewirtz & W. M. Kurtines (Eds.), *Intersections with attachment* (pp. 41–52). Hillsdale, NJ: Erlbaum.

Murdock, G. P., & White, D. R. (1969). Standard Cross-Cultural Sample. *Ethnology, 8,* 329–369.

Nakagawa, M., Lamb, M. E., & Miyake, K. (1992). Antecedents and correlates of the Strange Situation behavior of Japanese infants. *Journal of Cross-Cultural Psychology, 23,* 300–310.

Nakagawa, M., Teti, D. M., & Lamb, M. E. (1992). An ecological study of child–mother attachments among Japanese sojourners in the United States. *Developmental Psychology, 28,* 584–592.

Nsamenang, A. B. (1992). *Human development in cultural context: A Third World perspective.* Newbury Park, CA: Sage.

Oppenheim, D., Koren-Karie, N., & Sagi-Schwartz, A. (2007). Emotional dialogues between mothers and children at 4.5 and 7.5 years: Relations with children's attachment at 1 year. *Child Development, 78,* 38–52.

Oppenheim, D., Sagi, A., & Lamb, M. E. (1990). Infant–adult attachments on the kibbutz and their relation to socioemotional development four years later. In S. Chess & M. E. Hertzig (Eds.), *Annual progress in child psychiatry and child development, 1989* (pp. 92–106). New York: Brunner/Mazel.

Peterson, N. J., Drotar, D., Olness, K., Guay, L., & Kiziri-Mayengo, R. (2001). The relationship of maternal and child HIV infection to security of attachment among Ugandan infants. *Child Psychiatry and Human Development, 32,* 3–17.

Pike, K. L. (1967). *Language in relation to a unified theory of the structure of human behavior* (rev. ed.). The Hague: Mouton.

Posada, G., Gao, Y., Wu, F., Posado, R., Tascon, M., Schoelmerich, A., et al. (1995). The secure-base phenomenon across cultures: Children's behavior, mothers' preferences, and experts' concepts. In E. Waters, B. E. Vaughn, G. Posada, & K. Kondo-Ikemura (Eds.), *Caregiving, cultural, and cognitive perspectives on secure-base behavior and working models: New growing points of attachment theory and research. Monographs of the Society for Research in Child Development, 60*(2–3, Serial No. 244), 27–48.

Rabin, A. I., & Beit-Hallahmi, B. (1982). *Twenty years later.* New York: Springer.

Reed, G., & Leiderman, P. H. (1981). Age-related changes in attachment behavior in polymatrically reared infants: The Kenyan Gusii. In T. M. Field, A. M. Sostek, P. Vietze, & P. H. Leiderman (Eds.), *Culture and early interactions* (pp. 215–236). Hillsdale, NJ: Erlbaum.

Robertson, J., & Robertson, J. (1971). Young children in brief separation: A fresh look. *Psychoanalytic Study of the Child, 26,* 264–315.

Rothbaum, F., Weisz, J., Pott, M., Miyake, K., & Morelli, G. (2000). Attachment and culture. Security in the United States and Japan. *American Psychologist, 55,* 1093–1104.

Sagi, A., Koren-Karie, N., Gini, M., Ziv, Y., & Joels, T. (2002). Shedding further light on the effects of various types and quality of early child care on infant–mother attachment relationship: The Haifa study of early child care. *Child Development, 73,* 1166–1186.

Sagi, A., Lamb, M. E., Lewkowicz, K. S., Shoham, R., Dvir, R., & Estes, D. (1985). Security of infant–mother, –father, and –metapelet attachments among kibbutz-reared Israeli children. In I. Bretherton & E. Waters (Eds.), *Growing points of attachment theory and research. Monographs of the Society for Research in Child Development, 50*(1–2, Serial No. 209), 257–275.

Sagi, A., & van IJzendoorn, M. H. (1996). Multiple caregiving environments: The kibbutz experience. In S. Harel & J. P. Shonkoff (Eds.), *Early childhood intervention and family support programs: Accomplishments and challenges* (pp. 143–162). Jerusalem: JDC–Brookale Institute.

Sagi, A., van IJzendoorn, M. H., Aviezer, O., Donnell, F., & Mayseless, O. (1994). Sleeping out of home in a kibbutz communal arrangement: It makes a differ-

ence for infant –mother attachment. *Child Development, 65,* 992–1004.

Sagi, A., van IJzendoorn, M. H., Scharf, M., Joels, T., Koren-Karie, N., Mayseless, O., et al. (1997). Ecological constraints for intergenerational transmission of attachment. *International Journal of Behavioral Development, 20,* 287–299.

Sagi-Schwartz, A., & Aviezer, O. (2005). Correlates of attachment to multiple caregivers in kibbutz children from birth to emerging adulthood: The Haifa longitudinal study. In K. E. Grossmann, K. Grossmann, & E. Waters (Eds.), *Attachment from infancy to adulthood* (pp. 165–197). New York: Guilford Press.

Spangler, G., & Grossmann, K. E. (1993). Biobehavioral organization in securely and insecurely attached infants. *Child Development, 64,* 1439–1450.

Stafford, C. (1995). *The roads of Chinese childhood: Learning and identification in Angang.* Cambridge, UK: Cambridge University Press.

Takahashi, K. (1982). Attachment behaviors to a female stranger among Japanese two-year-olds. *Journal of Genetic Psychology, 140,* 299–307.

Takahashi, K. (1986). Examining the Strange Situation procedure with Japanese mothers and 12-month-old infants. *Developmental Psychology, 22,* 265–270.

Takahashi, K. (1990). Are the key assumptions of the 'Strange Situation' procedure universal?: A view from Japanese research. *Human Development, 33,* 23–30.

Tavecchio, L. W. C., & van IJzendoorn, M. H. (1987). *Attachment in social networks: Contributions to the Bowlby–Ainsworth attachment theory.* Amsterdam: North-Holland.

Thompson, R. A. (1993). Socioemotional development: Enduring issues and new challenges. *Developmental Review, 13,* 372–402.

Tomlinson, M., Cooper, P., & Murray, L. (2005). The mother–infant relationship and infant attachment in a South-African peri-urban settlement. *Child Development, 76,* 1044–1054.

Trivers, R. L. (1974). Parent–offspring conflict. *American Zoologist, 14,* 249–264.

Tronick, E. Z., Morelli, G. A., & Winn, S. (1987). Multiple caretaking of Efé (Pygmy) infants. *American Anthropologist, 89,* 96–106.

True, M. M. (1994). *Mother–infant attachment and communication among the Dogon of Mali.* Unpublished doctoral dissertation, University of California at Berkeley.

True, M. M., Pisani, L., & Oumar, F. (2001). Infant–mother attachment among the Dogon of Mali. *Child Development, 72,* 1451–1466.

Valenzuela, M. (1990). Attachment in chronically underweight young children. *Child Development, 61,* 1984–1996.

van IJzendoorn, M. H. (1990). Developments in cross-cultural research on attachment: Some methodological notes. *Human Development, 33,* 3–9.

van IJzendoorn, M. H. (1995). Adult attachment representations, parental responsiveness, and infant attachment: A meta-analysis on the predictive validity of the Adult Attachment Interview. *Psychological Bulletin, 117,* 387–403.

van IJzendoorn, M. H. (1996). Attachment patterns and their outcomes: Commentary. *Human Development, 39,* 224–231.

van IJzendoorn, M. H., Bakermans-Kranenburg, M. J., & Sagi-Schwartz, A. (2006). Attachment across diverse sociocultural contexts. The limits of universality. In K. Rubin & O. B. Chung (Eds.), *Parenting beliefs, behaviors, and parent–child relations: A cross-cultural perspective* (pp. 107–142). New York: Psychology Press.

van IJzendoorn, M. H., & De Wolff, M. S. (1997). In search of the absent father: Meta-analyses on infant–father attachment. A rejoinder to our discussants. *Child Development, 68,* 604–609.

van IJzendoorn, M. H., Dijkstra, J., & Bus, A.G. (1995). Attachment, intelligence, and language. *Social Development, 4,* 115–128.

van IJzendoorn, M. H., & Kroonenberg, P. M. (1988). Cross-cultural patterns of attachment: A meta-analysis of the Strange Situation. *Child Development, 59,* 147–156.

van IJzendoorn, M. H., & Sagi, A. (2001). Cultural blindness or selective inattention? *American Psychologist, 56,* 824–825.

van IJzendoorn, M. H., Sagi, A., & Lambermon, M. W. E. (1992). The multiple caretaker paradox: Data from Holland and Israel. *New Directions for Child Development, 57,* 5–24.

van IJzendoorn, M. H., Vereijken, C. M. J. L., Bakermans-Kranenburg, M. J., & Riksen-Walraven, J. M. (2004). Assessing attachment security with the Attachment Q-Sort: Meta-analytic evidence for the validity of the observer AQS. *Child Development, 75,* 1188–1213.

Vaughn, B. E., Stevenson-Hinde, J., Waters, E., Kotsaftis, A., Lefever, G. B., Shouldice, A., et al. (1992). Attachment security and temperament in infancy and early childhood: Some conceptual clarifications. *Developmental Psychology, 28,* 463–473.

Vaughn, B. E., & Waters, E. (1990). Attachment behavior at home and in the laboratory: Q-sort observations

and Strange Situation classifications of one-year-olds. *Child Development, 61,* 1965–1973.

Vereijken, C. M. J. L. (1996). *The mother–infant relationship in Japan: Attachment, dependency, and amae.* Unpublished doctoral dissertation, Catholic University of Nijmegen, The Netherlands.

Verweij-Tijsterman, E. (1996). *Day care and attachment.* Amsterdam: Academisch Proefschrift Vrije Universiteit.

Wang, Z. M. (1993). Psychology in China: A review dedicated to Li Chen. *Annual Review of Psychology, 44,* 87–116.

Waters, E. (1978). The reliability and stability of individual differences in infant–mother attachment. *Child Development, 49,* 483–494.

Weisner, T. S., & Gallimore, R. (1977). My brother's keeper: Child and sibling caretaking. *Current Anthropology, 18,* 169–190.

Wu, D. (1985). Child training in Chinese culture. In W. S. Tseng & D. Wu (Eds.), *Chinese culture and mental health* (pp. 113–134). Orlando, FL: Academic Press.

Yang, C.-F. (1988). Familism and development: An examination of the role of family in contemporary China mainland, Hong Kong, and Taiwan. In D. Sinha & H. S. R. Kao (Eds.), *Social values and development: Asian perspectives* (pp. 93–123). New Delhi: Sage.

Yang, K.-S. (1988). Will societal modernization eventually eliminate cross-cultural psychological differences? In M. H. Bond (Ed.), *The cross-cultural challenge to social psychology* (pp. 67–85). Beverly Hills, CA: Sage.

Zevalkink, J. (1997). *Attachment in Indonesia: The mother–child relationship in context.* Ridderkerk, The Netherlands: Ridderprint.

Zevalkink, J., Riksen-Walraven, J. M., & Van Lieshout, C. F. M. (1999). Attachment in the Indonesian caregiving context. *Social Development, 8,* 21–40.

Zhu, Z., & Lin, C. (1991). Research and application in Chinese child psychology. *Applied Psychology: An International Review, 40,* 15–25.

Ziv, Y., Oppenheim, D., & Sagi-Schwartz, A. (2004). Social information processing in middle childhood: Relation to infant–mother attachment, *Attachment and Human Development, 6,* 327–348.

CHAPTER 38

Attachment and Religious Representations and Behavior

PEHR GRANQVIST
LEE A. KIRKPATRICK

> Whenever the "natural" object of attachment behaviour is unavailable, the behaviour can become directed towards some substitute object. Even though it is inanimate, such an object frequently appears capable of filling the role of an important, though subsidiary, attachment "figure." Like the principal attachment figure, the inanimate substitute is sought especially when a child is tired, ill, or distressed.
>
> —BOWLBY (1969/1982, P. 313)

Although Bowlby's theorizing about attachment focused largely on the evolutionary origins of the attachment system and its manifestation in infant–mother relationships, he clearly believed from the beginning that the processes and dynamics of attachment have broad implications for social development and psychological functioning across the lifespan. One purpose of the present chapter is to demonstrate that with increased cognitive maturation, people may even develop attachments to unseen figures (e.g., God). More specifically, we argue that some core aspects of religious beliefs and behavior can be meaningfully and usefully interpreted in terms of attachment dynamics.

Serious students of attachment theory are well aware of the dangers inherent in extending the theory beyond its valid limits. Bowlby's choice of the term "attachment" was in one sense unfortunate, because of the word's much broader meaning in everyday language: People speak colloquially of feeling "attached" to many objects and persons in their lives, from important possessions (cars, homes, a favorite pen) to social groups to sports teams to the Grateful Dead to the World Trade Center. Whether such phenomena can be

understood properly in terms of attachment, as defined by Bowlby, remains disputable. Our own understanding is that they generally cannot.

Nevertheless, we wish to argue that some core aspects of religious belief and behavior represent real manifestations of attachment processes similar to those seen in infant–caregiver relationships. In fact, application of the attachment model to religious beliefs is in many ways more straightforward than its application to adult romantic relationships. The latter is complicated by a number of factors, including the reciprocal nature of adult relationships with peers, and the roles of sexuality and caregiving in romantic relationships (Mikulincer & Goodman, 2006; Weiss, 1982). Neither of these limitations is typically evident in adults' perceptions of their relationships with God, Allah, Jesus, or other supernatural figures. In some important ways, religious belief may provide a unique window into attachment processes in adulthood.

This chapter is divided into five major sections. The first brief section describes the observational points of departure used to launch the idea that God and other deities are often perceived as attachment figures. In the second section, we argue that an attachment model of religion provides more than an interesting analogy: Perceived relationships with God meet the defining criteria of attachment relationships reasonably well, and hence function psychologically much as other attachments do. The third major section examines maturational issues involved in the ontogenetic development of attachment and religion. These first three sections deal with normative aspects of attachment and religion. In the fourth section, we review the empirical connections between religion and individual differences in interpersonal attachments. This section is subdivided into two subsections—the first focusing on a "compensation" pathway to religion (via distress regulation in the context of insecure attachment and experiences from insensitive caregiving), and the second describing a "correspondence" pathway to religion (via secure attachment and experiences with sensitive and religious caregivers). Before we conclude, the final major section addresses some research findings and implications of the religion-as-attachment model with respect to psychological outcomes.

POINTS OF DEPARTURE

Religion as Relationship

The obvious starting point for the application of attachment theory to religion is the observation that central to monotheistic religions, particularly Christianity, is the belief in a personal God with whom believers maintain a personal, interactive relationship. Although diverse definitions of "religion" have been offered throughout the years, it may be helpful to consider its etymological roots. The word stems from the Latin *religare* or *relegere*, meaning "being bound" or "gather together" (see Ferm, 1945). This relationship connotation has a clear counterpart in how people evaluate their own faith. For example, when asked, "Which of the following four statements comes closest to your own view of 'faith': a set of beliefs, membership in a church or synagogue, finding meaning in life, or a relationship with God?," 51% of a national (U.S.) Gallup sample chose "a relationship with God" (compared to 19%, 4%, and 20% for the other alternatives, respectively; Gallup & Jones, 1989). Also, in a study of clergy, the most common response to the question "How does faith help you in daily life?" was "access to a loving God who is willing to help in everyday life" (Hughes, 1989). According to Greeley (1981, p. 18), "Just

as the story of anyone's life is the story of relationships—so each person's religious story is a story of relationships."

It is also important to note that other supernatural figures may fill this relationship role in addition to or instead of "God." In many Christian traditions, it is Jesus with whom one maintains an active day-to-day relationship, while "God the Father" remains a more distant background figure. In Roman Catholicism, Mary typically represents the "maternal functions" related to attachment (Wenegrat, 1989). Outside Christianity, the worlds of different groups of believers are populated by a variety of gods and other deities, many of whom function as attachment-like figures. Even in countries dominated by Eastern religions such as Hinduism and Buddhism, which Westerners tend to think of as abstract, godless philosophies, believers often focus on the more theistic components of the belief system and on personal gods imported from ancient folk religions (see Kirkpatrick, 1994, for a discussion). Throughout this chapter, we refer to "God" as an attachment-like figure, but it should be understood that in many cases another supernatural figure may fill this role.

Religion and Love

A second point of departure for discussing an attachment–religion connection is the centrality of the emotion of love in religious belief systems, and especially in people's perceived relationships with God. Bumper stickers proudly announce, "I [picture of a heart] Jesus," or, conversely, "Jesus loves me," or more broadly, "God is love." The powerful emotional experiences associated with religion are often expressed "in the language of human love," particularly in the writing of mystics (Thouless, 1923, p. 132).

The process of religious conversion has been likened frequently, by both scholars and religious writers, to falling in love (James, 1902; Pratt, 1920; Thouless, 1923). On the basis of her in-depth interviews with religious converts, Ullman (1989, p. xvi) wrote:

> What I initially considered primarily a change of ideology turned out to be more akin to a falling in love. … [C]onversion pivots around a sudden attachment, an infatuation with a real or imagined figure which occurs on a background of great emotional turmoil. The typical convert was transformed not by a religion, but by a person. The discovery of a new truth was indistinguishable from a discovery of a new relationship, which relieved, temporarily, the upheaval

of the previous life. This intense and omnipresent attachment discovered in the religious experience promised the convert everlasting guidance and love, for the object of the convert's infatuation was perceived as infallible.

(It is worth noting that despite her use of the term "attachment," Ullman never cited Bowlby or attachment theory in her struggle to find a theoretical perspective to explain her observations.)

The "love" experienced by a worshipper in the context of a relationship with God is of course qualitatively different from that experienced in adult romantic relationships; the latter typically includes sexuality, whereas the former usually does not. In fact, the form of "love" experienced in the context of a relationship with God resembles much more closely the prototypical attachment of a child to his or her mother. In Greeley's (1990, p. 252) words, "The Mary Myth's powerful appeal is to be found ... in the marvellous possibility that God loves us the way a mother loves her baby."

Images of God

The idea that God is experienced psychologically as a kind of parental figure is, of course, hardly new. Perhaps the most familiar version of this idea is Freud's (e.g., 1927/1961) characterization of God as an exalted father figure (see, though, Granqvist, 2006a, for a critical assessment of psychoanalytic theories of religion). Wenegrat (1989), however, observed that the deities of the oldest known religions were largely maternal figures, and that modern Protestantism is unusual in its lack of significant female deities.

Whether images of God more closely resemble maternal or paternal images has been a topic of much research in the psychology of religion, with decidedly mixed results. Some studies suggest that God images are more closely related to maternal than to paternal images (Godin & Hallez, 1965; Nelson, 1971; Strunk, 1959), whereas other studies suggest that God is perceived as more similar to one's preferred parent (Nelson & Jones, 1957). The most sensible conclusion from this research, however, seems to be that images of God combine elements of both stereotypically maternal and paternal qualities (Vergote & Tamayo, 1981): God is neither an exalted father figure nor an exalted mother figure, but rather an exalted attachment figure.

There is considerable evidence to support the notion that believers view God as a kind of

exalted attachment figure. One line of suggestive evidence comes from religious writings and songs. Wenegrat (1989) noted the striking degree of attachment imagery in the Psalms. Similarly, Young (1926) showed that a dominant theme of Protestant hymns is the "infantile return to a powerful and loving protector who shields humankind from all harm" (as summarized by Wulff, 1991, p. 304). In a word, God seems clearly to capture the very essence of the protective other that a parent represents to a child. As summarized by Kaufman (1981, p. 67), a theologian familiar with attachment theory, "The idea of God is the idea of an absolutely adequate attachment-figure. ... God is thought of as a protective and caring parent who is always reliable and always available to its children when they are in need."

Factor-analytic studies of God images consistently find a large first factor laden with attachment-related descriptors. For example, Gorsuch's (1968) first major factor (labeled "benevolent deity") included such descriptors as "comforting," "loving," and "protective," and the reverse of "distant," "impersonal," and "inaccessible"; Spilka, Armatas, and Nussbaum (1964) found a large general factor that included the items "comforting," "supporting," "protective," "strong," and "helpful"; and Tamayo and Desjardins (1976) found a first factor (labeled "availability") containing such items as "who gives comfort," "a warm-hearted refuge," "always ready with open arms," "who will take loving care of me," and "who is always waiting for me." In a factor analysis of diverse religious attitude and belief statements, the largest factor to emerge was "nearness to God": "Persons with high loadings on this factor would tend to feel that God was very real and constantly near and accessible. These persons feel they commune with God—'walk and talk' with Him" (Broen, 1957, p. 177).

BELIEVERS' PERCEIVED RELATIONSHIPS WITH GOD VIS-À-VIS ATTACHMENT RELATIONSHIP CRITERIA

The preceding section has suggested several parallels between religious belief and experience on the one hand, and attachment relationships on the other. Specifically, (1) perceived relationships with God are central to many people's religious beliefs and experiences; (2) the emotional bond experienced in this relationship is a form of love akin to the infant–caregiver attachment bond; and (3) images of God tend to parallel the characteristics of sensitive attachment figures. In this section we argue, using Ainsworth's (1985) and Bowlby's (1969/1982) criteria for distinguishing attachments from other types of relationships, that these resemblances are more than interesting analogies and in fact reflect genuine attachment processes. Our arguments in this section are based on religious phenomenology and empirical findings that accrued well before attachment theory was first applied to religion systematically (by Kirkpatrick, 1994, and Kirkpatrick & Shaver, 1990), as well as on results from more recent studies that were explicitly designed to test the religion-as-attachment model.[1]

Seeking and Maintaining Proximity to God

The biological function of the attachment system, as described by Bowlby (1969/1982), is the maintenance of proximity between an infant and a protective attachment figure. To achieve the objective of establishing physical proximity, infants engage in such behaviors as crying, raising arms (to be picked up), and clinging (however, see below for the "maturation" of the attachment system).

Religions provide various ways of enhancing perceptions about the proximity of God. A crucial tenet of most theistic religions is that God is omnipresent; thus one is always in "proximity" to God. God is frequently described in religious literature as always being by one's side, holding one's hand, or watching over one. Nevertheless, other, more concrete cues may be valuable in enhancing perceptions of proximity to God. For example, despite the presumption of God's omnipresence, virtually all religions provide places of worship where one can go to be closer to God. In addition, a diverse array of idols and symbols—ranging from graven images to crosses on necklaces to paintings and other art forms—seem designed to remind the believer continually of God's presence.

However, the most important form of proximity-maintaining attachment behavior directed toward God is prayer (Reed, 1978), which not coincidentally is also "the most often practiced form of religiosity" (Trier & Shupe, 1991, p. 354). Heiler (1932, p. 356) concluded from his classic study of prayer that a devout person who prays "believes that he speaks with a God, immediately present and personal," and that "The man who prays feels himself very close to this personal God." Among the major forms of prayer reviewed in the comprehensive psychology-of-religion text by Hood, Spilka, Hunsberger, and Gorsuch (1996,

pp. 394 ff.), two seem clearly related to proximity maintenance: "contemplative" prayer ("an attempt to relate deeply to one's God") and "meditational" prayer ("concern with one's relationship to God"). In many ways, prayer seems analogous to "social referencing" in young children—an intermittent checking back to make sure the attachment figure is still attentive and potentially available (Campos & Stenberg, 1981).

Finally, other religious behaviors provide interesting analogies to the proximal attachment behaviors of infants. For example, the uplifted arms and speaking in tongues commonly observed at Pentecostal services bear some resemblance to an infant reaching up expectantly, "babbling," and waiting to be picked up by his or her mother.

God as a Haven of Safety

A second defining criterion of attachment is that an attachment figure serves as a haven of safety in times of danger or threat, which fulfills the evolutionary function of protecting otherwise defenseless infants from injury or death. Bowlby (1969/1982) discussed three kinds of situations that activate the attachment system and thus elicit attachment behavior: (1) frightening or alarming environmental events; (2) illness, injury, or fatigue; and (3) separation or threat of separation from attachment figures.

As Freud (1927/1961) and many others have long speculated, religion does appear to be rooted at least partly in needs for protection and felt security. There are no atheists in foxholes, as the adage goes. Hood and colleagues (1996, pp. 386–387) concluded that people are most likely to "turn to their gods in times of trouble and crisis," listing three general classes of potential triggers: "illness, disability, and other negative life events that cause both mental and physical distress; the anticipated or actual death of friends and relatives; and dealing with an adverse life situation." This list bears a striking resemblance to Bowlby's (1969/1982) discussion of factors postulated to activate the attachment system.

Considerable evidence supports the view that people turn to religion particularly in times of distress and crisis, and it is important to note that they primarily turn at such times to *prayer*—a form of religious attachment behavior—rather than to *church* (Argyle & Beit-Hallahmi, 1975). Ross (1950) queried over 1,700 religious youth about why they prayed; the two reasons cited most frequently were "God listens to and answers your prayers" and "It helps you in time of stress and crisis." Pargament (1997) has outlined various religious coping strategies that people have employed in stressful situations, including such attachment-like responses as "experienced God's love and care," "realized God was trying to strengthen me," "let God solve my problems for me," and "took control over what I could and gave up the rest to God." Furthermore, research undertaken within a coping framework has documented that religious individuals are inclined to turn to God particularly when faced with threats (e.g., danger) and loss (e.g., death of a loved one) (Bjorck & Cohen, 1993; McCrae, 1984).

Frightening or Alarming Events

With respect to environmental stressors, empirical research suggests that there are indeed few atheists in foxholes: Combat soldiers do pray frequently (Stouffer, 1949). From his interviews with combat veterans, Allport (1950, p. 57) concluded: "The individual in distress craves affection and security. Sometimes a human bond will suffice, more often it will not." Of course, soldiers develop powerful attachments to their comrades under combat conditions, and attachments to individuals back home may continue to provide a source of strength, perhaps mitigating the likelihood of turning to God for strength and protection on the battlefield. As one combat veteran reported to Allport (1950, p. 56), "There were atheists in foxholes, but most of them were in love." Nevertheless, only an all-powerful deity can offer a truly safe haven once the bullets start flying.

Although warfare provides a clear (and extreme) example, other kinds of severe stressors can lead to emotional crises in which other attachment figures may be perceived as inadequate. A century of research supports the claim that sudden religious conversions are most likely during times of severe emotional distress and crisis (Clark, 1929; Galanter, 1979; Starbuck, 1899; Ullman, 1982). According to Strickland (1924), the turning point of the conversion process comes when one surrenders oneself to God and places one's problems— and one's faith—in God's hands. Hence even individuals who did not experience a relationship with God prior to a crisis may come to do so if sufficiently distressed. It is also noteworthy that the source of the distress precipitating religious conversions is often relationship-related; in our own studies, relationship problems with parents and romantic partners have been frequently cited

by respondents (Granqvist, 1998; Kirkpatrick & Shaver, 1990).

Moreover, recent studies suggest that appraisal of threat does not require conscious processing to result in increased God-related cognitions (Birgegard & Granqvist, 2004; Mikulincer, Gurwitz, & Shaver, 2007). For example, in an experimental study explicitly set up to test the religion-as-attachment model in a Jewish sample of Israeli college students, participants showed an increase in the psychological accessibility of God (or the concept of God) following subliminal exposure to threats (i.e., failure and death; Mikulincer et al., 2007).

Illness, Injury, Fatigue

Several studies show prayer to be an especially common method of coping with serious physical illnesses of various types (Duke, 1977; Gibbs & Achterberg-Lawlis, 1978; O'Brien, 1982). For example, O'Brien (1982) observed in his interviews with patients experiencing renal failure that many of them saw God as providing comfort, nurturance, and a source of personal strength for getting through this difficult time. Other studies have shown religion to be particularly helpful to people in coping with *chronic* illness (Mattlin, Wethington, & Kessler, 1990).

Separation and Loss

Research also suggests that religiousness and prayer tend to increase following the death of or (threat of) separation from loved ones, and that religious beliefs are correlated positively with successful coping at these times (Haun, 1977; Loveland, 1968; Parkes, 1972). Relevant research has focused mostly on effects of spousal separation/bereavement (i.e., the ending of the principal attachment relationship in adulthood). Loss of a principal attachment figure is a particularly powerful stressor: Not only is it a stressful event in itself, but it also eliminates the availability of the person to whom one would otherwise be likely to turn for support in a stressful situation. When a human attachment figure is lost, a perceived relationship with God may therefore become an appealing alternative.

We (Granqvist, 1998; Kirkpatrick & Shaver, 1990) noted that many of the crises reported retrospectively by religious converts involved relationship-focused difficulties including loss of or separation from attachment figures, particularly through relationship breakups and divorce. Similarly, in a prospective longitudinal study using a population-based sample of elders—some of whom were destined to suffer bereavement during the course of the study and some of whom were not—Brown, Nesse, House, and Utz (2004) found a prospective increase in the importance of the religious beliefs for the bereaved compared to the non-bereaved. (This study also showed that grief over the loss decreased as a function of the increased significance of the bereaved individual's religious beliefs.) None of these effects were obtained when church attendance rather than religious beliefs was used as the outcome (or predictor) variable, indicating that the attachment component of the individual's religiousness may be what is activated in such situations and contributes to a more favorable outcome (a topic to which we return in the final major section of the chapter).

The naturalistic research just reviewed was necessarily correlational in nature (nothing was manipulated) and concerned presumed effects of real-life losses and separations, not threats of loss or separation. However, in a recent attachment experiment, theistic believers who were primed with a subliminal separation threat ("Mother is gone") targeting their relationship with their mothers (i.e., the principal attachment figures in childhood), showed an increase in their wish to be close to God compared with participants in an attachment-neutral control condition (Birgegard & Granqvist, 2004). We suggest that the effects of loss and separation are due to two factors: (1) Loss of a loved one activates the attachment system, and thus gives rise to religious attachment behaviors such as prayer; and (2) bereaved/separated persons may find in God a substitute or surrogate attachment figure to replace the lost interpersonal attachment.

The safe-haven aspects of religious experience described above are clearly embedded in the religious individual's relationship with an anthropomorphically shaped and institutionally sanctioned deity. However, many seemingly spontaneous occurrences of "paranormal" experiences that are not sanctioned by institutionalized religion, such as extrasensory perception and out-of-body experiences, are also generally precipitated by significant turmoil (Irwin, 1993). Because such experiences may well occur in the absence of the individual's attributions to a divine power or any other form of sanctified, comforting presence, their occurrence does not require perceptions of the availability of any anthropomorphic safe haven. Later, we consider the possibility that religious experiences occurring in relation to perceptions of a comforting safe haven may have different correlates from those of the paranormal experiences occurring in the absence of such perceptions.

God as a Secure Base

Another defining characteristic of an attachment is that it provides a sense of felt security and a secure base for exploration of the environment. As noted previously, religious literature is replete with references to God's being "by my side" and "watching over me." Perhaps the best-known example is the 23rd Psalm: "Yea, though I walk through the valley of the shadow of death, I will fear no evil: for thou art with me; thy rod and thy staff they comfort me." Elsewhere in the Psalms, God is described or addressed as "a shield for me" (3:3), "my rock, and my fortress" (18:2), and "the strength of my life" (27:1).[2]

It is easy to imagine how an attachment figure who is simultaneously omnipresent, omniscient, and omnipotent can provide the most secure of secure bases. This is precisely what led Kaufman (1981) to his previously quoted conclusion that God represents an "absolutely adequate attachment-figure." It also led Johnson (1945, p. 191), a psychologist of religion, to write:

> The emotional quality of faith is indicated in a basic confidence and security that gives one assurance. In this sense faith is the opposite of fear, anxiety, and uncertainty. Without emotional security there is no relaxation, but tension, distress, and instability. Assurance is the firm emotional undertone that enables one to have steady nerves and calm poise in the face of danger or confusion.

This description of faith bears an almost uncanny resemblance to Bowlby's (1973) own later descriptions of the secure base and its psychological effects: "When an individual is confident that an attachment figure will be available to him whenever he desires it, that person will be much less prone to either intense or chronic fear than will an individual who for any reason has no such confidence" (p. 202).

In their zeal to study the effects of religious beliefs on other cognitions and behavior occurring in reaction to stressful events, researchers unfortunately have paid far less attention to the question of how religious beliefs affect behavior and cognition in the absence of such stressors. In other words, there exists considerably less direct evidence for a secure-base function of religion than for a safe-haven function. Nevertheless, several indirect lines of research bear on the issue. Some of this research is reviewed in the final major section of this chapter, when we examine psychological outcomes associated with "attachment to God." Suffice to say here that in a comprehensive review of empirical research on religion and mental health, intrinsic religiousness (i.e., religion as an end to itself, a "master-motive" in the individual's life) was found to be positively correlated with two conceptualizations of mental health: "freedom from worry and guilt" and "a sense of personal competence and control" (Batson, Schoenrade, & Ventis, 1993). Intrinsic religion is also associated with an active, flexible approach to problem solving (Pargament, 1997). Moreover, religious faith engenders a sense of optimism and hope with respect to both the long-term and the short-term future (Myers, 1992). These and similar findings suggest that at least some forms of religiousness are associated with the kind of confident, self-assured approach to life that a secure base is thought to provide.

Responses to Separation and Loss

We have noted in a previous section that certain aspects of religiousness become more salient in response to bereavement and (threatened or actual) separations from loved ones, and we have interpreted this result in terms of the safe-haven function of religious attachment. However, the fourth and fifth defining criteria of attachment, as outlined by Ainsworth (1985), concern responses to separation from, or loss of, the attachment figure per se: The threat of separation causes anxiety in the attached person, and loss of the attachment figure causes grief.

Determining whether God meets these criteria is a difficult matter, because one does not become separated from, or lose a relationship with, God as one might lose a human relationship partner. God does not die, sail off to fight wars, move away, or file for divorce. The potential for true separation from God is usually seen by believers to come only in the hereafter, at which time one spends eternity either with God or separated from God. It is noteworthy, however, that in most Christian belief systems, separation from God is the very essence of hell.

The most obvious approximation to separation from or loss of God is deconversion or apostasy—that is, abandoning one's religious beliefs. It is not clear, however, whether "losing" a

relationship with God in this way can be expected to engender grief, because it is the believer rather than God who is deliberately choosing to abandon the relationship. Nevertheless, there are instances in religious life when believers are unable to experience a previously felt communion with God, which may occur also in situations where the urge to feel such a communion is experienced as acute. In religious and mystical literature, such states are often referred to as a "wilderness experience" or a "dark night of the soul" (St. John of the Cross, 1990). Perhaps the best-known example is when Christ himself, nailed on the cross, cried out: "My God, my God, why hast thou forsaken me?" (Matthews 27:46). In an experimental paraphrase of this situation, Birgegard and Granqvist (2004) subliminally exposed theistic (mostly Christian) believers to either a separation prime targeting their God relationship ("God has abandoned me") or attachment-neutral control primes ("People are walking," "God has many names"), and examined whether the wish to be close to God would increase as expected from pre- to postexposure as a result of the separation-from-God priming. In other words, this was an attempt to create a conceptually analogous situation for adult believers to the separation situation in which infants studied in the Ainsworth Strange Situation find themselves (Ainsworth, Blehar, Waters, & Wall, 1978). Although modest support was obtained for the prediction, there were individual differences, similar to the ones seen in the Strange Situation, that moderated the effects of attachment activation on religious outcomes, as we discuss in more detail later.

Perceiving God as Stronger and Wiser

To highlight the inherently asymmetrical nature of attachment, Bowlby (1969/1982) used the term "attachment relationship" to denote the relationship that a weaker, less competent individual has with another individual perceived as stronger and wiser—prototypically, the mammalian offspring with its adult caregiver(s). As implied above, adult romantic relationships *qua* attachment relationships are somewhat compromised by the usually symmetrical nature of romantic relationships; neither partner is *typically* perceived as stronger or wiser, although such perceptions may admittedly arise in specific situations, such as when the attachment system of one of the two is activated.

Concerning believers' perceived relation with God, it should be clear that believers typically do perceive God as very much stronger and wiser than themselves. In fact, God is supposedly omnipotent, omniscient, and omnipresent—attributes that are difficult for any earthly caregiver, sensitive as he or she may be, to compete with.

MATURATIONAL ASPECTS IN THE DEVELOPMENT OF ATTACHMENT AND RELIGION

So far, we have mostly considered adult expressions of religious experience in relation to normative attachment processes. The story of attachment starts in early childhood, however, as does the story of how a perceived relationship with God develops. We argue here that the relationship with God develops in temporal conjunction with the maturation of the attachment system and the cognitive developments associated with this maturation. Furthermore, we demonstrate that situational experiences associated with heightened attachment activation are already associated in childhood with increased significance of the individual's relationship with God (see Granqvist & Dickie, 2006, for a more detailed overview).

As noted, the biological function of the attachment system is to maintain proximity between an infant and a protective attachment figure. With increasing cognitive abilities, older children are often satisfied by visual or verbal contact, or eventually by mere knowledge of an attachment figure's whereabouts (Bretherton, 1987). This observation led Sroufe and Waters (1977) to suggest that "felt security" is the set goal of the attachment system in older individuals. Likewise, the consideration of cognitive abilities was an important part of the "move to the level of representation" (Main, Kaplan, & Cassidy, 1985) that was undertaken in attachment research more than two decades ago. This move opens the door, we argue, to the possibility of a noncorporeal attachment figure (e.g., God) with whom actual physical contact is impossible.

Far from being cognitively able to grasp symbolic thought, the human infant's behavioral repertoire initially consists of a series of more or less reflexive behaviors that are necessary to obtain the biological set goals of nourishment and proximity to a protective caregiver. However, as attachment to primary caregivers increasingly moves toward goal-corrected partnerships in preschool, and as children develop an elementary capacity for symbolic thought (Bowlby, 1969/1982), they are able to withstand longer separations, presumably because of the emerging ability to represent their attachment figures symbolically. Already at this age, children are developing a concept of God that they describe or draw as a person (Heller, 1986). Common themes observed by Heller in his extensive study of children's images of God included "God, the therapist" ("an all-nurturant, loving figure"), "intimacy" (feelings of closeness to God), and "omnipresence" (God is "always there"). Interestingly, two other common themes observed by Heller seem to parallel insecure attachment patterns: "inconsistent God" and "God, the distant thing in the sky." Besides developing a general capacity for symbolic thought, preschool children start to elaborate a "theory of mind" (e.g., Wellman, 1985); that is, they begin to appreciate the fact that other people have intentions and goals that motivate their behavior.

It is easy to see how these two aspects of cognitive development—symbolic thought and theory of mind—may pave the way for an emerging understanding of God, particularly when adults provide information consonant with the existence (or at least the concept) of God. As children experience themselves thinking and planning, and imagine the intentions of their social interaction partners, they may also apply their increasingly sophisticated theory of mind to abstract, symbolic others. Although children's God concepts can be viewed as abstractions, they tend to be comparatively concrete and anthropomorphic by adult standards (cf. Piaget's [1954] concepts of preoperational egocentrism and animism). A child at this age may, for example, explain the rain as a result of God's need to pee. Once the requisite cognitive development has occurred, if a child's attachment system is highly activated—for example, during a separation—the child may draw on God as an abstract (yet anthropomorphized) attachment surrogate. In a related discussion, Rizzuto (1979) suggested that at this age children develop a "living" God representation, with God being an alternative safe haven.

In middle childhood, as children enter school and move even farther from their parents' immediate care, their God concepts become somewhat less anthropomorphic, although at the same time God is typically viewed as personally closer than in early childhood (Eshleman, Dickie, Merasco, Shepard, & Johnson, 1999; Tamminen, 1994). From early childhood on, empirical data indicate that God is definitely perceived as an available safe haven in times of stress. For example, Tamminen (1994) found that 40% of Finnish 7- to

12-year-olds reported that they felt close to God, particularly during emergencies (e.g., escaping or avoiding danger, dealing with death or sorrow) and periods of loneliness. In addition, Eshleman and colleagues (1999) found that American preschool and elementary school children placed a God symbol closer to a fictional child when the fictional child was in attachment-activating situations (e.g., being sick and in the hospital, having fallen from a bike, following the death of the child's dog) than when the fictional child was in situations that were less clear-cut as activators of the attachment system (e.g., the child had stolen an apple, stolen a ball, or hurt another child).

These findings have now been conceptually replicated in two studies: one conducted in Sweden with 5- to 7-year-old children from religious and nonreligious homes (Granqvist, Ljungdahl, & Dickie, 2007); and one conducted in the United States with children of the same ages, most of whose parents were highly religious (Dickie, Charland, & Poll, 2005). The results of these two studies were based on a clearer distinction between attachment-activating and non-attachment-activating situations. The attachment-neutral conditions included a fictional child being in good-mood, bad-mood, and neutral-mood situations. Even then, children placed God closer to the fictional child in the attachment-activating situations.

Adolescence and early adulthood have long been known to be periods of major religious transformations (e.g., Granqvist, 2003; James, 1902). These are the life periods most intimately associated with sudden religious conversions and other significant changes in one's relationship with God. Argyle and Beit-Hallahmi (1975, p. 59) referred to adolescence as "the age of religious awakening." It is well known that cult recruiters make teenagers and young adults primary targets of their proselytizing and recruitment activities. Because adolescence is a unique and complex developmental period, it is not surprising that a wide range of explanations has been offered for the prevalence of conversion at this time. These include postulated links to puberty and sexual instincts (Coe, 1916; Thouless, 1923); the increased need for meaning, purpose, and sense of identity (Starbuck, 1899); and self-realization (Hood et al., 1996). From an attachment perspective, however, it is important to note that adolescence represents a period of transition between principal attachment figures— usually from parents to peers (Zeifman & Hazan, 1997). According to Weiss (1982, p. 178), relin-

quishing one's parents as attachment figures has a number of predictable consequences, including vulnerability to emotional loneliness, which he defines as "the absence from one's internal world of an attachment figure." At such a time, adolescents may turn to God (or perhaps a charismatic religious leader) as a substitute attachment-like figure. As noted above, sudden religious conversions and other major religious changes are also typically precipitated by significant emotional turmoil, which is highly likely to keep the attachment system hyperactivated in this sensitive period of attachment transition (Granqvist, 1998; Kirkpatrick & Shaver, 1990).

Compared to the preceding age periods, middle adulthood is, normatively speaking, less associated with either attachment transitions or religious drama; it typically has more to do with the maintenance and transmission of the "religious habit" (James, 1902) to the next generation. However, there are notable exceptions, the most pronounced being marital separations and divorce. In old age, a person's relationship with God often regains importance, particularly when the person loses close friends or a spouse to death. As already noted, such attachment transitions have already been found to be associated with increased emphasis on one's relationship with God (e.g., Brown et al., 2004; Cicirelli, 2004; Granqvist & Hagekull, 2000; Kirkpatrick, 2005).

RELIGION AND INDIVIDUAL DIFFERENCES IN ATTACHMENT

An important characteristic of attachment theory is its virtually seamless integration of a dynamic normative model featuring a control system dynamic on the one hand, and a model of individual differences in the functioning of that system on the other. To be complete, a theory of religion as attachment must do the same. In the preceding sections, we have sketched a normative model within which many aspects of religious belief and behavior, and particularly perceived relationships with God, function psychologically as attachment processes. We turn in this section to the topic of relations between religion and individual differences in attachment. As it turns out, just as individual differences in attachment security modulate the behavioral and linguistic output of the attachment system in general, so do they modulate the effects of attachment activation in the context of believers' perceived God relations.

General Hypotheses

But the matter is not as straightforward as one might think. From the outset, Kirkpatrick (1994; Kirkpatrick & Shaver, 1990) noted that two somewhat opposing hypotheses could be derived from attachment theory concerning relations between religion and attachment security or insecurity. The development of these hypotheses is described next, before we discuss how they stand up to empirical tests.

The Compensation Hypothesis

According to Bowlby's control system model of attachment, the attachment system continually monitors internal states and external circumstances in relation to the question "Is the attachment figure sufficiently near, attentive, responsive, approving, etc.?" (Hazan & Shaver, 1994, p. 3). The set point of the system is variable, depending on expectancies (working models) concerning the attachment figure and perceived cues of environmental dangers. A negative answer to the question, according to the theory, activates a suite of potential attachment behaviors designed to restore an adequate degree of proximity. Under certain conditions, however, the individual may anticipate (based on prior experience and/or current circumstances) that efforts to achieve adequate proximity and comfort from the primary attachment figure are unlikely to be successful. It is in these cases that a search for an alternative and more adequate attachment figure seems likely to be initiated, and consequently that individuals are likely to turn to God as a substitute attachment-like figure. In the sections dealing with normative aspects of attachment and religion, we have noted a number of such situations—including loss of and separation from a primary attachment figure, as well as wartime and other extreme environmental situations during which any attachment figure might fail to induce adequate feelings of security in an attached person. In this section, we are concerned with whether individual differences in attachment history and attachment security are associated with a more habitual use of God and religion during distress.

Both Ainsworth (1985) and Bowlby (1969/1982) expected a history of unsatisfactory attachments to predispose a person to search for substitute attachment figures. Ainsworth (1985) argued that children who fail to establish secure attachments to parents are likely to seek surrogates, including teachers, older siblings, other relatives, or any stronger and wiser other who reliably proves to be accessible and responsive. Although Ainsworth (1985) did not include God in her list of potential surrogates, it seems reasonable to assume that God may fill this role for many people with insecure attachment histories. In a word, God may provide a kind of attachment relationship one never had with one's parents or other primary attachment figures. We hypothesize that regulation of distress is at the core of this surrogate use of God and religion. Prior to the application of attachment theory to religion, this idea had been supported—for example, by studies showing that religious converts, whose conversions were often preceded by emotional turmoil, reported more unfavorable childhood relationships with parents than a matched comparison group of nonconverts (Ullman, 1982).

The Correspondence Hypothesis

According to Bowlby's model, continuity of attachment patterns across time and transmission of attachment patterns across generations are traced to "internal working models" (IWMs; Bowlby, 1973; see also Bretherton & Munholland, Chapter 5, this volume; Collins & Read, 1994; Main et al., 1985). As a consequence of repeated experiences in interactions with their attachment figures, children develop beliefs and expectations (IWMs) about the availability and responsiveness of caregivers, and these models guide future behavioral, emotional, and cognitive responses in other social interactions. Moreover, the models of interaction partners are linked to models of the self—beliefs about the degree to which one sees oneself as worthy of love, care, and protection.

Although the level at which IWMs operate is a matter of debate, it seems likely that people maintain both (1) mental models of attachment figures in general and (2) mental models specific to particular relationships. Bretherton and Munholland (Chapter 5, this volume), as well as Collins and Read (1994), suggest that such models are hierarchically arranged: The top level comprises a highly general model of self and others; a second level comprises models of parent–child relationships as distinct from peer relationships; and so on (see Overall, Fletcher, & Friesen, 2003, for empirical results along these lines). We suggest that for many individuals, working models of God (or perceived relationships with God) hold an important place somewhere in this hierarchy. For example, it may be postulated that "religious relationships" constitute a third category at the second level of the Collins–Read hierarchy, next to "parent–child relationships" and "peer relationships"; under this general model may be found more specific mental models of "God the Father," Jesus, Mary, various saints, or other supernatural beings.

Whether or not various levels of attachment-relevant mental representations are arranged in this precise hierarchical structure, it seems certain that IWMs of various levels of generality are interconnected to at least some degree (e.g., Overall et al., 2003; Roisman, Sroufe, Madsen, & Collins, 2001). Consideration of the interrelatedness of attachment working models leads to a straightforward set of predictions, which we refer to as the "IWM aspect" of the correspondence hypothesis: Individual differences in religious beliefs and experience should correspond with individual differences in IWMs of attachment. Individuals who possess positive or "secure" generalized working models of themselves and their attachment figures may be expected to view God and other deities in similar terms. Likewise, an "avoidant" attachment may be expected to manifest itself in the religious realm as agnosticism or atheism, or in a view of God as remote and inaccessible. Finally, an "anxious" or "ambivalent" attachment may find expression in a deeply emotional, all-consuming, and "clingy" relationship to God. Prior to the application of attachment theory to religion, this idea had been supported—for example, in cross-cultural research showing that God is construed as more loving in cultures where parenting is warm and accepting, and as more distant in cultures marked by harsh, rejecting parenting behavior (Lambert, Triandis, & Wolf, 1959; Rohner, 1986).

A socially based aspect of religion (and religious membership) can be added to the IWM aspect of the correspondence hypothesis (Granqvist, 2002; Granqvist & Hagekull, 1999). Besides reflecting IWM correspondence, the religious beliefs and behaviors of people who are securely attached can be expected in part to reflect their sensitive attachment figures' (say, a loving parent's) religious standards. In contrast, insecure offspring can be expected to be less likely to adopt their relatively insensitive or unresponsive attachment figures' religious standards. This aspect of the correspondence hypothesis can be called "social correspondence" (Granqvist, 2002). Prior to its test in attachment-related research, this addition to the correspondence hypothesis had been indirectly supported by numerous studies showing that the religiosity

of offspring with more favorable offspring–parent relationships is more similar to their parents' religiosity than that of offspring with less favorable offspring–parent relationships (e.g., Batson et al., 1993; Spilka, Hood, Hunsberger, & Gorsuch, 2003). Such results also converge with findings in the attachment literature, indicating that securely attached offspring are more likely to adopt parental standards in general (e.g., Ainsworth, Bell, & Stayton, 1974; Kochanska, Aksan, Knaack, & Rhines, 2004; Richters & Waters, 1991).

Another reason for adding the concept of social correspondence was that *some* theoretical moderator was needed to avoid making the individual-difference aspect of the religion-as-attachment model nearly unfalsifiable (cf. Popper, 1959). Otherwise, the same outcome could have been predicted from opposing directions; for example, secure attachment (IWM correspondence) and insecure attachment (associated with a motive for compensation) would both predict perceptions of a personal relationship with a loving God. Thus, by adding the notion of social correspondence, we can expect securely attached individuals to become actively religious insofar as their parents were, in line with social correspondence; in this case, their perceived relations with God are expected to exhibit the attributes of security through IWM correspondence.[3]

Empirical Findings Regarding the Two Hypotheses

The compensation and correspondence hypotheses may be seen, then, as delineating two distinct developmental pathways to religion. One of these paths is via regulation of distress following experiences with insensitive caregivers (compensation), and one is via experiences with sensitive, religious caregivers (correspondence) (Granqvist, Ivarsson, Broberg, & Hagekull, 2007; Kirkpatrick, 2005). It is in this developmental-pathway sense that the compensation and correspondence hypotheses are conceptualized henceforth.

Below, findings supporting each of the pathways are reviewed. We describe findings from studies employing both self-reports (e.g., of romantic attachment) and more indirect, implicit assessments of attachment, such as the Adult Attachment Interview (AAI; George, Kaplan, & Main, 1984, 1985, 1996). Moreover, we argue that essentially the same conclusions can be drawn from the studies that have used different kinds of methods. In the empirical review, we focus on attachment security–insecurity in relation to aspects of traditional Western (theistic) religion, as well as in relation to a less orthodox domain of spirituality and associated paranormal experiences—namely, the New Age movement. We also give attention to some emerging findings on individual differences in attachment and religion among children. We hasten to add that none of the studies to be reported followed participants from infancy onward, although shorter-term longitudinal studies are included in the review.[4]

Empirical Findings Supporting the Compensation Pathway

Compensation and Traditional Western Religion. The need for compensation through religion was poignantly stated by Leo Tolstoy:

> During the whole course of this year, when I almost unceasingly kept asking myself how to end the business, whether by the rope or by the bullet, during all that time … my heart kept languishing with another pining emotion. I can call this by no other name than that of a thirst for God. This craving for God had nothing to do with the movement of my ideas … but it came from my heart. It was like a feeling of dread that made me seem like an orphan and isolated in the midst of all these things that were so foreign. And this feeling of dread was mitigated by the hope of finding the assistance of some one. (Tolstoy's *Confessions*, quoted in James, 1902, p. 156)

Some of the findings reported and arguments advanced in the normative attachment-and-religion sections of this chapter have been found to hold in particular for individuals who were likely to have experienced parental insensitivity while growing up, whether their attachment-related experiences were estimated with self-reports (e.g., Granqvist, 1998, 2002, 2005; Granqvist & Hagekull, 1999, 2003; Kirkpatrick & Shaver, 1990) or assessed with the AAI (Granqvist, Ivarsson, et al., 2007). For example, sudden religious conversions, the most pronounced examples of religious drama, are associated with estimates of parental insensitivity. This connection was reported in the first study of attachment and religion (Kirkpatrick & Shaver, 1990). Since then, these findings have been strongly supported by a meta-analysis of all studies conducted to date, including almost 1,500 participants (Granqvist & Kirkpatrick, 2004), and by scores on the "probable experience of parenting scales" used to score the AAI. For example, in an AAI study, participants whose parents were estimated by an independent coder to have been

relatively less loving self-reported more sudden and intense increases in religiousness (Granqvist, Ivarsson, et al., 2007).

Furthermore, regarding parental insensitivity in the meta-analysis, sudden converts not only outscored nonconverts but also individuals who had experienced a more gradual increase in religiousness. In addition, as would be expected given the distress-regulating aspect of sudden conversions, we found in the meta-analysis that sudden converts scored higher on a scale (the Emotionally Based Religiosity scale; Granqvist & Hagekull, 1999) that had been created to tap distress-regulating aspects of believers' perceived relations with God—a scale that focused explicitly on attachment aspects of the relationship (e.g., God being viewed as a safe haven and secure base).

Moreover, several studies have shown that the increases in religiousness reported by individuals whose parents were judged low in sensitivity, whether those increases amounted to full-blown conversions or not, were typically precipitated by significant emotional turmoil ("themes of compensation") that was typically relationship-related (e.g., Granqvist & Hagekull, 1999; Granqvist, Ivarsson, et al., 2007). These studies assessed religious changes retrospectively, but Granqvist and Hagekull (2003) showed that the association could also be obtained prospectively. That is, reports of parental insensitivity prospectively predicted increased religiousness—particularly an increased importance of the perceived relationship with God, following the breakup of a romantic relationship.

Similarly, insecure romantic attachment has reliably predicted essentially the same kinds of religious changes. For example, Kirkpatrick (1997) found that over a 4-year period, women with insecure (particularly anxious) attachments established a new relationship with God and reported religious experiences, such as being "born again" and speaking in tongues, to a larger extent than securely attached women did. Findings of prospectively predicted increases in the religiousness of adults reporting insecure romantic attachment were replicated in a second study by Kirkpatrick (1998b), this time over a 5-month period, and in both males and females. Unlike the 1997 study, which used Hazan and Shaver's (1987) three-category measure of attachment orientations, this study used Bartholomew and Horowitz's (1991) four-category model, based on two dimensions: positive versus negative model of self, and positive versus negative model of other. Again, increases in the image of a loving God and in a perceived personal relationship with God were predicted by ambivalent/preoccupied romantic attachment, but also by fearful-avoidant attachment, which is also characterized by a negative model of self.

In both of these studies, the magnitude of the effects was modest. However, when the contextual condition of romantic relationship breakup—possibly indicating an increased need to regulate distress via attachment—was considered in yet another sample, insecure romantic attachment prospectively predicted increases in aspects of religiousness somewhat more strongly (Granqvist & Hagekull, 2003).

One interpretation of the findings from these studies is that for people who view themselves as unworthy of love and care, turning to God may be possible because of God's unique characteristics as compared with other relationship partners. In most religious belief systems, God's love is either unconditional—so one need not be "worthy" of love to receive it—or available through particular courses of action (e.g., good deeds, prayer), which allow an otherwise "unworthy" person to "earn" God's love and forgiveness. We return later to the possibility that a process of positive change in the self-model of relatively insecure individuals may be initiated when they perceive themselves as having received God's love and forgiveness.

Although these studies might seem to suggest that individuals with insecure attachment patterns become increasingly religious over time, recall that this would be expected primarily in the context of a need to regulate distress. Accordingly, religiousness may also decrease for such individuals (Granqvist, 2002). As expected, this happens under conditions where the need to regulate distress through attachment surrogates is comparatively low, such as after establishing a new intimate human relationship (Granqvist & Hagekull, 2003).

In summary, the developmental pathway to religion in the case of parental insensitivity and insecure attachment is one marked by attachment system (hyper)activation, under conditions where a perceived relationship with God helps to regulate a believer's distress when no other sufficient attachment figures are available. This conclusion corresponds well with the general speculations about the use of attachment surrogates offered by Bowlby (1969/1982) and Ainsworth (1985). The possibility that some individuals engage in a somewhat opportunistic use of religion is further strengthened by findings showing that the relationship with God wanes when the need to regu-

late distress is low. As we have noted elsewhere (Granqvist, 2003; Granqvist & Hagekull, 1999; Kirkpatrick, 2005), this religious profile bears a striking resemblance to William James's (1902) century-old characterization of the religion of the "sick soul" (a prime candidate for which was Tolstoy, as the quotation above indicates).

However, whereas AAI judges' estimates of parental insensitivity during interviewees' childhoods did predict the interviewees' history of using religion to regulate distress, classifications of the interviewees' *current* attachment organization were generally unrelated to such compensatory use of religion (Granqvist, Ivarsson, et al., 2007). An intriguing possibility is that some individuals who suffered attachment-related adversities in the past may in fact have "earned" a certain degree of attachment security from their surrogate relationship with God. This interpretation is speculative at this point, but if it is supported in future studies, it would indicate that religion as compensation may sometimes be psychologically functional, not just reactive. We return to this possibility in the last major section of the chapter.

Compensation and Unorthodox Spirituality within the New Age. A large portion of the research on attachment and religion has been conducted in a country, Sweden, that is marked by a notable decline in traditional Western religiosity (Stark, Hamberg, & Miller, 2005). Yet at the same time there has been an internationally unparalleled increase in more private, less orthodox, and less institutionalized forms of religion-like spirituality, most notably in the New Age movement (Houtman & Aupers, in press). There has therefore been a great deal of interest in whether the New Age attracts individuals who might have sought out traditional religion if it had not become marginalized (Granqvist & Hagekull, 2001; Granqvist, Ivarsson, et al., 2007; see also Farias & Granqvist, 2007, for a review of psychological research on the New Age).

The term "New Age" refers to a wide range of beliefs and activities that typically combine esotericism/occultism, astrology, parapsychology, alternative medicine, outgrowths of humanist psychology, and Eastern thinking in a Western context. Whereas traditional Western religion has an attachment-like figure (i.e., a theistic God) at the doctrinal centre, the New Age movement typically does not. Instead, the New Age has been thought to represent a "celebration of the self" (Heelas, 1996), where individuals take pride in many of the attributes traditionally ascribed to the deity, and are free to pick any ingredient suitable to themselves from the diverse spiritual smorgasbord that characterizes the New Age. Hence a metaphysical self, rather than a metaphysical God, is typically at the center of New Age philosophies. Nevertheless, predictions from attachment theory and research are clear enough.

First, the increase in New Age spirituality cannot be accounted for as socially based in the early parental relationship with parents; nor can it be characterized in terms of IWM correspondence, as "New Agers" typically do not perceive a personal relationship with a loving God (see also Kirkpatrick, 2005). Hence parental sensitivity and security of attachment can be ruled out as attachment predictors of New Age spirituality.

Second, insecure attachment has been found to have correlates very similar to those implied in New Age spirituality in previous studies. More specifically, disorganized and anxious or ambivalent attachment have been considered the prime candidates for later involvement in the New Age. Regarding disorganization, disorganized behaviors such as freezing and stilling have been suggested to represent proto-dissociative states, already evident in infancy, that may protect an infant psychologically from the irresolvable approach–avoidance dilemma thought to characterize disorganized attachment (Hesse & Main, 2006). In other words, when the infant's attachment system is activated, instead of approaching the attachment figure—who is simultaneously the source of threat *and* of potential comfort—the infant "spaces out" or dissociates. If this becomes a habitual mode of responding when faced with stress, disorganized attachment should make the individual prone to later experiences of dissociative mental states (e.g., experiences of depersonalization, out-of-body experiences). Confirmatory evidence for this idea comes from studies linking infant disorganized attachment to later dissociative states throughout childhood and adolescence (e.g., Carlson, 1998), and adult disorganized attachment to a propensity to experience anomalous shifts in consciousness ("absorption"; Hesse & van IJzendoorn, 1999).

Dissociative states, such as out-of-body experiences, trance states, and responses to hypnotic suggestions, are not only present but even sanctioned and subjected to affirmative metaphysical interpretations within the New Age movement (Farias & Granqvist, 2007). Likewise, just as disorganized attachment is linked to experiences of abuse, so are many of the paranormal experiences associated with the New Age (e.g., Irwin, 1993). Moreover, Main and colleagues have found that unresolved/disorganized AAI discourse correlates with many of the central themes of New Age beliefs (e.g., belief in astrology, contact with the dead; Main & Morgan, 1996). In addition, George and Solomon (1996 and Chapter 35, this volume) have reported that mothers classified as disorganized tend to attribute supernatural powers to their offspring (e.g., psychic power, special connection with the deceased).

Similarly, anxious, preoccupied, or ambivalent attachment has been associated with difficulties in understanding the privacy of thought—a cardinal feature of the belief in telepathy—as well as with the attribution of psychic powers to some humans, most notably the self and the attachment figure (Main, 1991). Both kinds of beliefs are well represented within the New Age. Also, preoccupied attachment within the AAI is often expressed as preoccupying anger, wherein angry ranting against the attachment figure may occur in the presence of "authoritative" psychological statements marked by overused phrases and clinical jargon ("psychobabble"). This naturally brings some of the popular psychology literature of the New Age movement to mind (e.g., writings on "toxic," "dysfunctional" families and encounter groups).

As an initial step in testing the compensation predictions of an elevated identification with New Age practices and beliefs among insecure (particularly disorganized and preoccupied) individuals, a continuous questionnaire scale was created to tap New Age spirituality: the New Age Orientation Scale (NAOS; Granqvist & Hagekull, 2001). This scale has now been evaluated in diverse populations, drawn from both New Age settings and the general population. Although serious attempts were made to tap the *theoretical* heterogeneity of New Age-related beliefs and activities, all studies conducted to date indicate that scale scores *empirically* form one homogeneous factor that is highly internally consistent (Farias, Claridge, & Lalljee, 2005; Granqvist & Hagekull, 2001; Granqvist, Ivarsson, et al., 2007; Granqvist et al., 2005). In other words, although New Agers often emphasize the importance of formulating one's own philosophy of life, other New Agers come to form their own philosophies of life in essentially the same manner, resulting in greater homogeneity than might be expected. This also implies that individuals who affirm one set of beliefs (e.g., the possibility of fortunetelling, a seemingly fatalistic philosophy) tend to affirm other, theoretically unrelated, and even incompatible beliefs (e.g., unlimited individual freedom, as expressed in the idea that people choose their own parents). Finally, like unresolved/disorganized speech in the AAI (Hesse & van IJzendoorn, 1999), the NAOS correlates positively with absorption (Granqvist et al., 2005).

In line with predictions, all findings obtained to date on New Age spirituality in relation to estimates of parental sensitivity and security of attachment have supported the compensation hypothesis. First, regarding parental sensitivity, participants drawn from New Age settings reported lower parental sensitivity than those drawn from the general population (Granqvist & Hagekull, 2001). Also, NAOS scores are positively related to both self-reports of parental insensitivity (Granqvist & Hagekull, 2001) and AAI judges' independent estimates of "negative" probable experiences (Granqvist, Ivarsson, et al., 2007). Second, regarding romantic attachment, positive correlations have been found between fearful-avoidant romantic attachment (i.e., attachment characterized by high scores on both attachment anxiety and avoidance in romantic relationships)[5] and NAOS scores (Granqvist & Hagekull, 2001), and between preoccupied attachment and an interest in spirituality and esotericism books (Saroglou, Kempeneers, & Seynhaeve, 2003).

Third, concerning attachment-related states of mind within the AAI, higher NAOS scores have been associated, as expected, with independent judges' assignments of interviewees to the preoccupied and disorganized categories (both trauma-specific unresolved states and more globally disorganized "cannot classify" states[6]; Granqvist, Ivarsson, et al., 2007). Individuals assigned to the cannot classify category were particularly likely to score high in New Age spirituality. In other words, a globally incompatible stance with respect to attachment was paralleled by the embrace of an incompatible set of beliefs regarding life, the self, and the universe. Finally, in a 3-year longitudinal follow-up of the AAI study participants, a link was established between unresolved/disorganized states at the first measurement occasion and New Age spirituality at the second, and this link was mediated (as expected) by a propensity to experience anomalous shifts in consciousness (Granqvist & Fransson, 2007).

The findings from the AAI study are particularly noteworthy when we consider that AAI classifications are often unrelated to self-reports of external phenomena, although strongly related to behavioral observations and more indirect assessments of theoretically relevant constructs (see Hesse, Chapter 25, this volume). In addition, the findings from the AAI study show that whereas some individuals who have experienced parental insensitivity while growing up, and who have used God as a surrogate to regulate distress, *may* have earned a certain degree of attachment security from doing so; the same cannot be said for individuals drawn to the New Age. In fact, the most serious forms of *current* attachment insecurity seem to linger within these individuals. A speculative theoretical interpretation of these discrepancies between traditional religion and the New Age in relation to insecurity within the AAI system is that traditional religion may promote earned security through offering perceptions of a reparative attachment surrogate, conceived of as the perfect attachment figure, whereas such a figure is largely absent within the New Age perspective. Of course, it is also possible that only the most seriously insecure individuals, who have suffered more serious forms of parental insensitivity (potentially including abuse), are drawn to the New Age. If that is the case, it is also readily understandable why they would shy away from an attachment-like figure (e.g., the figure may be perceived as frightening).

Given that New Age spirituality typically does not revolve around God as an attachment-like figure, it is reasonable to question whether the attachment model in general and the compensation hypothesis in particular are at all conceptually applicable (see Kirkpatrick, 2005). We speculate that the adoption of New Age practices and beliefs is driven by motivation similar to that underlying religion as compensation, but that the generalization of IWMs of others (e.g., as frightening/threatening) restrict New Agers' use of God as an attachment surrogate. Note also that although the idea of a single theistic God is usually absent from New Age beliefs, the world of New Agers is often inhabited by imagined angels and spirits, as well as by human spiritual advisors and gurus who may fill some attachment-surrogate functions. Of course, the appeal of the New Age for disorganized and preoccupied individuals may also be due, at least in part, to its provision of metaphysical affirmations of these individuals' psychological states and experiences (e.g., of depersonalization, telepathy, contact with the dead, possession by abusive perpetrators). Prior to the individuals' introduction to the New Age, such states and experiences may well have been regarded by others as signs of "flakiness" or poor contact with reality.

Finally, and as emphasized elsewhere (Granqvist, Ivarsson, et al., 2007), it is important to note that identification with the New Age is only one example of the rejection of traditional beliefs in a particular context. It is an open question whether other examples might have similar correlates (e.g., Westerners' conversion to Hinayana Buddhism, aboriginals' conversion to "born-again" Christianity).

Empirical Findings
Supporting the Correspondence Pathway

The religion and spirituality of most people are far from fully represented by the characteristics described in the sections above on the compensation hypothesis. Consider this example:

> I observe, with profound regret, the religious struggles which come into many biographies, as if almost essential to the formation of the hero. I ought to speak of these, to say, that any man has an advantage, not to be estimated, who is born, as I was, into a family where the religion is simple and rational; who is trained in the theory of such a religion, so that he never knows, for an hour, what these religious or irreligious struggles are. I always knew God loved me, and I was always grateful to him for the world he placed me in. (James, 1902, p. 82)

Most religious people would probably not see themselves or the members of their religious community in descriptions of the "sick soul" or the psychologically abused. Psychologists who have studied religion would have to agree, based on the data.

Social Correspondence. In line with the social aspect of the correspondence hypothesis, individuals reporting experiences of being sensitively cared for by parents have been shown to score higher in religiousness than those reporting experiences of being less sensitively cared for, but only insofar as their parents also displayed high levels of religiosity (Granqvist, 1998, 2002; Granqvist & Hagekull, 1999; Kirkpatrick & Shaver, 1990). In addition, such people score higher on a scale created to assess religiosity as socially rooted in the parental relationship (Granqvist, 2002; Granqvist & Hagekull, 1999). Moreover, both sets of findings were supported in the AAI study, when coded estimates of parental sensitivity rather than direct self-reports were used (Granqvist, Ivarsson, et al., 2007). Similarly, in the case of romantic attachment, secure attachment is associated with scores on the scale measuring religiosity as socially based in the parental relationship (Granqvist, 2002).

We note that parental religiousness has often been portrayed in the psychology of religion as the single strongest predictor of offspring religiousness, especially by scholars who approach the topic from a social learning perspective (e.g., Batson et al., 1993; Spilka et al., 2003). However, the "effect" of parental religiousness is importantly moderated by the estimated quality of the offspring–parent attachment relationship. In fact, whereas parent–offspring correlations for retrospectively defined secure dyads have been large ($r \approx .50$), they have usually been nonsignificant and close to zero for insecure dyads (e.g., Granqvist, 1998; Kirkpatrick & Shaver, 1990). An implication of these findings for religious parents who wish their children to embrace their own religion is that religious teaching is not enough; in fact, it may be completely unsuccessful unless it is combined with placing a high priority on sensitive caregiving that meets the children's needs for protection and security. It is even possible that sensitive caregiving—in the absence of explicit religious training—suffices as long as a child has an opportunity to observe a caregiver engaging in religious speech and behavior.[7]

IWM Correspondence. Evidence for IWM correspondence in the interpersonal attachment and religious domains has also accrued in relation to attachment history as estimated through the AAI. Most notably, the AAI study described above revealed that coded estimates of probable experiences with loving parents were associated with participants' reports of a loving, as opposed to a distant, God image (Granqvist, Ivarsson, et al., 2007). Conversely, inferred experiences with rejecting and role-reversing parents were associated positively with a distant God image and negatively with a loving image of God.

Similar findings have recently been reported in an Italian AAI study (Cassibba, Costantini, & Gatto, 2007). This study contained two subsamples: a highly religious group (Catholic nuns, novitates, priests, and seminarists) and a comparison group of lay Catholic believers matched for gender. In further support of IWM correspondence, the highly religious group was coded significantly higher on loving experiences with mothers, as well as on a continuous dimension of current security/coherence of discourse. Finally—regardless of subsample—secure-autonomous participants reported a more loving God image than insecure-nonautonomous participants.

Although religious transformations are less frequent for individuals who have experienced sensitive caregiving, they sometimes do occur. When they do, the life context and the constituents of the change are very different from those reported in the sections on the compensation hypothesis. For example, prospectively predicted increases in religiousness occurred *not* following romantic relationship dissolution, but rather after the establishment of a new intimate relationship, for participants who reported sensitive parenting (Granqvist & Hagekull, 2003). Also, religious changes tended to occur at a comparatively early age for these individuals (Granqvist & Hagekull, 1999; Granqvist, Ivarsson, et al., 2007).

Regarding romantic attachment, IWM correspondence has typically been supported in contemporaneous relations between religious variables and romantic attachment security. For example, Kirkpatrick and Shaver (1992) found that people with a secure romantic attachment displayed a higher personal belief in and relationship with God, as well as perceptions of God as loving, whereas people reporting avoidant romantic attachment were agnostic or atheist to a larger extent. These findings have since been conceptually replicated in a number of studies (Byrd & Boe, 2000; Granqvist & Hagekull, 2000, 2003; Kirkpatrick, 1998; TenElshof & Furrow, 2000). For example, Byrd and Boe found that participants reporting secure romantic attachments engaged more in prayer that served to maintain closeness to God. Moreover, even in prospective analyses, IWM correspondence between romantic attachment security and religious change has been supported in expected contexts—for example, following the formation of a romantic relationship between assessments of religiosity (Granqvist & Hagekull, 2003).

Besides the correlational studies just reviewed, three sets of recent attachment and religion experiments or quasi-experiments involving direct attempts to activate attachment have been performed (Birgegard & Granqvist, 2004; Granqvist, Ljungdahl, et al., 2007; Mikulincer et al., 2007). The main effects of attachment activation observed in these studies have already been described. However, in all three sets of studies, the main effects were qualified, or moderated, by perceived attachment history or current attachment security in a manner that supports the IWM aspect of the correspondence hypothesis.

As we have seen, individuals who have experienced insensitive care are more likely to regulate distress through their perceived relationship with God than are those who have experienced sensitive care (i.e., a compensation effect). However, across the three experiments conducted by Birgegard and Granqvist (2004), an increase in the use of God to regulate distress was observed following subliminal separation primes among adult believers who had reported sensitive experiences with parents, thus supporting IWM correspondence instead. Because indirect assessments of religiosity (i.e., regression residuals from pre- to postpriming) were used in the context of *subliminal* priming, participants were unaware of attachment activation. Birgegard and Granqvist speculated that these conditions might have undermined the possibility of a "higher-order" compensatory use of religion in individuals who had experienced parental insensitivity, thus resulting in their withdrawal from God or (put differently) their defensive shift of attention away from attachment (e.g., Main et al., 1985). Conversely, presumably via automatic activation of IWMs, individuals with more sensitive experiences with caregivers drew upon God in this situation, or turned their attention to attachment, whereas they typically tend to rely on other means to regulate distress in the context of conscious attachment activation.[8]

In line with these speculations, the increase in the psychological accessibility of God concepts following subliminal threat exposures, observed by Mikulincer and colleagues (2007), was particularly notable in participants with a secure romantic attachment orientation. In a second experiment, Mikulincer and colleagues showed that participants with a secure romantic attachment style implicitly reacted with more positive affect following subliminal exposure to religion-related pictures (compared to neutral pictures). Hence not only did attention to God increase more for individuals reporting secure romantic attachment than for those reporting insecure attachment when faced with unconscious threat, but the former individuals were also more likely to benefit implicitly from being unconsciously exposed to religious material.

Finally, in the study of 5- to 7-year-old children who were asked to place a God symbol at a chosen distance from a fictional child who was in attachment-activating or attachment-neutral situations (Granqvist, Ljungdahl, et al., 2007), secure children placed God closer to the fictional child when the fictional child was in attachment-activating situations. However, the pattern was reversed when the fictional child was in attachment-neutral situations (i.e., insecure children placed God closer). Overall, the discrepancy in God proximity between the two types of situations was much larger in secure than in insecure children. Our interpretation of this interaction is that secure children's attention shifted to God following attachment activation, whereas insecure children's attention to God did not shift as a function of attachment activation. Importantly, this study used the adapted Separation Anxiety Test (SAT; Kaplan, 1987), an indirect (semiprojective) method, to measure security, and the God placement procedure was similarly semiprojective. (That is, the fictional child, not the study participants, was in different situations that were more or less likely to activate a child's attachment system.) As in the adult experiments using subliminal priming techniques, this semiprojective procedure may have undermined a higher-order compensatory use of religion in insecure children, and instead yielded automatic activation of IWMs and thus support for the correspondence hypothesis.

In sum, substantial empirical support has been obtained for the idea that the developmental pathway to religion for individuals with secure attachments runs through extensive experience with sensitive, religious caregivers and leads to the development of a security-enhancing image of a loving God. Moreover, in such cases God, like other good attachment figures (Mikulincer & Shaver, 2004), is implicitly seen as available in times of need, although secure individuals are unlikely to need to use the perceived relationship with God specifically to regulate distress.

ATTACHMENT TO GOD AND PSYCHOLOGICAL OUTCOMES

To the extent that having a secure base prevents or reduces fear and anxiety, as argued by Bowlby (1969/1982) and others, belief in God as an attachment figure should confer certain psychological benefits. The connections between religion and mental health and well-being, which are both very complex, multifaceted constructs, are immensely complex: It seems clear that religious belief and commitment can have highly positive, highly negative, or neutral effects on well-being as variously defined (see Paloutzian & Kirkpatrick, 1995, for examples). A thorough review of this literature is beyond the scope of this chapter, but in this final major section, we point to findings that seem particularly relevant to the claim that God functions psychologically like an attachment figure. We then turn our attention to the emerging topic of how individual differences in attachment to God relate to psychological outcomes.

A number of studies suggest that religious belief is related to the aspects of psychological well-being and mental health that are most obviously predicted from an attachment perspective. For example, religious commitment correlates inversely with trait anxiety (Baker & Gorsuch, 1982; McClain, 1978), and belief in a loving deity is positively correlated with self-esteem (Benson & Spilka, 1973; Spilka, Addison, & Rosensohn, 1975). Other studies suggest that the particular aspects of religious belief relating most strongly to psychological well-being are the ones consistent with the religion-as-attachment model. For example, Pollner (1989, p. 95) found in a large national sample that a dimension of religion he labeled "divine relationships" (defined as "psychological proximity of the divine other and the frequency and depth of interaction with that other") predicted psychological well-being more strongly than several other religion measures, even when numerous background variables (including church attendance) were statistically controlled for. In another large-scale national survey, Poloma and Gallup (1991) found that prayer, and particularly the "experience of God during prayer," were more strongly correlated than other religion variables with several measures of well-being. In a study of Unification Church members, Galanter (1979) reported that the two best predictors of emotional well-being were "My religious beliefs give me comfort" and "I feel a close connection to God."

A clear example of the differential relations between an attachment-relevant conception of well-being and attachment-relevant dimensions of religiosity comes from the literature on religion and loneliness. According to Weiss (1973), attachment relationships are important as a buffer against a particular form of loneliness he called "emotional isolation" (as opposed to "social isolation"). In a study by Schwab and Petersen (1990), loneliness was inversely related to "belief in a helpful God" and positively related to "belief in a wrathful God," but unrelated to "mere belief in God." Kirkpatrick, Shillito, and Kellas (1998) also found that belief in having a personal relationship with God predicted reduced loneliness even when other measures of interpersonal social support were statistically controlled for.

Research on religious conversion also indicates that turning to God as an attachment figure is associated with an improved sense of well-being. In the studies by Galanter (1979) and Ullman

(1982), for example, converts reported substantial reductions in anxiety, depression, and emotional distress after their conversions. Similarly, research on religion and coping (with stress) provides considerable support for the positive role of religion in this process. Investigations by Gibbs and Achterberg-Lawlis (1978), Maton (1989), and Pargament and colleagues (see Pargament, 1997) all provide empirical support for the assertion that certain religious variables and coping activities predict successful coping and positive psychological outcomes in dealing with stressful events ranging from health problems (both one's own and those of close others) to the 1990–1991 Gulf War. The importance of religion as a source of support is particularly well documented with respect to older adults (e.g., Koenig, George, & Siegler, 1988), perhaps—as suggested by findings reported by Brown and colleagues (2004)—in part because older adults are more likely to be without, and to have experienced the loss of, significant human attachments.

If believers' perceived relationships with God are actually attachment-like, then something analogous to security versus insecurity of attachment to God should be present, and should be linked to psychological outcomes in ways similar to the security–insecurity of attachment to parents and romantic partners. As part of the first study of adult attachment style and religion (described earlier in this chapter), Kirkpatrick and Shaver (1992) included several measures of psychological well-being. Of many religious variables included in the study, only one evinced significant and strong associations with these variables: a measure of "attachment style" with respect to God. Adults who described their perceived relationship with God as secure (God was seen as warm and responsive to the respondent), as opposed to avoidant (God was seen as distant and rejecting) or ambivalent (God was seen as inconsistent), scored significantly and substantially lower on measures of loneliness/depression, anxiety, and physical illness, and higher on general life satisfaction. Belavich and Pargament (2002) similarly documented associations between Kirkpatrick and Shaver's measure of attachment to God and styles of religious coping, suggesting that individuals who believe they have a secure attachment to God use more "positive" religious coping strategies to cope when a loved one is undergoing surgery.

These studies used a very simple measure of attachment to God consisting of three brief forced-choice paragraphs (similar to Hazan & Shaver's

[1987] early measure of romantic attachment style). More recently, however, researchers have developed somewhat more advanced multidimensional self-report instruments to assess attachment to God, focusing either on individual differences in avoidance and anxiety as these relate to attachment to God (Beck & McDonald, 2004; Rowatt & Kirkpatrick, 2002) or on the extent to which an attachment relationship with God is present (Sim & Loh, 2003). In these studies, lower attachment anxiety and avoidant attachment, as well as higher perceptions of having an attachment to God, were correlated with favorable psychological outcomes, such as optimism, positive affect, agreeableness, and (low) neuroticism—again, after the researchers controlled for such potential confounds as romantic attachment, attachment to parents, and social desirability.

In sum, correlates of attachment to God suggest, as in the case of attachment in general, that attachment security promotes psychological well-being and alleviates distress. However, in the case of attachment to God, it appears that this relatively straightforward conclusion is particularly applicable when other attachments are insufficient or other attachment figures are unavailable. This qualification is supported across several studies and, as it turns out, strikes at the heart of previous discrepancies between compensation and correspondence findings in the religion-as-attachment literature.

For example, in the study by Kirkpatrick and Shaver (1992), the effects of attachment to God on psychological outcomes were moderated by perceived attachment histories with mothers. Respondents who remembered their mothers as relatively insensitive but still had perceptions of a secure attachment to God appeared to benefit the most from their perceived relationship with God. In an intriguing parallel to these findings, Brown and colleagues (2004) found that increased religiousness following bereavement was particularly associated with attenuated grief for individuals whose "secular" attachment orientation was judged insecure. (These effects could not be accounted for by the potential confounds of social contact, past marital satisfaction with the deceased, or personality.) Similarly, the positive "effects" of religious variables more generally, such as those of religious coping and intrinsic religiousness, on mental health outcomes are typically moderated by levels of stress, so that religion confers its most beneficial effects in times of trouble (e.g., Smith, McCullough, & Poll, 2003).

Findings indicating a positive effect of religion on psychological outcomes in general are paralleled by two sets of findings (both briefly described above) suggesting that religion may also have positive effects on attachment. First, self-reported insecure attachment history and romantic attachment (in the latter case particularly, a negative self-model or a high degree of attachment anxiety) have been linked to increasing religiousness over time (longitudinal compensation), whereas self-reported secure attachment has been linked to higher religiousness at a given time (contemporaneous correspondence; see Kirkpatrick, 2005). Second, AAI-based estimates of parental insensitivity in the past have predicted a history of using religion as compensation for inadequate attachments, but current insecurity (incoherent attachment discourse) has been unrelated to religion as compensation (Cassibba et al., 2007; Granqvist, Ivarsson, et al., 2007). In some cases, therefore, religion as compensation may increase attachment security, which in turn may explain the increase in well-being that occurs when a person is coping with stress through religion. Although this interpretation is speculative at this point, it would make theoretical sense if the individual's perceived relationship with God actually functions as a compensatory attachment relationship. It would also be theologically plausible, given the portrayal of God as a sensitive secure base and haven of safety, which we have described in this chapter. In attachment terms, some aspects of religion may promote "earned security" (Main & Goldwyn, 1984; Main, Goldwyn, & Hesse, 2003)—possibly through a person's viewing him- or herself as worthy of love and care, thanks to perceiving God as a loving attachment figure.

Unfortunately, interpretation of the data collected so far is limited by several methodological problems. First, and perhaps most obvious, the causal direction of cross-sectional correlation between religion and various outcomes remains open to question. Second, the positive effects on mental health of religious conversions and religious experiences are based largely on retrospective accounts, so they are vulnerable to reconstructive memory processes (see Granqvist & Kirkpatrick, 2004, and Pargament, 1997, for overviews). Third, the (self-report) mode of measuring attachment to God and well-being in the studies reviewed here leaves us unable to exclude the possibility that (any combination of) self-deception, impression management, shared method variance, semantic overlap, and so on may be at least partly responsible for the associations obtained. Therefore, it is imperative to construct less explicit methods for evaluating individual differences in believers' perceived relationship with God. A longitudinal follow-up of the AAI-based study (Granqvist, Ivarsson, et al., 2007) is currently addressing this issue by using an interview (Granqvist & Main, 2003) concerning each individual's relationship with God, which was adapted from the AAI protocol. One aim in developing this interview is to be able to undermine some of the potential validity threats to the self-reports of attachment to God.

CONCLUSIONS AND FUTURE DIRECTIONS

In this chapter, we have marshaled evidence from various sources to support the hypothesis that many aspects of religious belief and experience, particularly those related to perceived relationships with God or other supernatural figures, reflect (at least in part) the operation of attachment processes. From a normative perspective, God evinces all of the usual defining characteristics of an attachment figure to whom people turn for a safe haven and secure base. We have also attempted to demonstrate that the attachment components of believers' perceived relations with God are far from surface aspects of religion, but instead are central components of their religion. Moreover, we have argued that people's perceived relationships with God develop in tandem with the maturation of their attachment systems and associated attachment working models. From an individual-differences perspective, we have described two attachment-related pathways relevant to the ontogenetic development of religion. One of these runs through experiences with insensitive caregivers and resulting attachment insecurity, in which case a relationship with God is sometimes used as a surrogate attachment useful in regulating distress (the compensation pathway). The other path runs through experiences with sensitive, religious caregivers and attachment security, in which case religion is socially rooted in the parental relationship and reflects a generalization of working models of the self as worthy of care and of others (including God) as willing and able to provide it (the correspondence pathway). We have also addressed attachment-related individual differences associated with less orthodox forms of spirituality (namely, the New Age movement), as well as ways in which such differences are linked to implicit/automatic versus explicit/controlled uses of religion. Finally, we have presented evidence suggesting that attachment to God may confer the kinds of psychological benefits associated with secure interpersonal attachments, especially in times of personal trouble when other attachment figures are insufficient or unavailable.

As we have seen, for some individuals, religious beliefs seem to reflect responses to insecure interpersonal attachments; for others, religious beliefs are established early in life, during childhoods characterized by secure attachment, in which cases they remain fairly constant across the lifespan. This distinction raises a host of interesting empirical questions. For example, do the religious beliefs emerging from these alternative processes differ qualitatively with respect to their effects on psychological outcomes? The prospective longitudinal findings from Brown and colleagues (2004), along with other lines of evidence, suggest that individuals who either are currently insecure or have suffered attachment-related difficulties in the past are particularly well served by religion. However, additional prospective longitudinal research is needed before a firm conclusion can be drawn. Such research should also aim to clarify whether—and if so, when and how—religion may be both a salutary factor and a risk factor for psychological outcomes in the context of insecure attachment and past attachment difficulties.

Besides the mental health and subjective well-being outcomes that have been considered in the studies to date, the time is now ripe to consider other psychological outcomes related to attachment to God. We believe that there are a number of situations (in history and today) in which believers are subjected to attachment system activation—for example, by fear or bereavement, in conjunction with religious "priming" of varying kinds. A believer whose attachment system is activated (e.g., by interpersonal losses due to war or terror-related killings) and who is also primed with an authoritarian attachment-like figure (e.g., "God punishes the evil") may become disposed to think, feel, and act in ways normally regarded as antisocial in relation to those considered "evil." On the other hand, a believer in a similar situation who is primed with a nurturant attachment-like figure (e.g., "God loves everyone") may be more likely to react in ways normally regarded as prosocial (cf. Mikulincer & Shaver, 2001; Mikulincer, Shaver, Gillath, & Nitzberg, 2005). Perhaps the presumed effects of various kinds of priming are moderated by individual differences in dispositional attachment security in relation to God, parents, or ro-

mantic partners. Related issues are currently under investigation in a cross-religion (Christianity and Judaism), cross-cultural (Sweden and Israel) project. Needless to say, more comparative research of this kind is needed.

A related set of questions concerns the interaction of correspondence and compensation processes within individuals across time. For example, in cases where religious change is motivated by insecure interpersonal attachment, does one's orientation toward interpersonal attachments change concomitantly? We have noted the possibility of "earned security" effects from religion for some individuals, but much remains to be done methodologically to secure such an interpretation, to predict for whom and under what conditions earned security might develop, and to pinpoint more precisely the psychological mechanisms involved. Increased knowledge in this area might provide a useful basis for the development of therapeutic strategies for dealing with relationship-related difficulties, particularly in religious populations.

Conversely, do changes in interpersonal attachments lead to concomitant changes in religious belief? For example, if an individual turns to a relationship with God in response to interpersonal difficulties, does the importance of these newly found religious beliefs then recede if the quality of his or her interpersonal relationships improves? We have noted that insecurity and reports of parental insensitivity predict increased religiousness for individuals who have experienced romantic relationship dissolution, and, conversely, predict decreased religiousness for (other) individuals who have experienced the formation of a new romantic relationship (Granqvist & Hagekull, 2003). However, to the best of our knowledge, no study has followed participants across multiple relationship formations and dissolutions. The general question of how the centrality of religious beliefs in people's lives may wax and wane in concert with, or inversely with, the ups and downs of their interpersonal relationships remains an important topic for research.

An additional aspect of correspondence and compensation processes that warrants future research is the distinction between implicit/automatic and explicit/controlled (or deliberate) uses of religion. Our expectation, based on the conclusions drawn from all of the studies reviewed here, is that when activation of the attachment system is consciously connected to its source, and its effects cause subjective distress, individuals with insecure attachment experiences with insensitive caregivers will be more inclined to regulate distress by turning to God. In other words, the compensation hypothesis refers to a deliberate, higher-order strategy of distress regulation through an attachment surrogate that may run counter to how the self and attachment figures are unconsciously represented by the individual. Another way to phrase this is to say that the relationship with God is not functional at the implicit level, due to an incoherent/multiple representation (Bowlby, 1973; Main, 1991) of God. In contrast, when attachment activation is not consciously connected to its source, and God is the only attachment figure available in the situation, automatic activation of IWMs and associated neural networks may lead individuals with secure attachment experiences with sensitive caregivers to experience God as psychologically accessible. Thus the IWM-aspect of correspondence may apply at an unconscious level, due to a coherent/singular representation (Bowlby, 1973; Main, 1991) of God.

Another conceptual challenge concerns the correspondence hypothesis itself. We have posited correspondence processes at two independent levels of operation: the level of IWMs, and the level of socialization or social learning. We have argued, reasoning from the bottom up, that both are needed to account for existing data on attachment and religion. However, thinking from the top down, we agree that much would be gained if the two aspects could somehow be integrated. To avoid an outdated and oversimplified view of development, this should be done in a manner that liberates the socialization/social learning concept from any presumption or implication that the offspring is a *tabula rasa* (Pinker, 2002).

Regarding limitations in the foci of attachment and religion studies to date, two are particularly important. First, although studies are underway, there are still no long-term longitudinal studies that have followed participants from early childhood, when their first attachments developed, to later in development, when their God relationship and other attachment relationships unfold. Second, very few attachment-and-religion studies have been conducted outside the Western world, and, to the best of our knowledge, none outside the major monotheistic traditions (other than the New Age beliefs discussed previously). The absence of such studies represents a clear limitation in the current attachment-and-religion database.

Concerning general theoretical issues, we have found in discussions with colleagues that a common misconception of the religion-as-

attachment model is that it would be built on, or even require, an adaptationist understanding of religion (i.e., an assumption that religion itself promoted inclusive fitness in the environments of evolutionary adaptation, or EEAs). This is a serious mistake. Our view has consistently been that religion is more likely to be an evolutionary by-product than a direct adaptation or set of adaptations. Hence, whereas the attachment system has a clear and very important biological function within its usual sphere of operation (promoting inclusive fitness through caregivers' protection and support of offspring), it is unlikely that a relationship with (an imagined) God increased inclusive fitness by systematically protecting the individuals who had it from danger in the EEAs. Although some theorists would suggest that the God relationship promoted inclusive fitness in some other ways, such as through sexual selection or group selection mechanisms, we believe that there are a number of good arguments against an adaptationist view of religion (see Kirkpatrick, 2005, for an extensive discussion; see also Hinde, 1999). Nevertheless, once a mechanism has established itself within the gene pool of a certain species, it may well continue to operate within individuals and in contexts that were not associated with its original biological function. Therefore, the question of religion's biological functionality is more or less orthogonal to the question of whether the relationship between a believer and God involves the attachment system and is an attachment relationship. As we have both argued elsewhere (Granqvist, 2006b; Kirkpatrick, 2005), corporations, institutions, and even religions and cultures may well capitalize on any behavioral system's operation outside the sphere of its biological function. As one example, pornography capitalizes on the sexual or reproductive system, but it is not the biological set goal of that system; hence pornography is one of the system's by-products. In an analogous way, we view religion as a by-product—a free rider on evolved mechanisms, one of which is the attachment system.

Another general issue is the conceptual limit of attachment theory in the psychology of religion. We have deliberately restricted most of our discussion to aspects of religion that we believe to be psychologically grounded in the attachment system per se—specifically, beliefs about certain kinds of supernatural beings and perceived relationships with these beings. Many other applications of attachment constructs to religion are tempting: "attachment" to human religious leaders (pastors, cult leaders, shamans); "attachment" to religious groups (congregations, cults, denominations); and the concept of "grasping attachment" in Buddhism—to name just a few. Although these and other religious phenomena may seem analogous to attachment in certain ways, we suspect that many reflect the operation of psychological processes and systems other than attachment. One of us (Kirkpatrick, 2005) has argued elsewhere, from the perspective of contemporary evolutionary psychology, that the attachment system is just one of numerous domain-specific psychological mechanisms underlying the diverse range of religious phenomena. For example, relationships with human leaders may be guided largely by mechanisms concerned with issues of status, power, and prestige, rather than (or in addition to) attachment; and relationships with religious groups may involve mechanisms concerned with social exchange or with coalition formation and maintenance. Hence we make no claim that attachment theory constitutes a comprehensive psychology of religion. What we do claim, however, is that attachment is one very central process underlying individuals' beliefs about, ways of relating to, and representations of God, particularly in Christianity.

Notwithstanding many unanswered questions, we submit that no model of adult interpersonal relationships in general, or attachment relationships in particular, will be complete without explicit acknowledgment of the role of God and other imaginary figures in people's relationship networks. Incorporating religious beliefs into research on adult relationships may be useful in addressing vexing questions in the attachment literature concerning such issues as the content, structure, and generality of IWMs, and the dynamic processes underlying change in attachment patterns and IWMs over time. In short, application of attachment theory to religion not only holds promise for the psychology of religion, but may also have much to offer for the study of attachment processes and individual differences across the lifespan.

ACKNOWLEDGMENTS

Preparation of this chapter was facilitated by a Swedish Research Council fellowship to Pehr Granqvist, and by a Faculty Semester Research Assignment from the College of William and Mary to Lee A. Kirkpatrick. The Swedish part of the research reported here was supported by a grant (Dnr 1999-0507:01,02) from the Bank of Sweden Tercentenary Foundation.

NOTES

1. Although it is doubtful that the most realistic or fruitful approach to deciding category membership is a definition based on necessary and sufficient conditions (philosophical "essentialism"), such criteria are implicitly applied in the following sections, for reasons of scientific convention. Very different approaches are suggested in Wittgenstein's (1953) notion of family resemblances and exemplar models of categorization (e.g., Juslin, Olsson, & Olsson, 2003). As applied to the category of attachment relationships, the infant–caregiver relationship would then constitute the category prototype. In order to add a new "family member," one would need to show that it bears convincing resemblance to the prototype, just as we will show that the believer–God relationship does.
2. All Biblical quotes are from the King James Version.
3. Although IWM correspondence and social correspondence are independent in principle, they are not so in practice. For example, insofar as a caregiver has an overtly expressed God image, a secure offspring is expected to adopt his or her caregiver's God image to a larger extent than an insecure offspring, even if the image is of, for example, a distant God (social correspondence). On the other hand, the secure offspring is anticipated to have a less distant God image, due to the operation of a generalized, positive set of working models (IWM correspondence). In practice, this is not a serious problem, because a reliably sensitive caregiver's God image is unlikely to be distant. Hence social and IWM correspondence will usually operate in concert rather than in opposition.
4. All attachment data reported in this chapter that required coding were, of course, coded by evaluators unaware of participants' religiousness and spirituality.
5. Notably, fearful-avoidant attachment has been considered a conceptual counterpart in the romantic relationship domain to disorganized attachment, as it is characterized by two incompatible sources of motivation: wanting closeness, but at the same time avoiding it because of being afraid of its consequences (Shaver & Clark, 1996).
6. The cannot classify category is most frequently assigned to interviewees who alternate between two incompatible discourse strategies—on the one hand dismissing the import of attachment experiences with parents (e.g., idealization), and on the other being preoccupied by these same experiences (e.g., involving anger) (see Main, Goldwyn, & Hesse, 2003).
7. One of us (Granqvist & Hagekull, 1999) originally proposed a "socialization" account of the origins of religiousness in individuals with memories of being sensitively cared for. The other of us (Kirkpatrick, 2005) disagreed, noting that "socialization" is a complex process itself in need of explanation. Although this was seemingly a genuine disagreement,

we reached our respective standpoints by different routes. Granqvist (1998; Granqvist & Hagekull, 1999) reached his socialization proposal by incorporating a replicated moderator effect into the religion-as-attachment framework while aiming to increase the falsifiability of predictions derived from that framework. Kirkpatrick (2005), on the other hand, was concerned with evolutionary psychology as well as with the integrity of scientific explanations more generally. In practice, we agree that "socialization" is not an explanation, but merely a description (often masked as an explanation) of similarities between parents and children. Likewise, we agree that level of parental religiousness does often interact with attachment history to affect religious outcomes.

8. In the social cognition literature, these distinctions are paralleled by distinctions between "contrast" (cf. compensation) and "assimilation" (cf. correspondence) effects (e.g., Wheeler & Petty, 2001). Contrast effects tend to occur when conditions or response modes require explicit processing (e.g., guided imagery, self-reports), whereas assimilation effects tend to occur when only implicit processes are operating (e.g., subliminal priming, lexical decision tasks).

REFERENCES

Ainsworth, M. D. S. (1985). Attachments across the life span. *Bulletin of the New York Academy of Medicine*, *61*, 792–812.

Ainsworth, M. D. S., Bell, S. M., & Stayton, D. J. (1974). Infant–mother attachment and social development: "Socialization" as a product of reciprocal responsiveness to signals. In M. P. M. Richards (Ed.), *The integration of a child into a social world* (pp. 99–137). Cambridge, UK: Cambridge University Press.

Ainsworth, M. D. S., Blehar, M. C., Waters, E., & Wall, S. (1978). *Patterns of attachment: A psychological study of the Strange Situation*. Hillsdale, NJ: Erlbaum.

Allport, G. W. (1950). *The individual and his religion*. New York: Macmillan.

Argyle, M., & Beit-Hallahmi, B. (1975). *The social psychology of religion*. London: Routledge & Kegan Paul.

Baker, M., & Gorsuch, R. (1982). Trait anxiety and intrinsic–extrinsic religiousness. *Journal for the Scientific Study of Religion*, *21*, 119–122.

Bartholomew, K., & Horowitz, L. M. (1991). Attachment styles in young adults: A test of a four-category model. *Journal of Personality and Social Psychology*, *61*, 226–244.

Batson, C. D., Schoenrade, P., & Ventis, W. L. (1993). *Religion and the individual: A social psychological perspective*. New York: Oxford University Press.

Beck, R., & McDonald, A. (2004). Attachment to God: The Attachment to God Inventory, tests of working model correspondence, and an exploration of faith

group differences. *Journal of Psychology and Theology*, *32*, 92–103.

Belavich, T. G., & Pargament, K. I. (2002). The role of attachment in predicting spiritual coping with a loved one in surgery. *Journal of Adult Development*, *9*, 13–29.

Benson, P. L., & Spilka, B. (1973). God image as a function of self-esteem and locus of control. *Journal for the Scientific Study of Religion*, *12*, 297–310.

Birgegard, A., & Granqvist, P. (2004). The correspondence between attachment to parents and God: Three experiments using subliminal separation cues. *Personality and Social Psychology Bulletin*, *30*, 1122–1135.

Bjorck, J. P., & Cohen, L. H. (1993). Coping with threats, losses, and challenges. *Journal of Social and Clinical Psychology*, *12*, 56–72.

Bowlby, J. (1969/1982). *Attachment and loss: Vol. 1. Attachment*. New York: Basic Books.

Bowlby, J. (1973). *Attachment and loss: Vol. 2. Separation: Anxiety and anger*. New York: Basic Books.

Bretherton, I. (1987). New perspectives on attachment relations: Security, communication, and internal working models. In J. D. Osofsky (Ed.), *Handbook of infant development* (2nd ed., pp. 1061–1100). New York: Wiley.

Broen, W. E., Jr. (1957). A factor-analytic study of religious attitudes. *Journal of Abnormal and Social Psychology*, *54*, 176–179.

Brown, S. L., Nesse, R. M., House, J. S., & Utz, R. L. (2004). Religion and emotional compensation: Results from a prospective study of widowhood. *Personality and Social Psychology Bulletin*, *30*, 1165–1174.

Byrd, K. R., & Boe, A. D. (2000). The correspondence between attachment dimensions and prayer in college students. *International Journal for the Psychology of Religion*, *11*, 9–24.

Campos, J. J., & Stenberg, C. (1981). Perception, appraisal, and emotion: The onset of social referencing. In M. E. Lamb & L. R. Sherrod (Eds.), *Infant social cognition: Empirical and theoretical considerations* (pp. 273–314). Hillsdale, NJ: Erlbaum.

Carlson, E. A. (1998). A prospective longitudinal study of attachment disorganization/disorientation. *Child Development*, *69*, 1107–1128.

Cassibba, R., Costantini, A., & Gatto, S. (2007 June). *The faith experience as attachment relationship: A comparison between Catholic religious and lays*. Paper presented at the 11° Congresso Internazionale: Attaccamento E Religione, Società Italiana di Psicologia della Religione, Milan, Italy.

Cicirelli, V. G. (2004). God as the ultimate attachment figure for older adults. *Attachment and Human Development*, *6*, 371–388.

Clark, E. T. (1929). *The psychology of religious awakening*. New York: Macmillan.

Coe, G. A. (1916). *Psychology of religion*. Chicago: University of Chicago Press.

Collins, N. L., & Read, S. J. (1994). Cognitive representations of attachment: The structure and function of working models. In K. Bartholomew & D. Perlman

(Eds.), *Advances in personal relationships: Vol. 5. Attachment processes in adulthood* (Vol. 5, pp. 53–90). London: Jessica Kingsley.

Dickie, J. R., Charland, K., & Poll, E. (2005). *Attachment and children's concepts of God.* Unpublished manuscript, Hope College, Hope, MI.

Duke, E. H. (1977). *Meaning in life and acceptance of death in terminally ill patients.* Unpublished doctoral dissertation, Northwestern University.

Eshleman, A. K., Dickie, J. R., Merasco, D. M., Shepard, A., & Johnson, M. (1999). Mother God, father God: Children's perceptions of God's distance. *International Journal for the Psychology of Religion, 9,* 139–146.

Farias, M., Claridge, G., & Lalljee, M. (2005). Personality and cognitive predictors of New Age practices and beliefs. *Personality and Individual Differences, 39,* 979–989.

Farias, M., & Granqvist, P. (2007). The psychology of the New Age. In D. Kemp (Ed.), *Handbook of New Age* (pp. 123–150). Leiden, The Netherlands: Brill.

Ferm, V. (1945). *The encyclopedia of religion.* Secaucus, NJ: Poplar.

Freud, S. (1961). *The future of an illusion* (J. Strachey, Trans.). New York: Norton. (Original work published 1927)

Galanter, M. (1979). The "Moonies": A psychological study of conversion and membership in a contemporary religious sect. *American Journal of Psychiatry, 136,* 165–170.

Gallup, G., Jr., & Jones, S. (1989). *One hundred questions and answers: Religion in America.* Princeton, NJ: Princeton Religious Research Center.

George, C., Kaplan, N., & Main, M. (1984). *Adult Attachment Interview protocol.* Unpublished manuscript, University of California at Berkeley.

George, C., Kaplan, N., & Main, M. (1985). *Adult Attachment Interview protocol* (2nd ed.). Unpublished manuscript, University of California at Berkeley.

George, C., Kaplan, N., & Main, M. (1996). *Adult Attachment Interview protocol* (3rd ed.). Unpublished manuscript, University of California at Berkeley.

George, C., & Solomon, J. (1996). Representational models of relationships: Links between caregiving and attachment. *Infant Mental Health Journal, 17,* 198–216.

Gibbs, H. W., & Achterberg-Lawlis, J. (1978). Spiritual values and death anxiety: Implications for counseling with terminal cancer patients. *Journal of Counseling Psychology, 25,* 563–569.

Godin, A., & Hallez, M. (1965). Parental images and divine paternity. In A. Godin (Ed.), *From religious experience to a religious attitude* (pp. 65–96). Chicago: Loyola University Press.

Gorsuch, R. L. (1968). The conceptualization of God as seen in adjective ratings. *Journal for the Scientific Study of Religion, 7,* 56–64.

Granqvist, P. (1998). Religiousness and perceived childhood attachment: On the question of compensation or correspondence. *Journal for the Scientific Study of Religion, 37,* 350–367.

Granqvist, P. (2002). Attachment and religiosity in adolescence: Cross-sectional and longitudinal evaluations. *Personality and Social Psychology Bulletin, 28,* 260–270.

Granqvist, P. (2003). Attachment theory and religious conversions: A review and a resolution of the classic and contemporary paradigm chasm. *Review of Religious Research, 45,* 172–187.

Granqvist, P. (2005). Building a bridge between attachment and religious coping: Tests of moderators and mediators. *Mental Health, Religion, and Culture, 8,* 35–47.

Granqvist, P. (2006a). On the relation between secular and divine relationships: An emerging attachment perspective and a critique of the depth approaches. *International Journal for the Psychology of Religion, 16,* 1–18.

Granqvist, P. (2006b). Religion as a by-product of evolved psychology: The case of attachment, and implications for brain and religion research. In P. McNamara & E. Harris (Eds.), *Where God and science meet: How brain and evolutionary studies alter our understanding of religion: Vol. 2. The neurology of religious experience* (pp. 105–150). Westport, CT: Praeger.

Granqvist, P., & Dickie, J. R. (2006). Attachment theory and spiritual development in childhood and adolescence. In P. L. Benson, E. C. Roehlkepartain, P. E. King, & L. Wagener (Eds.), *The handbook of spiritual development in childhood and adolescence* (pp. 197–210). Thousand Oaks, CA: Sage.

Granqvist, P., & Fransson, M. (2007, August). *Prospective links among unresolved/disorganized attachment, absorption, and New Age spirituality.* Paper presented at the 115th Annual Convention of the American Psychological Association, San Francisco.

Granqvist, P., Fredrikson, M., Unge, P., Hagenfeldt, A., Valind, S, Larhammar, D., et al. (2005). Sensed presence and mystical experiences are predicted by suggestibility, not by the application of weak complex transcranial magnetic fields. *Neuroscience Letters, 379,* 1–6.

Granqvist, P., & Hagekull, B. (1999). Religiousness and perceived childhood attachment: Profiling socialized correspondence and emotional compensation. *Journal for the Scientific Study of Religion, 38,* 254–273.

Granqvist, P., & Hagekull, B. (2000). Religiosity, adult attachment, and why "singles" are more religious. *International Journal for the Psychology of Religion, 10,* 111–123.

Granqvist, P., & Hagekull, B. (2001). Seeking security in the New Age: On attachment and emotional compensation. *Journal for the Scientific Study of Religion, 40,* 529–547.

Granqvist, P., & Hagekull, B. (2003). Longitudinal predictions of religious change in adolescence: Contributions from the interaction of attachment and relationship status. *Journal of Social and Personal Relationships, 20,* 793–817.

Granqvist, P., Ivarsson, T., Broberg, A. G., & Hagekull, B. (2007). Examining relations between attachment, religiosity, and New Age spirituality using the Adult Attachment Interview. *Developmental Psychology, 43*, 590–601.

Granqvist, P., & Kirkpatrick, L. A. (2004). Religious conversion and perceived childhood attachment: A meta-analysis. *International Journal for the Psychology of Religion, 14*, 223–250.

Granqvist, P., Ljungdahl, C., & Dickie, J. R. (2007). God is nowhere, God is now here: Attachment activation, security of attachment, and perceived closeness to God among 5–7 year-old children from religious and non-religious homes. *Attachment and Human Development, 9*, 55–71.

Granqvist, P., & Main, M. (2003). *The Attachment to God Interview*. Unpublished manuscript, Uppsala University, Uppsala, Sweden.

Greeley, A. (1981). *The religious imagination*. New York: Sadlier.

Greeley, A. (1990). *The Catholic myth: The behavior and beliefs of American Catholics*. New York: Scribner.

Haun, D. L. (1977). Perception of the bereaved, clergy, and funeral directors concerning bereavement. *Dissertation Abstracts International, 37*, 6791A.

Hazan, C., & Shaver, P. (1987). Romantic love conceptualized as an attachment process. *Journal of Personality and Social Psychology, 52*, 511–524.

Hazan, C., & Shaver, P. (1994). Attachment as an organizational framework for research on close relationships. *Psychological Inquiry, 5*, 1–22.

Heelas, P. (1996). *The New Age movement: The celebration of the self and the sacralization of modernity*. Oxford, UK: Blackwell.

Heiler, F. (1932). *Prayer*. New York: Oxford University Press.

Heller, D. (1986). *The children's God*. Chicago: University of Chicago Press.

Hesse, E., & Main, M. (2006). Frightened, threatening, and dissociative (FR) parental behavior as related to infant D attachment in low-risk samples: Description, discussion, and interpretations. *Development and Psychopathology, 18*, 309–343.

Hesse, E., & van IJzendoorn, M. H. (1999). Propensities towards absorption are related to lapses in the monitoring of reasoning or discourse during the Adult Attachment Interview: A preliminary investigation. *Attachment and Human Development, 1*, 67–91.

Hinde, R. A. (1999). *Why gods persist: A scientific approach to religion*. London: Routledge.

Hood, R. W., Jr., Spilka, B., Hunsberger, B., & Gorsuch, R. (1996). *The psychology of religion: An empirical approach* (2nd ed.). New York: Guilford Press.

Houtman, D., & Aupers, S. (in press). The spiritual revolution and the New Age gender puzzle. In G. Vincett, S. Sharma, & K. Aune (Eds.), *Women and religion in the West: Challenging secularization*. Aldershot, UK: Ashgate.

Hughes, P. J. (1989). *The Australian clergy: Report from the combined churches' survey for faith and mission*. Melbourne, Australia: Acorn Press.

Irwin, H. J. (1993). Belief in the paranormal: A review of the empirical literature. *Journal of the American Society for Psychical Research, 87*, 1–39.

James, W. (1902). *The varieties of religious experience*. New York: Longmans, Green.

Johnson, P. E. (1945). *Psychology of religion*. New York: Abingdon-Cokesbury.

Juslin, P., Olsson, H., & Olsson, A.-C. (2003). Exemplar effects in categorization and multiple-cue judgment. *Journal of Experimental Psychology: General, 132*, 133–156.

Kaplan, N. (1987). *Individual differences in 6-years olds' thoughts about separation: Predicted from attachment to mother at age 1*. Unpublished doctoral dissertation, University of California at Berkeley.

Kaufman, G. D. (1981). *The theological imagination: Constructing the concept of God*. Philadelphia: Westminster.

Kirkpatrick, L. A. (1994). The role of attachment in religious belief and behavior. In K. Bartholomew & D. Perlman (Eds.), *Advances in personal relationships: Vol. 5. Attachment processes in adulthood* (pp. 239–265). London: Jessica Kingsley.

Kirkpatrick, L. A. (1997). A longitudinal study of changes in religious belief and behavior as a function of individual differences in adult attachment style. *Journal for the Scientific Study of Religion, 36*, 207–217.

Kirkpatrick, L. A. (1998). God as a substitute attachment figure: A longitudinal study of adult attachment style and religious change in college students. *Personality and Social Psychology Bulletin, 24*, 961–973.

Kirkpatrick, L. A. (2005). *Attachment, evolution, and the psychology of religion*. New York: Guilford Press.

Kirkpatrick, L. A., & Shaver, P. R. (1990). Attachment theory and religion: Childhood attachments, religious beliefs, and conversion. *Journal for the Scientific Study of Religion, 29*, 315–334.

Kirkpatrick, L. A., & Shaver, P. R. (1992). An attachment theoretical approach to romantic love and religious belief. *Personality and Social Psychology Bulletin, 18*, 266–275.

Kirkpatrick, L. A., Shillito, D. J., & Kellas, S. L. (1999). Loneliness, social support, and perceived relationships with God. *Journal of Social and Personal Relationships, 16*, 13–22.

Kochanska, G., Aksan, N., Knaack, A., & Rhines, H. M. (2004). Maternal parenting and children's conscience: Early security as moderator. *Child Development, 75*, 1229–1242.

Koenig, H. G., George, L. K., & Siegler, I. C. (1988). The use of religion and other emotion-regulating coping strategies among older adults. *Gerontologist, 28*, 303–310.

Lambert, W. W., Triandis, L. M., & Wolf, M. (1959). Some correlates of beliefs in the malevolence and benevolence of supernatural beings: A cross-societal study. *Journal of Abnormal and Social Psychology, 58*, 162–169.

Loveland, G. G. (1968). The effects of bereavement on certain religious attitudes. *Sociological Symposium, 1*, 17–27.

Main, M. (1991). Metacognitive knowledge, metacognitive monitoring, and singular (coherent) vs. multiple (incoherent) models of attachment: Findings and directions for future research. In C. M. Parkes, J. Stevenson-Hinde, & P. Marris (Eds.), *Attachment across the life cycle* (pp. 127–159). London: Tavistock/Routledge.

Main, M., & Goldwyn, R. (1984). *Adult attachment scoring and classification system*. Unpublished manuscript, University of California at Berkeley.

Main, M., Goldwyn, R., & Hesse, E. (2003). *Adult attachment scoring and classification system*. Unpublished manuscript, University of California at Berkeley.

Main, M., Kaplan, N., & Cassidy, J. (1985). Security in infancy, childhood, and adulthood: A move to the level of representation. In I. Bretherton & E. Waters (Eds.), Growing points of attachment theory and research, *Monographs of the Society for Research in Child Development, 50*(1–2, Serial No. 209), 66–104.

Main, M., & Morgan, H. (1996). Disorganization and disorientation in infant Strange Situation behavior: Phenotypic resemblance to dissociative states. In L. Michelson & W. Ray (Eds.), *Handbook of dissociation: Theoretical, empirical, and clinical perspectives* (pp. 107–138). New York: Plenum Press.

Maton, K. (1989). The stress-buffering role of spiritual support: Cross-sectional and prospective investigations. *Journal for the Scientific Study of Religion, 28*, 310–323.

Mattlin, J. A., Wethington, E., & Kessler, R. C. (1990). Situational determinants of coping and coping effectiveness. *Journal of Health and Social Behavior, 31*, 103–122.

McClain, E. W. (1978). Personality differences between intrinsically religious and nonreligious students: A factor analytic study. *Journal of Personality Assessment, 42*, 159–166.

McCrae, R. R. (1984). Situational determinants of coping responses: Loss, threat, and challenge. *Journal of Personality and Social Psychology, 46*, 919–928.

Mikulincer, M., & Goodman, G. S. (Eds.). (2006). *Dynamics of romantic love: Attachment, caregiving, and sex*. New York: Guilford Press.

Mikulincer, M. Gurwitz, V., & Shaver, P. R. (2007, August). *Attachment security and the use of God as a safe haven: New experimental findings*. Paper presented at the 115th Annual Convention of the American Psychological Association, San Francisco.

Mikulincer, M., & Shaver, P. R. (2001). Attachment theory and intergroup bias: Evidence that priming the secure base schema attenuates negative reactions to out-groups. *Journal of Personality and Social Psychology, 81*, 97–115.

Mikulincer, M., & Shaver, P. R. (2004). Security-based self-representations in adulthood: Contents and processes. In W. S. Rholes & J. A. Simpson (Eds.), *Adult attachment: Theory, research, and clinical implications* (pp. 159–195). New York: Guilford Press.

Mikulincer, M., Shaver, P. R., Gillath, O., & Nitzberg, R. A. (2005). Attachment, caregiving, and altruism: Boosting attachment security increases compassion and helping. *Journal of Personality and Social Psychology, 89*, 817–839.

Myers, D. G. (1992). *The pursuit of happiness*. New York: Morrow.

Nelson, M. O. (1971). The concept of God and feelings toward parents. *Journal of Individual Psychology, 27*, 46–49.

Nelson, M. O., & Jones, E. M. (1957). An application of the Q-technique to the study of religious concepts. *Psychological Reports, 3*, 293–297.

O'Brien, M. E. (1982). Religious faith and adjustment to long-term hemodialysis. *Journal of Religion and Health, 21*, 68–80.

Overall, N., Fletcher, G. J. O., & Friesen, M. (2003). Mapping the intimate relationship mind: Comparisons between three models of attachment representations. *Personality and Social Psychology Bulletin, 29*, 1479–1493.

Paloutzian, R. F., & Kirkpatrick, L. A. (Eds.). (1995). Religious influences on personal and societal well-being [Special issue]. *Journal of Social Issues, 51*(2).

Pargament, K. (1997). *The psychology of religion and coping*. New York: Guilford Press.

Parkes, C. M. (1972). *Bereavement: Studies of grief in adult life*. New York: International Universities Press.

Piaget, J. (1954). *The construction of reality in the child*. New York: Basic Books.

Pinker, S. (2002). *The blank slate: The modern denial of human nature*. New York: Viking Penguin.

Pollner, M. (1989). Divine relations, social relations, and well-being. *Journal of Health and Social Behavior, 30*, 92–104.

Poloma, M. M., & Gallup, G. H., Jr. (1991). *Varieties of prayer: A survey report*. Philadelphia: Trinity Press International.

Popper, K. (1959). *The logic of scientific discovery*. London: Routledge & Kegan Paul.

Pratt, J. B. (1920). *The religious consciousness*. New York: Macmillan.

Reed, B. (1978). *The dynamics of religion: Process and movement in Christian churches*. London: Darton, Longman & Todd.

Richters, J. E., & Waters, E. (1991). Attachment and socialization: The positive side of social influence. In M. Lewis & S. Feinman (Eds.), *Genesis of behavior: Vol. 6. Social influences and socialization in infancy* (pp. 185–213). New York: Plenum Press.

Rizzuto, A. M. (1979). *The birth of the living God: A psychoanalytical study*. Chicago: University of Chicago Press.

Rohner, R. P. (1986). *The warmth dimension: Foundations of parental acceptance–rejection theory*. Newbury Park, CA: Sage.

Roisman, G., Sroufe, L. A., Madsen, S., & Collins, W. A. (2001). The coherence of dyadic behavior across parent–child and romantic relationships as mediated by the internalized representation of experience. *Attachment and Human Development, 3*, 156–172.

Ross, M. G. (1950). *Religious beliefs of youth*. New York: Association Press.

Rowatt, W. C., & Kirkpatrick, L. A. (2002). Two dimensions of attachment to God and their relation to affect, religiosity, and personality constructs. *Journal for the Scientific Study of Religion, 41,* 637–651.

Saroglou, V., Kempeneers, A., & Seynhaeve, I. (2003). Need for closure and adult attachment dimensions as predictors of religion and reading interests. In P. Roelofsma, J. Corveleyn, & J. van Saane (Eds.), *One hundred years of psychology and religion* (pp. 139–154). Amsterdam: VU University Press.

Schwab, R., & Petersen, K. U. (1990). Religiousness: Its relation to loneliness, neuroticism, and subjective well-being. *Journal for the Scientific Study of Religion, 29,* 335–345.

Shaver, P. R., & Clark, C. L. (1996). Forms of adult romantic attachment and their cognitive and emotional underpinnings. In G. G. Noam & K. W. Fischer (Eds.), *Development and vulnerability in close relationships* (pp. 29–60). Mahwah, NJ: Erlbaum.

Sim, T. N., & Loh, B. S. M. (2003). Attachment to God: Measurement and dynamics. *Journal of Social and Personal Relationships, 20,* 373–389.

Smith, T. B., McCullough, M. E., & Poll, J. (2003). Religiousness and depression: Evidence for a main-effect and the moderating influence of stressful life-events. *Psychological Bulletin, 129,* 614–636.

Spilka, B., Addison, J., & Rosensohn, M. (1975). Parents, self, and God: A test of competing individual-religion relationships. *Review of Religious Research, 16,* 154–165.

Spilka, B., Armatas, P., & Nussbaum, J. (1964). The concept of God: A factor-analytic approach. *Review of Religious Research, 6,* 28–36.

Spilka, B., Hood, R. W., Jr., Hunsberger, B., & Gorsuch, R. (2003). *The psychology of religion: An empirical approach* (3rd ed.). New York: Guilford Press.

Sroufe, L. A., & Waters, E. (1977). Attachment as an organizational construct. *Child Development, 48,* 1184–1199.

Starbuck, E. D. (1899). *The psychology of religion.* New York: Scribner.

Stark, R., Hamberg, E. M., & Miller, A. (2005). Exploring spirituality and unchurched religions in America, Sweden, and Japan. *Journal of Contemporary Religion, 20,* 3–23.

Stouffer, S. A. (1949). *The American soldier: Vol. 2. Combat and its aftermath.* Princeton, NJ: Princeton University Press.

St. John of the Cross. (1990). *Dark night of the soul.* New York: Doubleday.

Strickland, F. L. (1924). *Psychology of religious experience.* New York: Abingdon.

Strunk, O. (1959). Perceived relationships between parental and deity concepts. *Psychological Newsletter, 10,* 222–226.

Tamayo, A., & Desjardins, L. (1976). Belief systems and conceptual images of parents and God. *Journal of Psychology, 92,* 131–140.

Tamminen, K. (1994). Religious experiences in childhood and adolescence: A viewpoint of religious development between the ages of 7 and 20. *International Journal for the Psychology of Religion, 4,* 61–85.

TenElshof, J. K., & Furrow, J. L. (2000). The role of secure attachment in predicting spiritual maturity of students at a conservative seminary. *Journal of Psychology and Theology, 28,* 99–108.

Thouless, R. H. (1923). An introduction to the psychology of religion. New York: Macmillan.

Trier, K. K., & Shupe, A. (1991). Prayer, religiosity, and healing in the heartland, USA: A research note. *Review of Religious Research, 32,* 351–358.

Ullman, C. (1982). Change of mind, change of heart: Some cognitive and emotional antecedents of religious conversion. *Journal of Personality and Social Psychology, 42,* 183–192.

Ullman, C. (1989). *The transformed self: The psychology of religious conversion.* New York: Plenum Press.

Vergote, A., & Tamayo, A. (Eds.). (1981). *The parental figures and the representation of God.* The Hague: Mouton.

Weiss, R. S. (1973). *Loneliness: The experience of emotional and social isolation.* Cambridge, MA: MIT Press.

Weiss, R. S. (1982). Attachment in adult life. In C. M. Parkes & J. Stevenson-Hinde (Eds.), *The place of attachment in human behavior* (pp. 171–184). New York: Basic Books.

Wellman, H. M. (1985). The child's theory of mind: The development of conceptions of cognition. In S. R. Yussen (Ed.), *The growth of reflection* (pp. 169–206). Orlando, FL: Academic Press.

Wenegrat, B. (1989). *The divine archetype: The sociobiology and psychology of religion.* Lexington, MA: Lexington Books.

Wheeler, S. C., & Petty, R. E. (2001). The effects of stereotype activation on behavior: A review of possible mechanisms. *Psychological Bulletin, 127,* 797–826.

Wittgenstein, L. (1953). *Philosophical investigations.* Oxford, UK: Blackwell.

Wulff, D. M. (1991). *Psychology of religion: Classic and contemporary views.* New York: Wiley.

Young, K. (1926). The psychology of hymns. *Journal of Abnormal and Social Psychology, 20,* 391–406.

Zeifman, D., & Hazan, C. (1997). A process model of adult attachment formation. In S. Duck (Ed.), *Handbook of personal relationships* (pp. 179–195). Chichester, UK: Wiley.

CHAPTER 39

An Attachment-Theoretical Perspective on Divorce

BROOKE C. FEENEY
JOAN K. MONIN

There are few blows to the human spirit so great as the loss of someone near and dear.
—Bowlby (1979, p. 67)

Divorce is among the most significant of all life events because it involves the disruption of one of the strongest affectional bonds formed by adults. The significance of this disrupted bond is often compounded by its far-reaching implications— not only for the divorcing spouses, but also for their children, the extended family, and future relationships formed by the couple members and their children. In this chapter, we consider the processes and effects of divorce from an attachment-theoretical perspective, beginning with a discussion of attachment theory's relevance to the study of divorce and its aftermath. We then consider the effects of divorce on the couple members' postdivorce adjustment, which includes the effects on the individuals' physical and psychological health and on their relationship, which often continues well past the divorce. Later sections of the chapter deal with the effects of divorce on children. Throughout the chapter, we review relevant research and consider ways in which individual differences in attachment orientation affect the process and sequelae of divorce. We conclude by discussing important next steps for research.

THE RELEVANCE OF ATTACHMENT THEORY TO THE STUDY OF DIVORCE

Attachment theory provides an important perspective on divorce because divorce involves the disruption and often the termination of a powerful attachment bond. Although attachment theorists have not specifically focused on divorce, the theory has a great deal to say about separation from an attachment figure and the breaking of an attachment bond (Bowlby, 1973, 1979, 1980), both of which are core aspects of divorce.

In considering the relevance of attachment theory to divorce, it is important to emphasize that one of the most common attachment bonds formed in adulthood is the one formed with a romantic or marriage partner. According to the theory, neither love nor grief nor other forms of strong emotion are felt for just any person; instead, they are felt for particular individuals with whom one has established an attachment bond (Bowlby, 1969/1982, 1979). "Attachment bonds" are strong and persistent ties that cause each member of a dyad to maintain proximity to the other and to engage in

934

proximity-seeking behavior when greater protection or support is needed (see Cassidy, Chapter 1, this volume). The biological function of attachment bonds is protection, and the capacity to make and maintain bonds appropriate to each phase of life is as important for survival and reproductive fitness as are nutrition and reproduction (Bowlby, 1969/1982; see Simpson & Belsky, Chapter 6, this volume). Once formed, an attachment bond tends to endure, and its disruption is strongly resisted. Therefore, to the extent that dissolving a marriage requires the dissolution or reorganization of an attachment bond, divorce is a tremendously important life transition.

AN ATTACHMENT-THEORETICAL PERSPECTIVE ON WHY PEOPLE DIVORCE

Although attachment theory does not specifically delineate the factors that contribute to divorce, it provides an important foundation for understanding the mechanisms underlying this prevalent form of social disruption in adulthood. The theory stipulates two important criteria for healthy human functioning: First, every individual (throughout the lifespan) requires the presence and availability of a trustworthy figure who is willing and able to provide a safe haven (where the person can retreat for comfort and support in times of need) and a secure base (from which to engage in exploration of the world and the person's own capacities). Second, everyone must be able both to recognize when another person is a trustworthy attachment figure and to collaborate with him or her to maintain a mutually rewarding relationship (Bowlby, 1979). From an attachment perspective, the absence of one or both of these important features of a marriage—for one or both partners—sets the stage for dysfunctional relations and eventual separation and divorce. Theory regarding these potential reasons for divorce, and empirical evidence supporting them, are discussed below.

What Happens when a Spouse Fails to Function as a Trustworthy Attachment Figure?

Human beings of all ages are happiest and able to deploy their talents to best advantage when they are confident that, standing behind them, there are one or more trusted persons who will come to their aid should difficulties arise.
—Bowlby (1979, p. 103)

This proposition from attachment theory is obviously relevant to the stability and dissolution of marriages, because "trusted persons" in adulthood often include a person's spouse. As noted above, attachment theory specifies the characteristics of a trustworthy figure—one who enhances a person's safety and security by providing (1) a safe haven to which he or she can retreat in times of need, and (2) a secure base from which to explore (i.e., to learn, discover, work, play, engage in challenging activities, develop relationships with peers, and grow as an individual). According to the theory, an attachment figure who fosters security recognizes and respects the partner's needs and desire for a safe haven and secure base, and acts accordingly. Such an attachment figure understands, accepts, and respects both attachment behavior (proximity seeking in times of need) and exploratory behavior, and recognizes that one of the most common causes of negative emotion is frustration of the desires for love and care. Emotions such as anxiety and anger often stem from uncertainty about whether an attachment figure will be available and responsive to one's needs for support and exploration (Bowlby, 1979).

Of course, spousal provision of a safe haven and a secure base can vary considerably, and the ability to fulfill the role of reliable caregiver to a romantic or marital partner is often influenced by a person's attachment history. As Bowlby (1979) said, "Each of us is apt to do unto others as we have been done by" (p. 141). Attachment theory and research suggest that when spouses provide favorable conditions for each other (as just described), each is likely to feel secure and self-reliant, trusting, cooperative, and helpful in dealing with the other, as well as with their children. In contrast, spouses who do not provide favorable conditions for each other are likely to be insecure in their relationship and plagued by feelings of anxiety, hurt, anger, mistrust, resistance to cooperation, and frustrated personal growth (Bowlby, 1979, 1988).

To extrapolate from attachment theory, a spouse may encourage a partner's attachment anxiety or avoidance (compulsive or defensive self-reliance) by (1) being unresponsive to signals of need for care, (2) behaving in a rejecting and disparaging manner, (3) threatening to leave the partner or the family as a means of controlling the partner, and (4) not being consistently available to the partner (Bowlby, 1969/1982, 1979, 1988). Such experiences may cause the partner to live in constant anxiety regarding potential loss of the spouse, to have a low threshold for activation of attachment behavior, and to be overly solicitous or dependent (see also Feeney, 2007). Alternatively, the partner may react to inadequate spousal care by inhibiting attachment feelings and behavior, being deeply distrustful of the spouse, and insisting on extreme self-reliance.

According to attachment theory, all kinds of poor care are likely simultaneously to arouse anger toward one's attachment figure and to inhibit its expression (Bowlby, 1969/1982, 1979, 1988). The result is often underlying resentment that contributes to dysfunctional relations, because everyone— even a person who has learned to be what Bowlby (1969/1982) called "compulsively self-reliant"— needs love, care, and support. Moreover, when a person's attachment needs go unmet, he or she is more vulnerable to stress and less capable of dealing with it. In fact, unmet attachment needs may be expressed in aberrant forms of care-eliciting behavior (e.g., eating disorders, substance use, sexual infidelity), which are likely to take a great toll on marriage and family relations (Bowlby, 1979).

What Causes the Inability to Recognize a Trustworthy Attachment Figure and Collaborate in a Mutually Rewarding Relationship?

There is a strong causal relationship between an individual's experiences with his parents and his later capacity to make affectional bonds.
—BOWLBY (1979, p. 135)

According to attachment theory, a healthy person is able to trust and rely on others and to know who can be relied upon (Bowlby, 1969/1982, 1979, 1988). A healthy adult is also capable of exchanging roles when the situation calls for it— sometimes providing a secure base and safe haven from which a partner can operate, and at other times being able to rely on the partner to provide a secure base and safe haven in return. Each partner in a good relationship must have the capacity to adopt either role as circumstances require. Each must be able to express a desire for help or support in a direct and effective way, and each in turn must be able to give to the other and to their children (Bowlby, 1979, 1988).

The theory also stipulates that impairment of the ability to collaborate in a mutually rewarding relationship can take many forms and be present to varying degrees. For example, a person who has difficulty trusting his or her spouse may either be unable to express a desire for support when needed or do so in a demanding, aggressive way. Both kinds of behavior reflect lack of confidence that support will be forthcoming, dissatisfaction with what is given when provided, and inability to give

spontaneously to others. Marriage partners with these kinds of impairments are likely to exhibit anxious clinging and make excessive demands, or to be aloof, emotionally unavailable, and defiantly independent (Bowlby, 1979, 1988). According to attachment theory, these impairments stem from inadequate care from previous attachment figures (most often one's parents).

A major claim of the theory is that mental and behavioral patterns learned in prior attachment relationships tend to persist because people inevitably construct representational models of themselves and their attachment figures during childhood and adolescence, and new partners in attachment relationships get assimilated to these models, often despite extensive evidence that the model is no longer appropriate. These biased perceptions and expectations result in misconceptions of others, false expectations about the way people behave, and inappropriate actions intended to forestall expected negative experiences. For example, Bowlby (1979) said that

> a man who during childhood was frequently threatened with abandonment can easily attribute such intentions to his wife. He will then misinterpret things she says or does in terms of such intent, and then take whatever action he thinks would best meet the situation he believes to exist. Misunderstanding and conflict must follow. In all this he is as unaware he is being biased by his past experience as he is that his present beliefs and expectations are mistaken. (p. 142)

Bowlby (1979) further stated that inappropriate but persistent representational models often coexist with more appropriate ones: "A husband may oscillate between believing his wife to be loyal to him and suspecting her of plans to desert" (p. 142). Bowlby contended that the stronger the emotions aroused in a relationship, the more likely are the earlier and less conscious models to become dominant and guide perception and behavior. Thus, in order to collaborate in a mutually rewarding relationship with a marriage partner, an adult must consider how his or her prior experiences may influence needs, worries, expectations, and relational behavior. A major premise of attachment theory is that representational models and patterns of behavior based on them can be so entrenched that they continue unchecked, even when they are dysfunctional (see Bretherton & Munholland, Chapter 5, this volume).

For example, people who have learned a pattern of fault finding, punishment, revenge, guilt induction, or evasion tend to carry those patterns into their marriages, where they are likely to contribute to a destructive downward spiral that is difficult to break. Breaking such a negative interaction cycle may require (1) attempting to understand a partner's viewpoint and negotiate openly with him or her; (2) developing a capacity for empathy and for tolerating intense emotions; (3) discovering the specific situations (current or past) that may underlie the negative interaction patterns, and recognizing that negative interaction patterns are either responses to those situations or side effects of trying not to respond to them; (4) identifying the representational models of self and attachment figures that govern one's perceptions, predictions, and actions, often without conscious awareness or clarity; and (5) reevaluating relationships, modifying representational models in light of more recent experiences, and making deliberate changes in ways of treating others (Bowlby, 1979). Such changes are typically slow and patchy, and they require a great deal of motivation and effort (Bowlby, 1979; see Johnson, Chapter 34, this volume). Insecurity especially leaves people handicapped in all of these areas. This may explain why many marriages end despite couples having sought marital counseling.

An Attachment Theoretical Integration of Empirical Work Relevant to the Prediction of Divorce

Empirical work specifically linking attachment history and attachment orientation to the prediction of divorce is lacking. However, attachment theory offers a useful framework for explaining and integrating the processes that have been shown to predict marital dissolution. Personal characteristics and marital interaction patterns that predict divorce are all indicative of either (1) having a spouse who is not a trustworthy attachment figure, or (2) being unable to recognize, benefit from, and maintain a mutually rewarding relationship with a trustworthy figure.

As explained earlier, attachment theory stipulates that every individual builds experience-based "representational" or "working" models of self and others, which affect how he or she perceives events, forecasts the future, constructs plans, and selects strategies for interacting with others (Bowlby, 1969/1982, 1973, 1980; Bretherton, 1990; Bretherton & Munholland, Chapter 5, this volume; Collins, Guichard, Ford, & Feeney, 2004; Main, Kaplan, & Cassidy, 1985). These

working models are thought to underlie individual differences in attachment orientation or style. Such differences have proven strongly predictive of relationship dynamics, including conflict behaviors (e.g., Pietromonaco, Greenwood, & Barrett, 2004), social support and caregiving behaviors (e.g., B. C. Feeney & Collins, 2001; Kunce & Shaver, 1994; Simpson, Rholes, & Nelligan, 1992), biased information processing (e.g., Collins & Feeney, 2004; B. C. Feeney & Cassidy, 2003), coping strategies (e.g., Mikulincer & Florian, 1998; Ognibene & Collins, 1998), physiological responses to stress (e.g., B. C. Feeney & Kirkpatrick, 1996; Roisman, 2007), emotion regulation/ expression (e.g., Mikulincer & Shaver, 2005 and Chapter 23, this volume; Shaver & Mikulincer, 2007; Simpson, Collins, Tran, & Haydon, 2007), trust (e.g., Hazan & Shaver, 1987; Mikulincer, 1998), defensiveness (e.g., Fraley, Garner, & Shaver, 2000; Mikulincer & Orbach, 1995), and forgiveness (e.g., Mikulincer, Shaver, & Slav, 2006). Although surprisingly little of this research has examined the influence of attachment insecurity on interpersonal dynamics specifically within the context of marriage (for an exception, see J. A. Feeney's work and her Chapter 21 in this volume), some marital research does show that attachment insecurity (viewing oneself as unable to rely on others, and viewing others as unreliable or psychologically unavailable) is associated with relationship dissatisfaction, poor communication, poor emotion regulation, poor problem solving, and poor support behavior in marriage (Davila, Karney, & Bradbury, 1999; J. A. Feeney, Noller, & Callan, 1994; Kobak & Hazan, 1991).

In a happy, well-functioning relationship, the attachment system works so that both partners feel secure and protected, each is able to depend on the other, and each is unafraid of the other's dependence or both partners' interdependence (Fisher & Crandell, 1997). In securely attached couples this reciprocity is achieved, but in insecure couples there is rigidity (Reibstein, 1998). In an insecure relationship, protecting oneself is the primary objective, and it often overrides one's ability to respond empathically to one's partner (Reibstein, 1998). Insecure relationships include ones in which (1) both partners defensively avoid dependency, each fleeing or withdrawing in times of distress; (2) one partner feels deprived of responsive support, while the other feels overwhelmed by what seem to be the other's insatiable needs; and (3) one partner always occupies the dependent role, while the other is defensively accusatory and dismissive

(Fisher & Crandell, 1997). In all such cases, the attachment relationship, which ideally is supportive and rewarding, has become painful, conflictual, and unsatisfying. The defensive processes that ensue—the very ones delineated so well and extensively by Gottman and colleagues (e.g., Gottman, 1993, 1994; Gottman & Levenson, 1992, 2000)—are likely to result in marital dissolution.

Reibstein (1998), in particular, has noted that the behaviors stemming from insecure attachment are often defensive in nature. For example, in response to a partner's unavailability and inaccessibility (particularly in times of need), a spouse may shut the partner out, belittle him or her, or become dismissive. The partner may then defend him- or herself by becoming angry or withdrawing interest—responses that thwart the fulfillment of both couple members' attachment needs. One or both partners' feelings of attachment may lessen or cease to exist. This seems most likely to occur in individuals who were avoidant to begin with; consistent with this idea, some research has shown that avoidant attachment is a risk factor for multiple marriages (Ceglian & Gardner, 1999).

Attachment theory provides additional insight into the mechanisms underlying stability or instability of marriages. In a 4-year longitudinal study of newlyweds, Davila and Bradbury (2001) found that, compared with spouses in happy marriages and divorced spouses, spouses in stable but unhappy marriages showed the highest levels of attachment insecurity both initially and over time. It seems that insecurity causes spouses to be unhappy in and dissatisfied with their marriages, yet simultaneously keeps them tied to their marriages. Although dissatisfaction is a proximal predictor of divorce (Karney & Bradbury, 1995), many couples do remain together despite dissatisfaction. Because anxious-preoccupied individuals are chronically concerned about abandonment and their love-worthiness, they may attempt to maintain their relationships at almost any cost (Kirkpatrick & Davis, 1994), whereas avoidant individuals may view divorce as a suitable way to avoid intimacy.

EFFECTS OF DIVORCE ON COUPLE MEMBERS

Attachment theory conceptualizes the propensity of human beings to form strong emotional bonds with particular others, and it explains the many forms of emotional distress and personality disturbance (including anxiety, anger, depression, and emotional detachment) to which unwilling separation and loss can give rise (Bowlby, 1973, 1979).

Because attachment is an instinctive or evolved process that is elicited particularly during times of threat and stress (illness, injury, trauma, fear), the threat associated with losing an attachment figure is likely to intensify feelings of distress and to have adverse effects on a person's adjustment, health, and well-being—particularly if the decision to divorce is not mutual, and the attachment bond is therefore not broken for both couple members. These issues are explored in this section.

Psychological and Physical Health

Studies of divorce have focused primarily on adjustment to divorce and the effects of divorce on physical and psychological well-being. Most such studies have examined the link between marital status and various indicators of individual well-being, finding consistently that separated and divorced individuals have higher rates of physical and mental health disturbance than married individuals, and often higher rates even than widowed individuals (Blumenthal, 1967; Gove, 1973; Mirowsky & Ross, 2003; Verbrugge, 1979). Specifically, separated and divorced individuals experience increased rates of minor or acute illnesses (e.g., infectious diseases, respiratory illnesses), major and chronic physical illnesses (e.g., diabetes, heart disease), physical limitations and disabilities, depression and other psychopathology, suicide, homicide, violence, substance abuse (e.g., alcoholism), accidents and injuries, and disease-caused mortality (e.g., Aseltine & Kessler, 1993; Berkman & Breslow, 1983; Berkman & Syme, 1979; Bloom, Asher, & White, 1978; Booth & Amato, 1991; Bruce, 1998; Burman & Margolin, 1992; Chatav & Whisman, 2007; Hemstrom, 1996; Hu & Goldman, 1990; Kiecolt-Glaser et al., 1987; Lorenz, Wickrama, Conger, & Elder, 2006; Overbeek et al., 2006; Stack, 1990; Verbrugge, 1979; Wade & Pevalin, 2004; Williams & Umberson, 2004). Divorced individuals also report lower levels of happiness, life satisfaction, self-esteem, self-confidence, and competence (Amato, 2000; Glenn & Weaver, 1988; Kurdek, 1991; Lucas, 2005; Spanier & Casto, 1979; Weiss, 1979).

It is important to note that although divorced individuals are worse off than married people in general, if the divorced are compared with people in the most unhappy marriages, the divorced are seen to have higher morale; fewer physical problems and depressive symptoms; and greater life satisfaction, self-esteem, and overall health (Hawkins & Booth, 2005; Overbeek et al., 2006). Thus the more unhappiness and distress experienced in a marriage (i.e., the lower the marital quality), the greater the relief and potential benefit that may follow divorce (Coontz, 2007; Hawkins & Booth, 2005; Overbeek et al., 2006; Spanier & Thompson, 1984). Also consistent with the idea that divorce may not be uniformly harmful, research has shown that after a period of both emotional and physical upheaval, most adults cope successfully with divorce (Amato, 2000; Aseltine & Kessler, 1993; Booth & Amato, 1991; Hetherington & Kelly, 2002; Sbarra & Emery, 2005). Indeed, some report opportunities for growth, increased independence, and increased life satisfaction (Huddleston & Hawkings, 1991; Marks, 1996; Spanier & Thompson, 1984).

Nonetheless, a great deal of research indicates that divorce is generally very taxing and distressing. Although some studies have suggested that marital dissolution affects men more strongly than women (Berkman & Syme, 1979; Gove, 1973; Hu & Goldman, 1990; Kotler & Wingard, 1989), and some have suggested the reverse (Aseltine & Kessler, 1993; Gottman & Levenson, 1992; Kiecolt-Glaser et al., 1987, 1988), the effects of separation and divorce on psychological and physical health have been extensively documented for both sexes. It appears, however, that the processes responsible for the link between divorce and particular health outcomes may be somewhat different for women and men. For example, the health effects of marital loss have been attributed to the economic hardships and material conditions suffered by women when marriages dissolve (Lillard & Waite, 1995), and to the loss of social networks and social controls that encourage healthy living for men (Gove & Shin, 1989; Umberson, 1987; see Dupre & Meadows, 2007, for a review). Also, Gottman (1994) found that the health of women is directly affected by marital distress, whereas for men it is mediated through loneliness.

It is important to note, however, that most of the studies in this area provide little information about why or how marital status is related to health or well-being (Mirowsky & Ross, 2003). Most researchers explain their results in terms of the protective effects of marriage, which include a healthier lifestyle, higher socioeconomic status, more financial resources, and a stable social network. Other explanations include (1) a model of social selectivity or preexisting pathology, according to which people who divorce are less physically or psychologically fit for marriage; and (2) a crisis model, according to which divorce is a traumatic event that induces psychological distress and health problems, which lessen as a person

adjusts to a changed social situation (Bloom et al., 1978; Kitson, 1982; Lucas, 2005). The crisis model identifies the divorce-related stressors likely to affect health and well-being, such as the emotional strain of marital breakdown, continuing conflict with the ex-spouse, fewer material and economic resources, more risky behaviors (e.g., drinking, driving recklessly), less stringent health monitoring, loss of supportive social networks, loss of social status, social isolation, daily hardships associated with single parenthood, time constraints, role strain, and the need to rebuild one's life.

Attachment theory provides an integrative account of both perspectives by postulating that although separation anxiety and distress are normative responses to loss, some people are predisposed by previous experiences to react more strongly to losses (Kitson, 1982; Simos, 1979; Weiss, 1975). One attachment-theoretical explanation for links between divorce and poor health outcomes emphasizes continuing attachment to one's spouse, as discussed next.

Continuing Attachment

Although there are many problems and stressors with which divorced individuals must cope (e.g., economic problems, legal issues, property settlements, community and social network changes, concerns regarding children and coparenting, formation of new relationships; see Bohannon, 1970; Spanier & Casto, 1979), the loss of the marital relationship itself, combined with continuing contact and involvement with the ex-spouse, has sometimes been viewed as the most stressful part of the divorce experience (Bohannon, 1970; Hetherington, Cox, & Cox, 1982; Weiss, 1975, 1976). Separation from a spouse elicits conflicting and confusing emotions in both spouses—regardless of what led to the divorce (Weiss, 1976). These emotions include anger, contempt, regret, resentment, longing, affection, wish for reconciliation, guilt, anxiety, panic, sadness, and loneliness. This mixture of positive and negative emotions can be very confusing and is attributed to the persistence of the attachment bond when intimate relationships are disrupted (Berman, 1988a, 1988b; Weiss, 1975).

Studies have shown that many men and women going through divorce continue to have feelings of attachment to their ex-spouses (e.g., Berman, 1988b; Brown, Felton, Whiteman, & Manela, 1980; Goode, 1956; Kitson, 1982; Spanier & Casto, 1979; Weiss, 1975). "Attachment" was operationalized in these studies as preoccupation with an ex-spouse (e.g., spending a lot of time thinking about the spouse, feeling that one will never get over the divorce) or as continuing positive feelings for the ex-spouse. Although feelings of attachment are greatest when the divorce is recent and when the spouse was the one who initiated the divorce, attachment does not seem to be influenced by the length of marriage. This suggests that attachment bonds may be established fairly quickly but are broken slowly (Brown et al., 1980; Brown & Reimer, 1984; Kitson, 1982), and that the loss of an attachment bond is as difficult for those married a few years as for those married many years (Weiss, 1975). Once partners have significantly bonded, attachment often persists and resists dissolution—even in the face of anger, hurt, and knowledge that the relationship should be terminated (Aydintug, 1995; Davis, Shaver, & Vernon, 2003; Mazor, Batiste-Harel, & Gampel, 1998; Weiss, 1975).

These continued feelings of attachment for an ex-spouse have been considered (in both the clinical and empirical literature) to be a primary cause of the emotional and adjustment problems that follow separation (Berman, 1988a, 1988b; Brown et al., 1980; Kitson, 1982; Weiss, 1976). Although not consistently shown (Masheter, 1991; Spanier & Casto, 1979), continuing attachment to an ex-spouse has been linked with a variety of symptoms, including depression, anxiety, distress, loneliness, anger, lowered of self-efficacy, lack of social self-confidence, less autonomy, less life satisfaction, and poor self-rated adjustment (Brown & Reimer, 1984; Emery, 1994; Madden-Derdich & Arditti, 1999; Masheter, 1997).

This continuing attachment to an ex-spouse may be accounted for by the biological predisposition to use attachment figures as a safe haven and a secure base. The core idea in attachment theory is that strong and consistent support from an attachment figure, combined with encouragement and respect for one's autonomy, provides the conditions in which one can thrive. Losing an attachment figure eliminates these protective functions, and it both creates separation anxiety and activates the attachment system. First, both human and primate researchers have shown that separation from attachment figures elicits anxiety, protest, and depression (Bowlby, 1973, 1979). An undesired separation of a child from his or her parental attachment figure—or of an adult from his or her trusted companion—arouses fear and intensifies fears aroused by other conditions (Bowlby, 1973, 1979). Second, activation of the

attachment system and the proximity-seeking behavior it arouses are natural reactions to any threat (Bowlby, 1969/1982). The many challenges associated with divorce (e.g., beginning a new life, taking on new responsibilities, becoming a single parent, changing social networks) are stressors that are likely to intensify activation of the attachment system and create a desire for proximity to one's attachment figure (which may have been the spouse prior to the divorce). The process of detachment and reorganization (Bowlby, 1980) is likely to be more difficult than either spouse anticipates, because bonds of attachment are likely to be partly unconscious and sometimes masked by feelings of dissatisfaction with the spouse (Weiss, 1975, 1976). This idea is consistent with research indicating that partners are often unaware of their emotional investment in their relationship until the relationship is terminated (Berscheid, 1983). This may explain why 42% of couples headed for divorce separate and then reconcile at least once before ending the relationship (Kitson & Raschke, 1981); why some ex-spouses end up having sex and sleeping together overnight when they were intending only to transfer control of their children from one parent to the other for a few days (Davis et al., 2003); and why only a few years after their divorce, a majority of remarried men say that they regret having divorced their former wives (Reibstein & Bamber, 1997).

Because of the difficulty of detaching, Reibstein (1998) notes that a divorced individual often experiences a deep vulnerability to the former spouse, and thus may engage in defensive strategies to prevent the pain of reevoked attachment feelings. Regardless of who initiated the divorce, both couple members are likely to be vulnerable, and the process of detachment is likely to be slow and painful for both. In fact, Bowlby (1973) noted that before detachment occurs, the attachment bond may be reactivated if the attachment figure reappears and invites renewed attachment. Attachment feelings and behaviors can be easily reactivated by drawing the former spouse back into old behavior patterns—similar to the way in which attachment feelings and behaviors can be reactivated when adult children spend time with their parents (Reibstein, 1998). Consistent with these ideas, Mikulincer and Florian (1996) proposed that adaptation to loss of an attachment figure involves a dialectical interplay of two opposing forces: the desire to maintain proximity to the lost person, and the simultaneous desire to detach from the person to form new relationships.

Individual Differences in Adjustment

Because attachment theory predicts differential experiences of relationships, appraisals of threats, regulation of emotions, and coping strategies, depending on attachment styles (e.g., Mikulincer & Florian, 1998; Shaver & Mikulincer, 2007), there are likely to be systematic individual differences in adjustment to divorce. In fact, individual differences should be very evident in the context of divorce, because (1) divorce raises a core attachment issue, loss of an attachment figure; and (2) the stresses and challenges associated with divorce are likely to heighten activation of the attachment system. According to attachment theory, traumatic life events such as divorce should be particularly stressful for individuals with troubled attachment histories—that is, those with insecure attachment orientations (Bowlby, 1979). Insecure individuals are particularly likely to break down after loss or separation because the separation confirms their worst fears and expectations. The divorce is likely to reactivate earlier unresolved separations from attachment figures, and because insecure individuals lack the inner resources and coping strategies needed for adjustment to divorce, they are likely to have difficulty adjusting to the loss (Mikulincer & Florian, 1996).

When discussing bereavement in adult life, Bowlby (1979) noted that adults generally respond to separation and loss in a series of stages, including numbness, yearning and searching, disorganization and despair, and then reorganization. In addition, he identified characteristics of loss situations that interfere with healthy adjustment. These include (1) having been involved in a relationship that provided considerable self-esteem and role identity, which are less sustainable without the lost partner; (2) having no close relationship with another person, to whom the individual can transfer some of the feelings that were bound up with the lost spouse; and (3) having been in a marriage that was conflicted or ambivalent. Bowlby emphasized that in order for mourning to result in a favorable outcome, the bereaved person must be able to express his or her feelings (i.e., yearning, anger, sadness, fear of loneliness, desires for sympathy and support) and may need the support of another trusted person.

Attachment theory makes predictions regarding individual differences in adjustment to divorce. Theoretically, secure individuals (who hold representations of others as responsive and dependable, and of themselves as love-worthy and capable) possess the social and personal resources to cope with divorce. The divorce-related distress experienced by secure individuals is likely to be buffered by social and personal resources that facilitate coping (e.g., the ability to seek and elicit support from others; Vareschi & Bursik, 2005). In contrast, insecure individuals view stressors as more threatening. Those high in attachment anxiety view themselves as less capable of coping and report greater distress (Davis et al., 2003); those high in avoidant tendencies engage in distancing coping, do not turn to others for support, and report greater hostility (Mikulincer & Florian, 1998; Ognibene & Collins, 1998).

Very few studies have specifically examined divorcing adults' adjustment as a function of attachment orientation. Birnbaum, Orr, Mikulincer, and Florian (1997) examined the association between attachment style and reactions to divorce in Israel and found that dispositional attachment anxiety and avoidance were associated with greater divorce-related distress and poorer coping. Fraley and Bonanno (2004) studied a group of bereaved (not divorced) adults, and found differences between two kinds of avoidance (Bartholomew, 1990): Whereas some avoidant individuals (those who were also high in anxiety, or fearfully avoidant) had difficulty adapting to the loss of a loved one, those who were dismissingly avoidant seemed resilient in adapting to loss, perhaps because they were not as invested in their relationship before the loss. In extremely threatening situations in which it is impossible to maintain a defensively dismissive stance, both anxious and avoidant attachment are associated with symptoms (Mikulincer, Horesh, Eilati, & Kotler, 1999; Mikulincer & Shaver, 2007 and Chapter 23, this volume)—indicating that avoidant individuals are sometimes vulnerable to stress. However, because research is lacking in this area, it will be important to conduct more in-depth studies of the links between attachment security and adjustment specifically to the process of divorce.

Research not specifically focused on attachment or attachment orientations indicates that predictors of postdivorce adjustment include the presence of another intimate relationship (Berman, 1988a; Hetherington, Cox, & Cox, 1978); the presence of social and personal resources (e.g., supportive friends and family, resiliency, good mental health status) (Kitson, 1982; Price & McKenry, 1988; Spanier & Casto, 1979; Weiss, 1975); integration of the divorce experience into one's life trajectory (Hetherington & Kelly, 2002);

forgiveness (Mazor et al., 1998; Rye, Folck, Heim, Olszewski, & Traina, 2004); the ability to shift attention from the ex-spouse and marriage to a new lifestyle (Brown & Reimer, 1984; Weiss, 1975, 1976, 1979); the ability to develop a working relationship with the ex-spouse, particularly when children are involved (Berman, 1988b); and the ability to develop an identity that is separate from the former spouse and marriage (Booth & Amato, 1992; Bray & Hetherington, 1993; Madden-Derdich & Arditti, 1999). Secure individuals are most likely to possess these characteristics (e.g., Mikulincer et al., 2006; Vareschi & Bursik, 2005). In contrast, predictors of poor adjustment—which include preoccupation with the ex-spouse, lack of social and personal resources, lower initial self-esteem, social isolation, and unwanted separation (Berman, 1988a; Kitson, 1982; Spanier & Casto, 1979)—are likely to be more characteristic of insecure individuals.

POSTDIVORCE CONTACT BETWEEN EX-SPOUSES

Despite a large empirical literature on other aspects of the divorce experience, little is known about postdivorce relationships between ex-spouses. This is surprising, given that such relations are likely to have important effects on the entire family system (Cole & Cole, 1999). It was once assumed that all postdivorce relations reflect separation distress and should be avoided (e.g., Kressel, Lopez-Morillas, Weinglass, & Deutsch, 1978). Consistent with this idea, both clinical and empirical reports have shown that continued relations with a former spouse are often problematic (Aydintug, 1995; Kitson & Morgan, 1990), and that postdivorce harmony is rare, particularly when children are involved (Ambert, 1988; Buunk & Mutsaers, 1999). For example, research has shown that half of divorced women and a third of divorced men continue to be intensely angry at their former spouses, even 10 years after the breakup (Wallerstein & Blakeslee, 1989). Moreover, a study of remarried individuals found little continued friendship between former spouses (Buunk & Mutsaers, 1999). It has been claimed that few relationships offer as many opportunities for anger, blame, hatred, retaliation, desires for revenge, and violence as the ones between former spouses (Guisinger, Cowan, & Schuldeberg, 1989), particularly given that ex-spouses know each other's weaknesses and vulnerabilities. Remarriages may also contribute to poor postdivorce relations, because a close relationship with a former spouse may be threatening

to a new spouse and create conflicts in the new marriage (Buunk & Mutsaers, 1999).

Attachment theory provides a basis for explaining some of the negative ways in which former spouses behave toward each other. Bowlby (1969/1982) knew that behavior of an aggressive sort (protest, anger) often plays a role in maintaining affectional bonds. Anger can be functional when separation is perceived to be temporary, because it may hasten reunion and make it less likely that another separation will occur. This may help to explain why high levels of disagreement and conflict typically occur during the first year of marital separation (Toews, McKenry, & Catlett, 2003); why many women continue to suffer physical and verbal abuse after separation and divorce, typically from men who do not want the relationships to end (Arendell, 1995; Jasinski & Williams, 1998); and why many relationships without a history of violence often become violent at the time of separation (Ellis & DeKeseredy, 1989; Toews et al., 2003).

Although research has indicated the disadvantages of continuing attachment to one's ex-spouse, it is important to note that a majority of divorced individuals report at least occasional contact with their ex-spouses, and that continuing attachment (presumably relatively secure attachment) may be associated with healthy development as well (Masheter, 1990, 1991). For example, research on children's continued contact with both parents has acknowledged the benefits of postdivorce relationships between ex-spouses (e.g., Ahrons & Rodgers, 1987; Ahrons & Wallisch, 1986; Dozier, Sollie, Stack, & Smith, 1993). More specifically, cooperative postdivorce parenting can reduce role strain for custodial parents and the sense of estrangement and loss for noncustodial parents (Hetherington & Camara, 1984; Masheter, 1991). In fact, it has been argued that for couples with children (especially couples who share custody of the children and therefore see each other frequently), detachment can be only limited (Reibstein, 1998); therefore, some degree of attachment, if transferred effectively into constructive behavior, may be beneficial (Emery, 1988; Furstenberg & Cherlin, 1991; Madden-Derdich & Arditti, 1999; Masheter, 1991).

Reibstein (1998) has argued that, given the strength of the attachment bond, divorced spouses need protection from each other during and after divorce in the form of limited and rule-bound contact (i.e., agreed-upon rules of engagement and civility, to set limits on dysfunctional behavior that might reevoke attachment feelings). Just as children need clarity, predictability, and consistency in the divorce context, so do the divorcing adults. The challenge for ex-spouses is to redefine their relationship in a way that is mutually supportive while minimizing of behaviors that adversely affect adjustment (Madden-Derdich & Arditti, 1999). Given that the relationship between former spouses often determines the emotional climate in which family members function after a divorce (Ahrons & Rodgers, 1987; Hetherington et al., 1982), this redefinition process is likely to have significant implications for the functioning of the family in its new form.

Thus both theoretical analysis and empirical research on the redefinition process are needed. In some ways, this process may be similar to the reorganization of attachment representations following bereavement. At first Bowlby (1969/1982) viewed this as a case of "detachment," but in his later years (e.g., Bowlby, 1980, 1988) he viewed it as a matter of reorganization of attachment representations (see Shaver & Fraley, Chapter 3, this volume). Perhaps postdivorce attachments can be reorganized so that some of the earlier positive feelings and a new commitment to cooperative interdependence (e.g., in parenting) can be beneficial, whereas the disappointment and animosity engendered by the failed sexual and marital relationship can fade into the background of memory. This redefinition process may involve a process of transition from an attachment bond to an affiliative bond, which according to attachment theory relies on a separate behavioral system (see Cassidy, Chapter 1, this volume). This redefinition process also involves the coordination and maintenance of joint caregiving responsibilities toward the children, while recognizing that other aspects of the prior marital relationship (attachment, sexuality, and caregiving toward the spouse) no longer apply. Positive relations between ex-spouses serve the interests of both spouses' caregiving systems, thus enhancing the children's well-being and the divorced parents' reproductive fitness.

Divorcing parents with secure attachment orientations are at an advantage, because qualities associated with secure attachment (good communication skills, constructive coping strategies, ability to regulate and integrate emotions, and the ability to solve conflicts cooperatively and constructively) should enable them to share parenting while keeping their children's best interests in mind (Cohen & Finzi-Dottan, 2005). Interventions may assist in this redefinition process; for example, Vareschi and Bursik (2005) found that parenting workshops dramatically increased positive parental interactions and decreased negative parental interactions for insecure participants. These findings suggest that interventions can provide insecure individuals with previously unused or unfamiliar tools and strategies for diffusing conflict and facilitating cohesion and support in shared parenting.

EFFECTS OF DIVORCE ON CHILDREN

Not only does divorce present attachment-related challenges for children, but the divorce-related stressors experienced by parents frequently interfere with the parents' ability to respond adequately and consistently to their children's needs for safety and security (Page & Bretherton, 2001). In this section, we describe theory and research relevant to the effects of divorce on children's attachment security (presumably due to the quality of postdivorce relationships with their parents), their psychological and physical health, and their future relationship functioning.

Attachment Security

As described above, a major proposition of attachment theory is that people build representational or working models of themselves and others from their experiences with caregivers, and that these models are the essence of attachment security versus insecurity (Bowlby, 1969/1982, 1973, 1980). To the extent that divorce reduces a child's confidence in who and where his or her attachment figures are; in his or her perceived acceptability in the eyes of attachment figures; and in the availability, accessibility, and sensitive responsiveness of attachment figures (all core aspects of working models), divorce is likely to affect the child's attachment security. The mere fact that parents are living apart may undermine a child's feelings of security, because parental accessibility becomes more tenuous (Maccoby, Buchanan, Mnookin, & Dornbusch, 1993; Page & Bretherton, 2001). In fact, Bowlby (1980) noted that some children who have experienced loss of or separation from one parent may fear the loss of or separation from the other parent.

Infants and Children

Few studies have investigated the effects of divorce on infants' and young children's attachment patterns, and the few that have been conducted yielded mixed results. Nair and Murray (2005) found that 3- to 6-year-old children from divorced families had lower security scores on the Attachment Q-Sort (Waters & Deane, 1985). Clarke-Stewart, Vandell, McCartney, Owen, and Booth (2000) also found that children from divorced families were less secure as measured by the Strange Situation (Ainsworth, Blehar, Waters, & Wall, 1978) at 15 months, the Attachment Q-Sort at 24 months, and a modified Strange Situation at 36 months. Similarly, Solomon, George, and Wallerstein (1995; cited in Nair & Murray, 2005) found that infants from divorced families were more likely than infants from intact families to be classified as insecure in the Strange Situation. However, Kier and Lewis (1997), also using the Strange Situation, found no differences between infants from divorced families and infants from intact families. And Vaughan, Gove, and Egeland (1980) found only a trend for infants from nonintact families to be more anxiously attached to their mothers than children from intact families.

Investigators have identified several factors that moderate the association between divorce and attachment security in young children, and thus are likely to explain the inconsistent links. First, as predicted by attachment theory, quality of parenting moderates the link. For example, mothers from intact families are more likely than divorced mothers to have a positive/authoritative parenting style (involving sensitivity and responsiveness), which directly affects attachment security (Bray, 1988; Hetherington et al., 1982; Nair & Murray, 2005). Second, father visitation patterns influence mother–infant attachment. For example, repeated overnight separation from a primary caregiver, usually the mother, is associated with disruption in mother–infant attachment when the conditions of visitation are poor (e.g., when parents are unable to provide adequate psychological support to the child) (George & Solomon, 1999; Hodges et al., 1991). However, mothers who function as a secure base for their children promote attachment security, despite separations due to overnight visits with fathers (Solomon & George, 1999). Furthermore, mothers who provide psychological protection to their children in the context of father visitation (e.g., by being sensitively responsive to the children during the fathers' visitation) also promote secure attachment to the father (Solomon & George, 1999).

Third, maternal education and family income reduce the effects of divorce on attachment security (Clarke-Stewart et al., 2000), perhaps because better education and finances facilitate the kinds of parenting that foster attachment security.

Finally, a child's cognitive ability (associated with age) has been identified as a protective factor. Kier and Lewis (1997) tested two contradicting predictions about the effects of parental separation on infants' attachment to mother: Whereas the "early adversity" hypothesis predicts that infants will be adversely affected by negative life events and thus will become anxiously attached to their mothers, the "protective" hypothesis predicts that infants are resistant to stressors because of their limited cognitive ability. Results supported the protective hypothesis, suggesting that cognitive ability associated with age and incomplete attachment formation to fathers protected young children against the ill effects of divorce.

Overall, the research tends to support a context-sensitive view in which separation effects are moderated by the conditions of separation and reunion (Solomon & George, 1999). For example, observations of young children undergoing separations under varying circumstances (Heinicke & Westheimer, 1965; Robertson & Robertson, 1971) show, consistent with attachment theory, that a familiar and sensitive caretaking environment during separation can mitigate or even prevent infant distress and detachment (see Solomon & George, 1999). According to this view, separation is a risk factor for attachment insecurity that may be either potentiated by adverse conditions or prevented by conditions known to promote security.

Adolescents and Young Adults

A larger number of studies have investigated the impact of divorce on children's attachment later in life. With a few exceptions, the consensus is that adolescents and young adults from divorced families are more likely to be insecurely attached than those from intact families, with most evidence pointing toward a greater likelihood of becoming fearful or preoccupied (i.e., more anxiously attached) as adults. For example, Beckwith, Cohen, and Hamilton (1999) found that adverse life events through age 12, particularly parental divorce, reduced the likelihood of secure attachment representations and increased the likelihood of preoccupied representations at 18 years of age. In this investigation, attachment security was assessed via naturalistic observation in the home when children were very young, with a Q-sort procedure when children were 12, and with the Adult Attachment Interview (AAI; George, Kaplan, & Main, 1984, 1985, 1996) when children were 18. Consistent with these findings, other longitudinal investigations have shown that divorce is predictive of an insecure attachment status at 18 years as measured by the AAI (Lewis et al., 2000), and that stressful life events, which included divorce in some cases, were significantly related to the likelihood that an infant classified as secure in the Strange Situation would become insecure by early adulthood as assessed by the AAI (Waters, Merrick, Treboux, Crowell, & Albersheim, 2000). Similar results were obtained in a study using a self-report measure of attachment that assesses the quality of relationships with parents (Ruschena, Prior, Sanson, & Smart, 2005).

Other studies that have employed self-report adult attachment measures, such as the Relationship Scales Questionnaire (Griffin & Bartholomew, 1994) and Bartholomew's (1990) four attachment categories, indicate that adolescents and college students from divorced families more often develop a fearful attachment style than those from intact families do (Brennan & Shaver, 1998; Kilman, Carranza, & Vendemia, 2006; Ozen, 2003). Riggs and Jacobvitz (2002) also found that adults classified as preoccupied or unresolved (i.e., those who experience a brief collapse of mental organization during discussions of trauma) on the AAI were more likely than others to report a history of divorce or parental separation during childhood. Thus it appears that parental separation or divorce is linked with attachment anxiety, which underlies both fearful and preoccupied attachment orientations. Supporting this conclusion, Mickelson, Kessler, and Shaver (1997) found parental divorce or separation to be negatively associated with secure attachment and positively related to anxious attachment in a nationally representative study that employed both categorical and continuous attachment measures (see also McCabe, 1997; Shaver & Mikulincer, 2004; and Summers, Forehand, Armistead, & Tannenbaum, 1998, for evidence linking divorce to insecure attachment). The studies that do not support this conclusion found no relation between parental divorce and offspring's later attachment style (Brennan & Shaver, 1993; J. A. Feeney & Noller, 1990; Hazan & Shaver, 1987; Hazelton, Lancee, & O'Neil, 1998), as assessed with either a single-item measure of adult attachment (Hazan & Shaver, 1987) or the Reciprocal Attachment Questionnaire (West & Sheldon-Keller, 1992).

Although the majority of empirical evidence suggests that divorce has a negative impact on adolescents and young adults' attachment security, research has also shown that many factors may moderate this association. First, Brennan and Shaver (1993) found that parents' postdivorce marital

status was related to their offspring's attachment style. It seems that having either a mother or both parents remarry is associated with the best attachment outcome for a young adult. Second, researchers have shown that individuals who come from divorced families do not differ from those who come from unhappy/intact families in their attachment security, indicating that the quality of the parents' relationship is important (Sprecher, Cate, & Levin, 1998). Third, perceptions of the reasons for divorce are important (Walker & Ehrenberg, 1998). For example, young people who felt that they were not involved in their parents' decision to divorce scored higher on measures of attachment security, whereas those who felt they were involved were more likely to be preoccupied. Furthermore, those who felt that they were involved in their parents' decision to divorce and also viewed overt anger as leading to the marital breakdown scored high on measures of fearfulness. Fourth, gender of the child has sometimes been a moderator. Women from divorced families are less likely to be securely attached than are men from divorced families (Barber, 1998; Evans & Bloom, 1996). Even within a sample of men, gender identification affected the association between divorce and attachment, such that feminine men were more influenced by divorce than other sex-role groups (Sexton, Hingst, & Regan, 1985). The reason for these gender differences may be the quality of care the child receives from primary attachment figures.

In fact, the quality of parent–child relationships has been identified as a key mediator between parental divorce and children's later adjustment (Amato, 2000; Amato & Sobolewski, 2001). Because divorce entails significant changes in family structure, it has the potential to influence the sensitive responsiveness and accessibility (both physical and psychological) of attachment figures, and thus to affect the safe-haven and secure-base caregiving functions that parents normally provide for their children. Parents may fail to provide these protective functions following divorce by (1) inverting the parent–child relationship, so that the child becomes a major attachment figure for the parent; or (2) becoming psychologically and/or physically unavailable to the child (Bowlby, 1969/1982, 1979).

Not surprisingly, the influence of divorce on parent–child relationships has been an important topic in the research literature on divorce (e.g., Bretherton & Page, 2004; Buchanan, Maccoby, & Dornbusch, 1996; Bulduc, Caron, & Logue, 2007; Cohen & Finzi-Dottan, 2005; Fabricius &

Luecken, 2007; Heterington, 1999; Hetherington et al., 1978; Kilman et al., 2006; Kruk, 1992; Luedemann, Ehrenberg, & Hunter, 2006; Page & Bretherton, 2001, 2003). For example, studies indicate that father–child attachment is particularly affected by divorce (Hannum & Dvorak, 2004; Tayler, Parker, & Roy, 1995), and that boys are more distressed than girls by separation from (or loss of) their fathers because of their attachment to and strong identification with the same-sex parent (Hetherington et al., 1978). However, girls are more likely to feel a burden or responsibility for their fathers' well-being when the parents engage in conflict (see also Bretherton & Page, 2004; Bretherton, Ridgeway, & Cassidy, 1990; Page & Bretherton, 2001, 2003). The next section considers psychological and physical indicators of maladjustment, which from an attachment-theoretical perspective are most likely to arise when children's attachment and security needs are not met.

Psychological and Physical Health

Children of divorce may experience the effects of separation and loss to an even greater extent than the divorcing adults, because (1) children typically have no control over the decision, and (2) it often seems to them to occur suddenly and without warning. For children, the disruption of important attachment bonds occurs not only with regard to one or both parents, but often with regard to friends and extended family members (e.g., grandparents) as well (e.g., Johnson, 1988). The cumulative toll of these separations and losses, coupled with other divorce-related stressors (e.g., economic hardship, moving, changing schools, and parental remarriage), may complicate children's psychological development and influence adjustment (Amato, 2000).

Thus an enormous amount of research has focused on the effects of divorce on children's psychological health. There are some studies showing that divorce may have a positive effect on children's adjustment (e.g., Crosnoe & Elder, 2004; Hagerty, Williams, & Oe, 2002), and that children may benefit if stress decreases or resources increase following divorce (Amato, 1993). However, the majority of studies show that children from divorced families score lower on a wide range of outcome measures associated with well-being (including academic achievement, psychological adjustment, self-esteem, conduct, and social competence), and that they are at increased risk for developmental delays, psychopathology (e.g., anxiety, depression, phobia), and problematic behaviors such as aggression (Amato, 2000; see Amato & Keith, 1991, for a meta-analysis of 92 studies; Bray & Hetherington, 1993; Brennan & Shaver, 1998; Chase-Lansdale, Cherlin, & Kiernan, 1995; Clarke-Stewart et al., 2000; Hodges et al., 1991; Kilman et al., 2006; Sirvanli-Ozen, 2005; Wallerstein & Blakeslee, 1989; Zill, Morrison, & Coiro, 1993). Longitudinal studies suggest that the effects for some children may be quite large and enduring (Cherlin, Chase-Lansdale, & McRae, 1998; Gilman, Kawachi, Fitzmaurice, & Buka, 2003; Laumann-Billings & Emery, 2000; Rodgers, Power, & Hope, 1997; Wallerstein & Lewis, 2004).

Researchers have also begun to discover that physical health problems are associated with exposure to distressing parental divorce processes (Guidubaldi, Cleminshaw, & Perry, 1985; Katz & Gottman, 1997; Luecken & Fabricius, 2003; Mechanic & Hansell, 1989). For example, Troxel and Matthews (2004) highlighted five studies that demonstrated a link between parental divorce and increased physical health problems (Dawson, 1991; DeGoede & Spruijt, 1996; Guidubaldi & Clemenshaw, 1985; Maier & Lachman, 2000; Mauldon, 1990). Overall, research evidence indicates that parental divorce in childhood is associated with increased risk for unintentional injuries, illness, hospitalization, somatic symptoms, premature mortality, and suicide (e.g., Aro & Palosaari, 1992; de Jong, 1992; D'Onofrio et al., 2006; Schwartz et al., 1995; Tucker et al., 1997). Parental divorce has also been linked with poor or risky health-related behaviors, including irregular eating and sleeping patterns (Sirvanli-Ozen, 2005), substance abuse (Amato & Keith, 1991; Bray & Hetherington, 1993), alcohol use (Hope, Power, & Rodgers, 1998; Sartor, Lynskey, Heath, Jacob, & True, 2007), smoking (Isohanni, Moilanen, & Rantakallio, 1991), marijuana use (Hoffman, 1995), early sexual activity (Amato & Keith, 1991; Barber, 1998; D'Onofrio et al., 2006; Gabardi & Rosen, 1992), and teen pregnancy (Aseltine & Doucet, 2003).

Although children from divorced families are clearly at greater risk for psychological and physical problems, research has identified important moderating variables consistent with attachment theory's predictions that disruptions in important attachment bonds (and the protective functions that attachment bonds serve) adversely affect individual functioning (Rogers, 2004). First, the increased risk for children from divorced homes stems from discordant, conflictual relationships that precede or follow the losses associated with divorce (Cherlin et al., 1991; Rutter, 1994), and not from divorce itself. In fact, children experience better outcomes when parents in high-conflict marriages (in which conflict is intense, chronic, and overt) divorce rather than remain together (Amato & Booth, 2000; Amato & Keith, 1991; Booth & Amato, 2001; Emery, 1982; Hetherington, 1999). The quality of marital and familial relations is more predictive than marital status of health outcomes, including physical symptoms (Mechanic & Hansell, 1989; Sweeting & West, 1995), cancer (Duszynski, Shaffer, & Thomas, 1981; Shaffer, Duszynski, & Thomas, 1982), and mortality (Lundberg, 1993). Thus the overall toxicity of the home environment is a central factor in explaining the link between divorce and adverse outcomes (Emery, 1982).

Second, high levels of warmth and affection in the custodial mother–child relationship are negatively associated with postdivorce adjustment problems (e.g., Hetherington et al., 1992; Simons, Lin, Gordon, Conger, & Lorenz, 1999; Wolchik, Wilcox, Tein, & Sandler, 2000). Negative aspects of the mother–child relationship that contribute to adjustment problems include maternal depressive mood, which has been directly related to child and adolescent functioning (Forehand, McCombs, & Brody, 1987), and fear of abandonment, which mediates the link between mother–child relationship quality and both internalizing and externalizing problems (Wolchik, Tein, Sandler, & Doyle, 2002). This makes theoretical sense, given that the hallmark of secure attachment is open and relaxed communication between parent and child, as well as confidence in the availability and accessibility of attachment figures (Bowlby, 1969/1982).

Third, a strong social support network moderates the effects of divorce on children's well-being. For example, divorce mediation for the parents and extended family support (Emery, 1999) protect against maladjustment, particularly if a parent is psychologically unable to provide high-quality parenting following a divorce. For adolescents, peer support also moderates the effect of low parental support after divorce on internalizing symptoms (Rodgers & Rose, 2002). However, in a 3-year longitudinal investigation of divorcing families, Maccoby and colleagues (1993) found that the factors most powerfully associated with good adolescent adjustment were (1) having a close relationship with a residential parent who monitored the child and remained involved in decisions concerning his or her life, and (2) not feeling caught in the middle

of parental conflict. Noncustodial parent involvement (Furstenberg, Morgan, & Allison, 1987; Sirvanli-Ozen, 2005), strong father–child relations (Fabricius & Luecken, 2007), and attachment to the family home (Stirtzinger & Cholvat, 1991) have also been identified as potentially protective factors. These network supports may reduce negative feelings about parental divorce, which have been linked with hostility, somatic complaints, and illness reports—again indicating that it is the negativity of experiences associated with divorce (and not the divorce itself) that increases vulnerability (Luecken & Fabricius, 2003).

Consistent with this research and with attachment-theoretical predictions, Troxel and Matthews (2004) proposed that many health effects of divorce on offspring are mediated through disrupted parenting in general, and specifically through diminished warmth/sensitivity and reduced physical and/or psychological availability of parents. Inadequate parenting or physical absence of a parent, in turn, is hypothesized to cause a particular kind of distress in children—namely, emotional insecurity regarding their parents' love and ability to care for them (Davies & Cummings, 1994; Wolchik et al., 2002). Emotional insecurity is hypothesized to disrupt emotion regulation processes and render children susceptible to stress-related health problems. Some researchers have identified biopsychosocial pathways from the parental marital system to childhood health that require future study (Krantz & McCeney, 2002; Troxel & Matthews, 2004).

Future Romantic Relations

Attachment theory stipulates that working models of attachment and the forecasts derived from them, once developed, guide behavior, feelings, and the processing of information (attention, perception, memory, interpretation) in future relationships (Bowlby, 1980; Bretherton, 1990; Collins et al., 2004; Main et al., 1985). Because the construction of these working models is thought to be influenced by experiences of separation and loss, attachment theory predicts that (particularly unresolved) experiences of separation/loss should be linked to the quality of future romantic relationships.

Although some investigators have found that young adults from divorced versus intact families do not differ on measures of intimacy (Nelson, Hughes, Handal, Katz, & Searight, 1993; Sinclair & Nelson, 1998), dating behavior (Greenberg &

Nay, 1982), or quality of attachment to adult intimates (Olivas & Stoltenberg, 1997; Tayler et al., 1995), a majority of studies do find differences in later romantic relationship functioning between those who grew up in intact versus divorced families (see Amato, 1999, for a review). First, young adults from divorced families are likely to hold less positive attitudes toward marriage and relationships (Sirvanli-Ozen, 2005), to show less trust (Southworth & Schwartz, 1987; Sprague & Kinney, 1997), to have problems with dependency and control (Bolgar, Zweig-Frank, & Paris, 1995), to be less optimistic (Sprecher et al., 1998), and to believe that disagreement is destructive (Sinclair & Nelson, 1998; but see Coleman & Ganong, 1984, for an exception). Second, parental divorce increases the risk of marital instability and dissolution in offspring (e.g., Amato & DeBoer, 2001; Glenn & Kramer, 1987; McLanahan & Bumpass, 1988; Wolfinger, 2000) and of conflict in romantic relationships (Chen et al., 2006). The influential Virginia Longitudinal Study of Divorce and Remarriage indicates that both divorce and marital conflict in the family of origin contribute to couple instability in offspring (Hetherington, 2003). Third, a history of parental conflict and divorce predicts lower intimacy in romantic relationships (Ensign, Scherman, & Clark, 1998; Sprecher et al., 1998), avoidance of short-term relationships (Knox, Zusman, & DeCuzzi, 2004), and perpetration of teen dating violence (Banyard, Cross, & Modecki, 2006).

It is important to consider, however, that not all children from divorced families have the same risks for troubled romantic relationships in adulthood, and that not every child from a divorced family experiences later relationships in the same way. Closeness to parents and positive appraisals of parental divorce have been identified as protective factors (Coleman & Ganong, 1984; Shulman, Scharf, Lumer, & Maurer, 2001), whereas parental conflict associated with divorce has a particularly negative effect on children's later relationships. The significant differences between those from intact and divorced families are often due to dysfunctional family dynamics and not to the divorce per se (Sprecher et al., 1998). In support of this conclusion, Hayashi and Strickland (1998) found that college students who experienced protracted inter-parental conflict, parental rejection, or overprotective parents were more likely to report jealousy and fears of abandonment in their love relationships, regardless of whether their parents had divorced.

Although a number of explanations have been offered for the intergenerational transmission of relationship instability (e.g., Amato & DeBoer, 2001; Glenn & Kramer, 1987; Gottman & Notarius, 2000; Hetherington & Kelly, 2002; Jockin, McGue, & Lykken, 1996; McGue & Lykken, 1992; McLanahan & Bumpass, 1988), attachment theory offers a particularly comprehensive and complete explanation for why children from divorced families grow up to have more problems with relationships than children from intact families do (Brennan & Shaver, 1993). Because the process of divorce is so taxing on the separating parents (who are the primary, and perhaps only, attachment figures for their children), it is likely to have a huge influence on their caregiving capacity. As described above, the separation anxiety and attachment system activation that the separating adults often experience are likely to interfere with their caregiving systems. In fact, in the absence of personal and social resources for coping, simultaneous activation of the attachment and caregiving systems is likely to result in caregiving that is more self-focused than other-focused (Kunce & Shaver, 1994). These caregiving dynamics, coupled with parental modeling of poor marital communication, are likely to play an important role in shaping children's attachment orientations and experiences in romantic relationships (Brennan & Shaver, 1993).

CONCLUSIONS

The purpose of this chapter is to explore the relevance of attachment theory for understanding all aspects of divorce. Although divorce has received a great deal of attention because of its obvious importance to modern societies, the research on divorce lacks theoretical motivation and integration, and many aspects of divorce have not been thoroughly investigated. More work is needed to (1) specify the combinations of intrapersonal and interpersonal processes (both distal and proximal) that lead to divorce; (2) establish the mechanisms responsible for the strong and consistent links between divorce and health for both adults and children; (3) determine the benefits and costs of various forms of postdivorce contact between exspouses, particularly where children are involved; and (4) specify the connections between parental divorce and future romantic relationship functioning, particularly with regard to the intergenerational transmission of divorce.

Attachment theory provides an integrative framework for this research program, because it suggests that divorce is a *process* of disrupted attachment that has far-reaching roots in previous attachment relationships and profound implications for future relationships. Attachment theory is capable of linking all aspects of the divorce process and telling a coherent story about who is likely to divorce and why; the processes involved in ending or reorganizing attachment bonds; the effects of detachment and reorganization on divorcing adults, and the mechanisms underlying these effects; the impact of parental conflict and detachment on children, and the mechanisms that account for this impact; and the nature and quality of postdivorce relationships between former spouses and between them and their children. Because attachment, separation, and loss are core issues addressed by attachment theory, the consideration of the divorce process from an attachment perspective is important.

If an attachment-theoretical approach to divorce is to be developed, it will be necessary first to elaborate and test more detailed hypotheses concerning the normative processes involved in detaching or reorganizing attachment working models. Although Bowlby discussed separation and loss extensively, most of his insights came from observations of children who were separated from their attachment figures; he gave much less attention to separation in adult relationships, except in the case of bereavement. Because divorce often requires a continuing and evolving relationship with a living person, the issue of negotiated reorganization becomes important, along with the possibility of transforming what was a primary attachment with sexual components into an affiliative relationship. Surprisingly little research or theorizing has been focused on individual differences in attachment orientations that affect the divorce process. We know a great deal about the effects of attachment orientations on relationship dynamics; it is very likely that there are equally important effects on the divorce process and postdivorce adjustment, and that some of these effects are dyadic, not just intrapsychic.

Clinicians have taken on part of the necessary theoretical work, providing a preliminary formulation of the ways in which attachment patterns may affect the divorce process (Cohen, Finzi, & Avi-Yonah, 1999; Finzi, Cohen, & Ram, 2000; Johnson, 2003; Todorski, 1995). They propose that individuals with different attachment orientations deal differently with divorce, experi-

ence separation differently, have different coping capacities and strategies, and deal differently with ex-spouses as coparents. Based on clinical observations and prior attachment research, they describe hypothetical divorce dynamics for different kinds of couples (e.g., secure–secure, secure–avoidant, secure–anxious, anxious–avoidant, anxious–anxious, avoidant–avoidant) and offer general guidelines for clinical intervention (e.g., Finzi et al., 2000). These ideas are ripe for empirical testing.

In attachment theory, John Bowlby provided a foundation for identifying and understanding both intrapersonal and interpersonal processes involved in marital dissolution and postdivorce adjustment. It is now up to us to provide detailed theoretical elaborations specific to each aspect of the divorce process, and to test predictions derived from these elaborations. Given the significance of divorce for adults' and children's physical and psychological health, theory-guided investigations of divorce and postdivorce processes are of paramount importance. We hope that future research will reveal pathways that separating couples can take to ensure the health and well-being of all family members.

REFERENCES

Ahrons, C. R., & Rodgers, R. H. (1987). *Divorced families: A multidisciplinary development view*. New York: Norton.

Ahrons, C. R., & Wallisch, L. S. (1986). The relationship between former spouses. In S. Duck & D. Perlman (Eds.), *Close relationships: Development, dynamics, and deterioration* (pp. 269–296). Beverly Hills, CA: Sage.

Ainsworth, M. D. S., Blehar, M. C., Waters, E., & Wall, S. (1978). *Patterns of attachment: A psychological study of the Strange Situation*. Hillsdale, NJ: Erlbaum.

Amato, P. R. (1993). Children's adjustment to divorce: Theories, hypotheses, and empirical support. *Journal of Marriage and the Family, 55*, 23–38.

Amato, P. R. (1999). Children of divorced parents as young adults. In E. M. Hetherington (Ed.), *Coping with divorce, single parenting, and remarriage: A risk and resiliency perspective* (pp. 147–163). Mahwah, NJ: Erlbaum.

Amato, P. R. (2000). The consequences of divorce for adults and children. *Journal of Marriage and the Family, 62*, 1269–1287.

Amato, P. R., & Booth, A. (2000). *A generation at risk: Growing up in an era of family upheaval*. Cambridge, MA: Harvard University Press.

Amato, P. R., & DeBoer, D. D. (2001). The transmission of marital instability across generations: Relationship skills or commitment to marriage? *Journal of Marriage and the Family, 63*, 1038–1051.

Amato, P. R., & Keith, B. (1991). Parental divorce and the well-being of children: A meta-analysis. *Psychological Bulletin, 110*, 26–46.

Amato, P. R., & Sobolewski, J. M. (2001). The effects of divorce and marital discord on adult children's psychological well-being. *American Sociological Review, 66*, 900–921.

Ambert, A. (1988). Relationships between ex-spouses: Individual and dynamic perspectives. *Journal of Social and Personal Relationships, 5*, 327–346.

Arendell, T. (1995). *Fathers and divorce.* Thousand Oaks, CA: Sage.

Aro, H. M., & Palosaari, U. K. (1992). Parental divorce, adolescence, and transition to young adulthood: A follow-up study. *American Journal of Orthopsychiatry, 62*, 421–429.

Aseltine, R. H., Jr., & Doucet, J. (2003). The impact of parental divorce on premarital pregnancy. *Adolescent and Family Health, 3*, 122–129.

Aseltine, R. H., & Kessler, R. C. (1993). Marital disruption and depression in a community sample. *Journal of Health and Social Behavior, 34*, 237–251.

Aydintug, C. D. (1995). Former spouse interaction: Normative guidelines and actual behavior. *Journal of Divorce and Remarriage, 22*, 147–161.

Banyard, V. L., Cross, C., & Modecki, K. L. (2006). Interpersonal violence in adolescence: Ecological correlates of self-reported perpetration. *Journal of Interpersonal Violence, 21*, 1314–1332.

Barber, N. (1998). Sex differences in dispositions towards kin, security of adult attachment, and sociosexuality as a function of parental divorce. *Evolution and Human Behavior, 19*, 125–132.

Bartholomew, K. (1990). Avoidance of intimacy: An attachment perspective. *Journal of Social and Personal Relationships, 7*, 147–178.

Beckwith, L., Cohen, S. E., & Hamilton, C. E. (1999). Maternal sensitivity during infancy and subsequent life events relate to attachment representation at early adulthood. *Developmental Psychology, 35*, 693–700.

Berkman, L. F., & Breslow, L. (1983). *Health and ways of living: The Alameda County study.* Oxford, UK: Oxford University Press.

Berkman, L. F., & Syme, S. L. (1979). Social networks, host resistance, and mortality: A nine year follow-up study of Alameda County residents. *American Journal of Epidemiology, 109*, 186–204.

Berman, W. H. (1988a). The relationship of ex-spouse attachment to adjustment following divorce. *Journal of Family Psychology, 1*, 312–328.

Berman, W. H. (1988b). The role of attachment in the post-divorce experience. *Journal of Personality and Social Psychology, 54*, 496–503.

Berscheid, E. (1983). Emotions in close relationships. In H. H. Kelley, E. Berscheid, A. Christensen, J. Harvey, T. Huston, G. Levinger, et al. (Eds.), *The psychology of close relationships* (pp. 110–168). New York: Freeman.

Birnbaum, G. E., Orr, I., Mikulincer, M., & Florian, V.

(1997). When marriage breaks up: Does attachment style contribute to coping and mental health? *Journal of Social and Personal Relationships, 14*, 643–654.

Bloom, B. L., Asher, S. J., & White, S. W. (1978). Marital disruption as a stressor: A review and analysis. *Psychological Bulletin, 85*, 867–894.

Blumenthal, M. D. (1967). Mental health among the divorced: A field study of divorced and never divorced persons. *Archives of General Psychiatry, 16*, 603–608.

Bohannon, P. (1970). The six stations of divorce. In P. Bohannon (Ed.), *Divorce and after.* New York: Doubleday.

Bolgar, R., Zweig-Frank, H., & Paris, J. (1995). Childhood antecedents of interpersonal problems in young adult children of divorce. *Journal of the American Academy of Child and Adolescent Psychiatry, 34*, 143–150.

Booth, A., & Amato, P. (1991). Divorce and psychological stress. *Journal of Health and Social Behavior, 32*, 396–407.

Booth, A., & Amato, P. (1992). Divorce, residential change, and stress. *Journal of Divorce and Remarriage, 18*, 205–213.

Booth, A., & Amato, P. R. (2001). Parental predivorce relations and offspring postdivorce well-being. *Journal of Marriage and the Family, 63*, 197–212.

Bowlby, J. (1969/1982). *Attachment and loss: Vol. 1. Attachment.* New York: Basic Books.

Bowlby, J. (1973). *Attachment and loss: Vol. 2. Separation: Anxiety, and anger.* New York: Basic Books.

Bowlby, J. (1979). *The making and breaking of affectional bonds.* London: Tavistock/Routledge.

Bowlby, J. (1980). *Attachment and loss: Vol. 3. Loss: Sadness and depression.* New York: Basic Books.

Bowlby, J. (1988). *A secure base.* New York: Basic Books.

Bray, J. H. (1988). Children's development during early remarriage. In E. M. Hetherington & J. D. Arasteh (Eds.), *Impact of divorce, single parenting, and stepparenting on children* (pp. 279–298). Hillsdale, NJ: Erlbaum.

Bray, J. H., & Hetherington, E. M. (1993). Families in transition: Introduction and overview. *Journal of Family Psychology, 7*, 3–8.

Brennan, K. A., & Shaver, P. R. (1993). Attachment styles and parental divorce. *Journal of Divorce and Remarriage, 21*, 161–175.

Brennan, K. A., & Shaver, P. R. (1998). Attachment styles and personality disorders: Their connections to each other and to parental divorce, parental death, and perceptions of parental caregiving. *Journal of Personality, 66*, 835–878.

Bretherton, I. (1990). Open communication and internal working models: Their role in the development of attachment relationships. In R. A. Thompson (Ed.), *Nebraska Symposium on Motivation: Vol. 36. Socioemotional development* (pp. 57–113). Lincoln: University of Nebraska Press.

Bretherton, I., & Page, T. (2004). Shared or conflicting working models?: Relationships in postdivorce families seen through the eyes of mothers and their preschool children. *Development and Psychopathology*, *16*, 551–575.

Bretherton, I., Ridgeway, D., & Cassidy, J. (1990). Assessing internal working models of the attachment relationship: An attachment story completion task for 3-year-olds. In M. T. Greenberg, D. Cicchetti, & M. E. Cummings (Eds.), *Attachment in the preschool years: Theory, research, and intervention* (pp. 273–308). Chicago: University of Chicago Press.

Brown, P., Felton, B. J., Whiteman, V., & Manela, R. (1980). Attachment and distress following marital separation. *Journal of Divorce*, *3*, 303–317.

Brown, S. D., & Reimer, D. A. (1984). Assessing attachment following divorce: Development and psychometric evaluation of the Divorce Reaction Inventory. *Journal of Counseling Psychology*, *31*, 520–531.

Bruce, M. L. (1998). Divorce and psychopathology, In B. P. Dohrenwend (Ed.), *Adversity, stress, and psychopathology* (pp. 219–232). London: Oxford University Press.

Buchanan, C. M., Maccoby, E. E., & Dornbusch, S. M. (1996). *Adolescents after divorce*. Cambridge, MA: Harvard University Press.

Bulduc, J. L., Caron, S. L., & Logue, M. E. (2007). The effects of parental divorce on college students. *Journal of Divorce and Remarriage*, *46*, 83–104.

Burman, B., & Margolin, G. (1992). Analysis of the association between marital relationships and health problems: An interactional perspective. *Psychological Bulletin*, *112*, 39–63.

Buunk, B. P., & Mutsaers, W. (1999). The nature of the relationship between remarried individuals and former spouses and its impact on marital satisfaction. *Journal of Family Psychology*, *13*, 165–174.

Ceglian, C. P., & Gardner, S. (1999). Attachment style: A risk for multiple marriages? *Journal of Divorce and Remarriage*, *31*, 125–139.

Chase-Lansdale, P. L., Cherlin, A. J., & Kiernan, K. K. (1995). The long-term effects of parental divorce on the mental health of young adults: A developmental perspective. *Child Development*, *66*, 1614–1634.

Chatav, Y., & Whisman, M. A. (2007). Marital dissolution and psychiatric disorders: An investigation of risk factors. *Journal of Divorce and Remarriage*, *47*, 1–13.

Chen, H., Cohen, P., Kasen, S., Johnson, J. G., Ehrensaft, M., & Gordon, K. (2006). Predicting conflict within romantic relationships during the transition to adulthood. *Personal Relationships*, *13*, 411–427.

Cherlin, A. J., Chase-Lansdale, P. L., & McRae, C. (1998). Effects of parental divorce on mental health throughout the life course. *American Sociological Review*, *63*, 239–249.

Cherlin, A. J., Furstenberg, F. F., Chase-Lansdale, P. L., Kiernan, K. E., Robins, P. K., Morrison, D. R., et al. (1991). Longitudinal studies of effect of divorce on children in Great Britain and the United States. *Science*, *252*, 1386–1389.

Clarke-Stewart, K. A., Vandell, D. L., McCartney, K., Owen, M. T., & Booth, C. (2000). Effects of parental separation and divorce on very young children. *Journal of Family Psychology*, *14*, 304–326.

Cohen, O., Finzi, R., & Avi-Yonah, O. K. (1999). An attachment-based typology of divorced couples. *Family Therapy*, *26*, 167–190.

Cohen, O., & Finzi-Dottan, R. (2005). Parent–child relationships during the divorce process: From attachment theory and intergenerational perspective. *Contemporary Family Therapy*, *27*, 81–99.

Cole, C. L., & Cole, A. L. (1999). Boundary ambiguities that bind former spouses together after the children leave home in post-divorce families. *Family Relations*, *48*, 271–272.

Coleman, M., & Ganong, L. H. (1984). Effects of family structure on family attitudes and expectations. *Family Relations*, *33*, 425–432.

Collins, N. L., & Feeney, B. C. (2004). Working models of attachment shape perceptions of social support: Evidence from experimental and observational studies. *Journal of Personality and Social Psychology*, *87*, 363–383.

Collins, N. L., Guichard, A. C., Ford, M. B., & Feeney, B. C. (2004). Working models of attachment: New developments and emerging themes. In S. W. Rholes & J. A. Simpson (Eds.), *Adult attachment: Theory, research, and clinical implications* (pp. 196–239). New York: Guilford Press.

Coontz, S. (2007). The origins of modern divorce. *Family Process*, *46*, 7–16.

Crosnoe, R., & Elder, G. H., Jr. (2004). Family dynamics, supportive relationships, and educational resilience during adolescence. *Journal of Family Issues*, *25*, 571–602.

Davies, P. T., & Cummings, E. M. (1994). Marital conflict and child adjustment: An emotional security hypothesis. *Psychological Bulletin*, *116*, 387–411.

Davila, J., & Bradbury, T. N. (2001). Attachment insecurity and the distinction between unhappy spouses who do and do not divorce. *Journal of Family Psychology*, *15*, 371–393.

Davila, J., Karney, B. R., & Bradbury, T. N. (1999). Attachment change processes in the early years of marriage. *Journal of Personality and Social Psychology*, *76*, 783–802.

Davis, D., Shaver, P. R., & Vernon, M. L. (2003). Physical, emotional, and behavioral reactions to breaking up: The roles of gender, age, emotional involvement, and attachment style. *Personality and Social Psychology Bulletin*, *29*, 871–884.

Dawson, D. A. (1991). Family structure and children's health and well-being: Data from the 1988 National Survey of Child Health. *Journal of Marriage and the Family*, *53*, 573–584.

DeGoede, M., & Spruijt, E. (1996). Effects of parental divorce and youth unemployment on adolescent health. *Patient Education and Counseling*, *29*, 269–276.

de Jong, M. J. (1992). Attachment, individuation, and risk of suicide in late adolescence. *Journal of Youth and Adolescence*, *21*, 357–373.

D'Onofrio, B. M., Turkheimer, E., Emery, R. E., Slutske, W. S., Heath, A. C., & Madden, P. A. (2006). A genetically informed study of the processes underlying the association between parental marital instability and offspring adjustment. *Developmental Psychology, 42,* 486–499.

Dozier, B. S., Sollie, D. L., Stack, S. J., & Smith, T. A. (1993). The effects of postdivorce attachment on co-parenting relationships. *Journal of Divorce and Remarriage, 19,* 109–123.

Dupre, M. E., & Meadows, S. O. (2007). Disaggregating the effects of marital trajectories on health. *Journal of Family Issues, 28,* 623–652.

Duszynski, K. R., Shaffer, J. W., & Thomas, C. B. (1981). Neoplasm and traumatic events in childhood: Are they related? *Archives of General Psychiatry, 38,* 327–331.

Ellis, D., & DeKeseredy, W. D. (1989). Marital status and woman abuse: The DAD model. *International Journal of Sociology of the Family, 19,* 67–87.

Emery, R. E. (1982). Interparental conflict and the children of discord and divorce. *Psychological Bulletin, 92,* 310–330.

Emery, R. E. (1988). *Marriage, divorce, and children's adjustment.* Thousand Oaks, CA: Sage.

Emery, R. E. (1994). *Renegotiating family relationships: Divorce, child custody, and mediation.* New York: Guilford Press.

Emery, R. E. (1999). Postdivorce family life for children: An overview of research and some implications for policy. In R. A. Thompson & P. R. Amato (Eds.), *The postdivorce family: Children, parenting, and society* (pp. 3–27). Thousand Oaks, CA: Sage.

Ensign, J., Scherman, A., & Clark, J. J. (1998). The relationship of family structure and conflict to levels of intimacy and parental attachment in college students. *Adolescence, 33,* 575–582.

Evans, J. J., & Bloom, B. L. (1996). Effects of parental divorce among college undergraduates. *Journal of Divorce and Remarriage, 26,* 69–91.

Fabricius, W. V., & Luecken, L. J. (2007). Postdivorce living arrangements, parental conflict, and long-term physical health correlates for children of divorce. *Journal of Family Psychology, 21,* 195–205.

Feeney, B. C. (2007). The dependency paradox in close relationships: Accepting dependence promotes independence. *Journal of Personality and Social Psychology, 92,* 268–285.

Feeney, B. C., & Cassidy, J. (2003). Reconstructive memory related to adolescent–parent conflict interactions: The influence of attachment-related representations on immediate perceptions and changes in perceptions over time. *Journal of Personality and Social Psychology, 85,* 945–955.

Feeney, B. C., & Collins, N. L. (2001). Predictors of caregiving in adult intimate relationships: An attachment theoretical perspective. *Journal of Personality and Social Psychology, 80,* 972–994.

Feeney, B. C., & Kirkpatrick, L. A. (1996). Effects of adult attachment and presence of romantic partners on physiological responses to stress. *Journal of Personality and Social Psychology, 70,* 255–270.

Feeney, J. A., & Noller, P. (1990). Attachment style as a predictor of adult romantic relationships. *Journal of Personality and Social Psychology, 58,* 281–291.

Feeney, J. A., Noller, P., & Callan, V. J. (1994). Attachment style, communication and satisfaction in the early years of marriage. In K. Bartholomew & D. Perlman (Eds.), *Advances in personal relationships: Vol. 5. Attachment processes in adulthood* (pp. 269–308). London: Jessica Kingsley.

Finzi, R., Cohen, O., & Ram, A. (2000). Attachment and divorce. *Journal of Family Psychotherapy, 11,* 1–20.

Fisher, J. V., & Crandell, L. E. (1997). Complex attachment: Patterns of relating in the couple. *Sexual and Marital Therapy, 12,* 211–223.

Forehand, R., McCombs, A., & Brody, G. H. (1987). The relationship between parental depressive mood states and child functioning. *Advances in Behaviour Research and Therapy, 9,* 1–20.

Fraley, R. C., & Bonanno, G. A. (2004). Attachment loss: A test of three competing models on the association between attachment-related avoidance and adaptation to bereavement. *Personality and Social Psychology Bulletin, 30,* 878–890.

Fraley, R. C., Garner, J. P., & Shaver, P. R. (2000). Adult attachment and the defensive regulation of attention and memory: Examining the role of perspective and postemptive defensive processes. *Journal of Personality and Social Psychology, 79,* 816–826.

Furstenberg, F. F., Jr., & Cherlin, A. J. (1991). *Divided families: What happens to children when parents part.* Cambridge, MA: Harvard University Press.

Furstenberg, F. F., Morgan, S. P., & Allison, P. D. (1987). Paternal participation and children's well-being after marital dissolution. *American Sociological Review, 52,* 695–701

Gabardi, L., & Rosen, L. A. (1992). Intimate relationships: College students from divorced and intact families. *Journal of Divorce and Remarriage, 18,* 25–56.

George, C., Kaplan, N., & Main, M. (1984). *Adult Attachment Interview protocol.* Unpublished manuscript, University of California at Berkeley.

George, C., Kaplan, N., & Main, M. (1985). *Adult Attachment Interview protocol* (2nd ed.). Unpublished manuscript, University of California at Berkeley.

George, C., Kaplan, N., & Main, M. (1996). *Adult Attachment Interview protocol* (3rd ed.). Unpublished manuscript, University of California at Berkeley.

George, C., & Solomon, J. (1999). Attachment and caregiving: The caregiving behavioral system. In J. Cassidy & P. R. Shaver (Eds.), *Handbook of attachment: Theory, research, and clinical applications* (pp. 649–670). New York: Guilford Press.

Gilman, S. E., Kawachi, I., Fitzmaurice, G. M., & Buka, S. L. (2003). Family disruption in childhood and risk of adult depression. *American Journal of Psychiatry, 160,* 939–946.

Glenn, N. D., & Kramer, K. B. (1987). The marriages and divorces of the children of divorce. *Journal of Marriage and the Family, 49,* 811–825.

Glenn, N. D., & Weaver, C. N. (1988). The changing relationship of marital status to reported happiness. *Journal of Marriage and the Family, 50,* 317–324.

Goode, W. J. (1956). *After divorce.* Glencoe, IL: Free Press.

Gottman, J. M. (1993). A theory of marital dissolution and stability. *Journal of Family Psychology, 7,* 57–75.

Gottman, J. M. (1994). *What predicts divorce?: The relationship between marital processes and marital outcome.* Hillsdale, NJ: Erlbaum.

Gottman, J. M., & Levenson, R. W. (1992). Marital processes predictive of later dissolution: Behavior, physiology, and health. *Journal of Personality and Social Psychology, 63,* 221–233.

Gottman, J. M., & Levenson, R. W. (2000). The timing of divorce: Predicting when a couple will divorce over a 14-year period. *Journal of Marriage and the Family, 62,* 737–745.

Gottman, J. M., & Notarius, C. I. (2000). Decade review: Observing marital interaction. *Journal of Marriage and the Family, 62,* 927–947.

Gove, W. R. (1973). Sex, marital status, and mortality. *American Journal of Sociology, 79,* 45–67.

Gove, W. R., & Shin, H. (1989). The psychological well-being of divorced and widowed men and women: An empirical analysis. *Journal of Family Issues, 10,* 122–144.

Greenberg, E. F., & Nay, W. R. (1982). The intergenerational transmission of marital instability reconsidered. *Journal of Marriage and the Family, 44,* 335–347.

Griffin, D. W., & Bartholomew, K. (1994). Models of the self and other: Fundamental dimensions underlying measures of adult attachment. *Journal of Personality and Social Psychology, 67,* 430–445.

Guidubaldi, J., & Cleminshaw, H. K. (1985). Divorce, family health, and child adjustment. *Family Relations, 34,* 35–41.

Guidubaldi, J., Cleminshaw, H. K., & Perry, J. D. (1985). The relationship of parental divorce to health status of parents and children. *Special Services in the Schools, 1,* 73–87.

Guisinger, S., Cowan, P. A., & Schuldberg, D. (1989). Changing parent and spouse relations in the first years of remarriage of divorced fathers. *Journal of Marriage and the Family, 51,* 445–456.

Hagerty, B. M., Williams, R. A., & Oe, H. (2002). Childhood antecedents of adult sense of belonging. *Journal of Clinical Psychology, 58,* 793–801.

Hannum, J. W., & Dvorak, D. M. (2004). Effects of family conflict, divorce, and attachment patterns on the psychological distress and social adjustment of college freshmen. *Journal of College Student Development, 45,* 27–42.

Hawkins, D. N., & Booth, A. (2005). Unhappily ever after: Effects of long-term, low-quality marriages on well-being. *Social Forces, 84,* 451–471.

Hayashi, G. M., & Strickland, B. R. (1998). Long-term effects of parental divorce on love relationships: Divorce as attachment disruption. *Journal of Social and Personal Relationships, 15,* 23–38.

Hazan, C., & Shaver, P. R. (1987). Romantic love conceptualized as an attachment process. *Journal of Personality and Social Psychology, 52,* 511–524.

Hazelton, R., Lancee, W., & O'Neil, M. K. (1998). The controversial long term effects of parental divorce: The role of early attachment. *Journal of Divorce and Remarriage, 29,* 1–17.

Heinicke, C. M., & Westheimer, I. (1965). *Brief separation.* New York: International Universities Press.

Hemstrom, O. (1996). Is marriage dissolution linked to differences in mortality risks for men and women? *Journal of Marriage and the Family, 58,* 366–378.

Hetherington, E. M. (1999). Should we stay together for the sake of the children? In E. M. Hetherington (Ed.), *Coping with divorce, single parenting, and remarriage: A risk and resiliency perspective* (pp. 93–116). Hillsdale, NJ: Erlbaum.

Hetherington, E. M. (2003). Intimate pathways: Changing patterns in close personal relationships across time. *Family Relations, 52,* 318–331.

Hetherington, E. M., & Camara, K. A. (1984). Families in transition: The process of dissolution and reconstitution. In R. D. Parke (Ed.), *Review of child development: Vol. 7. The family* (pp. 398–440). Chicago: University of Chicago Press.

Hetherington, E. M., & Clingempeel, W. G. (1992). Coping with marital transitions: A family systems perspective. *Monographs of the Society for Research in Child Development, 57*(2–3, Serial No. 227, 1–238.

Hetherington, E. M., Cox, M., & Cox, R. (1978). The aftermath of divorce. In J. H. Stevens, Jr. & M. Matthews (Eds.), *Mother–child, father–child relationships* (pp. 149–176). Washington, DC: National Association for the Education of Young Children.

Hetherington, E. M., Cox, M., & Cox, R. (1982). The effects of divorce on parents and children. In M. Lamb (Ed.), *Nontraditional families* (pp. 233–288). Hillsdale, NJ: Erlbaum.

Hetherington, E. M., & Kelly, J. (2002). *For better or for worse: Divorce reconsidered.* New York: Norton.

Hodges, W. F., Landis, T., Day, E., & Oderberg, N. (1991). Infant and toddlers and post divorce parental access: An initial exploration. *Journal of Divorce and Remarriage, 16,* 239–252.

Hoffman, J. P. (1995). The effects of family structure and family relations on marijuana use. *International Journal of the Addictions, 30,* 1207–1241.

Hope, S., Power, C., & Rodgers, B. (1998). The relationships between parental separation in childhood and problem drinking in adulthood. *Addiction, 93,* 505–514.

Hu, Y. R., & Goldman, N. (1990). Mortality differentials by marital-status: An international comparison. *Demography, 27,* 233–250.

Huddleston, R. J., & Hawkings, L. D. (1991). A comparison of physical and emotional health after divorce in a Canadian and United States' sample. *Journal of Divorce and Remarriage, 15,* 193–207.

Isohanni, M., Moilanen, I., & Rantakallio, P. (1991). Determinants of teenage smoking, with special reference to non-standard family background. *British Journal of Addiction, 86,* 391–398.

Jasinski, J. L., & Williams, L. M. (Eds.). (1998). *Partner violence: A comprehensive review of 20 years of research.* Thousand Oaks, CA: Sage.

Jockin, V., McGue, M., & Lykken, D. T. (1996). Personality and divorce: A genetic analysis. *Journal of Personality and Social Psychology, 71,* 288–299.

Johnson, C. L. (1988). Active and latent functions of grandparenting during the divorce process. *The Gerontologist, 28,* 185–191.

Johnson, S. M. (2003). Attachment theory: A guide for couple therapy. In S. M. Johnson & V. E. Whiffen (Eds.), *Attachment processes in couple and family therapy* (pp. 103–123). New York: Guilford Press.

Karney, B. R., & Bradbury, T. N. (1995). The longitudinal course of marital quality and stability: A review of theory, methods, and research. *Psychological Bulletin, 118,* 3–34.

Katz, L. F., & Gottman, J. M. (1997). Buffering children from marital conflict and dissolution. *Journal of Clinical Child Psychology, 26,* 157–171.

Kiecolt-Glaser, J. K., Fisher, L. D., Ogrocki, P., Stout, J. C., Speicher, C. E., & Glaser, R. (1987). Marital quality, marital disruption, and immune function. *Psychosomatic Medicine, 49,* 13–34.

Kiecolt-Glaser, J. K., Kennedy, S., Malkoff, S., Fisher, L. D., Speicher, C. E., & Glaser, R. (1988). Marital discord and immunity in males. *Psychosomatic Medicine, 50,* 213–229.

Kier, C., & Lewis, C. (1997). Infant–mother attachment in separated and married families. *Journal of Divorce and Remarriage, 26,* 185–194.

Kilman, P. R., Carranza, L. V., & Vendemia, J. M. C. (2006). Recollections of parent characteristics and attachment patterns for college women of intact vs. non-intact families. *Journal of Adolescence, 29,* 89–102.

Kirkpatrick, L. A., & Davis, K. E. (1994). Attachment style, gender, and relationship stability: A longitudinal analysis. *Journal of Personality and Social Psychology, 66,* 502–512.

Kitson, G. C. (1982). Attachment to the spouse in divorce: A scale and its application. *Journal of Marriage and the Family, 44,* 379–393.

Kitson, G. C., & Morgan, L. A. (1990). The multiple consequences of divorce: A decade review. *Journal of Marriage and the Family, 52,* 913–924.

Kitson, G. C., & Raschke, H. J. (1981). Divorce research: What we know; what we need to know. *Journal of Divorce, 4,* 1–37.

Knox, D., Zusman, M., & DeCuzzi, A. (2004). The effect of parental divorce on relationships with parents and romantic partners of college students. *College Student Journal, 38,* 597–601.

Kobak, R. R., & Hazan, C. (1991). Attachment in marriage: Effects of security and accuracy of working models. *Journal of Personality and Social Psychology, 60,* 861–869.

Kotler, P., & Wingard, D. L. (1989). The effects of occupational, marital and parental roles on mortality: The Alameda County study. *American Journal of Public Health, 79,* 607–612.

Krantz, D. S., & McCeney, M. K. (2002). Effects of psychological and social factors on organic disease: A critical assessment of research on coronary heart disease. *Annual Review of Psychology, 53,* 341–369.

Kressel, K., Lopez-Morillas, M., Weinglass, J., & Deutsch, M. (1978). Professional intervention in divorce: A summary of the views of lawyers, psychotherapists, and clergy. *Journal of Divorce, 2,* 119–155.

Kruk, E. (1992). Psychological and structural factors contributing to the disengagement of noncustodial fathers after divorce. *Family and Conciliation Courts Review, 30,* 81–101.

Kunce, L. J., & Shaver, P. R. (1994). An attachment theoretical approach to caregiving in romantic relationships. In R. Bartholomew & D. Perlman (Eds.), *Advances in personal relationships: Vol. 5. Attachment processes in adulthood* (pp. 205–237). London: Jessica Kingsley.

Kurdek, L. A. (1991). The relations between reported well-being and divorce history, availability of a proximate adult, and gender. *Journal of Marriage and the Family, 53,* 71–78.

Laumann-Billings, L., & Emery, R. E. (2000). Distress among young adults from divorced families. *Journal of Family Psychology, 14,* 671–687.

Lewis, M., Feiring, C., & Rosenthal, S. (2000). Attachment over time. *Child Development, 71,* 707–720.

Lillard, L. A., & Waite, L. J. (1995). 'Til death do us part: Marital disruption and mortality. *American Journal of Sociology, 100,* 1131–1156.

Lorenz, F. O., Wickrama, K. A. S., Conger, R. D., & Elder, G. H., Jr. (2006). The short-term and decade-long effects of divorce on women's midlife health. *Journal of Health and Social Behavior, 47,* 111–125.

Lucas, R. E. (2005). Time does not heal all wounds: A longitudinal study of reaction and adaptation to divorce. *Psychological Science, 16,* 946–950.

Luecken, L. J., & Fabricius, W. V. (2003). Physical health vulnerability in adult children from divorced and intact families. *Journal of Psychosomatic Research, 55,* 221–228.

Luedemann, M. B., Ehrenberg, M. F., & Hunter, M. A. (2006). Mothers' discussions with daughters following divorce: Young adults reflect on their adolescent experiences and current mother–daughter relations. *Journal of Divorce and Remarriage, 46,* 29–55.

Lundberg, O. (1993). The impact of childhood living conditions on illness and mortality in adulthood. *Social Science and Medicine, 36,* 1047–1052.

Maccoby, E. E., Buchanan, C. M., Mnookin, R. H., & Dornbusch, S. M. (1993). Postdivorce roles of mothers and fathers in the lives of their children. *Journal of Family Psychology, 7,* 24–38.

Madden-Derdich, D. A., & Arditti, J. A. (1999). The ties that bind: Attachment between former spouses. *Family Relations, 48,* 243–249.

Maier, E. H., & Lachman, M. E. (2000). Consequences of early parental loss and separation for health and well-being in midlife. *International Journal of Behavioral Development, 24,* 83–189.

Main, M., Kaplan, N., & Cassidy, J. (1985). Security in infancy, childhood, and adulthood: A move to the level of representation. In I. Bretherton & E. Waters (Eds.), Growing points of attachment theory and research. *Monographs of the Society for Research in Child Development, 50*(1–2, Serial No. 209), 66–104.

Marks, N. F. (1996). Flying solo at midlife: Gender, marital status, and psychological well-being. *Journal of Family Issues, 58,* 917–932.

Masheter, C. (1990). Postdivorce relationships between exspouses: A literature review. *Journal of Divorce and Remarriage, 14,* 97–122.

Masheter, C. (1991). Postdivorce relationships between ex-spouses: The roles of attachment and interpersonal conflict. *Journal of Marriage and the Family, 53,* 103–110.

Masheter, C. (1997). Healthy and unhealthy friendship and hostility between ex-spouses. *Journal of Marriage and the Family, 59,* 463–475.

Mauldon, J. (1990). The effect of marital disruption on children's health. *Demography, 27,* 431–446.

Mazor, A., Batiste-Harel, P., & Gampel, Y. (1998). Divorcing spouses' coping patterns, attachment bonding and forgiveness processes in the post-divorce experience. *Journal of Divorce and Remarriage, 29,* 65–81.

McCabe, K. (1997). Sex differences in the long term effects of divorce on children: Depression and heterosexual relationship difficulties in the young adult years. *Journal of Divorce and Remarriage, 27,* 123–135.

McGue, M., & Lykken, D. T. (1992). Genetic influence on risk of divorce. *Psychological Science, 3,* 368–373.

McLanahan, S., & Bumpass, L. (1988). Intergenerational consequences of family disruption. *American Journal of Sociology, 94,* 130–152.

Mechanic, D., & Hansell, S. (1989). Divorce, conflict, and adolescents' well-being. *Journal of Health and Social Behavior, 30,* 105–116.

Mickelson, K. D., Kessler, R. C., & Shaver, P. R. (1997). Adult attachment in a nationally representative sample. *Journal of Personality and Social Psychology, 73,* 1092–1106.

Mikulincer, M. (1998). Attachment working models and the sense of trust: An exploration of interaction goals and affect regulation. *Journal of Personality and Social Psychology, 74,* 1209–1224.

Mikulincer, M., & Florian, V. (1996). Emotional reactions to interpersonal losses over the life span: An attachment theoretical perspective. In C. Magai & S. H. McFadden (Eds.), *Handbook of emotions, adult development, and aging* (pp. 269–285). San Diego, CA: Academic Press.

Mikulincer, M., & Florian, V. (1998). The relationship between adult attachment styles and emotional and cognitive reactions to stressful events. In J. A. Simpson & W. S. Rholes (Eds.), *Attachment theory and close relationships* (pp. 143–165). New York: Guilford Press.

Mikulincer, M., Horesh, N., Eilati, I., & Kotler, M. (1999). The association between adult attachment style and mental health in extreme life-endangering conditions. *Personality and Individual Differences, 27,* 831–842.

Mikulincer, M., & Orbach, I. (1995). Attachment styles and repressive defensiveness: The accessibility and architecture of affective memories. *Journal of Personality and Social Psychology, 68,* 917–925.

Mikulincer, M., & Shaver, P. R. (2005). Attachment theory and emotions in close relationships: Exploring the attachment-related dynamics of emotional reactions to relational events. *Personal Relationships, 12,* 149–168.

Mikulincer, M., & Shaver, P. R. (2007). Attachment, group-related processes, and psychotherapy. *International Journal of Group Psychology, 57,* 233–245.

Mikulincer, M., Shaver, P. R., & Slav, K. (2006). Attachment, mental representations of others, and gratitude and forgiveness in romantic relationships. In M. Mikulincer & G. S. Goodman (Eds.), *Dynamics of romantic love: Attachment, caregiving, and sex* (pp. 190–215). New York: Guilford Press.

Mirowsky, J., & Ross, C. E. (2003). *Education, social status, and health.* Hawthorne, NY: Aldine de Gruyter.

Nair, H., & Murray, A. D. (2005). Predictors of attachment security in preschool children from intact and divorced families. *Journal of Genetic Psychology, 166,* 245–263.

Nelson, W. L., Hughes, H. M., Handal, P., Katz, B., & Searight, H. R. (1993). The relationship of family structure and family conflict to adjustment in young adult college students. *Adolescence, 28,* 29–40.

Ognibene, T. C., & Collins, N. L. (1998). Adult attachment styles, perceived social support and coping strategies. *Journal of Social and Personal Relationships, 15,* 323–345.

Olivas, S. T., & Stoltenberg, C. D. (1997). Post-divorce father custody: Are mothers the true predictors of adult relationship satisfaction? *Journal of Divorce and Remarriage, 28,* 119–137.

Overbeek, G., Vollebergh, W., de Graaf, R., Scholte, R., de Kemp, R., & Engels, R. (2006). Longitudinal associations of marital quality and marital dissolution with the incidence of DSM-III-R disorders. *Journal of Family Psychology, 20,* 284–291.

Ozen, D. S. (2003). The impact of interparental divorce on adult attachment styles and perceived parenting styles of adolescents: Study in Turkey. *Journal of Divorce and Remarriage, 40,* 129–149.

Page, T., & Bretherton, I. (2001). Mother– and father–child attachment themes in the story completions of pre-schoolers from post-divorce families: Do they predict relationships with peers and teachers? *Attachment and Human Development, 3,* 1–29.

Page, T., & Bretherton, I. (2003). Representations of attachment to father in the narratives of preschool girls in post-divorce families: Implications for family relationships and social development. *Child and Adolescent Social Work Journal, 20,* 99–122.

Pietromonaco, P. R., Greenwood, D., & Barrett, L. F. (2004). Conflict in adult close relationships: An attachment perspective. In W. S. Rholes & J. A. Simpson (Eds.), *Adult attachment: Theory, research, and clinical implications* (pp. 267–299). New York: Guilford Press.

Price, S. J., & McKenry, P. C. (1988). *Divorce*. Thousand Oaks, CA: Sage.

Reibstein, J. (1998). Attachment, pain, and detachment for the adults in divorce. *Sexual and Marital Therapy, 13*, 351–360.

Reibstein, J., & Bamber, R. (1997). *The family through divorce: How you can limit the damage*. London: Thorsons.

Riggs, S. A., & Jacobvitz, D. (2002). Expectant parents' representations of early attachment relationships: Associations with mental health and family history. *Journal of Consulting and Clinical Psychology, 70*, 195–204.

Robertson, J., & Robertson, J. (1971). Young children in brief separation: A fresh look. *Psychoanalytic Study of the Child, 26*, 264–315.

Rodgers, B., Power, C., & Hope, S. (1997). Parental divorce and adult psychological distress: Evidence from a national birth cohort: A research note. *Journal of Child Psychology and Psychiatry, 38*, 867–872.

Rodgers, K. B., & Rose, H. A. (2002). Risk and resiliency factors among adolescents who experience marital transitions. *Journal of Marriage and the Family, 64*, 1024–1037.

Rogers, K. N. (2004). A theoretical review of risk and protective factors related to post divorce adjustment in young children. *Journal of Divorce and Remarriage, 40*(3–4), 135–147.

Roisman, G. I. (2007). The psychophysiology of adult attachment relationships: Autonomic reactivity in marital and premarital interactions. *Developmental Psychology, 43*, 39–53.

Ruschena, E., Prior, M., Sanson, A., & Smart, D. (2005). A longitudinal study of adolescent adjustment following family transitions. *Journal of Child Psychology and Psychiatry, 46*, 353–363.

Rutter, M. (1994). Family discord and conduct disorder: Cause, consequence, or correlate? *Journal of Family Psychology, 8*, 170–186.

Rye, M. S., Folck, C. D., Heim, T. A., Olszewski, B. T., & Traina, E. (2004). Forgiveness of an ex-spouse: How does it relate to mental health following divorce? *Journal of Divorce and Remarriage, 41*, 31–51.

Sartor, C. E., Lynskey, M. T., Heath, A. C., Jacob, T., & True, W. (2007). The role of childhood risk factors in initiation of alcohol use and progression to alcohol dependence. *Addiction, 102*, 216–225.

Sbarra, D. A., & Emery, R. E. (2005). Comparing conflict, nonacceptance, and depression among divorced adults: Results from a 12-year follow-up study of child custody mediation using multiple imputations. *American Journal of Orthopsychiatry, 75*, 63–75.

Schwartz, J. E., Friedman, H. S., Tucker, J. S., Tomlinson-Keasey, C., Wingard, D. L., & Criqui, M. H. (1995). Sociodemographic and psychosocial factors in childhood as predictors of adult mortality. *American Journal of Public Health, 85*, 1237–1245.

Sexton, T. L., Hingst, A. G., & Regan, K. A. (1985). The effect of divorce on the relationship between parental bonding and sex role identification of adult males. *Journal of Divorce, 9*, 17–31.

Shaffer, J. W., Duszynski, K. R., & Thomas, C. B. (1982). Family attitudes in youth as a possible precursor of cancer among physicians: A search for explanatory mechanisms. *Journal of Behavioral Medicine, 5*, 143–163.

Shaver, P. R., & Mikulincer, M. (2004). What do self-report attachment measures assess? In W. S. Rholes & J. A. Simpson (Eds.), *Adult attachment: Theory, research, and clinical implications* (pp. 17–54). New York: Guilford Press.

Shaver, P. R., & Mikulincer, M. (2007). Adult attachment strategies and the regulation of emotions. In J. J. Gross (Ed.), *Handbook of emotion regulation* (pp. 446–465). New York: Guilford Press.

Shulman, S., Scharf, M., Lumer, D., & Maurer, O. (2001). How young adults perceive parental divorce: The role of their relationships with their fathers and mothers. *Journal of Divorce and Remarriage, 34*, 3–17.

Simons, E. L., Lin, K.-H., Gordon, L. C., Conger, R. D., & Lorenz, F. O. (1999). Explaining the higher incidence of adjustment problems among children of divorce compared with those in two-parent families. *Journal of Marriage and the Family, 61*, 1020–1033.

Simos, B. G. (1979). *A time to grieve: Loss as a universal human experience*. New York: Family Services Association of America.

Simpson, J. A., Collins, W. A., Tran, S., & Haydon, K. C. (2007). Attachment and the experience and expression of emotions in romantic relationships: A developmental perspective. *Journal of Personality and Social Psychology, 92*, 355–367.

Simpson, J. A., Rholes, W. S., & Nelligan, J. S. (1992). Support seeking and support giving within couples in an anxiety-provoking situation: The role of attachment styles. *Journal of Personality and Social Psychology, 62*, 434–446.

Sinclair, S. L., & Nelson, E. S. (1998). The impact of parental divorce on college students' intimate relationships and relationship beliefs. *Journal of Divorce and Remarriage, 29*, 103–129.

Sirvanli-Ozen, D. (2005). Impacts of divorce on the behavior and adjustment problems, parenting styles, and attachment styles of children: Literature review including Turkish studies. *Journal of Divorce and Remarriage, 42*, 127–151.

Solomon, J., & George, C. (1999). The development of attachment in separated and divorced families: The effects of overnight visitation, parent and couple variables. *Attachment and Human Development, 1*, 2–33.

Southworth, S., & Schwartz, J. C. (1987). Post-divorce contact, relationship with father, and heterosexual trust in female college students. *American Journal of Orthopsychiatry, 57*, 371–382.

Spanier, G. B., & Casto, R. F. (1979). Adjustment to separation and divorce: An analysis of 50 case studies. *Journal of Divorce, 2*, 241–253.

Spanier, G. B., & Thompson, L. (1984). *Parting*. Beverly Hills, CA: Sage.

Sprague, H. E., & Kinney, J. M. (1997). The effects of interparental divorce and conflict on college students' romantic relationships. *Journal of Divorce and Remarriage, 27*, 85–104.

Sprecher, S., Cate, R., & Levin, L. (1998). Parental divorce and young adults' beliefs about love. *Journal of Divorce and Remarriage, 28*, 107–120.

Stack, S. (1990). New micro-level data on the impact of divorce on suicide, 1959–1980: A test of two theories. *Journal of Marriage and the Family, 52*, 119–127.

Stirtzinger, R., & Cholvat, L. (1991). The family home as attachment object for preschool age children after divorce. *Journal of Divorce and Remarriage, 15*, 105–124.

Summers, P., Forehand, R., Armistead, L., & Tannenbaum, L. (1998). Parental divorce during early adolescence in Caucasian families: The role of family process variables in predicting the long-term consequences for early adult psychosocial adjustment. *Journal of Consulting and Clinical Psychology, 66*, 327–336.

Sweeting, H., & West, P. (1995). Family life and health in adolescence: A role for culture in the health inequalities debate? *Social Science and Medicine, 40*, 163–175.

Tayler, L., Parker, G., & Roy, K. (1995). Parental divorce and its effects on the quality of intimate relationships in adulthood. *Journal of Divorce and Remarriage, 24*, 181–202.

Todorski, J. (1995). Attachment and divorce: A therapeutic view. *Journal of Divorce and Remarriage, 22*, 189–204.

Toews, M. L., McKenry, P. C., & Catlett, B. S. (2003). Male-initiated partner abuse during marital separation prior to divorce. *Violence and Victims, 18*, 387–402.

Troxel, W. M., & Matthews, K. A. (2004). What are the costs of marital conflict and dissolution to children's physical health? *Clinical Child and Family Psychological Review, 7*, 29–57.

Tucker, J. S., Friedman, H. S., Schwartz, J. E., Criqui, M. H., Tomlinson-Keasey, C., Wingard, D. L., et al. (1997). Parental divorce: Effects on individual behavior and longevity. *Journal of Personality and Social Psychology, 73*, 381–391.

Umberson, D. (1987). Family status and health behaviors: Social control as a dimension of social integration. *Journal of Health and Social Behavior, 28*, 306–319.

Vareschi, C. G., & Bursik, K. (2005). Attachment style differences in the parental interactions and adaptation patterns of divorcing parents. *Journal of Divorce and Remarriage, 42*, 15–32.

Vaughn, B., Gove, F., & Egeland, B. (1980). The relationship between out-of-home care and the quality of infant–mother attachment in an economically disadvantaged population. *Child Development, 51*, 1203–1214.

Verbrugge, L. M. (1979). Marital status and health. *Journal of Marriage and the Family, 41*, 267–285.

Wade, T. J., & Pevalin, D. J. (2004). Marital transitions and mental health. *Journal of Health and Social Behavior, 45*, 155–170.

Walker, T. R., & Ehrenberg, M. F. (1998). An exploratory study of young persons' attachment styles and perceived reasons for parental divorce. *Journal of Adolescent Research, 13*, 320–342.

Wallerstein, J. S., & Blakeslee, S. (1989). *Second chances: Men, women, and children a decade after divorce.* New York: Ticknor & Fields.

Wallerstein, J. S., & Lewis, J. M. (2004). The unexpected legacy of divorce: Report of a 25-year study. *Psychoanalytic Psychology, 21*, 353–370.

Waters, E., & Deane, K. E. (1985). Defining and assessing individual differences in attachment relationships: Q-methodology and the organization of behavior in infancy and early childhood. In I. Bretherton & E. Waters (Eds.), Growing points of attachment theory and research. *Monographs of the Society for Research in Child Development, 50*(1–2, Serial No. 209), 41–65.

Waters, E., Merrick, S., Treboux, D., Crowell, J., & Albersheim, L. (2000). Attachment security in infancy and early adulthood: A twenty-year longitudinal study. *Child Development, 71*, 684–689.

Weiss, R. S. (1975). *Marital separation*. New York: Basic Books.

Weiss, R. S. (1976). The emotional impact of marital separation. *Journal of Social Issues, 32*, 135–145.

Weiss, R. S. (1979). *Going it alone*. New York: Basic Books.

West, M., & Sheldon-Keller, A. (1992). The assessment of dimensions relevant to adult reciprocal attachment. *Canadian Journal of Psychiatry, 37*, 600–606.

Williams, K., & Umberson, D. (2004). Marital status, marital transitions, and health: A gendered life course perspective. *Journal of Health and Social Behavior, 45*, 81–98.

Wolchik, S. A., Tein, J.-Y., Sandler, I. N., & Doyle, K. W. (2002). Fear of abandonment as a mediator of the relations between divorce stressors and mother–child relationship quality and children's adjustment problems. *Journal of Abnormal Child Psychology, 30*, 401–418.

Wolchik, S. A., Wilcox, K. L., Tein, J.-Y., & Sandler, I. N. (2000). An experimental evaluation of theory-based mother and mother–child programs for children of divorce. *Journal of Consulting and Clinical Psychology, 68*, 843–856.

Wolfinger, N. H. (2000). Beyond the intergenerational transition of divorce: Do people replicate the patterns of marital instability they grew up with? *Journal of Family Issues, 21*, 1061–1086.

Zill, N., Morrison, D. R., & Coiro, M. J. (1993). Long-term effects of parental divorce on parent–child relationships, adjustment, and achievement in young adulthood. *Journal of Family Psychology, 7*, 91–103.

CHAPTER 40

Implications of Attachment Theory and Research for Child Care Policies

MICHAEL RUTTER

Attachment theory was derived in large part from insights gained through clinical observations of children in institutional care, as well as of children who had been separated from or who had lost one or both parents (Bowlby, 1951, 1969/1982). Initially, therefore, there was an explicit concern to improve child care policies (Rutter & O'Connor, 1999). However, it was equally the case that Bowlby sought to bring about a conceptual integration between the processes involved in normal and abnormal development, and an integration between biological and social influences. His approach to the development of attachment theory was revolutionary in several key respects.

First, despite his psychoanalytic background, Bowlby relied heavily on empirical findings from observational studies of both humans and other animals. He insisted on the importance of children's real-life experiences and not just their internal thought processes. More than anything else, this led to an initially extremely hostile response from the psychoanalytic camp (see Rutter, 1995, 2002).

Second, Bowlby gave primacy to a biologically based need for social relationships, rather than to feeding or to sexual motives—again bringing him into conflict with psychoanalysis. As he put

it in 1988, psychoanalysis was never more wrong than in its conceptualization of the processes involved in psychological development.

Third, Bowlby focused on the importance of love relationships as they develop over time between parent and child, rather than on the here-and-now perceptual stimulation or reinforcement favored by behaviorist theories (see, e.g., Casler, 1968; Gewirtz, 1972). This shift played a role in the initially critical response of many academic psychologists to attachment theory (see, e.g., O'Connor & Franks, 1960). Interestingly, Harlow's studies of rhesus monkeys (Harlow & Zimmerman, 1959) were as influential in supporting Bowlby's emphasis on mother love (see also Blum, 2002) as were the Robertsons' studies of children admitted to hospitals or residential nurseries (Robertson & Robertson, 1971).

However, Bowlby's development of attachment theory was revolutionary not just in its overall conceptual approach, but also in several key specifics. Most crucially, attachment theory replaced the general undifferentiated notion of "mother love" with a specific postulated biological mechanism by which early parent–child relationships might shape psychological development. Specifically, Bowlby proposed that the development of selective attachments serves a biological purpose in providing emotional support and protection against stress. He thereby differentiated attachment from other components of relationships. In particular, it was found that whereas anxiety intensifies attachment (in keeping with its hypothesized protective role), it inhibits play and playful social interactions. Research has broadly confirmed the validity of these tenets (Barrett, 2006; Rajecki, Lamb, & Obmascher, 1978; Rutter, 1981). In his emphasis on these special qualities, Bowlby indicated that attachment does *not* constitute the whole of social relationships. The success of attachment theory has sometimes led uncritical enthusiasts to neglect the rest of social interactions and relationships (see Dunn, 1993, and Sroufe, 1988, for warnings about this). As discussed below, this remains an issue with respect to child care policy implications.

A further revolutionary feature of attachment theory was the postulate that early infant–parent attachment is not just a transient feature of infantile dependency that is outgrown with further development; rather, it represents a psychological need that persists throughout the whole of life. It was argued that loving support is an important protective feature in old age just as much as in infancy. Attachment theory was a lifespan theory and not just an infancy theory. It was proposed that early child–parent selective attachments constitute the basis of all later intense reciprocal relationships—including love relationships and the relationship of providing parenting and not just receiving it. Of course, it was recognized from the outset that these later relationships differ in some crucial respects from the early selective attachments of infancy, but they were thought to share an essentially identical core. As discussed below, however, the issue of how to conceptualize and measure attachment security in the postinfancy years remains essentially unresolved.

Another important feature of attachment theory was its strong emphasis on cognitive processes to account for how the effects of early relationships may be carried forward into later life (Bowlby, 1973, 1980). Internal working models were proposed. Bowlby recognized that although initially attachment is a dyadic feature, nevertheless over time it comes to be a more general feature that characterizes people's functioning more broadly and not just with respect to one specific relationship. There is a good deal of support for the general proposition that people do indeed conceptualize their social relationships and thereby form

concepts about themselves and about other people (Bretherton, 1995; Bretherton & Munholland, 1999 and Chapter 5, this volume). But as Hinde (1988) pointed out, the concepts remain too general to be susceptible to critical testing. This is so despite considerable progress in the measurement of internal representations of relationships, as described in several chapters of this volume.

A crucial feature of attachment theory was that it postulated substantial differences in the qualities of different attachment relationships—with a focus on the extent to which a relationship provides security. Ainsworth's (1967; Ainsworth, Blehar, Waters, & Wall, 1978) development of the Strange Situation procedure provided an effective operationalized measure of these postulated qualities. Although it might seem too much to expect that a mere 25-minute period of observation could tap the essential qualities of attachment security, this assessment procedure has stood the test of time remarkably well (Barrett, 2006; Greenberg, 1999; Sroufe, 1983), despite concerns about cultural variations (discussed by van IJzendoorn & Sagi-Schwartz, Chapter 37, this volume). Nevertheless, in keeping with attachment theory's roots in detailed naturalistic observations, careful studies of extreme groups have led to a recognition of the need to tap other dimensions, such as "disorganization" (Main & Solomon, 1986, 1990), and to diagnose attachment disorders that involve qualities other than security versus insecurity (see Zeanah & Smyke, 2008; Zeanah et al., 2004). The issues that these new concepts have created for child care policies are crucially important but far from resolved.

EARLY EFFECTS OF ATTACHMENT CONCEPTS ON CHILD CARE POLICIES

Along with this historical background, mention must be made, before I turn to contemporary matters, of the early effects of attachment concepts on child care policies. Actually, the first main impact on child care came from Bowlby's (1951) World Health Organization (WHO) monograph, and not from his exposition of attachment theory some 18 years later (Bowlby, 1969/1982)—although the two were always closely linked in his own writings. People were shocked by the findings on children in institutions and were persuaded—not just by Bowlby's writings, but also by the Robertsons' films (Robertson & Robertson, 1971)—that the apathy and loss of interest shown by many young children in residential care represented a negative reaction and not contentment.

The link with attachment theory, as it later developed, lay in Bowlby's postulate that the damaging feature was the lack of personalized care and hence the lack of opportunity to develop selective attachments. Over time, this led to a virtual revolution in patterns of hospital care for children (Rutter, 1979) and in the use of residential nurseries as a means of caring for children who had experienced a breakdown in parenting (Triseliotis & Russell, 1984). After a period of foot dragging in medical circles, hospital policies were changed to allow first regular daily visiting by parents, then unrestricted visiting, and then encouragement for parents to stay overnight in hospitals with their young children.

Importantly, however, there was not a narrow reliance on attachment considerations; Bowlby was also concerned with broader aspects of hospital experiences. Play activities and schooling became more generally available in hospital units for children, and increasingly children were prepared psychologically for what hospital admission might involve. Furthermore, even when highly specialized medical and surgical wards were needed, pediatricians were given overall responsibility for general care with respect to all children's hospital experiences beyond the specialized treatment of their illness or injury. Parental pressure groups, as much as attachment theory, played a key role in these changes. Nevertheless, although it would be misleading to claim that all is well in all hospitals, patterns of hospital care in the 21st century could scarcely be more different from those prevailing half a century ago.

The second revolution concerned the virtual abandonment of residential nurseries and orphanages as a first-choice solution for young children whose parents could no longer care for them for one reason or another (Cliffe & Berridge, 1991). Instead, there was increasing use of long-term as well as short-term foster care. The aim, in line with attachment theory, was to provide personalized care in a family context that offered an opportunity for continuity over time in relationships. Unfortunately, the consequences were not as satisfactory as the aims. To begin with, although large orphanages providing group residential care have largely been phased out in most industrialized countries, this has not been the case worldwide (see Groark & McCall, 2008; Vorria, Rutter, Pickles, Wolkind, & Hobsbaum, 1998a, 1998b; Zeanah et al., 2003). Second, even when residential care has been pro-

vided in more individualized, family-style small groups (see King, Raynes, & Tizard, 1971; Tizard & Tizard, 1971), an extremely high level of staff turnover is the norm. Thus Tizard (1977) reported that in the nurseries she studied, each child had had an average of 24 different caregivers by the age of 2 years, and double that number by age 5. The problem has not been ignorance (or ignoring) of attachment theory, so much as a societal unwillingness to make the necessary investment in child care.

The third problem was that all too often, residential care staff adopted an emotionally detached style to prevent children from becoming too distressed when a staff member had to leave. This tendency stemmed from Bowlby's (1951) report in which the risks were conceptualized as stemming from separation. Bowlby's own research (Bowlby, Ainsworth, Boston, & Rosenbluth, 1956), as well as that of others, soon showed that the main risk did not derive from the separation as such; rather, it stemmed either from a lack of an ongoing attachment relationship or from family discord, conflict, disorganization, or neglect. Often it takes some years for new ideas to catch on, but frequently it takes even longer for them to be put aside when they are not supported by empirical research.

The fourth problem came from the observed very high rate of breakdown in foster family placements (Berridge & Cleaver, 1987; Parker, Ward, Jackson, Aldgate, & Wedge, 1991). The difficulty did not stem from limitations in attachment theory, but rather from a serious failure to deal with the numerous practical difficulties involved. Regrettably, there has been very little progress on this problem in recent years.

The fifth problem concerned the inappropriate generalization of findings on residential care to day care (see the WHO Expert Committee on Mental Health's [1951] warning on the supposedly permanent deleterious effects of day nurseries and crèches). The lesson here lies in the need to look closely at the research evidence, and not to jump to premature conclusions based on unwarranted extrapolations. Nevertheless, the controversies over day care have not gone away, as discussed below.

The third revolutionary effect of attachment theory on child care policies has concerned legal discussion of custody and contact following parental divorce or separation (Bretherton, Walsh, Lependorf, & Georgeson, 1997) and in relation to applications by social parents to adopt when the biological parents withdraw permission (Hale

& Fortin, 2008). In the past, especially in North America, psychoanalytic theory tended to provide the main basis for decisions (see, e.g., Goldstein, Freud, Solnit, & Goldstein, 1986); increasingly, however, attachment theory has come to replace it. The positive aspect of this shift has been the attention to the reality of ongoing relationships, but the negative aspect has been a tendency to focus on whether the children concerned are, or are not, "attached" or "bonded" to the various adults disputing who should care for the children. In part, this focus represents a failure to appreciate that attachment theory emphasizes the security of attachments and not just their presence. Also, however, it probably stems from the categorical nature of attachment security designations. This is an issue considered further below.

CURRENT INTERCONNECTIONS BETWEEN ATTACHMENT THEORY AND CHILD CARE POLICY

As noted, social policies concerning the care of children constituted a driving force in Bowlby's initial development of attachment theory (Bowlby, 1969/1982). Since then, despite its continuing relevance (see Schaffer, 1990), for quite some time there seems to have been a considerable weakening of the connections between the two. It is not that there has been any failure to appreciate the importance of attachment theory; on the contrary, it is widely invoked with respect to all sorts of social policy issues. Rather, the dilemma lies in the difficulties in applying attachment concepts in a vigorous and discriminating way to complicated issues of policy and practice (see Barrett, 2006; Kraemer & Roberts, 1996). Nevertheless, the last decade has seen an important resurgence in the study of attachment features in extreme situations, and hence in the more considered application of attachment concepts to key issues in policy and practice. In this substantial section of this chapter, therefore, I pay attention to nine main topics: (1) attachment disorders, (2) neural underpinnings, (3) attachment therapies, (4) measurement issues, (5) continuities and discontinuities over the lifespan, (6) group day care and other forms of nonmaternal care, (7) divorce and separation, (8) the search for biological parents by individuals not reared by them, and (9) assisted conception. In the tradition set by Bowlby, Ainsworth, and Main, I focus the discussion as much on the implications of research on unusual groups for attachment theory and attachment measures as on the implica-

tions of the theory and measures for treatment of particular groups. Similarly, and again in line with the thinking of the attachment theory pioneers, I consider the extent to which the social policy issues are best tackled by reference to attachment theory rather than through other theoretical and empirical approaches.

Attachment Disorders

From the very first studies of children being reared in institutions some 60 years ago, there has been an emphasis on the high frequency of markedly atypical and apparently maladaptive patterns of social relationships. Supposedly indiscriminate friendliness was the feature most emphasized in children who had been in institutions in infancy and had remained there (Wolkind, 1974). In many ways, the most influential of the early studies was Tizard's investigation of young children placed in residential nurseries in London in the 1960s (Tizard & Hodges, 1978; Tizard & Rees, 1975). When assessed at the age of 4 years, just under a third were emotionally withdrawn and unresponsive, and just over a third were indiscriminate in approaching and seeking attention from relative strangers as well as from familiar caregivers. In keeping with these findings, together with more extensive clinical reports, the diagnostic concept of two different forms of reactive attachment disorder (RAD)—the emotionally withdrawn/inhibited type and the indiscriminately social/disinhibited type—has been included in both the American Psychiatric Association (2000) and WHO (1992) psychiatric classifications. Zeanah and colleagues (2004) have suggested that the criteria for the inhibited variety should include (1) absence of a discriminated, preferred attachment figure; (2) lack of comfort seeking when distressed; (3) failure to respond when comfort is offered; (4) lack of social and emotional reciprocity; and (5) emotion regulation difficulties.

Smyke, Dumitrescu, and Zeanah (2002), studying children within a Romanian institution, found both types of RAD much more common than in a never-institutionalized community group attending child care. Part of the Bucharest Early Intervention Project (Zeanah et al., 2003) compared 95 children who had spent almost all their life in institutions with a sample of 50 Romanian children who had never been institutionalized and who were recruited from pediatric clinics. An interview to assess disturbances of attachment was used with caregivers; the first five items in the interview dealt with emotionally withdrawn/ inhibited RAD, and the next three items with indiscriminately social/disinhibited RAD. The Ainsworth Strange Situation was used for both groups and was scored both categorically and dimensionally. Children were assessed at a mean age of just below 2 years. The two samples were demographically similar, except for the relevant feature that a much higher proportion of the institutional group was Roma (32% vs. 6%). The scores for the institutional children were much higher than those of the never-institutionalized sample for both types of RAD. The between-group difference was greatest for the most abnormal scores. The findings therefore confirmed the postulate that both types of RAD were particularly common in children who had been reared in institutions from infancy. An organized or disorganized attachment, as assessed with the Strange Situation, was not significantly related to either type of RAD.

Nevertheless, there was an important difference between the two varieties of RAD in their correlates. Continuous ratings of attachment in the Strange Situation were moderately correlated ($r = -.44$) with withdrawn/inhibited RAD, but not with indiscriminately social/disinhibited RAD ($r = -.16$). Similarly, in the institutionalized group, the quality of caregiving was related to withdrawn/ inhibited RAD scores ($r = -.32$), but not to indiscriminately social/disinhibited RAD scores ($r = -.14$). The implication would seem to be that the inhibited variety of RAD is related to traditional concepts of attachment insecurity, but that the disinhibited variety of RAD has a different meaning, despite the fact that both types were more common in the institutional groups. It might be suggested that the disinhibited variety of RAD represents a relative failure to develop selective attachments, rather than the development of selective attachments that are insecure.

We (Rutter et al., 2007) similarly sought to examine the validity of the designation of disinhibited attachment. The study differed from the Bucharest study in that the children had all left the institutions by at least the age of 3½ years and had been adopted into generally well-functioning U.K. families. The study also differed in having longitudinal data extending from 6 to 11 years of age and in having a broader range of measures of psychopathology, as well as ratings based on a form of the Strange Situation modified for use in the home (O'Connor, Marvin, Rutter, Olrick, & Britner, 2003). In addition, there were investigator ratings of the children's observed behavior.

Several findings were important with respect to the validity of the concept. First, marked disinhibited attachment was much more common in the group of children who had been institution-reared in Romania than in a comparison group of noninstitutionalized children adopted within the United Kingdom before the age of 6 months. Mild evidence of disinhibited attachment was equally common in the two groups, but this seemed to have a quite different meaning in each group. In the institution-reared sample from Romania, both mild and marked forms of disinhibited behavior proved remarkably persistent from age 6 to age 11. By contrast, mild disinhibition in the comparison group did not persist and was usually followed by ratings of normal behavior at age 11. The investigator ratings showed that the children with disinhibited attachment in the institutional group tended to be unusually physically intrusive and to violate conventional social boundaries. The findings showed that disinhibited attachment was not just an unusual pattern of behavior that was particularly common in children reared in institutions; it was also associated with a much increased rate of psychopathology in other domains of functioning. The great majority of the children with this pattern had had either mental health services involvement, special educational provision, or (most often) both. Nevertheless, despite the association with other forms of psychopathology, the evidence indicated that the disinhibited attachment was not a consequence of other psychopathology. Thus, of the children who developed new emotional disorders or conduct problems between the ages of 6 and 11, scarcely any showed a pattern of disinhibited attachment.

The findings of these two studies taken together strongly suggest that the disinhibited variety of RAD is not only much commoner in institution-reared children than in other children; it is also a pattern associated with substantial malfunction, and one that follows a rather persistent course. In other words, unlike what would be expected of insecure attachment, it did not show responsiveness to the change from a seriously depriving institutional environment to a normal family upbringing. Both at age 4 (O'Connor et al., 2003) and at age 6 (Rutter et al., 2007), the study showed weak associations with insecurity of attachment as measured in the modified form of the Strange Situation. It was not that the children's behavior was normal in the situation, but rather that the abnormality lay in unusual features of the interaction with the stranger in a pattern designated "other-insecure." Although it was labeled as a variety of insecurity, the overall evidence suggests that this is a misleading descriptor. It is clearly an abnormal pattern, but it is not like ordinary varieties of insecurity. Similarly, in a Canadian study of institution-reared children adopted from Romania into Canadian families, measures of indiscriminate friendliness did not map well onto measures of security of attachment (see also Maclean, 2003).

Although it has been usual for attachment researchers to regard attachment security measured in the Strange Situation as the preferred, most adaptive pattern, there has been a recognition from the outset that attachment insecurity should not be considered as synonymous with any form of disorder (Ainsworth et al., 1978). When children from seriously adverse backgrounds were studied, it became clear that there were unusual patterns of attachment security that were not picked up by the traditional categorizations. The category of "disorganized" attachment (Main & Solomon, 1990) was developed to designate children who appeared to have impaired organization of a response to separation (and other forms of adversity). Main and Solomon (1986, 1990) highlighted sequential displays of contradictory behavior; misdirected or interrupted patterns, stereotypies, and anomalous postures; freezing; apprehension regarding the parent; and direct indices of disorganization. Crittenden (1985, 1988) similarly developed a way of coding such atypical patterns, but with somewhat different criteria.

High rates of disorganized attachment have been found in high-risk samples (usually well over half), as compared with a rate of about 15% in low-risk families (van IJzendoorn, Schuengel, & Bakermans-Kranenburg, 1999). Several studies, too, have shown that disorganized attachment tends to predict later psychopathology (for reviews, see Green & Goldwyn, 2002; Lyons-Ruth & Jacobvitz, 1999 and Chapter 28, this volume). Because of these findings, there has been some tendency to view disorganized attachment, although it is not an attachment disorder as such, as rather close to one. Vorria and colleagues (2003), in a study of 11- to 17-month-old infants in a Greek institution, found a rate of 66% disorganized attachment, as against 25% in a community comparison group. Similarly, Zeanah, Smyke, Koga, Carlson, and The Bucharest Early Intervention Project Core Group (2005), in their study of children in Romanian institutions, found that 65% showed disorganized attachment as compared with 22% in a never-institutionalized group. Because disorga-

nized attachment has been found in a wide range of high-risk families, it does not seem to have the highly specific association with an institutional rearing that RAD has. Clearly, it is a feature of some predictive importance, but there is still some uncertainty as to exactly what it is reflecting.

Because attachment insecurity of one sort or another has been associated with most forms of psychopathology, it might seem that there should be a very broad spectrum of attachment-related disorders. Although there is indeed good reason to suppose that disturbances in social relationships are implicated in the development of much psychopathology, the lack of diagnostic specificity would seem to argue against any concept of a broad spectrum of attachment disorders. The two varieties of RAD may reasonably be regarded as distinctive categories, although the evidence is greater in the case of disinhibited attachment. Although Zeanah (1996) raised queries over a decade ago as to whether RAD should legitimately be classified as an attachment disorder, the evidence would seem to justify it. Disinhibited attachment disorder differs from other forms of psychopathology with respect to the centrality of the disturbance of attachment behavior, and it warrants being distinguished from ordinary varieties of insecurity—both because of its lack of association with security as measured by the Strange Situation and because the high degree of persistence after the adoption of institution-reared children indicates an unusual lack of response to changed rearing circumstances.

The situation with respect to the inhibited variety of RAD is more complicated. Zeanah and colleagues (2004, 2005) produced good evidence for its association not only with an institutional rearing, but also with maltreatment (although, as always, independent replications are needed). It is not quite so obvious how it should be differentiated from the various forms of attachment insecurity. The lack of organization and the strong association with institutional care warrant its retention as a distinct classification, but further studies are needed to determine the processes involved in its development. Also, for the reasons given, it should not be conceptualized as an attachment disorder as such.

Neural Underpinnings

The last decade or so has seen an outpouring of claims regarding the supposed effects of experiences on the brain (see, e.g., Gerhardt, 2004; Schore,

1994, 2001a, 2001b). It is important to emphasize (1) that these claims represent speculative extrapolations from the findings of neuroscience, and not empirically demonstrated causal connections; and (2) that the supposition that all the "action" with respect to brain development takes place in the first 3 years is simply wrong (Bruer, 1999). Nevertheless, the findings on the disinhibited variety of RAD have raised important queries about a possible early sensitive period for the establishment of normal selective attachments (Rutter et al., 2007). The U.K. study of adoptees from profoundly depriving Romanian institutions found that although no persisting adverse sequelae were detectable in the case of children who came to the United Kingdom under the age of 6 months, there was a markedly increased rate of disinhibited RAD in children who left institutional care at ages over 6 months. It is crucial to emphasize, however, that the finding reflects the effects of prolonged institutional deprivation. It does *not* mean that normal selective attachments cannot develop after 6 months. In the first place, in all ordinary circumstances they do not usually become well established until the second half of the first year. Also, studies of children adopted after the age of 1 or 2 years have shown that the majority do develop attachment relationships with their adoptive parents, most of which appear secure (Hodges & Tizard, 1989a, 1989b; Vorria at al., 2006). Although there can be no doubt that the development of secure attachments has neural underpinnings, the evidence is not available to substantiate claims on either the presence or limits of a sensitive period, and certainly not to draw conclusions about implications for therapeutic practice.

Attachment Therapies

Numerous so-called "attachment therapies" have been developed, together with often strong claims regarding their supposed efficacy. Four main points stand out (Barrett, 2006; O'Connor & Zeanah, 2003). First, not only do most of them appear not to derive from the usually understood tenets of attachment theory, but some seem to use approaches that run directly counter to such tenets. This would apply, for example, to the forms of holding therapy that provoke anger in order to impose physical constraint. Second, such highly intrusive techniques carry real risks and have occasionally led to death. Third, these unconventional techniques are unevaluated and lack any evidence of their value. Fourth, there are a few psychological interventions

that do appear to reflect attachment principles and that have been subject to limited evaluations (Bakermans-Kranenburg, van IJzendoorn, & Jutter, 2003; Berlin, Ziv, Amaya-Jackson, & Greenberg, 2005; van IJzendoorn, Juffer, & Duyvesteyn, 1995). Thus Juffer, Bakermans-Kranenburg, and van IJzendoorn (2005) undertook a randomized controlled trial with 130 families, each with a 6-month-old adopted child. Video feedback focusing on maternal sensitivity was compared with booklet information. The main aim was to reduce disorganized attachment. The findings showed a significant reduction in disorganized attachment and an improvement in maternal sensitivity, although interestingly the latter effect did not mediate the former. The study was a good one and, together with other evidence (e.g., Cohen et al., 1999, 2002; Marvin, Cooper, Hoffman, & Powell, 2002; van den Boom, 1994; see Berlin, Zeanah, & Lieberman, Chapter 31, this volume) suggests the possible value of interventions focused on maternal sensitivity. Nevertheless, caution is indicated for several reasons: Babies adopted before the age of 6 months do not constitute a high-risk group; the initial rate of disorganized attachment was not much different from that found in normal general population samples; maternal sensitivity has only a weak association with disorganized attachment; and the children were not suffering from RAD. Clearly, the treatment of such disorders remains a substantial challenge for the future. What is surprising is that none of the interventions specifically intended to prevent disorganized attachment have focused on the frightening/frightened parental behaviors that are supposed to constitute the main risk factor (van IJzendoorn, Bakermans-Kranenburg, & Juffer, 2005). Such a focus would seem to be a logical next step, and it should be helpful that there are now measures of these parental behaviors (Abrams, Rifkin, & Hesse, 2006; Hesse & Main, 2006; Jacobvitz, Leon, & Hazen, 2006).

Somewhat similar issues apply to Cohen and colleagues' (1999, 2002) Watch, Wait, and Wonder (WWW) program, used with 10- to 30-month-old infants referred to a clinic for a variety of problems. The WWW approach focused on infant-led activities between mother and child, with the goal of helping mothers reflect on the interactions in order to become more appropriately responsive. WWW was compared, in a quasi-random assignment design, with a more parent-led approach. Both methods yielded behavioral gains, but the WWW method did so faster. The method follows attachment theory concepts, but the findings are limited by the fact that attachment disorders were not the main problem.

Howe and Fearnley (2003) have described the approach used in the U.K. Keys Attachment Centre. The method is said to provide a "corrective emotional experience" that approximates what should have occurred in the child's formative years, using nonabusive "bonding" behaviors. There is an equal focus on therapist–child and caregiver–child interactions, and cognitive restructuring is a key objective. Hart and Thomas (2000) urge the value of parent cotherapy for fostered and adopted children, on the grounds that the foster/adoptive parents have not been responsible for the attachment problems, but the need is for them to provide the appropriate rearing conditions to foster recovery.

Probably the fullest account of how attachment theory may be used to guide treatment methods when dealing with attachment-related problems is that provided by Brisch (2002), based on Bowlby's (1988) suggestions, and by the range of reports in Berlin and colleagues (2005). Brisch emphasized the need for child therapists to provide secure, caring interactions that can facilitate the development of secure attachments; to interpret and foster emotional expression in relation to attachment issues; and to integrate these with similar concerns in relation to parents. The approach is different from behavioral methods in focusing on relationships rather than maladaptive symptoms, and it differs from psychoanalytic methods in focusing on real-life experiences and on ongoing relationships rather than internal conflicts. It shows, however, a recognition of the need to be concerned with internal working models and mental sets.

As with the other approaches noted, Brisch's book deals mainly with a broad application of attachment concepts, rather than with the treatment of attachment disorders per se. The same is the case with many of the high-quality interventions described in Berlin and colleagues (2005), but there are three programs designed to deal with attachment disorders in fostered or adopted children (see Dozier, Lindhiem, & Ackerman, 2005; Zeanah & Smyke, 2005). These are discussed elsewhere in this volume (Dozier & Rutter, Chapter 29). It may be concluded that attachment concepts have been helpful in suggesting how psychological interventions might be adapted to deal with attachment disorders, but that up to now these interventions remain untested and unevaluated extrapolations.

Measurement Issues

The categorical conceptualization of attachment security according to B, A, and C patterns has become the standard method of scoring children's behavior in the Strange Situation. Nevertheless, the notion of discrete categories is not an essential part of attachment theory; most coders initially rate several interactive behavior dimensions, and Ainsworth and colleagues (1978) noted that 92% of their sample could be correctly classified on the basis of a linear combination of such behavioral ratings. Since then, there have been many other attempts to develop multidimensional scales (see Cassidy, 2003). The issues were brought to the fore by Fraley and Spieker's (2003a, 2003b) application of Meehl's taxometric techniques to the National Institute of Child Health and Human Development (NICHD) Early Child Care Research Network (1997) attachment data collected when children were 15 months of age. Fraley and Spieker argued that their findings suggested that variations in attachment security were largely continuous rather than categorical.

The measurement issues, however, are more complex than that. Moreover, a major strength of the attachment approach has been a reliance on observed behaviors, rather than predetermined theory or statistical modeling. Thus Main and Solomon (1986) noted anomalous responses to the Strange Situation that could not be encompassed by the B, A, and C categories. This led to the development of the "disorganized" (D) construct. This construct could be dealt with either categorically or dimensionally, but, most crucially, it was an important feature that was additional to the concept of security–insecurity. Further research showed that it also differed in having a stronger association with psychopathology (van IJzendoorn et al., 1999). More recently, studies of children in severely depriving institutions have shown that their responses to the Strange Situation are different in ways that are not well encompassed by either the standard B, A, and C categories *or* the D category, necessitating yet a further "other" category (O'Connor et al., 2003; Rutter et al., 2007). Fraley and Spieker (2003a, 2003b) argued for a two-dimensional approach, based first on proximity-seeking versus avoidant strategies and second on angry versus resistant strategies. These may well constitute useful dimensions, but the NICHD data did not allow consideration of either "disorganization" or "other" constructs. As Juffer and colleagues (2005) have shown, however, both "disorganization" and "security" can be reliably dimensionalized. Similarly, Zeanah and colleagues (2004) showed the same with the two varieties of RAD.

At least three other measurement issues are important. First, in order to study unusual samples that may be geographically scattered, there was a need to modify the Strange Situation for use in home settings. The procedure developed by Marvin (O'Connor et al., 2003) served that purpose. Second, the Strange Situation relies on the "press" provided by a separation–reunion procedure, and this becomes increasingly less relevant as children grow older. Various measures have been devised (see Barrett, 2006), including Waters's (1987) Q-sort based on observation sessions of caregivers with 1- to 5-year-old children. In addition, there are many questionnaire measures designed for adolescents and adults (see, e.g., Hazan & Shaver, 1987; Hazan & Zeifman, 1999; Mikulincer & Shaver, 2007). The limited available evidence suggests that there are only rather modest correlations between the Strange Situation and Waters's Q-sort categories (van IJzendoorn, Vereijken, Bakermans-Kranenburg, & Riksen-Walraven, 2004), and little is known about the extent to which the adult measures map onto childhood security categories. The Q-sort does not assess disorganization. The third issue concerns the shift from the dyadic Strange Situation measure to more generalized internal working models or mental sets that apply to individuals' views of themselves and their relationships with others more generally. The Adult Attachment Interview (AAI) devised by Mary Main and her colleagues (George, Kaplan, & Main, 1985) provides the prototype, but there are childhood procedures that are similar in their focus on mental representations rather than observed behaviors. These include the Slough and Greenberg (1990) separation anxiety test based on children's responses to pictures, and the Attachment Story Completion Task (ASCT) based on 3- to 7-year-old children's completion of stress-arousing stories (Bretherton, Ridgeway, & Cassidy, 1990; Hodges, Steele, Hillman, Henderson, & Kaniuk, 2003). The Vorria and colleagues (2006) comparison of adopted children and comparison children showed differences on ASCT responses, but these were unrelated to preadoption attachment security as measured in infancy.

It is good that a reasonable range of measures tapping key aspects of attachment are available. Nevertheless, the limited agreement among them, together with the fact that they tap rather different constructs, clearly makes for difficulties in assessing both continuities–discontinuities over the lifespan and the quality of functioning in clinical (or otherwise atypical) groups.

Continuities and Discontinuities across the Lifespan

The early writings on attachment security, almost always assessed with the Strange Situation, tended to emphasize the extent to which insecurity is a stable feature and mediates a wider range of later forms of maladjustment or psychopathology (see, e.g., Hamilton, 2000; Sroufe, 1983; Waters, Hamilton, & Weinfield, 2000). Because of the assumption that maternal sensitivity constitutes the main influence on security–insecurity, the implication drawn was of the great long-term importance of early parent–child relationships. This was reinforced by the evidence from one study (Fonagy, Steele, & Steele, 1991) showing that maternal representations of attachment during pregnancy predicted the organization of infant–mother attachment at 1 year of age. Recent research requires a substantial reassessment of the findings on both the role of maternal sensitivity and the stability of attachment security–insecurity. The meta-analysis undertaken by De Wolff and van IJzendoorn (1997) showed a correlation of only .24 for maternal sensitivity, and a later meta-analysis by Atkinson and colleagues (2000) similarly found a correlation of .27. The implication is clear that although the quality of parent–child relationships may well be crucial, the key qualities are by no means encompassed by the concept of sensitivity.

Comparable reassessments are needed with respect to the long-term stability of assessments of attachment security–insecurity, as shown by a most useful bringing together of the findings of the main long-term studies extending from infancy into adult life (Grossmann, Grossmann, & Waters, 2005; see also Sroufe, Egeland, Carlson, & Collins, 2005). The bottom-line message is that on its own, attachment security in infancy constitutes a very weak predictor of adult functioning, accounting for only some 5% of the variance. On the other hand, when combined with other social measures at somewhat later ages, social relationships in childhood constitutes a powerful predictor of adult functioning, accounting for nearly half of the total variance (Rutter, 2006). It may be concluded that early selective attachments play a significant role in the overall development of close social relationships in later life. What remain to be determined, however, are just how the different social relationship features come together, and what causal processes are involved.

These findings all apply to attachment security–insecurity as assessed in the traditional way, and it is necessary to ask similar questions about disorganized attachment. The van IJzendoorn and colleagues (1999) meta-analysis showed clearly that whereas it occurred in some 15% of low-risk samples, it was present in 40–50% of maltreated children. Moreover, some two-thirds of institution-reared children have been found to have disorganized attachment (Vorria et al., 2003; Zeanah et al., 2005). Accordingly, the contemporaneous association with serious abnormalities in childrearing is strong. But in view of the 15% rate in normal samples, disorganized attachment cannot sensibly be viewed as a disorder in its own right. Indeed, Crittenden and Claussen (2000) have even suggested that it might constitute an adaptive response to particularly difficult circumstances. Possibly in line with that suggestion is the (as yet to be replicated) finding by Vorria and colleagues (2006) that disorganized attachment in children being reared in institutions actually constituted a predictor of greater postadoption security. It is also noteworthy that maternal sensitivity has only a very weak association with disorganized attachment—.10 to .15 in the De Wolff and IJzendoorn (1997) and van IJzendoorn and colleagues meta-analyses. At present, there is no good reason to conclude that disorganized attachment differs in important ways from the ordinary forms of attachment insecurity, but we know little about its meaning and even less about its predictive validity.

Group Day Care and Other Forms of Nonmaternal Care

Despite a vast amount of research over the last century—including a particularly thorough, large-scale, multisite study in the United States (NICHD Early Child Care Research Network, 1997, 2003a, 2003b, 2003c)—controversy remains over whether nonmaternal care, especially in group settings in the first year of life, has deleterious effects on young children's social development (Belsky, 2001; Campbell, Ramey, Pungello, Sparling, & Miller-Johnson, 2002; Love et al., 2002; Sagi, Koren-Karie, Gini, Ziv, & Joels, 2002; Vandell, 2004). Nevertheless, certain reasonably firm conclusions are possible. First, poor-quality care, in or outside the maternal home, carries risks. Second, the great majority of children who experience good-quality

group day care cope well; moreover, children from disadvantaged backgrounds may actually benefit from nonmaternal care if the care provided is superior to that available from their own mothers (Borge, Rutter, Côté, & Tremblay, 2003; Côté, Borge, Rutter, & Tremblay, 2008; Geoffroy et al., 2007). There are few if any direct effects of day care on attachment security, but what remains a slightly open question is whether many hours or changing patterns of group day care (not just nonmaternal care) in the first year of life carries significant risks. The main messages are that the severe risks claimed in Bowlby's very early writings were clearly mistaken; that the quality of early care is certainly important; that whether maternal or nonmaternal care is preferable will depend on the quality of both; and that (at least for very young children) it may be quite difficult to provide really good-quality care in group settings in which caregiving is shared and not individualized.

It may be added that the situation in the first 3 months after birth may involve particular physical health considerations. The United States differs from most European countries in not providing statutory paid maternal leave, and data from the National Longitudinal Study of Youth indicate that a very early return to full-time work is associated with less regular medical checkups and less complete immunization, as well as a lower rate of breast feeding (Berger, Hill, & Waldfogel, 2005). European data similarly suggest health benefits from governmental expenditure on parental leave and other financial provisions (Tanaka, 2005).

Divorce and Separation

When a child's parents separate or divorce, and when the parents cannot agree on child care arrangements, professionals (both clinicians and judges) often need to advise on what would be best for the child. Old-fashioned attachment concepts might have suggested that the main weight should be attached to whichever of the parents the child has the more secure attachment to. That mechanistic approach should no longer provide the criterion. Research findings, as well as theory, indicate that it is usual for children to have security-providing selective attachments with both parents, and often with grandparents or other relatives as well. Judgments concerning child care need to take all of these into account—as well as to incorporate assessments of other aspects of parent–child relationships; of the child's own wishes; of the family situation as a whole;

and of the impact of stepparents, stepsiblings, and continuity in schooling (Dunn et al., 1998; Dunn, Davis, O'Connor, & Sturgess, 2000; Hetherington & Stanley-Hagan, 1995). Attachment theory has been crucially important in highlighting the essential role of social relationships, but, particularly as Bowlby's (1988) later writings emphasized, attachment needs to be considered in multipathway dynamic terms and not as a mechanical "bond" that is present or absent.

Searching for Biological Parents

One of the biggest changes with respect to adoption has been the shift from so-called "closed" to "open" adoptions. In the former, neither the adopted child nor the adopting parents had access to the biological parents; indeed, they were provided with no more than the most rudimentary information about the child's origin. With "open" adoption, both access and information are expected to be available. Of course, at present we are in the middle of a most interesting but complicated interim situation, in which individuals adopted under the "closed" system are now (with appropriate safeguards) able to search for their biological parents, or biological parents to search for their adopted-away children. It is far too early for any definitive evaluation of the effects of these changes on all concerned.

Probably the most systematic studies were those undertaken by Howe and Feast (2000) and by Triseliotis, Feast, and Kyle (2005). The second study was most distinctive in focusing on both the seekers of contact and the sought; on the 78 dyads of the adopted person and the birth mother; on the 86 dyads of the adopted person and the adoptive parents; and on the 38 triads of the adopted person, adoptive parents, and the birth mother. The researchers (especially Howe—see Howe, Brandon, Hinings, & Schofield, 1999) were strongly influenced by attachment theory, but it has to be said that it is not obvious quite how the theory informed the research.

The findings do not lend themselves to a succinct summary, and in any case, the adoptions took place in circumstances far different from those prevailing today. Most of the relationships between the two biological parents did not last long, and most of the mothers felt unsupported by their families. Some two-fifths of the mothers experienced a great sense of loss in giving up their babies, and a majority experienced some guilt. Despite that, their overwhelming thought was

the hope that their children were well and happy. The great majority viewed the search and renewed contact as positive; as one might have expected, however, there was substantial variation in the extent to which the biological mother and adopted child "hit it off," and great variation in whether contact continued.

About four-fifths of the adopted persons felt happy about being adopted, felt loved by their adoptive parents, and had a sense of belonging. For some, this was accompanied by a sense that they had been rejected by their biological parents, and in most cases the reunions helped in resolving this negative feeling. Some 8 years after that contact, some three-quarters continued to have contact. The majority of adopted persons reported a feeling of enhanced identity following the reunion. Interestingly, the most common description of the renewed relationship between the adopted person and his or her biological mother was of friendship rather than of a filial or parental relationship.

Obviously, the importance of this search would be expected on the basis of attachment theory. It is less obvious, however, whether the issues would have been illuminated to a greater extent by more use of attachment concepts (see Dozier & Rutter, Chapter 29, this volume). I doubt it. Attachment notions need to be embedded in broader aspects of psychopathology and not kept separate.

Assisted Conception

Comparable issues now arise with assisted conception, although there are also differences. Advances in assisted conception mean that babies can be born by egg donation (so that the social mother is not the biological mother), by sperm donation (so that the social father is not the biological father), and by surrogacy (so that there is no gestational link to the mother). Because there will be two social parents, it is possible for a child to have five parents (or more than that through divorce and remarriage). Through changes in the law, it is now permissible for individuals born through one of these techniques to search for and make contact with their biological parents. One key difference from, and contrast with, adoption is that it is unusual in the United Kingdom for children to be informed about their biological origins. We (Golombok, MacCallum, Goodman, & Rutter, 2002) found that none of a group of such children had been told by early school age, and only 8.6% by early adolescence. Because the social climate is somewhat different in Scandinavia, the proportion of children being informed there has tended to be higher (Gottlieb, Lalos, & Lindblad, 2000; Lindblad, Gottlieb, & Lalos, 2000). It may be higher in the United States (Leiblum & Aviv, 1997; Nachtigall, Pitcher, Tschann, Becker, & Szkupinski Quiroga, 1997), and almost certainly it is higher in New Zealand (Daniels & Lewis, 1996; Rumball & Adair, 1999). Surrogacy is yet more different, in that its existence is bound to be more generally known. The question is whether the different opportunities for the social mother to develop attachment representations before birth matters (Laxton-Kane & Slade, 2002; Slade, Belsky, Aber, & Phelps, 1999).

It is not at all obvious what attachment theory would predict in these circumstances. Presumably, evolutionary theory would predict a more troublesome or weaker parent–child relationship when there is not a genetic bond, whereas attachment theory would not. Family systems theory presumably would predict difficulties if there is secrecy, but would not place much reliance on the genetic link. Other psychological theories might place emphasis on whether or not the infertile partner experiences continuing resentments, and, either through that route or others, what the quality of the marital relationship is.

The need here would seem to be not so much the application of attachment theory, but rather the opportunity to use both comparisons among samples and contrasts in analytic strategies in testing competing explanations.

CONCLUSIONS

To a much greater extent than was the case when the first edition of this handbook was published, it is clear that there has been real progress in applying attachment concepts to child care policy issues. However, as the evidence shows, although the questions and issues are better understood, there is still a way to go in obtaining practical answers.

REFERENCES

Abrams, K. Y., Rifkin, A., & Hesse, E. (2006). Examining the role of parental frightened/frightening subtypes in predicting disorganized attachment within a brief observational procedure. *Development and Psychopathology, 18,* 345–361.

Ainsworth, M. D. S. (1967). *Infancy in Uganda: Infant care and the growth of love.* Baltimore: Johns Hopkins University Press.

Ainsworth, M. D. S., Blehar, M. C., Waters, E., & Wall, S. (1978). *Patterns of attachment: A psychological study of the Strange Situation.* Hillsdale, NJ: Erlbaum.

American Psychiatric Association. (2000). *Diagnostic and statistical manual of mental disorders* (4th ed., text rev.). Washington, DC: Author.

Atkinson, L., Niccols, A., Paglia, A., Coolbear, J., Parker, K. C. H., Poulton, L., et al. (2000). A meta-analysis of time between maternal sensitivity and attachment assessments: Implications for working models in infancy/toddlerhood. *Journal of Social and Personal Relationships, 17,* 791–810.

Bakermans-Kranenburg, M. J., van IJzendoorn, M. H., & Juffer, F. (2003). Less is more: Meta-analyses of sensitivity and attachment interventions in early childhood. *Psychological Bulletin, 129,* 195–215.

Barrett, H. (2006). *Attachment and the perils of parenting: A commentary and a critique.* London: National Family and Parenting Institute.

Belsky, J. (2001). Developmental risks (still) associated with early child care. *Journal of Child Psychology and Psychiatry, 42,* 845–859.

Berger, L. M., Hill, J., & Waldfogel, J. (2005). Maternity leave, early maternal employment and child health and development in the US. *Economic Journal, 115,* F29–F47.

Berlin, L. J., Ziv, Y., Amaya-Jackson, L., & Greenberg, M. T. (Eds.). (2005). *Enhancing early attachments: Theory, research, intervention, and policy.* New York: Guilford Press.

Berridge, D., & Cleaver, H. (1987). *Foster home breakdown.* Oxford, UK: Blackwell.

Blum, D. (2002). *Love at Goon Park: Harry Harlow and the science of affection.* Cambridge, MA: Perseus.

Borge, A. I. H., Rutter, M., Côté, S., & Tremblay, R. E. (2004). Early child care and physical aggression: Differentiating social selection and social causation. *Journal of Child Psychology and Psychiatry, 45,* 367–376.

Bowlby, J. (1951). *Maternal care and mental health.* Geneva: World Health Organization.

Bowlby, J. (1969/1982). *Attachment and loss: Vol. 1. Attachment.* London: Hogarth Press.

Bowlby, J. (1973). *Attachment and loss: Vol. 2. Separation: Anxiety and anger.* London: Hogarth Press.

Bowlby, J. (1980). *Attachment and loss: Vol. 3. Loss: Sadness and depression.* London: Hogarth Press.

Bowlby, J. (1988). *A secure base: Clinical implications of attachment theory.* London: Routledge.

Bowlby, J., Ainsworth, M. D. S., Boston, M., & Rosenbluth, D. (1956). The effects of mother–child separation: A follow-up study. *British Journal of Medical Psychology, 29,* 211–247.

Bretherton, I. (1995). A communication perspective on attachment relationships and internal working models: Commentary. In E. Waters, B. E. Vaughn, G. Posada, & K. Kondo-Ikemura (Eds.), Caregiving, cultural, and cognitive perspectives on secure-base behavior and working models: New growing points of attachment theory and research. *Monographs of the Society for Research in Child Development, 60*(2–3, Serial No. 244), 310–329.

Bretherton, I., Ridgeway, D., & Cassidy, J. (1990). Assessing internal working models of the attachment relationship: An Attachment Story Completion Task for 3-year-olds. In M. T. Greenberg, D. Cicchetti, & E. M. Cummings (Eds.), *Attachment in the preschool years: Theory, research, and intervention* (pp. 273–308). Chicago: University of Chicago Press.

Bretherton, I., & Munholland, K. A. (1999). Internal working models in attachment relationships: A construct revisited. In J. Cassidy & P. R. Shaver (Eds.), *Handbook of attachment: Theory, research, and critical applications* (pp. 89–111). New York: Guilford Press.

Bretherton, I., Walsh, R., Lependorf, M., & Georgeson, H. (1997). Attachment networks in postdivorce families: The maternal perspective. In L. Atkinson & K. J. Zucker (Eds.), *Attachment and psychopathology* (pp. 97–134). New York: Guilford Press.

Brisch, K. H. (2002). *Treating attachment disorders: From theory to therapy.* New York: Guilford Press.

Bruer, J. T. (1999). *The myth of the first three years.* New York: Free Press.

Campbell, F. A., Ramey, C. T., Pungello, E., Sparling, J., & Miller-Johnson, S. (2002). Early childhood education: Young adult outcomes from the Abecedarian Project. *Applied Developmental Science, 6,* 42–57.

Casler, L. (1968). Perceptual deprivation in institutional settings. In G. Newton & S. Levine (Eds.), *Early experience and behavior: The psychobiology of development* (pp. 573–626). Springfield, IL: Thomas.

Cassidy, J. (2003) Continuity and change in the measurement of infant attachment: Comment on Fraley and Spieker (2003). *Developmental Psychology, 39,* 409–412.

Cliffe, D., & Berridge, D. (1991). *Closing children's homes: An end to residential child care?* London: National Children's Bureau.

Cohen, N. J., Lojkasek, M., Muir, R., Parker, C. J., Barwick, M., & Brown, M. (1999). Watch, Wait, and Wonder: Testing the effectiveness of a new approach to mother–infant psychotherapy. *Infant Mental Health Journal, 20,* 429–451.

Cohen, N. J., Lojkasek, M., Muir, R., Parker, C. J., Barwick, M., & Brown, M. (2002). Six-month follow-up of two mother–infant psychotherapies: Convergence of therapeutic outcomes. *Infant Mental Health Journal, 23,* 361–380.

Côté, S., Borge, A. I. H., Rutter, M., & Tremblay, R. E. (2008). Non-maternal care in infancy and emotional/behavioral difficulties at 4 years: Moderation by family risk characteristics. *Developmental Psychology, 44,* 155–168.

Crittenden, P. M. (1985). Maltreated infants: Vulnerability and resilience. *Journal of Child Psychology and Psychiatry, 26,* 85–96.

Crittenden, P. M. (1988). Relationships as risk. In J. Belsky & T. Nezworski (Eds.), *Clinical implications of attachment* (pp. 136–174). Hillsdale, NJ: Erlbaum.

Crittenden, P. M., & Claussen, A. H. (Eds.). (2000). *The organisation of attachment relationships: Maturation, context, and culture.* Cambridge, UK: Cambridge University Press.

Daniels, K., & Lewis, G. M. (1996). Openness of information in the use of donor gametes: Developments in New Zealand. *Journal of Reproductive and Infant Psychology, 14,* 57–68.

De Wolff, M. S., & van IJzendoorn, M. H. (1997). Sensitivity and attachment: A meta-analysis on parental antecedents of infant attachment. *Child Development, 68,* 571–591.

Dozier, M., Lindhiem, O., & Ackerman, J. P. (2005). Attachment and Biobehavioral Catch-Up: An intervention targeting empirically identified needs of foster infants. In L. J. Berlin, Y. Ziv, L. Amaya-Jackson, & M. T. Greenberg (Eds.), *Enhancing early attachments: Theory, research, intervention, and policy* (pp. 178–194). New York: Guilford Press.

Dunn, J. (1993). *Young children's close relationships: Beyond attachment.* Newbury Park, CA: Sage.

Dunn, J., Davis, L. C., O'Connor, T. G., & Sturgess, W. (2000). Parents' and partners' life course and family experiences: Links with parent–child relationships in different family settings. *Journal of Child Psychology and Psychiatry, 41,* 955–968.

Dunn, J., Deater-Deckard, K., Pickering, K., O'Connor, T. G., Golding, J., & the ALSPAC Study Team. (1998). Children's adjustment and prosocial behaviour in step-, single-parent, and non-stepfamily settings: Findings from a community study. *Journal of Child Psychology and Psychiatry, 39,* 1083–1095.

Fonagy, P., Steele, H., & Steele, M. (1991). Maternal representations of attachment during pregnancy predict the organization of infant–mother attachment at one year of age. *Child Development, 62,* 891–905.

Fraley, R. C., & Spieker, S. J. (2003a). Are infant attachment patterns continuously or categorically distributed?: A taxometric analysis of Strange Situation behavior. *Developmental Psychology, 39,* 387–404.

Fraley, R. C., & Spieker, S. J. (2003b). What are the differences between dimensional and categorical models of individual differences in attachment?: Reply to Cassidy (2003), Cummings (2003), Sroufe (2003), and Waters and Beauchaine (2003). *Developmental Psychology, 39,* 423–429.

Geoffroy, M.-C., Côté, S., Borge, A. I. H., Larouche, F., Séguin, J. R., & Rutter, M. (2007). Association between early non-maternal care and children's receptive language skills prior to school entry: The moderating role of the socio-economic status. *Journal of Child Psychology and Psychiatry, 48,* 490–497.

George, C., Kaplan, N., & Main, M. (1984). *Adult Attachment Interview protocol.* Unpublished manuscript, University of California at Berkeley.

George, C., Kaplan, N., & Main, M. (1985). *Adult Attachment Interview protocol* (2nd ed.). Unpublished manuscript, University of California at Berkeley.

George, C., Kaplan, N., & Main, M. (1996). *Adult At-*

tachment Interview protocol (3rd ed.). Unpublished manuscript, University of California at Berkeley.

Gerhardt, S. (2004). *Why love matters: How affection shapes a baby's brain.* New York: Brunner-Routledge.

Gewirtz, J. L. (1972). Attachment, dependence, and a distinction in terms of stimulus control. In J. L. Gewirtz (Ed.), *Attachment and dependency* (pp. 139–177). Washington, DC: Winston.

Goldstein, J., Freud, A., Solnit, A. J., & Goldstein, S. (1986). *In the best interests of the child.* New York: Free Press.

Golombok, S., MacCallum, F., Goodman, E., & Rutter, M. (2002). Families with children conceived by donor insemination: A follow-up at age twelve. *Child Development, 73,* 952–968.

Gottlieb, C., Lalos, O., & Lindblad, F. (2000). Disclosure of donor insemination to the child: The impact of Swedish legislation on couples' attitudes. *Human Reproduction, 15,* 2052–2056.

Green, J., & Goldwyn, R. (2002). Annotation: Attachment disorganization and psychopathology: New findings in attachment research and their potential implications for developmental psychopathology in childhood. *Journal of Child Psychology and Psychiatry, 43,* 835–846.

Greenberg, M. T. (1999). Attachment and psychopathology in childhood. In J. Cassidy & P. R. Shaver (Eds.), *Handbook of attachment: Theory, research, and clinical applications* (pp. 469–496). New York: Guilford Press.

Groark, C. J., & McCall, R. B. (2008). Community-based interventions and services. In M. Rutter, D. Bishop, D. Pine, S. Scott, J. Stevenson, E. Taylor, et al. (Eds.), *Rutter's child and adolescent psychiatry* (5th ed., pp. 971–988). Oxford, UK: Blackwell.

Grossmann, K. E., Grossmann, K., & Waters, E. (Eds.). (2005). *Attachment from infancy to adulthood: The major longitudinal studies.* New York: Guilford Press.

Hale, B., & Fortin, J. (2008). Legal issues in the care and treatment of children with mental health problems. In M. Rutter, D. Bishop, D. Pine, S. Scott, J. Stevenson, E. Taylor, et al. (Eds.), *Rutter's child and adolescent psychiatry* (5th ed., pp. 95–110). Oxford, UK: Blackwell.

Hamilton, C. E. (2000). Continuity and discontinuity of attachment from infancy through adolescence. *Child Development, 71,* 690–694.

Harlow, H. F., & Zimmerman, R. R. (1959). Affectional responses in the infant monkey. *Science, 130,* 421–432.

Hart, A., & Thomas, H. (2000). Controversial attachments: The indirect treatment of fostered and adopted children via parent co-therapy. *Attachment and Human Development, 2,* 306–327.

Hazan, C., & Shaver, P. R. (1987). Romantic love conceptualized as an attachment process. *Journal of Personality and Social Psychology, 52,* 511–524.

Hazan, C., & Zeifman, D. (1999). Pair bonds as attachments: Evaluating the evidence. In J. Cassidy & P. R. Shaver (Eds.), *Handbook of attachment: Theory,*

research, and clinical applications (pp. 336–354). New York: Guilford Press.

Hesse, E., & Main, M. (2006). Frightened, threatening, and dissociative parental behavior: Theory and associations with parental adult attachment interview status and infant disorganization. *Development and Psychopathology, 18,* 309–343.

Hetherington, E. M., & Stanley-Hagan, M. M. (1995). Parenting in divorced and remarried families. In M. Bornstein (Ed.), *Handbook of parenting* (Vol. 3, pp. 233–254). Mahwah, NJ: Erlbaum.

Hinde, R. A. (1988). Continuities and discontinuities: Conceptual issues and methodological considerations. In M. Rutter (Ed.), *Studies of psychosocial risk: The power of longitudinal data* (pp. 367–383). Cambridge, UK: Cambridge University Press.

Hodges, J., Steele, M., Hillman, S., Henderson, K., & Kaniuk, J. (2003). Changes over attachment representations over the first year of adoptive placement: Narratives of maltreated children. *Clinical Child Psychology and Psychiatry, 8,* 351–367.

Hodges, J., & Tizard, B. (1989a). IQ and behavioural adjustment of ex-institutional adolescents. *Journal of Child Psychology and Psychiatry, 30,* 53–75.

Hodges, J., & Tizard, B. (1989b). Social and family relationships of ex-institutional adolescents. *Journal of Child Psychology and Psychiatry, 30,* 77–97.

Howe, D., Brandon, M., Hinings D., & Schofield, G. (1999). *Attachment theory, child maltreatment and family support: A practice and assessment model.* Basingstoke, UK: Palgrave.

Howe, D., & Fearnley, S. (2003). Disorders of attachment in adopted and fostered children: Recognition and treatment. *Clinical Child Psychology and Psychiatry, 8,* 369–387.

Howe, D., & Feast, J. (2000) *Adoption, search and reunion.* London: British Association for Adoption and Fostering.

Jacobvitz, D., Leon, K., & Hazen, N. (2006). Does expectant mothers' unresolved trauma predict frightened/frightening maternal behavior?: Risk and protective factors. *Development and Psychopathology, 18,* 363–379.

Juffer, F., Bakermans-Kranenburg, M. J., & van IJzendoorn, M. H. (2005). The importance of parenting in the development of disorganized attachment: Evidence from a preventive intervention study in adoptive families. *Journal of Child Psychology and Psychiatry, 46,* 263–274.

King, R. D., Raynes, N. V., & Tizard, J. (1971). *Patterns of residential care: Sociological studies in institutions for handicapped children.* London: Routledge & Kegan Paul.

Kraemer, S., & Roberts, J. (1996). *The politics of attachment: Towards a secure society.* London: Free Association Books.

Laxton-Kane, M., & Slade, P. (2002). The role of maternal prenatal attachment in a woman's experience of pregnancy and implications for the process of care. *Journal of Reproductive and Infant Psychology, 20,* 253–266.

Leiblum, S. R., & Aviv, A. L. (1997). Disclosure issues and decisions of couples who conceived via donor insemination. *Journal of Psychosomatic Obstetrics and Gynecology, 18,* 292–300.

Lindblad, F., Gottlieb, C., & Lalos, O. (2000). To tell or not to tell: What parents think about telling their children that they were born following donor insemination. *Journal of Psychosomatic Obstetrics and Gynecology, 21,* 193–203.

Love, J., Kisker, E. E., Ross, C. M., Schochet, P. Z., Brooks-Gunn, J., Paulsell, D., et al. (2002). *Making a difference in the lives of infants and toddlers and their families: The impacts of Early Head Start. Vol. 1. Final technical report.* Retrieved from *www.mathematica-mpr.com/PDFs/ehsfinalvol1.pdf*

Lyons-Ruth, K., & Jacobvitz, D. (1999) Attachment disorganization: Unresolved loss, relational violence, and lapses in behavioral and attentional strategies. In J. Cassidy & P. R. Shaver (Eds.), *Handbook of attachment: Theory, research, and clinical applications* (pp. 520–554). New York: Guilford Press.

Maclean, K. (2003). The impact of institutionalization on child development. *Development and Psychopathology, 15,* 853–884.

Main, M., & Solomon, J. (1986). Discovery of an insecure-disoriented attachment pattern. In T. B. Brazelton & M. W. Yogman (Eds.) *Affective development in infancy* (pp. 95–124). Norwood, NJ: Ablex.

Main, M., & Solomon, J. (1990). Procedures for identifying infants as disorganized/disoriented during the Ainsworth Strange Situation. In M. Greenberg, D. Cicchetti, & E. M. Cummings (Eds.), *Attachment in the preschool years: Theory, research, and intervention* (pp. 121–160). Chicago: University of Chicago Press.

Marvin, R., Cooper, B., Hoffman, K., & Powell, B. (2002). The Circle of Security project: Attachment-based intervention with caregiver–preschool child dyads. *Attachment and Human Development, 4,* 107–124.

Mikulincer, M., & Shaver, P. R. (2007). *Attachment in adulthood: Structure, dynamics, and change.* New York: Guilford Press.

Nachtigall, R. D., Pitcher, L., Tschann, J. M., Becker, G., & Szkupinski Quiroga, S. (1997). Stigma, disclosure and family functioning among parents of children conceived through donor insemination. *Fertility and Sterility, 68,* 83–89.

National Institute of Child Health and Human Development (NICHD) Early Child Care Research Network. (1997). The effects of infant child care on infant–mother attachment security: Results of the NICHD Study of Early Child Care. *Child Development, 68,* 860–879.

National Institute of Child Health and Human Development (NICHD) Early Child Care Research Network. (2003a). Does amount of time spent in child care predict socio-emotional adjustment during the transition to kindergarten? *Child Development, 74,* 976–1005.

National Institute of Child Health and Human Development (NICHD) Early Child Care Research Network. (2003b). Does quality of child care affect child outcomes at age 4½? *Developmental Psychology, 39,* 451–469.

National Institute of Child Health and Human Development (NICHD) Early Child Care Research Network. (2003c). Early child care and mother–child interaction from 36 months through first grade. *Infant Behavior and Development, 26,* 345–370.

O'Connor, N., & Franks, C. M. (1960). Childhood upbringing and other environmental factors. In H. J. Eysenck (Ed.), *Handbook of abnormal psychology* (pp. 393–416). London: Pitman.

O'Connor, T., & Zeanah, C. (2003). Attachment disorders: Assessment strategies and treatment approaches. *Attachment and Human Development, 5,* 223–244.

O'Connor, T. G., Marvin, R. S., Rutter, M., Olrick, J. T., & Britner, P. A. (2003). Child–parent attachment following early institutional deprivation. *Development and Psychopathology, 15,* 19–38.

Parker, R., Ward, H., Jackson, S., Aldgate, J., & Wedge, P. (1991). *Looking after children: Assessing outcomes in child care.* London: Her Majesty's Stationery Office.

Rajecki, D. W., Lamb, M. E., & Obmascher, P. (1978). Toward a general theory of infantile attachment: A comparative review of aspects of the social bond. *Behavioral and Brain Sciences, 1,* 417–464.

Robertson, J., & Robertson, J. (1971). Young children in brief separation: A fresh look. *Psychoanalytic Study of the Child, 26,* 264–315.

Rumball, A., & Adair, V. (1999). Telling the story: Parents' scripts for donor offspring. *Human Reproduction, 14,* 1392–1399.

Rutter, M. (1979). Separation experiences: A new look at an old topic. *Journal of Pediatrics, 95,* 147–154.

Rutter, M. (1981). *Maternal deprivation reassessed* (2nd ed.). Harmondsworth, UK: Penguin Books.

Rutter, M. (1995). Clinical implications of attachment concepts: Retrospect and prospect. *Journal of Child Psychology and Psychiatry, 36,* 549–571.

Rutter, M. (2002). Maternal deprivation. In M. H. Bornstein (Ed.), *Handbook of parenting: Vol. 4. Social conditions and applied parenting* (2nd ed., pp. 181–202). Mahwah, NJ: Erlbaum.

Rutter, M. (2006). Critical notice: Attachment from infancy to adulthood: The major longitudinal studies. *Journal of Child Psychology and Psychiatry, 47,* 974–977.

Rutter, M., Colvert, E., Kreppner, J., Beckett, C., Castle, J., Groothues, C., et al. (2007). Early adolescent outcomes for institutionally-deprived and non-deprived adoptees: I. Disinhibited attachment. *Journal of Child Psychology and Psychiatry, 48,* 17–30.

Rutter, M., & O'Connor, T. G. (1999). Implications of attachment theory for child care policies. In J. Cassidy & P. R. Shaver (Eds.), *Handbook of attachment: Theory, research, and clinical applications* (pp. 823–844). New York: Guilford Press.

Sagi, A., Koren-Karie, N., Gini, M., Ziv, Y., & Joels, T.

(2002). Shedding further light on the effects of various types and quality of early child care on infant–mother attachment relationship: The Haifa Study of Early Child Care. *Child Development, 73,* 1166–1186.

Schaffer, H. R. (1990). *Making decisions about children: Psychological questions and answers.* Oxford, UK: Blackwell.

Schore, A. N. (1994). *Affect regulation and the origin of the self: The neurobiology of emotional development.* Hillsdale, NJ: Erlbaum.

Schore, A. N. (2001a). Effects of a secure attachment relationship on right brain development, affect regulation, and infant mental health. *Infant Mental Health Journal, 22,* 7–66.

Schore, A. N. (2001b). Minds in the making: Attachment, the self-organizing brain, and developmentally-oriented psychoanalytic psychotherapy. *British Journal of Psychotherapy, 17,* 299–328.

Slade, A., Belsky, J., Aber, J. L., & Phelps, J. L. (1999). Mothers' representations of their relationships with their toddlers: Links to adult attachment and observed mothering. *Developmental Psychology, 35,* 611–619.

Slough, N. M., & Greenberg, M. T. (1990). Five-year-olds' representations of separation from parents: Responses from the perspective of self and other. *New Directions in Child Development, 48,* 67–84.

Smyke, A. T., Dumitrescu, A., & Zeanah, C. H. (2002). Disturbances of attachment in young children: I. The continuum of caretaking casualty. *Journal of the American Academy of Child and Adolescent Psychiatry, 41,* 972–982.

Sroufe, L. A. (1983). Infant–caregiver attachment and patterns of adaptation in preschool: The roots of maladaptation and competence. In M. Perlmutter (Ed.), *Minnesota Symposium on Child Psychology: Vol. 16. Development and policy concerning children with special needs* (pp. 41–83). Hillsdale, NJ: Erlbaum.

Sroufe, L. A. (1988). The role of infant–caregiver attachments in development. In J. Belsky & T. Nezworski (Eds.), *Clinical implications of attachment* (pp. 18–38). Hillsdale, NJ: Erlbaum.

Sroufe, L. A., Egeland, B., Carlson, E., & Collins, W. A. (2005). *The development of the person: The Minnesota Study of Risk and Adaptation from Birth to Adulthood.* New York: Guilford Press.

Tanaka, S. (2005). Parental leave and child health across OECD countries. *Economic Journal, 115,* F7–F28.

Tizard, B. (1977). *Adoption: A second chance.* London: Open Books.

Tizard, B., & Hodges, J. (1978). The effect of early institutional rearing on the development of eight year old children. *Journal of Child Psychology and Psychiatry, 19,* 99–119.

Tizard, B., & Rees, J. (1975). The effect of early institutional rearing on the behaviour problems and affectional relationships of four-year-old children. *Journal of Child Psychology and Psychiatry, 16,* 61–73.

Tizard, J., & Tizard, B. (1971). The social development of two-year-old children in residential nurseries. In

J. Schaffer (Ed.), *The origins of human social relations* (pp. 147–160). London: Academic Press.

Triseliotis, J., Feast, J., & Kyle, F. (2005). *The adoption triangle revisited: A study of adoption, search and reunion experiences.* London: British Association for Adoption and Fostering.

Triseliotis, J., & Russell, J. (1984). *Hard to place: The outcome of adoption and residential care.* London: Heinemann.

Vandell, D. L. (2004). Early child care: The known and the unknown. *Merrill–Palmer Quarterly, 50,* 387–414.

van den Boom, D. C. (1994). The influence of temperament and mothering on attachment and exploration: An experimental manipulation of sensitive responsiveness among lower-class mothers with irritable infants. *Child Development, 65,* 1457–1477.

van IJzendoorn, M. H., Bakermans-Kranenburg, M. J., & Juffer, F. (2005). Why less is more: From the dodo bird verdict to evidence-based interventions on sensitivity and early attachments. In L. J. Berlin, Y. Ziv, L. Amaya-Jackson, & M. T. Greenberg (Eds.), *Enhancing early attachments: Theory, research, intervention, and policy* (pp. 297–312). New York: Guilford Press.

van IJzendoorn, M. H., Juffer, F., & Duyvesteyn, M. G. (1995). Breaking the intergenerational cycle of insecure attachment: A review of the effects of attachment-based interventions on maternal sensitivity and infant security. *Journal of Child Psychology and Psychiatry, 36,* 225–248.

van IJzendoorn, M. H., Schuengel, C., & Bakermans-Kranenburg, M. J. (1999). Disorganized attachment in early childhood: Meta-analysis of precursors, concomitants, and sequelae. *Development and Psychopathology, 11,* 225–249.

van IJzendoorn, M. H., Vereijken, C. M. J. L., Bakermans-Kranenburg, M. J., & Riksen-Walraven, J. M. (2004). Assessing attachment security with the Attachment Q-Sort: Meta-analytic evidence for the validity of the observer AQS. *Child Development, 75,* 1188–1213.

Vorria, P., Papaligoura, Z., Dunn, J., van IJzendoorn, M. H., Steele, H., Kontopoulou, A., et al. (2003). Early experiences and attachment relationships of Greek infants raised in residential group care. *Journal of Child Psychology and Psychiatry, 44,* 1–13.

Vorria, P., Papaligoura, Z., Sarafidou, J., Kopakaki, M., Dunn, J., van IJzendoorn, M. H., et al. (2006). The development of adopted children after institutional care: A follow-up study. *Journal of Child Psychology and Psychiatry, 47,* 1246–1253.

Vorria, P., Rutter, M., Pickles, A., Wolkind, S., & Hobsbaum, A. (1998a). A comparative study of Greek children in long-term residential group care and in two-parent families: I. Social, emotional, and behavioural differences. *Journal of Child Psychology and Psychiatry, 39,* 225–236.

Vorria, P., Rutter, M., Pickles, A., Wolkind, S., & Hobsbaum, A. (1998b). A comparative study of Greek children in long-term residential group care and in two-parent families: II. Possible mediating mechanisms. *Journal of Child Psychology and Psychiatry, 39,* 237–245.

Waters, E. (1987). *Attachment Q-Set (Version 3.0)*. Unpublished manuscript, State University of New York at Stony Brook.

Waters, E., Hamilton, C. E., & Weinfield, N. S. (2000). The stability of attachment security from infancy to adolescence and early adulthood: General introduction. *Child Development, 71,* 678–683.

Wolkind, S. (1974). The components of 'affectionless psychopathy' in institutionalized children. *Journal of Child Psychology and Psychiatry, 15,* 215–220.

World Health Organization (WHO). (1992). *The ICD-10 classification of mental and behavioural disorders: Clinical descriptions and diagnostic guidelines.* Geneva: Author.

World Health Organization (WHO) Expert Committee on Mental Health. (1951). *Report on the Second Session, 1951.* Geneva: Author.

Zeanah, C. H. (1996). Beyond insecurity: A reconceptualization of attachment disorders in infancy. *Journal of Consulting and Clinical Psychology, 64,* 42–52.

Zeanah, C. H., Nelson, C. A., Fox, N. A., Smyke, A. T.,

Marshall, P., Parker, S. W., et. al. (2003). Designing research to study the effects of institutionalization on brain and behavioral development: The Bucharest Early Intervention Project. *Development and Psychopathology, 15,* 885–907.

Zeanah, C. H., Scheeringa, M., Boris, N. W., Heller, S. S., Smyke, A. T., & Trapani, J. (2004). Reactive attachment disorder in maltreated toddlers. *Child Abuse and Neglect, 28,* 877–888.

Zeanah, C. H., & Smyke, A. T. (2005). Building attachment relationships following maltreatment and severe deprivation. In L. J. Berlin, Y. Ziv, L. Amaya-Jackson, & M. T. Greenberg (Eds.), *Enhancing early attachments: Theory, research, intervention, and policy* (pp. 195–216). New York: Guilford Press.

Zeanah, C. H., & Smyke, A. T. (2008). Attachment disorders in relation to deprivation. In M. Rutter, D. Bishop, D. Pine, S. Scott, J. Stevenson, E. Taylor, et al. (Eds.), *Rutter's child and adolescent psychiatry* (5th ed., pp. 906–915). Oxford, UK: Blackwell.

Zeanah, C. H., Smyke, A. T., Koga, S. F., Carlson, E., & the Bucharest Early Intervention Project Core Group. (2005). Attachment in institutionalized and community children in Romania. *Child Development, 76,* 1015–1028.

Author Index

Subject Index

Page numbers followed by *f* indicate figure; *n*, note; and *t*, table